DIAGNOSIS

Primary Care Across the Lifespan

Primary Care Across the Lifespan

Denise Robinson, PhD, RN, ARNP
Professor
Northern Kentucky University
Director, MSN Programs
Highland Heights, Kentucky
Family Nurse Practitioner
Northern Kentucky Family Health Centers, Inc.
Covington, Kentucky

Pamela Kidd, PhD, RN, ARNP, CEN
Associate Professor
University of Kentucky College of Nursing
Director, Kentucky Injury Prevention and Research Center
Family Nurse Practitioner
St. Joseph Hospital Mobile Clinic
Lexington, Kentucky

Karen Mangus Rogers, MSN, ARNP
Family Health Center, Inc.
Louisville, Kentucky
Volunteer Faculty/Preceptor
University of Kentucky
Lexington, Kentucky
University of Louisville
Louisville, Kentucky

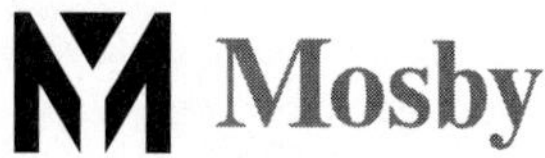

St. Louis Baltimore Boston Carlsbad Chicago Minneapolis New York Philadelphia Portland
London Milan Sydney Tokyo Toronto

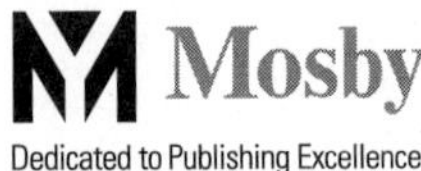

Dedicated to Publishing Excellence

Editor-in-Chief: Sally Schrefer
Senior Editor: Loren Wilson
Developmental Editor: Nancy L. O'Brien
Project Manager: Deborah Vogel
Production Editor: Mary Drone
Designer: Bill Drone

FIRST EDITION

NOTICE

Pharmacology is an ever-changing field. Standard safety precautions must be followed, but as new research and clinical experience broaden our knowledge, changes in treatment and drug therapy may become necessary or appropriate. Readers are advised to check the most current product information provided by the manufacturer of each drug to be administered to verify the recommended dose, the method and duration of administration, and contraindications. It is the responsibility of the treating physician, relying on experience and knowledge of the patient, to determine dosages and the best treatment for each individual patient. Neither the publisher nor the editor assumes any liability for any injury and/or damage to persons or property arising from this publication.

Mosby, Inc.
A Harcourt Health Sciences Company
11830 Westline Industrial Drive
St. Louis, Missouri 63146

Printed in the United States of America

Library of Congress Cataloging-in-Publication Data

Primary care across the lifespan / [edited by] Denise Robinson, Pamela Kidd, Karen Mangus Rogers. — 1st ed.
p. cm.
Includes bibliographical references and index.
ISBN 0-323-00148-3
1. Primary nursing. 2. Primary care (Medicine) 3. Nurse practitioners. I. Robinson, Denise L. II. Kidd, Pamela Stinson. III. Rogers, Karen Mangus.
[DNLM: 1. Primary Nursing Care—methods. 2. Nurse Practitioners. 3. Primary Health Care—methods. WY 101 P9511 1999]
RT90.7.P75 1999
610.73—dc21
DNLM/DLC
for Library of Congress 99-37349
CIP

99 00 01 02 03 GW/MVB 9 8 7 6 5 4 3 2 1

This book is dedicated to my family for their understanding and support.

DR

There were times when I thought I was going to go crazy and take my family with me while writing this book. My husband is a saint on earth. He is the calm in my storm. I am so thankful that he picked me to live with for all these years!

PK

This book is dedicated to my husband, Terry, and my son, Daniel. Thank you, Terry, for knowing when to encourage me and when to leave me alone. Your words, "I am proud of you," meant a lot to me. And to my twelve-year-old son, Daniel, thank you for your help on the computer. Your timing and your computer skills were greatly appreciated. I love you both.

KMR

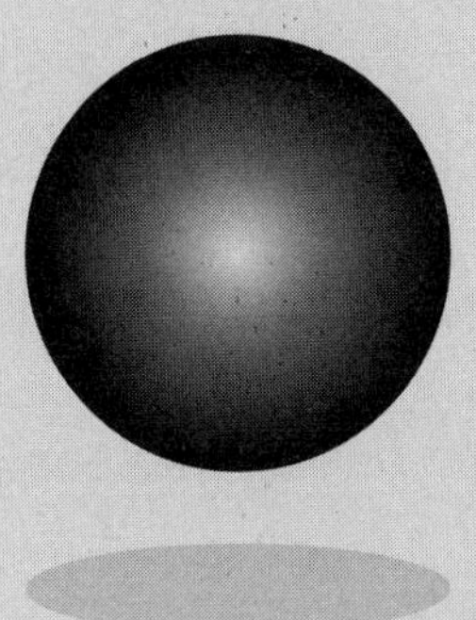

Contributors

Cindy M. Allison, MSN, RN, CNP
Pediatric Nurse Practitioner
Northeastern Pediatrics
Mason, Ohio
Well Child

Janet (Jan) Andrews, PhD, RNC, WHNP
Assistant Professor
School of Health Sciences
Georgia College and State University
Milledgeville, Georgia
Dysfunctional Uterine Bleeding, Pelvic Inflammatory Disease, Pregnancy Problems: Early and Late Bleeding, Pregnancy Problems: Hypertension

Alanna Conrad Andrus, MSN, PNP, FNP
Redwood City, California
Congenital Heart Defects, Developmental Dysplasia of the Hip

Ellen L. Bailey, MSN, CFNP
Family Nurse Practitioner
Bluegrass Regional Primary Care Centre
Frankfort, Kentucky
Bell's Palsy, Gout

Dorothy R. Baker, MSN, RN, ARNP
Family Nurse Practitioner
Alliance Primary Care
Covington, Kentucky
Seizure Disorders

Patricia C. Birchfield, DSN, RN, ANP, GNP
Associate Professor
Eastern Kentucky University
Richmond, Kentucky
Arthritis, Low Back Pain, Prostate Problems

Suzanne B. Black, MSN, RN, CS, FNP
Family Nurse Practitioner
Hematology/Oncology Pediatric Outpatient
Children's Hospital Medical Center
Cincinnati, Ohio
Clinical Instructor/Preceptor
Family Nurse Practitioner Program
Northern Kentucky University
Highland Heights, Kentucky
Anemia, Leukemia

Julie Mead Bogguss, MSN, RNC, FNP
Certified Family Nurse Practitioner
Randolph Pediatric Associates — PHA
Charlotte, North Carolina
Fifth Disease, Hand, Foot, and Mouth Disease

Lisa Dittami Bradshaw, MSN, RN, FNP
Family Nurse Practitioner
Internal Medicine Department
Veterans Administration Medical Center
Cincinnati, Ohio
Diverticulosis and Diverticulitis

Katherine L. Bushong, MSN, RN, FNP
Nurse Practitioner
Neurology Division
Riverhills Healthcare, Inc.
Crestview Hills, Kentucky
Tinea Infections, Trigeminal Neuralgia

Leslie M. Cooper, MSN, RN, CS, ARNP
Director of School Health Services
Boone County Schools
Florence, Kentucky
Family Nurse Practitioner
Warsaw Family Medicine, PSC
Warsaw, Kentucky
Chicken Pox, Fifth Disease, Mumps, Pertussis, Roseola, Rubella, Rubeola, Scarlet Fever

Rita A. Dello-Stritto, MSN, RN, CEN, CNS, ENP
Emergency Nurse Practitioner
Kelsey-Seybold Urgent Care Clinic
Houston, Texas
Dental Problems, Upper Respiratory Infections, Wound Management

Ann M. Dollins, PhD, MPH, MSN, CNM
Assistant Professor
Northern Kentucky University
Highland Heights, Kentucky
Primary Care Related to Pregnancy, Well Adult — Woman

Diane M. Enzweiler, MSN, RN-CS, ARNP
Adult Nurse Practitioner
Cardiology Associates, P.S.C.
Edgewood, Kentucky
Adjunct Faculty
Northern Kentucky University
Highland Heights, Kentucky
Congestive Heart Failure, Myocardial Infarction, Hyperlipidemia

Holly Yeatts Fox, MSN, RN, NP-C, COHN-S
Occupational Health Nurse Practitioner
ALCOA, Warrick Operations
Newburgh, Indiana
Carpal Tunnel Syndrome

Mary Gabriel, MSN, CPNP
Pediatric Nurse Practitioner
Infant Care Center
The Children's Hospital of Denver
Denver, Colorado
Breastfeeding Problems

Lisbeth Gabrielski, BSN, RN, IBCLC
Director, Lactation Support Service
The Children's Hospital of Denver
Centura Health St. Anthony Central Hospital
Denver, Colorado
Breastfeeding Problems

Lynette M. Galloway, MSN, RNC, PNP
Director, Student Health Services
Spalding University
Pediatric Nurse Practitioner
Jefferson County Health Department
Louisville, Kentucky
Eating Disorders

Bonnie Gance-Cleveland, PhD, RNC, PNP
Assistant Professor
University of Colorado Health Science Center
Denver, Colorado
Addison's Disease

Carrie Gordy, MSN, ARNP
Assistant Professor, College of Nursing
University of Kentucky
Lexington, Kentucky
Constipation, Diarrhea, Encopresis, Enuresis

Susan Hagedorn, PhD, RN, PNP, WHCNP
Assistant Professor
University of Colorado Health Sciences Center
Denver, Colorado
Delayed Puberty

Jerelen D. Hancox, MSN, RN, CEN, FNP
Instructor, Nursing Program
Cincinnati State College
Cincinnati, Ohio
Family Nurse Practitioner
Dearborn County Hospital Emergency Department
Lawrenceburg, Indiana
Corneal Abrasion/Foreign Body

Barbara A. Heidt, MSN, RN, CS
Psychiatric Clinical Nurse Specialist
Children's Hospital Medical Center
Cincinnati, Ohio
Attention Deficit Hyperactivity Disorder

Marilyn J. Jacobs, MSN, RNC, WHNP
Associate Professor
Missouri Southern State College
Women's Health Services, Student Health Center
Missouri Southern State College
Joplin, Missouri
Scabies

Delwin B. Jacoby, MSN, CFNP
Family Nurse Practitioner
Anderson Family Health Center
Lawrenceburg, Kentucky
Musculoskeletal Injuries: Ankle, Hand/Fingers, Knee, Wrist

Debra A. Johnsen, MSN, RN, ANP, GNP
Adult/Gerontological Nurse Practitioner
Northern Kentucky Family Health Centers, Inc.
Covington Medical Center
Covington, Kentucky
Alopecia, Blepharitis

Colleen Keller, PhD, RN, FNP
Professor, Department of Family Care Nursing
University of Texas Health Sciences Center
San Antonio, Texas
Obesity

Sandra Hall Kesner, MSN, FNP
Family Nurse Practitioner
North College Hill Medical Group
Cincinnati, Ohio
HIV/AIDS, Parkinson's Disease

Pamela Kidd, PhD, RN, ARNP, CEN
Associate Professor
University of Kentucky College of Nursing
Director
Kentucky Injury Prevention and Research Center
Family Nurse Practitioner
St. Joseph Hospital Mobile Clinic
Lexington, Kentucky
Abscess/Boil/Furuncle, Contact Dermatitis, Cystic Fibrosis, Dermatology, Diaper Rash, Eczema, Epididymitis, Fatigue, Folliculitis, Impetigo, Kawasaki Disease, Molluscum Contagiosum, Renal Failure, Rosacea, Skin Cancer, Tuberculosis, Varicose Veins

Pam King, MSN, RN, FNP
Instructor, School of Nursing and Health Sciences
Spalding University
Louisville, Kentucky
Anxiety, Cataract, Failure to Thrive, Glaucoma, Osgood-Schlatter Disease

Cheryl Pope Kish, EdD, RNC, WHNP
Professor and Coordinator
Graduate Programs in Health Science
Director, Family Nurse Practitioner Program
Georgia College and State University
Milledgeville, Georgia
Breast Problems: Masses and Pain, Breast Problems: Nipple Discharge and Inflammation, Lice, Ovarian Cysts, Premenstrual Syndrome

Deborah Bedner Kupecz, MSN, NP
Adult/Gerontological Nurse Practitioner
Veterans Affairs Medical Center
Adjunct Faculty
University of Phoenix
Regis University
Denver, Colorado
Diabetes

Linda Larson, PhD, FNP
Nurse Practitioner
Internal Medicine, Geriatrics, and Endocrinology
Adjunct Affiliate Faculty
Assistant Professor
University of Colorado
Denver, Colorado
Chest Pain, Syncope, Transient Ischemic Attacks

Mary Lavelle, MSN, RN, CWOCN, ARNP
Adult Nurse Practitioner, Certified
Veterans Administration Medical Center
Louisville, Kentucky
Lower Extremity Ulcers

Alice B. Loper, MN, RN-C, FNP
Family Nurse Practitioner, Certified
Assistant Professor of Nursing
Georgia College and State University
Milledgeville, Georgia
Dysmenorrhea

Lori McConlogue-O'Shaughnessy, MSN, RN, ARNP
Family Nurse Practitioner
Northern Kentucky Family Health Centers
Covington, Kentucky
Allergic Rhinitis, Amenorrhea, Bartholin Cyst, Chancroid, Chlamydia, Dysfunctional Uterine Bleeding, Endometriosis, Family Planning, Gonorrhea, Herpes, Menopause, Pelvic Pain, Post-Abortion Care, Proteinuria, Syphilis, Urinary Incontinence, Uterine Fibroids, Uterine Prolapse, Vaginitis, Warts

Kathleen K. McGee, MSN, RN, CPNP
Pediatric Nurse Practitioner
Children's Hospital Medical Center
Cincinnati, Ohio
Lead Poisoning

Susan M. McNiel, MN, ARNP, WHCNP, ANP
Women's Health and Adult Nurse Practitioner
UW Physicians, Woodinville Clinic
Woodinville, Washington
Hirsutism

Darcie Meierbachtol, MS, RN-C, ANP, FNP
Senior Instructor
University of Colorado Health Sciences Center
Denver, Colorado
Gastroesophageal Reflux Disease

Barbara Crosby Moseley, MSN, ARNP
Adult and Geriatric Nurse Practitioner
Veterans Administration Medical Center (formerly)
Lexington, Kentucky
Fibromyalgia

Louise Niemer, PhD, RN, PNP, CPNP
Assistant Professor
Northern Kentucky University
Highland Heights, Kentucky
Bronchiolitis, Bronchitis, Meningitis, Worms

Kathy J. Noyes, MSN, RN, CS, ARNP
Family Nurse Practitioner
Comprehensive Cardiology Consultants, Inc.
Cincinnati, Ohio
Dearborn County Hospital — Emergency Department
Lawrenceburg, Indiana
Edema, Hypertension

Carol A. Ormond, MSN, RN, CNAA, FNP
Assistant Professor
School of Health Sciences
Georgia College and State University
Milledgeville, Georgia
Cholecystitis and Cholelithiasis

Cindy Pastorino, RN, MSN
Gerontological Nurse Practitioner
Division of Geriatrics
University of Louisville
Louisville, Kentucky
Confusion

Betty M. Porter, MSN, EdD, ARNP, CFNP
Chair, Department of Nursing and Allied Health Sciences
Professor of Nursing
Morehead State University
Morehead, Kentucky
Headaches

Kathleen Reeve, MSN, RN, CS, ANP, AOCN
Assistant Professor, School of Nursing
Houston Health Science Center
University of Texas
Houston, Texas
Multiple Sclerosis, Systemic Lupus Erythematosus

Veronica Weaver Renfrow, MSN, RN, CS
Family Nurse Practitioner
Verterans Administration Medical Center
Cincinnati, Ohio
Substance Abuse

Angela Riley, MSN, RN-CS, NP-C, ARNP, CCRN
Cardiology Associates
Crestview Hills, Kentucky
Atrial Fibrillation

Kay T. Roberts, MSN, EdD, ARNP, CFNP, FAAN
Professor, School of Nursing
University of Louisville
Louisville, Kentucky
Alzheimer's Disease, Osteoporosis

Denise L. Robinson, PhD, RN, ARNP
Professor, Northern Kentucky University
Director, MSN Programs
Highland Heights, Kentucky
Family Nurse Practitioner
Northern Kentucky Family Health Centers, Inc.
Covington, Kentucky
Abdominal Pain, Acne, Allergic Reactions/Anaphylaxis, Appendicitis, Burns, CAD Management, Cirrhosis/Liver Disease, Conjunctivitis, Cough, Cytochrome P-450 Enzymes (Appendix D), Depression, DOT Physical Examination, Hearing Loss, Heart Murmur, Lifestyle Changes, Lower Extremity Pain/Limp in Children, Lymphadenopathy, Meniere's Disease, Mononucleosis, Muscular Dystrophy, Musculoskeletal Injuries (Ankle, Elbow, Foot, Knee, Shoulder, Wrist), NSAIDs (Appendix J), Otitis Externa, Otitis Media, Palpitations, Pancreatitis, Pediatric Antibiotics (Appendix L), Peripheral Neuropathy Lymphoma, Physical Examination (Sports), Preoperative Checklist, Rectal Bleeding, Red Eye, Sexual Dysfunction, Sleeping Disorders, Telephone Triage Guidelines (Appendix P), Temporal Mandibular Joint Disorder, Tendinitis/Bursitis, Thyroid Problems, Tinnitus, Urinary Tract Infections, Vertigo, Well Adolescent, Well Adult—Male, Wellness and Health Maintenance Guidelines

Karen Mangus Rogers, MSN, ARNP
Family Health Center, Inc.
Louisville, Kentucky
Voluntary Faculty/Preceptor
University of Kentucky
Lexington, Kentucky
University of Louisville
Louisville, Kentucky
Cellulitis, Cushing's Disease, Ear—Impacted Cerumen, Epistaxis, Fever, Folliculitis, Gastroenteritis, Hemorrhoids, Hernia, Immunizations During Pregnancy (Appendix H), Impotence, Infertility, Inflammatory Bowel Disease, Influenza, Irritable Bowel Syndrome, Medications Commonly Used During Pregnancy (Appendix E), Pneumonia, Scoliosis, Stomatitis, Strabismus, Testicular Mass, Toxic Shock Syndrome

Karen L. Ruschman, FNP-C
Family Nurse Practitioner
Patient First
Butler, Kentucky
Nurse Practitioner
Coordinator Nutrimed Program
St. Luke Hospital
Ft. Thomas, Kentucky
Hepatitis, Male Adult 65+

Carol Satterly, MSN, PNP
Pediatric Nurse Practitioner
College of Nursing
University of Kentucky
Lexington, Kentucky
Abuse, Asthma, Behavior Problems

Kristine A. Scordo, PhD, RN
Director, Acute Care Nurse Practitioner Program
Wright State University, College of Nursing and Health
Dayton, Ohio
Clinical Director, MVP Program of Cincinnati
Cincinnati, Ohio
Mitral Valve Prolapse

Cinda Crawford Simpson, MSN, ARNP
Nurse Practitioner, Primary Care
Veterans Administration Medical Center
Lexington, Kentucky
Chronic Obstructive Pulmonary Disease

Bernice "Bunny" Sornson, BSN, MSN, RN, ARNP
Family Nurse Practitioner
Winchester Quick Care
Winchester, Kentucky
Lyme Disease

Ann Stone, MSN, RNC, ANP, FNP
Adult/Family Nurse Practitioner
Internists of Fairfield
Fairfield, Ohio
Anticoagulation Therapy, Dyspnea, Hematuria, Sinusitis, Thrombophlebitis, Weight Loss (Unexplained)

Mary Kay Wooten, MSN, RN, CWOCN
Wound/Ostomy/Continence Clinical Nurse Specialist
Department of Veterans Affairs Medical Center
Durham, North Carolina
Lower Extremity Ulcers

Sadie S. Young-Hughes, BSN, MSN, NP
Adult Nurse Practitioner
Home Health Care Coordinator
Veterans Administration Medical Center
Cincinnati, Ohio
Peptic Ulcer Disease, Pityriasis, Psoriasis

Candace F. Zickler, MSN, RN, CPNP
Adjunct Faculty, Family Nurse Practitioner Program
College of Nursing and Health
Wright State University
Dayton, Ohio
Colic

Reviewers

Arlene M. Airhart, PhD, RN
Professor, College of Nursing
Northwestern State University
Shreveport, Louisiana

Lillian Kay Cowan, MHA, MSN, RN, CS, FNP-C
Certified Family Nurse Practitioner
Austin, Texas

Gail Hettermann, MS, RN, CS-FNP
Certified Family Nurse Practitioner
Coleman Medical Associates
Canton, Illinois

Steven B. Johnson, PharmD, BPharm, BS
Pharmacy Resident in Geriatrics
Washington State University College of Pharmacy
Elder Services of Spokane
Spokane, Washington

Judy A. Lidy, MSN, RNC, FNP
Certified Family Nurse Practitioner
Clinical Practice—Dr. Roger E. Bishop
Effingham, Illinois
Adjunct Faculty
Southern Illinois University
Edwardsville, Illinois

Cheryl McKenzie, MN, RNC, FNP
Associate Professor, Department of Nursing
Northern Kentucky University
Highland Heights, Kentucky
Family Nurse Practitioner
Northern Kentucky Family Health Center, Inc.
Dayton, Kentucky

Stephen M. Setter, PharmD, DVM, BPharm, BS
Assistant Professor, Pharmacy Practice
Washington State University College of Pharmacy
Elder Services of Spokane
Visiting Nurses Association
Spokane, Washington

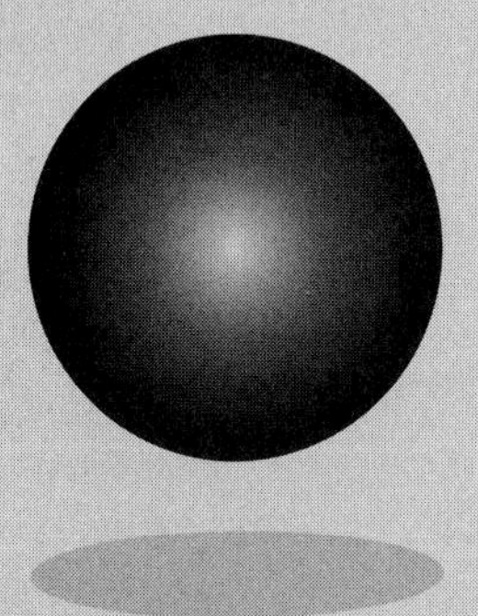

Preface

This book was written by a team of nurse practitioners who understand the complexity and diversity of chief complaints and conditions treated on a daily basis in a family practice setting. We searched long and hard for the perfect reference book—a book that was comprehensive, yet readable and useful; one that contained information to help us counsel patients as well as provide facts to empower the family to make good health decisions. Based on the reality of patients being scheduled every 10 to 15 minutes apart, we needed a book that was well organized and complete and had essential information that could be visually surveyed quickly. We did not want to have to look in several different books to obtain the information we needed. Although there are several family nurse practitioner guideline books available now, none captured all of the information we were looking for. So we wrote *Primary Care Across the Lifespan.* We are confident that it is a *good* book and that it will help all of us to be the most competent family nurse practitioners we can be. As you use this book, we hope you will provide us with feedback on what you think works and how you think the book can be improved.

What is different about *Primary Care Across the Lifespan*? It addresses common complaints, diseases, and wellness issues across the lifespan, using SOAPE format (subjective, objective, assessment, plan, and evaluation). What differentiates common complaints from disease states is that a complaint may be derived from multiple systems, such as the complaint of fatigue or dizziness. Often patients present with a complaint rather than a symptom of a known disease— the aim is to make an appropriate diagnosis. This book not only presents information about a disease state, but also provides data to help in the diagnostic process when a patient presents with only a symptom.

This book is comprehensive and targets the family. Thus you should rarely need another book to help you with pediatric, adult, reproductive health, or geriatric conditions. Pediatric, women's health, and geriatric issues are bolded within chapters so that the information can be located easily.

Tables are used generously in each chapter. Differential diagnosis tables contain supporting data for each possible diagnosis. Diagnostic test tables explain which diagnostic procedures will provide the best yield for the least buck. Approximate costs are included in the table so the patient has some degree of understanding and can be part of the decision-making process when options are available. The cost information was obtained from the *1998 Physicians Fee and Coding Guide,* which is updated yearly by HealthCare Consultants of America, Inc., Augusta, Georgia.

Pharmaceutical treatment tables are also included in each chapter. These tables organize essential and important information about treatment options, including dosing information, pregnancy category, possible side effects, and the approximate cost of the medication. Drug cost is given as cost per number of pills/capsules identified in parentheses (usually 100). Adjunct information related to P450 enzymes and pediatric dosing by weight are located in the appendices for easy accessibility. The pharmaceutical treatment tables can be used as an important teaching guide when considering the fiscal impact that medications may have on an individual's or family's lifestyle. Diet modification as a therapy option is discussed in each chapter.

Algorithms are included for most conditions to help cover the bases in diagnosis and treatment and to support consistency in practice. These are wonderful visual decision trees that can be reviewed quickly. Numerous drawings and photographs illustrate many conditions and procedures. We have also included sample policies for some of the "tough" situations that can occur in any practice, such as telephone triage guidelines and prescribing policies for controlled substances.

Patient education is addressed in each chapter. Actual handouts and educational materials are provided when appropriate. The Resources head appearing in many chapters provides telephone numbers, mail addresses, and Internet addresses for support groups and educational resources on the condition discussed in that chapter.

The extensive appendices include information that you use so much that you keep it with you at all times (e.g., pediatric antibiotic dosing tables) or information that is very hard to find when you need it because often you can't remember where you found it originally (e.g., preoperative antibiotic prophylaxis algorithm). These pages are screened for easy identification and fast accessibility.

The chapters were reviewed by other family nurse

practioners and by PharmDs to ensure that content was relevant and accurate. The contributors were recruited from across the United States, ensuring that content would reflect the diversity of family nurse practitioner practices and that regional differences would be minimized.

You work hard and you want to do your best. We hope that this book makes your life as a family nurse practitioner easier and that it affects the lives of student nurse practitioners, practicing nurse practitioners, and their patients in many positive ways.

Onward!

Denise Robinson
Pamela Kidd
Karen Rogers

Acknowledgments

Thanks to the nurse practitioners who willingly shared their knowledge and expertise to make this book a thorough and complete reference. Our thanks to Stephen Setter, PharmD, and Steven Johnson, PharmD, for reviewing the pharmacology information. Their attention to detail and their comments were invaluable. They did a great job. Thanks also to Pam and Karen who put in the time, effort, and creative juices needed to make this book a reality.

DR

This book was an extremely tough undertaking. Just when I felt overwhelmed, Karen and Denise picked me up. What a team! Many thanks to Mark Schneider who kept me from committing homicide with my computer.

PK

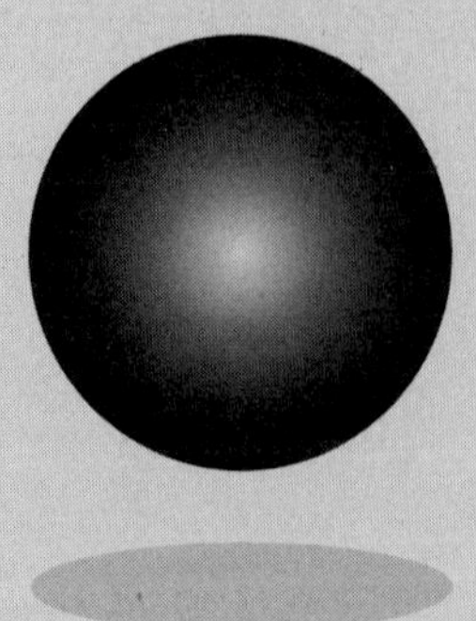

Contents

I

Common Complaints and Conditions

Abdominal Pain

ICD-9-CM

Abdominal Pain 789.0
Appendicitis 540.9
Acute Cholecystitis 575.0

OVERVIEW

Definition

The abdomen, the largest cavity in the body, may present with a variety of signs and symptoms that indicate disease, trauma, malfunction, or infection.

Acute abdomen refers to any acute condition within the abdomen that requires surgical attention; acute abdominal pain may be of nonabdominal origin and does not always require surgery.

Recurrent abdominal pain (RAP) is defined as three discrete episodes of abdominal pain occurring over 3 or more months. It is more common over the age of 5.

Incidence

Abdominal pain accounts for 5% of all Emergency Department (ED) visits and is one of the most frequently described reasons for ambulatory visits within general adult and family practice settings. Almost 50% of patients presenting with abdominal pain to an ED are found to have no identifiable cause. Of the remaining 50%, the most common diagnoses were medical, not surgical. Surgical conditions account for <15% of cases.

Pathophysiology

Pain impulses originate within the abdominal cavity and are transmitted via the autonomic and anterior/lateral spinothalamic tracts.

Common pathogenic mechanisms underlying acute (surgical) abdominal pain include *perforation* (hollow viscus), *obstruction* (intestinal, sigmoid volvulus), *ischemia* (mesenteric infarction), *inflammation* (diverticulitis with perforation, peritonitis), and *hemorrhage* (abdominal aneurysm, ulcers, ectopic pregnancy).

Nonsurgical causes may include hepatitis, cholecystitis, gastritis, nephrolithiasis, pneumonia, hernia, pelvic inflammatory disease (PID), pyelonephritis, endometriosis, and colon carcinoma.

Three major causes of pain exist:

Colic
Ischemia
Peritoneal inflammation

SUBJECTIVE DATA

History of Present Illness

Acute abdominal pain must be evaluated first to determine acuity level; the evaluation should only progress after nonemergent status is determined.

When the chief complaint is abdominal pain, the patient should be asked about:

Location
Onset
Radiation
Aggravating factors (movement, coughing, respiration)
Relieving factors (position, lying still, vomiting, antacids, food)
Mode of onset with progression (better, same, worse; abruptness of onset; duration)
Previous similar episodes of the pain, treatment, and resolution
Character (intermittent, steady, colicky) and pattern
Severity (rated on a 1/10 scale)
Last bowel movement
Stools (tarry or bloody)

Urinary pattern (frequency, urgency, dysuria, flank or back pain)

Women

Regardless of age, inquire about:

Vaginal bleeding, including last normal menses

In women of childbearing age ask about:

Sexual history
Obstetric history
Ectopic risk factors (PID, intrauterine contraceptive device [IUD], previous ectopic pregnancy, history of tubal and/or abdominal surgery), infertility treatment, history of endometriosis, Mittelschmertz. Ask about tubal ligation, date.

Men

Ask about urologic symptoms:

Hesitancy
Nocturia
Low urinary volume with frequency; lower abdominal distention
Sexual history

Children

Question child and/or parent about general indicators of illness: activity level, appetite, food intake, history of recent infections, and presence of fever.

Past Medical History

Ask about previous abdominal surgery, cardiovascular disease, analgesic use (acute, chronic), alcohol use, other substance abuse (tobacco, recreational drugs), weight change, past illness, risk factors (recent travel: travel history may direct the examiner to the possibility of gastroenteritis or dysentery), environmental exposure (immunologic suppression), allergies, social history indicating domestic violence.

Family History

Family history of appendicitis increases risk of a surgical problem.

Medication History

Anticoagulant therapy has been implicated in the development of abdominal hematomas.
Oral contraceptives have been associated with hepatic adenomas and with mesenteric infarction.
Corticosteroids may mask the symptoms of advanced peritonitis.
Previous surgery, especially abdominal or gynecologic operations, are common predisposing factors to bowel obstruction caused by adhesions. Previous surgery is also a risk factor for an ectopic pregnancy.
Laxative use

Review of Systems

A complete review of systems should be done as allowed by the patient's condition. Special attention should be given to cardiac, pulmonary, gynecologic, and genitourinary systems because abdominal pain may originate from these systems (e.g., angina, basilar pneumonia, PID, pyelonephritis).

Associated Symptoms

Ask about other symptoms that accompany the abdominal pain:

Gastrointestinal (GI) symptoms: Anorexia, nausea and vomiting, or diarrhea generally are nonspecific symptoms but are significant in the presence of abdominal pain. In an acute surgical abdomen, pain generally occurs after vomiting; the opposite is true in medical conditions. Patients with an acute developing abdomen usually have no desire for food. Diarrhea is usually associated with medical etiologies.

Patients with an acute abdomen often present with a paralytic ileus; thus it is important to determine if the subjective complaint of constipation is really obstipation (absence of both stool and flatus). True obstipation is strongly suggestive of a mechanical bowel obstruction, especially when accompanied by progressively increasing abdominal distention or repeated vomiting.

Fever and chills

OBJECTIVE DATA

Physical Examination

Perform a complete history and physical examination when possible. Include:

Vital signs with orthostatics
General appearance: Check for lymphadenopathy if concerned about mononucleosis and splenic rupture; note gait
Cardiac/pulmonary
Abdominal: Inspect abnormal pulsations, scars, character of skin, color, temperature
- Cullen's sign: periumbilical ecchymosis
- Grey turner's sign: flank ecchymosis
- Auscultation: bruits, bowel sounds, character of sounds heard
- Percussion: check for abdominal distention, shifting dullness in ascites
- Palpation: (ask patient to bend knees to relax musculature) (Notice facial grimacing or involuntary guarding, rebound tenderness, organomegaly, or abnormal masses.)

TABLE 1-1 Special Maneuvers for Physical Examination

Sign	Organ	Physical Findings	Meaning
Murphy's	Gallbladder	Temporary inspiratory arrest with palpation of right subcostal margin	Cholecystitis, cholelithiasis
Iliopsoas	Psoas abscess	Psoas muscle pain with active hip flexion or passive extension	Peritoneal irritation
Rebound tenderness	Peritoneal irritation	Increased pain on release of deep palpation	Appendicitis
Obturator	Obturator muscle	Pain with internal/external rotation of flexed thigh	Peritoneal irritation
Punch tenderness	Liver, spleen, or adjacent structures	Tenderness with firm palpation to lower costal margin	Hepatitis, splenic injury
CVA tenderness	Kidney	Tenderness over costal vertebral angle	Pyelonephritis

Adapted from Burkhardt C: Guidelines for the rapid assessment of abdominal pain indicative of acute surgical abdomen, *Nurse Pract* 17(6):43-46, 1992.
CVA, Costovertebral angle.

Rectal: Check for occult blood, fecal impaction, prostatic enlargement, tenderness or hemorrhoids; may need to do anoscopic examination with GI bleeding

Pelvic: Check for cervical motion tenderness, adnexal tenderness, abnormal masses, uterine organ size (Table 1-1)

Pediatric Abdominal Examination

As much as possible, examine the young child while the child is seated with the parent.

Place the child's hand over your hand for palpation, especially if the child is ticklish.

Normal abdomen in young child is rounded and scaphoid in the school-age and younger child.

Attempts to elicit psoas and obturator signs in the young child are seldom helpful.

Gentle percussion should be used instead of the usual test for rebound tenderness.

Kidney in the newborn and liver and spleen in all children should be palpated.

The inguinal canal should be examined for hernias.

Diagnostic Procedures

About 65% of acute surgical abdomen cases can be diagnosed by history and physical examination alone. However, supplemental examinations are necessary for diagnosis or exclusion of nonsurgical abdominal pain. Laboratory tests that should be ordered on all patients with severe abdominal pain include those shown in Table 1-2.

ASSESSMENT

The following findings are most closely correlated with a surgical abdomen (Figure 1-1):

Peritoneal signs

Markedly decreased or absent bowel sounds

Involuntary guarding

Pain <48 hours

Pain followed by vomiting

Advanced age

Prior surgery

The single most valuable test to rule out a possible surgical abdomen is repeated physical examinations by the same person over several hours.

Life-threatening diagnoses must be ruled out first (Table 1-3). Additional diagnoses to consider in abdominal pain are found in Tables 1-4 to 1-6 and Figures 1-2 to 1-5.

THERAPEUTIC PLAN

Pharmaceutical/Nonpharmaceutical

Minimally symptomatic patients may be managed initially with bed rest, clear liquids, and careful observation.

Therapy for moderate to severe pain and vomiting includes intravenous fluids, nasogastric suction, and correction of electrolyte imbalance. Antibiotics should be considered if the patient has fever. H_2 blockers (e.g., famotidine, ranitidine) or proton pump inhibitors (omeprazole, lansoprazole) may be indicated for the relief of gastritis and colicky pain. Serial abdominal examinations and laboratory tests cannot be overemphasized during the watchful waiting period.

Lifestyle/Activities

Careful observation may be needed if no acute signs and symptoms are found. If the patient does not appear toxic, close observation for 3 to 4 hours may provide some indication of diagnosis.

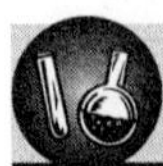

TABLE 1-2 Diagnostic Procedures: Abdominal Pain

Diagnostic Test	Findings	Cost ($)
CBC with differential	Indicates infection with elevated WBC with shift to the left (90% of appendicitis patients have ↑ WBCs; 80%; cholecystitis; 60%, intestinal obstruction; and 30%, no cause.)	18-23
Type and cross match	In preparation of surgery	74-129
Serial Hgb, Hct	Indicates continuing blood loss (When Hct is elevated, it suggests hemoconcentration and hypovolemia; when low, it suggests intraabdominal hemorrhage.)	Hgb: 11-14
U/A	Indicates infection, glucose, or bilirubinemia of hepatobiliary disease	15-20
Stool for occult blood/ova and parasites, and WBC	Check for bleeding, parasitic infestation, or infection; blood is usually seen with intussusception, late mesenteric vascular occlusion, and obstructing neoplasm or inflammatory lesions	13-17
Renal and liver function tests: BUN, creatinine, ALT, AST, alkaline phosphatase, GGT, amylase, lipase, bilirubin	Abnormalities may be seen with prolonged diarrhea and vomiting or with renal involvement.	Hepatic function panel: 29-41 Basic metabolic: 28-39
ECG	If there is a question as to cardiac origin, an ECG should be done.	56-65
Serum pregnancy	A necessity for females in childbearing ages	28-35 (qualitative) 51-65 (quantitative)
Chest x-ray	Rule out conditions that may mimic an acute abdomen, such as basilar pneumonia or pleural effusion	77-91
Flat and upright of abdomen	To detect the presence of free air (perforated viscus); is necessary before surgery; may also visualize AAA	142-169
Ultrasound of abdomen/gallbladder	Rule out gallstones, ectopic pregnancy, mass, appendicitis or bile duct dilation; best imaging choice for acute abdomen, unknown etiology, cholecystitis, AAA, appendicitis, biliary tract obstruction, ectopic pregnancy, ovarian cyst, solid organ pathology	351-419
CT	Best imaging choice for abscess, acute abdomen of unknown etiology, complicated appendicitis, biliary tract obstruction, multiple trauma, pancreatitis, perforated viscus, recent surgical incisions, retroperitoneal mass, solid organ pathology	807-956
IVP	Rule out kidney stones	280-333

Adapted from Trott A, Trunkey D, Wilson S: Acute abdominal pain: a guide to crisis management, *Patient Care* 29(15):119, 1995.

CBC, Complete blood count; *Hgb,* hemoglobin; *Hct,* hematocrit; *U/A,* urinalysis; *WBC,* white blood count; *BUN,* blood urea nitrogen; *ALT,* alanine aminotransferase; *AST,* aspartate aminotransferase (SGOT); *GGT,* gamma-glutamyl transferase; *ECG,* electrocardiogram; *CT,* computed tomography; *AAA,* abdominal aortic aneurysm; *IVP,* intravenous pyelogram.

Diet

If experiencing vomiting and nausea, allow only clear liquids.

If hungry, patient can probably eat lightly without problems.

Advise patient to avoid spicy, fatty, or gas-producing foods.

If patient is unable to retain fluids (see Chapter 57), especially for children.

A high-fiber diet may be helpful in RAP (not excessive fiber).

Patient Education

Discuss with patients and parents the rules for eating and return to hospital/clinic.

RAP: Discuss with parents theories of RAP and the existence of real pain.

Elimination of factors known to increase pain should help decrease frequency and severity of pain.

Child should go to school despite pain after a careful evaluation has been completed.

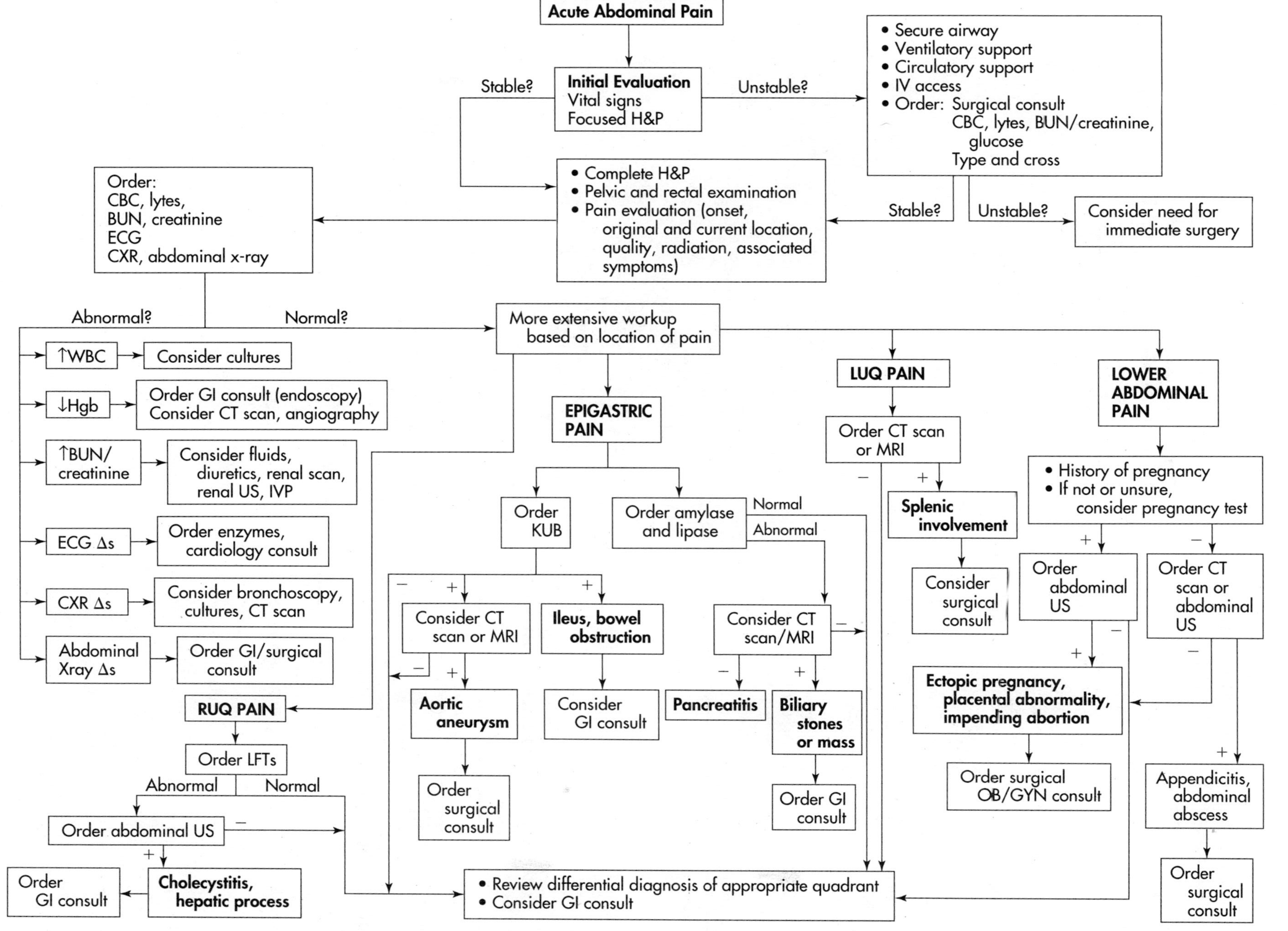

Figure 1-1 Diagnostic algorithm of acute surgical abdominal pain. *H&P,* History and physical; *CBC,* complete blood count; *BUN,* blood urea nitrogen; *ECG,* electrocardiogram; *CXR,* chest x-ray; *Hgb,* hemoglobin; *GI,* gastrointestinal; *CT,* computed tomography; *US,* ultrasound; *IVP,* intravenous pyelogram; *RUQ,* right upper quadrant; *LUQ,* left upper quadrant; *LFTs,* liver function tests; *KUB,* kidneys, ureter, bladder; *MRI,* magnetic resonance imaging; *IV,* intravenous; *OB/GYN,* obstetrics/gynecology. (Redrawn from Kelso L, Kugelman M: Nontraumatic abdominal pain, *AACN Clin Issues* 8(3):437-448, 1997.)

TABLE 1-3 Life-Threatening Diagnoses: Abdominal Pain

Diagnosis	Supporting Data
Abdominal aortic aneurysm	Tearing abdominal pain, severe mid to lower back pain; may radiate to genitals, sacrum, or flank; pulsatile mid to upper abdominal mass, lower-extremity ischemia
Bowel obstruction	No flatus, abdominal distention, vomiting, bowel sounds diminished or absent or have peristaltic rushes, abdominal x-ray film shows air
Ruptured ectopic pregnancy	Late or missed menses, breast tenderness, unexplained weight gain, lower-quadrant abdominal pain, vaginal spotting, +hCG
Splenic rupture	Shocky, hypotensive, left upper quadrant abdominal pain
Myocardial infarction	Gastritis, heartburn, nausea, diaphoresis, just doesn't feel right

hCG, Human chorionic gonadotropin.

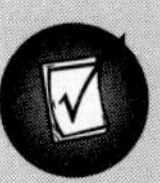

TABLE 1-4 Differential Diagnosis by Symptom

Symptom	Diagnosis*
Significant vomiting or diarrhea (Ch. 57)	Bowel obstruction, **gastroenteritis,** gastroparesis, **pregnancy** volvulus
Hematemesis or melena (Ch. 154)	Aortic enteric fistula, **diverticular disease, malignancy,** polyps, **peptic ulcer disease,** varices
Syncope (Ch. 172)	AAA, **ectopic pregnancy,** gastroenteritis, **gastrointestinal bleed, myocardial infarction**
Dysuria, urgency, frequency, hematuria (Ch. 87)	**Pyelonephritis, renal colic**
Constipation (Ch. 45)	Bowel ischemia, **bowel obstruction, volvulus,** diverticular disease
Rectal pain	Ovarian cyst, **prostatitis**

Adapted from ACEP: Clinical Policy, *Ann Emerg Med* 23(4), 1994.
*Most common diagnoses in bold.

TABLE 1-5 Most Common Causes of Acute Abdominal Pain by Age Group

Age	Common	Less Common
0-1	Intussusception Incarcerated hernia Gastroenteritis (Ch. 77) Hernia (Ch. 90)	Appendicitis Testicular torsion
2-5	Appendicitis (Ch. 14) Constipation Gastroenteritis Pneumonia Poisonings	Intussusception Urinary tract infection Testicular torsion
6-11	Appendicitis Pneumonia (Ch. 146) Constipation/encopresis Gastroenteritis (Ch. 77) Urinary tract infection (Ch. 187) Recurrent abdominal pain	Intussusception Testicular torsion Incarcerated inguinal hernia
12-21	Appendicitis Inflammatory bowel disease (IBD) (Ch. 100) Testicular torsion Pelvic inflammatory disease (Ch. 140) Mittelschmertz pregnancy Ectopic pregnancy Urinary tract infection (sexually active female)	Urinary tract infection Pneumonia Constipation Sickle cell crisis
21-55	Peptic ulcer disease (30-50) (Ch. 142) IBD Gastroenteritis Nonspecific abdominal pain (more common <40)	
>55	Intestinal obstruction Diverticulitis (Ch. 58) Cholelithiasis/cholecystitis (Ch. 36) Strangulated hernia Colon cancer Abdominal aortic aneurysm (40-70)	Pneumonia Congestive heart failure

Adapted with permission from Finelli L: *Pediatr Health Care,* 5(5):251-255, 1991.

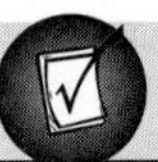

TABLE 1-6 Common Causes of Abdominal Pain

Diagnosis	Supporting Data
Appendicitis	Generalized abdominal pain that localizes to RLQ, acute to persistent pain, may have N/V, low-grade fever, slight ↑ WBCs, US shows appendix with inflammatory changes
Cholecystitis/biliary colic	Epigastric or RUQ pain with referral to right shoulder, gradual to acute onset, RUQ tenderness, + Murphy's sign, US shows inflammation and gallstones; clinical signs and symptoms are poor indicators in **elderly**
Diverticulosis/diverticulitis	Acute abdominal pain and fever, LLQ tenderness and mass, increased WBCs; N/V are frequent; constipation or loose stools may be present
Gastroenteritis	Crampy, diffuse abdominal pain that follows or coincides with a bout of diarrhea; cramping occurs primarily after meals
Pancreatitis (Ch. 136)	Epigastric pain boring to back; persistent, dull pain; epigastric tenderness; ↑ amylase; CT shows pancreatic inflammation
IBS/IBD	Diffuse abdominal pain, gradual onset of crampy pain, diarrhea common, may have fever; blood and WBCs in stool; abnormal results on scope
Intestinal ischemia	Acute mesenteric ischemia is a life-threatening emergency: acute onset, colicky pain. Distention and nausea may be seen. Chronic mesenteric ischemia may present as intestinal angina: postprandial abdominal pain that is crampy and located in the upper abdomen. Onset is 10-15 min after eating and lasts up to 3 hours. Caution **elderly** that, even with acute mesenteric ischemia, distention and localized tenderness may be minimal. Rebound tenderness and rigidity are late signs.
Renal colic	Sharp, abrupt CVA tenderness radiates into lower abdomen. Hematuria may be present, there may be flank tenderness, and IVP shows stones.
Pelvic inflammatory disease	There may be abdominal pain with CMT, guarding and adnexal tenderness; vaginal discharge; purulent cervicitis; and history of STD exposure, fever.
Peptic ulcer disease	There may be heartburn, indigestion, RUQ pain with variable relationship to meals. In **older patients** the first sign may be peritonitis caused by perforation or anemia.
Chronic nonspecific abdominal pain	This may be referred to as RAP in children. It is thought to be caused by interaction of physical and psychosocial stressors. Typical presentation is gradual onset of paroxysmal pain in periumbilical region. It is usually not related to meals or specific events, but it may be severe enough to interrupt normal activities of daily living. Diagnosis is by exclusion.

RLQ, Right lower quadrant; *N/V,* nausea/vomiting; *WBC,* white blood cells; *US,* ultrasound; *RUQ,* right upper quadrant; *LLC,* left lower quadrant; *IBS/IBD,* irritable bowel syndrome/inflammatory bowel disease; *CT,* computed tomography; *CVA,* costovertebral angle; *IVP,* intravenous pyelogram; *CMT,* cervical motion tenderness; *STD,* sexually transmitted disease.

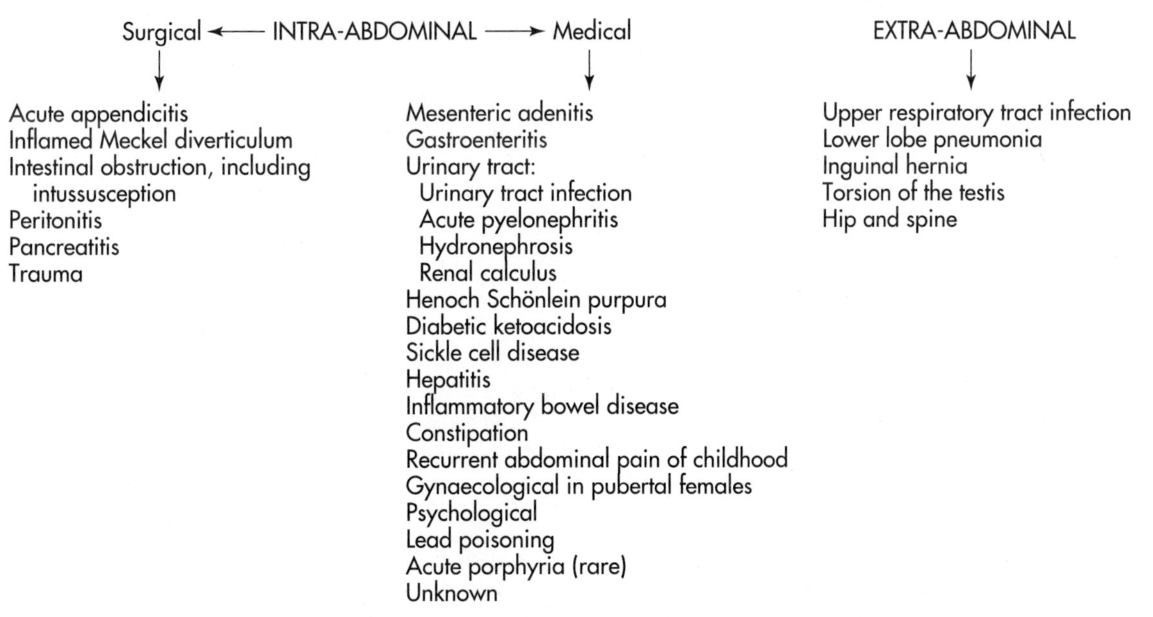

Figure 1-2 Causes of acute abdominal pain in children. (Redrawn from Lissauer T: *Illustrated textbook of paediatrics,* St Louis, 1996, Mosby.)

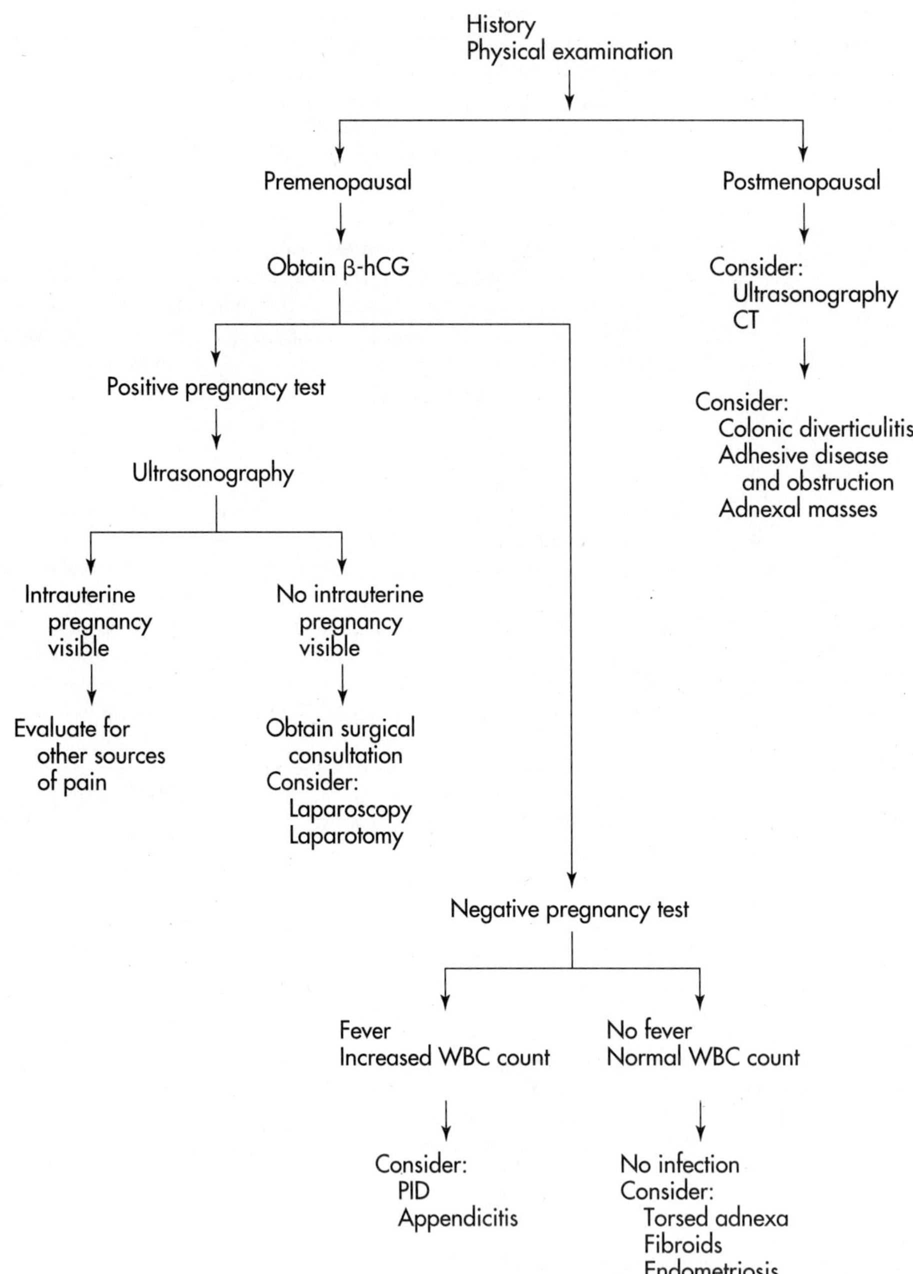

Figure 1-3 Female patient with acute abdominal pain. *hCG,* Human chorionic gonadotropin; *WBC,* white blood count; *PID,* pelvic inflammatory disease; *CT,* computed tomography. (Redrawn from Greene HL, Johnson WP, Lemcke D: *Decision making in medicine: an algorithmic approach,* ed 2, St Louis, 1998, Mosby.)

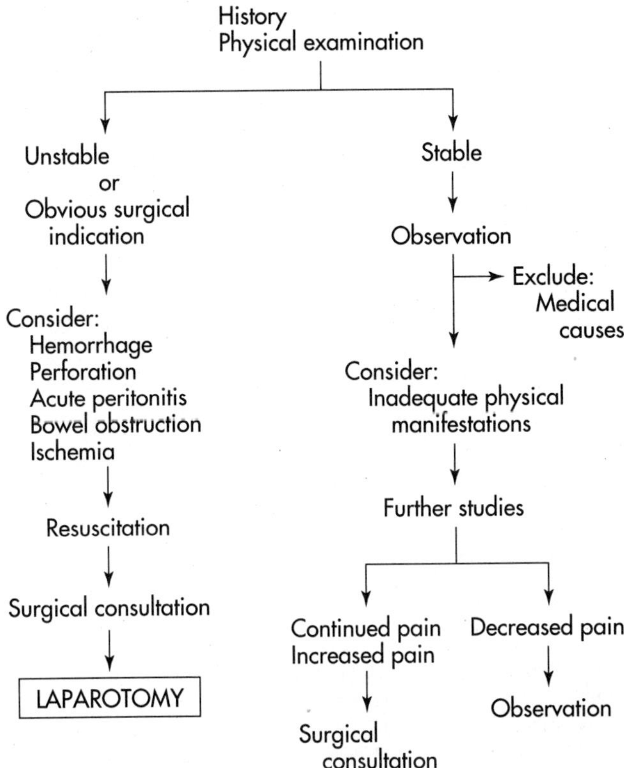

Figure 1-4 Adult patient with acute abdominal pain. (Redrawn from Greene HL, Johnson WP, Lemcke D: *Decision making in medicine: an algorithmic approach,* ed 2, St Louis, 1998, Mosby.)

Encourage parents of children with RAP to deal with it matter-of-factly. Do not give excessive attention, which only reinforces pain.

Family Impact

Having severe abdominal pain is frightening, both for the patient and/or parents. Giving them information to participate in the decision making and when to seek care empowers them.

Referral

Patients should be referred to the consulting physician for evaluation and probable admission:

Rigid abdomen
Peritoneal signs
Localized tenderness
Evidence of gastrointestinal obstruction
Bleeding
<2 and >65 years of age
Tender pulsatile mass
Uncontrolled vomiting and abdominal tenderness

Consultation

Consider a surgical consult if the patient has the following symptoms:

Fever >38° C
Tachycardia
>110: Adult
Child
Elevated white blood cell count with >75% shift in neutrophils
Peritoneal signs: tenderness to palpation, rebound tenderness, abdominal tenderness on coughing, guarding, rigidity
>65 years old
Consider consultation with collaborating physician when etiology of abdominal pain is not clear or history, physical examination, or diagnostic tests are contradictory.
Seek consultation if abdominal pain continues.

Follow-up

Follow-up abdominal pain in 1 week, sooner if the patient experiences fever or prostrating pain.
If no problems in 1 week, follow-up in 1 month, then 6 months.

EVALUATION

Advise adult patient to return immediately if:

Pain gets worse or is now only in one area
Bloody emesis or stool
Dizziness or syncope
Abdomen becomes swollen
Elevated temperature >102° F orally
Difficulty passing urine
Shortness of breath

Advise parent of pediatric patient to return immediately if:

Pain increases or is only in one specific area.
Child begins to vomit blood or blood in stool.
The child is walking bent over or holding his/her abdomen or refuses to walk.
Pain is in the testicle or scrotum.
Child's abdomen becomes swollen or quite tender to the touch.
Child has difficulty urinating.
Child is short of breath.

All patients should seek immediate care if:

A new symptom appears.
Current symptoms worsen.
Symptoms such as dizziness or dehydration develop.

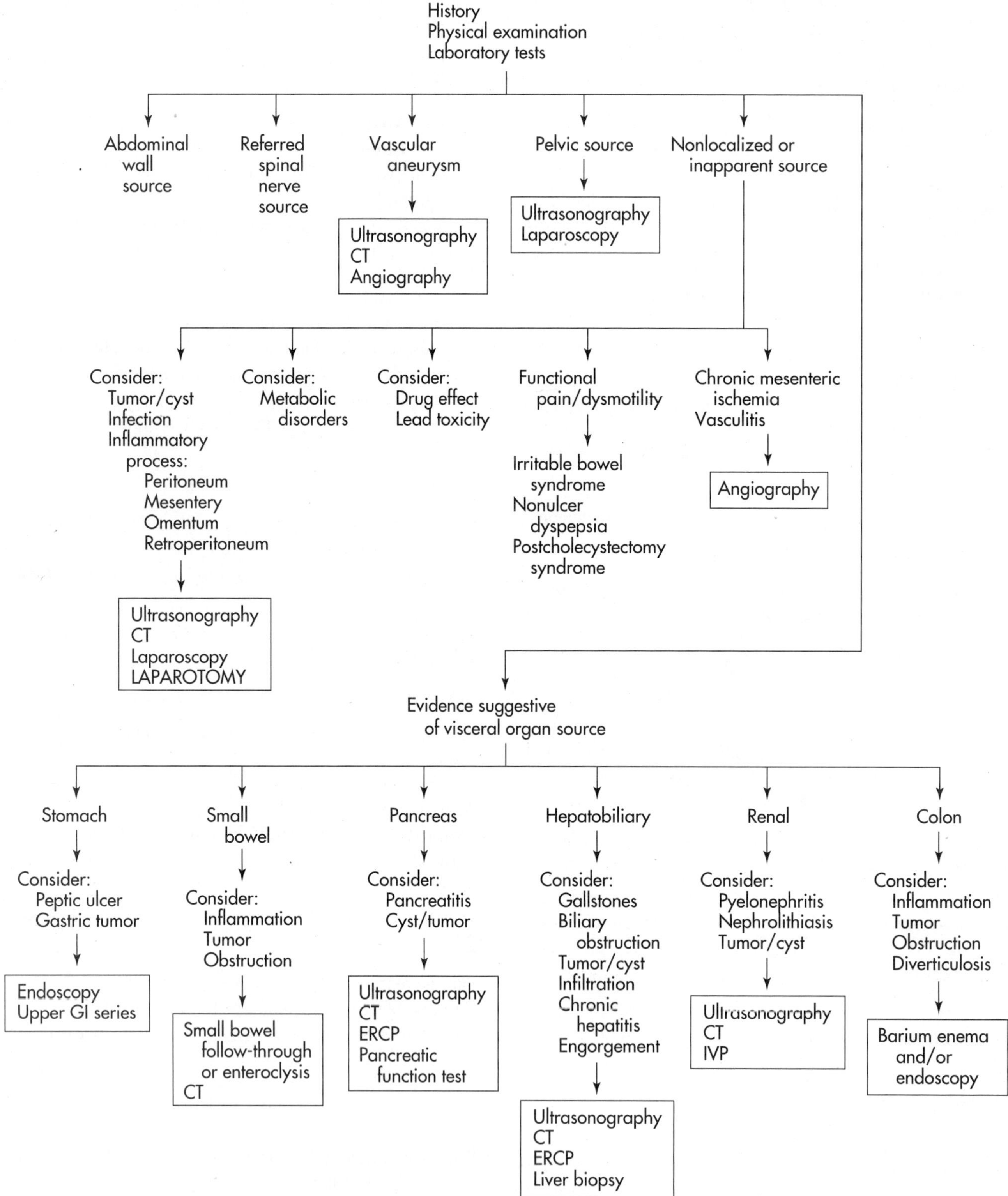

Figure 1-5 Adult patient with chronic abdominal pain. *CT,* Computed tomography; *GI,* gastrointestinal, *ERCP,* endoscopic retrograde cholangiopancreatography; *IVP,* intravenous pyelography. (Redrawn from Greene HL, Johnson WP, Lemcke D: *Decision making in medicine: an algorithmic approach,* ed 2, St Louis, 1998, Mosby.)

SUGGESTED READINGS

American College of Emergency Physicians: Clinical policy for the initial approach to patients with a chief complaint of nontraumatic acute abdominal pain, *Ann Emerg Med* 23(4):906-922, 1994.

Burkhardt C: Guidelines for the rapid assessment of abdominal pain indicative of acute surgical abdomen, *Nurse Pract* 17(6):43-46, 1992.

Clinical abstracts: Scoring system helps differentiate appendicitis from non-specific pain, *Modern Med* 66:20, 25, 1998.

Ellsworth A et al: *Mosby's 1998 medical drug reference*, St Louis, 1998, Mosby.

Finelli L: Evaluation of the child with acute abdominal pain, *J Pediatr Health Care* 5(5):251-256, 1991.

Healthcare Consultants of America: *1998 physicians fee and coding guide*, Augusta, Ga, 1998, Healthcare Consultants of America.

Hixson L: Chronic abdominal pain. In Greene H, Johnson W, Lemcke D, editors: *Decision making in medicine,* ed 2, St Louis, 1998, Mosby.

Kelso L, Kugelman M: Nontraumatic abdominal pain, *AACN Clinical Issues* 8(3):437-448, 1997.

Mead M: Detecting appendicitis, *Practice Nurse* 11(7):486-487, 1996.

Palley S: Acute abdominal pain. In Greene H, Johnson W, Lemcke D, editors: *Decision making in medicine,* ed 2, St Louis, 1998, Mosby.

Parker D, Evan S, Kingham J: Chronic abdominal pain, *Postgrad Med* 73:831-833, 1997.

Rice P: Abdominal pain: predicting who will need an operation, *Emerg Med* April:14-25, 1996.

Rothrock S: When appendicitis isn't "classic," *Emerg Med* 28(3):108-124, 1996.

Samuelson R: Acute abdominal pain in women. In Greene H, Johnson W, Lemcke D, editors: *Decision making in medicine,* ed 2, St Louis, 1998, Mosby.

Stone R: Primary care diagnosis of acute abdominal pain, *Nurse Pract* 21(12), 19-40, 1996.

Abscess/Boil/Furuncle

ICD-9-CM

Furuncle, Carbuncle 680.9
Skin Infection 686.9

OVERVIEW

Definition

Inflammation of a hair follicle or of cutaneous gland and surrounding tissue

Incidence

More common in adolescents with acne; can be recurrent problem in patients with diabetes and persons who are chronic nasal carriers of *Staphylococcus aureus*

Pathophysiology

A furuncle is usually caused by *S. aureus*. Inflammatory process causes swelling and pus formation. A form of furunculosis is related to obstruction of apocrine sweat glands.

Protective Factors Against

Intact immune system
Clean skin and nails

Factors That Increase Susceptibility

Diabetes
Injection drug use
Human immunodeficiency virus disease

SUBJECTIVE DATA

History of Present Illness

Pain and tenderness at site
Pruritus
Lesion usually on areas exposed to friction: buttocks, neck, face, axillae, groin, thighs, upper back

Past Medical History

Chronic illness
Prior history of furuncles

Medications

Noncontributory

Family History

Not usually significant

Psychosocial History

Not significant

Associated Symptom

Fever

OBJECTIVE DATA

Physical Examination

Have patient undress and check the patient all over for lesions.
Skin: Target the following areas: buttocks, neck, face,

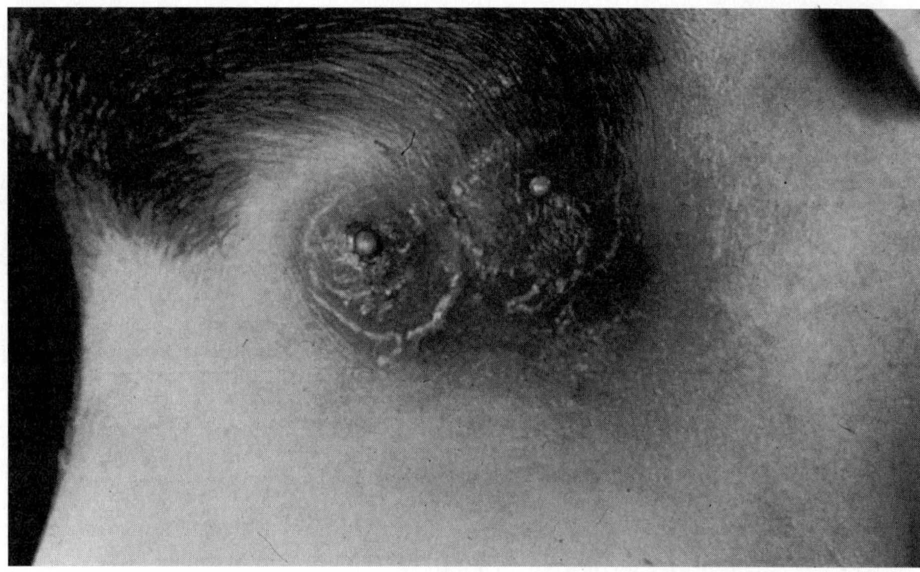

Figure 2-1 Pustular deep nodule on the posterior aspect of the right neck. (From Hooper BJ, Goldman MP: *Primary dermatologic care,* St Louis, 1999, Mosby.)

axillae, groin, thighs, upper back. There will usually be a lesion, 5-mm to 3-cm in size, that is erythematous and tender to palpation. Pus will be in the center of the lesion, and the skin will be thin over the center (Figure 2-1).

Lymph: Lymphadenopathy may be present if several follicles are infected and interconnected forming a carbuncle.

Diagnostic Procedures

Laboratory: Culture drainage ($31 to $39); consider culture of nares ($24 to $30) if chronic staphylococcal carriage is suspected (recurrent cutaneous infection)

ASSESSMENT

Differential diagnoses are included in Table 2-1.

TABLE 2-1 Differential Diagnosis: Abscess

Diagnosis	Supporting Data
Folliculitis	Painless, minor erythema, if present, most frequently involves face only
Epidermal inclusion cyst	History of small cyst in the same area, presence of visible cyst orifice, extrusion of cheesy material

THERAPEUTIC PLAN

Pharmaceutical

Antibiotics should be used in cases in which the patient has diabetes, multiple furuncles, or a carbuncle (Table 2-2).

Surgical

Incise and drain lesions greater than 1 cm in diameter, that are painful, or that do not drain spontaneously. Consider infiltrating with lidocaine 0.5% or 1% first. Consider packing with iodoform gauze for 1 to 2 days.

Lifestyle/Activities

In cases of recurrent furunculosis, the patient has to bathe and shampoo TID with hexachlorophene soap.

Diet

Noncontributory

Patient Education

Gently apply warm heat for 30 minutes QID to area.

Do not touch area.

Change bed and bath linens daily in cases of recurrent furunculosis.

Do not wear tight clothing.

Do not use antiperspirants but can use deodorants.

Avoid shaving axillae.

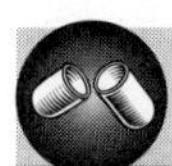

TABLE 2-2 Pharmaceutical Plan: Abscess/Boil/Furuncle

Drug	Dose	Comments	Cost
Dicloxacillin	1 g daily in divided doses × 10 days		\$20-\$94 \$16/Oral solution
Cephalexin	250 mg QID × 10 days		\$15-\$130
Erythromycin	333 mg TID × 10 days	Don't use in conjunction with lovastatin	\$14-\$20
Bacitracin ointment	TID or QID × 14 days, apply to nares	Use for recurrent furuncles	\$2-\$5
Mupirocin ointment	2%, apply BID × 5 days in nares	Use for recurrent furuncles	\$29/30 g

Family Impact

Extra washing of linens

Referral/Consultation

Consider referral to surgeon for incision and drainage of large areas.

Consultation with a dermatologist may be necessary for recurrent furunculosis.

Follow-up

Check open draining lesion or incised lesion for healing in 1 week.

EVALUATION

No systemic infection
No recurrence of furuncle
Negative nares culture for *S. aureus*

SUGGESTED READINGS

Berger T, Goldstein S, Odom R: Skin and appendages. In Tierney L, McPhee S, Papadakis M, editors: *Current medical diagnosis and treatment,* ed 36, Stamford, Conn, 1998, Appleton & Lange.

Pierce N: Bacterial infections of the skin. In Barker L, Burton J, Zieve P, editors: *Principles of ambulatory medicine,* ed 4, Baltimore, 1995, Williams & Wilkins.

3 Abuse

ICD-9-CM

Child Abuse 995.5
Physical 995.54
Adult/Spouse Abuse 995.81
Sexual 995.83

OVERVIEW

Definition

Abuse is a nonaccidental injury as a result of commission or omission on the part of a parent, guardian, spouse, or other caretaker. Harm may also occur as a result of neglect or inattention to physical, emotional, medical and financial needs in a dependent situation.

Types of Abuse

Physical: Inflicted injuries often a result of hitting, beating, shaking or burning; may be unusual for age of victim or incompatible with history

Sexual: **(Children and elders) assault, incest or exploitation for the sexual gratification of an adult caregiver; (women) forced sexual activity without the consent of the sexual partner**

- Nontouching offenses: Verbal sexual stimulation, exhibitionism, and invasion of privacy
- Touching offenses: fondling, masturbation, intercourse, sodomy, anal penetration, and/or oral genital contact

Emotional/psychological: An attack on the person's sense of self and social competence; concurrent with other forms of abuse

Types: Ignoring, rejecting, isolating, terrorizing, corrupting, verbally assaulting, and overpressuring

Financial: Exploitation of resources through misrepresentation, coercion, or theft (most likely to elderly)

Neglect: Failure of responsible person to provide adequate food, clothing, shelter, and/or medical care

Incidence: Numbers are known to be underreported/underrecognized in the United States.

- **Children:** >200,000 are abused; > 800,000 are neglected each year.
- **Women:** Approximately 2 million are victims of domestic violence each year, and more than 12 million will be abused at some time in their lives. 45% of wives of alcoholics have been assaulted.
- **Elderly:** As many as 2 million are abused each year; problems are expected to worsen as population ages.

Pathophysiology/Etiology

Often physical abuse is explained as an accident, but more likely it is the result of a stressful situation and a caretaker/partner with poor decision-making and/or coping skills.

Families under chronic strain from financial and health problems are particularly at risk.

Isolation/lack of social support may contribute.

There may be a history of psychopathology or substance abuse by the abuser.

The vulnerable or powerless **(children, women, elderly)** tend to be victims of abuse.

SUBJECTIVE DATA

Multiple health care providers and/or Emergency Department visits

Conflicting stories about how injuries occurred

Information possibly unknowingly revealed in the context of other questions (e.g., *Nurse Practitioner:* What was your last medicine for this condition? *Parent:* I didn't get that prescription filled; I thought she was better. OR

Elder: I don't have money in my checkbook anymore, so I didn't get it.

Caretaker affect inappropriate for situation (e.g., laughter, anger, lack of concern)

History of sleep disturbances, appetite changes, withdrawn behavior, aggressive behavior/violent outbursts, suicide attempts

Children: Temper tantrums, poor school performance, accident described inconsistent with child's developmental ability, delinquent behavior, knowledge and use of sexual terms, excessive masturbation or sex play, suspicious of adults

Women/elderly: Frequent requests for pain medication, frequent visits for somatic complaints, gastrointestinal disturbances, chronic pain of unclear etiology

OBJECTIVE DATA

Physical Examination

A complete examination is warranted, with particular focus on the following areas:

General: Responsiveness/affect, hygiene, nutritional status, appropriateness of dress, presence of unattended physical problems

Head/eyes/ears/nose/throat: Head trauma, patchy hair loss; PERRLA funduscopic: retinal hemorrhage, hemorrhage of sclerae, bleeding from ears/nose, blood behind tympanic membrane

Skin: Bruises in different stages of healing; burns; physical marks of an object (e.g., looped cord, belt buckle), restraint marks on extremities, neck or mouth, human bite marks

Abdomen: Tenderness, organomegaly, bruising

Musculoskeletal: Tenderness or swelling of joints, signs of fractures or dislocations

Neurological: Mental status, neurodevelopmental screening (children)

Genitalia: Genital, urethral, vaginal, or anal bruising or bleeding; swollen, red vulva or perineum; presence of foreign body in genital area

Accurate/thorough description of findings is vital (photos are helpful); significant negatives are required.

Diagnostic Procedures

Children: Growth measures (plotted on appropriate growth charts), height, weight, head circumference (2 yrs and under) (Flattening weight curve may indicate early signs of neglect or nonorganic failure to thrive, whereas flattening of curves in all growth parameters is indicative of a more serious condition.)

Other tests such as radiographs and laboratory as indicated by subjective and objective data.

ASSESSMENT

Differential Diagnoses

Women/elderly: Unintended injury, self-neglect, poverty

Children: Injury events, normal skin variations (e.g., mongolian spots), organic failure to thrive, blood dyscrasias (e.g., leukemia), osteogenesis imperfecta, cultural practices (e.g., Asian—cupping)

THERAPEUTIC PLAN

Nonpharmaceutical

Report any suspected abuse to appropriate social service agency. NOTE: Nurse practitioners (NPs) are considered mandated reporters and are required by law to report suspected cases of abuse. NPs incur some form of legal immunity (varies by state) if making a good faith report, but they are also subject to criminal charges if they fail to make a report in a case of suspected abuse.

Treat/refer identified medical conditions.

Ensure that victim does not return to hostile environment in case of life-threatening situations.

Initiate team approach including medical, social services, and law enforcement members as appropriate.

Prevention: Incorporate screenings into practice that would identify families at risk.

Patient Education

Patient education is most appropriate as a preventive measure.

Children

Teach positive attitudes toward child/pregnancy to prevent later abuse.

Teach behavioral expectations by developmental level.

Teach appropriate and inappropriate touch.

Teach parenting strategies for specific behaviors.

Address further knowledge deficits regarding child behavior and parenting as identified.

Stress that parents need time away from children.

Women/Elderly

Explain risk factors for abuse.

Familiarize families at risk with resources available.

Provide lists of shelters/referral sources if abuse does occur.

EVALUATION/FOLLOW-UP

Consultation with an MD may be mandatory in some states. Certification for nurse practitioners in the forensic evaluation of abuse is of a growing interest and demand.

Follow-up the same day by phone if returning to same environment.

Confirm social services investigation once a report is made (within 24 hours).

Monitor progress of case until resolution.

RESOURCE

Domestic Violence Assistance Guide available from: Violence Against Women Grants Office, Office of Justice Programs, U. S. Department of Justice.

SUGGESTED READINGS

Arvin AM et al, editors: *Nelson textbook of pediatrics*, ed 15, Philadelphia, 1996, WB Saunders.

Boyton RW, Dunn ES, Stephens GR, editors: *Ambulatory pediatric care*, ed 2, Philadelphia, 1994, JB Lippincott.

Fingerhood MI, Barker LR: Alcoholism and associated problems. In Barker LR, Burton JR, Zieve PD, editors: *Principles of ambulatory medicine*, ed 4, Baltimore, 1995, Williams & Wilkins.

Finucane TE, Burton JR: Geriatric medicine: special considerations. In Barker LR, Burton JR, Zieve PD, editors: *Principles of ambulatory medicine*, ed 4, Baltimore, 1995, Williams & Wilkins.

Lynch SH: Elder abuse: what to look for, how to intervene, *AJN* 97(1):26-32, 1997.

Monteleone JA: *Recognition of child abuse for the mandated reporter*, St Louis, 1994, G.W. Medical Publishing.

Schmitt, BD: Seven deadly sins of childhood: advising parents about difficult developmental phases, *Child Abuse Neglect* 11:421-432, 1987.

Uphold CR, Graham MV: *Clinical guidelines in child health*, Gainesville, Fla, 1994a, Barmarrae Books.

Uphold CR, Graham MV: *Clinical guidelines on family practice*, Gainesville, Fla, 1994b, Barmarrae Books.

Acne Vulgaris

ICD-9-CM

Acne Vulgaris 706.1

OVERVIEW

Definition

Acne is a chronic follicular eruption at the pilosebaceous unit that begins as a comedone. Papules, pustules, and cysts develop if an inflammatory reaction occurs. Other disorders such as neonatal acne and steroid acne have been labeled acne. These disorders, better labeled acneiform, originate with inflammation, missing the comedone stage.

Incidence

Acne vulgaris affects nearly 17 million people in the United States. The peak onset is puberty. Boys are affected more than girls; nearly 100% of boys will experience acne by age 16 years. The prevalence decreases in adulthood: 8% of adults 25 to 34 year old, and 3% of adults 35 to 44 years old. The incidence of mild to moderate acne among women ages 20 to 50 is increasing. It currently affects 40% to 50% of all adult women to some degree. Acne is the second most common diagnosis in black women ages 35 to 64 who visit dermatologists. Acne vulgaris usually improves during pregnancy; however, exacerbations may also occur.

Pathophysiology

The exact pathogenesis of acne is still not completely understood. The cause is multifactorial and is most influenced by:

Excessive sebum production: The rate of sebum production is determined genetically. The production of sebum is increased by the presence of androgens.

Comedogenesis: The follicle canal becomes blocked by the sebum, resulting in the formation of comedones—open comedones or blackheads and closed comedones or whiteheads. Acne can not occur without a hair follicle. Comedogenesis occurs in sebaceous follicles only.

Propionibacterium acnes: the presence of *P. acnes* causes the inflammatory aspects of acne. This bacteria is benign and resides on the skin at all times.

Factors That Contribute to Acne

Premenstrually increased progesterone during luteal phase of menstrual cycle is a cause.

Although diet has not been shown to be in a clear relationship to acne, most clinicians advise clients to avoid foods they believe increases their acne.

Pollution is a contributing factor.

Constant pressure such as heavy sweating, especially under athletic gear, is a cause.

Mechanical trauma, from picking at lesions or from rubbing of clothes can make acne worse.

Oil-based cosmetics and hair products can worsen acne.

Medications are a contributing factor to acne. Excessive or abrasive cleaning is not necessary. Acne is not caused by lack of cleanliness.

History of Present Illness

When did acne start?
(Adults) Did you have acne as a teenager?
Is the acne related to menses?
Are OTC medications used for skin?
Do you exercise regularly?
How many times a day do you wash your face?
Do you use moisturizers: how often and how much?

Hormonal Influences

Determine the timing of the onset of pubertal changes in relationship to the increase in acne. Females with cystic acne should be assessed for hirsutism and a history of irregular menses to rule out androgen production.

Family History

Parental and sibling history of acne

Medication History

Oral and injectable steroids; both prescribed and illicit
Lithium, isoniazid, and phenytoin are some of the most common drugs that cause drug-induced acne.
Oral and infectable contraceptives

Home Treatments

Type of soap used, frequency of face washing, over-the-counter treatments tried, use of cosmetics

Work History

For example, work in a fast-food restaurant over hot grease

Psychosocial History

Is the acne of concern to the client? Does the client's appearance inhibit social interactions?

TABLE 4-1 Differential Diagnosis: Acne Vulgaris

Diagnosis	Supporting Data
Acne conglobata	Severe cystic acne with more involvement of trunk than face; lesions include coalescing nodules, cysts, and abscesses
Rosacea	Chronic acneform disorder of the facial pilosebaceous units, ↑ reactivity of capillaries to heat, leading to flushing and telangiectasia; occurs in 30-50 y/o, predominantly females
Folliculitis	Infection of the upper portion of the hair follicle: follicular papule in beard, axillae, genital area from shaving
Tinea barbae	A dermaphyte trichomycosis involving the beard and moustache areas (ringworm of the beard); occurs in males only; pustular folliculitis surrounded by red inflammatory pustules or papules

SUBJECTIVE DATA

Description of Most Common Symptoms

Microcomedo, papules, pustules, or nodules, blackhead, whitehead; erythema lasting several months

OBJECTIVE DATA

Physical Examination

Assess skin on the face, chest, neck and upper back.
Adolescents: Assess pubertal stage and hirsutism in females with cystic acne.
Skin: Assess the severity of the lesions.
Assess for scarring.

Diagnostic Procedures

None

ASSESSMENT

Determine grade of acne.
- Grade I pure comedonal acne
- Grade II mild papular acne
- Grade II-III papulopustular and cystic acne
- Grade III-IV persistent pustulocystic acne
- Grade V pustulocystic nodular acne

Differential diagnosis includes acneform lesions such as *drug-induced acne,* or neonatal acne (Table 4-1).

THERAPEUTIC PLAN

Development of a treatment plan that will maximize improvement and compliance requires an accurate assessment of history, number of lesions, and lifestyle priorities (Figure 4-1).

Pharmaceutical

Treatment options depend on the severity of the acne lesions. Understanding the pathogenesis is the key to choosing the proper treatment. Treatment may need to be long term to avoid exacerbations (Table 4-2).

Lifestyle/Activities

Avoid use of oil-based cosmetics
Consider change in occupation if work environment is aggravating factor

Diet

Well-balanced

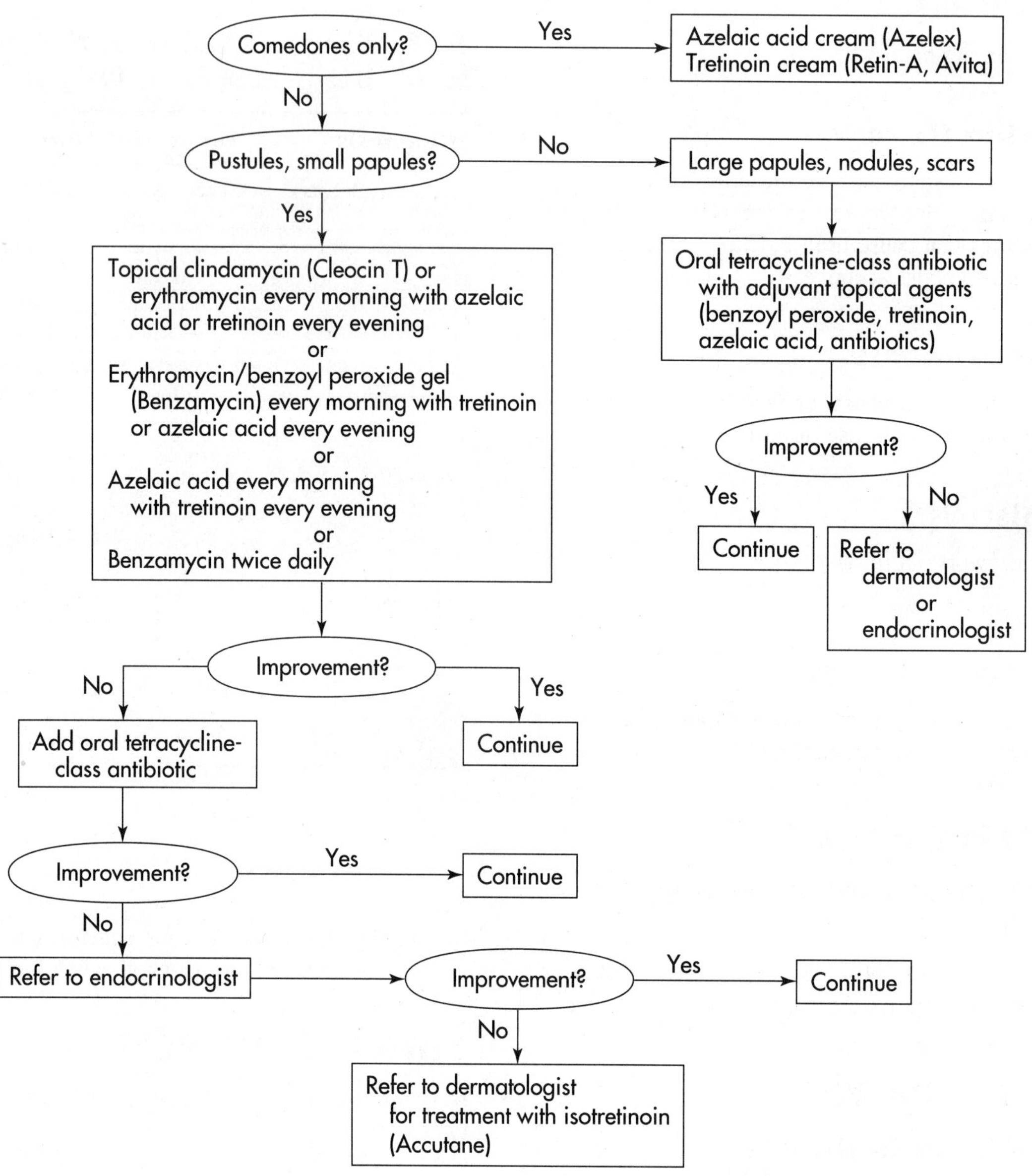

Figure 4-1 Treatment algorithm for acne vulgaris. (Redrawn from Sykes N, Webster G: Acne: a review of optimum treatment, *Drug* 48(1): 59-70, 1994.)

Patient Education

Type of diet eaten does not affect acne, but a well-balanced diet helps with healing.
Wash the skin twice daily with a gentle soap.
Use a moisturizer unless skin is very oily.
Avoid greasy hair products; keep hair off forehead.
All cosmetics should be removed nightly.
Instruct the client not to pick at lesions.
Warn the client that improvement will not be noted until 4 to 6 weeks of treatment.
Sunscreen and sun protection must be used with tretinoin, oral tetracycline, doxycycline, isotretinoin, and trimethoprim.
Effective and reliable contraceptive method is necessary if isotretinoin is used because of the potential for birth defects.
Cholesterol and triglyceride levels must be monitored during isotretinoin treatment.
Patients taking isotretinoin should be advised to avoid excessive alcohol consumption.

Family Impact

Parents should be aware of the impact acne may have on adolescents and their interaction with others, as well as self-esteem issues.

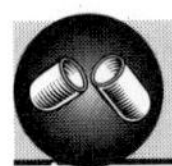

TABLE 4-2 Pharmaceutical Plan: Acne Vulgaris

Type of Acne	Drug	Dose	Comments	Cost
Pure comedomal	Tretinoin (Retin-A) Two new agents under investigation (tazarotene and adapalene) appear to be more effective and better tolerated	Several formulations exist with cream (0.025%, 0.05%, or 0.1% [the most mild]), followed by gel (0.01% or 0.025%), and liquid (0.05%)	To avoid overdrying of skin, treatment should be initiated on a QOD basis at bedtime Pregnancy: C SE: Redness and peeling of skin, temporary worsening of acne Sun sensitivity: Use sunscreen	\$26-\$32/20 g cream \$21/15 g gel \$43/28 ml liquid
Mild papular	Benzoyl peroxide Also available in combination with erythromycin (Benzamycin)	Available as 5% or 10% gel by Rx	Begin treatment slowly with QOD application to avoid overdrying of skin; wash with antibacterial soap AM and HS; follow with benzoyl peroxide Pregnancy: C May bleach clothing and fabrics	\$12/42.5 g gel 5% \$10-\$15/120 g cream 5%
Mild to moderate	Azelaic acid (Azelex) cream, 30 g	Wash and dry skin; massage thin film gently into affected areas BID; wash hands after use	Contains a comedolytic agent with antiinflammatory agent; helpful for those who do not want to use systemic antibiotic; may cause irritation and sun sensitivity Pregnancy: B SE: pruritis, burning, contact dermatitis greatest during first 4 weeks but decrease with continued use	\$27-\$81/60 ml lotion \$20/30 g gel \$13-\$23 solution
Papulopustular	Tretinoin and benzoyl		Each applied QD to skin Multiple products available with sulfur or salicylic acid	
	Tretinoin with topical clindamycin	Clindamycin available 1% in solution, lotion, or gel	Useful especially in inflammatory acne Pregnancy: B	
Grade III or IV	Tetracycline	500-1000 mg/day	↓ Gradually to a goal of 250 mg/day or QOD; erythromycin (pregnancy B), doxycycline (pregnancy D) and occasionally trimethoprim-sulfamethoxazole (pregnancy C) may be RX	\$6-\$19/500 mg (100)
Females: mild to moderate	OCPs: Combo with levonorgestrel, gestodene, and desogestrel Bromocriptine, spironolactone, gonadotropin-releasing hormone antagonists		↓ Endogenous androgen production and ↓ the bioavailability of the woman's circulating androgens Other hormonal approaches for acne; used for polycystic ovarian syndrome	\$15-\$23/pak

SE, Side effects.

Referral

Clients in need of isotretinoin treatment (dermatologist)
Females with cystic acne, irregular menses, and hirsutism for hormonal evaluation (OB/GYN)
Clients with significant depressive symptoms as a result of the acne (psychologist)

EVALUATION/FOLLOW-UP

Reevaluate at 4 to 6 weeks; assess for satisfaction with medication and problems with skin irritation. Note the number and type of lesions present. Consider combination treatment if current treatment is not decreasing the lesions.

SUGGESTED READINGS

Berson DS, Shalita AR: The treatment of acne: the role of combination therapies, *J Am Acad Dermatol* 32:S31-41, 1995.

Cooley S et al: Management of acne vulgaris, *J Pediatr Healthcare* 12(1):38-40, 1998.

Ellsworth A et al: *Mosby's 1998 medical drug reference,* St Louis, 1998, Mosby.

Fitzpatrick T et al: *Color atlas and synopsis of clinical dermatology*, ed 3, New York, 1997, McGraw Hill.

Habif T: *Clinical dermatology: a color guide to diagnosis and therapy*, ed 3, St Louis, 1996, Mosby.

Healthcare Consultants of America, Inc: *1998 Physicians fee and coding guide,* Augusta, Ga, 1998, Healthcare Consultants of America, Inc.

Hurwitz S: Acne treatment for the '90s, *Contemp Pediatr* 12:(8)19-32, 1995.

Kaminer MS, Gilchrest BA: (1995) The many faces of acne, *J Am Acad Dermatol* 32:S6-S14, 1995.

Leyden JJ: New understandings of the pathogenesis of acne, *J Am Acad Dermatol* 32:S15-25, 1995.

Lowe N: Managing acne in adult women, *Patient Care* 31(10):30-43, 1997.

Newton J et al: The effectiveness of acne treatment: an assessment by patients of the outcome of therapy, *Br J Dermatol* 137(4):563-567, 1997.

Peters S: Saving face: treating adolescents affected by acne vulgaris, *Advanced Nurse Practitioner* 5(3):43-46, 1997.

Rothman KF, Lucky AW: Acne vulgaris, *Adv Dermatol* 8:347-369, 1993.

Usatine R, Quan M, Strick R: Acne vulgaris: a treatment update, *Hosp Pract* 33(2):111-117, 1998.

Addison's Disease

Adrenocortical Insufficiency

ICD-9-CM

Corticoadrenal Insufficiency 255.4

OVERVIEW

Definition

Addison's disease is a rare endocrine disorder characterized by a variety of nonspecific symptoms such as malaise, anorexia, nausea that results from the lack of hormones produced in the adrenal cortex, including cortisol, aldosterone, and androgens.

Incidence

Incidence is 4 per 100,000; can occur **in all age groups**.
The majority of cases are between 30 and 50 years of age.
Females and children more likely to have autoimmune adrenal insufficiency.
Males more likely to have tuberculous adrenal insufficiency.

Etiology

Autoimmune adrenocortical insufficiency is the cause of 65% to 84% of cases of Addison's disease. Adrenal antibodies react with antigens in adrenocortical tissue and cause an inflammatory reaction that destroys all three layers of the adrenal cortex but not the medulla. Before signs and symptoms of the disease develop, 80% to 90% of both adrenal glands are affected. The disease may occur concurrently with other autoimmune endocrine disorders. The classification in Box 5-1 was developed to categorize autoimmune disease and Addison's disease.

Tuberculosis was the main cause of Addison's disease in the past, now accounting for approximately 18% of cases.

Fungal infections, including histoplasmosis, blastomycosis, cryptococcosis, occidiomycosis, have been shown to cause primary adrenal insufficiency.

Other causes seen less commonly include adrenal hemorrhage, certain medications, granulomatous diseases, and metastatic neoplasms that involve both adrenal glands. See Box 5-2 for a comprehensive list of etiologies.

Pathophysiology

The clinical picture of Addison's disease results from lack of cortisol, aldosterone, and androgens. Figure 5-1 describes the pathophysiology of Addison's disease.

SUBJECTIVE DATA

History of Present Illness

There is slow and insidious onset in majority of cases.

Patient reports gradual onset over a period of time or sudden hypotension, shock, or dehydration with acute trauma or surgery.

Chief complaints usually are nausea and vomiting, hypotension, shock, dehydration.

Cardinal features are weight loss, fatigue, and weakness.

Past Medical History

Ask about all the diseases listed in Box 5-2 on etiologies.

History may include other autoimmune disorders.

With a history of insulin-dependent diabetes mellitus (IDDM), patient may report that the usual insulin dose causes hypoglycemia.

Medications

Ask about medications listed under etiologies.

Family History

Ask about autoimmune endocrine disorders such as thyroid disease, IDDM, rheumatoid arthritis, Addison's disease.

Box 5-1

Autoimmune Adrenocortical Insufficiency Classifications

Polyglandular Autoimmune Syndrome (Type I)

Patient has at least two or three of the following: Addison's disease, hypoparathyroidism, chronic mucocutaneous candidiasis.

Disease occurs in children and young adults, with peak incidence of Addison's disease developing at age 10 years.

Associated diseases include chronic active hepatitis, malabsorption syndromes, juvenile onset pernicious anemia, gonadal failure, and alopecia.

Autoimmune thyroid disease and IDDM are less frequently seen.

Polyglandular Autoimmune Syndrome (Type II)

Patient has Addison's disease with autoimmune thyroid disease and/or IDDM.

Subjects do not have hypoparathyroidism or candidiasis.

There is a broad range for age of onset from childhood to late adulthood, with peak incidence of Addison's disease in midlife.

IDDM, Insulin-dependent diabetes mellitus.

Box 5-2

Etiologies of Adrenal Insufficiency

Primary Adrenal Insufficiency

Autoimmune destruction
Tuberculosis
Fungal infections
Hemorrhage
  Idiopathic thrombocytopenic purpura
  Sepsis
  Anticoagulation
  Coagulopathy
  Surgery
  Pregnancy
  Trauma
Familial
  Glucocorticoid deficiency
  Adrenoleukodystrophy
  Adrenomyeloneuropathy
Infarction
  Thrombosis
  Arteritis
Invasive disorders
  Cancer
  Sarcoidosis
  Amyloidosis
  Hemochromatosis
Congenital hypoplasia
Human immunodeficiency virus
Drugs that decrease steroid synthesis
  Aminoglutethimide
  Etomidate
  Ketoconazole
  Metyrapone
  Mitotane
Drugs that increase steroid catabolism
  Dilantin
  Rifampin
  Phenobarbital

Secondary Adrenal Insufficiency

Exogenous steroid administration
Pituitary disease
Hypothalamic disease
Adrenocorticotropic hormone deficiency
Surgery
  Adrenal
  Pituitary

Familial predisposition may be related to abnormal reactivity of patient's immune system.

Psychosocial History

Ask about depression, apathy, confusion.

64% to 84% of patients with Addison's disease present with or experience accompanying psychiatric symptoms.

Description of Most Common Symptoms

See Table 5-1.

Associated Symptoms

Craving salt
Nausea and vomiting
Diarrhea/constipation
Abdominal pain
Back pain
Possible syncope and anemia
Possible decreased libido due to diminished androgen levels (females)

OBJECTIVE DATA

Physical Examination

General: Assess the patient for mild fever, tachycardia, hypotension, weight loss, dehydration, lethargy, and orthostatic changes in pulse and blood pressure.

Children: Assess the weight on the growth chart, compare to previous weight, a drop on the child's growth chart curve is indicative of problems.

Skin: Observe for hyperpigmentation, especially of distal extremities exposed to sun. Hyperpigmentation also may occur on nipples, extensor surfaces of extremities, genitalia, buccal mucosa, tongue, palmar creases, knuckles, and face. Vitiligo is less common; when it is present,

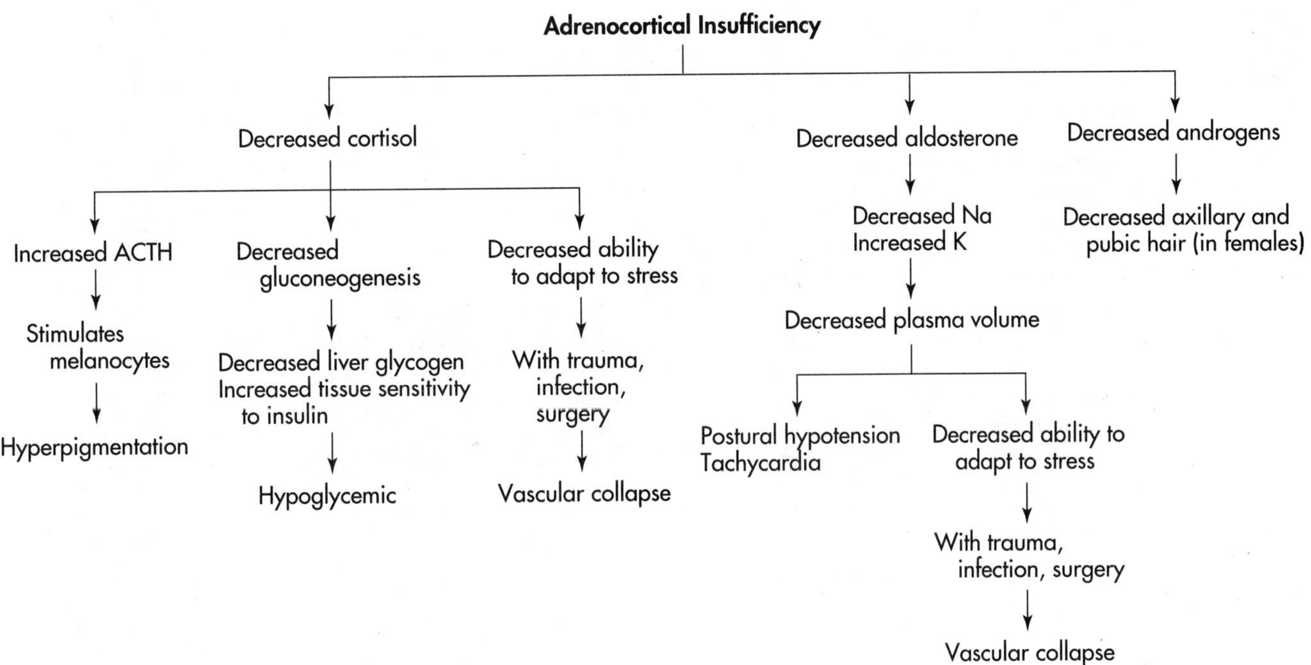

Figure 5-1 Pathophysiology of Addison's disease.

TABLE 5-1 Signs and Symptoms in Addison's Disease

Symptoms	%
Weakness and malaise	74-100
Weight loss	56-100
Hyperpigmentation	91-96
Hypotension	59-88
Psychiatric complaints	64-84
Hyponatremia	88-96
Hyperkalemia	52-64
Gastrointestinal symptoms	56-81
Postural dizziness	12
Adrenal calcification	9-33
Hypercalcemia	6-41
Muscle and joint pains	6
Vitiligo	4-20

it suggests autoimmune etiology with autoimmune destruction of melanocytes. Decreased skin turgor is evident with dehydration.

Children: Parents may report difficulty getting the child's elbows and knees clean, mistaking the hyperpigmentation for uncleanliness

Head/eyes/ears/nose/throat: Observe for calcification of external ear cartilage, which is seen rarely.

Cardiac: Observe for decreased pulses, pallor, and poor perfusion.

GI: Assess for generalized abdominal pain.

GU: Assess for decreased body hair in females.

Muscloskeletal: Assess for decreased muscle strength, muscle cramping, arthalgia.

Elderly: Elderly may experience increased osteoporosis due to decreased androgens.

Neurological: Assess for irritability, depression, confusion.

Diagnostic Procedures

When the nurse practitioner suspects Addison's disease, consultation with a physician and/or endocrinologist is essential to obtain appropriate diagnostic tests and initial therapy for the patient. See Table 5-2 for diagnostic protocol for adrenal insufficiency and Table 5-3 for diagnostic tests to confirm Addison's disease.

ASSESSMENT

Differential diagnoses are listed in Table 5-4. Figure 5-2 provides a diagnostic algorithm for adrenal insufficiency.

THERAPEUTIC PLAN

Acute Phase Management

Acute adrenal insufficiency requires consultation with a physician and/or endocrinologist and immediate hospitalization. Patients require intravenous fluids, electrolyte replacement, correction of metabolic acidosis, and intravenous Solu-Cortef.

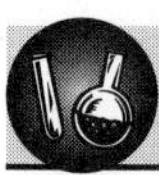

TABLE 5-2 Diagnostic Protocol for Addison's Disease

Diagnostic Test	Results with Addison's	Cost ($)
ACTH (serum)	Elevated	129-162
Cortisol (serum)	Decreased	60-76
Renin	Elevated	69-88
Aldosterone	Decreased	142-179
Electrolyte Panel	Decreased Na; elevated K	23-30
Comprehensive Metabolic Panel	Decreased bicarbonate; metabolic acidosis	32-42
Amylase	Increase with pancreatitis; may occur concurrently	24-30
CBC	Anemia, eosinophilia	18-23
Thyroid profile	WNL unless concurrent thyroid disease	47-61
Adrenal antibody test	Positive indicates autoimmune disease	43-53
PPD	Positive indicates may be TB adrenal insufficiency	18
KUB	May show enlarged adrenals	98

ACTH, Adrenocorticotropic hormone; *CBC,* complete blood count; *WNL,* within normal limits; *PPD,* purified protein derivative; *KUB,* kidney, ureter, and bladder; *TB,* tuberculosis.

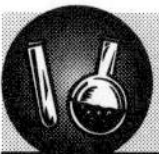

TABLE 5-3 Diagnostic Tests to Confirm Addison's Disease

Test	Finding/Rationale	Cost ($)
Rapid ACTH stimulation test (monitor serum cortisol levels @ 30, 60, 90 min after IV infusion of ACTH)	No increase in cortisol (normal response is double cortisol level) Differentiation between primary and secondary adrenal insufficiency is possible with the rapid corticotropin stimulation test. Low undetectable serum aldosterone and no response to ACTH indicates primary insufficiency. A rise in aldosterone and cortisol after the ACTH stimulation test indicates secondary insufficiency.	97-120
ACTH stimulation (measure urinary 17-hydroxycorticoid for 24-72 hours after IV infusion of ACTH	Increased cortisol with pituitary disease	73-95
CT scan	Enlarged adrenals with infection, hemorrhage, metastatic disease Atrophy with autoimmune disease Calcification with granulomatous disease	347-416

ACTH, Adrenocorticotropic hormone; *IV,* intravenous; *CT,* computed tomography.

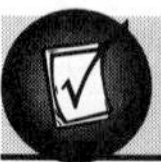

TABLE 5-4 Differential Diagnosis: Addison's Disease

Diagnosis	Supporting Data
Eating disorders	Weakness, muscle aches, sleep disturbances, constipation, bloating. Amenorrhea, weight loss
Thyroid disease	Fatigue, elevated or decreased thyroid-stimulating hormone
Diabetes	Elevated blood sugar, fatigue, polydipsia, polyuria, polyphagia
Pancreatitis	Severe abdominal pain, nausea and vomiting, weakness, sweating, abdominal tenderness
Failure to thrive (children)	Weight below the third percentile on standardized growth charts, decreased appetite, vomiting frequently

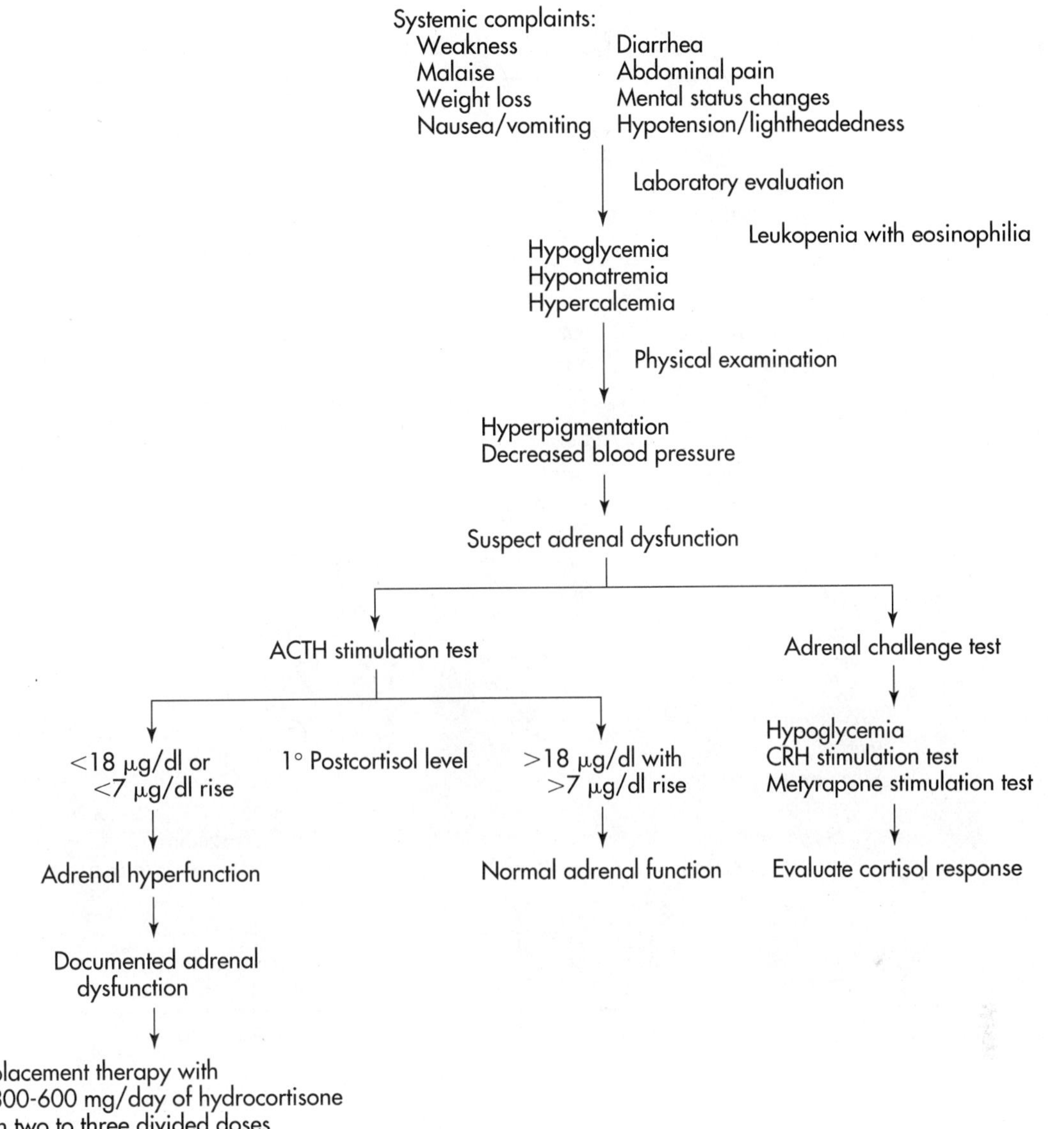

Figure 5-2 Diagnostic algorithm for adrenal insufficiency. *ACTH,* Adrenocorticotropic hormone; *CRH,* corticotropin-releasing hormone. (Redrawn from Curran P, Mazzone T: Case 10. In Grodzin C, Schwartz S, Bone R, editors: *Diagnostic strategies for internal medicine,* St Louis, 1996, Mosby.)

Pharmaceutical Management

A pharmaceutical plan is outlined in Table 5-5.

Lifestyle/Activities

Instruct patient to carry a medical identification bracelet and register with a national medical alerting system.

Diet

Instruct patients to add extra salt to diet when sweating, exercising, or during hot weather and gastrointestinal illness.

Patient Education

All patients should be instructed to adjust the steroid dose when they are ill. Patients should be instructed on self-administration of injectible hydrocortisone and have a supply on hand to administer if vomiting persists and there is a delay in seeking medical attention. Patients also need to increase cortisol before surgery and dental procedures.

Family/Impact

Families report a process of adaptation to this chronic disease, which involves adjusting to the diagnosis, seeking information on the disease, learning to manage the disease,

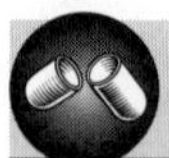

TABLE 5-5 Pharmaceutical Plan: Addison's Disease

Drug	Adult Dose	Child Dose	Comments	Cost
Hydrocortisone (cortisol replacement)	20 mg AM and 10 mg PM to duplicate normal circadian rhythm	12-15 mg/kg/day (⅔ in AM; ⅓ in PM)	Double or triple dose with stress and illness; repeat dose if vomits within 1 hour of medication	$20/5 mg (50); $6/10 mg (100) $7-$43/20 mg (100)
Cortisone (Cortone)	25 mg in AM and 12.5 mg in PM	Contraindicated in children <2 yrs; no solution available	Pregnancy: B (cortisone C) SE: Gastric upset, edema, HTN, hypokalemia, insomnia,	$7/5 mg (50) $24/10 mg (100) $9-$62/25 (100)
Prednisone (Deltasone)	5 mg in AM and 2.5 mg in PM	0.05-2 mg/kg/day divided as above BID	excitability, diabetes mellitus, weight gain Monitor weight, B/P, and ECG regularly	$3-$8/2.5 mg (100) $3-$8/5 mg (100)
Deoxycorticosterone trimethylacetate in oil	2-5 mg IM Q3-4 weeks		For mineralcorticoid loss	N/A
Fluohydrocortisone (Florinef)	0.05-0.2 mg given QD Increase by 0.05 When treating postural hypotension, decrease dose with edema, hypokalemia, CHF, and HTN		Increase with exposure to heat, increased sweating Replaces mineralcorticoids	$45/0.1 mg (100)
Depotestosterone	25 mg IM q4-6 weeks to treat decreased libido	Not indicated	Observe carefully for masculinization optional	$2-$5/25 mg/ml

CHF, Congestive heart failure; *ECG,* electrocardiogram; *HTN,* hypertension; *IM,* intramuscularly; *N/A,* not available.

needing support and acceptance, and maintaining the ability to live a normal life.

Children

Report not wanting to feel different, needing acceptance of peer group, and facing additional periods of adjustment as they progress to new developmental levels.

Referral/Consultation

The nurse practitioner should refer patients suspected to have Addison's disease to an endocrinologist. After initial stabilization the nurse practitioner may collaborate with the endocrinologist to provide primary care to the patient.

EVALUATION/FOLLOW-UP

Measurement of serum and urinary cortisol values and serum corticotropin values, along with the patient's report on how he or she is feeling, can be used to better control the dosage of cortisol. In primary adrenal insufficiency a patient experiencing an elevated adrenocorticotropic hormone and low cortisol levels while on cortisol replacement requires increased dosage or changing the times of administration of medication. An elevated urinary cortisol suggests that cortisol replacement dosage should be decreased. A low urinary cortisol suggests the cortisol replacement should be increased.

Children

Monitor growth—some may require growth hormone replacement.

SUGGESTED READINGS

Curran P, Mazzone T: Case 10. In Grodzin C, Schwartz S, Bone R, editors: *Diagnostic strategies for internal medicine,* St Louis, 1996, Mosby.

Davenport J et al: Addison's disease, *Am Family Physician* 43(4):338-342, 1991.

Derish M, Eckert K, Chin C: Reversible cardiomyopathy in a child with Addison's disease, *Intensive Care Medicine* 22(5):460-463, 1996.

Ellsworth A et al: *Mosby's 1998 Medical Drug Reference,* St. Louis, 1998, Mosby.

Healthcare Consultants of America, Inc: *1998 Physicians fee and coding guide,* Augusta, Ga, 1998, Healthcare Consultants of America, Inc.

Epstein CD: Fluid volume deficit for the adrenal crisis patient, *Dimensions Crit Care Nurs* 10(4):210-217, 1991.

Stoffer SS: Addison's disease: how to improve the patient's quality of life, *Postgrad Med* 93(4):265-266, 1993.

Werbel SS, Ober KP: Acute adrenal insufficiency. *Endocrinol Metabol Clin North Am* 22(2):303-328, 1993.

Allergic Reactions

ICD-9-CM

Angio Edema 995.1
Anaphylaxis 995.0

OVERVIEW

Definition

There are two types of generalized reactions: urticaria/angioedema (usually not life threatening) and anaphylaxis (life threatening).

Urticaria/angioedema consists of lesions (extravascular accumulation of fluid in dermis) resulting from exposure to an inciting substance.

Anaphylaxis is an acute systemic reaction manifested by sudden onset of pruritus, generalized flush, urticaria, respiratory distress, and vascular collapse (Griffith and Dambro, 1998). It results from an antigen exposure in a sensitized person.

Incidence

Urticaria occurs at some time in one fifth of the population.

Anaphylaxis occurs in 1 of 2700 hospitalized patients, and approximately 400 to 800 people die each year for anaphylactic reactions.

Hymenoptera causes allergic reactions in 0.4% of population.

Allergic reactions occur equally in males and females, and they occur in all ages.

Food allergies are much more common in **children** <3 years of age (8%).

Milk allergies: **Children** (2%); **older children** and **adults** (1% to 2%)

Pathophysiology

The underlying mechanism for both urticaria and anaphylaxis is a classic immunoglobulin E (IgE)–mediated allergy, causing an immune response in which chemical mediators (histamine and kinins) are released. Allergic prone individuals produce more IgE-specific antibodies; and they have a tendency to become allergic on repeated exposures.

Factors That Increase Susceptibility

Family history of allergies
Past history of allergic reaction
History of asthma, hay fever, or other allergic disorders

Common Items That Cause Allergic Reactions

Beta lactam antimicrobials (penicillin most common)
Insect stings: Honeybees/wasps
Foreign serum
Vaccines
Blood products
Hormones (e.g., aminocorticotropic hormone, insulin, estradiol)
Diagnostic chemicals (iodine)
Foods (peanuts, eggs, legumes, popcorn, seafood)
In **children:** Milk, chocolate
Nonsteroidal antiinflammatory drugs (NSAIDs), aspirin
Snake venom
Animal dander
Latex
Exercise

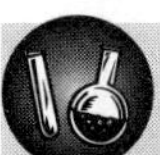

TABLE 6-1 Diagnostic Tests: Allergic Reactions

Diagnostic Test	Finding/Rationale	Cost ($)
Epicutaneous immediate-reacting IgE skin test	Using food extract method to determine the presence of food-specific IgE antibodies (This is a good screen for allergies. A positive result indicates the likelihood of allergy.)	12-14
In vitro test for allergen-specific IgE antibodies	Appropriate test in life-threatening allergies (A negative test rules out allergy.)	13-16
Food challenge	Only method to confirm the suspicion of food reaction, regardless of mechanism (A double-blind placebo-controlled food challenge is the gold standard.)	150-185
Food diet/diary and home challenges	Possibly helpful when reactions are not life threatening	N/A

IgE, Immunoglobulin E; *N/A,* not available.

SUBJECTIVE DATA

History of Present Illness

Determine type of bite, sting, or antigen
Determine location of antigen
Time of occurrence

Past Medical History

Ask about previous history of hives/urticaria/anaphylaxis.
Ask about hay fever or asthma.

Medication

Ask about medications: angiotensin-converting enzyme inhibitors (benazepril, captopril, enalapril, fosinopril, lisinopril, moexipril, quinapril, ramipril, trandolapril). They are frequently combined with other antihypertensive drugs and can cause a reaction with first dose or after prolonged treatment as a result of kinin-mediated reaction.
Ask specifically about NSAIDs, since many people do not think of them as a medication.
Ask about antibiotics taken recently.

Family History

Ask about family history of allergies or allergic reactions.

Psychosocial History

Environmental exposures: Animals, chemicals in the home or workplace
Physical agents, including light, exercise, or heat

Description of Most Common Symptoms

Quick treatment may be necessary, given signs and symptoms and past history. Foods associated with anaphylaxis will probably present a lifelong risk. In addition to peanuts, these foods include tree nuts (e.g., almonds, Brazil nuts, cashews) fish, shellfish (especially crab, crayfish, shrimp and lobster), and seeds (caraway and sesame).

Urticaria: Itching, transient hives on any part of the body, exposure proceeding symptoms, dysphagia
Anaphylaxis: Generalized itching, erythema of skin followed by sense of warmth and then generalized hives; rapidly progressive respiratory distress

Associated Symptoms

Ask about presence of systemic symptoms such as fever, chills, nausea, vomiting, and weakness.
Ask about shortness of breath, chest tightness, or facial swelling, throat tightness.

OBJECTIVE DATA

Physical Examination

A problem-oriented physical examination should be conducted with particular attention to:
Vital signs: Hypotension
Skin: Urticaria, cutaneous erythema, angioedema
Head/eyes/ears/nose/throat: Eyelid edema, facial edema, throat swelling, rhinitis, conjunctivitis
Respiratory: Dyspnea, wheezing, shallow respirations, increased secretions
Cardiovascular: Tachycardia, circulatory collapse
Gastrointestinal: Abdominal colic, nausea and vomiting/diarrhea
Central nervous system: Confusion, coma
Hematologic: Disseminated intravascular coagulation

Diagnostic Procedures

Diagnostic procedures are outlined in Table 6-1.

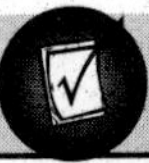

TABLE 6-2 Differential Diagnosis: Allergic Reactions

Diagnosis	Supporting Data	Management
Mild reaction	Characterized by urticaria that involves the superficial dermis; pruritic, well-circumscribed wheals that may coalesce	Acute (<6 weeks): treat symptoms. Antihistamines are usually effective (2-5 days), or a 4-5 day course of prednisone is effective.
Moderate reaction	Characterized by bronchospasm and angioedema, which is well-demarcated localized edema that involves the entire dermis and subcutaneous tissue; common sites: the skin, GI tract, and upper airway (GI angioedema can produce cramping abdominal pain, nausea and vomiting, and diarrhea.)	Give epinephrine 0.01 mg/kg (up to 0.3 to 0.5 mg) subcutaneously.
Severe reaction: anaphylaxis	Severe systemic reaction of multiple organ systems to IgE-driven mediator release in previously sensitized individuals. (Hypotension, bronchoconstriction, and upper airway obstruction are common.)	Oxygen: Monitor O_2 saturation. Give epinephrine: Dilute 0.5 ml (0.5 mg) of a 1:1000 (1 mg/ml) solution to 10 ml with 0.9% sodium chloride injection for IV administration. Repeat dose 2-3 min if needed. IV: volume expanders—crystalloids: Patients should be observed for at least 4-6 hrs after episode.

GI, Gastrointestinal; *IgE*, immunoglobulin E; *IV*, intravenous.

ASSESSMENT

Differential diagnoses include those listed in Table 6-2.

THERAPEUTIC PLAN

Pharmaceutical/Nonpharmaceutical

Treatment depends on severity of reaction. If there is a life-threatening systemic reaction, follow ABCs: airway, breathing, and circulation.

Life-threatening

Initiate emergency transport service (call 911).

Administer oxygen; assess need for intubation

Epinephrine (1:1000 solution) 0.5 mg given subcutaneously or intravenously (IV) (dilute 0.5 ml of 1 mg/ml in 10 ml normal saline solution) and repeated every 5 to 10 minutes as needed; can also be given via endotracheal tube

Intravenous fluids: Normal saline or Ringer's lactate

Aminophylline: For bronchospasm, 6 mg/kg IV over 10 to 20 minutes

Nonlife-threatening

Nonlife-threatening pharmaceutical treatment is outlined in Table 6-3.

Lifestyle/Activities

If an accidental exposure occurs, the parent or patient should use the epinephrine and then be taken to the nearest ED.

Treatment medication must be on hand at all times.

Diet

Avoid involved or suspected food indefinitely.

Patient Education

Emphasize need to have antihistamine or epinephrine on hand.

Avoid insects, food, or drugs that cause reaction.

Wear medical alert bracelet identifying allergy.

Use drugs carefully if there is a history of allergic disorders, hay fever, or asthma.

If there is an acute generalized reaction, there is a potential for life-threatening reaction in the future.

Wear shoes at all times; this is the single most important preventive measure.

Do not wear perfume or bright clothing when outside if allergic to Hymenoptera; consider pretreatment with antihistamines and corticosteroids.

Know how to use EpiPen.

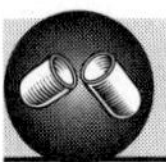

TABLE 6-3 Pharmaceutical Plan: Allergic Reactions

Drug	Dose	Comment	Cost
Epinephrine (1:1000 solution) (Adrenalin)	0.01 ml/kg 0.3 to 0.5 ml subcutaneously every 20-30 minutes for up to 3 doses	Pregnancy: C SE: Anxiety, H/A, fear, palpitations, local necrosis, pulmonary edema, HTN, cerebral hemorrhage	$5-$15/10 ml
EpiPen	0.3 mg single dose of 1:1000 solution	Emphasize the need to take ASAP after food or allergy exposure **Caution: do not take if suspension is pinkish or brownish in color:** indicates oxidation of epinephrine. See Epinephrine.	$25/1 pen
EpiPen JR	0.15 mg single dose of 1:2000 solution	As above	$25/1 pen
Sus-Phrine	0.15 to 0.25 ml (5 mg/ml)	Follow epinephrine with long-acting agent.	$5-$14
Diphenhydramine (Benadryl)	25 mg-50 mg q4-6h	May help shorten duration of reaction Pregnancy: B SE: drowsiness, dizziness, anticholinergic effects	Cap: $2-$22/ 25 mg (100) $2-$29/50 mg (100) Elixir: $2-$16/12.5/5 ml (450 ml)
H2 blocker: cimetidine (Tagamet)	300 mg intravenously	Useful for mild allergic reactions	$5-$18/300 mg/2 ml (8 ml)
Prednisone (Deltasone)	1-2 mg/kg/d for 4-5 days	If extensive swelling present in local reaction, consider adding a short course; delayed therapeutic effect: not effective for 4-6 hours after dosing; side effects minimal with short course of therapy Pregnancy: C SE: Masks infection, glaucoma, cataracts, should be minimal effects in 4-5 days	$12-$17/5 mg/5 ml (480 ml) $3-$6/1 mg (100) $3-$8/2.5 mg (100) $3-$8/5 mg (100) $4-$13/10 mg (100) $7-$18/20 mg (100)

SE, Side effects, *H/A,* headache; *HTN,* hypertension.

Referral

Referral for allergy testing to identify sensitizing agent if unknown and immunotherapy reduces likelihood of a similar reaction from 50% to 5%.

EVALUATION/FOLLOW-UP

Follow-up by phone call in 24 hours to client with moderate local reaction or mild allergic reaction.

Patients who experience an anaphylactic reaction should be closely monitored for 12 to 24 hours afterward.

RESOURCE

Food Allergy Network, 4744 Holly Ave, Fairfax, VA 22030, publishes an informative newsletter, *Food Allergy Awareness, Support and Training,* (800-929-4040, 513-683-8668; e mail: FAASTcin@aol.com).

REFERENCE

Griffith H, Dambro M: *The 5-minute clinical consultant,* ed 38, Philadelphia, 1998, Lea & Febiger.

SUGGESTED READINGS

Anderson J: Milk, eggs and peanuts: food allergies in children, *Am Family Physician* 56(5):1365-1374, 1997.

Ellsworth A et al: *Mosby's 1998 medical drug reference,* St Louis, 1998, Mosby.

Healthcare Consultants of America, Inc: *1998 Physicians fee and coding guide,* Augusta, Ga, 1998, Healthcare Consultants of America, Inc.

Kidd P, Sturt P: *Mosby's emergency nursing reference,* St Louis, 1996, Mosby.

O'Brien J: Allergic reactions: 10 questions physicians often ask, *Consultant* 38(4): 851-866, 1998.

Valentine M: Allergy and related conditions. In Barker L, Burton J, Zieve P, editors: *Principles of ambulatory medicine,* ed 4, Baltimore, 1995, Williams & Wilkins.

Allergic Rhinitis

ICD-9-CM

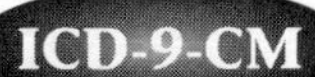

Allergic Rhinitis 477.9

OVERVIEW

Definition

Rhinitis is a hyperfunction of the nose that results in rhinorrhea and nasal obstruction. Allergic rhinitis often has a seasonal component or specific inciting agents such as animals or dust.

Incidence

Onset is most commonly between ages 10 and 20, rarely before 4 or after 40. It is a common disease that affects up to 30% of the population.

Pathophysiology

Atrophic patients produce excessive amounts of immunoglobulin E (IgE) antibodies. IgE binds to high-affinity receptors on the surface of the mast cells and basophils, thus serving as an allergen receptor. With reexposure there is binding of the allergen to the mast cell surface IgE, which triggers a cascade of cell activation.

Release of a number of inflammatory mediators (histamine, prostaglandin D_2, leukotriene C_4) are responsible for a number of the symptoms of rhinitis: sneezing, pruritus, congestion, rhinorrhea.

Seasonal Allergic Rhinitis

Ragweed: mid-August until the first frost
Tree pollen: March to May
Grass pollen: May to early July

Perennial Allergic Rhinitis

Dust mites
Molds
Animal dander or saliva
Cockroach antigen

Irritants and Other Stimuli May Trigger Symptoms

Smoke, air pollutants
Perfumes, deodorants, soaps
Solvents and fumes
Change in air temperature, light, or atmospheric pressure
Emotion

SUBJECTIVE DATA

History of Present Illness

Ask about:

- Onset, triggers, exposure.
- Onset, duration and progression of symptoms. (Explore relationship of symptoms to season, place, time of day and activity.)
- Nasal stuffiness, nasal obstruction, sensation of facial pressure around eyes, itching of eyes, sneezing.
- Mouth breathing, changes in hearing or smell acuity, snoring, fatigue.
- Self treatment, especially duration and use of nasal sprays.

In *seasonal allergic rhinitis,* usually caused by outdoor allergens, symptoms include:

- Itchy eyes
- Watery nasal discharge
- Nasal stuffiness
- Sneezing

In *nonseasonal allergic rhinitis,* usually caused by indoor allergens, the symptoms include:

- Red, itchy, watery eyes
- Watery nasal discharge
- Spasmodic sneezing
- Chronic nasal congestion with or without mucus

TABLE 7-1 Medications That Can Cause Symptoms That Mimic Allergic Rhinitis

Medication	Symptom
Aspirin	Rhinitis
Clonidine (Catapres)	Dry, itchy eyes, dry nasal mucosa
Guanabenz acetate (Wytensin)	Nasal congestion
Guanethidine monosulfate (Ismelin)	Nasal congestion
Hydralazine (Apresoline)	Lacrimation, nasal congestion
Labetalol (Normodyne, Trandate)	Nasal stuffiness
Methyldopa (Aldomet)	Nasal stuffiness
Oral contraceptives	Rhinitis
Prazosin (Minipress)	Nasal congestion
Propranolol (Inderal)	Nasal congestion, rhinitis
Reserpine (Serpasil)	Nasal congestion
Terazosin (Hytrin)	Nasal congestion, rhinitis

Past Medical History

Ask about frequent sinus infections and persistent middle ear infections in **children**.

Conditions that can cause or mimic allergic rhinitis symptoms are pregnancy, alcoholism, cocaine abuse, hypothyroidism, and eating spicy foods.

Medications

Ask about any medications taken; include oral contraceptive pills, prescriptions, and over-the-counter preparations for allergies or other conditions (Table 7-1).

Family History

Incidence of occurrence is about 26% if one parent has allergic rhinitis and 52% if both do.

Psychosocial History

Ask about smoking history.

Description of Most Common Symptoms

Nasal congestion (may lead to loss of taste or smell)
Nasal itching (may result in frequent nose rubbing: allergic salute; nasal crease)
Sneezing (often in the morning)
Clear rhinorrhea (may be perfuse or continuous)
Chronic postnasal drip may cause cough and/or sore throat
Palatal itching, dry mouth, and halitosis
Conjunctivitis causes ocular itching, redness, and tearing
General symptoms include fatigue and disrupted sleep

OBJECTIVE DATA

Physical Examination

Vital signs: Temperature should be normal; pulse and B/P may be elevated if sympathomimetic drugs were used.
Special attention should be paid to nose, eyes, ears, mouth, throat, heart, and chest.
Head/eyes/ears/nose/throat: Check eyes for "allergic shiners," tearing, conjunctival injection, lid edema.
Check ears to rule out otitis media, and to check for serous otitis.
Nares: Nasal mucosa is often pale blue and boggy with a clear mucus discharge, edematous turbinates; check sinuses for transillumination.
Pharynx: Check for tonsillar enlargement and inflammation, lymphoid hyperplasia in posterior oropharynx (cobblestoning).
Neck: Check for lymphadenopathy.
Heart: Check for abnormal heart sounds.
Lungs: Check to rule out concurrent asthma or lower airway infection

Diagnostic Procedures

Diagnosis is generally based on history and examination. However, if allergic rhinitis is suspected and immunotherapy is being considered, skin testing is necessary because treatment success depends on accurate evaluation of allergen sensitivities (Table 7-2).

ASSESSMENT

Diagnosis of a specific type of rhinitis is made based on:

History
Nature of presenting complaints
Onset of symptoms
Pattern of symptoms
Duration

Differential diagnosis includes those found in Table 7-3.

THERAPEUTIC PLAN

See Figure 7-1.

Pharmaceutical/Nonpharmaceutical

Drugs used in treatment of seasonal and perennial allergic rhinitis are found in Tables 7-4 to 7-10.

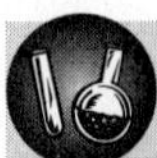

TABLE 7-2 Diagnostic Procedures: Allergic Rhinitis

Diagnostic Test	Finding/Rationale	Cost ($)
Nasal smear	The value of nasal smears is controversial. The results are reported as the eosinophil to neutrophil (E:N) ratio. A ratio of >1 suggests allergic rhinitis; a ratio of <1 suggests infectious rhinitis or sinusitis.	19-23

TABLE 7-3 Differential Diagnosis: Allergic Rhinitis

Diagnosis	Supporting Data
URI	Usually fever, purulent nasal discharge, inflamed nasal mucosa
Sinusitis	Purulent drainage, facial tenderness, fever, impaired transillumination
Otitis media	Bulging, immobile tympanic membrane, or conductive hearing loss associated with eustachian tube dysfunction
Nasal abnormalities	Septal deviations, nasal polyp, adenoid hypertrophy

URI, Upper respiratory infection.

- Lifestyle/environment control
- Identify triggers, avoid/control causes

Episodic (Intermittent) Symptoms (symptoms $<$3-4 times per week)

First generation antihistamine prn*

Decongestant, if needed

If symptoms persist, place on intranasal steroid

Continuous (Persistent) Symptoms (symptoms daily or near daily)

Daily intranasal corticosteroid

Add ocular antihistamines, if needed

Add decongestant, if needed

Refractory Symptoms (symptoms despite appropriate therapy)

Daily intranasal corticosteroid

Consider adding oral antihistamine

Consider adding decongestant, if indicated

If symptoms persist, consider a 3-5 day course of prednisone

Consider referral to allergist

* For oral antihistamines, unless there is a contraindication, recommend starting with a first generation antihistamine. If the sedative and cognitive side effects may be problematic, then change to a second generation, nonsedating antihistamine.

For nasal steroids, once clinical response is achieved, the dose can often be reduced.

Figure 7-1 Treatment of allergic rhinitis. (Courtesy Choice Care, Cincinnati, Ohio.)

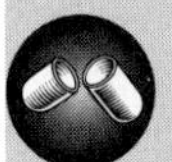

TABLE 7-4 Pharmaceutical Plan: Allergic Rhinitis

Drug Class	Symptoms Targeted
Intranasal corticosteroids	Sneezing, itching, rhinorrhea, nasal congestion
Antihistamines (systemic)	Sneezing, itching, rhinorrhea, ocular itching
Decongestants (systemic)	Nasal congestion
Mast cell stabilizers (Cromolyn sodium)	Nasal itching, sneezing, rhinorrhea
Ophthalmic mast cell stabilizers	Ocular itching
Ophthalmic antihistamines	Ocular itching

Modified from *American Pharmaceutical Association guide to drug treatment protocols—seasonal and perennial allergic rhinitis,* February 1996.

Immunotherapy

1. Specific allergens (identified by skin tests or RAST) are injected weekly or monthly.
2. It is reserved for patients with severe rhinitis who do not respond to or who cannot or will not take medications.
3. The best response is seen with seasonal allergies to pollen.

Patient Education

Avoidance of triggers is vital (Boxes 7-1 and 7-2)!

Close windows and use the air conditioner.

Wear a face mask for mowing the grass or doing factory work that produces dust.

Change furnace filters frequently.

Vacuum rather than sweep; vacuum furniture at least 2 times per week.

Use disposable bags in the vacuum cleaner.

Use a humidifier if the air is too dry or a dehumidifier if the air is too moist (Keep humidity to below 50%).

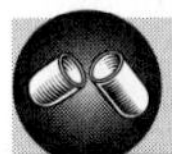

TABLE 7-5 Antihistamine Treatment

Drug	Dose	Comments	Cost
Over-the-Counter			
Brompheniramine (Dimetapp)	4 mg q4-6h (24 mg max) SR 8 mg q8-12h or 12 mg q12h Children: 6-11 y/o: 2 mg q4-6h	Not recommended <5 y/o Pregnancy: C SE: Drowsiness, sedation, constipation, excitability in children	\$3-\$20/elixir: 2 mg/5 ml (480 ml) \$2-\$9/tablet 4 mg (100)
Chlorpheniramine (Chlor-Trimeton)	4 mg q4-6h (24 mg max) 8 or 12 mg BID or 16 mg q24h Children: 6-11 y/o: 2 mg q4-6h	Not recommended <5 y/o Precaution: Pregnancy SE: Drowsiness, sedation, constipation, excitability in children	\$1-\$12/SR: 4 mg (100) \$4-\$11/4 mg (100) \$3-\$4/syrup: 2 mg/5 ml (120 ml)
Dexbrompheniramine + pseudophedrine (Drixoral)	6 mg q12h	Not recommended <12 y/o Precaution: Pregnancy SE: Drowsiness, sedation, constipation, excitability in children	N/A
Diphenhydramine (Benadryl Allergy)	25-50 mg q4-6h Children: 6-11 y/o: 12.5-25 mg q4-6h	Not recommended <6 y/o Precaution: Pregnancy SE: Drowsiness, sedation, constipation, excitability in children	\$2-\$22/25 mg (100) \$2-\$29/50 mg (100) \$2-\$15/elixir: 12.5/5 ml (480 ml)
Triprolidine (Actifed Cold and Allergy)	2.5 mg q4-6h Children: 6-11 y/o: 1.25 mg q4-6h	Not recommended <6 y/o Precaution: Pregnancy SE: Drowsiness, sedation, constipation, excitability in children, palpitations	\$5/syrup: 1.25 mg/5 ml (480 ml) \$3/2.5 mg (100)

Antihistamines: Effective in treating and preventing symptoms from the early phase of an allergic reaction. They do not block other mediators in the early phase reaction (leukotrienes, cytokines) so not all symptoms are eliminated. Helpful for symptoms of sneezing, itching, rhinorrhea, and allergic conjunctivitis. Not helpful for nasal congestion/sneezing. Use with caution with narrow-angle glaucoma, prostatic hypertrophy, central nervous system depressants.

SE, Side effects; *SR,* sustained release; *GI,* gastrointestinal; *H/A,* headache; *URI,* upper respiratory infection; *MDI,* metered-dose inhaler; *N/A,* not available.

Continued

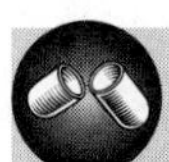

TABLE 7-5 Antihistamine Treatment—cont'd

Drug	Dose	Comments	Cost
Over-the-Counter			
Clemastine (Tavist)	1 mg tab BID, maximum 6 mg/d Children: 6-12: Rhinitis 0.5 mg BID Urticaria 1 mg BID, max. 3 mg/d	Not recommended <6 y/o Pregnancy: B SE: Drowsiness, dizziness, gastritis, anticholinergic effects, paradoxical excitement	$31-$64/1.34 mg (100) $17-$24/syrup: 0.67 mg/ 5 ml (120 ml)
Prescription			
Azatadine (Trinalin)	1 tab BID	Not recommended in children Pregnancy: C SE: Drowsiness, anticholinergic effects, GI upset, dizziness, anxiety, insomnia, thickening of bronchial secretions, palpitations	$91/1 mg (100)
Loratadine (Claritin) Tabs or liquid: 1 mg/ml	10 mg QD Redi-tabs: Dissolve on tongue without water	Not recommended for children <6 Pregnancy: B SE: H/A, dry mouth, nervousness, malaise, URI (children)	$194/10 mg (100)
Astemizole (Hismanal)	10 mg QD on empty stomach	Not recommended for children <12 Pregnancy: C **Contraindicated with concurrent: erythromycin, ketoconazole, itraconazole, mibefradil, quinine, cisapride, nefazodone** SE: Appetite increase, weight gain, fatigue, dry mouth, palpitations	$185/10 mg (100)
Fexofenadine (Allegra)	60 mg BID	Not recommended for children <12 Pregnancy: C SE: Viral infection, nausea, dysmenorrhea, drowsiness, dyspepsia, fatigue	$86/60 mg (100)
Azelastine (Astelin)	2 sprays in each nostril BID; not recommended in children	Antihistamine (caution with other antihistamines) Pregnancy: C SE: Bitter taste, somnolence, weight increase, nasal burning, sneezing	$43/spray: 1 mg (200 sprays/ twin pack)

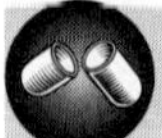

TABLE 7-6 Decongestants

Drug	Dose	Comments	Cost
Pseudoephedrine (Sudafed) Tabs: 30, 60 mg Liquid: 7.5 mg/ 0.8 ml; 15 mg/5 ml	Adult: 60 mg q4-6h (max 240 QD) Children 2-6 y/o: 15 mg (1.6 ml) q4-6h (max 4 doses/day) Children 6-12 y/o: 30 mg q4-6h	Not recommended <2 years of age Pregnancy: B Helpful for nasal congestion only SE: CNS overstimulation, H/A, palpitations, hypertension, nervousness, insomnia, tremor	$5-$7/syrup: 30 mg/5 ml (480 ml) $1-$11/30 mg (100); $3-$25/60 mg (100)

Decongestants are used to relieve symptoms of nasal congestion. They do not affect the underlying allergic process. Use with caution with patients with uncontrolled diabetes, hypertension, or hyperthyroidism.

CNS, Central nervous system; *H/A,* headache; *SE,* side effects.

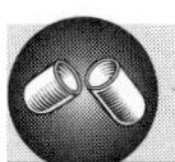

TABLE 7-7 Topical Nasal Corticosteroids

Drug	Dose	Comments	Cost
Beclomethasone dipropionate (Beconase AQ) 42 μg/spray: (200 sprays)	Children >6: 1-2 sprays in each nostril BID	Needs to maintain regular regimen; may use decongestants if needed Pregnancy: C SE: Nasal discomfort, sneezing, H/A, nausea, epistaxis, rhinorrhea	$34/spray: 42 μg (25 g) $17-$36/MDI nasal inhalant 6.7-7 g
Fluticasone propionate (Flonase) 50 μg/spray (120 sprays)	Initially 2 sprays in each nostril 1× daily or 1 spray BID; maintenance: 1 spray in each nostril QD Children >4 yrs: 1 spray in each nostril	Needs to maintain regular regimen; may use decongestants if needed Pregnancy: C Caution: CYP3A4 inhibitors (see CYP Chart in Appendix D) (ketoconazole) SE: Nasal discomfort, sneezing, H/A, nausea, epistaxis, rhinorrhea	$41/0.05 μg/ inhalation (16 g)
Triamcinolone acetonide (Nasacort AQ) 55 μg/spray (120 sprays)	2 sprays in each nostril QD Children 6-12: 1 spray in each nostril QD	Needs to maintain regular regimen; may use decongestants if needed Pregnancy: C SE: Nasal discomfort, sneezing, H/A, nausea, epistaxis, rhinorrhea	$39/55 μg (10 g)
Flunisolide (Nasalide) 25 μg/spray (200 sprays) (Nasarel)	Blow nose Adults: 2 sprays in each nostril BID (max 8 sprays/nostril/day) Children 6-14: 1 spray in each nostril TID or 2 sprays BID (max 4/nostril/day)	Needs to maintain regular regimen; may use decongestants if needed Pregnancy: C SE: Nasal discomfort, sneezing, H/A, nausea, epistaxis, rhinorrhea, septal perforation	$28/0.25 mg/ml (25 ml)
Mometasone furoate (Nasonex) 50 μg/spray (120 sprays)	2 sprays in each nostril QD Begin 2-4 weeks before anticipated start of pollen season	Needs to maintain regular regimen; may use decongestants if needed Pregnancy: C SE: Nasal discomfort, sneezing, H/A, nausea, epistaxis, rhinorrhea	N/A
Budesonide (Rhinocort) 32 μg/spray (200 sprays)	Blow nose Initially 2 sprays in each nostril BID or 4 sprays QD; gradually reduce to lowest effective dose	Needs to maintain regular regimen; may use decongestants if needed Pregnancy: C SE: Nasal discomfort, sneezing, H/A, nausea, epistaxis, rhinorrhea	$28/32 μg/spray (200 sprays)
Beclomethasone dipropionate (Vancenase AQ double strength) 84 μg/spray (120-200 sprays)	Children >6: 1-2 sprays in each nostril QD	Needs to maintain regular regimen; may use decongestants if needed Pregnancy: C SE: Nasal discomfort, sneezing, H/A, nausea, epistaxis, rhinorrhea, fungal overgrowth	$42/inhalation 84 μg (19 g)

H/A, Headache; *MDI*, metered-dose inhaler; *N/A*, not available; *SE*, side effects.

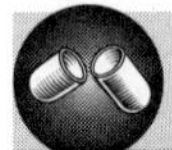

TABLE 7-8 Intranasal Decongestants

Drug	Dose	Comments	Cost
Naphazoline (Privine)	1-2 sprays of 0.05% solution in each nostril q6h PRN	Do not exceed 3-5 days Children <12 y/o: Not recommended Caution: Pregnancy	$4/0.05% (20 ml)
Oxymetazoline (Afrin)	2-3 sprays of 0.05% solution in each nostril in AM and PM PRN	Do not exceed 3-5 days Children <6 y/o: Not recommended Caution: Pregnancy SE: CNS stimulation, palpitations, HTN, H/A	$3/0.025% (20 ml)
Phenylephrine (Neo-Synephrine)	2-3 sprays of 1.0% or 0.5% in each nostril q4h PRN	Do not exceed 3-5 days Not recommended <2 y/o Caution: Pregnancy SE: Rebound congestion, HTN, nasal discomfort, insomnia, palpitations	$4/1% spray (15 ml)
Xylometazoline (Otrivin)	2-3 drops or sprays of 0.1% in each nostril q8-10h PRN (max 3 doses/24h or 3 days of use)	Not recommended <2 y/o Caution: Pregnancy SE: As above	$3-$5/0.01% (20 ml)

SE, Side effects; *CNS,* central nervous system; *HTN,* hypertension; *H/A,* headache.

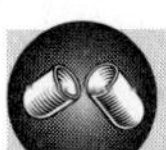

TABLE 7-9 Miscellaneous Drugs*

Drug	Dose	Comments	Cost
Ipratropium (Atrovent nasal spray)	2 sprays in each nostril 0.03%: BID/TID 0.06%: TID/QID	Anticholinergic, effective for rhinorrhea Caution: BPH or narrow-angle glaucoma Pregnancy: B SE: Epistaxis, nasal dryness, or irritation	N/A
Cromolyn sodium (Nasalcrom) OTC	One spray to each nostril TID/QID; can increase to one spray to each nostril 6× daily; begin use before expected contact with allergan	Mast cell stabilizer†—effective for all nasal symptoms of early- and late-phase reaction: nasal congestion, nasal pruritus, rhinorrhea, sneezing Pregnancy: B SE: Sneezing, nasal irritation	$23/5.2 mg/spray (100 sprays)

OTC, Over-the-counter; *BPH,* benign prostatic hypertrophy; *N/A,* not applicable.

*Drugs specific to eye symptoms are discussed in Chapter 43.

†Works by preventing the release of histamine and other mediators by stabilizing the mast cell wall and inhibiting the inflow of calcium ions into the mast cell, thereby preventing degranulation; generally considered less effective than antihistamines.

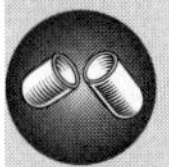

TABLE 7-10 Sedative and Anticholinergic Effects of First- and Second-Generation Antihistamines

Drug	Sedative Effects	Anticholinergic Effects
First-generation Antihistamines		
Cyproheptadine (Periactin)	Low	Moderate
Dexchlorpheniramine (Polaramine)	Low	Moderate
Diphenhydramine (Benadryl)	High	High
Hydroxyzine (Atarax, Vistaril)	Moderate	Low
Promethazine (Phenergan)	High	High
Clemastine (Tavist)	Moderate	High
Second-generation Antihistamines		
Cetirizine (Zyrtec)	Low to moderate	Low to none
Fexofenadine (Allegra)	Low to none	Low to none
Loratadine (Claritin)	Low to none	Low to none

Box 7-1

Pollen Avoidance Measures

Monitor pollen forecasts.
Stay inside the house when pollen count is high.
Limit outdoor activity when pollen count is high.
Use air conditioning when possible.
Use air conditioning in cars.
Use dust masks when mowing lawn and shower afterwards.
Rinse hair during high pollen season before going to bed.
Do not hang bed linens outside during high pollen season.

Box 7-2

Instructions on How to Use Nasal Sprays

Blow nose gently to clear nostrils.
Clean outer portion of nose with a damp tissue.
Shake medication container.
Keep head upright.
Press a finger against the side of your nose to close one nostril.
With mouth closed, insert into open nostril.
Sniff in through nostril while quickly and firmly dispensing medication.
Hold breath for a few seconds—then breathe out through your mouth.
Repeat for other nostril if so directed.
Rinse the dispenser with hot water. Wash your hands.

Dust the house daily with a moist cloth.
Do not allow anyone to smoke in the house.
Clean curtains monthly.
Encase mattress, box springs, and pillows in plastic or allergen impermeable material.
Remove feather pillows, woolen blankets—replace with synthetic.
Wash bedding weekly at 130° F.
Remove carpets.
Vent and clean bathrooms with fungicides.
Remove plants.
Install air filters or free-standing HEPA filters in commonly used rooms.
Keep closet doors shut.
Remove pets from the house or at least the bedroom.
Do not allow children to sleep with furry toys in their beds.
Toys should be vacuumed, tumble dried, or put in deep freeze (–20° F) overnight to reduce mites.

Referral

If response to treatment is poor and an anatomic or a secondary disorder is a consideration, refer to an MD.

EVALUATION/FOLLOW-UP

As needed

SUGGESTED READINGS

Brunton S: Allergic rhinitis: breaking the cycle of disease and treatment, *Fam Practice Recertification* 19(9):14-31, 1997.
Busse W: Current research and future needs in allergic rhinitis and asthma, *J Allergic Clin Immunol* 101(2):S424-426, 1998.
Choice Care: *Treatment of allergic rhinitis,* Cincinnati, 1997, Choice Care.
Cornell S: Allergic rhinitis in children: it's nothing to sneeze at, *Adv Nurse Pract* 5(2):30-32, 1997.
Ferguson B: Cost-effective pharmacotherapy for allergic rhinitis, *Otolaryngol Clin North Am* 31(1): 91-110, 1998.
Ellsworth A et al: *Mosby's 1998 medical drug reference,* St Louis, 1998, Mosby.

Healthcare Consultants of America, Inc: *1998 Physicians fee and coding guide,* 1998, Augusta, Ga, Healthcare Consultants of America, Inc.

Kaiser H et al: The anticholinergic agent, ipratropium bromide, is useful in the treatment of rhinorrhea associated with perennial allergic rhinitis, *Allergy Asthma Procedures* 19(1):23 29, 1998.

Lemanske R: A review of current guidelines for allergic rhinitis and asthma, *J Allergic Clin Immunol* 101(2):S392-S396, 1998.

Meltzer C: Treatment options for the child with allergic rhinitis, *Clin Pediatr* 37(1): 1-10, 1998.

Rachelefsky G: Pharmaceutical management of allergies and rhinitis, *J Allergic Clin Immunol* 101 (2Pt2), S367-369, 1998.

Slavin R: Comparison of allergic rhinitis: implications for sinusitis and asthma, *J Allergic Clin Immunol* 101(2): S357-360, 1998.

Alopecia

ICD-9-CM

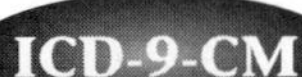

Alopecia Areata 704.1

OVERVIEW

Definition

Alopecia is hair loss from any part of the body where hair normally grows. There are two classifications: scarring (cicatricial) and nonscarring (noncicatricial).

Incidence

Alopecia areata: Lifetime incidence rate of 2%, with the same rate in males as in females; ⅓ to ½ of all cases occur by the age of 20; relapses are frequent

Pathophysiology

Often the exact etiology is unknown. However, the mechanisms appear to be caused by the destruction of the hair matrix by physical agents and infectious or immunologically mediated inflammation.

Scarring

Scar tissue formation resulting from inflammation and tissue destruction. The hair follicle is destroyed with no potential for regrowth.

Injury: Burns, physical trauma

Traction: Tight braiding or hair rolling

Infection: Bacterial (e.g., cellulitis), fungal (e.g., *Trichophyton schoenleinii*), viral (e.g., herpes simplex or zoster)

Dermatologic processes: Discoid lupus erythematous, scleroderma, lichen planus, cutaneous neoplasm

Nonscarring: There are several types of nonscarring alopecia with separate etiologies.

Male-pattern baldness—androgenic alopecia

Female-pattern baldness—caused by androgenic excess secondary to polycystic ovary disease, hyperprolactinemia, and androgen-producing ovarian and adrenal tumors.

Alopecia areata—unknown etiology, round patches of hair loss with small hair shafts at the periphery that taper toward the skin surface (exclamation point hairs); can progress to alopecia totalis (loss of *all* scalp hair) or alopecia universalis (loss of facial and body hair as well)

Telogen effluvium—(loss of resting hair) postpartum alopecia with resolution within 18 months

Infectious diseases—tinea capitis, folliculitis, secondary syphilis, typhoid, or pneumonia (following high fevers)

Anagen effluvium—caused by chemotherapy affecting hair follicles in the growing phase

Thyroid disorders/iron deficiency/collagen vascular diseases

Trichotillomania—self-induced hair loss, can affect the hair or eyebrows

SUBJECTIVE DATA

History of Present Illness

Ask about onset, duration, and severity of symptoms. Is the hair loss specific or generalized? Ask about any recent physical trauma or use of curlers, hair dyes, straightening agents, or hot combs. Ask if there is a previous history of hair loss. Ask about recent weight loss or gain, dieting, or increase in stress. Ask about any recent febrile illness. Ask about current birth control, including levonorgestrel implant (Norplant system) and /or medroxyprogesterone (Depo-Provera).

Adults: Higher incidence of male-female pattern baldness

Women: Postpartum hair loss (telogen effluvium)

Children/adolescents: Higher incidence of alopecia areata with ⅓ to ½ of all cases starting by age 20; increased incidence of trichotillomania, tinea capitis

Past Medical History

Ask about crash diets, postpregnancy status, trauma, infection, tinea capitis, collagen vascular disease, neoplasms, thyroid disease.

Medications

Commonly used medications that can cause alopecia include beta-blockers, tricyclic antidepressants, anticonvulsants, warfarin anticoagulants, allopurinol, antithyroid medications, quinine, verapamil, indomethacin, sulfasalazine, haloperidol, excessive doses of vitamin A, progesterones, and several anti-neoplastic agents.

Family History

Ask about a family history of male-female pattern baldness or arthritis.

Psychosocial History

Ask about crash diets, vitamin A supplements

Ask about any recent increase in stress, self-induced hair loss (trichotillomania)

Description of Most Common Symptoms

Occasional antecedent paresthesia or tenderness, pruritus

OBJECTIVE DATA

Physical Examination

The extent of the physical examination depends on the suspected underlying cause. It is important to distinguish between scarring and nonscarring alopecia. A problem-oriented physical examination should be conducted. Obtain vital signs, general appearance, and weight.

Scalp: Close examination for pattern (local, diffuse, androgenic), extent of hair loss, including eyebrows. Assess for inflammation, cellulitis, folliculitis, scarring. Assess for fungal infection (Wood's light will produce fluorescent glow if fungal). Short broken hairs suggest pulling or twirling (trichotillomania). Check for scratching.

Assess the hair shaft. Assess for a well-circumscribed oval or circular nonscaly patch of nonscarring hair loss with proximally tapering exclamation point peripheral hairs (alopecia areata). Check for follicular plugging.

Nails: Presence of Beau's lines may correlate with a systemic process. Based on history and scalp examination, a complete physical examination may be indicated.

Diagnostic Procedures

Diagnostic procedures are outlined in Table 8-1.

ASSESSMENT

Differential diagnoses include:

Nonscarring alopecia: Androgenetic, alopecia areata, postfebrile infection, tinea capitis, thyroid disease, iron deficiency, systemic lupus erythematosus, secondary syphilis, medications (including antineoplastic), psychiatric disorders, crash diets, postpartum, trichotillomania

Scarring alopecia: Physical trauma, severe bacterial folliculitis, formation of kerion secondary to tinea capitis or discoid lupus, lichen planus (Table 8-2)

THERAPEUTIC PLAN

Pharmaceutical

The underlying cause must be determined before pharmaceutical treatment is begun.

Alopecia areata can be treated with intralesional injections, topical steroids, and systemic steroids in extreme cases, although systemic steroids are not recommended.

Androgenetic alopecia is treated with minoxidil.

Tinea capitis requires systemic antifungal agents. Occasionally the addition of prednisone for inflammation and antibiotic therapy for secondary bacterial infection is indicated (Tables 8-3 and 8-4). See tinea chapter for more details.

Lifestyle/Activities

Learn stress management/relaxation.

Encourage contact with local alopecia support groups.

Diet

Assess vitamin A intake and decrease as indicated (vitamin A 400U QD).

Eat a well-balanced diet.

Patient Education

Instruct about etiology and treatment, if known.

Instruct about medication for regrowth if nonscarring alopecia areata.

Caution to avoid caustic agents for hair, avoid alkaline shampoos.

Instruct to comb hair, avoid excessive brushing.

Caution to avoid excessive dieting.

Give advice on wigs or hairpieces.

Reassure, help patient and family come to terms with hair loss.

Make patient aware of hair transplants.

Family Impact

This is an extremely sensitive issue for children/adolescents because of the cultural emphasis and peer pressure on young

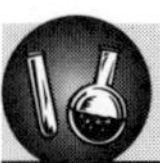

Table 8-1 Diagnostic Procedures: Alopecia

Diagnostic Test	Findings/Rationale	Cost ($)
KOH examination or culture	Rule out fungal infestation	15-19
Scalp biopsy for suspected inflammation	Identification of underlying inflammatory process	93-111
CBC with differential, serum iron	Identification of underlying systemic disease	18-23
Thyroid function tests	Rule out thyroid dysfunction	47-61
ANA titer	Rule out connective tissue disorders	42-52
RPR or VDRL	Rule out secondary syphilis, which can cause alopecia	18-122
Women: Free Testosterone and dehydroepiandrosterone sulfate (DHEA-S)	Identification of increased male hormones in Women	83-103/testosterone; 78-98/DHEA
Lymphocyte T or B—cell count	Sometimes low in alopecia areata	78-97/T

KOH, Potassium hydroxide; *CBC*, complete blood count; *ANA*, antinuclear antibody; *RPR*, rapid plasma reagin; *VDRL*, Venereal Disease Research Laboratories.

Table 8-2 Differential Diagnosis: Alopecia

Diagnosis	Supporting Data
Alopecia areata	Diagnosed clinically; rapid onset; circumscribed oval or circular nonscaly patch of nonscarring hair loss with broken, proximally tapering exclamation point peripheral hairs; antecedent paresthesia or tenderness; normal TSH, CBC, FE
Trichotillomania	Diagnosed clinically; manually pulling out hair causes fractured hairs of unequal length; possible underlying psychiatric disturbance
Tinea capitis (Ch. 179)	Most likely found in young children, black more often than white; scalp pruritus, with hair loss having a "moth eaten" appearance; black dots visible within larger patches; positive fungal culture or Wood's lamp for dermatophytes
Androgenetic alopecia	Symmetrical, beginning in frontoparietal scalp Older, genetic predisposition Permanent: Scalp hairs replaced by fine unpigmented vellus hairs Female: Hirsutism, PCO syndrome, hyperprolactinemia (↑ levels of free testosterone and DHEA)

TSH, Thyroid-stimulating hormone; *CBC*, complete blood count; *FE*, iron; *PCO*, polycystic ovary; *DHEA*, dehydroepiandrosterone sulfate.

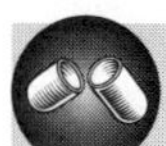

Table 8-3 Drug Therapy for Alopecia Areata

Drug	Adult Dose	Comments	Cost
Triamcinolone acetonide (Aristacort) intralesional, 25 mg/ml, 5-ml vials	Up to 1 mg as needed, max 12.5 mg/site Children: Not recommended	Pregnancy: C SE: HPA axis suppression, masking of infection, glaucoma, PUD, atrophy at site	$9/3 mg/ml (5 ml)
Betamethasone dipropionate Halbetasol propionate (ultra potent steroids) (15 g, 50 g)	Apply topically BID Children: Not recommended	Pregnancy: C SE: Burning, itching, dryness, folliculitis, hypopigmentation	$5-$20/ointment: 0.05% (20 g) $3-$20/cream: 0.05% (15/g)
Prednisone oral pulse therapy	300 mg q week, minimum 4 weeks Children: Not recommended	Pregnancy: C	$12-$17/solution: 5 mg/5 ml (480 ml) $3-$6/tablets: 1 mg (100); $3-$8/2 mg (100); $3-$8/5 mg (100)
Anthralin (Drithoscalp) 0.25%, 0.5%, (50 g)	Apply thin coat QD Children: Not recommended	Begin with 0.25%; apply sparingly, massage, wash area thoroughly; apply only to lesions Pregnancy: C SE: Irritation of normal skin; may stain hair, skin, or fabrics	$21/0.1% (50 g) $22-$23/0.25% (50 g) $25/0.05% (50 g) $29/0.1% (50 g)

HPA, Hypothalamic-pituitary-adrenal; *SE*, side effects; *PUD*, peptic ulcer disease.

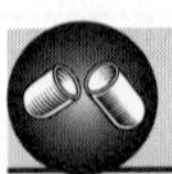

Table 8-4 Drug Therapy for Androgenetic Alopecia

Drug	Adult Dose	Children	Comments	Cost
Topical minoxidil (Rogaine) 5% concentration recommended (only 2% available in United States) (60 ml)	Apply 1 ml to affected scalp area BID	Not recommended	Results seen over long treatment time; hair loss resumes if drug stopped; not recommended during pregnancy or nursing Assess for systemic SE: Chest pain, tachycardia, dizziness 1 mo after starting SE: Dermatitis	$60/solution 2% (60 ml)
Finasteride (Propecia) Type II 5-alpha reductase specific inhibitor	1 mg QD	Not recommended	Men only Pregnancy: X (pregnant women should not handle drug) SE: ↓ Libido, erectile dysfunction, ejaculation disorder (all rare)	N/A

N/A, Not available; *SE,* side effects.

adults regarding appearance. The need for support groups for alopecia persists. Contacting a counselor at school may be helpful.

Male pattern baldness compromises self-image and self-confidence. It is advantageous to maintain a sense of humor.

Referral

For intralesional injections (dermatologist)
For trichotillomania (counselor)

Consultation

Not indicated

EVALUATION/FOLLOW-UP

Children with tinea capitis on griseofulvin, about every 2 weeks

Others can return every month for several months to monitor hair growth, then on an as needed basis.

RESOURCES

Refer to local support group or to National Alopecia Areata Foundation, P.O. Box 150760, San Rafael, CA 94915-4644; Tel: (415) 456-4644, Fax: (415) 456-4274.

SUGGESTED READINGS

Ellsworth AJ et al: *Mosby's 1998 medical drug reference,* St Louis, 1998, Mosby.

Forgarty M, Golitz L: Disorders of the nails and hair. In Mladenovic J, editor: *Primary care secrets,* Philadelphia, 1995, Hanley & Belfus.

HealthCare Consultants of America, Inc: *1998 Physicians fee and coding guide,* Augusta, Ga, 1998, HealthCare Consultants of America, Inc.

Lewis E, Lam M: Some common—and uncommon—causes of hair loss, *Patient Care* 31(20): 50-67, 1997.

Schleicher S, Vacher P: Alopecia areata, *Emerg Med* 29(10)20-27, 1997.

Shellow W: Approach to the patient with hair loss. In Goroll A, May L, Mulley A Jr, editors: *Primary care medicine,* Philadelphia, 1995, JB Lippincott.

Alzheimer's Disease and Related Disorders

ICD-9-CM

Senile Dementia 290.0

Definition

Alzheimer's Disease

Alzheimer's disease (AD) is a slow, progressive deterioration of the brain leading to death. It is marked by changes in behavior and personality and by an irreversible decline in intellectual abilities. Problems with memory are the hallmark of AD (Box 9-1).

Dementia

Dementia is an acquired syndrome that erodes intellectual abilities enough to erode daily life in an alert person. AD is the most common type of dementia.

Delirium

Delirium is a potentially reversible syndrome of acquired cognitive impairment of attention, alertness, and perception. It develops over hours to days and exhibits fluctuations in cognitive function. Hallucinations and visual illusions are frequent. It is usually caused by a general medical condition such as infection, metabolic disturbance, or pharmacological toxicity. Drug toxicity is the most common cause of delirium in the elderly.

Incidence

Approximately 6% to 8% of all persons over age 65 have AD. The prevalence doubles every 5 years after age 60. About 30% of persons over age 85 and 50% over age 90 have AD. Higher rates among women may reflect longevity. Two to 4 million Americans are affected at any one time. Costs associated with the disease are almost $100 billion/year.

Box 9-1

Diagnostic Criteria for Alzheimer-type Dementia

A. The development of multiple cognitive deficits manifested by both
   1. Memory impairment (impaired ability to learn new information or to recall previously learned information)
   2. One (or more) of the following cognitive disturbances
      a. Aphasia (language disturbance)
      b. Apraxia (impaired ability to carry out motor activities despite intact motor function)
      c. Agnosia (failure to recognize or identify objects despite intact sensory function)
      d. Disturbance in executive functioning (i.e. planning, organizing, sequencing, abstracting)

B. The cognitive deficits in Criteria A1 and A2 each cause significant impairment in social or occupational functioning and represent a significant decline from a previous level of functioning.

C. The course is characterized by gradual onset and continuing cognitive decline.

D. The cognitive deficits in Criteria A1 and A2 are not due to any of the following:
   1. Other central nervous system conditions that cause progressive deficits in memory and cognition (e.g., cerebrovascular disease, Parkinson's disease, Huntington's disease, subdural hematoma, normal-pressure hydrocephalus, brain tumor)
   2. Systemic conditions that are known to cause dementia (e.g., hypothyroidism, vitamin B_{12} or folic acid deficiency, niacin deficiency, hypercalcemia, neurosyphilis, HIV infection)
   3. The deficits do not occur exclusively during the course of a delirium.
   4. The disturbance is not better accounted for by another axis I disorder (e.g., major depressive disorder, schizophrenia).

Reprinted with permission from the American Psychiatric Association: *Diagnostic and statistical manual for mental disorders,* ed 4, Washington DC, 1994, American Psychiatric Association.

HIV, Human immunodeficiency virus.

Pathophysiology

Cells in the hippocampus and cerebral cortex are destroyed, leading to problems with memory, language, and reasoning. Amyloid plaques and neurofibrillary tangles appear to be related to cell destruction.

Amyloid (neuritic) plaques are thought to either initiate or be an early finding in a slow, multistep process that leads to brain cell malfunction. Beta-amyloid may be toxic to neurons, disrupt potassium channels, reduce choline levels, and/or cause a combination of these effects. Neurofibrillary tangles result as Tau (a protein) twists into paired helical filaments and microtubules that carry nutrients collapse.

Protective Factors Against

Possible protective factors are postmenopausal estrogen replacement therapy, long-term use of nonsteroidal anti-inflammatory drugs, cigarette smoking, higher education, and occupation. The role of vitamins E and C and ginko biloba in preventing AD is under investigation.

Factors That Increase Susceptibility

Well-established risk factors: **Aging,** presence of Down's syndrome, family history of AD

Other possible risk factors: Severe head injury with loss of consciousness, low level of education and/or occupation, **female sex**

SUBJECTIVE DATA

Early detection of AD reduces the likelihood of inappropriate treatment, hazardous situations, and unnecessary stress

Triggers That Indicate the Need for Assessment for AD

Concerns about cognitive decline or function by the patient, family, or others

Living alone, having Down's syndrome, socially isolated

History of Cognitive Decline

Obtain the history from the patient *and* a reliable informant. It is preferable to include more than one informant. Interview the patient alone first, and tell the patient that others will be interviewed. Interview the informants away from the patient, and be aware of possible questionable motives.

Obtain a detailed description of the chief complaint, including (1) when symptoms began, (2) if symptoms had an abrupt or gradual onset or occurred in a stepwise of continuous progression, and (3) whether they are worsening, fluctuating, or improving.

Ask if there are signs of confusion, delirium, or dysphoric mood (e.g., depression)

Past Medical History

Ask about relevant systemic diseases, psychiatric disorders, head trauma, and other neurological disorders.

Ask about alcohol and other substance abuse and exposure to environmental toxins (e.g., occupational toxins).

Ask about infectious or metabolic illness such as pneumonia, urinary tract infection, diabetes, or acute or chronic renal disease.

Medication History

Ask about prescription and nonprescription drugs.

Medications commonly causing delirium are anticholinergic agents, antipsychotic agents, antidepressants, digoxin, H_2 blockers, and antihypertensive agents.

Encourage patient to bring all (over-the-counter, herbal, and prescription) medications to each visit.

Family History

Ask about family history of early and late-onset AD, Down's syndrome, Huntington's disease or other genetic conditions leading to dementia.

Psychosocial History

Ask about education, literacy, socioeconomic, ethnic, and cultural background.

Ask about recent life events and social support (may affect risk for dementia and performance on mental status examinations).

Description of Most Common Symptoms

Difficulty learning and retaining new information, performing complex tasks, reasoning ability, spatial ability, and orientation, such as getting lost in familiar places

Difficulty with language (e.g., finding words)

Failure to arrive at the right time for appointments

Difficulty discussing current events

Changes in behavior or dress

Agitation

Mood disturbances and/or psychotic symptoms such as hallucinations

Symptoms increase in severity as the disease progresses.

Associated Symptoms

Decline in functional ability and the ability to manage personal affairs

Depression

OBJECTIVE DATA

Physical Examination

Do a brief neurological examination.
Assess for life-threatening or rapidly progressing etiologies such as mass lesions, vascular lesions, and infections.
Measure blood pressure and pulse, supine and standing.
Assess vision and hearing.
Evaluate for evidence of cardiac failure, poor respiratory function, or problems with mobility or balance.
Assess for caregiver abuse or neglect.

Functional Assessment

Conduct a functional assessment (e.g., the *Functional Activities Questionnaire*) (Box 9-2).

Mental Status Assessment

Assess abstract reasoning and judgment (e.g., ask patient what he or she would do if the house was on fire).
Administer a mental status examination (e.g., the *Mini-Mental Status Examination*) (see Tables 40-2 and 40-3).

Assess for Delirium

Observe for evidence of decreased attention span, alterations in level of consciousness, and perceptual disturbances.

Assess for Depression

Administer a depression scale (e.g., the *Geriatric Depression Scale*) (see Boxes 40-1 and 40-2).

Diagnostic Procedures

If the patient demonstrates impairment in multiple domains that represents a decline from previous levels, delirium, depression, and/or confounding factors such as lower education:

Obtain: CBC ($13 to $16), sedimentation rate ($16 to $20), comprehensive metabolic profile ($32 to $42), liver function tests ($29 to $41), urinalysis ($14 to $18), thyroid-stimulating hormone ($56 to $70), vitamin B_{12} ($53 to $67), rapid plasma reagent or Venereal Disease Research Laboratories ($18 to $22), and human immunodeficiency virus ($58 to $72) if indicated by risk factors.

If indicated by the history and physical examination, obtain an electrocardiogram ($56 to $65), chest x-ray ($77 to $91), or psychiatric evaluation.

Consult re: CT scan ($990 to $1175) or MRI ($1781 to $2004) to exclude mass lesions, assess vascular changes, and determine regional atrophy; positron emission tomography; electroencephalogram (EEG) to exclude Creutzfeldt-Jakob disease or epilepsy; or lumbar puncture with rapidly progressing symptoms that indicate inflammation.

Box 9-2

Functional Activities Questionnaire (FAQ): Administration and Scoring

The Functional Activities Questionnaire (FAQ) is an informant-based measure of functional abilities. Informants provide performance ratings of the target person on 10 complex, higher-order activities.

Individual Items of the Functional Activities Questionnaire

1. Writing checks, paying bills, balancing a checkbook
2. Assembling tax records, business affairs, or papers
3. Shopping alone for clothes, household necessities, or groceries
4. Playing a game of skill, working on a hobby
5. Heating water, making a cup of coffee, turning off the stove
6. Preparing a balanced meal
7. Keeping track of current events
8. Paying attention to, understanding, discussing a TV show, book, or magazine
9. Remembering appointments, family occasions, holidays, medications
10. Traveling out of the neighborhood, driving, arranging to take buses

The levels of performance assigned range from dependence to independence and are rated as follows:

- Dependent = 3
- Requires assistance = 2
- Has difficulty but does by self = 1
- Normal = 0

Two other response options can also be scored:

- Never did (the activity), but could do it now = 0
- Never did and would have difficulty now = 1

A total score for the FAQ is computed by simply summing the scores across the 10 items. Scores range from 0 to 30; the higher the score, the poorer the function (i.e., the greater the impairment). A cutpoint of "9" (dependent in three or more activities) is recommended.

Pfeffer R et al: Measurement of functional activities of older adults in the community, *J Gerontology* 37:323-329, 1992.

Clinical Note

To avoid errors in test results, give clear, continuous information about the various diagnostic procedures, and be sure that caregivers are aware of restrictions in food and drink.

Diagnostic Decisions

See Figure 9-1 for additional and follow-up clinical evaluation.

ASSESSMENT

Differential Diagnoses

The most common differential diagnoses related to dementia are vascular dementia; acquired immune deficiency syndrome–related dementia; diffuse Lewy Body (DLB) disease; and Parkinson's, Pick's, Creutzfeldt-Jakob, and Huntington's disease.

The most common differential diagnoses related to delirium are depression, drug and alcohol toxicity, normal pressure hydrocephalus, metabolic changes, hepatic disease, hyponatremia, calcium disorders, vitamin B_{12} deficiency, thyroid disease, and hypoglycemia.

Clinical Notes

Vascular dementias account for 15% of dementias and are associated with hypertension and cardiovascular disease. The clinical course is stepwise and variable. Focal motor and sensory signs, except fluent aphasia and apraxia, suggest vascular dementia.

Dementia associated with DLB may account for 25% of dementias. A positive diagnosis of DLB requires a finding of dementia and at least one of three core symptoms: detailed visual hallucinations, parkinsonian signs, and alterations in alertness or attention. Parkinsonian rigidity and bradykinesia accompanying the onset of dementia suggest DLB. (Parkinsonian signs, especially pill rolling tremor in years predating cognitive decline, usually are indicative of Parkinson's disease, not DLB; see also Chapter 139.)

Pick's disease is a rare brain condition of unknown cause. Atrophy occurs in a relatively circumscribed area of the brain, usually the frontal and temporal regions. It occurs in the age range of 40 to 60 and rarely in old age.

Creutzfeldt-Jakob disease may be caused by a slow-acting virus. Once expressed, it is progressive and fatal, with death usually occurring in 2 years. It is found in middle-age women and men and produces ataxia, muscle spasms, seizures, incontinence, psychotic behavior, and visual symptoms. An EEG will show a characteristic pattern.

THERAPEUTIC PLAN

Pharmaceutical

Cholinesterase Inhibitors

Cholinesterase inhibitors (prevent degradation of endogenously released acetylcholine) to improve memory

Tacrine hydrochloride (Cognex) (**At time of publication, this drug was "falling out of favor"; however, it is still available and may be encountered in the clinical setting.)**

Drug improves cognitive functioning in 20% to 30% of persons with AD in the mild to moderate stage.

Start with 10 mg 4 times a day (increase to maximum of 40 mg 4 times daily).

Obtain baseline alanine aminotransferase before initiating and every week times 16 weeks. Modify dosage according to manufacturer's directions if elevations are greater than 2 times the upper limits of normal.

Take with meals to decrease gastrointestinal irritation.

Treat for a minimum of 3 months to assess therapeutic response.

Donepezil hydrochloride (Aricept)

Donepezil has a longer duration of action than tacrine and greater specificity for brain tissue.

Start with 5 mg/QD and increase if needed to 10 mg/QD after 1 month.

Side effects of nausea, vomiting, and diarrhea are increased with a more rapid increase in dosage.

Prescribe HS with or without food.

Clinical Note

Administer baseline and follow-up mental status and functional status examinations to provide a quantitative comparison of functioning.

Other Medications in Clinical Trials With Inconclusive Evidence

Estrogen, nonsteroidal antiinflammatory drugs, ginko biloba, vitamin B_{12}, selegiline, vitamins E and C

Antidepressants

Consider antidepressant medication in patients with depressive symptoms, even if they fail to meet criteria for a depressive syndrome.

Refer patients with suicidal ideation and signs of major depressive symptoms to geropsychiatry.

Selective serotonin reuptake inhibitors (fluoxetine, paroxetine, and sertraline) are considered first-line by many specialists.

Tricyclic antidepressants can cause significant anticholinergic activity and orthostatic hypotension or cardiac conduction abnormalities. Do not prescribe. They are contraindicated in Alzheimer's disease because lack of acetylcholine is the presumed pathologic cause of Alzheimer's disease. All medications with anticholinergic activity should be avoided. Check before prescribing.

Monoamine oxidase inhibitors can cause postural hypotension and have complex drug and food interactions.

Lifestyle/Activities

The *goal* is to maintain normal activities as long as possible with attention to safety. Suggest an *exercise routine* to continue safe ambulation as long as possible. Add supervision to walks and the use of door locks or electronic guards to prevent wandering in the later stages.

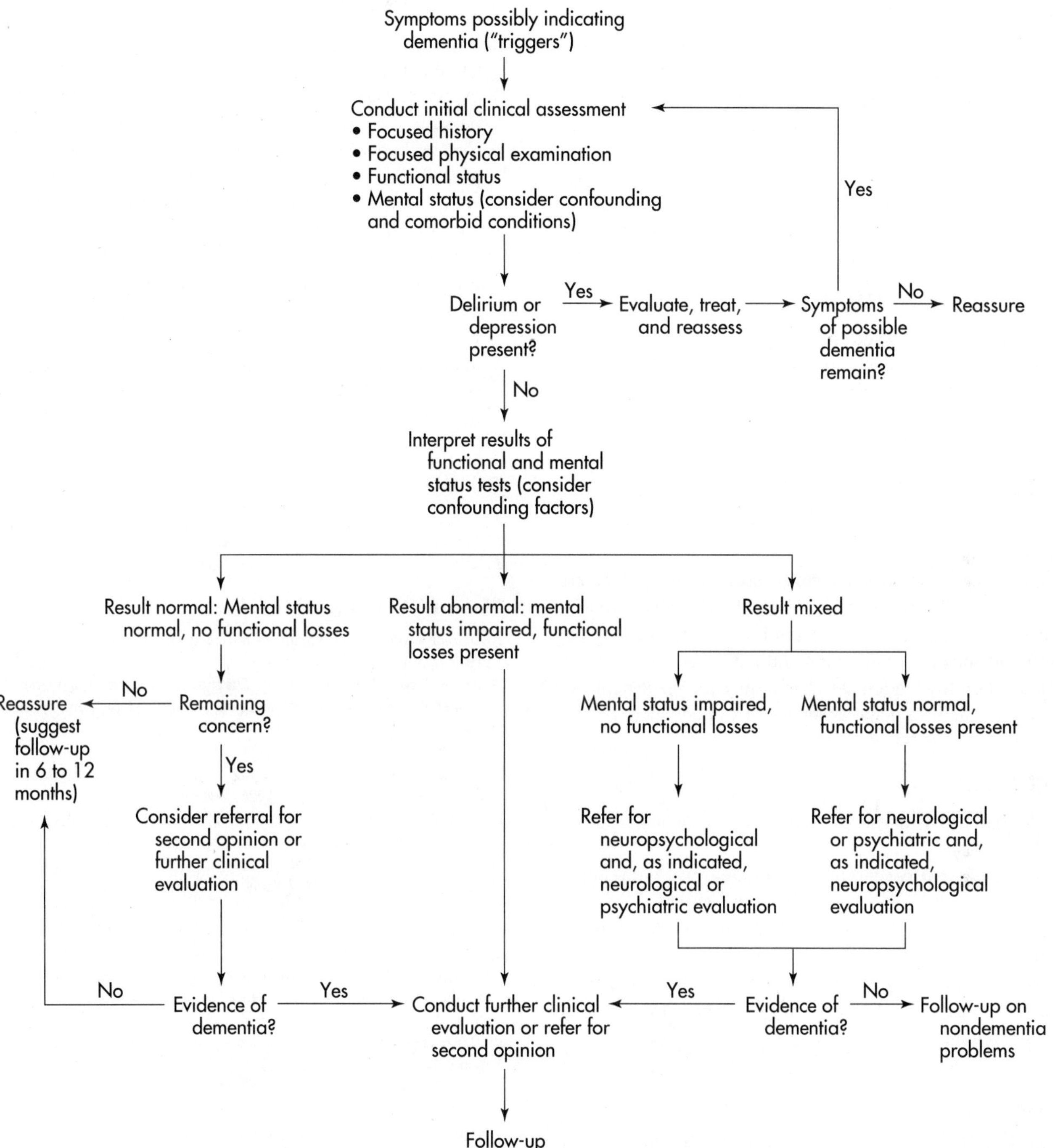

Figure 9-1 Algorithm for recognition and initial assessment of Alzheimer's disease and related dementias. (Redrawn from US Department of Health and Human Services: Early identification of Alzheimer's disease and related dementias [AHCPR Publication No-97-0703], Rockville, Md, 1996, US Department of Health and Human Services.)

Evaluate activities for *safety issues to prevent injuries* (e.g., the use of power tools that may cause injury—putting one's hand in the area of the blade without shutting off electricity—with memory loss).

Discuss *driving issues* early and help patient and family decide when driving a car should be stopped. Examine state laws regarding AD driving. Patients with advanced dementia should not be driving.

Encourage patients to maintain *social and intellectual activities* as tolerated.

Help caregivers formulate a routine to establish predictability; stimulate memory through clocks, calendars, written lists, newspapers, radios, and television. Too much stimulation in the environment often increases confusion.

Diet

Finger foods may be helpful in maintaining nutrition during the later stages.

Patient Education

Help patients understand the disease process and management regime according to their tolerance for knowledge.

Assist them to put their personal affairs in order during the mild stages of AD.

Family Impact

Establish and maintain a close working relationship with caregivers.

Establish a health maintenance program for caregivers.

Help caregivers establish medical and legal advance directives. Suggest a trusted family member cosign any important financial transaction and pay bills.

Help families anticipate long-term care placement and encourage them to make arrangements in advance.

Referral

Refer patients with major depression, psychosis, and/or violent behavior to geropsychiatry.

Consider clinical psychologists for caregivers with adjustment problems not helped by support groups.

Refer to social workers for assistance in securing community resources.

Consider physical therapists to assist with physical activity and occupational therapists for strategies to maximize functioning.

Consultation (See Figure 9-1)

Consult with geriatrician or geriatric psychiatrists regarding pharmaceutical management of mild agitation or aggression.

Consult with neurologist regarding patients with parkinsonism-type symptoms, focal neurological signs, rapid progression, or abnormal neuroimaging findings.

Consult with neuropsychologists to clarify uncertainties in diagnosis and the degree and type of impairment.

Follow-up

Schedule patient surveillance and health maintenance visits every 3 to 6 months.

EVALUATION

Schedule office visits every 3 to 6 months for ongoing surveillance and more often as needed for problems.

The goal of care for the patient is to maintain the highest possible level of wellness for the longest possible time. This will entail helping the patient complete the grieving process, complete personal affairs, avoid excess disability, live in a supportive environment, and to die with dignity and with the highest possible physical and emotional comfort.

The goal of care for the family is that they will provide the highest level of physical and emotional care to the patient while maintaining their personal health and well-being, maintain a positive relationship with the patient, experience satisfaction with their caregiving role, and successfully complete the grieving process.

RESOURCES

Alzheimer's Association Support Groups (800) 272-3900
Alzheimer's Disease Education and Referral Center (800) 438-4380
American Geriatric Society (212) 308-1414

SUGGESTED READINGS

Alzheimer's Association: *Advances in Alzheimer's research,* 7:1A-4A, 1-7, 1997.

American Psychiatric Association: Diagnostic and statistical manual of mental disorders. (4th ed). Washington, DC, 1994, American Psychiatric Association.

Buckwalter K, Hall G: Alzheimer's disease. In McBride A, Austin J: *Psychiatric mental health nursing: Integrating the behavioral and biological sciences,* Orlando, 1996, WB Saunders.

Edwards AJ: *Dementia,* New York, 1992, Plenum Press.

Ellsworth AJ et al: *Mosby's medical drug reference,* St Louis, 1998, Mosby.

Healthcare Consultants of America, Inc: *1998 Physicians fee and coding guide,* Augusta, Ga, 1998, Healthcare Consultants of America, Inc.

Knapp M et al: A 30-week randomized controlled trial of high-dose tacrine in patients with Alzheimer's disease, *JAMA* 271:985-991, 1994.

McKhann G et al: Clinical diagnosis of Alzheimer's disease: report of the NINCDS-ARDRA work group under the auspices of Department of Health and Human Services Task Force on Alzheimer's disease, *Neurology* 34:939-944, 1984.

Pfeffer R et al: Measurement of functional activities of older adults in the community, *J Gerontology* 37:323-329, 1992.

Small GW et al: Diagnosis and treatment of Alzheimer disease and related disorders: General consensus statement of the American Association of Geriatric Psychiatry, the Alzheimer's Association, and the American Geriatric Society, *JAMA* 278(16):1363-1372, 1997.

Strub R, Black F: *The mental status exam in neurology,* ed 3, Philadelphia, 1993, FA Davis.

US Department of Health and Human Services: Early identification of Alzheimer's disease and related dementias (AHCPR Publication No-97-0703), Rockville, Md, 1996, U.S. Department of Health and Human Services.

US Department of Health and Human Services: Progress report on Alzheimer's disease (NIH Publication No. 95-3994), Rockville, Md, 1995, US Department of Health and Human Services.

US Department of Health and Human Services: Quick reference guide for clinicians: Early identification of Alzheimer's disease and related dementias, *Am Acad Nurse Pract* 9:85-87, 1997.

Yanagihara T, Petersen R, editors: *Memory disorders: research and clinical practice,* New York, 1991, Marcel Dekker.

Amenorrhea

ICD-9-CM

Amenorrhea (Primary or Secondary) 626.0
Amenorrhea Due to Ovarian Dysfunction 256.8

OVERVIEW

Definition

Amenorrhea is the absence of menstrual bleeding. There are essentially two types of amenorrhea: primary and secondary.

Primary amenorrhea is defined as no bleeding by age 16, regardless of the presence of normal growth and development with the appearance of secondary sex characteristics.

Secondary amenorrhea occurs in a woman who has been previously menstruating and misses at least 3 menstrual cycles.

Incidence

Secondary amenorrhea affects a large number of women at some time during their reproductive years.

Pathophysiology

Amenorrhea is caused either by failure of the hypothalamic-pituitary-gonadal axis, by the absence of end organs, or by obstruction of the outflow tract.

Common Causes of Primary Amenorrhea

Gonadal dysgenesis: There is a lack of mature breast/pubic hair development, but small amounts of secondary sex characteristics are present (Tanner stage 2 or 3).
Mullerian anomalies: Normal breast/pubic hair development occurs.
Hypothalamic/pituitary disorders: Normal breast/pubic hair does not occur.
Constitutional delay secondary to an immature hypothalamic-pituitary axis, short stature (under 5 ft. at age 14)

Common Causes of Secondary Amenorrhea

Pregnancy
Prolactin-secreting pituitary adenomas
Hypothalamic amenorrhea secondary to excessive stress, weight loss, and/or exercise
Polycystic ovarian disease
Hypothyroidism
Hyperprolactinemia

SUBJECTIVE DATA

History of Present Illness

Ask about:
Lifestyle practices: Eating habits, athletic training, aerobics
Headaches
Visual disturbances

Primary Amenorrhea

Ask about growth and development and any recent growth spurts.
Ask about any pubertal signs, when they began, and how far have they progressed.

Secondary Amenorrhea

Include a careful menstrual, sexual and pregnancy history. Include age at menarche, regularity of cycles and frequency of missed cycles. Ask about any complications of pregnancies or difficulties becoming pregnant. Ask about any diagnosis of fibroids or endometriosis.
Question about any past or present serious illnesses, including any radiation or chemotherapy.
Ask about last menstrual period.
Question about any physical changes that may be taking

Box 10-1

Drugs Associated with Amenorrhea

Phenothiazines	**Haloperidol**
Tricyclic antidepressants	Calcium channel blockers
Methyldopa	Digitalis
Marijuana	Fluorouracil
Oral contraceptives	Depo-Provera/Norplant
Busulfan	Cisplatin
Cytoxan	

place: growth of facial hair, loss of scalp hair, deepening of voice.
Question about any recent loss or added weight in the past year.
Ask about methods of contraception.

Past Medical History

Chronic illness
Central nervous system trauma
Congenital anomalies

Medications

Ask about any medications taken in the past year (Box 10-1).

Psychosocial History

Ask about exercise patterns, any special training for an upcoming event.
Ask about body image, history of eating disorders.
Any chronic or recent stress should be noted.

Description of Most Common Symptoms

Patients should be questioned about breast discharge, hirsutism, and signs and symptoms of hypothyroidism.

OBJECTIVE DATA

Physical Examination

Primary Amenorrhea

Height and weight
Signs of gonadal dysgenesis: Neck folds, setting of ears, chest configuration, short fourth metacarpal, cubitus, valgus
Body hair (see Figure 93-1)
Skin pigmentation
Assessment of Tanner stage of breast and pubic hair development
Speculum examination for the presence of a vagina, uterus, and enlarged clitoris and a bimanual examination for any adnexal masses

Secondary Amenorrhea

Height and weight
Skin examination for acne, hirsutism (The absence of both axillary and pubic hair in a phenotypically normal female suggests complete androgen insensitivity.)
Neck assessment for enlarged thyroid gland, nodes
Breast examination for staging, any galactorrhea
Abdominal striae on a nulliparous woman may indicate hypercortisolism (Cushing's syndrome)
Speculum examination for assessment of rugation, type of cervical mucus (amount, stretching pattern, and ferning when dried on a glass slide) (A vaginal septum may cause a blockage of the outflow tract and prevent menstruation, as will an imperforate hymen.)
Bimanual examination for masses, especially unilateral ovarian masses, fundal enlargement
Deep tendon reflexes; check to assess thyroid status

Diagnostic Procedures

Minimal workup should include tests listed in Table 10-1.

ASSESSMENT

Primary Amenorrhea

Identified by lack of menses by age 16; requires further workup because of possibility of significant organ dysfunction

Secondary Amenorrhea

Common causes of secondary amenorrhea are found in Box 10-2 and Figure 10-1.

General Management

Obtain a pregnancy test. If the pregnancy test is negative, thyroid-stimulating hormone (TSH) and prolactin levels should be drawn, a progesterone challenge (10 mg Provera for 5 to 10 days) administered. If bleeding occurs 3 to 5 days after completing the Provera, and TSH and prolactin levels are normal, the amenorrhea is due to anovulation rather than to hypothalamic-pituitary insufficiency or ovarian failure (Table 10-2).

If no bleeding occurs, it indicates either an incompetent outflow tract, nonreactive endometrium, or inadequate estrogen stimulation. To rule out an abnormality of the outflow tract, a combined oral contraceptive pill (OCP) (see family planning chapter for specific details of OCP therapy)

TABLE 10-1 Diagnostic Tests: Amenorrhea

Diagnostic Test	Finding/Rationale	Cost ($)
Urine HCG	First line test to r/o pregnancy. Most common cause of amenorrhea.	17-23
TSH and Prolactin Level	Helps to determine if problem is due to lack of pituitary stimulation	47-61/thyroid panel 70-89/prolactin
FSH, LH, estradiol	Helps indicate if hormonal stimulation is occurring A serum FSH/LH is then drawn to localize the problem to the follicle, pituitary or hypothalamus. High gonadotropin levels and a low estrogen level indicate ovarian failure.	62-78/ FSH 61-76/LH 85-107/estradiol
Prolactin	Increased prolactin level can be caused by medications, pituitary tumor	70-80
Secondary Tests		
Thyroid antibodies	Helps determine if thyroid failure is the cause of amenorrhea	64-81
Cortisol	Helps to determine if premature ovarian failure is the cause of amenorrhea	60-76
Calcium, phosphorus	Secondary tests to determine cause of amenorrhea	18-23/calcium 16-20/phosphorus
Complete blood count		18-23
ESR		16-20
Antinuclear antibodies		42-56
Rheumatic factors		25-32
Total protein		22-27/protein
Albumin		18-23/albumin
Progesterone		59-73

HCG, Human chorionic gonadotropin; *TSH*, thyroid-stimulating hormone; *FSH*, follicle-stimulating hormone; *LH*, luteinizing hormone; *ESR*, erythrocyte sedimentation rate.

Box 10-2

Most Common Causes of Secondary Amenorrhea

Pregnancy
Chronic anovulation
Asherman's syndrome: Partial or total endometrial obliteration by adhesions
Hypogonadotropic hypogonadism (pituitary or hypothalamic dysfunction)
Adrenal failure (congenital adrenal hyperplasia and Cushing's syndrome [Ch. 49])
Ovarian failure (persistent corpus luteum cysts, premature ovarian failure, and polycystic ovary [Ch. 135])

is then initiated (or estrogen 1.25 mg on days 1 to 21, with medroxyprogesterone 5 to 10 mg on days 16 to 21). Withdrawal bleeding confirms the presence of a normal outflow tract and a normal endometrium. If bleeding occurs, the problem is localized to the hypothalamic-pituitary axis or ovaries, and anatomic causes are excluded.

A woman who does not have withdrawal bleeding after the progesterone challenge test but does bleed after using either the combined oral contraceptive pill or the estrogen/Provera pills is considered to have hypoestrogenic amenorrhea.

If the prolactin level is elevated (hyperprolactinemia), review the patient's medications for possible causes of increased prolactin. Instruct the patient to avoid any breast stimulation. Repeat the test with the patient in a relaxed, fasting state because prolactin levels may be increased by stress, exercise, anxiety, sleep, and food ingestion.

Amenorrheic women with a history of galactorrhea and/or an elevated prolactin level should have magnetic resonance imaging done to rule out a pituitary tumor.

In patients who have prolonged amenorrhea with signs of androgen or estrogen excess, an endometrial biopsy should be considered before withdrawal bleeding is induced.

THERAPEUTIC PLAN

Amenorrhea Caused by Chronic Anovulation

A change in lifestyle may be sufficient to stimulate ovulation (reduce stress, adequate nutrition).

Treatment must include cyclic progesterone to induce withdrawal bleeding.

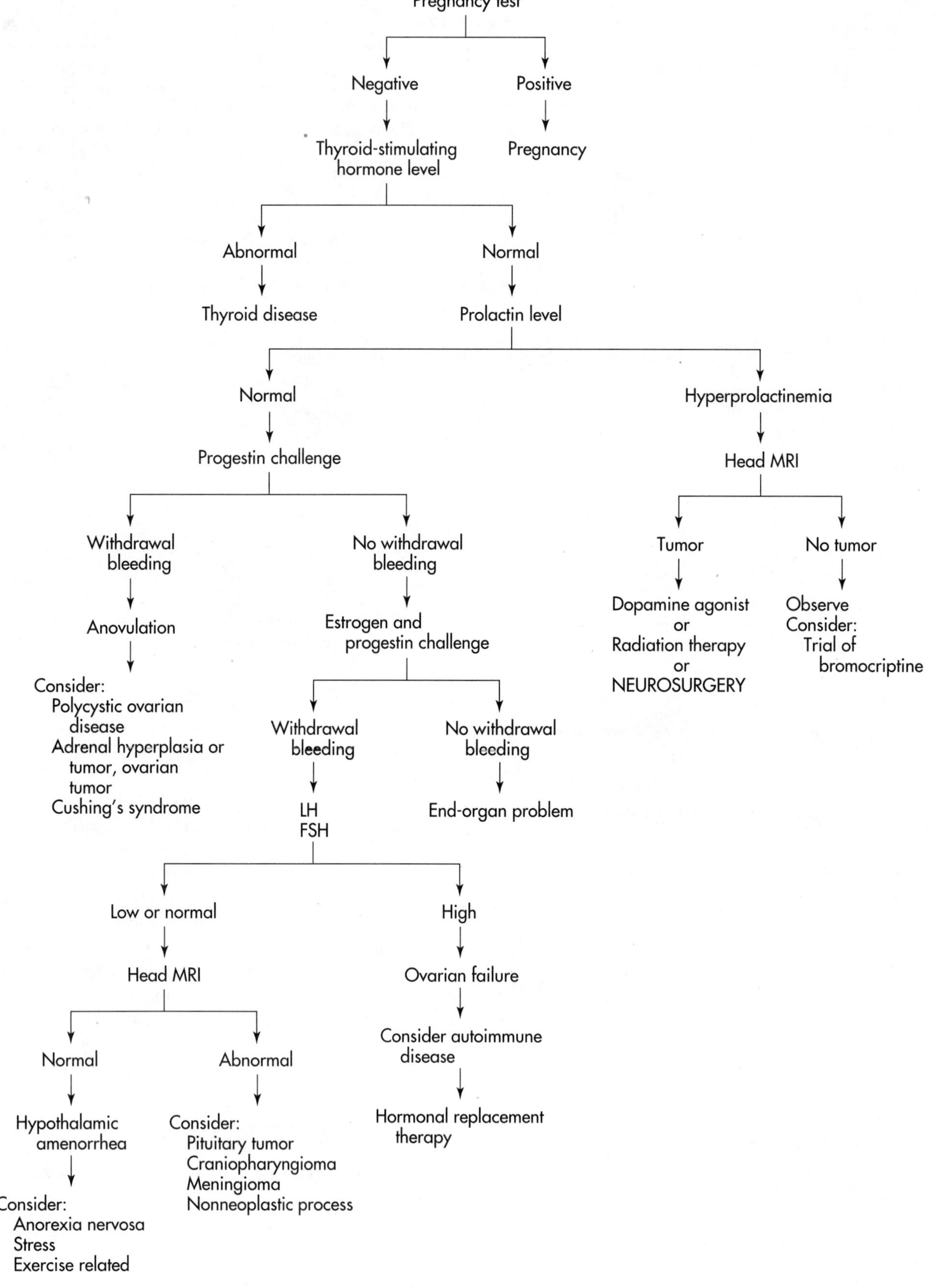

Figure 10-1 Algorithm for the patient with secondary amenorrhea. *MRI,* Magnetic resonance imaging; *LH,* luteinizing hormone; *FSH,* follicle-stimulating hormone. (Redrawn from Greene HL, Johnson WP, Lemcke D: *Decision making in medicine: an algorithmic approach,* ed 2, St Louis, 1998, Mosby.)

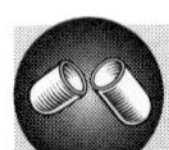

TABLE 10-2 Progesterone Challenge: Amenorrhea

Drug	Dose	Comment	Cost
Medroxyprogesterone (Provera)	10 mg for 5-10 days	Pregnancy: D SE: headache, nausea, increased weight, amenorrhea, breakthrough bleeding, gynecomastia	\$29-\$35/2.5 mg (100) \$44-\$53/5 mg (100) \$11-\$66/10 mg (100)

Medroxyprogesterone 10 mg/day for the first 7 to 10 days of each month should be prescribed. Newer studies are suggesting that cycling a woman every 3 months is sufficient to decrease the risk of endometrial cancer secondary to unopposed estrogen.

If pregnancy is desired, ovulation may be induced with clomiphene (Clomid) (see infertility chapter).

Amenorrhea Secondary to Hypothalamic Dysfunction

No withdrawal bleeding from a progesterone challenge but a positive response to combined oral contraceptives.

This type of amenorrhea usually results from psychological stress, depression, severe weight loss, anorexia nervosa, or strenuous exercise.

Athletic-related amenorrhea is usually reversible within a few months of decreased training. In anorexic patients amenorrhea may be more persistent despite weight gain.

These patients are at greater risk of developing osteoporosis and cardiovascular disease.

Hormonal therapy should be prescribed for all hypoestrogenic women.

Calcium supplements (1500 mg/day) is also recommended (\$1-\$7/500 mg [60]).

Oral contraceptives are more appropriate than cyclic hormone replacement therapy (HRT) to prevent bone loss.

If cyclic HRT is preferred or necessary because of risk factors (e.g., smokers >35 years of age), the patient should take conjugated estrogen 0.625 mg with medroxyprogesterone 2.5 mg/day every day of the month in a continuous manner.

Contraceptives should be used by sexually active women who do not desire pregnancy because pregnancy may occur in up to 10% of cases.

Management of Disorders of the Ovary

Ovarian failure should be considered if menopausal symptoms occur, especially hot flushes or dyspareunia.

Women who are diagnosed with premature ovarian failure who are less then 30 years of age should undergo karyotyping to rule out the presence of a Y chromosome. If a Y chromosome is detected, the patient should be evaluated for the presence of testicular tissue, and, if present, the testicular tissue should be removed.

Women between the ages of 30 and 40 years of age with ovarian failure can usually be assumed to have premature ovarian failure and normal chromosomes.

Twenty percent to 40% of cases of premature ovarian failure are associated with autoimmune disorders. Therefore an evaluation for autoimmune diseases is recommended for patients diagnosed with premature ovarian failure.

Laboratory Workup of Patients With Premature Ovarian Failure

Recommended: TSH, free T_4, thyroid antibodies, morning cortisol levels, calcium and phosphorus

Consider: Complete blood count, erythrocyte sedimentation rate, antinuclear antibody, rheumatoid factor, total protein, albumin:globulin ratio

Adrenal failure can follow ovarian failure; thus adrenal function surveillance should be considered.

Patients with ovarian failure should be prescribed estrogen 0.625 mg with progesterone QD with 1500 mg of calcium (see menopause chapter for specific dosage/cost information).

Patient Education

It takes 1 to 2 years for adolescents to establish a regular and cyclic pattern of menstruation.

Family Impact

Patients with primary amenorrhea are most likely to have serious causes.

Psychologic trauma can be severe; counseling is recommended.

Referral/Consultation

Referral to an gynecologist who specializes in endocrine abnormalities is appropriate for primary amenorrhea

EVALUATION

If menstruation is absent for 3 months (assuming cycle has been regular), investigation is in order.

SUGGESTED READINGS

Curosh N: Secondary amenorrhea. In Greene H, Johnson W, Lemcke D, editors: *Decision making in medicine,* ed 2, St Louis, 1998, Mosby.

Dunnihoo DR: *Amenorrhea: fundamentals of gynecology and obstetrics,* ed 2, JB Lippincott, 1992, Philadelphia.

Ellsworth A et al: *Mosby's 1998 medical drug reference,* St Louis, 1998, Mosby.

Fogel C: Endocrine causes of amenorrhea, *Lippincott's Primary Care Pract* 1(5):507-518, 1997.

Glaiser A: *Gynecologic problems in the family planning consultation: handbook of family planning and reproductive health,* ed 3, New York, 1995, Churchill Livingstone.

Glass RH: *Amenorrhea. Office Gynecology,* ed 4, Baltimore, 1993, Williams & Wilkins.

Hawkins JW, Roberto-Nichols DM, Stanley-Haney JL: *Protocols for nurse practitioners on gynecologic settings,* ed 5, New York, 1995, Tiresias Press.

Healthcare Consultants of America, Inc: *1998 Physicians fee and coding guide,* Augusta, Ga, 1998, Healthcare Consultants of America, Inc.

Johnson CA: *Women's health care handbook,* St Louis, 1996, Mosby.

Laughlin G, Dominquez C, Yen S: Nutritional and endocrine-metabolic aberrations in women with functional hypothalamic amenorrhea, *J Clin Endocrinol Metabol* 83(1):25-32, 1998.

Marantides D: Management of polycystic ovary syndrome, *Nurse Pract* 22(12):34-38, 1997.

McIver B, Romanski S, Nippoldt T: Evaluation and management of amenorrhea, *Mayo Clin Proc* 72(12):1161-1169, 1997.

Anemia

ICD-9-CM

Anemia 285.9
Other and Unspecified Anemia (chronic disease) 285
Iron-Deficiency Anemia, Unspecified 280.0
Aplastic Anemia 284
Autoimmune Hemolytic Anemia 283.0
Sickle Cell Anemia, Unspecified 282.60
Pernicious Anemia 281.0
Other Vitamin B_{12} Anemia 281.1
Folate Deficiency Anemia 281.2
Thalassemia 282.4

OVERVIEW

Definition

Anemia is a condition in which the concentration of hemoglobin or the number or volume of red blood cells (RBCs) is reduced below normal. This may be caused by impaired production of RBCs, increased destruction of RBCs, or rapid loss of RBCs.

Incidence

Anemia occurs most frequently in young **children, women** of reproductive age, and **elderly** persons. The most common cause of anemia in the United States is iron deficiency. The prevalence of iron deficiency is currently estimated to be about 3% for **children** 1 to 5 years old. About 9% of women 15 to 44 years old have low hemoglobin levels, and anemia is especially common in **pregnant** patients. The prevalence of anemia in persons older than 65 years of age is 2.3% in men and 5.5% in women.

Sickle cell anemia affects more than 70,000 blacks; one third of the affected individuals are between 2 and 16 years old.

Pathophysiology

The physiological defect caused by the anemia is a decrease in the oxygen-carrying capacity of the blood and a reduction in the oxygen available to the tissues. The signs and symptoms of anemia are a result of failure to oxygenate tissues and the degree of acuity (the gradual onset of anemia allows time for compensatory mechanisms to increase oxygenation). Anemias can be classified either by causative (etiological) mechanisms or by red blood cell morphology.

Etiologically, anemia results from:

Acute or chronic hemorrhage
An increased loss or destruction of red blood cells
Production of abnormal hemoglobin, which leads to anemia, and tissue damage from vascular blockage by trapped, abnormal RBCs; RBCs assume a crescent shape when oxygen tension is lowered (sickle cell)
Impaired hemoglobin and red blood cell formation (resulting from nutritional causes, bone marrow infiltration, or chronic disease)

The morphological classification of anemia includes:

Normocytic/normochromic (resulting from blood loss, hemolytic anemia, chronic disease, or bone marrow infiltration)
Microcytic/hypochromic (resulting from iron deficiency, presence of lead, thalassemias)
Macrocytic/normochromic (resulting from vitamin B_{12} or folate deficiency, use of certain drugs, or bone marrow failure)

Risk Factors

Age

Newborns: The most common causes of anemia include blood loss, isoimmunization, congenital infection, and congenital hemolytic anemia.

3- to 6-month-old infants: Anemia results from congenital disorders of hemoglobin synthesis or hemoglobin structure; anemia in this age-group is almost never the result of nutritional iron deficiency in an otherwise normal full-term infant; prematurity predisposes to early development of iron deficiency.

Older infants/toddlers: Anemia can result from a nutritional iron deficiency in babies who have been switched to whole cow's milk.

Women: Menstrual bleeding or other blood loss can lead to anemia.

Elderly: Gastrointestinal bleeding and/or poor iron intake can cause anemia.

Race/Ethnic Origin

Hemoglobin S and C are more common in blacks.

Beta-thalassemia is more common in persons of Mediterranean heritage.

Alpha-thalassemia is more common among the black and Oriental races.

Diet

Decreased intake of iron, folate, vitamin B_{12}, or vitamin E increases the risk of anemia.

Drugs

Administration of anticonvulsants or undergoing chemotherapy increases the risk of anemia.

Types of Anemia

Microcytic/Hypochromic

Iron deficiency

Caused by increased physiological requirements, decreased intake of iron, or chronic blood loss

Presence of lead leads to aminolevulinic acid synthetase, which leads to deficient hemoglobin synthesis

Thalassemias

Genetic cause, secondary to deficient synthesis of one or more of the polypeptide chains of hemoglobin

Major: Lack of B-chain synthesis, intramedullary hemolysis

Minor: Heterozygous state

Alpha: Deletion of one or more alpha genes

Normocytic/Normochromic

Hemolytic

Reduced survival of circulating RBCs secondary to destruction in the circulation (intravascular) or within the phagocytic cells of the liver, spleen, or bone marrow (extravascular)

Intrinsic red cell defects

Congenital spherocytosis: Abnormality of RBC membranes secondary to spectrin deficiency

G-6-PD deficiency: Deficient enzyme concentration does not allow detoxification of oxygen free radicals by nicotinamide adenine dinucleotide (reduced form) (NADH), precipitating hemolysis

Hemoglobinopathies: Hemoglobin SS, hemoglobin C

Extrinsic red cell defects

Immune mediated

Hemolytic disease of the newborn—ABO incompatibility

Anemia of chronic disease: Resulting from chronic infection, osteomyelitis, tuberculosis, pyelonephritis, chronic inflammatory disorders (rheumatoid arthritis, systemic lupus erythematosus, inflammatory bowel disease)

Macrocytic

Aplastic anemia/Fanconi's anemia

Causes include idiopathic, hepatitis, chemicals, pregnancy

Vitamin B_{12} or folate deficiency

Caused by inadequate intake, malabsorption, increased body requirements

SUBJECTIVE DATA

Past Medical History

Determine whether there is a history of symptoms related to anemia, including irritability, dyspnea, fatigability, palpitations, headache, edema, jaundice, bleeding, pallor, infection, heart murmur, chronic illness, drug use, bone pain, and past viral infections.

Ask about anemia with previous pregnancies.

Family History

Ask about ethnic origin, travel, history of gallstones, or splenectomy in other family members.

Diet

Diet, any recent weight gain or loss, anorexia, nausea/vomiting, decreased intake, diarrhea

Medication History

Ask about the patient's use of anticonvulsant medications.

Psychosocial History

Alcohol intake

Ask about environmental exposures at home and in the workplace (lead, chemicals, heavy metal).

OBJECTIVE DATA

Physical Examination

Perform a complete physical examination, with increased attention to:

Vital signs, weight, height

In mild anemia (hemoglobin level 10 to 14 g/dl) and even moderate anemia (6 to10 g/dl), few clinical manifestations may be seen. Most commonly palpitations and dyspnea are the first symptoms seen.

In severe anemia (hemoglobin <6 g/dl), the following may be seen:

General: Sensitivity to cold, weight loss, lethargy

Skin: Jaundice, bleeding, pallor, petechiae, purpura

Cardiovascular: Tachycardia, murmur, or gallop, angina, myocardial infarction, congestive heart failure

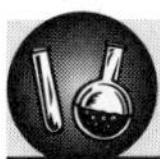

TABLE 11-1 Diagnostic Tests: Anemia

Test	Finding/Rationale	Cost ($)
CBC	Include all indices, MCV, MCH, MCHC	18-23
Hgb	Indicates the oxygen-carrying pigment of the RBC	11-14
HCT	Volume of packed RBCs; reflects total mass of RBCs	
Blood smear	Size (anisocytosis, microcytes or macrocytes) Inclusions: basophilic stippling, Howell-Jolly bodies, polychromasia	Review by hematologist 54-68
Reticulocyte count	Normal 0.5%-1.5%; reflects state of erythroid activity of bone marrow	17-21
Bone marrow	Evalutes number of RBC precursors and maturation; used to rule out infiltration	401-499
Direct/indirect bilirubin	Helps to rule out hemolytic anemia; increased indirect bilirubin (unconjugated) in hemolytic anemia	23-30
LDH, SGOT, uric acid, total iron, vitamin B_{12}, vitamin E, folic acid levels	SGOT ↑ In hemolytic anemia, total iron ↓ in iron deficiency anemia, vitamin B_{12} ↓ in megaloblastic anemia, folic acid levels ↓ in megaloblastic anemia	20-25/LDH 18-23/SGOT, uric acid 23-28/total Fe 96/vitamin B_{12} 46-55/vitamin E 49-62/folic acid
TIBC	↑ In iron deficiency anemia, ↓ in anemia of chronic disease	33-41
Ferritin	Serum ferritin <10 μg/ml in iron-deficient state, ↑ in anemia of chronic disease	48-60
FEP	Sometimes ↑ in lead poisoning, anemia of chronic disease, and iron deficiency anemia	42
Direct/indirect Coombs' test	Rule out hemolytic disease	16-20/direct 21-26/indirect

CBC, Complete blood cell count; ↓, decreased; Fe, iron; *FEP,* free erythrocyte protoporphyrin; *HCT,* hematocrit level; *Hgb,* hemoglobin level; ↑, increased; *LDH,* lactate dehydrogenase; *MCV,* mean corpuscular volume; *MCH,* mean corpuscular hemoglobin; *MCHC,* mean corpuscular hemoglobin concentration; *RBC,* red blood cells; *SGOT,* serum glutamic oxaloacetic transaminase; *TIBC,* total iron-binding capacity.

Abdominal: Hepatosplenomegaly or other masses; lymphadenopathy; anorexia
Respiratory: Tachypnea
Musculoskeletal: Bone pain
HEENT*: Mouth: glossitis, angular stomatitis
Eyes: Eyelid edema, retinal hemorrhage
Neurological: Headache, vertigo, irritability, depression, impaired thought processes

Diagnostic Procedures

Diagnostic tests for anemia are presented in Table 11-1.

ASSESSMENT

The patient's hemoglobin and hematocrit levels should be compared with a set of standards appropriate for age (see Appendix I). The mean corpuscular volume (MCV) and reticulocyte count should be analyzed to suggest a potential cause of the anemia (Figure 11-1).

Differential Diagnosis

Autoimmune pancytopenia, marrow infiltration with a solid tumor, marrow suppression secondary to drug toxins or infections, bleeding colitis, osteomyelitis, pyelonephritis, blood loss, hemolysis, chronic inflammatory bowel disease, rheumatoid arthritis, systemic lupus erythematosus, leukemia

Age-Specific Differential Diagnosis

Newborns: Blood loss, hemolysis
Infant: Iron-deficiency anemia, GI bleeding, thalassemia, sickle cell anemia, lead exposure, spherocytosis
Toddlers/school-age children: Fanconi's anemia, aplastic anemia, anemia of chronic disease, G-6-PD deficiency, transient erythroblastopenia following viral illness

**HEENT,* head, eyes, ears, nose, and throat.

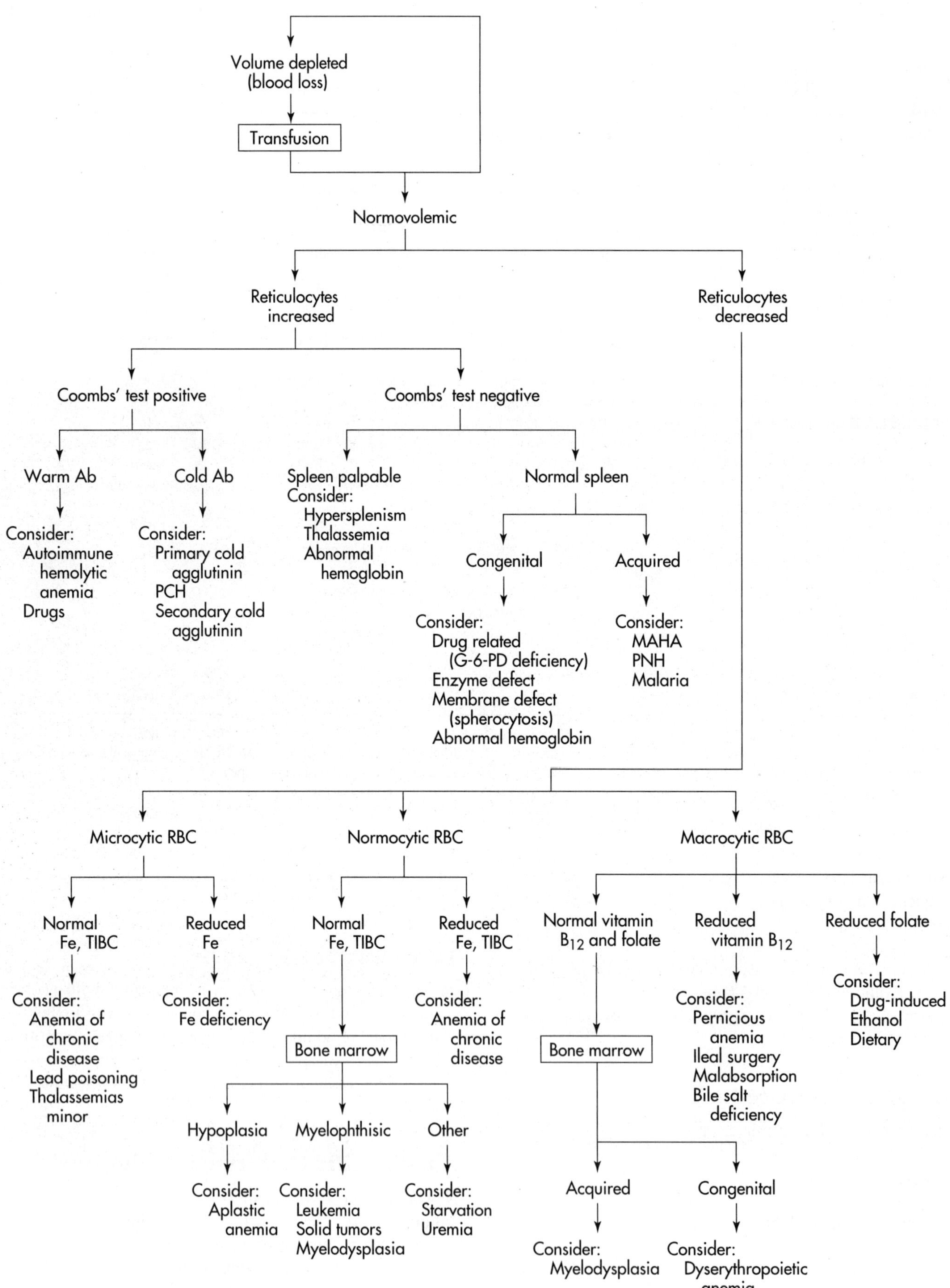

Figure 11-1 Algorithm for treatment of a patient with anemia (decreased red blood cell [RBC] mass). *Ab,* antibodies; *Fe,* iron; *MAHA,* microangiopathic hemolytic anemia; *PCH,* paroxysmal cold hemoglobinuria; *PNH,* paroxysmal nocturnal hemoglobinuria; *TIBC,* total iron-binding capacity. (Redrawn from Taetle R: Patient with anemia. In Greene HL, Johnson WP, Lemcke D, editors: *Decision making in medicine,* ed 2, St Louis, 1998, Mosby.)

Adolescents: Iron-deficiency anemia, aplastic anemia, autoimmune hemolysis, sickle cell anemia

Adult: Folic acid deficiency, pernicious anemia, iron-deficiency anemia, autoimmune hemolysis, aplastic anemia

Pregnant woman: Acute blood loss, iron-deficiency anemia, folic acid deficiency

Further considerations for age-specific differential diagnoses are outlined in Table 11-2.

THERAPEUTIC PLAN

The goal of treatment is to eradicate the anemia and its cause.

Pharmaceutical

Iron-Deficiency Anemia (Table 11-3)

In an adult, iron deficiency anemia is almost always the result of blood loss. Treatment consists of identifying and correcting the source of blood loss.

Adults

Mild anemia: 900 mg elemental iron replacement

Moderate anemia (hemoglobin 10 g/dl): 1500 to 2000 mg elemental iron replacement

Children

Mild to moderate iron deficiency: 3 mg/kg/day in one dose or two divided doses

Severe iron deficiency: 4 to 6 mg/kg/day in three divided doses

Prophylaxis: 1 to 2 mg/kg/day

Sickle Cell Anemia (Table 11-4)

Prevent infection by standard immunizations.

Treat febrile episodes for sepsis.

Begin prophylactic administration of penicillin at 2 to 3 months of age.

Pernicious Anemia

The pharmaceutical treatment for pernicious anemia is outlined in Table 11-5.

Aplastic Anemia

The treatment for patients who are less than 45 years old is a bone marrow transplant.

The treatment for patients older than 45 years of age is cyclosporin ($42/25 mg [30 tablets]).

Thalassemia

Major thalassemia: Treatment consists of transfusions, chelating agents for hemosiderosis; a splenectomy may be considered.

Minor thalassemia: No medical therapy; genetic counseling and psychosocial support are recommended.

Folic Acid Deficiency

Nutrition assessment and counseling are recommended. The pharmaceutical plan for folic acid deficiency is outlined in Table 11-6.

Patient Education

Iron Deficiency Anemia

Identify the causes of low iron and explain the appropriate treatment plan.

Teach the family about a diet high in iron and the side effects of iron therapy.

Sickle Cell Anemia

Identify the causes of sickle cell crisis and its disease process; early recognition of possible complications

Priapism

Temperature of 101° F requires immediate attention

Make the family aware of precipitating factors:

- Cold exposure
- Decreased fluid intake
- Exercise at high altitude
- Overexertion, emotional or physical stress
- Increased blood viscosity
- Viral, bacterial infections
- Surgery, blood loss

Need for routine health care, including penicillin prophylaxis (Consider pneumovax.)

Outline pain management plan for crises

Well-balanced diet with folic acid supplementation

Psychosocial support

Genetic counseling

Avoidance of high-dose estrogen oral contraceptives

Pernicious Anemia

Etiology and nature of disease

Need for lifelong vitamin B_{12} replacement

Review side effects of vitamin B_{12} injection

Referral/Consultation

Recommend referral/consultation with a hematologist for a multidisciplinary approach and management for chronic anemias.

EVALUATION/FOLLOW-UP

Evaluation of Treatment Response

Iron-Deficiency Anemia

Infants

The reticulocyte count will be increased in 2 to 3 days.

Hemoglobin levels should be rechecked in 2 to 3 weeks when indices have returned to normal.

Table 11–2 Differential Diagnosis: Anemia

Age	Diagnosis	Supporting Data
Infants and children	Iron deficiency anemia	Serum ferritin <10 mg/ml CBC with RBC indices decreased; MCV <83 mm Serum iron <30 mEq/dl Reticulocyte count may be low, normal, or slightly elevated Blood smear shows RBC microcytic, hypochromic
Adults	Iron deficiency anemia	Hemoglobin <14 g/dl in men and <12 g/dl in women, hematocrit <42% men and <36% in women Low MCV (microcytic) and low MCHC (hypochromic) Low RBC count Increased RDW Low serum iron (<50 mg/ml) TIBC elevated
All ages	Sickle cell anemia	Tests: Hemoglobin electrophoresis, solubility test Peripheral smear: Target cells, poikilocytes, and sickled cells LFT abnormal Decreased ESR Increased platelets
All ages	Thalassemia	Hemoglobin electrophoresis: Increased hemoglobin A (minor) and decreased or absent hemoglobin A (major) CBC: Microcytosis in minor; hypochromic microcytic in major Peripheral smear shows coarse basophilic stippling in minor; target cells and stippling in major
Adults	Pernicious anemia	Hemoglobin/hematocrit levels decreased RBCs decreased Reticulocytes normal or low MCV >100 mm, MCHC WNL Serum vitamin B_{12} decreased (0.1 μg/ml) Increased LDH Serum folate +/or RBC level normal or low Serum bilirubin increased U/A: Increased urobilinogen
All	Aplastic anemia	Hypoplastic, fatty bone marrow (pancytopenia) Decreased WBCs, RBCs, platelets
Pregnant women	Folic acid deficiency	Hemoglobin/hematocrit decreased MCV increased (megaloblastic anemia) Decreased serum Fe TIBC increased Serum folate <165 ng/ml

CBC, Complete blood cell count; *LDH,* lactate dehydrogenase; *LFT,* liver function test; *MCHC,* mean corpuscular hemoglobin concentration; *MCV,* mean corpuscular volume; *RBCs,* red blood cells; *RDW,* red cell distribution width; *TIBC,* total iron-binding capacity; *WBCs,* white blood cells; *ESR,* erythrocyte sedimentation rate; *WNL,* within normal limits.

Iron therapy should be continued for 2 to 3 months to replenish iron stores once hemoglobin levels are in the normal range.

Adults

Hemoglobin should be rechecked in 4 weeks.

Iron therapy should be continued for 3 months after hemoglobin levels return to normal to replenish the body's iron stores.

Pernicious Anemia

Follow up with **elderly** patients and those with a cardiac condition in 48 hours (a rapid increase in RBC production can lead to hypovolemia).

Consider iron supplementation.

Check the initial hematological response in 4 to 6 weeks, then every 6 months for hematocrit and stool for occult blood (the incidence of gastric cancer increases with pernicious anemia).

Folic Acid Deficiency

Repeat hemoglobin and hematocrit evaluation in 2 to 4 weeks (should expect increased by 2 points within 1 month).

Refer to collaborating MD or hematologist if anemia is severe.

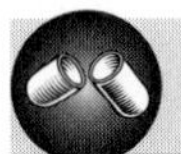

Table 11-3 Pharmaceutical Plan: Iron-Deficiency Anemia

Drug	Dose	Comments	Cost
Ferrous sulfate (Feosol) Iron 65 mg	1 tab TID/QID pc and hs Children: 6-12 yr: 1 tab TID pc >1 yr: 2.5-5 ml TID between meals; mix with water or juice	Doses can be reduced as needed for GI symptoms, or taken with meals (may reduce delivery by 50%) Special iron formulations and compounds are expensive and reduce symptoms only as they reduce the delivery of iron. Pregnancy: B Iron is highly toxic; keep out of reach of children SE: Cause black BM, GI upset	\$2-\$10/325 mg (100)
Ferrous gluconate (Fergon) Iron 36 mg	1 tab QD		\$2 \$4/300 mg (100)
Ferrous polysaccharide (Niferex) Iron 50 mg	1-2 tabs QD Children: 6-12 yr: 1-2 tabs QD <6 not recommended		N/A
Slow FE Iron 50 mg	1-2 tabs QD (tab must be swallowed whole) Children: 6-12 yr: 1 tab QD <6: not recommended		\$2-\$6/150 mg (100)
Fer-In-Sol Iron: 18 mg/5 ml	Adults: 5 ml QD Children: >4 yr: 5 ml QD <4 yr: drops, 0.6 ml QD		Approximately \$20

BM, Bowel movement; *FE,* iron; *GI,* gastrointestinal; *SE,* side effects; *N/A,* not available.

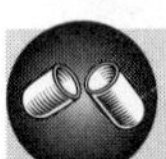

Table 11-4 Pharmaceutical Plan: Sickle Cell Anemia

Drug	Dose	Comments	Cost
Amoxicillin (Amoxil)	<3 yr: 125 mg BID >3 yr: 250 mg BID	Continue indefinitely Use erythromycin if patient is allergic to penicillin SE: GI upset, urticaria, superinfection, hyperactivity	\$3-\$5/125 mg/5 ml (150 ml) \$4-\$8/20 250 mg/5 ml (150 ml)

SE, Side effects; *GI,* gastrointestinal.

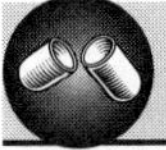

Table 11-5 Pharmaceutical Plan: Pernicious Anemia

Drug	Dose	Comments	Cost
Vitamin B_{12} (cyanocobalamin)	100-200 μg subcutaneously Administer QD for first week, then weekly for 1 month, then monthly	Injections required lifelong	\$2-\$7/1 μg/ml (30 ml)
Cyanocobalamin (Nascobal)	1 spray (500 μg) in one nostril 1×/wk	Used only when hematological parameters are within normal range Allow 1 hr before or after ingestion of hot foods or liquids Not recommended for children Pregnancy: C SE: Headache, nausea, rhinitis	N/A

SE, Side effects; *N/A,* not available.

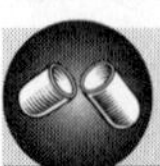

TABLE 11-6 Pharmaceutical Plan: Folic Acid

Drug	Dose	Comments	Cost
Folate (Folvite)	1 mg QD	For pregnant women: Included in all prenatal vitamins	\$1-\$8/1 mg (100)

SUGGESTED READINGS

Bates B: *Physical exam and history taking,* ed 2, Philadelphia, 1995, JB Lippincott.

Children's Hospital Medical Center Formulary, Cincinnati, Ohio, 1995.

Cunningham F et al: Hematological disorders. In Cunningham G et al: *Williams obstetrics,* ed 20, Norwalk, Conn, 1997, Appleton & Lange.

Ellsworth AJ et al: *Mosby's 1998 medical drug reference,* St Louis, 1998, Mosby.

Healthcare Consultants of America, Inc: *1998 Physicians fee and coding guide,* Augusta, Ga, 1998, Healthcare Consultants of America, Inc.

Hay W et al: Anemias. In *Current pediatric diagnosis and treatment,* Norwalk, Conn, 1995, Appleton & Lange.

Jandl J: The anemias. In *Blood, textbook of hematology*, ed 3, Boston, 1987, Little, Brown.

Kalinyak K: Anemias. In Arceci R, editor: *Hematology oncology stem cell transplant handbook,* ed 2, Cincinnati, 1997, Hematology Oncology Division, Children's Hospital Medical Center.

Miller D: Anemias: general considerations. In Miller D, Baehner R, Miller L, editors: *Blood diseases in infancy and childhood,* ed 7, St Louis, 1989, Mosby.

Mitus A, Rosenthal D: History and physical examination of relevance to the hematologist. In Handlin R, Lux S, Stossel T, editors: *Blood: principles and practice of hematology,* Philadelphia, 1995, JB Lippincott.

Taetle R: Patient with anemia. In Greene H, Johnson W, Lemcke D, editors: *Decision making in medicine,* ed 2, St Louis, 1998, Mosby.

Oral Anticoagulant Therapy

ICD-9-CM

Not Available

OVERVIEW

Definition

Anticoagulants are drugs that disrupt the coagulation cascade thereby suppressing production of fibrin. The most widely prescribed oral anticoagulant is crystalline warfarin sodium (Coumadin). Oral anticoagulants are medications with a narrow therapeutic index.

Incidence

Venous thromboembolism, which includes both venous thrombosis and pulmonary embolism, is a common clinical problem that is both serious and potentially fatal. It is estimated that approximately 800,000 cases of venous thromboembolism occur each year in the United States. Massive pulmonary embolism causes 5% to 10% of all hospital deaths. As new indications for anticoagulant therapy become established and the population ages, the use of anticoagulants is likely to become more frequent.

Pathophysiology

Factors That Increase the Risk for Thromboembolism

A number of factors, both inherited and acquired, may place a patient at risk for development of thromboembolism. These include but are not limited to immobility or paralysis, heart disease, malignancy, surgery, systemic lupus erythematosus (SLE), anticoagulant and estrogen use, obesity, varicosities, and venous stasis. Inherited risks include sickle cell anemia, polycythemia, and coagulopathies such as activated protein C resistance, antithrombin III deficiency, Protein S deficiency and protein C deficiency.

Clinical Indications

Anticoagulants are the standard therapeutic choice for the treatment and prophylaxis of thromboembolic disorders. In addition, oral anticoagulants are used to prevent systemic embolism in conditions such as valvular heart disease, acute myocardial infarction, atrial fibrillation, accompanying valve replacement surgery, and to prevent venous thrombosis after hip, total knee, or major gynecological surgery.

Mechanism of Action

Six clotting factors (factors II, VII, IX, X, and proteins C and S) require vitamin K for their synthesis. Warfarin suppresses coagulation by acting as an antagonist of vitamin K, thereby decreasing the production of active vitamin K–dependent clotting factors. Warfarin is used to prevent new clot formation or further clot propagation.

Monitoring

Unlike other drugs, there is no "typical" dose that is considered effective for most patients. Dosing is highly individualized and is guided by the prothrombin time (PT) to an established therapeutic range specific to the patient's indication. Standardization of the PT has been accomplished with the international normalized ratio (INR) system for monitoring anticoagulant therapy. The World Health Organization and the American College of Chest Physicians recommend use of the INR in evaluating therapy. Research suggests use of the INR for monitoring oral anticoagulant therapy has reduced hemorrhagic complications.

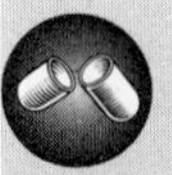

Table 12-1 Pharmaceutical Plan: Anticoagulation Therapy With Warfarin Sodium

Drug	Dosage	Comments	Cost
Warfarin sodium (Coumadin)	Patient dependent	Pregnancy: X SE: Hepatotoxicity, systemic cholesterol microembolization, necrosis or gangrene of skin and other tissues, red-orange urine	$47/2 mg (100) $31-$50/5 mg (100) $75/10 mg (100)

SE, Side effects.

Making the Decision to Anticoagulate

Initial Assessment

The decision to initiate anticoagulation therapy is based on the patient's diagnosis and an assessment of the following bleeding risks and contraindications:

The risk of hemorrhage outweighs the potential clinical benefits of therapy
Pregnancy
Uncontrolled alcoholism or drug abuse
Unsupervised dementia/psychosis
Uncontrolled hypertension
Gait disturbances
Severe liver disease
Aortic aneurysm
Recent surgery of the nervous system, spine, or eye
Noncompliance

Children

Administration of anticoagulants to **children** is difficult because of their variable responses to therapy.

Children's medical care should be managed by a physician.

Instituting Therapy

Rapid Anticoagulation Required

Consider overlapping a brief course of heparin (e.g., 4 to 5 days) if a rapid anticoagulant effect is required. There is no benefit to giving a loading dose of warfarin; the effect of warfarin is delayed while active vitamin K-dependent clotting factors become depleted. This usually takes 2 to 3 days. Once the INR is within the therapeutic range for 2 to 3 days, heparin therapy is usually discontinued (Table 12-1).

When Initiation of Therapy Is Nonurgent

Begin with an anticipated maintenance dose of warfarin: 4 mg/day to 5 mg/day. This will result in a steady-state anticoagulant effect in 10 to 14 days.

*General Guidelines**

The intensity and duration of therapy will depend on the indication (Table 12-2).
Obtain a baseline INR and blood profile.
Low initiation doses are recommended for **elderly** or debilitated patients or others with a potentially increased responsiveness to warfarin.
Patients should not alternate between manufacturers of warfarin products; the therapeutic index is too narrow.
Repeat the INR every 3 days until INR is stable and therapeutic.
Once the INR is stable, check weekly for 4 weeks, then monthly thereafter.
If the INR is not stable or therapeutic and dosage adjustments are made, check the INR more frequently.

Maintenance Therapy

Anticipate that a lower maintenance dose will be necessary in **elderly** patients.
Avoid overreacting to minor INR changes, including values just outside the therapeutic range.
The dose-response curve of warfarin is not linear. Changes in therapy should be based on a percent, usually 5% to 20% of the total weekly dose and spread out over several days. This is because warfarin has a long half-life. A protocol for adjustment of outpatient anticoagulation therapy is shown in Table 12-3.
INR should not be rechecked for at least 2 or 3 days after a change in dose.
Monitor INR every 4 weeks once therapy is stabilized.
Prescribe a single-strength warfarin tablet if possible. Select a tablet strength that allows for flexibility in dosage adjustment (e.g., 2.5-mg or 5-mg tabs).
Provide the patient with a calendar to record the number of tablets per day and dates of blood tests. (A sample calendar is shown in Box 12-1.)
Use INR to monitor anticoagulation.

*Adapted from Bridgen ML: Oral anticoagulant therapy: practical aspects of management, *Postgrad Med* 99(6):81-102, 1996.

TABLE 12-2 Therapeutic Ranges for Oral Anticoagulant Therapy

Indication	Recommended INR
Prophylaxis and/or treatment of venous thrombosis and its extension	2.0-3.0
Pulmonary embolism	2.0-3.0
Prophylaxis and/or treatment of thromboembolic complications associated with atrial fibrillation	2.0-3.0 Below 2.5 if used in an older patient (>70 yr) who has atrial fibrillation
Adjunctive therapy in the prophylaxis of systemic embolism after myocardial infarction	2.0-3.0 for at least 3 months
Tissue valves	2.0-3.0
Cardiac valve replacement with mechanical valves	2.5-3.5
Infants and children with homozygous protein C or protein S deficiency	3 to 4.5

Adapted from Du Pont Pharmaceuticals: *A team approach to clinical management of Coumadin,* Wilmington, Del., 1997.
INR, International normalized ratio.

TABLE 12-3 Protocol for Warfarin Dosage Adjustments in Outpatients with a Target INR of 2.0 to 3.0

INR	Adjustment
1.1-1.4	*Day 1:* Add 10%-20% of TWD *Weekly:* Increase TWD by 10%-20% *Repeat PT/INR:* 1 week
1.5-1.9	*Day 1:* Add 5%-10% of TWD *Weekly:* Increase TWD by 5%-10% *Repeat PT/INR:* 2 weeks
2.0-3.0	*Day 1:* No change *Weekly:* No change *Repeat PT/INR:* 4 weeks
3.1-3.5	*Day 1:* Subtract 5%-10% of TWD *Weekly:* Reduce TWD by 5%-10% *Repeat PT/INR:* 2 weeks
3.6-4.0	*Day 1:* No warfarin *Weekly:* Reduce TWD by 10%-15% *Repeat PT/INR:* 1 week
4.1-5.0	*Day 1:* No warfarin *Day 2:* No warfarin *Day 3:* Monitor PT/INR until INR 3.0, reinstitute at reduced TWD of 10%-20% *Repeat PT/INR:* 1 week after reinstitution
>5.0	Stop warfarin therapy; monitor INR until a level of 3.0 is achieved; reinstitute at lower TWD, decrease by 20%-50% *Repeat PT/INR:* Daily

Adapted from Bridgen ML: Oral anticoagulant therapy: practical aspects of management, *Postgrad Med* 99(6):81-102, 1996.
PT, Measurement of prothrombin time; *TWD,* total weekly dose of warfarin. A patient taking 2.5 mg on Monday, Wednesday, and Friday and 5 mg on the remaining days would have a TWD of 27.5 mg.

Warfarin is best taken at the same time every evening to allow for absorption of the prior dose and return of laboratory results.

When it is necessary to initiate a course of a medication that causes a known drug interaction with warfarin (especially antibiotics and antifungals), consider monitoring the INR every second day during initial stages of combined drug therapy, with subsequent appropriate adjustments in warfarin dosage.

Problems in Management

Unstable Prothrombin Times

The majority of patients on long-term warfarin therapy experience minor fluctuations in prothrombin times (PTs). However, some patients pose a major challenge because they have widely oscillating PTs. Careful management of narrow therapeutic index therapies requires controlling as many variables as possible. Abnormal product performance, using warfarin products from various manufacturers, and adopting the INR system of PT standardization are among the variables that can be controlled. In addition, numerous factors such as travel, environment, and physical state may influence the patient's response to warfarin. Concurrent illnesses such as heart failure, diarrhea, and liver disease lower anticoagulant requirements.

Sometimes changes in the vitamin K content of foods are responsible (salads in the summer, poor vitamin K intake as a result of illness or intravenous fluids without vitamin K supplements). Drug interactions (especially antibiotics) and alcohol are causes of instability. In fact, more food and drug-drug interactions are reported with warfarin therapy than any other drug. Viral illnesses in **children** often cause an increase in the INR. However, poor compliance, even when only it is slightly erratic, is the most common reason for unexpected fluctuations in anticoagulant control.

Intercurrent Surgical or Dental Procedures

Surgical or invasive diagnostic procedures such as dental extractions, biopsies, and gastrointestinal endoscopy can often be safely performed by allowing the INR to drift toward 1.5. This takes approximately 4 days in almost all patients. Once the INR reaches 1.5, surgery can be safely performed. After warfarin therapy is restarted, it takes about

Box 12-1

Sample Patient Coumadin Calendar

Name:
Date:
Tablet color:
Tablet strength:
My INR today is:
My INR therapeutic range should be between:
Next protime evaluation is due:

Day of Week	Sunday	Monday	Tuesday	Wednesday	Thursday	Friday	Saturday
Number of Tablets							

3 days for the INR to reach 2.0. Therefore, if warfarin therapy is withheld for 4 days before surgery and treatment is restarted as soon as possible after surgery (within 12 hours if there is no significant bleeding), patients can be expected to be at a subtherapeutic level for approximately 4 days (2 days before and 2 days after surgery). Patients at high risk for thrombotic complications may require conversion to heparin, which would be discontinued within hours of the surgical procedure.

Pregnancy and Lactation

Oral anticoagulants are not recommended during **pregnancy** (FDA Pregnancy Category X). Maternal warfarin therapy does not pose a problem for nursing infants, as long as they do not have a vitamin K deficiency.

Side Effects and Complications

Hemorrhage

Hemorrhage is the most serious complication of anticoagulant therapy. The risk of hemorrhage is related to the level of intensity and duration of anticoagulant therapy, patient characteristics, and the use of drugs that interfere with hemostasis. If bleeding occurs from the GI or genitourinary (GU) tract while the INR is within the therapeutic range, an underlying cause should always be sought. See Table 12-4 for management of excessively anticoagulated patients.

Early Clinical Manifestations of Excess Anticoagulation

Hematuria
Melena
Ecchymoses
Excessive uterine or menstrual bleeding
Petechiae
Persistent oozing from superficial injuries
Bleeding from gums or other mucous membranes

Skin Necrosis and Purple Toe Syndrome

Skin necrosis usually occurs between the third and tenth day after warfarin therapy is initiated. It typically affects subcutaneous tissues and presents as a localized, painful erythematous or ecchymotic skin lesion. Purple toe syndrome consists of bilateral painful peripheral discoloration of the plantar or lateral aspects of the toes. In both instances, these conditions are contraindications to continued warfarin therapy.

Lifestyle/Activities

Regular exercise is beneficial, but the patient should be cautioned to avoid contact sports and activities that may result in a serious fall or injury.

Diet

Recommend a healthy, well-balanced diet. The amount of vitamin K in the patient's diet should remain constant rather than be changed. Vitamin K dietary sources include green leafy vegetables such as broccoli, cabbage, collard greens, kale, lettuce, and spinach, and to a lesser extent, dairy products or meats. Vitamin K is also included in multiple vitamins or nutritional supplements.

Patient Education

Studies indicate that warfarin patients who understand their therapy frequently achieve better therapeutic outcomes. The patient and family should understand the following:

Action of anticoagulants
Alcohol intake
Complication of warfarin therapy
Dental work and dental surgery
Diet: Maintenance of stable diet, in particular, foods high in vitamin K

Table 12-4 Guidelines for Management of Excessively Anticoagulated Patients With and Without Bleeding

Clinical Presentation	Action
INR > therapeutic range and <6 and no clinical evidence of bleeding	Discontinue warfarin therapy until INR is in therapeutic range; reinstitute warfarin at lower TWD
INR >6 and <10 with no clinical evidence of bleeding	Discontinue warfarin therapy; administer vitamin K, 1-2 mg SQ; reduction of INR should occur within 8 hr If INR at 24 hr is still high, a second dose of vitamin K can be repeated When therapeutic range is reached, warfarin therapy should be resumed at lower TWD
INR >10 but <20 and there is no bleeding	Discontinue warfarin; administer vitamin K, 2.5-5 mg SQ; INR should be reduced substantially at 6 hr INR should be checked every 6-12 hr and vitamin K repeated as necessary; when therapeutic range reached, warfarin should be restarted at lower TWD
Major warfarin overdose (e.g., INR >20) or rapid reversal of an anticoagulant effect is required because of serious bleeding	Vitamin K, 10 mg by slow IV infusion; check INR q6h Vitamin K may be repeated q12h and supplemented with plasma transfusion or factor concentrate depending on the urgency of the situation
Life-threatening bleeding or serious warfarin overdose	Institute replacement with factor concentrates as indicated, supplemented with vitamin K, 10 mg by slow IV infusion Vitamin K may be repeated as necessary, depending on INR

Adapted from Hirsh J, Poller L: The international normalized ratio: a guide to understanding and correcting its problems, *Arch Intern Med* 154:282-288, 1994.

INR, International normalized ratio; *IV,* intravenous; *SQ,* subcutaneous; *TWD,* total weekly dose.

Dosing schedule: Missed doses and improper dosing
Indications for anticoagulation
Invasive diagnostic or surgical procedures
Medication interactions with warfarin
Monitoring effects of therapy with PT/INR
Need for strict compliance with prescribed doses
Need to report falls, injuries, and bleeding
Physical activities
Pregnancy avoidance
Self-monitoring for and response to bleeding
Starting and stopping additional medications, including over-the-counter drugs
Tablet identification
Use of medical alert bracelet or card
Warfarin is best taken at the same time every evening

Family Impact

Families must understand the information included under patient education.

Referral

All children, pregnant women, and patients who require rapid anticoagulation with heparin or rapid reversal of the anticoagulation effects of warfarin with intravenous vitamin K should be referred to an MD.

Consultation

For patients with unstable prothrombin times, consult with an MD.

EVALUATION/FOLLOW-UP

Prothrombin times should be measured at least monthly and more often as indicated. At each visit the patient should be questioned about missed doses, concurrent medications, early manifestations of excessive anticoagulation, and signs and symptoms of thromboembolism.

SUGGESTED READINGS

Becker R, Ansell J: Antithrombotic therapy: an abbreviated reference for clinicians, *Arch Intern Med* 155:149-161, 1995.

Brigden M: Oral anticoagulant therapy: practical aspects of management, *Postgrad Med* 99: 81-102, 1996.

Du Pont Pharmaceuticals: *A team approach to clinical management of Coumadin,* Wilmington, Del, 1997.

Ellsworth A et al: *Mosby's 1998 medical drug reference,* St Louis, 1998, Mosby.

Healthcare Consultants of America, Inc: *1998 Physicians fee and coding guide,* Augusta, Ga, 1998, Healthcare Consultants of America, Inc.

Hathaway W, Goodnight S: *Disorders of hemostasis and thrombosis: a clinical guide,* New York, 1993, McGraw-Hill.

Hirsh J et al: Oral anticoagulants: mechanism of action, clinical effectiveness and optimal therapeutic range, *Chest* 108:2315-2346S, 1995.

Hirsh J, Poller L: The international normalized ratio: a guide to understanding and correcting its problems, *Arch Intern Med* 154:282-288, 1994.

Kearon C, Hirsh J: Management of anticoagulation before and after elective surgery, *N Engl J Med* 336:1506-1511, 1997.

Kornblit P et al: Anticoagulation therapy: patient management and evaluation of an outpatient clinic, *Nurs Pract* 15:21-32, 1990.

Landefeld C, Beyth R: Anticoagulant-related bleeding: clinical epidemiology, prediction and prevention, *Am J Med* 95:315-328, 1993.

McPherson M, Grace K: Anticoagulant therapy: what. to consider in practical management, *Adv Nurs Pract* 5:33-39, 1997.

Oertel LB: Internationalized normalized ratio (INR): an improved way to monitor anticoagulant therapy, *Nurs Pract* 20:15-22, 1995.

Weibert R et al: Correction of excessive anticoagulation with low-dose oral vitamin K_1, *Ann Intern Med* 126:959-962, 1997.

13 Anxiety

ICD-9-CM

Anxiety States 300.00

OVERVIEW

Definition

Anxiety is a subjective feeling of uneasiness that often accompanies other emotions, such as anger, shame, fear, and guilt. It is an uncomfortable feeling of apprehension and/or dread usually that is often accompanied by psychological, physiological, or behavioral symptoms. Anxiety serves to alert the individual to real or perceived threats. Anxiety occurs when a person's coping skills are insufficient to deal with the perceived threat. The person experiencing anxiety may not know the specific source of the anxiety. Mild anxiety can be productive, spurring the person to action, but greater levels of anxiety often prevent individuals from performing routine activities. Anxiety is considered pathological when the anxiety reaction is out of proportion to the actual experience of the threat, and impaired social or intellectual functioning and psychosomatic symptoms occur.

Incidence

Anxiety is extremely common. Anxiety disorders are more common in **women** than in men and represent one of the most prevalent mental health problems in the United States today. Anxiety is often categorized into different types, as shown in Table 13-1.

Pathophysiology

Neuroregulators have been implicated in the cause of anxiety. These include neurotransmitters: norepinephrine, dopamine, and serotonin; neuromodulators: endorphins; and neurohormones: antidiuretic hormone, angiotensin II, and somatostatin.

Patients who experience anxiety have an excessive autonomic reaction with an increased release of catecholamines (sympathetic response). Decreased gamma-aminobutyric acid (GABA) causes central nervous system (CNS) hyperactivity (GABA inhibits CNS ability). An increase in serotonin level causes anxiety, increased dopaminergic activity is also associated with anxiety. The hyperactive center is in the temporal cerebral cortex. The lucus ceruleus, center of noradrenergic neurons, becomes hyperactive in anxiety states.

Conditioned learning may also play a role in the development of anxiety disorders.

Protective Factors Against

Defense mechanisms and coping behaviors help relieve anxiety. Defense mechanisms may include the following:

Compensation
Denial
Displacement
Dissociation
Projection
Rationalization
Repression

Coping behaviors may be categorized as follows:

Adaptive	Maladaptive
Prayer	Drugs and/or alcohol
Exercise	Excessive eating
Relaxation techniques	Social isolation
Problem solving	Self-injury

Factors That Increase Susceptibility

Recurrent anxiety stimuli that exceed coping abilities
Maladaptive coping mechanisms
Abnormal blood levels of norepinephrine and lactate
Family history of anxiety

TABLE 13-1 Types of Anxiety and Their Characteristics

Type	Characteristics
Generalized anxiety disorder (GAD)	Excessive or unrealistic anxiety that lasts 6 mo or longer. Generalized anxiety syndrome occurs in 2% to 5% of the population each year. It typically occurs in individuals 16 to 40 years old. Its incidence increases threefold among persons with a family history of anxiety.
Panic disorder	Periods of intense fear accompanied by somatic symptoms, including diaphoresis, dyspnea, dizziness or a feeling of faintness, paresthesias, and palpitations. Panic disorders occur in 1.4% of the population. It is most common in persons 17 to 30 years old.
Phobia	Fear of a situation, activity, or object that is out of proportion to the actual threat. Phobias occur in 15% to 20% of the population. They may start in the early teens. The most common phobias are of animals, storms, heights, illness, and death.
Posttraumatic stress disorder (PTSD)	A series of symptoms of anxiety characterized by flashbacks to a situation that involved an overwhelming stressor. Usually generated by experiencing an extremely traumatic event, such as military combat, rape, or natural disaster. Posttraumatic stress disorder affects 0.5% to 1% of the population. It is most common among **young adults.**
Obsessive-compulsive disorder (OCD)	Obsession refers to constantly recurring thoughts; compulsion refers to repetitive actions. In OCD the irrational idea or impulse persistently intrudes into awareness. Anxiety is relieved only by the ritualistic performance of the action. The individual's primary concern is to maintain control of the recurring thoughts. OCD occurs in 2% to 3% of the population; its distribution is equal in males and females.

Common Causal Factors

Developmental crises, such as **adolescence** or **aging**
Trauma, such as rape, incest, abuse
Threats to safety and security, such as assaults/abuse and natural disasters
Loss, such as death, divorce, major illness, and disability
Threats to self-esteem and integrity
Guilt

SUBJECTIVE DATA

History of Present Illness

Most persons with anxiety give a long history of symptoms.

Past Medical History

Persons with anxiety often have had previous bouts of anxiety during times of stress.

Clinician should ask about similar symptoms in the past.

Medications

Medications that cause anxiety symptoms, such as:

Amphetamines
Diet aids
Pseudoephedrine
Medications, foods/drink with caffeine
Withdrawal from some medications, especially sedatives, may cause symptoms

Family History

There is a high incidence of anxiety occurring in other family members.

Psychosocial History

Inquire about recent life changes, both positive and negative, including:

Marriage or divorce
Birth of a child
Loss
Job change or promotion
Entering school
Change in residence
Be aware that alcohol is the most commonly used over-the-counter (OTC) drug used to treat anxiety.
Consider CAGE screening test for alcohol abuse/dependence (see Chapter 171).

Description of Most Commonly Reported Symptoms (in order of increasing anxiety)

Selective inattention and hesitation
Diminished problem-solving ability
Rapid speech with frequent change of topic
Muscle tension and restlessness
Fear that they cannot control the symptoms or prevent symptoms from escalating
Tachycardia, dyspnea, hyperventilation

Fear of loss of control and impending doom
Chest pain and feeling of choking

Associated Symptoms

Restlessness and irritability
Difficulty sleeping /awakening frequently during the night, significant changes in eating (anorexia, overeating)
Chronic fatigue
Feelings of apprehension, guilt, dread
Acting out behaviors (violence, truancy, alcohol and drug abuse)
Somatic complaints (stomach ache, nausea and vomiting, headache)

Evaluation

The mental health evaluation should:

Attempt to identify the precipitating factor or event as perceived by the patient
Determine the patient's perception of when the problem started and its duration, when it first started, and when it started this time
Questions that may assist in screening for anxiety include:
Would you describe yourself generally as a nervous person?
Are you a worrier?
Have you ever had a sudden onset of rapid heartbeat? A rush of intense fear, anxiety, or nervousness?
Some people have strong fears about things like heights, flying, or bugs. Do you have any strong fears?
Some people are bothered by doing something over and over that they can't resist—has anything like that been a problem for you?
Have you ever seen or experienced a traumatic event in which you thought your life was in danger, or someone else's life was in danger? What happened? (Levinson and Engel, 1997)
What has worked in the past to decrease your symptoms?

OBJECTIVE DATA

Physical Examination

A complete physical should be performed, with particular attention to the cardiovascular, respiratory, and neuroendocrine systems.

Complete a mental status examination, observing:

Behavior and appearance
Level of consciousness, cognitive functioning, and memory
Thought processes, concentration, speech patterns
Insight
Whether the patient has suicidal or homicidal ideation

TABLE 13-2 Psychological Tests

Test	Purpose
Hamilton Anxiety Scale	Brief semistructured interview, helps to quantify the clinical assessment of anxiety symptoms
Zung Anxiety Scale	Self-report measure
Primary Care Evaluation of Mental Disorders (Prime-MD)	Two-stage assessment: questionnaire that screens for anxiety and other mental disorders in primary practice; and structured interview that provides diagnostic information in the identified problem areas. (This process takes about 8 minutes to complete [Spitzer, 1994].)

The use of various psychological tests may assist in gathering data about the anxiety (Table 13-2).

Diagnostic Tests

Laboratory tests are primarily ordered to rule out physiological causes for the presenting symptoms and may include those shown in Table 13-3.

ASSESSMENT

Differential diagnoses must first rule out possible physiological causes, including those shown in Table 13-4.

Once physiological causes have been ruled out, it is helpful to classify the anxiety according to the specific type anxiety as shown in Table 13-5.

THERAPEUTIC PLAN

Figure 13-1 presents an algorithm for the treatment of patient with anxiety. Pharmaceutical and nonpharmaceutical options and plans are presented in Tables 13-6 to 13-8.

Lifestyle/Activities

For generalized moderate anxiety, assist the patient in problem solving to facilitate the identification of stressors and development of effective coping skills. Various relaxation techniques can be used in combination with medication or alone, such as exercise and rest, guided imagery, and other stress-reduction techniques. The mainstay of therapies is deep-breathing techniques; all other relaxation mechanisms accompany this. The patient should have adequate sleep and should engage in leisure activities that are relaxing and enjoyable.

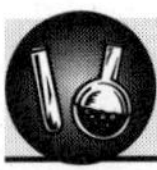

TABLE 13-3 Diagnostic Tests: Anxiety

Test	Finding/Rationale	Cost ($)
Cardiovascular workup: ECG, CXR, electrolyte levels	Rule out hypoxia/coronary insufficiency	56-65/ECG 77-91/CXR 23-30/electrolytes
Thyroid profile, TSH	Rule out hyperthyroidism	47-61/thyroid profile
CBC	Rule out anemia	18-23/CBC
Drug screen	Identify agents which may cause symptoms of anxiety such as amphetamines, cocaine	57-72/drug screen
Pulse oximetry	Rule out pulmonary disease	28-33/pulse oximetry

CBC, Complete blood cell count; *CXR,* chest x-ray; *ECG,* electrocardiogram, *TSH,* thyroid-stimulating hormone.

TABLE 13-4 Differential Diagnosis: Anxiety

System/Cause	Diagnosis	Supporting Data
Cardiovascular	Angina	Chest pain on exertion; ECG shows ST depression; crushing chest pain with MI Anxiety pains usually are sharp and more superficial
	Arrhythmias	Irregular pulse; ECG abnormalities
	CHF	Pedal edema; JVD; rales; SOB
	HTN	Elevated blood pressure
Dietary	Caffeine	History of high intake of coffee, tea, caffeinated soft drinks, some drugs
	MSG sensitivity	Anxiety related to food ingestion
	Drug-induced anticholinergic toxicity	Use of anticholinergics; dry mouth
	Digitalis toxicity	Use of digoxin, elevated serum levels; arrhythmias; nausea and vomiting
	Use of hallucinogens/illicit drugs and/or withdrawal	Use of LSD, PCP; altered liver enzymes, enlarged liver; needle marks; history of cellulitis
	Stimulants	Use of pseudoephedrine, crack cocaine, amphetamines
Hematological	Anemia	Low hemoglobin levels; SOB; tachycardia
Immunological	Anaphylaxis	Wheezing; cyanosis; altered blood gases
Metabolic	Hypoglycemia	Low glucose levels; nausea, headache; diaphoresis; decreased concentration
	Hyperthyroidism	Decreased TSH; elevated T_3 and T_4; nervousness; decreased heat tolerance; weight loss
Neurological	Encephalopathies, CNS tumors, seizures	History of alcohol use; neurological changes, EEG changes, headache
Respiratory	Asthma, COPD, pulmonary embolus	Wheezing; low oxygen saturation; CXR changes; SOB; chest pain; hemoptysis; hypoxia
Secreting tumors	Pheochromocytoma, insulinoma	Elevated B/P, elevated catecholamines, low glucose levels
Psychiatric disorders	Depression	50% to 70% of depressed patients have anxiety Depressed mood, lack of concentration, lack of interest in activities; decreased or increased eating and sleeping
	Hyperventilation syndrome	History of rapid, deep respirations; circumoral pallor, carpopedal spasm; responds to rebreathing in paper bag
	Bipolar disorder	A period of abnormally and persistently elevated mood with distractibility, flight of ideas, and decreased sleep; patient more talkative than usual

CHF, Congestive heart failure; *CNS,* central nervous system; *COPD,* chronic obstructive pulmonary disorder; *ECG,* electrocardiogram; *EEG,* electroencephalogram; *HTN,* hypertension; *JVD,* jugular venous distention; *LSD,* D-lysergic acid diethylamide; *MI,* myocardial infarction; *MSG,* monosodium glutamate; *PCP,* phencyclidine (angel dust); *CXR,* chest x-ray; *SOB,* shortness of breath; *TSH,* thyroid-stimulating hormone.

TABLE 13-5 Classification of Types of Anxiety Disorders

Type	Supporting Data
GAD	Excessive anxiety and worry occurring for at least 6 mo Restlessness, fatigue, difficulty concentrating, irritability, muscle tension, sleep disturbance, impaired social function
Panic disorder	Sudden intense, unpredictable anxiety attacks; debilitating physical symptoms, including dyspnea, dizziness, increased heart rate, sweating, choking, nausea, numbness, sensation of throat closing Debilitating emotional symptoms, including fear of dying and/or of "going crazy"
PTSD	Recurrent reexperiencing of a traumatic event; examples include natural disasters, rape, major accidents, and military combat Substance abuse and depression are common means of dealing with emotional pain.
Phobia	Irrational fear of specific places or situations; agoraphobia is fear of open places; social phobia is fear of appearing inept in the company of others
OCD	Persistent thoughts and impulses Repetitive behaviors (hand washing, checking) or mental acts (praying, counting, repeating words silently)

GAD, Generalized anxiety disorder; *PTSD,* posttraumatic stress disorder; *OCD,* obsessive-compulsive disorder.

Diet

The patient should avoid foods containing stimulants such as caffeine, which may precipitate anxiety symptoms.

A well-balanced diet should be maintained; some symptoms may be result of poor nutrition.

Patient Education

Belly breathing

- Assist the patient to focus on slowing breathing, inhaling and exhaling from the diaphragm; to help calm the anxious patient.
- Demonstrate stress-reduction exercises.

Discuss effective coping behaviors.

Review appropriate use of medication.

Instruct the patient

- Not to ignore fears or worries when they interfere with activities of daily living
- Not to perform any one activity to excess but to maintain a balance in work, rest and play
- Not to use alcohol to calm nerves

Family Impact

Anxiety may have a significant impact on the family unit; the degree will depend on the type of anxiety disorder. Examples of the impact on the family include:

Frequent medical visits
Inability to leave home or face others
Substance abuse
Discuss benefits of Al-Anon with family
Hypervigiliance, irritability
Inability to be involved in family member's activities

Referral

Refer a patient to a mental health professional for inpatient or outpatient evaluation and treatment if the patient seems to be a threat to himself or herself or others.

Psychotic paranoid thought processes, panic level of anxiety, or escalation of symptoms to the point of refusal of treatment warrants referral.

Patients who require increasingly larger doses of medication or those unresponsive to medical therapy should be referred.

Refer to Alcoholics Anonymous or Narcotics Anonymous if alcohol or drug abuse is a contributing factor.

When a patient is referred to mental health professional for counseling and treatment of an anxiety disorders, such therapy may include one of the therapies outlined in Table 13-9.

Consultation

May be indicated if therapy with benzodiazepines is indicated, unless clinician is comfortable with their use and able to prescribe controlled substances.

May also be indicated in recurrent episodes of anxiety or to help rule out cardiac pathology.

EVALUATION/FOLLOW-UP

Frequent follow-up is indicated to assess coping mechanisms and the effectiveness of therapy and to give encouragement and reassurance.

The patient is able to recognize early signs of his or her own anxiety response.

Text continued on p. 84.

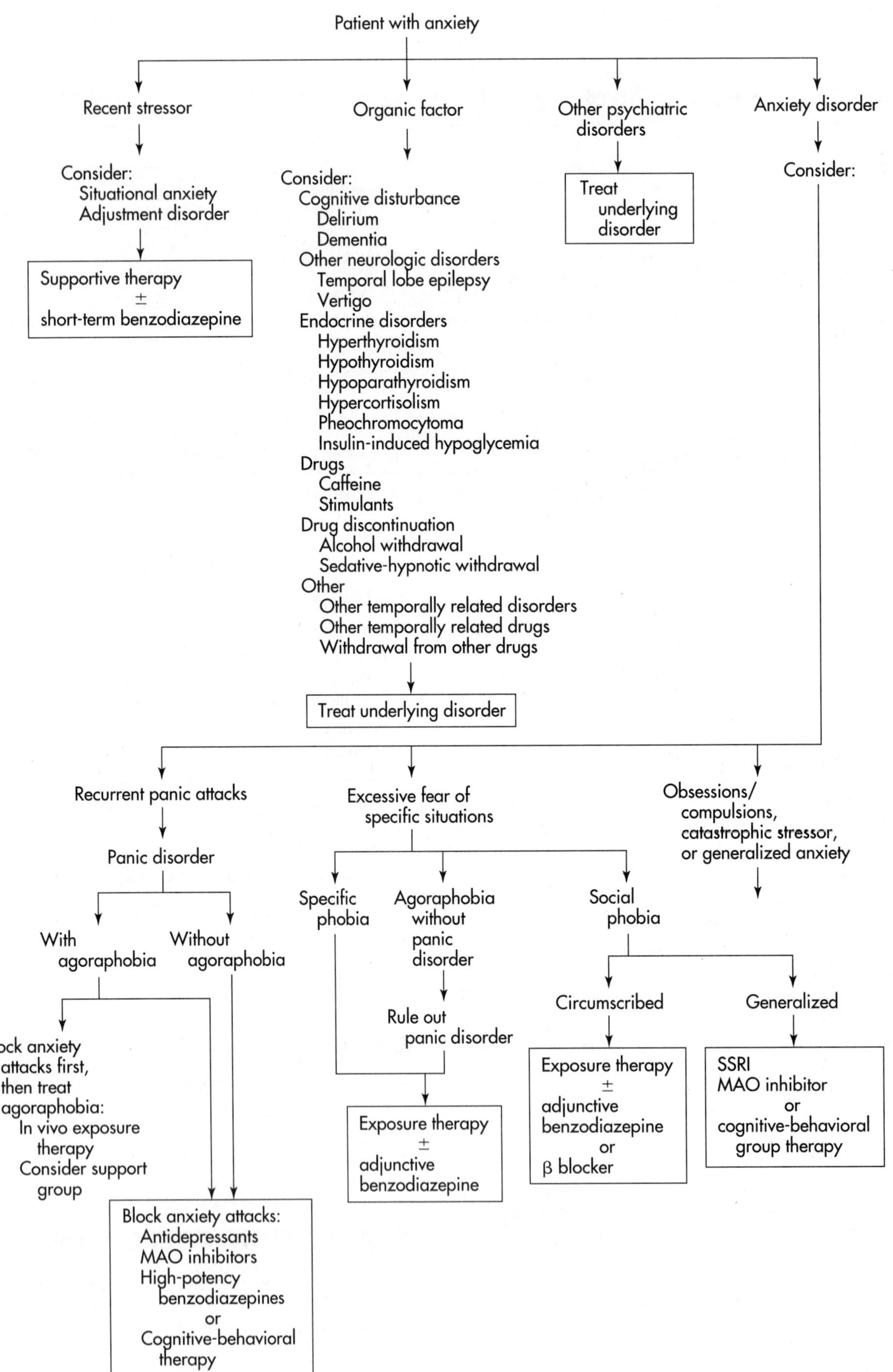

Figure 13-1 Algorithm for a patient with anxiety. *SSRI,* Selective serotonin reuptake inhibitors; *MAO,* monoamine oxidase. (Redrawn from Reiman E: Anxiety. In Greene H, Johnson W, Lemcke D, editors: *Decision making in medicine,* ed 2, St Louis, 1998, Mosby.)

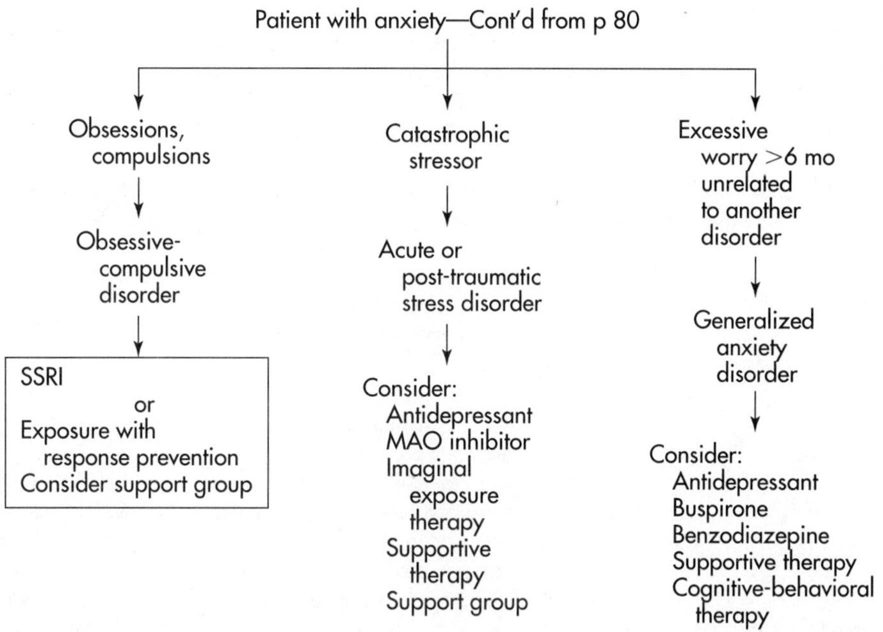

Figure 13-1, cont'd For legend see opposite page.

TABLE 13-6 Advantages and Disadvantages of Drugs by Class

Class of Drug	Advantages	Disadvantages
Benzodiazepines	Relieve symptoms rapidly, within first week of treatment; wide therapeutic index	Potential for misuse and dependence High incidence of rebound panic attacks when medication is discontinued Drugs need to be weaned over 1-3 mo
Tricyclic antidepressants SSRIs Buspirone	Take 3-4 wk or longer to reach maximum effectiveness	Not associated with dependence but may increase anxiety symptoms in first 1-2 wk of treatment

SSRI, Selective serotonin reuptake inhibitor.

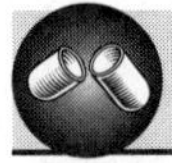

TABLE 13-7 Pharmaceutical Plan: Anxiety

Drug	Dosage	Comments	Cost
Alpazolam (Xanax) (CS)	0.75-4 mg/24 hr in 3 divided doses	Use short-term only while other treatment modalities are initiated Use for 3-4 wk while increasing other drugs Withdraw by 0.25 to 0.50 mg/wk if drug is stopped Pregnancy: D SE: CNS depression, drowsiness, dizziness, ataxia, dry mouth, tremors	$5-$66 /0.25 mg (100); $6-$80/0.5 mg (100); $8-$113/1 mg (100); $21-$168/2 mg (100)
Chlordiazepoxide (Librium) (CS)	15-100 mg/24 hr in 4-6 divided doses	Benzodiazepine; often used for alcohol withdrawal Pregnancy: Not recommended SE: Abuse potential, CNS depression, ataxia, extra pyramidal effects	$34/5 mg (100); $48/10 mg (100)
Diazepam (Valium) (CS)	2-10 mg BID-QID	20-50h ½ life; withdraw by 5 mg/wk Pregnancy: Not recommended SE: Abuse potential, CNS depression drowsiness, memory impairment	$2-$43/2 mg (100); $2-$66/5 mg (100); $3-$109/10 mg (100)
Lorazepam (Ativan) (CS)	2-3 mg BID or TID	Pregnancy: Not recommended SE: Abuse potential, drowsiness, memory impairment, CNS depression, agitation	$2-$74/0.5 mg (100); $2-$83/1 mg (100); $2-$136/2 mg (100)
Oxazepam (Serax) (CS)	10-15 mg TID or QID	Pregnancy: Not recommended SE: Abuse potential, CNS depression, dizziness, memory impairment, ataxia	$6-$70/10 mg (100); $8-$89/15 mg (100); $10-$128/30 mg (100)
Buspirone (Buspar)	5 mg TID, increase in 5 mg increments to a maximum daily dose of 60 mg	Not associated with tolerance, withdrawal, or dependence Appears to be more effective when used in patients not requiring long-term therapy and those who have not tried benzodiazepines Pregnancy: B SE: Dizziness, nausea, H/A, lightheadedness, dream disturbances, nasal congestion	$57/5 mg (100); $100/10 mg (100); $83/15 mg (100)
Clonazepam (Klonapin) (CS)	0.25 mg BID; increase after 3 days to 1 mg/day Usual 4 mg/day	Pregnancy: D SE: Abuse potential, somnolence, depression, dizziness, nervousness, ataxia, hypersalivation Interaction with CYP3A drugs: azole antifungals (see Appendix D)	$57-$72/0.5 mg (100); $65-$83/1 mg (100); $90-$114/2 mg (100)
SSRIs Fluoxetine (Prozac) Paroxetine (Paxil) Sertaline (Zoloft)	 20-80 mg QD 20-50 mg QD 50-200 mg QD	Initiate at half the antidepressant dose; continue antidepressants for minimum of 6 mo, although longer treatment is often necessary Pregnancy: Prozac: B Zoloft: C Paxil: C SE: Sweating, dry mouth, headache, insomnia, ejaculatory problems, impotence Interaction with CYP2D6/CYP450 drugs	Prozac: $214-$262/ 10 mg (100); $220/20 mg (100) Paxil: $57/10, 20, 30 mg (100) Zoloft: $176/50 mg (100); $100-$181/100 mg (100)

CNS, Central nervous system; *CS*, controlled substance; *SE*, side effects; *H/A*, headache; *SSRI*, selective serotonin reuptake inhibitor.

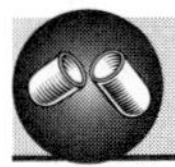

Table 13-8 Pharmacological Options by Disorder

Anxiety Disorder	Pharmacology Options	Comments
Panic	1. Antidepressant: Imipramine 25 mg QD; increase up to 150-200 mg QD, to a maximum of 300 mg QD or Paroxetine 20 mg QD; increase up to 60 mg QD 2. Use benzodiazepine during first 3-4 wk only while titrating antidepressants	Paroxetine may be started in smaller dose for elderly Panic may be increased during initial treatment Imipramine: $2-$36/10 mg (100); $2-$43/25 mg (100) $3-$74/50 mg (100)
Phobias	1. Beta blocker: Propranolol (Inderal) 10-40 mg before anticipated exposure 2. Benzodiazepine prn for infrequent exposure 3. SSRIs may be effective for those with social phobias	$1-$33/10 mg (100) $2-$35/20 mg (100) $2-$60/40 mg (100) SSRIs reserved for those who cannot tolerate other medications
OCD	1. Clomipramine (Anafranil) 25 mg QD; increase to 100 mg over 2 wk or Fluoxetine (Prozac) initially 20 mg in morning; increase in several weeks if clinical improvement seen to a maximum of 80 mg/day Fluvoxamine (Fluvox) 50 mg at hs Increase dose in 50-mg increments every 4-7 days to a maximum of 300 mg/day Paroxetine (Paxil) initially 20 mg in morning Increase by 10 mg/day at intervals of 7 days 40 mg is recommended dosage for OCD	Treatment is often chronic Higher doses than used in major depression Clomipramine: $78/25 mg (100) Fluvoxamine: $184/50 mg (100)
GAD	1. Buspirone, 5 mg TID; increase in 5-mg increments, to a maximum dosage of 60 mg/day 2. Low-dose benzodiazepines may be needed (lorazepam 1-5 mg QD, divided)	Tricyclic antidepressants may be effective, especially in those with coexisting depression

Adapted from Levinson W, Engel C. Anxiety. In Feldman M, Christensen J, editors. *Behavioral medicine in primary care,* Norwalk, Conn, 1997, Appleton & Lange. *SSRI,* Selective serotonin reuptake inhibitor; *GAD,* generalized anxiety disorder; *OCD,* obsessive-compulsive disorder.

Table 13-9 Treatment Modalities for Anxiety

Therapies	Purpose
Cognitive therapy	Short-term, active, directive, collaborative model of psychotherapy that has as its goal behavioral change; process-focused; helps patient reorganize way of thinking
Behavior modification	Systematic desensitization to gradually introduce small amounts of the feared stimulus; guided imagery may be used, along with muscle relaxation, distraction, rehearsal, graded tasks, scheduling
Cognitive-behavioral therapy	Provider guides patient into testing the faulty belief Thought-stopping may also be appropriate: blocking out intrusive thoughts with repeated silent mental command for obsessions to stop
Adjunct Therapies	
Eye movement desensitization and reprocessing (EMDR)	Therapeutic intervention for traumatic stress using eye movements to help reprocess the traumatic event
Thought field therapy (TFT)	Therapeutic intervention that reduces or eliminates perturbations that cause negative emotions in a thought field
Hypnosis	Communicative interaction that elicits a trance in which other than conscious processes effect therapeutic changes in the subject's mind/body system; hypnosis can be other- or self-induced
Biofeedback	Computer-assisted measurement of physiological changes for the purpose of training the patient to bring them into voluntary control
Meditation	Time to thoroughly recognize and experience our inner states; can be a valuable process in the transition to self-control and the core of one's personal philosophy

The patient is able to recognize current life stressors that trigger an anxiety response.

The patient attempts to eliminate maladaptive coping behaviors.

The patient implements adaptive coping behaviors.

RESOURCES

www.nimh.nih.gov/anxiety

SUGGESTED READINGS

American Psychiatric Association: *Diagnostic and statistical manual of mental disorders,* ed 4, Washington, DC, 1994, The Association.

Aguilera DC, Messick JM: *Crisis intervention theory and methodology,* St Louis, 1990 Mosby.

Aromando L: *Mental health and psychiatric nursing,* ed 2, Springhouse, Pa, 1995, Springhouse/Reed-Elsevier.

Blackburn I, Davidson K: *Cognitive therapy for depression and anxiety,* Blackwell Scientific, 1995, Oxford, England.

Burgess A: *Psychiatric nursing promoting mental health,* Norwalk, Conn, 1997, Appleton & Lange.

Ellsworth A et al: *Mosby's 1998 medical drug reference,* St Louis, 1998, Mosby.

Healthcare Consultants of America, Inc: *1998 Physicians fee and coding guide,* Augusta, Ga, 1998, Healthcare Consultants of America, Inc.

The Harvard Mental Health Letter, Anxiety and antidepressant drugs, Harvard Medical School, Jan 1993.

Levinson W, Engel C: Anxiety. In Feldman M, Christensen J, editors: *Behavioral medicine in primary care,* Norwalk, Conn, 1997, Appleton & Lange.

Mengel M: *Ambulatory medicine,* ed 2, Norwalk, Conn, 1996, Appleton & Lange.

Reiman E: Anxiety. In Greene H, Johnson W, Lemcke D, editors: *Decision making in medicine,* ed 2, St Louis, 1998, Mosby.

Spitzer R et al: Utility of a new procedure for diagnosing mental disorders in primary care: the prime-MD 1000 study, *JAMA* 272:1749, 1994.

14 Appendicitis

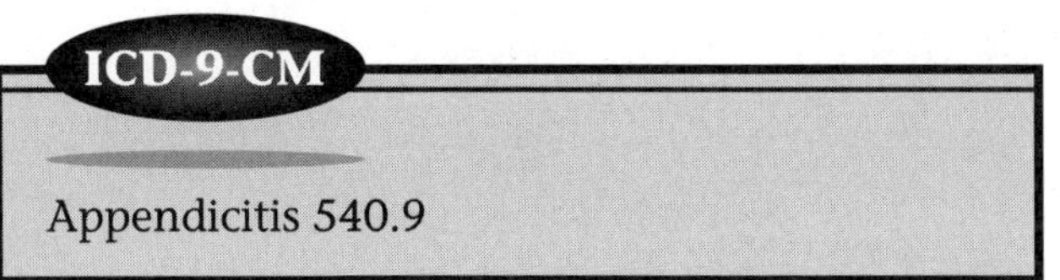
ICD-9-CM

Appendicitis 540.9

OVERVIEW

Definition

Appendicitis is an inflammation of the appendix resulting from bacterial infection.

Incidence

In the United States appendicitis develops in approximately 1 in 15 persons. The incidence rises after age 3 until it peaks during the late teen years; 69% of cases occur in persons younger than 30 years old. Appendicitis is the most common surgical condition, with the greatest incidence in the **pre-adolescent, adolescent,** and **early adult** age groups.

Males are more often affected than females by a ratio of 1.5 to 1. Up to two thirds of cases occur between October and May. Persons with a family history of appendicitis are at increased risk.

Pathophysiology

Appendicitis arises from obstruction of the appendiceal lumen, usually by a fecalith, but also by foreign bodies such as seeds, barium, bones, wood, metal fragments, or plastic. Conditions that can induce obstruction include Crohn's disease, respiratory infections, measles, mononucleosis, amebiasis, and bacterial gastroenteritis. Obstruction prevents emptying of the intraluminal fluid into the cecum. The fluid accumulates and distends the appendix. The increased luminal pressure inhibits lymphatic and venous drainage. Luminal bacteria multiply and then invade the appendiceal wall.

Risk Factors for Abdominal Pain

Dietary factors (fatty diet)
Medications (erythromycin, theophylline, amoxicillin with clavulanate)
Sexual activity
Consumption of contaminated food
Dysfunctional coping methods
Stressful situations

Protective Factors Against

Dietary fiber lessens the risk of obstruction of the appendiceal lumen by decreasing the viscosity of feces, reducing bowel transit time, and subsequently diminishing the likelihood that a fecalith will form.

Common Pathogens

Escherichia coli
Bacteroides
Enterococcus
Pseudomonas

SUBJECTIVE DATA

History of Present Illness

Determine the time of onset and the duration of pain.
Describe the character of the pain.
Ask whether the patient has had nausea, vomiting, or diarrhea.
Ask whether fever is present.
Determine whether there is a history of trauma.
Ask about the last bowel movement and passing of flatus.
Ask about the patient's interest in eating.
Ask about activities, such as running and jumping (versus lying still).
Ask about the patient's typical diet and what he or she has eaten in the past 24 to 48 hours.

Past Medical History

Ask about intestinal problems: diverticulitis, constipation, inflammatory bowel disease.
Ask about previous abdominal surgeries.

Medications

Ask whether the patient is taking these medications: erythromycin, theophylline, amoxicillin with clavulanate.

Family History

Ask whether family members have had appendicitis.

Psychosocial History

Ask about tobacco dependence.
Ask about alcohol ingestion.

Description of Most Common Symptoms

Abdominal tenderness
- Not always dull at first, then intense and persistent later on.
- Migration of pain from the umbilical area to right lower quadrant (RLQ) occurs in only 50% to 65% of patients.
- **After age 2**, clinical symptoms of appendicitis become more typical.
  - Right-sided abdominal pain
  - At first vague, progressing to a more intense and persistent pain
  - In a **child**, RLQ tenderness should never be considered insignificant, no matter how mild it is
- **Elderly** patients have few or no prodromal symptoms.

Nausea
- Nausea is a common but not universal symptom.

Emesis
- Emesis almost always follows the onset of pain, except in a few **children.**
- **Children** may be systemically ill with vomiting rather than presenting with abdominal pain and tenderness.

Anorexia
- Ten percent to 40% have no loss of appetite.

OBJECTIVE DATA

Physical Examination

Problem oriented, with particular attention to:
- Vital signs: Low-grade fever
- Heart and lungs
- Abdomen: Bowel sounds, guarding, distention, tenderness, masses; inability to jump, walk, and cough without pain
- Rectal area: Especially note tenderness on the right
- Pelvic examination is indicated for **females** who are sexually active.
- NOTE: In **pregnant** patients the appendix is displaced to a higher position, with pain and tenderness outside the classic position.

In very young children:
- The abdomen is commonly distended, and the **child** appears to be in a toxic state. The child is usually lethargic, with irritability and vomiting.
- In acute appendicitis the **child** is likely to exhibit guarding and to lie on his or her left side with the legs drawn up to reduce tension on the rectus muscle.
- Suspect appendicitis in any patient with nonspecific complaints who is taking corticosteroids.

Diagnostic Procedures

Diagnostic procedures include those listed in Table 14-1.

ASSESSMENT

Differential diagnosis for appendicitis includes those presented in Table 14-2.

A scoring system is being tested in Sweden to help differentiate appendicitis from nonspecific abdominal pain. A score of –2 or higher supports a diagnosis of appendicitis and a decision to operate (sensitivity of 0.73 and a specificity of 0.87 for predicting appendicitis). A score of –17 or lower indicates nonspecific abdominal pain. The scoring system is outlined in Table 14-3.

THERAPEUTIC PLAN

Whenever appendicitis is suspected, a prompt surgical consultation is critical.

Preoperative Care

Before an emergency appendectomy, start intravenous fluid replacement.
Do not give the patient anything by mouth.
Rectal metronidazole may be given 3 hours before surgery to prevent infection.
Give broad-spectrum antibiotics immediately if the patient appears septic.

In **children** use single-dose cefoxitin.

The accepted therapy for perforation or abscess formation includes administration of an aminoglycoside (gentamicin) (always obtain a baseline creatinine before starting this drug), with one or more of the following: ampicillin, clindamycin, metronidazole, and cefoxitin.

An alternative therapy for gentamicin is ticarcillin with clavulanate or cefotaxime with clindamycin.

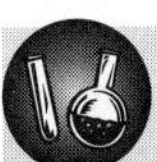

TABLE 14-1 Diagnostic Tests: Appendicitis

Test	Finding/Rationale	Cost ($)
WBC	Usually normal during the first 24 hours of symptoms; leukocytosis >15,000 cells/mm^3 may be seen	18-23/CBC
Flat and upright x-ray examination of abdomen	Plain abdominal films are of little value except in patients (usually **children**) with a calcified fecalith in the right lower quadrant.	142-169
FOB	Blood in the stool suggests that abdominal pain originates in the gut; blood is seen with intussusception, mesenteric vascular occlusion, and obstructing neoplasm or inflammatory lesions	13-17
Amylase, lipase, alkaline phosphatase	Rule out biliary or pancreas involvement	24-30/amylase 28-35/lipase 19-24/alkaline phosphatase
Ultrasound of abdomen	80%-90% sensitive and 90%-100% specific for appendicitis; can be used safely during pregnancy	351-419
CT scan of abdomen	Rule out other abdominal conditions	807-956
U/A	Used to exclude genitourinary conditions in patients of all ages	15-20
Pregnancy	Rule out ectopic pregnancy	51-65/quantitative 28-35/qualitative

CBC, Complete blood cell count; *CT,* computed tomography; *FOB,* fecal occult blood; *U/A,* urinalysis; *WBC,* white blood cell count.

TABLE 14-2 Differential Diagnosis: Appendicitis

Differential Diagnosis	Supporting Data
Crohn's disease	Insidious onset; intermittent episodes of fever, diarrhea, and RLQ pain An RLQ mass and tenderness may also be present X-ray evidence of ulceration, strictures of small colon
Diverticulitis	In elderly patients: Acute abdominal pain and fever, with LLQ abdominal tenderness and mass Leukocytosis
Gastroenteritis	Nausea and vomiting, low-grade fever, diarrhea Pain is more generalized, with tenderness less localized
Henoch-Schönlein purpura	Rash, arthritis, abdominal colic, and renal involvement Usually follows URI in school-age **children**
Pneumonia	Pain in the abdomen or lower chest after a URI Cough, fever
In young women, appendicitis is most often confused with gynecological problems	PID: Abdominal pain, CMT, fever, purulent vaginal discharge Mittelschmerz: Sudden onset of lower abdominal pain in the middle of the menstrual cycle Dysmenorrhea: Lower abdominal pain associated with menstrual period Tubal pregnancy: Sudden severe abdominal pain with diffuse pelvic tenderness and shock, positive pregnancy test, and positive pelvic ultrasound; a pregnancy test and pelvic ultrasonography are necessary to confirm Ovarian torsions, ruptured cysts, ruptured ovarian follicles with bleeding: sudden severe pain in RUQ or LUQ
Appendicitis	Appendicitis is the most common atraumatic abdominal surgical emergency in **pregnant** women Whenever a **pregnant** woman complains of right-sided abdominal pain, a surgical consultation should be ordered, especially in a patient in her second or third trimester Think of appendicitis in every **child,** regardless of age, who has GI or other abdominal complaints Early: Periumbilical pain Late: RLQ pain and tenderness; anorexia, nausea and vomiting, obstipation, low-grade fever, and leukocytosis

CMT, Cervical motion tenderness; *GI,* gastrointestinal; *LLQ,* lower left quadrant; *LUQ,* left upper quadrant; *PID,* pelvic inflammatory disorder; *RLQ,* right lower quadrant; *RUQ,* right upper quadrant; *URI,* upper respiratory infection.

TABLE 14-3 Scoring System for Suspected Appendicitis

Symptom/Sign	Indicator	Score
Constant		−10
Sex	Male	+8
	Female	−8
WBC	<8.9	−15
	9.0-13.9	+2
	>14.0	+10
Duration of pain	<24 hr	+3
	24-48 hr	0
	>48 hr	−12
Progression of pain	Yes	+3
	No	−4
Relocation of pain	Yes	+7
	No	−9
Vomiting	Yes	+7
	No	−5
Aggravation by coughing	Yes	+4
	No	−11
Rebound tenderness	Yes	+5
	No	−10
Rigidity	Yes	+15
	No	−4
Tenderness outside RLQ	Yes	−6
	No	+4

From Fenyo G, Lindberg G, Blind P: Diagnostic decision support in suspected acute appendicitis: validation of a simplified scoring system, *Eur J Surg* 163:831-838, 1997.
RLQ, Right lower quadrant; *WBC,* white blood cell count.

Referral

Seek early consultation with a surgeon for a **child** with a gastrointestinal or abdominal complaint when the child appears to have a toxic condition.

Obtain an obstetrical consultation for a **pregnant** woman with right-sided abdominal pain, especially in the second and third trimester.

EVALUATION/FOLLOW-UP

Schedule routine postoperative visits at 2 and 6 weeks.

The postoperative follow-up is normally limited to checking the wound and providing a work release. The most common complication is wound infection, which may require antibiotic therapy, dressings, or packings.

SUGGESTED READINGS

A one-antibiotic regimen for ruptured appendix, *Emerg Med* 24:742, 1992.

Ellsworth A et al: *Mosby's 1998 medical drug reference*, St Louis, 1998, Mosby.

Fenyo G, Lindberg G, Blind P: Diagnostic decision support in suspected acute appendicitis: validation of a simplified scoring system, *Eur J Surg* 163:831-838, 1997.

Finelli L: Evaluation of the child with acute abdominal pain, *J Pediatr Healthcare* 5:251-256, 1991.

Fox J: *Primary health care of children,* St Louis, 1997, Mosby.

Griffith H, Dambro M: *The five-minute clinical consult,* ed 5, Malvern, Penn, 1998, Lea & Febiger.

Healthcare Consultants of America, Inc.: *1998 Physician's fee and coding guide,* Augusta, Ga, 1998, Healthcare Consultants of America, Inc.

Mead M: Detecting appendicitis, *Pract Nurse* 11:486-487, 1996.

Rothrock S: When appendicitis isn't "classic," *Emerg Med* 28:108-124, 1996.

Arthritis

Osteoarthritis and Rheumatoid Arthritis

ICD-9-CM

Juvenile Rheumatoid Arthritis 714.30
Osteoarthritis 715.9
Rheumatoid Arthritis 714.0
Septic Arthritis 711.0

OVERVIEW

Definition

Osteoarthritis (OA) is a degenerative disease of the cartilage of joints with reactive formation of new bone at the articular margins.

Primary OA is the most common form of OA. It is of unknown cause. Primary OA most commonly affects the distal interphalangeal joints (DIPs) and less commonly, the proximal interphalangeal joints (PIPs), the metatarsophalangeal and carpometacarpal joints of the hip and knee, the metatarsophalangeal joint of the great toe, and the cervical and lumbar spine.

Secondary OA may occur in any joint as a result of articular injury (fracture, overuse of joint, or metabolic disease), from either intraarticular (including rheumatoid arthritis) or extraarticular causes.

Rheumatoid arthritis (RA) is an immunologically mediated chronic inflammatory disease of unknown cause that primarily affects joints but may have generalized manifestations.

Juvenile RA (JRA) has three major presentations: (1) an acute febrile form with salmon macular rash, arthritis, splenomegaly, leukocytosis, and polyserositis; (2) a polyarticular (five or more joints involved) pattern that resembles adult disease, with chronic pain and swelling of many joints, and (3) pauciarticular disease (less than five joints affected), characterized by chronic arthritis of a few joints, often the large weight-bearing joints, in asymmetric distribution. Up to 30% of children 1 to 16 years old with this form of disease develop iridocyclitis, which can cause blindness if untreated.

Incidence

OA is the most common form of arthritis, affecting approximately 20 million Americans. Ninety percent of people will have radiographic evidence of OA by age 40 in weight-bearing joints.

RA affects approximately 7 million Americans; females more than males, based on diagnostic criteria. The incidence increases with age and peaks in the fourth decade of life. **The onset of JRA is between 2 and 4 years of age; the rate of JRA in girls is almost twice that of boys.**

Pathophysiology

Protective factors:
- Normal weight
- Male gender

Factors That Increase Susceptibility

Obesity
Positive family history
Posttraumatic injury
Fracture/immobilization
Increasing age
Female gender
History of gout, hemochromatosis, psoriasis, avascular necrosis, congenital hip dysplasia
Intraarticular corticosteroid overusage
Metabolic abnormalities (Wilson's disease, acromegaly)

SUBJECTIVE DATA

History of Present Illness

Ask about duration of symptoms, morning stiffness, pain, systemic symptoms

OA: Insidious onset, morning stiffness of less than 30 minutes, pain on movement, limitation of movement

RA: Prodromal systemic symptoms of malaise, fever, weight loss; morning stiffness lasting 30 to 60 minutes

Children: Nonmigratory, one or more joints affected; arthropathy, tending to involve larger joints or PIPs, lasting more than 3 months with systemic manifestations of fever, rash, nodules, leukocytosis; onset related to age of child, with systemic involvement; more likely in younger children

Past Medical History

Corticosteroid articular injections, occupational/leisure activity and/or injuries, history of metabolic, endocrine, autoimmune, or other musculoskeletal diseases (postural or developmental defects, joint instability, past meniscectomy)

Inquire how condition has affected or is affecting activities of daily living (ADL)

Children: Past medical history may be unremarkable

Medications

Use of antiinflammatory or analgesic agents (results, any other prescribed or over-the-counter medications)

Family History

Ask about family history of OA, RA, musculoskeletal, endocrine, autoimmune, or metabolic diseases.

Psychosocial History

Adults/elderly: Inquire how OA or RA affects their ADL or instrumental activities of daily living (IADL)

Children: Consider how RA may affect their daily life and school performance

Diet History

Perform overall nutritional assessment with emphasis on weight reduction, if necessary

Associated Symptoms

OA: Crepitus, pain relieved by rest, joint instability, edema and joint swelling minimal (or absent), slight erythema/warmth, nocturnal pain after vigorous exercise, joint deformity, such as bony enlargement, Heberden's nodes, flexion contracture/valgus or varus deformity of knee, quadriceps atrophy

RA: Articular inflammation with swelling, pain, erythema, and warmth; progression of joint involvement is centripetal and symmetric; tenosynovitis, rheumatoid nodules; be alert for systemic manifestations, such as vision loss, conjunctivitis, pain associated with pleural effusion, carpal tunnel, cutaneous lesions, rashes, neuropathies, and vasculitis

JRA: Characteristic salmon-colored maculopapular rash seen in 25% to 50% of children; rash may be intermittent, associated with fever spikes, and increased splenomegaly; may precede joint symptoms by 3 years

OBJECTIVE DATA

Physical Examination

A problem-oriented physical examination should be conducted. The examiner should keep in mind potential systemic manifestations of RA (e.g., dermatological conditions, pleurisy, splenomegaly, ocular manifestations) that might necessitate a complete physical examination.

Vital signs: Weight, blood pressure, and pulse; also general appearance, gait, and activity level.

Musculoskeletal

- Inspect affected joints for deformities, nodes, number of affected joints, symmetry of affected joints, and erythema.
- Observe affected joints in active and passive range of motion (ROM).
- Palpate affected joints for warmth, tenderness, crepitus, edema.
- Assess muscle strength.
- Assess joint stability.

Diagnostic Procedures

There are no definitive tests for either OA, RA, or JRA; however, some diagnostic tests may help to include or exclude the diagnosis (Table 15-1).

OA

- First line: None
- Second line: Radiographic evidence of narrowing of joint space, soft tissue swelling, and marginal osteophytes
- Third line: Erythrocyte sedimentation rate (ESR), complete blood cell count (CBC), and electrolyte measurements may be ordered to support OA as a diagnosis of exclusion.

RA

- First line: None
- Second line: ESR (Westergren method) provides useful but nonspecific information in confirming inflammatory disease; an ESR greater than 60 mm/hr indicates

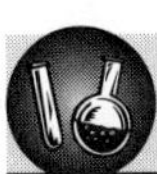

TABLE 15-1 Diagnostic Tests: Arthritis

Symptoms	Findings	Diagnostic Tests	Cost ($)
OA			
Slow onset, morning stiffness <30 min, pain on movement, limited movement, pain relieved with rest, pain after exercise	Crepitus, joint instability, absence of deformity, Heberden's nodes, valgus/varus deformities, absence of joint effusion, quadriceps atrophy	First line: None	None
		Second line: Joint x-ray evaluation	67-151/Depends on site
		Third line:	
		CBC	13-16
		ESR	16-20
		Electrolytes	23-30
RA			
Prodrome with fever, malaise, weight loss, morning stiffness of >30 min, joint pain, warmth	Joint edema, erythema, warmth, nodules, joint involvement is centripetal and symmetrical, tenosynovitis	First line: None	None
		Second line: ESR	See above
		Third line:	
		ANA	42-52
		Rheumatoid factor	22-28
		CBC	See above
JRA			
Fever with rash, five or more or five or fewer joints with swelling, migratory joint involvement, pain	Macular salmon-colored rash, or joint edema, erythema, effusion	First line: None	None
		Second line:	
		Rheumatoid factor	See above
		Third line: ESR, ANA	See above

ANA, Antinuclear antibody; *CBC*, complete blood cell count; *ESR*, erythrocyte sedimentation rate; *ANA*, antinuclear antibody.

severe inflammation. The ESR, useful in following response to treatment, is not useful when inflammatory disease is in remission.

Third line: Rheumatoid factor is not pathognomonic of RA but is present in 70% to 80% of persons meeting the criteria for RA. A significant titer is a finding of 1:80 or greater, although it may yield a negative result in early disease. Antinuclear antibodies (ANAs) are present in 20% to 30% of persons with RA; ANAs are more common in those with extraarticular manifestations of RA and in those with a high titer of rheumatoid factor. CBC: The white blood cell count (WBC) is normal or slightly elevated and may reveal normocytic, hypochromic anemia; platelet count is often elevated.

Children: Rheumatoid factor is positive by latex fixation in about 15% of cases; ANAs may be present in pauciarticular disease; may have normal ESR in presence of active disease.

ASSESSMENT

Differential Diagnoses (Figure 15-1 and Table 15-2)

OA: Because articular inflammation or minimal and systemic manifestations are absent, OA is seldom misdiagnosed. However, diagnosis is not always straightforward. In these instances, the following conditions may be included in the differential diagnoses of OA: rheumatoid arthritis, gout, pseudogout, psoriatic arthritis, septic arthritis, malignancy, osteoporosis, tendinitis (bursitis).

RA: Osteoarthritis, polymyalgia rheumatica, systemic lupus erythematosus (SLE), Sjögren's syndrome, vasculitis, gout, pseudogout, scleroderma, septic arthritis, psoriatic arthritis, Lyme disease, malignancy, polymyositis

JRA: Rheumatic fever, Osgood-Schlatter disease, fracture, slipped capital femoral epiphysis, Schönlein-Henoch purpura, infections, SLE, Lyme disease, neoplasms (leukemia, lymphoma, neuroblastoma), syndromes of psychoorganic origin

THERAPEUTIC PLAN

Pharmaceutical (Figure 15-2 and Table 15-3)

The objectives of therapy are to restore function, relieve pain, and maintain joint motion. Often analgesics such as acetaminophen and aspirin are adequate to control the pain associated with OA. Use of enteric-coated aspirin to reduce gastrointestinal upset is recommended. Because the role of inflammation is not well defined, the use of stronger nonsteroidal antiinflammatory drugs (NSAIDs) should be considered a second-line therapy.

In RA and JRA, aspirin is effective, inexpensive, and

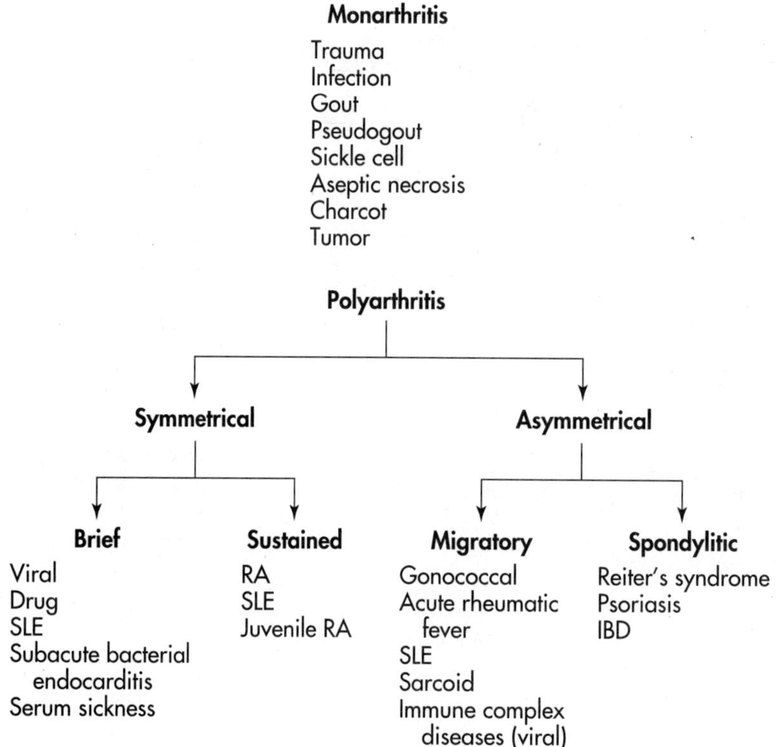

Figure 15-1 Common causes of joint pain. *IBD,* Inflammatory bowel disease; *RA,* rheumatoid arthritis; *SLE,* systemic lupus erythematosus. (Redrawn from Barth WF: Office evaluation of the patient with musculoskeletal complaints, *Am J Med* 102:3-10S, 1997.)

may be the first NSAID used. If NSAIDs fail to provide relief in 2 to 3 months, disease-modifying antirheumatic drugs (DMARDs) such as antimalarials, corticosteroids, cytotoxic drugs, and gold salts may be effective. DMARDs are used in persons with RA who show evidence of progressive joint involvement, persistent inflammation, elevated ESR/RF, and changes as demonstrated on x-ray evaluation. The use of DMARDs early in the course of the disease in these patients may prevent disability and morbidity, since 90% of erosive changes can occur within 2 years of onset. Use of DMARDs almost always accompanies the use of NSAIDs; this should be done in consultation with the collaborating physician and may necessitate a referral to a rheumatologist.

NOTE: Gastropathy associated with the use of NSAIDs is a major health problem in the United States. Risk factors for GI hemorrhage include advanced age, prior or present peptic ulcer disease, prior GI hemorrhage, alcoholism, concomitant use of anticoagulant medications or high-dose corticosteroids. Nonacetylated salicylates produce the least inhibition of platelet aggregation.

Children: Consider consultation with a pediatric rheumatologist at the time of diagnosis. NSAIDs in liquid form have replaced salicylates as the drugs of choice for pediatric patients. NSAIDs have a decreased dosage frequency and fewer side effects than salicylates; thus compliance is more likely. The following drugs are equally effective: naproxen 7.5 mg/kg BID, ibuprofen 10 mg/kg QID, and tolmetin sodium 10 mg/kg TID.

Aspirin 75 to 100 mg/kg in three divided doses is equally effective (but aspirin should not be given if the child has been exposed to chicken pox or Asian flu). For children who fail to respond to NSAIDs, methotrexate ($79/injection) is a second-line medication (5 to 10 mg/m^2/wk). Injectable gold salts are an alternative. Children with ophthalmic involvement should be referred to an ophthalmologist.

Elderly: Elderly have an increased risk of NSAID-induced gastropathy as well as other serious side effects (renal failure, fluid retention) from long-term NSAID use. As with other pharmaceutical treatments, it may be necessary to start with a lower dosage and titrate upward until symptoms are controlled.

Lifestyle/Activities

Weight loss, if needed, to desirable weight
Exercise to maintain ROM and increase strength
Periods of rest during the day
Proper posture
Assistive aids: canes, walkers, crutches

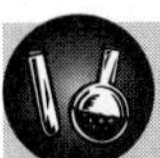

TABLE 15-2 Differential Diagnosis: Arthritis

Diagnosis	Supporting Data
Gout/pseudogout	Acute onset, typically nocturnal, monoarticular Hyperuricemia Asymptomatic between episodes Quick response to NSAIDs Pseudogout: Acute, recurrent, but not chronic, involving principally knees and wrists
Psoriatic arthritis	Psoriasis precedes arthritis in 80% of cases Asymmetric arthritis No rheumatoid factor present Commonly sacroiliac joint involvement Usually, lack of osteoporosis May have ankylosing spondylitis
Septic arthritis	Sudden onset Usually monarticular, often in weight-bearing joints Infection with causative organisms elsewhere in body Large joint effusions
Osteoporosis	Spontaneous fractures Loss of height Demineralization, especially of hip, spine, pelvis
Polymyalgia rheumatica	Age usually >50 Pain and stiffness in shoulder and pelvic girdle Frequently accompanied by fever Anemia and increased ESR
Systemic lupus erythematosus	Occurs primarily in young women Rash over areas exposed to sunlight 90% of patients experience joint symptoms + ANA Decreased hemoglobin, WBC, platelet count
Osgood-Schlatter disease	Young athletes Prepatellar bursa swelling Anterior tibial tuberosity tenderness
Lyme disease	Headache, stiff neck Arthralgias, arthritis, myalgias; often chronic and recurrent Flat or slightly raised red lesion that expands with central clearing Wide geographic distribution

ANA, Antinuclear antibody; *ESR*, erythrocyte sedimentation rate; *NSAIDs*, nonsteroidal antiinflammatory drugs, *WBC*, white blood cell count.

Diet

None, unless weight reduction is desirable

Patient Education

Selective rest of affected joints to prevent contractures (e.g., splinting at night)
Heat and cold to relieve muscle spasm and provide pain relief
Physical therapy
Proper posture
Assistive devices: canes, walkers, crutches
Surgery in some cases

Family Impact

In children, a diagnosis of JRA can influence socialization with peers, and activities may be curtailed to some extent. Children's activities that can be performed with a diagnosis of JRA should be encouraged. Proper management in children can result in less morbidity as an adult.

A diagnosis of OA or RA is lifelong and will require intermittent treatment. Because of this, adults may experience interruptions with their job and/or family life, which can result in economic difficulties. Safety in performing everyday activities may also become an issue, and plans to ensure a safe environment need to be made accordingly.

Referral

For children and adults who do not respond to therapy or have severe disease, treatment must be by a team approach and should include referrals for nutritional counseling, physical and/or occupational therapy, and surgery when necessary.

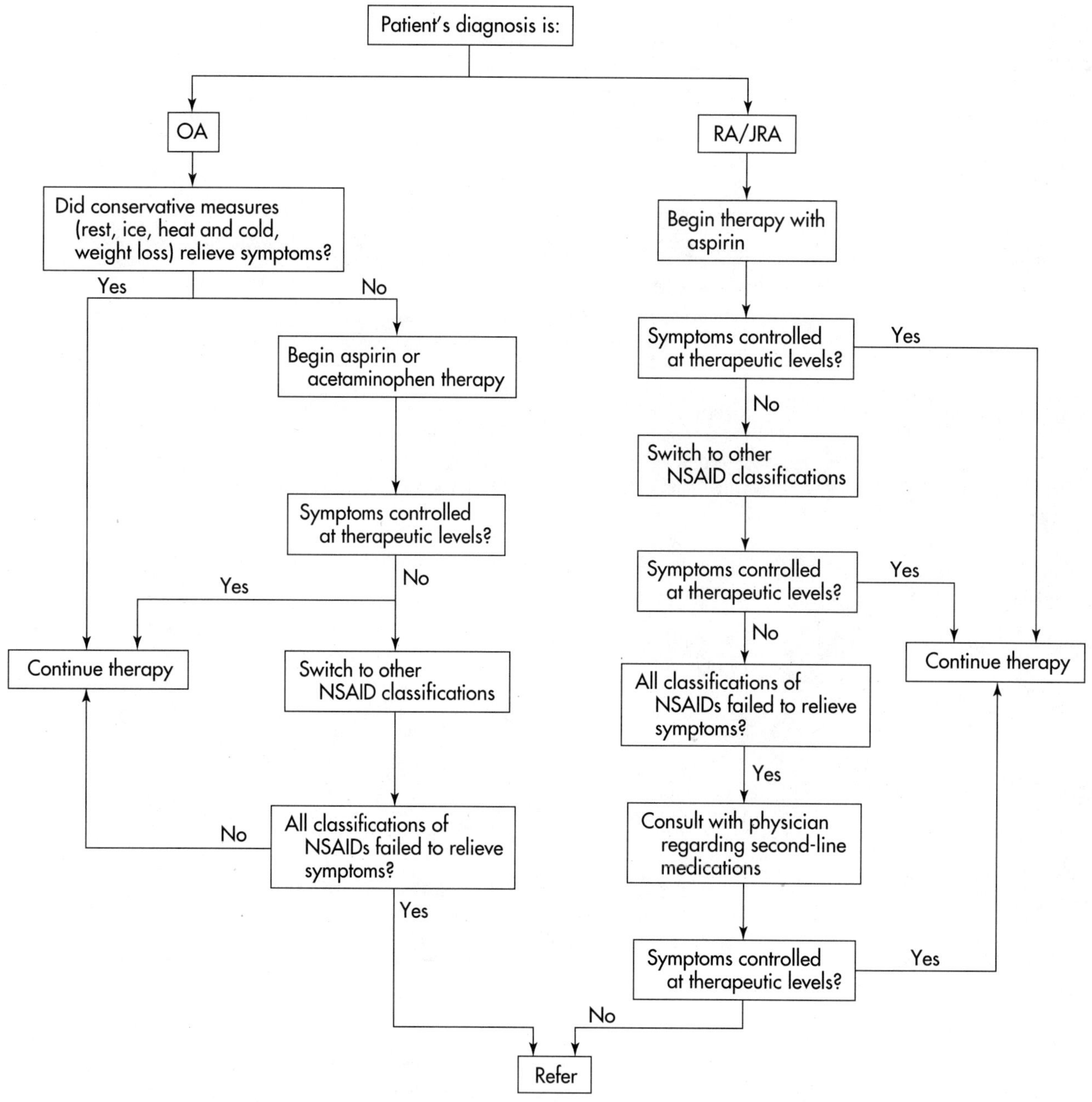

Figure 15-2 Pharmacological management of osteoarthritis and rheumatoid arthritis. *JRA*, Juvenile rheumatoid arthritis; *OA*, osteoarthritis; *RA*, rheumatoid arthritis; *NSAID*, nonsteroidal antiinflammatory drug.

Consultation

Consult with the physician on any patient with an initial diagnosis of arthritis and if treatment with first-line medications fails.

Follow-up

Follow-up will depend on the severity of the patient's disease. If medications are to be advanced weekly, laboratory evaluations should be performed and patients should be seen on a weekly basis until symptoms are controlled. At follow-up visits, patient education measures should be reinforced and the patient's psychosocial adaption and ability to cope with the disease should be assessed.

EVALUATION

Children: Disease activity progressively diminishes with age and, in 95% of cases, ceases by puberty. In a few cases, disease will persist into adulthood. Problems after

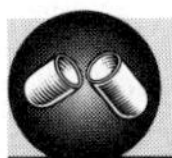

TABLE 15-3 Pharmaceutical Plan: Arthritis

Generic Name	Trade Name	Adult Dose	Child Dose	Maximum Daily Dosing/Cost
Acetaminophen	Tylenol	2 tablets q4-6h	15 mg/kg q4h	$4-$6/Children: 60 mg/kg/day; adults: 8 tablets in 24 hours

Refer to nonsteroidal antiinflammatory drug table in Appendix J for further dosing information.

puberty relate to joint damage, but RA presenting in adolescence may precede adult disease. If JRA is stable, children may be seen on a routine basis that meets both the family's and the provider's needs. Laboratory studies, such as CBC, appropriate for medication regimen and disease process should be obtained to follow progress of the disease and to observe for side effects of medications.

Adults: Once the disease is stable, adults may also be evaluated on a routine basis. Laboratory studies should be done as appropriate based on symptoms of the disease and medication regimen; the results will allow monitoring both disease progress and medication side effects.

SUGGESTED READINGS

Barker LR, Burton JR, Zieve PD: *Principles of ambulatory medicine,* ed 4, Baltimore, 1995, Williams & Wilkins.

Burns CE et al: *Primary pediatric care: a handbook for nurse practitioners,* Philadelphia, 1996, WB Saunders.

Bynum DT: Clinical snapshot: gout, *AJN* 97:36-37, 1997.

Cornell S: New directions in rheumatoid arthritis, *Adv Nurs Pract* 5:61-64, 1997.

Ellsworth AJ et al: *Mosby's 1998 medical drug reference,* St Louis, 1998, Mosby.

Gorroll AH, May LA, Mulley AG: *Primary care medicine,* Philadelphia, 1995, JB Lippincott.

Healthcare Consultants of America, Inc: *1998 Physicians fee and coding guide,* Augusta, Ga, 1998, Healthcare Consultants of America, Inc.

Hery WW et al, editors: *Current pediatric diagnosis and treatment,* Norwalk, Conn, 1997, Appleton & Lange.

Hooker RS: Osteoarthritis of the hip and knee: managing a common joint disease, *Clin Rev* 6(1):54-67, 1996.

Hurst JW: *Medicine for the practicing physician,* Norwalk, Conn, 1996, Appleton & Lange.

Peters S: Osteoarthritis options: new guidelines for primary care, *Adv Nurs Pract* 4(12):41-50, 1996.

Ross C: A comparison of osteoarthritis and rheumatoid arthritis: diagnosis and treatment, *Nurse Pract* 22:20-41, 1997.

Tierney LM, McPhee SJ, Papadakis MA: *Current medical diagnosis and treatment,* Norwalk, Conn, 1996, Appleton & Lange.

Uphold C, Graham M: *Clinical guidelines in family practice,* Gainesville, Fla, 1994, Barmarrae Books.

16 Asthma

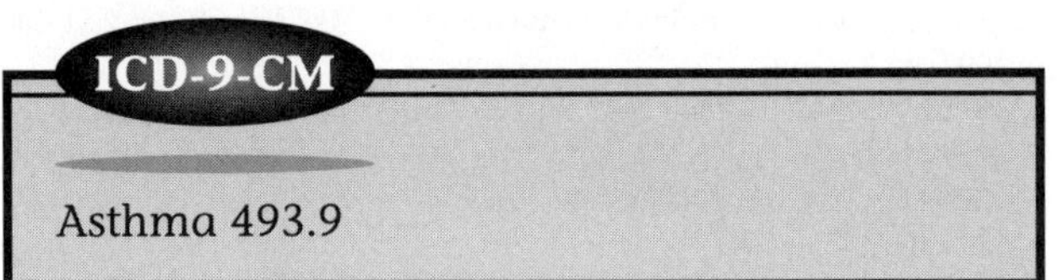

OVERVIEW

Definition

Asthma is a chronic inflammatory disorder of the airways causing airway hyperresponsiveness and obstruction. Airway obstruction may reverse spontaneously or require treatment. Inflammation also increases existing bronchial hyperresponsiveness to a variety of stimuli. The classic syndrome of symptoms includes recurrent wheeze, cough (particularly at night), and mild to severe respiratory distress. Recent evidence suggests that sub-basement membrane fibrosis may occur in some patients with asthma and this results in persistent abnormalities in lung function.

Incidence

More than 15 million people in the United States have been diagnosed with asthma.

10% of all **children** with asthma are under 20 years old (most common).

Asthma is a major cause of outpatient visits and hospitalizations for all ages.

There is a high incidence among adolescent and young adult blacks.

Underdiagnosis and inappropriate therapy are major contributors to asthma morbidity and mortality.

More than 5000 deaths annually in the United States can be attributed to asthma.

Pathophysiology

Bronchial obstruction as a result of acute airway constriction, airway edema, and mucus plug formation.

Characterized by erosion of the airway epithelium, deposition of collagen beneath the basement membrane, edema, mast-cell activation and infiltration by inflammatory cells

Epidemiology

Atopy is the strongest predisposing factor associated with asthma (IgE-mediated response to allergens manifested as rash, or upper respiratory symptoms).

Development of asthma is also associated with sensitivity to nonsteroidal antiinflammatory drugs, presence of nasal polyps, and/or chronic sinusitis; viral respiratory illness may also act as a trigger.

Environmental exposures are highly associated with development of asthma.

Children: The most common environmental triggers are cigarette smoke, animal proteins, and house dust mites.

Adults: Occupational exposures can lead to asthma; these include organic chemicals and wood dusts.

SUBJECTIVE DATA

History of Present Illness

Cough (especially nocturnal)
Recurrent wheeze
Recurrent trouble breathing (dyspnea)
Recurrent chest tightness

Description of Most Common Symptoms

Symptoms occur or worsen in the presence of certain factors:

- Airborne dust or chemicals
- Animals with fur or feathers
- Exercise
- Weather changes
- House dust
- Mold
- Pollen

TABLE 16-1 Classification of Asthma Severity*

Category	Symptoms	Nocturnal Symptoms	Lung Function
Step 4			
Severe persistent	Continuous symptoms Limited activity Frequent exacerbations	Frequent	Peak flow 60% or less of predicted; >30% variability
Step 3			
Moderate persistent	Daily symptoms Daily use of inhaled short-acting beta-agonist Exacerbations affect activity Exacerbations >2×/wk	>1×/wk	Peak flow 60%-80% of predicted; >30% variability
Step 2			
Mild persistent	Symptoms <1×/day, but >2×/wk Exacerbations may affect activity	>2×/mo	Peak flow 80% of predicted; 20%-30% variability
Step 1			
Mild intermittent	Symptoms <2×/wk Asymptomatic between exacerbations Brief exacerbations Exacerbations vary in intensity	2×/mo or less	Peak flow at least 80%; <20% variability Normal peak flow between exacerbations

**Instructions:* Begin at bottom of table and move upward (step up) as symptoms progress.

Smoke (tobacco or wood)
Stress/emotional response
Viral infection

OBJECTIVE DATA

Physical Examination

Targeted: Other systems as individually indicated
General: Vital signs, responsiveness, signs of distress
Eyes: Allergic shiners (dark circles under the eyes), infection, watery discharge
Ears **(children):** Concurrent signs of otitis media (acute or with effusion)
Nose: Polyps, congestion, discharge
Mouth: Infection of throat, postnasal discharge
Skin: Signs of atopy (eczema, dermatitis)
Chest: Observation—use of accessory muscles, retractions, breathing effort
Auscultation: Wheeze (end expiratory), air movement (decreased or absence of air movement is a sign of a more severe condition)
Percussion: Resonance

Diagnostic Procedures

Lung function (peak expiratory flow rate): A 20% variation between first morning measurement (before medications) and early afternoon measurement (after taking a short-acting inhaled beta-adrenergic agonist) is indicative of asthma (see Appendix L) for a chart of predicted flow rates for men, women, and children.
Asthma diagnosis is also based on symptom history, identifiable triggers, and reversibility of airway obstruction.
Provocation testing: May be completed if diagnosis is unclear.

ASSESSMENT

See Table 16-1 for classification of severity of asthma.

Differential Diagnosis

Allergic rhinitis
Heart disease
Gastroesophageal reflux
Sinusitis
Vocal cord dysfunction

Infants and Children

Aspiration
Bronchopulmonary dysplasia
Cystic fibrosis
Foreign body
Laryngeotracheomalacia
Tracheal stenosis
Vascular rings

TABLE 16-2 Action Guide for Medication Adjustment*

	Daily Medications for Long Term Control	Medications for Quick Relief
Step 4		
Severe Persistent	Two daily medications	
Refer to specialist	Antiinflammatory agent (high dose) and/or Long-acting bronchodilator and/or Oral glucocorticoid	Short-acting inhaled beta-agonist (Daily use or increasing use indicates need for additional long-term therapy.)
Step 3		
Moderate Persistent	One or two daily medications	
Refer to specialist (children)	Antiinflammatory agent (medium dose) and/or long-acting bronchodilator plus medium-dose inhaled glucocorticoid	Short-acting inhaled beta-agonist (Daily use or increasing use indicates need for additional long-term therapy.)
Step 2		
Mild Persistent	One daily medication	
	Antiinflammatory agent (low-dose inhaled glucocorticoid, cromolyn, or necromil) or sustained-release theophylline	Short-acting inhaled beta-agonist (Daily use or increasing use indicates need for additional long-term therapy.)
Step 1		
Mild Intermittent	No daily medications	Short-acting inhaled beta-agonist (Use more than 2×/wk may indicate the need to initiate long-term therapy.)

**Instructions:* Begin at bottom of table and move upward (step up) as symptoms progress.

Adults

Chronic obstructive pulmonary disease
Congestive heart failure

THERAPEUTIC PLAN

Therapeutic Management

Management of the patient's condition is carried out in consultation with a physician (especially during the diagnostic phase).

Control acute exacerbation.
- Correct significant hypoxia.
- Reverse airway obstruction.
- Reduce inflammation and risk of recurrence by intensifying therapy.

Manage coexisting illness or disease.
Determine patient's personal best peak expiratory flow rate (PEFR) once condition is stabilized.
- Record PEFR two to four times/day for 2 to 3 weeks for consistent pattern.
- Personal best measure is established as 100% PEFR; other parameters for identification of worsening symptoms and medication adjustments are based on this measure.

Establish individualized written action plan in partnership with patient/family.
Consider allergy testing and immunotherapy once unavoidable allergens are determined.

Pharmacological Management

A stepped-care approach to pharmacological management of asthma is outlined in Table 16-2, following the same levels of severity detailed in Table 16-1.

Step up if control is not maintained after confirmation of medication technique, compliance, and environmental control.
Step down gradually if review of status (see Table 16-1) indicates that reduction of medications is possible.

Types of Medication

Long-Term Control. Long-term medications are given on a daily basis and are not to be given to relieve an attack (Table 16-3). Their benefit is in reducing the likelihood of an attack over time. This group includes corticosteroid medications (e.g., Prednisone, $3 to $8), cromolyn sodium (Intal, $23 to $60), nedocromil (Tilade, $27 to $50), long-acting beta-agonists (e.g., salmeterol/Serevent, $50), sustained-release theophylline ($6 to $27),

Table 16-3 Dosing of Long-Term Asthma Control Medications*

Drug Class or Drug and Route of Administration	Selected Dosage Forms and Strengths† (brand names)	Usual Adult Dosage	Usual Pediatric Dosage for Children 6-12 Years Old
Oral Corticosteroids			
Methylprednisolone	2-, 4-, 8-, 16-, 32-mg tablets (Medrol)	Long-term treatment: 7.5-60 mg/day as single daily dose or in four divided doses as needed for control Short-course "burst" therapy: 40-60 mg/day as single daily dose or in two divided doses for 3-10 days	Long-term treatment: 0.25-2 mg/kg/day as single daily dose or in four divided doses as needed for control Short-course "burst" therapy: 1-2 mg/kg/day, not to exceed 60 mg/day, as single daily dose or in two to four divided doses, for 3-10 days
Prednisolone	5-mg tablets, 5-, 15-mg/ml oral liquid (Delta-Cortef, Prelone)	Same as for methylprednisolone	Same as for methylprednisolone
Prednisone	1-, 2.5-, 5-, 10-, 20-, 25-mg tablets, 5-mg/ml oral liquid (Deltasone, Orasone, others)	Same as for methylprednisolone	Same as for methylprednisolone
Other Antiinflammatory Agents*			
Cromolyn sodium inhalation	800-µg/puff pMDI (Intal Aerosol Spray)‡	2-4 puffs three or four times daily‡	1-2 puffs three or four times daily‡
Nedocromil inhalation	1.75-mg/puff pMDI (Tilade)	2-4 puffs two to four times daily‡	1-2 puffs two to four times daily‡
Long-Term β_2-Agonists			
Salmeterol inhalation	21-µg/puff pMDI (Serevent)	2 puffs every 12 hr‡	1-2 puffs every 12 hr‡
Oral albuterol	4-mg sustained-release tablets (Proventil Repetabs, Volmax)	4 mg every 12 hr	0.3-0.6 mg/kg/day, not to exceed 8 mg/day
Methylxanthine			
Theophylline	Oral liquid, sustained-release tablets and capsules of various strengths (various brands)	10 mg/kg/day (not to exceed 300 mg) initially; titrate to serum concentration of 5-15 µg/mL (usual maximum 800 mg/day)	10 mg/kg/day initially; titrate to serum concentration of 5-15 µg/mL, not to exceed 16 mg/kg/day in patients at least 1 year old§
Leukotriene Modifiers			
Zafirlukast	20-mg tablets (Accolate)	40 mg/day in two divided doses	Not indicated
Zileuton	300-, 600-mg tablets (Zyflo)	2400 mg/day in four divided doses	Not indicated

From American Pharmaceutical Association: New Product Bulletin: Pulmicort Turbuhaler, Washington, DC, 1998, American Pharmaceutical Association.
*See Table 16-4 for information about inhaled corticosteroids.
†Other dosage forms may be available but may not be indicated for long-term asthma control (e.g., albuterol pMDI, which is used for quick relief). *pMDI*, Pressurized aerosol metered-dose inhaler.
‡Consult prescribing information or reference 3 for dosage used as prophylaxis for nocturnal and exercise-induced symptoms.
§Not to exceed $(0.2 \times \text{age in weeks}) + 5$ mg/kg/day in infants less than 1 year old. For example: $(0.2 \times 20 \text{ wk}) + 5$ mg/kg/day = 9 mg/kg/day.

Box 16-1

Special Considerations for Children Younger Than 5 Years Old

Trials of inhaled bronchodialators and antiinflammatory medications for diagnostic purposes. (Symptomatology is difficult to evaluate in patients this age; performance on spirometry is inconsistent or impossible to measure.)
Symptoms that occur two or more times per week require long-term control by medication.
Cromolyn and nedocromil are good choices because they produce very limited side effects. If the patient is using a corticosteroid inhaler, consider prescribing budesonide since it is a dry powder inhaler (DPI) and is easier to use. Do not use a spacer with a DPI.
Close monitoring is critical, especially until control of symptoms is achieved.
The parents can maintain an asthma diary for the child, with symptom severity criteria to help them determine appropriate medication adjustment (similar red/yellow/green stoplight categories to diaries with PEFR measures).
These children require more frequent follow-up, especially during a period of exacerbation (days versus weeks).
Refer the patient to a specialist at step 3 (moderate persistent) and consider referral at the step 2 level of care.

and leukotriene modifiers. Zafirlukast (Accolate) and Zileuton (Zyflo) are leukotriene modifiers that have the same efficacy as inhaled cromolyn. Symptoms should improve within 1 week.

Quick Relief. The second category of medications is given as needed for relief of exacerbations (acute symptoms) and prevention of exercise-induced bronchospasm. This group includes short-acting beta-agonists (e.g., Albuterol, $22 to $24), anticholinergics (Ipratropium, $29; the inhaler is not FDA approved for use in asthma), and systemic corticosteroid medications.

Special Considerations for Children

Box 16-1 outlines special management considerations for children. Table 16-4 compares high to low dosage of orally inhaled corticosteroid medications.

Patient Education

Patient education is an ongoing process. Continuity with a primary provider is important so that a partnership can develop between the patient and the provider, with each having a sense of accountability to the partnership. This continuity also provides opportunities for the care provider

TABLE 16-4 Orally Inhaled Corticosteroid Therapy for Adults and Children* with Asthma

Drug	Amount Released per Actuation and Delivery Device† (brand name)	Low Dosage (µg/day)	Medium Dosage (µg/day)	High Dosage (µg/day)
Beclomethasone dipropionate	42, 84 µg/puff pMDI (Beclovent, Vanceril, Vanceril DS)	Adults: 168-504 Children: 84-336	Adults: 504-840 Children: 336-672	Adults: >840 Children: >672
Budesonide	200 µg/inhalation with inhalation-driven, dry powder inhaler (Pulmicort Turbuhaler)†	Adults: 200-400 Children: 100‡-200	Adults: 400-600 Children: 200-400	Adults: >600§ Children: >400§
Flunisolide	250 µg/puff pMDI (Aerobid, Aerobid-M)	Adults: 500-1000 Children 500-750	Adults: 1000-2000 Children: 1000-1250	Adults: >2000 Children: >1250
Fluticasone	44, 110, 220 µg/puff pMDI (Flovent)	Adults: 88-264 Children: 88-176	Adults: 264-660 Children: 176-440	Adults: >660 Children: >440
Triamcinolone	100 µg/puff pMDI (Azmacort)	Adults: 400-1000 Children: 400-800	Adults: 1000-2000 Children: 800-1200	Adults: >2000 Children: >1200

From American Pharmaceutical Association: New Product Bulletin: Pulmicort Turbuhaler, Washington, DC, 1998, American Pharmaceutical Association.
*6-12 years of age.
†The delivery device for budesonide inhalation powder (Pulmicort Turbuhaler) has been shown to deliver approximately twice as much drug to the airway compared to the pMDI. No resultant effect is implied with regard to clinical efficacy. One strength of Pulmicort Turbuhaler is available: 200 µg per metered dose, which delivers approximately 160 µg from the mouthpiece to the patient.
‡This strength is not available in the United States.
§The recommended maximum daily dose is 1600 µg for adults and 800 µg for children.
pMDI, Pressurized aerosol metered-dose inhaler.

to reinforce and confirm the patient's knowledge base at each visit in the important areas discussed in the following paragraphs.

Basic asthma facts (overview)
Role of medications: Emphasis on the difference between quick relief and long-term control
Medication administration: Use of inhalers/spacers; nebulizers; cleaning of equipment
Self-monitoring
- Recognizing signs and symptoms of an attack
- Lung function—peak expiratory flow
- Tracking of condition with an asthma diary

Use of Asthma Self-Monitoring Plan (see plan on p. 101)
Medication adjustment according to symptoms and response
Emergency plan: "Rescue steps"
- Give initial home treatment of quick-relief medication
- Contact provider, according to response
  - Good response: PEFR >80% (green)—call for follow-up
  - Incomplete response: PEFR 50% to 80% (yellow)—call today for appointment
  - Poor response: PEFR <50% (red)—go to Emergency Department (ED) of the hospital

Referral

Patients with a severe persistent condition (step 4 care), as well as any patient whose asthma cannot be reliably controlled with a maintenance regimen, should be referred to an asthma/allergy specialist.

EVALUATION/FOLLOW-UP

The timing to the initial follow-up depends on the severity of exacerbation (1 day to 3 weeks).
Regular follow-up visits should be scheduled for 1- to 6-month intervals.
Successful therapy based on:
- Preventing symptoms such as cough
- Maintaining near-normal pulmonary function
- Maintaining regular activities
- Preventing exacerbations (no hospitalizations or visits to ED)

SUGGESTED READINGS

Arvin AM et al, editors: *Nelson textbook of pediatrics*, ed 15, Philadelphia, 1996, WB Saunders.

Boyton RW, Dunn ES, Stephens GR, editors: *Ambulatory pediatric care*, ed 2, Philadelphia, 1994, JB Lippincott.

Milgrom H et al: Noncompliance and treatment failure in children with asthma, *J Allergy Clin Immunol* 98:1051-1057, 1996.

National Asthma Education and Prevention Program: Expert panel report II: guidelines for the diagnosis and management of asthma, Bethesda, Md, 1997, National Heart, Lung and Blood Institute, NIH.

National Asthma Education and Prevention Program: Nurses: partners in asthma care, Bethesda, Md, 1995, National Heart, Lung and Blood Institute, NIH.

Pharmacists' Letter: New Drug: Budesonide inhalation powder, Document 13092, 1998.

Plaut TF: *One-minute asthma*, ed 3, Amherst, Mass, 1996, Pedipress.

Uphold CR, Graham MV: *Clinical guidelines in child health*, Gainesville, Fla, 1994, Barmarrae Books.

Uphold CR, Graham MV: *Clinical guidelines in family practice*, Gainesville, Fla, 1994, Barmarrae Books.

Wise RA, Liu MC: Obstructive airway diseases: asthma and chronic pulmonary obstructive disease. In Barker LR, Burton JR, Zieve PD, editors: *Principles of ambulatory medicine*, ed 4, Baltimore, 1995, Williams & Wilkins.

Asthma Self-Monitoring Plan

Name____ **Date**______________________

For everyday use when feeling well. No cough or wheeze. Peak flow normal levels (__________)

______________________puffs/cc ________times per day **GREEN ZONE**

______________________puffs/cc ________times per day **PF 80%-100%**

For increasing symptoms or decrease in peak flow (__________). Continue at this level until symptom-free for 4 or 5 days and peak flow returns to the GREEN zone.

______________________puffs/cc ________times per day **YELLOW ZONE**

______________________puffs/cc ________times per day **PF 65%-80%**

Further increase in cough, wheezing, shortness of breath. Peak flow (__________). CALL.
May need to be seen in office.

______________________puffs/cc ________times per day **LOW YELLOW**

______________________puffs/cc ________times per day **PF 50%-65%**

If severe shortness of breath, wheezing, cough, chest tightness, difficulty walking or talking, peak flows less than (__________) 50% of predicted. Use ____________ puffs. CALL NOW!

RED ZONE
PF less than 50%

For exercise, use two puffs ______________ and/or ____________15 minutes before exercise.

I have been instructed on this plan and understand it.

________________________________Self/guardian____________Date

________________________________Provider ____________Date

Atrial Fibrillation

ICD-9-CM

Atrial Fibrillation and Flutter 427.3
Atrial Fibrillation 427.31
Atrial Flutter 427.32

OVERVIEW

Definition

Atrial fibrillation (AF) is a cardiac arrhythmia associated with a rapid impulse origination in the atria and disorganized atrial depolarization without effective atrial contraction. The ventricular response varies and is usually grossly irregular.

Incidence

Atrial fibrillation is frequently cited as the most commonly occurring cardiac rhythm disorder. It is seen in up to 5% of person over 65 years old. It is the most common cause of ischemic stroke among **elderly** persons. The 5-year incidence of stroke from AF is 44% in patients 60 to 70 years old, 80% in patients 71 to 80 years old, and 63% in patients 81 to 90 years old (Chrzanowski, 1998).

Pathophysiology

Atrial fibrillation is not caused by a single factor; many factors have been cited, and in some incidences the etiological factors remain unknown. Some mechanisms known to be associated with AF are abnormal automaticity, reentry, and other abnormal electrophysiological patterns. In addition, other pathophysiological factors that promote AF include increased atrial size, reduced refractory period, and decreased conduction velocity. Whatever the cause, the outcome is a chaotic, rapid firing of multiple atrial ectopic foci without complete atrial depolarization.

Occasionally an impulse gets through the AV node and stimulates the ventricle but the ventricular stimulation is irregular, allowing time for pooling of blood and potential thrombus formation. Dislodgement of these potential thrombi or the presence of extremely rapid ventricular rates causes the most dangerous and life-threatening sequela of atrial fibrillation. These complications include (but are not limited to) hemodynamic instability, congestive heart failure, pulmonary edema, and cerebral vascular accident.

There are two sequelae to AF:

Controlled ventricular response (rate 60 to 100 beats/min)
Uncontrolled ventricular response (rate >100 beats/min)
  Symptoms include anxiety, palpitations, syncope, angina.
  There may be an inadequate ventricular filling time, leading to decreased cardiac output.
Chronic AF is associated with cardiovascular diseases, including congestive heart failure, (CHF), rheumatic heart disease, cardiomyopathy, mitral valve disease, and chronic lung disease.

SUBJECTIVE DATA

Symptoms

The patient may be asymptomatic or may have severe, debilitating, and potentially life-threatening symptoms. Atrial fibrillation may be discovered as a incidental finding during a physical examination or may be the reason for an acute onset of chest pain, palpitations, or dyspnea. Other symptoms include angina, heart failure, palpitations, dizziness, fatigue, and syncope.

History of Present Illness

Ask the patient about the onset of symptoms.
Determine whether similar episodes have ever occurred.

Onset is *very* important in determining the appropriate treatment.

Ask whether the following have been noted:

- Palpitations
- Angina
- Fatigue
- Dizziness
- Weight loss
- Hair loss
- Mood changes
- Emotional stress
- Drug or alcohol use
- Cough
- Hemoptysis
- Respiratory distress

Past Medical History

Ask about thyroid disorders, rheumatic fever, history of murmurs, congenital heart problems, recent infections, dental work, myocardial infarction, coronary artery bypass graft, enlarged heart, CHF, chronic obstructive pulmonary disease, hypertension, diabetes, valve replacements, or recent surgery.

Medications

List all current medicines including prescription, over-the-counter, and illicit drugs.

Family History

Ask about family history of heart problems, hypertension, cardiomyopathy, and thyroid problems.

Psychosocial History

Stress: Physical or emotional

Diet: Increased ingestion of caffeine or salt

Alcohol: Customary level of consumption, alcoholism, binging

Nicotine use: Cigars, cigarettes, smokeless tobacco

Soaking in hot tub in combination with consumption of alcohol

Description of Most Common Symptoms

Ask about dizziness, lightheadedness, chest pain, palpitations, dyspnea, exertional dyspnea, orthopnea, and cough.

Associated Symptoms

Associated symptoms may include diaphoresis, loss of consciousness, weakness of extremities, orthostatic hypotension, and dependent edema.

OBJECTIVE DATA

Physical Examination

A complete physical should be conducted with particular attention to:

- Vital signs, including orthostatic changes
- Weight
- General appearance, general hydration status
- Neck: Neck vein distention, bruits
- Chest: Adventitious sounds
- Cardiovascular: Extra heart sounds, murmur
- Abdominal: Bowel sounds, hepatojugular reflex
- Extremities: Edema, pulses
- Neurological: Alertness, level of consciousness

Diagnostic Procedures

Diagnostic procedures are outlined in Table 17-1. Diagnostic tests to consider when patient presents with various symptoms are shown in Table 17-2.

ASSESSMENT

Differential Diagnosis

Differential diagnoses for AF are outlined in Table 17-3.

THERAPEUTIC PLAN

NOTE: **Treatment of atrial fibrillation requires physician collaboration or referral. Initial treatment usually requires hospitalization and cardiac monitoring (Box 17-1).**

Pharmaceutical

Tables 17-4 through 17-7 list drugs that are potential choices for treatment of AF. However, there is no simple algorithm for treating AF. The existence of concomitant disease processes and potential imposter arrhythmias (such as Wolff-Parkinson-White syndrome) need to be taken into consideration.

It is imperative to keep in mind the goals of restoring sinus rhythm, controlling heart rate, and reducing cardiovascular risk when choosing the appropriate pharmacological treatment for AF. The drugs described in the tables are divided into groups according to the goal each might be used to achieve.

Nonpharmaceutical

Electrical cardioversion

- Emergent for rapid decompensation
- Elective procedure

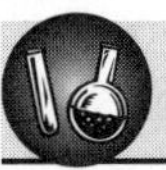

TABLE 17-1 Diagnostic Tests: Atrial Fibrillation

Diagnostic Test	When to Order	Finding/Rationale	Cost ($)
CBC, electrolytes	On presentation	Baseline data; identify potential etiologies for arrhythmias, such as anemia, leukocytosis	18-23/CBC; 23-30/Electrolytes
Thyroid function tests	On presentation	Rule out thyroid dysfunction; in a study with newly diagnosed AF patients, 3.3% had hyperthyroidism, and 4.8% had hypothyroidism	47-61
Renal function	On presentation	Baseline data to identify renal functioning	17-21/BUN 18-24/CR
CXR	On presentation	Identify underlying lung disease, signs of CHF, or cardiomegaly	77-91
ECG	On presentation	Identify arrhythmias and determine whether any changes are the result of MI	56-65
Echocardiogram	Soon after presentation with new onset AF	Identify valvular problems, chamber enlargement, or wall motion abnormalities, as well as identifying potential embolization of cardiac origin	675
Transesophageal echocardiogram	If heart is poorly visualized on transthoracic echocardiogram; also used if atrial fibrillation is new onset < 48 hr and electrocardioversion is being considered	May be indicated if there is a potential for electrical cardioversion to be needed or to identify thrombi in the left atrium or aortic arch; also evaluates valves and chamber size, and left atrial appendage (If thrombus is present, cardioversion is contraindicated until patient has undergone sufficient anticoagulation therapy.)	878-1035
Magnesium	On presentation, especially if chemical cardioversion with Corvert is a potential treatment	Hypomagnesemia	20-25
Prothrombin time, partial thromboplastin time	On presentation	As baseline before initiating anticoagulation therapy	22-27/PT; 23-29/PTT

CBC, Complete blood count; *AF*, atrial fibrillation; *BUN*, blood urea nitrogen; *CR*, creatinine; *CXR*, chest x-ray; *ECG*, electrocardiogram; *CHF*, congestive heart failure; *MI*, myocardial infarction.

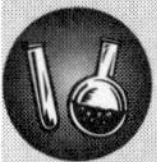

TABLE 17-2 Diagnostic Tests Based on Presenting Symptoms: Atrial Fibrillation

Symptoms	Findings	Diagnostic Tests	Cost($)
Irregular heart rate	Arrhythmias	ECG, event monitor, Holter monitor, echocardiogram	ECG: 56-65 ECHO: 675
Palpitations	Arrhythmias	ECG, event monitor, Holter monitor	CXR: 77-91
Cough (pulmonary congestion)	Adventitious lung sounds (crackles), decompensation secondary to atrial fibrillation with altered ventricular response	CXR, auscultation	
Dizziness	Hypotension	ECG, event monitor, Holter monitor, BP measurement	

CXR, Chest x-ray; *ECG*, electrocardiogram.

TABLE 17-3 Differential Diagnosis: Atrial Fibrillation

Diagnosis	Supporting Data
AF (new onset)	Acute onset of symptoms, previous documentation of sinus rhythm, evidence of AF on ECG (irregular supraventricular complexes with no obvious P waves)
Chronic AF	Documentation of AF on ECG, with previous documentation of AF on ECG
Hyperthyroidism	Decreased levels of TSH
CHF secondary to AF and altered ventricular response	Documentation of AF on ECG, CHF on CXR, dependent crackles in lungs on auscultation
Pericarditis	Low-grade fever, pain on deep inspiration, cardiac friction rub, pericardial effusion on echocardiogram
Pulmonary emboli	Dyspnea, hypoxemia, positive ventilation perfusion scan, positive pulmonary angiogram
Mitral valve stenosis	Diastolic murmur, mitral stenosis on echocardiogram, enlarged left atrium

AF, Atrial fibrillation; *ECG,* electrocardiogram; *TSH,* thyroid-stimulating hormone; *CHF,* congestive heart failure; *CXR,* chest x-ray.

Box 17-1

Therapeutic Goals for Atrial Fibrillation

Rate Control

The goal should be a resting heart rate of 60-80 beats/min, not exceeding 100 beats/min with slight exercise.

Risk Reduction

Prevent formation of emboli through anticoagulation therapy.

Prevention of Electrical Remodeling

Prevent electrical remodeling by conversion to sinus rhythm if possible.

Prolonged atrial fibrillation (AF) causes cardiac anatomical changes that perpetuate AF, such as fibrotic changes in the sinus node, atrial enlargement, disruption of the sarcoplasmic reticulum, increases in mitochondrial size, and decreases in atrial refractoriness.

New Onset Fibrillation

Transient Atrial Fibrillation

A paroxysm lasting less than 48 hours

Persistent Atrial Fibrillation

An episode of AF lasting more than 48 hours but with the potential to be converted to sinus rhythm

Treatment Plan

Consult with collaborating MD and/or cardiologist.
Hospitalize the patient and initiate heparin therapy.
Rule out myocardial infarction or ischemia.
Evaluate laboratory results and vital signs.
Control heart rate.
Correct precipitating events (abnormal thyroid hormone levels, fever, pain, fluid overload).

Consult with Cardiologist Concerning Treatment Options

Consider chemical cardioversion with ibutilide fumarate (Corvert) if new onset occurred less than 48 hours ago.
Consider electroshock cardioversion.
Consider consultation with an electrophysiologist.
A pacemaker may be indicated if the heart rate cannot be controlled without symptomatic bradycardia.

Chronic Atrial Fibrillation

AF is permanent.
Continue anticoagulation therapy and monitor the results (unless the use of anticoagulants is contraindicated).
Attempt rate control through pharmaceutical agents.

Maintenance of sinus rhythm
- Catheter ablation
- Surgery
- Atrial pacing
- Atrial defibrillation

Rate control
- Catheter ablation

Lifestyle/Activities

If risk is deemed low, heart rate is controlled, and sinus rhythm is maintained, no specific limitations in activity are indicated. If risk reduction is maintained by anticoagulation therapy, activities that could put the patient at high risk for bleeding should be limited. **Elderly** patients with a high risk for falling or medical noncompliance have to be

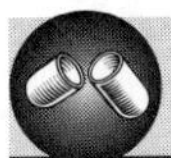

TABLE 17-4 Pharmaceutical Therapy to Restore Sinus Rhythm

Drug	Usual Adult Dosage	Comment	Cost
Adenosine (Adenocard)	IV: 6 mg (rapid IV push and flush; central line preferable)	If no response in 1-2 min, repeat with 12 mg; third dose of 12 mg can be given PRN Half-life is 10 sec	N/A
Ibutilide fumarate (Corvert)	>60 lb: 1 mg IV over 10 min (may repeat ×1) <60 lb: 0.01 mg/kg over 10 min (may repeat ×1)	Pregnancy: C SE: Sustained ventricular tachycardia; must correct hypokalemia or hypomagnesemia before administration; cardiac monitoring needed Proarrhythmic: If arrhythmias develop with this therapy electrical cardioversion and electrolyte therapy are treatment of choice Avoid use of other antiarrhythmics	$150/0.1 mg (10 ml)
Class IA (quinidine, Norpace, procainamide)	PO Procainamide: 17 mg/kg (total loading dose)	Pregnancy: C New or exacerbated arrhythmias, heart block, diarrhea, headache, syncope, flushing, hepatic dysfunction	$14/80 mg/ml (10 ml)
Amiodarone (Cordarone)	150 mg IV over 10 min, then 1 mg/min ×6 hr, then 0.5 mg ×18 hr PO load after IV is done and patient is converted PO load: 800-1600 mg/day for 1-3 wk, then 600-800 mg/day for 1 mo Maintenance: 200-600 mg/day	Pregnancy: C SE: Sinus arrest, arrhythmias, pulmonary fibrosis Interactions with many drugs: check before treatment Use sunscreen; take with food	$307/200 mg (100); $69/IV 50 mg/ml (3 ml)
Class IC Flecainide (Tambocor)	300-400 mg PO as a single bolus dose; 50-150 mg BID for maintenance (not first-line therapy) Reserve for resistant arrhythmia resulting from proarrhythmic effects	Pregnancy: C SE: Dizziness, lightheadedness, headache, fatigue, nausea, constipation	$67/50 mg (100); $122/100 mg (100); $168/150 mg (100)

N/A, Not available; *SE,* side effects.

thoroughly evaluated for risk/benefit of anticoagulation therapy.

Patients should also be counseled about smoking cessation, limiting alcohol intake, and avoiding the use of stimulants.

Diet

A 2-g sodium diet should be introduced if the AF is associated with CHF.

A step II diet should be introduced if the AF is associated with coronary artery disease.

For patients undergoing anticoagulation therapy with warfarin, the diet needs to be consistent, and foods high in vitamin K should be avoided.

Patient Education

Emphasize the importance of compliance with the medication regimen.

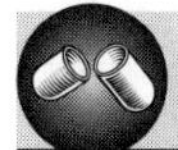

Table 17-5 Pharmaceutical Therapy to Maintain Sinus Rhythm

Drug	Dose	Comments	Cost
Amiodarone (Cordarone) Class III	After loading dose, usual maintenance dose is 200 mg QD; see Table 17-4 for loading information	Pregnancy: C Correct potassium and magnesium deficiencies before administering SE: Pulmonary fibrosis, increased arrhythmias, heart block, optic neuropathy, photosensitivity, thyroid disorders, malaise, peripheral neuropathy, GI upset Monitor digoxin levels when used concurrently, thyroid, CXR, liver function test	$307/200 mg (100); $69/IV 50 mg/ml (3 ml)
Disopyramide (Norpace) Class IA	400-600 mg/day in divided doses	**Must be used with negative ionotrope to prevent increased AV conduction** Pregnancy: C Adjust dose for renal impairment Avoid in CHF or heart block SE: Dry mouth, urinary retention, blurred vision, GI upset, fatigue, impotence, heart failure, edema, hypoglycemia, hypokalemia Monitor renal and glucose functions	$11/100 mg (100); $40-$80/150 mg (100)
Propafenone (Rythmol) Class 1C	150 mg TID Max daily dose: 900 mg/dl	Pregnancy: C Reduce dose if patient is in hepatic failure Watch for bradycardia, proarrhythmic events, hypotension, or bronchospasm Avoid in severe CHF SE: Fatigue, dizziness, GI upset, dyspnea, rhinitis, myalgia, elevated ANA titers Monitor digoxin and INR	$46/7.5 mg (100); $23-$70/15 mg (100)
Flecainide (Tambocor) Class 1C	50-200 mg BID Max daily dose: 400 mg/day	Reduce dose in renal impairment Not first-line therapy Pregnancy: C Correct potassium or magnesium levels before administration Precaution with CHF SE: new or exacerbated arrhythmias, headache, tremor, chest pain, GI upset, cardiac arrest, conduction defects, dizziness, lightheadedness, ↑CPK Monitor pacing thresholds, blood levels	$67/50 mg (100); $122/100 mg (100); $168/150 mg (100)

ANA, Antinuclear antibody; *AV,* atrioventricular; *CHF,* congestive heart failure; *CPK,* creatine phosphokinase; *CXR,* chest x-ray; *GI,* gastrointestinal; *INR,* international normalized ratio; *LFT,* liver function test; *SE,* side effects.

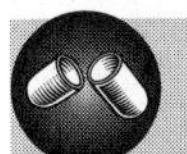

TABLE 17-5 Pharmaceutical Therapy to Maintain Sinus Rhythm—cont'd

Drug	Dose	Comments	Cost
Sotalol (Betapace) Nonselective beta-adrenergic blocker Class III	160-320 mg QD in divided doses Max daily dose: 640 mg/dl	Pregnancy category: B SE: New or exacerbated arrhythmias, bradycardia, chest pain, edema, palpitations, dyspnea, asthma, syncope, headache, GI upset, rash Cardiac monitoring with attention to Q-T interval	$161/80 mg (100); $215/120 mg (100); $269/160 mg (100)
Quinidine (Quinaglute) Class 1A	Maintenance dosage: 200-400 mg TID or QID	**Must be used in combination with digoxin or other agent to prevent increasing AV conduction** Pregnancy category: C SE: New or exacerbated arrhythmias, widening of QRS complex, anemia, thrombocytopenia, fever, flushing, impaired hearing and vision Monitor: Digoxin level (may need to decrease dose of digoxin), LFT	$8-$23/200 mg (100); $14-$31/300 mg (100)
Moricizine (Ethmozine) Class 1	200-300 mg PO TID	Pregnancy category: B Avoid in patients with right bundle-branch block and left hemiblock who do not have a pacemaker Watch for proarrhythmias, CHF, cardiac death	$97/200 mg (100); $116/250 mg (100); $132/300 mg (100)

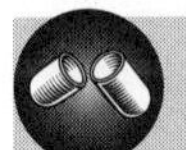

TABLE 17-6 Pharmaceutical Therapy for Rate Control

Drug	Adult Dose	Comments	Cost
Digoxin (Lanoxin) (cardiac glycoside and positive ionotrope)	0.125-0.25 mg daily after digitalization, then dosage managed based on digoxin level and symptoms	Pregnancy: C SE: Bradycardia, anorexia, nausea, heart block, visual disturbances Monitor digoxin level yearly unless toxic symptoms develop, change in rate/rhythm	$8-$11/0.125 mg (100); $20/0.5 mg (100); $8-$11/0.25 mg (100)
Diltiazem (Cardizem) Class IV (also can use verapamil) (Calan)	30 mg QID up to 360 mg/dl in divided doses or in 180-240 mg sustained-release form (can also be given IV at 0.25 mg/kg [load]) May repeat ×1 at 0.35 mg/kg if needed Continuous infusion to a maximum of 15 mg/hr	Pregnancy: C SE: Bradycardia, constipation, hypotension Monitor digoxin level closely if added	$71-$92/60 mg (100); $81-$105/90 mg (100); $96-$136/120 mg (100)
Esmolol (Brevibloc) Class II	Load 500 μg/kg IV over 1 min, then infuse 56-200 μg/kg/min Half-life is 9 min	Pregnancy: C SE: bradycardia, second- or third-degree heart block, hypotension, nausea, asthma Monitor B/P, HR	$5/250 mg/ml (10 ml); $11/10 mg/ml (10 ml)
Beta blockers metoprolol (Lopressor) atenolol (Tenormin)	Used for rate control (non-FDA approved use) Met: 2.5-5 mg IV bolus over 2 min, up to 3 doses	Pregnancy: B (met); C (aten) SE: Fatigue, dizziness, lethargy Multiple drug interactions: check before treatment	met, slow release: $45/50 mg (100); $67/100 mg (100); aten: $9-$88/25 mg (100); $5-$90/50 mg (100)

B/P, Blood pressure; *HR*, heart rate; *SE*, side effects.

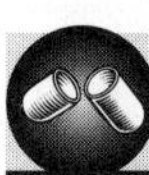

TABLE 17-7 Miscellaneous Pharmaceutical Therapy

Drug	Dose	Comments	Cost
Warfarin sodium (Coumadin)	Dosage titrated to goal INR of 2-3 If in AF <48 hr, risk of embolic event is low; if > 48 hr, should be treated with anticoagulants for 3 weeks before pharmacological or electrical cardioversion is attempted	Prevention of clots/CVA (see Chapter 12) Pregnancy: X SE: Multiple drug interactions, hemorrhage, rash	$47/2 mg (100); $30-$50/5 mg (100); $73/7.5 mg (100)

INR, International normalized ratio; *AF,* atrial fibrillation; *CVA,* cardiovascular accident.

Patient and family should be instructed in the anticoagulation purposes, side effects, and risk factors related to anticoagulation therapy.

Patient and family should be educated as to when to seek emergency treatment.

Provide information about the signs of complications: weight gain, dyspnea, dizziness, rapid heart rate, palpitations, and exertional dyspnea.

Family Impact

Families can assist patients by watching for signs of complications or subtle signs of decompensation, such as progressive dyspnea or edema. The family should also be aware of symptoms of drug toxicity or side effects.

Referral/Consultation

Refer for new onset AF, tachycardic or bradycardic arrhythmias, or hemodynamic instability.

Referral to a cardiologist and electrophysiologist may be appropriate.

Follow-up

If the patient is not hospitalized, he or she should return for a follow-up within 24 to 48 hours for evaluation or 4 to 6 weeks after stabilization in hospital, then every 3 to 6 months.

Follow-up laboratory tests should be scheduled for regulation of anticoagulation therapy. Potassium and digoxin levels should be monitored.

EVALUATION

Rate control

Absence of dizziness, syncope, CHF, embolic events

Periodic reevaluation by echocardiography

RESOURCES

Commercial web site for atrial fibrillation, 1-800-462-6687; http://www.incontrol.com/atrial/welcome.htm

American Heart Association, http://www.amhrt.org

SUGGESTED READINGS

Anderson JL: Acute treatment of atrial fibrillation and flutter, *Am J Cardiol* 78(8A):17-21, 1996.

Antman EM: Maintaining sinus rhythm with antifibrillatory drugs in atrial fibrillation, *Am J Cardiol* 78(Suppl 4):67-72, 1996.

Chrzanowski D.: Managing atrial fibrillation to prevent its major complication: ischemic stroke, *Nurs Pract* 23:26-42, 1998.

Coumel P, Thomas O, Leenhardt A: Drug therapy for prevention of atrial fibrillation, *Am J Cardiol* 77:3A-9A, 1996.

Dell'Orfano J et al: Drugs for conversion of atrial fibrillation, *Am Family Physician* 58:471-480, 1998.

Dubin D: Rapid interpretation of EKGs (pocket reference), Tampa, 1996, *Cover,* pp 159-161.

Ellenbogen KA et al: Efficacy of ibutilide for termination of atrial fibrillation and flutter, *Am J Cardiol* 78 (Suppl 8A):42-45, 1996.

Ellsworth A et al: *Mosby's 1998 medical drug reference,* St Louis, 1998, Mosby.

Gottlieb SH: Arrhythmias. In Barker LR, Burton JR, Zieve PD, editors: *Principles of ambulatory medicine,* Baltimore, 1995, Williams & Wilkins.

Healthcare Consultants of America, Inc: *1998 Physicians fee and coding guide,* Augusta, Ga, 1998, Healthcare Consultants of America, Inc.

Howard PA: Amiodarone for the maintenance of sinus rhythm in patients with atrial fibrillation, *Ann Pharmacother* 29:569-602, 1995.

Kowey PR, WanderLugt JR, Luderer JR.: Safety and risk/ benefit analysis of ibutilide for acute conversion of atrial fibrillation/flutter, *Am J Cardiol* 78 (Suppl 8A):46-52, 1996.

Zipes DP: Specific arrhythmias: diagnosis and treatment. In Braunwald E, editor: *Heart disease: a textbook of cardiovascular medicine,* Philadelphia, 1992, WB Saunders.

Attention-Deficit Hyperactivity Disorder

ICD-9-CM

Attention Deficit Disorder 314.00
Attention Deficit Disorder with Hyperactivity 314.01

OVERVIEW

Definition

Attention-deficit hyperactivity disorder (ADHD) is the current term applied to a specific developmental disorder of both children and adults that is characterized by deficits in sustained attention, impulse control, and the regulation of activity level to situational demands. ADHD, has had a variety of labels, including: hyperkinetic disorder of childhood, minimal brain dysfunction, attention deficit disorder (with or without hyperactivity).

Incidence

ADHD is one of the most common disorders of childhood, affecting 3% to 5% of **children.** The disorder occurs much more frequently in males than in females; the male-to-female ratios range from 4/1 to 9/1, depending on the setting (i.e., general population or clinics). It is estimated that one child in every classroom in the United States needs help for the disorder.

Pathophysiology

There are many different theories about the cause of ADHD. There may be a biological basis—an imbalance in brain chemistry, especially neurotransmitters such as dopamine, norepinephrine, and serotonin. ADHD has a genetic component in that 30% to 40% of children diagnosed with ADHD have relatives with similar difficulties. Cerebral blood flow studies show frontal hypoperfusion; thus frontal lobe dysfunction is suspected.

The following is a list of environmental toxins that have been incorrectly identified as causes of ADHD. There is no scientific proof to render these toxins responsible for the development of ADHD:

Food additives
Food dyes
Preservatives
Salicylates
Refined sugar
Fluorescent lighting

Factors that have been linked to ADHD include:

Prenatal and postnatal exposure to lead
Cigarette smoking during pregnancy
Alcohol consumption during pregnancy
Drug abuse during pregnancy
Poor maternal prenatal nutrition
Brain injuries during and after birth
Infections
ADHD may be a side effect of sedatives or anticonvulsants
Prematurity

SUBJECTIVE DATA

History of Present Illness

Ask about the onset of symptoms. ADHD onset is usually identified as occurring before the patient is 7 years old, with a duration of symptoms greater than 6 months. Ask the parents to list the behaviors that concern them and identify when they first noticed each behavior.

Psychiatric History

Ask the parents if the child has received mental health or psychiatric services for behavior difficulties before the current situation.

Ask whether the child has ever been evaluated by a mental health professional.

Ask whether members of the extended family have had behavior problems, mental illness, or ADHD.

Family History

Develop a list of all members of the household.
Ask whether there have been changes in who lives in the household—when, who, and why.
Ask about physical and sexual abuse.
Elicit information about how the child gets along with siblings.

School History

Inquire about the child's entire school history, from the first school experience, including preschool and day care.
Ask about school changes—when and why.
Ask about the child's attitude toward school, academic performance, relationship with teacher, what subjects are liked and disliked, and any instructional modifications that have occurred.
Ask whether the child is in special programs or receiving support services at the school.

Peer Relationships

Ask the child about friends at school and in the neighborhood and what the child likes to do with friends.
Ask whether the child has friends of the same age.
Ask about drug/alcohol abuse/use and sexual activity.

Past Medical History

Obtain the child's prenatal history, including exposure to lead, cigarette smoking, alcohol consumption, drug abuse, and prenatal nutrition. Other areas to explore include:

Brain injuries during and after birth
Infections
Chronic health problems
History of accidents
Allergies

Medications

Ask whether the child is taking or ever has taken any of the following:
methylphenidate (Ritalin), dextroamphetamine (Dexedrine), pemoline (Cylert), Adderall, tranquilizers, anticonvulsants, antihistamines, antidepressants, other prescription drugs

Psychosocial History

Ask questions about involvement with the police and custody issues.

Observe interaction between the parent and the child:
Parents of hyperactive children are more likely to give commands to their children.
Parents may be more negative toward the child and less likely to respond to the social initiatives of the child toward them.
Hyperactive children are more negative, less compliant, and less able to sustain compliance to parental commands.

Developmental History

Ask about the completion of developmental milestones.
Children with ADHD demonstrate behavioral characteristics during developmental stages:
Infancy: Sleep problems, crying, feeding problems
Preschool: Increased gross motor activity
School: Restlessness, inattention, impulsiveness
Adolescence: Rebelliousness and antisocial behaviors

Description of Most Common Symptoms

Uninhibited behavior, demonstrated by lack of ability to regulate behavior by awareness of rules and consequences
Inability to sustain attention; easily bored with repetitive tasks, loss of concentration during lengthy tasks, and failure to complete tasks or activities without supervision
Impaired impulse control; inability to stop and think about consequences before acting, interrupting conversations, not able to wait one's turn, needing immediate rewards rather than being able to wait for a long-term reward
Displaying excessive movements; typically "on the move," fidgeting, restless, can't sit still, "bouncing off the walls" (Box 18-1)

OBJECTIVE DATA

Physical Examination

Conduct a complete physical examination of the child, including hearing and vision testing. Determine whether the child has any developmental or learning difficulties such as problems with motor skills, motor coordination, memory, remembering sequences, listening and speaking, and recognizing and reproducing pictures and symbols.

Behavioral Assessment

Obtain information about the child's behavior in a variety of settings: school, play, at home, organized sports, youth organizations, and after school programs. Use any of the available "checklists" or behavior rating scales to have teachers and others who observe the child's behavior assess the child's behavior in different environments. Two straightforward and easy-to-use tools are those developed by Connors and Taylor (see the assessment form on p. 118).

Box 18-1

DSM IV Criteria

A. Either 1 or 2:
  1. Six (or more) of the following symptoms of inattention have persisted for at least 6 months to a degree that is maladaptive and inconsistent with developmental level:
     Inattention
     a. Often fails to give close attention to details or makes careless mistakes in schoolwork, work, or other activities
     b. Often has difficulty sustaining attention in tasks or play activities
     c. Often does not seem to listen when spoken to directly
     d. Often does not follow through on instructions and fails to finish schoolwork, chores, or duties in the workplace (not due to oppositional behavior or failure to understand instructions)
     e. Often has difficulty organizing tasks and activities
     f. Often avoids, dislikes, or is reluctant to engage in tasks that require sustained mental effort (such as schoolwork or homework)
     g. Often loses things necessary for tasks or activities (e.g., toys, school assignments, pencils, books, or tools)
     h. Is often easily distracted by extraneous stimuli
     i. Is often forgetful in daily activities
  2. Six (or more) of the following symptoms of hyperactivity-impulsivity have persisted for at least 6 months to a degree that is maladaptive and inconsistent with developmental level:
     Hyperactivity
     a. Often fidgets with hands or feet or squirms in seat
     b. Often leaves seat in classroom or in other situations in which remaining seated is expected
     c. Often runs about or climbs excessively in situations in which it is inappropriate (in adolescents or adults, may be limited to subjective feelings of restlessness)
     d. Often has difficulty playing or engaging in leisure activities quietly
     e. Is often "on the go" or often acts as if "driven by a motor"
     f. Often talks excessively
     Impulsivity
     g. Often blurts out answers before questions have been completed
     h. Often has difficulty awaiting turn
     i. Often interrupts or intrudes on others (e.g., butts into conversations or games)

B. Some hyperactive-impulsive or inattentive symptoms that caused impairment were present before age 7 years.
C. Some impairment from the symptoms is present in two or more settings (e.g., at school [or work] and at home).
D. There must be clear evidence of clinically significant impairment in social, academic, or occupational functioning.
E. The symptoms do not occur exclusively during the course of a pervasive developmental disorder, schizophrenia, or other psychotic disorder and are not better accounted for by another mental disorder (e.g., mood disorder, anxiety disorder, dissociative disorder, or personality disorder).

From American Psychiatric Association: *Diagnostic and statistical manual of mental disorders,* ed 4, Washington, DC, 1994, The Association.

Diagnostic Procedures

There are currently no laboratory tests available to make the diagnosis of ADHD, although a battery of tests may be ordered to rule out other neurodevelopmental illnesses.

ASSESSMENT

Use the DSM IV criteria to make diagnosis based on history, questionnaires, and physical examination (Table 18-1).

Differential diagnoses include:
- Oppositional defiant disorder (ODD)
- Conduct disorder (CD)
- Generalized anxiety disorder
- Learning disorders
- Mental retardation
- Understimulating environment
- Developmentally appropriate behaviors in active children

Comorbidity frequently occurs:
- ADHD + ODD
- ADHD + CD
- ADHD + Depression
- ADHD + Anxiety disorders

THERAPEUTIC PLAN

Pharmaceutical/Nonpharmaceutical Plan

Central nervous system stimulants are very effective for the management of symptoms, primarily attention span and impulse control. (These medications are schedule II drugs and in most states must be prescribed by a physician; Table 18-2.) Changes in other behaviors are most likely the result of the improvement in attention span and impulse control. School performance will also show improvement as a result

Table 18-1 Differential Diagnosis: Attention-Deficit Hyperactivity Disorder

Diagnosis	Supporting Data
Oppositional defiant disorder (ODD)	Characteristic behavior is negativistic, hostile, and defiant, lasting at least 6 months. These **children** and **adolescents** demonstrate persistent stubbornness, resistance to directions, and unwillingness to compromise or negotiate with peers or adults.
Conduct disorder (CD)	Characteristic behavior includes a repetitive and persistent pattern of violating the basic rights of others or major age-appropriate societal norms. **Children** or **adolescents** with CD are quick to initiate aggressive behavior toward others as well as react aggressively toward others.
Generalized anxiety disorder (GAD)	Behavior is characterized by excessive anxiety and worry that occurs on more days than not and lasts for at least 6 months. **Children** with GAD will demonstrate restlessness, feeling keyed up or on edge, difficulty concentrating, and irritability.
Learning disorder (LD)	Child's demonstrated achievement on standardized tests in reading, math, or written expression is substantially below the expected scores for age, schooling, and intelligence. (These tests must be individually administered to be valid.) These **children** and adolescents demonstrate demoralization, low self-esteem, and poor social skills.
Mental retardation	Child demonstrates significantly subaverage general intellectual functioning accompanied by limited adaptive functioning.
Neurological abnormalities	Need to rule out the presence of neoplasms or other intracranial assault/abnormalities that might be causing hyperactivity.

of medication. Medication is only part of the treatment, and if this is all the child receives, the results may be less than desired.

Psychological and Behavioral Approaches

Parents must be educated about ADHD, including a review of symptoms, its course, and what is known about causative factors. Training the parents in the use of techniques for dealing with the child's behavior is one of the best therapeutic approaches, when done properly. Behavior management skills help the parents to reduce negative behaviors and promote positive behaviors. Parents need guidance on modifying the environment rather than the child. The child with ADHD functions best in a highly structured environment with clear rules, limits, and consequences. Parents will benefit from counseling in the areas of acceptance of ADHD and the potential for grief reaction.

Psychotherapy may be needed to help some children with ADHD to cope with the anxiety, depression, and self-esteem issues they are experiencing. Family therapy is helpful to improve communication within the family and help siblings deal with their concerns. Social skills training and peer relationship training may be beneficial to children with ADHD, because they demonstrate problems in social situations and are at high risk for peer rejection.

Educational/School Interventions

Teacher and staff education on ADHD
Teacher training in classroom management of ADHD
Work with the teacher to develop educational approaches and ensure consistency between home and school

Diet

Recent reliable research supports a reduction in the use of artificial additives and the intake of simple sugars, showing an improvement in 50% of the children in the study.

Referral

All children with ADHD need to be assessed and evaluated by a mental health professional. NOTE: Because not all mental health professionals work with children or specifically with ADHD, it is important to know who you are referring to and how they can help the child and family.

A child requiring a combination of medications should be referred to a child psychiatrist/NP. The psychiatric clinical nurse specialist can be helpful with monitoring medication and providing counseling services. The child psychologist and social worker may not have pharmacological privileges but can be helpful in providing counseling services.

Consultation

Be aware of state laws with regard to who can prescribe stimulant medications, and seek consultation when side effects are reported.

EVALUATION

Treatment of ADHD is long term, adjustments in medications must be made as the child grows. Work with the child

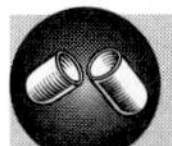

TABLE 18-2 Pharmaceutical Plan: Attention-Deficit Hyperactivity Disorder

Medication	Dose	Comments	Cost
Methylphenidate (Ritalin) (schedule II)	Initial: 0.3 mg/kg/dose or 2.5-5 mg/dose BID, dose given early morning and midday TID dose given early morning, midday, after school Increase by 0.1 mg/kg/dose or 5-10 mg/day at weekly intervals Usual dose: 0.5-1 mg/kg/day Maximum dose not to exceed 60 mg/day Dosage form: tablet: 5 mg, 10 mg, 20 mg	Caution: Pregnancy SE: Nervousness, insomnia, weight loss, headache, tachycardia, abdominal pain	\$25-\$31/5 mg (100); \$35-\$45/10 mg (100); \$50-\$64/20 mg (100)
Methylphenidate (Ritalin) SR	One dose/day effective 8 hours Dosage form: tablet: 20 mg SR	Same SE as above Response less predictable	\$79-\$98/SR (100)
Dextroamphetamine sulfate (Dexedrine) (schedule II)	3-5 years old: 2.5 mg/day given every morning Increase by 2.5 mg/day in weekly intervals until optimal response is obtained Usual range is 0.1- 0.5 mg/kg/dose every morning Maximum dose 40 mg/day 6 years and older: 5 mg once or twice daily Increase in increments of 5 mg/day at weekly intervals until optimum response is reached Usual range is 0.1-0.5 mg/kg/dose every morning Maximum dose 40 mg/day Dosage form: tablet: 5 mg, 10 mg	Pregnancy: C SE: Palpitations, ↑ B/P, overstimulation, restlessness, insomnia, headache, weight loss	\$18-\$20/5 mg (100); \$30-\$31/10 mg (100)
Dextroamphetamine sulfate (Dexedrine) spansule long-acting	One dose/day Dosage form: capsule: 5 mg, 10 mg, 15 mg	Same SE as above Better absorbed and more predictable than Ritalin SR	\$21-\$30/5 mg (50); \$27/10 mg (50); \$34/15 mg (50)
Adderall	3-5 years old: initial dose 2.5 mg/day Increase in increments of 2.5 mg/day at weekly intervals until optimal response is reached 6 years and older: initial dose 5 mg 1-2 times/day Increase in increments of 5 mg/day at weekly intervals until optimal response is reached Dosage form: tablet: 5 mg, 10 mg, 20 mg, 30 mg	Pregnancy: C SE: High abuse potential, hypertension, tachycardia, CNS overstimulation, dry mouth, GI disorders, anorexia, urticaria (mixture of dextro-amphetamine sulfate and saccharate, and amphetamine aspartate and sulfate)	\$4/5 mg (100); \$6/10 mg (100); \$75/20 mg (100)

SE, Side effects; *SR,* sustained release; *B/P,* blood pressure; *CNS,* central nervous system; *GI,* gastrointestinal; *FDA,* Food and Drug Administration; *CV,* cardiovascular.

Continued

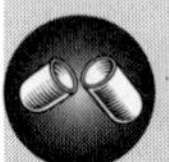

TABLE 18-2 Pharmaceutical Plan: Attention-Deficit Hyperactivity Disorder—cont'd

Medication	Dose	Comments	Cost
Pemoline (Cylert) (schedule IV)	Initial: 37.5 mg in the morning, ↑ weekly if needed by 18.75 mg daily, maximum 112.5 mg/day Not recommended <6 years old	Pregnancy: B Less effective than other drugs; requires liver function tests q 6mo SE: Insomnia, anorexia, CNS effects, dizziness, headache, hepatic dysfunction	$129/37.5 mg (100); (chewable) tablet: $75/18.75 mg (100); $75-$204/37.5 mg (100)
Clonidine (Catapres)	Initial: 0.05 mg at HS Begin gradual titration every week by 0.05 mg Max dose 0.2 mg	Pregnancy: C Not FDA-approved for ADHD; may be useful for children who cannot take stimulants. It may help with frustration tolerance and disinhibition. CAUTION: **Do not stop giving medication suddenly. Do not use if the patient has a history of CV disease or depression.** SE: Dry mouth, drowsiness, sedation, agitation, arrhythmias	$2-$5/0.1 mg (100); $2-$86/0.2 mg (100); $3-$108/0.3 mg (100)
Imipramine (Tofranil)	Initial dose, >6 years of age: 0.5 mg/kg/day, up to 25 mg day Gradually ↑; BID dosing recommended	Not FDA-approved for ADHD, but may be helpful if depression or anxiety is present. SE: Sedation, anticholinergic and orthostatic hypotension; titrate slowly	$2-$26/10 mg (100); $2-$44/25 mg (100); $3-$74/50 mg (100)

and the family will change as the child and family changes. It was previously thought that children "outgrow" ADHD, now it is more widely accepted that ADHD has an inborn biological basis and that parents and children can learn how to cope with the behavioral difficulties rather than cure them. The core symptoms of ADHD are carried into adulthood by 50% to 80% of the children diagnosed with ADHD.

RESOURCES

Attention Deficit Information Network
617-455-9895
www.5mcc.com

Attention Deficit Disorder Advocacy Group
430 W. Park Blvd, Plano TX 75-93
303-690-7548

SUGGESTED READINGS

Adderall: the newest available option: ADHD, *Adv Nurs Pract* 5:73-74, 1997.

American Psychiatric Association: *Diagnostic and statistical manual of mental disorders,* ed 4, Washington, DC, 1994, The Association.

Barkley RA: *Attention-deficit hyperactivity disorder: a handbook for diagnosis and treatment,* New York, 1990, Guilford Press.

Barkley RA: *Attention-deficit hyperactivity disorder: a clinical workbook,* New York, 1991, Guilford Press.

Biederman J et al: Is childhood oppositional defiant disorder a precursor to adolescent conduct disorder? Findings from a four-year follow-up study of children with ADHD, *J Am Acad Child Adolesc Psychiatry* 35:1193-1204, 1996.

Biederman J et al: A prospective 4-year follow-up study of attention-deficit hyperactivity and relate disorders, *Arch Gen Psychiatry* 53:437-446, 1996.

Biederman J et al: Predictors of persistence and remission of ADHD into adolescence: results from a four-year prospective follow-up study, *J Am Acad Child Adolesc Psychiatry* 35:343-351, 1996.

Bpscj J: ADHD, *J Pediatr Healthcare* 11:306, 1997.

Cantwell D: ADHD through the lifespan: role of bupropion in treatment, *J Clin Psychiatry* 59(Suppl 4): 92-94, 1998.

Connors C et al: A new self-report scale for assessment of adolescent psychopathology: factor structure, reliability, validity and diagnostic sensitivity, *J Abnorm Child Psychol* 25:487-497, 1997.

Dahl RE: The impact of inadequate sleep on children's daytime cognitive function, *Semin Pediatr Neurol* 3:44-50, 1996.

Ellsworth A et al: *Mosby's 1998 medical drug reference,* St Louis, 1998, Mosby.

Healthcare Consultants of America, Inc: *1998 Physicians fee and coding guide*, Augusta, Ga, 1998, Healthcare Consultants of America, Inc.

Hellerman S, Seibold E: Learning disabilities. In Fox F, editor: *Primary health care of children,* St Louis, 1997, Mosby.

Javorsky J: An examination of youth with attention-deficit/hyperactivity disorder and language learning disabilities: a clinical study, *J Learn Disabil* 29:247-258, 1996.

Kendall J: The use of qualitative methods in the study of wellness in children with attention deficit hyperactivity disorder, *J Child Adolesc Psychiatr Nurs* 10:27-38, 1997.

MacDonald VM, Achenback TM: Attention problems versus conduct problems as six-year predictors of problem scores in a national sample, *J Am Acad Child Adolesc Psychiatry* 35:1237-1246, 1996.

Murphy KR, Barkley RA: Parents of children with attention-deficit/hyperactivity disorder: psychological and attentional impairment, *Am J Orthopsychiatry* 66:93-102, 1996.

Nemeth M: ADHD: a guide to diagnosis and treatment, *Adv Nurs Pract* 5:22-25, 1997.

Ricchini M: Self esteem and ADHD: too important to overlook, *Adv Nurs Pract* 5(5):59, 1997.

Taylor E et al: Hyperactivity and conduct problems as risk factors for adolescent development, *J Am Acad Cild Adolesc Psychiatry* 35:1213-1226, 1996.

CHILDREN'S HOSPITAL MEDICAL CENTER
PEDIATRIC PRIMARY CARE CLINIC

Behavior/Activity Assessment

Child's Name: ______________________ **Date:** ____________

Teacher: ______________________ **School Grade:** ____________

Physician Requesting Form: ______________________

Part I: Connors

Behavior	Not At All (0)	Little (1)	Pretty Much (2)	Very Much (3)
1. Restless (overactive)	______	______	______	______
2. Excitable, impulsive	______	______	______	______
3. Disturbs other children	______	______	______	______
4. Fails to finish things he starts (short attention span)	______	______	______	______
5. Fidgeting	______	______	______	______
6. Inattentive, distractable	______	______	______	______
7. Demands must be met immediately	______	______	______	______
8. Cries	______	______	______	______
9. Mood changes quickly	______	______	______	______
10. Temper outbursts (explosive and unpredictable behavior)	______	______	______	______

Part II: Taylor

Activity	More Like This (0)	No Trend (1)	More Like This (2)	Activity
1. Quiet when sitting				Noisy and talkative when sitting
2. Voice volume soft or average				Voice is generally too loud
3. Few mouth or body noises				Makes lots of clicks, whistles, and sounds with mouth/body
4. Walks at appropriate times				Runs and jumps rather than walks
5. Keeps hands to self				Pokes, touches, feels, and grabs
6. Appears calm, can be still				Always something moving; fidgets with hands or feet; jumpy

Continued

Part II: Taylor (cont'd) **Activity**	**More Like This (0)**	**No Trend (1)**	**More Like This (2)**	**Activity**
7. Can just sit				Has to be doing something when sitting to occupy self
8. Concentrates, blocks out distractions				Gets distracted by noises, people, etc.
9. Slow to react, thinks before acting				Quick to react, reacts on impulse
10. Finishes one thing before starting on another				Starts many new things without finishing any
11. Obeys directions and follows orders				Disobeys and needs supervision or reminding
12. Avoids joining into others' mischief				Attracted by and gets drawn into other's mischief
13. Understands why others are displeased after misbehavior				Expects others not to be displeased by misbehavior, or does not realize that misbehavior has occurred
14. Thinks ahead to later consequences				Acts without considering consequences, doesn't plan ahead
15. Cooperates, obeys and enforces rules				Wants rules changed, wants to be the exception
16. Concerned about punishments and consequences				Pretends to have an "I don't care" attitude if threatened or punished
17. Constant mood with mild or slow mood changes				Rapid and extreme mood changes, happy one minute and hostile the next, moody
18. Gives up when denied by parent or teacher				When denied, child pesters, harps on it, doesn't give up
19. Easy going, can accept frustration, can take no for an answer				Irritable, can't accept frustration, can't take no for an answer
20. Doesn't try to bother or hurt others with words				Needles, teases, picks on others with words
21. Emotions don't disrupt relationships, are reasonably restrained				Emotions are extreme rather than moderated; child seems ruled by them; very hostile or very affectionate

Office use only.

1. Connors Total Score ______________
   (0-30)
2. Taylor Total Score ______________
   (0-42)

Norms:	Connors	0-14
	Taylor	0-27

____

NAME OF PERSON COMPLETING FORM

■ TEACHER ■ PARENT/GUARDIAN

DATE OF COMPLETION: ______________

Bartholin Cyst

ICD-9-CM

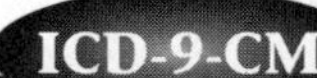

Bartholin Cyst 616.2

OVERVIEW

Definition

The Bartholin glands are a pair of pea-sized glands embedded in the erectile tissue of the bulb of the vestibule of the vagina. They are drained by a 2-cm duct and open into the vestibule at the junction of the labia minora and the hymen. They function to maintain moisture of the nonkeratinized epithelium of the vestibule, but they contribute very little to vaginal lubrication during intercourse. A Bartholin cyst arises from this gland or its ducts.

Incidence

Unknown

Pathophysiology

Bartholin cysts arise from intraluminal expansion of trapped mucus resulting from blockage of the major duct or one of its larger branches, possibly by one of the following:

Accidental or obstetrical trauma
Congenital atresia
Epithelial hyperplasia
Infection with secondary edema

Most cysts result from simple obstruction from unknown causes, remain smaller than 4 cm, and are not infected. However:

Infected cysts are often extremely painful, which signals infection instead of a simple blockage.
Most contain mixed vaginal flora.
Ten percent of infected Bartholin cysts are positive for either gonorrhea or chlamydia; prior infection with either organism may result in scarring, blockage, or abscess formation.

SUBJECTIVE DATA

History of Present Illness

Patient generally complains when acute symptoms signal infection.
Patient presents with pain and tenderness of the vaginal area with dyspareunia; often sits off to one side because of pain.
The surrounding tissue becomes edematous and inflamed.
A unilateral mass is palpable in the vaginal opening.
Additional pertinent information:
- Onset and duration of the symptoms
- Relieving factors
- History of sexually transmitted diseases (STDs)
- History of recent trauma
- History of diethylstilbestrol exposure

Past Medical History

Prior problems with infections or masses around the vagina

Medications

Current medications

Family History

Not applicable

Psychosocial History

Ask about previous STDs, current relationship with partner, if partner has symptoms

OBJECTIVE DATA

Physical Examination

Vital signs, including temperature and blood pressure
Inguinal lymph nodes

Benign Noninfectious Cysts

Small, noninflamed cysts are often asymptomatic and of little consequence unless progressive enlargement compromises the vaginal introitus or acute infection occurs.

Infected Bartholin cysts

External genitalia
- A tender, fluctuant mass is palpable at the introitus.
- Surrounding tissue may be erythematous and edematous.

Pelvic examination
- An examination with use of a speculum is often impossible because of pain

Diagnostic Procedures

Diagnostic procedures are outlined in Table 19-1.

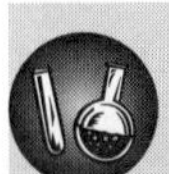

TABLE 19-1 Diagnostic Tests: Bartholin Cyst

Diagnostic Test	Finding/ Rationale	Cost ($)
Culture of secretions from gland	Rule out gonorrhea, chlamydia, or other pathogens	31-39/ gonorrhea 49-62/ chlamydia

ASSESSMENT

Differential Diagnosis (Table 19-2)

Differential diagnoses include:
- Vulvar lesions: Sebaceous cyst, hematoma, fibroma, lipoma, endometriosis, accessory breast tissue, leiomyoma, adenocarcinoma
- Vaginal lesions: Vaginal inclusion cyst, endometriosis, adenosis, leiomyoma, inguinal hernia

THERAPEUTIC PLAN

Pharmaceutical

In most cases antibiotics are not necessary, unless *Neisseria gonorrhoeae* or *Chlamydia* or other organisms are evident on culture.

Severe symptoms with pain, edema, or cellulitis may require therapy with antibiotic agents that are effective against streptococci and staphylococci.

Nonpharmaceutical

Small, benign cysts in women under 40 years old may be observed unless bothersome.

Large or tender cysts can be treated by simple incision and drainage, although these cysts tend to recur.

Recurrence requires creation of a fistulous tract from dilated duct to vestibule.

Simple incision and drainage with gauze packing relieves acute abscess pain.

Definitive therapy with marsupialization, excision, or insertion of a Word catheter is often necessary.

TABLE 19-2 Differential Diagnosis: Bartholin Cyst

Diagnosis	Supporting Data
Vulvar Lesions	
Sebaceous cyst	A cystic mass that is firm, globular, movable, and nontender; seldom causes discomfort unless infected
Hematoma	A localized mass of extravasated blood that is confined within a space, usually with history of trauma
Lipoma	Overgrowth of adipose tissue, nontender soft, well-circumscribed, lobulated, freely movable, painless masses in subcutaneous tissue; usually also on trunk or arms; typically expand downward along course of labia majora
Endometriosis	Cyclic pain 5-7 days before menses
Adenocarcinoma	Must be ruled out in a woman >40 years old who presents with a Bartholin cyst mass
Vaginal Lesions	
Endometriosis	Cyclic pain 5-7 days before menses
Adenosis	General name for any condition of a gland
Leiomyoma	Muscular benign tumor, may grow to >6 cm
Inguinal hernia	Narrow outpouching within vaginal walls
Vulvar carcinoma	Vulvar mass is the most common symptoms, usually occurring in women >65, bleeding, pain, or burning may also be noted

Lifestyle/Activities

Warm soaks may be helpful

Diet

Not applicable

Patient Education

Discuss the possibility that the symptoms may recur, since the duct outlet is distended.
Emphasize the need for immediate attention if an abscess forms.
The surgical site will heal slowly.
Emphasize the use of barrier contraceptives to protect against STDs.

Family Impact

A painful and swollen Bartholin duct will interfere with sexual activities, as well as activities of daily living, depending on the size of the abscess.

Referral

To rule out malignancy, all women over 40 years old and all postmenopausal women presenting with a cyst should be referred to a gynecologist for a complete excision under general anesthesia to rule out carcinoma.

Consultation

None

EVALUATION/FOLLOW-UP

None needed for nonsymptomatic cysts
Follow-up on weekly basis after incision and drainage

SUGGESTED READINGS

Ellsworth A et al: *Mosby's 1998 medical drug reference,* St Louis, 1998, Mosby.

Healthcare Consultants of America, Inc: *1998 Physicians fee and coding guide,* Augusta, Ga, 1998, Healthcare Consultants of America, Inc.

Hawkins J, Roberto-Nichols D, Stanley-Haney J: Bartholin cyst. In *Protocols for nurse practitioners in gynecologic settings,* ed 5, New York, 1995, The Tiresias Press.

Hill A, Lense J: Office management of Bartholin gland cysts and abscesses, *Am Family Physician* 57:1611-1616, 1998.

Newkirk G: Bartholin gland infections. In Johnson C, editor: *Women's health care handbook,* St Louis, 1996, Mosby.

Behavior Problems: Child

ICD-9-CM

Child Behavior Problems V71.02

OVERVIEW

Definition

A behavior problem is a behavior that is perceived by a supervising adult to deviate from acceptable norms. Common behavior problems include temper tantrums, hitting, kicking, biting, noncompliance, back-talk, fighting, arguing, yelling, and refusing to go to bed.

Incidence

First years of life through adolescence: Most children will display one or more problematic behaviors.
Preschool years: Highest—90% of mothers report at least mild concern.
Often undiagnosed (i.e., not addressed during health care visits).

Pathophysiology/Etiology

Unclear and irregular enforcement of parental expectations for behavior is the primary cause.
The temperament of the child and the quality of parenting skills are also contributing factors.
Research has demonstrated an association between a child's having behavior problems and maternal smoking, increased family stress, increased family size, illness in the family, socioeconomic status, and maternal marital status.

SUBJECTIVE DATA

Family History

Birth order, family composition, family dynamics, discipline techniques, illness, developmental milestones, family history of behavior problems
Description of misbehavior(s), parent response and its effectiveness
Consider:
- Age and sex appropriateness
- Persistence
- Life circumstance and precipitating events
- Setting/situation specificity
- Extent of disturbance
- Type, severity, and frequency of symptoms
- Change in behavior

OBJECTIVE DATA

Physical Examination

Complete physical examination (rule out illness or other physical etiology for behavior change)
Focus on the following areas:
- General: Observation of parent/child interaction; child's response to direction and correction; child's affect and behavior during play
- Neurological: Neurodevelopmental screen; vision and hearing screen

Diagnostic Procedures

Denver developmental screening tests (DDSTs)
Behavior rating scale
- Select scale according to age and complaint

Scales may be completed by supervising adults other than parents (e.g., teachers); school counselors have these scales; practitioner can request evaluation.
Helpful to differentiate the psychologically disturbed child

ASSESSMENT

Common (Minor) Behavior Problems

Differential Diagnosis

Normal behavior of childhood
Major behavior problem
Psychological disturbance
Learning disorder
Ineffective parenting
Dysfunctional parenting
Child abuse

THERAPEUTIC PLAN

Therapeutic Management

Establish a relationship with the child's family.
Acknowledge how difficult developmental issues can be to resolve.
Initiate a behavior management system as appropriate.
Refer for parenting classes, parent-support groups, and/or social services as needed.
Maintain open communication and support during the process of implementing the behavior management system; it may take weeks to notice any consistent change.

Patient Education

Developmental stages
- Expected behaviors according to developmental level
- Parents discuss and agree early in child's life what constitutes misbehavior (e.g., cute to some is misbehaving to others)

Discuss appropriate parenting strategies, including a system for behavior modification:
- Clear expectations
- Consequences (punishment) for misbehavior (Box 20-1 and Table 20-1)
- Positive reinforcement of appropriate behavior

Reinforce consistency as key to a successful system:
- Between parents and all caretakers
- Applicable across circumstances

Identify parents as role models (and encourage a consciousness for own behavior in all situations)
HELP—My Child Keeps Changing! on p. 126 can help facilitate discussion between practitioner and patient.

Box 20-1

Guidelines for Using Punishment

Use punishment sparingly.
Use mild punishment (avoid physical punishment).
Punish quickly after the misbehavior.
Punish only if you are in control of yourself.
Provide a brief reason for the punishment.

TABLE 20-1 Comparison of Mild Punishment

Method	Description	Applicable Ages
Distraction	Removal from situation by providing alternative site for attention (e.g., another toy if one is in dispute)	Infants and toddlers
Time out	Interrupt disruptive or aggressive behavior by immediate isolation at onset; few words; boring place; timed for a minute per year of age	2-12 years
Scolding/disapproval	Naming misbehavior (stern voice) and expressing dissatisfaction	All ages
Natural consequences	Result occurs without intervention from parent and allowed only if does not jeopardize safety (e.g., play too roughly with cat—get scratched)	All ages
Logical consequences	Punishment determined by parent and logically connected to misbehavior (e.g., ride bike without helmet — no bike riding for 1 week)	3 years to adolescence
Behavioral penalty	Loss of privileges for misbehavior that has no clear consequence (e.g., refusal to do chores—"grounded" for the weekend)	5 years to adolescence

Consultation/Referral

Consult with the physician regarding aggressive or self-destructive behaviors.

Report any suspected cases of child abuse to appropriate authorities.

Refer complicated (multiple types) and/or major behavior problems (persistent, inappropriate for age/sex, increasing severity or frequency of symptoms) for psychiatric evaluation.

EVALUATION/FOLLOW-UP

Follow-up by telephone in 1 to 2 weeks (encourage the parent to call sooner if there are any questions or difficulties with implementing behavior management).

Schedule a return visit in 4 to 6 weeks:

Repeat the neurodevelopmental screen if any developmental lags/deficits are noted or if misbehavior is still unmanaged after 4 weeks of implementing a management system.

Consider a 6-month interval between well-child visits until stability is maintained.

SUGGESTED READINGS

Arvin A et al: *Nelson textbook of pediatrics,* ed 15, Philadelphia, 1996, WB Saunders.

Boynton RW, Dunn ES, Stephens GR, editors: *Ambulatory pediatric care,* ed 2, Philadelphia, 1994, JB Lippincott.

Clark L: *SOS! Help for parents,* Bowling Green, Ky, 1985, Parents Press.

Coleman WL: Family-focused pediatrics: solution-oriented techniques for behavior problems, *Contemp Pediatr* 14:121-134, 1997.

Herman-Staab B: Screening, management, and appropriate referral for pediatric behavior problems, *Nurs Pract* 19:40-49, 1994.

Schmitt BD: Time-out: intervention of choice for the irrational years, *Contemp Pediatr* 10:64-71, 1993.

Schmitt BD: Seven deadly sins of childhood: advising parents about difficult developmental phases, *Child Abuse Negl* 11:421-432, 1987.

HELP—MY CHILD KEEPS CHANGING!!
(CHILD BEHAVIOR—WHAT TO EXPECT AS A PARENT)

Behavior could be defined as actions or conduct that carry a message. How a child behaves from an early age is one way he or she communicates feelings. Parents can use behavior as a gauge for how their child is doing as well as a guide for a need for action on their part.

First Year. Expect drastic changes. Your child will move from being totally dependent on you for everything to starting to do things on his own by 11 or 12 months of age. Groundwork is laid during this first year of infancy for managing your child's behavior. This system for behavior management (discipline) needs to be established in your family as early as possible in the life of your child.
Highlights:

Determine your child's temperament.
Establish a relationship of *Trust.*
You are responsible for meeting the needs of your child.
The awesome responsibility of being a role model begins now!

Toddler Years. Your child will become more interactive with you and with the environment. Toddlers tend to resist attempts to modify behavior and to learn through repetition rather than reasoning. Mood swings are common and somewhat unpredictable and have a direct effect on behavior. Children between 1 and 3 years most likely "misbehave" by testing limits that have been established. Firm boundaries are actually needed for the child to feel secure. Parents' actions and reactions to child's behavior develop patterns that children recognize. Consistency is key. Frustration for the toddler is also common when physical skills do not match the will or desire of the child. It is a hard job for the parent to judge when and if to intervene, as unwanted help may only add to the frustration level.
Highlights:

Toddler enjoys and seeks more independence—allow as much as possible.
Parents may notice connections between behavior and temperament.
Remember that toddlers have minimal ability to control impulses.
Reinforce positive behaviors of the toddler.
Be consistent with behavior management system across caregivers.

Preschool Years. Prepare for the developing imagination. Preschool years can be such a joy, but also a challenge. Preschoolers are less dependent on parents for everyday tasks. Children during this time begin to think abstractly and are eager to soak up new experiences. Your child will learn the basics of reasoning, but without a good grasp of the logic component. Conflict among siblings is common and may be manifested as jealousy if birth of a baby is involved. This is a good time to establish household rules. Socialization begins as your child is exposed to people and interactions outside the home.
Highlights:

Child is more independent with self-care.
Seek new opportunities and experiences for child.
Develop basic household rules.
Give child reasonable choices.
Model respect in all interactions.

School-age Years. Children during the middle years of childhood are focused on interacting with others. Relationship standards (values) learned at home are played out in various social settings. As cognitive abilities grow, the child learns to understand the world and how he or she "fits in." Achievement at school often depends on the family's value on learning as well as parental encouragement. Peer approval emerges as important to children. Children are like sponges during these early school years and are greatly influenced by teachers, other supervising adults, and TV and other media. Caution should be used that children are not overextended with extracurricular activities (e.g., a child who is pulled in a different direction everyday after school is *likely* to act or display forms of misbehavior).
Highlights:

Help children get along with others.
Child wants to be like friends.
Adult approval/acceptance is highly sought.
Parents need to hold firm with rule enforcement.
Though children are very independent, they still need guidance.

Adolescent Years. The later years of childhood are often viewed negatively—most likely because of lack of preparation for still further behavior changes. Other factors such as puberty, an emerging adult body, and limited decision-making ability related to idealistic thinking aggravate behaviors and may lead to disastrous outcomes. On the other hand, if a positive relationship built on respect has been established between the child and parent, these potentially explosive factors can be addressed in positive ways. The time can be overwhelming for children in teen years—they are faced with choosing a vocation or career, whether or not to go to college, and financial implications—adult issues without life experience on which to base decisions. Close communication and assessment by parents are helpful to divert negative interactions and outcomes. Adolescents should be allowed to make decisions on their own and understand responsibility for their actions. This time in life is a transition to adulthood, yet is still under the guidance of parents.
Highlights:

Peers are major influence and their acceptance is critical to the adolescent.
On the surface, adult approval is not important.
Parents may need to alter rules, but enforcement of limits is critical.
Monitoring a child's behavior may help to identify problems that require attention.

Try to Remember . . .

Show *love* constantly.
Get *control* of yourself first—never discipline when you are angry.
Establish *rules* early and enforce them.
Model behaviors/habits that you want to see in your child.
Behaviors may be unacceptable, but the *child is not bad.*
Reinforce good behaviors.
Avoid mixed messages—*consistency* between parents and situations is key!

NOTE TO PRACTITIONER: Use highlights as "talking points." Parents may voice frustration with change at any point in the child's development. Recalling past accomplishments with transitions might provide encouragement for making it over the next transition.

21 Bell's Palsy

ICD-9-CM

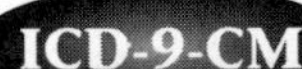

Bell's Palsy 351.0

OVERVIEW

Definition

Bell's palsy is an acute idiopathic unilateral paralysis of the facial muscles innervated by the seventh cranial nerve.

Incidence

Bell's palsy occurs in 20 per 100,000 persons worldwide each year. It is the most common of all facial neuropathies, accounting for 60% to 80% of all cases. It affects all age groups, and its frequency increases with age; onset in the middle years is most common. **Under age 50, women are more often affected, with men more likely to be affected after age 50.**

The problem encompasses all races. Seasonally, Bell's palsy is more common in winter. Higher risk groups include **pregnant women**, persons with diabetes mellitus, and those with hypothyroidism, hypertension, a family history of Bell's palsy, and persons in lower socioeconomic groups. Bell's palsy may be an early manifestation of human immunodeficiency virus infection.

Pathophysiology

Acute inflammation of the seventh cranial nerve causes edema, which produces compression and entrapment, resulting in hypoxia, ischemia, and degeneration of the nerve. The process is progressive over 7 to 10 days with nerve conduction altered approximately 3 days after nerve degeneration. Improvement with neuropraxia will occur within 3 to 6 weeks, but with axon degeneration, improvement is prolonged to 3 to 6 months. Aberrant regeneration of the nerve during healing occasionally results in excessive tearing with chewing ("crocodile tears") as the new nerve tendrils stimulate the lacrimal ducts instead of the salivary glands. The cause of Bell's palsy is unknown, but clinical and research evidence implicates the herpes viruses. The herpes simplex virus is most often the causal agent, although herpes zoster oticus (Ramsay Hunt syndrome) can cause similar symptoms. Other causal theories include autoimmune processes and inflammatory diseases, such as sarcoidosis and Lyme disease.

SUBJECTIVE DATA

History of Present Illness

Ask about the onset and speed of progression and the duration of symptoms.

Past Medical History

Ask whether the patient is currently pregnant.

Ask about a history of diabetes mellitus, hypothyroidism, hypertension, trauma, infection, rash, or tick bite.

Ask about risk factors for heart disease or stroke.

Approximately three of four patients will have had an upper respiratory infection preceding the facial paralysis.

Medications

Obtain a list of the patient's current medications. Note whether the patient is already taking prednisone or acyclovir for other conditions.

Family History

Ask about any family history of Bell's palsy.

Psychosocial History

Consider the impact of facial paralysis on the individual.

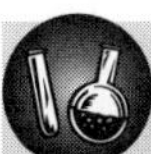

TABLE 21-1 Primary Diagnostic Tests: Bell's Palsy

Diagnostic Test	Diagnostic Value	Considerations	Cost ($)
Audiometric screen	Objectively screens complaint of hearing impairment	Provides baseline of audiometric acuity; hearing loss inconsistent with Bell's Palsy	24-29/4 puretones; 119-154/comprehensive
Lyme serology	Rule out Lyme disease	Endemic area; history of rash	34-42
HIV screen	Rule out HIV	Risk factors for HIV	58-72

HIV, Human immunodeficiency virus.

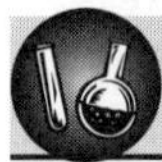

TABLE 21-2 Secondary Diagnostic Tests: Bell's Palsy

Diagnostic Test	Diagnostic Value	Considerations	Cost ($)
X-ray	Rule out fracture of temporal bone	Obtain if history of blunt trauma; CT scan may be more helpful	
Laboratory: ESR TFT Electrolyte profile	Limited diagnostic value	Help identify associated conditions	13-16/CBC 16-20/ESR 23-30/electrolytes
EMG	Help predict outcome in severe cases	Obtain at least 72 hours after onset, preferably 7-10 days from onset	
MRI	Evaluate facial nerve and rule out other causes such as tumor or stroke	Obtain if no improvement in 6 months	

CBC, Complete blood count; *EMG,* electromyelogram; *ESR,* erythrocyte sedimentation rate; *TFT,* thyroid function test; *MRI,* magnetic resonance imaging.

Description of Most Common Symptoms

Onset of unilateral facial paralysis is sudden, usually over a few hours, with progression over 1 to 3 days. Persons affected may wake up and notice the problem of unilateral facial weakness and numbness. Malaise and low-grade fever are possible at onset.

Associated Symptoms

Dry eye on the affected side
Mild transient post auricular pain
Tinnitus
Slightly decreased hearing for a few hours at onset
Increased sensitivity to sound (hyperacusis)
Altered taste on the anterior two thirds of the tongue (dysgeusia)

OBJECTIVE DATA

Physical Examination

Check vital signs, noting any elevation of temperature or blood pressure. Observe general appearance and gait. Note facial asymmetry, with loss of voluntary and involuntary movement in both upper and lower portions of the face. The forehead is unilaterally smooth, the nasolabial fold is flattened, and the eyelid on the affected side does not close. The palpebral fissure is widened. Weakness of the muscles around the eye can result in an exaggerated upward curve of the eyelid with lid closure; this sign is known as *Bell's phenomenon.*

Inspect the skin for:

Zosteriform lesions behind the ear or in the ear canal
Expanding target lesion, erythema chronicum migrans, or Lyme disease
Neurofibroma and café-au-lait lesions
Ear: Look for cholesteatoma (pressure on the facial nerve) and otitis media (invasive infection)
Nose/jaw: Observe for trauma, palpate jaw for tenderness or parotid mass
Neck: Check for lymphadenopathy
Lungs: Auscultate for adventitious sounds (sarcoidosis)
Neurological: Neurological examination with assessment of cranial nerves (corneal reflex may be decreased); a facial nerve grading system, such as the House-Brackmann scale, can be used to specifically document facial asymmetry and diminished voluntary movement

TABLE 21-3 Differential Diagnoses: Bell's Palsy

Diagnosis	Supporting Data
Surgery	There is past history of middle ear or mastoid surgery—damage to facial nerve.
Neoplasms	Tumors or cholesteatoma put pressure on or invade the facial nerve; onset is slower, some branches of facial nerve may be spared; tics/spasms are frequent; MRI/CT scan is positive.
Blunt trauma	Fracture of the temporal bone may damage the seventh nerve; x-ray/CT scan findings are positive.
Herpes zoster oticus; Hunt and Ramsay	There is facial paralysis with vesicles in ear; diminished hearing syndrome and dizziness are possible; there is poorer prognosis for facial recovery.
Middle ear infection	Acute or chronic otitis media with facial palsy requires surgery, cultures, and intravenous antibiotic therapy.
Sarcoidosis	Sites of granulomatous infiltration may occur in the parotid gland and produce facial weakness.
Guillain-Barré syndrome	Demyelinating neuropathy can cause facial weakness, usually bilateral; progressive paralysis moves upward from extremities.
Stroke	There is unilateral facial weakness, spastic hemiparesis resulting from cerebrovascular accident.

MRI, Magnetic resonance imaging; *CT,* computed tomography.

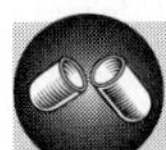

TABLE 21-4 Pharmaceutical Plan: Bell's Palsy

Medication/Action	Drug/Dose	Considerations	Cost ($)
Prednisone	Adults: 1 mg/kg/day, average 30-40 mg BID for 5-10 days with taper over 5-10 more days Children: 2 mg/kg/day for 1 week, then 1 mg/kg for another week	Begin treatment as soon as possible after onset of symptoms; review contraindications to corticosteroid therapy.	3-19
Acyclovir (Zovirax)	Adults: 400 mg 5 times a day for 5-10 days	Pregnancy: C **Not approved for children under age 2**	97
or			
Famciclovir (Famvir)	500 mg TID for 10 days	**Not approved for children under 18 years of age**	116

Diagnostic Procedures

No diagnostic procedures are required, unless the diagnosis is uncertain; selected testing may be done in the instances outlined in Tables 21-1 and 21-2.

ASSESSMENT

Differential Diagnosis

Differential diagnoses include:
Surgery, neoplasms, blunt trauma
Infections (including herpes zoster, sarcoidosis, Guillain-Barré syndrome)
Elderly: Stroke (Table 21-3)

THERAPEUTIC PLAN

Pharmaceutical Management

A pharmaceutical plan for the treatment of Bell's palsy is outlined in Table 21-4. A double-blind trial randomized two groups of patients with Bell's palsy; one group took prednisone plus acyclovir, 400 mg five times a day for 10 days, and the other group took prednisone plus a placebo. The prednisone/acyclovir group had better facial-recovery than the prednisone/placebo group (Bauer and Coker, 1996).

Because of the defective healing that is common in up to 40% of cases of Bell's palsy, more aggressive treatment with antiinflammatory intravenous infusion therapy using a combination of three drugs has been advocated by some neurologists (Stennert and Sittel, 1997).

Nonpharmaceutical Management

On the opposite end of the treatment spectrum, some internists and neurologists do not treat the patient with any medication. Selected patients who have no voluntary movement on examination or voluntary motor unit potentials on electromyelogram may require surgical decompression of the nerve within 14 days of the onset of symptoms (Hughes, 1998). Surgical decompression of the nerve has also been recommended for recurrent facial palsy (Stennert and Sittel, 1997).

Physical Therapy

Electrical stimulation can lead to irreversible facial contractures and should be used cautiously, if at all. Safer alternatives are massage and facial exercises, which may be helpful during the recuperative phase.

Lifestyle/Activities

Eye care is of extreme importance. The patient should use artificial tears twice a day and at bedtime to prevent drying of the cornea; the eyelid may need to be taped shut at night. A moisture chamber over the eye at night may be helpful. Instruct the patient to report symptoms of eye pain or visual problems, to wear safety glasses when working with tools or in the yard, and to wear sunglasses when driving.

Diet

None

Patient Education

Discuss symptoms that might be expected, such as altered taste, hypersensitive hearing, and decreased tearing and saliva production. Individuals experiencing these symptoms in association with significant facial paralysis and increased age have a poorer prognosis for complete recovery. Overall, the prognosis is generally considered favorable, but with varying rates of recovery, ranging from 60% to 90%, with children having the best outcome. Symptoms usually resolve within 3 to 6 weeks.

Family Impact

Explain the transient nature of Bell's palsy and reasonable chances for a favorable recovery.

Referral

URGENT: Refer the patient to a physician for any facial palsy associated with an acute otitis media, because this indicates an invasive process.

Referral to a neurologist is indicated for facial palsy in which the diagnosis is not clearly Bell's palsy.

Evaluate for signs of corneal abrasion and refer the patient to an ophthalmologist if indicated.

Consultation

Consider consultation with a physician before starting treatment with prednisone and consultation with an obstetrician before treating a pregnant patient with acyclovir.

REFERENCES

Bauer CA, Coker NJ: Update on facial nerve disorders, *Otolaryngol Clin North Am* 29:445-455, 1996.

Stennert E, Sittel C: Acute peripheral facial paralysis. In Rakel R, editor: *Conn's current therapy,* Philadelphia, 1997, WB Saunders.

SUGGESTED READINGS

Billue JA: Bell's palsy: an update on idiopathic facial paralysis, *Nurs Pract* 22:88-105, 1997.

Bonner JS, Bonner JJ: *The little black book of neurology,* ed 2, St Louis, 1991, Mosby.

Ellsworth A et al: *Mosby's 1998 medical drug reference,* St Louis, 1998, Mosby.

Healthcare Consultants of America, Inc: *1998 Physicians fee and coding guide,* Augusta, Ga, 1998, Healthcare Consultants of America, Inc.

Hughes GB: Acute peripheral facial paralysis. In Rakel R, editor: *Conn's current therapy*, Philadelphia, 1998, WB Saunders.

Pruitt AA: Management of Bell's palsy. In Goroll AH, May LA, Mulley AG, editors: *Primary care medicine,* ed 3, Philadelphia, 1995, JB Lippincott.

Uphold CR, Graham MV: *Clinical guidelines in family practice,* Gainesville, Fla, 1994, Barmarrae Books.

22 Blepharitis

ICD-9-CM

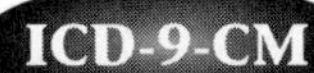

Blepharitis 373.00

OVERVIEW

Definition

Blepharitis is an inflammation of the eyelid margin, resulting in redness, scaling, and crusting.

Incidence

Blepharitis is more common in fair-skinned people and adults. It is associated with seborrhea or rosacea of the face and scalp. It is a chronic condition, with acute flare-ups. Incidence is equal in men and women.

Adults: Seborrheic dermatitis is common after the second decade of life and affects 5% of adults.

Infants: Seborrheic dermatitis is common.

Pathophysiology

Ulcerative blepharitis: Caused by staphylococcal bacterial infection

Seborrheic (nonulcerative) blepharitis: Causative factor is often obscure but associated with seborrheic dermatitis; increased skin shedding with sebaceous gland dysfunction

SUBJECTIVE DATA

History of Present Illness

Ask about onset and duration of symptoms, previous occurrences

Ask about contact lens use, use of eye makeup, eye pain, tearing, and visual disturbances

Past Medical History

Ask about history of seborrheic dermatitis.

Ask about repeated incidence of styes (hordeolum) and chalazia.

Medications

Ask about use of any over-the-counter drugs or current medications.

Family History

Not applicable

Psychosocial History

Not applicable

Description of Most Common Symptoms

Itching, burning, redness of lid margins, lid edema, loss of lashes, conjunctival irritation with increased lacrimation and photophobia

OBJECTIVE DATA

Physical Examination

Depends on underlying cause

Staphylococcal blepharitis: May cause conjunctivitis; crusting and bleeding surface when removed; may progress to shallow ulcers

Seborrheic blepharitis: Associated with greasy, easily removable scales on lid margins and eyelashes

Check visual acuity

Diagnostic Procedures

None; however, may need culture of discharge if condition does not resolve in 1 month

ASSESSMENT

Differential Diagnosis

Differential diagnoses include those outlined in Table 22-1.

THERAPEUTIC PLAN

Pharmaceutical

Antibiotic treatment for prophylaxis is for 3 to 9 weeks. An antistaphylococcal antibiotic medication is used (Table 22-2).

Nonpharmaceutical

Lid hygiene: Dilute Johnson's baby shampoo with water 50/50.
Use cotton balls to scrub the eyelids well. Rinse with water; apply hot compress to closed lids 5 to 10 minutes.

Lifestyle/Activities

Patient may need to refrain from using eye makeup, specifically mascara.
Reinforce good hygiene.
Refrain from contact lens use during acute exacerbations.

Diet

Not applicable

Patient Education

Disease process and treatment, use of ophthalmic antibiotics and side effects
Good hygiene/eyelid cleansing (see Nonpharmaceutical)
Treatment for seborrheic dermatitis

Family Impact

Not applicable

TABLE 22-1 Differential Diagnosis: Blepharitis

Diagnosis	Supporting Data
Chalazion	Granulomatous inflammation of meibomian gland Tender, mildly inflamed, quiet, discrete mass on the conjunctival side of lid, not the lid margin
Hordeolum	Acute staphylococcal infection of sebaceous, apocrine, or meibomian gland Diffuse erythema, tenderness, edema Superficial lid infection called preseptal cellulitis **Children** affected more often than adults
Dacryocystitis	Infection in the nasolacrimal sac Mucopurulent reflux from the superior and inferior puncta
Lice infestation	White or black specks seen attached to hair shaft; may appear as dry flakes May indicate sexual abuse in children
Cellulitis	Erythema, edema, pain, fever, skin warm to touch
Carcinoma: basal cell, squamous cell, sebaceous cell	Any of the above symptoms, with no resolution in 1 month's time

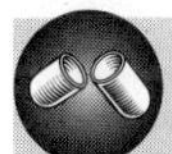

TABLE 22-2 Pharmaceutical Plan: Blepharitis

Drug	Dose	Comments	Cost
Erythromycin ophthalmic ointment 0.5% (⅛ oz)	Apply to lid margin 4-6 times daily Instill ophthalmic ointment in the inferior fornix; rub excess onto eyelid base	Pregnancy: B SE: Local irritation	\$2-\$5/5 mg/g (3.5 g)
Sulfacetamide ointment (3.5 g)	See erythromycin	Pregnancy: C SE: Local irritation	\$1-\$16/ointment: 10% (3.5 g) \$3-\$19/solution: 10% (15 ml)
Natamycin (Natacyn)	1 gtt 4-6 times daily	Use for fungal blepharitis Pregnancy: C SE: Temporary visual haze, conjunctival chemosis	\$93.75/5% (15 ml)

SE, Side effects.

Referral

Refer the patient to an ophthalmologist if blepharitis proves treatment resistant.

Refer the patient to a dermatologist if seborrheic dermatitis is poorly controlled.

Consultation

None

EVALUATION/FOLLOW-UP

If not resolved in 1 month, send for biopsy.

Squamous cell, basal cell, and sebaceous cell cancers can masquerade as blepharitis, styes, or chalazions. This is known as masquerade syndrome.

Possible complications include scarring of eyelid margin, corneal infection.

SUGGESTED READINGS

Beaty L, Herting R: Ophthalmology. In Graber M, Toth P, Herting R, editors: *The family practice handbook,* St Louis, 1997, Mosby.

Carter S: Eyelid disorders: diagnosis and management, *Am Fam Physician* 57:2695-2702, 1998.

Ellsworth A et al: *Mosby's 1998 medical drug reference,* St Louis, 1998, Mosby.

Healthcare Consultants of America, Inc: *1998 Physicians fee and coding guide,* Augusta, Ga, 1998, Healthcare Consultants of America, Inc.

Riordan-Eva P, Vaughan D: Eye. In Tierney L, McPhee S, Papadakis M, editors: *Current medical diagnosis & treatment,* Stamford, Conn, 1998, Appleton & Lange.

Breast Disorders: Masses and Pain

ICD-9-CM

Mastalgia 611.71
Diffuse Cystic Mastopathy 610.1
Malignant Neoplasm Female Breast 174
Malignant Neoplasm Male Breast 175

OVERVIEW

Definitions

Breast mass: A three-dimensional dominant palpable lump or area of thickening can be appreciated, distinct from surrounding breast tissue and generally asymmetrical when compared with the opposite breast.

Mastalgia (breast pain): Pain that occurs either cyclically or noncyclically in a woman's breast. Cyclical pain, which occurs premenstrually and is generally relieved with the onset of menses, is more common with fibrocystic changes in the breast. Some women experience mastalgia initially with oral contraceptives or hormone replacement therapy.

Noncyclic mastalgia is not related to the menstrual cycle, occurring in a poorly defined pattern; there is usually no discrete mass. The primary cause is mammary duct ecstasia.

Incidence

Four of five breast masses are benign, but breast cancer must always be ruled out. According to the American Cancer Society, a woman has a lifetime risk of breast cancer of 1 in 8 and a lifetime risk of dying from breast cancer of 1 in 28. The incidence of breast cancer is 100 times more common in women. Gynecomastia occurs in 40% or more of **prepubertal/pubertal males.** Mastalgia occurs in 70% of females at some point during their lifetimes.

Pathophysiology

Masses: Most common benign breast disorders associated with masses—fibrocystic changes and fibroadenoma—represent normal glandular responses to fluctuating levels of estrogen.

Fibrocystic changes: Alterations in breast tissue associated with fluid-filled cysts within the glandular structure; these cysts, with areas of thickness and nodularity, are cyclic in nature.

Fibroadenoma: Abnormal growth of fibrous and ductal tissue under hormonal influence. An excessively large fibroadenoma—cystosarcoma phyllodes—grows rapidly and may stretch skin to the point of ulceration; these are usually benign, but 1% become cancerous.

Lipoma: Benign fatty tumor of the breast.

Gynecomastia: Benign proliferation of the glandular portion of the breast resulting from estrogen stimulation, occurring in **newborns** of both genders, **prepubertal and pubertal boys,** and **involutional men** 50 to 80 years old. Pathological gynecomastia is associated with cancer of the testes, adrenal gland, and lungs; with liver disease, renal disease, and thyroid disease; and with hypogonadism, androgen insensitivity, malnutrition, and certain drugs. Neonatal gynecomastia is caused by transplacental maternal estrogen influence.

Intraductal papilloma: Benign, small, wartlike growth in the lining of the mammary duct near the nipple.

Fat necrosis: Benign mass often associated with trauma (in half of cases), including trauma associated with surgical procedures. Many women cannot recall the traumatic episode. Fat necrosis has many of the clinical features of cancer.

Duct ecstasia: Results from dilation of the subareolar ducts with fibrosis and inflammation behind the nipple and areola area; it is a benign condition.

Breast cancer, the second leading cause of cancer death in women, involves malignant cells that invade the breast tissue with potential for spread. Paget's disease is a type of breast cancer that affects the epidermis of the areola and nipple.

Protective Factors Against Breast Cancer and Some Benign Masses

Breastfeeding
First pregnancy at an early age before 30 years old
Oral contraceptives
Bilateral oophorectomy
Daily serving of green or yellow vegetables (carotene)
Men: Biological fatherhood
Lower than average rate of breast cancer in the following groups of women: Hispanics, blacks, Japanese, Filipino, Native Americans, Seventh Day Adventists, and Mormons

Factors That Increase Susceptibility to Breast Cancer

Being female
Being over 50 years old
Personal history of breast cancer
Family history of breast cancer, especially in first-degree female relatives
History of fibrocystic disease with epithelial hyperplasia
Early menarche (under 12 years old) and late menopause (older than 55 years old)
Nulliparity
Over age 30 at first pregnancy
Exposure to ionizing radiation
Prolonged unopposed estrogen replacement therapy (without progestins)
Excess alcohol intake
Smoking
Increased intake of dietary fat
Obesity
Exposure to diethylstilbestrol
Ashkenazi Jewish heritage (increased probability of inherited gene mutation for breast cancer)
Inheritance of BRCA 1 or BRCA 2 gene (accounts for 5% to 10% of breast cancer)
Men: Infertility, genital disease, injury, Klinefelter's syndrome
Eighty-five percent of women who get breast cancer do not have risk factors

Factors That Increase Susceptibility to Gynecomastia

Being a neonate, prepubescent or pubescent male, or involutional male
Early maturity of adolescent male
Klinefelter's syndrome
Testicular failure, gonadal failure (i.e., decreased testosterone)
Severe illness with malnutrition and weight loss

Factors That May Increase Susceptibility to Mastalgia

Dietary intake of caffeine or methylxanthines

SUBJECTIVE DATA

Breast pain is a common presenting complaint.
The majority (probably 80%) of breast masses are discovered by the patient.

History of Present Illness

Ask questions to determine the following:

Description of the mass or pain and its location
When the mass or pain in the breast was first noticed
Whether the mass has increased or decreased since first noticed
What the relationship is, if any, between the complaint and her menstrual cycle
Whether there have been changes in the size, contour, or skin of the breast or changes in the areola or nipple
What makes the symptoms better or worse
How the symptoms have affected lifestyle
Whether there are any associated symptoms
Whether the patient performs breast self-examination
Last menstrual period
Current method of contraception
Age at menarche or menopause (if applicable)
Evidence of risk factors for breast cancer
Soreness in axilla or awareness of enlarged lymph nodes in axilla

Past Medical History

Has there has been a previous history of breast mass (obtain details), trauma, biopsy, or surgery?
When was the most recent mammography, ultrasonography, and/or clinical breast examination?
Is there a history of chronic illness, including cancer?
Boys: Ask about recent history of serious illness

Medications

Current medications, especially oral contraceptives, hormone replacement therapy, or drugs associated with nipple discharge and mastalgia (Boxes 23-1 to 23-3).

Family History

Ask about family history of breast problems, history of cancer of the breast, ovaries, and colon or rectum (especially significant in first-degree maternal relatives and occurring before menopause).
Boys: Ask about family history of gynecomastia.

Box 23-1

Drugs That Cause Nipple Discharge

Tricyclic antidepressants	Digoxin
Phenothiazides	Reserpine
Corticosteroids	Methyldopa
Phenytoin	Contraceptives
Diuretics	Neuroleptics

Not an exhaustive list; consult drug references based on drug history of patient.

Box 23-2

Drugs That Increase Mastalgia

Anacin	Midol
Dristan	Empirin
No Doz	Fiorinal
Theophylline	Hormones
Percodan	

Not an exhaustive list; consult drug references based on drug history of patient.

Box 23-3

Common Medications that Predispose to Gynecomastia

Androgens	Digoxin
Anabolic steroids	Metronidazole
Cimetidine	Ketoconazole

Not an exhaustive list; the nurse practitioner should consult drug references based on patient history.

Psychosocial History

Ask about leisure drug use, smoking, and alcohol intake.

Boys: Ask about weight lifting and other athletic pursuits that increase pectoral muscle size, which might complicate diagnosis.

Inquire how symptoms are affecting school and athletic activities. Note any evidence of limitations in activities with other males out of embarrassment.

Diet

Ask about increased intake of caffeine, methylxanthines (coffee, tea, cola, and chocolate), vegetables with carotene, and fat.

Ask about sodium intake and potential relationship to mastalgia.

Description of Most Common Symptoms

Use of a symptom chart or calendar for two or three menstrual cycles can assist in distinguishing the nature of symptoms.

Mastalgia is characterized by cyclic diffuse heaviness and tenderness in the breast. It is commonly more.noticeable in the upper outer quadrants and may radiate to the axilla, upper arm, and/or elbow. Noncyclic mastalgia is usually characterized by sensations of drawing, burning, aching, and throbbing in the medial half of the breast beneath the areola, unrelated to the menstrual cycle.

Gynecomastia is characterized by enlargement and heaviness of the breast with tenderness.

The characteristics of breast masses differ, depending on the type of lesion.

Associated Symptoms

Nipple Discharge

Record findings on color and consistency, duration, persistence, whether the discharge occurs spontaneously or is elicited, its relationship to the patient's menses, its relationship to sexual activity, whether it is unilateral or bilateral, and whether one or more ducts are involved.

OBJECTIVE DATA

Physical Examination

Problem-Oriented Physical Examination for Females and Males

Note the general appearance of breasts, axillae, and supraclavicular and infraclavicular lymph nodes.

With the patient sitting on the examination table with arms at sides, observe the uncovered breasts for symmetry, contour, and change in vascular pattern. Note discoloration or peau d'orange skin, dimpling, inversion or retraction of nipple, crusting of areola or nipple, and local edema.

Repeat this observation with the patient's arms behind the head and with hands pressing against the hipbones.

With the patient supine, inspect the breasts and skin. Begin palpation on the side opposite the identified mass. Palpate the entire breast for masses, including the tail of Spence. Palpate for axillary, supraclavicular, and infraclavicular lymphadenopathy.

Check for nipple discharge by compressing the nipple-areola complex between thumb and index finger, "milking" toward the nipple from three or four directions. Dot any discharge with white tissue or linen and note the color of fluid at the margins for accurate assessment. (If there is a nipple discharge, check the discharge fluid for guaiac with Hemoccult or Hemostix at the completion of the examination.)

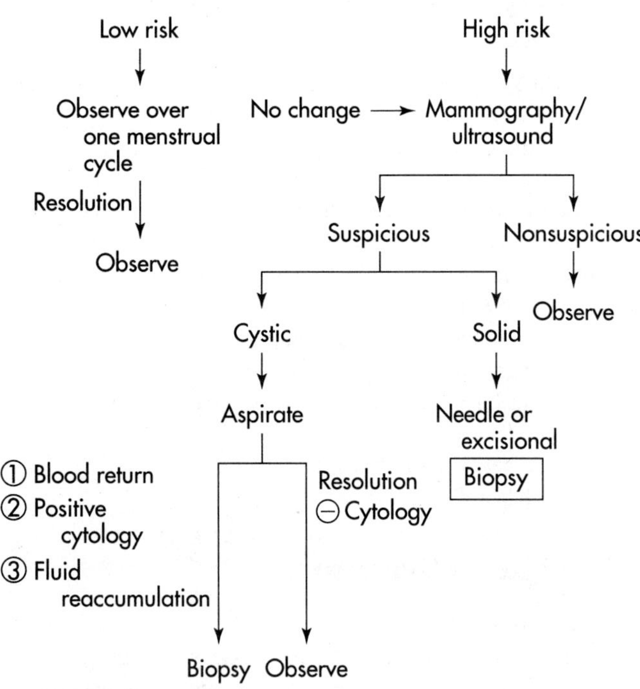

Figure 23-1 Diagnostic algorithm for a solitary breast mass. (From Grodzin CJ, Schwartz SC, Bone RC: *Diagnostic strategies for internal medicine,* St Louis, 1996, Mosby.)

Palpate the axilla with the patient's arm relaxing on your arm. Press nodes toward the chest wall, noting size, number, and characteristics. (A node of less than 1 cm that is soft and mobile would prompt a low level of suspicion.)

For a patient with large, pendulous breasts, consider having the patient turn on the side while you palpate half the breast before completing examination with the patient supine. Pendulous breasts can also be examined between the examiner's hands.

For **males,** the examination is the same.

Boys: To differentiate gynecomastia from fatty enlargement of breast tissue, with the boy supine, the examiner should grasp the breast between the thumb and forefinger and gently move toward the nipple; a concentric mound is noted between the nipple and areola in gynecomastia. The genitals should be examined, and Tanner staging should be done (gynecomastia usually occurs at Tanner stage 3 or 4).

Diagnostic Procedures

See Figure 23-1 and Tables 23-1 and 23-2 for diagnostic procedures.

ASSESSMENT

Differential diagnoses include premenstrual breast tissue, fibrocystic disease, fibroadenoma, mammary duct ecstasia, fat necrosis, lipoma, gynecomastia, cyclic or noncyclic mastalgia, mastitis, costal cartilage disorder (Tietze's syndrome), breast cancer, and Paget's disease (Table 23-3).

THERAPEUTIC PLAN

Pharmaceutical

A pharmaceutical plan is appropriate for mastalgia; initially may try:

Evening primrose oil: 3 g/day; may cause mild nausea
Vitamin E: 400 to 600 IU/day

Other drugs (danazol [Danocrine], bromocriptine mesylate, tamoxifen citrate) may be ordered in consultation with the physician if mastalgia is unresponsive to lifestyle changes and these drugs; if drugs are used, the woman must be educated about the use of barrier methods of birth control, since these drugs are teratogens.

Lifestyle/Activities

Avoid breast trauma.
Wear supportive brassiere, especially while exercising.
Eliminate risk factors for breast cancer.

Diet

Decrease caffeine, methylxanthines, and fat in diet.
Increase intake of carotene-containing vegetables (green and yellow).
Decrease sodium intake to reduce breast pain, especially premenstrually.

Patient Education

Teach breast self-examination and reinforce need for performing this monthly, beginning at age 20.

Stress need for clinical breast examination every 3 years from ages 20 through 40 and yearly after age 40. Advise the patient to schedule mammography in accordance with national guidelines: baseline at age 40; every 2 years after age 40; annually after age 50.

Teach signs and symptoms of breast cancer.

For mastalgia:

Suggest mild analgesics (but see Box 23-2) and warm compresses for comfort.

Reassure that it does not predispose to breast cancer.

For gynecomastia:

Reassure boy and family when condition is nonpathologi-

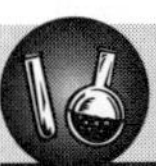

TABLE 23-1 Diagnostic Procedures: Breast Masses

Test	Findings/Rationale	Cost ($)
Mammography	Used to locate suspicious lesions; can localize mass <1 cm (smallest clinically detectable lesion), thus increasing survival potential and decreasing likelihood of necessary extensive surgery Cannot diagnose benign versus malignant 10% appear normal on mammogram with actual breast cancer; 20% false-negative rate; even higher false-positive rate Indications: Ages 40—baseline Ages 40-50—every other year Ages 50 and older—every year If patient has first-degree relative who developed breast cancer before menopause, schedule baseline mammogram 5 to 10 years before age at which relative was diagnosed	99-125
Breast ultrasonography	Differentiates cystic and solid masses; more effective detecting lesions in denser breast tissue of those <30 years old	277-327
Fine-needle aspiration	Aspiration of fluid and sample cells from cystic mass using sterile technique with or without local anesthesia, followed by cytological analysis by pathologist; accuracy is 90+% in diagnosing cancer; NOTE: Papanicolaou test of breast fluid produces inconclusive results and is of little value	260-301
Breast biopsy	Excision of breast mass with operative procedure performed with patient under anesthesia; considered both diagnostic and therapeutic	522-620
Stereotactic guided biopsy	X-ray-guided location and biopsy of suspicious lesion found through mammography; performed with breast placed in hole in table, where lesion is targeted for tissue removal; takes 1-2 hr	1194-1775
Genetic studies: BRCA 1 and BRCA 2	Genetic tests that locate abnormal genes located on chromosomes 17 and 13, respectively—genes transmitted by autosomal-dominant inheritance pattern	1000-3000

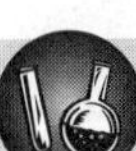

TABLE 23-2 Diagnostic Tests for Boys with Gynecomastia*

Test	Findings/Rationale	Cost ($)
Serum hCG	Normal hCG, LH, T, and E_2 levels: Cause is idiopathic High hCG: Order testicular ultrasonography to rule out tumor; refer to specialist if tumor found; refer if normal (may order CT abdomen and CXR sent to referral physician)	28-35/(qual); 51-65/(quan)
LH	Normal or low LH and low T levels: Order tests of serum prolactin level; if prolactin high, order CT to rule out pituitary tumor or empty sella turcica; if prolactin normal, cause is probably secondary hypogonadism; refer	61-76
T	Normal or low LH and high E_2 levels: Order testicular ultrasonography; refer if mass found; if normal, refer (may order adrenal CT or MRI sent to referral physician)	83-103
E_2	High LH and high T levels: Order TSH and T_4 tests to rule out thyroid condition; if normal, cause probably androgen resistance; if TSH low and T_4 high, cause is hyperthyroidism High LH and low T levels: Primary hypogonadism; refer	85-107

*Order tests in consultation with physician.

CT, Computed tomography; *CXR,* Chest x-ray evaluation; E_2, estradiol level; hCG, human chorionic gonadotropin; *LH,* luteinizing hormone; *MRI,* magnetic resonance imaging; *T,* testosterone level; T_4, thyroxine; *TSH,* thyroid-stimulating hormone.

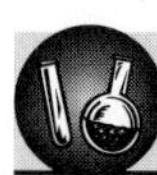

TABLE 23-3 Differential Diagnosis: Breast Masses

Disorder	Description of Mass	Associated Findings	Typical Age	Treatment
Fibrocystic changes	Areas of thickening, soft rubbery nodularity; may note gross lumpiness or fine granular feeling; both breasts symmetrical	Mass noted 7-14 days before menses; tender; axillary adenopathy possible	10% <age 21: Some degree of changes; usually age 30-55; cease at menopause without ERT	Lifestyle changes most important and effective; medications are secondary treatment
Fibroadenoma	Single, round or lobular; distinct margins; freely moveable; 2-3 cm; nontender	Noncyclic; 10%-20% recurrence; size increases in high-estrogen states	Age 20-40; rare in postmenopausal patients	Surgery
Intraductal papilloma	2-5 mm wartlike growth in lining of mammary duct; usually near nipple; palpable mass in half of cases	Bloody, serous, or cloudy discharge from nipple; usually spontaneous	Age 45-55	Surgery
Fat necrosis	Painless, small, firm, rounded mass; smooth or irregular; fixed	Ecchymosis and nipple retraction possible	Any age	Biopsy considered if mass cannot be directly linked to a traumatic injury
Lipoma	Small smooth mobile; distinct		Any age	Biopsy possible
Breast cancer	Usually solitary mass; irregular or stellate; fixed; not clearly distinct from surrounding tissue; firm to rock-hard	Nipple retraction or inversion; bloody discharge; prominent vascular pattern; dimpled or peau d' orange skin	Age 30-80; significant increase after menopause	Surgery; adjuvant therapy—radiation, chemotherapy
Paget's disease	Subareolar mass may be palpable	Nipple/areola eczema-like rash; excoriation or scaling; itching and burning of nipple and areola; exacerbated by cold	Usually postmenopausal patient	Surgery
Gynecomastia	<4 cm firmness, subareola	Tenderness	Neonatal, 10-14, 50+	Resolves spontaneously; drugs may be used; surgery if causing significant life problems

ERT, Estrogen replacement therapy.

cal; transient in nature; prepare for any diagnostic tests to differentiate idiopathic from pathological causes.

Family Impact

Mastalgia can affect sexual relationships, work performance, sleep, and leisure activities as well as home maintenance management activities.

Gynecomastia can affect a boy's body image, lead to isolation from his peers, and limit his engaging in athletics or other activities because of being teased. A boy may worry about his sexual identity, and this may also concern his parents.

Breast masses contribute to feelings of anxiety and uncertainty. Few findings are as alarming to women and their partners as detection of a breast mass, since the potential for malignancy always exists. Many fear the consequences of a diagnosis of cancer and the inherent risk of pain, mutilation, and death. Breast surgery potentially affects the woman's body image and intimate relationships. Adjuvant therapy, radiation, and chemotherapy all have negative consequences on life activities, a sense of wellness, and family life.

Referral

Referral to general surgeon for gynecomastia persisting beyond age 18 months or causing undue stress

Masses clinically suspicious for cancer or solid, palpable lymph nodes, positive mammography findings, cystic masses persist after aspiration or 1 week after next menses

Consultation

Mastalgia unresponsive to conservative therapy

Any patient about whom you have concerns or whose prospective treatment is outside the usual scope of nurse practitioner practice

Gynecomastia associated with physical abnormalities; breast enlargement >4 cm, patient >18 years of age

Follow-up

Ideal time for clinical breast examination: 7 to 9 days after menses

If a mass found on clinical examination during premenstrual phase, follow up in 2 to 3 weeks for reexamination

For a soft, mobile mass or thickening with suspicion of fibrocystic change in low-risk women, consider reexamination 1 week after next menses terminates; refer to OB/GYN or general surgeon if mass persists

Plan for follow-up of cystic mass:

- Fine-needle aspiration with resolution of cyst—recheck in 6 weeks; if it recurs, refer to OB/GYN or general surgeon
- Fine-needle aspiration with persistence of cyst—refer
- Gynecomastia: Reevaluate pubertal males every 6 months

EVALUATION

BSE is performed by woman monthly, clinical breast examinations are performed annually, and mammography is performed according to national guidelines or clinician advice based on history.

Successful outcome includes resolution of gynecomastia and mastalgia; management of fibrocystic changes or masses; prevention or early recognition of breast cancer; and, when cancer is diagnosed, treatment plan that prolongs survival and quality of life.

Treatment of breast cancer usually involves breast-conserving surgery, with or without breast reconstruction. Systemic treatment with adjuvant therapy, radiation, and/or chemotherapy usually follows. Special attention is paid to the increased risk of recurring breast cancer and/or bowel, ovarian, or endometrial cancer in this patient population.

SUGGESTED READINGS

Bowman, MA et al: Who are you screening for cancer—and when? *Patient Care* 30:54-87, 1996.

Carlson KJ et al: *Primary care of women,* St Louis, 1996, Mosby.

Chin HG: *On call obstetrics & gynecology,* Philadelphia, 1997, WB Saunders.

Conry C: Evaluation of a breast complaint: is it cancer? *Am Fam Physician* 49:445-452, 1994.

Ellsworth A: *Mosby's 1998 medical drug reference,* St Louis, 1998, Mosby.

Healthcare Consultants of America, Inc: *1998 Physicians fee and coding guide,* Augusta, Ga, 1998, Healthcare Consultants of America, Inc.

Fiorica JV, Schorr SJ, Sickles EA: Benign breast disorders—first rule out cancer, *Patient Care* 31:140-154, 1997.

Fogel CI, Woods NF: *Women's health care: a comprehensive handbook,* Thousand Oaks, Calif, 1995, Sage.

Fullerton JT, Lanz, J, Sadler GR: Breast cancer among men: raising awareness for primary prevention, *J Am Acad Nurse Pract* 9:211-216, 1997.

Hindle WH: Other benign breast problems, *Clin Obstet Gynecol* 37:916-923, 1994.

Lawrence HC: History, physical examination, and education in breast self-examination, *Clin Obstet Gynecol* 37:881-886, 1994.

Lichtman R, Papera S: *Gynecology: well woman care,* Norwalk, Conn, 1990, Appleton & Lange.

Ma JC, Easter DW: Current guidelines for breast cancer screening, *Contemp Nurse Pract* 1:10-17, 1995.

Reifsnider E: Educating women about benign breast disease, *AAOHNJ* 38:121-125, 1990.

Schwartz S, Schwartz G: Diagnostic algorithm for a solitary breast mass. In Grodzin C, Schwartz S, Bone R, editors: *Diagnostic strategies for internal medicine,* St Louis, 1996, Mosby.

Smith RP: *Gynecology in primary care,* Baltimore, 1997, Williams & Wilkins.

Spiegel KK: On your markers—research advances in breast cancer in women, *AWHONN Lifelines* 1:33-38, 1997.

Star WL, Lommel LL, Shannon MT, editors: *Women's primary health care—protocols for practice,* Washington, DC, 1995, American Nurses Publishing.

White GL et al: Breast cancer: reducing mortality through early detection, *Clin Rev* 6:77-106, 1996.

Youngkin EQ, Davis MS: *Women's health: a primary care guide,* Norwalk, Conn, 1994, Appleton & Lange.

Breast Disorders: Nipple Discharge and Inflammation

ICD-9-CM

Galactorrhea 676.6
Abscess 611.0
Mastitis 611

OVERVIEW

Definitions

Nipple discharge: Serous, bloody, milky, or multicolored fluid from the nipple that occurs spontaneously or is intentionally expressed. The discharge may be physiological or pathological. It increases with sexual stimulation of the breasts, frequent breast self-examination (BSE), or frequent attempts to elicit the discharge to see "if it is still there." Milky nipple discharge is called *galactorrhea.* "Witches milk," or galactorrhea in newborns, is a benign and transient condition caused by maternal estrogen and progesterone crossing the placental barrier and affecting the newborn's breast tissue. No treatment is necessary for this; an appropriate intervention is to reassure the parents of its normalcy.

Chiari-Frommel syndrome: Persistent amenorrhea and galactorrhea after pregnancy.

Forbes-Albright syndrome: Galactorrhea and amenorrhea caused by pituitary tumor.

Galactocele: Overdistended or obstructed milk duct that becomes cystic and milk-filled after weaning a breast-fed baby or, rarely, with oral contraceptive pills. Galactocele is associated with a painless periareolar or subareolar mass. Removal of the fluid via fine-needle aspiration is both diagnostic and therapeutic.

Lactational (puerperal) mastitis: Infection of connective tissue of the lactating breast, typically occurring 2 to 4 weeks postpartum. The usual causative organisms are *Staphylococcus aureus* and streptococcal species.

Nonlactational mastitis: Infection of the breast that is unrelated to lactation; usually caused by mixed aerobes and anaerobes. Occasionally, nonlactational mastitis is associated with such other infections as tuberculosis, syphilis, typhoid, cancer, and *Actinomyces* infection.

Incidence

Nipple discharge is the presenting breast complaint in 3% to 10% of women—much fewer than with breast masses. Most nipple discharges represent benign conditions; galactorrhea occasionally occurs at menarche or premenopausally secondary to physiological hormone alterations. At times it may be drug induced.

Fewer than 10% of breast biopsies performed to confirm the cause of nipple discharge reveal breast cancer. **Males** with a nipple discharge are more likely to have a malignancy.

Mastitis develops in about 2.5% of nursing mothers. Nonlactational mastitis is relatively rare.

Pathophysiology

Protective Factors Against Nipple Discharge

None

Factors That Increase Susceptibility to Nipple Discharge

Vigorous stimulation of the breasts and nipples through sexual activity or frequent manipulation of breasts (from BSE) or attempts to elicit discharge

Current use of oral contraceptives or other drugs that contribute to nipple discharge by suppressing dopamine or stimulating prolactin release (Box 24-1)

Being a neonate under the influence of transplacental maternal hormones

Box 24-1

Drugs Known to Cause Nipple Discharge

Methyldopa	Corticosteroids
Reserpine	Digoxin
Phenytoin	Diuretics
Opiates	Metoclopramide
Phenothiazines	Contraceptives
Tricyclic antidepressants	Neuroleptics

This is not an exhaustive list; consult a drug reference for more details.

Disorders of the hypothalamus
Thyroid disease
Chest lesions (burns, cancer, trauma)
Renal disease
Nonpituitary: Prolactin-secreting tumor (lung, kidney)
Pituitary tumor

Protective Factors Against Mastitis

Use of positioning and techniques to ensure correct latch-on and sucking by breastfeeding infant, thereby preventing nipple trauma
Bottle-feeding infant
Good nipple hygiene

Factors That Increase Susceptibility to Mastitis

Breastfeeding problems, especially that lead to traumatized nipples or milk stasis
Breast abnormality or previous surgery, including implants
Inverted nipples
History of previous mastitis
Diabetes mellitus
Steroid therapy
Smoking
Infant colonized with staphylococcal or streptococcal organisms

SUBJECTIVE DATA

History of Present Illness

Nipple Discharge

Note discharge from one or more ducts on the nipple of one or both breasts that either occurs spontaneously or is elicited.
Ask whether patient finds dried stains on night clothing or linens.
Ask about color and consistency of discharge, whether unilateral or bilateral, whether one duct or several are involved.
Ask whether mass has been palpated.
Ask whether there are skin problems in the breast area where drainage may be confused with discharge from the nipples.

NOTE: *Presence of unilateral bloody, serous, serosanguineous, or watery discharge from a single duct and/or associated with a mass is indicative of breast cancer in males or females.*

Galactocele

Determine recent initiation of oral contraceptive pills.
Ask about sudden cessation of breastfeeding.
Ask whether the patient has gradually weaned a breastfed infant.
Ask about color and consistency of fluid, one or both breasts, spontaneous or expressed, one or more ducts involved.

Mastitis

Note date of childbirth and account of breastfeeding experience thus far.
Note specifics and duration of symptoms.
Ask what makes the symptoms better or worse; ask about associated symptoms.
Determine how symptoms have affected lifestyle of woman and baby.
Ask about fever, chills, and flulike aching and malaise.
Ask about breast and nipple pain before symptoms occurred.
Ask about fatigue level and stress.

Past Medical History

Inquire about chronic illnesses and allergies.
Note serious acute illnesses and surgical procedures.
Record menstrual and contraceptive history.
Note previous breast problems, trauma, surgeries, and implants.
Ask about current use of medications, especially those that cause nipple discharge.
If patient is in the postpartum period, inquire about postpartal course and any problems in breastfeeding.

Family History

Ask about chronic illness with familial tendencies.
Ask about history of breast problems.

Psychosocial History

Ask about use of leisure/street drugs, especially marijuana and opiates.

Diet History

None

TABLE 24-1 Types of Nipple Discharge

Type of Discharge	Number of Ducts Involved	Color of Discharge
Lactational	Multiple ducts—bilateral	Yellow, sticky, opaque: colostrum "Skim-milk" gray-white: breast milk Bloody: Rare variation
Nonlactational	Multiple ducts—unilateral	Purulent: Duct ecstasia or Inflammation of involved breast
	Single duct—unilateral	Bloody, serous, or watery: possible benign condition; **Probable cancer**
	Multiple ducts—bilateral	Milk: Physiological or pathological galactorrhea; Green, yellow, gray, or brown: usually benign condition
	Unilateral or bilateral with eczema-like condition of nipple and/or areola	Variable Usually Paget's disease

Description of Most Common Symptoms and Associated Symptoms

Nipple discharge: Color and subtleties of discharge are less significant than whether it is bilateral and from multiple ducts or unilateral and a single duct (Table 24-1).

OBJECTIVE DATA

Physical Examination

Problem-oriented physical examination should be conducted with particular attention to:

General appearance, vital signs, thyroid, heart, lungs

If galactorrhea noted, check visual fields by a test of confrontation

Breast examination:

Observe breast with woman sitting with arms at sides, with arms behind head, and with hands pressing against hips

Palpate both breasts carefully, including tail of Spence

Palpate for axillary, supraclavicular, and infraclavicular lymph nodes

Elicit discharge (or have woman do so) by compressing nipple-areola complex between thumb and index finger and "milking" toward nipple from three or four directions

Dot fluid onto white tissue or linen to check margins for most accurate color; may not be otherwise apparent

Use of a magnifying glass may enhance visualization of discharge and localization of ducts involved; wetting the breast sometimes eases expression of discharge

Diagnostic Procedures

Diagnostic procedures will be based on findings of the history and physical examination and suspected underlying cause (i.e., TSH and T_4 if a thyroid disorder is suspected; computed tomography or magnetic resonance imaging [cranial/sella turcica] if pituitary tumor is suspected). Mammography and/or breast ultrasound may be ordered.

Procedures used to evaluation of nipple discharge or inflammation of the breast are outlined in Table 24-2.

ASSESSMENT

Differential Diagnosis

Differential diagnoses of nipple discharge include physiological galactorrhea, pathological galactorrhea, Paget's disease, lactation, breast cancer, duct ecstasia, dermatological conditions (i.e., eczema, excoriation, trauma) of breast with associated drainage confused with nipple discharge (Figure 24-1).

Differential diagnoses of mastitis include puerperal or lactational mastitis, ductal ecstasia/periductal/nonlactational mastitis (Table 24-3).

THERAPEUTIC PLAN

Pharmaceutical Management

Nipple Discharge

Drug of choice: Dopamine agonist bromocriptine (Parlodel)

Dosage: 1.25 to 2.5 mg/day for 1 week at supper, then 1.25 to 2.5 BID (2.5 mg [100] $108-$158)

Nurse practitioners generally prescribe this medication in consultation with a physician.

If nipple discharge does not respond to lifestyle changes and/or bromocriptine and is creating problems for the woman's social and sex life, surgery may be indicated.

Mastitis

Antibiotic treatment of mastitis may be based on results of culture and sensitivity study of breast milk.

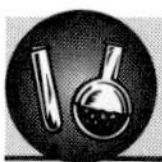

TABLE 24-2 Diagnostic Tests: Nipple Discharge or Inflammation of the Breast

Test	Findings/Rationale	Cost ($)
Microscopic analysis of fluid	Examine sample of fluid under microscope; with evidence of leukocytosis, send sample for culture and sensitivity; with suspicion of galactorrhea, check for evidence of fat globules to confirm or send sample for fat stain and thin-layer chromatography	15-18
Check for blood	Check sample of discharge for occult blood (may use Hemoccult or Hemastix)	15-20
Fat stain of nipple discharge	Microscopic examination of nipple discharge for the presence of fat globules to aid in a diagnosis of galactorrhea	15-19
Thin-layer chromography	Procedure that tests for lactose level in a sample of nipple discharge	N/A
Prolactin radioimmunoassay	Test on blood that indicates level of prolactin; *normal <20 ng/ml;* blood test should be performed between 8 AM and 12 noon for most exact results The following factors are known to elevate prolactin levels and should be considered when interpreting results: excessive breast or nipple stimulation, stress, pelvic examination, coitus, extended sleep, high-protein diet *(Hyperprolactinemia is associated with pituitary tumors, Addison's disease, hypothyroidism, and decreased prolactin clearance secondary to decreased renal or liver function; this factor suggests additional diagnostic procedures when prolactin level is elevated.)*	70-89
Culture and sensitivity of breast milk	Microbiological test of nipple discharge, colostum, or breast milk expressed from the nipple(s) or withdrawn from galactocele by fine-needle aspiration to confirm organism causing infection and identify which antibiotics are likely to be effective as treatment Mastitis diagnosed with leukocytes 1 million/ml and bacterial count >1000/ml	31-39
Galactography/ ductography	Imaging study of breast ductal system Using aseptic technique, and contrast medium to enhance visualization, small catheter or thin probe inserted into the duct(s)	164-198

N/A, Not available.

Since the most common causes are *Staphylococcus aureus* and streptococcus and culture/sensitivity testing is expensive, presumptive treatment may be used (Table 24-4).
If the infection is unresponsive to drug therapy or an abscess forms, incision and drainage may be necessary.

Lifestyle/Activities

Warn women that overstimulation of the breasts contributes to nipple discharge.
Teach women appropriate nipple hygiene.
Suggest clean white handkerchief or cut squares of sanitary napkins as breast pads, stressing the need for avoiding plastic-lined breast pads and prolonged wet pads in contact with nipples to minimize irritation.

Diet

Decreasing caffeine, methylxanthines, salt, and saturated fats may decrease swelling and discomfort in the breasts.

Patient Education

Teach BSE to be initiated monthly from age 20, stressing the importance of scheduling 2 or 3 days after menstrual period ends to decrease hormonal effects. After normal clinical breast examination, suggest the woman examine her breasts the same day to recognize "normal" as a subsequent baseline.
For nonmenstruating women, advise selection of a particular day each month for examination (e.g., the first of the month, the fifteenth of the month). For women using oral contraceptives, suggest BSE when beginning a new pill pack.
Advise women to schedule clinical breast examination every 2 years from ages 20 to 40, every other year between ages 40 and 50, and annually over age 50.
Teach signs and symptoms of breast cancer.
Advise importance of mammograms according to national guidelines: baseline at age 40, every other year between ages 40 and 50, annually after age 50 (American Cancer Society Recommendations, 1997).
In women in whom first-degree female relative had breast

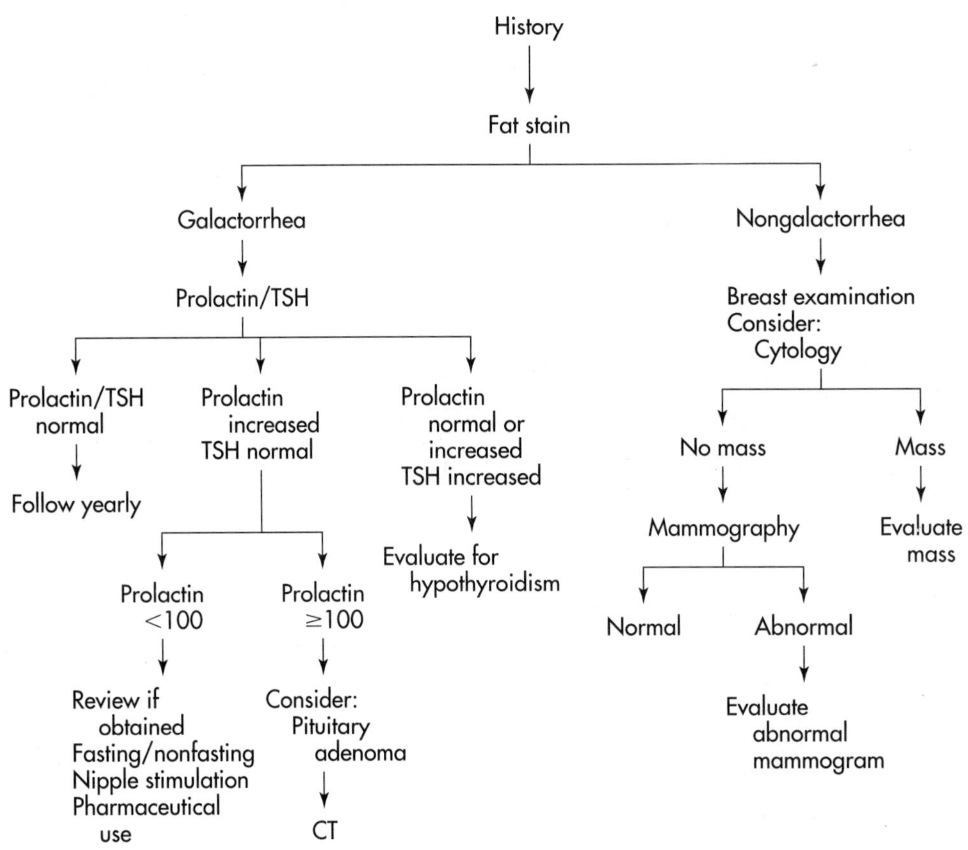

Figure 24-1 Algorithm for the treatment of patient with a nipple discharge. (From Greene HL, Johnson WP, Lemcke D, editors: *Decision making in medicine,* ed 2, St Louis, 1998, Mosby.)

TABLE 24-3 Differential Diagnoses: Mastitis

Disorder	Common Symptoms	Associated Symptoms	Age
Nonlactational mastitis	Erythema, warmth, tenderness, induration Possible abscess	No fever or flulike symptoms; no malaise	Any
Periductal mastitis/ ductal ecstasia	Inflamed breast with possible abscess 1-2 cm wormlike or tubular firm, tender mass; burning or stinging pain exacerbated by exposure to cold	Unilateral or bilateral nipple discharge (thin and watery in young women; thick, pasty, and sticky in older women); spontaneous, intermittent Color of discharge: cream, brown, gray, green, or bloody	45-55
Lactational mastitis	Inflamed breast: Reddened, warm, tender, edematous Possible abscess Due to septal distribution of connective tissue—inflammation may appear in wedge-shaped pattern	Chills and fever, malaise, flulike aching Milk culture reveals causative organism and increased WBCs	Childbearing age

WBC, White blood cell count.

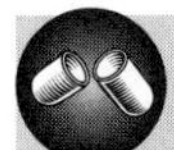

TABLE 24-4 Pharmaceutical Plan: Mastitis

Antibiotic	Dosage	Cost
Amoxicillin/clavulonate (Augmentin)	250 mg PO q8h ×10 days	$57/250 mg (30)
Erythromycin (If allergic to penicillin)	250-500 q6h or EES 400 mg q8h ×7-10 days	$23-$51/250 mg (100)
Dicloxacillin (for penicillin-resistant staphylococcal organisms)	125-250 mg q6h	$13/125 mg (24) $19-$94/250 mg (100)
Vancomycin (for methicillin-resistant staphylococcal organisms)	250-500 mg q6h	$189/250 mg (20)
Cephalosporins (cephalexine [Keflex], cephadrins [Anspor, Velosef]) may also be used		Varies

EES, Erythromycin ethyl succinate.

TABLE 24-5 Considerations for Persistent Spontaneous Nonlactational Nipple Discharge

Question to Ask	Yes/No	Action
Are there skin changes on nipples or areola indicative of Paget's disease?	Yes	Refer for punch biopsy to rule out breast cancer and need for possible surgical treatment
Is the discharge unilateral, heme positive, or grossly bloody or watery?	Yes	Refer for biopsy
	No	Is discharge bilateral and milky? Check fat stain and thin-layer chromography
Suspicious for cancer?	No	Consider endocrine or physiological cause; order testing for verification
Could drugs be causing nipple discharge?	Yes	Discontinue if possible; reevaluate
	No	Consider endocrine or physiological cause; order testing for verification
Is discharge yellow, gray, green or brown?	Yes	Suspect benign condition; follow closely
Is discharge sticky and multicolored?	Yes	Suspect duct ectasia; reassure patient; advise use of PhisoHex or betadine washes to area
Is discharge purulent?	Yes	Check for abscess; refer for incision and drainage if needed; order antibiotics and teach nipple hygiene if no abscess
Does it recur?	Yes	Refer to OB/GYN or surgeon

cancer, advise need for mammography 10 years earlier than age of the relative's diagnosis (i.e., if the mother was diagnosed at age 39, the patient should undergo mammography at age 29).

Nipple Discharge

Reassure patient that nipple discharge is usually not associated with breast cancer (Table 24-5).

Advise about relationship between breast stimulation and increasing discharge.

For any discharge other than suspected malignancy-related discharge, teach appropriate lifestyle changes.

Mastitis

Recognize that most women will be discharged from the maternity unit before experiencing signs of mastitis.

Teach all new nursing mothers signs and symptoms and preventive strategies—correct positioning for nursing that minimizes nipple trauma, good hand washing before handling breasts, frequent breastfeeding to minimize probability of milk stasis.

Advise wearing a support bra without underwires 24 hours a day.

Advise rest for several days, increasing fluid intake, use of heat or cold packs on breasts for comfort, and analgesics.

Advise no need to discontinue breastfeeding unless mother feels too ill. If woman decides to temporarily discontinue nursing because she feels too ill, teach procedure for pumping breasts to continue lactation process. Teach about antibiotic therapy.

Family Impact

To the woman and her family, nipple discharge may inevitably be associated with breast cancer; this misperception can cause unnecessary anxiety and may prolong initiation of treatment. For a breastfeeding woman and her family, there may well be concerns about the baby's nutrition, discontinuation of desired breastfeeding, and the mother's health status.

Referral

Refer the patient to surgeon when:
- Mammography results are abnormal
- Suspicious palpable mass present
- Serous or bloody fluid, heme-positive fluid present (particularly if unilateral)
- Nonlactational mastitis suspected
- Breast abscess present

For breastfeeding woman with mastitis:
- Consider referral to lactation specialist or La Leche League for support

Consultation

Moderate to severe nonlactational mastitis/duct ecstasia
Pathological galactorrhea and use of bromocriptine therapy

Follow-up

Heme-negative discharge: 1 to 2 months
Galactocele: 1 month
Mastitis: 10 to 14 days

EVALUATION

Positive outcomes include reassurance about and treatment of benign conditions; early recognition and treatment of a malignancy contibuting to nipple discharge; and resolution of inflammatory conditions without sequelae.

SUGGESTED READINGS

Bowman MA et al: Who are you screening for cancer—and when? *Patient Care* 30:54-87, 1996.

Carlson KJ et al: *Primary care of women,* St Louis, 1996, Mosby.

Chin HG: *On call obstetrics & gynecology,* Philadelphia, 1997, WB Saunders.

Conry C: Evaluation of a breast complaint: is it cancer? *Am Fam Physician* 49:445-452, 1994.

Ellsworth A et al: *Mosby's 1998 medical drug reference,* St Louis, 1998, Mosby.

Healthcare Consultants of America, Inc: *1998 Physicians fee and coding guide,* Augusta, Ga, 1998, Healthcare Consultants of America, Inc.

Fiorica JV, Schorr SJ, Sickles, EA: Benign breast disorders—first rule out cancer, *Patient Care* 31:140-154, 1997.

Fogel CI, Woods, NF: *Women's health care: a comprehensive handbook,* Thousand Oaks, Calif, 1995, Sage.

Fullerton JT, Lanz J, Sadler GR: Breast cancer among men: raising awareness for primary prevention, *J Am Acad Nurse Pract* 9:211-216, 1997.

Hindle WH: Other benign breast problems, *Clin Obstet Gynecol* 37:916-924, 1994.

Lawrence HC: History, physical examination, and education in breast self-examination, *Clin Obstet Gynecol* 37:881-886, 1994.

Lichtman R, Papera S: *Gynecology: well woman care,* Norwalk, Conn, 1990, Appleton & Lange.

Ma JC, Easter DW: Current guidelines for breast cancer screening, *Contemp Nurs Pract* 1995, pp 10-17.

Reifsnider E: Educating women about benign breast disease, *AAOHNJ* 38:121-125, 1990.

Smith RP: *Gynecology in primary care,* Baltimore, 1997, Williams & Wilkins.

Spiegel KK: On your markers—research advances in breast cancer in women, *AWHONN Lifelines* 1:33-38, 1997.

Star WL, Lommel, LL, Shannon MT, editors: *Women's primary health care—protocols for practice,* Washington, DC, 1995, American Nurses Publishing.

White GL et al: Breast cancer: reducing mortality through early detection, *Clin Rev* 1996, pp 77-106.

Youngkin EQ, Davis MS: *Women's health: a primary care guide,* Norwalk, Conn, 1994, Appleton & Lange.

Breastfeeding Problems

Disturbances in the Production and Transfer of Human Milk

ICD-9-CM

Puerperal, Postpartum 675.1

OVERVIEW

Definition

Breastfeeding problems are the perceived or actual lack of adequate lactation to sustain an infant. The causes of breastfeeding problems include multiple interrelated psychosocial and physiological elements.

Incidence

The perceived or actual instances of inadequate lactation are the leading cause of cessation of breastfeeding in mothers worldwide. These instances are seen equally in urban and rural settings and in women of various socioeconomic backgrounds. Reportable percentages in the first 6 months of breastfeeding vary from 35% to 80%.

Pathophysiology

The process of lactogenesis begins with stimulation of the hypothalamus by the infant's suckling at the breast. This in turn produces secretion and release of prolactin and oxytocin from the pituitary gland into the bloodstream. The presence of oxytocin in the circulation stimulates milk synthesis and release into the alveoli and the lactiferous sinuses. Anything that inhibits the removal of milk from the breast will inhibit the lactation process.

Psychosocial Factors That May Influence Lactation

Maternal time restraints, such as home or work responsibilities

Temperament of infant (e.g., a fussy baby is often interpreted as hungry, so the mother questions her milk supply and begins to use supplement)

Decreased suckling time of the infant at the breast will lead to decreased stimulation and therefore decreased milk supply

Physical Factors That May Influence Lactation

Maternal discomfort, including breast engorgement, nipple tenderness, pain from incision or episiotomy

Poor nutrition/inadequate fluid intake of mother

Inadequate rest or excessive anxiety in mother

History of breast surgery that resulted in the severing of the nerves and/or the lactiferous ducts

Minimal or no breast enlargement during pregnancy

Drug/alcohol or tobacco use

Maternal illness

Inadequate time at breast

Inadequate suckling ability of infant

SUBJECTIVE DATA

History of Present Illness

Ask mother why she feels her milk supply is inadequate. Determine:

- Number of breastfeedings per day and the length of time at each breast vs. actual suckling time
- Use of breast pump
- Use of supplements
- Voiding and stooling pattern of infant

Past Medical History

Ask about:

Complications of the pregnancy and delivery, including the postpartal course

The mother's past history of breast disease or breast surgery

Previous experiences with breastfeeding

Medications

Ask about recent use of medications, in particular oral or injectable contraceptives or anticholinergic drugs.

Family History

Explore the family history of breastfeeding:

Is it an acceptable feeding method?

Has the mother had previous experiences with breastfeeding?

Psychosocial History

Ask the mother when in her pregnancy she decided to breastfeed.

Does the mother have the support of her family in her efforts at breastfeeding?

Is the mother comfortable with the concept of breastfeeding?

Inquire about the infant's temperament.

Inquire about the mother's home and work responsibilities.

Description of Most Common Symptoms

Psychosocial

Ambivalence and/or lack of confidence in her ability to breastfeed

Lack of education about breastfeeding

Physical (Mother)

Breast engorgement

Inverted or flat nipples

Nipple tenderness

Illness in mother such as anemia, mastitis, or other infections

Minimal or no change in breast size during pregnancy

Physical (Infant)

Borderline premature infant (36 to 37 weeks)

Small for gestational age infant

Intrauterine growth retardation infant

Infant with oral clefts

Infant with dysfunctional sucking

Jaundiced infant

Infant with systemic disease

Infant with low energy

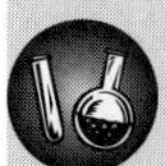

TABLE 25-1 Diagnostic Tests: Breastfeeding Problems

Test	Findings/Rationale	Cost ($)
Culture and sensitivity	Obtain swab of nipple before breastfeeding and specimen of expressed milk	31-39

OBJECTIVE DATA

Physical Examination

A problem-oriented physical examination should be conducted, with particular attention to vital signs, weight, general appearance, general hydration status.

Breasts

Nipples/integument: Observe for cracks, fissures, ulcers, inflammation or severe tenderness to light touch

Nipple adequacy: Inverted or flat nipples

Glandular tissue: Observe for fullness, symmetry, vascularity, palpate for masses

Observe infant suckling at breast

Milk volume:

Does mother report that her breast feels full and firm before feeding?

Does she feel empty after nursing?

Does she use an electric pump, and what are her average yields?

Diagnostic Procedures

Diagnostic procedures are outlined in Table 25-1.

ASSESSMENT

Differential diagnoses include those listed in Table 25-2.

THERAPEUTIC PLAN

Pharmaceutical

Treatment for suspected fungal or documented bacterial infection of nipples

Concurrent treatment of mother and baby is necessary to eradicate a persistent fungal infection (Table 25-3 and Box 25-1.)

TABLE 25-2 Differential Diagnosis: Breastfeeding Problems

Diagnosis	Supporting Data
Psychosocial issues	Supplementing several times a day because of perceived lack of milk supply or fussy baby; mother with no or minimal support systems; mother returning to work; mother extremely fatigued; sexual abuse
Breast engorgement	Distended, hard, painful breasts; increased vascularity present; 2-4 days postpartum; obstruction of expressed milk
Sore nipples*	Poor positioning: Soreness on top or tip of nipple; poor latch-on Bruised, scabbed, or blistered nipples with pain on underside; mother presenting nipple up to infant; infant stokes underside of nipple Infection: Nipples cracked with fissures, ulcers, general inflammation Afebrile, severe tenderness to light touch Infant <1 month old, positive culture and sensitivity for *Staphylococcus aureus* or *Streptococcus* group B Probable *Candida albicans:* Inflamed, fissures, burning, itching, tender to touch with shooting pain in breast, usually hurts between feedings History of antibiotic use in postpartum period; positive history of oral thrush in infant Some women may have no visible signs but experience the pain and tenderness
Inadequate feeding methods	Rigid feeding schedules, short, restricted suckling times, absence of night feedings, mother-infant separation, use of supplementation, poor positioning, and/or inadequate areolar grasp
Breast anomalies	Flat/inverted nipples, history of breast surgery, history of minimal enlargement of breasts during pregnancy (normally, breasts approximately double in size)
Maternal illness/ poor nutrition	Anemia, infection such as UTIs, URIs, or mastitis Inadequate caloric intake or fluid intake
Maternal drug/ alcohol/smoking	Smoking decreases prolactin; large amounts of alcohol decrease milk ejection Use of oral contraceptives or anticholinergic medications (both can cause a decrease in milk production)

*Most women experience some degree of nipple soreness with associated breakdown of skin integument during the first week of breastfeeding.
UTI, Urinary tract infection; *URI,* upper respiratory infection.

Lifestyle/Activities

Pacifiers: Discourage use until breastfeeding is well established. Sterilize or change pacifiers daily if *Candida* infection suspected.

Bras: Change daily, add bleach to wash cycle.

Diet

Breastfeeding mothers require a balanced diet of fruits, vegetables, whole grains, calcium-rich dairy products and protein-rich food. The caloric increase required is approximately 500 kcal/day. It is normal for nursing mothers to demonstrate an increase in appetite and in thirst.

Patient Education

Psychosocial

Provide the mother with education and encouragement. Assist her in identifying a support person (husband, mother, or friend). Provide her with information concerning local support groups such as La Leche League; Nursing Mothers Counsel; and local Women, Infants, and Children (WIC) agency.

Sore Nipples

Teach the mother proper positioning for breastfeeding. Demonstrate traditional cradle hold, side-lying, and football positions. Mother needs to be in a comfortable position. She will introduce her breast by placing her thumb above the areola and her other fingers below the breast for support. The nipple will project straight ahead or slightly downward. The infant needs an adequate grasp of the areola for proper suckling. Anhydrous lanolin may be applied after feeding for cracked, raw nipples with or without bleeding and free from infection. Pain inhibits the letdown reflex; therefore consider the use of analgesics.

Flat or Inverted Nipples

This condition may require the use of a breast shell (i.e., a clear plastic device placed over the areola/nipple to help the infant latch on to the nipple) between feedings to draw out the nipple. Instruct the mother to compress the areola and breast between her fingers to protrude the nipple as much as possible when offering it to the infant. Use of an electric or manual pump for several minutes before the feeding session will also facilitate nipple protrusion. Severe nipple inversion may prohibit feeding at the breast.

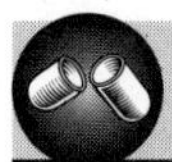

TABLE 25-3 Pharmaceutical Plan: Infections

Organism	Drug	Adult Dose	Infant Dosage	Cost
Candida albicans	First line: Mycostatin cream 100,000 U	Apply to nipples after feeding, TID until resolved (14 days minimum)	Nystatin suspension 100,000 U; swab 1 ml in mouth QID	$3-$22/100,000 U/ml (480 ml)
	Second line: If no response after 14 days, start fluconazole (Diflucan); continue topical treatment	Loading dose of 200 mg, then 100 QD for 15 days If yeast persists, increase dose to 200 mg QD for 15 days (monitor liver function) Max: 600 mg/day Pregnancy: C SE: Nausea and vomiting, headache, abdominal pain, diarrhea		
Staphylococcus aureus	Dicloxacillin sodium (Dynapen)	250 mg QID for 7 days Pregnancy: B SE: Nausea and vomiting, abdominal pain Take with water on empty stomach		$19-$94/250 mg (100)
	Ibuprofen for pain (see Appendix J for complete NSAID information)	400 mg q4-6h as needed Pregnancy: B (D in third trimester) SE: Anorexia, nausea and vomiting, GI bleeding		$3-$9/200 mg (100)

SE, Side effects; *NSAID*, nonsteroidal antiinflammatory drug; *GI*, gastrointestinal.

Engorgement

Instruct mother to apply warm, moist heat to both breasts 5 to 10 minutes before nursing. Hand express some milk to soften the areola. Gently massage breasts before and during feeding. Apply cold compresses after feeding to relieve discomfort and decrease swelling. The mother needs to offer both breasts at each feeding. If the infant cannot latch on because nipples are flattened by engorgement, it may help to use an electric pump to draw out the nipples before the feeding. Consider use of an analgesic (ibuprofen or acetaminophen) for pain. Engorgement usually resolves within 48 hours.

Adequate Breastfeeding

Newborns: Breastfed infants will have more rapid stomach-emptying time than bottle-fed infants; therefore frequent feedings are to be expected. The newborn should nurse 8 to 12 times per day with a minimum of 10 to 15 minutes per breast. As the infant recovers his birthweight, generally between 10 and 14 days, a mature suckling pattern will emerge and the infant will decrease demand to every 2 to 3 hours and eventually 3 to 4 hours as the mother's milk supply increases. Mothers with large milk supplies may satisfy the infant with nursing 15 to 20 minutes on one breast. These mothers should offer the opposite breast at the next feeding.

Older infants: Infants may increase demand during periods of growth spurts, 2 to 3 weeks, 6 weeks, 3 months, and 6 months of age. Advise the mother to breastfeed more often to build her milk supply. If fussiness in between feedings persists, the mother should be advised to explore other reasons for the discomfort, such as overstimulation, tiredness, otitis media.

Rest/Diet

The mother should be advised to nap when the infant naps and attempt to plan nap time for other young children at the same time. Mother needs a well-balanced diet with an approximate increase of 500 kcal/day. Suggest minimizing caffeine intake and discourage use of alcohol, especially during the newborn period.

Box 25-1

Medications That Affect Breastfeeding

Antibiotics Excreted in Breast Milk

Aminoglycosides
Chloramphenicol
Erythromycin
Metronidazole
Trimethoprim-sulfamethoxazole

Antibiotics Excreted in Trace Amounts

Acyclovir
Cephalosporins
Clindamycin
Nitrofurantoin
Penicillins

Drugs Contraindicated During Breastfeeding

Bromocriptine
Cimetidine
Clemastine
Cyclophosphamide
Drugs with potential for abuse
Ergotamine
Gold salts
Methimazole
Thiouracil

Breastfeeding May Be Resumed After Drugs Eliminated From Body

Cascara
Lithium
Metronidazole
Radiopharmaceuticals
- Gallium-69
- Iodine-125
- Iodine-131
- Radioactive sodium
- Technetium-99m

Not an exhaustive list; consult a more specific drug reference as needed.

Milk Supply

The mother should be taught that the best indicator of adequate milk supply is appropriate weight gain and an appropriate voiding and stool pattern of the infant. During the first 6 weeks of life the infant will have 6 to 8 wet diapers a day and 2 to 5 yellow, seedy stools. The infant will achieve birthweight by 2 weeks and gain 4 to 7 ounces per week. The infant will feed frequently and appear healthy. Things that will inhibit milk ejection reflex or milk supply include strict feeding schedules, use of formula or water as a supplement, maternal stress, and use of drugs or contraceptives, smoking, or excessive alcohol intake.

Family Impact

Fathers occasionally will have feelings of jealousy of the physical and emotional closeness of the mother and infant. Advise the mother to involve the father in her decision to breastfeed. Encourage his participation in the baby's care. Siblings will also have questions about their mother's breastfeeding. It is best to breastfeed openly in front of older children and answer their questions honestly.

Referral

A mother with true insufficient milk supply as documented by indicators of a failure-to-thrive infant should be referred to a lactation specialist.

A mother with a history of breast surgery and/or no change in glandular tissue should be referred to a lactation specialist.

Consultation

Consult with the infant's primary care physician for any child in whom you suspect dehydration or failure to thrive.

Follow-up

Mothers with positive cultures or have clinical symptoms of a candidal infection should be reassessed at 1 week to evaluate the response to medication.

EVALUATION

Place weekly calls to assess mother's confidence level and review general health status.

Follow up weekly with mothers who continue to have sore nipples.

SUGGESTED READINGS

Amir L et al: *Candida albicans:* is it associated with nipple pain in lactating women? *Gynecol Obstet Invest* 41:30-34, 1996.

Bodley V, Powers D: Long-term treatment of a breastfeeding mother with fluconazole—resolved nipple pain caused by yeast: a case study, *J Hum Lact* 13:307-311, 1997.

Committee on Drugs: The transfer of drugs and other chemicals into human milk, *Pediatrics* 93:137-150, 1994.

Driscoll JW: Breastfeeding success and failure: implications for nurses, *NAACOG Clin Issues* 3:565-569, 1992.

Ellsworth A et al: *Mosby's 1998 medical drug reference,* St Louis, 1998, Mosby.

Healthcare Consultants of America, Inc: *1998 Physicians fee and coding guide,* Augusta, Ga, 1998, Healthcare Consultants of America, Inc.

Hill P: Insufficient milk supply syndrome, *NAACOG Clin Issues* 3:605-612, 1992.

Hurst N: Lactation after augmentation mammoplasty, *Obstet Gynecol* 87(1):30-34, 1996.

Lawrence R: *Breastfeeding: a guide for the medical professional,* ed 4, St Louis, 1994, Mosby.

Livingstone V, Willis C, Berkowitz J: *Staphylococcus aureus* and sore nipples, *Can Family Physician* 1996, pp 654-659.

Main Trail Collaboration Group: Preparing for breastfeeding: treatment of inverted and non-projectile nipples in pregnancy, *Midwifery* 1994, pp 200-214.

Mozingo J: Empowering women to breastfeed, *Adv Nurse Pract* 4:43-65, 1996.

Neifert M: Breastfeeding after breast surgical procedure or breast surgery, *NAACOG Clin Issues* 3:673-682, 1992.

26 Bronchiolitis

ICD-9-CM

Bronchiolitis 466.19

OVERVIEW

Definition

Generalized inflammation of the bronchioles

Incidence

Bronchiolitis usually accompanies a respiratory viral infection. Respiratory syncytial virus (RSV) accounts for about 80% of all cases. Influenza and parainfluenza viruses, adenoviruses, and allergies are less commonly implicated.

Bronchiolitis usually affects **children under the age of 3 years,** with a peak incidence around **2 to 3 months**. Its seasonal clustering during late winter and early spring can create annual epidemics. Bronchiolitis also occurs infrequently in school-age children and is usually caused by *Mycoplasma pneumoniae*.

Pathophysiology

Etiologic organisms are transmitted by respiratory secretions and/or droplet contamination. Inflammation, excess mucus secretion, and epithelial hyperplasia and necrosis contribute to narrowing and blockage of the small airways of the bronchioles. The resultant obstruction contributes to increased airway resistance, air trapping, and respiratory compromise. The smaller bronchioles in infants exacerbate these processes and account for the higher mortality and morbidity in this age group.

Factors That Increase Susceptibility

Premature infants, especially those with bronchopulmonary dysplasia are at risk.

Infants with congenital heart disease are at particularly highest risk for severe RSV infection.

Immunocompromised children and adults are also more susceptible to RSV infections.

SUBJECTIVE DATA

History of Present Illness

Question about onset, fever, prodromal and associated symptoms. Ask about recent exposures to respiratory illness.

Past Medical History

Assess for allergies/atopy; immune disorders; prematurity; and/or bronchopulmonary dysplasia, congenital heart disease, and foreign body aspiration. Determine immunization status.

Activity/Lifestyle

Ask about feeding and sleeping difficulties, infant's general behavior.

Family Medical History

Assess for allergies, asthma, immune disorders.

Description of Most Common Symptoms

Abrupt onset of wheezing and difficulty breathing; prodromal history of mild rhinitis and cough/coryza for 1 to 2 days is common; fever may be low-grade or absent.

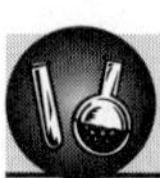

TABLE 26-1 Diagnostic Tests: Bronchiolitis

Diagnostic Test	Findings	Cost ($)
CBC: Not usually needed	WBC usually normal or very slightly elevated; eosinophilia may be seen	18-23
CXR: Not usually needed; may obtain with consultation	Typically reveals hyperinflation, ↑ bronchovesicular markings and mild interstitial infiltration	77-91
RSV throat culture: Not usually done	Positive if RSV is present; rapid diagnosis if detection of antigen by nasopharyngeal wash	45-57

CBC, Complete blood count; *WBC,* white blood count; *CXR,* chest x-ray; *RSV,* respiratory syncytial virus.

Associated Symptoms

Parent may report a hacking/gagging cough, difficulty feeding and sleeping, and lethargy. Very young and/or premature infants may present with apnea.

OBJECTIVE DATA

Physical Examination

Vital signs: Fever usually low-grade or absent; increased respiratory and heart rate typical (see Appendix S)
General: Toxic appearance with diminished sensorium and mild to marked signs of respiratory distress—rapid, shallow breathing; nasal flaring; cyanosis and retractions if severe
Observe the parent feeding the infant. Monitor for feeding difficulties.
Skin: Pallor/mottling, cyanosis, delayed capillary refill, decreased skin turgor and dryness of lips and mouth (may indicate dehydration)
Head/eyes/ears/nose/throat: Possibly concomitant infections (e.g., conjunctivitis, otitis media)
Lungs: Increased respiratory effort (paradoxical or "seesaw" respirations require immediate referral), grunting, and prolonged expiration; hyperresonance; diminished breath sounds with scattered crackles/rales and symmetric expiratory wheeze
Heart: Tachycardia (see Appendix S for norms)
Abdomen: May be able to palpate liver and spleen (due to hyperinflation of lungs)

Diagnostic Tests

Diagnostic tests include those found in Table 26-1.

ASSESSMENT

Diagnosis is based on history of abrupt onset of wheezing and difficulty breathing. Physical examination findings that support hyperinflation of the lungs corroborate the diagnosis.

Differential diagnoses include asthma, bronchitis, foreign body aspiration, gastroesophageal reflux disease, pneumonia, tuberculosis, and viral croup (Table 26-2).

THERAPEUTIC PLAN

Pharmaceutical

Empirically administer antibiotics only if a secondary infection is suspected (uncommon) and analgesics for fever and/or discomfort or to relieve anxiety and promote rest. Use analgesics cautiously in an infant. They may mask a fever, which may confuse the clinical presentation.
Aerosolized bronchodilators may provide transient improvement of the airway obstruction.
Aerosolized antiviral (Ribavirin) has been demonstrated to shorten the clinical course for severe bronchiolitis (20 mg/ml for 12 to 18 hours/day for 3 to 7 days), but its use remains controversial.
Immunoglobulin therapy has been used on an experimental basis (both intravenous and aerosol), and the data thus far are encouraging. Pharmaceutical choices for bronchiolitis are found in Table 26-3.

Lifestyle/Activity

Rest, quiet, comfort are recommended; increased environmental humidity will facilitate loosening and clearing of secretions.

Dietary

Ensure adequate fluid intake—smaller amounts more frequently while the infant is very ill; percussion and postural drainage are advised before eating.

Education

Instruct parents regarding signs of respiratory distress; parents may need to be taught how to use a bulb syringe

TABLE 26-2 Differential Diagnosis: Bronchiolitis

Diagnoses	Supporting Data
Bronchitis	Bronchitis is a generalized inflammation of the major bronchi. It usually is preceded by rhinitis and URI. The hallmark symptom is a dry hacking, nonproductive cough which is frequently paroxysmal. A low-grade fever may be present. Breath sounds are usually normal, although occasional wheezes may be heard.
Pneumonia	Infections typically occur in the late winter and spring. It presents with abrupt onset of fever, restlessness, and respiratory distress after an URI. Auscultation of the lungs reveals diminished breath sounds and crackles on the affected side. Dullness on percussion may also be present. WBCs usually range from 15,000 to 40,000.
Asthma/RAD	Reactive airway has been recognized as one of the most common causes of cough in children. Expiratory wheezing may be noted along with recurrent coughing, and accessory muscle use. PEFR is frequently less than expected for age/height. Dramatic improvements are noted with use of bronchodilator.
Croup/bacterial tracheitis	Symptoms usually begin as viral URI followed by barking cough. The fever is usually higher, and the patient more ill appearing with tracheitis than croup. Upper airway obstruction may develop rapidly.
Pertussis	Paroxysms of cough are followed by a characteristic inspiratory whoop. Consider in children >5 years, or in older children or adults who present with coughing for >10 days (the whoop may not be present).
Tuberculosis	Symptoms may be initially absent for 4 to 6 weeks after infection. The client may complain of night sweats and productive coughing, hemoptysis, malaise and fatigue, and weight loss.

URI, Upper respiratory infection; *WBC,* white blood cell count; *RAD,* reactive airway disease; *PEFR,* peak expiratory flow rate.

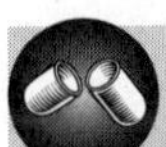

TABLE 26-3 Pharmaceutical Plan: Bronchiolitis

Drug	Dose	Comments	Cost
Acetaminophen (see Pediatric Dosing in Appendix L)	10-15 mg/kg q4-6h	Pregnancy: B SE: Rash, hepatotoxicity	$2/drops: 80 mg/0.8 ml (15 ml) $2/elixer: 160 mg/5 ml (120 ml)
Albuterol	Nebulizer: 5 mg/ml, 0.10-0.15 mg/kg in 2 ml of NS q4-6h; max. 5 mg/day	Pregnancy: C SE: Tachycardia, nervousness, tremor, GI upset, cough	$1-$2/0.083% (3 ml)
Metaproterenol	Nebulizer: 50 mg/ml, 0.25-0.50 mg/kg in 2 ml of NS q4-6h, max. 15 mg/day	Pregnancy: C SE: Tachycardia, nervousness, tremor, GI upset, cough	$17-$42/0.4%, 0.6%/ 2.5 ml (25)

SE, Side effects; *NS,* normal saline; *GI,* gastrointestinal.

to clear secretions or how to administer percussion and postural drainage.

Family Impact

Parents are usually very frightened and anxious and need support and reassurance.

Consultation/Referral

Hospitalization and mechanical ventilation are needed for 1% to 2% of infants with bronchiolitis. Medical consultation/referral is warranted if the infant is in respiratory distress and/or has a respiratory rate >60/min; has apnea; is under 3 months of age or under 6 months of age with a history of prematurity, bronchopulmonary dysplasia, or congenital heart disease; feeds with difficulty and/or shows signs of dehydration. Also consult/refer if there has been no resolution in 3 weeks or if bronchiolitis reoccurs (other pathology may be present).

Follow-up

Telephone call within 24 hours and daily thereafter until symptoms of respiratory distress have abated

Return visit in 48 hours if there is minimal or no improvement with supportive therapy

Return visit in 1 week if symptoms are still present

EVALUATION

The prognosis for bronchiolitis is good, and most infants fully recover within 2 weeks. However, as many as half of these will experience recurrent episodes of wheezing and coughing over 3 to 5 years. Very rarely the illness is so severe that permanent airway damage occurs.

SUGGESTED READINGS

Andral M et al: Acute otitis media in children with bronchiolitis, *Pediatrics* 101(4PI):617-619, 1998.

Chang A, Jasel J, Masters B: Postinfection bronchiolitis obliterans: clinical, radiological, and pulmonary function sequelae, *Pediatr Radiol* 28(1): 23-29, 1998.

Couriel J: Respiratory disorders. In Lissauer T, Clayden G, editors: *Illustrated textbook of pediatrics,* St Louis, 1997, Mosby.

D'Auria JP: Respiratory system. In Fox JA, editor: *Primary health care of children,* St Louis, 1997, Mosby.

Ellsworth A et al: *Mosby's 1998 medical drug reference,* St Louis, 1998, Mosby.

Healthcare Consultants of America, Inc., *1998 Physicians fee and coding guide,* Augusta, Ga, 1998, Healthcare Consultants of America, Inc.

Hashmay R, Shandera W: Infectious diseases: viral & rickettsial. In Tierney L, McPhee S, Papadakis M, editors: *Current medical diagnosis & treatment,* ed 36, Stamford, Conn, 1997, Appleton & Lange.

Larsen G et al: Respiratory tract and mediastinum. In Hay W et al, editors: *Current pediatric diagnosis and treatment,* ed 4, Stamford, Conn, 1997, Appleton & Lange.

27 Bronchitis

ICD-9-CM

Acute Bronchitis 466.0
Chronic Bronchitis 491.9

OVERVIEW

Definition

Bronchitis is a generalized inflammation of the major bronchi and trachea resulting in a productive cough. Acute bronchitis is an episodic presentation. Chronic bronchitis is said to be present when there is a productive cough for at least 3 months in 2 consecutive years.

Etiology/Incidence

Inflammation of acute bronchitis can occur at any age and is usually associated with a viral or bacterial infection involving the upper respiratory tract. It most typically occurs in the winter and early spring. Chronic bronchitis occurs more typically in smoking adults and is a form of chronic obstructive pulmonary disease (COPD). Although it may appear in early adulthood, it is typically diagnosed during middle years.

Pathophysiology

Bronchitis results from irritation and subsequent inflammation of the mucosal lining of the tracheobronchial tree. There is increased airway swelling, excess mucus secretion, and ciliary impairment.

Acute Bronchitis

Viruses are implicated in acute bronchitis, which is usually self-limiting. Common pathogens include influenza viruses, adenoviruses, and rhinoviruses. Common bacterial agents include *Streptococcus pneumoniae, Hemophilus influenzae,* and *Mycoplasma pneumoniae.*

Chronic Bronchitis

Chronic bronchitis is most commonly associated with smoking or exposure to a respiratory irritant. Resultant airway swelling, excess mucus production, and ciliary dysfunction contribute to increased expiratory airway resistance, which can induce right-sided heart failure. Excessive mucus production also predisposes the individual to superimposed respiratory infections.

Factors That Increase Susceptibility

Children of parents who smoke have more frequent episodes that last for longer periods of time. Subsequent bacterial infections, chronic bronchitis, and respiratory infections occur more frequently in individuals who smoke, are frequently exposed to respiratory irritants and/or air pollution, or have compromised pulmonary function.

SUBJECTIVE DATA

History of Present Illness

Symptoms include those found in Table 27-1.

Past Medical History

Inquire about history of asthma, chronic cardiorespiratory disease (e.g., cystic fibrosis, COPD), and immune disorders.
Inquire about immunization and influenza vaccination status and tuberculin test results.

Environmental/Lifestyle

Elicit a history related to upper respiratory symptoms if this was not identified above. Assess the patient's history of smoking or exposure to a respiratory irritant. Identify changes, such as decreased appetite and/or unexplained weight loss, sleeping positions, and fatigue, which would be associated with progressive shortness of breath.

TABLE 27-1 Symptoms: Bronchitis

	Acute Bronchitis	Chronic Bronchitis
Onset:	Usually preceded by rhinitis, upper respiratory infection	Insidious; cold may herald symptoms; may experience exertional dyspnea
Cough:	Initially dry, hacking, nonproductive cough for 4-6 days (often worse at night) that progresses to a loose productive cough; cough frequently paroxysmal	Productive cough, copious sputum
Fever:	Afebrile or low-grade; may experience chills and/or myalgia	Afebrile (unless infection present); purulent mucus may indicate a superimposed infection
Other:	May complain of substernal chest pain	May complain of difficulty breathing

TABLE 27-2 Physical Findings: Bronchitis

	Acute Bronchitis	Chronic Bronchitis
General:	Unless bronchitis is severe, patients may not appear acutely ill; may have mild shortness of breath	Appears short of breath, especially when speaking; uses accessory muscles
Skin:	Normal	Pedal edema; may be pale, gray, or cyanotic
HEENT:	Rhinitis, dry coarse cough	Frequent productive cough
Lungs:	Resonance; normal breath sounds with scattered rales or rhonchi; expiratory wheeze	Resonance to hyperresonance; rhonchi and expiratory wheeze; prolonged expiration
Heart:	Normal; mild tachycardia if febrile or dehydrated	Jugular venous distention; a third heart sound may be heard if right-sided heart failure is present

HEENT, Head, ears, eyes, nose, and throat.

OBJECTIVE DATA

Physical Examination

Physical examination findings commonly associated with acute and chronic bronchitis are described in Table 27-2.

Diagnostic Procedures

Diagnostic tests for bronchitis are found in Table 27-3.

ASSESSMENT

Differential diagnoses include bronchiolitis, pneumonia, tuberculosis, viral croup, bacterial tracheitis, foreign body aspiration, emphysema, and congestive heart failure (Table 27-4).

THERAPEUTIC PLAN

Pharmaceutical/Nonpharmaceutical

Treatment for acute bronchitis is primarily palliative for fever/discomfort and cough. If mucus production is purulent and heavy and other systemic symptoms associated with infection are present, antibiotics should also be administered. Trials of antibiotics in the treatment of acute bronchitis show little benefit on most outcomes, although a recent study (King, 1996) showed that treated patients returned to work earlier than untreated patients.

Pharmaceutical treatment for acute bronchitis is outlined in Table 27-5.

Lifestyle/Activities

Rest, a cool mist humidifier, ample fluids, and avoidance of respiratory irritants may also help to alleviate symptoms.

Diet

Noncontributory

Patient Education

Family members should be encouraged to stop smoking or refrain from smoking in the vicinity of the patient.

If the patient's occupation exposes her or him to respiratory irritants, advocate the use of protective face masks.

Referral/Consultation

Medical referral/consultation is warranted for patients in significant respiratory distress, patients who appear toxic and whose symptoms worsen or fail to improve within 72

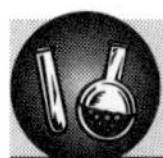

TABLE 27-3 Diagnostic Tests: Bronchitis

Diagnostic Test	Findings	Cost ($)
Sputum culture: Not necessary unless sputum is purulent or pneumonia is suspected	Identify causative organism (i.e., pertussis or mycoplasma)	31-39
PEFR: Identifies peak expiratory flow; assesses whether there might be a reactive airway	Based on height and age Men: 350-650 Women: 250-450 Children: See Appendix L for a predicted peak flow rate for all ages Usually <60% normal in chronic bronchitis	N/A
CBC: Not indicated unless the clinical presentation is unclear	WBC usually normal or slightly elevated; may see ↑ hematocrit in chronic bronchitis	18-23
ECG: Not indicated in acute bronchitis unless the clinical presentation is unclear	In advanced chronic bronchitis, the ECG may show atrial arrhythmias and right ventricular hypertrophy	56-65
CXR: Not indicated unless diagnosis is not clear	Usually normal or may show hyperinflation from old pulmonary disease or long-term smoking; diaphragm is rounded	77-91

CBC, Complete blood count; *CXR,* chest x-ray; *ECG,* electrocardiogram; *N/A,* not available; *PEFR,* peak expiratory flow rate; *WBC,* white blood count.

TABLE 27-4 Differential Diagnosis: Bronchitis

Diagnoses	Supporting Data
Bronchiolitis	Inflammation of the bronchioles, usually the result of a viral (RSV most common) illness Characterized by cough, low-grade fever, rapid respirations (50-60), chest retractions, and wheezing **Child:** Thick tenacious secretions **Infants** 2-6 months of age: bronchiolitis a major cause of hospitalization, usually late fall and winter
Pneumonia	Infections typically occur in the late winter and spring. Pneumonia presents with abrupt onset of fever, restlessness, and respiratory distress, after an URI. Auscultation of the lungs reveals diminished breath sounds, as well as crackles on the affected side. Dullness on percussion may also be present. WBCs usually range from 15,000 to 40,000.
Asthma/RAD	Reactive airway has been recognized as one of the most common causes of cough in **children.** Expiratory wheezing may be noted, along with recurrent coughing and accessory muscle use. PEFRs are frequently less than expected for age/height. Dramatic improvements are noted with use of bronchodilator. Asthma should be considered in repetitive episodes of bronchitis.
Occupational exposures	Coughing and symptoms worsen during work week, but tend to improve with weekends, holidays, vacations.
Croup/ bacterial tracheitis	Symptoms usually begin as viral URI, followed by barking cough. Fever is usually higher, and the patient more ill appearing with tracheitis than croup. Upper airway obstruction may develop rapidly.
Common cold	Upper airway inflammation, no evidence of bronchial wheezing
Pertussis	Paroxysms of cough followed by a characteristic inspiratory whoop Consider in children >5 years or in older children or adults who present with coughing for >10 days (the whoop may not be present)
CHF	Basilar rales, orthopnea, wheezing, cardiomegaly, S_3 gallop, tachycardia
GERD	Intermittent symptoms that worsen when lying down, indigestion, heartburn
Bronchogenic tumor	Chronic cough, sometimes with hemoptysis; constitutional symptoms: fatigue, weight loss

RSV, Respiratory syncytial virus; *URI,* upper respiratory tract infection; *WBC,* white blood count; *RAD,* reactive airway disease; *PEFR,* peak expiratory flow rate; *CHF,* congestive heart failure; *GERD,* gastroesophageal reflux disease.

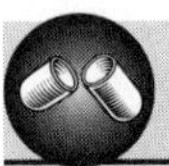

TABLE 27-5 Pharmaceutical Plan: Bronchitis

Drug	Dose	Comments	Cost
Analgesia, Antipyretica			
Acetaminophen	325-650 mg po q4-6h; max 4 g/day	Pregnancy: B SE: Rash, hepatic toxicity, nausea and vomiting	$3-$8
Cough Suppressants			
Dextromethorphan (Robitussin, Vicks Formula 44)	Adult: 10-20 mg q4h, ER: 60 mg BID, max 120 mg/day **Children** 2-6 yr: 2.5-5 mg (½ tsp) q6-8h ER: 15 mg BID, max 30 mg/day **Children** 6-12 yr: 5-10 mg q6-8h ER: 30 mg BID, max: 60 mg/day	Pregnancy: C SE: dizziness, nausea	$3/3.5 mg/ml (120 ml); $2/7.5 mg/ml (60 ml); $3/15 mg/5 ml (120 ml); ER: $6/30 mg/5 ml (90 ml)
Expectorants			
Guaifenesin	Adults: 100-400 mg q4-6h *or* 600 mg SR q12h, max 2.4 g/day **Children** 2-6 yr: 50-100 mg q4h, max 600 mg/day **Children** 6-12 yr: 100-200 mg q4h, max 1.2 g/day	Pregnancy: C SE: Gastrointestinal upset, drowsiness, rash, headache	$72/liquid: 100 mg/5 ml (480 ml); tablets: $11-$27/200 mg (100); SR: $19-$80/600 mg (100)
Antibiotics			
Amoxicillin	Adults: 250-500 mg TID **Children:** 40 mg/kg TID	Consider using if patient smokes or has underlying pathology. Clinical trials concluded there is no evidence to support the use of antibacterials for treatment of acute bronchitis (O'Brien et al, 1998). If pertussis is suspected, treat with macrolide or tetracycline in child >8 yr.	amox: $3-$5/125/5 ml (150 ml); $4-$8/250 mg/5 ml (150 ml); $8-$27/250 mg (100); $17-$49/ 500 mg (100)
Erythromycin	Adults: 500 mg BID **Children:** 30-50 mg/kg/day q6h		eryth: susp: $13-$27/200 mg/5 ml (480); tablets: $18-$40/500 mg (100)
TMP-SMZ	Adults: 1 DS tab BID **Children:** 8 mg/kg trimethoprim and 40 mg/kg sulfamethoxazole BID		TMP-SMZ: $7-$74/RS (100); $9-$121/DS (100)
Bronchodilators			
Albuterol MDI for short-term use	Albuterol MDI 2 puffs QID or nebulizer in children <5 yr	Most effective when bronchial inflammation is present (Hueston, 1998)	$22-$24/0.09 mg/inhalation (17 g)

ER, Extended relief; *DS,* double strength; *MDI,* metered-dose inhaler; *RS,* regular strength; *SE,* side effects; *TMP-SMZ,* trimethoprim-sulfamethoxazole.

hours, and patients who are **elderly** and/or debilitated or have an existing chronic pulmonary illness.

Follow-up

Return immediately if symptoms of respiratory distress occur and in 1 week if symptoms do not resolve (2 to 3 days if the patient has a chronic pulmonary or cardiorespiratory disease). If the cough persists for >3 weeks, consider a further workup.

EVALUATION

Acute bronchitis is usually self-limiting and without sequelae. Consider asthma if the client has recurrent acute bronchitis episodes.

REFERENCES

Hueston W, Mainous A: Acute bronchitis, *Am Fam Physician* 57(6), 1270-1276, 1998.

King D et al: Effectiveness of erythromycin in the treatment of acute bronchitis, *J Fam Practice* 42(6):601-605, 1996.

O'Brien K et al: Cough illness/bronchitis: principles of judicious use of antimicrobial agents, *Pediatrics* 101(1) (Suppl) 178-181, 1998.

SUGGESTED REFERENCES

Ellsworth A et al: *Mosby's 1998 medical drug reference*, St Louis, 1998, Mosby.

D'Auria JP: Respiratory System. In Fox JA, editor: *Primary health care of children*, St Louis, 1997, Mosby.

Healthcare Consultants of America Inc: *1998 Physicians fee and coding guide,* Augusta, Ga, 1998, Healthcare Consultants of America, Inc.

Larsen G et al: Respiratory tract and mediastinum. In Hay W et al, editors: *Current pediatric diagnosis and treatment*, ed 4, Stamford, Conn, 1997, Appleton & Lange.

Seidel H et al: *Mosby's guide to physical examination,* ed 3, St Louis, 1995, Mosby.

Sommers M, Johnson S: Bronchitis. In *Davis' manual of nursing therapeutics for diseases and disorders,* Philadelphia, 1997, FA Davis.

Burns

ICD-9-CM

Burns Confined to Eye and Adnexa 940
Burns of Face, Head and Neck 941
Burn of Trunk 942
Burn, any Degree, <10% BSA 948
Burn, Unspecified Degree 949.0
Burn, 1° 949.1
Burn, 2° 949.2
Burn, 3° 949.3

OVERVIEW

Definition

Burns are a tissue injury caused by heat, chemicals, electricity, or irradiation. The depth of the burn is the result of the intensity of the heat and the duration of the exposure. Minor burns are considered to be <10% of the body surface area (BSA), involving <2% full-thickness injury.

Incidence

There are 2 to 5 million burns/year; 1,000,000 patients require hospitalization; 12,000 die.

Children: Burns are the leading cause of death in children. All ages are affected.

Rate of occurrence in men and women is equal.

Pathophysiology

Burns occur as a result of excessive heat energy transferred to the skin, causing cellular protein coagulation and destruction of enzyme systems.

Partial Thickness—Superficial (First Degree) Burns

Erythema; skin blanches with pressure, may be tender; devitalization of superficial layers of epidermis, congestion of intradermal vessels

Partial Thickness—Deep (Second Degree) Burns

Erythema with blisters, skin very tender; coagulation of varying depths of epidermis, vesicles, skin appendages intact

Full Thickness (Third Degree) Burns

Destruction of all skin elements with destruction of subdermal layers, burned skin tough and leathery, not tender, may be black or white; necrosis of all skin elements

Factors That Increase Susceptibility

Hot water heaters set too high (>120)
Workplace exposure to chemicals, electricity, or irradiation
Young children and the **elderly** more susceptible to burns because of thin skin
Carelessness with cigarettes
Inadequate or faulty wiring
Use of alcohol or drugs
Wearing flammable clothing

Causes of Burns

Open flame and hot liquid: Most common
Caustic chemicals: May show little damage for the first days
Electricity: May cause significant damage, with little damage seen on the surface
Excessive sun exposure

SUBJECTIVE DATA

History of Present Illness

Exposure to cause
Ask about being in an enclosed location for smoke inhalation
Type of burning agent
Prior treatment
Use of alcohol or drugs
Concurrent trauma

Past Medical History

Previous skin damage or burns

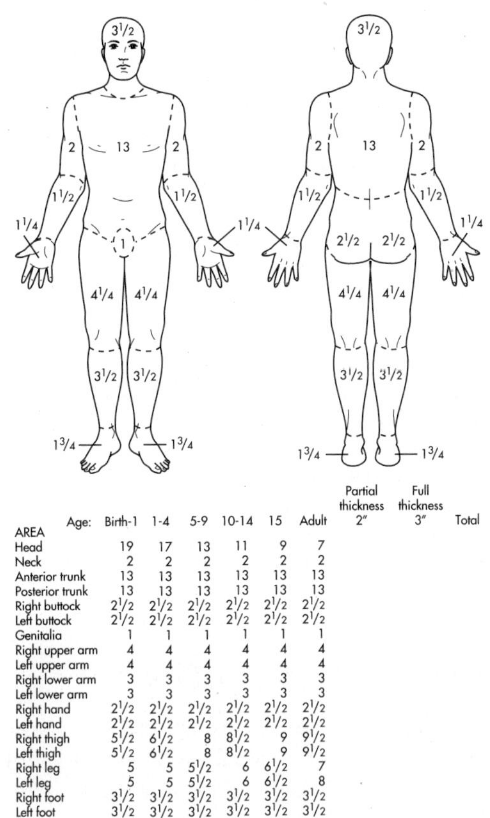

AREA / Age:	Birth-1	1-4	5-9	10-14	15	Adult	Partial thickness 2″	Full thickness 3″	Total
Head	19	17	13	11	9	7			
Neck	2	2	2	2	2	2			
Anterior trunk	13	13	13	13	13	13			
Posterior trunk	13	13	13	13	13	13			
Right buttock	2½	2½	2½	2½	2½	2½			
Left buttock	2½	2½	2½	2½	2½	2½			
Genitalia	1	1	1	1	1	1			
Right upper arm	4	4	4	4	4	4			
Left upper arm	4	4	4	4	4	4			
Right lower arm	3	3	3	3	3	3			
Left lower arm	3	3	3	3	3	3			
Right hand	2½	2½	2½	2½	2½	2½			
Left hand	2½	2½	2½	2½	2½	2½			
Right thigh	5½	6½	8	8½	9	9½			
Left thigh	5½	6½	8	8½	9	9½			
Right leg	5	5	5½	6	6½	7			
Left leg	5	5	5½	6	6½	8			
Right foot	3½	3½	3½	3½	3½	3½			
Left foot	3½	3½	3½	3½	3½	3½			

Figure 28-1 Estimating surface area in burns. (Adapted from Nussbaum MS, editor: *The Mont Reid handbook,* St Louis, 1994, Mosby. Used with permission.)

Medications

Determine if patient is taking any regular medications.

Family History

Not applicable

Diet History

Time of last meal eaten

Description of Most Common Symptoms

Complaint of pain, redness, or blisters

Associated Symptoms

Shortness of breath: smoke inhalation (may occur up to 72 hours after fire)
Palpitations
Nausea/vomiting
Chills
Headache

OBJECTIVE DATA

Physical Examination

A problem-oriented physical should be conducted, with particular attention to:
- Vital signs
- Weight
- General appearance
- Skin: Determine extent of burn using BSA (Figure 28-1)
- ENT/chest evaluation: Rule out possible smoke inhalation (carbon particles, singed nasal hair)

Cardiovascular: For electrical burns
Check for circulation and neurological status distal to burn

Diagnostic Procedures

Determined by extent of burn; may need extensive laboratory workup for serious burns
Electrocardiogram if electrical burn ($56-$65)

ASSESSMENT

Differential diagnoses include those listed in Table 28-1.

THERAPEUTIC PLAN

Pharmaceutical (Table 28-2)

Prophylactic antibiotics not usually needed unless history of valvular heart disease
Tetanus prophylaxis

Nonpharmaceutical

Remove all rings to avoid tourniquet affect.
Flush chemical burn copiously with water.
Do not apply ice to site.
Apply cold compress.

Initial care of first- and second-degree burns is as follows: gentle cleansing with a mild detergent (such as Ivory) and water, followed by debridement of broken blisters or dead skin. Blisters that are intact can be left alone. The burned areas should be covered with a thin layer of silver sulfadiazine cream and a fluffy dressing that will absorb drainage.

Lifestyle/Activities

Smoking and alcohol cessation
Proper storage of flammable substances
Smoke detectors
Development of evacuation plan for family

TABLE 28-1 Differential Diagnosis: Burns

Diagnosis	Supporting Data
Scalded skin syndrome	Adverse cutaneous reaction to an ingested drug characterized by formation of solitary or multiple bullae
Abuse	Circumferential burns of foot, lower legs, or buttocks are suspicious for person being forced into water; deep round lesions: cigarette burns; discrepancies in stories, delay of treatment

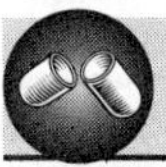

TABLE 28-2 Pharmaceutical Plan: Burns

Drug	Dose	Comments	Cost ($)
Silver sulfadiazine 1% cream (Silvadene)	Apply to burned area QD BID	Effective against gram-positive and gram-negative organisms Pregnancy: B SE: Burning, rash, skin discoloration	28-68/400 g

SE, Side effects.

Diet

Not applicable

Patient Education

Instruct about care of burn at home: cleanse burn of old cream 2 times day, dry well, and reapply cream and then dressing. Keep dressings clean and dry.
Instruct about signs and symptoms of infections.
Use sunscreens to avoid future burns.
Identify risk of skin changes in future: monitor skin of area carefully.
Decrease temperature of hot water heater to <120° F.
Store household chemicals in safe place, away from children.
Do not smoke in bed.

Referral

Hospitalize all patients with second-degree burns over 10% BSA or any third-degree burn. Patients with any of the following burns should also be hospitalized:

Any second-degree burns of hands/feet or perineum
Electrical or lightning burns
Inhalation burns
Chemical burns
Circumferential burns

EVALUATION/FOLLOW-UP

First-degree burns: Complete resolution
Second-degree burns: Epithelialization in 10 to 14 days; deep second-degree may require skin grafts
Third-degree burns: Skin graft required

Follow up initially in 48 hours and closely thereafter to make sure healing is taking place.

Consider child or elder abuse if burns seen in a "dipping" pattern, or cigarette or iron burns.

SUGGESTED READINGS

Dunn S: *Primary care consultant,* St Louis, 1998, Mosby.

Ellsworth A et al: *Mosby's 1998 medical drug reference,* St Louis, 1998, Mosby.

Healthcare Consultants of America, Inc: *1998 Physicians fee and coding guide,* Augusta, Ga, 1998, Healthcare Consultants of America, Inc.

Fultz J, Messer M: *Mosby's emergency nursing reference,* St Louis, 1996, Mosby.

Graber M, Allen R, Levy B: Estimating surface area in burns. In Graber M: *University of Iowa family practice handbook,* ed 2, St Louis, 1994, Mosby.

Griffith H, Dambro M: *The five-minute clinical consult,* Philadelphia, 1997, Lea & Febiger.

Latchaw L: Burns: the outpatient treatment. In Dershewitz R: *Ambulatory pediatrics,* Philadelphia, 1993, JB Lippincott.

Carpal Tunnel Syndrome

ICD-9-CM

Carpal Tunnel Syndrome 354.0

OVERVIEW

Definition

Carpal tunnel syndrome (CTS) is compression of the median nerve at the wrist with associated symptoms of tingling, numbness or pain of affected fingers, wrist. Found in occupations/hobbies with frequent repetitive motion of wrist.

Incidence/Epidemiology

Common wrist-hand disorder
Occurs three to five times more in women than men
Highest frequency in age group of 30 to 60
Hormones and fluid retention may have role in women
Increasing incidence in industry with repetitive forceful flexion-extension, vibration, or awkward positioning of wrist without sufficient rest

Pregnancy

There is an increased incidence of CTS in pregnancy, typically third trimester. Most cases resolve after childbirth.

Childhood

Not typically found in children

Statistics

The National Institute of Occupational Safety and Health (NIOSH) estimates there are 20 million workers at risk for CTS, 23,000 new cases/year. 100,000 CTS release surgeries are performed annually. CTS treatment is expensive; including surgery, it ranges from $25,000 to $30,000.

Pathophysiology

The median nerve is easily compressed as it runs through the carpal tunnel of the wrist (Figures 29-1 and 29-2). The tunnel is made of carpal bones on the dorsal side and the transverse carpal ligament (flexor retinaculum) on ventral (volar) side. The median nerve lies in this 2- to 3-m tunnel, along with the nine flexor tendons of the fingers. Any swelling, trauma, or systemic metabolic process can affect the tunnel and cause compression on the median nerve with accompanying symptoms. Frequent wrist flexion/extension causes increased friction of tendons against the carpal bones or ligaments with inflammation and swelling. The median nerve supplies sensory fibers to the thumb, second, third, and radial side of fourth finger. Pressure on the nerve produces symptoms of paresthesia with tingling, numbness, pain. CTS caused by repetitive factors can take weeks to years to develop, with intermittent symptoms.

Risk Factors to Develop CTS

Causes of CTS are complex and multicausal; not everyone with exposure develops CTS. There are three categories of causes.

Work/Hobby Repetitive Flexion/Extension

Major types: Computer keyboard typists, checkout clerks, meatcutters, seamstress, hairdressers, vibrating tool use, musicians, mailhandlers-sorters, domestic, cooks, bowlers, knitters, gardeners, painters

Trauma

Fractures, dislocations, blow to wrist, structural defects

Metabolic/Pregnancy-Related

The following conditions have shown an increased incidence of CTS; diabetes, rheumatoid arthritis, gout, hypo-

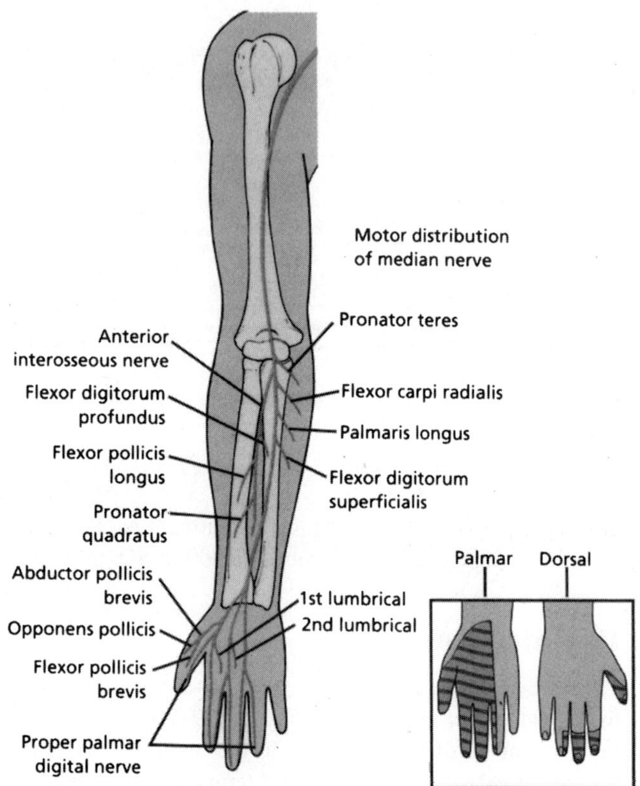

Figure 29-1 Innervation of median nerve of right arm. (From Fortunato NM, McCullough S: *Plastic and reconstructive surgery,* St Louis, 1998, Mosby.)

thyroidism, birth control pill use, degenerative joint disease, congenital defects of wrist. It is frequently seen in pregnancy.

SUBJECTIVE DATA

History of Present Illness

Ask patient:

- Does CTS wake him/her up at night?
- What aggravates it?
- What impact does it have on life activities?
- Is there a problem with sensation, weakness, fine motor tasks, discomfort while driving a car?
- What is the length of symptoms? Are they intermittent or continuous? Are they getting worse?
- Has there been any recent trauma to the wrist?

Past Medical History: Metabolic/Trauma

Ask about:

- Diabetes (most commonly associated risk factor)
- Thyroid disease

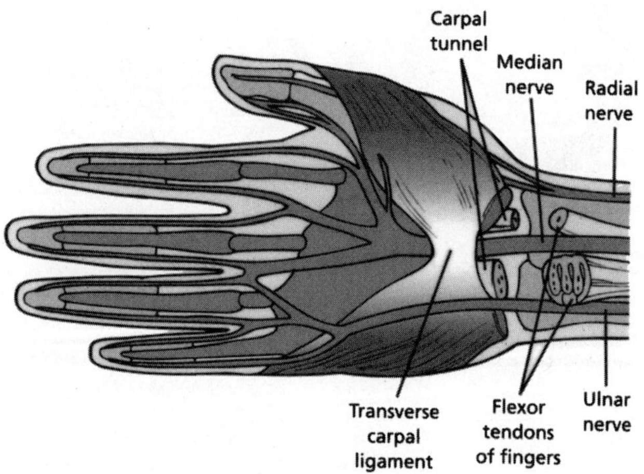

Figure 29-2 Diagram of carpal tunnel, palmar view. (From Fortunato NM, McCullough S: *Plastic and reconstructive surgery,* St Louis, 1998, Mosby.)

- Any similar past problems during prior pregnancies
- Arthritis
- Oral contraceptives
- Medications/hormones
- Cancer
- Trauma (e.g., fracture to wrist or carpal bones)

Occupational/Hobbies

Ask about:

- Past job/work history and extensive current job description; history of repetitive forceful work, vibration, small tools, keyboard
- Length of rest periods, breaks, demonstrate postures, motions
- Discomfort: Does it decrease when away from work or on vacation?
- Hobbies, how often performed, discomfort level

Medications

Current medications: Impact on fluid retention
Identify medication tried, trial of NSAIDs, and results

Family History

There is some indication of familial association, with familial thickening of transverse carpal ligament.

Description of Most Common Symptoms

Most common symptoms include paresthesia with numbness, tingling, pain to thumb, second, third, and fourth finger of affected hand; it most often wakes person at

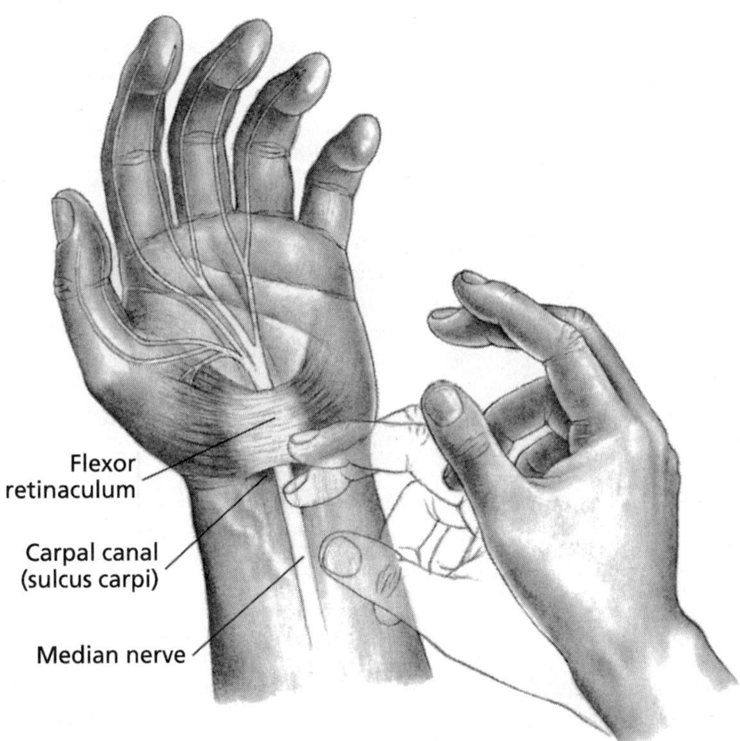

Figure 29-3 Elicitation of Tinel's sign. (From Seidel HM et al: *Mosby's guide to physical examination,* ed 4, St Louis, 1999, Mosby.)

night; onset is insidious, symptoms may be intermittent for months

Associated Symptoms

Wrist, forearm, and shoulder pain

Chronic/late stages: Thenar wasting (muscle pad of thumb), weakness of hand with decreased grip strength, and decreased sensitivity of fingers

OBJECTIVE DATA

Physical Examination

Always do comparative examination.

Inspect for swelling, thenar wasting, changes to skin (skin of affected area may be dry).

Palpate carpal bones, ligament to localize pain.

Check pulses (rule out thoracic outlet syndrome).

Assess grip strength; active and passive range of motion; two-point discrimination of 6-mm distance along fingertips (normal is able to discriminate at 6 mm or less, questionable reliability and is late symptom).

Specific Maneuvers

Tinel's Sign. Tap at the volar surface of wrist; results are positive if reproduced symptoms or tingling into median nerve distribution. Maneuver has a 50% accuracy (Figure 29-3).

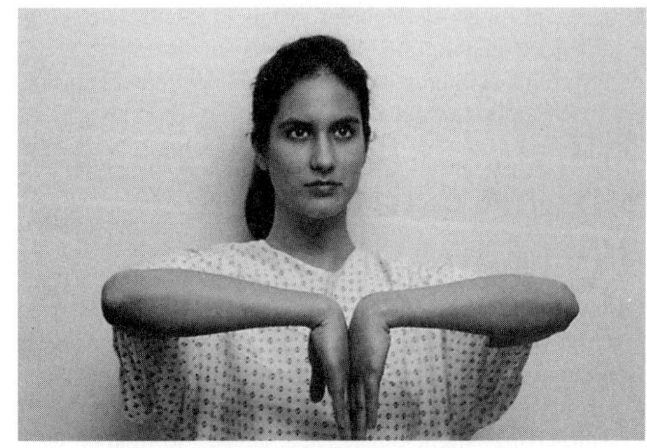

Figure 29-4 Phalen's test for carpal tunnel syndrome. (From Thompson JM, Wilson SF: *Health assessment for nursing practice,* St Louis, 1996, Mosby.)

Phalen's Test. Most sensitive physical test. Flex wrists maximally and hold 60 seconds; results are positive if reproduced symptoms (Figure 29-4).

Carpal Compression. New test: With examiner's thumbs, apply direct compression to median nerve at wrist for 30 seconds; results are positive if reproduced symptoms. Preliminary results show more sensitivity and specificity than Tinel's or Phalen's sign.

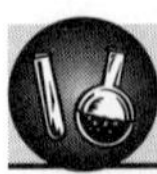

TABLE 29-1 Diagnostic Tests: Carpal Tunnel Syndrome

Diagnostic Test	Finding/Rationale	Cost ($)
Nerve conduction test	Used as a standard to confirm clinical diagnosis; EMG/nerve conduction studies will show abnormality in time/velocity of nerve conduction; 90% sensitive and 60% specific; aids confirmation of clinical diagnosis; considered first line test	393-475
Quantitative grip and pinch studies	Measure loss of strength; considered first line test	46-56
Laboratory work	Indication is history of or suspected metabolic disorder: CBC, thyroid, glucose, renal, uric acid, ERS, rheumatoid factor	12-250, depending on extent
Radiographic	Used to assess trauma, fracture, tumor, structural defect; MRI may be useful for detailed studies	1485-1755/MRI wrist; 1489-1758/MRI neck; 102-121/x-ray wrist

CBC, Complete blood count; *EMG*, electromyelogram; *ERS*, erythrocyte sedimentation rate; *MRI*, magnetic resonance imaging.

Diagnostic Procedures

The following examinations may be considered. Diagnosis can be made based on history and physical examination, with further studies used to confirm (Table 29-1).

ASSESSMENT

Differential diagnosis includes metabolic/connective tissue disorders or generalized nervous system disorders, **pregnancy** with swelling in canal. The more common diagnoses are listed in Table 29-2.

THERAPEUTIC PLAN

Noninvasive

Conservative treatment 50% to 75% effective if started early, without thenar wasting, severe pain, or weakness

Limitation of activities/work that stress wrist; specific work restrictions if necessary; cock-up splint to affected wrist with wrist in slight extension; should be worn at night to prevent hyperflexion in sleep

May be used in day, if activity is restricted

Application of cold to wrist to decrease inflammation

Nonsteroidal antiinflammatory drugs (NSAIDs) taken with food daily 4 to 8 weeks

May consider physical therapy, in conjunction with above; bioconductive therapy, interference currents, cold therapy

Treatment of concurrent conditions: diabetes mellitus, thyroid, arthritis

Pregnancy: Avoid repetitive activities; splinting most effective; cold therapy to wrist helpful; educate that most CTS symptoms abate after delivery

See Appendix J for detailed prescribing information on NSAIDs

Invasive

Steroid injection into carpal tunnel may provide temporary relief; there is risk of infection, damage to nerve, scarring.

Surgical intervention may be necessary for continued pain, thenar wasting, and progressive weakness. Surgery is highly successful, with 90% to 95% improvement in symptoms (if not chronic disease). The transverse carpal ligament is incised, which opens the tunnel and releases pressure.

Two procedures: Open procedure with ability to visualize and explore tunnel; and endoscopic procedure, which provides less visualization but faster recovery

Postoperative care: Splinting for 1 week or more, continued job restriction, sutures out in 10 to 14 days; continued restriction of limb for up to 4 to 6 weeks; restriction may be lessened based on healing and activities/work

Lifestyle/Activities

Refrain from repetitive motion of wrist in work and hobbies.

Diet

None (If excessive salt intake, advise no added salt diet when actively symptomatic.)

Patient Education

Prevention is the key. Modify environment for proper joint alignment at worksite. Advise to seek ergonomic assessment from company of work tasks, tools. This strategy is important, especially in high-risk jobs. Conditioning exercises for hands and wrists with mild stretching and strengthening may help prevent in nonsymptomatic patients.

TABLE 29-2 Differential Diagnosis: Carpal Tunnel Syndrome

Diagnosis	Supporting Data
Carpal tunnel syndrome	Positive Phalen's, Tinel's, carpal compression, EMG
Guyans canal: Ulnar nerve compression at wrist	Paresthesia fifth and ulnar side only fourth fingers
Cubital tunnel syndrome: Ulnar nerve compression at elbow	As above
Metabolic/connective tissue/nervous system disorders	Diabetes mellitus, peripheral neuropathy, lupus, RA, multiple sclerosis
DeQuervain's: Tenosynovitis of abductor pollicis longus/extensor pollicis brevis (tendons of thumb)	Positive Finkelstein's test: patient makes fist with thumb inside fingers; stabilize forearm and ulnarly deviate wrist; pain over tendons is positive
Cervical radiculopathy: pressure on the nerve root as it exits the C-spine	Cervical spine x-rays, MRI: rule out disk lesions, nerve root palsy, cervical disk herniation or protrusion
Thoracic outlet syndrome: Compression of nerves and vessels (neurovascular bundle) in shoulder/neck region of brachial plexus	Paresthesia all 5 digits unilateral; pain in arm; abduction of arm may increase symptoms; pulses may be unequal, weaker in affected side
Median nerve compression proximally	Symptoms of CTS; may be more proximal in limb Cause: Trauma/tumor/injury

EMG, Electromyelography; *RA,* rheumatoid arthritis; *MRI,* magnetic resonance imaging.

Advise that it takes a long time to heal following treatment regimen, possibly months. If activities are not modified, symptoms will return.

Wear splint at night. Avoid use of splint during work day. It may be worn if it does not interfere with activities.

Pregnancy cases usually resolve. If symptoms continue after delivery and patient is not nursing, initiation of NSAIDS and referral may be considered.

Family Impact

Affected limb will have restricted use during treatment or postoperative recovery time.

Family will need to assist with responsibilities, housekeeping, activities of daily living.

Referral

If symptoms are no better after 1 to 2 months of conservative treatment, refer to orthopedic hand specialist for surgical evaluation.

Consultation

Consult for complicated, nonprogressing, or worsening cases; allergy or intolerance of NSAIDs, renal disease.

EVALUATION/FOLLOW-UP

Initial follow up is 2 to 4 weeks for noninvasive treatment.

Expect to see some improvement in symptoms 2 weeks after compliant noninvasive treatment and avoidance of cause.

It may take 4 to 8 weeks to achieve results with conservative treatment.

If CTS is work related, specific job restrictions will be needed (e.g., typing for no more than 20 minutes every 2 hours). It may be necessary to work closely with nurse at worksite.

Usually there is a resolution of symptoms following surgical intervention, if caught early. If patient returns to same activity following surgery without modification and correct joint positioning, symptoms may recur.

RESOURCES

Association for Repetitive Motion Syndromes, 707-571-0397

National Institute for Occupational Safety and Health (NIOSH), 800-356-4674

Websites:

NIOSH http://www.cdc.gov.niosh.homepage

American Academy of Orthopaedic Surgeons http://www.aaos.org

SUGGESTED READINGS

Agur AM, Lee MJ: *Grant's atlas of anatomy,* ed 9, Baltimore, 1991, Williams & Wilkins.

Bhattacharya A, McGlothlin JD, editors: *Occupational ergonomics, theory, and application,* New York, 1996, Marcel Dekker.

Dionne ED: "Carpal tunnel syndrome. Part 1: the problem," *National Safety News,* March, 1984, pp 143-146.

Dorwart BD: Carpal tunnel syndrome: a review, *Semin Arthritis Rheum* 14(2):134-139, 1984.

Ellsworth A et al: *Mosby's 1998 medical drug reference,* St Louis, 1998, Mosby.

Healthcare Consultants of America, Inc: *1998 Physicians fee and coding guide,* Augusta, Ga, 1998, Healthcare Consultants of America, Inc.

Hoppenfeld S: *Physical exam of spine and extremities,* Norwalk, Ct, 1976, Appleton & Lange.

Magee DJ: *Orthopedic physical assessment,* Philadelphia, 1987, WB Saunders.

Miller BK: Carpal tunnel syndrome: a frequently misdiagnosed common hand problem, *Nurse Pract* 18(12): 52-56, 1993.

National Institute of Occupational Safety and Health: Carpal tunnel syndrome selected references, Cincinnati, March, 1989, Department of Health and Human Services Publication (No. 1992-648-179/60023).

Putz-Anderson V, editor: *Carpal tunnel disorder: a manual for musculo-skeletal diseases of the upper limbs,* Pennsylvania, 1988, Taylor & Francis.

Siebenaler MJ, McGovern P: Carpal tunnel syndrome, *Am Assoc Occup Health Nurs* 40(2):62-71, 1992.

Tomal DR: Reduce carpal tunnel syndrome through safety training, *Am Assoc Safety Engineers,* December, 1992, pp 27-29.

Williams K: Doing business with carpal tunnel syndrome, *Work* 2(4):2-7, 1992.

Wright PE: Carpal tunnel and ulnar tunnel syndromes and stenosing tenosynovitis. In Crenshaw AH, editor: *Campbell's operative orthopedics,* ed 9, St Louis, 1998, Mosby.

30 Cataracts

ICD-9-CM

Age-related Cataracts 366.19
Congenital Cataract 743.30

OVERVIEW

Definition

Cataracts are defined as unilateral or bilateral opacification of the crystalline lens of the eye. They usually result in functional impairment due to visual disturbances.

Incidence

Cataracts are the leading cause of preventable blindness in adults in the United States. Incidence increases with age, with an incidence of approximately 50% in individuals after age 75. Senile cataracts are typically bilateral, but progression may vary between eyes. **Pediatric cataracts are rare.** They are generally a result of congenital factors.

Pathophysiology

The lens is posterior to the iris and suspended from the ciliary body. It is normally a transparent structure with an elastic capsule. The lens is avascular and acellular and lacks innervation. Transparency of the lens depends on active metabolism of the epithelium. If the epithelium becomes traumatized, opacity to the lens may result. Density of the lens fibers increase with age, and chemical changes in protein of the lens occur. Both of these factors contribute to cataract formation. Cataracts may be either nuclear (central) or cortical (peripheral/sunflower shape). Nuclear cataracts are most common, especially in the **aged.**

Protective Factors Against Cataract Formation

Measures are needed to protect the visual lens from harm from irritants, smoke, or sun damage. Therefore such measures as protective eyeware, including sunglasses when appropriate, may help protect against cataract development.

Factors That Increase Susceptibility

Trauma
Eye disease
Drug therapy
A consequence of metabolic disease such as diabetes
Aging process (most common cause)

Susceptibility to Specific Types of Cataracts

Congenital cataracts occur as a result of inheritance of an autosomal-dominant gene for cataracts. Many Down's syndrome infants may have congenital cataracts. Infants also develop cataracts as a consequence of prematurity. Intrauterine factors such as maternal malnutrition, infection (cytomegalovirus/rubella), metabolic disease (diabetes), or medication ingestion (steroids) may lead to congenital cataract development.

Traumatic cataracts result from such factors as eye injury, recurrent exposure to ultraviolet rays, ocular foreign bodies, or scratches to the crystalline lens.

Secondary cataracts occur as a result of a variety of eye disorders, including retinal dystrophy or detachment, atrophy of the iris, glaucoma, neoplasia, or ischemia. Medications, including corticosteroids and radiation, also may predispose one to cataracts. Metabolic diseases leading to cataracts include diabetes mellitus, Wilson's disease, and hypoparathyroidism.

SUBJECTIVE DATA

History of Present Illness

Patients will describe a slow onset of symptoms, particularly the gradual worsening of vision over time.

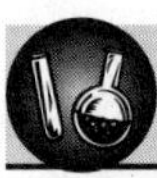

TABLE 30-1 Diagnostic Tests: Cataracts

Diagnostic Tests	Findings/Rationale	Cost ($)
Visual acuity with Snellen	Determine ability to see distance	N/A
Slit-lamp examination	Allows magnified view of structures in eye	108-133
Visual field	Determines the extent of peripheral vision	47-56 (using computerized equipment)

N/A, Not available.

Past Medical History

Ask about:

Long-term steroid use for immunosuppressive therapy for transplants
Frequent steroid use for treatment of chronic inflammation
Former eye injury or recurrent eye trauma
Systemic diseases:
- Diabetes
- Wilson's disease
- Hypothyroidism

Medications

Corticosteroid use or radiation results in edema of the lens, leading to cataract development.

Family History

Ask about a positive family history of cataracts, including congenital cataracts.

Psychosocial History

Recreational or occupational exposure to ultraviolet B rays has been linked with cataract development. Ask about history of being outdoors in sun or in area of high reflections such as snow, beaches, or water.

Part of the subjective evaluation should include an assessment of the degree of lifestyle impairment as a result of this condition and social isolation because of visual difficulties.

Description of Most Common Symptoms

Patients often complain of a constant fog over their eyes and rings or halos around lights and objects.
Many patients complain of glare especially affecting vision in bright light situations.
Vision may be described as more blue or yellow, and distant vision becomes impaired.
The location of the cataract will determine the extent of visual loss.

Associated Symptoms

Persons with central opacities will report improved vision in low light as a result of pupillary dilation leading to a larger portion of the lens being available for viewing.
Typically there is no pain with this disorder.

OBJECTIVE DATA

Physical Examination

General appearance: Vital signs, height, weight
HEENT: Eye
- Visual acuity
- Red reflex
- Directed visual examination
- Funduscopic examination
- Peripheral fields

Diagnostic Procedures

Diagnostic procedures include those found in Table 30-1.

ASSESSMENT

Differential diagnoses include those found in Table 30-2.

THERAPEUTIC PLAN

Surgical lens extraction improves visual acuity in 95% of cases. However, the decision to pursue surgery is a highly individualized one. Before recommending surgical correction, the clinician must rule out other possible causes for visual impairment. Evaluation of the effects of visual impairment on activities of daily living and the probability of improvement with surgery should be considered as part of the decision regarding undergoing surgery.

Standard means of adaptation for the visually impaired should be pursued. Magnification, modification of spectacles, large print, tactical cues may allow patients to delay or forego surgery altogether.

If the patient decides to proceed with surgery, preoperative evaluation for surgery should address stabilization of chronic disease, including hypertension and diabetes, the availability of a caregiver after surgery, and an understand-

TABLE 30-2 Differential Diagnosis: Cataract

Diagnosis	Supporting Data
Macular degeneration	Loss of central vision in the **elderly** Neovascularization of the eye Exudates, drusen bodies, and holes in the macula
Retinal detachment	Sudden impairment of vision in one eye "A curtain dropping over the eye" Loss of a portion of the visual fields Flashing lights and floaters Associated with a blow to the head or eye trauma (Detached retina is visible on funduscopy.)
Glaucoma (chronic, wide-angle)	Loss of peripheral vision, "tunnel vision" Increased intraocular pressure per tonometry
Presbyopia, myopia	Bilateral visual disturbance Visual fields not affected Vision may improve with use of corrective lens
Cataracts	Absence of red reflex in **children** Gray-white opacity of the lens on direct lighted visual examination Black against the red reflex on funduscopic examination Spokelike shadows that point inward (peripheral cortical cataract) Eye redness is *not* present.

ing of patient expectations of surgery. Anticoagulants are not generally stopped since their benefit in preventing possible surgical complications outweighs risks of bleeding during this minimally invasive surgery.

Pharmaceutical

Mydriatics (atropine) are occasionally used to improve vision by dilating the pupil and allowing for increased light to enter the lens. Mydriatic drops are relatively inexpensive. These should be prescribed by an ophthalmologist.

Lifestyle/Activities

Patients should be advised to wear sunglasses to protect against further cataract development from ultraviolet B radiation.

Diet

Cataracts are unaffected by diet, with the possible exception of diabetic patients who require effective glucose control to reduce likelihood of cataract development.

Patient Education

Clients may help with the decision to pursue surgery (Figure 30-1). Patient education for patients not choosing surgery include the lifestyle recommendations discussed in previous paragraphs. In discussing surgery, the patient is advised that the surgery is usually done on an outpatient basis. The most common surgical procedure is extracapsular extraction of opaque lens. Intracapsular extraction removes the lens through a small incision. In phacoemulsification (ultrasonic) the lens is broken up by vibration and removed extracapsularly, generally avoiding the need for sutures. Surgery also usually involves reimplantation of intraocular lens. Aphakic glasses and contact lens have been used in the past to restore vision, but are rarely used now.

General postoperative instructions usually include the following:

An eye shield should be worn at night, and glasses during the day to protect the eye.
Patients should avoid bending, stooping, or lifting heavy objects for 3 to 4 weeks after surgery.
Patients should not take showers or wash hair for 2 weeks after surgery.
Strenuous or excessive physical activity should be avoided for 4 weeks after surgery.

Family Impact

The patient may need family care or additional care for a short period after surgery, usually 7 to 14 days, although full healing will take 6 to 8 weeks.

Referral

Candidates for surgery will require ophthalmology referral.

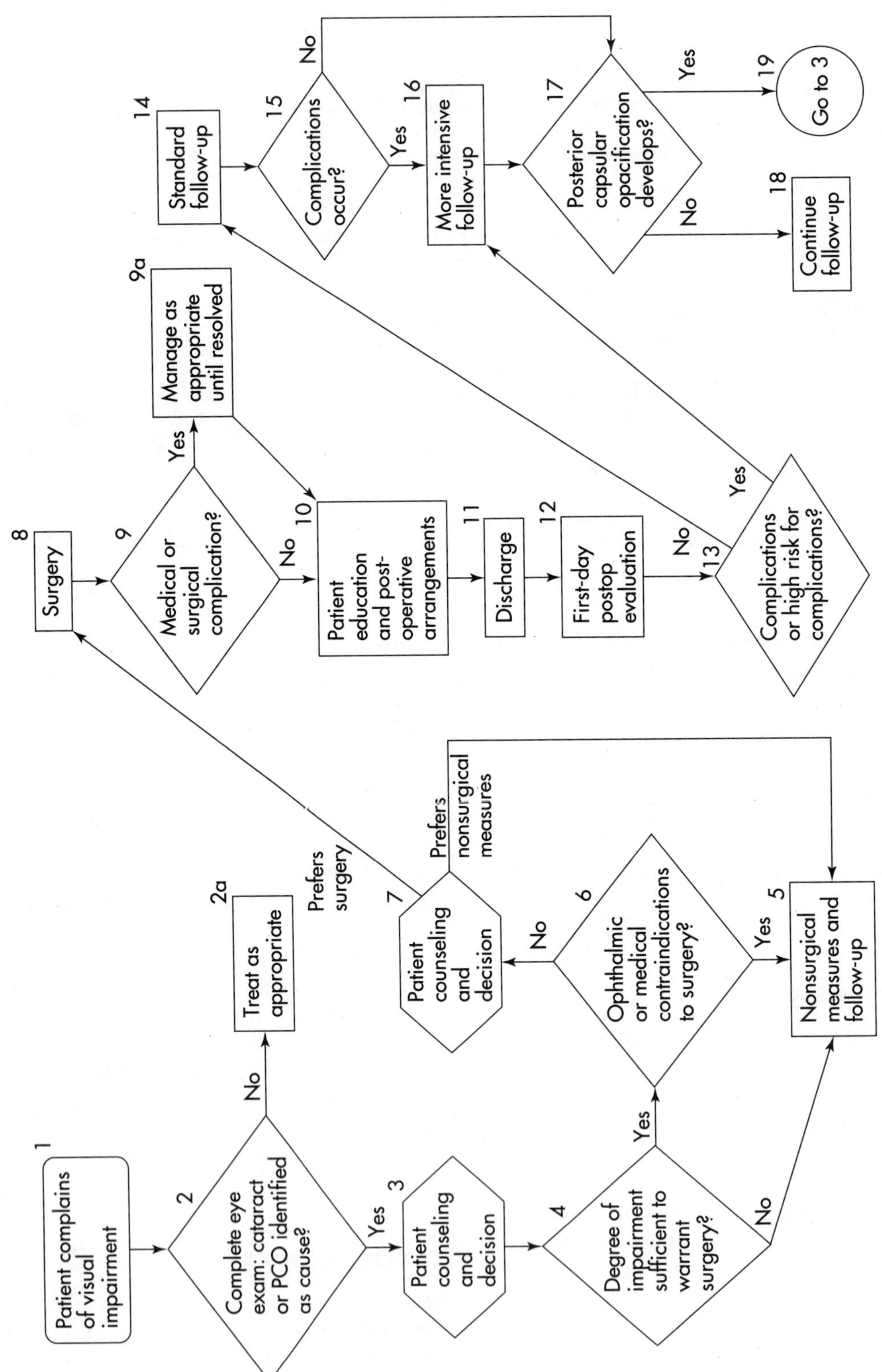

Figure 30-1 Cataract in adults. *c/o*, Complains of; *PCO*, posterior capsular opacification. (From US Department of Health and Human Services: Clinical practice guideline: cataract in adults, AHCPR Publication No. 93-0542, 1993.)

Consultation

Ophthalmology evaluation is indicated for most patients to help the patient compare options for therapy and determine risks/benefits of surgical correction of cataracts.

Follow-up

If surgery is undertaken, the patient will be primarily followed by ophthalmology care. Primary care providers should be aware of signs and symptoms of postoperative complications, including altered lens adjustment, red eye, or discharge, indicating inflammation/infection; and delayed opacification of the posterior capsule, sometimes referred to as "after-cataracts." Retinal detachment, macular edema, and glaucoma may also occur; therefore screening for these conditions are part of postoperative evaluation.

EVALUATION

If surgery is delayed or avoided, continued assessment of the client's functional capacity as related to visual impairment should be assessed. Patients having surgery unilaterally should be assessed for development of cataracts in the opposite eye.

SUGGESTED READINGS

Barker R: *Principles of ambulatory medicine,* Baltimore, 1995, Williams & Wilkins.

Ellsworth A et al: *Mosby's 1998 Medical drug reference,* St Louis, 1998, Mosby.

Healthcare Consultants of America, Inc: *1998 Physicians fee and coding guide,* Augusta, Ga, 1998, Healthcare Consultants of America, Inc.

Javitt JC: Cataract surgery in one eye or both, *Ophthalmology* 102:1583, 1995.

Schein OD: Predictors of outcome in patient who underwent cataract surgery, *Ophthalmology* 102:817, 1995.

US Department of Health and Human Services: Clinical practice guideline: cataract in adults, AHCPR Publication No. 93-0542, 1993.

31 Cellulitis

OVERVIEW

Definition

Cellulitis is an acute, diffuse, inflammatory infection of the dermis and subcutaneous tissue.

Pathophysiology

Cellulitis is usually caused by a group A streptococcus.

It can also be caused by nongroup A streptococcus, *Staphylococcus aureus, Haemophilus influenzae type B,* or *Campylobacter fetus.*

Other organisms that cause cellulitis include *Pseudomonas aeruginosa,* which may be present in puncture wounds. *Pasteurella multocida* may be present with bite wounds.

Cellulitis is often precipitated by a break in the integrity of the skin from trauma, burns, bites, and puncture wounds. It may also result from scratches, insect bites, and stings. Tinea pedis with fissures has been implicated as potential portal of entry in some cases.

SUBJECTIVE DATA

History of Present Illness

Ask about the presence and duration of erythema, warmth, edema, and pain.

Ask about port of entry and whether an injury or break in the skin occurred.

Investigate associated symptoms of fever, chills, malaise, and recent pharyngitis.

Past Medical History

History of recurrent cellulitis
Diabetes
Peripheral vascular disease
Saphenous venectomy for coronary arterial bypass grafting

OBJECTIVE DATA

A physical examination of the skin is performed to evaluate for:

Warm, tender, erythematous plaques
Lesions not well demarcated or elevated
Purulent or serous drainage or superficial blisters
Break in the integrity of the skin or other identifiable port of entry
Regional adenopathy or lymphadenitis with red streaking along lymphatics
Concurrent pathological condition of the extremities, as with peripheral vascular disease
- Absent or diminished pulses
- Cool to touch
- Decreased hair
- Decreased sensation
- Dermatitis
- Discoloration
- Edema
- Increased capillary refill
- Pain
- Varicose veins
- Ulcers

Diagnostic tests for cellulitis are outlined in Table 31-1.

ASSESSMENT

Differential Diagnosis

Differential diagnoses include (Table 31-2):
- Cellulitis
- Erysipelas

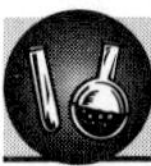

TABLE 31-1 Diagnostic Procedures: Cellulitis

Test	Finding/Rationale	Cost ($)
Wound culture	Culture and sensitivity; aids in selection of antimicrobial treatment	31-39
Complete blood count	Evaluate systemic response; leukocytosis with left shift is consistent with bacterial infection	13-16
Blood culture	Rule out bacteremia; cellulitis in patient who appears ill, is febrile, and has elevated WBC is at risk for bacteremia	37-45
X-ray film of site	Rule out osteomyelitis; gas may present under skin	75-151/Based on site
Erythrocyte sedimentation rate (ESR)	Nonspecific inflammatory response; ↑ESR consistent with inflammation	16-20

TABLE 31-2 Differential Diagnosis: Cellulitis

Disorder	Associated Findings
Erysipelas	Distinct form of superficial cellulitis that usually occurs on the cheek; caused by beta-hemolytic streptococci; edematous, spreading; well-circumscribed, hot, painful, erythematous lesions with possible vesicular or bulla formation; systemic involvement of fever, chills, and adenitis
Contact dermatitis	Allergic or irritative reaction to a specific agent, resulting in erythematous, edematous, often pruritic lesions with vesicles or bullae; can become weepy, crusted, or lead to a secondary infection
Impetigo	Autoinoculable infection caused by staphylococci or streptococci, usually on the face; lesions consist of macules, vesicles, bullae, pustules, and honey-colored crusted areas; when removed leave denuded red areas
Ecthyma	Deeper form of impetigo with ulceration and scarring; occurs frequently on legs
Abscess	Erythematous, firm, tender nodule with ill-defined borders that occurs deep in the skin, at bottom of a follicle or an apocrine gland
Scalded skin syndrome, also known as toxic epidermal necrolysis	Toxic or hypersensitive reaction of skin characterized by erythema, superficial necrosis, and skin erosions resulting in scalded appearance of skin
Candidal infections	Superficial fungal infection of the skin causing beefy red, pruritic, areas, with and without satellite lesions, typically in body folds, vulva, and perianal areas
Necrotizing fasciitis	Resembles cellulitis; caused by group A beta-hemolytic streptococci; spreads rapidly, associated with severe pain and marked systemic toxicity; as the infection progresses the involved skin loses normal sensation secondary to destruction of nerves
Venous stasis dermatitis	Caused by venous insufficiency of lower extremities and presents as edema, dermatitis with pruritus, hyperpigmentation, and skin breakdown; ulcers may develop
Thrombophlebitis	Partial or complete occlusion of a vein by a thrombus, with secondary inflammation in the wall of the vein; can present as calf pain, swelling, erythema, with a palpable cord
Gout	Erythema, pain, and swelling over a septic joint
Fifth disease or erythema infectiosum	Acute, benign infectious disease caused by the human parvovirus, mainly of children; causes fever and an erythematous, lacy, maculopapular rash on the cheeks, spreading to the arms, thighs, buttocks, and trunk; child is described as having a "slapped cheek" appearance

THERAPEUTIC PLAN

Cellulitis of an Extremity in a Child or Adult

Most often caused by group A beta-hemolytic streptococci
Expanding, red, swollen, painful plaques with indefinite borders, bullae, suppurates
Possible associated symptoms of fever, chills, or malaise
Diagnosis based on clinical presentation
Empirical treatment appropriate if there is no evidence of systemic involvement

Pharmaceutical

The antibiotic of choice is penicillin:

Amoxicillin oral suspension 125 mg/5 ml or 250 mg/5 ml ($3-$5); tablets 250 mg or 500 mg ($8-$27)
- **Children:** 20-40 mg/kg/day divided doses every 8 hours for 10 days
- **Adults:** 250-500 mg PO every 8 hours for 10 days

Pen Vee K oral suspension 125 mg/5 ml or 250 mg/5 ml ($1-$5); tablets 250 mg or 500 mg ($11-$88)
- **Children:** 30-60 mg/kg/day in divided doses every 6 hours for 10 days
- **Adults:** 250 to 500 mg PO every 6 hours for 10 days

For patients allergic to or intolerant of penicillin, consider one of the following:

Cephalexin
- **Children:** 50 mg/kg/day in two divided doses for 10 days ($5-$48)
- **Adults:** 250 mg to 500 mg PO every 6 to 12 hours for 10 days ($32-$95)

Erythromycin ethylsuccinate
- **Children:** 30 to 50 mg/kg/day in three divided doses for 10 days ($20-$30)
- **Adults:** 400 mg PO every 6 hours for 10 days ($13-$49)

Azithromycin 500 mg PO on first day, then 250 mg PO for 4 days for adults ($31)

Nonpharmaceutical

Children with cellulitis, fever, and an elevated WBC are at greater risk for bacteremia; blood cultures should be considered.
Osteomyelitis is a potential complication in some cases. The diagnosis is established by isolating *S. aureus* from the blood or bone of any patient with signs and symptoms of focal bone infection.
Consider concurrent peripheral vascular disease in adults with other findings.
Reevaluate the patient in 24 to 48 hours if there is no improvement in his or her condition; if drainage from the wound or systemic symptoms develop; or if the patient has peripheral vascular disease, diabetes, recent surgery or is immunocompromised.

Cellulitis With an Associated Puncture Wound

Pharmaceutical

Consider treatment with ciprofloxacin 500 to 750 mg PO every 12 hours for 7 to 10 days (for adults) for a puncture wound, especially of the foot, for coverage of *P. aeruginosa.*
Consider a tetanus–diphtheria toxoid (Td) booster, depending on the wound and the patient's immunization status.

Cellulitis of the Head, Face, or Neck in a Child With *Haemophilus Influenzae*

Child typically 6 months to 3 years of age
Rapid onset of cellulitis with fever
No obvious portal of entry
Usually involves one cheek and (less often) the orbit
Purple-red discoloration
Concurrent unilateral or bilateral otitis media
Meningitis is a possible complication and evaluation of cerebrospinal fluid should be considered in children with fever, irritability, and nuchal rigidity
Wound, middle ear, and/or nasopharyngeal cultures should be considered if diagnosis uncertain
Complete blood count and blood cultures should be considered to rule out bacteremia
Consult with physician for hospital admission, the necessity of intravenous antibiotics, and further evaluation
Antibiotics of choice are penicillins and cephalosporins; erythromycin does not cover *H. influenzae*
Consider prophylaxis for family members and/or close contacts in day care
Children over 3 years of age who have an identifiable portal of entry such as a laceration, insect bite, eczema, dental infection, or other obvious trauma can be treated for presumptive staphylococcus or streptococcus cellulitis

Cellulitis of the Head, Neck or Face in an Adult Caused by *Haemophilus Influenzae*

Adult typically >50 years of age
Appears to be in a toxic state and possibly in danger of airway compromise
Cellulitis preceded by pharyngitis, followed by a high fever, rapidly progressive anterior neck swelling, tenderness, and erythema with dysphagia
Blood and respiratory cultures will confirm the presence of *H. influenzae*
Consult with a physician regarding hospital admission, the use of intravenous antibiotics, and further testing
Same antibiotics of choice as for the child

Erysipelas of the Face in Adults

It is caused by group A beta-hemolytic *Streptococcus.*
Trauma or a surgical wound may precipitate erysipelas, but most cases occur without a portal of entry.
Differs from cellulitis in that lymphatic involvement in the form of streaking may be present, lesions can be elevated with more definite borders, and the color becomes dark fiery red with vesicles appearing at the advancing border.
Pain can be moderate to severe.
Associated systemic symptoms of nausea, vomiting, fever, chills, and malaise are common.
Treatment is the same for streptococcal cellulitis.

Orbital vs. Periorbital Cellulitis

Periorbital cellulitis is more common than orbital cellulitis.
Infection is limited to the eyelid and presents with edema and erythema of the lid and conjunctiva.
Sinusitis, upper respiratory infections, and trauma are the most common predisposing factors.
Staphylococci and streptococci are the most common pathogens in adults.
H. influenzae is the most common pathogen in children.
Aggressive treatment is indicated to prevent progression to orbital cellulitis or spreading to the brain. A consultation with the physician is warranted.
Orbital cellulitis causes proptosis, orbital pain, and restricted eye movement, as well as erythema and edema of the eyelid and conjunctiva.
Concurrent complications include sinusitis, abscess formation, sinus thrombosis, visual disturbance, limited movement, diplopia, blindness, and meningitis.
Blood cultures yield positive results in 10% to 60% of cases.
Immediate consultation and hospitalization are indicated.

Perianal Cellulitis in a Child

Caused by group A beta-hemolytic streptococci
Often misdiagnosed as candidiasis
Presents as bright perianal erythema that extends 2 to 3 cm into surrounding skin
Accompanied by painful defecation, tenderness, soilage from oozing, blood-streaked stools, perianal itching
May be preceded by pharyngitis, but children not typically systemically ill

Cellulitis After Saphenous Venectomy for Coronary Artery Bypass Grafting

Fever, erythema, and swelling may occur for months to years after stripping the veins in the legs or arms for coronary bypass surgery.
Cellulitis is caused by group C, G, or B beta-hemolytic streptococci.
Concurrent tinea pedis may permit portal of entry of bacteria.
Immediate hospitalization should be considered in any patient with the following emergent conditions:
Extensive cellulitis with systemic involvement
Diminished pulses in a cool, swollen, infected extremity
Presence of cutaneous necrosis
Periorbital and/or orbital cellulitis (because of the proximity to the brain)
Immunocompromised or diabetic patient

Patient Education

Fever care instructions
Wound care instructions
Return to clinic if no improvement in 24 to 48 hours
Stress that hospitalization may be necessary
Smoking cessation if peripheral vascular disease a concurrent problem

Consultation/Referral

Consult with an MD about any patient who has decreased responsiveness, an extremely elevated white blood count, or peripheral vascular disease or is immunocompromised.
If osteomyelitis is evident on x-ray evaluation or bone scan, refer to an orthopedic surgeon for surgical debridement to prevent further complications.

EVALUATION/FOLLOW-UP

Recheck the patient's status 24 to 48 hours after starting antibiotic therapy if there is no improvement.
Recheck at the end of the antibiotic course when the patient's condition has improved to ensure resolution.

SUGGESTED READINGS

Barker L, Burton J, Zieve P: *Principles of ambulatory medicine,* Baltimore, 1995, Williams & Wilkins.
Bisno A. Streptococcal infections of the skin and soft tissue, *N Engl J Med* 334:240-245, 1996.
Callen I: *Current practice of dermatology*, Philadelphia, 1995, Current Medicine.
Dershewitz RA: *Ambulatory pediatric care,* ed 2, Philadelphia, 1993, JB Lippincott.
Habif T: *Clinical dermatology,* ed 2, St Louis, 1990, Mosby.
Raz R, Miron P: Oral ciprofloxacin for treatment of infection following nail puncture wounds, *Clin Infect Dis* 21:194-195.
Sanford J, Gilbert D, Sande M: *The Sanford guide to antimicrobial Therapy,* Dallas, 1996, SmithKline Beecham Pharmaceuticals.

32 Chancroid (Genital Ulcer Disease)

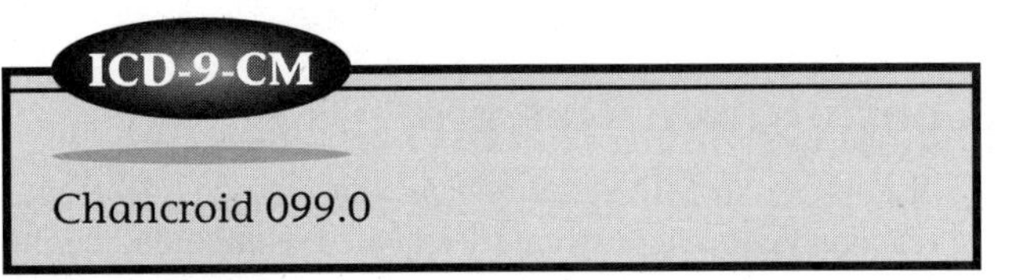

ICD-9-CM

Chancroid 099.0

OVERVIEW

Definition

Chancroid or genital ulcer disease (GUD) is a bacterial infection of the genitals in which rapidly growing, painful, ulcerative lesions form on external genitalia.

Incidence

In the United States chancroid is endemic in Florida and New York, rare in other parts of the country.

Pathophysiology

Common Pathogen

The causative organism is *Haemophilus ducreyi*, a gram-negative *Streptobacillus*. This organism is known to enhance transmission of human immunodeficiency virus (HIV). It is found primarily in prostitutes who then transmit the organism into the general public. It is prevalent in tropical and semitropical environments.

GUD is known to be a cofactor in HIV transmission, with particular attenuation with chancroid infection. Ten percent of people with GUD are also coinfected with *Treponema pallidum* or herpes simplex virus. The incubation is generally 4 to 5 days.

SUBJECTIVE DATA

History of Present Illness

The patient usually complains of a painful lesion on the external genitalia. He or she may also complain of enlarged and tender lymph nodes as well as pain with voiding or defecating.
There may be rectal bleeding.
Dyspareunia is a common complaint.
Ask if the patient is sexually active and how long he or she has been with current partner.
Ask about the number of partners in past 6 months.
Ask about the patient's last sexual contact.
Did the partner complain of "sores" or tender areas?
Sexual preference: male, female, or both?
When was the patient's last menstrual period?
Method of birth control; use of barrier methods.
Any vaginal or urethral discharge?
Any associated pain?

Past Medical History

History of sexually transmitted infections or pelvic inflammatory disease
Previous vaginal infections
Recent urinary tract infection

Medications

Any medications (antibiotics may mask symptoms)

Family History

Not applicable

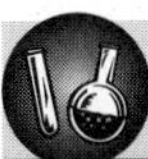

TABLE 32-1 Diagnostic Tests: Chancroid

Test	Findings/Rationale	Cost ($)
Culture: *H. ducreyi* or herpes	Culture for *H. ducreyi* is the preferred method; however, the organism is very difficult to culture Consult with laboratory for appropriate culture medium (usually defibrinated rabbit's blood or patient's own serum); even cultures using these media have a sensitivity of <80% Positive culture will show gram-negative *Streptobacillus* in chains or clusters with "school of fish" appearance. Culture for herpes may need to be run to rule out genital herpes	31-39/culture; 61-75/herpes
RPR	CDC recommends that all patients with genital ulcers should include a test for syphilis	18-22
HIV	CDC recommends HIV testing for anyone who has genital ulcers caused by *H. ducreyi;* chancroid is a cofactor for HIV transmission	41-52

CDC, Centers for Disease Control and Prevention; *HIV,* human immunodeficiency virus; *RPR,* rapid plasma reagin.

TABLE 32-2 Differential Diagnosis: Chancroid

Diagnosis	Supporting Data
Chancroid	Combination of a painful ulcer and tender inguinal lymphadenopathy suggests a diagnosis of chancroid
Chancre (syphilis)	Clean, painless ulcer with a hard base
Herpes	Multiple, painful vesicles that rupture, leaving an ulcerated base
Lymphogranuloma venereum	Begins with an initial ulcerative or vesicular lesion, often unnoticed; lymph node enlargement, softening and suppuration with draining sinuses, positive groove sign

OBJECTIVE DATA

Physical Examination

Vital signs: Blood pressure, temperature, pulse

Inguinal lymphadenopathy, size and tenderness of palpated nodes

Determine whether any nodes feel "matted together" (fluctuant abscess?)

Examine external genitalia looking for macules, papules

Men: Prepuce, coronal sulcus, frenulum

Women: Labia, anogenital skin, vagina, cervix, fourchette, clitoris

Look for painful, deep ulcers with a soft consistency

Appearance like an Erlenmeyer flask, opening at skin surface

Look for shallow, nonindurated, painful ulcers with ragged, undetermined edges, varying in size and often coalesced

Look for new lesions on opposite surfaces (from autoinoculation)

Vaginal speculum examination: Observe for lesions in the vagina or cervix

Bimanual examination

Diagnostic Procedures

Diagnostic tests for genital ulcer disease are outlined in Table 32-1.

ASSESSMENT

A presumptive diagnosis may be made on:

One or more painful ulcers, regional lymphadenopathy

No evidence of *T. pallidum* infection by serology performed 7 days after appearance of ulcers

No evidence, either clinically or by test results, of herpes simplex virus (HSV) (Table 32-2)

THERAPEUTIC PLAN

Pharmaceutical

Successful treatment cures the infection, resolves the clinical symptoms, and prevents transmission to others (Table 32-3). Patients who are uncircumcised and HIV infected may not respond as well to treatment.

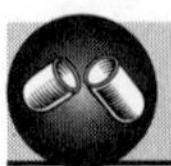

TABLE 32-3 Pharmaceutical Plan: Chancroid

Drug	Dosage	Comments	Cost
Azithromycin (Zithromax)	1 g PO in a single dose	Pregnancy: B Avoid taking with antacids SE: GI upset, abdominal pain, angioedema	$31/250 mg (100)
Ceftriaxone (Rocephin)	250 mg IM in a single dose	Treatment of choice in pregnant women SE: Local reactions, eosinophilia, rash, diarrhea, anaphylaxis, superinfection	$12/250 mg/vial
Ciprofloxacin (Cipro)	500 mg PO BID for 3 days	Contraindicated for pregnant women or for persons <18 years of age Pregnancy: C SE: Superinfection, rash, Stevens-Johnson syndrome, local reactions	$335/500 mg (100)
Erythromycin	500 mg PO QID for 7 days	Pregnancy: B Interaction with drugs metabolized by CYP450 (see Appendix D for complete list of cytochrome P-450 isozymes) Avoid use with statins SE: GI upset, abdominal pain, anorexia, rash	$26-$40/250 mg (100) $25-$154/500 mg (100)

GI, Gastrointestinal; *SE,* side effects.

Management of Sex Partners

Partners should be examined and treated, regardless of whether symptoms are present, if they had sexual contact with the patient within 10 days of onset of the infection.

Lifestyle/Activities

Use barrier contraceptive protection.

Diet

Not applicable

Patient Education

All patients who are diagnosed with chancroid should be tested for HIV and syphilis at the time of initial diagnosis and 3 months later.

Emphasize the need to use barrier protection with new partners.

Family Impact

None specific, other than the stigma associated with sexually transmitted disease (STD)

Referral

None needed, unless no response is obtained from treatment

Consultation

None needed, unless patient is allergic to recommended drugs

Follow-up

Patients should be reexamined 3 to 7 days after initiation of therapy.

Repeat syphilis and HIV testing 3 months after the chancroid was diagnosed.

EVALUATION

If treatment is successful, ulcers will improve symptomatically and objectively within 7 days. If no improvement is evident, consider that (1) the diagnosis is incorrect, (2) the patient is coinfected with another STD, (3) the patient is infected with HIV, (4) the treatment was not taken as directed, or (5) the *H. ducreyi* is resistant to the antimicrobial agent prescribed.

Complications include balanitis and phimosis.

SUGGESTED READINGS

Centers for Disease Control and Prevention: Guidelines for treatment of sexually transmitted diseases, *MMWR* 47(No. RR-1):59-69, 1998 (www.cdc.gov).

DiCarlo R, Martin D: The clinical diagnosis of genital ulcer disease in men, *Clin Infect Dis* 25:292-298, 1997.

Ellsworth A et al: *Mosby's 1998 medical drug reference,* St Louis, 1998, Mosby.

Healthcare Consultants of America, Inc: *1998 Physicians fee and coding guide*, Augusta, Ga, 1998, Healthcare Consultants of America, Inc.

Erbelding E, Quinn T: The impact of antimicrobial resistance on the treatment of sexually transmitted diseases, *Infect Dis North Am* 11:889-903, 1997.

Glass RH: *Sexually transmitted infection: office gynecology,* ed 4, Baltimore, 1993, Williams & Wilkins.

Hawkins JW, Roberto-Nichols DM, Stanley-Haney JL: *Chancroid protocols for nurse practitioners in gynecologic settings,* ed 5, New York, 1995, Tiresias Press.

Larson M: Chancroid. In Johnson C, Murray J, Johnson B: *Women's health care handbook,* St Louis, 1996, Mosby.

Ronald A: Genital ulceration and clinical acumen, Clin Infect Dis 25:299-300, 1997.

33 Chest Pain

ICD-9-CM

Angina 413.9
Myocardial Infarction 410.9
Pleurisy 511.0
Respiratory Distress 786.09

OVERVIEW

Definition

Chest pain is most closely associated with cardiac and pulmonary events. Coronary artery disease remains one of the most common causes of death in our society accounting for about 50%. In the 35- to 65-year-old age group, coronary artery disease accounts for about 33% of deaths. The most predictive risk factors for coronary artery disease include hypertension, smoking, and hyperlipidemia. Other factors that may play a part are diabetes mellitus type II, obesity, sedentary lifestyle, psychosocial factors (e.g. stress), and heavy alcohol consumption. Unmodifiable risk factors include advanced age, genetic predisposition, male gender, race (particularly black and oriental), and diabetes mellitus type I.

SUBJECTIVE DATA

History of Present Illness

Onset, duration, intensity, aggravating and alleviating factors, location, and quality are critical components to differentiate chest pain

Past Medical History

Hypertension, diabetes, hyperlipidemia, cardiovascular or peripheral vascular disease, gout, angina, previous or recent deep venous thrombosis (DVT), cancer (associated hypercoagulability), chronic obstructive pulmonary disease, previous spontaneous pneumothorax, previous or recent surgery (particularly orthopedic or trauma), **recent delivery of baby**

Medications

Use of antihypertensives or vasoactive medications, birth control pills
Include all over-the-counter medications the patient may have taken in the past 2 weeks

Family History

History of cardiovascular disease, history of pulmonary disease, history of hypercoagulability, blood dyscrasias

Psychosocial History

Smoking, increased stress levels, increased alcohol intake

Diet History

High-fat diet

Associated Symptoms

If a patient complains of diaphoresis, pain radiating down the left arm and/or into the jaw, shortness of breath, midsternal pain with exercise, or shortness of breath with exercise, consider this to be cardiac in nature until proven otherwise. Pain with inspiration indicates a pleuritic component.

OBJECTIVE DATA

Physical Examination

General appearance: Obvious pallor, diaphoresis
Vital signs: Hydration status, orthostatic changes
Neck: Listen to carotid arteries for bruits, check for diminished or absent carotid pulsations

TABLE 33-1 Differential Diagnosis: Chest Pain

Diagnosis	History/Physical Findings	Evaluation
Pulmonary embolus	Sudden onset chest pain Pleuritic in nature Dyspnea Tachypnea Pulse rate >100 beats/min Hemoptysis History of recent surgery, trauma, oral contraceptive usage, recent childbirth Phlebitis/deep venous thrombosis	12-lead ECG O_2 saturation Consider pulmonary function test Consider VQ lung scan Consider assessing ABGs
Pleurisy	Chest pain Dyspnea Pleuritic chest pain Friction rub	12-lead ECG O_2 saturation Consider pulmonary function test Consider CXR
Congestive heart failure (Ch. 42)	Chest pain Dyspnea Jugular venous distention Crackles in the base of the lungs Peripheral edema Gallop heart rhythm	12-lead ECG O_2 saturation CXR Consider echocardiogram Electrolyte panel
Pneumonia (Ch. 146)	Chest pain Dyspnea Adventitious breath sounds Temp >100° F Productive cough	12-lead ECG O_2 saturation CXR
Pneumothorax/ hemothorax	Chest pain Dyspnea History of trauma, smoking Diminished breath sounds	12-lead ECG O_2 saturation CXR Consider assessing ABGs
Angina	Chest pain: Relieved by rest, nitroglycerin and <20 min in duration Stable: No change in frequency, severity or duration of episodes Unstable: Increasing frequency, severity, or duration; often occurs at rest Radiation of pain to neck, left arm, jaw Dyspnea	12-lead ECG O_2 saturation
MI (Ch. 130)	Chest pain with or without radiation, lasting >20 min Dyspnea Diaphoresis	12-lead ECG O_2 saturation
Pericarditis	Chest pain: May be pleuritic or may be constant and resemble angina Typically pain decreases with leaning forward or sitting History of recent MI Friction rub Dyspnea	12-lead ECG O_2 saturation
Endocarditis	Chest pain Patient usually presents acutely ill Fever History of deformed or damaged valve History of recent dental procedure, instrumentation of GU or GI tract	12-lead ECG O_2 saturation Troponin I CPK isoenzymes
GERD (Ch. 78)	Chest pain May have radiation of pain into neck Nausea	12-lead ECG O_2 saturation

ABG, Arterial blood gas; *CPK,* creatine phosphokinase; *CXR,* chest x-ray; *ECG,* electrocardiogram; *GERD,* gastroesophageal reflux disease; *GI,* gastrointestinal, *GU,* genitourinary; *MI,* myocardial infarction; *O_2,* oxygen; *VQ,* ventilation quantitation.

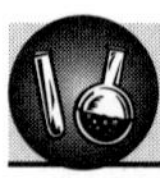

TABLE 33-2 Diagnostic Tests: Chest Pain

Diagnosis	O_2 Saturation	Electrocardiogram	Chest X-ray Evaluation
Pulmonary embolus	Decreased	Inferior ST elevation or ST shifts V1-V3	May appear normal
Pleurisy	Normal	Normal	Normal
Congestive heart failure	Normal or decreased	Normal or no changes	Pulmonary edema
Pneumonia	Normal or decreased	Normal	Infiltrate
Pneumothorax/hemothorax	Decreased	Normal	Pneumothorax or hemothorax
Angina	Normal	Normal or nonspecific changes	Normal
Myocardial infarction	Normal or decreased	ST elevations in inferior, lateral, anterior, or subendocordial leads	Normal
Pericarditis	Normal	ST elevation in almost all leads	Normal, or may show effusion if present
Endocarditis	Normal or decreased	Normal, varying degrees of AV block ST elevation indicative of MI may also occur secondary to endocarditis and should be treated as an acute MI	Normal
GERD	Normal	Normal	Normal

AV, Atrioventricular; *GERD,* gastroesophageal reflux disease; *MI,* myocardial infarction.

Cardiovascular: Listen for irregular rhythms, S_3 and/or S_4 murmurs, artificial heart valves

Pulmonary: Adventitious breath sounds, diminished or absent

Extremities: Check extremities for possible signs of DVT, pretibial edema

Diagnostic Procedures

Special tests: Electrocardiogram (ECG) ($56-$65), oxygen saturation ($28-$33), stress testing (graded exercise test [GXT]); consider ordering a thallium test ($825-$866) or Cardiolite GXT ($249-$305) if the patient has a bundle branch block because ECG findings are nondiagnostic in the presence of the block, consider doing a dipyridamole thallium stress test if the patient is unable to walk on the treadmill

Laboratory tests: Complete blood count ($13-$16), Biochemical survey 19 (includes glucose, $16-$20), electrolytes ($23-$30), lipid profile ($49-$62), and creatine phosphokinase isoenzymes ($43-$55), troponin I ($34-$46) (>0.04 is considered positive; 0.4-0.9 are highly indicative of impending myocardial infarction [MI], >0.9, MI has occurred); if MI must be ruled out, troponin I is a more sensitive indicator of an MI than cardiac isoenzymes

Radiological tests: Chest x-ray ($77-$91), consider ventilation quantitation (VQ) scan if possible to assess for pulmonary embolus; consultation with physician should occur before this is undertaken

ASSESSMENT

Differential diagnoses include angina, myocardial infarction, endocarditis, pericarditis, pulmonary embolus, pneumonia, pleurisy, pneumothorax, hemothorax if related trauma, gastroesophageal reflux disease (GERD); patients sometimes have difficulty in distinguishing cardiac and epigastric pain and chest wall pain (Table 33-1).

Diagnostic procedures for evaluating the patient with chest pain are outlined in Table 33-2.

THERAPEUTIC PLAN

The therapeutic plan for a patient presenting with chest pain depends on the selected diagnosis. Patients with acute life-threatening or potential life-threatening problems should be referred to a physician or a consultation with a physician should be sought.

A nonlife-threatening condition may require further evaluation over the next several days, but the patient may not require hospitalization. For example, patients with intermittent chest pain that has occurred several times recently but the pain is not noted at present can be evaluated for coronary artery disease as outpatients. However, if there is a strong indication that such a pain is cardiac in nature, the patient should be sent home with nitroglycerin tablets and a careful explanation of how and when to use them and who to contact. If a patient's cardiac evaluative tests all yield negative results yet the pain persists, a GI workup should be initiated for GERD and gastritis.

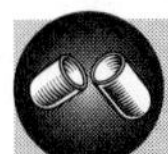

TABLE 33-3 Pharmaceutical Plan: Treatment of Chest Pain

Diagnosis	Treatment
Pulmonary embolus	Consult with physician for admission to the hospital.
Pleurisy	NSAID, such as Relafen 500 mg ($103) BID, can be given. Be aware of possible GI problems and warn the patient accordingly. Heat may also be helpful.
Congestive heart failure	If the CXR shows mild congestion and the patient is not in acute distress, the patient may be treated on an outpatient basis with diuretics. If the patient is not receiving any diuretic medication, this can be started with HCTZ 25 mg QD ($2-$13). If the patient is on a diuretic, this may need to be switched to furosemide or another loop diuretic (e.g., torsemide). An alternative is to add metolazone (Zaroxolyn). Loop diuretics need to be given in more frequent doses than other diuretics, but not necessarily in higher doses. The combination of a loop diuretic and a thiazide diuretic may be effective when a loop diuretic alone is not. Consult with the physician.
Pneumonia	Depending on the age and condition of the patient and the severity of the pneumonia, the patient may be treated on an outpatient basis with antibiotics. Consult physician for admission.
Pneumothorax/ hemothorax	Consult physician. The patient will probably need to be admitted to have a chest tube placed.
Angina	Stable: A graded exercise tolerance test (GXT) should be performed if not done recently. Aspirin 81 mg (enteric coated in the elderly) QD, Nitrostat 1/150 grain sublingual q5min for a total of three for pain. If the patient is not presently on a nitrate regimen, a nitroglycerin patch 0.2 mg/hr ($7-$16) could be ordered, to be put on in the morning and removed at bedtime. The dosage can be increased up to 0.6 mg/hr via the patch. Some patients do not tolerate the patch and may need to be placed on an oral form such as Ismo 20 mg in the morning and 20 mg 7 hours later. Unstable: The patient may need hospital admission for a nitroglycerin drip. Increasing the dosage of the patient's current nitrate therapy could be considered. The patient will definitely need a thallium GXT and possibly a cardiac catheterization procedure.
Myocardial infarction	Consult physician for immediate admission. Aspirin 81 mg ($1-$3) can be administered STAT if the patient has not received any previously.
Pericarditis	Consult physician for admission to the hospital.
Endocarditis	Consult physician for admission to the hospital.
GERD	Pain is often burning in nature, related to eating a large meal, lying down or bending over, and is relieved with antacid or food. If this cannot be distinguished from angina, the patient may need to be admitted for further evaluation, with administration of ranitidine (Zantac) 150 mg BID ($95-$100) or similar agent, or a proton pump inhibitor such as omeprazole 20 mg QD ($109). Omeprazole may be more efficacious, compared with histamine$_2$-receptor antagonists.

CXR, Chest x-ray; *GERD,* gastroesophageal reflux disease; *GI,* gastrointestinal; *GXT,* graded exercise test; *HCTZ,* hydrochlorothiazide; *NSAID,* nonsteroidal antiinflammatory drug.

Pharmaceutical

If a cardiac origin of chest pain is suspected, platelet aggregation should be inhibited with aspirin 81 mg ($1-$3) daily; enteric coated is best in elderly patients.

A pharmaceutical plan for the treatment of patients with chest pain is outlined in Table 33-3.

EVALUATION/FOLLOW-UP

Schedule return visit for 1 to 2 weeks, depending on the diagnosis. If indicated, a GXT should be scheduled as soon as possible. Have the patient document symptoms and notify you if there are any new symptoms or there is a change in the symptoms.

SUGGESTED READINGS

Brater, DC: Diuretic therapy, *Drug Therap* 339:387-395, 1998.

McCance K, Huether S: *Pathophysiology: the biologic basis for disease in adults and children,* ed 3, St Louis, 1998, Mosby.

Reuben D, Yoshikawa T, Besdine R, editors: *Geriatrics review syllabus,* New York, 1995, American Geriatrics Society.

Uphold CR, Grahman MV: *Clinical guidelines in family practice,* ed 2, Gainesville, Fla, 1994, Barmarrae Books.

Wilson J et al, editors: *Harrison's principles of internal medicine,* ed 12, New York, 1991, McGraw-Hill.

Woodley M, Whelan A, editors: *Manual of medical therapeutics,* ed 27, Boston, 1992, Little, Brown.

Chickenpox (Varicella Zoster)

ICD-9-CM

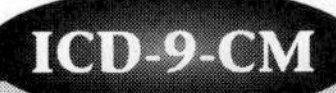

Varicella Without Mention of Complications
052.9

OVERVIEW

Definition

Chickenpox is an acute, generalized viral infection of the Herpes family.

Incidence

Occurs in late winter and early spring
Worldwide occurrence
Incubation period is 10 to 21 days; average is 14 days
Contagious 1 or 2 days before and 5 days after lesions appear
Common in children between **5 and 10 years old**

Pathophysiology

Transmission is person to person, spread by direct contact and airborne droplets. Universal susceptibility among those not previously infected. In metropolitan communities at least 90% of the population has had chickenpox by age 15 and 95% by young adulthood.

Infection confers long immunity. Second attacks are rare. Viral infection remains latent and may recur as herpes zoster (shingles) in **older adults,** occasionally **children.**

SUBJECTIVE DATA

History of Present Illness

Sudden onset of fever lasting 1 to 3 days with upper respiratory symptoms, anorexia, and followed by a pruritic, vesicular rash usually starting on the trunk and spreading to face and extremities

Past Medical History

Previous infection
Immunization history including Varivax after 12 months of age
Recent exposure to infected individual

Medications

Current/new medications

Family History

Recent infection among family members, infection of family members by this entity, especially siblings

Psychosocial History

Not applicable

Description of Most Common Symptoms

Rash is maculopapular for a few days, vesicular for 3 or 4 days, then forms a scab. Lesions appear in crops; new crops appear for 3 or 4 days. Lesions of varying size and stage are diagnostic.

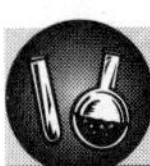

TABLE 34-1 Diagnostic Tests: Chickenpox

Test	Finding/Rationale	Cost ($)
Varicella virus culture (Tzanck smear)	Virus can be isolated from vesicular lesions during the first 3-4 days; not usually done for most patients	24-30
Varicella titer	Determines whether antibodies are present for varicella	48-59

TABLE 34-2 Differential Diagnosis: Chickenpox

Diagnoses	Supporting Data
Impetigo	Honey-crusted lesions at the site of broken or irritated skin; frequently around the mouth, nose, or hands; not associated with fever
Roseola	Erythematous, maculopapular rash; appears on the trunk following a fever as high as 106º F; spreads to the extremities, neck and face; rash fades within 24 hr
Rubella	Erythematous, maculopapular, discrete rash; generalized lymphadenopathy; slight fever
Rubeola	Erythematous, maculopapular rash; begins on face, becomes generalized; sometimes ends in branny desquamation; prodromal fever, conjunctivitis, coryza, cough, and Koplik spots on buccal mucosa

Associated Symptoms

Illness is more severe in adolescents and adults.

Immunocompromised children may exhibit progressive varicella, characterized by continued eruptions of lesions and high fever into second week of illness.

Pneumonia can develop in older persons and immunocompromised children.

Reye's syndrome is often preceded by clinical chickenpox.

OBJECTIVE DATA

Physical Examination

Skin: Observe trunk, head, face, legs for lesions.

More abundant on covered areas of body, scalp, axilla, mucous membranes of mouth and respiratory tract, conjunctiva, and areas of irritation (sunburn, diaper rash).

Diagnostic Procedures

Diagnostic procedures are not usually needed to make the diagnosis of chickenpox, but they may include those listed in Table 34-1.

ASSESSMENT

Differential diagnoses are outlined in Table 34-2.

THERAPEUTIC PLAN

Pharmaceutical

Symptomatic care for chickenpox is outlined in Table 34-3.

Lifestyle/Activities

Exclude from school or day care until all lesions are crusted (usually 5 to 6 days after onset of rash).

Provide supportive care.

Diet

Regular as tolerated; encourage fluid intake with fever.

Patient Education

Cut nails.

To relieve pruritus, apply calamine or cetaphil lotion to lesions.

Daily baths with baking soda or Aveeno to relieve pruritus and prevent bacterial superinfection.

Discuss administration of Varivax vaccine for children >1 year of age (Table 34-4).

Stress that aspirin (salicylates) not be used for fever/pain control.

Discuss link with Reye's syndrome.

Teach patients to identify potential complications.

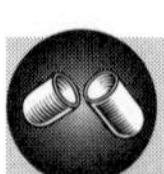

TABLE 34-3 Pharmaceutical Plan: Chickenpox

Drug	Dosage	Comments	Cost
Acyclovir (Zovirax)	Children over 2 yr: 20 mg/kg Adults: 800 mg PO 5 times a day for 5 days (max 800 mg/dose) Children: Not recommended in children under 2 yr	Initiate at earliest sign (not recommended for use in children in uncomplicated cases) Pregnancy: C	$98/200 mg (100) $189/400 mg (100) $368/800 mg (100)
Diphenhydramine (Benadryl)	Adults: 25-50 mg PO (max 300 mg /day) Children: 2-6 yr: 6.25 mg (max 37.5 mg/day) 6-12 yr: 12.5-25 mg (max 150 mg/day)	q4-6h for itching Neonates: Not recommended Pregnancy: B in second and third trimester; may cause idiosyncratic excitement in children	$2-$22/25 mg (100) $2-$15/elixir: 12.5/5 ml (120)
Acetaminophen	Adults: 325-650 mg Infants/children: See Appendix M, Pediatric Dosing	q4-6h (max 5 doses/day) Pregnancy: B	$2/drops: 80 mg /0.08 ml (15 ml) $2/elixir: 160/5 mg (120)
Postexposure prophylaxis: varicella-zoster immune globulin	125 U/10 kg 625 U maximum for patient >50 kg	Used in pregnant women or immunocompromised patients; provides passive immunity for 3 wk	$62-$80

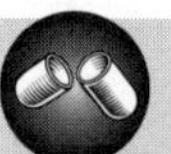

TABLE 34-4 Pharmaceutical Plan: Chickenpox Vaccination

Drug	Dosage	Comments	Cost
Varicella vaccine (live virus)	Adults >12 years old: 0.5 ml SQ in two doses (second dose 4-8 wk after first) Children >12 mo: 0.5 ml SQ in 1 dose	Wait 5 wk if immune globulin (VZIG) has been given Do not give to immunocompromised patients, those with active tuberculosis, or any febrile illness Pregnancy: C	$51-$64

Family Impact

Previously uninfected household members are at risk of exposure.
Can develop in infants born to mothers with active varicella.
The need for ill-child care for the duration of the outbreak may pose a problem for working parents.

Referral

Neonates (fatality rate of up to 30%)
Children with acute leukemia, including those in remission after chemotherapy
Pregnant women who have not had chickenpox

Consultation

Immunocompromised patients and those who develop complications

Follow-up

Not necessary, unless complications develop

EVALUATION

In addition to Reye's syndrome, complications include bacterial superinfection (pneumonia in adults), thrombocytopenia, arthritis, hepatitis, encephalitis, meningitis and glomerulonephritis.

SUGGESTED READINGS

American Academy of Pediatrics: Varicella-zoster infections. In Peter G, editor: *1997 Red Book: report of the committee on infectious disease,* ed 24, Elk Grove Village, Ill, 1997, The Academy.

American Public Health Association: *Control of communicable diseases manual,* ed 16, Washington, DC, 1995, The Association.

Ellsworth A et al: *Mosby's 1998 medical drug reference,* St Louis, 1998, Mosby.

Healthcare Consultants of America, Inc: *1998 Physicians fee and coding guide,* Augusta, Ga, 1998, Healthcare Consultants of America, Inc.

35 Chlamydia

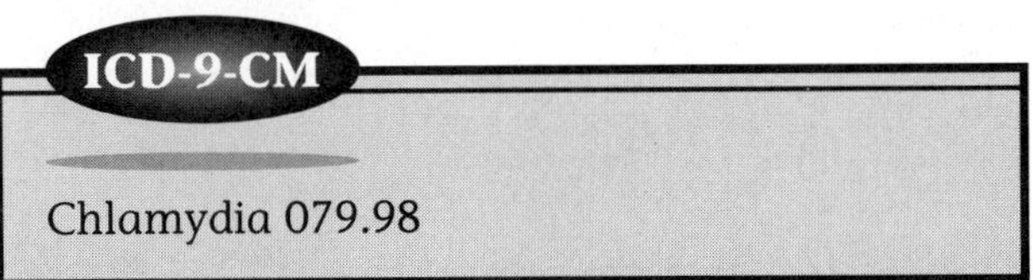

OVERVIEW

Definition

Chlamydia is a sexually transmitted disease of the mucous membranes of the reproductive tract caused by the bacterium *Chlamydia trachomatis.*

Incidence

The most common sexually transmitted disease in the United States among sexually active adolescents and young adults.

Prevalence

Eight percent to 12% sexually active **adolescent males** are affected.

Eleven percent to 23% sexually active inner-city **adolescent females** are affected.

Adolescents: The rate of recurrence for previously infected adolescent females is 40% within 14 months.

There is a 5% occurrence rate among college students.

It frequently occurs among patients who have gonococcal infections.

In **pregnancy,** transmission to the infant occurs in 70% of untreated women.

Pathophysiology

Chlamydia infects the genital tract of women at the transformation zone of the endocervix. In men it is found along the urethral tract. It possesses properties of both viruses and bacteria. Infections may be symptomatic or asymptomatic; however, even asymptomatic infections may cause significant damage to the reproductive tract.

Factors That Increase Susceptibility to Chlamydia

Sexual promiscuity/multiple partners
No use of barrier contraceptives
Lower socioeconomic status
Inversely related to age
Oral contraceptive (possible mediation through extension of columnar epithelium to exocervix)
Pregnancy
History of another sexually transmitted disease (STD) (especially gonorrhea)
Adolescents:
- Extension of columnar epithelium to the exocervix
- Perceived lack of risk
- Inadequate knowledge about STDs
- Increased risk in adolescent if:
  - First intercourse occurred at an early age
  - Her pattern of partner selection is poor
  - She uses drugs or alcohol
- African-American youths more at risk than white or Hispanic teens

Common Pathogens

The organism responsible for chlamydial infections is *Chlamydia trachomatis*, which is classified as a bacterium. It is an obligate intercellular parasite that infects columnar epithelium. Chlamydia may cause serious complications in women, including pelvic inflammatory disease, which can lead to ectopic pregnancy and infertility.

SUBJECTIVE DATA

History of Present Illness

Adults: Obtain information regarding sexual practices, use of barrier methods of contraception, changes in partners or in number of partners.

Children:

Ask about baby-sitters, daycare staff, any person who is with the child alone.

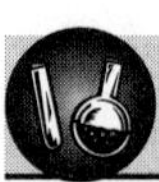

TABLE 35-1 Diagnostic Tests: Chlamydia

Test	Finding/Rationale	Cost ($)
Wet prep	Increased WBCs and decreased normal vaginal flora	15-19
Chlamydia culture	There are several laboratory tests available; sensitivities and specificities may vary; cultures for gonorrhea should be obtained at the same time; routine screening of young adult women is currently recommended, particularly those not using a barrier method of birth control or who have new or multiple partners	49-62
Gonococcus culture	Also should be done when Chlamydia culture is obtained	61-79
Syphilis/HIV testing	Consider testing for HIV and syphilis if the history indicates	18-22/RPR 41-52/HIV
Eye culture	Specimens specific for ophthalmia neonatorum must contain conjunctival cells, not exudate alone; specimens should be obtained from the everted eyelid using a Dacron-tipped swab Ocular exudate from infants should also be tested for *Neisseria gonorrhoeae*	31-39
Nonculture methods of testing for chlamydia (DNA probes)	Nonculture methods of diagnosing chlamydia should not be used in children under 12 years old because of the possibility of false-positive results; high specificity of cell cultures is required; DNA probes also have poorer clinical performance in adolescents than other methods	61-79

DNA, Deoxyribonucleic acid; *HIV,* human immunodeficiency virus; *RPR,* rapid plasma reagin; *WBC,* white blood count.

Ask about changes in behaviors.

Ask whether there is any redness or discharge around the child's genitals.

Past Medical History

Ask about previous infections and treatment.

Ask about recent sexual contacts.

Medications

Ask about current medications, oral contraceptives.

Family History

Not applicable

Associated Symptoms

Women: The disease is often asymptomatic, although if the condition is left untreated, the woman may complain of abdominal pain, vaginal pain, dysuria, postcoital bleeding, and dyspareunia.

Men: May also be asymptomatic; however, more often they complain of a thick, cloudy penile discharge with dysuria.

OBJECTIVE DATA

Physical Examination

Vital signs should be measured, including blood pressure, pulse, and temperature.

Lymph nodes should be palpated, checking for size and tenderness.

Men: Should include examination of the penis, including "milking" of the shaft, to assess for presence of a discharge, and examination of the testes for edema and tenderness. A rectal examination should be performed to assess for prostate enlargement. Collect cultures before a urinalysis in male patients.

Women: Should focus on the abdomen (checking for guarding and rebound tenderness), genitalia (looking for excoriation, lesions, ulcerations). A speculum examination is then performed, checking for any pain with insertion of the speculum. The cervix should be assessed, looking for inflammation and any mucopurulent discharge. A bimanual examination is performed to check for any cervical motion tenderness, adnexal tenderness, or fundal fullness. If anal intercourse is practiced, the anus should be assessed for redness and discharge.

Children (neonates): Chlamydia infections in the neonate is most often recognized by conjunctivitis that develops 5 to 12 days after birth (ophthalmia neonatorum).

TABLE 35-2 Differential Diagnosis: Chlamydia

Diagnosis	Supporting Data
Gonorrhea	Considerable overlap with chlamydia
Appendicitis	Abdominal pain with rebound tenderness and guarding; may begin as vague, periumbilical abdominal pain radiating to RLQ; fever
Cystitis	Dysuria, frequency, urgency
Men	
Urethritis	Dysuria and mucoid discharge one week after exposure. The d/c becomes purulent.
Epididymitis	Acute scrotal pain, fever, dysuria, urethral discharge
Proctitis	Anorectal pain, mucopurulent or bloody discharge, tenesmus, perianal excoriation
Women	
Pelvic inflammatory disease, cervicitis	CMT, adnexal pain, fever, abdominal pain, vaginal discharge, postcoital bleeding
Bartholinitis	Vaginal pain, erythema at Bartholin glands
Children (neonate)	
Conjunctivitis	Thin mucoid discharge, eyelids edematous with matting on awakening, burning, tearing, photophobia, enlarged preauricular lymph nodes
Pneumonitis	Persistent cough, tachypnea, nonspecific abnormalities on CXR, usually preceded by conjunctivitis in the first 2 mo after birth

CMT, Cervical motion tenderness; *CXR,* chest x-ray; *RLQ,* right lower quadrant.

Diagnostic Procedures

Diagnostic tests to confirm a chlamydial infection are outlined in Table 35-1.

ASSESSMENT

Differential diagnoses are outlined in Table 35-2.

THERAPEUTIC PLAN

Pharmaceutical

Recommended and alternative pharmaceutical plans are outlined in Tables 35-3 and 35-4.

Recommended Regimens for Neonates

Erythromycin 20 mg/kg/day PO in two divided daily doses for 10 to 14 days.

Topical antibiotic therapy alone is inadequate for treatment of chlamydial infections and is unnecessary when systemic therapy is administered.

A positive culture for chlamydia of the neonate confirms the need for treatment of the infant's mother and her partner (or partners).

Recommended Regimens for Children

Children who weigh <45 kg:

Erythromycin base 50 mg/kg/day divided into four doses daily

NOTE: The effectiveness of treatment with erythromycin is approximately 80%; a second course of therapy may be required

Children who weigh ≥45 kg but are <8 years of age:

Azithromycin 1 g PO in a single dose

Children ≥8 years of age:

Azithromycin 1 g PO in a single dose *or*

Doxycycline 100 mg PO BID for 7 days

Azithromycin should be available to the health care provider to treat patients in the clinic or office for whom compliance is in question.

Lifestyle/Activities

Counsel adults that they should refrain from sexual intercourse until 7 days after completing treatment, whether a single-dose treatment or a 7- to 12-day course.

Discuss the role of barrier methods to protect against sexually transmitted infections.

Provider should consider supplying condoms to patients.

Diet

Not applicable

Patient Education

Counsel in a nonjudgmental, compassionate, and respectful way regarding the need for prevention: abstinence, barrier contraception.

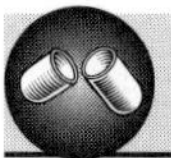

TABLE 35-3 Pharmaceutical Plan (Adults): Chlamydia

Drug	Dosage	Comments	Cost
Recommended Regimens			
Azithromycin (Zithromax)	1 g PO in single dose	Pregnancy: B Avoid taking with antacids SE: GI upset, abdominal pain, angioedema	$16/1 g sachet
or			
Doxycycline (Vibramycin)	100 mg PO BID for 7 days	Pregnancy: D SE: Photosensitivity, GI upset, enterocolitis, rash	$6-$123/100 mg (50)
Alternative Regimens			
Erythromycin base	500 mg PO QID for 7 days	Pregnancy: B Multiple drug interactions to CYP 450 Avoid use with statins (e.g., atorvastatin [Lipitor], HMG-CoA reductase inhibitors) SE: GI upset, abdominal pain, anorexia, rash	$25-$154/500 mg (100)
or			
Erythromycin ethylsuccinate	800 mg PO QID for 7 days		$21-$31/400 mg (100)
or			
Ofloxacin (Floxin)	300 mg PO BID for 7 days	Contraindicated for pregnant women or for children <18 years old Pregnancy: C SE: Superinfection, rash, Stevens-Johnson syndrome, local reactions	$366/300 mg (100)

GI, Gastrointestinal; *SE*, side effects.

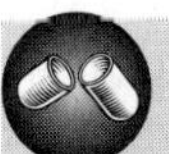

TABLE 35-4 Pharmaceutical Plan: Chlamydia in Pregnant Women

Drug	Dosage	Comment	Cost
Recommended Regimen			
Erythromycin	500 mg PO QID for 7 days	See Table 35-3	See Table 35-3
Amoxicillin (Amoxil)	500 mg PO TID for 7 days	Pregnancy: B SE: Superinfection, GI upset, urticaria, anaphylaxis	$17-$49/500 mg (100)
Alternative Regimen			
Erythromycin base	250 mg PO QID for 14 days	See Table 35-3	
or			
Erythromycin ethylsuccinate	800 mg PO QID for 7 days	See Table 35-3	
or			
Erythromycin ethylsuccinate	400 mg PO QID for 14 days	See Table 35-3	
or			
Azithromycin	1 g PO in a single dose	See Table 35-3	

Discuss how teens can obtain condoms, negotiate their use with partners, and use them correctly.
Provide written information.

Family Impact

The diagnosis of an STD is a traumatic event for all involved. Encourage the patient to share this information with parents or partner as appropriate and to seek counseling as needed.

Referral/Consultation

Any **child** in whom sexual abuse is suspected should be referred to a center or provider experienced in collecting specimens, as well as in providing appropriate therapy. Any suspicion of child abuse should also be reported to Child Protective Services.

EVALUATION/FOLLOW-UP

Adults: A "test of cure" is not necessary if recommended regimens have been used and both partners treated. Screen for compliance or possible reexposure. All sexual contacts should be tested and treated, especially those who have had sexual contact in the past 2 months or the most recent sexual contact, even if it has been longer than 2 months.

Pregnant women: A "test of cure" is recommended 3 weeks after treatment if erythromycin or amoxicillin has been used; if azithromycin is used, a follow-up test is not necessary. Pregnant women should be screened at the initial visit and at 36 weeks' gestation.

Neonates and children: Follow-up cultures should be performed.

SUGGESTED READINGS

Augenbraun M: Compliance with doxycycline therapy in STD clinic, *Sex Transm Dis* 25:1-4, 1998.

Bonny A, Biro F: Recognizing and treating STDs in the adolescent, *Contemp Nurse Pract* 3:15-24, 1998.

Centers for Disease Control and Prevention: Guidelines for treatment of sexually transmitted diseases, *MMWR* 47(No. RR-1):59-69, 1998 (www.cdc.gov).

Ellsworth AJ et al: *Mosby's 1998 medical drug reference,* St Louis, 1998, Mosby.

Hawkins JW, Roberto-Nichols DM, Stanley-Haney JL: *Protocols for nurse practitioners in gynecologic settings,* ed 5, New York, 1995, Tiresias Press.

Healthcare Consultants of America, Inc: *1998 Physicians fee and coding guide,* Augusta, Ga, 1998, Healthcare Consultants of America, Inc.

Johnson C: *Women's health care handbook,* St Louis, 1996, Mosby.

McMillan A: *Handbook of family planning and reproductive health,* ed 3, New York, 1995, Churchill Livingstone.

Reddy S, Yetura S, Sleepik R: Chlamydia trachomatis in adolescence: a review, *J Pediatr Adolesc Gynecol* 10:59-72, 1998.

Cholecystitis and Cholelithiasis

ICD-9-CM

Acute Cholecystitis 575.0
Cholecystitis 575.1
Choledocholithiasis with Cholecystitis 574.4
Choledocholithiasis 574.5
Cholelithiasis 574.5

OVERVIEW

Definition

Cholecystitis is an inflammation of the gallbladder caused by cystic duct irritation or obstruction. Cholelithiasis is stone formation with or without obstruction. Gallbladder disease may be asymptomatic or can be accompanied by recurrent bouts of abdominal discomfort. With asymptomatic disease the probability that biliary pain will develop is less than 20% in a patient 20 years old. However, when silent gallstones are present, 18% to 33% of patients will become symptomatic, most often within 1 to 2 years of discovery of stones.

Incidence

More than 24 million persons in the United States have gallstones. In 60% to 80% of cases the gallstones do not cause symptoms. The costs associated with the treatment of gallbladder disease exceed $3 billion each year in the United States. Gallbladder disease is more common in **women** than in men; among affected women, the condition is more common in overweight women over 40 years of age. However, gallbladder disease also occurs in young, thin to normal-weight women. In men and women 65 years old, the incidence is equal. The incidence among male patients older than 70 years and diabetic patients is growing. Blacks have the lowest incidence; 75% of Native American women over 25 years old and 90% over 60 years old have gallstones. The risk of gallbladder disease increases with age in all populations.

Pathophysiology

Gallbladder disease is caused by cystic duct irritation or obstruction, usually from stone or inflammation. Bile becomes supersaturated with cholesterol. A tiny nucleus of cholesterol crystals can form and ultimately grow into macroscopic stone.

Protective Factors Against Cholecystitis or Cholelithiasis

Normal-weight individual with low-calorie diet
No family history of gallbladder disease or diabetes
No history of use of thiazide diuretics or estrogen replacement therapy
Gallbladder disease not a frequent find in young people, however, rare cases have been found

Factors That Increase Susceptibility

Obesity
Female
Age (over 40)
Family history
Hyperlipidemia
Ileal disease
Degree of parity
Rapid weight loss on very low caloric diet
Insulin-dependent and noninsulin-dependent diabetes
Fasting while receiving total parenteral nutrition

Common Pathogens

Pigmented stones are associated with infection; the stones tend to be black or brown. The most common pathogens found are *Escherichia coli* and *Klebsiella pneumoniae,* but *Pseudomonas, Enterococcus,* and *Proteus* are also common. Candidal cholecystitis has been described rarely.

SUBJECTIVE DATA

History of Present Illness

Right upper quadrant (RUQ) pain with sudden or gradual onset, belching, nausea, pain in the right shoulder
History of a recent high caloric intake
Previous gastric or gallbladder surgery
Children: Rare, but symptoms similar to adult onset
Elderly: Most have typical signs and symptoms; some may have vague abdominal pain, no previous episodes; may or may not have elevated white blood count and fever; may present with altered mental state; second most common cause of abdominal pain in the elderly; more prone to ascending cholangitis, disseminated intravascular coagulation, subphrenic and liver abscess, small bowel obstruction

Past Medical History

Ask about:
Diabetes
Estrogen or progesterone therapy
Thiazide diuretic use
Frequent starvation diets or recent high-calorie meal
Prior episodes of gallbladder problems or RUQ pain
Use of calcium supplements
Patient on parenteral nutrition
History of gastric surgery or resection, ulcerative colitis, or ileal disease also risk factor

Medications

Ask specifically about:

Estrogen, progesterone, thiazides, clofibrate (should be discontinued or dosage decreased to avoid stone formation)
Calcium supplements have also been implicated in stone formation

Family History

Family or ethnic history of gallbladder disease

Psychosocial History

Social use of alcohol may decrease incidence of gallstones

Description of Most Common Symptoms

Cholecystitis

Sudden pain that builds over time, localized to the right upper quadrant with radiation possible to right or left scapula, lasting 2 to 4 hours
Pain may be associated with nausea and vomiting
Fever, itching or yellow skin
Elderly patients may describe vague symptoms

Cholelithiasis

Same as above, or may be asymptomatic
Elderly: Abdominal pain, fever, altered mental status; symptoms may be vague

Associated Symptoms

Nausea, vomiting, fever
Bloating, frequent belching, indigestion
Itching skin
Jaundice

OBJECTIVE DATA

Physical Examination

A thorough screening examination should be performed to assess:

General: Vital signs
Skin: Jaundice may or may not be present
Cardiovascular: May have slight tachycardia
Abdominal: Colicky RUQ tenderness with guarding or rigidity; respiratory pause with deep inspiration and palpation (positive Murphy's sign)

Diagnostic Procedures

Diagnostic tests are outlined in Table 36-1.

ASSESSMENT

Differential Diagnosis

Biliary disease, peptic ulcer disease, bowel obstruction, pancreatitis, diverticular disease, mesenteric ischemia, cardiovascular disease, urogenital, pneumonia, pulmonary emboli, pneumothorax, CHF with hepatic congestion, herpes zoster, diabetic ketoacidosis, porphyria, hypercalcemia, gastroesophageal reflux with or without hiatal hernia. Selected differential diagnoses are outlined in Table 36-2 and Figure 36-1.

THERAPEUTIC PLAN

Refer any symptomatic patient to a surgeon for evaluation.

Pharmaceutical

Referral to or consultation with a physician is recommended before therapy is initiated (Table 36-3).

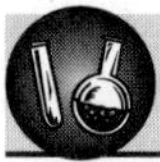

TABLE 36-1 Diagnostic Tests: Cholecystitis and Cholelithiasis

Test	Finding/Rationale	Cost ($)
CBC with differential	Indicates infection, anemia (elevation indicates cholangitis)	18-23;
Total bilirubin, alkaline phosphatase		19-24/bilirubin; 19-24/alkaline phosphatase
Transaminases (AST and ALT), GGTP	Elevated levels indicate obstruction of biliary tree	18-23/AST; 17-23/ALT
PT and PTT	Evaluate vitamin K synthesis or absorption, possibly suggesting hepatic damage	18-23/PT; 23-29/PTT
Serum amylase and lipase	Diagnose or rule out pancreatitis	24-30/amylase; 28-35/lipase
Urinalysis	Presence of bilirubin suggests hyperbilirubinemia	15-20
ECG	In patients over 50 yr old	56-65
Abdominal ultrasound	Confirms diagnosis; first choice for imaging	358
HIDA	HIDA scan also confirms diagnosis	750
Elderly		
ECG: Upright, chest	Sometimes detects air in the wall of the gallbladder which indicates emphysematous cholecystitis	77-91/CXR;
KUB		98/KUB

ALT, Alanine transaminase; *AST,* aspartate aminotransferase; *CBC,* complete blood cell count; *CXR,* chest x-ray; *ECG,* electrocardiogram; *GGTP,* gamma-glutamyl transpeptidase; *HIDA,* hepatic 2,6-dimethyliminodiacetic acid; *KUB,* kidneys, ureter, and bladder; *PT,* prothrombin time; *PTT,* partial thromboplastin time.

TABLE 36-2 Differential Diagnosis: Cholecystitis and Cholelithiasis

Diagnosis	Supporting Data
GERD	Indigestion, heartburn; worse after eating and lying down after eating
Appendicitis	Abdominal pain, worse after vomiting; rebound tenderness, guarding of abdomen; ↓ appetite, ↑ WBC
Diverticulitis	Acute abdominal pain and fever, LLQ abdominal tenderness
Pneumothorax	Acute onset of ipsilateral chest pain; dyspnea, diminished breath sounds
Pancreatitis	Abrupt deep epigastric pain that may radiate to back; nausea and vomiting, sweating, ↑ amylase and lipase
Bowel obstruction	Abdominal pain, distention; nausea and vomiting; diminished bowel sounds or high-pitched tinkling bowel sounds
Mesenteric ischemia	Crampy, steady epigastric and periumbilical pain; ↑ WBC; hypotension; abdominal distention
IBS/IBD	Chronic cramping abdominal pain, diarrhea, usually RLQ pain

GERD, Gastroesophageal reflux disease; *IBD,* inflammatory bowel disease; *IBS,* irritable bowel syndrome; *LLQ,* left lower quadrant; *RLQ,* right lower quadrant; *WBC,* white blood count.

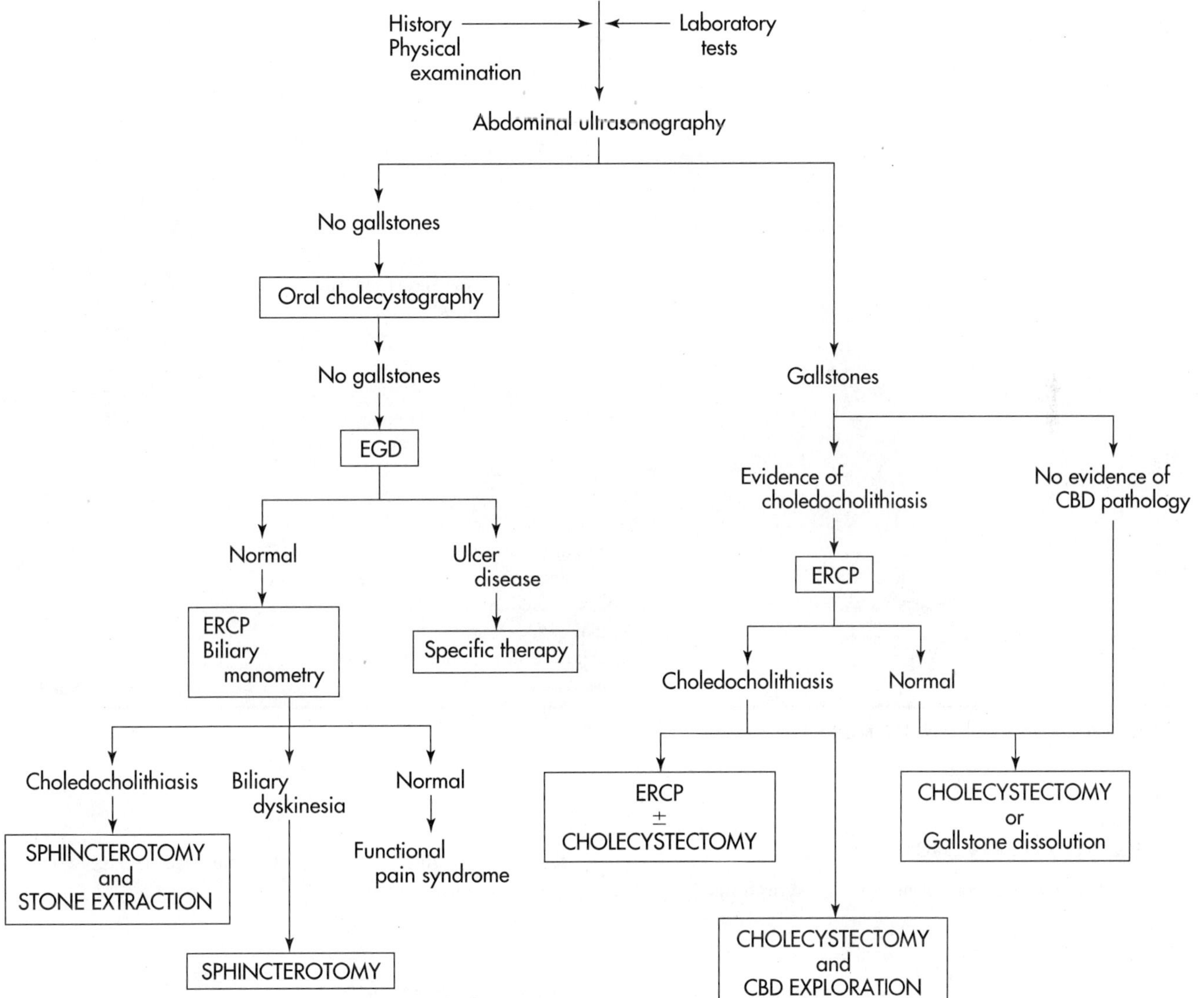

Figure 36-1 Algorithm for assessment of suspected biliary colic. *CBD,* Common bile duct; *EGD,* esophagogastroduodenoscopy; *ERCP,* endoscopic retrograde cholangiopancreatography. (Modified from Jaffe P: Biliary colic. In Greene H, Johnson W, Lemcke D, editors: *Decision making in medicine*, ed 2, St Louis, 1998, Mosby.)

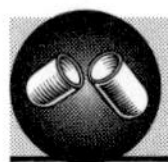

TABLE 36-3 Pharmaceutical Plan: Cholecystitis and Cholelithiasis

Drug	Dosage	Comments	Cost
Indomethacin (Indocin)	Usual dose is 25 mg 2-3×/day	NSAIDs have been shown to relieve pain and prevent stones in some cases Contraindicated in children under 14 yr old Pregnancy: Not recommended SE: GI ulcers, upset, nephrotic syndrome, headache, dyspepsia, CNS symptoms (hallucinations, confusion)	\$3-\$56/25 mg (100)
Ursodiol (Actigall)	8-10 mg/kg/day in 2 or 3 divided doses; also used at 300 mg BID as preventive therapy in obese patients experiencing rapid weight loss	Used for oral dissolution therapy Not recommended in children Criteria for treatment of gallstones with ursodiol include: Functioning gallbladder Stones <15 mm in diameter Stones that float (as shown on oral cholecystogram or are lucent) Patients who are poor candidates for or refuse surgery Symptoms are mild Single stone or multiple stones but patient is receiving long-term NSAID therapy Pregnancy: B Decreases the effectiveness of oral contraceptives, clofibrates	\$207/300 mg (100)
Monoctanoin (Moctanin)	Administered through biliary tract via T tube	Usually requires 2-10 days for elimination of or reduction in stones Pregnancy C SE: Abdominal pain, nausea, vomiting, diarrhea, anorexia	

CNS, Central nervous system; *NSAID*, nonsteroidal antiinflammatory drug; *SE*, side effects.

Lifestyle/Activities

May be limited or curtailed because of symptoms

Diet

Avoid fasting or starvation diets
Restricting fat/cholesterol of little benefit

Patient Education

Asymptomatic gallstones do not grow rapidly, and they rarely dissolve or pass spontaneously; generally surgery is not performed unless patient is symptomatic.

Gradually lose weight through caloric restriction; avoid fasting or starvation diets.

Notify health care providers of previous presence of gallstones.

Know signs and symptoms of acute disease and when to seek emergency help.

Be aware of therapy options.

Family Impact

Possible loss of income during illness
Anxiety and stress

Referral

Symptomatic patients

Children: Refer symptomatic patients for definitive testing and treatment.

Elderly: Refer for definitive diagnosis and treatment; mental status changes or poor social support in the elderly require hospitalization.

Pregnant women: Refer for definitive diagnosis and treatment

Consultation

When gallstones are found incidentally
For symptomatic patients

EVALUATION/FOLLOW-UP

If surgery is performed or the patient had a cholecystectomy previously, ask about symptoms at each visit because of the possibility of new stone formation in duct.

RESOURCES

National Institute of Diabetes and Digestive and Kidney Diseases (part of the National Institutes of Health [NIH]): http://www.niddk.nih.gov/health/health.htm

SUGGESTED READINGS

Barnes W: Cholecystitis, *Austr J Emerg Care* 2:18-22, 1995.

Birnbaumer D: Abdominal emergencies in later life, *Emerg Med* 25(5): 74-82, 1993.

Ellsworth A et al: *Mosby's 1998 medical drug reference*, St Louis, 1998, Mosby.

Gruber PJ: Presence of fever and leukocytosis in acute cholecystitis, *Ann Emerg Med* 28:273, 1996.

Healthcare Consultants of America, Inc: *1998 Physicians fee and coding guide,* Augusta, Ga, 1998, Healthcare Consultants of America, Inc.

Jaffe P: Biliary colic. In Greene H, Lemcke D, Maricic M, editors: *Decision making in medicine,* ed 2, St Louis, 1998, Mosby.

Nahrwold, D: Update: diagnostic dilemmas, therapeutic options, *Consultant* 33:27-29, 1993.

Rhodes V, Madison J: Gallbladder disease: confirming the diagnosis, *Acad Phys Assist* 4:457-469, 1991.

Schade R, Cattano C: Trends in gallbladder disease and its treatment (Part 2), *Hosp Med* 28(11):30-45, 1992.

Shaw B: Primary care of women, *J Nurse-Midwifery* 42:155-167, 1996.

Shaw B: Current management of symptomatic gallstones, *Postgrad Med* 93:183-187, 1993.

Stone R: Primary care diagnosis of acute abdominal pain, *Nurse Pract* 21:19-39, 1996.

Van Ness M, Chobanian S: *Manual of clinical problems in gastroenterology,* ed 2, New York, 1994, Little, Brown.

Yee J: Gallbladder sonography: review and update, *Appl Radiol* 24(11): 51-53, 1995.

Chronic Obstructive Pulmonary Disease

ICD-9-CM

Chronic Bronchitis 491.8
Emphysema 492.8
Asthma with COPD 493.2

OVERVIEW

Definition

Chronic obstructive pulmonary disease (COPD), also referred to as *chronic airflow limitation,* is a complex syndrome of decreased pulmonary function. All three components (bronchitis, emphysema, and asthma) are caused in part by oxidative and elastase-mediated lung damage of the small airways and alveoli. They are characterized by obstruction or limitation of expiratory airflow that fails to reverse completely following the use of bronchodilators.

Chronic Bronchitis

A diagnosis of chronic bronchitis is based on clinical criteria (a chronic productive cough for 3 consecutive months in 2 successive years). Hypertrophy and hypersecretion occur in the goblet cells and bronchial mucous gland cells, thus producing increased amounts of sputum, bronchial congestion, and narrowing of bronchioles and small bronchi. When the hypersecretion leads to chronic obstructive bronchitis, rapid deterioration of pulmonary function results.

Emphysema

Emphysema, based on morphological features, is the irreversible dilation and destruction of alveolar ducts and air spaces distal to the terminal bronchiole. This results in air trapping and decreased gas exchange caused by the derangement of lung elastin by the neutral proteases.

Asthma

Asthma is the increased responsiveness of the trachea bronchi to various stimuli, inflammation, and reversible airway obstruction (see Chapter 16).

Incidence

Sixteen million persons are affected, usually diagnosed after an acute exacerbation. There are approximately another 16 million people who are asymptomatic and undiagnosed.

COPD statistics:
- Fifth leading cause of death
- Mortality has risen substantially in 20 years
- Men affected more often than women
- Mortality higher in whites than other races

Pathophysiology

Preclinical stage: A 20- to 40-year period during which the patient is asymptomatic, but lung damage accumulates and function declines; the forced expiratory volume in 1 second (FEV_1) is <50% predicted for physical or body size

Middle stage: Cough and shortness of breath (SOB); FEV_1 <35% to 49% predicted for size

Late stage: Long-term oxygen therapy necessary; FEV_1 <35% predicted for size

Predisposing factors
- Cigarette smoking
- Recurrent infections, allergies
- Exposure to irritants
- Genetic factor: Congenital homozygous α_1-antitrypsin deficiency (AAT)

SUBJECTIVE DATA

History of Present Illness

Ask about risk factors, symptoms, and the patient's overall quality of life—ability to perform activities of daily living.

Cough: What time of day, when was the onset, and for how long have you had it?

Productive cough: What is the type, character, color, and amount of sputum produced?

Is there any audible wheezing or has there been any hemoptysis?

Dyspnea is frequently the most disabling symptom of COPD; it is important to know the onset, duration, and degree it interferes with activity.

What were/are the patient's past or present smoking habits? Is the patient exposed to passive smoking?

Any weight lost or gained? Weight loss has a deleterious effect on respiratory function and is a predictor of poor outcome.

Ask about the relationship of the symptoms with exercise and sexual activity.

Has there been any exposure to irritants or noxious materials?

It is essential to assess associated cardiac symptoms.

Past Medical History

Ask about allergies, previous respiratory diagnosis, and recurrent pulmonary disease, hypertension, obesity, congestive heart failure, peptic ulcer disease, cor pulmonale.

Are morning headaches a problem?

Medications

What medications and over-the-counter drugs does the patient presently take? It is best to have the patient bring in all medications for review to detect polypharmacy. This will also allow evaluation of the patient's technique with inhaled medication.

Family History

Ask about family history of COPD and AAT.

Psychosocial History

Passive smoke exposure

Smoking history

- Has the patient ever smoked? If so, at what age did he or she start, and what is the current smoking status?
- Calculate total pack-years

Alcohol or drug usage

If the patient is at a late stage of the disease, it is important to ask questions about:

- The patient's wishes concerning intubation, resuscitation
- Living will, power of attorney

It is important to screen patients for anxiety, depression, cognitive changes, and coping skills

Description of Most Common Symptoms

A nighttime cough may suggest asthma or gastroesophageal reflux in addition to COPD.

Morning cough may be caused by cigarette smoking.

Daily sputum volume rarely exceeds 60 ml in patients with COPD.

The interval between wheezing and production of purulent sputum grows shorter as COPD progresses.

Hemoptysis can be caused by acute bronchitis, yet the possibility of lung cancer must be investigated.

Morning headaches may suggest hypoxemia or hypercapnia, often present in end-stage COPD.

Signs and Symptoms of Infection

Emphysema: Progressive dyspnea/dyspnea on exertion, mild hypoxia, cough with clear sputum, muscle wasting, weight loss

Chronic bronchitis: Intermittent dyspnea, severe productive cough of mucopurulent sputum, cyanosis

COPD more common in obese patients

OBJECTIVE DATA

Physical Examination

Vital signs: Height, weight, respirations (tachypnea), pulse (tachycardia), blood pressure, pulsus paradoxus (a pulse that markedly increases during inspiration)

Major emphasis placed on observation and auscultation

Important to note the ability to follow simple commands

General appearance (cachexia, diaphoresis): Is there difficulty talking in full sentences?

Unusual body positions to relieve SOB?

Dependent edema?

Head/eyes/ears/nose/throat: Pursed-lip breathing; dry and pale, bluish mucous membranes; or perioral cyanosis

Neck: Jugular vein distention

Chest: Increased anteroposterior diameter, low diaphragmatic positions, retractions, and accessory muscle use; expect to hear expiratory wheezes, if crackles present, suspect accompanying heart failure; emphysema: Barrel chest, hyperresonance, diminished breath sounds

Bronchitis: Wheezes, rhonchi

Heart: Right ventricular heave, S_3 gallop or premature atrial contractions; atrial fibrillation if cor pulmonale is present; both heart and breath sounds are generally diminished in COPD

Abdomen: Palpate for organomegaly, liver engorgement (cor pulmonale)

TABLE 37-1 Relationship of History, Physical Examination, and Diagnostic Test

Symptoms	Findings	Diagnostic Tests
Cough, dyspnea	Decreased breath sounds, hyperresonance	Spirometry Expiratory peak flow
Productive cough, fever, dyspnea	Crackles; dry, pale mucous membranes	Chest x-ray

Extremities: Note peripheral edema and pulses, cyanosis, clubbing
Neurological: Mental status (somnolence, confusion)

Diagnostic Procedures (Table 37-1)

Spirometry ($96 to $117) is the most important technique for diagnosing COPD. This test should be performed at least once in every smoker 40 years old or older and in all patients who wheeze, cough, or have SOB.

Pulmonary function tests are helpful to determine the severity, reversibility, and prognosis of obstruction. Tidal volume (TV) is the volume of air inspired or expired during normal breathing. Vital capacity (VC) is the volume of air blown off after maximal inspiration to full expiration. The volume of air left in the lung after maximal expiration is the residual volume (RV). The volume of air left after a normal expiration is functional residual capacity (FRC). Total lung capacity (TLC) is the vital capacity plus the residual volume. Patients with COPD have difficulty with expiration and thus tend to have a decreased VC, increased RV, and a normal TLC. The single most useful test for ventilatory dysfunction is forced expiratory volume (FEV); it is considered the gold-standard test for determining reversibility of airway disease and bronchodilator efficiency. Loss of forced expiratory volume or compromise of forced volume capacity is associated with compromised airflow. This is measured by having a patient exhale into a spirometer as forcefully and completely as possible after maximal inspirations. Healthy persons can generally exhale 75% to 80% of VC in 1 second and almost all in 3 seconds. An FEV of more than 3 seconds, coupled with decreased vital capacity and expiratory flow rates, is seen in patients with COPD. An exhaled percentage of less than 75% is the hallmark of obstruction of airflow. Increased respiratory volume and total lung capacity are seen in emphysema. After initial spirometry testing, give the patient an inhaled bronchodilator and repeat the spirometry test in 15 to 20 minutes to determine the effectiveness of treatment. Box 37-1 outlines the three stages of COPD.

Other tests include the following:

Complete blood count (CBC) ($13 to $16): Polycythemia in advanced stages of chronic bronchitis resulting from chronic hypoxemia
Comprehensive metabolic profile ($32 to $42)

Box 37-1

Three Stages of COPD

Stage I

FEV_1 <50% of predicted for body size
Minimal impact on health-related quality of life
Typically managed by primary care physician
May progress to severe dyspnea, requiring added diagnostic studies and evaluation by a pulmonologist
Severe hypoxemia usually not present
Arterial blood gas measurements not required

Stage II

FEV_1 35% to 49% of predicted for body size
Significant impact on health-related quality of life
Typically managed by a respiratory subspecialist
Arterial blood gas measurements needed

Stage III

FEV_1 <35% of predicted for body size
Profound impact on health-related quality of life
Typically managed by a respiratory subspecialist
Arterial blood gas measurements needed

From Celli R et al: COPD: step by step through the workup, *Patient Care* January 1998, pp 20-52.

Electrocardiogram (advanced COPD: right atrial hypertrophy) ($56 to $65)
Chest x-ray examination ($77 to $91): Emphysema will show hyperaeration of lungs, a low, flat diaphragm, increased retrosternal airspace, and a narrow heart silhouette; in chronic bronchitis, enlarged heart and arteries will be seen on film
Pulse oximetry ($28 to $33) can be used in the office to screen for hypoxemia; if oxygen saturation is 90% or less at rest, it will be necessary to perform an arterial blood gas evaluation
Blood gases ($78 to $98): If FEV_1 is <50% (usually 1 L), this indicates hypoxemia in varying degrees, respiratory alkalosis (early), acidosis (late), hypoxia, and hypercapnia (CO_2 retention)
Mild to moderate: All test results within normal limits except spirometry
Severe: CBC (polycythemia)

An AAT concentration determination indicated for patient less than 50 years old who has COPD and a positive family history of emphysema

ASSESSMENT

Differential diagnoses include:

Cardiac causes:
- Congestive heart failure (CHF)
- Infarction
- Arrhythmia

Pulmonary causes:
- Acute bronchitis
- Pulmonary embolism
- Lung cancer
- CHF
- COPD
- Tuberculosis
- Pneumonia
- Pneumothorax
- Atelectasis

Other causes:
- Deconditioning
- Obesity
- Psychogenic factors
- Anemia
- Gastroesophageal reflux disease
- Postnasal drip
- Chronic aspiration
- Aspiration
- Anaphylaxis
- Epiglottitis

Figure 37-1 is a flowchart for diagnosing COPD. Table 37-2 addresses the most common differential diagnoses.

THERAPEUTIC PLAN

Goals of therapy are to prevent progression of the disease, improve symptoms, and control infection. Patient education and participation are critical.

Pharmaceutical (Figures 37-2 and 37-3)

Figures 37-2 and 37-3 illustrate stepped care approaches to the treatment of COPD.

Level 1 (least severe): All symptomatic patients—anticholinergic (ipratropium bromide [Atrovent]) metered-dose inhaler (MDI) with spacer, 3 to 6 puffs QID

Level 2: Inhaled β_2-selective agonist (albuterol [Ventolin] or metaproterenol sulfate [Alupent]) MDI with spacer, 2 to 6 puffs q3-6 h; can use nebulizer solutions (plus level 1 therapy)

Level 3: Inhaled corticosteroid (beclomethasone dipropionate, triamcinolone, or flunisolide) MDI, 2 puffs BID; rinse mouth after each use (plus levels 1 and 2 therapy)

Level 4: Extended-release theophylline, 300 to 900 mg/day (serum level 8 to 12 µg/ml) (plus levels 1 to 3 therapy)

Level 5: Extended-release inhaled albuterol (salmeterol [Serevent]) MDI, 2 puffs BID (plus levels 1 to 4 therapy); formulations may benefit selected patients with nocturnal symptoms

Level 6 (most severe): Oral corticosteroid (prednisone), 40 mg/day for 14 days, then reduce corticosteroids to a minimum; possible 0 to 10 mg QD or QOD (plus levels 1 to 5 therapy)

Table 37-3 summarizes drug therapy. It is important to avoid sedatives, antihistamines, and beta blockers.

Infection Control (Acute Exacerbation)

Educate the patient regarding factors that contribute to upper respiratory infections. *Streptococcus pneumoniae, Haemophilus influenzae, Mycoplasma pneumoniae,* and *Moraxella catarrhalis* are the most common organisms of infection. Signs and symptoms are increased cough, thick/odorous sputum production, change of sputum color, increased SOB, fatigue, chest congestion, and fever and chills.

Treatment

Broad-spectrum antibiotics covering common organisms for 7 to 10 days

Sulfamethoxazole/trimethoprim (Bactrim) DS one tablet PO BID

Erythromycin 250 mg QID ($14 to $18) or azithromycin (Zithromax) ($31), (if compliance with frequent medication dosing is a problem)

Amoxicillin 250 to 500 mg oral TID ($8 to $50)

Cough with difficulty in clearing secretions—mucolytic agents such as benzonatate (Tessalon) ($47-$84), Guaifenesin ($10-$27)

Oxygen Therapy and Safety Issues

Oxygen therapy will help control symptoms and improve quality of life. A low flow rate (2 L or less) has been shown to improve survival in COPD patients. Home oxygen therapy is prescribed when the Pao_2 is less than 55 mm Hg or O_2 saturation is less than 85%. O_2 is not used within 6 feet of an open flame. Also there is a need for a fire extinguisher and a smoke alarm in a home where oxygen is being used.

Lifestyle/Activities

Smoking cessation will immediately improve declining lung function. Usually after 5 years, lung function will return to that of a nonsmoker.

A pulmonary rehabilitation program (purse-lip breathing

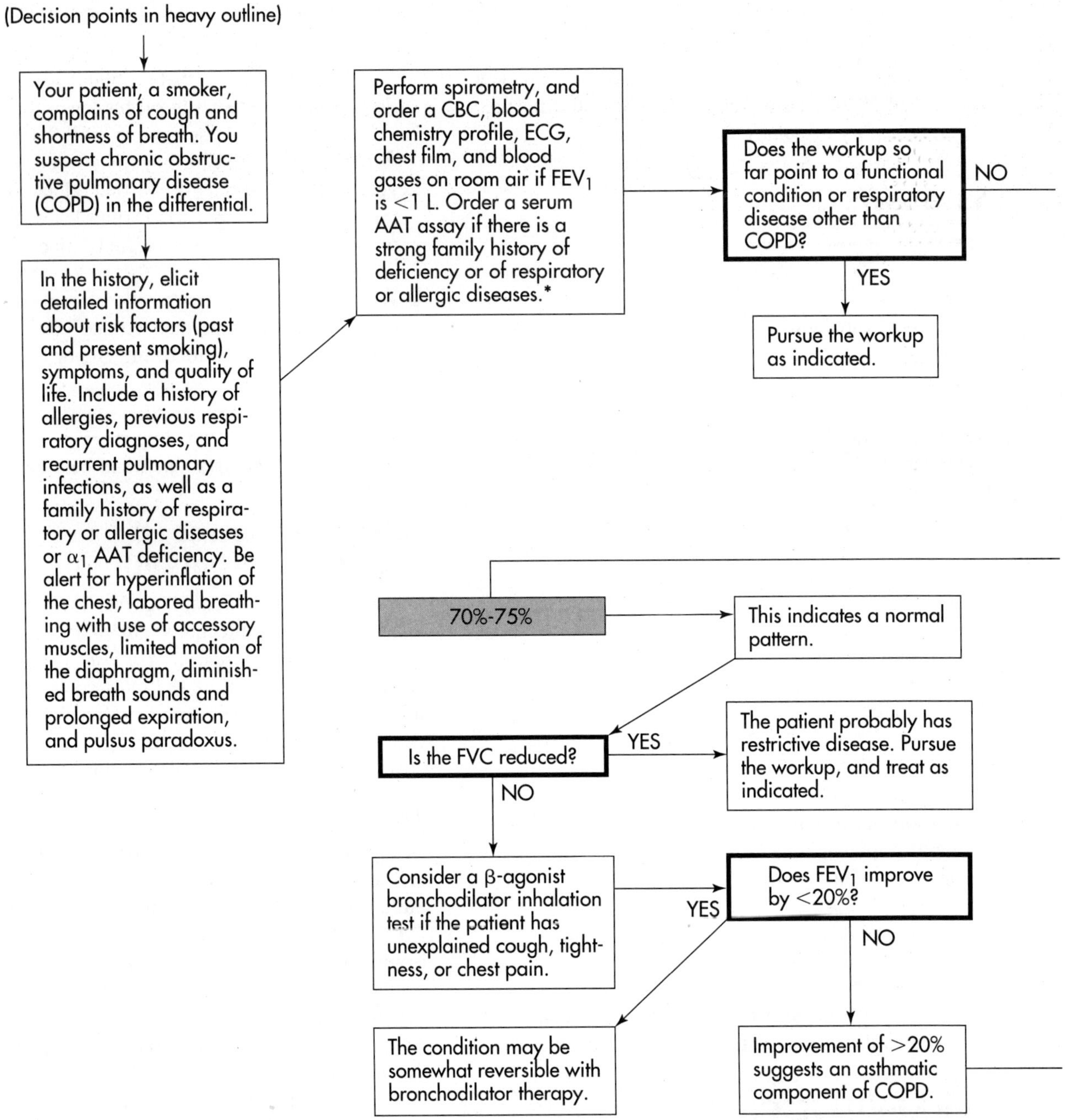

(Decision points in heavy outline)

Your patient, a smoker, complains of cough and shortness of breath. You suspect chronic obstructive pulmonary disease (COPD) in the differential.

In the history, elicit detailed information about risk factors (past and present smoking), symptoms, and quality of life. Include a history of allergies, previous respiratory diagnoses, and recurrent pulmonary infections, as well as a family history of respiratory or allergic diseases or α_1 AAT deficiency. Be alert for hyperinflation of the chest, labored breathing with use of accessory muscles, limited motion of the diaphragm, diminished breath sounds and prolonged expiration, and pulsus paradoxus.

Perform spirometry, and order a CBC, blood chemistry profile, ECG, chest film, and blood gases on room air if FEV_1 is <1 L. Order a serum AAT assay if there is a strong family history of deficiency or of respiratory or allergic diseases.*

Does the workup so far point to a functional condition or respiratory disease other than COPD?

NO

YES

Pursue the workup as indicated.

70%-75%

This indicates a normal pattern.

Is the FVC reduced?

YES

The patient probably has restrictive disease. Pursue the workup, and treat as indicated.

NO

Consider a β-agonist bronchodilator inhalation test if the patient has unexplained cough, tightness, or chest pain.

Does FEV_1 improve by <20%?

YES

The condition may be somewhat reversible with bronchodilator therapy.

NO

Improvement of >20% suggests an asthmatic component of COPD.

Figure 37-1 Diagnosing COPD. *Other findings that should prompt an AAT assay include bronchiectasis, age <40, predominance of basilar emphysema, unremitting asthma, and cirrhosis without risk factors. Therapy involves AAT replacement. *AAT,* α_1-antitrypsin; *COPD,* Chronic obstructive pulmonary disease; *CBC,* complete blood count; *ECG,* electrocardiogram; *FEV_1,* forced expiratory volume during the first second; *FVC,* forced vital capacity. (Modified from Celli R et al: COPD: step by step through the workup, *Patient Care,* January 1997, pp 20-52.)

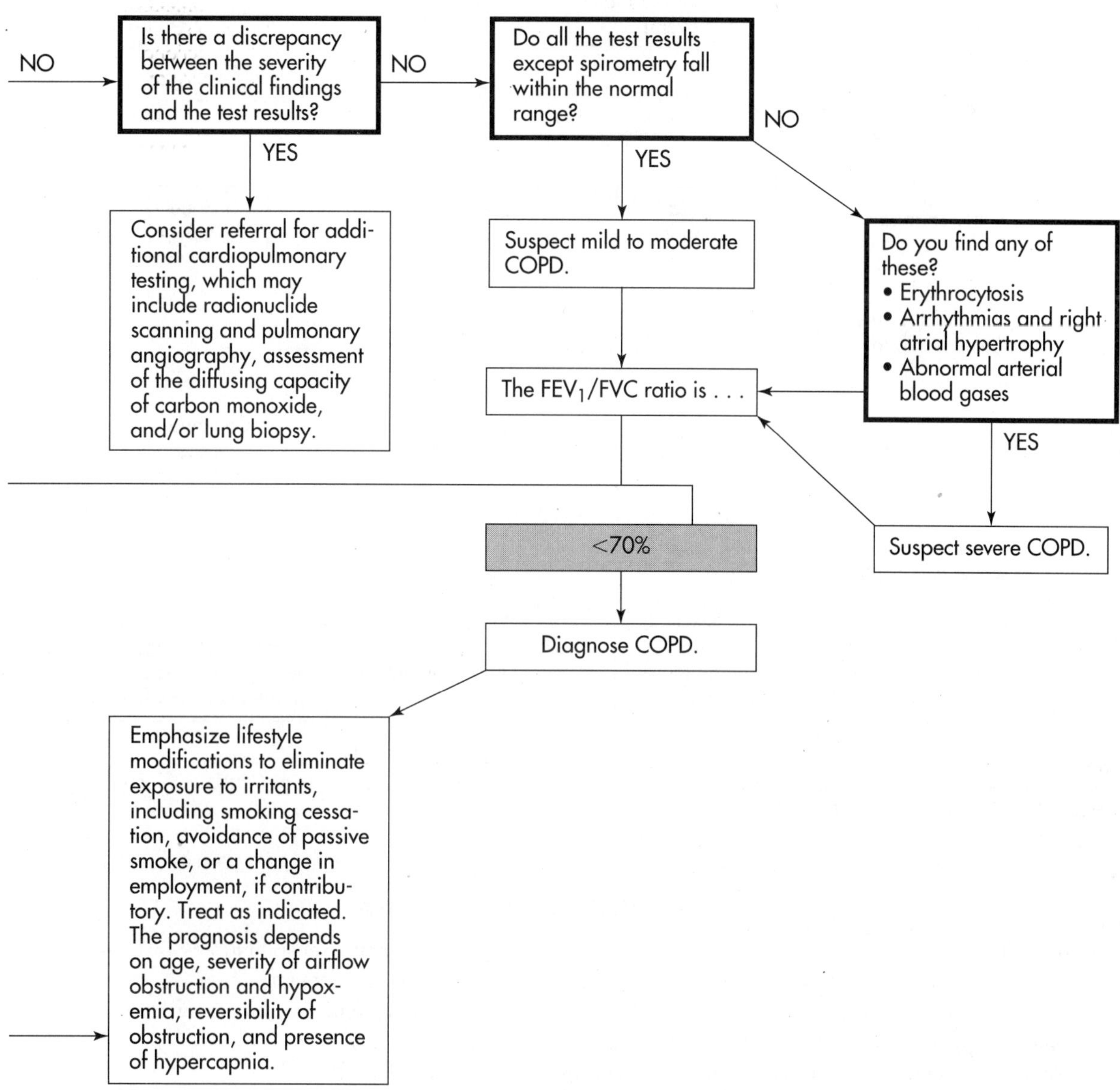

Figure 37-1, cont'd For legend see opposite page.

TABLE 37-2 Differential Diagnosis: COPD

Diagnosis	Supporting Data
Emphysema	Cough, little or no sputum, SOB with exertion, barrel chest
Chronic bronchitis	SOB, cough, infection, mucus production at least 3 months a year for a minimum of 2 years; lying down at night worsens condition
Lung cancer	Frequent bouts of pneumonia or lung infection, weight loss, fever, SOB, bloody sputum, chest pain
Bronchiectasis	Chronic sinusitis, chronic cough, heavy sputum, serious frequent respiratory infections, usually starting in childhood

SOB, Shortness of breath.

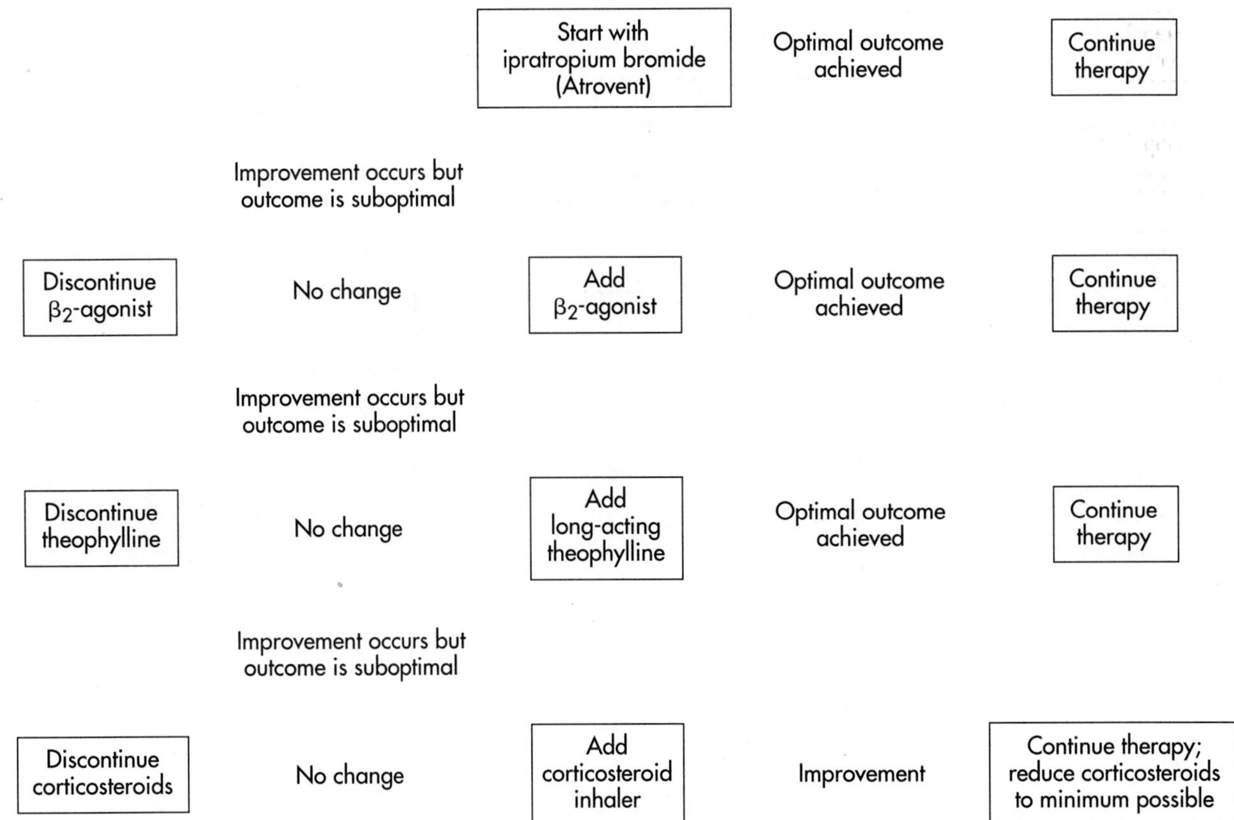

Figure 37-2 Treatment protocol for COPD. *COPD,* Chronic obstructive pulmonary disease; *MDI,* metered-dose inhaler (Modified from Ferguson GT et al: Current concepts: management of COPD, *N Engl J Med* 328:1017-1022, 1993.)

and diaphragmatic exercises) is extremely important. Prolonged inactivity leads to increased disability. Encourage exercise to increase activity tolerance at a lower oxygen consumption; upper extremity training can lessen diaphragmatic work. Occupational therapy, vocational rehabilitation, and physical therapy should be recommended or a consultation sought.

Diet

Good nutrition is important for timely response of the lungs to hypoxemia and hypercapnia. A healthy diet will help to maintain the immune system for fighting infection. It is important to drink at least 8 to10 glasses of fluid, preferably water, daily.

It is important to avoid foods that increase bronchospasm and sputum (alcohol, spicy food, dairy products). Encourage the patient to eat frequent small meals, since large meals can cause abdominal distention and impair diaphragmatic function. Six small, calorically dense meals helps to conserve energy and prevent abdominal distention. Dental status needs evaluation for poor hygiene or improperly fitted dentures, which will have an impact on nutrition.

Patient Education

Multidisciplinary pulmonary rehabilitation: Instruct on coughing: deep breath, then cough

Effects of COPD on lung function, breathing techniques, and coping skills

Education in use of inhaler (Box 37-2)

Counsel patient about advance directives

Review signs and symptoms of respiratory infections

Avoidance of extremes in temperature (or wear a mask)

Home humidification and ingestion of 2 to 3 L of water per day

Prevention of infection with yearly influenza vaccine

Pneumovax every 6 to 10 years

Smoking cessation and reducing exposures to airway irritants

Reduction of airflow obstruction with avoidance of sedatives, antihistamines, and beta-blockers

Family Impact

COPD has considerable impact on the patient's family and friends as the disease runs its course and the patient becomes debilitated and increasingly dependent. The diag-

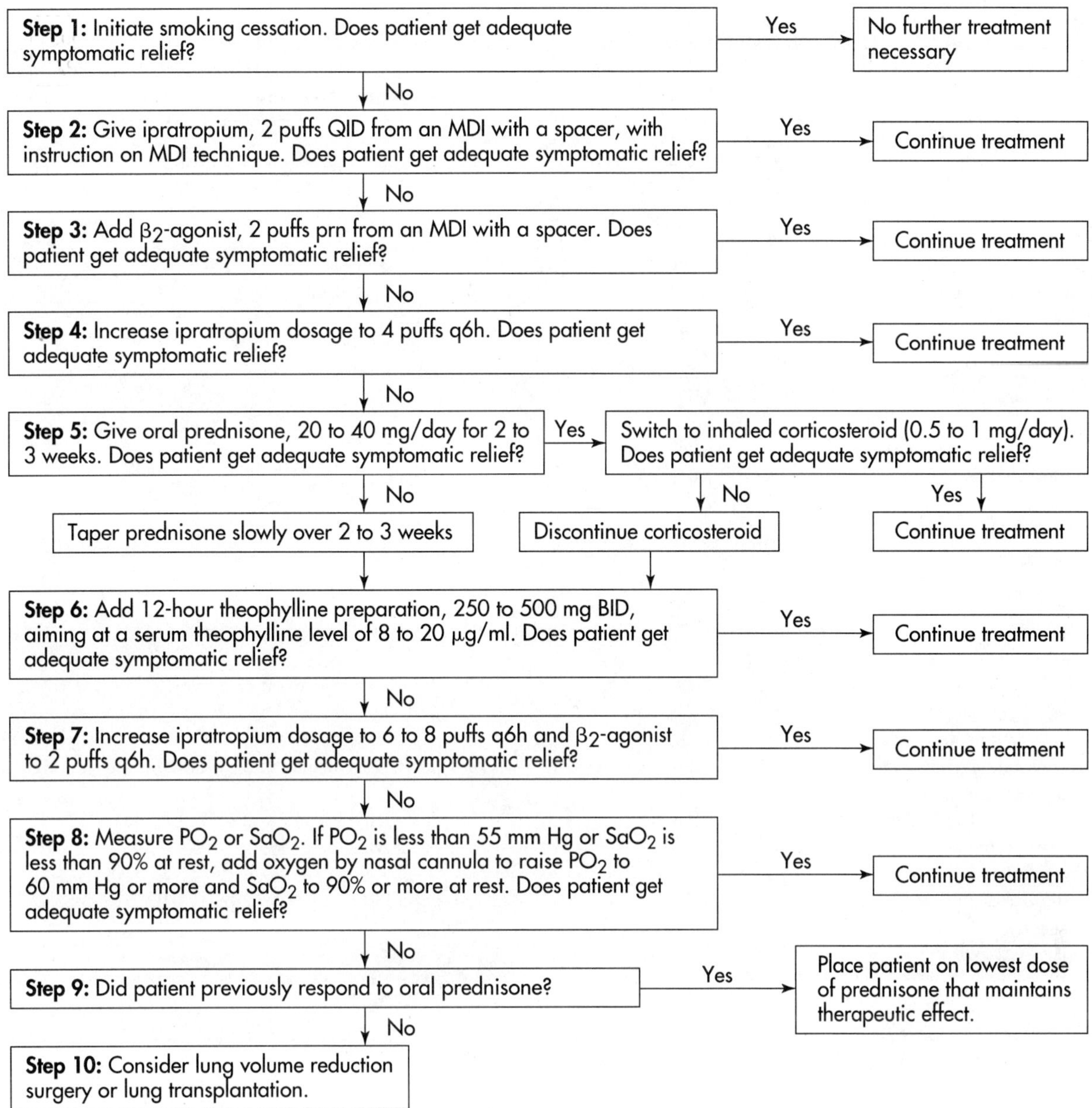

Figure 37-3 A step-care plan for patients with COPD. *COPD,* Chronic obstructive pulmonary disease; *MDI,* metered-dose inhaler; *PO_2,* arterial oxygen tension; *SaO_2,* arterial oxygen saturation. (Modified from Boyars MC: COPD: a step-care approach when FEV_1 is deteriorating, *Consultant,* June 1997, pp 1673-1687.)

nosis and prognosis should be shared with people involved in the patient's life—with appropriate consent obtained from the patient.

Elderly persons are at higher risk for developing COPD, because they grew up in an age when smoking was fashionable and the dangers of second-hand smoke and pollution were not recognized. They may ignore symptoms of fatigue, SOB, and cough because of embarrassment or denial of nicotine addiction. They also may attribute these symptoms to normal aging. A list of support agencies is given in Resources at the end of the chapter.

Referral

AAT deficiency: Refer to endocrinologist
Cor pulmonale: Refer to pulmonologist
End-stage lung disease: Referral to/consultation with cardiothoracic surgeon for single- or double-lung transplant

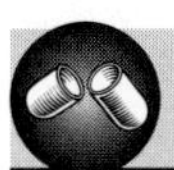

TABLE 37-3 Pharmaceutical Plan: Chronic Obstructive Pulmonary Disease

Drug	Form	Usual Adult Dosage	Cost ($)
Anticholinergic			
Ipratropium bromide (Atrovent)	MDI	2 puffs QID	29
β_2-Agonists			
Albuterol (Proventil, Ventolin)	MDI	1-2 puffs q4-6h	22-24
	Solution (0.5%)	2.5 mg 3-4 times/day	
Metaproterenol sulfate (Alupent, Metaprel)	Oral	10-20 mg q6-8h	N/A
	MDI	2-3 puffs q3-4h	
	Solution (5%)	0.2-0.3 ml 3-4 times/day	
Pirbuterol acetate (Maxair)	MDI	2 puffs q4-6h	10-34
Salmeterol xinafoate (Serevent)	MDI	2 puffs BID	50
Terbutaline sulfate (Brethaire)	MDI	2 puffs q4-6h	21
Terbutaline sulfate (Brethine, Bricanyl)	Oral	2.5-5.0 mg q6h	25-42
Methylxanthines			
Theophylline	Oral	10-12 mg/kg/day in 4 divided doses	6-37
Corticosteroids			
Methylprednisolone	Oral	40-48 mg/day in divided doses for 10-14 days	46
Prednisone/prednisolone	Oral	40-60 mg/day for 10-14 days	3-19
Beclomethasone dipropionate (Beclovent, Vanceril)	MDI	2-4 puffs QID; reduce to 2 puffs BID	17-43
Flunisolide (AeroBid, AeroBid-M)	MDI	2-4 puffs BID; reduce to 2 puffs BID	49
Fluticasone propionate (Flovent inhalation aerosol)	MDI	2-4 puffs BID	37-72
Triamcinolone acetonide (Azmacort)	MDI	2-4 puffs QID; reduce to 2 puffs BID	43
OTC Preparation			
Epinephrine inhaler (Bronkaird Mist, Primatene Mist)	MDI	1-4 puffs q4-6h	9

MDI, Metered-dose inhaler; *NA,* not available; *OTC,* over the counter.

and lung volume reduction surgery if the patient is younger than 60 years old

Consultation

Consult with a physician for any patient using home nebulizers, when home oxygen is needed, or hospitalization is required.

Consult with a respiratory therapist regarding pulmonary rehabilitation.

Nutritional management by a registered dietitian is often necessary to evaluate the patient's caloric intake, identify potential psychosocial impediments to adequate nutrition, and devise meal plans.

Follow-up

Acute attacks: Phone contact 24 to 48 hours

If on theophylline, measure drug levels 2 weeks after initiation of therapy (target level 10 to 20 mg/dl)

Follow-up visits every 3 to 6 months for stable, chronic disease

Stress importance of early recognition of respiratory infection or distress

EVALUATION

Spirometry should be performed at least once in every smoker older than 40 years. Early detection is most important. Treatment will maximize the reversible compo-

Box 37-2

Using an Inhaler: Instructing and Reinstructing

The metered-dose inhaler releases a fixed, measured dose of medication. Each puff delivers a small amount, and inadequate technique can result in serious underdosing.
Shake the canister.
Hold the canister upright with the mouthpiece below.
Hold the mouthpiece at the widely opened mouth.
Inhale slowly, discharging the puffer at midinspiration; continue the inhalation slowly until full inspiration is reached.
Hold the breath for 10 seconds; exhale.
Using an MDI is not as simple as it may seem, because the patient has to coordinate hand movement with inhalation. Patients, especially the elderly, often have to be instructed and reinstructed.

From Celli R et al: COPD: step by step through the workup, *Patient Care,* January 1997, pp 20-52.

nents of the disease process, improve the course of the disease, control symptoms, and improve quality of life.

RESOURCES

Alpha$_1$ National Association
4220 Old Shakopee Road
Minneapolis, MN 55437-2974
(800) 425-7421 (recorded message)
(612) 703-9979 (recorded message
http://www.alpha1.org
This is an excellent organization that offers support and information for people with AAT deficiency.

American Cancer Society
1599 Clifton Road
Atlanta, GA 30329
(404) 320-3333
Smoking cessation

American College of Cardiology
9111 Old Georgetown Road
Bethesda, MD 20814
(800) 257-4740
FAX: (301) 897-9745

American Heart Association
7472 Greenville Avenue
Dallas, TX 75231
(214) 373-6300
FAX: (214) 706-1341

American Lung Association
1740 Broadway
New York, NY 10019-4374
(800) 586-4872 (800-LUNG-USA)
http://www.lungusa.org
The American Lung Association is very responsive and offers a wide range of information and services, including Open Airways for Schools, an education program for teachers and parents.

Call the American Lung Association for the following client education pamphlets:
#1230C Around the Clock with COPD
#4001 Help Yourself to Better Breathing
#0301 Facts About Emphysema
#0222 Facts About AAT-Related Symptoms
#0139 Facts About Chronic Bronchitis
#2555 Understanding Lung Medications
#2326 Using Medicines Wisely

American Thoracic Society
1740 Broadway
New York, NY 10019
(212) 315-8863
FAX: (212) 315-6498
http://www.thoracic.org

Canadian Thoracic Society
1900 City Park Drive
Suite 508
Gloucester, Ontario
Canada K1J 1A3
(613) 747-6776
FAX: (613) 747-7430

National Heart, Lung, and Blood Institute
P.O. Box 30105
Bethesda, MD 20824-0105
Write for information, or visit their site on the Internet:
http://www.nhlbi.nih.gov/nhlbi/nhlbi.htm

National Jewish Center for Immunology and Respiratory Medicine
1400 Jackson Street
Denver, CO 80206
(800) 222-5864 (800-222-LUNG)"The Lung Line"
(303) 355-5864 (303-355-LUNG)"The Lung Line"
(800) 552-5864 (800-552-LUNG)"Lung Facts"
FAX: (303) 270-2162
http://www.njc.org
This excellent organization publishes a number of booklets for the public and offers an information line staffed by trained nurses. They also have a service called Lung Facts which offers specific recorded messages about allergies, asthma, and other lung problems.

Society of Thoracic Surgeons
http://www.sts.org

Internet link for respiratory problems:
http://www.xmission.com/~gastown/herpmed/respi.htm

SUGGESTED READINGS

Boyars MC: COPD: a step-care approach when FEV$_1$ is deteriorating, *Consultant,* June, 1997, pp 1673-1687.
Carlile PV et al: Practice guidelines and clinical pathway for chronic obstructive pulmonary disease, *Fed Pract* 15:S26-S31, 1998.
Celli R et al: COPD: step by step through the workup, *Patient Care* January 1997, pp 20-52.
Chen P: Diagnostic history and physical exam in medicine, Fountain Valley, Calif, 1993, Current International Clinical Strategies Publication, p 20.
Davis A et al: When chronic bronchitis turns acute, *Patient Care,* January 1996, pp 124-127.

Gammon B, Bailey WC: COPD: steps to improve pulmonary function and quality of life, *Patient Care,* July 1995, pp 939-950.

Hoole A et al: *Patient care guidelines for nurse practitioners,* Philadelphia, 1995, JB Lippincott.

Johannsen J: Chronic obstructive pulmonary disease: current comprehensive care for emphysema and bronchitis, *Nurse Pract* 19:59-67, 1994.

Tierney LM, McPhee SJ, Papadakis MA: *Current medical diagnosis and treatment 1997,* Norwalk, Conn, 1997, Appleton & Lange.

Uphold C, Graham M: *Clinical guidelines in family practice,* Gainesville, Fla, 1994, Barmarrae Books.

Witta K: COPD in the elderly, *Adv Nurse Pract,* July 1997, pp 18-27, 72.

Cirrhosis/Liver Disease

ICD-9-CM

Alcoholic Cirrhosis 571.2
Cirrhosis of Liver without Mention of Alcohol 571.5

OVERVIEW

Definition

Cirrhosis is a chronic disease in which the liver architecture is disrupted by diffuse fibrosis. It is the end stage of many different disease processes that affect the liver.

Incidence

Alcoholic hepatitis is the most common precursor of cirrhosis in the United States. The frequency of cirrhosis caused by alcohol is estimated to be about 8% to 15% among persons who consume an average of 120 g of alcohol (8 oz of 100-proof whiskey, 30 oz of wine, or eight 12-oz cans of beer) daily for more than 10 years. Cirrhosis is the eleventh leading cause of death in the United States, with more than 45% of cases related to alcohol use. Hepatitis B and C also can lead to cirrhosis.

Pathophysiology

Chronic liver disease evolves over months or years. The process by which the liver becomes nonfunctioning depends on the extent histological changes in the liver. Chronic persistent hepatitis describes a stage of chronic liver injury in which inflammatory infiltration is limited largely to portal triads. This is a very gradual process of cell destruction. In chronic active hepatitis, the inflammatory cells spread beyond the triad and into adjacent parenchyma. This process likely leads to progressive and clinically overt liver damage.

Cirrhosis is the term describing the distortion of normal hepatic cells from progressive necrosis, compensatory liver cell proliferation, and associated fibrosis.

Factors That Increase Risk of Liver Disease

Genetic disposition
Women (more susceptible because of a lower gastric mucosal alcohol dehydrogenase level)

SUBJECTIVE DATA

History of Present Illness

Jaundice
Pruritus
Fever
Abdominal pain
Pale, chalky stools
Anorexia and nausea
Weight loss
Usually a vague onset
Weakness, fatigue, muscle cramps
Menstrual abnormalities
Loss of libido
Enlarged breasts in men
Variceal bleeding
Ascites
Hematemesis

Past Medical History

History of hepatitis

Medications

Chlorpromazine
Isoniazid
Estrogen
Acetaminophen

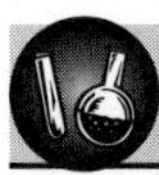

Table 38-1 Diagnostic Tests: Cirrhosis/Liver Disease

Test	Finding/Rationale	Cost ($)
Urine bilirubin	Perhaps the best way to detect early jaundice	15-20
Serum bilirubin: direct, indirect, total	↑ Unconjugated (indirect) suggests either an increase in pigment load present in liver or a defect in the uptake or conjugation of bilirubin; ↑ In conjugated (direct) is evidence of a defect in the excretory pathway of bilirubin	23-30
Serum aminotransferase levels (AST [SGOT], ALT [SGPT])	Found in large quantities in the hepatocytes, ↑ when these cells are injured; elevation of the transaminases for >6 mo defines chronic hepatitis; ALT is more specific for the liver than AST, but an AST at least 2× the ALT is typical of alcoholic liver injury	18-23/SGOT 17-23/SGPT
Serum alkaline phosphatase level	Group of isoenzymes made by the liver, bone, intestine, and placenta; ↑ when liver diseases involve obstruction of the bile ducts	19-24
CBC platelets	Anemia and moderate thrombocytopenia commonly seen	18-23
Serum ammonia	Increased ammonia seen in encephalopathy	45-57
Prothrombin time	Measure of the clotting factors, some of which are produced by the liver	22-27
Total serum protein with albumin and globulin fractions	The liver produces the majority of serum proteins, including albumin, fibrinogen, and globulins; serum albumin is usually low in patients with chronic liver disease	42-53
Ultrasound of liver	Useful in evaluating patients with hepatomegaly or unexplained elevation in alkaline phosphatase; can detect dilation of the bile ducts or lesions within the liver; can also guide FNA and identify ascites; in cirrhosis the liver is altered in size and contour, presence of ascites, splenomegaly, and portosystemic venous collaterals	259-319
Needle biopsy of the liver	Used to make a differential diagnosis of hepatomegaly and hepatocellular disease; can assess the effect of therapy in chronic liver disease; may be used to stage the level of cirrhosis; contraindicated in severe coagulopathy	307-363

CBC, Complete blood count; *FNA*, fine-needle aspiration.

Family History

Wilson's disease
α_1-Antitrypsin deficiency
Hemochromatosis
Alcoholism

Psychosocial History

Alcohol ingestion/abuse
Intravenous drug use
Occupational exposure: Environmental toxins; health care worker—exposure to blood/blood products
Sexual history: Sexual contacts

OBJECTIVE DATA

Physical Examination

If liver disease is suspected, a thorough examination should be performed with particular attention to:

Vital signs
General appearance: Wasting
Skin: Tan, jaundiced; palmar erythema, spider angiomas on face/chest
Head/eyes/ears/nose/throat: Lacrimal gland enlargement, glossitis, cheilosis
Chest: Gynecomastia
Abdominal: Splenomegaly, hepatomegaly, dilated abdominal veins, ascites (shifting dullness)
- Percuss the liver size.
- Identify the edge of the liver: soft, enlarged versus hard, nodular/smooth.
- In 79% of cases with cirrhosis, the liver is enlarged, palpable, and firm.
- Listen for a bruit.
- Check for Murphy's sign.

Extremities: Edema, ecchymosis
Genitals: Testicular atrophy
Neurological: Asterixis, hyperreflexia, lowered level of consciousness, diminished intellect

Diagnostic Procedures

Diagnostic tests are outlined in Table 38-1. (See also Figure 38-1)

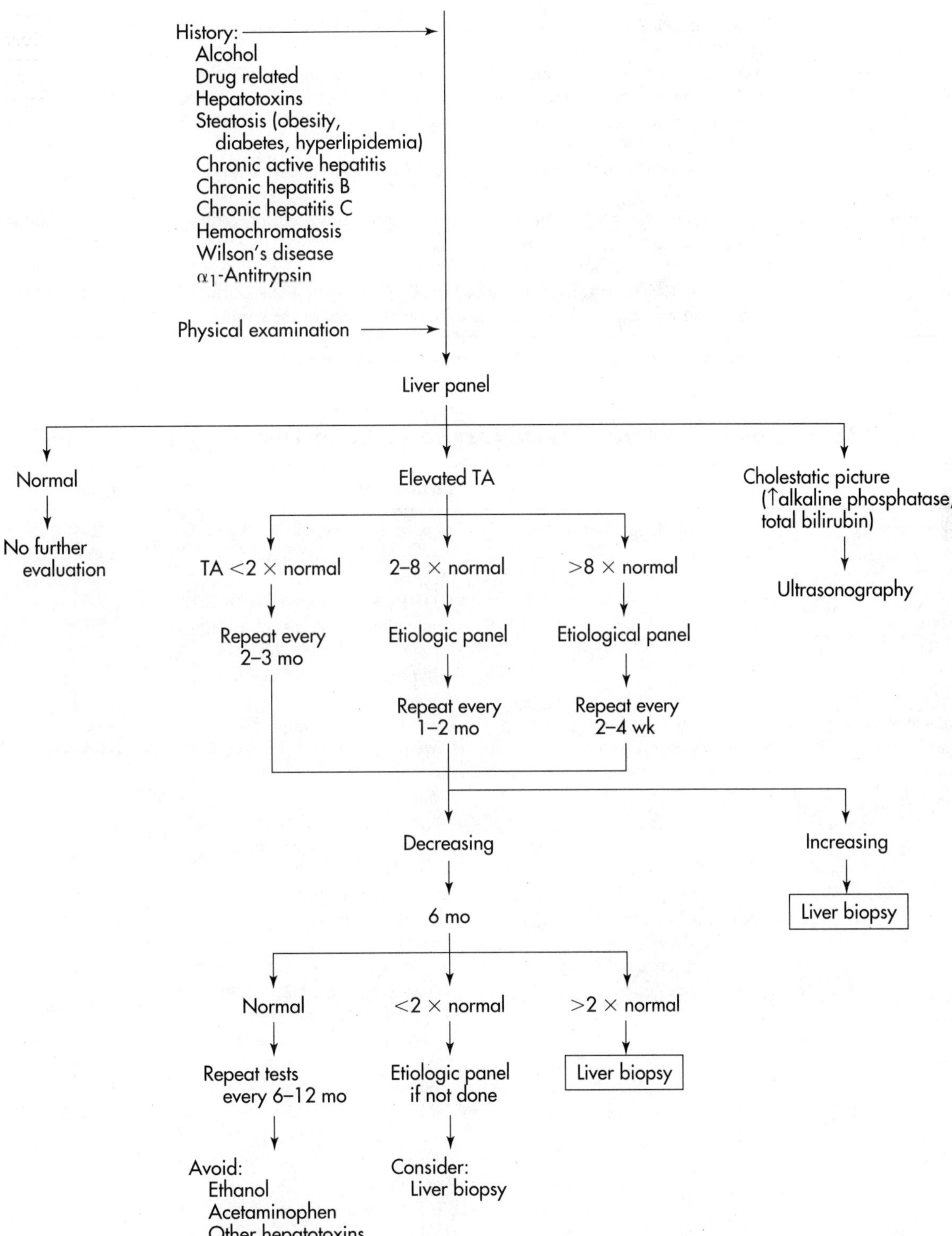

Figure 38-1 Algorithm for the treatment of a patient with asymptomatic increased transaminase level. *TA*, Transaminase. (Modified from Greene HL, Johnson WP, Lemcke D: *Decision making in medicine*, ed 2, 1998, St Louis, Mosby.)

TABLE 38-2 Differential Diagnosis: Cirrhosis/Liver Disease

Diagnosis	Supporting Data
Cirrhosis	Confirmed with liver biopsy; presentation includes ↓ platelets, hepatic encephalopathy, ascites, hypoalbuminemia, hypergammaglobulinemia, ↑ prothrombin time
Viral hepatitis	Inflammation of the liver caused by various viruses; symptoms include fatigue, nausea, flulike illness, and low-grade fever; 10 days later, dark urine, pruritus, and jaundice may be seen
Alcoholic hepatitis	Acute or chronic inflammation and parenchymal necrosis of the liver induced by alcohol use; usually a long history of alcohol drinking, macrocytic anemia, ↑ AST, ↑ alkaline phosphatase, ↑ bilirubin, ↑ GGTP, and ↑ MCV
Cholecystitis/ cholelithiasis	Abdominal pain, Murphy's sign, jaundice, mild fever, nausea and vomiting
Hemachromatosis	Bronzing of the skin, >50% saturation of serum transferrin or serum ferritin levels above the upper limit of normal
Wilson's disease	Rare disorder of copper metabolism (autosomal-recessive disorder); it should be suspected in children and young adults with cirrhosis; characteristic finding is Kayser-Fleisher rings, which are greenish-brown rings found on the posterior surface and in the periphery of the cornea

AST, Aspartate transaminase; *GGTP,* gamma-glutamyltranspeptidase; *MCV,* mean corpuscular volume.

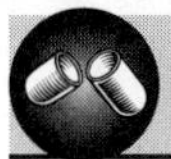

TABLE 38-3 Pharmaceutical Plan: Cirrhosis/Liver Disease

Drug	Dose	Comments	Cost
Methylprednisolone (Medrol)	Variable dosing (long taper if on high dose)	Appears to be beneficial in patients with alcoholic hepatitis Pregnancy: C SE: HPA axis suppression, masks infection, glaucoma, cataracts, hypokalemia, hypocalcemia, hypertension, weight gain, peptic ulcer	\$46-\$64/16 mg (50); \$46/32 mg (25)
Spironolactone (Aldactone)	100 mg QD, increased by 100 mg q3 days, up to a maximum of 400 mg	Used in patients with ascites for weight loss of 1-1.5 lb per day if sodium retention treatment does not work Pregnancy: Not recommended SE: Hyperkalemia, hyponatremia, gynecomastia, GI upset, menstrual changes	\$71/50 mg (100); \$119/100 mg (100)
Iron	100-200 mg of elemental iron in divided doses (ferrous gluconate, ferrous polysaccharide, ferrous sulfate)	Given for anemia Pregnancy: B SE: Black stools; nausea and vomiting; abdominal pain; constipation	\$5/63 mg (40)
Propranolol (Inderal) or nadolol (Corgard)	20-40 mg BID 40 mg QD	Helps prevent initial hemorrhage in patient with large esophageal varices by lowering the portal pressure gradient; titrate to produce a 25% reduction in the heart rate or heart rate between 55 and 60 beats/min Pregnancy: C SE: Fatigue, depression, dizziness, GI upset, bronchospasm	\$1-\$33/10 mg (100); \$2-\$35/20 mg (100); \$2-\$60/40 mg (100); \$85-\$105/Corgard: 40 mg (100)
Lactulose (Chronulac or Duphalac)	20-30 ml TID to QID	Reduces blood ammonia levels; effective only when it increases frequency of stools Pregnancy: B SE: Flatulence, diarrhea, intestinal cramps	\$12-\$37/10 g/15 ml (480 ml)

GI, Gastrointestinal; *HPA,* hypopophysial pituitary axis; *SE,* side effects.

ASSESSMENT

Differential diagnoses include those outlined in Table 38-2.

THERAPEUTIC PLAN

Pharmaceutical

Pharmaceutical treatment is outlined in Table 38-3.

Lifestyle/Activities

Discontinue all alcoholic beverages
Rest, decrease activity

Diet

Well-balanced diet, with sufficient carbohydrates and calories to reduce protein catabolism (at least 75 to 100 g/day)
Restriction of sodium intake if edema or ascites present; limit sodium to 1 to 2 g/day
In the presence of hepatic encephalopathy, reduction of protein intake 60 g/day, with the majority of protein coming from vegetable sources

Patient Education

Discuss the implications of continued alcohol drinking:
- Progression to portal hypertension, cirrhosis, with a 10 times greater death rate than among those who do not drink; in most patients, dramatic improvement of liver function with alcohol cessation

Weigh daily; keep record of weight.
Tips and support for alcohol cessation: Alcoholics Anonymous
Caution patients about use of drugs that are degraded in the liver

Referral/Consultation

Refer to a gastroenterologist (GE) or hepatologist.

Follow-up

In most cases, the GE will follow this patient. Liver biopsy is often indicated.

EVALUATION

Prevention of esophageal varices/bleeding

RESOURCES

The liver in health and disease: www.mediconsult.com/liver
Liver disease center of Scripps Clinic: www.nerdworld. com/users/dstein/nw4726.html
American Association for the Study of Liver Diseases: http://hepar-sfgh.UCSF.edu
American Liver Foundation: www.giUCSF.edu/ALF/pubs.html
Children's Liver Disease Foundation: www. yahoo.co.UK/healthdiseases_and_conditions/liver

SUGGESTED READINGS

Dunn S: *Mosby's primary care consultant,* St Louis, 1998, Mosby.
Ellsworth A et al: *Mosby's 1998 medical drug reference,* St Louis, 1998, Mosby.
Healthcare Consultants of America, Inc: *1998 Physicians fee and coding guide,* Augusta, Ga, 1998, Healthcare Consultants of America, Inc.
Friedman L: Liver, biliary tract and pancreas. In Tierney L, McPhee S, Papadakis M, editors: *Current medical diagnosis and treatment,* Stamford, Conn, 1999, Appleton & Lange.
McGuire B, Bloomer J: Complications of cirrhosis, *Postgrad Med* 103:209-224, 1998.
Sechopoulos P, Jensen D: Case 3. In Grodzin C, Schwartz S, Bone R, editors: *Diagnostic strategies for internal medicine,* St Louis, 1996, Mosby.

39 Colic

ICD-9-CM

Abdominal Pain 789.0
Infantile Colic 789.0
Urinary Tract Stone Disease 592.9
Calculus of Bile Duct without Mention of Cholecystitis 574.5
Calculus of Bile Duct with Acute Cholecystitis 547.3

OVERVIEW

Definition

The word colic implies that it pertains to the colon. Colic is acute, paroxysmal, abdominal pain. This is thought to be caused by spasmodic contractions of the intestines, or other abdominal organs.

Infant Colic

Infant colic is a poorly defined syndrome of paroxysmal infant crying that occurs in an infant who is 3 months of age or younger, cries more than 3 hours a day, and cries in this manner 3 or more days in a week. Other names used are 3-month colic, evening colic, or paroxysmal fussing.

Biliary Colic

Biliary colic is a sudden-onset, steady, localized, right upper quadrant abdominal pain that lasts 2 to 4 hours and results from gallstones passing through the bile ducts.

Renal Colic

Renal colic is a unilateral, abrupt-onset pain and is localized to the flank when a kidney stone is lodged or is passing through the tube in the upper renal tract.

Incidence

Infant colic is said to occur in 13% of the population, with equal rates in males and female infants (Lehtonen and Korvenranta, 1995). Biliary colic is estimated to occur in 20 million Americans each year. Nearly one quarter of these will require surgery to resolve the condition. Eighty percent of gallstones are cholesterol stones. Approximately 20% are pigment stones composed of bilirubin and calcium salts. Many persons with stones in their gallbladder are asymptomatic and require no treatment. Renal colic is predicted to have a 1% to 3% occurrence rate. It has an increased incidence in white males. The highest incidence is in **men 30 to 60 years old**. The annual frequency for nephrolithiasis is estimated to be 1 per 1000 population. Most stones pass spontaneously, but 10% to 30% will not and require surgery (Fang, 1995). Following the first occurrence of renal colic, the recurrence rate for renal colic is approximately 10% the first year, 33% 5 years, and 50% by 10 years from the initial diagnosis (Fang, 1995).

Pathophysiology

Infant Colic

Infant colic has no specifically known cause but is thought to have component physiological, psychological, and social factors. Physiologically there may be a predisposition for this syndrome, since it is known to occur in family members. Psychologically it is thought that the infants' temperament may play a part, especially those infants described as difficult and those described as having a low sensory threshold. Socially the infant with colic tends to have parents who demonstrate anxiety and frustration at dealing with the excessive crying behavior.

Protective Factors Against Infant Colic

Infants with an "easy" temperament
Parents who are very "easy" in their own temperament characteristics and those who are not stressed by the crying

Factors That Increase Susceptibility

Infants on a cow's milk–based formula (10% to 15% of colicky infants may have IgE-mediated hypersensitivity)
Infants who are poor feeders and never seem satisfied
Infants with neurological deficits
Infants affected by prenatal drug abuse
A genetic predisposition, such as a family history of parents or other siblings with similar symptoms as an infant
Difficult temperament in the infant
Anxious/nervous parents

Biliary Stones

Eighty percent of gallstones are the result of cholesterol, a normal constituent of bile, precipitating out of solution and forming small crystals. One theory suggests that the gallbladder becomes sluggish and works ineffectively. Another theory suggests that the gallbladder secretes a higher than normal amount of cholesterol, or the amount of bile salts is decreased or lower than normal when the precipitation occurs (Rhoades and Pflanzer, 1992). The stones that are large enough to become lodged in the biliary ducts are the ones that cause the biliary colic. Major complications of untreated gallstones that result in blockage of passage of the bile through the ducts includes jaundice, cholangitis, and pancreatitis.

Protective Factors Against Biliary Colic

Being male, until age 60, when the risk is the same for both sexes
Eating a diet calorically appropriate for body build
A normal body weight for age/ build also decreases risk

Factors That Increase Susceptibility to Biliary Colic

Women 20 to 60 years old are twice as likely to develop gallstones as men
Pregnant women
Women on birth control pills or estrogen replacement therapy
Native Americans, Hispanics
Persons who are overweight
Persons who go on crash diets
Men and women over the age of 60

Renal Stones

Renal stones are the result of crystals of poorly soluble substances from the urine that precipitate out of solution and form stones. Seventy-five percent of kidney stones are made up of calcium salts (calcium oxalate or calcium phosphate), and the rest are composed of ammonium magnesium phosphate, uric acid, or cystine. When urinary flow is low, the increased concentration of poorly soluble salts favors stone formation. Some renal stones (particularly the staghorn calculi that extend from one renal calix to another) can get quite large and cause backup and stagnation of urine flow. When the stones are large enough to become lodged in the ureters, the associated pain is called renal colic.

Protective Factors Against Renal Colic

Female
Young age
Drinking adequate fluids daily
Persons with no anatomical abnormalities

Factors That Increase Susceptibility to Renal Colic

Males living in highly industrialized areas
Males who tend to drink inadequate quantity of fluids daily
Persons with a family history of renal stones, such as rare genetic disorders (xanthine oxidase deficiency)
High oxaluric acid levels, as occurs when coexistent small bowel disease (Crohn's disease) exists, predisposes to renal stone formation
Medications that put a person at risk for increased stone formation are vitamins A, C, D; loop diuretics (furosemide, ethacrynic acid, and bumetanide), calcium-containing medications (antacids), acetazolamide (Diamox, used in treating open angle glaucoma), ammonium chloride, and acid- and alkaline-based medications
Persons with primary hyperparathyroidism (women are at increased risk), sarcoidosis, pyridoxine deficiency, immobilization, distal renal tubular acidosis, secondary gout (e.g., in patients undergoing chemotherapy), neoplastic disorders such as myeloproliferative disease, and urinary tract infection from urea-splitting organisms

SUBJECTIVE DATA

Infant Colic

Infant colic is seen in infants only, not in older children or adults. Symptoms present at 1 to 2 weeks of age and persist to approximately 3 months of age. The condition is considered to be self-limiting.

Patient history should include onset of symptoms, crying and associated behaviors such as drawing up of knees, and frequency of the crying. It is important to determine the stool patterns, such as the frequency and consistency of bowel movements.

Determine feeding patterns, how formula is mixed, how long feedings last, and how much is taken in by the baby. Determine comfort measures used by the family, any tactics that work, and those that do not work. The nurse practitioner should try to determine how long the crying lasts and what time of day it occurs.

The caretakers should also elicit information on who (mother, father, grandparent) is the caretaker when the colic usually occurs. A few specific and direct questions regarding caretaking practices will help rule out any suspicion of child neglect or abuse.

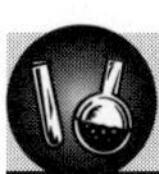

TABLE 39-1 Diagnostic Tests: Infant Colic

Symptoms	Findings	Tests	Costs
Cyclical, intense crying; infant stiffens legs or draws up knees onto abdomen; clenches fists	Infant is growing well and gaining weight; no overt abnormalities on physical examination	None indicated; may do an immune globulin subclass profile if immune deficiency is strongly suspected	Cost of visit and time spent may range from $65-$115 for an initial evaluation and $22-$35.00 for follow-up appointment; immune globulin subclass will cost approximately $194 and will take 2 weeks to get results

Past Medical History

Thoroughly analyze the labor, delivery, and postpartal periods.

Identify medications or elicit drugs taken by the mother prenatally, natally, or presently.

Is there history of allergies in the family? Who has these allergies?

Assess mother's breastfeeding technique in the office, if applicable.

Assess general caretaking and feeding techniques that are used in caring for the infant.

Biliary Colic

Children

Cholelithiasis occasionally seen in **school-age children and teens** and should be considered when a child presents with vague or colicky upper quadrant pain (Holcomb, 1997).

Assess severity of pain and location of greatest intensity.

Ask about frequency of the pain episodes.

Assess meals and caloric intake in diet.

Adults

Document onset and duration of pain symptoms, location and frequency of pain.

Identify any medications that were taken to relieve the symptoms.

Document diet history to determine the quantity and quality of food items eaten.

Elderly

Determine whether the person has any associated symptoms that would indicate biliary cancer (e.g., weight loss, unexplained bleeding, change in bowel habits).

Determine whether the elderly adult is a good historian or whether a caretaker needs to assist with giving data.

Past Medical History

Recognize pregnancy and length of gestation.

Ask about any previous illnesses such as hepatitis or biliary obstruction, surgeries, or liver problems.

Determine whether the patient has been on a crash diet or has lost excessive weight in the last several months.

Identify whether the woman is menopausal or postmenopausal, whether she is receiving estrogen replacement therapy, and obtain dosage.

Medications

Note any medications that the person is presently taking, whether prescription or over the counter.

Identify any allergies to medications.

Note any medications used to relieve gastrointestinal symptoms.

Psychosocial History

Determine whether there is a history of excessive consumption of alcohol, excessive intake of calories, or an excessively fatty diet is consumed.

Family History

Document any family history of a colicky disorder.

Identify whether there is Hispanic or Native Indian heritage.

Renal Colic

Children

Renal stones are rarely seen before age 30; however, this should not be ruled out if the pain is unilateral and of the right flank.

Adults

The history of the present illness should include onset and duration of pain symptoms, location of pain.

Determine whether this pain has occurred previously and if so, when.

A brief history of liquid intake and diet should reveal the quantity and quality of the items eaten.

Past Medical History

Ask the patient to recall any previous hospitalizations, illnesses that were kidney/bladder related, and any chronic illnesses such as diabetes or hypertension.

Elderly: Determine whether the older adult is a good historian or whether a caretaker needs to help answer the questions.

Medications

Identify any medications that are taken, whether prescription or over-the-counter.

Ask about allergies to medications.

Determine which medications were taken to relieve the symptoms.

Family History

Should include information about any family members with similar symptoms or diagnoses.

Description of Most Common Symptoms

Infant Colic

Typical symptoms are excessive, inconsolable crying. The infant draws up the knees onto the abdomen or may stiffen the extremities. These babies tend to keep their hands fisted tightly during crying spells. The infant also demands frequent feedings and has excess gas (flatus).

Biliary Colic

The patient typically has recurrent pain with sudden onset that builds to a maximum within an hour, is unrelenting, and is localized in the right upper quadrant or epigastrium. The pain may last up to 4 hours and occasionally radiates to the scapular area. There is accompanying belching, bloating, nausea, and vomiting. The patient may also complain of dyspepsia.

Renal Colic

The patient will describe pain that started abruptly, was constant and intense, unilateral, and localized to the flank (if the stone is lodged in the upper tract), or the groin (if the stone is in the lower portion of the ureter). The patient may have accompanying nausea and vomiting. There are reported cases of hip pain that were actually renal colic (referred pain).

OBJECTIVE DATA

Infant Colic

Physical Examination

Vital signs/growth: Measure temperature, pulse, respirations, weight, length, and head circumference; plot the growth parameters on the growth grids to see the trends.

General: Assess overall appearance, hydration, skin integrity, and any special features that you note about the baby's overall appearance.

A problem-focused examination with special emphasis on the abdomen is indicated.

Head/eyes/ears/nose/throat: Check the mouth for intact palate.

Abdominal: Assess for bowel sounds, masses, hepatosplenomegaly.

Because of the complaint of excessive crying, assess carefully for any bruises or abrasions that may indicate abuse.

Diagnostic Procedures

None indicated. (In fact, the more testing that is done tends to reinforce the parent's belief that the baby has a physical problem that can be treated medically.)

The diagnostic procedures for infant colic are outlined in Table 39-1.

Biliary Colic

Physical Examination

Vital signs: Measure temperature, pulse, respirations, blood pressure, height, and weight.

General: Assess general appearance, hydration status, degree of pain, and level of pain tolerance.

Abdominal: Assess for bowel sounds and determine general size of the liver; locate the liver edge and measure if enlarged. Rebound tenderness on deep palpation in the right upper quadrant of moderate to severe intensity, with normalized liver is presumptive evidence for cholecystitis. Murphy's sign: Abrupt cessation of inspiration on palpation of the gallbladder represents cholecystitis.

Diagnostic Procedures

Real-time ultrasonography of the gallbladder is the test of choice for evaluation of biliary colic symptoms. If ultrasonography is not diagnostic, then scintigraphy with radionuclide HIDA is done.

Table 39-2 outlines diagnostic procedures for biliary colic.

Renal Colic

Physical Examination

Vital signs: Measure temperature, pulse, respirations, height, weight, and blood pressure.

General: Assess general appearance, hydration status, and degree of pain tolerance.

Chest: Assess heart and lungs.

Lymph: Lymphadenopathy may be indicative of systemic disease such as sarcoidosis.

Abdominal: Assess with light and deep touch all four quadrants of the abdomen for bowel sounds and any masses that may be palpable. Assess for rebound tenderness

Back: Unilateral costovertebral angle tenderness.

Diagnostic Procedures

Diagnostic procedures for renal colic are outlined in Table 39-3.

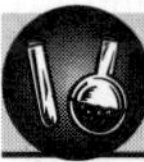

TABLE 39-2 Diagnostic Tests: Biliary Colic

Tests	Symptoms	Findings/Rationale	Cost ($)
Routine CXR may be done; Real-time US of the gallbladder	May be asymptomatic and be an incidental finding on x-ray evaluation	Overweight, vital signs normal, bowel sounds present, RUQ pain	77-91/CXR 358/real-time US of gallbladder
Assess liver functions by obtaining SGOT, SGPT, PTT; if patient vomiting for long time, may check electrolytes	If symptomatic, patient has episodic, recurrent pain in RUQ; pain may radiate to epigastrium and scapular area; may have nausea and vomiting	Sudden onset, pain increases for ~1 hr, is steady, and usually lasts 2-4 hr	29-41/liver function panel; 26-32/ coagulation panel; 18-23/ CBC; 23-30/ electrolytes; 98/ KUB; 750/real-time scintigraphy with radionucleotide HIDA

CXR, Chest x-ray; *KUB,* kidney-ureter-bladder; *PTT,* partial prothrombin time; *RUQ,* right upper quadrant; *SGOT,* serum glutamic oxaloacetic transaminase (aspartate aminotransferase); *SGPT,* serum glutamic pyruvic transaminase (alanine aminotransferase); *US,* ultrasonography.

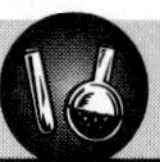

TABLE 39-3 Diagnostic Tests: Renal Colic

Test	Symptoms	Findings/Rationale	Cost ($)
UA and urine culture; CBC, BUN, creatinine, calcium, electrolytes, KUB	Abrupt onset, unilateral sharp lower quadrant pain that is localized	UA to assess pH, presence of bacteria or sediment/crystals is necessary; strain urine after obtaining specimen for culture; 24-hr urine sample should be obtained to determine creatinine, calcium, uric acid, oxalate levels of urine if stones found on UA Bloodwork: Serum calcium, uric acid, BUN, creatinine KUB of abdomen and IVP provide evidence of stones, renal abnormalities, and level of obstruction; obtain renal US if hydronephrosis suspected	15-20/ UA; 31-39/ Urine culture; 98/KUB
IVP to assess for stones also	Fever and chills or significant dehydration require hospitalization		280-333/IVP; 18-23/CBC; 28-39/metabolic panel

BUN, Blood urea nitrogen; *CBC,* complete blood cell count; *IVP,* intravenous pyelogram; *KUB,* kidney-ureter-bladder; *UA,* urinalysis, *US,* ultrasonography.

TABLE 39-4 Differential Diagnosis: Infant Colic

Diagnosis	Supporting Data
Diaper dermatitis	Erythema, papules, oozing, ulcerations in diaper area
Otitis media	Fever, usually history of URI, ear pain, discomfort, may have diarrhea, restless or diminished sleeping
Meningitis	Young infants: Onset is generally acute, with nonspecific symptoms of temperature instability or hypothermia, irritability, lethargy, poor feeding, unusual cry, jitteriness and/or hypotonia Older infants, children, and adults: Onset is usually acute, though sometimes subacute; prodromal febrile illness rapidly progresses to vague complaints of irritability, listlessness, or general malaise; older children and adults may complain of photophobia, myalgia, headaches, stiff neck, and vomiting; seizures may also occur Associated symptoms: Diffuse macular, maculopapular, or purpuric rash may occur, depending on the type of infection; abdominal pain and diarrhea may also be present if the offending agent is an enterovirus
Gastroenteritis	May have elevated temperature, decreased consistency of stools, crampy abdominal pain, localized abdominal pain
Child abuse/injury	Unexplained bruises in many areas in different stages of healing, human bites, unexplained burns, suspicious of adults, excessively withdrawn, lies quietly during examination, FTT, excessive crying, sleep disorders

FTT, Failure to thrive; *URI,* upper respiratory infection.

TABLE 39-5 Differential Diagnosis: Biliary Colic

Diagnosis	Supporting Data
GERD	Esophageal irritation and heartburn (substernal burning, often radiating to the neck) increased after meals, bending or recumbency
Constipation	Decrease in frequency of stools, stools hard or dry, pain with bowel movement, recurrent abdominal pain
Hepatitis	Hepatitis A: Signs and symptoms will appear at end of prodromal period: fatigue, weakness, mild gastrointestinal disturbances; a striking aversion to cigarettes may occur; some may have joint pain, fever, hepatomegaly, lymphadenopathy, and jaundice Hepatitis B: General malaise, joint swelling, rash pruritus, hepatomegaly, gastrointestinal symptoms; jaundice presents with more nausea and vomiting Hepatitis C: Acute illness with fever, chills, malaise, nausea and vomiting
Alcoholic cirrhosis	History of alcohol ingestion; symptoms range from asymptomatic to enlarged liver, anorexia and nausea, abdominal pain and tenderness, ascites, fever, and splenomegaly
Pancreatitis	Abrupt onset of deep epigastric pain with radiation to back, nausea and vomiting, abdominal tenderness and distention, fever, leukocytosis, elevated serum amylase and lipase levels
Pneumonia	Productive cough, fever, dyspnea, pleuritic chest pain that may mimic abdominal pain, consolidating lobar pneumonia seen on CXR

CXR, Chest x-ray; *GERD,* gastroesophageal reflux disease.

ASSESSMENT

Differential Diagnosis

Differential diagnoses for infant, biliary, and renal colic are outlined in Tables 39-4 to 39-6.

THERAPEUTIC PLAN

Infant Colic

See Figure 39-1.

Pharmaceutical

None indicated.

Lifestyle/Activities

Decrease environmental stimulation during feedings or stressful crying periods.

Diet

Dietary changes not initially indicated if diarrhea and vomiting are not present and all physical findings are within normal limits for age.

TABLE 39-6 Differential Diagnosis: Renal Colic

Diagnosis	Supporting Data
Constipation	Decrease in frequency of stools, stools hard or dry, pain with bowel movement, recurrent abdominal pain
PID	Lower abdominal pain, adnexal and cervical motion tenderness, fever may be present, cervical or vaginal discharge, positive gonorrhea or chlamydia cultures
Epididymitis	Fever, irritative voiding symptoms, painful enlargement of epididymis; pain may reflect to flank area
UTI/pyelonephritis	Dysuria, frequency, suprapubic tenderness, positive CVA tenderness, fever, positive urine culture, leukocytosis with left shift, WBC casts in urine
Crohn's disease	Gradual onset, intermittent bouts with low-grade fever, diarrhea, and RLQ pain, RLQ mass and tenderness, x-ray showing ulceration, strictures, or fistulas of small intestine
Pneumonia	Productive cough, fever, dyspnea, pleuritic chest pain that may mimic abdominal pain, consolidating lobar pneumonia on CXR

CVA, Costovertebral angle; *CXR,* chest x-ray; *PID,* pelvic inflammatory disease, *RLQ,* right lower quadrant; *UTI,* urinary tract infection.

History and examination
Specific cause identified
No specific cause
What is crying like? (crying diary)
Frequent, consolable crying
High-intensity crying, inconsolable, cramping, gas
Breastfed
Formula-fed
Trial of maternal milk–free diet
Trial of soy-based formula
No effect
No effect
Trial of hydrosylate formula
No effect
Behavioral interventions

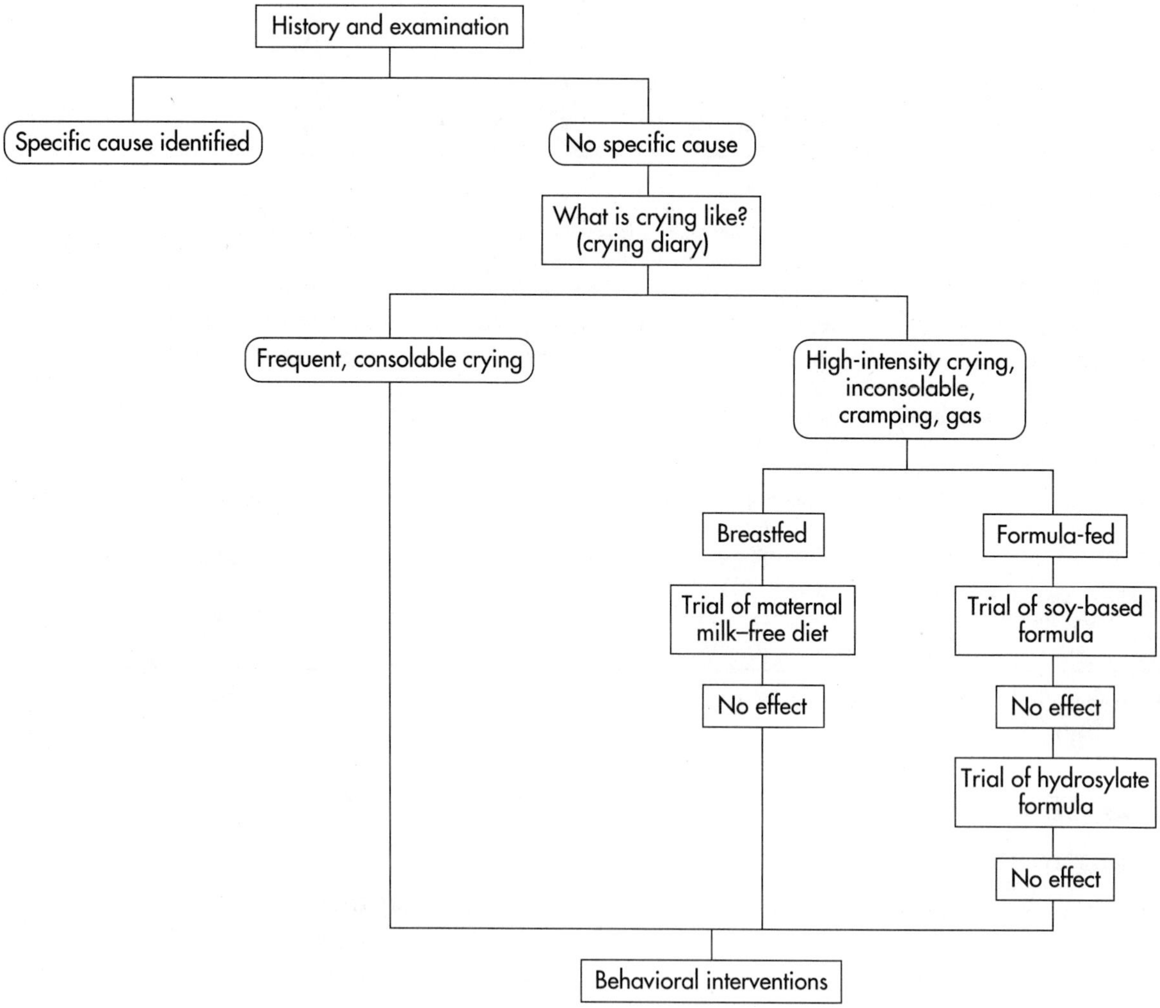

Figure 39-1 A clinical approach to colic. (Adapted from Geertsma M, Hyams JS: Colic: a pain syndrome of infancy? *Pediatr Clin North Am* 89:905, 1989. Adapted with permission.)

Patient Education

Reassure the parents that the condition is self-limited. Teach comfort measures such as swaddling, holding close during feedings, rubbing the tummy, burping frequently, feeding smaller quantities more frequently. Encourage caretakers to have someone come in and help care for infant when crying is likely to occur.

Family Impact

May increase stress and marital discord. Parents need to be able to verbalize their frustrations. There is a risk for child abuse if crying continues for more than 2 hours.

Referral/Consultation

None indicated.

Follow-up

Encourage the family to call with a report in 1 to 2 weeks; otherwise see them at regularly scheduled visits and reassess at that time.

Biliary Colic

Pharmaceutical

Pharmaceutical management is contraindicated for stones larger than 20 mm, bile pigment stones, or radiopaque stones (Table 39-7). Some stones may recur within 5 years in 50% of patients.

Frail patients such as chronically ill, debilitated, and elderly patients may benefit from nonsurgical approaches to care, such as oral dissolution medications: Ursodiol (Actigall) or chenodiol (Chenix). It often takes months to years to dissolve stones. Morphine or meperidine (Demerol) injected intramuscularly may relieve pain.

Lifestyle/Activities

If the patient is asymptomatic, advise weight loss by decreasing calories, giving up drinking alcoholic beverages, increasing exercise to improve overall well-being.

Diet

Patient can decrease excessive calories in diet and may need to decrease fats if eating them tends to aggravate symptoms.

Patient Education

Discuss the causes of biliary colic and the probable need for surgery. Explain surgical options, such as conventional open cholestectomy, laparoscopic cholecystectomy, and medical therapies available. Explain ultrasonography and the patient's preparation for test.

Family Impact

Treatment will require inpatient or outpatient surgery and a period of time with limited activity. This may interfere with family responsibilities. The condition may be costly if the patient has no insurance.

Referral

Refer the patient to an obstetrician if she is **pregnant.** The patient should be referred to a general surgeon for surgery if ultrasonography yields a positive result, the individual's risk is low, and surgery could be tolerated.

Consultation

If the patient is **pregnant,** consult with high-risk obstetrician to determine testing and immediacy of referral.

Follow-up

Send the patient for real-time ultrasonography of the gallbladder; then schedule an office visit to review findings. Schedule the patient for postsurgical follow-up if surgery is required.

Renal Colic

Pharmaceutical

Morphine or meperidine (Demerol) injected intramuscularly may help control pain.

Lifestyle/Activities

Encourage the patient to drink more fluids and void more frequently.

Diet

Discourage the patient from eating licorice, chocolate, and nuts.

Patient Education

If the stone did not pass during the office visit, teach the patient to strain the urine with cheesecloth and to save all stones in a jar. Encourage the patient to drink fluids regularly, carrying liquids with them at all times. Explain the symptoms and possible need for surgery or lithotripsy. Explain x-ray tests for kidneys, ureter, and bladder (KUB) and intravenous pyelography and preparation for these.

Family Impact

Because the condition may require hospitalization, there may be a disruption of family routines.

Referral

None indicated.

Consultation

Consult with a urologist or general surgeon if the stone is too big to pass.

Follow-up

Order KUB, bloodwork, and urinalysis. Schedule the patient to come back to the office afterward to review findings. If surgery is required, see the patient for annual KUB and metabolic studies as indicated.

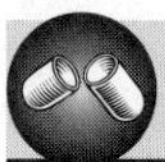

TABLE 39-7 Pharmaceutical Plan: Biliary Colic

Drug	Dose	Comments	Cost
Ursodiol (Actigall)	8-10 mg/kg/day in 2-3 divided doses Maintenance: 250 mg qhs for 6-12 mo	Pregnancy: B Monitor response q6 mo by US SE: Headache, fatigue, cough, dry skin, sweating, alopecia	$208/300 mg (100)
Chenodiol (Chenix)	250 mg BID for 2 wk, then increase to a maximum of 16 mg/kg/day	Pregnancy: X SE: Same as above Monitor LFT, CBC, cholesterol	$107/250 mg (100)

CBC, Complete blood count; *LFT,* liver function test; *SE,* side effects; *US,* ultrasound.

EVALUATION

Infant Colic

Infant colic is self-limited and should resolve on its own. Telephone follow-up periodically should assist the parents in coping with this stressful time. Reassess at each office visit.

Biliary Colic

Children

The symptoms/problem will be resolved by medical management or surgery.

Adults

Evaluate resolution of the symptoms, loss of weight, and/or surgical removal of the gallbladder.

Elderly

Evaluate the relief of symptoms through medical management and confirm dissolution of stones by ultrasound.

Pregnant Women

Pregnant women can be evaluated following referral to the obstetrician/gynecologist for management of gallbladder dysfunction.

Renal Colic

Adults/elderly: Evaluate resolution of pain, passage of the stone, and that KUB are stone free.

REFERENCES

Fang LS: Approach to the patient with nephrolithiasis. In Goroll AH, May LA, Mulley AG: *Primary care medicine: office evaluation and management of the adult patient,* ed 3, Philadelphia, 1995, JB Lippincott.

Holcomb GW III: Minimally invasive surgery. In Hoekelman, RA: *Primary pediatric care,* ed 3, St Louis, 1997, Mosby.

Lehtonen L, Korvenranta H: Infantile colic: seasonal incidence and crying profiles, *Arch Pediatr Adolesc Med* 149:533-536, 1995.

Rhoades R, Pflanzer R: *Human physiology,* ed 2, Philadelphia, 1992, WB Saunders.

SUGGESTED READINGS

Bromberg DI: Colic. In Hoekelman, RA: *Primary pediatric care,* ed 3, St Louis, 1997, Mosby.

Ellsworth AJ et al: *Mosby's 1998 medical drug reference,* St Louis, 1998, Mosby.

Geertsma M, Hyams JS: Colic: a pain syndrome of infancy? *Pediatr Clin North Am* 36:905, 1989.

Goroll AH, May LA, Mulley AG: *Primary care medicine: office evaluation and management of the adult patient,* ed 3, Philadelphia, 1995, JB Lippincott.

Healthcare Consultants of America, Inc: *1998 Physicians fee and coding guide,* Augusta, Ga, Healthcare Consultants of America, Inc.

Jarvis C: *Physical examination and health assessment,* ed 92, Philadelphia, 1996, WB Saunders.

Petersen-Smith AM: Gastrointestinal disorders. In Burns CE et al, editors: *Pediatric primary care: a handbook for nurse practitioners,* Philadelphia, 1996, WB Saunders.

40 Confusion

ICD-9-CM

Confusion 298.9
Delirium 780.09
Senile Dementia 290.3
Drug-induced Delirium 292.81

OVERVIEW

Definition

Confusion is an imprecise term describing some change in the level of mental status. Most often, confusion can better be defined as either delirium or dementia. Delirium is a reversible alteration in awareness that usually has an acute onset. Delirium has identifiable physiological causes and can be reversed with appropriate treatment. It is characterized by a sudden onset, fluctuating periods of awareness, perceptual disturbances, disturbed sleep/wake cycle, changes in level of psychomotor activity, and changes in cognitive and functional ability (Ham, 1997). Dementia is a progressive deterioration of mental status that occurs gradually, as in Alzheimer's, or somewhat stepwise, as in vascular dementia, and encompasses a declining level of awareness, memory, cognitive, visual/spatial, language, calculation, and judgment skills.

Etiology/Risk Factors

Delirium can be caused by hypoxia, infection, dehydration, acute metabolic disturbance, trauma, pathological conditions of the central nervous system, endocrinopathies, myocardial infarction, toxins, and drug withdrawal. Medicines implicated in the development of delirium include anticholinergic agents, antipsychotic and antidepressant medications, digoxin, histamine blocking agents, anticonvulsants, nonsteroidal antiiflammatory drugs (NSAIDs), H_2 blockers, narcotics, corticosteroids, and antihypertensive agents. Risk factors include **age over 80,** impaired vision and hearing, dementia, history of previous delirium, multiple medications, and multiple coexistent diseases (Simon, 1997).

Although there are many types of dementia, Alzheimer's dementia can account for approximately 70% of dementias (Geldmacher and Whitehouse, 1996) (see also Chapter 9). Risk factors for Alzheimer's dementia include **advanced age (more than 85 years old)** (Hebert et al., 1995), a family history of Alzheimer's dementia, and possibly a history of trauma to the head. Vascular dementia accounts for at least 10% of dementias seen (Geldmacher and Whitehouse, 1996), but vascular and Alzheimer's dementia may overlap (Hamm, 1997). Risk factors associated with vascular dementia include vasculitis, high blood pressure, the presence of atherosclerotic vessel disease, and a history of stroke. Many other types of dementia have been identified, each with differing presentation.

Other types of dementia include the dementia associated with acquired immunodeficiency syndrome, frontal lobe dementia (characterized by disinhibition and disordered initiation and goal setting), and parkinsonism (characterized by movement disorder) (Geldmacher and Whitehouse, 1997).

SUBJECTIVE DATA

History of Present Illness

Determine the mode of onset (abrupt or gradual), the progression (fluctuating, continuous decline, improving), and the duration of symptoms. Delirium and dementia can be differentiated by the time course of the symptoms. Delirium occurs over a relatively short period. The symptoms tend to fluctuate, there is disorientation, disturbance in attention, a change in the level of consciousness, and perceptual disturbances (i.e., hallucinations).

Dementia occurs over months and years, and the symptoms tend to worsen or become more noticeable over time. There is cognitive impairment in multiple areas: memory, short-term recall, abstract thinking, judgment, aphasia, apraxia, agnosia, constructional ability, concentration, orientation and visual/spatial ability. Determining independence in activities of daily living (ADLs) (dressing, bathing, eating, ambulation, and toileting) and the instrumental ADLs (e.g., handling finances, shopping, taking medicines) is probably the most important indicator of presence and degree of dementia.

Past Medical History

Determine whether there has been alcohol abuse, toxin exposure, or any neurological events or diagnoses. A history of delirium of any cause may predate other symptoms of dementia. A history of hypertension and other vascular diseases may support the differential diagnosis of vascular dementia rather than dementia of Alzheimer type. A history of alcoholism, toxin exposure, and head injury is significant.

Medications

Numerous medications have been associated with changes in cognitive status or delirium, including antiarrhythmics, antibiotics, anticholinergics, antidepressants, antiemetics, antihypertensives, antineoplastics, antimania agents, cardiotonics, steroids, H_2 antagonists, immunosuppressives, narcotics, muscle relaxants, NSAIDs, radiocontrast agents, and sedatives. It is important to determine the relationship between any change in medication and the onset of delirious symptoms.

Family History

Determine the presence of any dementia-type illnesses in the parents, siblings, and children of the patient.

Psychosocial History

Determining the patient's level of education, lifelong occupation and hobbies, and characteristics of his or her personality before this illness are important to an understanding of the deviation from the individual's normal level of functioning.

Diet History

Delirium may be related to an inadequate intake of food and fluid (e.g., in dehydration associated with acute urinary tract infection). Of importance in dementia is the history of weight loss as it relates to the patient's remembering to shop, prepare food, and ability to stay on the task of eating.

Description of Most Common Symptoms

Symptoms of cognitive decline include increasing memory loss, wandering or getting lost, and a decline in the ability to perform activities of daily living, decline in the ability to learn new tasks, and behavior or personality changes, such as apathy or increased irritability. Since dementia is a gradual process, the family may not be aware of the extent to which they have taken over activities for their loved one. Patients may be unable to answer questions and may skillfully redirect the conversation to socially appropriate "small talk." Unexplained weight loss and unkempt appearance are clues to possible dementia.

Associated Symptoms

The presence of associated complaints can give a clue as to the cause of delirium. For example, new incontinence associated with delirium may suggest the presence of a urinary tract infection; shortness of breath may indicate an exacerbation of congestive heart failure. The onset of delirium after a medication is added or changed suggests medications contribute to the alteration in awareness. It may be difficult to determine whether the symptoms being reported are a change from baseline symptoms because of the overlying confusion. It is important to note how the symptoms differ from the usual for the patient, how rapidly the symptoms are progressing, and how the symptoms have varied over time.

Important symptoms associated with dementia are a gradual decline in the ability to perform instrumental ADLs, as well as a change in memory, decreased ability to learn new information, decreased ability to handle complex tasks, reasoning ability, spatial ability and orientation, language, and behavior (e.g., use of inappropriate words, nonsensical sentences, unpredictable behavior) (Costa et al, 1996).

OBJECTIVE DATA

Physical Examination

It is important to identify the cause of delirium, since virtually any illness may trigger a delirium in a susceptible individual. Because the cause of delirium may be difficult to determine, a complete examination is warranted. In dementia, eliminate any reversible cause of change in mental status, such as hypothyroidism or vitamin deficiency. Perform a complete neurological examination, being especially observant for focal neurological deficits. In mild to moderate Alzheimer's dementia, the neurological examination may not show any focal neurological deficits. In other types of dementia, motor signs such as bradykinesia and rigidity may be noted (Geldmacher and Whitehouse, 1997).

Diagnostic tests for assessing objective data related to confusion are outlined in Table 40-1.

Diagnostic Procedures

Evaluation of Mental Status (Tables 40-2 and 40-3). The Mini-Mental State Examination can be admin-

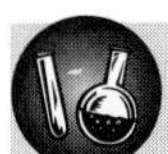

TABLE 40-1 Diagnostic Tests: Confusion

Symptoms	Findings/Examples	Test	Cost ($)
Delirium	Neurological changes: CVA, TIA, seizure	CT (head)	990-1175
		MRI (head)	1781-2004
		Lumbar puncture	172-208
		EEG	N/A
	Infection: Identify source	CBC	13-16
		CXR	77-91
		UA	14-18
		Urine and sputum culture	31-39/culture
		AFB	23-28
		HIV	58-72
	Cardiovascular: MI, arrhythmia, hypotension, DVT, CHF	ECG	56-65
		N/A	ECHO
		N/A	Doppler
		Cardiac isoenzymes	43-55
	Metabolic: Renal failure, liver failure, diabetes, hypothyroidism, anemia	Electrolytes	23-30
		TSH	56-70
		CBC	13-16
		UA	14-18
		Guaiac stool	13-17
	Pulmonary: Infection, COPD, PE, hypoperfusion	CXR	77-91
		ABGs	78-98
		Ventilation/perfusion scan	N/A
		Pulmonary function tests	96-227
	Miscellaneous: Pain, drug effects, occult fractures	Drug levels	N/A
		X-ray evaluation of suspected fracture	N/A
Dementia	Progressive cognitive decline	CT	990-1175
		MRI	1781-2004
		CBC	13-16
		Multiple chemical analyses	N/A
		UA	14-18
		RPR	18-22
		TSH	56-70
		B_{12} folate levels	N/A

From Luremberg J: Delirium. In Lonergan E, editor: *Geriatrics,* Norwalk, Conn, 1996, Appleton & Lange.

ABGs, Arterial blood gases; *AFB,* acid-fast bacteria; *CBC,* complete blood cell count; *CHF,* congestive heart failure; *COPD,* chronic obstructive pulmonary disease; *CT,* computed tomography; *CVA,* cerebrovascular accident; *CXR,* chest x-ray evaluation; *DVT,* deep venous thrombosis; *ECG,* electrocardiography; *ECHO,* echocardiography; *EEG,* electroencephalography; *HIV,* human immunodeficiency virus; *MRI,* magnetic resonance imaging; *N/A,* not available; *PE,* pulmonary embolus; *RPR,* rapid plasma reagin; *TIA,* transient ischemic attack; *TSH,* thyroid-stimulating hormone; *UA,* urinalysis.

istered (Table 40-2). Education, culture, and command of English may all influence the individual's score on this evaluation. A highly educated individual may test "unimpaired" (false negative), whereas an individual with little education may test "impaired" (false positive) (Costa et al, 1996). The diagnosis of dementia is not based solely on a score on this test, but rather on this test plus the patient history and the results of other tests. Further neurocognitive testing may be beyond primary care office capabilities, and an appropriate referral should be made.

Depression Inventory. This test helps to determine whether depression is contributing to the patient presentation of confusion. The Geriatric Depression Scale is a 10-minute yes/no questionnaire that is useful in determining the extent of depression in elders (Boxes 40-1 and 40-2).

Genetic Testing. Genetic testing can be conducted to determine whether the Alzheimer genetic marker apolipoprotein E4 is present, which increases the likelihood that the person has Alzheimer's disease. The absence of the gene does not mean that the individual does not have the disease (Small, 1996). Thus, although this test may provide a greater precision in making the Alzheimer's diagnosis, it cannot be used to provide absolute confirmation of the disease at this time (Mayeux et al, 1998). When specific

TABLE 40-2 Mini-Mental State Exam

Maximum Score	Score	
		ORIENTATION
5	( )	What is the (year) (season) (date) (month)?
5	( )	Where are we: (state) (country) (town) (hospital) (floor)
		REGISTRATION
3	( )	Name 3 objects: 1 second to say each. Then ask the patient all 3 after you have said them. Give 1 point for each correct answer. Then repeat them until he learns all 3. Count trials and record. Trials
		ATTENTION AND CALCULATION
5	( )	Serial 7's. 1 point for each correct. Stop after 5 answers. Alternatively, spell "world" backwards.
		RECALL
5	( )	Ask for the 3 objects repeated above. Give 1 point for each correct.
		LANGUAGE
5	( )	Name a pencil, and watch (2 points) Repeat the following "No ifs, ands or buts." (1 point) Follow a 3-stage command: *"Take a paper in your right hand, fold it in half, and put it on the floor"* (3 points) Read and obey the following: CLOSE YOUR EYES (1 point) Write a sentence (1 point) Copy design (1 point)
______		Total score
		ASSESS level of consciousness along a continuum ______ Alert Drowsy Stupor Coma

INSTRUCTIONS FOR ADMINISTRATION OF MINI-MENTAL STATE EXAMINATION

ORIENTATION

(1) Ask for the date. Then ask specifically for parts omitted, e.g., "Can you also tell me what season it is?" One point for each correct.

(2) Ask in turn "Can you tell me the name of this hospital?" (town, country, etc.). One point for each correct.

REGISTRATION

Ask the patient if you may test his memory. Then say the names of 3 unrelated objects, clearly and slowly, about 1 second for each. After you have said all 3, ask him to repeat them. This first repetition determines his score (0-3) but keep saying them until he can repeat all 3, up to 6 trials. If he does not eventually learn all 3, recall cannot be meaningfully tested.

ATTENTION AND CALCULATION

Ask the patient to begin with 100 and count backwards by 7. Stop after 5 subtractions (93, 86, 79, 72, 65).

Score the total number of correct answers.

If the patient cannot or will not perform this task, ask him to spell the word "world" backwards. The score is the number of letters in correct order, e.g., dlrow = 5, dlorw = 3.

RECALL

Ask the patient if he can recall the 3 words you previously asked him to remember. Score 0-3.

LANGUAGE

Naming: Show the patient a wristwatch and ask him what it is. Repeat for pencil. Score 0-2.

Repetition: Ask the patient to repeat the sentence after you. Allow only one trial. Score 0-1.

3-Stage command: Give the patient a piece of plain blank paper and repeat the command. Score 1 point for each part correctly executed.

Reading: On a blank piece of paper print the sentence "Close your eyes," in letters large enough for the patient to see clearly. Ask him to read it and do what it says. Score 1 point only if he actually closes his eyes.

Writing: Give the patient a blank piece of paper and ask him to write a sentence for you. Do not dictate a sentence, it is to be written spontaneously. It must contain a subject and verb and be sensible. Correct grammar and punctuation are not necessary.

Copying: On a clean piece of paper, draw intersecting pentagons, each side about 1 in., and ask him to copy it exactly as it is. All 10 angles must be present and 2 must intersect to score 1 point. Tremor and rotation are ignored.

Estimate the patient's level of sensorium along a continuum, from alert on the left to coma on the right.

Mini-Mental State: a practical method for grading the cognitive state of patients for the clinician, *J Psychiatr Res* 12:189-198, 1975.

TABLE 40-3 Median Mini-Mental State Examination Score by Age and Educational Level

	Education				
	0-4 y	5-8 y	9-12 y	>12 y	Total
18-24	23	28	29	30	29
25-29	25	27	29	30	29
30-34	26	26	29	30	29
35-39	23	27	29	30	29
40-44	23	27	29	30	29
45-49	23	27	29	30	29
50-54	22	27	29	30	29
55-59	22	27	29	29	29
60-64	22	27	28	29	28
65-69	22	27	28	29	28
70-74	21	26	28	29	27
75-79	21	26	27	28	26
80-84	19	25	26	28	25
≥85	20	24	26	28	25
Total	22	26	29	29	29

From Crum RM, et al: Population-based norms for the mini-mental state examination by age and educational level, *JAMA* 269:2386-2391, 1993.

treatment is available, this test may be more useful in differentiating the type of dementia. Apolipoprotein E (APOE) genotyping is not predictive of the onset of disease or the course of the disease. There remains ethical concerns about the individual's right to genetic privacy; for example, if a person is shown to have the genetic marker, could she or he be denied health insurance (Prost, 1997). Other chemical markers are now being identified in urine and cerebrospinal fluid.

CT and MRI Scanning. Scans can be performed to determine the presence of small vessel disease, brain focal abnormalities, evidence of stroke, or hydrocephalus. Positron emission tomography (PET) and single photon emission computed tomography (SPECT) can provide information on the biochemical functioning of the brain (Small, 1996). These studies are largely investigational and not widely available at this time. Figure 40-1 summarizes the clinical approach to a patient with memory loss and confusion.

ASSESSMENT

Major criteria for delirium: See Table 40-4
Major criteria for dementia: See Table 40-4
Minor criteria for delirium: Change in baseline functioning, identifiable cause
Minor criteria for dementia: Supportive data from the physical examination; social history; past medical history that suggests the type of dementia

THERAPEUTIC PLAN

Pharmaceutical

Delirium is a medical emergency. Treat the identified cause of delirium: treat infection, modify the drug regimen, etc. The decision to refer is based on the severity of the presenting symptoms, the ease of identification of probable cause, and the experience of the provider.

Pharmacological symptom management of problematic/confusional behaviors associated with both delirium and dementia include the use of short-acting benzodiazepines and antipsychotic and neuroleptic medications. These are used for targeted behaviors when environmental modifications have been unsuccessful; they are meant to be short-term treatment measures.

Consider treatment with donepezil (Aricept) or another acetylesterase uptake inhibitor if the diagnosis is early dementia of the Alzheimer type. These drugs do not correct the underlying pathology of Alzheimer's disease but may help stabilize the patient and promote a more gradual rate of decline. A common side effect of donepezil is nausea, so bedtime dosing is advised.

Treat depression if applicable. The side effect profile and drug interactions of each of the major categories of antidepressants must be considered when choosing an antidepressant for a specific patient.

Table 40-5 outlines the pharmaceutical plan for treatment of confusion.

Box 40-1

Geriatric Depression Scale

Test items may be administered in oral or written format. If the latter is used, have the patient read the first few items out loud and answer them in your presence to ensure that he/she understands the instructions.

1. Are you basically satisfied with your life? (No)
2. Have you dropped many of your activities and interests? (Yes)
3. Do you feel that your life is empty? (Yes)
4. Do you often get bored? (Yes)
5. Are you hopeful about the future? (No)
6. Are you bothered by thoughts you cannot get out of your head? (Yes)
7. Are you in good spirits most of the time? (No)
8. Are you afraid that something bad is going to happen to you? (Yes)
9. Do you feel happy most of the time? (No)
10. Do you often feel helpless? (Yes)
11. Do you often get restless and fidgety? (Yes)
12. Do you prefer to stay home at night, rather than do new things? (Yes)
13. Do you frequently worry about the future? (Yes)
14. Do you feel that you have more problems with memory than most? (Yes)
15. Do you think it is wonderful to be alive now? (No)
16. Do you often feel downhearted and blue? (Yes)
17. Do you feel pretty worthless the way you are now? (Yes)
18. Do you worry a lot about the past? (Yes)
19. Do you find life very exciting? (No)
20. Is it hard for you to get started on new projects? (Yes)
21. Do you feel full of energy? (No)
22. Do you feel that your situation is hopeless? (Yes)
23. Do you think that most people are better off than you are? (Yes)
24. Do you frequently get upset over little things? (Yes)
25. Do you frequently feel like crying? (Yes)
26. Do you have trouble concentrating? (Yes)
27. Do you enjoy getting up in the morning? (No)
28. Do you prefer to avoid social gatherings? (Yes)
29. Is it easy for you to make decisions? (No)
30. Is your mind as clear as it used to be? (No)

Scoring: Score 1 point for each response that matches the yes or no answer after the question.
Interpreting scores: Scores greater than 5 indicate probable depression.

From Yesavage JA, Brink TL: Development and validation of a geriatric depression screening scale: a preliminary report, *J Psychiatr Res* 17:41, 1983. Copyright 1983, Pergamon Journals Ltd.

Box 40-2

Geriatric Depression Scale (Short Form)

Test items may be administered in oral or written format. If the latter is used, have the patient read the first few items out loud and answer them in your presence to ensure that he/she understands the instructions.

1. Are you basically satisfied with your life? (No)
2. Have you dropped many of your activities and interests? (Yes)
3. Do you feel that your life is empty? (Yes)
4. Do you often get bored? (Yes)
5. Are you in good spirits most of the time? (No)
6. Are you afraid that something bad is going to happen to you? (Yes)
7. Do you feel happy most of the time? (No)
8. Do you often feel helpless? (Yes)
9. Do you prefer to stay home at night, rather than do new things? (Yes)
10. Do you feel that you have more problems with memory than most? (Yes)
11. Do you think it is wonderful to be alive now? (No)
12. Do you feel pretty worthless the way you are now? (Yes)
13. Do you feel full of energy? (No)
14. Do you feel that your situation is hopeless? (Yes)
15. Do you think that most people are better off than you are? (Yes)

Scoring: Score 1 point for each response that matches the yes or no answer after the question.
Interpreting scores: Scores greater than 5 indicate probable depression.

From Yesavage JA: Geriatric depression scale, *Psychopharmacol Bull* 24:709-710, 1988.

Lifestyle/Activities

The patient should be assisted to do the following:

Maintain social contacts and cognitive and sensory stimulation and hobbies as long as possible

If delirious, reduce the level and intensity of activity and stimulation until treatment of cause of delirium is completed

Patient Education

Determine the patient's safety needs: Independent living capabilities, cooking, driving.

If the patient is delirious, discuss with the family or caregiver specific treatments and therapies needed to correct the delirium. Once it is corrected, teach the family/caregiver the symptoms to report.

Discuss specific nonpharmacological/environmental modifications for the management of problematic behaviors. Examples include providing consistency of routine, avoiding overstimulation and understimulation, installing child-safe locks on cabinets where household cleaning supplies are kept, assisting with scheduled toileting, and providing visual cues related to the functions of the rooms in the house, especially the bathroom.

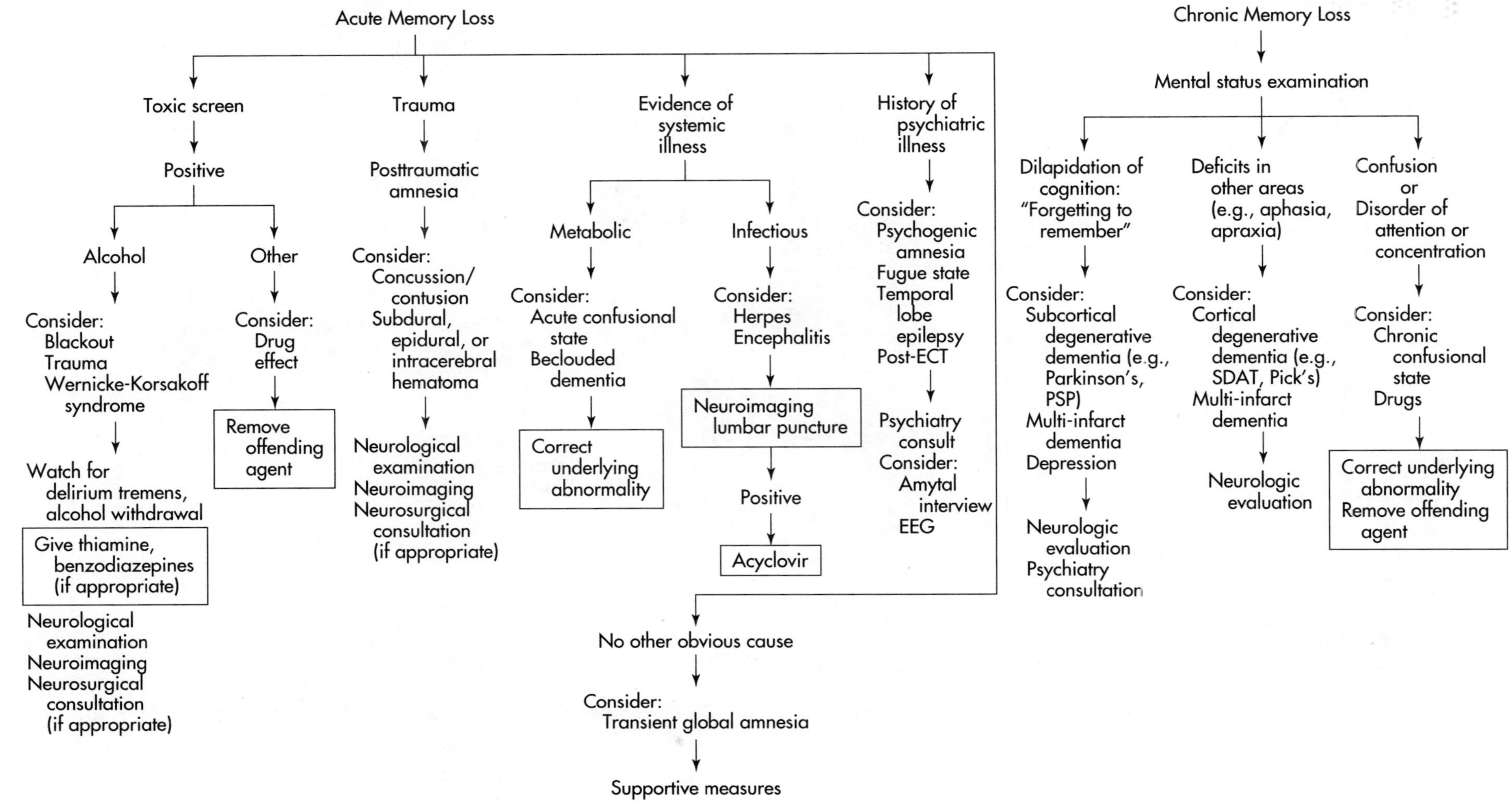

Figure 40-1 Algorithm for the treatment of a patient with memory loss. (*ECT,* electroconvulsive therapy; *EEG,* electroencephalography; *SDAT,* senile dementia, Alzheimer type.) (From Greene HL, Johnson WP, Lemcke D: *Decision making in medicine,* ed 2, St Louis, 1998, Mosby.)

TABLE 40-4 Differential Diagnosis: Confusion

Diagnosis	Supporting Data
Delirium	Sudden onset, fluctuating course, fluctuating level of awareness, disturbed attention, sleep/wake cycle disturbance, change in psychomotor behavior, physiological changes indicating cause of delirium (e.g., infection, cardiovascular event)
Dementia	Gradual onset, progressive decline, decline in functional capability, initially affects instrumental activities of daily living, memory loss

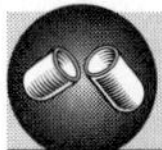

TABLE 40-5 Pharmaceutical Plan: Confusion

Drug	Adult Dose	Comments	Cost
Dementia			
Donepezil	5-10 mg	Administer at bedtime to lessen GI side effects. Advise keeping a diary to describe impact on functional ability. Most beneficial effects seen in mild to moderate Alzheimer dementia. Does not affect disease progression but may slow rate of apparent decline.	N/A
Estrogen, antioxidants, NSAIDs		Investigational at this time.	N/A
Depression			
SSRI (e.g., fluoxetine, paroxetine, sertraline) NOTE: TCAs are not recommended for use in elderly patients		Start at the lowest possible dose, titrate slowly, and monitor for side effects, such as nausea, insomnia, diarrhea (selective serotonin reuptake inhibitors), sedation, and orthostatic hypotension.	$215-$220/ fluoxetine; $57-$65/paroxetine; $176-$181/sertraline
Problematic Behavior			
Antipsychotic agents (e.g., haloperidol), atypical antipsychotic agents (e.g., risperidone, olanzaprine [Zyprexa]), antidepressant medications (e.g., trazodone, SSRIs), antianxiety medications (e.g., lorazepam), anticonvulsant agents (e.g., valproic acid)		Initiate only when environmental and behavioral methods have proved unsuccessful, or the individual is at great risk for injury to self or others. Identify targeted behaviors. Choose the drug most likely to modify those targeted behaviors. Start with the lowest possible dose; doses used for problematic behaviors in delirium and dementia are much lower than for treatment of psychiatric illness. A geropsychiatric evaluation may be helpful. Monitor the patient closely for side effects.	$2-$83/haloperidol; $190-$315/risperidone; $2-$75/lorazepam; $14-$116/valproic acid

Adapted from Tariot PN: Treatment strategies for agitation and psychosis in dementia, *J Clin Psychiatr* 57(Suppl 14):21-29, 1996; and Ham, RJ: Confusion, dementia and delirium. In Ham RJ, Sloane, PD, editors: *Primary care geriatrics: a case-based approach,* St Louis, 1997, Mosby.

GI, Gastrointestinal; *SSRI,* selective serotonin reuptake inhibitor; *N/A,* not available; *NSAID,* nonsteroidal antiinflammatory drug; *TCA,* tricyclic antidepressant.

Discuss effects and side effects of pharmacological interventions for problematic behaviors.

Family Impact

Link the family with community resources such as the Alzheimer's Association (see Resources at the end of this chapter) for availability of day programs, emotional support, and planning for continued care.

Referral

Referral to a physician may be indicated for patients with delirium, based on the degree of confusion and intensity of symptoms. Individuals with acute confusional states are likely to be hospitalized to expedite evaluation and treatment.

In dementia, consider referral to a geriatric evaluation center for formal mental status testing and individual and family counseling and education. Refer to support groups and social agencies as indicated.

Referral to a geropsychiatrist may be indicated for management of problematic behaviors.

Consultation

Determine the level of stress and burden on the patient's caregiver. Be alert for suspicion of abuse.

Refer to family counseling if needed.

EVALUATION/FOLLOW-UP

Follow-up for patients with delirium must be frequent until the episode resolves.

For dementia, ask the patient and family to return to the office every 3 to 6 months to monitor changes and provide support and information to caregivers.

Monitor the effectiveness of any medicine or treatment prescribed.

Monitor the effectiveness of home care systems to ensure safety and that nutrition is adequate.

Monitor for signs of caregiver stress.

Monitor for subtle signs of changes in health status, because the patient may not be able to report changes.

Monitor for the resolution of delirium. If the delirium is mild and the cause is readily identifiable, the patient or caregiver should be contacted in 24 hours for a status report.

Monitor for the progression of dementia.

RESOURCES

Alzheimer's Association: 800-272-3900; web site: http://www.alz.org

Administration on Aging (Department of Health and Human Services): 202-619-0724; web site: http://www.aoa.dhhs.gov

American Association of Retired Persons (AARP): 800-424-3410; web site http://www.aarp.org

Early Alzheimer's Disease, Patient and Family Guide, Clinical Practice Guideline Number 19; AHCPR Publication No. 96-0704; or call 800-358-9295

Medicare Hotline: 800-638-6833

REFERENCES

Costa PT Jr et al: Early identification of Alzheimer's disease and related dementias. Clinical practice guideline, quick reference guide for clinicians No 19, Rockville, Md, November 1996, U.S. Department of Health and Human Services, Public Health Service, Agency for Health Care Policy and Research. AHCPR Publication No. 97-0703.

Geldmacher D, Whitehouse PJ: Differential diagnosis of Alzheimer's disease, *Neurology* 48(Suppl 6):2-9, 1997.

Geldmacher D, Whitehouse PJ: Evaluation of dementia, *N Engl J Med* 335:330-335, 1996.

Ham RJ: Confusion, dementia and delirium. In Ham RJ, Sloane PD, editors: *Primary care geriatrics: a case-based approach,* St Louis, 1997, Mosby.

Hebert LE et al: Age specific incidence of Alzheimer's disease in a community population, *JAMA* 273:1354-1359, 1995.

Mayeux R et al: Utility of the apolipoprotein E genotype in the diagnosis of Alzheimer's disease. *N Engl J Med* 338:506-511, 1998.

Prost S et al: The clinical introduction of genetic testing for Alzheimer's disease, *JAMA* 277:832-836, 1997.

Simon L, Jewell N, Brokel J: Management of acute delirium in hospitalized elderly: a process improvement process, *Geriatr Nurs* 18: 150-154, 1997.

Small GW: Neuroimaging and genetic assessment for early diagnosis of Alzheimer's disease, *J Clin Psychiatr* 57(Suppl 14):9-13, 1996.

SUGGESTED READINGS

Ellsworth AJ et al: *Mosby's medical drug reference,* St Louis, 1998, Mosby.

Greene HL, Johnston WP, Lemcke D: *Decision making in medicine,* ed 2, St Louis, 1998, Mosby.

Healthcare Consultants of America, Inc: *1998 Physicians fee and coding guide,* Augusta, Ga, 1998, Healthcare Consultants of America, Inc.

Luremberg J: Delirium. In Lonergan, E, editor: *Geriatrics,* Norwalk, Conn, 1996, Appleton & Lange.

Tariot PN: Treatment strategies for agitation and psychosis in dementia, *J Clin Psychiatr* 57 (Suppl 14):21-29, 1996.

Congenital Heart Defects

Acyanotic Lesions and Cyanotic Congenital Heart Defects

ICD-9-CM

Complete Transposition of the Great Vessels 745.10
Ventricular Septal Defect 745.4
Patent Ductus Arteriosus 747.0
Coarctation of the Aorta 747.1
Tetralogy of Fallot 745.2
Tricuspid Valve Atresia 746.1
Congenital Primary Pulmonary Stenosis 746.02
Atrial Septal Defect 429.71

OVERVIEW

Definition

A *congenital heart defect* is a cardiac lesion present in neonates.

Incidence

Approximately 0.8% of all **neonates** are born with a congenital heart defect. This includes lesions diagnosed later in life.

Types

Acyanotic Heart Defects

Congenital heart defects in which *no* deoxygenated or poorly oxygenated blood enters the systemic circulation are *acyanotic*. Types include the following:

Left-to-right shunting through abnormal opening:
- Patent ductus arteriosus (PDA)
- Atrial septal defect (ASD)
- Ventricular septal defect (VSD)

Obstructive lesions that restrict ventricular outflow:
- Aortic valvular lesions
- Pulmonary artery stenosis
- Coarctation of the aorta

Cyanotic Heart Defects

Congenital heart defects in which deoxygenated blood enters the systemic circulation are *cyanotic*. Types include the following:

Right-to-left shunting:
- Tetralogy of Fallot
- Tricuspid atresia
- Transposition of great arteries (TGA)
- Truncus arteriosus
- Hypoplastic left heart syndrome
- Total anomalous pulmonary venous communication

Risk Factors

Fetal and maternal infection during the first trimester (especially rubella)
Maternal alcoholism
Maternal use of other drugs with teratogenic effects
Maternal age older than 40 years
Maternal dietary deficiencies
Maternal insulin-dependent diabetes
Other congenital defects

ACYANOTIC LESIONS

Patent Ductus Arteriosus

OVERVIEW

Definition

Patent ductus arteriosus is the persistent patency of the fetal structure bridging the pulmonary artery and the descending aorta. Two types of shunting are possible. One is *left-to-right shunting*, in which congestive heart failure (CHF) is possible, depending on the size of the PDA. The other is *right-to-left shunting*, in which oxygenation is a problem.

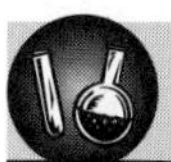

TABLE 41-1 Diagnostic Procedures Patent Ductus Arteriosus

Diagnostic Test	Finding/Rationale	Cost ($)
Echocardiography	Shows structural defect with persistent flow or color flow mapping in the PA or descending aorta for confirmation. Direction of flow should be determined using the Doppler mode. An enlarged left atrium is usually seen.	592-755
Chest x-ray	Dependent on the direction of the flow across the PDA and on the degree of shunt. For example, the heart size is normal for small shunt PDAs, however, cardiomegaly may exist for large shunt PDAs. Pulmonary edema may be seen with large left to right shunts, but not right to left shunts.	77-91
Electrocardiogram	Normal, or LVH in small to moderate PDA	56-67

PA, Pulmonary artery; *PDA,* pulmonary ductus arteriosus; *LVH,* left ventricular hypertrophy.

Incidence

In term infants the ductus arteriosus usually closes at birth. PDA accounts for between 2% and 5% of symptomatic cardiac diseases seen in the first 28 days. Premature infants of less than 34 weeks' gestational age have a significantly higher incidence of PDA in conjunction with respiratory distress syndrome.

Pathophysiology

Factors that influence ductal patency include the following:
- Muscle mass
- Low oxygen tension
- Low pH
- Acetylcholine
- Prostaglandin E_2
- Catecholamines
- Bradykinin

SUBJECTIVE DATA

Infants with significant heart malformations:
- Tire easily, especially when feeding
- May have excessive sweating
- Have persistent tachypnea
- Have central cyanosis in the lips, oral mucosa, extremities, and trunk
- Have abnormal growth patterns, especially decreased weight in relation to age

Children may have syncopal episodes.

OBJECTIVE DATA

Physical Examination

A physical examination should be conducted, with particular attention to the following:

Blood pressure of the upper and lower extremities
Pulse pressure of the upper and lower extremities (should be palpated simultaneously)
Vital signs
- Assess for tachypnea
- Weight and weight gain

General appearance
- Assess for stigmata associated with specific genetic syndromes
- Assess for cyanosis
- May need to watch infant feed (while infant is quiet)

Abdominal
- Hepatosplenomegaly

Respiratory and cardiac status

Circulatory Status

Bounding pulses with wide pulse pressure, hyperactive precordium, enlarged heart, and pulmonary edema can all be signs of decompensation.

Cardiac Status

A continuous, "machinery" grade I to IV/VI murmur may also be audible at the upper left sternal border or left interclavicular area.

Urinary Status

Decreased urinary output may be seen.

Diagnostic Procedures (Table 41-1)

Echocardiography with Doppler detects the structural defect.
Chest x-ray findings are dependent on the direction of flow across the PDA and on the degree of the shunt.
Electrocardiogram findings may be normal or reveal left ventricular hypertrophy in small-to-moderate PDAs.

ASSESSMENT

Differential diagnosis includes the following:
- Noncardiogenic pulmonary edema
- Respiratory distress syndrome

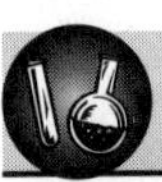

TABLE 41-2 Diagnostic Procedures: Atrial Septal Defects

Diagnostic Test	Finding/Rationale	Cost ($)
Electrocardiogram	Right axis deviation, right ventricular hypertrophy, right atrial enlargement	56-65
Chest x-ray	Demonstrates cardiac enlargement with the main pulmonary artery dilated; increased pulmonary vascular markings are frequently seen	77-91
Echocardiography	Shows paradoxical motion of the ventricular septal wall and a dilated right ventricular cavity	675
Cardiac catheterization	Reveals a significant increase in oxygen saturation at the atrial level; pulmonary pressures normal or elevated	N/A

N/A, Not available.

ASD
VSD

THERAPEUTIC PLAN

Patient may be free of symptoms and in hemodynamically stable condition with a small PDA; this would require no immediate intervention.

Patient should be closely monitored for any respiratory or hemodynamic instability.

In patients with symptoms and hemodynamic instability, surgical ligation is the treatment of choice.

Atrial Septal Defects

OVERVIEW

Definition

An *ASD* is an opening between the two atria that permits the shunting or mixing of blood.

Incidence

ASD occurs in approximately 10% of patients with congenital heart disease. It is twice as common in females as in males.

Pathophysiology

There is no pressure differential between the right and left sides of the heart during the first month of life as a result of relatively elevated pulmonary artery pressures. As the right-sided pressures begin to fall, more blood is shunted along the path of least resistance from both atria into the right ventricle and pulmonary vessels. This creates an increased volume load on the right ventricle. Excessive flow passes through the pulmonic valve, creating a relative pulmonic stenosis with a concomitant murmur. It also leads to right-sided heart failure. In addition, through time this may lead to pulmonary hypertension as a result of high blood flow through the pulmonary arteries.

SUBJECTIVE DATA

Patient may have no symptoms or may demonstrate varying degrees of right-sided heart failure. Older children are seen with fatigue, shortness of breath, and poor growth and development.

OBJECTIVE DATA

Physical Examination

A physical examination should be conducted with particular attention to general appearance and cardiac status.

General Appearance

Failure to thrive; cyanosis only with pulmonary hypertension

Cardiac Status

Arterial pulses are normal and equal; the heart is hyperactive, with heave best felt at left lower sternal border. S2 is widely split and fixed at pulmonic area, with no thrills. A grade I to IV/VI systolic ejection murmur (SEM) is heard best at the left sternal border.

Diagnostic Procedures (Table 41-2)

Electrocardiogram shows right axis deviation, right ventricular hypertrophy, and right atrial enlargement.

Chest x-ray demonstrates cardiac enlargement, with the main pulmonary artery dilated.

Echocardiography shows paradoxical motion of the ventricular septal wall and a dilated right ventricular cavity.

Cardiac catheterization reveals a significant increase in

oxygen saturation at the atrial level. Pulmonary pressures are normal or elevated.

THERAPEUTIC PLAN

Surgery is recommended for patients with a ratio of pulmonary to systemic blood flow greater than 2:1. Elective surgery is performed in patients between 2 and 4 years. Early surgery is recommended for infants with CHF or critical pulmonary hypertension.

Ventricular Septal Defects

OVERVIEW

Definition

A *VSD* is an opening between the two ventricles that permits the shunting or mixing of blood. Defects may occur in the membranous, muscular, or apical portions of the ventricular septum.

Incidence

VSD is the most common form of congenital cardiac heart defect, representing 20% to 25% overall. Thirty percent to 50% of all VSDs close spontaneously. Sixty percent to 70% of small defects also close.

Pathophysiology

There is only a slight pressure difference between the right and left ventricles during the first month of life as a result of relatively elevated pulmonary artery pressures. Therefore there is little flow across the VSD, and only a slight murmur is heard. As the right-sided pressures begin to fall, more blood is shunted along the path of least resistance from the left ventricle into the right ventricle and pulmonary vessels. As the pressure gradient increases, turbulence of circulation between the two ventricles increases and creates a louder murmur. It also creates an increased volume load on the right ventricle and left atrium. This leads to biventricular failure or right-sided heart failure. In addition, in time this may lead to pulmonary hypertension as a result of high blood flow through the pulmonary arteries.

SUBJECTIVE DATA

Past Medical History

Ask about frequent respiratory infections, as noted previously.

Diet History

Inquire about feeding intolerance and high salt intake if edema is present.

Associated Symptoms

Acyanosis
Frequent respiratory infections during infancy or early childhood
Dyspnea
Exercise or feeding intolerance
Edema
Abdominal distention
Fatigue

OBJECTIVE DATA

Physical Examination

A problem-oriented physical examination should be conducted with particular attention to vital signs and weight, general appearance, respiratory status, and cardiac status.

General Appearance

Many children demonstrate failure to thrive, with slow growth and poor weight gain. Some may even demonstrate developmental delay. This is predominately a result of CHF, which develops between 1 to 4 months.

Respiratory Status

Signs of respiratory distress include grunting, flaring, retracting, and increased respiratory rate. Inspiratory rales and expiratory wheezing may occur.

Cardiac Status

The degree of symptoms varies depending on the size of the shunt.

Small left-to-right shunts
- Grade II or III pansystolic murmur, left sternal border

Moderate left-to-right shunts
- Grade III to IV/VI harsh, pansystolic murmur, lower left sternal border at fourth intracostal space
- No heaves, lifts, or thrills

Diagnostic Procedures (Table 41-3)

Electrocardiogram is normal in most cases.
Chest x-ray may also vary according to the size of the shunt.
Echocardiography only will identify VSD ≥4 mm.
Angiography shows normal to increased left atrial pressures.
Pulmonary vascular resistance varies from normal to markedly increased.

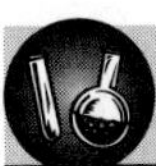

TABLE 41-3 Diagnostic Procedures: Ventricular Septal Defects

Diagnostic Test	Finding/Rationale	Cost ($)
Electrocardiogram	Normal in most cases. RVH or biventricular hypertrophy may occur as shunting worsens. With the development of CHF, right axis deviation and right atrial enlargement may also be seen.	56-65
Chest x-ray	May vary according to the size of the shunt. Small shunts: pulmonary vascular markings may be slightly increased. Large shunts: cardiac enlargement involving left and right ventricle, as well as the left atrium; a small to normal size aorta; pulmonary artery is dilated with increased pulmonary vascular markings.	77-91
Echocardiography	Cannot always be used for diagnostic purposes in identifying VSDs unless the defect is 4 mm or larger. Newer techniques may show smaller lesions.	675
Angiography	Shows normal to increased left atrial pressures. Pulmonary vascular resistance varies from normal to markedly increased. The shunt may be seen between the left ventricle and right ventricle if contrast is introduced directly into the ventricles.	N/A

N/A, Not available.

ASSESSMENT

Differential diagnosis may include the following:

- ASD
- Tetralogy of Fallot (the acyanotic type, "pink tet")
- PDA

THERAPEUTIC PLAN

If the patient does not respond to selective therapy or has increasing pulmonary hypertension, surgery is indicated. Age at elective surgery ranges from younger than 2 to 5 years.

Obstructive Lesions: Coarctation

OVERVIEW

Definition

Coarctation is a constricture of the aorta, most commonly surrounding the insertion site of the ductus arteriosus into the descending thoracic aorta.

Incidence

Coarctation occurs in 0.2 per 1000 live births, with a male predominance of almost 2:1. As the eighth most common defect among all age groups, it is seen frequently in infancy when collateral circulation is poor.

Pathophysiology

Left ventricular outflow tract obstruction occurs with development of left ventricular hypertrophy and eventually CHF.

Factor Increasing Risk of Recurrence

One parent with coarctation.

Other Associated Defects Occurring With Coarctation

- Bicuspid aortic valve
- VSD
- PDA
- TGA
- Hypoplastic left ventricle

SUBJECTIVE DATA

Description of Most Common Symptoms

- Dyspnea
- Tachypnea
- Irritability
- Feeding difficulties
- Tachycardia
- Failure to thrive
- Cool lower extremities with decreased pulses
- Ashen color
- Cyanosis

These symptoms are typically not present until 2 weeks of age. Circulatory shock, as demonstrated by oliguria, anuria, or any of the preceding symptoms, may not appear

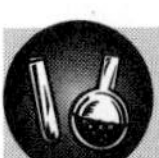

TABLE 41-4 Diagnostic Procedures: Coarctation of the Aorta

Diagnostic Test	Finding/Rationale	Cost ($)
Electrocardiogram	Reveals LVH for mild cases and right axis deviation, with RVH in more severe forms	56-65
Chest x-ray	Shows normal or enlarged heart. Classic figure of 3 sign on overpenetrated films and notched ribs in children >5 years old. Also classic is the "E sign" on barium swallow	77-91
Echocardiography	2 D echocardiography shows a shelflike narrowing of descending aorta in periductal region. Doppler flow will demonstrate turbulence in the same area.	675
Cardiac catheterization	Measures increased pressure gradient or pressure drop across the coarctation. This pressure gradient depends on patency of the ductus arteriosus, severity of the coarctation, and intrapulmonary shunting.	N/A

LVH, Left ventricular hypertrophy; *N/A,* not available; *RVH,* right ventricular hypertrophy.

until 2 to 6 weeks of age. Relatively symptom-free children may only report leg pains.

OBJECTIVE DATA

Physical Examination

Attention should focus on four-extremity blood pressure, vital signs, weight, and general appearance.

Respiratory: Pulmonary rales
Circulatory: Mild periorbital edema, dorsum hand and feet edema
Cardiac: SEM most common at left sternal border; frequent hypertension from poor renal perfusion; typically upper extremity blood pressure higher than that of lower extremities by >10 mm Hg
Hepatic: Hepatosplenomegaly
Renal: Oliguria or anuria

Diagnostic Procedures (Table 41-4)

Electrocardiogram reveals left ventricular hypertrophy for mild cases and right axis deviation with right ventricular hypertrophy in more severe forms.
Chest x-ray shows normal or enlarged heart.
Two-dimensional (2D) echocardiography shows shelflike narrowing of descending aorta.
Cardiac catheterization measures an increased pressure gradient or pressure drop across the coarctation.

ASSESSMENT

Differential diagnosis includes the following:

Hypoplastic left heart syndrome
CHF

THERAPEUTIC PLAN

Plan of care depends on whether a patient has symptoms or not. Observe for increasing symptoms. In some cases balloon angioplasty may be necessary. The surgical option of choice includes resection of the coarctated segment with an end-to-end anastomosis.

CYANOTIC CONGENITAL HEART DEFECTS

Transposition of the Great Arteries

OVERVIEW

Definition

TGA is defined as a switch of the origin of the great arteries from their normal ventricular origins so that the aorta originates from the right ventricle and the pulmonary artery arises from the left ventricle.

Incidence

Prevalence is 2 in 10,000 live births, representing the second most common defect in the first year of life.

Pathophysiology

Associated Factors

Male (3:1)
Normal to slightly increased birth rate
No maternal or fetal distress

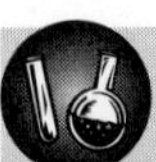

TABLE 41-5 Diagnostic Procedures: Transposition of the Great Vessels

Diagnostic Test	Finding/Rationale	Cost ($)
Chest x-ray	Indicates right axis deviation/right ventricular hypertrophy. CHF may be present if presence of VSD, PA, or PS. In addition, the chest x-ray may show an egg-shaped silhouette resulting from the CHF, with a slender mediastinum due to the abnormal alignment of the great vessels.	77-91
Echocardiography	2 D echocardiography reveals two circular structures. (Normal configuration of great vessels resembles a circle and sausage.)	675
Electrocardiogram	Right ventricular hypertrophy in more severe form.	56-65

CHF, Congestive heart failure; *PA,* pulmonary atresia; *PS,* pulmonary stenosis; *VSD,* ventricular septal defect.

Associated Defects

VSD
Tricuspid regurgitation
Pulmonic stenosis

OBJECTIVE DATA

Physical Examination

General Status

Infant is normal or large at birth; however, a growth and developmental delay is seen if the condition remains undetected.

Circulatory Status

Baseline cyanosis increases with crying and has little or no response to increased inspired oxygen. Clubbing of the digits is seen.

Cardiac Status

The S2 is single and loud. When auscultating, no murmur is audible if ventricular septum is intact. CHF may be present.

Diagnostic Procedures (Table 41-5)

Chest x-ray indicates right axis deviation and right ventricular hypertrophy, "egg on a string" appearance.
Electrolytes: Hypoglycemia, hypocalcemia, and acidosis.

ASSESSMENT

Differential diagnosis includes the following:

Truncus arteriosus
Hypoplastic right ventricle syndrome
Hypoplastic left ventricle syndrome
Double-outlet right ventricle
Double-outlet left ventricle

THERAPEUTIC PLAN

Before surgical intervention, temporizing measures include infusion of prostaglandin E1, to maintain patency of the ductus arteriosus, and treatment of CHF.

Tetralogy of Fallot

OVERVIEW

Definition

Tetralogy of Fallot is a congenital heart disease consisting of four different abnormalities, including pulmonary stenosis or atresia, VSD, right ventricular hypertrophy, and overriding or dextroposition of aorta.

Incidence

Tetralogy of Fallot accounts for 10% to 15% of all congenital heart disease, representing the most prevalent form of heart disease beyond infancy. Incidence is the same for males and females.

Pathophysiology

Severe right ventricular outflow tract obstruction coupled with a large VSD results in a right-to-left shunt at the ventricular level, with subsequent desaturation of arterial blood. The size of the shunt determines the degree of desaturation and amount of cyanosis. The greater the obstruction, the larger the VSD; the lower the systemic

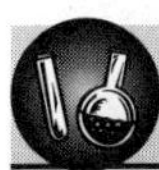

TABLE 41-6 Diagnostic Procedures: Tetralogy of Fallot

Diagnostic Test	Finding/Rationale	Cost ($)
Electrocardiogram	Shows right axis deviation, right ventricular hypertrophy. Rhythm disturbances occasionally occur	56-65
Chest x-ray	Shows decreased pulmonary vascular markings. Heart size is overall normal, but CHF may be present if acyanotic. The classic finding of a boot-shaped heart is due to a normal heart size with significant right ventricular hypertrophy, and upturning of the apex of the heart. Right aortic arch may be present in 25%.	77-91
Echocardiography	2 D echocardiography reveals a large PDA, and overriding of the aorta. Doppler studies confirm antegrade pulmonary flow and/or continuous or diastolic pulmonary flow. A VSD is also seen.	

CHF, Congestive heart failure; *PDA,* pulmonary ductus areriosus; *VSD,* ventricular septal defect.

vascular resistance, the greater the right-to-left shunt noted. Therefore right ventricular pressure cannot surpass left ventricular pressure, but they may be equal.

Associated Defects

Right-sided aortic arch, 25%
ASD, 15%

SUBJECTIVE DATA

Description of Most Common Symptoms

Dyspnea on exertion or squatting
Cyanosis, especially during vagal maneuvers

OBJECTIVE DATA

Physical Examination

A physical examination should be conducted, with particular attention to vital signs, weight, general appearance, and the following:

Respiratory Status

Patient may have hypoxic spells, peaking at 2 to 4 months. These begin with rapid and deep respirations, followed by irritability with crying. Cyanosis and heart murmur intensity decrease. An intense spell can lead to limpness, seizures, cerebrovascular accident (CVA), or even death. Death during a cyanotic spell is extremely rare.

Cardiac Status

Thrill at lower left sternal border, aortic ejection click, normal S_1, loud and single S2, III to V/VI SEM at middle to upper left sternal border
Complete blood count shows polycythemia, iron deficiency anemia with normal hematocrit, coagulopathies

Diagnostic Procedures (Table 41-6)

Electrocardiogram shows right axis displacement and right ventricular hypertrophy.
Chest x-ray shows decreased pulmonary vascular marking. Heart size is normal overall, but CHF may be present in acyanotic patients.

ASSESSMENT

Differential diagnosis includes the following:

- Severe valvular pulmonic stenosis with intact ventricular septum
- Truncus arteriosus with decreased pulmonary flow
- Double-outlet right ventricle
- TGA with subpulmonic stenosis, VDS, and tricuspid atresia

THERAPEUTIC PLAN

Diagnose and treat iron deficiency anemia because patients are predisposed toward CVAs.

Palliative Treatment

Detect and treat hypoxic spells.
Propranolol decreases heart rate and may increase stroke volume.
Prostaglandin E_1 is indicated with severe cyanosis and ductal dependence in infancy.
Atrial septostomy is performed by means of cardiac catheterization.
Surgical procedure is shunt to allow flow to bypass the obstructive lesion to the lungs.

Definitive Treatment

Closure of VSD with removal of ventricular outflow obstruction frequently results in rhythm disturbances.

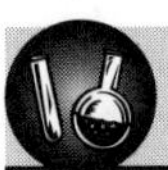

TABLE 41-7 Diagnostic Procedures: Truncus Arteriosus

Diagnostic Test	Finding/Rationale	Cost ($)
ABGs	Shows mild desaturation with little improvement with hyperoxia	75
Electrocardiogram	Shows electrographic signs of CHF in 70% of cases	56-65
Chest x-ray	Shows cardiomegaly (biventricular and left atrial enlargement), narrow mediastinum, and increased pulmonary blood flow (Right aortic arch is present 50% of the time.)	77-91
Echocardiography	Reveals large PDA right under truncal valve	675

CHF, Congestive heart failure; *PDA,* pulmonary ductus arteriosus.

Truncus Arteriosus

OVERVIEW

Definition

Truncus arteriosus is a condition in which the arterial trunk arises out of both ventricles in fetal life and later divides into the aorta and the pulmonary artery with the development of the bulbar septum.

Incidence

Truncus arteriosus accounts for less than 1% of all congenital heart disease. Occurrence is 3 in 100,000 live births, with frequency more in females than in males.

Pathophysiology

Associated defects include the following:
- Large VSD
- Right aortic arch in 50% of cases
- DiGeorge syndrome should be considered in any infant with this defect.

OBJECTIVE DATA

Physical Examination

A physical examination should be conducted, with particular attention to vital signs, weight, general appearance, and the following:

Circulatory Status

Variable degrees of cyanosis may be present after birth.

Respiratory Status

Signs of CHF may develop within several weeks.

Cardiac Status

A harsh grade II to IV/VI systolic murmur, similar to VSD, that can go into diastole may be present at the upper left sternal border. An apical diastolic rumble with or without gallop may be present if pulmonary blood flow is large. A constant ejection click, bounding pulses, and wide pulse pressure may be present.

Diagnostic Procedures

Diagnostic procedures are outlined in Table 41-7.

Assessment

Differential diagnosis includes the following:
- TGA
- Hypoplastic right ventricle syndrome
- Hypoplastic left ventricle syndrome
- Double-outlet right ventricle
- Double-outlet left ventricle

THERAPEUTIC PLAN

Diuretics and digoxin are required to decrease pulmonary congestion.

Cardiac catheterization demonstrates the abnormal anatomy, as well as the hemodynamics and pressures. It can determine the size and branching pattern of the main pulmonary artery. An aortogram rules out truncal insufficiency and major stenosis in pulmonary arteries.

Early surgical repair is the treatment of choice. Most infants die of CHF between 6 and 12 months unless surgery is performed.

GENERAL CARE STRATEGIES FOR CONGENITAL HEART DEFECTS

When caring for a patient with a congenital heart defect in either the preoperative or postoperative period, some simple principles should be followed to ensure optimized care. The three major areas of concern are worsened CHF, increased shunt, and inadequate surgical correction. These can be easily followed up with careful histories and physical examinations. Parents should also be alerted to the same signs so that they can seek the earliest possible care to correct the problem. If an infant is experiencing hypoxic spell, place infant over the shoulder in the knee-chest position.

SUBJECTIVE DATA

The history should concentrate on the following:

Respiratory Status

Shortness of breath
Dyspnea
Inability to feed
Cyanosis (at rest or exacerbating factors)
Cough
Retractions
Grunting
Flaring

Cardiovascular Status

Sweating
Cyanosis
Pallor
Increased facial ruddiness
Increasing head size
Limb discrepancies
Mottling
Increasing edema

Abdominal Status

Increased abdominal girth
Vomiting
Constipation
Diarrhea

Renal Status

Decreased wet diapers or decreased urination.

Neurologic Status

Lethargy
Irritability
Seizures
Disorientation
Developmental delay (inability to achieve milestones)

OBJECTIVE DATA

Physical Examination

The physical examination should concentrate on the following:

Vital Signs/General Status

Failure to thrive/poor weight and height gain
Tachypnea
Tachycardia
Hypotension
Hypertension

Respiratory Status

Shortness of breath
Dyspnea
Cyanosis (at rest or exacerbating factors)
Cough
Retractions
Grunting
Flaring
Inspiratory rales
Wheezing

Cardiovascular Status

Murmur changes
Decreased pulses
Decreased capillary refill
Sweating
Cyanosis
Pallor
Increased facial ruddiness
Increasing head size
Limb discrepancies, mottling, and edema

Abdominal Status

Hepatosplenomegaly
Neurologic status
Lethargy
Irritability
Seizures
Disorientation
Developmental delay (inability to achieve milestones)

EVALUATION/FOLLOW-UP

During follow-up appointments, the patient must always be evaluated for recurrence of symptoms.

Consultation

All children with congenital heart lesions are followed by a pediatric cardiologist. A genetic evaluation may also be indicated if a genetic cause is suspected.

SUGGESTED READINGS

Kempe CH et al: *Current pediatric diagnosis and treatment,* Norwalk, Conn, 1997, Appleton & Lange.

Korones S, Bada-Ellzey H: *Neonatal decision making,* St Louis, 1993, Mosby.

Long W: *Fetal and neonatal cardiology,* Philadelphia, 1990, WB Saunders.

Park M: *The pediatric cardiology handbook,* St Louis, 1991, Mosby.

42 Congestive Heart Failure

ICD-9-CM

Left Ventricular Failure 428.1
Right Ventricular Failure 428.0
Hypertensive Heart Failure 402.91

OVERVIEW

Definition

Congestive heart failure (CHF) occurs when the heart is unable to maintain an output adequate to meet the metabolic demands of the body.

Incidence

Two million Americans have CHF.
400,000 new cases are diagnosed each year.
The 5-year mortality is greater than 50%.
CHF patients are six to nine times more likely to die from sudden cardiac death (Konstam and Dracup, 1994).
CHF is the most common inpatient diagnosis.

Pathophysiology

Symptoms occur as a result of organ hypoperfusion and inadequate tissue oxygen delivery due to a decreased cardiac output, decreased cardiac reserve, and pulmonary and venous congestion.

Systolic Dysfunction

Inotropic abnormalities
Decreased systolic emptying
Causes include myocardial infarction, cardiomyopathy, valvular disorder

Diastolic Dysfunction

Impaired ability of ventricle to accept blood due to abnormal ventricular filling
Causes include hypertension, coronary artery disease, left ventricular (LV) hypertrophy
Systolic and diastolic dysfunction may occur together (Guthery, 1998)
Compensatory mechanisms: Left ventricular dilation and hypertrophy, increase in systemic vascular resistance secondary to activation of the sympathetic nervous system and an increase in catecholamines, activation of the renin-angiotensin system

Precipitating Risk Factors

Coronary artery disease
Hypertension
Valvular disorder
Anemia (severe)
Thyroid disease
Cardiomyopathy
Arrhythmias
Infection
Pregnancy
Volume overload
Medications (e.g., beta-blockers, nonsteroidal antiinflammatory drugs [NSAIDs])
Decreased patient compliance

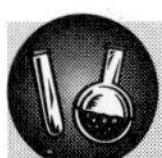

TABLE 42-1 Diagnostic Procedures: Congestive Heart Failure

Diagnostic Test	Findings	Cost ($)
Chest x-ray	Cardiomegaly, pulmonary congestion	77-91
Electrocardiogram	Evidence of ischemia, arrhythmias, LVH	56-65
Complete blood count	Anemia	18-23
Electrolytes/serum Creatinine/liver enzymes	Hyponatremia/renal abnormality/elevated AST and/or ALT due to passive congestion	23-30/electrolytes 18-24/creatinine 29-41/liver function
Thyroid function test	Hypothyroidism; check TSH in all patients ≥65 who present with heart failure and no obvious etiology	47-61/thyroid panel (without TSH); 86-109/with TSH
Serum albumin	Low albumin may cause an increase in extravascular volume	18-23
Urinalysis	Proteinuria, RBCs	15-20
Echocardiogram/radionuclide ventriculography	Measures left ventricular function (systolic vs. diastolic dysfunction)	675/echo 271-327/myocardial perfusion study

ALT, Alanine aminotransferase; *AST,* aspartate aminotransferase; *LVH,* left ventricular hypertrophy; *TSH,* thyroid-stimulating hormone; *RBC,* red blood cell.

SUBJECTIVE DATA

Past Medical History

Ask about listed risk factors.

Assess for coronary artery disease, chronic obstructive pulmonary disease, renal disease, diabetes, hypertension, previous myocardial infarction, valvular disease.

Medication

Recent use of beta-blockers, NSAIDs, calcium channel blockers

Family History

Ask about family history of heart disease, hypertension, diabetes mellitus. (CHF occurs as a result of an underlying pathology.)

Diet History

Recent increase in use of sodium

Increased consumption of fluids in patients with previous decompensated heart failure and known LV dysfunction

Description of Most Common Symptoms

Dyspnea on exertion, orthopnea/paroxysmal nocturnal dyspnea, edema, decreased exercise capacity, dry hacky cough, fatigue, recent weight gain, bloating-abdominal fullness, change in mental status (mainly in the **elderly**)

OBJECTIVE DATA

Physical Examination

A thorough examination should be performed, with attention to:

Vital signs, weight, general appearance: may be hypotensive, normotensive, or hypertensive. Pulse rate may be tachycardic. Weight may be increased (it is important to assess the time span over which the weight gain occurred).

Neck: Jugular venous distention

Chest: Basilar rales that do not clear with cough, wheezes

Cardiac: S3 gallop, S4 gallop, laterally displaced point of maximal impulse, murmur

Abdomen: Hepatomegaly, hepatojugular reflex, ascites

Extremities: Peripheral edema

The most specific diagnostic physical findings in a patient with symptoms include elevated jugular venous pressure, third heart sound and displaced PMI (Konstam and Dracup, 1994).

Diagnostic Procedures

Diagnostic procedures include those found in Table 42-1.

ASSESSMENT

List New York Heart Association functional class (I-IV).

Class I: No dyspnea with exertion

Class II: Dyspnea with maximal exertion

Class III: Dyspnea with minimal exertion

Class IV: Dyspnea at rest

TABLE 42-2 Differential Diagnosis: Congestive Heart Failure

Differential Diagnosis	Supporting Data
Pneumonia	Fever, cough, with or without sputum production, dullness or rales, and dyspnea Chest x-ray: Infiltrates Sputum: Purulence, hemoptysis, Gram stain
Myocardial infarction	Chest pain: Associated with or without activity ECG: Evidence of ischemia Laboratory data: Elevated CPKs, troponin
Arrhythmias	Palpitations, near syncope/syncope ECG: Evidence of bradycardia or tachycardia Electrolytes: Hypokalemia
Cirrhosis	Anorexia/nausea, jaundice, fatigue, weakness Ascites, hepatosplenomegaly, GI bleeding Anemia (microcytic secondary blood loss, macrocytic secondary iron deficiency), hyponatremia, prolonged protime

CPK, Creatine phosphokinase; *ECG,* electrocardiogram; *GI,* gastrointestinal.

Differential diagnosis include pulmonary disease, pneumonia, myocardial infarction, arrhythmias, cirrhosis, nephrotic syndrome (Table 42-2 and Figure 42-1).

THERAPEUTIC PLAN

The goal is to improve quality of life; treatment is aimed at the underlying etiology and symptom control.

Pharmaceutical

Systolic Dysfunction

Angiotensin-converting enzyme inhibitor
Decrease mortality and prolong survival in patients with CHF
Should be prescribed for all patients with systolic dysfunction unless contraindicated
Contraindications include intolerance or side effects, K^+ >5.5, signs of hypotension (Table 42-3)
Starting doses may need to be adjusted in the **elderly**

If cough or angioedema develops with an angiotensin-converting enzyme (ACE) inhibitor, an alternative may be the use of angiotensin II antagonists. These drugs have not received the same recommendation as ACE inhibitors in terms of CHF mortality and morbidity, although they have been used for that purpose (Table 42-4).

Diuretics

Diuretics decrease preload, dyspnea on exertion, orthopnea/PND, and edema (Table 42-5).

Increased doses may be needed in patients with renal failure, and decreased doses may be necessary in the **elderly.**
Use loop diuretics when a rapid response is needed (acute presentation of CHF). CAUTION: overdiuresis may lead to renal insufficiency or hypotension.
Complications of diuretic usage includes electrolyte imbalances and carbohydrate intolerance.

Digoxin

Digoxin increases the force of ventricular contraction in patients with LV systolic dysfunction. It should be used in conjunction with diuretics and ACE-I in patients with severe heart failure (0.125 to 0.25 mg QD; normal starting dose 0.25 mg QD).

Hydralazine and Isosorbide

If ACE inhibitors are contraindicated, an alternative may be the combination of hydralazine and isosorbide (Konstam and Dracup, 1994) (Table 42-6).

Beta-blockers

Ongoing research regarding use of beta-blockers in CHF is showing that there is a decrease in mortality in patients already stable on ACE inhibitors, diuretics, and digoxin. However, caution should be used when prescribing beta-blockers. Recurrent symptoms should be monitored closely. Carvedilol has been approved for use in mild to moderate CHF. Starting dose is 3.125 mg BID and should be titrated to tolerance (Massie and Amidon, 1998). Response may be less in African Americans (Table 42-7).

See Figure 42-2 for a summary of CHF (systolic dysfunction) pharmaceutical management.

Diastolic Dysfunction

Diastolic dysfunction pharmaceutical therapy includes the use of a negative inotrope such as a beta blocker or calcium channel blocker. Caution must be used with

Text continued on p. 254.

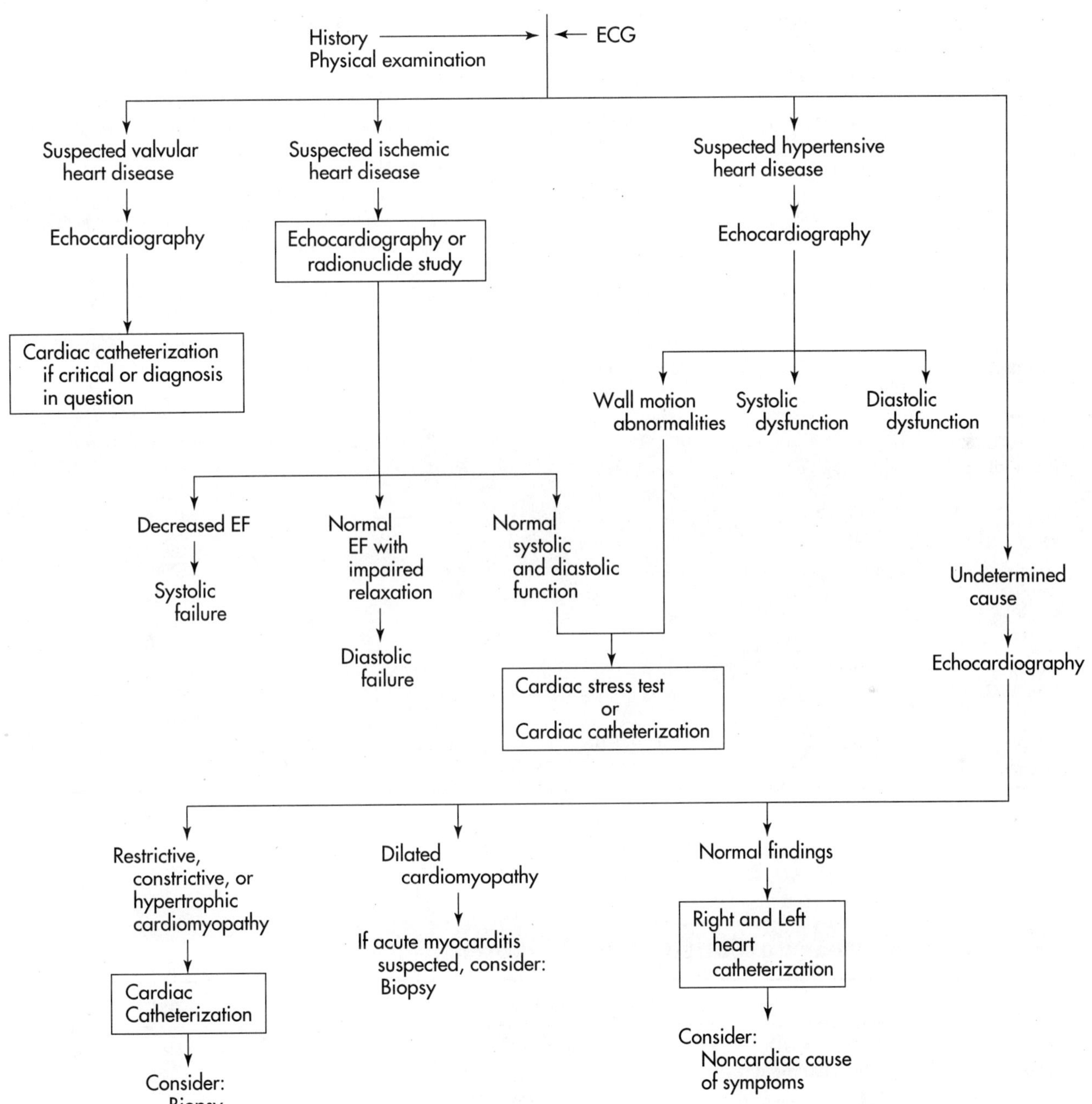

Figure 42-1 Algorithm for patient with congestive heart failure. *ECG,* Electrocardiogram; *EF,* ejection fraction. (From Greene HL, Johnson WP, Lemcke D: *Decision making in medicine,* ed 2, St Louis, 1998, Mosby.)

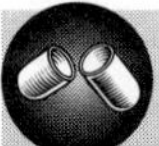

TABLE 42-3 Pharmaceutical Plan: Angiotensin-converting Enzyme Inhibitors

ACE Inhibitor	Initial Dose	Target Dose	Comments	Cost
Captopril (Capoten)	12.5 mg BID/TID	50 mg TID Max: 100 mg TID	Pregnancy: C first trimester, D second and third trimesters SE: Cough, angioedema, hyperkalemia, hypotension, elevated creatinine	$63-$67/12.5 mg (100); $68-$73/25 mg (100); $116-$124/50 mg (100)
Benazepril (Lotensin)	10 mg QD	40 mg QD Max: 80 mg/day	As above	$63/10-40 mg (100);
Moexipril (Univasc)	7.4 mg QD	15 mg QD Max: 30 mg/day	As above	$40/7.5, 15 mg (100)
Ramipril (Altace)	2.5 mg QD	5 mg BID Max: 10 mg BID	As above	$69/2.5 mg (100); $74/5 mg (100); $86/10 mg (100);
Trandolapril (Mavik)	1-2 mg QD	4 mg QD Max: 8 mg/day	As above	$63/1-4 mg (100)
Fosinopril (Monopril)	10 mg QD	20 mg QD Max: 40 mg/day	As above	$71/10 mg (100); $76/20 mg (100); $22/40 mg (30)
Enalapril (Vasotec)	2.5 mg BID	10 mg BID Max: 20 mg BID	As above	$72/2.5 mg (100); $91/5 mg (100); $96/10 mg (100)
Lisinopril (Prinivil/Zestril)	5 mg QD	20 mg QD Max: 40 mg QD	As above	$79/5 mg (100); $81/10 mg (100); $87/20 mg (100)
Quinapril (Accupril)	5 mg BID	20 mg BID Max: 20 mg BID	As above	$91/5-40 mg (100)

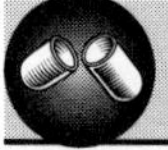

TABLE 42-4 Pharmaceutical Plan: Angiotensin II Antagonists

Drug	Dose	Comments	Cost
Losartin (Cozaar)	25-50 mg QD Max: 100 mg/day	Pregnancy: C first trimester, D second and third trimesters SE: Dizziness, insomnia, nasal congestion	$110/25, 50 mg (100)
Valsartan (Diovan)	80 mg QD Max: 320 mg/day	Pregnancy: As above SE: Dizziness, H/A	$114/80, 160 mg (100)

SE, Side effects; *H/A,* headache.

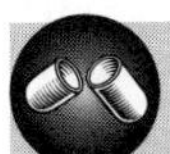

TABLE 42-5 Pharmaceutical Plan: Diuretics

Drug	Dose	Comments	Cost
Potassium Sparing		(Monitor K levels for hyperkalemia)	
Spironolactone (Aldactone)	25-200 mg/day in 4-5 divided doses Children: 1-3/kg/day in divided doses	Take with meals or milk Pregnancy: D SE: Diarrhea, vomiting, rash, pruritus, hyperkalemia Not recommended for children	$5-$39/25 mg (100); $71/50 mg (100); $119/100 mg (100)
Triamterene (Dyrenium)	25-100 mg /day Max: 300 mg/day Children: 2-4 mg/kg/day	Pregnancy: D SE: Diarrhea, weakness, nausea, fatigue, hyperkalemia	$32-$34/50 mg (100); $34/100 mg (100)
Amiloride (Midamor)	5-10 mg QD Max: 20 mg/day	Pregnancy: B SE: H/A, orthostatic hypotension, nausea, diarrhea, anorexia, hyperkalemia	$26-$46/5 mg (100)
Thiazide Type			
Chlorothiazide (Diuril)	250-500 mg QD/BID	Pregnancy: B SE: Adverse lipid values, photosensitivity, hypokalemia, hyponatremia	N/A
Hydrochlorothiazide (e.g., HCTZ, Esidrix)	12.5-50 mg QD	Pregnancy: B SE: Adverse lipid values, photosensitivity, hypokalemia, hyponatremia	$2-$13/25 mg (100); $2-$21/50 mg (100)
Metolazone (Zaroxolyn)	5 mg QD Max: 20 mg/day	Pregnancy: B SE: Hypokalemia, hyponatremia, hyperglycemia, hyperuricemia, gout, blurred vision	$53/2.5 mg (100); $59/5 mg (100); $68/10 mg (100)
Other:			
Indapamide (Lozol)	2.5 mg QD; after 1 week may increase to 5 mg/day	Pregnancy: B SE: H/A, nausea, rash, hypokalemia	$65/1.25 mg (100); $66-$85/2.5 mg (100)
Loop Diuretics			
Bumetanide (Bumex)	0.5-1 mg IV/IM 0.5-2 mg PO (1 mg Bumex is roughly = 40 mg furosemide)	Pregnancy: C SE: Muscle cramps, H/A, ototoxicity, electrolyte imbalance, hyperuricemia	$37-$45/1 mg (100); $63-$72/2 mg (100)
Ethacrynic acid (Edecrin)	0.5-1 mg/kg up to 50 mg IV 25-100 mg PO QD/BID Children: 25 mg QD	Use in infants not recommended Pregnancy: B SE: Fluid/electrolyte imbalance, ototoxicity, deafness, vertigo, tinnitus, GI upset, H/A, rash	$20/IV: 50 mg/vial; $30/25 mg (100); $43/50 mg (100)
Furosemide (Lasix)	1 mg/kg up to 20-40 mg IV 20-80 mg QD/BID PO Children: PO: 2 mg/kg/day as single dose	Pregnancy: C SE: Photosensitivity, xanthopsia, vertigo, paresthesia, jaundice, tinnitus, photosensitivity, hypokalemia	$2-$16/20 mg (100); $3-$22/40 mg (100); $6-$37/80 mg (100)
Torsemide (Demadex)	5-20 mg IV/PO QD	Pregnancy: B Interactions with Amphotericin B, anticoagulants, hypokalemia-causing medications, lithium, salicylates (high-dose) SE: Constipation, dizziness, GI upset, H/A	$53/5 mg (100); $49/10 mg (100); $53/20 mg (100); 100 (100) $216

GI, Gastrointestinal; *H/A,* headache; *N/A,* not available; *SE,* side effects.

Continued

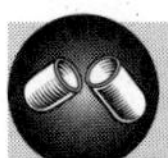

TABLE 42-5 Pharmaceutical Plan: Diuretics—cont'd

Drug	Dose	Comments	Cost
Combination Diuretics			
Triamterene, HCTZ (Dyazide)	1-2 caps QD	Pregnancy: C SE: Drowsiness, muscle cramps, weakness, H/A, GI upset, dry mouth, impotence, urine discoloration	N/A
Spironolactone + HCTZ (Aldactazide)	Used for maintenance: 4 tabs in single or divided doses	Pregnancy: Not recommended SE: Hyperkalemia, gynecomastia, H/A, menstrual changes, photosensitivity, GI disturbances	N/A

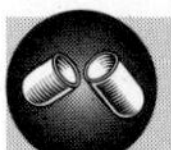

TABLE 42-6 Alternatives to ACE Inhibitors

Drug	Initial Dose	Maximum Dose	Side Effects	Cost
Hydralazine (Apresoline)	10-25 mg TID	100 mg TID	Pregnancy: C SE: Tachycardia, hypotension, dizziness, lupuslike syndrome, angina, palpitations, anorexia, N/V/D	\$2-\$21/10 mg (100) \$2-\$29/25 mg (100); \$3-\$44/50 mg (100)
Isosorbide dinitrate (Iso-Bid, Isordil)	10 mg TID	40 mg TID	Pregnancy: C SE: H/A, hypotension, dizziness	\$1-\$31/10 mg (100); \$2-\$50/20 mg (100)

From Konstam M, Dracup K:1994 Heart failure: evaluation and care of patients with left ventricular systolic dysfunction, Clinical Practice Guideline No. 11, AHCPR Publication 94-0612, Silver Springs, Md, 1994, Agency for Health Care Policy and Research, Public Health Service, US Department of Health and Human Services.

H/A, Headache; *N/V/D,* nausea, vomiting, diarrhea; *SE,* side effects.

TABLE 42-7 Pharmaceutical Plan: Beta-blockers

Drug	Initial Dose	Target Dose	Comments	Cost
Carvedilol (Coreg)	3.125 mg BID	25 mg BID	Beta blocker with alpha-1 blocking activity and antioxidant effects. Patient must not be fluid overloaded or hypotensive and must be on stable therapy for CHF. Give with food 2 hrs before ACE. Pregnancy: C SE: Dizziness, bradycardia, syncope	N/A

ACE, Angiotensin-converting enzyme; *CHF,* congestive heart failure; *N/A,* not available; *SE,* side effects.

diuretics to prevent overdiuresis; therefore they are not first-line agents. Aggressive blood pressure control is important.

Lifestyle/Activities

Weigh daily and record. Weight gain of 2 to 4 lb over a 2- to 3-day period should be reported.

Regularly exercise and stay active to improve functional capacity.

Stop smoking if appropriate.

Diet

Dietary restrictions: 2 g sodium diet, fluid restriction if appropriate, and decrease in alcohol consumption.

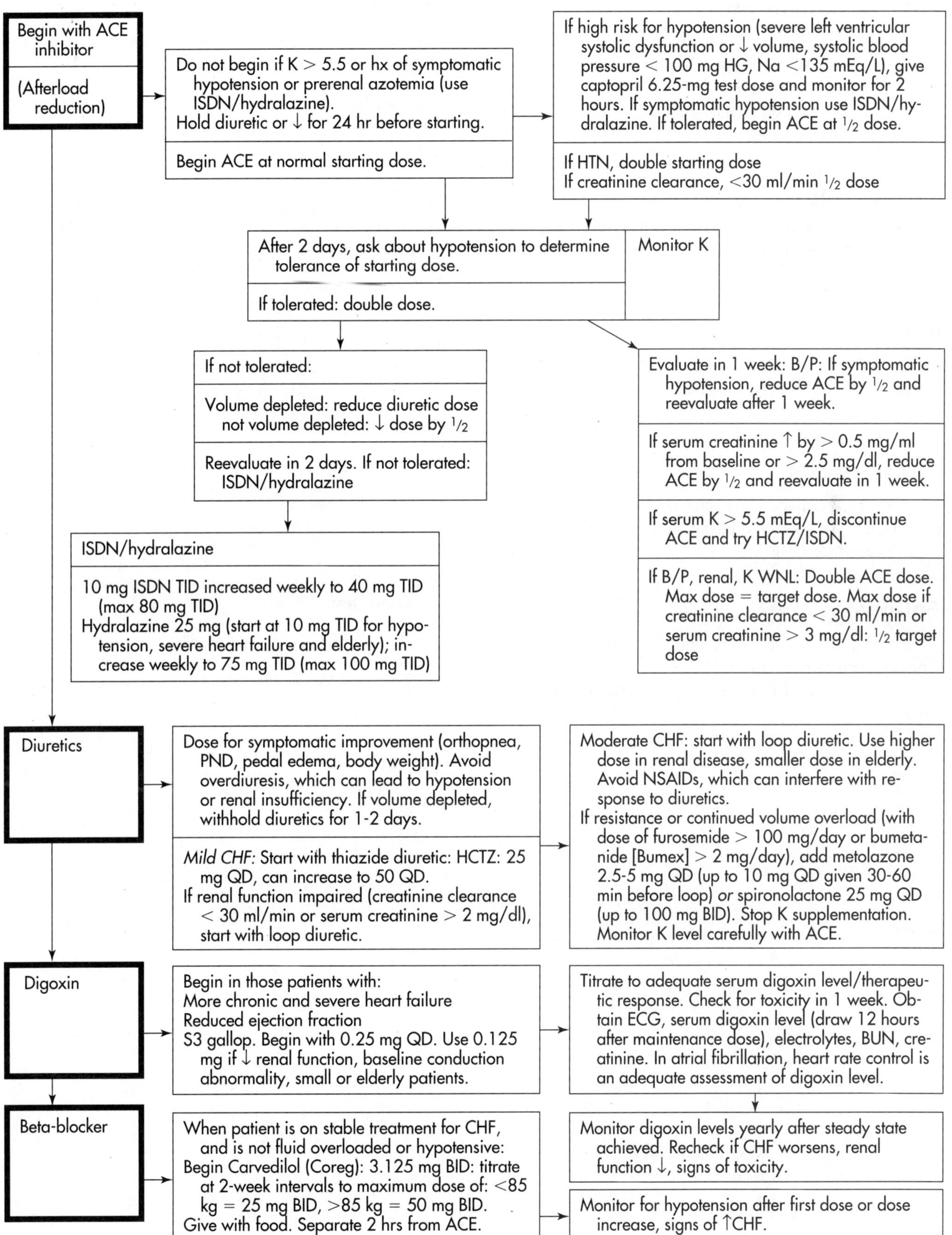

Figure 42-2 Algorithm for congestive heart failure (systolic dysfunction) medical management. *ACE*, Angiotensin-converting enzyme; *BUN*, blood urea nitrogen; *ECG*, electrocardiogram; *HCTZ*, hydrochlorothiazide; *HTN*, hypertension; *ISDN*, isosorbide; *Na*, sodium; *PND*, paroxysmal nocturnal dyspnea; *WNL*, within normal limits.

Patient Education

Patient and family education includes explanation of the diagnosis, prognosis, and symptoms of worsening heart failure and resultant interventions.

Medications and compliance include rationale for medications and side effects.

Family Impact

Chronic illness requires change in lifestyle in some instances, depending on how severe; may cause an alteration in family economics

Referral

Refer to physician: Cases of new onset heart failure or heart failure refractory to conventional therapy, **children** with CHF

Consultation

Discuss with collaborating physician before beginning digoxin. Carvedilol should be initiated by cardiologist since it can exacerbate CHF.

Follow-up

Return to clinic as necessary until CHF is compensated. Once compensated, routinely follow up every 1 to 3 months. Refer to physician if CHF refractory to intervention.

EVALUATION

Each visit to reevaluate for progressive or worsening symptoms

REFERENCES

Guthery D: Congestive heart failure, *J Am Acad Nurse Pract* 10 (1):31-38, 1998.

Konstam M, Dracup K:1994 Heart failure: evaluation and care of patients with left ventricular systolic dysfunction, Clinical Practice Guideline No. 11, AHCPR Publication 94-0612, Silver Springs, Md, 1994, Agency for Health Care Policy and Research, Public Health Service, US Department of Health and Human Services.

Massie BM, Amidon IH: Heart. In Tierney LM, McPhea SJ, Papadakiss MA, editors: *Current medical diagnosis and treatment,* ed 38, Stamford, Conn, 1998, Appleton & Lange.

SUGGESTED READINGS

Deedwania P, Carbajal E: Congestive heart failure. In Crawford M, editor: *Current diagnosis and treatment of cardiology,* Norwalk, 1995, Appleton & Lange.

Ellsworth A et al: *Mosby's 1998 medical drug reference*, St Louis, 1998, Mosby.

Healthcare Consultants of America, Inc: *1998 Physicians fee and coding guide*, Augusta, Ga, 1998, Healthcare Consultants of America, Inc.

Hoole A et al: *Patient care guidelines for nurse practitioners,* ed 4, Philadelphia, 1995, Lippincott.

Kern K: Congestive heart failure. In Greene H, Johnson W, Lemcke D, editors: *Decision making in medicine,* ed 2, St Louis, 1998, Mosby.

Miller M: Current trends in the primary care management of chronic congestive heart failure. *Nurse Prac: Am J Prim Health Care* 19(5):64-70, 1994.

Smith T, Braunwald E, Kelly R: The management of heart failure. In Braunwald E, editor: *Heart disease: a textbook of cardiovascular medicine,* ed 4, Philadelphia, 1992, WB Saunders.

43 Conjunctivitis

ICD-9-CM

Conjunctivitis 372.30
Acute Atopic Conjunctivitis 372.5
Other Chronic Allergic Conjunctivitis 372.14

OVERVIEW

Definition

Conjunctivitis is an inflammation of the conjunctiva. Ophthalmia neonatorum is conjunctivitis that occurs in the first month of life.

Incidence

Infection is common in **children**, less common in the adult population. Children are at increased risk because of physical contact with large groups of other children, inadequate hand washing, increased incidences of upper respiratory infection and acute otitis media. Several studies have concluded that bacteria are the most frequent cause of conjunctivitis followed by viruses.

Pathophysiology

Conjunctiva is a thin transparent mucous membrane covering the globe of the eye and the inner surface of the eye lids. Irritants that include bacteria, viruses, chemicals, allergens, and foreign bodies can result in inflammation of this tissue. Incubation for bacterial conjunctivitis is 2 to 3 days; for viral conjunctivitis it is 5 to 14 days.

Protective Factors Against

Tears continually wash the eye, inhibiting colonization and diluting/flushing irritants (Tears do not develop in infants to approximately 1 month of age.)

Factors That Increase Susceptibility

Poor hand washing
Exposure to someone with conjunctivitis
Exposure to impetigo
Presence of upper respiratory infection
Presence of allergens
Lack of tears/moisture in eye

Pathogenesis

Bacterial

Haemophilus influenza (40% to 50% of cases in **children**), often concurrent with acute otitis media
Streptococcus pneumoniae (10% of cases in **children**)
Moraxella catarrhalis
Staphylococcus aureus (most common in **adults**)
Proteus
Neisseria gonorrhea (hyperacute bacterial conjunctivitis)
Chlamydia trachomatis

Viral

Adenovirus: Most common
Enterovirus
Coxsackie virus
Herpes simplex: Complication: Optic neuritis

Ophthalmia Neonatorum

Neisseria gonorrhea
Complication: Destruction and/or perforation of the cornea

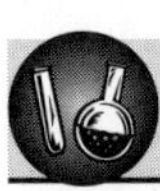

TABLE 43-1 Diagnostic Tests: Conjunctivitis

Diagnostic Test	Finding/Rationale	Cost
Culture/Gram stain	Culture and Gram stain are not usually necessary unless infection is severe, recurring, or resistant to routine treatment. Cultures should always be done on **infants** less than 1 month of age. Cultures of the eye and nasopharynx should be done concurrently. Cultures should be done for chlamydial trachomatis, gonorrhea, and bacteria. If a child has gonococcal or chlamydial ophthalmia neonatorum, both parents need to be screened for gonococcal and chlamydial infection (Baker, 1996).	\$31-\$39
Fluorescein stain	Fluorescein stain with examination under cobalt blue light source for corneal abrasion or trauma. Epithelial abrasion is brilliant green; deeper injuries are darker.	\$37/0.6 mg (360)

Chlamydia trachomatis
- Leading cause of ophthalmia neonatorum
- Complication: Conjunctival scarring

Herpes simplex
- Complications: Cataracts, keratitis, optic neuritis

Other listed bacteria

Antibiotics
- Primarily silver nitrate and erythromycin

Allergic/Vernal

Chemical: Irritant chemicals

Medications: Antibiotics: Gentamicin, neomycin, tobramycin, atropine, and eye drop preservatives

SUBJECTIVE DATA

History of Present Illness

Photophobia
Itching of eyes
Burning of eyes
Discharge from eyes
Eyelids stick together
Ask about visual changes

Associated Symptoms

Upper respiratory infection (URI), fever, ear pain, acute otitis media, throat pain

Past Medical History

Ask about history of:

Previous ear infection
Eye diseases
Recent illness or concurrent illness
Allergies
Recent swimming in chlorinated pool or contaminated pond
Recent herpes simplex infection or exposure to someone with herpes
Exposure to someone with conjunctivitis or impetigo
Use of contact lenses
History of sexually transmitted disease (STD) of self or partner(s)
Recent eye trauma or foreign body
Collagen vascular disease: Alert to the possibility of dry eyes
Infants: Ask mothers about treatment during pregnancy for STD.

Medications

Recent use of antibiotics or any eye preparations
Diuretics or antidepressants: May cause dry eyes
If corneal abrasion/trauma suspected, ask about tetanus immunity status

Family History

Ask about family history of eye diseases or atopic diseases such as allergic rhinitis, eczema, or asthma.

OBJECTIVE DATA

Physical Examination

Use a problem-oriented approach to physical examination.

Vital signs: Temperature, heart rate, respiratory rate, blood pressure in everyone over age 3 years
Skin: Color, character, herpes simplex or herpes zoster lesions
Ear, nose, throat: Looking for concurrent URI and acute otitis media (AOM)

TABLE 43-2 Differential Diagnosis: Conjunctivitis

Diagnosis	Supporting Data
Trauma/cornea abrasion	Watery discharge, usually unilateral, photophobia of infected eye, exposure to trauma or foreign body
Bacterial conjunctivitis	Presence of mucopurulent discharge; eyes matted on wakening, itching of the affected eye, mild pain, injection of conjunctival vessels, unilateral involvement that often becomes bilateral after 48 hours, less frequently mild photophobia *Chlamydia trachomatis:* Discharge thinner, more mucoid; pronounced photophobia; not self-limited, can persist for months Gonococcal: Hyperacute conjunctivitis: copious yellow-green purulent d/c, marked conjunctival injection, excessive edema, lid swelling and tender preauricular adenopathy.
Viral conjunctivitis	Watery discharge, eyes matted upon waking, presence of upper respiratory infection, bilateral eye involvement Herpes simplex: Possible presence of fever blister, vesicles on eyelids
Allergic conjunctivitis	Mild to moderate inflammation of conjunctiva, severe itching, marked burning, rhinorrhea, drainage watery, bilateral involvement, seasonal presentation, conjunctiva of the eyelids may have cobblestone appearance, symptoms are often reported to be more severe than clinical presentation
Iritis	Moderate pain, no discharge, diminished vision, poor pupillary reaction
Uveitis	Photophobia, pain, decreased vision
Chemical conjunctivitis	Discharge watery, injected conjunctiva, photophobia, marked burning, history of exposure to irritant
Ophthalmia neonatorum	Gonococcal infection: Presentation 24 to 48 hours after birth; dramatic symptoms: erythremic, edematous conjunctiva, perfuse purulent discharge, usually bilateral *Chlamydia trachomatis:* Presentation 5 to 12 days after birth; bilateral or unilateral, moderate inflammation, mucopurulent discharge Herpes simplex: Presents 48 hours to 14 days after birth; marked inflammation, mucoid drainage, herpetic vesicles Chemical: Presents within the first 24 hours of life; usually related to instillation of silver nitrate and to a lesser extent erythromycin, both used as chlamydial and gonococcal prophylaxis; mild injection, mucopurulent discharge; self-limited, usually resolved in 24 to 48 hours
Dacryocystitis	Infection of the lacrimal sac; caused by obstruction of the nasolacrimal system; common in infants and persons >40 years; unilateral presentation; tearing, discharge, pain, redness, swelling can be present; *Staphylococcus aureus,* ß-hemolytic streptococci, and *Streptococcus pneumoniae* often causative organisms

Eyes: Determine visual activity in school age and over. Assess visual fields, extraocular movements and pupillary functions. Examine sclera and conjunctiva for inflammation edema and discharge. Examine cornea for clarity and ulceration. Examine eyelid margins. Do funduscopic examination on all, although this may not be possible on **infants** and **small children**.

Heart sounds

Breath sounds: Looking for concurrent URI

Lymphatics: Focus on head and neck. Enlarged preauricular nodes are often present in viral and chlamydial conjunctivitis.

Diagnostic Procedures

Diagnostic procedures for conjunctivitis are listed in Table 43-1.

ASSESSMENT

Differential diagnoses include bacterial conjunctivitis, viral conjunctivitis, allergic conjunctivitis, chemical conjunctivitis, corneal abrasion/trauma, iritis, glaucoma, herpes simplex blepharitis (Table 43-2).

Table 43-3 compares different types of conjunctivitis.

THERAPEUTIC PLAN

Pharmaceutical

In general, ointments are better for **small children** since there is less blurring of vision. Most **adults** and **adolescents** prefer solutions (Table 43-4).

Concurrent Acute Otitis Media

It is best to use a betalactamase-resistant drug. There is no need to use topical antibiotics concurrently.

Table 43-3 Comparison of Different Types of Conjunctivitis

Type	Discharge	Conjunctiva	Unilateral vs Bilateral Itching	Pain/Photophobia/ Blurred Vision
Bacterial	Purulent/ mucopurulent	Mildly injected to markedly inflamed	Unilateral initially	Not usually a feature of typical conjunctival inflammatory process; consider more serious disease process: uveitis, keratitis, acute glaucoma, or orbital celulitis; Blurred vision is rarely associated with conjunctivitis
Viral	Serous or mildly mucopurulent	Hyperemic	Unilateral initially	
Allergic	Watery or stringy mucoid	Edematous or moderately inflamed	Itching bilateral	
Chemical	Serous	Inflamed and edematous	Depends on exposure	

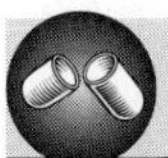

Table 43-4 Bacterial Conjunctivitis

Drug	Dosage	Comments	Cost
Sodium sulfacetamide 10% (Sulamyd or Bleph-10)	0.5-10 cm ointment in conjunctival sac QID for 7 days or 10% solution 2 gtts every 2 to 3 hours while awake	Effective, well tolerated, and inexpensive; weak to moderate activity against many gram-positive and gram-negative organisms Pregnancy: C Rare potential SE: Stevens-Johnson syndrome	$1-$16/oint: 10% (3.5 g); $2-$19/sol: 10% (15ml)
Bacitracin-polymixin (Polysporin)	0.5-1 cm in conjunctival sac QID for 7 days	Pregnancy: C Treat for 7 days Good coverage for gram-positive and gram-negative organisms	$2-$5/500 U/g (3.5 g)
Tobramycin (Tobrex) ointment or solution	Severe: Initially 2 gtts or ½ cm q3-4h Mild to moderate: 1-2 gtts or ½ cm q4h	Pregnancy: B Good coverage for gram-negative organisms, but poor coverage for gram-positive organisms	$10-$20/solution: 0.3% (5 ml); $20/oint: 0.3% (3.5 g)
Trimethoprim, polymyxin B (Polytrim)	1 gtt q3h for 7-10 days; max 6 doses/day	Not for infants <2 mos Pregnancy: C Good coverage for gram-positive and gram-negative organisms	N/A
Erythromycin ointment or solution (Ilotycin)	Small amount of ointment 1 or more times daily	Pregnancy: B SE: Superinfection, local irritation	$2-$5/oint: 5 mg/g (3.5 g)
Gentamicin, neomycin		Options for use, but have higher incidence of allergic reaction; not recommended as first choice Pregnancy: C	
Ciprofloxacin (Ciloxan); ofloxacin (Occuflox); norfloxacin (Chibroxin)	1-2 gtts q2h while awake for 2 days; then 1-2 gtts q4h while awake	High cost Poor coverage of *Streptococcus* species; potential for developing resistant pathogens; reserve for more severe ocular infections: bacterial keratitis Pregnancy: C SE: Superinfection, burning, lid margin crusting, pruritus, foreign body sensation, bad taste	$11/0.3% (2.5 ml)

N/A, Not available; *SE,* side effects.

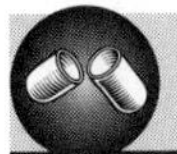

TABLE 43-5 Concurrent Otitis Media and Conjunctivitis Treatment

Drug	Dosage	Comments	Cost
TMP/SMX (Bactrim)	TMP: 8 mg/kg/day; SMX: 40 mg/kg/day in 2 divided doses	Children >2 mos Pregnancy: C SE: GI distress, crystalluria, hepatic or renal toxicity	$27-$43/susp: 200 SMX/ 40 SMX (480 ml)
Amoxicillin + clavulanate (Augmentin)	25 mg/kg/day (dose based on amoxicillin component)	Category B SE: GI upset, rash, urticaria, vaginitis, anaphylaxis	$27/amox: 125 mg/$31.25/5 ml (150 ml); $52/amox + clav: 250 mg/62.5 mg/5 ml

GI, Gastrointestinal; *SE*, side effects; *susp*, suspension; *TMP-SMZ*, trimethoprim-sulfamethoxazole.

Gonococcal conjunctivitis: Ceftriaxone (Rocephin) is drug of choice. Since over 30% of patients also have concurrent chlamydial STD, it is advisable to treat with supplemental oral antibiotics that are effective against chlamydia.

Table 43-5 outlines treatment for concurrent otitis media and conjunctivitis.

Opthalmia Neonatorum/Hyperacute Bacterial Conjunctivitis (Adults). Refer to ophthalmologist.

Gonococcal Conjunctivitis. Ceftriaxone 50 mg/kg/day IM as single dose. If organism is sensitive to penicillin, give aqueous penicillin G 100,00 U/kg/day (Baker, 1996). The client may need frequent eye irrigation with sterile normal saline to clear discharge.

Chlamydia Trachomatis. Erythromycin suspension 30 to 40 mg/kg/day PO in three divided doses.

Viral Conjunctivitis. Treatment is supportive. Cold compresses and topical vasoconstrictors may provide symptomatic relief. Topical antibiotics are rarely necessary since secondary bacterial infection is uncommon.

Topical antiviral agents can help to manage ocular herpes simplex or herpes zoster such as trifluridine (Viroptic).

Allergic Conjunctivitis (Table 43-6). Treatment should include allergen avoidance, cold compresses, topical vasoconstrictors, and antihistamine drops. See allergic rhinitis chapter for additional drug information.

All ages: Do not prescribe ophthalmic corticosteroids. They are associated with increased incidence of cataracts and glaucoma as well as uncontrolled virus proliferation.

Lifestyle/Activities

Comfort Measures

Wet compresses, cool or warm per patient's preference. Use cotton balls.

Children: May need distraction to keep from rubbing eyes.

Infection control

Patient and family should practice good hand washing.

Patient should keep hands away from face and eyes.

Patient's face, clothes, and towels should be kept separate from others. Use these linens one time only.

Patient should refrain from wearing contact lenses for 24 hours.

Patient should clean contact lenses and storage case with appropriate disinfectant.

Monitor other family members, especially siblings, for symptoms of conjunctivitis.

Children should stay home from school/day care until inflammation and discharge are gone, 24 to 48 hours after treatment begins.

Diet

No changes required

Patient Education

Medication Administration

Clean eye before medication administration.

To apply or instill: Gently separate eyelids, pull down lower lid toward the center of the eye. Place the drops or a thin line of ointment in pocket that is formed (Boynton, Dunn, and Stephens, 1994).

Infection should respond to treatment in 2 to 3 days.

Call if poor response to medication after 48 hours.

Instruct to call if symptoms worsen or vision decreases.

Referral/Consultation

Refer to an ophthalmologist.

Children: Infants under 1 month of age.

All ages: Corneal ulcer

Extensive corneal defect

Corneal inflammation

Suspected gonococcal infection (left untreated rapid and severe corneal involvement is inevitable, leading to ulceration/perforation and loss of vision)

Suspected herpes simplex infection

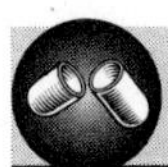

TABLE 43-6 Treatment of Allergic Rhinitis

Drug	Dose	Comments	Cost
Diphenhydramine (Benadryl)	Children: 5 mg/kg/day for 4 days in four divided doses. Adults: 25-50 mg TID for 4 day.	Systemic antihistamine Pregnancy: B SE: Sedation, anticholinergic effects: Dry mouth, constipation, blurred vision	\$2-\$15/elix: 12.5 mg/5 ml (480 ml) \$2-\$22/cap: 25 mg (100)
Cromolyn sodium ophthalmic solution 4% (Crolom) or	1-2 gtts four to six times per day	Mast cell stabilizer Not recommended <4 yrs (Crolom)	\$35/4% (10 ml)
Lodoxamide (Alomide)	1-2 gtts QID for up to 3 mos	Not recommended <2 yrs (Alomide) Contraindicated with soft contact lenses wear Pregnancy: B SE: Transient burning	
Levocabastine (Livostin)	1 gtt QID	Topical antihistamine well tolerated, rapid onset of action Not recommended for children Contraindicated: Soft contact wearers Pregnancy: C SE: Mild transient stinging, H/A, visual disturbances, cough, nausea, eye lid edema	N/A
Ketorolac tromethamine (Acular), diclofenac sodium (Voltaren)	1 gtt QID	Topical NSAIDS Well tolerated, rapid onset of action Not recommended for children Soft contact wear not recommended Pregnancy: C Transient stinging, superficial keratitis, allergic reactions, increased ocular bleeding	\$26-\$28/0.5% (5 ml)

H/A, Headache; *N/A*, not available; *NSAID*, nonsteroidal antiinflammatory drug; *SE*, side effects.

Any irregularities in pupil size or reaction
No improvement after 48 hours of treatment
Patient complains of any of the following: Moderate to severe pain, severe photophobia, decreased visual acuity

EVALUATION/FOLLOW-UP

Bacterial infection: No follow-up is necessary if patient responds to treatment.

Practitioner may want to follow up with severe cases.

Viral infection: Follow up for persistent symptoms.

Allergic conjunctivitis: Follow up for persistent symptoms. Possible referral to allergist or ophthalmologist may be necessary.

Ophthalmia neonatorum: Follow up as advised by referred physician.

REFERENCES

Baker RC: *Handbook of pediatric primary care,* Boston, 1996, Little Brown.

Boynton RW, Dunn ES, Stephens GR: *Manual of ambulatory pediatrics,* ed 4, Philadelphia, 1998, JB Lippincott.

SUGGESTED READINGS

Barker LR, Burton J, Zieve P: *Principles of ambulatory medicine,* Baltimore, 1995, Williams & Wilkins.

Dambro M: *Griffith's 5-minute clinical consult,* Baltimore, 1996, Williams & Wilkins.

Ellsworth A et al: *Mosby's 1998 medical drug reference,* St Louis, 1998, Mosby.

Healthcare Consultants of America, Inc: *1998 Physicians fee and coding guide,* Augusta, Ga, 1998, Healthcare Consultants of America, Inc.

Merenstein GB, Kaplan DW, Rosenberg AA: *Handbook of pediatrics,* Norwalk, 1994, Appleton & Lange.

Morrow G, Abbott R: Conjunctivitis, *Am Family Phys* 57(4):735-746, 1998.

Pellerano R, Bishop V, Silber T: Gonococcal conjunctivitis in adolescents: recognition and management, *Clin Pediatr* 33(2):114-116, 1994.

Ruppert SD: Differential diagnosis of pediatric conjunctivitis, *Nurse Pract* 21(7):12-26, 1996.

Weiss A, Brinser JH, Nazar-Stewart V: Acute conjunctivitis in childhood, *J Pediatr* 22(1):10-14, 1993.

Weiss A: Acute conjunctivitis in childhood, *Curr Probl Pediatr* 24(1), 4-11, 1994.

44 Constipation

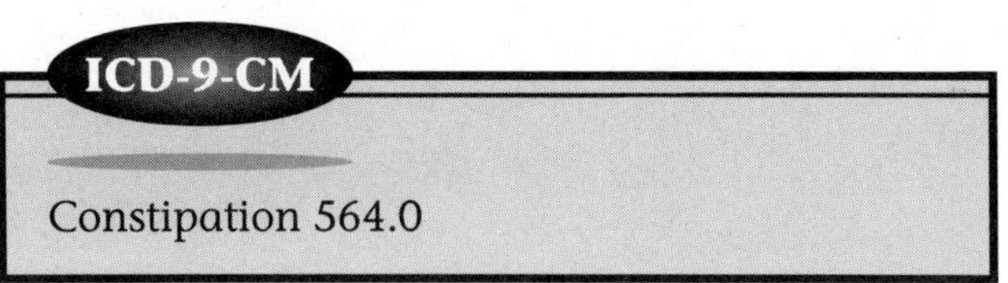

ICD-9-CM

Constipation 564.0

OVERVIEW

Definition

Constipation is a decrease in the frequency, size, and/or liquid content of bowel movements. The term refers more to the consistency than to the frequency of stools. Constipated stools are small, hard, and dry.

Incidence

Constipation is common among **children, adolescents,** and the **elderly.** Accounts for 2.5 million health care visits annually and **4% of all pediatric visits.**

Pathophysiology

Most constipation is functional (a disturbance in function with no change in the organ or system itself) with no organic cause. Contributing factors are low fiber in the diet, sedentary lifestyle, and voluntarily ignoring the urge to defecate because of lack of privacy or painful anal fissures or hemorrhoids.

Organic causes: Hirschsprung's disease, strictures, anal-rectal stenosis, and volvulus

Neuromuscular defects: Spinal cord lesions

Metabolic causes: Hypokalemia, dehydration, and hypothyroidism

Adverse drug effects: Narcotics, psychoactive drugs, and antidepressants

Eating disorders: Anorexia nervosa

SUBJECTIVE DATA

History of Present Illness

Decrease in number of stools (normal stooling pattern: newborns: >4×/day; 4-month-old: 2 stools per day; 4-year-old to adult: 1 stool per day. Stool size increases with age.

Hard, dry, small stools

Straining required to push stool out

Pain with defecation

Children: Nausea, vomiting, excessive urination, blood in stools, soiling of underclothes, and behavioral problems

Adults: Abdominal pain, blood in stools, weight loss, depression, diarrhea

History should include client's definition of constipation, usual bowel pattern, including recent changes, dietary recall, activity level, and current or recent use of medications, including laxatives.

OBJECTIVE DATA

Physical Examination

Abdominal examination: Distended with a palpable mass in the midline or left lower quadrant. Auscultation of bowel and percussion for dullness over fecal mass.

Rectal examination: Check for fissures, hemorrhoids, irritation, fecal impaction, and sphincter tone. NOTE: Clients with functional constipation usually have normal sphincter tone and large rectal vaults.

Children should be screened for urinary tract infections (UTIs) when constipation is present. Decreased fluids, which cause constipation, may also result in UTIs.

Diagnostic Procedures

Usually no diagnostic tests are necessary. Abdominal x-ray ($149-$162) may be necessary to help estimate the amount of stool retained or identify obstruction. In adults stools for occult blood should be obtained ×6. Figure 44-1 illustrates a typical workup for patients with heme-positive stools.

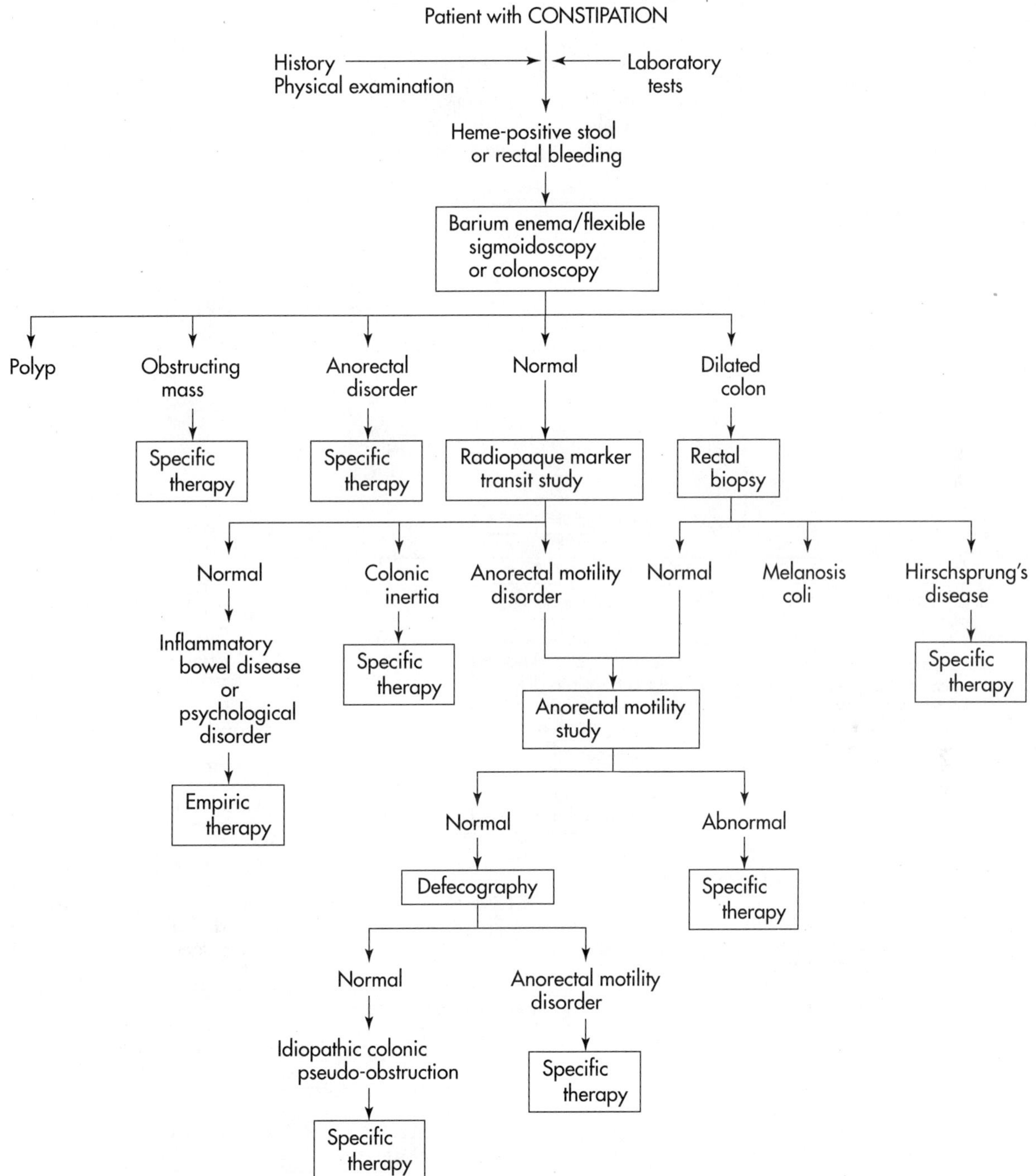

Figure 44-1 Algorithm for patient with constipation. (From Greene HL, Johnson WP, Lemcke D: *Decision making in medicine,* ed 2, St Louis, 1998, Mosby.)

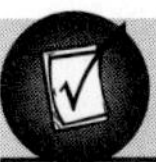

TABLE 44-1 Differential Diagnosis: Constipation

Diagnosis	Supporting Data
Functional constipation	History of holding or resistance to stooling, diet low in fiber and fluids, sedentary lifestyle
Toilet training resistance	History of traumatic toilet training attempts (e.g., being spanked or forced to sit on the toilet until stool is produced)
Normal straining of infancy	Soft stool
Hirschsprung's disease	Constipation from birth, rectal ampule empty, no meconium in first week of life
Partial bowel obstruction	Vomiting, abdominal pain
Rectal fissures or hemorrhoids (Ch. 88)	Bright red rectal bleeding, pain associated with stooling, fissures or hemorrhoids found on rectal examination
Hypothyroidism (Ch. 178)	Adults: Fatigue, dry skin, weight gain, heavy menses, cold intolerance, hair loss, sleeping more
	Decreased activity, poor growth and development, limb length reduction with increased upper to lower body segment ratio
Encopresis (Ch. 66)	Chronic constipation, which results in fecal impaction and involuntary soiling of underwear; common in school-age children.

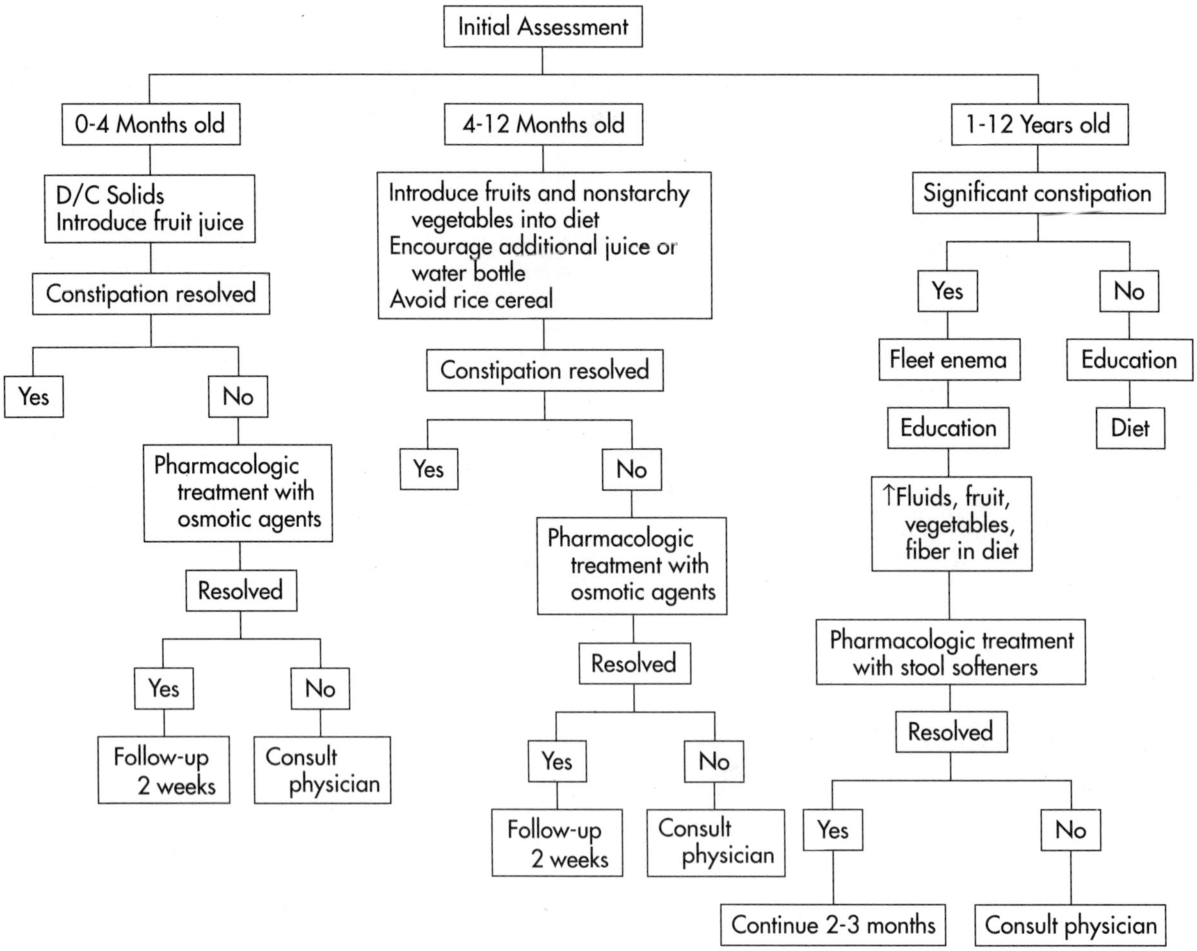

- Initial Assessment
  - 0-4 Months old
    - D/C Solids / Introduce fruit juice
    - Constipation resolved
      - Yes
      - No
        - Pharmacologic treatment with osmotic agents
        - Resolved
          - Yes: Follow-up 2 weeks
          - No: Consult physician
  - 4-12 Months old
    - Introduce fruits and nonstarchy vegetables into diet / Encourage additional juice or water bottle / Avoid rice cereal
    - Constipation resolved
      - Yes
      - No
        - Pharmacologic treatment with osmotic agents
        - Resolved
          - Yes: Follow-up 2 weeks
          - No: Consult physician
  - 1-12 Years old
    - Significant constipation
      - Yes
        - Fleet enema
        - Education
        - ↑Fluids, fruit, vegetables, fiber in diet
        - Pharmacologic treatment with stool softeners
        - Resolved
          - Yes: Continue 2-3 months
          - No: Consult physician
      - No
        - Education
        - Diet

Figure 44-2 Pediatric constipation treatment algorithm.

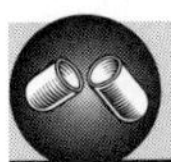

TABLE 44-2 Medications for Constipation or Impaction

Drug	Dose
Osmotic Agents	
Karo syrup	1-2 tsp/8 oz bottle/day ×3 days
Lactulose	Adult: 0.5-1 ml/kg/dose (max dose 3 oz) usually 30 ml HS but can be given BID to QID and titrated to effect
Stool Softener:	
Mineral oil	1-2 ml/kg/dose BID (max dose 8 oz)
	Adult: 100 mg PO QD or BID
Colace (docusate sodium) ($2-$87)	Child: <3 years of age, 10-40 mg/dose 3 to 6 years of age, 20-60 mg/dose
Peri-Colace (contains stimulant plus docusate)	Adult: 1-2 tabs or 15-30 ml PO QHS Child: 5-15 ml/dose
Laxatives	
MOM (magnesium hydroxide)	Adult: 5-15 ml q6h prn (400 mg/5 ml)
Senokot (senna)	Adult: 2 tabs or 1 tsp granules or 10-15 ml syrup PO QHS (max dose 8 tsp or 30 ml/day) Child: <5 years: 1-2 tsp >5 years: 2-3 tsp (max dose 2.5 tbsp)
Dulcolax (Bisacodyl) ($2-$4)	<5 years: 5 mg >5 years: 10 mg (max dose 4 tabs)
Suppositories	
Glycerin Dulcolax (bisacodyl) ($2-$10)	1 adult or pediatric suppository PR >2 years: 10 mg suppository
Enemas	
Mineral oil	Adult: 5-45 ml PO QHS
Sodium phosphate (Fleet)	Child: 5-20 ml PO/dose 1 adult or pediatric enema PRN
Fiber	
Metamucil (psyllium) ($5-$11)	1 tbsp/ 8 oz liquid QD
Citrucel (methyl-cellulose) ($12)	1 tbsp/ 8 oz liquid QD/BID/TID

ASSESSMENT

Diagnosis of functional constipation is made by detailed history and physical examination. Differential diagnoses include (Table 44-1):

Normal straining of infancy-soft stools
Hirschsprung's disease: Constipation from birth, rectal vault empty
Encopresis
Partial bowel obstruction
Irritable bowel syndrome
Rectal fissures or hemorrhoids
Hypothyroidism

THERAPEUTIC PLAN (Figure 44-2)

Child

Pharmaceutical

Stool softeners: Use only if other measures fail:
- Docusate sodium (Colace), 5 mg/kg/day, or
- Maltsupex
  - Age 1-5 years, 1 tsp BID; may increase to 2 tbsp BID
  - Age 5-15 years, 2 tsp BID; may increase to 2 tbsp BID
- Reduce daily dose once stools are soft.
- Continue for 2 to 3 months until regular bowel habits are established.

If there is significant constipation at presentation, give a pediatric fleet enema.

Pharmaceutical treatment for both adults and children is included in Table 44-2.

Diet

Infant (0-12 months): Introduce fruits and nonstarchy vegetables into diet. Encourage an occasional juice or water bottle. Avoid rice cereal. May be necessary to use Maltsupex 1-2 tsp TID.

Child (1-12 years): Encourage an increase of fiber, fluids, vegetables, and fruit.

Lifestyle/Activities

Child (1-2 Years): Retrain bowels: Have the child sit on the toilet for 20 minutes after meals. Educate child and parents about gastrocolic reflex.

Toddlers: If not completely potty trained, put the child back in diapers and remove all pressure related to toileting.

Adult (>12 years)

Pharmaceutical

Pharmacological measures: Use if general measures fail.

Stool softener:

Docusate sodium (Colace) 50 to 300 mg QD or docusate calcium (Doxidan) 240 mg QD. Short-term use only (up to 3 months)

Bulk-forming agents: Polycarbophil (Fibercon), methylcellulose (Citrucel), or psyllium (Effer-Syllium); begin with 1 tbsp daily and increase as needed to 3 tbsp daily; must be accompanied by plenty of fluids; may be used long term (see also Chapter 66).

Diet

Increase fluid intake to 1.5 to 2 L daily.

Increase fiber in the diet: Fresh fruits and vegetables, bran cereals, whole grain breads.

Patient Education

Increase daily exercise. Retrain bowel habits: Sit on the toilet ×15 minutes after meals. Do not ignore the urge to defecate.

Instruct the client to avoid chronic laxative use.

EVALUATION/FOLLOW-UP

Schedule follow-up visits every 2 weeks until normal bowel function resumes.

Refer any child who has a poor response to therapy or who exhibits emotional problems.

Refer adults over 50 with recurrent constipation presenting a change from their usual pattern.

Refer any client who has hemoccult-positive stools.

SUGGESTED READINGS

Arvin AM et al, editors: *Nelson textbook of pediatrics*, ed 15, Philadelphia, 1996, WB Saunders.

Boynton RW, Dunn ES, Stephens GR, editors: *Manual of ambulatory pediatrics*, ed 3, Philadelphia, 1994, JP Lippincott.

Dershewitz RA, editor: *Ambulatory pediatric care*, ed 2, Philadelphia, 1993, JP Lippincott.

Goepp JG, Santosham M: Oral rehydration therapy. In Oski MD, McMillan JA, editors: *Principles and practice of pediatrics updates*, Philadelphia, 1993, JP Lippincott.

Groothuis JR et al, editors: *Current pediatric diagnosis and treatment*, ed 12, Norwalk, Conn, 1995, Appleton & Lange.

McCargar LJ, Hotson BL, Nozza A: Fibre and nutrient intakes of chronic care elderly patients, *J Nutr Elderly* 15(1):13-31, 1995.

Rosenthal M: Diarrhea organisms are becoming media stars, *Infect Dis Child* 10(1):10-11, 1997.

Straughn A, English B: Oral rehydration therapy: a neglected treatment for pediatric diarrhea, *MCN* 6(5):1-5, 1996.

Uphold CR, Graham MV: *Clinical guidelines in family practice*, Gainesville, Fla, 1994, Barmarrae Books.

Contact Dermatitis

ICD-9-CM

Contact Dermatitis 692.9
Rash 782.1

OVERVIEW

Definition

Contact dermatitis is an eruption of the skin related to contact with an irritating substance or allergen. Secondary bacterial infection can occur, increasing inflammation.

Incidence

Contact dermatitis occurs in all ages and both sexes. There is no ethnic predisposition to the condition.

Pathophysiology

The epidermal reaction is caused by sensitized T lymphocytes after contact with an antigen or irritating substance. If produced by an antigen, it is considered a type IV delayed hypersensitivity reaction that takes several hours to manifest.

Protective Factors Against

Avoid known antigens

Factors That Increase Susceptibility

Jewelry
Cosmetics
Travel
Nickel
Rubber, latex
Plants
Detergents

SUBJECTIVE DATA

History of Present Illness

Rash 10-12 hours after exposure
Pruritus
Edema and erythema
Stinging, burning, and pain

Past Medical History

History of previous allergen exposure followed by pruritic rash

Medications

Recent use of an antimicrobial agent, topical antihistamine, topical anesthetics

Family History

Not usually significant

Psychosocial History

Occupation and exposures
Hiking, grass cutting
New clothes, perfume, detergent, food

Associated Symptoms

Fever

OBJECTIVE DATA

Physical Examination

Undress patient and check entire body for lesions.
Skin: Erythematous macules, papules, and vesicles (Figure 46-1). May have bullae with drainage. Secondary lesions

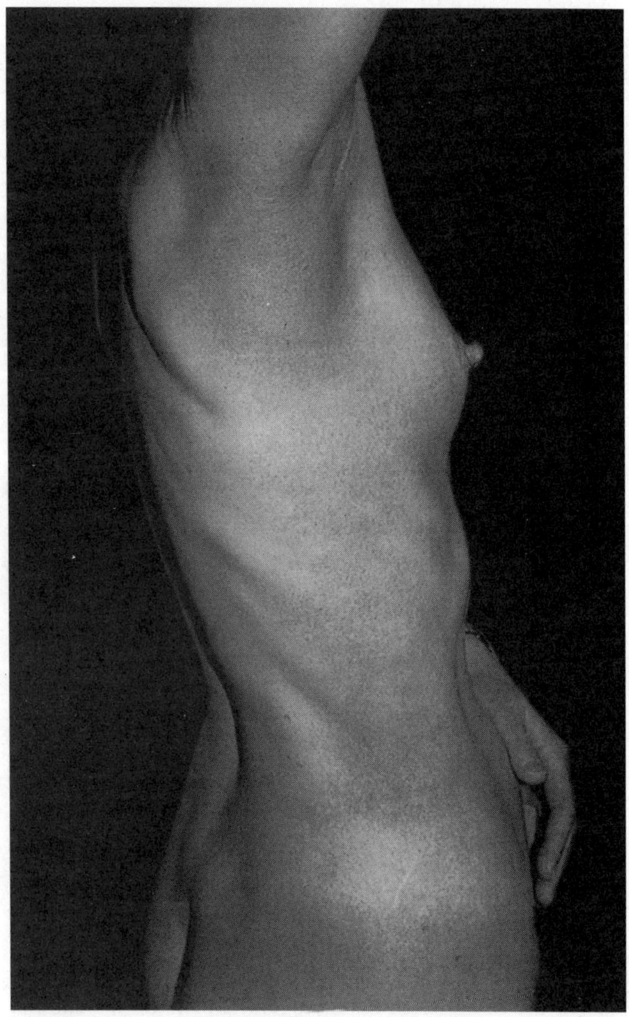

Figure 45-1 Diffuse allergic reaction occurring in a patient allergic to poison ivy who has ingested raw cashew nuts, the oil of which cross-reacts with the oleoresin of poison ivy. (From Habif TP: *Clinical dermatology,* ed 3, St Louis, 1994, Mosby.)

with crusting, excoriation, and lichenification may be present.

Lesions are on exposed parts and have bizarre distribution patterns. Swelling may be present.

The location of the rash helps provide clues to the offending antigen:

- Generalized: Airborne (paint, ragweed), bath oil, soap, powder, topical medications
- Scalp: Hair dyes, sprays, shampoos, hair preparations
- Forehead: Hat bands
- Eyelids: Eye makeup (e.g., eye shadow, eyeliner, mascara)
- Earlobes: Nickel in earrings
- Face: Cosmetics
- Perioral: Lipstick, toothpaste, mouthwash
- Neck: Perfumes
- Hands: Soap, nickel, lotion, chemicals, fingernail polish or remover (can inflame cuticle)
- Arms: Wristbands, soap, poison ivy or other plant, chemicals, new unwashed clothing
- Axilla: Deodorants
- Trunk: New unwashed clothing, nickel or rubber in clothing (belts, bra straps)
- Anogenital: Menstrual pads, contraceptives (condoms, foam, gels), plant/poison ivy (camping without rest-room facilities)
- Feet: powders, shoes, athlete foot medicine

TABLE 45-1 Differential Diagnosis: Contact Dermatitis

Diagnosis	Supporting Data
Tinea	Linked with heat and humidity; rash is more round than seen in contact dermatitis; usually affects face, neck, and arms
Impetigo	**Classically occurs in children;** history of other children/family member with similar lesions; poor hygiene may be evident; often described as a honey-colored crusted lesion; often seen on the face, under the nose, or on the chin; can occur elsewhere

Diagnostic Procedures

Laboratory Tests

None may be necessary.

Gram stain ($26 to $32) and culture ($22 to $28) will rule out impetigo.

Skin scraping will rule out scabies.

Potassium hydroxide (KOH) prep test ($19 to $23) will rule out tinea.

Patch test will help patient to know what to avoid in the future.

ASSESSMENT

Differential diagnoses for contact dermatitis include those outlined in Table 45-1.

THERAPEUTIC PLAN

Pharmaceutical

Pharmaceutical treatment is outlined in Table 45-2.

Antihistamine of choice may be used for itching and to decrease edema.

Antibiotics may be used for secondary infection (refer to Chapter 97, for choices).

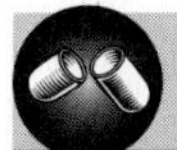

TABLE 45-2 Pharmaceutical Plan: Contact Dermatitis

Drug	Dose	Comment	Cost ($)
Topical corticosteroids	Midpotency (fluocinonide gel 0.05% BID or TID; or triamcinolone 0.1%) to high-potency corticosteroids (amcinonide 0.1%; or desoximetasone 0.25%)	Use for localized involvement only and *never* on the face or in body folds Taper number of applications per day	21-25/fluocinonide 4-27/triamcinolone 16/Amcinonide 10-16/desoximetasone
Tars	Fototar or LCD 10%	Use for chronic dermatitis with lichenification only	N/A
Prednisone	60 mg for 4 days, 40 mg for 5 days, 20 mg for 5 days		7-31

NOTE: For more information about prescribing topical corticosteroids, please refer to Appendix R.
LCD, Liquor carbonis detergens (coal tar solution); *N/A,* not available.

Lifestyle/Activities

Avoid irritant/antigen if known.

Diet

Usually noncontributory

Patient Education

Cool, moist compresses or tub bath with colloidal oatmeals
Calamine lotion to area
Can bandage areas with wet dressings several times a day

Family Impact

None

Referral/Consultation

Refer the patient to a dermatologist for patch testing.
Consult with the dermatologist if there is no improvement.

Follow-up

See the patient until symptoms subside.

EVALUATION

Patient is lesion free.
No further episodes because of avoidance of allergen or irritant

REFERENCES

Boynton R, Dunn E, Stephens G: *Manual of ambulatory pediatrics,* ed 4, Philadelphia, 1998, JB Lippincott.

SUGGESTED READINGS

Berger T, Goldstein S, Odom R: Skin and appendages. In Tierney L, McPhee S, Papadakis M, editors: *Current medical diagnosis and treatment,* ed 36, Norwalk, Conn, 1998, Appleton & Lange.
Ellsworth AJ et al: *Mosby's medical drug reference,* St Louis, 1998, Mosby.
Habif TP: *Clinical dermatology,* ed 3, St Louis, 1994, Mosby.
Healthcare Consultants of America, Inc: 1998 Physicians fee and coding guide, Augusta, Ga, 1998, Healthcare Consultants of America, Inc.
Pierce N: Bacterial infections of the skin. In Barker L, Burton J, Zieve P, editors: *Principles of ambulatory medicine,* ed 4, Baltimore, 1995, Williams & Wilkins.

46 Corneal Abrasion/ Foreign Body

ICD-9-CM

Corneal Abrasion 918.1
Abrasion Due to Contact Lenses 371.82

OVERVIEW

Definition

A corneal abrasion is a disruption in the epithelial surface of the cornea, resulting in tearing, blepharospasm, and severe pain.

Incidence

Corneal abrasions are one of the most frequent of eye emergencies and the most common sports related eye injury seen.

Anatomy/Pathophysiology

The cornea is the transparent outer "window" and primary focusing element of the eye (Figure 46-1). The cornea has five distinct layers. From the outermost layer inward, these are the epithelium, Bowman's membrane, stroma, Descemet's membrane, and the endothelium. Normally no blood vessels exist within the cornea. Its nutrition is chiefly derived from the vascular limbus and atmospheric oxygen. Lymphatic drainage is absent.

Mechanical or chemical factors that disrupt the epithelium result in a corneal abrasion. Because of the exposure of sensory nerve endings, even the smallest injuries are painful.

Protective Factors Against Corneal Abrasion

The corneal epithelium is made up of transparent cells that have the ability to regenerate quickly. The epithelium prevents organisms from entering the eye.

Factors That Increase Susceptibility

Persons who wear contact lenses have a higher incidence of corneal abrasions.

SUBJECTIVE DATA

History of Present Illness

It is essential to ask the following questions:

What was the time and mechanism of injury? (Use of high-speed drills, and grinders should raise the suspicion of an intraocular foreign body.)
What are the present complaints?
Does he or she normally wear glasses or contact lenses?
Has there been any visual loss?

Past Medical History

Document allergies, tetanus immunization status, and history of eye disease or surgery.

Medications

Eye medications (e.g., over-the-counter antibiotics, moisturizers, tears)

Family History

Not applicable

Psychosocial History

It is important to ascertain whether the patient is living with someone or has a family member or friend if he or she will need assistance with medications or follow-up.

Description of Most Common Symptoms

A corneal abrasion may produce significant pain, tearing, light sensitivity, foreign body sensation, and blepharospasm and possible alterations in vision.

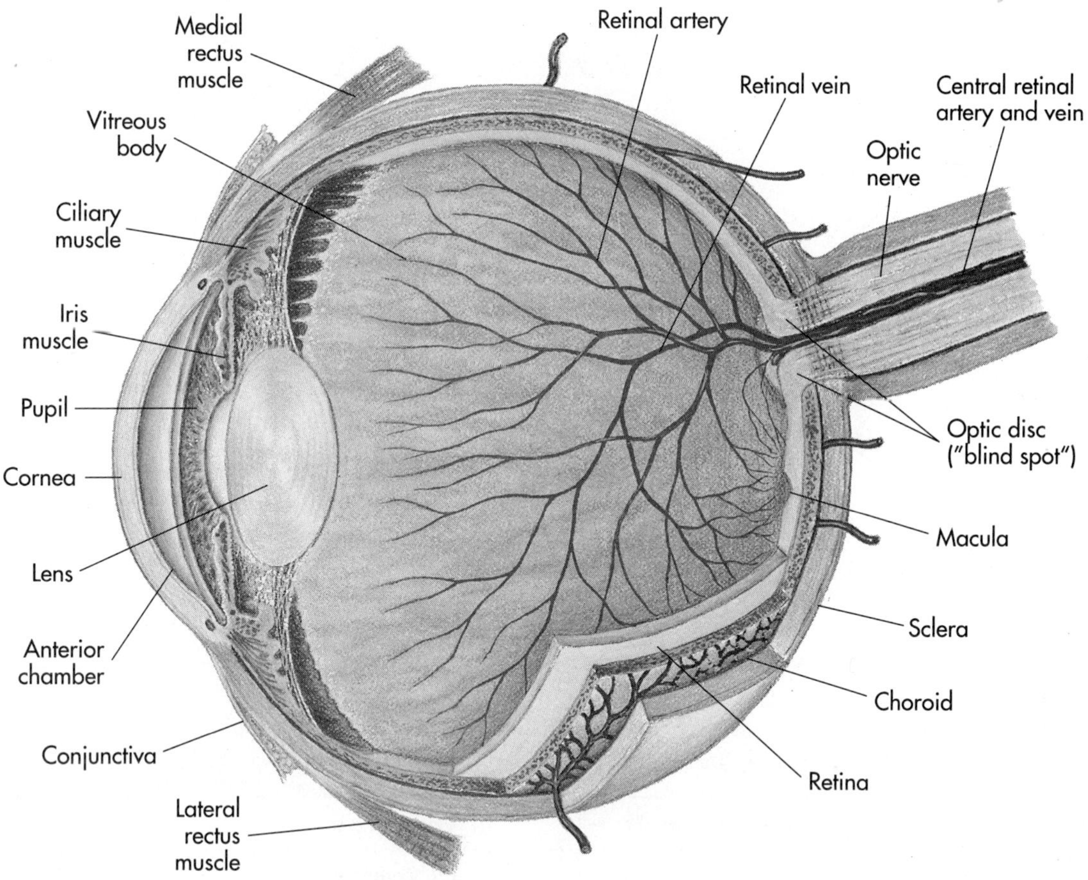

Figure 46-1 Anatomy of the human eye. (From Seidel HM et al: *Mosby's guide to physical examination,* ed 4, St Louis, 1999, Mosby.)

Associated Symptoms

Rhinorrhea

OBJECTIVE DATA

Physical Examination

For eye injuries, it is essential to measure visual acuity. Visual acuity may be decreased if the corneal abrasion is large or lies in the visual axis. A rapid-onset, short-acting topical anesthetic should be administered before beginning the physical examination. The cornea may be examined with a penlight, checking for clarity and the presence of a foreign body or laceration. Conjunctival injection, tearing, and blepharospasm are commonly seen.

The eyelid should be everted to check for a foreign body (Figure 47-2). The patient looks down, and the examiner gently grasps the upper eyelashes and positions a cotton-tipped applicator horizontally at the superior border of the tarsal plate. The lid is everted by applying gentle traction to the eyelid and slight downward pressure on the cotton applicator, moving the eyelid outward and upward. Foreign bodies are often found in the superior temporal cul-de-sac of the orbit and can usually be removed with a sterile moistened cotton tip applicator.

A slit lamp facilitates the eye examination if one is readily available. Illumination with blue light following staining with a fluorescein strip identifies the corneal abrasion.

Diagnostic Procedures

Diagnostic procedures are outlined in Table 46-1.

If a corneal foreign body is seen, the initial attempt at removal should be with a stream of sterile saline solution. If this fails, the foreign body should be removed using a commercial eye spud or 25-gauge needle with a 1- to 3-ml syringe as a handle, and magnification. The patient must be totally cooperative and have his or her head firmly stabilized. Use of a cotton-tipped applicator on the cornea is not recommended, because it may further disrupt the corneal epithelium.

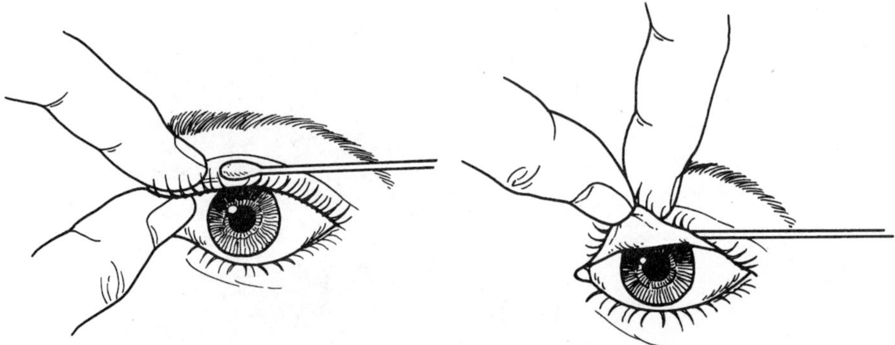

Figure 46-2 Everting the eyelid. (From Pfenninger JL, Fowler GC: *Procedures for primary care physicians,* St Louis, 1994, Mosby.)

TABLE 46-1 Diagnostic Procedures: Corneal Abrasion

Procedure	Findings/Rationale	Comments	Cost
Fluorescein staining is important to assess for integrity of the corneal epithelium	The following technique is used: Instill one or two drops of a topical anesthetic (proparacaine or tetracaine). Wet a fluorescein strip with sterile saline, and pulling down the lower eyelid, touch the strip to the inside of the lid. (Do not rub the strip across the front surface of the eye, because this may cause a corneal abrasion.) Ask the patient to blink to spread the stain over the ocular surface. If a corneal abrasion is present, the fluorescein is taken up by the affected area, which will appear bright green when a penlight illuminates it. When a cobalt blue filter is used over the penlight, the corneal abrasion is more easily visualized.	Pregnancy: C Temporary yellowing of eye, fades in 6-12 hr; may discolor urine for 24-36 hr; will stain contact lenses; wait at least 1 hr before reinserting lenses	$37/0.6 mg (300)
Slit lamp	Provides a magnified view of the anterior structures; allows for better depth perception of injury or foreign body		$108-$133

ASSESSMENT

Differential Diagnosis

Differential diagnoses include those outlined in Table 46-2.

THERAPEUTIC PLAN

Pharmaceutical

Treatment is designed to foster rapid healing, relieve the patient's pain, and prevent secondary infection. The pharmaceutical plan is outlined in Table 46-3.

Cycloplegic medications paralyze the ciliary muscles and cause dilation of the pupil. They are sometimes used to augment pain relief. Appropriate tetanus prophylaxis needs to be given if it has been more than 5 years since the patient has had a booster. Patients usually require oral analgesics for home use, but **topical anesthetics are absolutely contraindicated;** repeated use may delay healing and cause permanent corneal damage.

Lifestyle/Activities

Although eye patching has been traditionally recommended, recent studies refute the long-held belief that patching reduces the pain and improves the healing of corneal abrasions. Since no benefit has been proved, and the practice may actually cause harm in some patients, practitioners should feel confident about not using patches with superficial traumatic corneal abrasions. It is essential that contact lens wearers with corneal abrasions not be patched. Patching may increase the chance of infection, especially with *Pseudomona* or other gram-negative organisms.

Diet

Not applicable

Patient Education

If the patient is wearing an eye patch, it is important to tell him or her not to drive because of the loss of binocular vision. Prevention of infection in the affected eye should be stressed. Describe or demonstrate how to instill eye drops or ointment if appropriate.

Family Impact

The patient will probably need assistance with administration of eyedrops. Emphasize that follow-up in 24 hours is crucial.

Referral

All eye injuries should be referred to an ophthalmologist if healing has not occurred within 24 to 48 hours.

Consultation

True ophthalmological emergencies that require immediate consultation include acute visual loss, chemical burns, and penetrating eye trauma. Deeply imbedded or iron-containing foreign bodies should also be seen by an ophthalmologist for immediate treatment.

Follow-up

Patients should be reevaluated for corneal healing in 24 hours.

EVALUATION

The cornea has healed when reepithelialization has occurred and potential for infection no longer exists.

TABLE 46-2 Differential Diagnosis: Corneal Abrasion

Diagnosis	Supporting Data
Herpetic keratitis	Single or multiple dendrites seen on fluorescein staining
Corneal laceration	Deep injury through the cornea
Corneal ulcer	Whitening of underlying corneal stroma

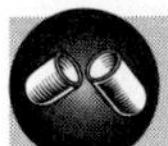

TABLE 46-3 Pharmaceutical Plan: Corneal Abrasion

Drug	Dosage	Comments	Cost
Gentamicin	One drop QID	Good gram-negative coverage	$4-$15/3 mg (5 ml)
Sulfacetamide 10%	One drop QID	Rare incidence of hypersensitive reactions	$3-$19/10% (15 ml)

SUGGESTED READINGS

Bresler M, Sternbach G: *Manual of Emergency Medicine,* St Louis, 1998, Mosby.

Clini D et al: *Emergency Medicine*, ed 4, New York, 1996, McGraw-Hill.

Ellsworth A et al: *Mosby's 1998 medical drug reference,* St Louis, 1998, Mosby.

Healthcare Consultants of America, Inc: *1998 Physicians fee and coding guide,* Augusta, Ga, 1998, Healthcare Consultants of America, Inc.

Kaiser PK: A comparison of pressure patching versus no patching for corneal abrasions due to trauma or foreign body removal, *Ophthalmology* 102:1936-1942, 1995.

Newell FW: *Ophthalmology: principles and concepts*, ed 8, St Louis, 1996, Mosby.

Rosen P, Barker R: *Emergency medicine,* ed 4, St Louis, 1997, Mosby.

Vaughn DG, Asbury RE: *General ophthalmology,* Norwalk, Conn, 1995, Appleton & Lange.

Zagelbaum B: Treating corneal abrasions and lacerations, *Physician Sports Med* 25:38-44, 1997.

Cough

ICD-9-CM

Cough 786.2
Smoker's Cough 491.0

OVERVIEW

Definition

Cough can be acute or chronic. An acute cough is generally defined as being present for less than 3 weeks. Chronic cough is one that lasts longer than 3 weeks. Cough is a physiological reflex to protect the airways by clearing secretions and foreign particles.

Incidence

In the nonsmoking population, persistent cough is reported in 14% to 23%. For adults who smoke half a pack per day, 25% report a chronic cough. In those who report more than two packs per day, 50% report a chronic cough. Cough is the fifth most common symptom seen in outpatient clinics, resulting in 30 million visits annually.

Pathophysiology

The cough reflex has five components:

1. Cough receptors
2. Afferent nerves (vagus, trigeminal, glossopharyngeal, and phrenic)
3. A cough center located in the medulla and separate from the respiratory center
4. Efferent nerves (vagus, phrenic, intercostal, lumbar, trigeminal, facial, and hypoglossal)
5. Effector organs (diaphragm, intercostal and abdominal muscles, and muscles of the larynx, trachea, and bronchi, as well as upper airway and accessory respiratory muscles)

An effective cough has three components:

1. Rapid inhalation of a large volume of air followed by closure of the glottis
2. Elevation of intrathoracic pressures as a result of the contraction of abdominal and thorax muscles
3. As the pressure increases, the glottis opens suddenly and expels the trapped air, thus producing the cough

SUBJECTIVE DATA

History of Present Illness

Ask the patient about the following:

Was the onset of the cough sudden?
How long has the cough been present?
Is the cough productive or nonproductive?
If productive, is it clear, mucoid, or purulent?
Description of cough: harsh, barking, or coarse?
Was the cough preceded by an upper respiratory infection or a lower respiratory infection, exposure to an allergen, or a choking/feeding episode?
Is the cough present during the day or night?
Is it worse at night or morning?
Does any associated shortness of breath or wheezing accompany the cough?
In a **child** (especially age 1-3 years): Is there the possibility of a foreign body?
Are there alleviating or precipitating factors?
- Cough worse after exercise
- Seasonal variation
- Decrease in cough with use of metered-dose inhalers or antibiotics
- Exposure to irritants (smoking, pollen, dust, chemicals, perfumes)
- Recent weight loss: Indicator of systemic disease

Associated Symptoms

Other symptoms may help to lead to the diagnosis (Table 47-1).

Past Medical History

Ask the patient about the following:

Asthma
Chronic obstructive pulmonary disease
Congestive heart failure
Gastroesophageal reflux disease
Postnasal drainage syndromes:
- Allergic rhinitis
- Acute sinusitis
- Chronic sinusitis
- Vasomotor rhinitis
- Primary nasal polyposis

Psychiatric illnesses

Medication

Ask the patient about the following:
- Angiotensin-converting inhibitor therapy
- Frequent use of antacids
- Cough syrups and drops

Family History

Cystic fibrosis
Asthma/COPD
Allergies
Smokers

Psychosocial History

Tuberculosis exposure
Smoker/exposed to smoke
Occupational/environmental exposure
Ask about current and past jobs
- Specific tasks performed
- Exposures to chemicals, fumes, dusts
- Exposure to asbestos, silica dust, or coal dust

Diet History

Food allergies
Eating late at night or lying down after meals

OBJECTIVE DATA

Physical Examination

General appearance: Comfort level, use of accessory muscles, spontaneous coughing dyspnea, cyanosis, chronically ill appearance
Head/eyes/ears/nose/throat: Signs of sinusitis, postnasal drainage, boggy nasal membranes, cobblestoning of pharyngeal mucosa, lymphadenopathy, jugular venous distention, position of trachea
Lungs: Wheezes, rhonchi, crackles, AP diameter, decreased breath sounds
Cardiovascular: Murmurs, rubs, gallops, extra heart sounds
Abdominal: Organomegaly, epigastric tenderness
Extremities: Edema, digital clubbing

Diagnostic Procedures

Diagnostic procedures are outlined in Table 47-2.

ASSESSMENT

Differential Diagnosis

Differential diagnoses are outlined in Table 47-3 and Figure 47-1.

THERAPEUTIC PLAN

General measures for acute cough include:

Smoking cessation
Avoiding environmental irritants
Air humidification
Cough suppressants
Inhaled beta agonists (if wheezing present)
Avoid toxins

Pharmaceutical

The pharmaceutical plan for patients with a cough are outlined in Table 47-4.

Treatment for chronic cough depends on the suspected diagnosis. A stepwise approach is suggested by Philip (1997).

Step 1: Treat empirically for postnasal drip with first-generation antihistamine/decongestant
- If symptoms improve but persist, add nasal steroids
- CT of sinuses if cough remains uncontrolled after 2 weeks
- If chronic sinusitis is identified, treat with antibiotics, decongestant spray, and combination antihistamine/decongestant drug. Consider referral to ear-nose-throat specialist if no improvement

Step 2: Evaluate for asthma:
- FEV_1/FVC (reduced ratio)
- FEV_1 before and after bronchodilator (improvement by 15% in asthma)
- If asthma confirmed: Avoid allergens, treat asthma appropriately (see Chapter16)

Step 3: If asthma is not confirmed (if not already done):
- CXR
- CT of sinuses

Step 4: Empirical treatment for GERD: High-dose proton

TABLE 47-1 Associated Symptoms: Cough

Associated Symptoms	Considerations for Possible Diagnosis
DOE or orthopnea	CHF
Bloody sputum, weight loss	Lung cancer or TB
Substernal burning, indigestion, regurgitation of digested material, hoarseness, bitter taste in mouth	GERD
Paroxysmal dry hacking cough made worse by cold air, exercise, laughing, or allergen exposure	Asthma
Tickle in throat, sensation of secretions in throat, frequent clearing of throat	Postnasal discharge and allergic rhinitis
Disappears with sleep, worse when attention drawn to it	Psychogenic cough (rare)
Children with recurrent URIs, poor weight gain, fatty stools	Cystic fibrosis
High fever, dyspnea, productive cough	Pneumonia
Acute onset with URI	Bronchitis
Dry cough after bronchitis	RAD secondary to allergies
Fever	Infections, especially TB, sarcoidosis, connective tissue lung disease

CHF, Congestive heart failure; *DOE,* dyspnea on exertion; *GERD,* gastroesophageal reflux disease; *RAD,* reactive airway disease; *TB,* tuberculosis; *URI,* upper respiratory infection.

TABLE 47-2 Diagnostic Tests: Cough

Test	Findings/Rationale	Cost ($)
CXR	Rule out pneumonia, CHF, TB, unexplained cough, lung mass; evaluate for gas trapping, peribronchial thickening, alveolar infiltrates, cardiomegaly. When patient with chronic productive cough has normal CXR, most likely causes are asthma, bronchitis, or bronchiectasis. A dry cough may be caused by primary lung cancer, treatment with ACE inhibitors or inhaled foreign body. All **children** with chronic cough should have a CXR.	77-91
PFT	COPD, often normal even with a diagnosis of asthma, helpful in **children >5 yr old;** low VC suggests restrictive defect; reduction in FEV_1 suggests COPD.	27-323
PEFR	Quick measurement of FEV (see Appendix L)	N/A
Sputum for AFB	Rule out TB	30-37
Barium swallow	Rule out GERD	201-240
24-hr esophageal probe	Rule out GERD	340-407
Nasal smear	Postnasal drainage syndrome	60-71
Sweat test	Cystic fibrosis	16-20
PPD	TB	15-18
Bronchial provocation test	Asthma	130-157
Nasopharyngeal swab	Pertussis	N/A

ACE, Angiotensin-converting enzyme; *AFB,* acid-fast bacillus; *CHF,* congestive heart failure; *COPD,* chronic obstructive pulmonary disorder; *CXR,* chest x-ray evaluation; *FEV,* forced expiratory volume; FEV_1, forced expiratory volume in 1 second; *GERD,* gastroesophageal reflux disease; *N/A,* not available *PFT,* pulmonary function test; *PPD,* purified protein derivative; *TB,* tuberculosis, *VC,* ventilatory capacity.

TABLE 47-3 Differential Diagnosis: Cough

Diagnosis	Supporting Data
Acute Cough	
URI/LRI	Upper and lower respiratory infections are the most common causes of acute cough. Rhinorrhea, fever, crackles (pneumonia)
FB aspiration (**children**)	Sudden onset of cough and SOB, wheezing
Allergy/irritant exposure	Allergic shiners, cobblestoning of mucus membranes, allergic salute
Chronic Cough	
Postnasal drainage	Frequent clearing of throat, or use of antihistamines (may be concurrent with allergic rhinitis), excess mucus production, smoking
Smoking	Smoke >½ packs/day
Asthma (Ch. 16)	Diffuse, polyphonic, musical wheezes most consistent with asthma.
GERD (Ch. 78)	Heartburn, coughing at night
Recurrent viral infections	Rhinorrhea, low grade temperatures, laryngitis, croup
Cystic fibrosis (Ch. 49)	Recurrent infections of lower respiratory tract, GI manifestations: steatorrhea, diarrhea, and FTT
TB (Ch. 184)	Chronic productive cough lasting >3 wks, fever, night sweats, chills, anorexia, weight loss, fatigue
Pneumoconiosis	Persistent, progressive cough, and SOB, end inspiratory "Velcro" crackles
Carcinoma	Symptoms may be late in clinical picture; early symptoms are caused by encroachment on airways (cough, sputum, hemoptysis), or pain, or weight loss
CHF (Ch. 42)	Dyspnea, fatigue, edema, cough, nocturia, nocturnal angina
Medications	ACE inhibitors

ACE, Angiotensin-converting enzyme; *CHF,* congestive heart failure; *FTT,* failure to thrive; *GERD,* gastroesophageal reflux disease; *GI,* gastrointestinal; *SOB,* shortness of breath; *TB,* tuberculosis.

pump inhibitor (80 mg omeprazole) to ensure complete suppression (sensitivity of 83% to 90%)
Lifestyle changes: Medications, raise head of bed
If no improvement: Endoscopy or 24-hour esophageal pH monitoring

Step 5: No improvement: Bronchoscopy
Negative findings: Repeat step 1 and consider less common diagnosis (< 6% of patients have one of these less common diagnoses)
Any **child** who coughs and has a history of recurrent pneumonia or FTT should have a sweat chloride test; also consider PPD and nasopharyngeal swab for pertussis
An evaluation for HIV is also appropriate at this time

Lifestyle/Activities

Avoid smoking/use smoking cessation strategies

Diet

Not applicable

Patient Education

Smoking cessation
Identify and treat allergies
Preventive gear for occupational exposures

Family Impact

Depends on diagnosis, and extent of interference with ADLs

Referral

If coughing continues, consider referral for bronchoscopy.

Consultation

Discuss possible diagnostic strategies with MD or pulmonary specialist.

EVALUATION

Acute cough syndromes should resolve within 3 weeks as the underlying illness resolves. If cough persists longer than 3 to 4 weeks, begin workup for chronic cough. If treating

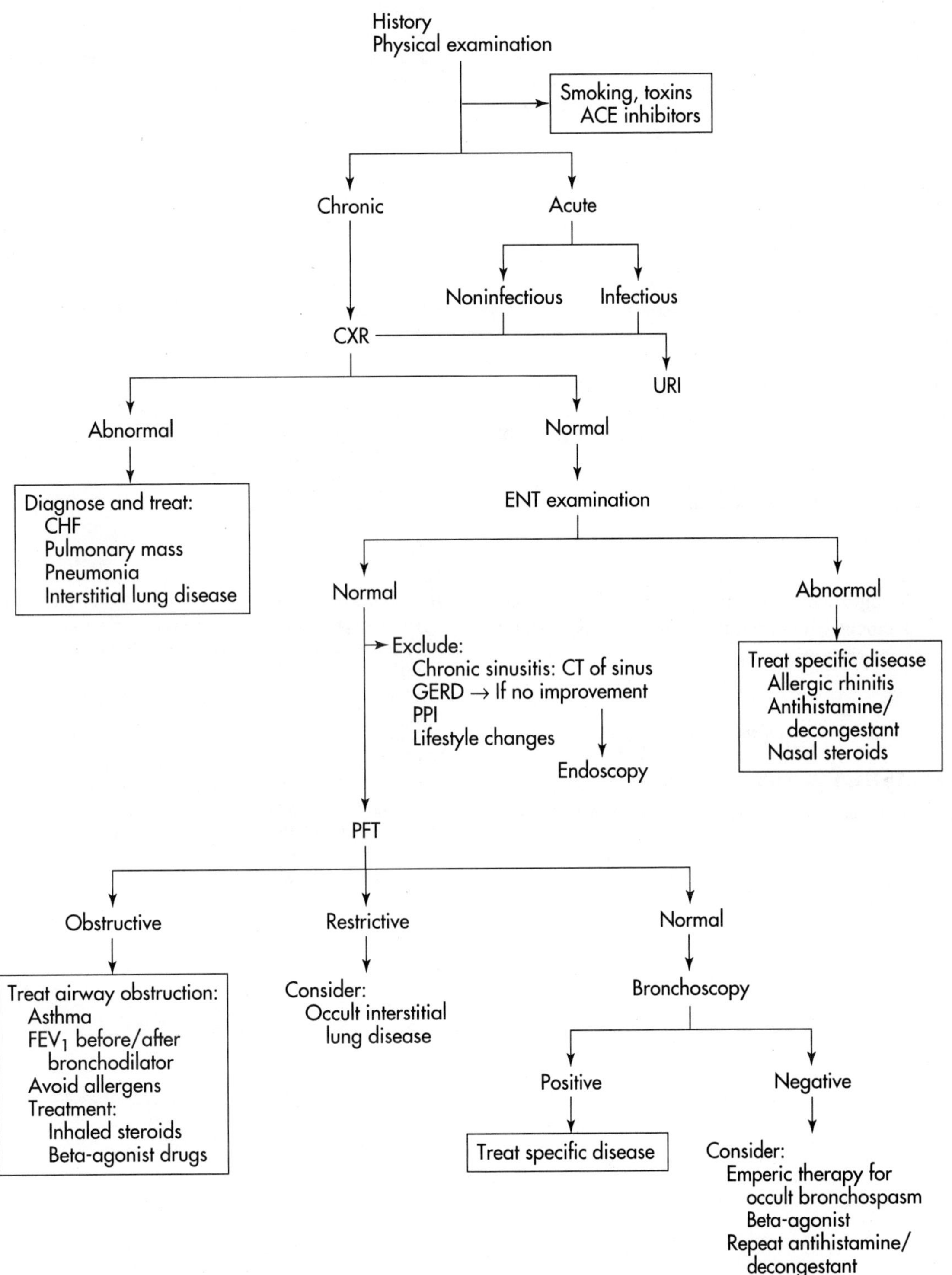

Figure 47-1 Algorithm for a patient with a cough. *ACE,* Angiotensin-converting enzyme; *CHF,* congestive heart failure; *CT,* computed tomography; *ENT,* ear, nose, throat; *FEV,* forced expiratory volume 1 second; *GERD,* gastroesophageal reflux. (Adapted from Greene HL, Johnson WP, Lemcke D: *Decision making in medicine,* ed 2, St Louis, 1998, Mosby.)

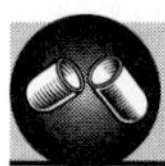

TABLE 47-4 Pharmaceutical Plan: Cough

Drug	Dosage	Comments	Cost
Dextromethorphan antitussive (Robitussin, Vicks Formula, Delsym [sustained action])	Adults: 10-30 mg q6-8h Child: 2-6: 2.5-7.5 mg q4-8h 6-8 (maximum 30 mg/24h) 6-12 yr: 5-10 mg q4h or 15 mg q6-9h Sustained release: Adult: 60 mg q12h 6-12 yr: 30 mg q12h 2-6 yr: 15 mg q12h	Pregnancy: C SE: Dizziness, nausea	$2/lozenges: 2.5 mg (20) $3/syrup: 3.5 mg/5 ml (120 ml)
Guaifenesin expectorant (Humibid, Robitussin)	Adult: 200-400 mg q4h 6 mo-2 yr: 25-50 mg 2-6 yr: 50-100 mg 6-12 yr: 100-200 mg	Pregnancy C SE: GI upset, dizziness, H/A, rash	$72/liquid: 100 mg/5 ml (480 ml)
Benzonatate (Tessalon Perles)	>10 yr: 1 perle (100 mg) TID, maximum 600 QD	Pregnancy C SE: Sedation, H/A, dizziness, GI upset, pruritus, skin eruptions, nasal congestion	$47-$84/100 mg (100)

chronic cough empirically for GERD, asthma, or allergies and no improvement occurs within 4 to 6 weeks, consult with or refer to a specialist.

REFERENCE

Philip E: Chronic cough, *Am Family Physician* 56:1395-1404, 1997.

SUGGESTED READINGS

Collins R: *Algorithmic diagnosis of symptoms and signs,* New York, 1995, Igaku-Shoin.

Corrao W: Chronic persistent cough: diagnosis and treatment update, *Pediatr Ann* 25:162-168, 1996.

Ellsworth A et al: *Mosby's 1998 medical drug reference,* St Louis, 1998, Mosby.

Healthcare Consultants of America, Inc: *1998 Physicians fee and coding guide,* Augusta, Ga, 1998, Healthcare Consultants of America, Inc.

Knoper S: Cough. In Greene H, Johnson H, Lemcke D, editors: *Decision making in medicine,* St Louis, 1998, Mosby.

Newman K: Chronic cough: a step by step diagnostic workup, *Consultant* 35:1535-1542, 1995.

Smith P, Britt E, Terry P: Common pulmonary problems: cough, hemoptysis, dyspnea, chest pain, and the abnormal chest x-ray. In Barker L, Burton J, Ziever P, editors: *Principles of ambulatory medicine,* ed 4, Philadelphia, 1995, Williams & Wilkins.

Wilmott R, Dato M: Respiratory diseases. In Rudolph A, Kamei R, editors: *Rudolph's fundamentals of pediatrics,* ed 2, Norwalk, Conn, 1998, Appleton & Lange.

Cushing's Disease

ICD-9-CM

Cushing's Disease 255.0

OVERVIEW

Definition

Cushing's disease is a result of extended glucocorticoid excess (hypercortisolism).

Incidence

Occurs in 2 to 4 persons per million per year
More common in **women 20 to 50 years old**
Rare in **children**

Physiology/Pathophysiology

Adrenal Gland

Controls the body's adjustment to an upright position
Permits accommodation to intermittent rather than a constant intake of food
Influences immune reactivity, blood cell formation, cerebral function, protein synthesis, and many other body processes

Cortisol

Principal glucocorticoid excreted by the adrenal gland
Influences appetite and well-being
Maintains blood sugar concentrations by promoting hepatic glucogenesis
Indirectly affects heart rate and pumping force by controlling synthesis of epinephrine in the adrenal medulla
Critical in the physiological response to stress and illness

Hypercortisolism

Hypercortisolism or Cushing's disease is a result of a pathological condition of the pituitary gland or the adrenal cortex.
Most cases of Cushing's disease result from hypersecretion of the adrenocorticotropic hormone (ACTH) from the pituitary gland with resultant bilateral adrenal hyperplasia.
Almost all of these cases result from pituitary microadenomas; a smaller number are caused by adrenal adenomas or carcinoma.
Cushing's syndrome results from a pathological condition of the adrenal gland.
An iatrogenic cause of Cushing's syndrome is long-term corticotropic or glucocorticoid use; this is the most common cause in **children.**

SUBJECTIVE DATA

Past Medical History

Hypertension
Diabetes
Osteoporosis
Amenorrhea
Medical conditions associated with glucocorticoids, including but not limited to

Rheumatoid arthritis
Asthma
Lymphoma
Skin disorders
Chronic obstructive pulmonary disease
Allergic disorders

Medications

Ask about use of glucocorticoids

Family History

Autoimmune disorders
Hypertension
Diabetes

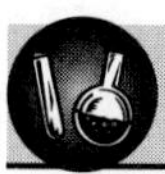

TABLE 48-1 Diagnostic Tests: Cushing's Disease

Test	Findings/Rationale	Comments	Cost ($)
Dexamethasone suppression test	Screening test to exclude diagnosis of Cushing's syndrome; used when diagnosis seems unlikely or the presentation is vague; more false positives than with the urinary free cortisol test; normal <5 μg/dl; if value >5 μg/dl, workup for Cushing's disease is indicated	Obesity, acute stress, agitated depression, and alcoholism can affect results Dexamethasone 1 mg is given PO at 11:00 PM, then plasma cortisol level is drawn at 8:00 AM	210-270/suppression test; 60-76/plasma cortisol
24-hr urinary excretion of cortisol (free cortisol)	Normal <120 μg; screening test used when diagnosis of Cushing's seems likely; urinary cortisol more widely used; using both urinary and plasma tests is advisable at times	Minimal elevations of plasma cortisol result in marked elevations in urinary cortisol; not affected by obesity	73-95/urinary excretion
Dexamethasone 0.5 mg PO every 6 hr for 2 days	This test is more definitive and used if results of screening tests are positive	<3.5 mg on the second day or plasma cortisol level <5 μg/dl on third day rules out Cushing's syndrome	73-95/24-hr 17-OHS level

Laboratory precision of the above values is imperative.

Psychosocial History

Depression
Insomnia
Mood swings
Confusion
Suicidal ideation
Anxiety

Diet History

Weight gain
Nausea

Description of Most Common Symptoms

Weight gain
Increased deposition of fat in upper body resulting in classic moon face, buffalo hump, and truncal obesity
Plethora or beefy red discoloration of the face
Muscle wasting as evidenced by thin extremities
Muscle weakness
Fatigue
Hypokalemia
Skin changes including telangiectasia over the face
Atrophy and thinning of the skin with easy or spontaneous bruising
Ecchymoses
Acne
Hyperpigmentation
Poor wound healing
Hypertension and diabetes mellitus

Associated Symptoms

Development of purplish abdominal striae
Menstrual irregularities including amenorrhea and oligomenorrhea
Hirsutism and slight balding in women
Impotence and decreased libido
Bone mineral loss, producing osteoporosis and back pain
Crush fractures of the vertebrae
Hip or wrist fractures may occur after minimal trauma

Lability of mood, depression, insomnia, anxiety, mania, and/or psychoses

OBJECTIVE DATA

Physical Examination

A complete physical examination should be performed, with particular attention to the following:

Vital signs: Blood pressure
Weight: Gain
Body habitus: Increased subcutaneous fat in the upper body: moonface, buffalo hump, truncal obesity
Cardiovascular: Edema
Musculoskeletal: Muscle wasting, muscle weakness
Skin: Telangiectasia over the face, atrophy and thinning with bruising, ecchymoses, purplish abdominal striae
Hair: Thinning, coarse, hirsutism

Diagnostic Procedures

Diagnostic procedures are outlined in Table 48-1.

Additional testing should include a comprehensive metabolic panel ($28 to $39) to identify hypokalemia, hypernatremia, or hyperglycemia.

ASSESSMENT

Figure 48-1 is a decision tree for assessing a patient for Cushing's disease.

The patient should be evaluated for the following:

Obesity
Diabetes mellitus
Hypertension
Depression

THERAPEUTIC PLAN

Nonpharmaceutical

If the screening and diagnostic testing is equivocal and clinical features strongly suggest Cushing's disease, referral to an internist or endocrinologist is indicated to confirm the presence of hypercortisolism and establish a plan of care.

The internist or endocrinologist will distinguish an ACTH-dependent from a non–ACTH-dependent source of the hypercortisolism.

If the ACTH level is normal or high, computed tomograph or magnetic resonance imaging evaluation of the pituitary is indicated to rule out the presence of a tumor. If the ACTH level is suppressed, evaluation should focus on the adrenal glands.

The primary treatment for Cushing's disease in **adults** resulting from excess pituitary ACTH is transsphenoidal microadenomectomy. The cure rate is as high as 90%, with a recurrence rate between 5% and 20%.

External irradiation, not adenomectomy, is the treatment of choice in **children.**

Bilateral adrenalectomy has also been used for years in the treatment of **adults** but has significant operative mortality and morbidity. All patients experience adrenal insufficiency after an adrenalectomy and risk the development of an enlarging pituitary adenoma accompanied by hyperpigmentation known as Nelson's syndrome.

Pharmaceutical

Pharmaceutical therapy includes the use of mitotane, which is an inhibitor of adrenal synthesis and is used alone or in combination with pituitary irradiation.

Patient Education

Development of signs and symptoms
Diagnosis
Treatment
Medication
Complications, including symptoms of adrenal insufficiency after treatment
Emotional support to improve body image and self-esteem

Consultation/Referral

Consultation with an internist or endocrinologist is indicated for evaluation and treatment.

EVALUATION/FOLLOW-UP

Schedule follow-up appointments every 3 months to monitor blood pressure, electrolytes, and symptoms of adrenal insufficiency.

Signs and symptoms of adrenal insufficiency are:

Weakness
Anorexia
Weight loss
Hypotension
Hypovolemia
Hyperpigmentation concentrated over palmar and other body creases, over pressure points, and around the areolas
Hyperkalemia
Hyponatremia
Hypoglycemia
Blood-urea-nitrogen elevation

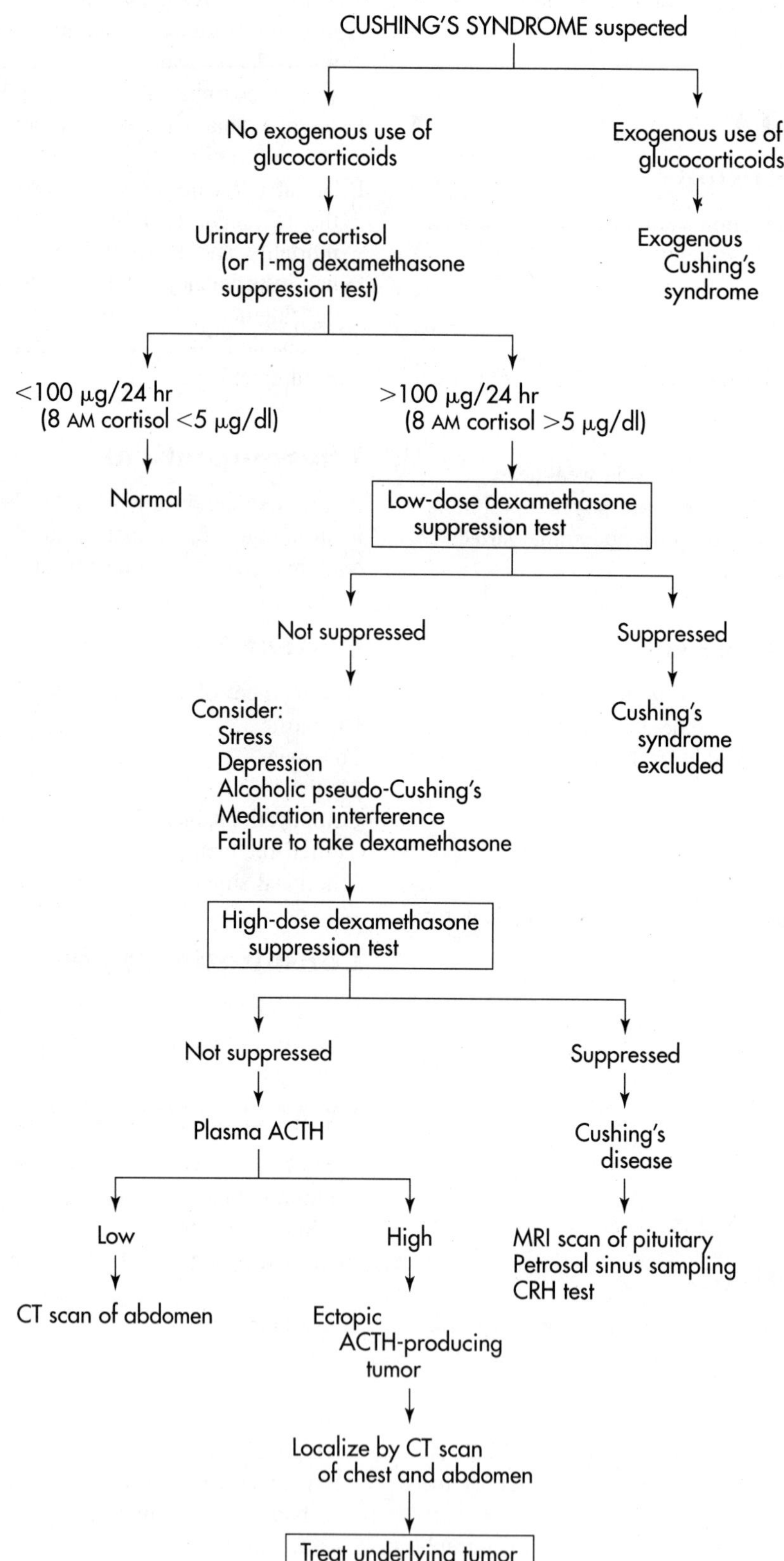

Figure 48-1 Algorithm for patient with suspected Cushing's disease. *ACTH,* Adrenocorticotropic hormone; *CRH,* corticotropic-releasing hormone; *CT,* computed tomography; *MRI,* magnetic resonance imaging. (From Greene HL II, Johnson WP, Lemcke D: *Decision making in medicine: an algorithmic approach,* St Louis, 1998, Mosby.)

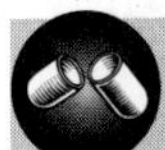

TABLE 48-2 Pharmaceutical Plan: Cushing's Disease

Drug	Dosage	Comments	Cost
Aminoglutethimide (Cytadren)	250 mg PO QID at 6-hr intervals, not to exceed 2 g/day	Usually used as an interim measure until surgery	$100
Ketoconazole (Nizoral)	Adults: 200-400 mg PO QD; higher doses for Cushing's	High doses used for Cushing's syndrome; **not FDA approved**	N/A

N/A, Not available.

SUGGESTED READINGS

Barker LR, Burton JR, Zieve PD: *Principles of ambulatory medicine,* Baltimore, 1995, Williams & Wilkins.

Davis-Martin S: Disorders of the adrenal glands, *J Am Acad Nurse Pract* 8:323-326, 1996.

Ellsworth AJ et al: *Mosby's 1998 medical drug reference,* St Louis, 1998, Mosby.

Gumowski J, Loughran M: Diseases of the adrenal gland, *Nurs Clin North Am* 31:747-768, 1996.

Hay W et al: *Current pediatric diagnosis & treatment*, Norwalk, Conn, 1997, Appleton & Lange.

Healthcare Consultants of America, Inc: 1998 Physicians fee and coding guide, Augusta, Ga, 1998, Healthcare Consultants of America, Inc.

Loriaux T: Endocrine assessment: red flags for those on the front lines, *Nurs Clin North Am* 31:695-712, 1996.

Price S, Wilson L: *Pathophysiology: clinical concepts of disease processes,* St Louis, 1997, Mosby.

Rusterholtz A: Interpretation of diagnostic laboratory tests in selected endocrine disorders, *Nurs Clin North Am* 31:715-724, 1996.

Scientific American Endocrine IV 3:1-17, 1997.

Cystic Fibrosis

ICD-9-CM

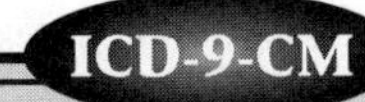

Cystic Fibrosis 277.0

OVERVIEW

Definition

Cystic fibrosis is a multisystem disorder characterized by chronic obstructive pulmonary disorder (COPD), maldigestion, and excessive sodium chloride excretion in sweat and saliva.

Incidence

Autosomal recessive gene located on chromosome 7

Cystic fibrosis is the most common genetic disorder among the white population

Occurs in 1 of every 3000 live births among whites and 1 of every 17,000 live births among blacks

70% present before 1 year of age

Pathophysiology

Respiratory tract: Defective chloride ion transport in respiratory epithelial cells leads to cellular dehydration, causing bronchial secretions to become viscous and difficult to clear. Glycoprotein secretions on cell surfaces adhere to *Pseudomonas* and *Staphylococcus aureus* organisms, increasing susceptibility to infection.

Digestive tract: Increased viscosity of mucous gland secretions obstruct the pancreatic ducts, producing pancreatic fibrosis. Pancreatic enzymes are unable to reach the duodenum, so the digestion of nutrients is impaired. Intrahepatic bile ducts become blocked with viscous secretions, producing biliary cirrhosis.

Reproductive system: Cervical glands become distended with mucus, and the cervical canal is filled with copious amounts of mucus. Endocervicitis occurs. In males, the epididymis, vas deferens, and seminal vessels become occluded.

Cystic fibrosis is a chronic, progressive disease. Persons with this disease have a life expectancy of 30 to 35 years.

SUBJECTIVE DATA

History of Present Illness

Newborn:

Meconium ileus (failure to pass meconium within 48 hours of birth)

Infant:

- Chronic cough
- Chronic diarrhea
- Abdominal distension
- Persistent vomiting with cough
- Salty taste to skin when kissed

Child:

- Frequent bulky, foul-smelling stools that float

Adolescent/Adult:

- Rarely diagnosed this late
- Delayed puberty

Past Medical History

Recurrent upper respiratory infection (URI) or bronchiolitis

Prolonged neonatal jaundice

Failure to thrive

Poor weight gain

Pansinusitis (older child)

Dyspnea

Family History

Family history of cystic fibrosis

Psychosocial History

Exercise intolerance

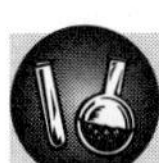

TABLE 49-1 Diagnostic Tests: Cystic Fibrosis

Test	Finding	Cost ($)
Sweat chloride test	A finding of 60 mEq/L or less is diagnostic for cystic fibrosis	N/A
CXR	Early findings are hyperinflation and increased peribronchial markings; later findings are infiltrates and bronchial thickening, patchy atelectasis	77-91
Sputum culture	Positive for bacteria	31-39
Pulmonary function tests	Not reliable until age 6; decreased midmaximal flow rate and increased residual volume and capacity	Up to 323, depending on how many tests are done; e.g., spirometry is 96-117
Serum glucose	Elevated	16-20
Serum amylase	Elevated	24-30

CXR, Chest x-ray; *N/A,* not available.

OBJECTIVE DATA

Physical Examination

A physical examination should be performed to assess the following.

Newborn:
- Jaundice
- Absent bowel sounds
- Abdominal distention

Infant:
- Abdominal distention
- Use of accessory muscles to breathe

Child:
- Rales, rhonchi, wheezes
- Digital clubbing
- Barrel chest
- Rectal prolapse
- Nasal polyps

Adolescent:
- Same signs as in child, plus portal hypertension, sterility in males

Diagnostic Procedures

Diagnostic procedures are outlined in Table 49-1.

ASSESSMENT

Differential diagnoses are many and differ based on age. The most common differential diagnoses are shown in Table 49-2. Other diagnoses to consider are:

TABLE 49-2 Differential Diagnosis: Cystic Fibrosis

Diagnosis	Supporting Data
Tuberculosis	Positive tuberculin skin test; night sweats; known exposure to person with active TB; crowded living conditions
Asthma	Cough in asthma is tight, nonproductive, and responsive to bronchodilators; the cystic fibrosis cough is deep, resonant, and strenuous enough to produce vomiting and rib fractures
Bronchiolitis	Mild, episodic URI with rhinitis and cough progressing to wheezing; difference is in duration—cystic fibrosis has repeated episodes of bronchiolitis plus other nonrespiratory symptoms

TB, Tuberculosis; *URI,* upper respiratory infection.

Infant:
- Chlamydial *(C. psittaci)* pneumonitis, gastroesophageal reflux with aspiration, immunodeficiency syndromes, gastrointestinal allergies

Child:
- Allergies

Adolescent:
- Allergies, acquired immunodeficiency syndrome

THERAPEUTIC PLAN

Goals of treatment are to: (1) prevent bronchial obstruction and respiratory infection, (2) optimize nutrition, and (3) promote a positive psychosocial climate to allow the patient to lead as normal a life as possible.

Table 49-3 Pancreatic Enzyme: Dosage by Age

Age	Oral Dosage
6 mo to 1 yr	2000 U/meal
1 to 6 yr	4000-8000 U with each meal, 4000 U with each snack
7-12 yr	4000-12,000 U with each meal and snack
Adolescent/adult	4000-8000 U with each meal and snack

Pharmaceutical

Aerosol Bronchodilators. The value of bronchodilators is controversial. They should be reserved for use in patients who have an increase of 10% or greater in forced expiratory volume in 1 second (FEV_1) in response to bronchodilator inhalation (Ramsey, 1996). Refer to Chapter 16 for dosage and costs.

Antibiotics. Chloramphenicol is the most effective antibiotic against *Staphylococcus aureus* or beta-lactamase–producing strains of *Haemophilus influenza*. Dosage is 50 to 100 mg/kg/day in divided doses q6h for adults or 50 to 75 mg/kg/day in divided doses every 6 hours for children; the cost is $37 to $125. Because of the toxicity associated with chloramphenicol, it should be prescribed only in consultation with a physician. Aerosolized antibiotics (e.g., tobramycin) may be more effective than oral forms, because increased concentrations can be delivered to the site of infection with decreased systemic side effects. Combinations of intravenous antibiotics are frequently necessary. Because the volume of distribution and clearance of antibiotics are often increased in patients with cystic fibrosis, serum antibiotic levels must be monitored closely. Ordering intravenous antibiotics for these patients is usually restricted to nurse practitioners working in a specialty practice. Refer to a current pharmacology text for specific dosage information.

Theophylline. Theophylline may be used for patients with an inadequate response to other forms of bronchodilator therapy. Cystic fibrosis patients have increased clearance of theophylline unless they are receiving antibiotics that decrease its clearance. Serum theophylline levels must be monitored carefully.

Corticosteroids. Oral corticosteroids are usually administered on a QOD schedule, although their efficacy is in question (prednisolone [Prednisone] [children: 0.1 to 0.2 mg/kg/day PO; $3 to $19 for tablets, $52 for syrup, $15 for liquid])

Recombinant Human Deoxyribonuclease. Dornase alfa (recombinant human deoxyribonuclease; DNase, Pulmozyme) by nebulizer to break down extracellular DNA in sputum; decreases viscosity of secretions and subsequent respiratory infections that would require intravenous antibiotics; 2.5 mg in nebulizer QD ($972), comes in 1 mg/1ml solution, approved for age 5 and older.

Pancreatic Enzyme Capsules. Enteric-coated pancreatic enzyme capsules (pancrelipase, $26 to $58); dosage based on age (Table 49-3).

Vitamins. Fat-soluble vitamins A, D, and E: twice the recommended daily dosage; vitamin K: supplementation weekly for the first 2 years of life.

Nonpharmaceutical

Chest physical therapy
High-frequency chest compression using an inflatable vest

Diet

Infants need predigested formula (e.g., Pregestimil or Portagen)
High-calorie foods of choice, multiple small meals throughout the day are easier to digest with the enzyme supplements and help meet the increased caloric requirements for breathing

Patient/Family Education

Teach parents to recognize early signs of respiratory infection and to act on these signs (e.g., increase dosage of bronchodilator, increase caloric intake and fluids, and start antibiotic therapy as agreed on by the pulmonary specialty team).

Stress importance of administering pancreatic enzyme supplements with EVERY meal and snack.

Referral

Every child with cystic fibrosis should be referred to an accredited cystic fibrosis center. These centers provide families with financial assistance as well as educational and psychological support. Because the complications of cystic fibrosis affect several body systems, referral to specialists should occur early in treatment. Most children with cystic fibrosis are managed by an adult or pediatric pulmonary disease specialist. The nurse practitioner (NP) may be involved with the initial workup of a child suspected of having cystic fibrosis, or the NP may be part of the pulmonary specialty team caring for the child.

These children should not be managed by the primary care provider only. A referral to a nutritionist is indicated in cases of poor weight gain. A referral to a psychologist is indicated to counsel an adolescent regarding sexual maturation and potential reproductive problems. The stress of chronic illness may produce the need for mental health support for all family members. Genetic counseling is indicated.

EVALUATION/FOLLOW-UP

Children with cystic fibrosis usually remain at or are below the 5th percentile for weight. However, a loss of weight or failure to gain for an extended period warrants a follow-up by a nutritionist. Monthly weight checks should be done if the child is not followed by a nutritionist. Seasonal immunizations (e.g., flu) are essential.

REFERENCE

Ramsey B: Management of pulmonary disease in patients with cystic fibrosis, *N Engl J Med* 335:179-188, 1996.

SUGGESTED READINGS

Arvin AM et al, editors: *Nelson's textbook of pediatrics,* ed 15, Philadelphia, 1996, WB Saunders.

Bindler RM, Howry LB: *Pediatric drugs and nursing implications,* ed 2, Norwalk, Conn, 1997, Appleton & Lange.

Dershewitz RA: *Ambulatory pediatric care,* ed 2, Philadelphia, 1993, WB Saunders.

Duffield RA: Cystic fibrosis and the gastrointestinal tract, *J Pediatr Care* 10:31-52, 1996.

Ellsworth AJ et al: *Mosby's 1998 medical drug reference,* St Louis, 1998, Mosby.

Groothuis JR et al: *Current pediatric diagnosis and treatment,* ed 12, Norwalk, Conn, 1995, Appleton & Lange.

Healthcare Consultants of America, Inc: *1998 Physicians fee and coding guide,* Augusta, Ga, 1998, Healthcare Consultants of America, Inc.

Neglia LP et al: The risk of cancer among patients with cystic fibrosis, *N Engl J Med* 332:494-499, 1995.

White RR, Munro CL, Pickler RH: Therapeutic implications of recent advances in cystic fibrosis, *Am J Maternal Child Nurs* 20:304-308, 1997.

Wilmott RW, Fielder MA: Recent advances in the treatment of cystic fibrosis, *Pediatr Clin North Am* 41:431-451, 1994.

50 Delayed Puberty

ICD-9-CM

Short Stature 783.4
Delayed Puberty 259.0

OVERVIEW

Definition

Delayed puberty is defined as development of reproductive organs that falls two or more standard deviations below the mean for age. Delayed puberty may be considered when onset of puberty is markedly later than in other members of the family, and in the following gender specific situations.

Male

A male may be considered to have delayed puberty if he has no androgen signs by 14 years of age (i.e., genital development at Tanner genital stage 1). Delayed puberty in males may be considered if pubic hair stage 1 persists beyond 15.1 years of age or more than 5 years have elapsed between initiation and completion of genital development.

Female

A female may be considered to have delayed puberty if she has no estrogen signs by 13 years of age (i.e., Tanner stage 1 breast development). Delayed puberty in females may be considered if pubic hair stage 1 persists beyond 14.4 years, there is a failure to menstruate beyond 15.5 years of age, or if more than 5 years have elapsed between initiation of breast growth and menarche.

Incidence

Delayed puberty is relatively rare, affecting 1% to 2.5% of children in the United States.

Pathophysiology

The etiological factors underlying delayed puberty are constitutional in 95% of cases. Relevant pathophysiology is related to deficiency of androgen or estrogen or their receptors in boys and girls, respectively. The hypothalamic pituitary-gonadal axis is affected by the issues outlined in Box 50-1.

SUBJECTIVE DATA

History of Present Illness

Chief concern: "No growth," "behind other children in growth"

Reports that the child has not developed secondary sex characteristics or has had growth in height that has not kept up with his or her peers; it is more common for concern to be expressed regarding boys' growth and development

Past Medical History

Growth record essential
Head size since birth
Identify chronic systemic illness
Review of systems:

- Head/eyes/ears/nose/throat: Vision problems, headache, vomiting
- Ability to detect odors
- Skin: Ichthyosis, increased tanning (adrenal insufficiency)
- Need for deodorant, hair-washing frequency
- Genital: Small genitalia at birth

Family History

More than 60% of patients with constitutional delay of puberty have a positive family history

Box 50-1

Causes of Delayed Puberty

Pubertal Delay without Short Stature

Constitutional delay of puberty (no causative factor found)
Acquired gonadotropin deficiency
- Tumors
- Trauma
- Infections: Tuberculosis, viral encephalitis

Isolated gonadotropin deficiency
- Kallman's syndrome
- LH or FSH deficiency

Acquired gonadal disorders
- Infections (i.e., gonorrhea, viral)
- Postradiation or chemotherapy

Congenital gonadal disorders
- Kleinfelter's syndrome
- Anorchism

Androgen receptor defects
- Testicular feminization
- Reinfenstein's syndrome

Chronic disease
- Heart disease
- Asthma
- IBD
- JRA
- SLE
- Anorexia nervosa
- Hyperthyroidism
- Hyperprolactinemia
- Chronic renal failure
- Sickle cell anemia
- Diabetes mellitus
- Cystic fibrosis
- Human immunodeficiency virus

Pubertal Delay with Short Stature

Constitutional delay of puberty and normal variant short stature
Panhypopituitarism
Congenital syndromes
- Turner's (female)
- Prader-Willi
- Noonan's

Glucocorticoid excess

Hypergonodal Conditions

Variants of ovarian and testicular dysgenesis
Gonadal toxins (antimetabolite and radiation treatments)
Enzyme defects (17 alpha-hydroxylase deficiency in genetic male or female and 17 ketosteroid reductase deficiency in the genetic male)
Androgen insensitivity (testicular feminization)

Hypogonadal Conditions

Multiple tropic hormone deficiency
Isolated growth hormone deficiency
Isolated gonadotropin deficiency
Polycystic ovarian disease

FSH, Follicle-stimulating hormone; *IBD,* inflammatory bowel disease; *JRA,* juvenile rheumatoid arthritis; *LH,* luteinizing hormone; *SLE,* systemic lupus erythematosus.

History of late puberty in other family members, heights of parents, siblings, and grandparents
Age of menarche for mother and siblings
Final height for mother and siblings
Was father small as a teenager in relation to classmates? Did he grow after getting his driver's license? Did he grow after graduating from high school? What was his final height?
At what age did father begin to shave?

Psychosocial History

Emotional distress can result from a delay in adolescent sexual development. Ask about:

- Depression
- Psychosomatic complaints (e.g., abdominal pain)
- Poor self-esteem
- Regression or withdrawal from peer contact
- Poor school performance
- Decreased sports activity
- Increased school absenteeism

Exercise: Carefully assess exercise patterns to rule out anorexia nervosa
Nutritional history: Have patient complete a 3-day diet recall; ask about decreased intake, or symptoms of eating disorder
Habits: Ask about smoking, alcohol use, other drugs that may influence eating/growth

OBJECTIVE DATA

Physical Examination

A full physical examination should be performed to assess for underlying disease:
- Vital signs: Especially temperature and blood pressure
- Nutritional status
- General: Body measurements, including height, weight, arm span, upper/lower body segment ratios

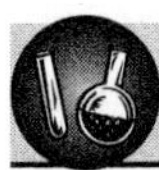

TABLE 50-1 Diagnostic Tests: Delayed Puberty

Test	Finding/Rationale	Cost ($)
Bone age	Will help determine the severity of pubertal delay	129-154
CBC with diff, ESR, sickle cell, glucose, creatinine, CA, phosphorus, albumin, LFT	Identification of underlying systemic illness	18-23/ CBC; 16-20/ESR; 16-20/glucose; 18-24/creatinine; 18-23/CA; 23-30/electrolytes; 16-20/phosphate; 29-41/LFT; 19-24/sickle cell; 18-23/albumin
U/A	Identifies renal problems	15-20
Thyroid function	Identifies thyroid disorders	47-51
Prolactin	May be increased in some conditions that cause amenorrhea	70-89
Upper GI series	Helps to rule out IBD	275-328
LH and FSH	Measurement of basal plasma	61-76/LH
	Gonadotropins: If elevated, patients have hypergonadotropic hypogonadism (primary ovarian or testicular failure); if low or normal, patient has constitutional delay or hypogonadotropic hypogonadism	62-78/FSH
GnRH response test	Evaluates LH response to administration of synthetic gonadotropin-releasing hormone; those with constitutional delay will respond	315-495
Growth hormone	Detects growth hormone deficiency	58-74
Gonadotropin-releasing hormone	Detects hypothalamic failure	N/A
Pubertal development scale (Peterson et al, 1988)	Objective measure of pubertal development	
Males		
DHEAS, testosterone	Identifies testosterone levels	83-103
Female		
Estradiol	Identifies estrogen levels	85-107
Vaginal smear	Evaluates estrogen effect	31-38
Karyotype	Rules out Turner's or Klinefelter's syndromes	315-695

CA, Cancer; *CBC with diff,* complete blood count with differential blood count; *DHEAS,* dehydroepiandrosterone sulfate; *ESR,* erythrocyte sedimentation rate; *FSH,* follicle-stimulating hormone; *GI,* gastrointestinal; *GnRH,* gonadotropin-releasing hormone; *IBD,* inflammatory bowel disease; *LFT,* liver function test; *LH,* luteinizing hormone; *U/A,* urinalysis.

Skin: Pigment, including café-au-lait spots, tanning, skinfold thickness, ichthyosis and androgen signs

Head/eyes/ears/nose/throat: Visual fields, ability to detect odors, fundi, teeth (persistent deciduous teeth), thyroid for goiter

Cardiopulmonary system

Abdomen

Genitalia: Tanner staging

- Estrogen effect on vaginal mucosa can be assessed visually

Neurological: Deep tendon reflexes, mental status

Growth Charts

Growth patterns vary according to the cause of pubertal delay (e.g., girls with constitutional delay and short stature usually have height and weight that remain at or below the 5th percentile). Girls with prematurity or deprivation states will gradually catch up from measurements well below the 5th percentile, whereas decreasing height and markedly decreased weight will be evident in children with chronic illness states. Children with Cushing's syndrome or hypothyroidism may exhibit decreased height and increased weight, whereas markedly decreased weight

TABLE 50-2 Differential Diagnosis: Delayed Puberty

Diagnosis	Supporting Data
Gonadotropin deficiency	Low FSH and LH, particularly if bone age is WNL Low response to GnRH if pituitary failure present Low testosterone in males History of neurological symptoms Absence of smell (Kallmann's syndrome)
Gonadal disorder	History of genital radiation Castrate levels of FSH and LH Abnormal karyotype Arm span exceeds height by >2 inches Gynecomastia in males Small testes in males
Turner's syndrome	Short stature in girls Streak gonads Absent pubertal growth Webbing of neck Low hairline Less breast than pubic hair development with normal vagina, cervix, and uterus
Chronic illness	Abnormal findings on review of systems or physical examination Falling-off height and weight curves at onset of disease Abnormal CBC, ESR, U/A, or chemistry panel results

CBC, Complete blood cell count; *ESR,* erythrocyte sedimentation rate; *FSH,* follicle-stimulating hormone; *GnRH,* gonadotropin-releasing hormone; *LH,* luteinizing hormone; *U/A,* urinalysis; *WNL,* within normal limits.

and normal height increments are seen in girls with anorexia nervosa.

Diagnostic Procedures

Diagnostic tests include those found in Table 50-1.

ASSESSMENT

Although the vast majority (90% to 95%) of teens with delayed puberty have constitutional delay of puberty, it is a diagnosis of exclusion. Consider the following when making a diagnosis:

Is there any evidence of systemic disorder?

How much has skeletal maturation progressed?

Is there evidence of interruption in either gonadal or hypothalamic-pituitary function?

Is the chromosomal sex consistent the genital sex of the child?

The differential diagnosis for delayed puberty includes those listed in Table 50-2.

THERAPEUTIC PLAN

Pharmaceutical

The cause of pubertal delay needs to be addressed. Treatment for chronic illness or Turner's syndrome must be provided (Table 50-3).

Lifestyle/Activities

If delayed puberty is affected by excessive exercise, counsel the child to reduce exercise. If delayed puberty affects the child's psychosocial adaptation, encourage the child to identify and participate in school activities and other activities. Moderate exercise increases the benefits of sex steroids for children being treated with medications.

Diet

Because pubertal development is partially associated with the percentage of body fat, it is recommended that children consume reasonable amounts of fat in their diet. The pyramid food plan offers well-balanced choices.

Patient Education

Discuss causes of constitutional or organic pubertal delay with child and family.

Identify plan of care, with expectations for eventual growth.

If there is a positive family history for delayed puberty, use information from that history in the description of projected outcomes.

Family Impact

Delayed puberty in a child may be a traumatic experience. Reassurance and support is essential.

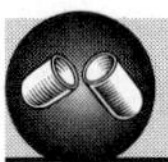

TABLE 50-3 Pharmaceutical Plan: Delayed Puberty

Drug	Dosage	Comments	Cost
Males			
Oxandrolone (Oxandrin)	0.05-0.25 mg/kg/day available in 2.5 mg tablets	Males with no androgen signs by age 14 may benefit from androgen therapy; start and maintain on lowest effective dose to minimize potential for adverse effects.	$375/2.5 mg (100)
Methyltestosterone (Android)	10-50 mg QD	Use a low dose, limit to 6 mo Pregnancy: X SE: premature epiphyseal closure, gynecomastia, priapism, acne, headache, depression	$43-$130/10 mg (100) $30-$130/tablets: 10 mg (100)
Testosterone (Androderm)	Transdermal patch 5 mg QHS on clean, dry skin (apply to nonscrotal skin)	Not recommended for males <15 yr old Pregnancy: X SE: Local itching, blistering, prostate abnormalities, depression	$98/2.5 mg/24 hr (60) $60/4 mg or 8 mg/ 24 hr (60)
Testosterone enanthate	25 mg IM q2wk or 50 mg q4wk for 6 mo	As above	$11/100 mg/ml (10 ml)
Females			
Estrogen	Conjugated estrogens (Premarin) of 0.15 to 0.3 mg/day for 6 mo	Girls with no estrogen signs by age 13 Pregnancy: X SE: BTB, headache, nausea, breast soreness, abdominal cramps, depression	$28/0.3 mg (100)

BTB, Breakthrough bleeding; *SE,* side effects.

Referral

It is appropriate to refer a child with suspected nonconstitutional pubertal delay to a pediatric endocrinologist.

Follow-up

If constitutional delay is identified, the child's growth and development and psychosocial adjustment should be monitored every 3 months. If delay continues beyond two standard deviations below mean for age, refer the patient to a pediatric endocrinologist.

EVALUATION

Delayed puberty is caught up when:

- Growth adheres to child's overall curve on growth charts
  - Secondary sexual characteristics develop
- Child functions well in social sphere

REFERENCE

Peterson A et al: A self-report measure of pubertal status: reliability, validity and initial norms, *J Youth Adolesc* 17:117-133, 1988.

SUGGESTED READINGS

Arslanian S, Supraingsin C: Testosterone in adolescents with delayed puberty: changes in body composition protein fat and glucose metabolism, *J Clin Endocrinol Metabol* 82:3213-3220, 1997.

Cronau H, Brown R: Growth and development: physical mental and social aspects, *Growth Primary Care* 25:23-47, 1998.

Emans S, Goldstein D: *Pediatric and adolescent gynecology,* ed 3, Boston, 1990, Little Brown.

Ellsworth A et al: *Mosby's 1998 medical drug reference,* St Louis, 1998, Mosby.

Healthcare Consultants of America, Inc: *1998 Physicians fee and coding guide,* Augusta, Ga, 1998, Healthcare Consultants of America, Inc.

Kerlin H et al: Diversity of pubertal testosterone changes in boys with constitutional delay in growth and/or adolescence, *J Pediatr Endocrine Metabol* 10:395-400, 1997.

Kliegman R: *Practical strategies in pediatric diagnosis and therapy,* Philadelphia, 1996, WB Saunders.

McArnarney E et al: *Textbook of adolescent medicine,* Philadelphia, 1992, WB Saunders.

Neinstein L: *Adolescent health care: a practical guide,* ed 3, Baltimore, 1996, Williams & Wilkins.

Speroff L, Glass R, Kase N: *Clinical gynecologic endocrinology and infertility,* Baltimore, 1994, Williams & Wilkins.

Dental Problems

Candidiasis, Gingivitis, Acute Necrotizing Ulcerative Gingivitis, Aphthous Ulcers, and Tooth Fracture

ICD-9-CM

Oral Candidiasis (Thrush) 112.0
Gingivitis 523.1
Acute Necrotizing Ulcerative Gingivitis 101.0
Aphthous Ulcers 528.2
Tooth Fracture 873.63

CANDIDIASIS (THRUSH)

OVERVIEW

Definition

Candidiasis is an oral pharyngeal infection of the mucous membranes caused most commonly by the yeastlike fungus *Candida albicans*.

Incidence

50,000 to 10,000 per year in the United States
May occur in any age group
Commonly seen in **infants** during first weeks of life
In **older children** most commonly associated with antibiotic use; inhaled corticosteroid use in asthmatic child
Seen most commonly in patients with debilitating diseases, diabetes, and cancer
Frequently occurs in patients receiving antibiotics, corticosteroid therapy, radiation therapy, and immunosuppressive drugs
Very common in patients with human immunodeficiency virus (HIV)

Pathophysiology

Protective Factors Against Thrush

Good oral hygiene
Good nutrition

Factors That Increase Susceptibility to Thrush

Poor oral hygiene
Poor nutrition
Radiation therapy to head or neck
Corticosteroid use
Antibiotic use
Immunosuppressive drug therapy

Common Pathogens

Candida albicans is most common cause

SUBJECTIVE DATA

Past Medical History

Is there a history of diabetes, cancer, HIV, or other chronic disease states?
Last dental examination, or dental examination pattern
Does the female patient have a vaginal discharge?
Did the male patient have intimate oral sexual contact with a woman with a vaginal discharge?

Is there a report of recent diaper rash in the infant?
Allergies
Last menstrual period

Medications

Antibiotics
Chemotherapy agents
Corticosteroids: Oral and inhaled
Radiation therapy

Family History

Others in household with the same symptoms?
Diabetes
HIV

Psychosocial History

Consider the possibility of sexual abuse in young children with no predisposing factors.

Diet History

Poor nutritional intake

Description of Most Common Symptoms

White "spots" in mouth
Mouth pain
Difficulty eating
Weight loss

Infants

Increased irritability
Difficulty feeding
Mother with possible history of vaginal candidiasis

OBJECTIVE DATA

Physical Examination

A problem-oriented examination should be conducted, with particular attention to:

General appearance: Does the patient appear healthy or ill?
Hydration status: May become dehydrated related to decreased oral intake
Oral membranes: White plaques that scrape off easily with a tongue blade to reveal erythematous areas
Genital/rectal: Female patients with a complaint of vaginal discharge should have a complete pelvic examination
Inspect area in children in whom sexual abuse is suspected
Infants should be evaluated for diaper rash

Diagnostic Procedures

None indicated for typical oral candidiasis
Potassium hydroxide (KOH) preparation ($19 to $23) of the scraping demonstrates budding yeast without hyphae

ASSESSMENT

Differential Diagnosis

Leukoplakia
Geographic tongue
Stomatitis
Milk products left on tongue

THERAPEUTIC PLAN

Pharmaceutical

Oral Antifungal Agents

Nystatin (Mycostatin) ($3 to $22) oral suspension 100,000 U/m
Infants: Place 1 ml in each cheek q6h for 7 to 10 days. May also paint lesions with a cotton swab.
Older children and adults: 2 or 3 ml in each cheek, then swish and swallow q6h for 7 to 10 days.
Adolescents and adults: Nystatin troches (Mycostatin Pastilles) ($30) 200,000 U/ml. Slowly dissolve 1 or 2 troches in mouth q5-6h for 7 to 10 days.

or

Clotrimazole (Lotrimin) ($53) buccal troches, 10 mg. Slowly dissolve 1 troche in mouth q5h for 14 days.
Ketoconazole 200 to 400 mg ($13 to $34) PO each morning with breakfast for 7 to 14 days. For better absorption of this medicine, the stomach must be acidic.

or

Fluconazole 100 mg PO ($206) each morning for 7 to 14 days.

NOTE: A troche is a lozenge-like tablet that is dissolved in the mouth.

Denture wearers must add:
Nystatin powder 100,000 units/g applied to dentures q6-8h for several weeks.

Patient Education

Rinse mouth with small amount of water before using medication.

Remove large plaques gently with cotton swabs moistened with water.
Wash hands thoroughly after changing baby's diaper.
Wash hands thoroughly after using the bathroom.

Infants and Small Children

Prevent reinfection by washing toys and sterilizing nipples and pacifiers.
Breastfeeding mothers should wash nipples with mild soap and water, then allow to air dry.

Referral

If thrush is persistent or recurrent or if there is no improvement in 5 days, consider a referral to an immunologist to evaluate immunological status.
Infants and small children should be referred to a pediatrician if failure to thrive is identified.

EVALUATION/FOLLOW-UP

Older children and adults should return in 5 to 7 days if there is no improvement.
Infants should be reevaluated if:
They refuse liquids, bottle, or breast
Symptoms do not improve or get worse

GINGIVITIS

OVERVIEW

Definition

Gingivitis is inflammation of the gingiva. It is caused by tooth-borne bacteria (plaque) build-up, which activates lymphocyte proliferation and activates cytokines. This results in destruction of the periodontal ligament and the alveolar bone, the supporting structures of the teeth.

Incidence

Pandemic; occurs in 90% of the population
Occurs in up to 50% of **children;** increases in severity with age
May lead to tooth and bone loss if untreated

Pathophysiology

Protective Factors Against Gingivitis

Good oral hygiene
Good nutrition

Factors That Increase Susceptibility to Gingivitis

Increased bacterial plaque buildup with an acute inflammatory response at the junctional epithelium (the attachment of the gingiva to the enamel surface of the tooth)

Systemic Factors

Drugs may cause hyperplasia:
Phenytoin (Dilantin)
Calcium channel blockers
Cyclosporine

Pregnancy leads to exaggerated inflammatory response, especially in third trimester
Vitamin C deficiency
Diabetes mellitus

Local Factors

Food impaction
Trauma
Smoking
Mouth breathing, which leads to drying of the gingiva

Common Pathogens

Gram-positive filamentous rods
Actinomyces is most common

SUBJECTIVE DATA

Past Medical History

Mouth breather
Dental hygiene habits
Treatment for malocclusion
Poor dental restorations: Poorly done or deteriorated
Diabetes
Pregnancy
Last menstrual period
HIV exposure
Access to dental care: Last dental examination or pattern for dental examinations
Smoking history

Medications

Antibiotics
Oral contraceptives
Dilantin
Corticosteroids: Oral and inhaled
Insulin
Chemotherapy

Family History

Diabetes
Periodontal disease

Psychosocial History

Economic status: Patient with low economic status often has less access to dental care

Diet History

Poor nutritional intake

Description of Most Common Symptoms

Early

Bleeding gums after brushing or flossing
"Bad breath"
Red gum
Painless gum swelling

Late

Sensitivity to sweets and hot and cold
Dull throbbing pain after eating and when awakening

OBJECTIVE DATA

Physical Examination

A problem-oriented examination should be conducted, with particular attention to:

General appearance: Does the patient look healthy or ill?
Gingiva: Inflammation and redness surrounding the neck of the tooth, erosion, presence of plaque, hyperplasia or recession of gums

Diagnostic Procedures

No tests indicated

ASSESSMENT

Differential Diagnosis

Dental abscess
Pericoronitis
Periodontitis
Stomatitis
Drug reaction
Impacted food particles

THERAPEUTIC PLAN

Pharmaceutical

None

Nonpharmaceutical

Removal of plaque and other irritants
Warm saline and water rinses 2 or 3 times a day

Patient Education

Brush and floss teeth between each meal
Rinse mouth with antibacterial mouthwash
Regular dental and hygienist check-up
Improve nutrition, especially vitamin C intake
Stop smoking

Referral

These patients must be referred to the dentist for treatment and further education. This usually results in the restoration of healthy gingiva.

EVALUATION/FOLLOW-UP

Close follow-up by the dentist and oral hygienist is essential for continued gingival health.
It is recommended that patients should see the oral hygienist every 6 months.
Pregnant women should visit the oral hygienist every 3 months.
Children should have their first dental examination between 12 and 18 months.

ACUTE NECROTIZING ULCERATIVE GINGIVITIS (TRENCH MOUTH, VINCENT'S INFECTION)

OVERVIEW

Definition

Acute necrotizing ulcerative gingivitis (ANUG) is a bacterial infection of the gingival tissue. It usually begins between the teeth and then spreads laterally. ANUG may lead to tooth and bone loss.

Incidence

Most common in **adolescents** and **young adults** who are usually under physical or psychological stress
First described by the early Romans
During World War I this inflammation was known as "trench mouth"

Protective Factors Against ANUG

Good oral hygiene especially when under severe stress

Factors That Increase Susceptibility to ANUG

Stress: Physical and psychological
Systemic diseases
Poor oral hygiene

Common Pathogens

It is believed that both of the following pathogens are present.

Fusospirochetal Complex

Fusobacterium fusiforme

Forms:
- Vibrios
- Streptococci
- Diplococci
- Filamentous

Spirochete

Borrelia vincentii

SUBJECTIVE DATA

Past Medical History

Recent emotional or physical stressors
Diabetes
HIV
Dental hygiene habits; date of last dental examination

Medications

Corticosteroids: Oral or inhaled
Chemotherapy agents
Immunosuppressive therapy

Family History

Others in household with same
Diabetes
HIV

Psychsocial History

Recent stressors: Major life change events
Patients with lower socioeconomic status are less likely to receive regular dental care

Diet History

Poor nutritional status, especially the lack of vitamin C intake
Recent decrease in oral intake related to pain in mouth

Description of Most Common Symptoms

Sudden onset of acute gingival pain
Bleeding gums with minimal stimulation
"Bad" taste: Foul metallic
Breath odor
Increased salivation
Fever
Malaise
Loss of appetite

OBJECTIVE DATA

Physical Examination

A problem-oriented examination should be conducted, with particular attention to:
- General appearance: Does the patient look ill?
- Hydration status: May become dehydrated as a result of decreased oral intake related to pain
- Gingiva: Classic triad
  - Intense pain
  - "Punched-out" interdental papillae, covered with a white pseudo-membrane
  - Foul mouth odor
- Vital signs: Fever, tachycardia
- Neck: Lymphadenopathy

Diagnostic Procedures

CBC ($12 to $16) if elevated fever and lymphadenopathy are present
Electrolytes ($23 to $30) if patient is dehydrated
Consider blood cultures ($37 and $45) if high fever is present to rule out systemic infection

ASSESSMENT

Differential Diagnosis

Acute viral or bacterial infections
Herpetic gingivostomatitis
Leukemic gingivitis

THERAPEUTIC PLAN

Pharmaceutical

Penicillin V 250 to 500 mg ($5 to $42) q6h for 10 days
  Children: 25 to 50 mg/kg/24 hours in four divided doses
Erythromycin 250 mg ($14 to $20) q6h for 10 days
  Children: 30 to 40 mg/kg/day in 4 divided doses
Rinse mouth with chlorhexidine gluconate 0.12% and warm water

Topical anesthetic
3% Hydrogen peroxide–soaked cotton pellets to debride lesions 3 or 4 times a day

Patient Education

Good oral hygiene
Smoking cessation
Improve dietary intake, especially vitamin C
Regular dental hygienist and dentist visits
Stress relieving exercises

Referral

If patient appears ill (i.e., febrile, dehydrated, experiencing severe pain), the patient should be admitted for IV antibiotic and rehydration
Must be seen by a dentist immediately for definitive care.

EVALUATION/FOLLOW-UP

The patient must be followed closely by a dentist for continued care; this is usually two to four visits, until healthy gingiva is restored.
Nutritional status must be monitored.

APHTHOUS ULCERS (CANKER SORES)

OVERVIEW

Definition

Aphthous ulcers (canker sores) are superficial ulceration of the mucous membranes of the mouth and lips.
Occasional aphthae: A single lesion that occurs at intervals of months or years. They usually heal without complications.
Acute multiple aphthae: Associated with gastrointestinal disorders. An acute episode may last for weeks. The lesions develop sequentially at different sites in the mouth.
Chronic recurrent aphthae: One or more lesions that are always present for years.

Incidence

Twenty percent to 50% of **adults**
Females are affected more often than males
Familial tendencies
More common during the winter and spring months

Protective Factors Against Aphthous Ulcer

Good oral hygiene
Avoiding oral exposure to others with aphthous ulcer

Common Pathogens

Once thought to be herpes simplex virus (HSV), but actual cause in not known

SUBJECTIVE DATA

Past Medical History

Allergies to chocolate, nuts, tomatoes, or other foods
Autoimmune disease
Recent trauma
Drugs: Possible reaction
Stressors: Physical or emotional

Medications

Antibiotics
Corticosteroids: Especially inhaled

Family History

History of canker sores
Autoimmune diseases

Psychosocial History

Recent life stressors

Diet History

Recent decrease in oral intake because of pain

Description of Most Common Symptoms

Burning sensation 1 to 48 hours before eruption of ulcer
Pain
Swelling
Erythema

OBJECTIVE DATA

Physical Examination

A problem-oriented examination should be conducted with particular attention to:
General appearance: Does the patient look ill?

Hydration status: May become dehydrated because of decreased oral intake

Oral membrane: Characteristic lesions found on buccal or labial mucosa, pharynx, or lateral tongue:

- One or more
- Small: Less than 10 mm
- Superficial, shallow, and oval
- Light yellow to grey fibrinoid center
- Red ridges

Diagnostic Procedures

An incisional biopsy of the lesion can be ordered if the cause of the lesion is uncertain or if the lesions become larger or change color in a manner that is inconsistent with previous aphthous ulcers in this patient.

ASSESSMENT

Differential Diagnosis

Herpes simplex virus
Drug allergies
Behçet's disease
Inflammatory bowel disease
Squamous cell carcinoma

THERAPEUTIC PLAN

Pharmaceutical

Topical corticosteroids:

- Triamcinolone acetonide, 0.1%, ($4 to $27)
- *or*
- Fluocinonide ointment 0.05% in an adhesive base (Orbase Plain); applied to lesions 3 times a day

Mouth coating:

- Mixture of diphenhydramine hydrochloride (Benadryl) suspension (5 mg/ml) ($2 to $15) and Maalox or Mylanta in equal parts
- Viscous lidocaine (Xylocaine) ($2 to $16), 15 ml swished in mouth every 4 hours for patients over 12 years, 3 to 5 ml for **children 5 to 12 years**

Mouth rinse:

- Tetracycline 250 mg capsule ($7 to $20) opened and the powder mixed in 30 to 50 ml of water, applied 3 or 4 times a day for 5 to 7 days.
- Tetracycline tends to abort the lesions and prevent secondary infections
- *Should not be used during pregnancy*
- Chloraseptic mouthwash every 2 hours for **children over 6 years**

Patient Education

Use of topical corticosteroid at first sign of tingling may abort eruption of aphthae.

Topical anesthetics should be applied directly to a lesion that has been dried.

Do not eat within 1 hour of using anesthetic.

A bland, soft diet should be eaten during lesion eruptions.

The patient should be encouraged to drink clear liquids.

Lesions can recur.

Referral

If the patient, especially a child, becomes dehydrated, he or she may require hospitalization.

Infants with multiple lesions should be referred to a pediatrician.

EVALUATION/FOLLOW-UP

Children should be reevaluated within 24 to 48 hours, especially if multiple lesions are present, to ensure the patient does not become dehydrated.

Routine follow-up is not always indicated.

SUMMARY

Table 51-1 presents pharmaceutical and nonpharmaceutical treatments for oral infections.

TOOTH FRACTURE

OVERVIEW

Definition

A fracture of the tooth is caused by blunt trauma to the tooth. There is a classification system for anterior teeth fractures (Figure 51-1).

Ellis I fracture: Fracture of the enamel resulting in a rough edge to the tooth

Ellis II fracture: Fracture that penetrates the dentin, leading to exposure of the pulp

Ellis III fracture: Full-thickness fracture of the tooth; involves the enamel, dentin, and pulp; pink tissue or blood will be seen in the fracture

Avulsed fracture: Tooth removed from the socket; may have bone involvement

Table 51-1 Pharmaceutical and Nonpharmaceutical Treatments for Oral Infections

Infection	Organism	Presentation	Medications	Other Treatments
Candidiasis (Thrush)	*Candida albicans*	White plaques on oral membranes that scrape off easily to reveal erythematous area	Nystatin (B*), or Clotriamzole (B*), or Ketoconazole (C*), or Fluconazole (C*)	Remove excess plaque with cottton swabs
Gingivitis	Gram-positive filamentous rods	Bleeding gums Red gums Sensitivity to sweets, hot, and cold	None	Tooth plaque removal by dentist Warm saline and water rinses 2-3 times/day
Acute necrotizing ulcerative gingivitis (ANUG)	Fusospirochetal complexes and spirochetes	Classic triad: Intense pain "Punched-out" interdental papillae covered with white pseudo-membranes Foul mouth odor Fever, tachycardia	Penicillin V (B*), or erythromycin (B*), or Topical anesthetics: Chlorhexidine gluconate 0.12% (B*)	Increase vitamin C intake Regular dental hygienist care
Aphthous ulcer (canker sore)	Herpes simplex virus	Burning sensation 1-48 hr before eruption; pain; swelling; redness; small oval lesion <10 mm	Topical corticosteroids: Triamanolone acetonide 0.1% (C*), or fluocinonide ointment 0.05% (C*)	Mouth rinse: Benadryl/Maalox (B*) Viscous lidocaine (B*) Tetracycline (D*) Chloraseptic (B*)

*Pregnancy safety category.
See text for cost estimates.

Pathophysiology

Protective Factors Against Tooth Fractures

Protective mouth equipment during contact sports activity
Environment safe from falls

SUBJECTIVE DATA

Past Medical History

Recent mouth trauma
Dental work: Caps, dentures, partial bridges, etc.
Tetanus status, especially if laceration of lips, tongue, or gums is noted
Allergies to medications
Chronic diseases such as diabetes and HIV
Last menstrual period
Oral hygiene status

Medications

Aspirin products: Increased bleeding tendencies
Corticosteroids, especially inhaled: Associated with gum disease, which increases risk of tooth loss to trauma

Family History

Noncontributory

Psychosocial History

Activities in which the patient is involved, especially contact sports
Use of safety equipment, such as mouth guards

Diet History

Good nutritional status (fractures can occur from biting down on ice or a hard food such as candy, especially if there is gum disease)

Description of Most Common Symptoms

Tooth pain
Bleeding gum line
Swelling of gum line
Paresthesia
Jaw pain
Difficulty opening or closing mouth

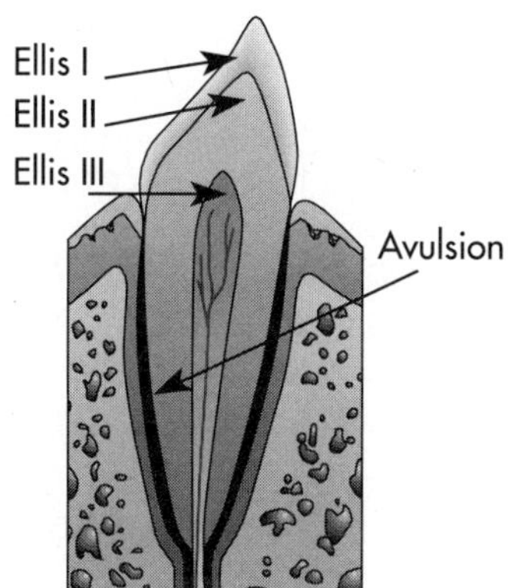

Figure 51-1 Ellis classification of tooth fractures. (From Kidd P, Robinson D: *Family nurse practitioner certification review,* St Louis, 1998, Mosby.)

OBJECTIVE DATA

Physical Examination

A problem-oriented examination should be conducted, with particular attention to:

- Neurological: Rule out possible head injury from trauma
- Oral cavity: Evaluate possible laceration to tongue or gum line and to evaluate for pieces of broken tooth
- Cervical spine: Ensure that no injury to spine has occurred as a result of trauma to the mouth
- Airway: Ensure that tooth fragments have not been aspirated or block airway
- Assess for loose teeth
- Assess for instability of maxillary bone

Diagnostic Procedures

X-ray evaluation: Facial, cervical spine, mandibular as indicated to rule out fractures of the bones

Chest x-ray: To rule out aspiration of missing tooth fragments

ASSESSMENT

Differential Diagnosis

Fracture of mandible
LeFort fractures
Malocclusion injuries
Closed head injury
Newly erupting tooth
Dental infection

THERAPEUTIC PLAN

Pharmaceutical

Narcotic pain medication if no head injury
Nonnarcotic pain medication if head injury is suspected

Nonpharmaceutical

Ice to area
Pressure dressing to bleeding socket
Placement of dislodged tooth in saline or milk

Patient Education

Use of proper safety equipment (correctly fitted mouth guard) during contact sports

Close follow-up by dentist is essential

Soft diet until injury resolves

Good oral hygiene

Avoidance of injury by doing home safety evaluation, prevent further falls

Referral

All tooth fractures must be followed up by a dentist.

Ellis I: Needs referral to a dentist within 24 hours to have crown filed to remove rough edges.

Ellis II: Needs urgent referral to dentist within 24 hours to have crown placed to prevent bacterial contamination of the pulp.

Ellis III: Needs urgent referral to an oral surgeon for probable tooth extraction or root canal.

Avulsion: Needs emergent referral to an oral surgeon within 2 hours for possible tooth reimplantation and root canal.

EVALUATION/FOLLOW-UP

Close follow-up by an oral surgeon or dentist is essential.

SUGGESTED READINGS

Abrams RB, Mueller WA: Oral medicine & dentistry. In *Current pediatric diagnosis and treatment,* ed 12, Norwalk, Conn, 1995, Appleton & Lange.

Belanger GK, Casamassimo PA: Dental injuries. In Barkin RM, Rosen P, editors: *Emergency pediatrics: a guide to ambulatory care,* ed 4, St Louis, 1994, Mosby.

Belanger GK, Casamassimo PA: Ear, nose, and throat disorders. In Barkin RM, Rosen P, editors: *Emergency pediatrics: a guide to ambulatory care,* ed 4, St Louis, 1994, Mosby.

Boynton RW, Dunn ES, Stephens GR: *Manual of ambulatory pediatrics,* ed 3, Philadelphia, 1994, JB Lippincott.

Dambro MR, Griffth J, Cann C: *Griffith's 5-minute clinical consult,* Baltimore, 1997, Williams & Wilkins.

Ellsworth AJ et al: *Mosby's 1998 medical drug reference,* St Louis, 1998, Mosby.

Healthcare Consultants of America, Inc: *1998 Physicians fee and coding guide,* Augusta, Ga, 1998, Healthcare Consultants of America, Inc.

Hoole AJ et al: *Patient care guidelines for nurse practitioners,* ed 4, Philadelphia, 1995, JB Lippincott.

Jackler RK, Kaplan MJ: Ears, nose, and throat. In Tierney LM, McPhee SJ, Papadakis MA, editors: *Current medical diagnosis and treatment,* Norwalk, Conn, 1996, Appleton & Lange.

MacLeod DK: Common problems of the teeth and oral cavity. In Baker LR, Burton JR, Zieve PD, editors: *Principles of ambulatory medicine,* ed 4, Philadelphia, 1995, Williams & Wilkins.

Rund DA: Facial and oral trauma. In Rund DA et al, editors: *Essentials of emergency medicine,* ed 2, St Louis, 1996, Mosby.

Sonis ST: Lesions of the mouth. In Branch WT, editor: *Office practice of medicine,* ed 3, Philadelphia, 1994, WB Saunders.

Uphold CR, Graham MV: *Clinical guidelines in family practice,* ed 2, Gainesville, Fla, 1994, Barmarrae Books.

52 Depression

ICD-9-CM

Depressive Disorder, Not Elsewhere Classified 311.0
Major Depressive Disorder, Single Episode 296.2
Major Depressive Disorder, Recurrent Episode 296.3

OVERVIEW

Definition

Depression is a disturbance in mood or affect. Depressive disorders are classified as follows:

Major depression, dysthymic disorder, or adjustment disorder depression
- A major depressive disorder is defined as symptoms of depression that last for at least 2 weeks.
- Dysthymia is defined as symptoms of depression that are less intense but of longer duration (at least 2 years) with impaired functioning.
- Adjustment disorder depression is defined as the onset of depression symptoms in response to an identifiable event (within 3 months). This does not include posttraumatic stress disorder (PTSD) or bereavement.

Incidence

Depression is the most common reason for a person to seek mental health treatment. It is the admitting diagnosis for 75% of hospitalized psychiatric patients and 6% to 8% of all outpatients in a primary care setting. At any given time 10 to 14 million Americans are suffering from some form of a mood disorder.

Depression is twice as common in **women** as in men, except in bipolar disorders, in which the incidence is about equal. It is believed that 8% to 12% of men and 18% to 25% of women will suffer a major depression in their lifetime. Depression is more common in young women and tends to decrease with age. In men, the incidence tends to increase with age. There is an increased incidence of depression in **older adults** who are living in long-term facilities. Older adults are at high risk for depression because of the multiple losses and health problems that frequently occur at this stage of life.

Etiology/Pathophysiology

Various theories have been formulated to explain the cause and dynamics of mood/affective disorders. It is believed that these disorders are a syndrome with common features and a variety of causative factors. The most common theoretical perspectives are these:

Biochemical/neurobiological: There is a functional deficiency of the neurotransmitters serotonin (5-HT), dopamine, norepinephrine, and acetylcholine, with a probable genetic component.
Psychodynamic: This theory focuses on perceived loss and the unresolved grieving that occurred in the early child-parent relationship. The unresolved grieving is accompanied by repressed anger resulting in anger turned against the self.
Cognitive: Schemas direct the way people experience others and themselves. Those who are depressed ignore the positive and focus on the negative messages, thus contributing to a view of self as unworthy, incompetent, and unlovable. When this occurs, cognitive distortions result.

Factors That Increase Incidence of Depression

Marital status: Single and divorced persons
Seasonal: Increase in spring and fall
Previous episode: Prior episodes with depression increase chance of another episode
Age (under 40 years old)
Postpartum
Physical illness

Inadequate social support
Substance abuse
Ineffective psychosocial functioning; i.e., ineffective coping skills (increases exposure to stressors)

Factors That Increase Risk of Suicide

Problems/trauma or loss
Patient is white
Physical illness
Substance abuse
Male
Increasing age
Living alone
Previous suicide attempts/gestures
Adolescent with events perceived as extremely distressing
Less education
Relationship conflict
Mental disorder
Family or significant other suicide
Impaired impulse control
Hopelessness
Loss of income/employment
Depressed **elder**

SUBJECTIVE DATA

The clinical interview is the most effective method for detecting depression.

History of Present Illness

Determine the level of depression and severity of symptoms.
Identify when the symptoms began, and what increases or improves symptoms.

Past Medical History

Ask about the following:

Panic attacks, depression, and /or suicide attempts
History of cerebrovascular accident, myocardial infarction, or other chronic debilitating illness

Medications

Identify all medications the patient might be taking, including OTC and herbal remedies (e.g., St. John's Wort).

Medications reportedly associated with depression are listed in Box 52-1.

Family History

Ask about family history of depression/suicide attempts, mental illness.
If positive, ask about treatment obtained.

Box 52-1

Medications Reportedly Associated With Depression

Cardiovascular Drugs

Alpha-methyldopa
Reserpine
Propranolol
Guanethidine
Clonidine
Thiazide diuretics
Digitalis

Hormones

Oral and injectable contraceptives
ACTH (corticotropin)
Glucocorticoids
Anabolic steroids

Psychotropics

Benzodiazepines
Neuroleptics

Anticancer Agents

Cycloserine

Antiinflammatory/Antiinfective Agents

NSAIDs
Ethambutol
Disulfiram
Sulfonamides
Baclofen
Metoclopramide

Others

Cocaine (withdrawal)
Amphetamine (withdrawal)
L-dopa
Cimetidine
Ranitidine

From Rush AJ: Depression in primary care: Clinical Practice Guideline No 5 (AHCPR 93-0550), Rockville, Md, 193, US Department of Health and Human Services, Public Health Services, Agency for Health Care Policy and Research.

ACTH, Adrenocortocotropic hormone; *NSAIDs,* nonsteroidal antiinflammatory drugs.

Psychosocial History

Identify the following:

Support systems and coping techniques
Substance abuse: Illegal or legal drug use and alcohol use
Perceived losses and current stressors

Suicide risk must be critically assessed. Specific and clear questions should be asked by the clinician regarding:

Suicidal thoughts and history of past attempts
Having a plan for suicide

TABLE 52-1 Lethality Assessment Scale

Danger to Self	Indicators
No predictable risk of immediate suicide	No notion of suicide, no history of attempts, satisfactory social support network, close contact with significant others
Low risk of immediate suicide	Person has considered suicide with low lethal method, no history of attempts or recent serious loss, has satisfactory support network, no alcohol problems, basically wants to live
Moderate risk of immediate suicide	Has considered suicide with high lethal method but no specific plan or threats or has plan with low lethality, history of low lethal attempts; has tumultuous family history and reliance on benzodiazepines for stress relief; is weighing the odds between life and death
High risk of immediate suicide	Has current high lethal plan, obtainable means, history of previous attempts, has a close friend but is unable to communicate with him or her; has a drinking problem; is depressed, wants to die
Very high risk of immediate suicide	Has current high lethal plan with available means, history of high lethal suicide attempts, is cut off from resources; is depressed and uses alcohol to excess, and is threatened with a serious loss, such as unemployment or divorce or failure in school

From Hoff LA: *People in crisis,* ed 4, San Francisco, 1995, Jossey Bass.

Access to a means or weapon for suicide
The more specific and structured the plan the greater the risk

Use mnemonic SAL:
S: Specific?
A: Available?
L: Lethal?

A guideline for assessing the lethality of a patient's suicidal intent is provided in Table 52-1.

Description of Most Common Symptoms

Symptoms most frequently associated with depression include:

Emotional
- Feelings of sadness, guilt, low self-esteem, worthlessness, apathy, pessimistic thoughts
- Suicidal thoughts, gestures, and attempts
- Tearfulness, anxiety, and irritability

Behavioral
- Poor hygiene, psychomotor retardation
- Anhedonia: Loss of interest or pleasure in activities that were previously enjoyed
- Decreased libido

Physical
- Headache
- Fatigue
- Constipation
- Sleep disturbances (insomnia or hypersomnia)
- Changes in appetite, with either weight gain or loss

Cognitive
- Memory loss
- Impaired concentration
- Obsessive thoughts
- Indecisiveness
- Impaired cognitive reasoning: All-or-nothing thinking, jumping to conclusions, mental filtering, personalization, and "should" statements
- Recurrent thoughts of death or suicide

Box 52-2 presents symptoms that are likely to be seen by age group.

Associated Symptoms

Ask about the following:
- Headache: Recent onset or change
- Vision: Deterioration, blurring, or spots
- Speech: Recent changes
- Writing: Recent changes
- Memory: Change in short- or long-term
- Gait: Ataxia, waddling, limping
- Sensation: Pins and needles, paresthesia
- Strength: Weakness or asymmetry, clumsiness
- Consciousness: History of blackout or loss of consciousness

OBJECTIVE DATA

Physical Examination

The physical examination should be thorough, with particular attention to:

General appearance: Poor eye contact, tearful, downcast, inattentive to appearance; speech—little or no spontaneity, monosyllabic, long pauses, soft, low, monotone
Mental status: Memory, affect, judgment, cognitive abilities,

Box 52-2

Age-Defined Symptoms: Depression

Children

Loss of appetite
Stomach aches
Headaches
Fatigue
Conduct problems
Aggression
Irritability
Anhedonia
Fear of separation from caregiver or fear of caregiver
Failure to achieve developmental tasks
Academic problems
School refusal
Antisocial behaviors

Adolescents

Isolation
Self-destructive behavior
Sexual promiscuity
Antisocial behavior
Negative thinking
School refusal
Academic problems
Increased sensitivity to rejection
Poor hygiene

Adults

Fatigue, headache
Chest pain
Alteration in bowel and bladder function
Amenorrhea
Nausea and vomiting
Psychomotor agitation or retardation

Elderly

Fatigue, anorexia, bowel/bladder problems often attributed to "old age"; they may also manifest symptoms that must be differentiated from those of dementia:
Disorientation
Impaired memory
Inability to concentrate
Anhedonia

thought content; preschool and school age children appear sad
Thyroid enlargement
Cardiovascular
Neurological

Diagnostic Procedures

Currently, there are no conclusive diagnostic physical examination findings or laboratory tests for depression. Usually a limited number of tests must be conducted to detect potential general medical causes for depression (Table 52-2). However, certain abnormal results have been noted in a few tests that are characteristic of a depressed state. They should not be used as a routine evaluation measure for primary care patients.

Rating scale instruments designed to measure the patient's mood aid in the identification of the depressed patient. These measures identify nearly every patient with a major depressive disorder but are not very specific. Costs for psychological testing range from $133 to $155 an hour. These include the tests shown in Box 52-3.

ASSESSMENT

Establish a differential diagnosis using the following steps:

1. Conduct a clinical interview for nine specific signs and symptoms according to DSM-IV.
2. Investigate the possibility of concurrent substance or alcohol abuse.
3. Conduct a medical review of systems to identify a medical disorder.
4. Identify the presence of another concurrent psychiatric disorder.
5. Exclude alternative causes.

Differential Diagnosis

Organic mood disorder, schizophrenia, grief, dysthymia, major depression, adjustment disorder, bipolar disorder, delirium, dementia, substance abuse, endocrine disorders, liver failure, chronic fatigue, renal failurc, concurrent anxiety disorder (Table 52-3 and Figures 52-1 to 52-3).

THERAPEUTIC PLAN (Figure 52-4)

1. The initial and primary goal is to provide for the safety of the patient. Determine the lethality of the patients suicidal ideation/plan. Remember that suicide is most likely when a patient is going into or emerging from depression.
2. Avoid excessive cheerfulness which might be perceived as diminishing the significance of the patient's feelings.
3. Establish a no-suicide contract with the patient. If the patient is unable or unwilling to sign a permanent no suicide contract, limit the contract to 24 or 48 hours and then renew.
4. Assist the patient in contacting immediate support systems.
5. If the patient is clearly suicidal and unwilling to contract not to harm himself or herself, immediate hospitalization must be considered. If the patient is considered a threat to himself or herself or someone else, he or she may be hospitalized involuntarily for 48 hours until further evaluation is completed.

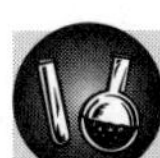

TABLE 52-2 Diagnostic Tests: Depression

Test	Findings	Cost ($)
EEG	Abnormal sleep EEG seen in about 50% of all outpatients with depression.	97-119
DST	In a nondepressed person, the production and secretion of cortisol by the adrenal gland is suppressed. If the person is depressed, the suppression of cortisol is slight and/or the recovery from the effects of the DST is quite rapid.	210-270
Thyroid function studies	Elevated TSH, lowered T_4 (hypothyroidism) Consider when patient is female and >50	47-61
Screening tests as appropriate	CBC	18-23/CBC
	Chemistry panel	32-42
	ESR	16-20
	ECG (for patients over 40 years old to rule out conduction disturbances or before tricyclic antidepressant therapy is started).	56-65

CBC, Complete blood cell count; *DST,* dexamethasone suppression test; *ECG,* electrocardiogram; *EEG,* electroencephalogram; *ESR,* erythrocyte sedimentation rate; *TSH,* thyroid-stimulating hormone.

Box 52-3

Rating Scales: Depression

Self-Rating Scales

Center for Epidemiological Studies–Depression Scale (CES-D)
Beck Depression Inventory (Beck et al, 1961)
Zung Scale (Zung, 1965)
PRIME-MD (two-part instrument to assess five DSM-IV disorders commonly seen in primary care: depression, anxiety, substance abuse, somatization, and eating disorders; consists of self-rating scale and interview) (Spitzer et al, 1994)
DSM-IV-PC focuses on diagnostic criteria and assessment approaches for nine categories of common mental disorders seen in primary care

Clinician-Completed Scales

Hamilton Rating Scale for Depression (HRS-D) (Hamilton, 1968)
The Inventory for Depressive Symptomatology—Clinician Rated (IDS-C) (Rush et al, 1986)
Bech-Rafaelsen Depression Scale (BRDS) (Wing et al, 1967)

6. Mobilizing is the process of helping the patient to develop a plan of action to follow, starting with the first visit. Identify a daily plan that provides structure. Even simple plans such as getting out of bed and dressed by a certain time, going for a walk, and meeting a friend can be effective (Oakley, 1997). The plan should include the following: interaction with supportive others, sleep and rest, restorative recreation, exercise, work, doing something for someone else, and limited time spent alone.
7. Use the acronym *SPEAK* (Christensen, 1997) for office counseling. The SPEAK method is not meant to replace psychotherapy, but it might be helpful as a first approach:
   *S*chedule: Counteracts the inertia that accompanies depression. Frontal lobe activities such as planning, organizing are often impaired by depression. Patient should plan ahead and develop a schedule, and then follow it even if he or she doesn't feel like it.
   *P*leasurable activities: The plan should include pleasurable activities to counteract lethargy and inertia.
   *E*xercise: Exercise is a short-term mood enhancer; the patient should exercise several times a week.
   *A*ssertiveness: Assertiveness is a key behavior in depression because of its positive effect on self-esteem. Encourage being direct with others about feelings, opinions and intentions. Reading *Your Perfect Right* (Alberti and Emmons, 1970) may be helpful.
   *K*ind thoughts about oneself: The patient should try to replace self-punishing thoughts. This may be the most challenging element of SPEAK. Use of the ABCD method of thought analysis may help the patient in review of emotions and beliefs (Feldman and Christensen, 1997).

Pharmaceutical (Tables 52-4 and 52-5)

See Figure 52-4 for an overview of therapy for depression. The choice of medication is based on:

History of prior treatment and response (including past family response)
Type of depression

TABLE 52-3 Differential Diagnosis: Depression

Diagnoses	Supporting Data
Delirium/dementia	Delirium is alteration of the mental state to one of acute confusion. Dementia presents with disorientation, memory loss, and distractibility.
Substance abuse	Mood disorder caused by drug or toxin: Cocaine, amphetamine, propranolol, steroids.
Endocrine disorders	Hypothyroidism: Fatigue, flat affect.
Major depression	Dysphoria, weight loss or gain, insomnia or hypersomnia, restlessness or slowness, fatigue, feelings of worthlessness, decreased concentration, thoughts of death or suicide.
Dysthymia	Symptoms fewer and less intense but longer than major depression. Depressed mood on a regular basis for at least 2 years, poor appetite or overeating, insomnia or hypersomnia, low energy, low self-esteem, poor concentration, feelings of hopelessness, symptoms free periods no longer than 2 months.
Adjustment disorder	Symptoms fewer and milder than major depression, and not as long as dysthymia but moderate rather than mild symptoms. Occurs as a response to event within last 3 months.
Bipolar disorder	Severe mood disorder defined by episodes of elation and depression, with depression usually lasting longer than manic episodes. Rapid thoughts and speech are seen in mania, while negativity, fatigue and dysphoria are seen with depression.
Grief	Presentation may be similar to depression but remits with time. Absence of suicidal ideation or profound feelings of worthlessness. Usually resolves within 1 year; can develop into major depression in predisposed persons.
Anxiety disorder	Coexists in 10%-30% of patients with depression.
Chronic fatigue syndrome	Excessive fatigue, aching muscles and joints, headache, sore throat, painful lymph nodes, muscle weakness, sleep disturbance, mental fatigue, difficulty concentrating, emotional lability, and sadness.

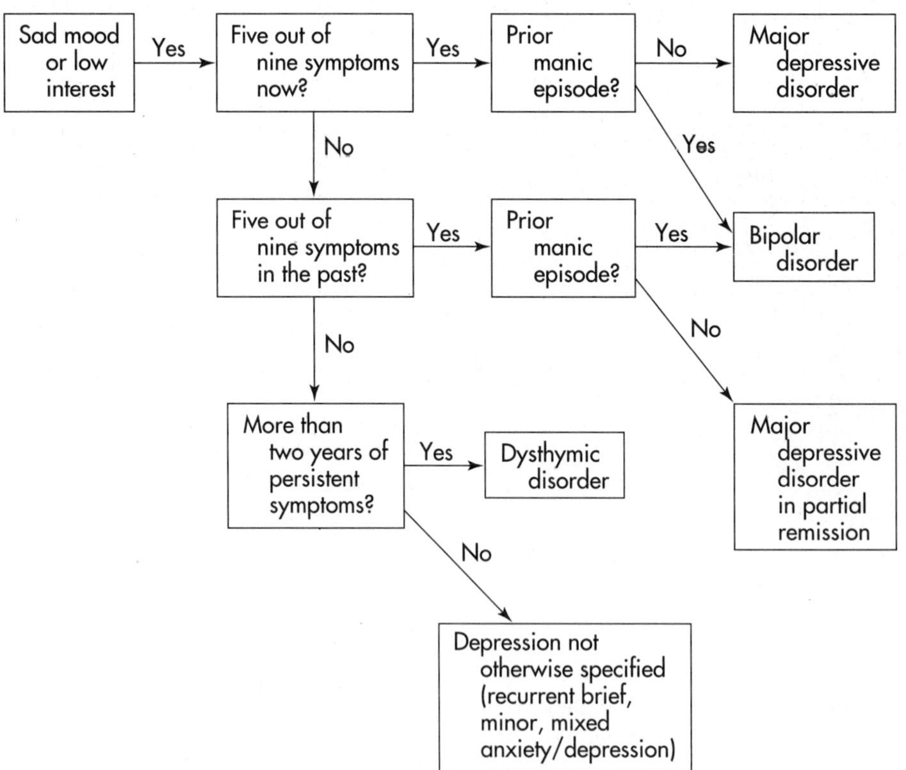

Figure 52-1 Differential diagnosis of primary mood disorders. (From Depression Guideline Panel: *Depression in primary care, vols 1 and 2, clinical practice guidelines no. 5,* Rockville, Md, US Dept of Health and Human Services, Public Health Service, Agency for Health Care Policy and Research. Publication No 93-0550, April 1993.)

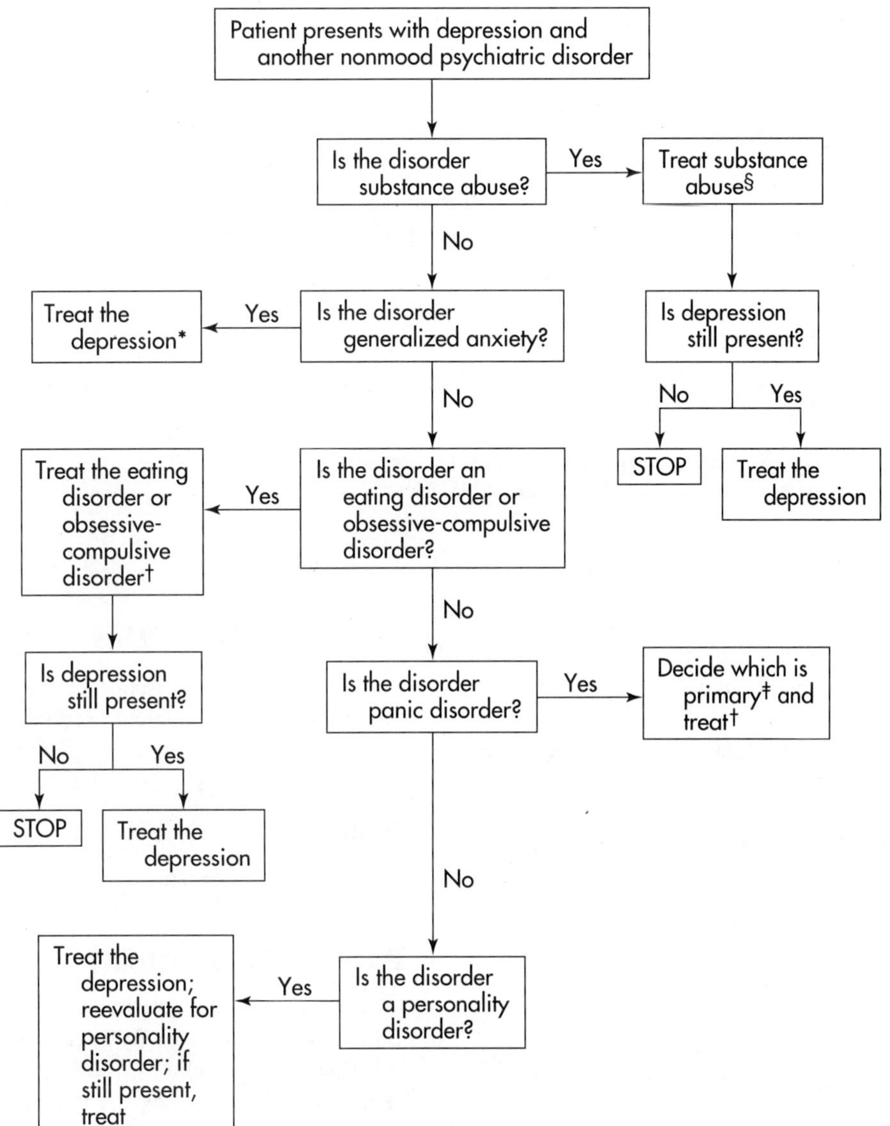

Figure 52-2 Relationship between major depressive and other concurrent psychiatric disorders. *When the depression is treated, the anxiety disorder should resolve as well.
†Choose medications known to be effective for both the depression and the other psychiatric disorder.
‡Primary is the most severe, the longest standing by history, or the one that runs in the patient's family.
§In certain cases (based on history), both major depression and substance abuse may require simultaneous treatment. (From Depression Guideline Panel: *Depression in primary care, vols 1 and 2, clinical practice guidelines no. 5,* Rockville, Md, US Dept of Health and Human Services, Public Health Service, Agency for Health Care Policy and Research, Publication No 93-0550, April 1993.)

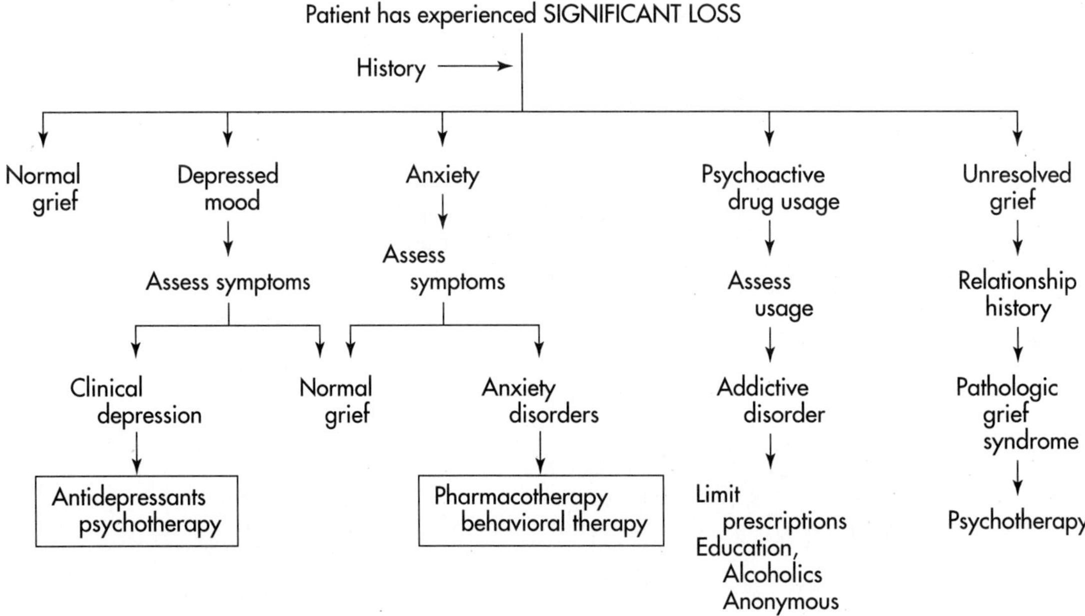

Figure 52-3 Patient has experienced significant loss. (From Greene H, Johnson W, Lemcke D: *Decision making in medicine,* ed 2, St Louis, 1998, Mosby.)

Potential side effects of the medication
Other medications the patient may be taking

In general, the dose for **elderly** patients should be approximately 50% of normal starting dose.

Strategies for Initial Antidepressant Therapy

Consider using selective serotonin reuptake inhibitors or venlafaxine as first-line therapy

Begin fluoxetine or paroxetine (10 mg at breakfast); 3 to 5 days later increase to 20 mg at breakfast
Sertraline: 50 mg QD; after 5 to 7 days increase to 100 mg
Venlafaxine: 37.5 mg QD (with food); 7 days later increase to 75 mg (sampled as starter pack with 7 days of 37.5 and 7 days of 75 mg)

Some improvement should be noted after 2 weeks. If not:

Fluoxetine or paroxetine: Increase to 40 mg; increase to 60 mg QD if patient is still moderately depressed after 4 to 6 weeks on 40 mg dose
Venlafaxine: Increase to 150 mg QD (Norman, 1998)
May take up to 12 weeks before improvement is noted in **elderly** patients

Psychotherapy or counseling is recommended for the treatment of depression, either alone or in combination with medication. Individual and group therapy are both effective modalities.

Lifestyle/Activities

Encourage activities; discourage time spent alone
Recommend that the patient exercise at least three times per week

Diet

No special diet needed

Patient Education

Describe medication actions and side effects.
Outline dietary and activity restrictions related to the medication, as appropriate.
Teach the family and the patient to report increasing signs of depression or suicidal thoughts.
Reinforce effective coping behaviors, nutrition, exercise, rest, and socialization.
Emphasize that depression can be an aggressive and invasive disorder that, left untreated, can invade all parts of persons life.

Family Impact

Families with a member who is suffering depression frequently report the following:

Grief over the loss of the person they once knew

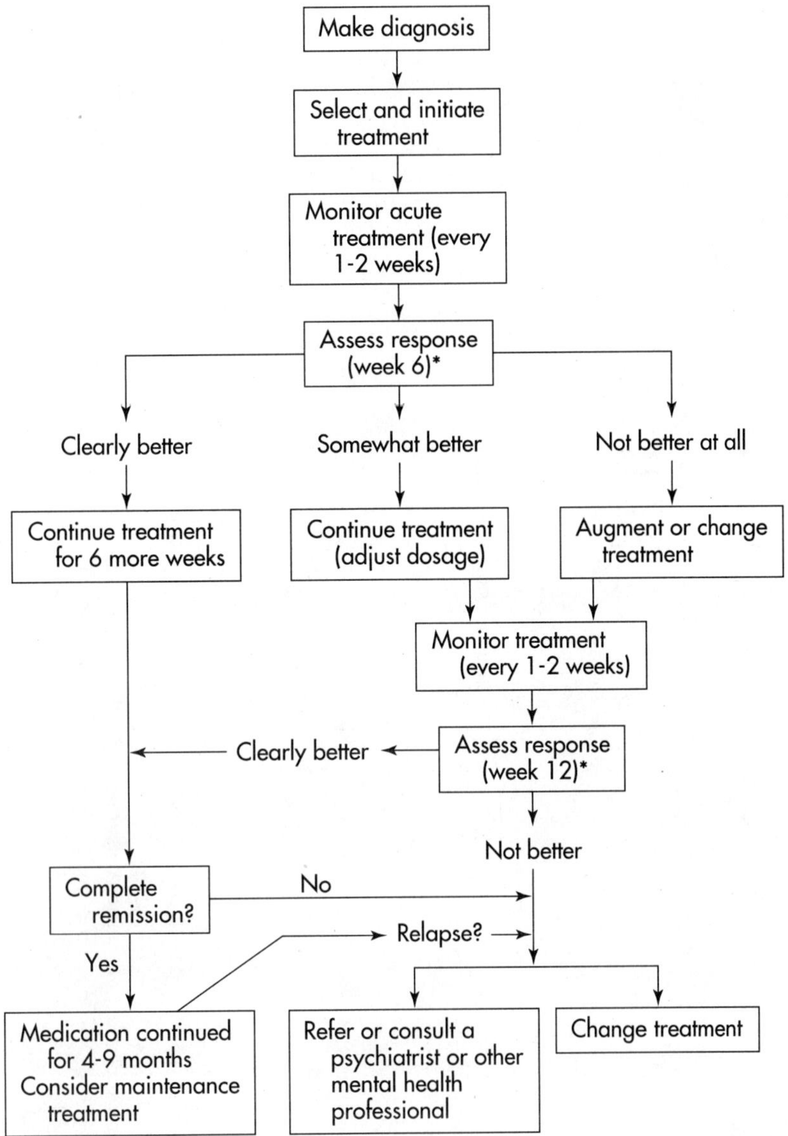

Figure 52-4 Overview of treatment for depression.
*Note that times of assessment (weeks 6 and 12) rest on very modest data. It may be necessary to revise the treatment plan earlier for patients failing to respond at all. (From Depression Guideline Panel: *Depression in primary care, vols 1 and 2, clinical practice guidelines no. 5,* Rockville, Md, US Dept of Health and Human Services, Public Health Service, Agency for Health Care Policy and Research. Publication No 93-0550, April 1993.)

Guilt at their part in the illness
Anger at the patient's behaviors/actions (or lack of)
Powerlessness
Concern that the depression may become a lifelong illness
Fear of the unknown
Changes in family dynamics may be seen
Altered communication/interaction patterns
Altered roles and responsibilities

Interventions for the family may include:
Family/marital counseling
Community support
Encouragement of "normal" family roles and routines as much as possible
Family meetings
Having crisis or hotline number available if needed

Referral

The following patients should be referred to a psychiatrist:
- Bipolar disorders
- Patients who do not improve even with maximal drug therapy and/or counseling

TABLE 52-4 Pharmaceutical Plan: Depression

Class	Drug	Beginning Dose	Maximum Dose	Comments	Cost
SSRI and other compounds	Fluoxetine (Prozac)	20 mg QD **Elderly:** 5-40 mg/day	80 mg	**Elders** tolerate SSRIs better than they do tricyclics. Good choice to avoid anticholinergic effects. Not FDA approved in **children.** Prozac comes in liquid form 20 mg/5 ml. Interactions with CYP 450 and CYP3A4, CYP2D6. SE: GI, headache, insomnia, nervousness, sexual dysfunction Prozac: Pregnancy: B Paxil and Zoloft: Pregnancy: C Do not combine with TCAs unless patient is under supervision of psychiatrist	$220/20 mg (100)
	Paroxetine (Paxil)	20 mg QD **Elderly:** 10-40/ day	50 mg QD		$57/20 mg (30) $64/40 mg (30)
	Sertraline (Zoloft)	50 mg QD, ↑ 1-week intervals **Elderly:** Start with 12.5-25 mg	200 mg QD **Elderly:** 150 mg		$176/50 mg (100) 100 mg $181 (100)
	Citalopram (Celexa)			Will be released soon.	
	Venlafaxine (Effexor) inhibits S, N, and to lesser extent D	37.5-75 mg BID **Elderly:** 37.5; a sustained-release form is available for QD dosing	↑ days q 4 in 75-mg increments; max 375 mg/day TID	Not recommended for patients under 18 years old. Effective in patients with refractory depression, lack of P450 inhibition, may have more rapid onset. SE: Nausea, insomnia, headache, mild ↑ in B/P, sweating, ↑ HR	$95/25 mg (100) $98/37.5 mg (100) $114/50 mg (100)
	Trazodone (Desyrel)	50 mg TID with food	Increase by 50 mg q 3-4 days; max: 600	Significant sedative properties: No anticholinergic effects, safety in OD SE: Sedation, orthostatic hypotention, dizziness, headache, nausea; can induce priapism in men	$5-$139/50 mg (100) $12-$242/100 mg (100)
Phenylpiperazine	Nefazodone (Serzone)	100 mg BID **Elderly:** 100-400 mg/day	↑ by 100-200 mg at 1 wk interval range 300-600 mg	Not recommended for patients under 18 Do not use with astemizole, cisapride or terfenadine. Interferes with P450-3A4 isoenzymes. Pregnancy: C	$50/All mg (100)

Aminoketone (Unicyclic) Weak effects N, S, D	Bupropion (Wellbutrin) Also SR	100 mg BID for 4-7 days **Elderly:** 50-450 mg/day; SR: 150 in morning, ↑ 150 BID	↑ to 100 mg TID Can ↑ to 375-450 mg QD SR: max: 200/BID	SR: Avoid bedtime dosing. No sexual dysfunction. Pregnancy: B Low doses can be combined with SSRI. Precaution: Seizure disposition—give only 150 mg of regular wellbutrin per dose; can give 200 mg of SR form/dose	$56/75 mg (100) $75/100 mg (100)
	Mirtazepine (Remeron)	15 mg at HS, ↑ in 15-mg increments QO week **Elderly:** 15-45 mg/day	45 mg	Strong sedative effects, but weak anticholinergic effects; does *not* block CYP450 isoenzymes; considered second- or third-line at this time SE: Somnolence, weight gain, and dizziness	N/A
Tricyclics	Amitriptyline (Elavil)	25-50 mg BID/TID	150 mg	Potential for overdose; narrow therapeutic range.	$2-$19/Elavil: 10 mg (100)
	Desipramine* (Norpramin)	75 mg QD	300 mg	Decrease doses in **elderly** and adolescents; not recommended in **children**	$3-$69/50 mg (100) $4-$91/100 mg (100)
	Doxepin (Sinequan)	75 mg QD	150 mg	Give in split doses until side effects are better tolerated; if give QD dosing, give at HS	
	Imipramine (Tofranil)	25 mg TID/QID	200 mg	Lower seizure threshold; class 1 antiarrhythmic effects	
	Nortriptyline* (Pamelor)	75 mg BID/TID	150 mg	Avoid use of TCAs in **elderly:** nortriptyline or desipramine are preferred if TCAs used	
	Trimipramine (Surmontil)	200 mg QD	200 mg QD	SE: Anticholinergic effects: dry mouth, constipation, urinary retention, blurred vision, sinus tachycardia, antihistamine effects, orthostatic hypotention	
MAO inhibitors	Phenelzine (Nardil) Tranylcypromine (Parnate)	15 mg TID 30 mg QD	↑ To max of 60 mg	Not recommended in patients under 16 years old Multiple drug/food interactions; third-line agent; should be used in collaboration with psychiatrist	

*Better side effect profile.
BP, Blood pressure; *D*, dopamine; *HR*, heart rate; *MAO*, monoamine oxidase inhibitors; *max*, maximum; *N*, Norephinephrine; *N/A*, not available; *S*, serotonin; *SE*, side effects; *SR*, slow release; *SSRI*, selective serotonin reuptake inhibitor; *TCA*, tricyclic antidepressants.

TABLE 52-5 Side-Effect Profiles of Antidepressant Medications

	Side Effect*						
		Central Nervous System		Cardiovascular		Other	
Drug	Anticho-linergic†	Drows-iness	Insomnia/Agitation	Orthostatic Hypo-tension	Cardiac Arrhythmia	Gastro-intestinal Distress	Weight Gain (over 6 kg)
Amitriptyline	4+	4+	0	4+	3+	0	4+
Desipramine	1+	1+	1+	2+	2+	0	1+
Doxepin	3+	4+	0	2+	2+	0	3+
Imipramine	3+	3+	1+	4+	3+	1+	3+
Nortriptyline	1+	1+	0	2+	2+	0	1+
Protriptyline	2+	1+	1+	2+	2+	0	0
Trimipramine	1+	4+	0	2+	2+	0	3+
Amoxapine	2+	2+	2+	2+	3+	0	1+
Maprotiline	2+	4+	0	0	1+	0	2+
Trazodone	0	4+	0	1+	1+	1+	1+
Bupropion	0	0	2+	0	1+	1+	0
Fluoxetine	0	0	2+	0	0	3+	0
Paroxetine	0	0	2+	0	0	3+	0
Sertraline	0	0	2+	0	0	3+	0
Monoamine oxidase inhibitors	1	1+	2+	2+	0	1+	2+

From: Depression Guideline Panel. *Depression in Primary Care. Volume 1 and 2, Clinical Practice Guidelines*. No. 5, Rockville, MD. US Dept of Health and Human Services, Public Health Service, Agency for Health Care Policy and Research. AHCPR Publication No. 93-0550. April 1993.
*0 = Absent or rare.
1+
2+ = In between.
3+
4+ = Relatively common.
†Dry mouth, blurred vision, urinary hesitancy, constipation.

Consultation

Seek immediate consultation for a patient who is actively suicidal

Follow-up (Figures 52-5 and 52-6)

Patients who are depressed and taking antidepressant medications should return weekly for evaluation. After 5 to 6 weeks, when improvement is seen, the follow-up can go to two times per month, then monthly, and so forth. It is critical to have the patient in counseling and receiving antidepressant therapy to see optimal improvement.

Each successive episode of depression suggests that psychosocial events play little or no role in subsequent episodes as disorder becomes firmly established.

Sudden discontinuation symptoms can occur when medication is suddenly stopped; taper all medications gradually.

Most common reasons for continuing depression are prescribing too low a dose, not treating long enough, or an underlying substance abuse or medical condition.

Maintain the patient on medication for at least 4 to 9 months for first episode. Some recommend 1 to 2 years for a second episode, and lifelong for three or more episodes.

Treat patients indefinitely over 40 with more than two episodes or one episode after the patient is 50 years old.

EVALUATION

Improvement is noted when:

The patient verbalizes and demonstrates compliance with treatment plan.

The patient experiences no suicidal thoughts and does not have a suicidal plan.

The patient verbalizes positive feelings about the future.

The patient demonstrates resolution of presenting symptoms.

Complete symptomatic response?*
Yes
Normal psychosocial function?
Yes
No
Go to continuation treatment
Chronic severe psychosocial dysfunction?
Yes
No
Add psychotherapy*
Reevaluate at 12 weeks* (If still present, add psychotherapy)

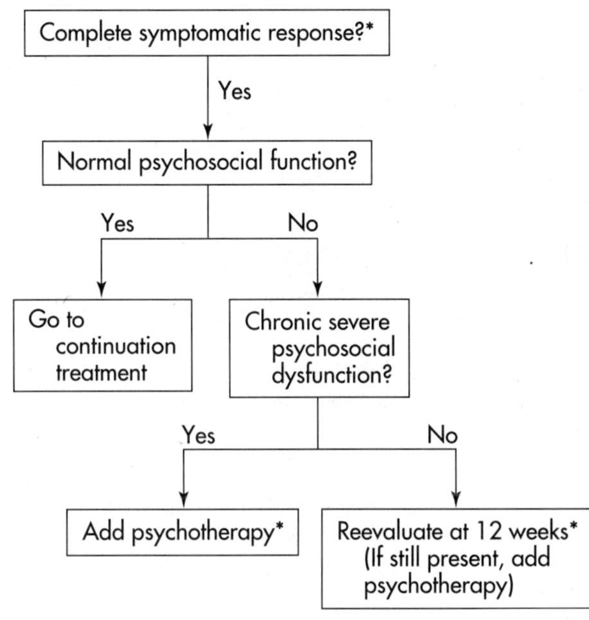

Figure 52-5 Six-week evaluation: Patients who respond to medication. Complete response—with no or very few symptoms. *These suggestions are based on indirectly relevant data, logical inference, and clinical experience. (From Depression Guideline Panel: *Depression in primary care, vols 1 and 2, clinical practice guidelines no. 5,* Rockville, Md, US Dept of Health and Human Services, Public Health Service, Agency for Health Care Policy and Research, Publication No 93-0550, April 1993.)

No or partial response at 6 weeks
Diagnosis correct?
No
Treat primary problem
Yes
Treatment adequate?
No
Adjust dosage, counsel adherence
Yes
Evaluate degree and nature of response
NONE*
PARTIAL†
PARTIAL†
Change medication
Augment medication
Consultation/ referral
(Largely cognitive symptoms remain)
(Largely vegetative symptoms remain)
Reevaluate at 12 weeks‡
Change or augment medication
Complete response
Partial response
To continuation treatment
Change medication
Add psycho- therapy
Augment medication
Consultation/ referral

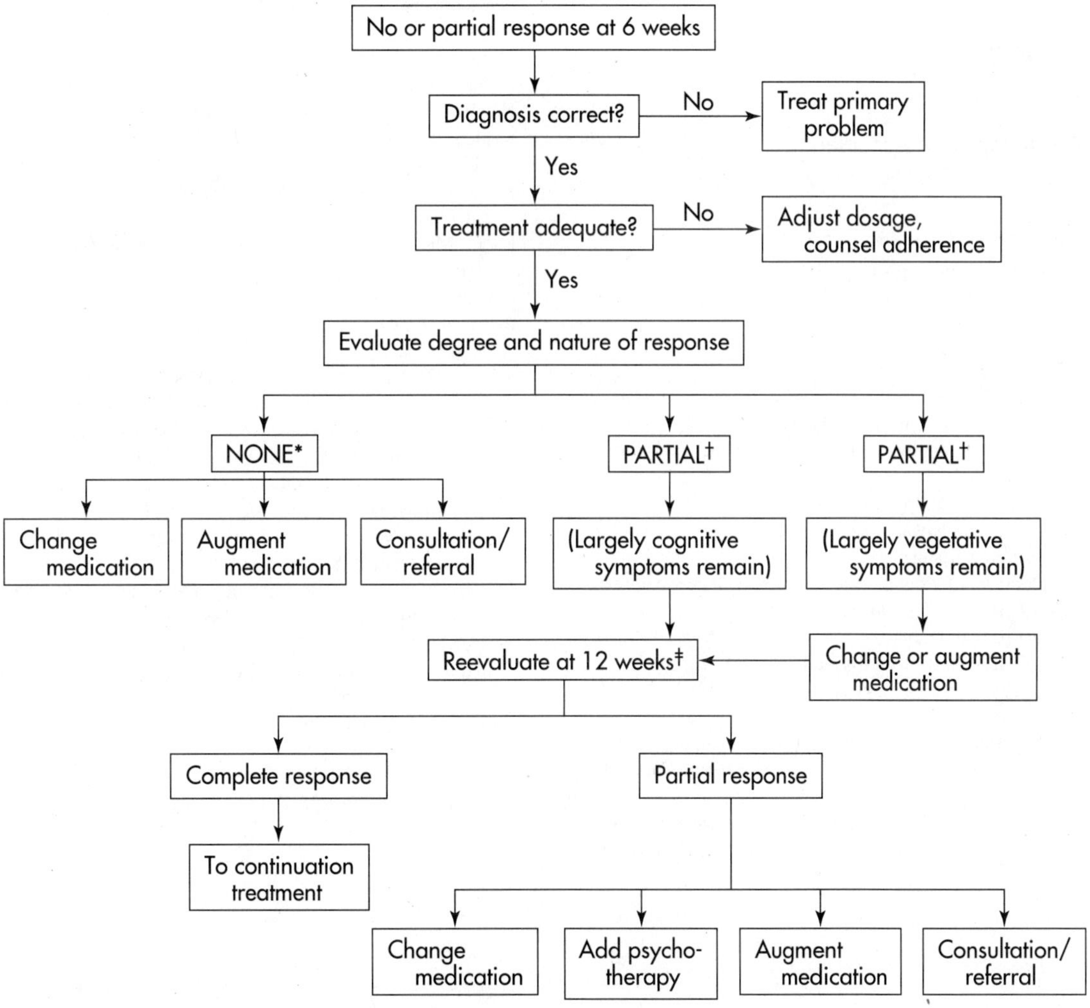

Figure 52-6 Six-week evaluation: Patients who partially respond and who do not respond to medication.
*No response—patient is nearly as symptomatic as at pretreatment.
†Partial response—patient is clearly better than at pretreatment, but still has significant symptoms. Consultation or referral may be valuable before proceeding further.
‡Suggestions for management are based on some indirectly relevant studies, logic, and clinical experience. (From Depression Guideline Panel: *Depression in primary care, vols 1 and 2, clinical practice guidelines no. 5,* Rockville, Md, US Dept of Health and Human Services, Public Health Service, Agency for Health Care Policy and Research, Publication No 93-0550, April 1993.)

Best criterion for full recovery: Minimum of 1 year of symptom remission and effective psychosocial functioning.

Relapse rate during the first 6 to 18 months is approximately 50%.

RESOURCES

National Institute of Mental Health
1-800-421-4211

National Depressive and Manic Association (NDMDA)
Chicago, IL 312-642-0049
1-800-82-NDMDA

National Foundation for Depressive Illness
1-800-248-4344

National Mental Health Association
1-800-969-6642

Information Referral and Crisis Hotline
1-800-233-4357

American Psychological Association
202-336-6062

Local Family Support Groups
National Alliance for the Mentally Ill
1-800-950-NAMI

REFERENCES

Alberti R, Emmons M: *Your perfect right: a guide to assertive behavior,* San Luis Obispo, Calif, 1970, Impact Publishers.

Christensen J: The SPEAK approach and pleasant events inventory. In M Feldmen M, Christensen J, editors: *Behavioral medicine in primary care,* Norwalk, Conn, 1997, Appleton & Lange.

Feldman M, Christensen J: *Behavioral medicine in primary care,* Stamford, Conn, 1997, Appleton & Lange.

Hamilton M: Development of a rating scale for primary depressive illness, *Br J Social Clin Psychol* 6:278-296, 1968.

Norman D: Recognizing and treating depression, 1998, *Advanced Practice Nurse Information Services* (www.information2.com).

Oakley L, Potter C: *Psychiatric primary care,* St Louis, 1997, Mosby.

Rush AJ: Depression in primary care: Clinical Practice Guideline No 5 (AHCPR 93-0550), Rockville, Md, 1993, US Department of Health and Human Services, Public Health Services, Agency for Health Care Policy and Research.

Sheikh J, Yesavage J: Geriatric depression scale: recent evidence of development of a shorter version, *Clin Gerontol* 5:165-172, 1998.

Wing J et al: Reliability of a procedure for measuring and classifying "present psychiatric state," *Br J Psychiatry* 113:499-515, 1967.

Zung WW, Richards C, Short M: Self-rating depression scale in an outpatient clinic: further validation of the SDS, *Arch Gen Psychiatry* 13(6)508-573, 1965.

SUGGESTED READINGS

American Psychiatric Association: *Diagnostic and statistical manual of mental disorders (DSM-IV),* ed 4, Washington, DC, 1994, The Association.

Beck AT et al: Screening for major depression disorders in medical inpatients with the Beck Depression Inventory for Primary Care, *Behav Res Ther* 35:785-791, 1997.

Bushfield-Kahan M: Managing adolescent depression in a primary care setting, *J Am Acad Nurse Pract* 9:235-240, 1997.

Eisendrath S: Psychiatric disorder. In Tierney L, McPhee S, Papadakis M, editors: *Current medical diagnosis and treatment,* ed 37, Norwalk, Conn, 1998, Appleton & Lange.

Ellsworth A et al: *Mosby's 1998 medical drug reference,* St Louis, 1998, Mosby.

Healthcare Consultants of America, Inc: *1998 Physicians fee and coding guide,* Augusta, Ga, 1998, Healthcare Consultants of America, Inc.

Fenstermacher K, Hudson B: *Practice guidelines for family nurse practitioners,* Philadelphia, 1997, WB Saunders.

Flowers ME: Recognition and psychopharmacologic treatment of geriatric depression, *J Am Psychiatr Nurse Assoc* 3:32-39, 1997.

Hoff LA: *People in crisis,* ed 4, San Francisco, 1995, Jossey Bass.

Kaplan H, Sadock B: *Pocket handbook of clinical psychiatry,* ed 2, Baltimore, 1996, Williams & Wilkins.

Kornstein S: Gender differences in depression: implications for treatment, *J Clin Psychiatry* 58 (Suppl 15):12-18, 1997.

Laraia M: Current approaches to the psychopharmacologic treatment of depression in children and adolescents, *J Child Adolesc Psychiatr Nurs* 9:15-26, 1996.

Robinson D: *Clinical decision making for nurse practitioners,* Philadelphia, 1998, JB Lippincott.

Schwartz G: Grief. In Greene H, Johnson W, Lemcke D, editors: *Decision making in medicine,* ed 2, St Louis, 1998, Mosby.

Spitzer et al: Utility of a new procedure for diagnosing mental disorders in primary care, *JAMA* 272:1749-1756, 1994.

The Harvard Mental Health Letter: *Update on mood disorders—part 1,* Harvard Medical School, Dec 1994, pp 1-4.

The Harvard Mental Health Letter: *Update on mood disorders—part 2,* Harvard Medical School, Jan 1995, pp 1-4.

The Harvard Mental Health Letter (November 1996) *Suicide—part 1,* Harvard Medical School, Nov 1996, pp 1-4.

Troxler M, Grogg S: Guide to family practitioners for the diagnosis and treatment of depression in children and adolescents, *J Am Osteopath Assoc* 97:280-285, 1997.

Wilson H, Kneisl C: *Psychiatric nursing,* ed 5, Reading, Mass, 1996, Addison-Wesley.

Workman C, Prior M: Depression and suicide in young children, *Issues Comp Pediatr Nurs* 20(2):125-132, 1997.

53 Dermatology

SUBJECTIVE DATA

History of Present Illness

Onset: Days, weeks, months, years
Location
Duration
Pruritus, pain, paresthesia
Relationship to seasons, travel, heat, cold, drug ingestion, occupation, hobbies, menses, pregnancy
Aggravating and relieving factors
Treatment (include prescribed treatment as well as OTC)

Past Medical History

Drugs taken
Allergies
Radiation treatments
Chronic illness or immunosuppression

Medications

New drugs being used
Corticosteroids

Family History

Allergies
Skin cancer

Psychosocial History

Hobbies
Occupational exposure to sun, chemicals
Use of tanning beds
Unprotected sex

Associated Symptoms

Systemic symptoms

OBJECTIVE DATA

Physical Examination

Vital signs
General appearance
Look for incidental findings (as opposed to chief complaint)
Examination of all skin
Describe *type* of lesion (primary/secondary) (Tables 53-1 and 53-2, Figure 53-1)
- Color
- Palpate for:
  - Consistency
  - Deviation in temperature
  - Mobility
  - Presence of tenderness
- Estimate depth of lesion
  - Shape
  - Margination
  - Arrangement of multiple lesions: Grouped/disseminated
  - Distribution/extent: Isolated, localized, regional, generalized
  - Pattern: Symmetrical, exposed areas, sites of pressure
  - Characteristic patterns: Secondary syphilis, lupus erythematosus, varicella zoster

Also examine hair, nails, mucous membranes
General medical examination

If possible, include a family member or responsible person in the examination and point out normal or worrisome lesions so they can help patient monitor the patient's skin.

TABLE 53-1 Primary Lesions

Lesion	Description
Macules	Up to 1 cm and circumscribed, flat discolorations of skin (e.g., freckles, flat nevi)
Patches	Larger than 1 cm, circumscribed, flat discolorations of skin (e.g., vitiligo, senile freckles, measles rash)
Papules	Up to 1 cm, circumscribed, elevated, superficial, solid lesions (e.g., elevated nevi, warts, lichen planus) Wheal is a type of papule that is edematous and transitory; size varies (e.g., hives, insect bites)
Plaques	Larger than 1 cm, circumscribed, elevated, superficial, solid lesions (e.g., mycosis fungoides, lichen simplex chronicus)
Nodules	Range to 1 cm, solid lesions with depth, above, level with, or below surface (e.g., xanthomas, epitheliomas)
Tumors	Larger than 1 cm, solid lesions with depth, above, level with, or below surface (e.g., tumor stage of mycosis fungoides, larger epitheliomas)
Vesicles	Up to 1 cm, circumscribed elevations of the skin containing serous fluid (e.g., early chickenpox, zoster, contact dermatitis)
Bullae	Larger than 1 cm, circumscribed elevations of the skin containing serous fluid (e.g., pemphigus, second-degree burns)
Pustules	Vary in size, circumscribed elevations of skin containing purulent fluid (e.g., acne, impetigo)
Petechiae	Range to 1 cm, circumscribed deposits of blood or blood pigment (e.g., certain insect bites, drug eruptions)
Purpura	Larger than 1 cm circumscribed deposit of blood or blood pigment

TABLE 53-2 Secondary Lesions

Lesion	Description
Scales	Shedding, dead epidermal cells that may be greasy or dry (e.g., dandruff, psoriasis)
Crusts	Variously colored masses of skin exudates (e.g., impetigo, infected dermatitis)
Excoriations	Abrasions of skin, usually superficial and traumatic (e.g., scratched insect bite, scabies)
Fissures	Linear breaks in skin, sharply defined, with abrupt walls (e.g., congenital syphilis, athletes foot)
Ulcers	Irregularly sized and shaped excavations in skin extending into corium (e.g., stasis ulcers, tertiary syphilis)
Scars	Formations of connective tissue replacing lost tissue through injury or disease
Keloids	Hypertrophic scars
Lichenification	Diffuse area of thickening and scaling with resultant increase in skin lines and markings
Special Lesions	
Comedones/ blackheads	Plugs of whitish or blackish sebaceous and keratinous material lodged in pilosebaceous follicle, usually seen on face, chest, or back, rarely on upper part of arms (e.g., acne)
Milia	Whitish nodules, 1-2 mm in diameter, no visible opening in skin.
Telangiectasis	Dilated superficial blood vessels (e.g., spider angiomas)
Burrows	Very small and short (scabies) or tortuous and long tunnels in the epidermis

TABLE 53-3 Seasonal Skin Disease

Season	Disease
Winter	Atopic eczema, contact dermatitis of hands, psoriasis, seborrheic dermatitis, nummular eczema, winter itch, dry skin (xerosis)
Spring	Pityriasis rosea, erythema multiforme, acne
Summer	Contact dermatitis (poison ivy), tinea of feet and groin, candidal intertrigo, miliaria or prickly heat, impetigo, actinic dermatitis, insect bites, tinea versicolor
Fall	Winter itch, senile pruritus, atopic eczema, pityriasis rosea, contact dermatitis (ragweed), tinea of scalp, acne

Diagnostic Procedures

Noninvasive, Augmented Inspection

Wood's lamp examination: Used to detect fungi and hypopigmentation

Ultraviolet light to inspect hair and skin

Findings: Bright, yellow-green indicates *Microsporum* (a type of organism responsible for some tinea capitis infections)

Yellow indicates tinea versicolor

Diascopy: Used to differentiate erythema from purpura

Press slide against lesion

Findings: If the redness is the result of erythema, blanching will occur; purpura or petechiae will persist

Epiluminescence microscopy: Skin surface microscope with battery handle that magnifies and illuminates skin lesions

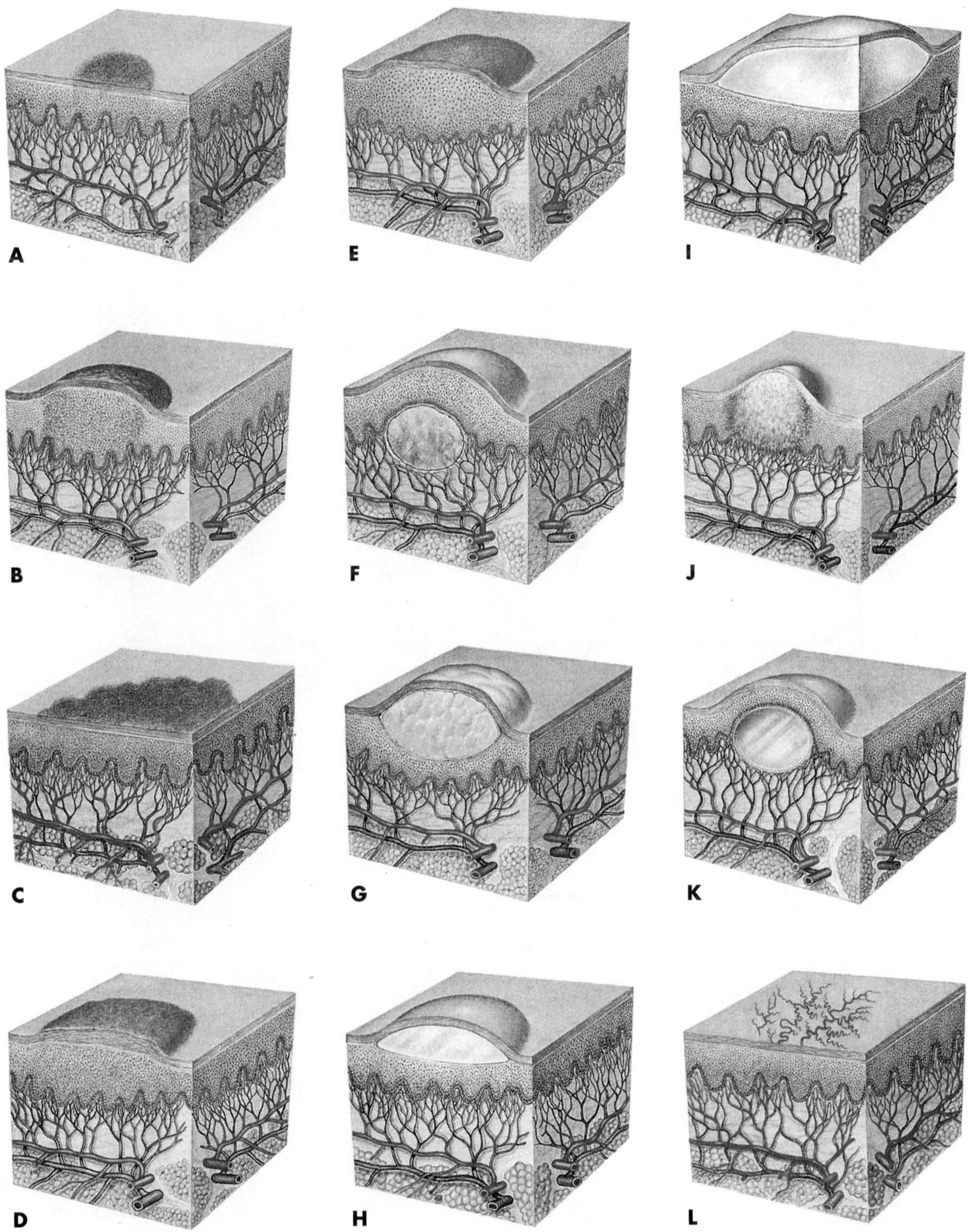

Figure 53-1 Primary skin lesions. **A**, Macule; **B**, papule; **C**, patch; **D**, plaque; **E**, wheal; **F**, nodule; **G**, tumor; **H**, vesicle; **I**, bulla; **J**, pustule; **K**, cyst; **L**, telangiectasia. (Adapted from Seidel HM et al: *Mosby's guide to physical examination,* ed 4, St Louis, 1999, Mosby.)

TABLE 53-4 Quantity of Cream to Apply and Dispense

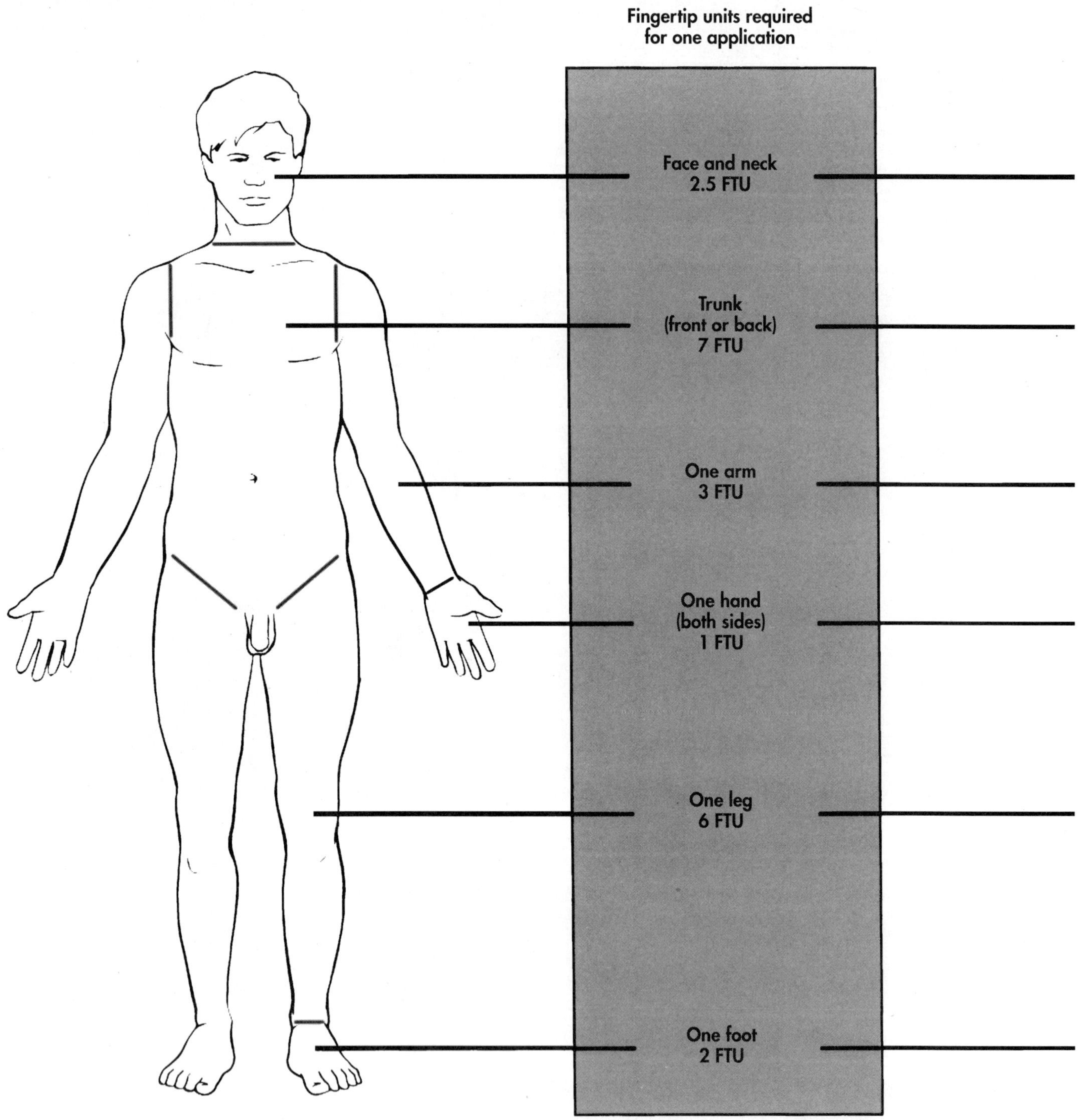

Adapted from Long CC, Finlay AY: The fingertip unit: a new practical measure, *Clin Exp Dermatol* 16:444-447, 1991.

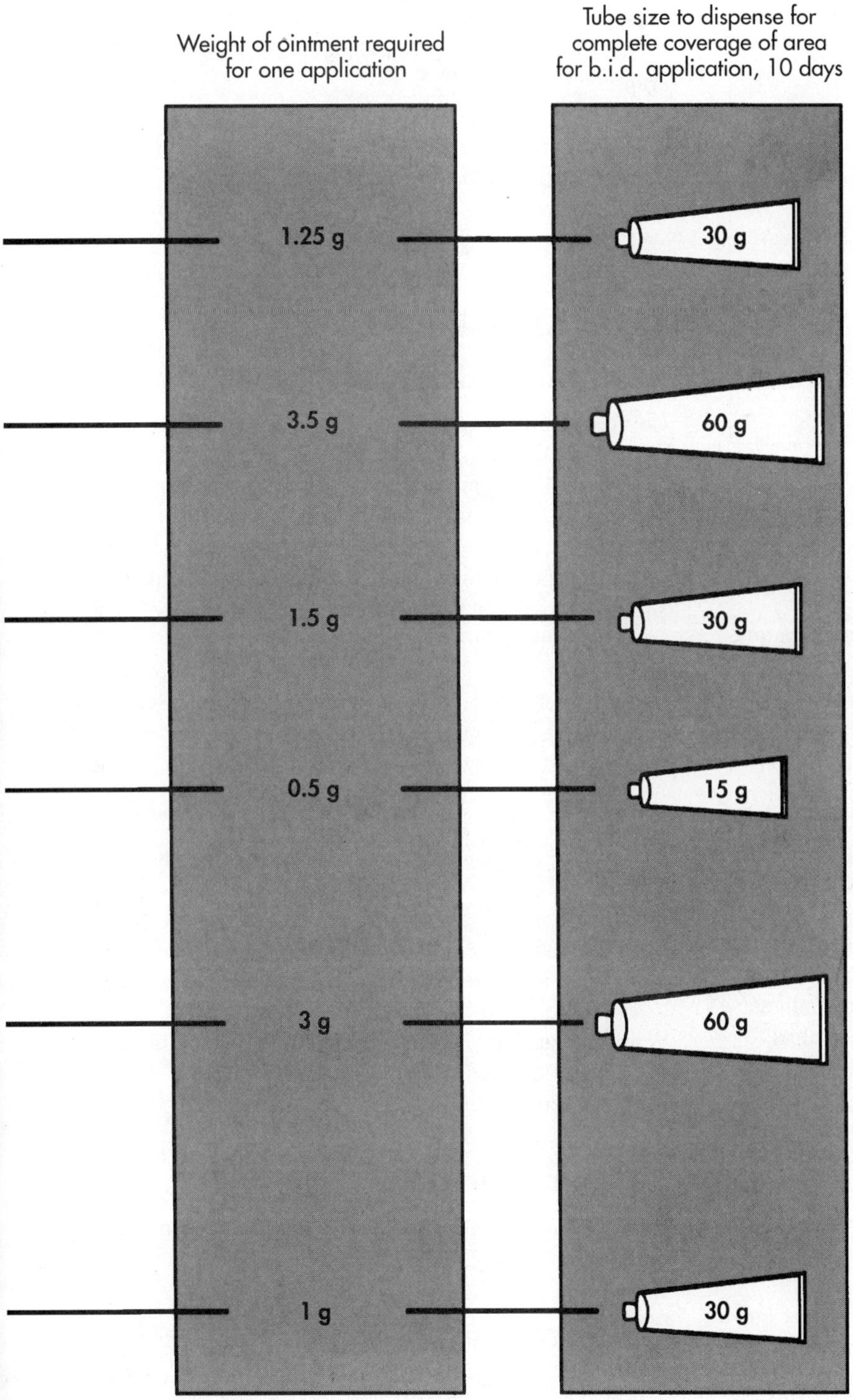

Weight of ointment required for one application	Tube size to dispense for complete coverage of area for b.i.d. application, 10 days
1.25 g	30 g
3.5 g	60 g
1.5 g	30 g
0.5 g	15 g
3 g	60 g
1 g	30 g

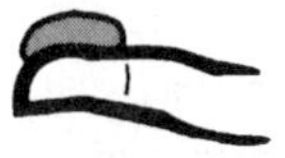

Fingertip Unit (FTU)

The amount of ointment expressed from a tube applied to the fingertip. One FTU weighs about 0.5 g.

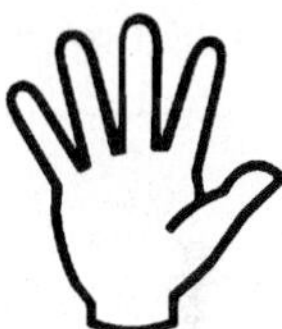

Hand Unit (one side of the hand)

$^{1}/_{2}$ FTU covers 1 side of the hand
$^{1}/_{2}$ FTU weighs 0.25 g

0.25 g × number of hand units = weight of cream required for one application

Laboratory Tests

Skin tests: To determine degree of reaction (allergy) to testing agents (antigens)
- Type: Intracutaneous
- Findings
  - Immediate reaction: Urticaria, atopic dermatitis
  - Delayed reaction: Tuberculosis, histoplasmosis
- Scratch
- Patch

Potassium hydroxide preparation ($19 to $23): Used to detect fungus and yeast infection
- Scrape skin lesion with knife blade; if blister, scrape blister roof

Box 53-1

Dermatoses of Blacks

Acne keloidalis
Actinic keratoses
Annular form of secondary syphilis
Dermatosis pupulosa nigra
Granuloma inguinale
Ingrown hairs on beard
Keloids
Mongolian spots
Pigmentary disorders: hypopigmentation, hyperpigmentation
Psoriasis
Pyoderma of legs in children
Seborrheic dermatitis: Grease on hair
Squamous cell or basal cell
Traumatic marginal alopecia (braids)

- Deposit on slide, cover with potassium hydroxide, add coverslip
- Can heat, or let sit for 15 to 60 minutes, and examine under microscope
- Findings: Oval and budding yeasts suggests *Candida*
- Short and long hyphae with clustered spores suggests *Pityrosporum* (tinea versicolor)
- Long, branched hyphae suggests dermatophyte

Biopsies: Surgical excision; use lidocaine 1% for anesthetic
- Types
  - Punch: Performed with tubular instrument that removes 3 to 4 mm circular core down to the subcutaneous tissue; bleeding is stopped with pressure or suture
  - Shave: Usually adequate for benign and malignant lesions; must be an elevated lesion; use scalpel
  - Excisional: Used for atypical pigmented lesions (performed by dermatologist)

Tzanck smear ($15 to $19): Use to help confirm a viral cause, with blister-type rash
- Select early lesion: Remove top with scalpel; blot excess fluid, gently scrape floor with scalpel blade—avoid bleeding; thin smear of cells on glass slide; stain with Wright's stain
- Findings: Multinucleated giant cells indicate virus; only viral culture of drainage will diagnosis type of virus

Scabies preparation
- Dip scalpel blade in mineral oil, scrape "burrows" (fine linear tracts), usually between fingers; if burrow cannot be located, scrape a nonexcoriated papule; transfer to slide
- Findings: Mite, eggs, feces under microscope

ASSESSMENT

Table 53-3 helps differentiate common seasonal dermatological diagnoses. Box 53-1 lists dermatoses common to blacks.

Always consider the following in rather generalized skin eruption:

- Allergic response to a medication
- Contact dermatitis
- Infectious disease: Acquired immunodeficiency syndrome, secondary syphilis

THERAPEUTIC PLAN

Pharmaceutical

Corticosteroids (topical): Do not use for longer than 2 weeks. May be absorbed systemically and can produce Cushing-like symptoms. Fluorinated (more potent) steroidal medications are more likely than nonfluorinated to cause these symptoms. Application where the skin is thinner (face, genitalia) will also increase the likelihood of symptoms. Table 53-4 illustrates the quantity of topical corticosteroids to apply and dispense.

Topical preparations
- Creams: Easier to apply, nongreasy; greater cosmetic acceptability but may dry skin
- Ointments: Greater penetration into the skin; reduces dryness

Surgical

Lesion is removed by cryosurgery or electrosurgery.

Photograph lesions before you remove them (date, name, location, and size of lesion should be recorded on photo) and place photo in patient's file.

Warn patient that removal of lesion and biopsy of lesions produces minor scarring.

Have consent signed.

Patient Education

Have a family member or other responsible person to check the patient monthly for new lesions and changes in existing lesions.

SUGGESTED READINGS

Butler J: Playing detective: assessing skin lesions in primary care, *Advance Nurse Pract* 5:42-43, 1997.

Davis L: Dermatologic testing. In Greene H, editor: *Clinical medicine,* ed 2, St Louis, 1996, Mosby.

Little J, Menscer D: Common skin problems. In Sloane P, Slatt L, Curtis P, editors: *Essentials of family medicine,* ed 2, Baltimore, 1993, Williams & Wilkins.

Developmental Dysplasia of the Hip

ICD-9-CM

Dyplasia of Hip, Congenital 755.63
With Dislocation 754.30

OVERVIEW

Definition

Developmental dysplasia of the hip (DDH) is defined as displacement of the femoral head with respect to normal orientation with the acetabulum.

Other Terms

Dislocatable: Hips that completely move out of the socket, referred to as a "clunk."

Subluxable: Hips that have movement within a joint; feels like popping out or a click.

Incidence

1 to 2 per 1000 births, females more than males, unilateral dislocation twice as frequent as bilateral.

Genetics

Unknown genetic link; association of first-born females with positive family history of affected first-degree relatives

Pathophysiology

In utero, the acetabulum starts as a flat surface that later cups around the head of the femur. This developmental process is completed during the first months of extrauterine life. DDH is the failure of formation of this normal cup around the head of the femur.

Factors That Increase Susceptibility to DDH

Congenital dislocation can be divided into two types: idiopathic and teratogenic.

Idiopathic

More frequent and often related to family history; can range from subluxed to dislocated and reducible to dislocated and irreducible

Abnormal intrauterine positioning

Relaxing effect of hormones acting on soft tissue during pregnancy

History of breech presentation—exhibits generalized increased ligamentous laxity

Teratogenic

More severe form of the disorder

Associated congenital anomalies are common in **infants;** significant association with club foot deformities and neuromuscular conditions

SUBJECTIVE DATA

History of Present Illness

Ask whether hip click has previously been noted.

Inquire about asymmetric use of lower extremities.

Past Medical History

Infant

Ask about birth order, family history, abnormal intrauterine positions, infant with congenital deformities, muscle disorder, or progress of ambulation.

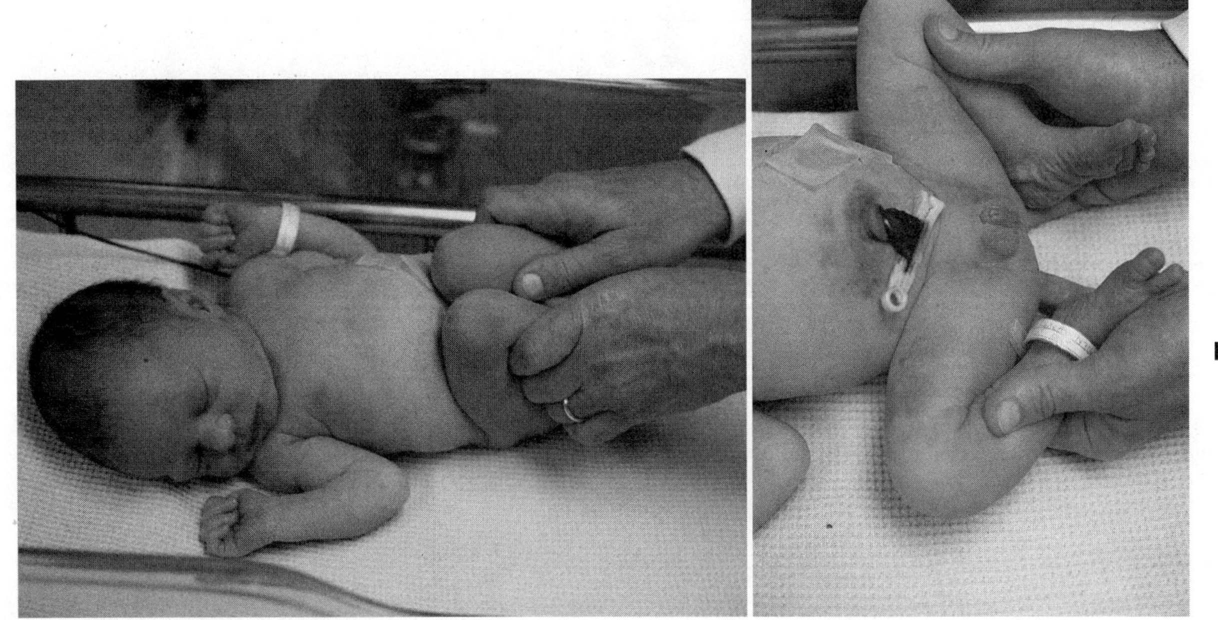

Figure 54-1 Barlow-Ortolani maneuver to detect hip dislocation. **A,** Phase I, adduction. **B,** Phase II, abduction. (From Seidel HM et al: *Mosby's guide to physical examination,* ed 4, St. Louis, 1999, Mosby.)

Children

Listen to parent complaints of abnormal gait, uneven length of legs, difficult diapering. Include questions asked about infant.

Medications

Vitamin D; hormone (Estrogen) supplements

Psychosocial History

Noncontributory

Diet History

Inquire into possible calcium- or vitamin D–deficient diets to rule out coxa vara secondary to rickets.

Family History

DDH is more common in patients with parents or first-degree relatives with history of hip dysplasia.

Description of Most Common Symptoms (DDH)

Infant

Holds leg in adduction and external rotation
Asymmetry of skin folds of thighs and buttocks, present 30% of the time; not true of bilateral dislocation
Limited abduction
Irritability on leg motion

Children

Gait disturbance
Inability to crawl
Hip or medial knee pain
Low activity level

Associated Symptoms

Motor delay and irritability.

OBJECTIVE DATA

Physical Examination

A problem-oriented physical should be conducted with particular attention to:

Height, general appearance
Skin: Assess for asymmetry of skin folds of thighs and buttocks.

Infants

Lower extremities: Do complete examination of legs and hips. Perform Barlow-Ortolani, and Galeazzi maneuvers.
Barlow test: Have infant supine with pelvis on flat surface. Adduct and internally rotate hips. Palpable clunk confirms hip dislocation (Figure 54-1, *A*).

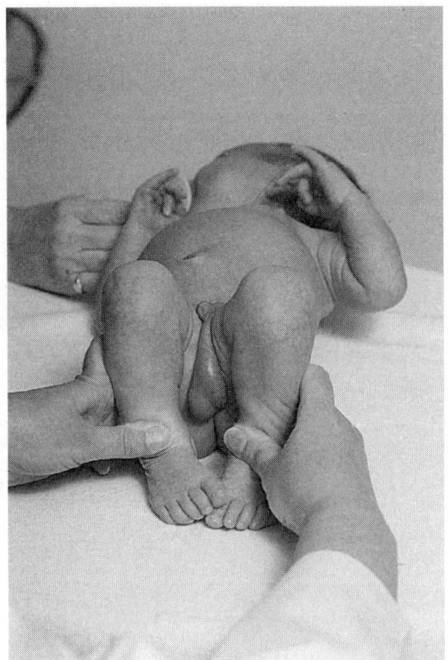

Figure 54-2 Examination for the Allis sign: unequal upper leg length would indicate a positive sign. (From Seidel HM et al: *Mosby's guide to physical examination,* ed 4, St. Louis, 1999, Mosby.)

Ortolani test: Have infant supine with pelvis on flat surface. Abduct and externally rotate hip. Middle finger of examiner should be over the greater trochanter. A palpable clunk confirms reduction of the dislocated hip (Figure 54-1, *B*).

Children

Assess gait status for limping, swayback, toe walking, lurch gait (Trendelenburg), or delay of ambulation.
Skin: Assess for excessive thigh or buttocks folds.
Galeazzi sign: Have child supine with knees fully adducted and held together. Test is positive if one femur is shorter than the other (Figure 54-2).

Diagnostic Procedures

The choice of diagnostic procedures largely depends on the age of the child and severity of the problem (Table 54-1).

First line: Repeat clinical examination, ultrasound
Second line: Pelvic radiograph, computed tomography (CT)
Third line: CT, magnetic resonance imaging

ASSESSMENT

Differential diagnoses include those found in Table 54-2.

THERAPEUTIC PLAN

The child should be referred to a pediatric orthopedic surgeon for evaluation

Pharmaceutical/Nonpharmaceutical

Therapy depends on the age of the child at the time of diagnosis and the duration of the abnormality on clinical examination (Figure 54-3)
Initially, if an infant is detected with mild hip laxity in the first 3 days of life, immediate treatment may not be necessary as maternal hormones decrease.
Reevaluate infant in 3 to 5 days.
Prognosis is excellent if treated early. Failure to diagnose early can result in more extensive management and less favorable outcome.
For age-dependent treatment, refer to Table 54-3.

Complications

If untreated, complications include:

No stable reduction
Avascular necrosis of the femoral head
Decreased range of motion

Lifestyle/Activities

Pavlik Harness

Diet

Not applicable

Education

Despite traditional use of double and triple diapering, there is no clinical evidence to support the benefit of these treatments. These therapies are not recommended since they promote hip extension, which is detrimental to normal hip development.
Pavlik harnesses should stay in place during all sleep and wake hours, with the exception of bathing. Harness straps should be adjusted by medical professional only.
Without harness therapy the DDH will result in permanent degenerative changes of the hip that will eventually lead to arthritis.

Family Impact

The use of the Pavlik harness requires special attention of all family members who change diapers. Incorrect placement of the device can cause injury. Extra time for changing diapers must be allowed.
Spica casts affect family life to an even greater degree, as the child must be carried everywhere, and diaper care is

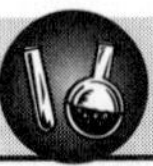

Table 54-1 Diagnostic Tests: Developmental Dysplasia of the Hip

Age	Symptom	Finding	Diagnostic Test	Cost ($)
Newborn	No risk factors	+Ortolani +Barlow	Repeat clinical examination If hip reduces, then hip U/S in 2-4 wk	84 368-460
Newborn	+Risk factors	+Ortolani +Barlow	Hip U/S in 2-4 wk	368-460
6 mo	Difficulty diapering	Difference in ROM; limited abduction; asymmetric buttocks folds	Pelvic AP (x-ray); AP and frogleg	127-151 117-139
Onset of walking	Gait asymmetry	Intoeing/Out-toeing Asymmetric buttocks folds; leg length discrepancy; limited abduction	Pelvic AP (x-ray); pelvic frogleg; CT of hip	127-151 117-139 835-984
>18 mo-5 yo (Walking)	Limp	Hyperlordosis	CT of hip	835-984
	Waddling gait Increased arch in back	Severely dysplastic hip	MRI of hip MRI of hip	1415-1670
>5 yo	Painful limp	Decreased abduction	CT of hip MRI of hip	835-984 1415-1610

AP, Anterior/posterior; *CT,* computed tomography; *MRI,* magnetic resonance imaging; +, positive; *ROM,* range of motion; *U/S,* ultrasound.

Table 54-2 Differential Diagnosis: Developmental Dysplasia of the Hip

Diagnosis	Supporting Data
Meningomyelocele with spina bifida	Abnormal neurologic examination of the lower extremities Urinary and bowel retention/incontinence Shortened lower limbs Midline defect of lumbosacral spine
Arthrogryposis	Contractures of all extremities, predominantly ankles, wrists, knees, and elbows
Neonatal Marfan's syndrome	Hyperextensible joints Bilateral lens dislocations Murmur: Aortic insufficiency and aneurysms
Septic joint/ osteomyelitis	Fever Point tenderness Warm to the touch Pain on range of motion Refusal to bear weight Erythema over affected joint Increased WBC count with left shift; Increased ESR; increased CRP
Slipped capital femoral epiphysis	Pain: Medial aspect of the knee Limited abduction and internal rotation Acute slip: May see inability to walk or bear weight
Coxa vara	Physical findings indistinguishable from hip dislocation, except there is no ligamentous laxity noted; make special note of past medical history and diet history to rule out rickets

CRP, C-reactive protein; *ESR,* erythrocyte sedimentation rate; *WBC,* white blood count.

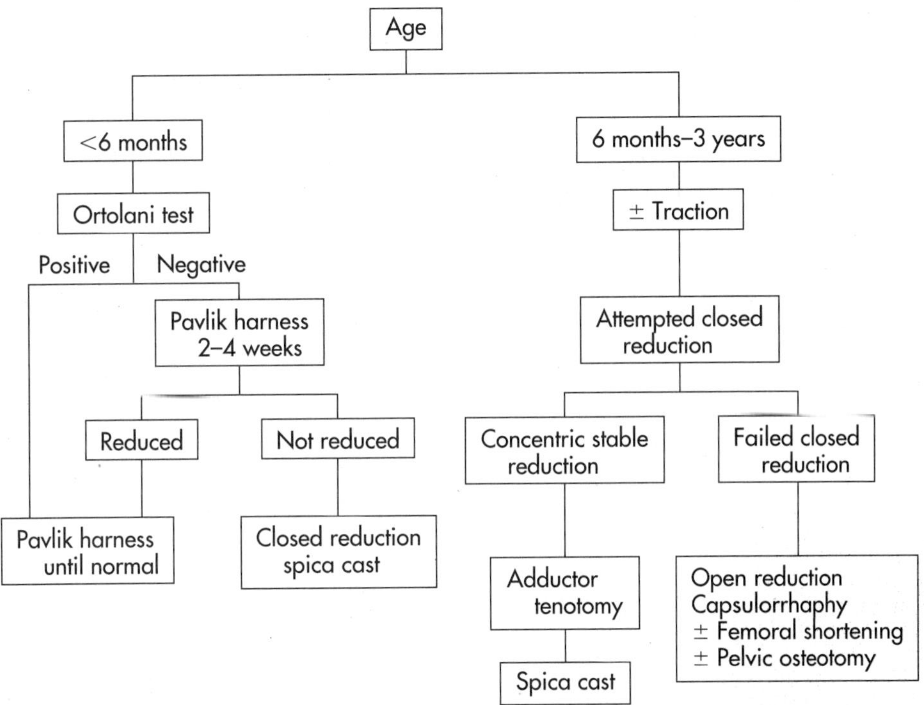

Figure 54-3 Algorithm for treatment of developmental dysplasia of the hip. (From Rudolph A, Kamei R: *Rudolph's fundamentals of pediatrics,* ed 2, Stamford, Conn, 1998, Appleton & Lange.)

TABLE 54-3 Treatment Plan: Developmental Dysplasia of the Hip

Age	Treatment	Duration
Birth-6 mo	Pavlik harness*	Minimum of 6 weeks, with adjustments every 2 weeks to maintain ideal position and prevent femoral head necrosis
6 mo-18 mo	Pavlik harness*	See above
	Skin traction	Generally used for 3 weeks; possible home treatment
	Closed reduction with spica cast	First cast change 4-6 weeks; hip spica casts are used; changed every 6 weeks; usually requires two to three casts
>18 mo	Open reduction	May require multiple cast changes

*Pavlik harness is a splint that permits a relaxed motion of the hip while maintaining a flexed and abducted position for natural development of joint space until the capsule tightens at approximately 6 weeks of age. Approximate cost is $115.

not an insignificant task. Special attention must be paid to neurovascular status of the lower extremities and to possible breaks in the skin at the edges of the cast. May use skin moisturizer in areas of strap erosions.

EVALUATION/FOLLOW-UP

Even though spontaneous reduction of the hip may occur in 6 weeks, it is recommended that the Pavlik stirrups should be continued for several months until the hips are stable. Spica casts should be changed every 4 to 6 weeks to allow for the child's growth. The spica cast should not be used for longer than 6 months.

SUGGESTED REFERENCES

Aronsson D et al: Developmental dysplasia of the hip, *Pediatrics* 94(2):201-208, 1994.

Behrman R, Vaughan V: *Nelson textbook of pediatrics,* ed 14, Philadelphia, 1997, WB Saunders.

Donaldson J, Feinstein K: Imaging of developmental dysplasia of the hip, *Pediatr Clin North Am* 44(3):591-614, 1997.

Ellsworth et al: *Mosby's 1998 medical drug reference,* St Louis, 1998, Mosby.

Healthcare Consultants of America, Inc: *1998 Physicians fee and coding guide,* Augusta, Ga, 1998, Healthcare Consultants of America, Inc.

Novacheck T: Developmental dysplasia of the hip, *Pediatr Clin North Am* 43(4):829-848, 1996.

Skinner S: Orthopedic problems in childhood. In Rudolph A, editor: *Rudolph's pediatrics,* ed 20, Stamford, Conn, 1996, Appleton & Lange.

Smith J: (1998) Orthopedic problems. In Rudolph A, Kamei R, editors: *Rudolph's fundamentals of pediatrics,* ed 2, Stamford, Conn, 1998, Appleton & Lange.

Swartz MW: *The 5-minute pediatric consult,* Baltimore, 1997, Williams & Wilkins.

Zitelli B, Davis H: *Atlas of pediatric physical diagnosis,* ed 2, London, 1994 Mosby-Wolfe.

55 Diabetes Mellitus

ICD-9-CM

Diabetes Mellitus 250.0
Diabetes Mellitus without Complications, Juvenile 250.01
Diabetes Mellitus with Ketoacidosis, Juvenile 250.11
Diabetes Mellitus with Renal Manifestation, Juvenile 250-41
Diabetes Mellitus with Hyperosmolarity 250-2
Diabetes Mellitus with Renal Manifestations 250.40
Diabetes Mellitus with Neurological Manifestations 250.50
Diabetes Mellitus with Peripheral Circulation Manifestations 250.70

OVERVIEW

Definition

Diabetes mellitus (DM) is a group of metabolic diseases with the primary manifestation of hyperglycemia. It is characterized by a lack of insulin secretion, increased cellular resistance to insulin, or both. The degree of hyperglycemia may change over time, depending on the extent of the underlying disease process. The chronic hyperglycemia of diabetes is associated with long-term damage, dysfunction, and failure of various organs, especially the eyes, kidneys, nerves, heart, and blood vessels. Diabetes is classified in five distinct categories, as outlined in Table 55-1.

Incidence

It is estimated that 16 million people in the United States have diabetes, primarily type 1 and type 2, but only half of these cases are diagnosed. The prevalence of diagnosed and undiagnosed diabetes is about 6% in the general population. Type 1 accounts for approximately 10% of cases and type 2 for 80% to 90%. Specific subgroups with certain attributes or risk factors have a much higher prevalence of type 2 diabetes mellitus. Gestational diabetes complicates about 4% of all **pregnancies** in the United States, resulting in approximately 135,000 cases annually.

Diagnostic Criteria

Standards have been established for the diagnosis of DM, impaired glucose tolerance, and gestational diabetes mellitus as shown in Table 55-2.

TYPE 1 DIABETES MELLITUS

Pathophysiology

In type 1 diabetes there is a genetic susceptibility plus an environmental "trigger" (either viral infection or toxin exposure) that initiates a cell-mediated autoimmune destruction of the beta cells of the pancreas. Markers of the immune destruction include islet cell antibodies, autoantibodies to insulin, autoantibodies to glutamic acid decarboxylase, and autoantibodies to the tyrosine phosphatases. One or more of the autoantibodies is present in 85% to 90% of individuals when fasting hyperglycemia is initially detected. This destruction occurs over time and causes progressive and ultimately absolute insulin deficiency. This deficiency results in hyperglycemia for two primary reasons: (1) increased hepatic production of glucose via accelerated glycogenolysis and gluconeogenesis and (2) decreased peripheral utilization of glucose by insulin-responsive tissues such as skeletal muscle.

Ketoacidosis may occur as a result of insulin deficiency and an increase in glucagon and other counterregulatory hormones, such as cortisol, growth hormone, and catechol-

Table 55-1 Classification of Diabetes

Classification	Definition
Type 1 diabetes mellitus (DM)	Absolute insulin deficiency as a result of islet cell loss. Ketosis prone. Often associated with specific human leukocyte antigens, with predisposition to viral insulitis or autoimmune phenomena. Occurs at any age, but most common in youth. The term IDDM is now eliminated.
Type 2 diabetes mellitus	May range from predominantly insulin resistance with relative insulin deficiency to a predominantly secretory deficit with insulin resistance. Ketosis resistant. May be seen in family groups as an autosomal dominant genetic trait. More frequent in adults but may be seen at any age. May require insulin for control of either acute or chronic hyperglycemia. The term NIDDM is now eliminated.
Diabetes mellitus associated with certain conditions or syndromes	Hyperglycemia occurring in relation to other disease states, such as pancreatic diseases, drug-induced diabetes, endocrinopathies, insulin-receptor disorders, certain genetic syndromes.
Impaired fasting glucose (IFG)	Abnormality in glucose levels (fasting plasma glucose [FPG] ≥ 110 mg/dl but ≤ 126 mg/dl). Abnormalities may improve, worsen, or remain unchanged on serial testing. The stage of impaired glucose tolerance (IGT) is retained, defined as oral glucose tolerance test of ≥ 140 mg/dl but < 200 mg/dl. Both IFG and IGT refer to metabolic stages of impaired glucose homeostasis that are intermediate between normal and overt diabetes. Although not clinical entities (in the absence of pregnancy), they are risk factors for future diabetes and cardiovascular disease.
Gestational diabetes mellitus (GDM)	Any degree of glucose intolerance with onset or recognition during pregnancy. High-risk groups include women over age 40, those with a family history of DM, those with a body mass index greater than 25 before pregnancy, smokers, Hispanics, Native Americans, Asian-Americans, and blacks. Euglycemia can be achieved by diet or insulin therapy. In the majority of cases, glucose regulation will return to normal after delivery. A small portion of patients may develop either type 1 or type 2 diabetes or impaired glucose tolerance later in life.

IDDM, Noninsulin-dependent diabetes mellitus.

amines. These hormones affect both glucose and lipid metabolism and can cause a widened anion gap.

SUBJECTIVE DATA

History of Present Illness

Duration of symptoms may be several days to several weeks, with significant weight loss and lethargy in newly recognized patients. Symptoms, results of laboratory tests, and previous treatment programs should be recorded for patients with long-standing diabetes.

Children: Symptoms may be vague; parents may report decreased physical activity, increased urination and thirst, bed wetting.

Adults: Usually occurs by age 40, although anecdotal cases have been reported at age 50. Rare in **elderly** patients.

Past Medical History

Ask about recent illnesses, infections, stress, exposure to toxins, weight change.

Assess diet and exercise patterns in previously diagnosed patients.

Assess cardiovascular risk factors, such as hypertension, hyperlipidemia, and tobacco use.

Complications may be present in individuals with long-standing diabetes; ask about problems of the eyes, kidneys, nerve, genitourinary system, bladder, and feet as well as cardiac and sexual problems.

Children: Include developmental history in children, adolescents, and young adults.

Adults: Include gestational history in females.

Medications

Young patients are unlikely to use long-term medications.

Inquire about use of over-the-counter or recreational drugs.

Use of steroids or adrenergic agonists increases the risk of ketoacidosis.

Family History

Commonly there is no family history of diabetes.

Include family history of other autoimmune diseases (Hashimoto's thyroiditis, Graves' disease, myasthenia gravis, Addison's disease, pernicious anemia, premature gonadal failure) and cardiovascular disease.

TABLE 55-2 Diagnostic Criteria

Classification	Criteria
Diabetes mellitus (DM)	Casual plasma glucose concentration ≥200 mg/dl with the classic symptoms of polyuria, polydipsia and unexplained weight loss. Casual is any time of day without regard to time since last meal. Fasting plasma glucose greater than or equal to 126 mg/dl. Fasting is defined as no caloric intake for at least 8 hours. Two-hour plasma glucose greater than or equal to 200 mg/dl during an oral glucose tolerance test (OGTT), using a glucose load containing the equivalent of 75 g anhydrous glucose dissolved in water. OGTT is not recommended for routine clinical use.
Impaired fasting glucose	Fasting plasma glucose >110 mg/dl but <126 mg/dl.
Impaired glucose tolerance	Two-hour plasma glucose ≥140 mg/dl and <200 mg/dl/
Gestational diabetes mellitus	When a diagnosis of DM is established by any of above criteria before pregnancy, no additional tests are needed. Routine screening for GDM should be performed between 24 and 28 weeks' gestation using a 50-g 1-hour OGTT. The test is positive if the 1-hour plasma glucose is greater than or equal to 140 mg/dl. If the 1-hour OGTT is greater than or equal to 140 mg/dl, a 3-hour OGTT should be performed, using a 100-g OGTT. This test is considered positive and diagnostic of gestational diabetes if the fasting plasma glucose level is elevated or any two of the following values: fasting—105 mg/dl; 1 hour—190 mg/dl; 2 hour—165 mg/dl. Screening for GDM may not be necessary in pregnant women who meet all the following criteria: Less than 25 years of age Normal body weight No first degree relative with diabetes Not Hispanic, Native American, Asian-American, or black

Psychosocial History

Include occupation, economic resources, and use of tobacco or alcohol.

Diet History

May indicate consumption of food and fluids in newly recognized patient.

Description of Most Common Symptoms

Polyuria, polydipsia, and orthostasis are common because of the increased renal excretion of glucose, osmotic diuresis, and obligate water loss.

Polyphagia and weight loss occurs as insulin deficiency produces a starvation-like catabolic state in uncontrolled diabetes.

In an established patient receiving insulin therapy, symptoms of hypoglycemia include confusion, tremors, increased diaphoresis and may lead to coma if untreated.

Associated Symptoms

Nausea, vomiting, blurred vision, abdominal pain, and pruritus may occur.

In the late stages of undetected type 1 diabetes, there may be altered sensorium with ketoacidosis.

OBJECTIVE DATA

Physical Examination

Findings on examination may be entirely normal. A complete physical examination should be conducted, with attention to the following:

General
- Orthostatic hypotension, tachycardia, and decreased skin turgor may be present with dehydration.
- Loose skinfolds or ill-fitting clothes may indicate recent weight loss. With significant hyperglycemia, there may be decreased visual acuity or decreased peripheral nerve or position threshold.

Height and weight

Children: Compare with norms

Blood pressure (with orthostatic measurement when indicated)

Skin examination, including insulin injection sites

Head/eyes/ears/nose/throat
- Oral examination
- Xanthomas
- Visual acuity (may be decreased with significant hyperglycemia)
- Ophthalmoscopic examination
- Thyroid palpation

Cardiovascular: Evaluation of pulses (by palpation and auscultation)

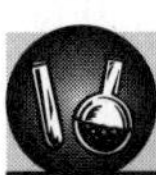

TABLE 55-3 Diagnostic Tests: Type 1 Diabetes Mellitus

Symptoms	Findings	Diagnostic Tests	Cost ($)
Polyuria, polydipsia	Decreased skin turgor, loose skinfolds, dry oral cavity	Urinalysis: Positive for glucose, ketones may be present in newly diagnosed or poorly controlled patient. Check for protein and sediment.	15-20
Polyphagia, weight loss	Same as for polyuria	Plasma glucose >126 mg/dl in newly diagnosed patient and often >200 mg/dl in the symptomatic patient.	16-20
		Glycosylated hemoglobin >7% (normal range is 4% to 6%)	34-43

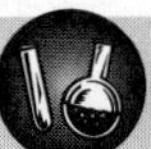

TABLE 55-4 Essential Diagnostic Tests for Patients with Diabetes Mellitus

Test	Findings/Rationale	Cost ($)
Fasting lipid profile	Diabetics frequently have dysfunction in lipid metabolism.	49-62
Renal function	Check creatinine in adults; in **children** if proteinuria present.	28-39/ metabolic panel
Thyroid function	Type 1 patients have an increased incidence of autoimmune disorders, especially thyroid disease.	47-61
Urine culture	If urinalysis result is abnormal, if sediment is present, or if there are signs of infection.	31-39
Urinary microalbumin	Check in all patients who have had DM for >5 years; Figure 55-1 illustrates the protocol for screening for microalbuminuria	19-24/dip 25-33/quan
ECG	In adults, perform ECG as a baseline.	56-65

ECG, Electrocardiogram.

Neurological: Sensation
  Position sense present with dehydration
Extremities
  Hand/finger examination
  Foot examination (see Table 55-14)
Genital: Sexual maturation staging (if patient is prepubertal)

Diagnostic Procedures

Diagnostic procedures for type 1 diabetes mellitus are shown in Tables 55-3 to 55-5.

ASSESSMENT

Differential Diagnosis

Differential diagnosis must primarily be made between type 1 and type 2 diabetes mellitus. Subjective data that favor type 1 include:

Age less than 40 at onset
Lean body habitus (at or below ideal body weight)
Ketosis-prone: Recurrent ketoacidosis by history or fasting ketonuria that does not clear postprandially

If the diagnosis remains unclear, laboratory tests may be performed; however, these tests are not always available and are expensive. Table 55-6 outlines differential diagnoses for type 1 diabetes mellitus; Table 55-7 lists the subjective and objective data for confirming the diagnosis.

THERAPEUTIC PLAN

Pharmaceutical

Exogenous insulin is required for patients with type 1 diabetes mellitus. The goal for insulin therapy is to achieve as near normal blood glucose levels as possible without excessive hypoglycemia. There are several insulin preparations available with varying onset and duration of action. Human insulin or insulin analogs are most commonly used; 70:30 insulin is not appropriate for type 1 diabetes unless the patient is unable to mix two preparations.

Table 55-8 outlines the pharmaceutical plan for type 1 diabetes mellitus.

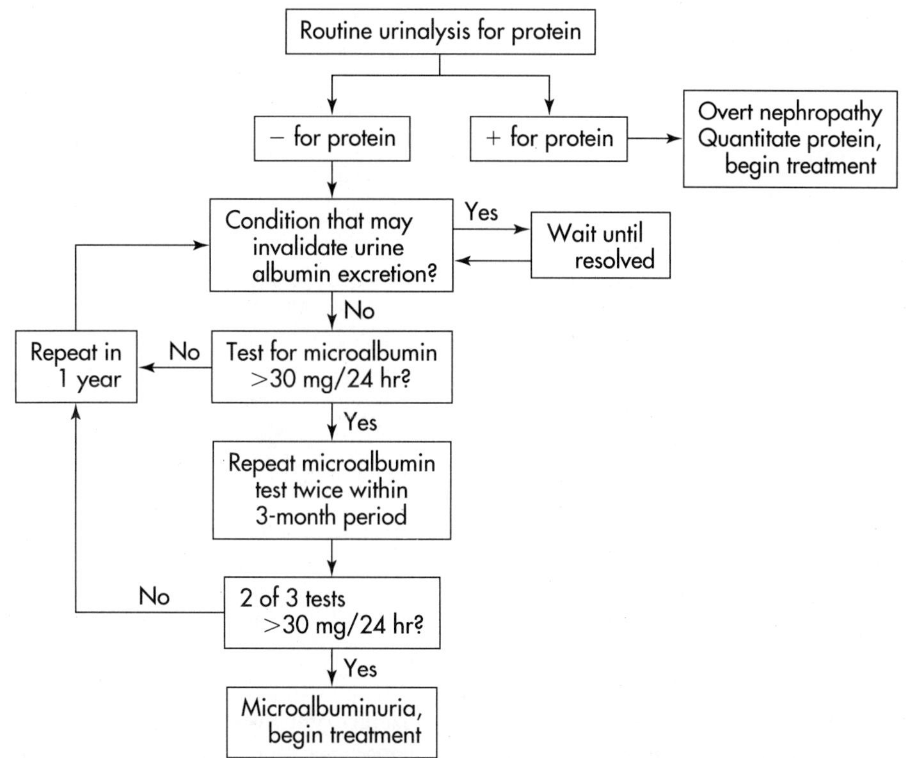

Figure 55-1 Screening for microalbuminuria. (From American Diabetes Association: Screening for microalbuminuria, *Diabetes Care* 20[Suppl 1]:526, 1997.)

TABLE 55-5 Comparative Values

$aHbA_{1c}$	Average Glucose Level
4	60
5	90
6	120
7	150
8	180
9	210
10	240
11	270
12	300

Adapted from Goldstein D et al: The test with a memory, *Diabetes Forecast* 5:22-26, 1994.

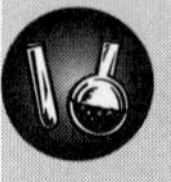

TABLE 55-6 Objective Data for Definitive Diagnosis: Type 1 Diabetes Mellitus

Test	Findings/Rationale	Cost ($)
Islet cell autoantibodies	Positive in 80% of new onset patients	43-56
Serum C peptide	Marker of endogenous insulin, less than detectable 5 min after IV administration of 1 mg glucagon is positive for type 1 diabetes mellitus	56-71

Goals for Glycemic Control

Target goals for glycemic control must be established with the patient. The desired outcome of glycemic control is to lower glycosylated hemoglobin and achieve maximum prevention of complications. Recommended goals include those found in Table 55-9.

Insulin Regimens

The insulin regimen should be balanced with the patient's diet and lifestyle. The first step in starting insulin therapy is to determine the patient's total daily dose (TDD). This can be calculated using approximately 0.6 U/kg/day. Alternatively, the patient's current TDD can be used by adding all insulin doses in a usual day. Table 55-10 describes the advantages and disadvantages of various regimens. The patient's lifestyle and willingness to intensify the regimen will dictate the selection of the regimen.

Insulin Adjustment

Patients may be instructed in adjusting insulin dosages based on results of glucose testing. The adjustment should be based on the patient's body weight, caloric intake, activity level, and home glucose monitoring results. A sample adjustment is shown in Table 55-11.

Lifestyle/Activities

Exercise should be encouraged to improve cardiovascular fitness and psychological well-being. Many variables, including level of fitness, duration, intensity, and time of exercise in relation to food intake and insulin injection will affect metabolic response to exercise. There is an increased risk of hypoglycemia with intense physical activity. Self-monitoring of glucose should be incorporated into the exercise regimen so the patient may adjust his or her calories or insulin dosage.

Children: Participation in competitive sports is possible. Children should be encouraged to eat a light snack before exercise and have a simple carbohydrate available during activity. They should be instructed to wear protective equipment as appropriate.

Tobacco use should be strongly discouraged because of the increased risk of cardiovascular complications.

The same precautions regarding alcohol use in the general population apply to diabetic patients. Blood glucose levels will not be affected by moderate use of alcohol. Reduction of abstention from alcohol may be advisable for patients with diabetes who have other medical problems such as pancreatitis, dyslipidemia, or neuropathy. If alcohol is consumed, it should only be ingested with a meal. Alcohol may increase the risk of hypoglycemia.

Individual treatment goals should take into account the patient's capacity to understand and carry out the treatment regimen, the risks of hypoglycemia, and other factors that may increase risk or decrease benefit. Self-management training and problem solving should be designed based on treatment goals.

Table 55-7 Confirmation of Type 1 Diabetes Mellitus

Subjective Date	Objective Data
Age <40	Positive islet cell autoantibodies
Lean body habitus	Serum C peptide not detectable
Ketosis prone	Positive HLA association

HLA, Human leukocyte antigens.

Diet

There is no single diabetic diet. A meal plan based on the patient's usual food intake should be used as a basis for integrating insulin therapy into the diet and exercise plan. The Food Guide Pyramid summarizes the guidelines for diabetic patients. It is recommended that patients eat at consistent times synchronized with the time-action of the insulin regimen. A nutrition assessment should include the items listed in Box 55-1.

Goals of nutrition therapy are:

Maintenance of as near-normal blood glucose levels as possible
Optimal serum lipids
Adequate calories for maintaining or achieving ideal body weight
Prevention of short-term and long-term complications

Patient Education

Basic pathophysiology of diabetes
Insulin injection technique

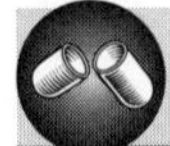

Table 55-8 Pharmaceutical Plan: Type 1 Diabetes Mellitus

Insulin Preparation	Onset of Action	Peak Action	Duration of Action	Cost ($) (10 ml)
Humalog (Lyspro)—insulin analog of recombinant DNA origin	10 to 15 min	30 to 90 min	4 hr	26
Regular	30 to 60 min	2 to 4 hr	5 to 7 hr	16-23
NPH	60 to 120 min	6 to 14 hr	24+ hr	16-23
Lente	60 to 180 min	6 to 14 hr	24+ hr	16-23
Ultralente	6 hr	18 to 24 hr	36+ hr	13-17
70:30 (70% NPH, 30% Regular)	70%: 60 to 120 min 30%: 30 to 60 min	70%: 6 to 14 hr 30%: 2 to 4 hr	70%: 24+ hr 30%: 5 to 7 hr	17-21

DNA, Deoxyribonucleic acid; *NPH,* neutral protamine Hagedorn (insulin).

Symptoms and treatment of hypoglycemia and hyperglycemia

Children: Most children under the age of 7 have a form of "hypoglycemic unawareness" and lack the cognitive capacity to recognize and respond to hypoglycemic episodes. Glycemic goals may have to be modified to prevent hypoglycemia. Teachers, friends, and family members should be taught to recognize and treat symptoms.

Frequent home glucose monitoring, recommended 3 to 4 times daily, before meals and bedtime. Monitoring should be individualized according to clinical circumstances. Patients should be instructed to check for urine ketones if glucose monitoring results are >300 mg/dl. Use of a logbook should be encouraged. Patients should be taught to use the results to adjust diet, exercise and insulin regimens.

Foot care, including daily inspection, hygiene, proper footwear, avoidance of foot trauma, need to stop smoking and actions to take if problems develop.

Sick-day management should include temporary adjustments for hyperglycemia with intercurrent illnesses.

For women of childbearing age, contraception should be discussed with an emphasis on the need for optimal blood glucose control before conception and during pregnancy. Self-management skills essential of preparation for pregnancy are listed in Box 55-2.

TABLE 55-9 Goals for Glycemic Control

Biochemical Index	Non-diabetic	Goal	Action Needed
Preprandial plasma glucose (mg/dl)	<115	80 to 120	<80 or >140
Bedtime plasma glucose (mg/dl)	<120	100-140	<100 or >160
Glycosylated hemoglobin (%)	<6	<7	>8

Family Impact

Diabetes is a chronic disease that affects all family members. Family members should be included in all patient education. They must be able to recognize and treat both hypoglycemia and hyperglycemia. Patients and family members should know and have access to the necessary tools for good diabetes care (Box 55-3). Some patients may experience depression related to their diagnosis and altered family roles. Care of children and adolescents requires integration of diabetes management with other complicated physical and emotional growth needs.

TABLE 55-10 Advantages and Disadvantages of Various Insulin Regimens

Regimen	Patient	Pros	Cons	Guidelines
Split/mix NPH/Regular Two injections	Type 1 patient who needs simple regimen	Requires only two injections daily. Regular before breakfast and supper can be adjusted based on home glucose monitoring	Low flexibility, forced lunch on time and snacks to avoid hypoglycemia; taking NPH at supper may cause hypoglycemia in predawn period	Start with ⅔ TDD before breakfast, divided as ⅔ NPH, ⅓ Regular. Give remaining ⅓ TDD before supper divided as ½ NPH, ½ Regular.
Split/Mix NPH/Regular Three injections	Type 1 child or adult who needs simple regimen but willing to do three injections	No injection required during the day, good for children who could not inject self during school day. Taking NPH at bedtime prevents predawn hypoglycemia and improves fasting level.	Requires three injections daily. NPH during day may not adequately cover lunch. Low flexibility, forced lunch on time and snacks to avoid hypoglycemia	Start with ⅔ TDD before breakfast, divided as ⅔ NPH, ⅓ Regular. Remaining ⅓ TDD as ½ NPH, ½ Regular. Give Regular before supper, NPH at bedtime.

NPH, Neutral protamine Hagedorn (insulin), *TDD,* total daily dose.

Continued

Table 55-10 Advantages and Disadvantages of Various Insulin Regimens—cont'd

Regimen	Patient	Pros	Cons	Guidelines
Basal/Bolus Ultralente/ Regular Three injections	Type 1 adolescent or adult who desires flexibility with schedule and food and willing to do home glucose monitoring 4 times daily	Allows flexibility to eat or not eat and cover food with boluses of Regular. Decreases hypoglycemia in predawn time.	Requires frequent home glucose testing and patient decision making re: mealtime doses. Ultralente has less predictable action and may peak as late as 10 to 12 hours after injection. May cause unexpected hypoglycemia.	Calculate total Ultralente dose: Weight in kg × 0.3 (female) or 0.4 (male). Give 40% prebreakfast and 60% presupper. Calculate meal coverage: Regular as 0.3 × weight in kg, then divide to cover three meals. Create a sliding scale based on home glucose monitoring until patient learns to cover food with Regular.
Basal/bolus NPH or Lente/ Regular Four injections	Type 1 adolescent or adult who desire flexibility with schedule and food and willing to do home glucose monitoring 4 times daily	Allows flexibility to eat or not eat and cover food with boluses of Regular. Good for achieving tight control since multiple doses of Regular may be used for fine tuning	Requires frequent home glucose testing and patient decision making regarding mealtime doses. Must have Regular injection every 4 to 5 hours during day. May have wide fluctuation in day.	Give 25% of TDD at bedtime as NPH or Lente. Remaining 75% of TDD is spread among three meals using a slide scale based on home glucose monitoring. Patient must be taught to cover food with insulin, understanding that about half of mealtime Regular is covering basal needs and half is covering caloric intake.
Basal/bolus Regular Insulin pump	Type 1 pt who desires max flexibility with schedule and food and willing to test QID. Must have finely tuned basal dose to avoid hypoglycemia. Must have financial resources for supplies.	Allows maximum flexibility to eat or not eat and cover food with boluses of Regular; good for tight control because multiple doses of Regular may be used for fine-tuning.	Requires frequent testing and patient decision making regarding mealtime doses. Patient must change needle site every 48 to 72 hours and wear external pump continuously. Expensive—initial cost approximately $4000, monthly supplies $75.	Pump uses Regular insulin only. Basal rate started at about 0.3 U/kg spread over 24 hours. Remaining 0.3 U/kg is given as bolus to cover three meals using a sliding scale. Pump initiation requires significant patient education, ideally before start.

TABLE 55-11 Adjustment of Insulin Based on Glucose Monitoring Results

Home Glucose Monitoring Results	Regular Insulin Dose
Fasting glucose >140	Increase evening or supper intermediate insulin
Prelunch glucose >140	Add or increase Regular insulin at breakfast
Presupper glucose >140	Increase morning intermediate insulin
Bedtime glucose >140	Add or increase Regular insulin at supper
Fasting glucose <75	Add snack at bedtime or decrease intermediate insulin at bedtime or supper
Glucose <75 after exercise	Snack before exercise or decrease previous dose of Regular insulin

Box 55-1

Nutritional Assessment

Weight and height
Home glucose monitoring results
Glycosylated hemoglobin results
Lipid panel
Blood pressure
Renal status
Cultural and ethnic background
Financial resources
Willingness to comply

Referral

Dietician may provide additional nutritional counseling as needed.

An ophthalmologist should be seen annually for dilated funduscopic examination for all patients 12 years old and older who have had diabetes for 5 years, all patients over 30 years old, and any patient with visual symptoms or abnormalities.

A podiatrist may be consulted for chronic foot problems or in high-risk patients. Risk factors for foot ulcers include neuropathy, vascular disease, structural deformities, abnormal gait, skin or nail deformities, and history of previous ulcers or infections.

Referral to a psychologist or mental health specialist may be indicated if symptoms of depression are present.

Box 55-2

Preparation for Pregnancy

Using an appropriate meal plan
Timing meals and snacks
Planning physical activity
Choosing time and site of insulin injections
Using carbohydrate and glucagon for hypoglycemia
Reducing stress, coping with denial
Home glucose monitoring
Self-adjusting insulin doses

Box 55-3

Tools for Good Diabetes Care

Medications

Oral agents
Insulin
Insulin syringes (1/3ml [30 U], 1/2ml [50 U], 1ml [100 U]) or pen.

For Blood Glucose Self-monitoring

Blood glucose meter
Test strips
Alcohol pads
Cotton balls
Lancet device and lancets
Logbook
Software for downloading and analysis of data

For Hypoglycemia

Glucose tablets, glucose gel, cake frosting, juice, or soft candy
Glucagon, injectable, for some

For Illness

Urine strips to test for ketones
Short-acting insulin (Regular, Semilente)

From Noble J: *Textbook of primary care medicine*, ed 2, St. Louis, 1996, Mosby.

Consultation

An internist or endocrinologist may be consulted if there is no improvement in glycemic control or the patient requires hospital admission. Consultation is appropriate in the cases outlined in Table 55-12.

Follow-up

Contact frequency is dependent on the duration of diabetes. Daily contact may be necessary for initiation of insulin or a change in regimen. Routine diabetic visits should be

TABLE 55-12 Consultation Criteria

Conditions Requiring Consultation	Signs and Symptoms
Acute metabolic complications	Diabetic ketoacidosis (blood glucose >250 mg/dl with arterial pH <7.35, venous pH <7.30, or serum bicarbonate level <15 mEq/L and ketonuria or ketonemia) Hyperosmolar nonketotic state (impaired mental status and elevated plasma osmolality >315 mOsm/kg and glucose >400); Hypoglycemia with neuroglycopenia (blood glucose <50 and treatment has not resulted in prompt recovery of sensorium; coma, seizures, or altered behavior; hypoglycemia has been treated but responsible adult cannot be with patient for 12 hours or the hypoglycemia was caused by a sulfonylurea drug)
Uncontrolled diabetes	Hyperglycemia associated with dehydration Persistent refractory hyperglycemia with metabolic deterioration Recurring fasting hyperglycemia >300 mg/dl is refractory to outpatient therapy or a glycosylated hemoglobin of 13% or greater Recurring severe hypoglycemia despite intervention Metabolic instability with frequent swings between hypoglycemia and fasting hyperglycemia Recurring diabetic ketoacidosis without precipitating trauma or infection Repeated absence from school or work due to severe psychosocial problems that cannot be managed on an outpatient basis
Complications of diabetes or other acute metabolic conditions	Diabetes is a confounding factor for acute condition (e.g., severe infections) Rapid initiation of tight control can improve outcome (e.g., pregnancy) Primary medical intervention can cause deterioration of diabetes (e.g., intravenous steroid use) Acute onset of retinal, renal, neurological, or cardiovascular complications

scheduled every 3 months for those patients not meeting their goals for glycemic control. Stable patients should be seen at least every 6 months. See sample diabetes flow sheet on p. 343.

The treatment regimen should be assessed at every visit, including the components listed in Box 55-4.

At every regular diabetes visit the physical examination should include:
- Height (until maturity)
- Weight
- Blood pressure
- Foot examination (Tables 55-13 and 55-14)
- Sexual maturation (periodically in peripubertal patients)
- Previous abnormalities on the physical examination

Tables 55-13 and 55-14 show the components of the foot examination. The sensory testing device used with the Foot Screen is a nylon monofilament mounted on a holder that has been standardized to deliver a 10-g force when properly applied. A patient with any abnormality should be referred to a podiatrist. If any ulcer or blister is present, the patient needs to be seen immediately.

Laboratory evaluations should be done on the schedule outlined in Table 55-15.

EVALUATION

The management plan should be evaluated at every visit, including the components indicated in Box 55-5.

The patient's knowledge of diabetes and self-management skills should be evaluated annually.

TYPE 2 DIABETES MELLITUS

Pathophysiology

In type 2 diabetes, insulin resistance is the primary defect that can be detected before deterioration of glucose tolerance occurs. The pancreatic beta cells normally respond to peripheral insulin resistance by increasing basal and postprandial insulin secretion, thereby maintaining normal or impaired glucose tolerance. Eventually the beta cells can no longer compensate for insulin resistance by increasing insulin secretion. At this stage, glucose-induced insulin secretion fails, resulting in the deterioration of glucose homeostasis, and frank diabetes occurs. The developmental stages of type 2 diabetes are illustrated in Figure 55-2.

Several components make up a syndrome known as syndrome X: hyperglycemia, hyperinsulinemia, dyslipidemia, and hypertension. This syndrome leads to coronary artery disease and stroke, may result from a genetic defect producing insulin resistance, especially when the patient is obese. While the mechanism for the develop of this

Diabetes Flow Sheet								
Date								
Vital signs								
Weight								
Height								
BP								
HR								
Laboratory Results								
A1c (q 3 mo)								
Glucose (q 6 mo)								
Creatinine (q 12 mo)								
UA (q 12 mo)								
Microalbumin (q 12 mo)								
Cholesterol (q 12 mo)								
TGL								
HDL/LDL								
HBGM Results High Low Range Frequency								
Foot Examination								
Pulses								
Sensation								
Eye Examination (date)								
Medications								
Insulin AM Lunch Supper HS								
Oral Agents AM PM								
BP Medications								
Other Medications								

Box 55-4

Treatment Regimen Assessment

Frequency and severity of hypoglycemia and hyperglycemia
Home glucose monitoring results
Patient regimen adjustments
Compliance problems
Lifestyle changes
Symptoms of complications
Other medical illnesses
Medications
Psychosocial issues

TABLE 55-13 Diabetic Foot Examination

Diabetic Foot Screen	Normal	Abnormal
Ulcer/blister/callus (present or past)	No/Normal	Yes/Abnormal
Fixed toe deformity (cannot straighten toe with gentle pressure)	No/Normal	Yes/Abnormal
Sensation in the foot (feel the monofilament)	Yes/Normal	No/Abnormal
Palpable foot pulse(s)	Yes/Normal	No/Abnormal

TABLE 55-14 Foot Assessment and Recommendations

Characteristics	Present	Absent	Recommendations
Skin			
Foot ulcer			If present, refer to podiatrist immediately
Macerated interspaces			Keep feet clean and dry; wear cotton or wool socks; antifungal cream, powder or spray; may use lamb's wool
Dry skin			Daily emollients, but not between toes
Toenails			
Improper trimming			Instruct patient or family member in proper technique
Fungal nails			Antifungal drops
Ingrown toenails			Refer to podiatrist
Foot deformity			
Prominent metatarsal heads or callus			Wear shoes with cushioned insoles; gently file or buff callus with emery board or pumice; apply emollients daily
Claw toes, hammer toes, or corns			Wear shoes with plenty of toe room; do not use OTC callus/corn removers; do not cut corns or calluses; refer to podiatrist as needed
Charcot foot			Recommend custom foot wear
Footwear			
Adequate shoes			Recommend shoes with cushioned insoles
Neurovascular			No tobacco, any form
Pulses			If absent, recommend vascular evaluation; wear socks if feet are cold
Sensation (using monofilament)			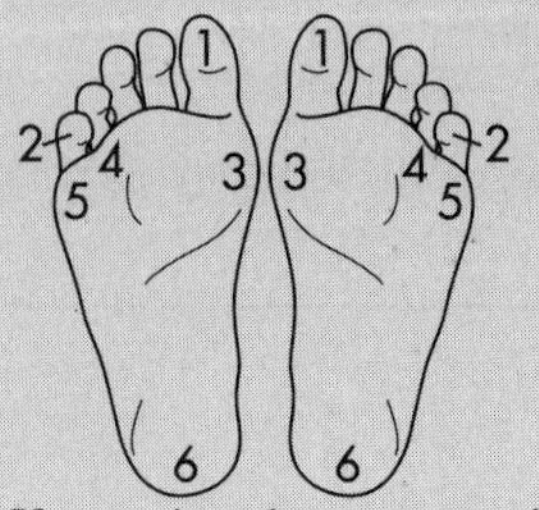 1 2 3 4 5 6 / 1 2 3 4 5 6
Circle number where sensation is absent			If sensation absent at any site, recommend daily visual or manual inspection

OTC, Over the counter.

TABLE 55-15 Follow-up Laboratory Tests

Test	Timing
Glycosolated hemoglobin (normal 4%-6%)	Every 3 months if treatment changes or not meeting goals Every 6 months if stable
Fasting glucose	Optional
Fasting lipid profile	Every 5 years if normal Annually if abnormal Every 3 months if treated with medication
Urinalysis for protein	Annually
Urinary microalbumin	Annually if urinalysis negative for protein Beginning with puberty and after 5 years' duration of diabetes, do annually

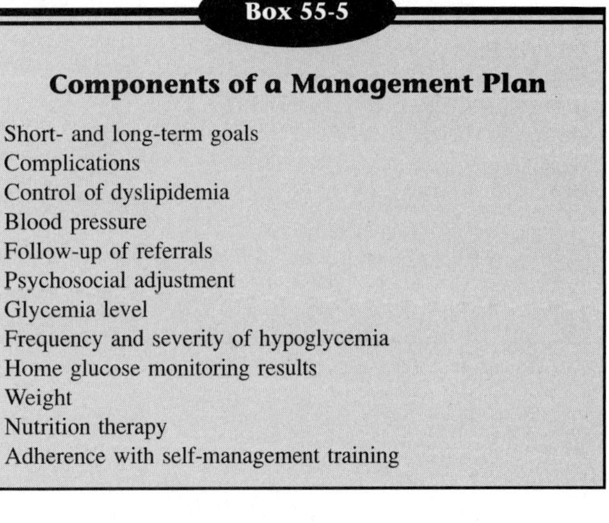

Box 55-5

Components of a Management Plan

Short- and long-term goals
Complications
Control of dyslipidemia
Blood pressure
Follow-up of referrals
Psychosocial adjustment
Glycemia level
Frequency and severity of hypoglycemia
Home glucose monitoring results
Weight
Nutrition therapy
Adherence with self-management training

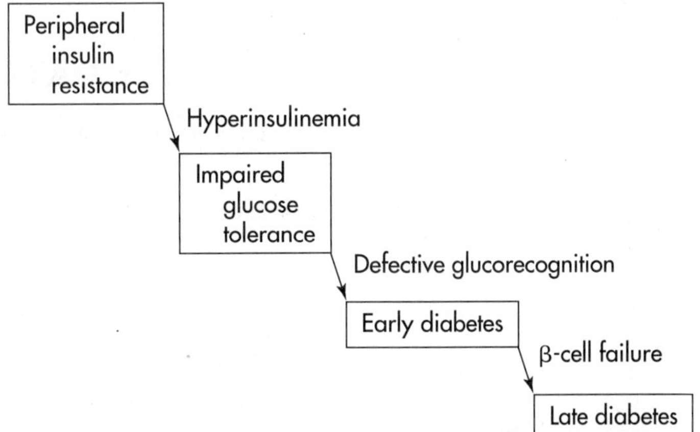

Figure 55-2 Metabolic staging of type 2 diabetes mellitus, showing the progression of metabolic abnormalities leading to the development of type 2 diabetes. Prospective epidemiological studies across several population groups have indicated that insulin resistance may be the primary defect in type 2 diabetes, because it can be detected long before deterioration of glucose tolerance occurs — often at a time when insulin secretion is actually increased. Thus, in many populations and patient groups, insulin resistance and hyperinsulinemia precede the development of type 2 diabetes and can be identified in most prediabetic persons. Beta cells normally respond to peripheral insulin resistance by increasing basal and postprandial insulin secretion to compensate for the insulin-resistant state, thus maintaining normal or impaired glucose tolerance but preventing frank deterioration of glucose homeostasis and type 2 diabetes. Eventually the beta cells can no longer compensate for insulin resistance by increasing insulin secretion. At this stage, glucose-induced insulin secretion falls (defective glucorecognition), resulting in deterioration of glucose homeostasis and subsequently leading to frank diabetes. (From Saltiel AR, Olefsky JM: *Diabetes* 45:1661-1669, 1996.)

Box 55-6

Risk Factors for Type 2 Diabetes

Family history of diabetes
Obesity
Race, including Hispanics, Native Americans, Asian-Americans, Pacific Islanders, and blacks
Previously identified IGT
Hypertension
HDL cholesterol ≤35 mg/dl and a triglyceride level ≥250 mg/dl
Physical inactivity
Women with a history of GDM or delivery of babies greater than 9 lb

GDM, Gestational diabetes mellitus; *HDL,* high-density lipoprotein; *IGT,* impaired glucose tolerance.

syndrome is unknown, it serves to remind us that treatment is to not only reduce hyperglycemia, but also to manage hypertension and dyslipidemia to prevent cerebrovascular and cardiovascular mortality.

Type 2 diabetes is more frequent in adults, but may occur at any age. Obesity accompanies 80% of cases, and there is a strong genetic component. Significant risk factors are outlined in Box 55-6.

SUBJECTIVE DATA

History of Present Illness

Patients have a gradual onset of frequent urination that may prevent recognition of symptoms and may not be able to pinpoint when symptoms began.
Nocturia over past 2 months and weight loss despite increased food intake are common.
Patients may present in a nonketotic, hyperosmolar state.

Past Medical History

Hypertension and dyslipidemia are common and are components of syndrome X, along with hyperglycemia and insulin resistance.

Medications

Several drugs may induce hyperglycemia, including glucocorticoids, furosemide, thiazides, estrogen-containing products, beta-blockers. and nicotinic acid.

Family History

Frequent strong positive family history of diabetes.
Identify family history of hypertension, dyslipidemia, and cardiovascular disease.

Psychosocial History

Include occupation, economic resources, use of tobacco or alcohol.

Diet History

May indicate consumption of food and fluids in newly recognized patient.

Description of Most Common Symptoms

Polyuria, polydipsia and fatigue are the cardinal symptoms.

Associated Symptoms

Chronic skin infections
Blurred vision
Paresthesias
Nausea
Gastroparesis
Yeast vaginitis

In long-standing untreated cases, patients may present with diabetic complications, including impotence, neuropathic pain, and/or angina.

OBJECTIVE DATA

Physical Examination

The physical examination should follow the guidelines listed for type 1 diabetes mellitus.

Diagnostic Procedures

Type 2 diabetes requires the same diagnostic procedures as for type 1 (Table 55-16).

Screening for type 2 diabetes should proceed as follows:

ASSESSMENT

Differential Diagnosis

Differential diagnoses include those listed in Tables 55-17 and 55-18.

THERAPEUTIC PLAN

Pharmaceutical

When diet and exercise are insufficient for glycemic control, medications may be added to the regimen. There are a variety of oral agents that act on various stages of insulin resistance and glucose metabolism. Sulfonylureas are the most widely used agents and should be tried first. If

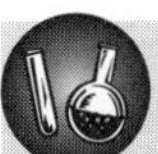

TABLE 55-16 Diagnostic Tests for Type 2 Diabetes Mellitus

Test	Asymptomatic Individuals	At-Risk Individuals	Cost ($)
Fasting plasma glucose	Test all asymptomatic, undiagnosed individuals beginning at age 45 and at 3-year intervals	Testing should be considered at a younger age in individuals who: Are obese: BMI ≥27 kg/m^2 Have first-degree relative with DM Are members of high-risk ethnic group (black, Hispanic, Native American, Asian) Delivered a baby weighing >9 lb or were diagnosed with GDM Are hypertensive Has an HDL cholesterol level ≤35mg/dl and or a triglyceride level ≥250 mg/dl Has had IGT or IFG on previous testing	16-20

FPG, Fasting plasma glucose; *HDL,* high-density lipoproteins; *IFG,* impaired fasting glucose; *IGT,* impaired glucose tolerance.

TABLE 55-17 Differential Diagnosis: Type 2 Diabetes Mellitus

Diagnosis	Supporting Data
Drug toxicity	Beta blockers, thiazides, phenytoin, possibly calcium channel blockers, and clonidine interfere with insulin secretion. Glucocorticoids, estrogen and nicotinic acid induce insulin resistance. Pentamidine is toxic to islet beta cells and cyclosporine affects glucose tolerance by a variety of mechanisms.
Endocrine disorders	Counterregulatory hormone overproduction in Cushing's syndrome, glucagonoma, acromegaly, and pheochromocytoma may induce hyperglycemia.
Addison's disease	Weakness, easy fatigability, anorexia, weight loss, nausea and vomiting, diarrhea, abdominal pain, increased skin pigmentation, hypotension
Diabetes insipidus	Polyuria, polydipsia, decreased urine specific gravity <1.006
Type 1 diabetes mellitus	See Table 55-18

glycemic control is not achieved in 6 to 9 months, a second agent may be added. If there is inadequate control on a combination of oral agents, insulin may be added to the regimen, either alone or in combination with one or more oral agents. Table 55-19 illustrates the advantages and disadvantages of various medical regimens, Figure 55-3 outlines the choice of drug therapies, and Table 55-20 provides details on pharmaceutical therapy.

Drug Interaction

Several drugs interact with oral agents used in diabetes. Patients should be cautioned about potential hypoglycemic events if these drugs are used concurrently (Table 55-21 and Box 55-7).

Lifestyle/Activities

Exercise enhances insulin sensitivity and aids in weight loss. Recommendations should be based on the ability of the

TABLE 55-18 Comparison of Type 1 and Type 2 Diabetes Symptoms

Symptoms	Type 1	Type 2
Polyuria and thirst	Yes	Some
Weakness or fatigue	Yes	Some
Polyphagia with weight loss	Yes	No
Recurrent blurred vision	Some	Yes
Vulvovaginitis or pruritus	Some	Yes
Peripheral neuropathy	Some	Yes
Nocturnal enuresis	Yes	No
Often asymptomatic	No	Yes
Ketosis	Yes	No

Adapted from Karam J: Diabetes mellitus an hypoglycemia. In Tierney L, McPhee S, Papadakis M, editors: *Current medical and treatment,* ed 37, Norwalk, Conn, 1998, Appleton & Lange.

patient. Advise patients to use proper footwear, avoid exercise in extreme heat or cold, inspect feet daily after exercise and avoid exercise during periods of poor metabolic control. Patients should have a preexercise evaluation to evaluate undiagnosed hypertension, neuropathy, retinopathy, nephropathy or ischemic heart disease. An exercise-stress test is recommended in patients over 35 years old. Components of the exercise program should include:

Aerobic exercise at 50 to 50% of maximum O_2 uptake
Twenty to 45 minutes duration, at least 3 days per week
Low-intensity warm-up and cool down phase
Exercise precautions are indicated as described for type 1 patient
Guidelines for alcohol, tobacco use and self-management training are the same as described for the type 1 patient

Diet

Diet is the most important aspect of treatment in type 2 diabetes. Weight loss and hypocaloric diets improve short-term glycemic control and have the potential to improve long-term control. Guidelines from the Food Guide

TABLE 55-19 Advantages and Disadvantages of Various Medical Regimens

Regimen	Patient	Pros	Cons	Guidelines
Oral agent: Sulfonylurea (first generation: chlorpropamide [not recommended for initiation of therapy; use only if patient currently taking], tolazamide, tolbutamide; second generation: glyburide [DiaBeta, Micronase], glipizide [Glucotrol], glimepiride [Amaryl])	Type 2 patient failing diet and exercise; hemoglobin A_{Ic} >9%	Easy, acceptable to patients. Increases endogenous insulin (also may be a *con* in that it can lead to earlier pancreatic burnout).	Patient must have adequate endogenous insulin production. May promote weight gain. Contraindicated in women planning pregnancy. Pregnancy: C	Start with small dose daily for one-week trial. Increase as tolerated. May be added to metformin or troglitazone. May add bedtime insulin to correct for high fasting glucose level. Second generation sulfonylureas should be used first, based on safety profile. Chlorpropamide should only be used in patients <65 years old who are already on it and stable.
Oral agent: Biguanide (metformin) (Glucophage)	Type 2 patient failing diet and exercise; hemoglobin A_{Ic} >9%. Obese patient with sedentary lifestyle may have greater benefit.	Easy, acceptable to patients. Does not increase endogenous insulin, no hypoglycemic effect. Patients may lose weight and improve serum lipids. Pregnancy: B	About 30% of patients have nausea or diarrhea beyond 1st week of therapy. May need addition of sulfonylurea for adequate control. Serum creatinine levels must be 1.4 (females) or 1.5 (males) mg/dl and must be monitored every 3 to 6 months. May cause lactic acidosis in patients with renal insufficiency and CHF. Must discontinue drug for hospitalization or IV contrast studies.	May start with 500 mg dose daily with gradual increase to maximum of 2000 mg. Diarrhea and nausea often resolve in 2 to 3 weeks. If fasting glucose is elevated, add sulfonylurea or insulin to regimen. Take with food to decrease side effects. Avoid use of alcohol, which may potentiate the risk of lactic acidosis.

TABLE 55-19 Advantages and Disadvantages of Various Medical Regimens—cont'd

Regimen	Patient	Pros	Cons	Guidelines
Oral agent: Alpha-glucosidase (acarbose) (Precose)	Type 2 patient failing diet and exercise and with high postprandial plasma glucose	Does not increase endogenous insulin. May improve glycemic control when used with a sulfonylurea. May decrease serum triglycerides. Pregnancy: B	Significant flatulence as a result of the delayed digestion of starch, sucrose and maltose in the small intestine. Flatulence limits patient tolerability. Liver functions must be monitored every 3 months during 1st year. Contraindicated in patient with renal or hepatic impairment.	Starting dose is 50 mg TID. Instruct patient to take dose with the first bite of each meal. May see better tolerance by starting with 25 mg QD for 1 month, then 25 mg BID for 1 month, then 25 mg TID for 1 month, then 50 mg TID. Discontinue if no improvement in glycemic control in 3 to 6 months.
Oral agent: Thiazolidinediones (troglitazone) (Rezulin)	Type 2 patient failing diet and exercise and other oral agents. Hemoglobin A_{Ic} >9%	Easy, acceptable. Does not increase endogenous insulin. Pregnancy: B	Expensive: about $4/day. No effect for first 2 weeks while drug acts to alter genes. May affect liver function and cause slight decrease in hemoglobin. Ovulation may resume in premenopausal, anovulatory women. Caution regarding use of oral contraceptive pill.	Start with 200 mg QD if added to sulfonylurea or insulin. Monotherapy should be initiated at 400 mg QD and may be increased to a maximum of 600 mg if no improvement in first 2 to 3 months. If no improvement noted at 600 mg in 6 to 8 wks, discontinue drug. Give with meals.
Oral agent: Repaglinide (Prandin)	Type 2 patient failing diet and exercise and other oral agents. Hemoglobin A_{Ic} >9%	Quick onset of action, increases endogenous release of insulin	Requires careful monitoring of renal or hepatic insufficiency. Interaction with P-450 system see Appendix D). Can cause hypoglycemia if taken without meals. Pregnancy: C	Starting dose: if HbA_{Ic} is <8%, begin with 0.5 mg. If HbA_{Ic} is >8%, initial dose is 1-2 mg. Adjust dose each week, maximum daily dose is 16 mg. Give before meals.
Oral agent and insulin: Sulfonylurea, metformin or troglitazone and NPH insulin at bedtime	Type 2 patient poorly controlled on maximum doses of oral agents, diet, and exercise	NPH insulin at bedtime will suppress excess hepatic glucose production without requiring daytime insulin which may cause hunger and weight gain. Oral agents used to increase endogenous insulin or decrease insulin resistance.	Patient must be willing to take insulin injection. Adding insulin increases weight gain potential.	Start with 10 U NPH at bedtime and increase 4 to 5 U weekly until fasting glucose is 140 mg/dl. Continue oral agents at previous doses. If fasting glucose is acceptable but random glucoses elevated throughout day, patient may need to start full insulin coverage or switch to a different oral agent.

Continued

TABLE 55-19 Advantages and Disadvantages of Various Medical Regimens—cont'd

Regimen	Patient	Pros	Cons	Guidelines
Insulin: Split/Mix NPH/Regular or 70:30 Two injections	Type 2 patient who needs simple regimen and 24 hour insulin coverage	Requires only 2 injections daily. Regular and NPH mixed provide quicker onset and less peak action later for smoother, intermediate coverage.	Low flexibility, forced lunch on time and snacks to avoid hypoglycemia. NPH at supper may cause hypoglycemia in pre-dawn period although hypo-glycemia in type 2 patients is rare.	Select TDD 20 to 50 U depending on body weight. Start with ⅔ TDD before breakfast with ⅔ as NPH and ⅓ as Regular. Give remaining ⅓ TDD before supper. Increase only evening dose until fasting glucose is <140 mg/dl before adjusting morning dose. Discontinue oral agents.
Insulin: Split/Mix NPH/Regular Three injections	Type 2 patient who needs simple regimen and additional coverage to achieve fasting glucose <140 mg/dl.	No injection required during daytime. Taking NPH at bedtime prevents predawn hypo-glycemia and improves fasting glucose levels.	Requires 3 injections daily. NPH during day may not adequately cover lunch. Low flexibility, forced lunch on time and snacks to avoid hypoglycemia.	Select TDD 20 to 50 U depending on body weight. Start with ⅔ TDD before breakfast, divided as ⅔ NPH and ⅓ Regular. Remaining ⅓ TDD is divided as ½ NPH, ½ Regular. Give Regular at supper, NPH at bedtime. Increase only bedtime dose of NPH until fasting glucose is 140 mg/dl before adjusting morn-ing dose.
Insulin: Basal/bolus NPH or Lente and Regular Four injections	Type 2 patient who desires flexibility with food and willing to do home glucose monitor-ing QID	Allows flexibility to cover food with boluses of Regular; good for achieving tight control, because multiple doses of Regular allow for fine-tuning.	Requires frequent home glucose monitoring and patient decision making re: mealtime doses. Type 2 patient may be able to eliminate testing at lunch meal, may have wide fluctuations during day.	Give 25% of TDD at bedtime as NPH or Lente. Remaining 75% of TDD spread among 3 meals using sliding scale. Patient should be taught to cover food with insulin. Increase NPH or Lente until fasting glucose is <140 mg/dl.

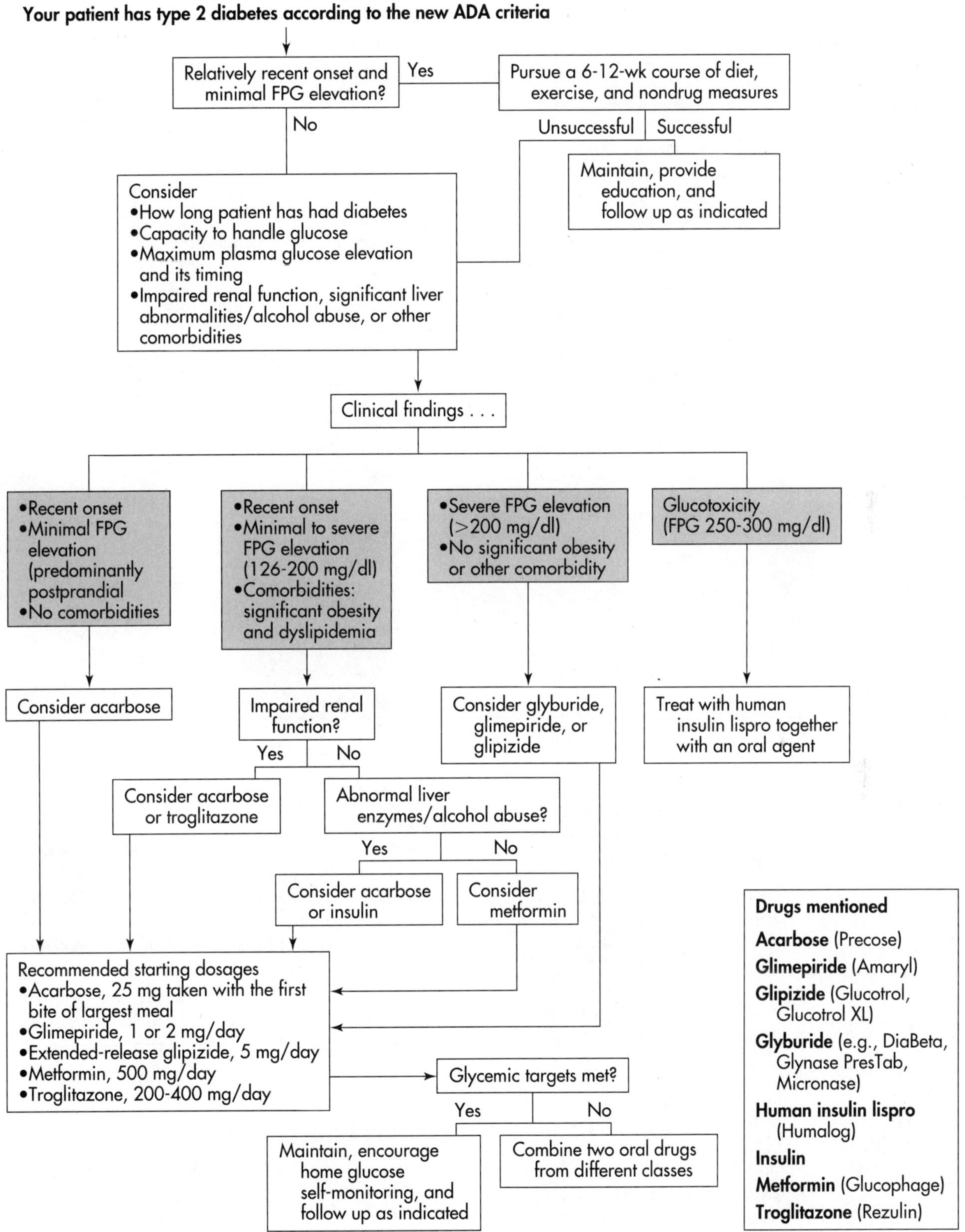

Figure 55-3 Choosing oral drug therapy for type 2 diabetes. *FPG*, Fasting plasma glucose. (From Patient care flowchart: *Patient Care Nurse Pract* March 1998, p. 22.)

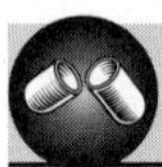

TABLE 55-20 Pharmaceutical Plan: Type 2 Diabetes Mellitus

Drug	Dose	Comments	Cost
Glyburide (Diabeta, Micronase)	1.25-5 mg QD (0.75-3 mg for micronized formulas) with breakfast or main meal Maximum: 20 mg/day (12 mg for micronized)	Pregnancy: B SE: Nausea, hypoglycemia, mild to moderate elevations in BUN and creatinine	$40-$55/3 mg (100)
Glimepiride (Amaryl)	1-2 mg QD with breakfast or the first main meal Maximum: 8 mg/day	Pregnancy: C SE: Weakness, fatigue, hypoglycemia, nausea, elevated LFTs	$23/1 mg (100); $37/2 mg (100); $69/4 mg (100)
Glipizide (Glucotrol, Glucotrol XL)	2.5-5 mg 30 min before breakfast; adjust dose in 2.5-mg increments Maximum: 40 mg/day	Pregnancy: B SE: Nausea, hypoglycemia, mild to moderate elevations in BUN and creatinine	$27-$35/5 mg (100); $50-$65/10 mg (100)
Metformin (Glucophage)	500 mg BID with morning and evening meals; increase by 500 mg weekly Maximum: 2550 mg/day	Pregnancy: B SE: Headache, diarrhea, nausea, vomiting, abdominal bloating, flatulence, anorexia, lactic acidosis	$46/500 mg (100); $79/850 mg (100)
Acarbose (Precose)	25 mg TID taken with meal; increase after 6-8 wk to 50-100 mg TID	Pregnancy B SE: Flatulence (70%), abdominal distention, diarrhea	$46/50 mg (100); $59/100 mg (100)
Troglitazone (Rezulin)	200 mg BID	Pregnancy: Not recommended SE: Nausea and vomiting, diarrhea, abdominal fullness *Need to monitor LFTs on regular basis; deaths have been reported in patients who have not been followed closely*	$104/200 mg (30) $160/400 mg (30)

BUN, Blood urea nitrogen; *LFT,* liver function tests; *SE,* side effects.

TABLE 55-21 Drug Interactions

Oral Agent	Drugs That Interact
Sulfonylureas	Acarbose, alcohol, monoamine oxidase inhibitors, chloramphenicol, warfarin, clofibrate, salicylates, sulfonamides, probenecid
Biguanides	Cimetidine, furosemide, nifedipine
Thiazolidinediones	Cholestyramine (decreases the action of Thiazolidinediones) Causes decreased effectiveness of: Oral contraceptives and terfenadine
Metformin	Nifedipine (increased plasma metformin) Cationic drugs (amiloride, digoxin, procainamide, quinidine, quinine, ranitidine, triamterene, trimethoprim, and vancomycin): compete for renal transport systems causing an increase in metformin (has been noted with cimetidine, others should be monitored carefully)

Pyramid (see Figure 199-2) should be followed with a reduction in total fats, especially saturated fats. Meal plans should be individualized as recommended for the type 1 patient. The goals of nutrition therapy are identical to those of the type 1 patient.

Weight loss should be attempted in obese patients by a moderate decrease in caloric intake and an increase in caloric expenditure. Initially advise the patient to decrease his or her usual caloric intake by 250 to 500 calories per day. In patients with refractory obesity, gastric reduction surgery may be considered.

Patient Education

Patients with type 2 diabetes should be instructed in the same areas as type 1 patients with some modifications:

Patients on oral agents may need less frequent home glucose monitoring. Concurrent medical conditions such as arthritis, poor vision, or poor motor coordination may limit patient's ability to test. Frequency and timing should be based on individual needs.

Box 55-7

Drugs Associated With Hyperglycemia

Alcohol	Asparaginase
Beta-adrenergic agents	Diazoxide
Calcium channel blockers	Diuretics
Corticosteroids	Glycerol
Lithium salts	Niacin
Pentamidine	Phenytoin
Rifampin	Sympathomimetics

Drugs Associated With Hypoglycemia

Anabolic steroids	Chloramphenicol
Beta-adrenergic blockers	Warfarin
Chloroquine	Clofibrate
Disopyramide	Ethanol
Pentamidine	Phenylbutazone
Salicylates	Sulfonamides

Strict glycemic control has increased risks in the **elderly** and may produce significant morbidity resulting cerebrovascular accident. The **elderly patient** may also experience hypoglycemic unawareness that prevents recognition and treatment of hypoglycemia. Use of beta-blockers may also produce unawareness.

Infections and other acute illnesses may produce significant hyperglycemia in the patient on oral agents. Insulin injections may be required during intercurrent illnesses.

Family Impact

Type 2 diabetes impacts the family in a manner similar to that for families of type 1 patients. Additionally, elderly patients may have concurrent illnesses or decreased functional abilities that limit their ability to control hyperglycemia and its complications. Limited financial resources may also limit ability to purchase necessary tools for gooddiabetes care. A thorough home assessment is sometimes required for elderly type 2 patients who live alone.

Referral

Same as in type 1 patients.

Consultation

Same as in type 1 patients.

Follow-up

Same as in type 1 patients.

EVALUATION

Same as in type 1 patients.

SUGGESTED READINGS

American Diabetes Association: Clinical practice recommendations: 1997, *Diabetes Care* 20(Suppl 1):51-70, 1997.

Brietzke S: Diabetes mellitus type I. In Rakel R, editor: *Saunders manual of medical practice,* Philadelphia, 1996, WB Saunders.

Chipkin SR et al: Diabetes mellitus. In Noble J, editor: *Primary care medicine,* St Louis, 1996, Mosby.

Goldstein D et al: The test with a memory, *Diabetes Forecast* 5:22-26, 1994.

Karam J: Diabetes mellitus and hypoglycemia. In Tierney L, McPhee S, Papadakis M, editors: *Current medical diagnosis and treatment,* ed 37, Norwalk, Conn, 1998, Appleton & Lange.

Saltiel AR, Olesky JM: Perspectives on diabetes: thiazolidenediones—treatment of insulin resistance and type 2 diabetes, *Diabetes* 45:1661-1669, 1996.

Wilson BE: Diabetes mellitus Type II. In Rakel R, editor: *Saunders manual of medical practice,* Philadelphia, 1996, WB Saunders.

56 Diaper Rash

ICD-9-CM

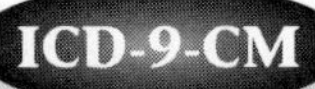

Diaper Dermatitis 691.0

OVERVIEW

Definition

Diaper dermatatis is erythema, scaling, vesicles, or ulceration of skin in the diaper area.

Incidence

Exact incidence is not known. It can present **from 2 weeks of life until child is toilet trained.**

Pathophysiology

Dermatitis results from prolonged contact of urine and feces with skin leading to skin irritation. Some cases may be caused by *Candida* and passed to child from mother through a maternal vaginal candidiasis during birth.

Protective Factors Against

Frequent diaper changing

Factors That Increase Susceptibility

Tightly applied diapers
Use of rubber or plastic pants over the diaper
Diarrheal stools

SUBJECTIVE DATA

History of Present Illness

Rash in diaper area
Irritability
Cries when voiding

Past Medical History

Prior episodes of rash (suggests neglect, carelessness)

Medications

Use of neomycin ointment has created allergic contact dermatitis in infants
Recent antibiotic use suggests candidal infection

Family History

Maternal vaginal candidiasis

Psychosocial History

History of abuse or neglect
Cultural differences in hygiene
Parents' low education level

Associated Symptoms

Eczema or other skin lesions may be present
Oral thrush

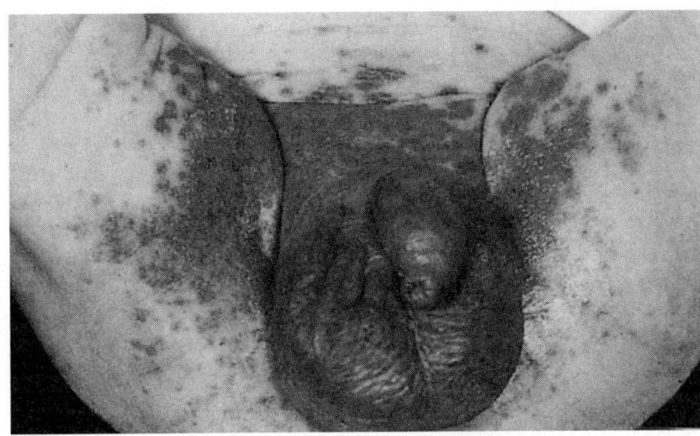

Figure 56-1 Diaper candidiasis, demonstrating confluent erythema and satellite lesions beyond the main area of the eruption. (From Cox NH, Lawrence CM: *Diagnostic problems in dermatology,* St Louis, 1998, Mosby.)

TABLE 56-1 Differential Diagnosis: Diaper Rash

Diagnosis	Supporting Data
Intertrigo	Appears in skin folds as erythema with maceration and erosions; may be found at neck, axillae, crease of buttocks
Psoriasis	Scaling papules, plaques with erythema; positive family history

OBJECTIVE DATA

Physical Examination

Genitalia: Erythema, papules or vesicles, ulcerations may be present. There may be drainage from lesions. Skin may have a burned or scalded appearance or a shiny appearance if caused by contact with irritant. Skin folds are spared. If rash is caused by *Candida,* it is intensely red, and inguinal folds are involved. If bullae or yellow crusts are present, suspect a secondary bacterial infection *(Staphylococcus aureus)* (Figure 56-1).

Diagnostic Procedures

Laboratory

Culture ($31-$39) of drainage to rule out *S. aureus* or *Candida*
KOH ($19-$23) will reveal yeast cells and pseudohyphae if *Candida*

ASSESSMENT

Differential diagnoses include those listed in Table 56-1.

THERAPEUTIC PLAN

Pharmaceutical

Pharmaceutical treatment is outlined in Table 56-2.

Lifestyle/Activities

Noncontributory.

Diet

Increase fluids
Cranberry juice if child is 1 year or older
Exclude other juices

Patient Education

Avoid petroleum products because they trap in moisture.
Change diapers frequently.
Cleanse diaper area with water at each diaper change.
Change brand of disposable diapers.
Wash hands carefully.

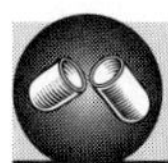

Table 56-2 Pharmaceutical Plan: Diaper Rash

Drug	Dose	Comment	Cost ($)
Zinc oxide (A&D ointment)	Apply at each diaper change.		
Clotrimazole, miconazole, nystatin	Apply to area BID × 3 weeks	Use for candidal infection	15-22/clotrimazole; 2-13/miconazole; 3-22/ystatin
Hydrocortisone ointment	1%, apply to area BID; dosage not established in children under 2 years	DO NOT use fluorinated corticosteroid preparation; causes skin atrophy DO NOT apply to macerated tissue to prevent systemic absorbance	5-11

Avoid packaged wipes, or, if used, do not reuse wet wipes.
Let infant go without diapers as much as possible.
Avoid talcum powder; it may produce aspiration pneumonitis

Family Impact

If candidal infection is diagnosed, mother should be examined (maternal mastitis or vaginal infection).

Referral/Consultation

If patient fails to respond in 1 week, cases should be referred to dermatologist.
If condition worsens and *Candida* is identified, refer to pediatrician or internal medicine specialist. An immunodeficiency may be indicated.

FOLLOW-UP

Return in 48 hours for recheck or follow-up by phone.

EVALUATION

No secondary bacterial infection

SUGGESTED READINGS

Boynton R, Dunn E, Stephens G: *Manual of ambulatory pediatrics,* ed 4, Philadelphia, 1998, JB Lippincott.
Healthcare Consultants of America, Inc: *1998 Physicians fee and coding guide,* Augusta, Ga, 1998, Healthcare Consultants of America, Inc.
Paller A: Diaper rash. In Dershewitz R, editor: *Ambulatory pediatric care,* ed 2, Philadelphia, 1993, JB Lippincott.

57 Diarrhea

ICD-9-CM

Acute Diarrhea 787.91
Chronic Diarrhea 558.9

OVERVIEW

Definition

Diarrhea is defined as an increase in the frequency and fluid content of stools.

Incidence

Accounts for approximately 20% of all pediatric office visits in the United States

Affects approximately 10% of all **infants** <1 year old in the United States

Incidence varies with age, causative organism, geographic location, seasons, and host susceptibility

Pathophysiology

Acute
- Infections, viral or bacterial
- Lactose intolerance
- Overfeeding
- Medications: Antibiotics, laxatives, antacids

Chronic
- Malabsorption
- Acquired immunodeficiency syndrome (AIDS)
- Hyperthyroidism
- Fecal impaction
- Functional bowel disease

Factors That Increase Susceptibility

Poor hand washing, improper food handling, recent antibiotics, immunocompromised host, poor sanitation, recent antibiotics, and recent travel

SUBJECTIVE DATA

History of Present Illness

May or may not have an elevated temperature

Anorexia

Lethargy

Sudden or gradual increase in number and liquidity of stools

Crampy abdominal pain

Ask about: Onset, description of stools, frequency of stools, usual pattern of elimination, associated symptoms such as vomiting or localized abdominal pain, current or recent drugs, exposure to others with diarrhea, detailed dietary history, including introduction of new foods, recent travel, psychological upsets, treatments tried, and urinary output

Past Medical History

Any history of digestive or metabolic disease

In **children** and **adolescents**, determine risk factors for human immunodeficiency virus

Medication

Many medications may induce diarrhea (Box 57-1)

Ask about current or recent medications

Box 57-1

Drug-induced Diarrhea

Laxatives
Antacids (magnesium-containing)
Antibiotics
- Clindamycin
- Tetracyclines
- Sulfonamides
- Any broad-spectrum antibiotic

Antihypertensives
- Reserpine
- Guanethidine
- Methyldopa
- Guanabenz
- Guanadrel

Cholinergics
- Bethanechol
- Metoclopramide
- Neostigmine

Cardiac agents
- Quinidine
- Digitalis
- Digoxin

Family History

Ask about other family members with similar symptoms.

OBJECTIVE DATA

Physical Examination

A problem-oriented physical examination should be completed, with particular attention to:

- Weight
- Hydration status: Mucous membranes, skin turgor, urine output, fontanel, tears, heart rate, level of consciousness, orthostatic blood pressure readings
- Temperature elevation: May be related to dehydration or infection
- Abdominal examination: Distention, hyperactive bowel sounds, diffuse tenderness, increased tympany to percussion, splenomegaly (bacterial)
- Look for other infections that can produce diarrhea and vomiting: Streptococcal pharyngitis, pneumonia, otitis media

Diagnostic Procedures

Diagnosis can usually be made by careful history alone.

Duration <48 hours: No tests are needed. Figure 57-1 illustrates a typical work up for acute diarrhea. Figure 57-2 illustrates a typical workup for chronic diarrhea.

Wet prep for WBCs ($15-$19), stool for O&P ($31-$38), stool culture ($37-$45) for enteric pathogens (Table 57-1).

ASSESSMENT

Differential diagnosis for acute diarrhea include (Table 57-2):
- Viral gastroenteritis (see Chapter 77)
- Bacterial gastroenteritis (see Chapter 77)
- Diarrhea induced by food or drug sensitivities
- Starvation diarrhea
- Parenteral infections: Urinary tract infection, upper respiratory infection

Differential diagnoses for chronic diarrhea include (Table 57-3):
- Malabsorption: Cystic fibrosis, lactose deficiency, celiac disease
- Reye's syndrome
- AIDS
- Inflammatory bowel disease
- Food allergies
- Hyperthyroidism
- Iatrogenic causes
- Toddler's chronic nonspecific diarrhea

THERAPEUTIC PLAN

Infants and Children

Diarrhea is usually self-limiting and requires no aggressive therapy. The treatment plan should be based on careful assessment of the degree of dehydration. Treat as follows (Figure 57-3).

- Diarrhea without dehydration:
  - Continue breast milk, formula, or age appropriate diet.
  - Give PO fluids at a rate of 150 ml/kg/day.
  - Follow each stool with 10 ml/kg of Pedialyte or Infalyte.
- Mild dehydration:
  - Provide oral rehydration therapy (ORT) with a solution containing 75 to 90 mEq/L of sodium. World Health Organization rehydration salts: Give 40 to 50 ml/kg over 4 hours.
  - Reassess hydration status q2-4 hours.
  - When dehydration is corrected, move to maintenance therapy.
- Moderate dehydration:
  - ORT at 100 ml/kg over 4 hours.
  - Reassess hydration status q2-4h.
  - When dehydration is corrected, move to maintenance therapy.
- Maintenance therapy:
  - Resume breast milk, formula, or age-appropriate diet.
  - Push PO fluids at a rate of 150 ml/kg/day.

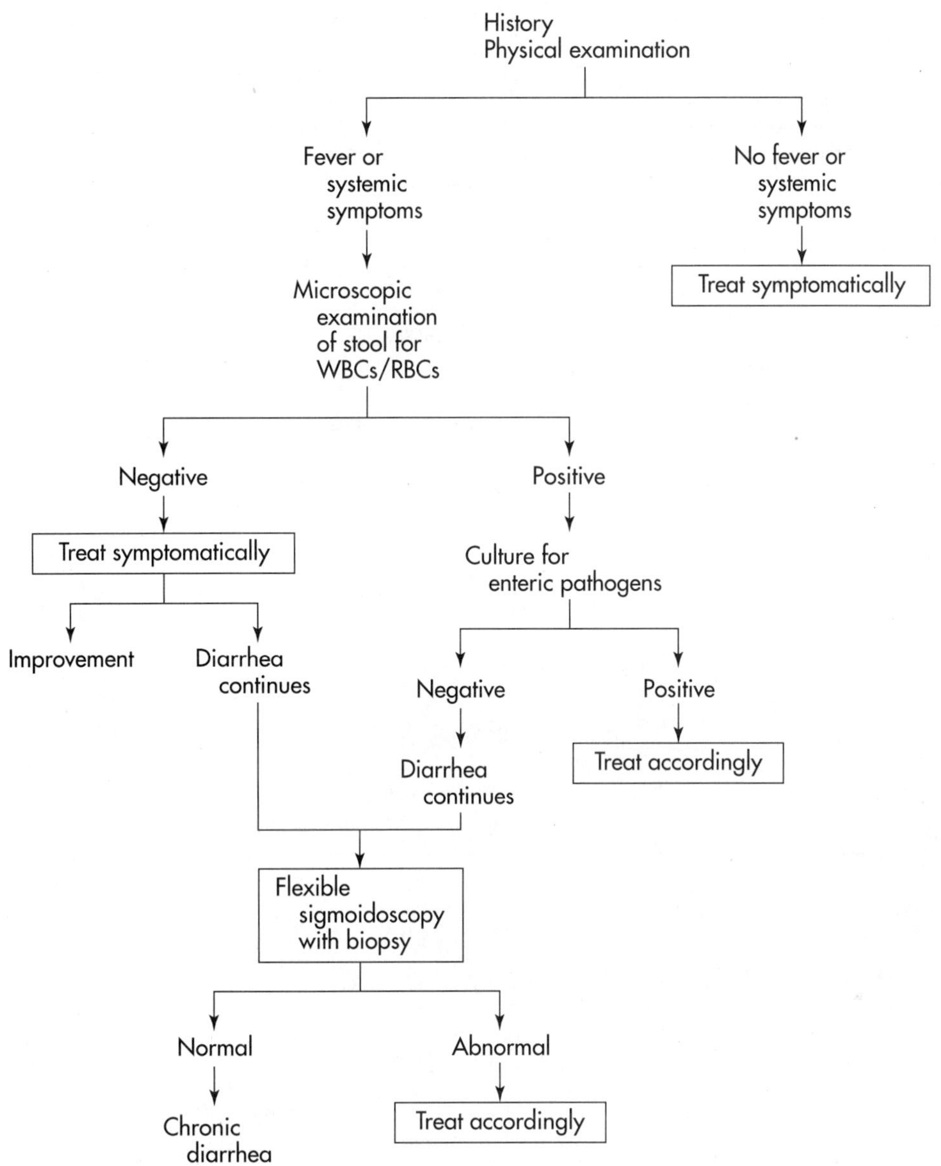

Figure 57-1 Algorithm for patient with acute diarrhea. *WBC,* White blood cell; *RBC,* red blood cell. (From Greene HL, Johnson WP, Lemcke D: *Decision making in medicine,* ed 2, St Louis, 1998, Mosby.)

Follow each stool with a solution containing 40 to 60 mEq of sodium per liter (Pedialyte or Infalyte) at 10 ml/kg and each emesis with 2 ml/kg.

Severe dehydration:

Consult physician and refer for hospitalization and intravenous rehydration.

Pharmaceutical

Pharmacological therapy is usually not indicated and at times may prolong the course; it may be used in severe cases to shorten course, prevent complications, or decrease excretion of the causative agent.

Parental Education (see also Chapter 77)

Teach signs and symptoms of dehydration; dry mouth, no tears, less moisture in diaper, lethargy, weight loss, irritability and sunken fontanel.

Oral Rehydration Therapy

Children <2 years old: Give ½ cup of ORT solution every hour.

Children >2 years: Give ½ to 1 cup ORT solution every hour.

If vomiting occurs, give 1 tsp of the ORT solution every 2 to 3 minutes until vomiting stops; then continue ORT as above.

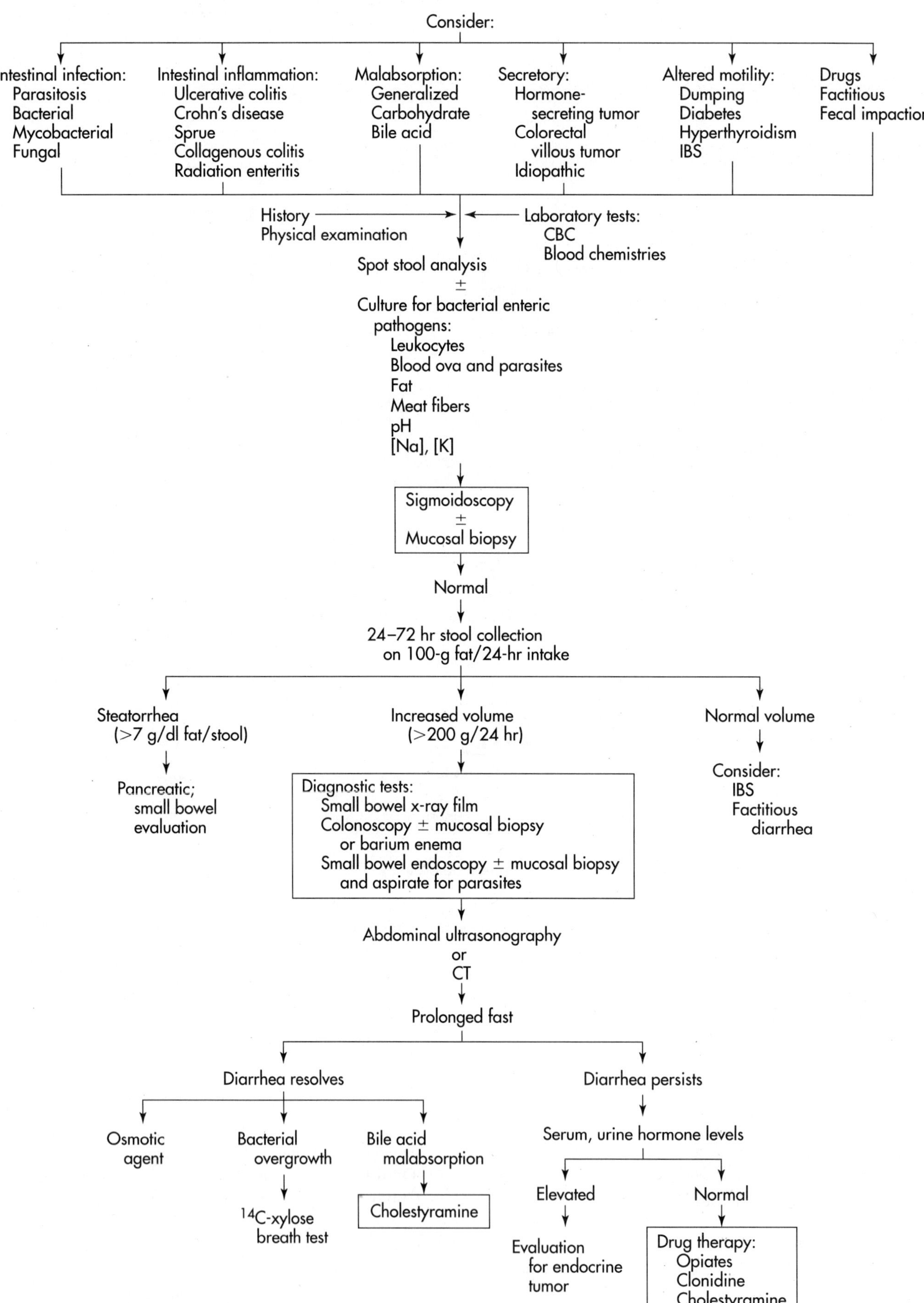

Figure 57-2 Algorithm for client with chronic diarrhea. *CBC,* Complete blood count; *CT,* computed tomography; *IBS,* irritable bowel syndrome. (From Greene HL, Johnson WP, Lemcke D: *Decision making in medicine,* ed 2, St Louis, 1998, Mosby.)

TABLE 57-1 Stool Characteristics in Acute Diarrhea

Agent	Age	Source	Symptoms	Stool Characteristics
Viral				
Rotavirus Norwalk, adenovirus, *Enterovirus*	Any	Food, person-to-person contact	Nausea, vomiting, low-grade fever may precede diarrhea, URI	Large liquid stools, variable odor, negative for blood and leukocytes
Bacterial				
Campylobacter jejuni	Any; most common bacterial diarrhea in ages **1-5 years**	Fecal, oral, food and water, person-to-person	Vomiting, fever	Profuse bloody, watery stools, with mucus in streaks, positive for blood and leukocytes
Salmonella	Any	Fecal, oral, animal or human source, food	Vomiting, fever, abdominal pain	Loose, slimy green stools with "rotten egg" odor, positive for leukocytes and blood
Shigella	Any; peaks at **2-10 years**	Fecal; oral, rarely food	Vomiting, fever, abdominal pain	Watery, yellow-green, mucoid, bloody stools; no change in odor; positive for blood and leukocytes
Escherichia coli (leading cause of traveler's diarrhea)	Any; peaks **<1 year**	Fecal, oral, food and water, undercooked beef	Low-grade fever, abdominal cramps, gradual onset of diarrhea	Green, slimy, foul-smelling stools, positive for leukocytes
Parasitic				
Giardia lamblia	Any; **peaks at 4 years**	Waterborne; seen in day care centers and communities with inadequate water treatment	Nausea, vomiting, anorexia, abdominal distention, and cramping	Pale, bulky, greasy stools, with foul odor; negative for blood and leukocytes, 30%-60% are positive for cysts

URI, Upper respiratory infection. (From Stephen TC: Outpatient management of diarrhea in infants, PCC News, vol 21, no 11, Louisville, 1994, University of Louisville publishers funded by a grant from the Department of Maternal/Child Health and The Cabinet for Health Services, Commonwealth of Kentucky.)

Have parent notify the family nurse practitioner if diarrhea is not improved in 24 hours, if there is an increase in the frequency or amount of vomiting or diarrhea, or if blood appears in either the stool or the emesis.

Avoid using antidiarrheal agents, including over-the-counter preparations.

Adults (Figure 57-4)

For acute episodes; discontinue solids for 12 hours.

Reintroduce food as soon as possible and advance as tolerated.

Pharmaceutical

Pharmacologic therapy is usually not indicated. It may be used in severe cases to shorten course, prevent complications, or decrease excretion of the causative agent (Tables 57-4 and 57-5).

Kaolin-pectin (Kaopectate) ($2-$3) 60 ml PO q3-4h; use not to exceed 2 days

Loperamide (Imodium) ($3-$6) 4 mg PO initially; then 2 mg after each loose stool to a maximum dose of 16 mg/24 hours; use not to exceed 2 days

TABLE 57-2 Differential Diagnoses in Acute Diarrhea

Diagnosis	Supporting Data
Viral	
Rotavirus Norwalk, adenovirus, *Enterovirus*	Large liquid stools, variable odor, negative for blood and leukocytes
Bacterial	
Campylobacter jejuni	Profuse bloody, watery stools, with mucus in streaks, positive for blood and leukocytes
Salmonella	Loose, slimy green stools with "rotten egg" odor, positive for leukocytes and blood
Shigella	Watery, yellow-green, mucoid, bloody stools; no change in odor; positive for blood and leukocytes
Escherichia coli (leading cause of traveler's diarrhea)	Green, slimy, foul-smelling stools, positive for leukocytes
Parasitic	
Giardia lamblia	Pale, bulky, greasy stools, with foul odor; negative for blood and leukocytes, 30%-60% are positive for cysts
Starvation diarrhea	Weight loss, poor food intake
Systemic infections, urinary tract infections (Ch. 187)	Urinalysis: Positive blood, nitrites, and leukocytes
Upper respiratory infections (Ch. 185)	Runny nose, cough, adventitious breath sounds, erythematous, bulging tempanic membrane, throat culture or screen positive for *Streptococcus*

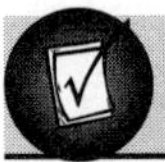

TABLE 57-3 Differential Diagnoses in Chronic Diarrhea

Diagnosis	Supporting Data
Malabsorption: Cystic fibrosis (Ch. 49), lactose deficiency, celiac disease	Weight loss, growth retardation, frequent upper respiratory infection
Reye's syndrome	Lethargy, drowsiness, hyperpnea, behavior changes, progressive stupor
Acquired immunodeficiency syndrome (Ch. 94)	Positive human immunodeficiency virus culture; opportunistic infections
Inflammatory bowel disease (Ch. 100)	Bloody diarrhea and pain with stooling, weight loss, pain in umbilical region and right lower quadrant, obstructive symptoms associated with eating
Food allergies	Other systemic symptoms of allergy, diarrhea associated with ingestion of certain foods
Iatrogenic causes	Diet history of excessive fluid intake, especially fruit juices, and/or insufficient intake of fat
Toddler's chronic nonspecific diarrhea	Loose, mucoid stools with food particles, symptoms increase with environmental stress
Hyperthyroidism (Ch. 178)	Enlarged thyroid, increased heart rate

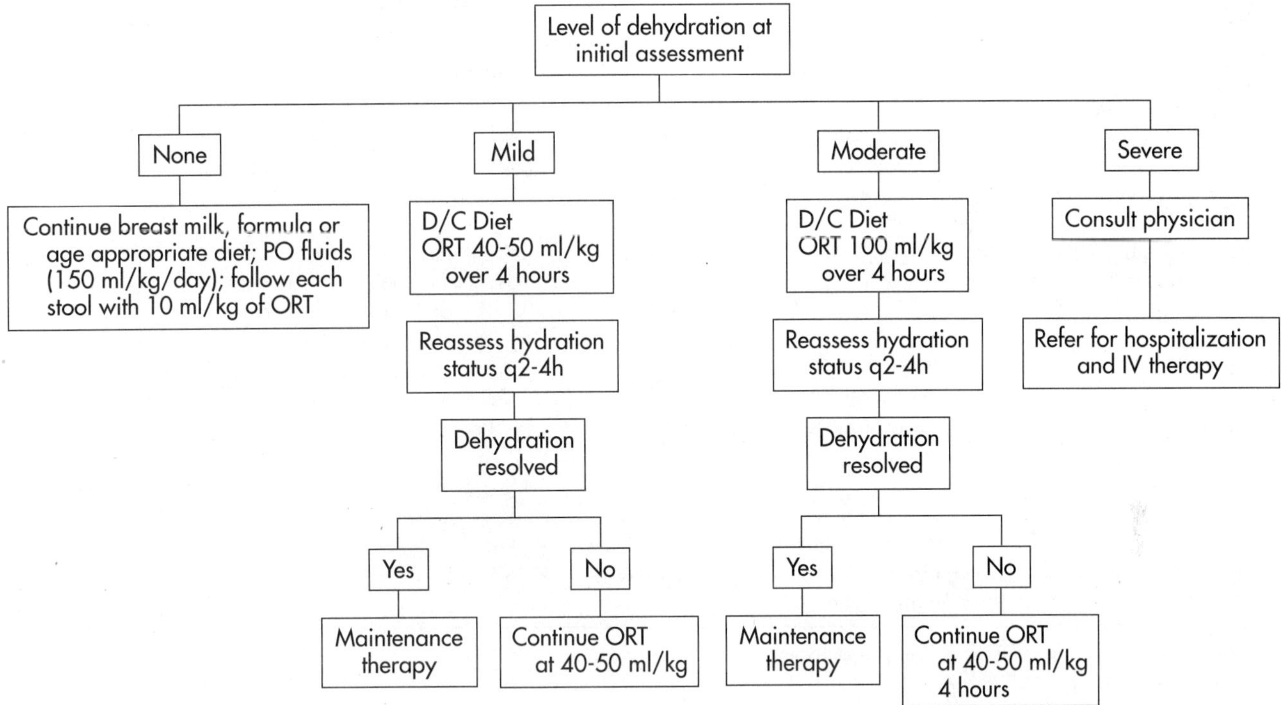

Figure 57-3 Treatment algorithm for diarrhea in infants and small children. *D/C,* Discontinue; *IV,* intravenous; *ORT,* oral rehydration therapy.

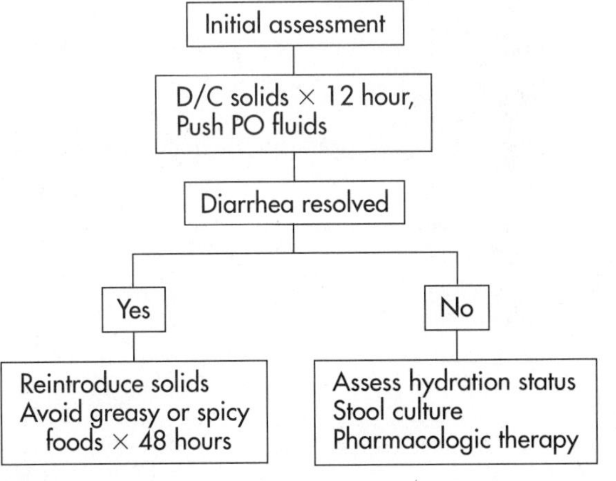

Figure 57-4 Treatment algorithm for diarrhea in adolescents and adults.

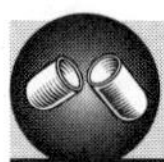

TABLE 57-4 Pharmaceutical Treatment in General Diarrhea

Drug	Dosage	Comments	Cost ($)
Kaolin-Pectin	A: 60 cc PO q3-4h or after each loose stool C: 15-50 cc PO after each loose stool	Pregnancy: C SE: Constipation ↓ Plasma and quinidine level	2-3
Loperamide	A: 4 mg po initially, then 2 mg PO after each loose stool C: 13-20 kg, give 1 mg TID; 20-30 kg, give 2 mg BID; >30 kg, give 2 mg TID	Pregnancy: B SE: N/V, dry mouth, constipation	3-6
Bismuth subsalicylate (Pepto-Bismol)	A: 2 tabs or 30 cc PO q1h up to 8 doses in 24 hours C: 5 cc PO 3-6 years of age; 10 cc PO 6-9 years of age	Pregnancy: C SE: Dark stools, numerous drug interactions, check reference for particular drug in question	2-35
Diphenoxylate (Lomotil)	A: 5-10 mg PO QID; do not exceed 20 mg/day C: >2 years of age 0.3-0.4 mg/kg/d divided into 4 doses	Pregnancy: C SE: Sedation, drowsiness, dizziness, dry mouth, blurred vision	2-47
Lactase	1-2 Capsules or 3-4 gtts taken with milk or dairy products	Pregnancy: Unknown SE: NA	N/A
Lactobacillus	2 Tablets or 1 granule packet TID to QID with milk, juice, or water; NOT useful in antibiotic-induced diarrhea	Pregnancy: Unknown SE: NA	N/A

A, Adult; *C*, child; *NA*, not available; *N/V*, nausea and vomiting; *SE*, side effects.

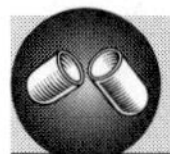

TABLE 57-5 Drugs to Treat Infectious Diarrhea

Drug	Dose	Comments	Cost ($)
Ciprofloxacin	500 mg PO BID	Pregnancy: C SE: Rash, numerous drug interactions; do not take antacids with this drug or within 2 hr	290-335
Doxycycline	100 mg PO BID	Pregnancy: D SE: N/D; photosensitivity; numerous drug interactions; do not take with antacids; take with food	3-123
Norfloxacin	400 mg PO BID	Same as for Ciprofloxacin	57
Tetracycline	250 mg PO QID	Pregnancy: D SE: N/V/D; rash; urticaria; photosensitivity; avoid antacids/milk within 2 hr of taking dose; do not use in children younger than 8 years of age because of tooth discoloration	6-10
Trimethoprim	100 mg PO BID	Pregnancy: C SE: N/V, rash	16-75
Metronidazole	250 mg PO TID	Pregnancy: B SE: Nausea, anorexia, dry mouth, metallic taste; avoid alcoholic beverages	3-131
Quinacrine	100 mg PO TID	Pregnancy: Unknown SE: N/A	N/A

N/A, Not available; *N/V/D*, nausea, vomiting, and diarrhea; *SE*, side effects.

Referral

Consult and/or refer to a collaborative MD, a pediatrician or internist, or an infectious disease specialist as appropriate.

Infants <3 months old
Severe dehydration
Diarrhea persisting over 3 days in **children** and over 2 weeks in adults
Bloody diarrhea or emesis

EVALUATION/FOLLOW-UP

Infants and small children: Follow up by telephone in 12 hours and then daily until diarrhea has subsided.

Infants need weight checks daily.

Instruct caregiver to call if fluids are refused or continually vomited.

Adults: Return to clinic/center/office in 3 days if diarrhea not resolved.

SUGGESTED READINGS

Arvin AM et al, editors: *Nelson textbook of pediatrics*, ed 15, Philadelphia, 1996, WB Saunders.

Boynton RW, Dunn ES, Stephens GR, editors: *Manual of ambulatory pediatrics*, ed 3, Philadelphia, 1994, JP Lippincott.

Dershewitz RA, editor: *Ambulatory pediatric care*, ed 2, Philadelphia, 1993, JP Lippincott.

Goepp JG, Santosham M: Oral rehydration therapy. In Oski MD, McMillan JA, editors: *Principles and practice of pediatrics updates,* Philadelphia, 1993, JP Lippincott.

Groothuis et al, editors: *Current pediatric diagnosis and treatment,* ed 12, Norwalk, Conn, 1995, Appleton & Lange.

McCargar LJ, Hotson BL, Nozza A: Fibre and nutrient intakes of chronic care elderly patients, *J Nutr Elderly* 15(1):13-31, 1995.

Rosenthal M: Diarrhea organisms are becoming media stars, *Infect Dis Children* 10(1):10-11, 1997.

Straughn A, English B: Oral rehydration therapy: a neglected treatment for pediatric diarrhea, *Am J Matern Child Nurs* 6(5):144-147, 1996.

Uphold CR, Graham MV: *Clinical guidelines in family practice,* Gainesville, Fla, 1994, Barmarrae Books.

58 Diverticulosis and Diverticulitis

ICD-9-CM

Diverticulosis of Colon without Mention of Diverticulitis 562.10
Diverticulitis of Colon 562.11

OVERVIEW

Definition

Diverticulosis is the presence of abnormal herniations or saclike protrusions (diverticula) of the intestinal mucosa through the muscle layer of the colon wall; this is often asymptomatic. Diverticulitis is an inflammation of the diverticula resulting from an infection, which may begin when food or fecal matter is caught in the diverticula.

Incidence

Diverticulosis

Diverticulosis is one of the most common illnesses in Western civilization. It affects men and women equally, and there is no known genetic pattern. The incidence increases with age, affecting **30% of the population over 50 years old, 50% of those over 70 years old, and 75% of those 80 years old and older.** It most commonly occurs in Europe and North America, where diets typically are low in fiber.

Diverticulitis

Diverticulitis occurs in 10% to 25% of individuals with diverticulosis; 33% of those treated for diverticulitis will probably have subsequent episodes. Two or three occurrences of diverticulitis in a 1- to 2-year period is usually indication for consideration of surgical removal of the affected portion of the colon.

Pathophysiology

The precise pathogenesis of diverticular disease is unknown. Aging, increased intraluminal colonic pressure, and a diet low in fiber appear to contribute to the formation of diverticula. Prolonged transit time in the colon and decreased stool volume cause contraction of the circular musculature, resulting in increased intraluminal pressure and herniation of the colonic wall. These saclike outpouchings occur at weak segments of the colon, often where arteries penetrate the tunica muscularis. Most diverticula occur in the sigmoid colon, where the lumen is narrow and the intraluminal pressure is high. Diverticulitis can occur when food or feces become trapped in the diverticular sacs, resulting in infection.

Complications

Fatal complications of diverticulosis occur in less than 1 in 10,000 cases. Complications of diverticulitis include fistula formation, most commonly to the bowel, bladder, skin, and vagina. Other complications include obstruction, perforation, abscess formation, and bleeding.

SUBJECTIVE DATA

History of Present Illness

Ask about the duration of symptoms; location and quality of discomfort, including what provides relief; bowel habits; nausea or vomiting; fever or chills; flatulence; and rectal bleeding.

Past Medical History

Ask about prior episodes of diverticulitis or severe abdominal pain.

Medications

Inquire about current medications, including laxative and oral corticosteroid use.

Psychosocial History

Not applicable

Diet History

Ask about the amount of fiber in the patient's diet (e.g., How many servings of vegetables or fruit do you eat per day? What kind of cereal do you eat?).
Ask about fluid intake.

Description of Most Common Symptoms

Diverticulosis

Symptoms may be vague or absent; 80% to 85% of individuals are asymptomatic.
Intermittent left lower quadrant abdominal discomfort, worse after eating, relieved with bowel movements or flatulence.
Mild cramps, constipation, diarrhea, or alternating bouts of both.

Diverticulitis

Abrupt onset of abdominal pain, usually localized to the left lower quadrant; most commonly described as severe and colicky
Fever and chills, nausea and vomiting, anorexia, constipation or diarrhea, rectal bleeding
Patient may complain of polyuria, dysuria, or pyuria
Elderly patients and persons taking corticosteroids may present with only mild symptoms, no fever, no elevation in leukocyte count, and only vague complaints of abdominal pain
Noting a prior history of diverticular disease is helpful with these individuals

OBJECTIVE DATA

Physical Examination

A problem-oriented physical should be conducted, with particular attention to:

Vital signs (including temperature and orthostatics) and general appearance.

Diverticulosis

Examination may be unremarkable.
Abdomen: Abdomen may be distended and tympanic.
Rectal: Digital rectal examination may reveal a palpable mass in the left lower quadrant, firm and tender to palpation. Rectal bleeding may be noted.

Diverticulitis

Remember that the examination may be unremarkable in **elderly** patients or those on corticosteroids.
Patient may be febrile and/or tachycardic.
Abdomen
Bowel sounds may be hyperactive, normal, or absent. The abdomen may be distended and tympanic. The patient may demonstrate guarding. A firm, fixed, palpable abdominal mass may be present in the left lower quadrant. Check for signs of peritonitis by having the patient cough and determine if and where the cough produced pain. Check for rebound tenderness.
Perform the iliopsoas muscle test (when supine, ask patient to raise leg while you exert pressure downward against it).
Check for obturator sign (abdominal pain in response to passive internal rotation of the right hip from 90-degree hip/knee flexion position).
Rectal: May note a tender mass in the cul-de-sac. Twenty-five percent of patients will have occult blood on examination.

Diagnostic Procedures

Diagnostic procedures include those listed in Table 58-1.

ASSESSMENT

Differential Diagnosis

Differential diagnoses include irritable bowel syndrome, ulcerative colitis, carcinoma of the colon, appendicitis, pelvic inflammatory disease, cholecystitis, lactose intolerance, gastroenteritis, fecal impaction, ectopic pregnancy, urinary tract infection, renal disease, small bowel obstruction, and peritonitis (Table 58-2).

THERAPEUTIC PLAN

Pharmaceutical

Diverticulosis

Pharmaceutical treatment will not alter the underlying pathogenesis but may help manage symptoms (Table 58-3).

Diverticulitis

Most mild to moderate cases can be treated on an outpatient basis (temperature <101° F, WBC 13,000 to 15,000).

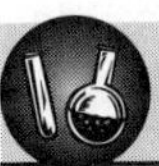

TABLE 58-1 Diagnostic Tests: Diverticulosis and Diverticulitis

Test	Findings/Rationale	Cost ($)
CBC with differential	May reveal elevated WBC with immature polymorphs with diverticulitis, low hemoglobin if bleeding is present	18-23
Erythrocyte sedimentation rate (ESR)	May be elevated with diverticulosis or diverticulitis	16-20
Flat plate and upright abdominal x-ray evaluation	Good initial first step; may be useful in detecting an ileus, obstruction, masses, ischemia, or perforation	142-169
Barium enema	When diagnosis is in doubt, water-soluble contrast medium may be used Double-contrast enema increases diagnostic yield but also increases the risk of diverticular perforation because air is injected under pressure Useful in diagnosing diverticulosis, but use is controversial when diverticulitis suspected	394-471
CT scan	Test of choice to evaluate acute diverticulitis; although expensive, it has been shown to be as good as or better than barium enema examination in diagnosis of diverticulitis, as well as in evaluation for other diseases	807-956
Colonoscopy and flexible sigmoidoscopy	Expensive, and there is risk of perforation Useful if patient is experiencing rectal bleeding or anemia and carcinoma, Crohn's disease, or ischemic bowel is suspected	799-956/colon 254-302/sig

CBC, Complete blood cell count; *CT,* computed tomography; *WBC,* white blood cells.

TABLE 58-2 Different Diagnosis: Diverticulosis and Diverticulitis

Diagnosis	Supporting Data
Irritable bowel syndrome	May be symptomatically identical to diverticulosis; both are treated similarly, and invasive testing to differentiate the two (i.e., barium enema) may not be cost effective
Ulcerative colitis	Symptoms: Persistent diarrhea, bloody stools Colonoscopy: Rectal ulceration and inflammation
Carcinoma of the colon	Symptoms: Rectal bleeding common Barium enema: Reveals a short strictured area with disruption of the mucosa (diverticular stricture is usually longer with the mucosa intact) Colonoscopic biopsy shows carcinoma
Appendicitis	Incidence: Usually afflicts **young adults** (diverticular disease is more common in the **elderly**) Examination: Pain more common in the right lower quadrant
Pelvic inflammatory disease	Incidence: Most common in young adult women History: Sexually active, denies condom use, vaginal discharge Examination: Mucopurulent cervicitis, adnexal tenderness, cervical motion tenderness Laboratory results: Positive cultures for *Neisseria gonorrhoeae* or *Chlamydia trachomatis* common

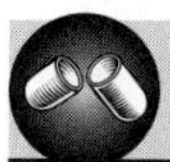

TABLE 58-3 Pharmaceutical Plan: Diverticulosis

Drug	Dose	Comments	Cost
Dicyclomine (Bentyl)	Initially 20 mg QID; may increase to 40 mg QID if tolerated	Used for abdominal discomfort (use with caution; may increase risk of constipation) Pregnancy: B SE: Confusion, stimulation in elderly, blurred vision, dry mouth, constipation, hesitancy, retention	\$3-\$35/20 mg (100)
Loperamide (Imodium); Diphenoxylate (Lomotil)	4 mg initially, then 2 mg after each diarrhea stool PRN to a maximum of 16 mg/day Lomotil 1-2 tabs or 5-10 ml QID PRN to a maximum of 20 mg/day (contains 2.5 mg diphenoxylate and 0.025 mg atropine)	Used for diarrhea Loperamide: Pregnancy: B SE: Drowsiness, dry mouth, constipation Diphenoxylate: Pregnancy: C SE: Sedation, drowsiness, dizziness, dry mouth, blurred vision	\$25-\$80/loperamide: 2 mg (100); \$3-\$5/OTC: 2 mg (12); \$2-\$47/diph: 2.5 mg/ 0.025 mg (100)
Psyllium products (Metamucil)	1 Tbsp in 8 oz of liquid followed by 8 oz of more liquid BID or TID	Used for constipation	\$5-\$12/varies by form
Simethecone (Flatulex, Mylicon, Gas-X)	40-125 mg 1-4 times/day and QHS	Used for flatulence (may turn stools black) Pregnancy: C SE: Belching, rectal flatus	\$2/80 mg (12)

SE, Side effects.

A pharmaceutical plan for diverticulitis is outlined in Table 58-4.

If the patient fails to show signs of improvement within this time frame, the patient needs immediate referral for consideration of hospitalization and/or surgical management.

Analgesics: mild (nonopiate) analgesics may be prescribed for pain.

Lifestyle/Activities

Regular exercise to increase peristalsis and decrease constipation.

Diet

Diverticulosis

A high-fiber diet is recommended to improve symptoms and slow the progression of the diverticular disease process. It is recommended that persons with diverticulosis take in 20 to 35 g of fiber per day (average American intake, 15 to 20 g per day). Box 58-1 outlines some high-fiber foods.

Patients should increase their fluid intake when they increase the fiber content of their diet. They should take in about 2500 ml or 10 8-ounce glasses of fluid a day. Consider adding a fiber supplement such as Metamucil (1 or 2 tbs in 8 ounces of water BID or TID) for patients who travel, eat away from home often, or find it difficult to get enough fiber through diet alone.

Diverticulitis

For patients with diverticulitis a clear liquid diet is prescribed, gradually increasing to soft foods as symptoms improve. Eventually these patients should be placed on a high-fiber diet when they have fully recovered.

Patient Education

Avoid constipation through a high-fiber diet, adequate fluid intake, and regular physical activity.

Avoid laxatives, enemas, and opiates because they can lead to chronic constipation.

Signs and symptoms of complications: Severe abdominal pain, fever >101° F, hard or firm abdomen, sudden change in bowel habits, frank rectal bleeding.

Family Impact

Include family members in teaching when appropriate.

Referral

Very ill patients with a history of diverticulosis (especially the elderly)

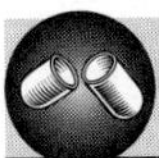

TABLE 58-4 Pharmaceutical Plan: Diverticulitis

Drug	Dose	Comments	Cost
Cefoxitin (Mefoxin)	2 g q8h for 7 days	For milder cases of diverticulitis Pregnancy: B SE: Local reactions, diarrhea, elevated liver enzymes	$17/IVPB 100 mg (7) $238
Or			
Metronidazole (Flagyl)	250-500 mg q8h for 7 days	For milder cases of diverticulitis Pregnancy: B SE: Seizures, peripheral neuropathy, GI upset, metallic taste, dysuria	$9-$131/250 mg (100); $7-$238/500 mg (100)
Plus			
Amoxicillin	500 mg q8h	For more severe cases Pregnancy: B SE: GI upset, urticaria, hyperactivity	$8-$27/500 mg (100)
Or			
TMP-SMX	160-180 mg for 7 days	For more severe cases Pregnancy: C SE: Hepatic or renal toxicity, pseudomembranous syndrome, GI distress, ataxia	$7-$74/RS: (100); $9-$121/DS: (100)

Most patients should respond to antibiotic therapy within 48-72 hours.
GI, Gastrointestinal; *DS*, double strength; *RS*, regular strength; *SE*, side effects.

Box 58-1

Foods High in Fiber

Cereals	Grains	Fruits	Vegetables
Branflakes, oatmeal, shredded wheat	Bran muffins, brown rice, whole-wheat bread	Artichokes, apples, blackberries, blueberries, dates, figs, oranges, pears, prunes, raspberries, tomatoes	Beans (baked, black, kidney, lima, pinto), broccoli, brussels sprouts, carrots, chick peas, green peas, lentils, pumpkin, rutabaga, winter squash

Failure of symptoms to resolve in 48 to 72 hours
Brisk rectal bleeding
Consider immediate hospitalization if the patient's condition worsens, temperature is >101° F, there is a marked change in abdominal pain, if the WBC count continues to increase, or if signs of peritonitis develop
Two or more episodes of diverticulitis during a 1- to 2-year period may indicate need for surgical referral

Consultation

If symptoms do not improve regardless of management regimens, consider a GI and/or surgical consultation.

EVALUATION/FOLLOW-UP

Diverticulosis

Follow up 1 to 2 weeks after diagnosis, then every 3 months to yearly as needed.
May repeat barium enema every 3 to 5 years (if no symptoms) followed by a colonoscopy if needed.
Patients over 50 should have a flexible sigmoidoscopy every 5 years for cancer screening.

Diverticulitis

Telephone follow-up for 24 to 72 hours; if symptoms do not improve, the patient will need to be seen for further evaluation. If recovery has progressed as expected, the patient may be seen in 10 days to 2 weeks, then in 1 to 3 months and then to once a year, based on symptoms.

RESOURCES

American College of Gastroenterology
www.acg.gi.org

Intestinal Disease Foundation
412-261-5888 3570

Intestinal Disease Research Programme GI links
www.fhs.mcmaster.ca/idrp/gi-sites.htm

National Institute of Diabetes, Digestive, and Kidney Information
www.niddk.nih.gov/health/health.htm

National Digestive Diseases Information Clearinghouse
2 Information Way
Bethesda, MD 20892-3570
www.niddk.nih.gov/health/digest/nddic.htm

SUGGESTED READINGS

Deckman RC, Cheskin LJ: Diverticular disease in the elderly, *J Am Geriatr Soc* 40:986-993, 1993.

Elfrink RJ, Miedema BW: Colonic diverticula, *Postgrad Med* 92:97-108, 1992.

Ellsworth A et al: *Mosby's 1998 medical drug reference,* St Louis, 1998, Mosby.

Freeman SR, McNally PR: Diverticulitis, *Med Clin North Am* 77:1149-1165, 1993.

Goroll A, May L, Mulley A, editors: *Primary care medicine: office evaluation and management of the adult patient,* Philadelphia, 1995, JB Lippincott.

Gray DS: The clinical uses of dietary fiber, *Am Family Physician* 51:419-425, 1995.

Haubrich WS et al: *Gastroenterology,* ed 5, Philadelphia, 1995, WB Saunders.

Healthcare Consultants of America, Inc: *1998 Physicians fee and coding guide,* Augusta, Ga, Healthcare Consultants of America, Inc.

Hurst JW: *Medicine for the practicing physician,* Norwalk, Conn, 1996, Appleton & Lange.

Isselbacher K: *Harrison's principles of internal medicine,* ed 13, New York, 1994, McGraw-Hill.

Lonergan E, editor: *Geriatrics: a clinical manual,* Norwalk, Conn, 1996, Appleton & Lange.

Rakel R, editor: *Textbook of family practice,* ed 5, Philadelphia, 1995, WB Saunders.

Dysfunctional Uterine Bleeding

ICD-9-CM

Postclimacteric Bleeding 627.1
Disorders of Menstruation and Other Abnormal Bleeding From Female Genital Tract 626.8

OVERVIEW

Definitions

Dysfunctional uterine bleeding (DUB) is abnormal uterine bleeding with no readily identifiable cause. The diagnosis is by exclusion among numerous etiological factors.
Adenomyosis is growth of endometrial tissue within and under the myometrium.
Leiomyoma is characterized by benign, slow-growing tumors made up of smooth muscle; these tumors develop in the uterus during the individual's reproductive years.
Metrorrhagia is irregular bleeding or bleeding between menstrual periods.
Menorrhagia is heavy or prolonged bleeding.
Polymenorrhea is characterized by menstrual cycles of less than 22 days.
Anovulation is the absence of ovulation.
Contact bleeding is postcoital bleeding.
Dysmenorrhea is painful menstruation.

Incidence

Dysfunctional uterine bleeding usually occurs around either end of the reproductive time frame—puberty (20%) or menopause (40%) (Gerbie, 1994). The exact incidence is unknown (Skrypzak, 1995).

Pathophysiology

Protective Factors Against

Ovulatory cycles, use or nonuse of contraception

Factors That Increase Susceptibility to DUB

Sometimes a cause cannot be identified.
Reproductive system-related factors:
- Anovulation (without a surge of luteinizing hormone [LH] or with insufficient progesterone, endometrial lining begins to shed), as with menarche or menopause
- Spontaneous abortion
- Endometritis
- Polycystic ovaries
- Leiomyoma
- Sexually transmitted diseases (STDs)
- Malignancy
- Contraception
- Ovarian dysfunction

Other:
- Trauma
- Obesity
- Hyperthyroidism
- Hypothyroidism
- Coagulation disorder
- Medications
- Hypothalamic disorder
- Pituitary or dysfunction

SUBJECTIVE DATA

History of Present Illness

Ask about duration and pattern of symptoms. Ask the patient to describe the abnormal bleeding pattern. If she is saturating one pad per hour for 7 days, blood loss is significant.

Ask about vaginal discharge, pelvic pain, or bleeding after intercourse. It may prove useful to have the patient keep a menstrual bleeding calendar (see p. 377).

Past Medical History

Ask about menstrual history (menarche, cycle length, and duration), birth control method, history of liver disease, diabetes, hypertension, obesity, thyroid disorder, blood dyscrasia, or coagulation abnormality, dysmenorrhea, date

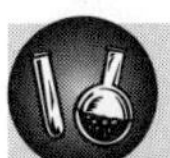

TABLE 59-1 Diagnostic Tests: Dysfunctional Uterine Bleeding

Diagnostic Test	Findings/Rationale	Cost ($)
Endometrial biopsy	Rules out endometrial carcinoma or hyperplasia, especially in perimenopausal or menopausal patients	142-170
Ultrasonography	Identifies leiomyomas, polyps, or adnexal mass; not useful with adenomyosis	235-295
Other Tests*		
Urine HCG	If pregnancy suspected	17-23
Thyroid function studies	Identifies hyperthyroidism and hypothyroidism	47-61
Hgb and Hct	If excessive bleeding	11-14/each
FSH level	If menopause suspected (levels >40/ml suggest menopause) If patient takes oral contraceptives, draw after fifth day of placebo pills	62-78
Coagulation studies	Any **woman under 35 years old** with excessive bleeding and a Hgb <10	26-32

*The tests chosen depend on the patient's age, history, and results of the physical examination.
FSH, Follicle-stimulating hormone; *HCG,* human chorionic gonadotropin; *Hgb,* hemoglobin; *Hct,* hematocrit; *H&P,* history and physical examination.

of last sexual contact, number of sexual partners, date of last Papanicolaou (Pap) smear, past Pap smear results.

Medications

History of use of major tranquilizers, anticoagulants, oral contraceptives, steroids, chemotherapy, medroxyprogesterone acetate (Depo-Provera), levonorgestrel (Norplant)

Family History

Ask about family history of leiomyomas.
Ask about age of her mother at menopause.

Psychosocial History

Ask about history of psychiatric illness.
Ask about smoking (smoking decreases the chance of leiomyoma).

Diet

Ask about diet history (particularly if obese).

Description of Most Common Symptoms

Menorrhagia: May have single occurrence of heavy bleeding or recurrent heavy bleeding, prolonged; patient may or may not complain of pelvic pain

Metrorrhagia: May have spotting, hemorrhage, or bleeding between menses, perimenopausally, or with use of oral contraceptives, Norplant (most often at midcycle), and Depo-Provera

Leiomyoma: Pelvic heaviness, low abdominal pressure, constipation, urinary incontinence, dysmenorrhea, spotting throughout cycle

Adenomyosis: Dysmenorrhea, menorrhagia, premenstrual spotting

OBJECTIVE DATA

Physical Examination

Every physical examination for DUB should include a thorough pelvic examination with careful Pap smear.

Bimanual examination: May suggest adenomyosis (globular, boggy enlargement of uterus), pregnancy (even, smooth enlargement), leiomyoma (smooth, spherical, firm masses). Note amount of bleeding coming through cervical os and presence of polyps. Cervical culture ($30-$79) and/or microscopic evaluation if indicated. If the patient is using an intrauterine device (IUD), visualize the strings. Palpate the thyroid.

Neck: Assess thyroid for masses and enlargement.

Abdomen: Assess for masses, tenderness, hepatosplenomegaly.

Diagnostic Procedures

Diagnostic procedures include those listed in Table 59-1.

ASSESSMENT

Differential Diagnosis

Differential diagnoses include pregnancy, uterine or cervical polyps, leiomyomas, carcinoma, STDs, adenomyosis, an-

TABLE 59-2 Differential Diagnosis: Dysfunctional Uterine Bleeding

Diagnosis	Supporting Data
Pregnancy	Cessation of menses for a period of time before bleeding began May be heavy bleeding/cramping HCG levels + (may be low) Pelvic heaviness and adnexal mass if ectopic pregnancy
Uterine polyps	Menorrhagia, dysmenorrhea; uterus not enlarged
Leiomyoma	Pelvic heaviness, low abdominal pressure, constipation, urinary incontinence, dysmenorrhea, spotting throughout cycle, uterus with smooth, spherical, firm masses
Carcinoma	Heavier menstrual bleeding than usual, bleeding after menopause, lower abdominal cramps, uterus enlarged with advanced disease
STD	Vaginal discharge, dyspareunia, bleeding with intercourse
Adenomyosis	Dysmenorrhea, menorrhagia, premenstrual spotting, even, globular, boggy enlargment of uterus
Anovulation	Irregular bleeding, patient may also be obese Usually occurs in adolescence or perimenopause
Coagulation disorder	Pale sclera and gums, multiple bruises, menorrhagia, abnormal values on coagulation studies

STD, Sexually transmitted disease.

ovulation, endocrine disorders, thyroid disorder, coagulation disorders (Table 59-2).

THERAPEUTIC PLAN

Treatment depends on the specific cause of DUB. Figure 59-1 is an algorithm from treatment of abnormal vaginal bleeding.

Pharmaceutical

If bleeding is severe, a consultation with a gynecologist is in order, with hospitalization for intravenous conjugated estrogens and/or dilation and curettage (D&C).

Oral therapy includes iron therapy and dietary adjustment if anemia identified.

Thyroid replacement if indicated.

Give hormonal therapy if no contraindications (Figure 59-2).

Use of nonsteroidal antiinflammatory drugs decreases endometrial blood flow through antiprostaglandin effect and may increase bleeding through antiplatelet effect.

Antibiotics are indicated for STD or endometritis.

Lifestyle/Activities

Change in contraceptives may be necessary.

May need to adjust lifestyle to accommodate bleeding episodes until they resolve.

Diet

Diet modification to achieve weight loss or may need to increase iron in patient's diet to correct anemia.

Patient Education

Stress the importance of safe sex practices. Explain side effects of medications, treatment plan options, and signs and symptoms that should be reported. Stress importance of scheduled Pap smears and gynecological examinations. Discuss fertility concerns and/or patient concerns surrounding menopause. If she chooses myomectomy for leiomyomas, the risk of recurrence is unknown. Polyps often return after removal. Hysterectomy is often successful for carcinoma, depending on type of cancer, metastasis, and other factors.

Referrals

Refer the patient to OB/GYN if abnormal bleeding resumes after being controlled (suspect malignancy), if you suspect ectopic pregnancy (which is a potential surgical emergency), if bleeding occurs 6 or more months after menopause (suspect malignancy), or if bleeding is severe or uncontrolled.

Refer to gynecologist if leiomyoma is larger than 12-week size, if it is rapidly increasing in size, if significant anemia is present, or if adenomyosis is suspected.

Consultation

Consider consulting an OB/GYN a collaborative MD in cases of heavy bleeding, significant anemia, or suspected pregnancy or malignancy.

EVALUATION/FOLLOW-UP

Repeat Pap smears per protocol for abnormal Pap result

Return visit 3 months after hormonal treatment

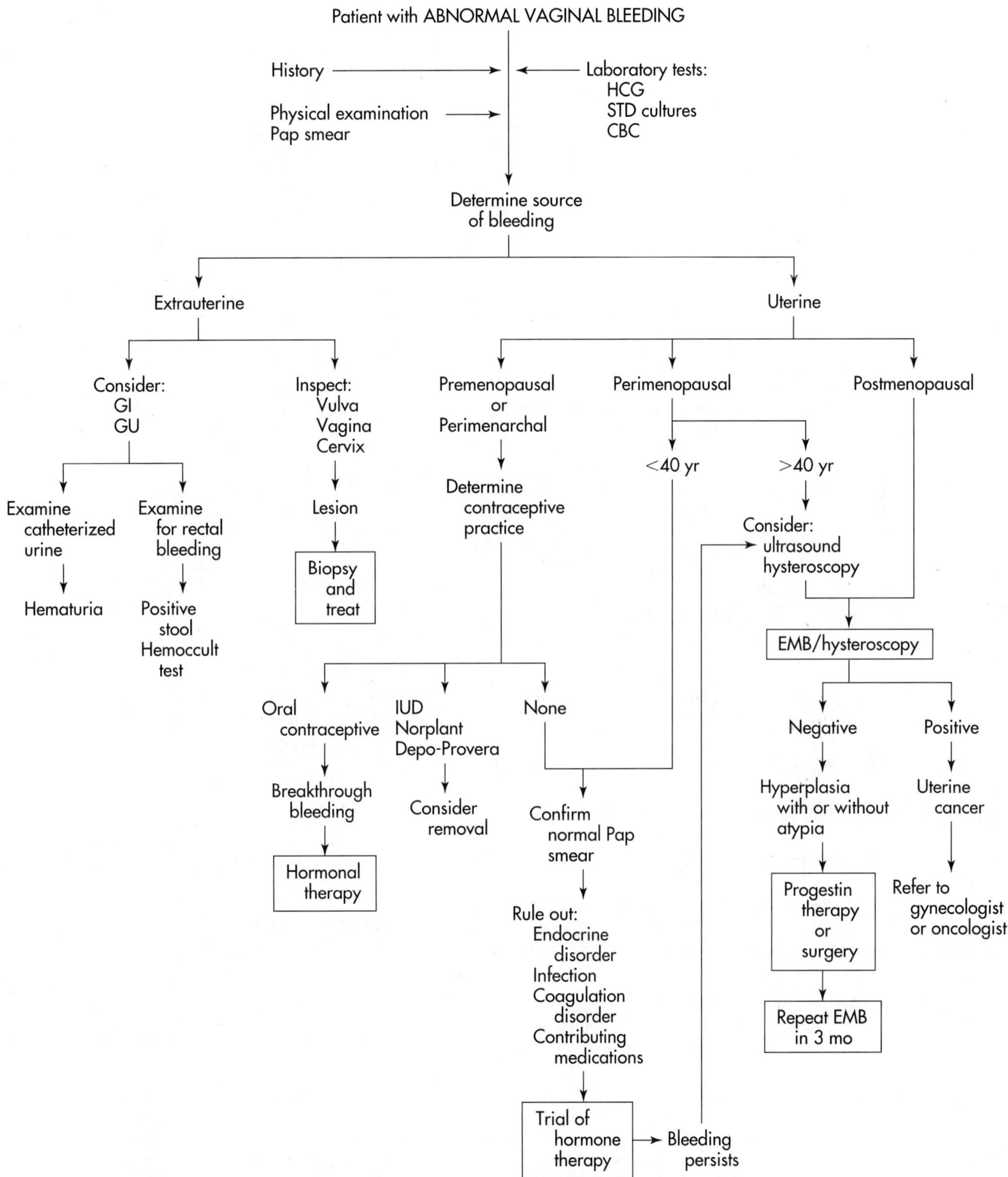

Figure 59-1 Algorithm for treatment of a patient with abnormal vaginal bleeding. *CBC,* Complete blood count; *EMB,* endometrial biopsy; *GI,* gastrointestinal; *GU,* genitourinary; *HCG,* human chorionic gonadotropin; *IUD,* intrauterine device; *STD,* sexually transmitted disease. (From Greene HL, Johnson WP, Lemcke D: *Decision making in medicine,* ed 2, St Louis, 1998, Mosby.)

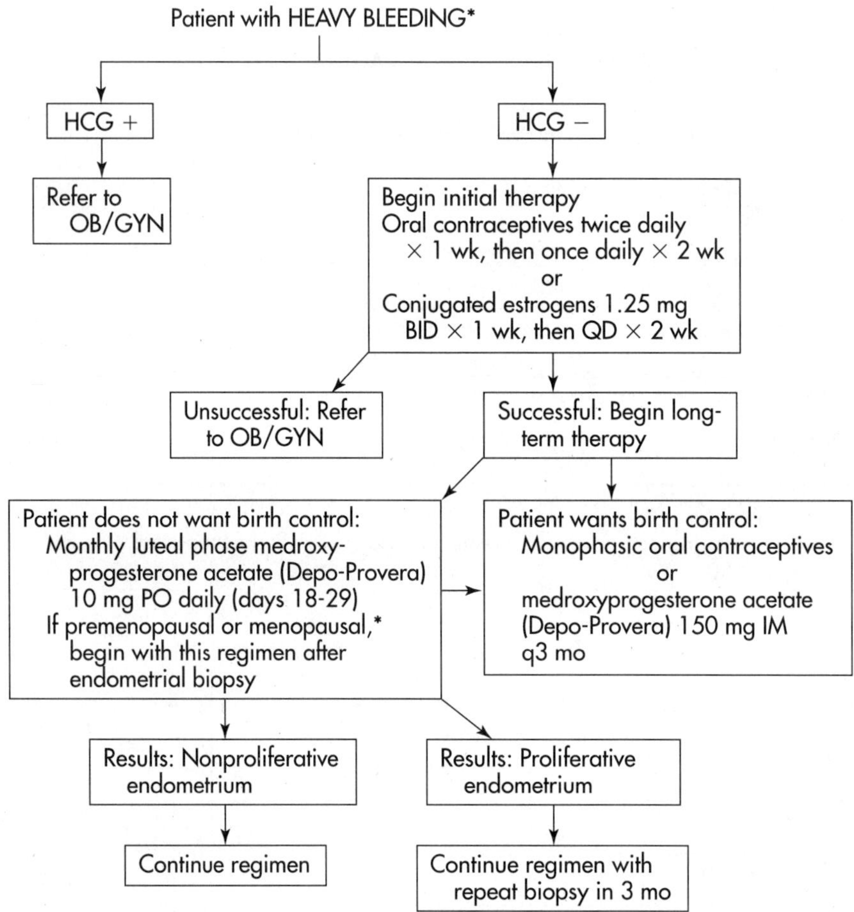

Figure 59-2 Algorithm for treatment of a patient with heavy bleeding. *If bleeding occurred after 6 months of absent menses, *immediate referral to an OB/GYN is indicated. CBC,* Complete blood cell count; *EMB,* endometrial biopsy; *GI,* gastrointestinal; *GU,* genitourinary; *HCG,* human chorionic gonadotropin; *IUD,* intrauterine device; *STD,* sexually transmitted disease.

SPECIAL CONSIDERATIONS

Leiomyomas may mask malignant uterine tumors (leiomyosarcoma).

Any bleeding 6 months or more after menopause suggests malignancy.

Postcoital bleeding may indicate *either* an STD or a malignancy.

Leiomyomas usually resolve with menopause.

Never overlook the possibility of sexual abuse in **children** (Smith, 1995).

REFERENCES

Gerbie MV: Complications of menstruation: abnormal uterine bleeding. In DeCherney A, Pernoll ML, editors: *Current obstetric & gynecologic diagnosis & treatment,* Norwalk, Conn, 1994, Appleton & Lange.

Skrypzak B: Approach to abnormal vaginal bleeding. In Lemcke D et al, editors: *Primary care of women,* London, 1995, Prentice-Hall.

Smith CB: Abnormal uterine bleeding: guide to management throughout a woman's lifetime, *Consultant* 3:339-349, 1995.

SUGGESTED READINGS

Brown JS, Crombleholme W: *Handbook of gynecology & obstetrics,* Norwalk, Conn, 1993, Appleton & Lange.

Ellsworth AJ et al: *Mosby's 1998 medical drug reference,* St Louis, 1998, Mosby.

Fogel CI, Woods NF: *Women's health care,* Thousand Oaks, Calif, 1995, Sage.

Healthcare Consultants of America, Inc: *1998 Physicians fee and coding guideline,* Augusta, Ga, Healthcare Consultants of America, Inc.

Miller H: Abnormal vaginal bleeding. In Greene H, Johnson W, Lemcke D, editors: *Decision making in medicine,* ed 2, St Louis, 1998, Mosby.

Strickland K: Primary care management of leiomyoma-induced abnormal bleeding *J Am Acad Nurse Pract* 8:541-545,

SAMPLE

Menstrual Bleeding Calendar

Patient Name *Jane Individual*

This calendar will assist your health provider in tracking the occurrence and character of your symptoms. Begin by filling in your name and the month in which you begin to keep track. Circle the date of the first day you are charting. Put a check mark (√) over each date as it passes. Please mark on the calendar using the following symbols:

Number of pads used in 24 hours; X for spotting — I = Intercourse, D = Discharge

Use the comments section to describe additional information.

MONTH 1: *August 1998*

1	2	3	4	5	6	7
8	9	10	11	12	13	14
15	16 (circled, √) I	17 √	18 √ X	19 √ X	20 √ 2	21 √
22 √ 12	23 √ 12	24 √ 8	25 √ 10	26 √ 5	27 √ X	28
29	30	31				

Comments:

Cramping on 1/22, ibuprofen taken.

Primary and Secondary Dysmenorrhea

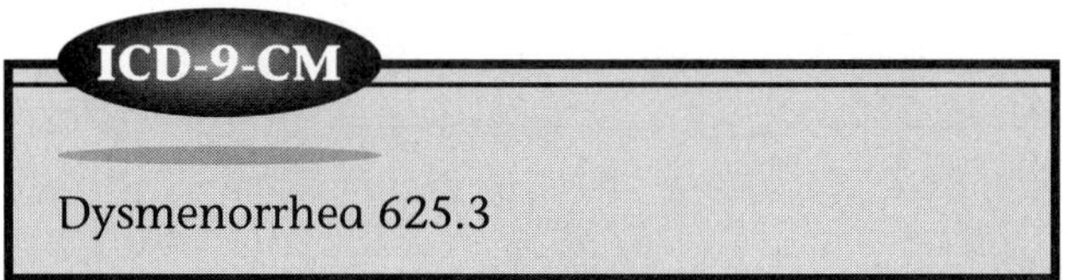

ICD-9-CM

Dysmenorrhea 625.3

OVERVIEW

Definition

Primary dysmenorrhea is painful menstruation, occurring with ovulatory menstrual cycles and in the absence of a pathological condition of the pelvis. Secondary dysmenorrhea is painful menstruation resulting from a pathological condition of the pelvis (endometriosis is the most common cause).

Incidence

Primary Dysmenorrhea

Primary dysmenorrhea is the most common medical problem in **young women** and the most common gynecological problem. It is estimated that 50% of all menstruating women have dysmenorrhea with 10% having symptoms severe enough to interfere with school, work, and/or activities. The onset is usually at least 6 to 12 months after menarche, or when ovulatory cycles begin. The incidence increases and peaks in the **late teens and early twenties**, then gradually declines with age.

The incidence of primary dysmenorrhea is increased in women who:
- Are obese
- Smoke
- Are sexually inactive
- Are nulliparous or who delay child-bearing

Secondary Dysmenorrhea

Incidence unknown

Onset usually after age 25 to 30; gradually increases with age

Pathophysiology

Primary Dysmenorrhea

Primary dysmenorrhea results from increased levels of prostaglandins during the luteal phase of the menstrual cycle, causing increased myometrial muscle tone, uterine contractions, and vasopression of uterine vessels, which results in ischemic pain and associated symptoms. Prostaglandin synthesis varies from woman to woman, as does the degree of pain, but pain can be severe. The severity of the pain is related to the amount of prostaglandin produced. The tendency to synthesize prostaglandin tends to be hereditary, so daughters of mothers with primary dysmenorrhea are more likely than others to have primary dysmenorrhea. Women with anovulatory cycles do not have luteal increases in prostaglandins and thus do not have primary dysmenorrhea.

Secondary Dysmenorrhea

Secondary dysmenorrhea is associated with pathological conditions of the pelvis, frequently endometriosis, but can result from many other causes, including but not limited to:

Extrauterine
- Congenital malformation
- Endometriosis
- Ovarian diseases, ectopic pregnancy
- Pelvic inflammatory disease
- Adhesive disease, secondary to surgery or infection

Intrauterine
- Endometriosis
- Adenomyosis
- Leiomyomas
- Polyps
- Malignant tumors
- Pregnancy/complication of pregnancy
- Congenital malformation
- Intrauterine device

Cervical
- Congenital malformation
- Polyps
- Stenosis

Rarely there may be cases of dysmenorrhea for which no cause is determined.

SUBJECTIVE DATA

History of Present Illness

Ask about onset and duration of symptoms.

Obtain detailed menstrual and gynecological history, including menarche, frequency, and duration of menses.

Ask about pain associated with the onset of menses, associated symptoms.

Obtain sexual and obstetrical history (e.g., treatment of sexually transmitted diseases, Pap history, contraceptive method, symptoms associated with sexual intercourse, gravity, parity).

Past Medical History

Hospitalizations, surgery/procedures, liver/renal disease, other chronic medical conditions, allergic reactions.

Medications

Any current prescription drugs, all over-the-counter medications, allergies

Prior use of analgesics

Family History

Positive family history for dysmenorrhea, other gynecological problems

Psychosocial History

Assess support systems, coping skills, prior coping mechanisms with pain

Diet History

Assess for diet high in refined sugar, salt, excessive caffeine. Complete nutritional history in the obese.

Description of Most Common Symptoms

Primary Dysmenorrhea

Crampy, spasmodic lower abdominal and pelvic pain

May radiate to the upper thighs, groin, and/or low back

Symptoms usually begin several hours before or at onset of menses, lasting 24 to 72 hours, at which time they begin to abate

Pain may be moderate to severe, with some women having more severe pain than with labor

Associated Symptoms. Symptoms may include nausea, vomiting, diarrhea, constipation, headache, fatigue, weakness, diaphoresis, flushing, anxiety, tension, depression, bloating with weight gain, and breast tenderness. In severe cases the patient may experience dizziness and fainting.

Secondary Dysmenorrhea

Symptoms are more variable than in primary dysmenorrhea, depending on cause.

Pain may occur at any time during menstrual cycle and tends to increase with age.

Detailed menstrual and gynecological history can often differentiate primary from secondary dysmenorrhea.

Additional diagnostic tests and usually referral to a physician are necessary to diagnose secondary dysmenorrhea.

Associated Symptoms. Associated symptoms of secondary dysmenorrhea depend on the cause.

OBJECTIVE DATA

Physical Examination

A problem-oriented physical examination should be conducted, with particular attention to:

- General appearance, vital signs, and weight
- Abdomen: Assess for masses, tenderness, other abnormalities
- Pelvic: Speculum visualization of cervix; bimanual examination to assess for cervical motion tenderness, adnexal tenderness and abnormality, and uterine tenderness, enlargement, and/or irregularity

Primary Dysmenorrhea

The physical examination may yield normal findings, yet the patient may have some uterine and cervical tenderness if she is examined when symptomatic. If the patient is being evaluated for the first time for this complaint, rule out pregnancy and pelvic infection.

Secondary Dysmenorrhea

A pathological condition of the pelvis may or may not be found on examination; diagnosis is a process of exclusion. Additional tests will be necessary to confirm the diagnosis.

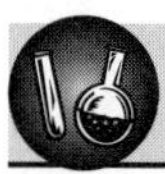

TABLE 60-1 Diagnostic Tests: Secondary Dysmenorrhea

Test	Findings/Rationale	Cost ($)
CBC, ESR	Rule out infection	18-23/CBC 16-20/ESR
RPR	Rule out syphilis	18-22
Vaginal D/C wet mount	Rule out BV, trichomoniasis, candidiasis	15-19
GC culture	Rule out gonorrhea	39-51
Chlamydia	Rule out chlamydial infection	39-51
Pap smear	Screen for cervical cancer	25-51
Vaginal ultrasonography	Rule out ectopic, confirm intrauterine pregnancy; assess uterus/ovaries	271-323
Endometrial biopsy	Rule out endometrial cancer	142-170
Laparoscopy	Diagnostic or treatment	1186-1398
Hysteroscopy	Diagnostic or treatment	665-820
D&C	Diagnostic	683-805
Endometrial ablation	Treatment	1410-1705

BV, Bacterial vaginosis; *CBC,* complete blood cell count; *D&C,* dilation and curettage; *ESR,* erythrocyte sedimentation rate; *GC,* gonorrhea culture; *RPR,* rapid plasma reagin test.

Diagnostic Procedures

Primary dysmenorrhea: None

Secondary dysmenorrhea: Based on physical findings and symptoms, the appropriate diagnostic tests may include those listed in Table 60-1.

ASSESSMENT

Differential Diagnosis

Differential diagnoses may include those listed in Table 60-2.

Other possible diagnoses include:

- Congenital abnormality of reproductive tract
- Gastrointestinal (GI) pathology (inflammatory bowel disease, irritable bowel syndrome, appendicitis, gastroenteritis, diverticulitis)
- Renal/biliary colic

THERAPEUTIC PLAN

Pharmaceutical

Primary Dysmenorrhea

Nonsteroidal antiinflammatory drugs (NSAIDs) effective in 75% to 90% of cases; try various ones for 6 months before considering treatment failure.

Treat 2 or 3 days when symptomatic; best relief with treatment before onset of pain; may treat 1 or 2 days before onset of menses if:

- Menses are regular
- Patient is not pregnant
- No indication of side effects associated with this NSAID (assess for sensitivity to NSAIDs before administration)
- No contraindications to the medication
- Patient should take with food or milk to lessen GI side effects
- Table 60-3 lists some NSAIDs used in the treatment of dysmenorrhea (also see Appendix J for specific instructions regarding use).

Oral contraceptives

- Combined estrogen/progesterone pill is the drug of choice if the patient also desires contraception and there are no contraindications
- Provide effective pain relief in 90% of cases

Antiemetics if nausea and vomiting are major symptoms

Vitamin E, B_1, B_6, omega-3 fatty acids recommended by some, but not approved for use in treatment of symptoms of primary dysmenorrhea

Calcium channel blockers show promising effects in experimental use, but likewise are not yet approved for treatment of symptoms of primary dysmenorrhea.

Lifestyle/Activities

Apply local heat, gentle abdominal massage, pelvic tilt, and stretching to increase uterine blood flow and decrease muscle spasm.

Use transcutaneous electrical nerve stimulation unit to stimulate release of endorphins.

Exercise aerobically three or four times a week for 20 to 30 minutes to suppress prostaglandin release, increase endorphin release, promote fitness and weight loss, improve overall sense of well-being.

Learn and use stress reduction, relaxation techniques.

Stop smoking.

TABLE 60-2 Differential Diagnosis: Dysmenorrhea

Diagnosis	Supporting Data
Endometriosis	Pelvic pain, beginning 1-2 days before menses; premenstrual dyspareunia, pelvic heaviness, low back pain, or pain radiating to legs Pelvic examination may be normal but may reveal bluish endometrial lesions on labia, cervix, or vaginal walls Adnexal tenderness or a mass or cul-de-sac nodularity may be found in the premenstrual interval May exhibit painful defecation and rectal pressure
Adenomyosis	Enlarged globular uterus, tender at time of menses Dysmenorrhea increases with severity, associated with menorrhagia and midline, deep dyspareunia Typically seen in multiparas, 35-50 yr old
Leiomyoma	Irregular, enlarged tender uterus; hypermenorrhea, metrorrhagia
PID	Pelvic pain, uterine and adnexal tenderness, cervical motion tenderness, vaginal discharge; may have fever and ↑ WBC
IUD	Confirm presence; may have slight uterine tenderness
Cervical stenosis	Scant menstrual flow; severe menstrual cramping
Ovarian cyst/neoplasm	Tender pelvic mass, may be unilateral; GI symptoms with advancing disease

GI, Gastrointestinal; *IUD,* intrauterine device; *PID,* pelvic inflammatory disease; *WBC,* white blood cell count.

TABLE 60-3 Nonsteroidal Antiinflammatory Drugs for Treatment of Primary Dysmenorrhea

Drug	Dosage	Frequency	Maximum Daily Dosage
Ibuprofen* (Motrin, other analogs)	200-800 mg PO	q6-8h	3200 mg
Naproxen Sodium* (Anaprox)	550 mg. PO, then 275 mg PO	q12h	
1375 mg Mefenamic acid (Ponstel)	500 mg PO, then 250 mg PO	q6h	Maximum treatment 2-3 days
Meclofenamate† (Meclomen)	50-100 mg PO	q6-8h	400 mg
Ketoprofen (Orudis)	50-75 mg PO	q8h	300 mg
Diclofenac (Cataflam)	50 mg PO	q8-12h	150 mg

*Available in lower-dose over-the-counter formulation.
†Not approved for use in dysmenorrhea.

Sexual activity: Sexual arousal and orgasm cause arteriolar vasodilation in uterus, decreasing ischemic pain.
Pregnancy: Reduces number of adrenergic nerves with only partial regeneration after delivery, resulting in decreased pain perception.

Secondary Dysmenorrhea

Treatment depends on cause.

Diet

Decreased salt, caffeine, alcohol, refined sugar; increased complex carbohydrates, foods that cause diuresis; moderate amount of protein; weight loss if obese

Patient Education

Primary Dysmenorrhea

Explain cause of symptoms in relation to menstrual cycle changes
Teach purpose, dosage, expected results, and potential effects of medications; contraindications, compliance with recommended timing and dosages
Nonpharmaceutical treatment options
Proper diet/exercise
Teach warning signs associated with oral contraceptive use
Keep record of menses, symptoms, effects of medications; a sample diary is included on p. 383
Encourage follow-up with health care provider

Secondary Dysmenorrhea

Educational needs determined by cause and treatment

Family Impact

Spouse/family members should understand cause of and cyclic nature of symptoms in relation to menstrual cycle.
They should be urged to be supportive and encourage compliance with recommended treatment.

Referral

Refer the patient to a gynecologist if secondary dysmenorrhea is suspected.

Consultation

Consider consultation with physician for further evaluation if the patient fails to improve with the treatment outlined here.
Refer the patient to a consultant for additional tests such as:
- Vaginal/pelvic ultrasonography
- Laparoscopic examination
- Hysteroscopy
- Hysterosalpingogram

Rarely, surgery is done for severe cases (e.g., presacral neurectomy, laser uterosacral nerve ablation [LUNA], hysterectomy)

Follow-up

Primary Dysmenorrhea

After initial evaluation, have the patient return in 2 months and at 4 months to evaluate the effectiveness of therapy, then annually for Pap smear and pelvic examination if symptoms are controlled. If there is no relief from symptoms, have the patient return for reevaluation.

Secondary Dysmenorrhea

Have the patient follow up with a gynecologist for continued monitoring

EVALUATION

Primary Dysmenorrhea

Monitor symptom control. The goal is improvement/relief of symptoms. Have the patient return for an annual Pap smear and pelvic examination. Return to clinic with new or worsening symptoms.

Secondary Dysmenorrhea

Monitor symptom control. Treatment and prognosis are dependent on the cause. Have the patient return for an annual Pap smear and pelvic examination and as indicated by the symptoms.

SUGGESTED READINGS

Baker S: Menstruation and related problems and concerns. In Youngkin E, Davis M: *Women's health care: a primary care clinical guide,* Norwalk, Conn, 1994, Appleton-Lange.

Beck W Jr: *The national medical series for independent study: obstetrics and gynecology,* ed 3, Philadelphia, 1993, Harwal Publishers.

Coupey S: Menstrual disorders in adolescents, *Emerg Med* 26(4): 20-2, 27-29, 33-36, 1994.

Gerbie M: Complications of menstruation: abnormal uterine bleeding. In DeCherney A, Pernoll M, editors: *Current obstetric and gynecologic diagnosis and treatment,* ed 8, Norwalk, Conn, 1994, Appleton & Lange.

Ellsworth A et al: *Mosby's 1998 medical drug reference,* St Louis, 1998, Mosby.

Healthcare Consultants of America Inc: *1998 Physicians fee and coding guide,* Augusta, Ga, 1998, Healthcare Consultants of America Inc.

Harel Z et al: Supplementation with omega-3 polyunsaturated fatty acids in the management of dysmenorrhea in adolescents, *Am J Obstet Gynecol* 174:1335-1338, 1996.

Harlow S, Park M: A longitudinal study of risk factors for the occurrence duration and severity of menstrual cramps in a cohort of college women, *Br J Obstet Gynecol* 103:1134-1142, 1996.

Havans C, Sullivan N, Tilton P, editors: *Manual of outpatient gynecology,* ed 2, Boston, 1992, Little Brown & Co.

Hawkins J, Roberto-Nichols D, Stanley-Haney J: *Protocols for nurse practitioners in gynecologic settings,* ed 5, New York, 1995, Tiresias Press.

Jamieson D, Steege J: The prevalence of dysmenorrhea dyspareunia pelvic pain and irritable bowel syndrome in primary care practice, *Obstet Gynecol* 87: 55-58, 1996.

Klotz M: Dysmenorrhea endometriosis pelvic pain. In Lemcke D et al, editors: *Primary care of women*, Norwalk, Conn, 1995, Appleton & Lange.

Murphy J: Dysmenorrhea. In Star W, Lommel L, Shannon M, editor: *Women's primary health care: protocols for practice,* Washington DC, 1995, American Nurses Publishing.

Stoll S: Dysmenorrhea. In Frederickson H, Wilkins-Haug L: *OB/Gyn secrets,* St Louis, 1991, Mosby.

Uphold C, Graham M: *Clinical guidelines in family practice,* ed 2, Gainesville, Fla, 1994, Barmarrae Books.

Webb T: Common menstrual disorders, *Adv Nurse Pract* 4:21-23, 1996.

DYSMENORRHEA DIARY

Name: ______________________ Age: ______ Month: ____________

SYMPTOM GRADING:

MENSES GRADING

1: None
2: Slight
3: Moderate
4: Heavy

CRAMPING GRADING

1: None
2: Slight
3: Moderate, present and interferes with activities
4: Severe, disabling, unable to function

MEDICATION RELIEF

1: None
2: Slight
3: Moderate pain relief
4: Pain gone

Symptom	Days of Month																														
	1	2	3	4	5	6	7	8	9	10	11	12	13	14	15	16	17	18	19	20	21	22	23	24	25	26	27	28	29	30	31
Cramping																															
Back pain																															
Nausea/ vomiting/ diarrhea																															
Relief with medication																															

INSTRUCTIONS:
Indicate symptoms experienced during menstrual period by placing menses and symptom grading (1-4) and medication relief (1-4) in appropriate day of month when they occur.

61 Dyspnea (Shortness of Breath)

ICD-9-CM

Dyspnea 786.09
Asthmatic Dyspnea 493.9
Cardiac Dyspnea 428.1
Functional Dyspnea 300.11

OVERVIEW

Definition

Dyspnea or shortness of breath (SOB) is the abnormal uncomfortable sensation or awareness of breathing. Dyspnea is very subjective, like pain, and depends on the individual's limit for discomfort and on the specific circumstances that provoke SOB. Dyspnea is a common symptom and can be caused by many different conditions, although the cardiac and pulmonary systems are the most frequently involved.

There are two types of dyspnea—acute and chronic. Dyspnea of sudden onset is usually easier to assess, but the workup must proceed more quickly. Evaluation of chronic dyspnea can usually be accomplished more slowly in an ambulatory setting.

Pathophysiology

Ventilation is related to the metabolic demands of oxygen consumption and carbon dioxide elimination. The carotid and aortic bodies and chemoreceptors respond to the partial pressure of oxygen and carbon dioxide, the pH of the blood, and cerebrospinal fluid. When stimulated the receptors cause changes in the rate and pattern of breathing. Also influencing the rate and pattern of breathing are neural receptors in the lung parenchyma, large and small airways, respiratory muscles, and chest wall.

The four systems that are primarily involved in dyspnea are outlined in Box 61-1.

SUBJECTIVE DATA

History of Present Illness (Table 61-1)

Ask about descriptive characteristics of the respiratory sensation, onset, frequency, intensity, and duration of symptoms, and activities or conditions that may precipitate breathlessness.

Absence of activity limitations and lack of exacerbation on exercising are important to know.

Determine whether SOB occurs at night or during the daytime.

Inquire about foreign body aspiration.

During the home-heating season or in certain industrial settings, questions about the possibility of carbon monoxide intoxication are appropriate.

It is important to know whether the onset of dyspnea occurs while the patient is at rest and whether it is accompanied by a sense of chest tightness, suffocation, or inability to take in air.

Ask about sleep at night and coughing.

Past Medical History

Inquire about:

- Past history of chronic cough
- Sputum production
- Recurrent respiratory infections
- Deep vein thrombosis
- Environmental allergies
- Multiple bodily complaints and history of emotional difficulties
- Asthma
- Coronary artery disease
- Congestive heart failure
- Valvular heart problems

Medications

Use of hormone replacement therapy and oral contraceptives increases the risk of deep venous thrombosis.

Box 61-1

Four Body Systems Associated With Dyspnea

Cardiac	Pulmonary	Mixed Cardiac or Pulmonary	Noncardiac or Nonpulmonary
CHF	Obstructive COPD	COPD with pulmonary	Metabolic conditions, acidosis, DKA
CAD	Asthma	Hypertension or cor pulmonale	Pain
MI	Restrictive	Deconditioning	Neuromuscular disorders
Cardiomyopathy	Obesity	Chronic pulmonary emboli	Muscular dystrophy
Valvular dysfunction	Spine or chest deformities	Trauma	MS
LVH	Interstitial fibrosis		Otorhinolaryngeal disorders
Asymmetric septal hypertrophy	Hereditary lung disorders		Polyps
Pericarditis	Pneumothorax		Septal deviation
Arrhythmias			Functional
			Anxiety
			Panic disorders
			Hyperventilation

Adapted from Morgan W, Hodge H: Diagnostic evaluation of dyspnea, *American Family Physician* 57:711-716, 1998.

CAD, Coronary artery disease; *CHF,* congestive heart failure; *COPD,* chronic obstructive pulmonary disease; *DKA,* diabetic ketoacidosis; *LVH,* left ventricular hypertrophy; *MI,* myocardial infarction; *MS,* multiple sclerosis.

TABLE 61-1 Historic Findings That May Lead to a Diagnosis of Dyspnea

Findings	Condition
Dyspnea on exertion	Cardiac or pulmonary disease, deconditioning
Dyspnea at rest	Severe cardiopulmonary disease or noncardiopulmonary disease
Orthopnea, PND, edema	CHF (Ch. 42) COPD (Ch. 37)
Medications	Beta blockers may exacerbate bronchospasm or limit exercise tolerance. Pulmonary fibrosis is a rare side effect of some medications
Smoking	Emphysema, chronic bronchitis (Ch. 27), asthma (Ch. 16)
Allergies, wheezing, +FH of asthma	Asthma
CAD	Dyspnea as anginal equivalent
Hypertension	LVH, CHF
Anxiety	Hyperventilation, panic attack
Lightheadedness, tingling in fingers and perioral area	Hyperventilation
Recent trauma	Pneumothorax, chest wall pain limiting respiration, rib fractures
Occupational exposure to dust, asbestos or chemicals	Interstitial lung disease

From Morgan W, Hodge H: Diagnostic evaluation of dyspnea, *American Family Phys* 57:711-716, 1998.

CAD, Coronary artery disease; *CHF,* congestive heart failure; *COPD,* chronic obstructive pulmonary disorder; *+FH,* positive family history; *LVH,* left ventricular hypertrophy; *PND,* paroxysmal nocturnal dyspnea.

Use of beta blockers, including ophthalmic beta blocker preparations, can cause severe bronchospasm.
Angiotensin-converting enzyme inhibitors may aggravate cough in patients with bronchial hyperresponsiveness.
The patient's use of antianxiety agents, antidepressants, and the like may point to an anxiety-induced SOB. These agents also may be introduced only after an acute COPD episode to reduce the anxiety associated with not being able to breathe. The breathing disorder is the underlying cause of dyspnea.

Family History

A family history of chronic health problems should be elicited:

Sickle cell anemia
Asthma
Cystic fibrosis
Heart disease (e.g., coronary artery disease, congestive heart failure, myocardial infarction, hypertension, valve problems)
Lung problems: Chronic bronchitis, bronchiectasis, serous pulmonary infections
Allergies
Hay fever

Psychosocial History

Factors that may contribute to SOB include:
Cigarette smoking
Occupational exposure (e.g., asbestos, silicone, coal dust)
Exposure to inhalants, animals, or birds

Significant life changes, lack of support networks, and psychiatric disorders can increase anxiety and may induce episodes of dyspnea.

Diet

Excessive salt intake and excessive weight gain may contribute to SOB.

Associated Symptoms

Ask the patient about the following areas:

Paroxysmal nocturnal dyspnea
Orthopnea and the number of pillows the patient uses
Platypnea (dyspnea in the upright position relieved by recumbency)
Repopnea (dyspnea that occurs in one lateral position but not the other)
Associated respiratory symptoms such as wheezing, cough, sputum production, and pleuritic chest pain
Leg edema, hemoptysis, pregnancy, recent major gynecological procedures, or abdominal, hip, or knee surgery
Chest pain or palpitations
Tingling in the fingers or mouth during dyspnea.

OBJECTIVE DATA

Physical Examination

A complete physical examination is indicated (Table 61-2), with special attention to:

Vital signs:
Check for tachycardia, tachypnea, fever, and hypertension
Weight gain
Head/eyes/ears/nose/throat: Nasal passages, pharynx
Neck: Masses, thyromegaly, bruits
Lungs: (A/P) Lateral diameter, respiratory rate, spinal deformities, use of accessory muscles; identify any adventitious sounds
Cardiac murmurs, extra heart sounds, point of maximal impulse, rate, rhythm
Abdomen: Hepatosplenomegaly, bruits
Extremities: Assess pulses, capillary refill, edema, hair growth pattern

Diagnostic Procedures

Diagnostic procedures for dyspnea are outlined in Table 61-3 and Figure 61-1.

THERAPEUTIC PLAN

In most patients the cause or causes of dyspnea can be determined via the history and physical examination to identify common cardiac or pulmonary causes. Both acute and chronic dyspnea management relies on treating the underlying cause as well as relieving the dyspnea. If the patient has a pulmonary emboli, myocardial ischemia, or pneumothorax, hospital admission is necessary. Supplemental oxygen is always indicated when oxygen saturation levels are low (<90%).

Pharmaceutical

Bronchodilators, anticholinergics, theophyllines, corticosteroids, antimediators, and antileukotrienes are used for obstructive airway disease (see appropriate chapters). Nitrostat is helpful for cardiac conditions that cause dyspnea. Respiratory tract infections need treatment with antibiotics. Psychogenic dyspnea patients may benefit from treatment with anxiolytic agents such as buspirone HCl (BuSpar), alprazolam (Xanax), or lorazepam (Ativan). Angiotensin-converting enzyme (ACE) inhibitors are used

TABLE 61-2 Physical Findings Indicating Causes of Dyspnea

System	Findings	Condition
Facial expression, manner, affect	Multiple body complaints, frequent sighing, hyperventilation, nervousness in any otherwise normal examination	Anxiety attack, psychogenic dyspnea
Skin, sclera, conjunctiva	Pale skin and conjunctiva Icteric sclera, jaundiced skin	Anemia, liver disease, right-sided heart failure
HEENT	Nasal polyp, septal deviation	Dyspnea resulting from nasal obstruction
	Postnasal discharge	Allergies, asthma
Neck	JVD	Left-sided heart failure, pulmonary hypertension, left-sided heart murmur
Chest	Contraction of accessory muscles, retraction of the supraclavicular fossa, pursed-lip breathing, prolonged expiratory phase	Severe difficulty, tracheal stenosis, significant outflow obstruction: COPD
	Dullness, hyperresonance, wheezes, crackles, decreased air movement, moist cough	Asthma, bronchitis, pneumonia, CHF, FB aspiration, pneumothorax
	Increased A/P diameter, retraction of intercostal muscles on inspiration	COPD/emphysema, chronic bronchitis
	Chest deformity	Kyphoscoliosis or ankylosing spondylitis
Heart	Systolic regurgitant murmur, accentuated and delayed P_2, right ventricular heave, right ventricular S_3	CHF, pulmonary hypertension
	Tachycardia	Anemia, hypoxia, CHF, hyperthyroidism
Abdomen	Hepatojugular reflux, ascites	Right-sided heart failure Liver disease
Extremities	Edema, pain, + Homans' sign, clubbing	CHF, DVT, cystic fibrosis, sickle cell anemia
	Decreased pulse or bruits	PVD with CAD

CAD, Coronary artery disease; *CHF*, congestive heart failure; *COPD*, chronic obstructive pulmonary disease; *DVT*, deep venous thrombosis; *FB*, foreign body; *HEENT*, head/eyes/ears/nose/throat; *JVD*, jugular venous distention, *PVD*, peripheral vascular disease.

for low ejection fractions (use cautiously in patients with concomitant renal failure—e.g., elevated creatinine, renal artery stenosis). Other medications may be used, depending on the underlying cause of the dyspnea.

Lifestyle/Activity

Lifestyle and activity are determined by the underlying cause of the patient's SOB.

Smoking cessation is a must!

Selected cardiac and pulmonary patients may benefit from an exercise program.

Pulmonary disease as a result of occupational exposure may require a change in job or occupation or use of specialized mask.

Patients with asthma will benefit from environmental control.

Diet

Not applicable

Patient Education

Depends on condition identified as cause of SOB

Referral

Appropriate referrals for the patient with dyspnea include a pulmonologist, cardiologist, psychiatrist, and/or infectious disease specialist.

Follow-up

Schedule patient for a return visit in 1 week.

EVALUATION

Evaluation is determined by the underlying cause. Monitoring peak flow readings is useful in asthma. Oxygen saturation readings and spirometry testing help monitor the clinical course during treatment when the cause of dyspnea is known. Subjective description of increased physical tolerance is beneficial.

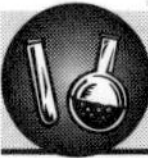

TABLE 61-3 Diagnostic Tests: Dyspnea

Test	Findings/Rationale	Cost ($)
CXR	First-level test for basic screening: Safely and easily accomplished: skeletal abnormalities, mass lesions, CHF, COPD, pneumonia, atelectasis, elevated hemidiaphragm, pleural effusion, pneumothorax, increased cardiac silhouette	77-91
ECG	First-level test to identify myocardial ischemia, injury, or infarction, electrical voltage, arrhythmias, pericarditis, chamber size, effusion, or obstructive lung disease	56-65
Fingerstick Hgb or CBC	Quantify the severity of suspected anemia	11-14/Hgb 18-23/CBC
Thyroid panel	Although thyroid diseases rarely present with dyspnea, a TSH can determine the presence of thyroid disease	86-109
Pulse oximetry	First-line test uses infrared light source to determine the hemoglobin oxygen saturation Valuable since rapid measurement can be done, non-invasive, accurate in most clinical situations	29-33
ABGs	First-level test helpful in assessing acid/base status, altered pH or the adequacy of tissue oxygen delivery More commonly used for acute dyspnea; normal ABGs do not exclude cardiac or pulmonary disease as a cause of dyspnea, invasive	78-98
PFT, spirometry, FVC, FEV_1, TLC	Second-line test if initial testing inconclusive, differentiate obstructive from restrictive Obstructive: FEV_1 ↓↓, FVC ↓ or normal, TLC ↑ Restrictive: FEV_1 ↓ or ↓↓, FVC ↓ or ↓↓, TLC ↓ Dependent on patient effort; coaching needed	27-323, depending on what tests are performed
Echocardiography	Second-line test to identify structural abnormalities of the heart; also identifies chamber size, hypertrophy, and left ventricular ejection fraction	675
Ventilation-perfusion scan	Second-line test to identify pulmonary embolism	269-376
Carbon monoxide diffusing capacity	Third-line test to help differentiate when suspicious of occupational interstitial disease	127-155
Bronchoprovocation testing	Third-line test to identify reactive airway disease	130-157
Exercise treadmill testing	Targets ischemia as a cause of dyspnea; used when symptoms are atypical May be limited by client's ability to perform a treadmill test because of poor conditioning or lower extremity pathological condition Relatively safe: 1 in 10,000 patients die of malignant arrhythmias, 1 in 10,000 patients have serious but nonfatal arrhythmias Negative results suggest that dyspnea is caused by something other than CAD	249-305

Adapted from Seamens C, Wrenn K: Breathlessness: strategies aimed at identifying and treating the cause of dyspnea. *Postgrad Med* 98:215-227, 1995; and Morgan W, Hodge H: Diagnostic evaluation of dyspnea, *Am Family Physician* 57:711-716, 1998.

ABG, Arterial blood gas; *CAD*, coronary artery disease; *CBC*, complete blood cell count; *CXR*, chest x-ray evaluation; *ECG*, electrocardiogram; FEV_1, forced expiratory volume in 1 second; *FVC*, forced vital capacity; *Hgb*, hemoglobin; *PFT*, pulmonary function test; *TLC*, total lung capacity; *TSH*, thyroid-stimulating hormone.

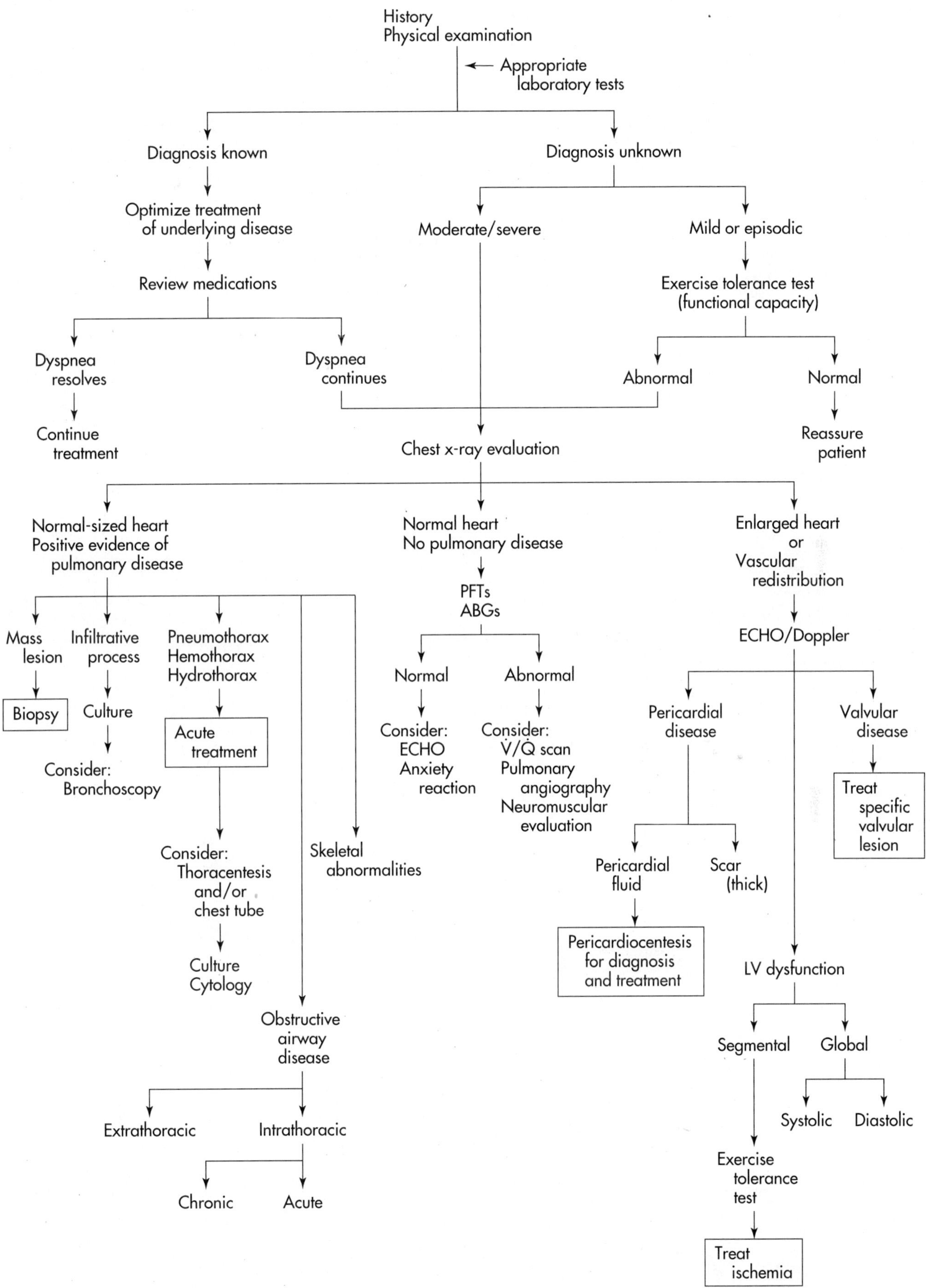

Figure 61-1 Algorithm for client with dyspnea. *ABG,* Arterial blood gas; *ECHO,* echocardiogram; *PFT,* pulmonary function test; *V/Q,* ventilation/perfusion scan. (From Greene HL, Johnson WP, Lemcke D: *Decision making in medicine,* ed 2, St. Louis, 1998, Mosby.)

SUGGESTED READINGS

Bone RC: Goals in asthma management: a step-care approach, *Chest* 109:1056, 1996.

Drugs for asthma, *Med Lett Drug Ther* 37:1, 1996.

Ellsworth A et al: *Mosby's 1998 medical drug reference*, St Louis, 1998, Mosby.

Framm D, Fenster P, Kern K: Patient with dyspnea. In Greene H, Johnson W, Lemcke D, editors: *Decision making in medicine,* ed 2, St Louis, 1998, Mosby.

Healthcare Consultants of America, Inc: *1998 Physicians fee and coding guide,* Augusta, Ga, 1998, Healthcare Consultants of America, Inc.

Morgan W, Hodge H: Diagnostic evaluation of dyspnea, *Am Family Physician* 57:711-716, 1998.

Seamens C, Wrenn K: Breathlessness: strategies aimed at identifying and treating the cause of dyspnea, *Postgrad Med* 98: 215-227, 1995.

Spector D: Common pulmonary problems. In Barker L, Burton J, Zieve P, editors: *Principles of ambulatory medicine,* ed 4, Baltimore, 1995, Williams & Wilkins.

Stauffer J: Lung. In Tierney L, McPhee S, Papadakis M, editors: *1998 Current medical diagnosis & treatment,* ed 37, Norwalk, Conn, 1997, Appleton & Lange.

Weisman IM, Zeballow RJ: Clinical exercise testing, *Clin Chest Med* 15:173 (Entire issue), 1994.

Ear: Impacted Cerumen

ICD-9-CM

Ear: Impacted Cerumen 380.4

OVERVIEW

Definition

Impacted cerumen is obstructive earwax of the external ear canal.

Incidence

Unknown

Pathophysiology

Cerumen is a protective secretion produced by the ceruminous gland of the outer portion of the ear canal.

The ear canal is self-cleansing through the body's natural mechanisms.

Cerumen impaction is often a result of cleaning attempts, usually with a cotton-tipped swab, which only pushes the cerumen down into the ear canal.

Total occlusion may cause conductive hearing loss.

SUBJECTIVE DATA

History of Present Illness

Most individuals will be asymptomatic; however, some may complain of pain, itching, or a sensation of fullness in the ear.

Ask about hearing loss.

OBJECTIVE DATA

Physical Examination

Use an otoscope to examine both ears.

Attempt to visualize the tympanic membrane around the earwax.

Assess the ear canal and the consistency of the earwax (hard or soft, superficial or deep).

No diagnostic testing is indicated.

ASSESSMENT

Differential Diagnoses

Foreign body
Otitis media
Otitis externa

THERAPEUTIC PLAN

Pharmaceutical

Diluted hydrogen peroxide 1:1 is effective, and earwax-softening drops are available to soften and remove wax.

Nonpharmceutical

It may be necessary to remove cerumen to visualize the tympanic membrane adequately.

Cerumen may be removed mechanically by a curette or irrigation.

Be gentle when using a curette to remove cerumen. Visualization with a good light and/or the otoscope is important. If the patient is a child, hold him or her securely. Let the **child** know in advance that the procedure could be uncomfortable.

Irrigate the canal with warm water (to avoid nausea and dizziness). The stream should be directed at the side of the ear canal to avoid trauma. A bulb syringe may be used; Water Piks are no longer recommended because of the risk of perforation of the eardrum.

Irrigation should not be performed if perforation is suspected.

Cerumen removal may cause irritation to the ear canal. Isopropyl alcohol may be used afterward to promote drying of the ear canal.

Patient Education

Recommend routine cleaning with a washcloth wrapped over the index finger.

Discourage the use of cotton-tipped swabs (e.g., Q-tips) down in the ear canal.

Educate the patient about the purposes of earwax.

Consultation/Referral

Refer the patient to a specialist:

- If the impaction does not respond to routine measures
- If the patient has a history of chronic otitis media
- If there is a perforated tympanic membrane

EVALUATION/FOLLOW-UP

Follow-up is indicated by the difficulty of the cerumen removal, the age of the child, and the frequency of the impaction.

The parents may want to continue with diluted hydrogen peroxide or softening drops to prevent a recurrence.

SUGGESTED READINGS

Graham MV, Uphold CR: *Clinical guidelines in child health,* Gainesville, Fla, 1994, Barmarrae Books.

Tierney LM, McPhee SJ, Papadakis MA, editors: *Medical diagnosis & treatment,* Norwalk, Conn, 1996, Appleton & Lange.

Eating Disorders: Anorexia Nervosa and Bulimia

ICD-9-CM

Anorexia Nervosa 307.1
Bulimia 307.51

OVERVIEW

Definition

Anorexia nervosa is the intentional loss of weight and refusal to maintain a body weight at or above 85% of a normal weight for age and height. Bulimia nervosa is characterized by recurrent episodes of binge eating and purging by use of vomiting, laxatives, or enemas. Binge eating disorder is defined as episodes of uncontrolled eating, without purging.

Incidence

Five percent of **adolescent** and **adult women** have an eating disorder, whereas only 1% of **men** have an eating disorder. Two percent of all adults in the United States are affected by binge eating disorder. Anorexia nervosa has the highest mortality rate of any mental health diagnosis (20%). More than 5 million people in the United States have some type of eating disorder.

Pathophysiology

Factors That Increase Susceptibility to Eating Disorders

Overemphasis on weight control and dieting
Depression
Mood disorders
Stress—psychological
Hormone imbalances

SUBJECTIVE DATA

History of Present Illness

Ask about eating habits:
"Are you satisfied with your eating patterns?"
"Do you ever eat in secret?"
Symptoms may be vague
Depression, mood swings, anxiety, feelings of loss of control, antisocial behavior

Anorexia Nervosa

Usual age of onset: **12 to 13** and **age 17**
Intense fear of gaining weight, even if significantly underweight
Unusual eating rituals like cutting food into tiny pieces
Fainting spells
Distorted image of body
Obsessed with food and weight
Strict exercise routines

Associated Symptoms

Amenorrhea in women
Constipation
Impotence in men
Heart tremors
Shortness of breath

Bulimia Nervosa

Usual age of onset: **Late adolescence to early adulthood**
Frequent bingeing episodes
Fear of gaining weight
Purging by use of vomiting, laxatives, or exercise
Stealing or hiding food, eating in private

Associated Symptoms

Weakness, exhaustion
Constipation
Indigestion

Binge Eating Disorder

Bingeing at least 2 days a week for at least 6 months
Eating in private

Table 63-1 Common Symptoms of Eating Disorders

Symptoms	Anorexia Nervosa	Bulimia Nervosa	Binge Eating Disorder
Excessive weight loss in relatively short period of time	*		
Continuation of dieting although bone-thin	*		
Dissatisfaction with appearance; belief that body is fat, even though severely underweight	*		
Loss of monthly menstrual periods	*	*	
Unusual interest in food and development of strange eating rituals	*	*	
Eating in secret	*	*	*
Obsession with exercise	*	*	
Serious depression	*	*	*
Bingeing—consumption of large amounts of food		*	*
Vomiting or use of drugs to stimulate vomiting, bowel movements, and urination		*	
Bingeing but no noticeable weight gain		*	
Disappearance into bathroom for long periods of time to induce vomiting		*	
Abuse of drugs or alcohol		*	*

From National Institutes of Health: Eating disorders, US Department of Health and Human Services, NIH Publication No 94-3477, 1994.
*Some individuals suffer from anorexia and bulimia and have symptoms of both disorders.

Obesity
Eating compulsively when not hungry
Guilt after eating

Table 63-1 summarizes assessment findings for each of these eating disorders.

OBJECTIVE DATA

Physical Examination

Anorexia Nervosa

Growth of fine body hair on arms, legs, and other body parts
Dry skin, brittle nails, pruritus
Loss of muscle; hollow cheeks
Alopecia
Hypotension
Irregular heartbeat, bradycardia
Decreased reflexes
Hypothermia
Cardiac arrest

Bulimia Nervosa

Usually weight is normal
Dental caries or loss of tooth enamel
Dry, flaky skin
Lymphadenopathy—parotid glands
Dysphagia, dyspepsia
Arrhythmias
Cathartic colon
Sores in mouth or on fingers
Broken blood vessels of face

Binge Eating Disorder

Obesity-related illnesses: Diabetes, gallbladder disease, heart disease
Hypertension

Diagnostic Procedures (General)

Laboratory studies performed for eating disorders include the following:
- CBC ($13-$16)
- Transferrin ($43-$54)
- Basic metabolic panel, including glucose ($28-$39)
- Liver enzymes ($29-$41)
- Creatine ($18-$23)
- Thyroid profile ($47-$61)
- Electrocardiogram ($56-$65)

Typical findings from diagnostic procedures are listed in Box 63-1.

Box 63-1

Findings from Diagnostic Procedures

Anorexia Nervosa

Hypocalcemia	Hypokalemia

Bulimia Nervosa

Pancreatitis	Hypokalemia
Hypoglycemia	Hypomagnesemia
Dehydration	Hyponatremia

Binge Eating Disorder

High cholesterol

ASSESSMENT

Differential Diagnoses

Differential diagnoses include:

Depression as a common co-diagnosis
Hyperthyroidism
Pregnancy
Human immunodeficiency virus/acquired immunodeficiency syndrome
Inflammatory bowel disease
Cancer
Substance abuse
Systemic lupus erythematosus
Diabetes

THERAPEUTIC PLAN

The therapeutic approach (Figure 63-1) depends on the severity of the eating disorder. Diagnosis is difficult because of the patient's secrecy or denial of disease. Treatment is long and includes psychological and physiological management. A mental health referral and follow-up are necessary because of the social nature of the eating disorder.

Pharmaceutical

Eating disorders may be treated with antidepressants. To get the best response, it may be necessary to try or combine several antidepressants before achieving results. Pharmaceutical intervention is usually monitored by a psychiatrist or mental health clinician. Table 63-2 outlines a pharmaceutical plan for a patient with an eating disorder. Please note that these drugs should be started at low doses, divided BID and TID. Once side effects are tolerated, one large dose at HS may be used.

Patient Education

Self-esteem workshops
Nutrition counseling
Assertiveness training

Family Impact

Eating disorders disrupt the entire family system. Families must understand their role in treatment and support to the individual affected by the eating disorder. The family must also realize that an estimated 42% of anorexics relapse after one hospitalization.

Referral and Consultation

Consult with a psychiatrist with experience in treating patients with eating disorders. The family should be involved in the treatment program. Therapy should include group, family, and individual counseling. Hospitalization may be required to ensure nutrition plan (because of excessive weight loss, risk of suicide, or severe bingeing and purging). A nutritionist should also be consulted to work with the patient and family to develop a nutrition plan.

EVALUATION/FOLLOW-UP

Patients with eating disorders should be monitored. Treat accompanying physical complications (Figures 63-2 and 63-3) as needed, such as diabetes, edema, anemia, and cardiac problems.

Complete physical examinations should be performed at least every 6 months without an emphasis on weight, until end of therapy, then yearly examinations may be performed.

Drug therapy should be monitored closely for side effects and interactions. Suspected noncompliance should be monitored by plasma levels. Therapy should continue, based on the patient's psychological needs.

RESOURCES

Academy for Eating Disorders
c/o Division of Adolescent Medicine
Montefiore Medical School
111 East 210th Street
Bronx, NY 10467

American Anorexia/Bulimia Association, Inc.
165 W. 46 Street #1108
New York, NY 10036
1-800-994-WOMAN

Anorexia Nervosa and Related Eating Disorders (ANRED)
P.O. Box 5102
Eugene, OR 97405
1-514-344-1144

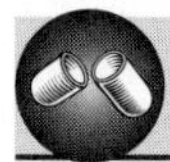

TABLE 63-2 Pharmaceutical Plan: Eating Disorders

Drug*	Initial Adult Dosage†	Dosage After 4-6 Weeks	Cost ($)
Desipramine (Norpramin)	50-150 mg/day	75-200 mg/day	15-50
Imipramine (Tofranil)	50-150 mg/day	100-200 mg/day	2-74
Fluoxetine (Prozac)	20 mg/day	20-40 mg/day	215-220

*Of desipramine and imipramine, desipramine is the safer drug choice.
†Doses may be given in single or divided doses, depending on the drug and the patient.

History
Physical examination
Bulimia
Anorexia nervosa
Atypical presentations
Evaluate for life-threatening complications:
Fluid or electrolyte disorder
Cardiac disorder
Esophageal rupture
Yes
No
Hospitalize and stabilize
Rule out other causes of low weight
Thyroid function tests
Sedimentation rate (for autoimmune disease)
Glucose (for diabetes)
Evaluate for life-threatening complications or weight below acceptable limit
Yes
No
Hospitalize and stabilize
Refeed in slow step wise fashion
Psychotherapy
Referral to nutritionist
Contractual agreement with patient
Frequent monitoring of weight
Bone density study
Estrogen replacement if indicated
Antidepressant if indicated

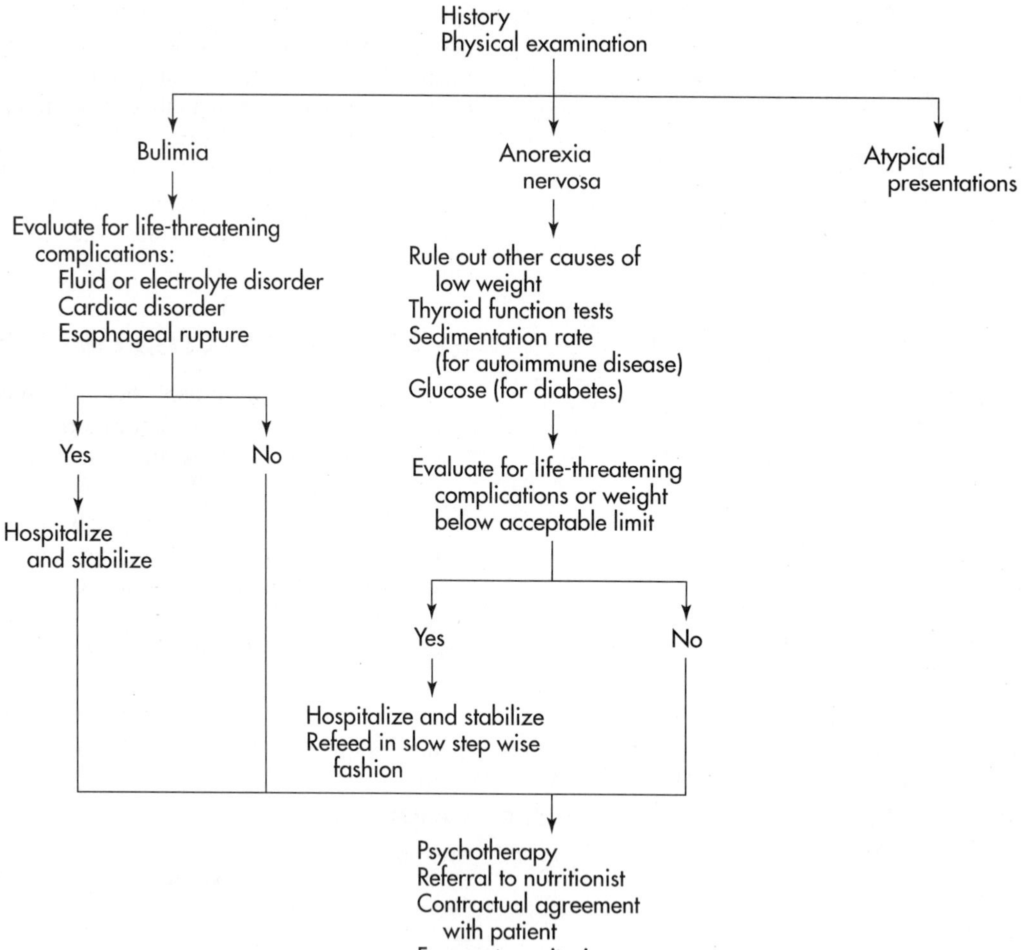

Figure 63-1 Algorithm for treatment of a patient with an eating disorder. (Adapted from Greene HL, Johnson WP, Lemcke D: *Decision making in medicine,* ed 2, St Louis, 1998, Mosby.)

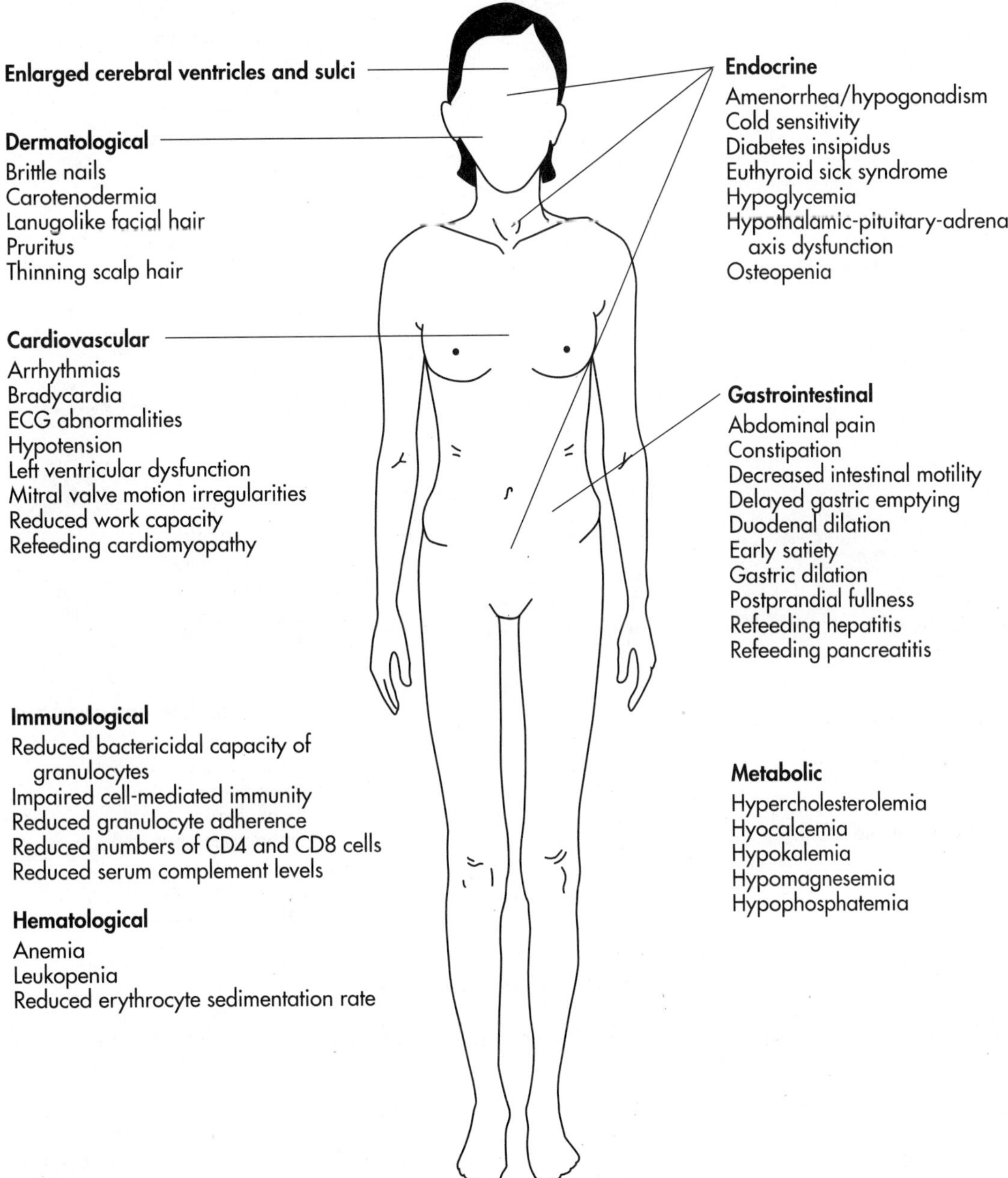

Figure 63-2 Signs, symptoms, and complications of anorexia nervosa. *ECG,* Electrocardiogram. (From Mehler P: Eating disorders: 1. Anorexia nervosa, *Hosp Pract* 31:109-118, 1996.)

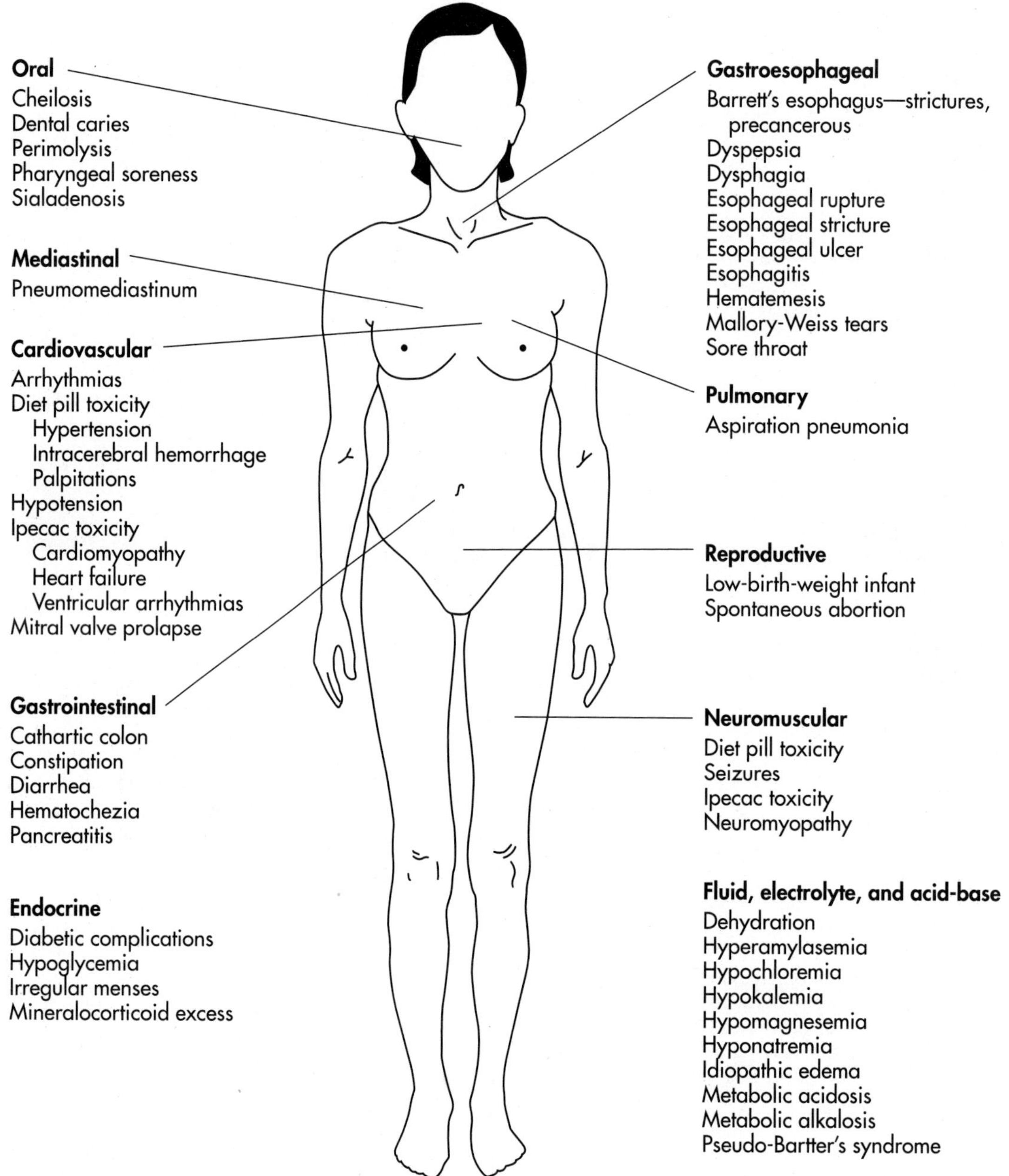

Figure 63-3 Selected complications of bulimia nervosa. (From Mehler P: Eating disorders: 2. Bulimia nervosa, *Hosp Pract* 31:107-126, 1996.)

Overeaters Anonymous, Inc.
PO Box 44020
Rio Rancho, NM 87174-4020
1-505-891-2664

SUGGESTED READINGS

Barker L, Burton J, Zieve P: *Principles of ambulatory care,* Baltimore, 1995, Williams & Wilkins.

Burns C et al: *Pediatric primary care: a handbook for nurse practitioners,* Philadelphia, 1996, WB Saunders.

Ellsworth AJ et al: *Mosby's 1998 medical drug reference,* St Louis, 1998, Mosby.

Healthcare Consultants of America, Inc: 1998 Physicians fee and coding guide, Augusta, Ga, 1998, Healthcare Consultants of America, Inc.

Lehne R: *Pharmacology for nursing care,* ed 2, Philadelphia, 1994, WB Saunders.

Mehler P: Eating disorders: 1. Anorexia nervosa, *Hosp Pract* 31:109-118, 1996.

Mehler P: Eating disorders: 2. Bulimia nervosa, *Hosp Pract* 31:107-126, 1996.

National Eating Disorders Screening Program: One Washington Street #304, Wellesley Hills MA 02181, 1998.

Palla B, Litt I: Medical complications of eating disorders in adolescents, *Pediatrics* 81:613-623, 1988.

Schwitzer A et al: Eating disorders among college women: prevention education and treatment responses, *J Am Coll Health* 46:199-207, 1997.

Eczema/Atopic Dermatitis

ICD-9-CM

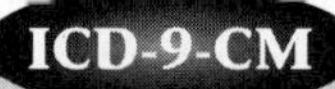

Eczema/Atopic Dermatitis 691.8

OVERVIEW

Definition

Eczema is a genetically determined chronic skin disorder with a relapsing pattern.

Incidence

Eczema affects 1.9% to 5% of the population. It is **more common in children;** 80% of cases are detected **before 1 year of age,** and most cases are detected by **age 5.** The condition **affects 1 in 10 children.**

Pathophysiology

The cause of eczema is not completely understood. Defects in cell-mediated immunity are present in these patients.

Protective Factors Against Eczema

Intact immune system

Factors That Increase Susceptibility to Eczema

Family history of asthma, allergic rhinitis, atopic dermatitis

SUBJECTIVE DATA

History of Present Illness

Infantile Stage

Occurs at 2 to 6 months of age, resolving by 3 years of age

Characterized by pruritus, redness, and blisters on cheeks, forehead, scalp, and extensor aspects of arms and legs

Childhood Stage

Occurs at 4 to 10 years of age

Characterized by dry, scaly, rash on antecubital, popliteal regions, flexures of wrists, ankles, neck, buttock-thigh creases (Figure 64-1)

Less pruritic

Adolescent or Adult Stage

Occurs on face, neck, and body

Characterized by scaling skin with xerosis and lichenification

Past Medical History

Hayfever

Asthma

Food allergies

Other skin disorders

Medications

Determine whether a new medication, particularly a topical agent, is being used (rule out contact dermatitis).

Family History

Hayfever

Asthma

Food allergies

Other skin disorders

Psychosocial History

Consider the stigma of having a visible skin disorder

Psychological stressors are triggers

Assess living conditions and exposure to dust mites

Associated Symptoms

Wheezing

Runny nose

Tearing of eyes

OBJECTIVE DATA

Physical Examination

Undress the patient and check the entire body for lesions.

Skin: As the condition progresses with aging, there is a change in the type of lesion.
- **Infants** will have more vesicles with exudation and scarring, extensor surfaces involved.
- **Children** will have less exudate and crusting and more papular, well-circumscribed patches.
- **Adults** will have more scaling and lichenification of flexures.
- Acute flare-ups may be in the form of red patches that are weepy, shiny, or lichenified.
- Hypopigmentation occurs in dark-skinned persons.
- Palms may have hyperlinear, xerotic creases.

Head
Facial pallor with infraorbital darkening may be noted.
Fissures can occur under the earlobes.

Diagnostic Procedures

None usually necessary but if performed, eosinophilia may be noted. Serum IgE levels ($53 to $67) will be elevated.
Cultures of drainage ($31 to $39) may help in ruling out other causes.

Assessment

Differential diagnoses include those listed in Table 64-1.

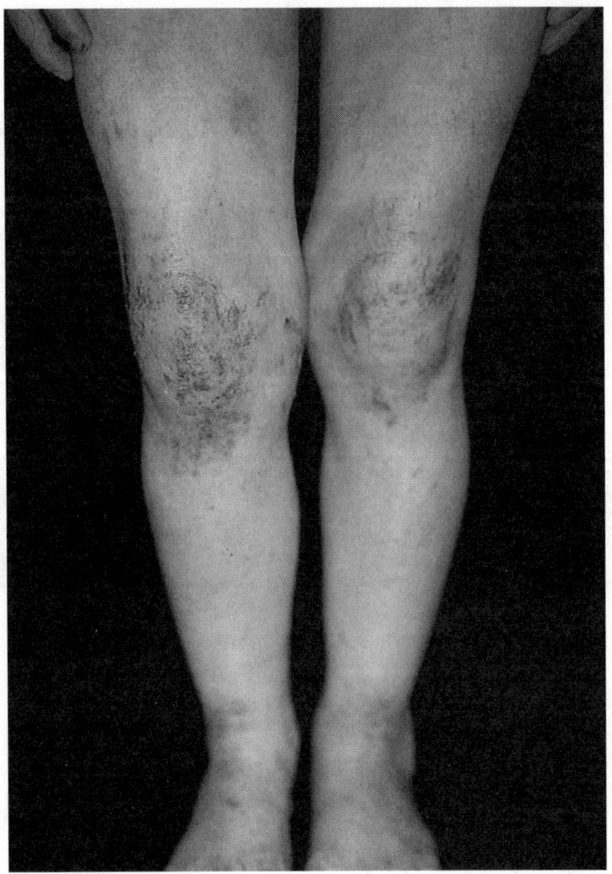

Figure 64-1 Inflammation in the flexural areas is the most common presentation of atopic dermatitis in children. (From Habif TP: *Clinical dermatology: a color guide to diagnosis and therapy*, ed 3, St Louis, 1996, Mosby.)

TABLE 64-1 Differential Diagnosis: Eczema

Diagnosis	Supporting Data
Psoriasis	Silvery scales on red plaques on knees, elbows, scalp. Separation of nail from nail bed is common (onycholysis).
Contact dermatitis	No characteristic distribution or chronic course. Usually linear pattern. Vesicles may occur at any age.

THERAPEUTIC PLAN

Pharmaceutical

A pharmaceutical plan for eczema is outlined in Table 64-2.

Treatment Considerations

Use water-miscible corticosteroid creams, not ointments.
Use mildest corticosteroids on face.
Use moderate corticosteroids on other parts of body and change to mild potency as the condition improves.
Oral corticosteroids should be avoided because of the potential for steroid dependency from the relapsing nature of the disease.
Antihistamines can be used for pruritus. Hydroxyzine produces less sedation than diphenhydramine.

Lifestyle/Activities

Avoid pets.
Avoid dry environments.
Avoid exposure to dust mites (post carpet cleaning).

Diet

Eliminate one food at a time to determine triggers. Food accounts as a trigger in 30% of the cases.
Dairy products and wheat are common triggers.

Patient Education

Teach the patient to avoid anything that dries or irritates the skin (e.g., skin preparations with alcohol).

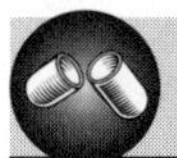

TABLE 64-2 Pharmaceutical Plan: Eczema

Drug	Dosage	Comment	Cost
Triamcinolone	0.1%—apply 2-4 times/day sparingly and rub in well	Never use on face; taper to avoid rebound flares; use for short period of time in children	$4-$27
Doxepin cream	5%—apply 4 times/day to lesions	Treats pruritus	$21/30 g
Tar preparations (LCD)	5% in Aquaphor; apply to area	Best for thickened, lichenified lesions when topical steroids are not helping	N/A
Burow's solution	Apply 4-6 times/day for 10 min each time using wet compresses	Best for acute, weeping lesions	
Salicylic acid solution	3%-5%—apply to area	Used more in chronic phase	$9-$16

NA, Not available.

The symptoms may be worse in winter, when humidity is low.
The patient should bathe minimally and avoid using bubble bath or sitting in the tub for prolonged periods.
Washcloths and brushes should not be used.
Soap should be used only on the armpits, groin, and feet. A mild soap (e.g., Neutrogena, Dove)
Pat skin dry and apply emollient.
Avoid scratchy material (wool).
Avoid overheating since perspiration can trigger itching.
Consider removing pet from the environment.

Family Impact

Exacerbations are frequent, increasing family stress.
Generally improves as **child** ages. Signs of poor prognosis for improvement are early onset, generalized lesions, and concomitant asthma.

Referral/Consultation

Referral to dermatologist is needed if there is minimal or no response to basic management measures.
Refer to dermatologist for skin testing (will detect dust mite allergy).

Follow-up

Follow up frequently (every 2 to 3 days) during a flare-up.

EVALUATION

Herpes simplex infection may occur from improper use of corticosteroids; if this occurs, treat with acyclovir.
No secondary infection of lesions.
Fewer primary lesions.

SUGGESTED READINGS

Berger T, Goldstein S, Odom R: Skin and appendages. In Tierney L, McPhee S, Papadakis M, editors: *Current medical diagnosis and treatment,* ed 36, Norwalk, Conn, 1998, Appleton & Lange.

Boynton R, Dunn E, Stephens G: *Manual of ambulatory pediatrics,* ed 4, Philadelphia, 1998, JB Lippincott.

Ellsworth AJ et al: *Mosby's 1998 medical drug reference,* St Louis, 1998, Mosby.

Healthcare Consultants of America, Inc: *1998 Physicians fee and coding guide,* Augusta, Ga, 1998, Healthcare Consultants of America, Inc.

Kolmer H et al: Effect of combined antibacterial and antifungal treatment in severe atopic dermatitis, *J Allergy Clin Immunol* 98:702-706, 1996.

Pierce N: Bacterial infections of the skin. In Barker L, Burton J, Zieve P, editors: *Principles of ambulatory medicine,* ed 4, Baltimore, 1995, Williams & Wilkins.

Roth M, Grant-Kels J: Diagnostic criteria for atopic dermatitis, *Lancet* 348:769-770, 1996.

65 Edema

ICD-9-CM

Edema 782.3

OVERVIEW

Definition

Edema is defined as an increase in interstitial fluid volume. Depending on the cause, edema may be classified as localized or generalized. Localized edema is usually confined to a single area (e.g., extremity), whereas generalized edema presents in more than one area (e.g., face, extremities, and abdomen). Localized edema may be caused by an inflammatory or hypersensitivity response, and venous or lymphatic obstruction. Generalized edema may be caused by advanced cardiac, renal, hepatic, or nutritional disorders.

Ascites is an excess of fluid in the peritoneal cavity. Hydrothorax is an excess of fluid in the pleural cavity. Anasarca refers to gross, generalized edema. Angioedema is the swelling of the lips, tongue, hands, and periorbital area and may involve laryngeal edema which can result in acute respiratory distress.

Incidence

Cardiopulmonary disease and peripheral vascular disease is the leading cause of edema in **adults**. Renal disease is the leading cause of generalized edema in **children.**

Pathophysiology

The fluid volume within the extracellular space consists of plasma volume and the volume within the interstitial space. The hydrostatic pressure of the vascular system and interstitial fluid helps regulate the flow of fluid into and out of the vascular system. The colloid oncotic pressure created by theplasma proteins in the interstitial and vascular fluid also regulates the flow between the vascular and interstitial compartments. Changes in either the oncotic or hydrostatic pressures result in the net movement of fluid from one compartment to another. Edema results when the oncotic pressure decreases as a result of decreased plasma proteins or when the hydrostatic pressure within the capillary membranes of the vascular system increases. Increased venous pressure is the most common cause of edema.

SUBJECTIVE DATA

History of Present Illness

Symptoms include localized or diffuse generalized swelling of body tissue. The following considerations help to differentiate localized versus generalized edema.

Where the edema is found?
  Localized edema may be unilateral or bilateral, whereas generalized edema is usually symmetrically seen in the face, extremities, and/or abdomen.

How long the edema has been present?
  The duration and progression of edema is indicative of the rate of fluid shifting, also known as "third spacing."

Has the area been injured recently?
  Edema may result from injury to the capillary endothelium, permitting protein to escape into the interstitial compartment. This may be caused by chemical, bacterial, thermal, or mechanical trauma, such as a burn, insect bite, or sprain. This type of edematous response will usually present as localized swelling, with other signs of inflammation.

Past Medical History

Ask about:

- Thyroid disease (Graves' disease)
- Cardiac disease (myocardial infarction, hypertension, congestive heart failure, valvular disease)
- Deep venous thrombosis
- Cancer (breast, prostate, ovarian, uterine, bone)
- Gastrointestinal or liver disease (cirrhosis)
- Renal failure or nephrotic syndrome
- Recent trauma or exposure to possible allergens
- Note all surgeries and hospitalizations

Medication and Diet History

Note all recently prescribed and over-the-counter (OTC) drugs. Also note dietary habits, because protein-deficient diets seen in starvation or malnutrition may produce edema. Drugs that may cause edema include those listed in Box 65-1.

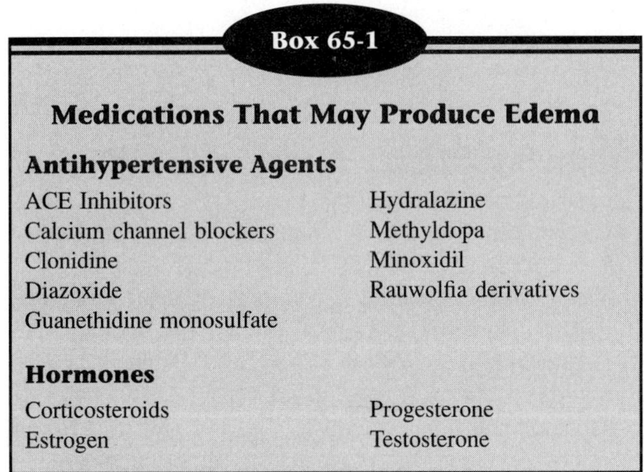

Box 65-1

Medications That May Produce Edema

Antihypertensive Agents	
ACE Inhibitors	Hydralazine
Calcium channel blockers	Methyldopa
Clonidine	Minoxidil
Diazoxide	Rauwolfia derivatives
Guanethidine monosulfate	
Hormones	
Corticosteroids	Progesterone
Estrogen	Testosterone

ACE, Angiotensin-converting enzyme.

Family History

Ask about anyone in the family with a history of diseases of the heart, kidneys, liver, or thyroid.

Associated Symptoms

The associated symptoms help to distinguish the underlying primary etiological factors. If the patient complains of dyspnea, orthopnea, increased fatigue, change in appetite, or change in urination patterns, consider cardiopulmonary disease. If the patient complains of decreased urination and increased thirst, consider renal disease. If the patient complains of appetite changes, nausea, vomiting, and changes in skin color, thickness, or sensitivity, consider hepatic, metabolic, or a pathological nutritional state. For a female patient, ask about her last menstrual period to rule out pregnancy. Angioedema is associated with an allergic reaction to medications, such as ACE inhibitors or foods.

OBJECTIVE DATA

Physical Examination

A complete physical examination is necessary with a chief complaint of generalized edema. This examination should include vital signs, height, weight, and a comprehensive examination of the heart, lungs, and abdomen. If pregnancy is suspected, a pelvic/rectal examination should be performed. In **children,** a complete physical examination should include head circumference, abdominal girth, and assessment of the labia or scrotum.

For localized edema the physical examination should focus on that specific area, including a musculoskeletal and neurovascular examination. Figure 65-1 illustrates assessment for pitting edema.

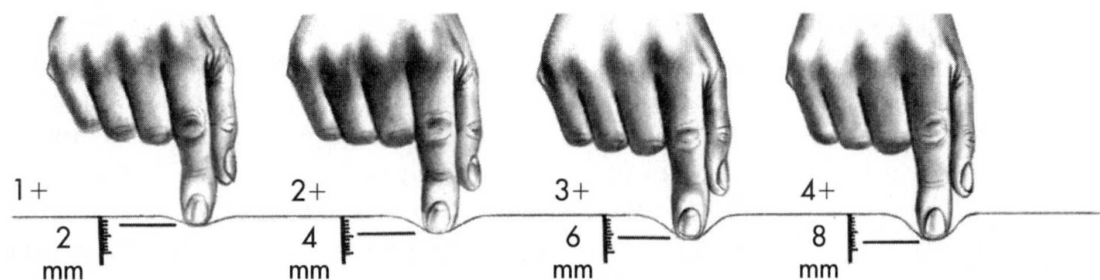

Figure 65-1 Assessing for pitting edema. The severity of edema may be characterized by grading 1+ through 4+. Any concomitant pitting can be mild or severe, as evidenced by the following: 1+, slight pitting, no visible distortion, disappears rapidly; 2+, a somewhat deeper pit than in 1+, but again no readily detectable distortion, and it disappears in 10-15 seconds; 3+, the pit is noticeably deep and may last more than a minute; the dependent extremity looks fuller and swollen; 4+, the pit is very deep, lasts as long as 2 to 5 minutes, and the dependent extremity is grossly distorted. (From Canobbio MM: *Cardiovascular disorders,* St Louis, 1990, Mosby.)

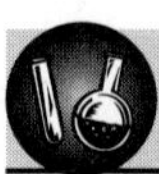

TABLE 65-1 Diagnostic Tests: Edema

Test	Findings/Rationale	Cost ($)
Generalized Edema		
Serum electrolytes	To detect renal failure or nephrotic syndrome	23-30
Serum albumin	To detect kidney or chronic liver disease	18-23
Serum protein	To detect chronic liver disease, infections and carcinoma	22-27
Serum HCG	To detect pregnancy	28-35/qual 51-65/quan
Echocardiography	To detect LVH	675
CXR	To detect cardiomegaly, heart failure, pulmonary edema	77-91
Liver enzymes	To detect cirrhosis, liver failure	29-41
Thyroid studies	To detect hypothyroidism	47-61
U/A	To detect proteinuria	12-16
Localized Edema		
CXR	To detect trauma	114-134
Venous Doppler studies	To detect venous obstruction	257-300
CBC	To assess presence of cellulitis	29-36
Lymphangiography	Differentiate lymphedema from venous insufficiency	1100-1206

CXR, Chest x-ray examination; *HCG,* human chorionic gonadotropin; *LVH,* left ventricular hypertrophy; *U/A,* urinalysis.

Diagnostic Procedures

For generalized and localized edema, consider the tests listed in Table 65-1. In **children,** urinalysis is essential. If results are positive for proteinuria, perform a 24-hour urine collection and evaluate for protein and creatinine levels. Also run panels for serum electrolytes, protein, albumin sedimentation rate, and complete blood count. Sickle cell screening should be performed in black children.

ASSESSMENT

Differential Diagnosis

Localized Edema

Localized edema may result from:

Venous/lymphatic obstruction: Thrombophlebitis, chronic lymphangitis, lymph node resection, cellulitis, vascular ulceration (Chapter 109), tumor, vasculitis

Children: Impaired lymphatic flow may be caused by genetic Turner's syndrome (an endocrinological disorder primarily of females characterized by short stature resulting from a growth-hormone deficiency), lymphoma (Chapter 113), intestinal lymphangiectasia, and filariasis

Trauma/injury: Sprains, burns, insect bites or stings, allergies, infection, Baker's cyst

Children (in addition): Scarlet fever (Chapter 162), mononucleosis (Chapter 119), roseola (Chapter 158), Rocky Mountain spotted fever, mumps (Chapter 121)

Generalized Edema

Generalized edema may result from:

Cardiopulmonary disease: Pulmonary edema, congestive heart failure (Chapter 42), pericardial effusion

Renal disease: Nephrotic syndrome, hypoalbuminemia, acute glomerulonephritis

Hepatic disease: Cirrhosis (Chapter 38), hepatitis (Chapter 89)

Metabolic/nutritional disease: Hypothyroidism (Chapter 178), malnutrition, pregnancy, systemic lupus erythematosus (Chapter 110), protein-losing enteropathy

Medications: Hormones, steroids, calcium antagonists, ACE inhibitors

Children (in addition): Kawasaki's disease (Chapter 103), cystic fibrosis (Chapter 49), celiac disease, nephrotic syndrome, biliary atresia, Chiari's syndrome (a disorder of the pituitary gland that causes persistent galactorrhea and amenorrhea caused by excessive prolactin and deficient gonadotropins), hydrops fetalis (in newborns), Henoch-Schönlein purpura, sinusitis (Chapter 166)

Table 65-2 outlines the differential diagnoses for edema. Figure 65-2 presents an algorithm for regional edema.

THERAPEUTIC PLAN

The treatment selected depends on the underlying pathological condition.

TABLE 65-2 Differential Diagnosis: Edema

Diagnosis	Supporting Data
Congestive heart failure (Ch. 42), venous or pulmonary edema	Pulmonary rales, elevated jugular distention, abnormal S_3 and S_4 heart sounds, peripheral edema, hepatomegaly
Nephrotic syndrome	Severe hypoalbuminemia, proteinuria, hyperlipidemia, generalized edema, oliguria
Cirrhosis (Ch. 38)	Ascites, jaundice, spider angiomas, hepatojugular reflex, hepatomegaly, abdominal tenderness, elevated hepatic enzymes
Hypothyroidism (myxedema) (Ch. 178)	Periorbital and facial puffiness, generalized edema, bradypnea, hypotension, bradycardia, sparse hair growth, large tongue, pale, cool skin that feels rough, thick, and doughy; stupor, coma, and respiratory arrest can occur
Venous/lymphatic obstruction	Unilateral edema, localized tenderness, erythema, and fever may be present

Pharmaceutical

Diuretic therapy may be appropriate for generalized or bilateral leg edema resulting from systemic causes (e.g., congestive heart failure ([CHF], renal insufficiency, cirrhosis, or venous insufficiency). Potassium-sparing or loop diuretics should be used to promote diuresis of 0.5 to 1 kg body weight loss per day. Use caution in **children** and **elderly patients** or individuals with rising creatinine levels or hypoproteinuria. Lower doses are generally effective, and as doses need to be increased, combination therapy is warranted. A single dose given in the morning tends to be more effective than moderate doses given BID. As dosage increases, monitor electrolytes more vigilantly.

Table 65-3 outlines a plan of diuretic therapy for edema.

Allergies

Corticosteroids or antihistamines may be necessary for allergic reactions (see Chapter 6).

Corticosteroids are the primary treatment in nephrotic syndrome (Table 65-4).

Thrombolytic therapy is necessary for patients with deep venous thrombosis for 3 to 6 months.

Antibiotic therapy may be necessary for infectious disease. See Chapter 31 for specific drug therapy.

Lifestyle/Activities Modification

For localized edema: Elevation, rest, and ice may decrease swelling and inflammation.

Compression leg stockings may facilitate lymph and blood circulation in the lower extremities.

Children: Activities should *not* be restricted.

Diet

A salt-restricted diet should be implemented. Usually a "no added salt" diet will be sufficient. Protein and albumin replacement may be necessary.

Patient Education

Avoidance of allergen or infectious agent
No added salt or salt-restricted diet
High-protein diet for hypoproteinemia
Use of compression stockings (for venous/lymphatic disease)
Medication precautions and side effects

Family Impact

Edema can be disfiguring as well as restrictive in physical activities; therefore issues of body image, self-esteem, and social isolation must be considered. Neurovascular and musculoskeletal function must also be protected to prevent decreased independence. The family may be required to assist with ambulation and therapeutic modalities. The financial impact of therapies and/or hospitalization should be considered.

Referral

Immediate referral is indicated for all patients:

- Unresponsive to diuretic therapy
- With elevated creatinine or hepatic enzymes
- With cardiomegaly or respiratory distress
- With acute infectious process unresponsive to antibiotics
- With vascular or lymphatic obstructions
- **Children:** With proteinuria >50 mg/kg/24 hours or 2 g/24 hours or protein: creatinine ratio of >3.5

Consultation

Consider consultation with a physician for children with acute infectious process (e.g., cellulitis), which may require hospitalization. Consider consultation with vascular specialists or dermatologists for vascular ulcerations.

EVALUATION/FOLLOW-UP

Follow-up depends on the severity of edema and underlying disease. For generalized edema, follow-up with diagnostic

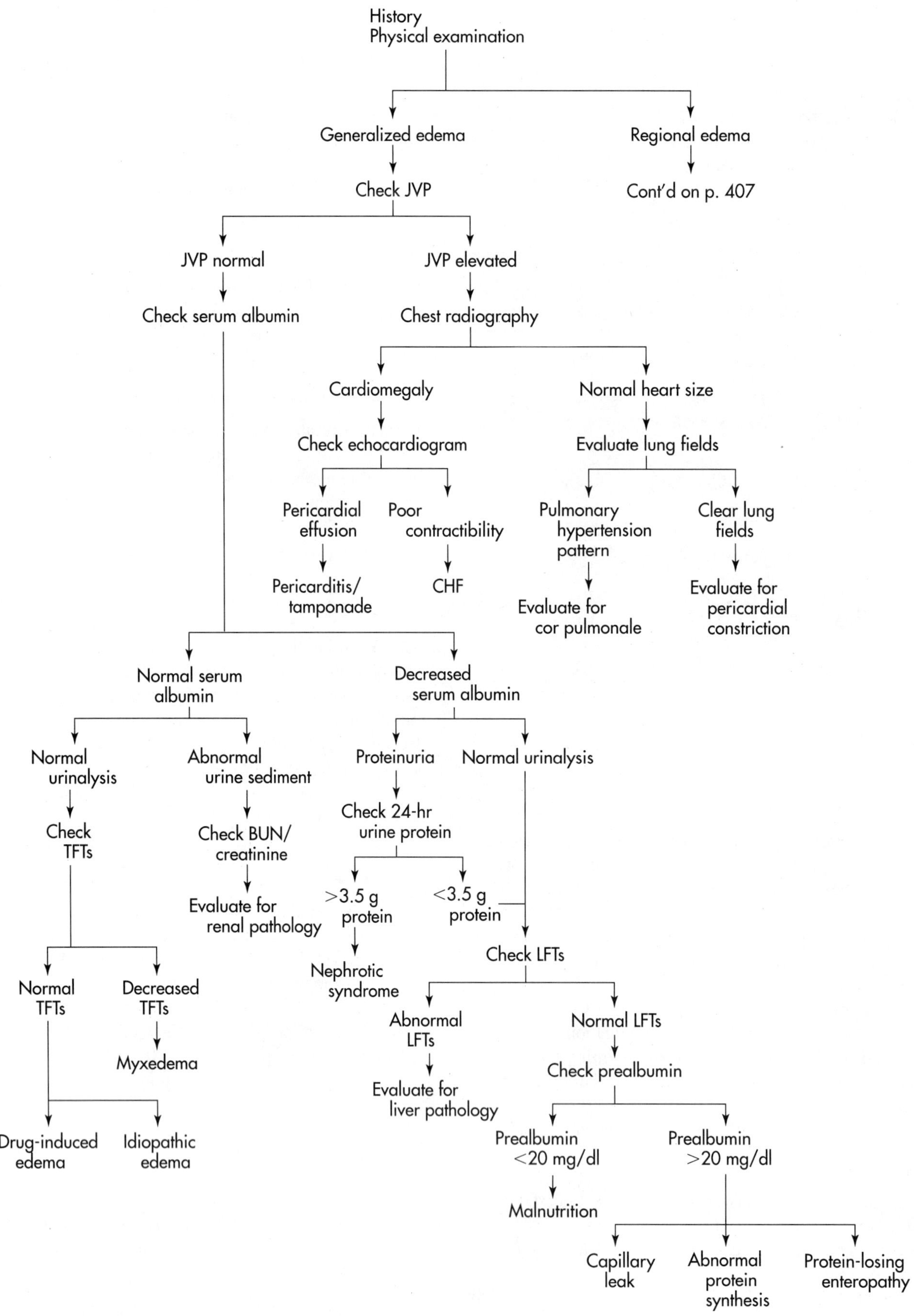

Figure 65-2 Algorithm for the treatment of a patient with edema. *BUN,* Blood urea nitrogen; *CHF,* congestive heart failure; *CT,* computed tomography; *CXR,* chest x-ray; *JVP,* jugular venous pressure; *LFT,* liver function test; *TFT,* thyroid function test. (Adapted from Greene HL, Johnson WP, Lemcke D: *Decision making in medicine,* ed 2, St Louis, 1998, Mosby.)

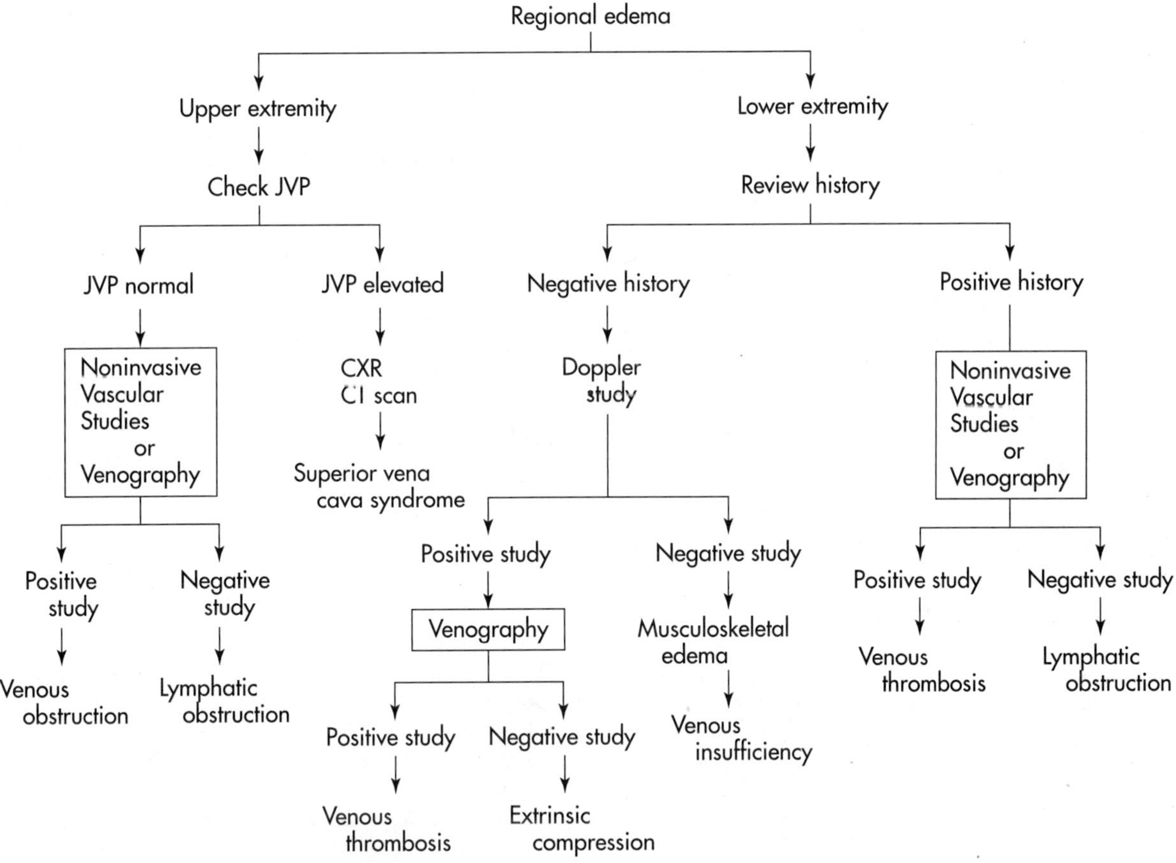

Figure 65-2, cont'd For legend see opposite page.

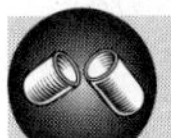

TABLE 65-3 Pharmaceutical Plan: Edema

Drug	Dosage	Comments	Cost
Potassium Sparing		Monitor potassium levels for hyperkalemia	
Spironolactone (Aldactone)	25-200 mg/day in 4-5 divided doses Children: 1-3/kg/day in divided doses	Take with meals or milk Pregnancy: D SE: Diarrhea, vomiting, rash, pruritus, hyperkalemia	$5-$39/25 mg (100); $71/50 mg (100); $119/100 mg (100)
Triamterene (Dyrenium)	25-100 mg /day Max. 300 mg/day Children: 2-4 mg/kg/day	Not recommended for children Pregnancy: D SE: Diarrhea, weakness, nausea, fatigue, hyperkalemia	$32-$34/50 mg (100); $34/100 mg (100)
Amiloride (Midamor)	5-10 mg QD Maximum: 20 mg/day	Pregnancy: B SE: Headache, orthostatic hypotension, nausea, diarrhea, anorexia, hyperkalemia	$26-$46/5 mg (100)
Thiazide Type			
Chlorothiazide (Diuril)	250-500 mg QD/BID	Pregnancy: B SE: Adverse lipid values, photosensitivity, hypokalemia, hyponatremia	N/A

GI, Gastrointestinal; *HCTZ*, hydrochlorothiazide; *N/A*, not available. *SE*, side effects.

Continued

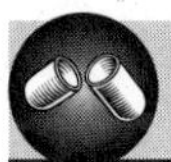

TABLE 65-3 Pharmaceutical Plan: Edema—cont'd

Drug	Dosage	Comments	Cost
Hydrochlorothiazide (HCTZ, Esidrix)	12.5-50 mg QD	Pregnancy: B SE: Adverse lipid values, photosensitivity, hypokalemia, hyponatremia	\$2-\$13/25 mg (100); \$2-\$21/50 mg (100)
Metolazone (Zaroxolyn)	5 mg QD, maximum 20 mg/day	Pregnancy: B SE: Hypokalemia, hyponatremia, hyperglycemia, hyperuricemia, gout, blurred vision	\$53/2.5 mg (100); \$59/5 mg (100); \$68/10 mg (100)
Other: Indapamide (Lozol)	2.5 mg QD; after 1 week may increase to 5 mg QD	Same as for metolazone	\$65/1.25 mg (100); \$66-\$85/2.5 mg (100)
Loop Diuretics			
Bumetanide (Bumex)	0.5-1 mg IV/IM 0.5-2 mg PO (1 mg bumetanide ≅ 40 mg furosemide)	Pregnancy: C SE: Muscle cramps, headache, ototoxicity, electrolyte imbalance, hyperuricemia	\$37-\$45/1 mg (100); \$63-\$72/2 mg (100)
Ethacrynic acid (Edecrin)	0.5 -1 mg/kg, up to 50 mg IV 25-100 mg PO QD/BID Children: 25 mg QD	Use in infants not recommended Pregnancy: B SE: Fluid/electrolyte imbalance, ototoxicity, deafness, vertigo, tinnitus, GI upset, headache, rash	\$20/50 mg/vial IV; \$30/25 mg (100); \$43/50 mg (100)
Furosemide (Lasix)	1 mg/kg up to 20-40 mg IV 20-80 mg qd/BID Children: PO: 2 mg/kg/day as single dose	Pregnancy: C SE: Photosensitivity, xanthopsia, vertigo, paresthesia, jaundice, tinnitus, photosensitivity, hypokalemia	\$2-\$16/20 mg (100); \$3-\$22/40 mg (100); \$6-\$37/80 mg (100)
Torsemide (Demadex)	5-20 mg IV/PO QD	Pregnancy: B Interactions with amphotericin B, anticoagulants, hypokalemia causing medications, lithium, salicylates (high dose) SE: Constipation, dizziness, GI upset, headache	\$53/5 mg (100); \$49/10 mg (100); \$53/20 mg (100); \$216/100 (100)
Combination Diuretics			
Triamterene, HCTZ (Dyazide)	1-2 caps QD	Pregnancy: C SE: Drowsiness, muscle cramps, weakness, headache, GI upset, dry mouth, impotence, urine discoloration	N/A
Spironolactone + HCTZ (Aldactazide)	Used for maintenance: 4 tablets in single or divided doses	Pregnancy: Not recommended SE: Hyperkalemia, gynecomastia, headache, menstrual changes, photosensitivity, GI disturbances	N/A

TABLE 65-4 Corticosteroid Therapy: Edema

Drug	Dosage	Comments	Cost
Prednisone (Deltasone)	Initially 5-60 mg/day for children and adults	Pregnancy: C SE: Hyperglycemia, PUD, weight gain, cushingoid facies, striae, infection	$3-$8/5 mg (100) $4-$13/10 mg (100)
Prednisolone (Prelone)	Initially 5-60 mg/day for children and adults	Pregnancy: C SE: Hyperglycemia, PUD, weight gain, cushingoid facies, striae, infection	$3-19/5 mg (100) $52/liquid: 5 mg/5 ml (240 ml)

PUD, Peptic ulcer disease; *SE,* side effects.

testing results should be within 1 week, if not hospitalized. For systemic diseases associated with generalized edema who are not hospitalized, follow-up should be scheduled weekly until edema is resolved or within 1 week following hospital discharge. Schedule return visit in 2 to 3 weeks for complaints associated with localized edema.

SUGGESTED READINGS

Braunwald E: *Harrison's principles of internal medicine,* New York, 1994, McGraw-Hill.

Ciocon J, Fernandez B, Ciscon D: Leg edema: clinical clues to differential diagnosis, *Geriatrics* 48:34-45, 1993.

Dershewitz R: *Ambulatory pediatric care,* Philadelphia, 1993, JB Lippincott.

Ellsworth AJ et al: *Mosby's 1998 medical drug reference,* St Louis, 1998, Mosby.

Gibson D, Greene H: Edema. In Greene H, Johnson W, Lemcke D, editors: *Decision making in medicine,* St Louis, ed 2, 1998, Mosby.

Healthcare Consultants of America, Inc: *1998 Physicians fee and coding guide,* Augusta, Ga, 1998, Healthcare Consultants of America, Inc.

Judge R, Zuidema G, Fizgerald F: *Clinical diagnosis,* Boston, 1989, Little Brown & Co.

Murphy J, editor: *Nurse practitioner's prescribing reference,* New York, 1997, Prescribing Reference, Inc.

Rakel R, editor: *Conn's current therapy,* Philadelphia, 1997, WB Saunders.

Seller R: *Differential diagnosis of common complaints,* Philadelphia, 1996, WB Saunders.

Uphold C, Graham M: *Clinical guidelines in family practice,* Gainesville, Fla, 1994, Barmarrae Books.

Washington University Department of Medicine: *The Washington manual,* Boston, 1995, Little Brown.

66 Encopresis

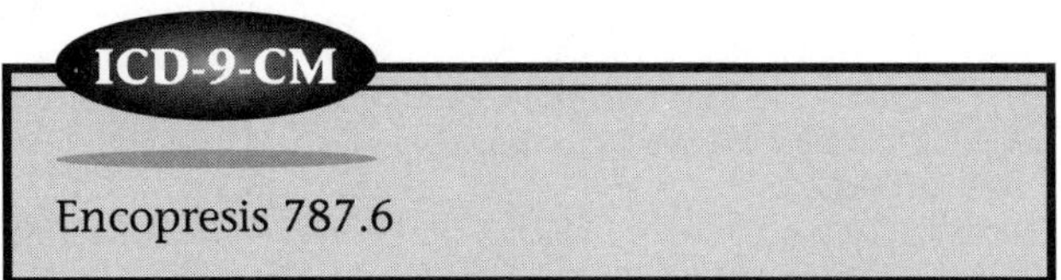

OVERVIEW

Definition

Encopresis is repeated fecal soiling in the absence of an organic defect or illness in **children older than 4 years.** The condition is usually secondary to constipation or incomplete defecation.

Incidence

Encopresis occurs in **2% to 3% of preschool and elementary school-age children.** There is a **greater incidence in boys than in girls.**

Pathophysiology

Encopresis frequently results from voluntary withholding of stool, which creates a functional megacolon. The defecation reflex occurs when the walls of the rectum become distended with stool, stimulating mass peristalsis. When stool is retained through voluntary constriction of the external sphincter, the rectum relaxes, decreasing peristalsis and the urge to defecate. The megacolon requires progressively larger stools to stimulate defecation. As the rectal vault becomes enlarged, control of the external sphincter is lost, and liquid stool involuntarily seeps past the fecal bolus.

SUBJECTIVE DATA

History of Present Illness

Ask about the following:

- "Dribbling" stool
- Staining of underpants, and when, where, and how often the staining occurs
- Duration and frequency of symptoms (is the child aware of the soiling?) and any nocturnal episodes
- Abdominal pain and distention
- Associated symptoms such as anorexia, enuresis
- Usual pattern of elimination, description of stools, including frequency
- Dietary history
- Use of laxatives, any treatments tried, and effectiveness
- Availability of bathrooms, including degree of privacy
- Any psychosocial factors
- Problems with or changes in gait

Past Medical History

- Complete history of bowel pattern in infancy; delayed passage of meconium (greater than 24 hours), constipation, small-caliber stools
- Any chronic illness or surgery, especially bowel surgery?
- Hypothyroidism?
- Complete history of toilet training

Medications

Current or recent medications with emphasis on laxatives and narcotics

TABLE 66-1 Differential Diagnosis: Encopresis

Diagnosis	Supporting Data
Hirschsprung's disease	Failure to pass meconium in first week of life, poor weight gain, chronic constipation
Neuromuscular defect: spinal cord lesion, cerebral palsy	Abnormalities found on neurological examination, midline abnormalities, gait difficulties, delayed motor skills
Hypothyroidism	Adults: Fatigue, dry skin, weight gain, heavy menses, cold intolerance, hair loss, increased sleep Children: Decreased activity, poor growth and development, reduced limb length with increased ratio of upper- to lower-body segment
Stress	History of stressful event, such as divorce, birth of sibling, death or other loss, or sexual or physical abuse
Anal stricture/fissure	Bright red rectal bleeding pain associated with defecation Fissures or hemorrhoids found on rectal examination
Lead poisoning	History of possible exposure Serum lead level >10 μg/dl
Chronic diarrhea	Empty rectal vault; abdominal x-ray evaluation negative for impaction
Crohn's disease	Fever, weight loss, arthralgias/arthritis in large joints, symptoms associated with meals, abdominal pain (umbilical and right lower quadrant), and bloody, painful stools
Ulcerative colitis	Fever, weight loss, arthralgias/arthritis in large joints, anorexia, abdominal pain (lower abdominal and left lower quadrant), bloody mucoid stools; pain increases before defecation or passing of flatus; oral ulcers

Family History

Assess for family history of similar problems and hypothyroidism.

Psychosocial History

Assess the child's emotional state, history of abuse, relationship with peers, parental reaction to the soiling

OBJECTIVE DATA

Physical Examination

A complete physical examination should be conducted, with emphasis placed on the following:

Abdomen: Usually normal; may reveal soft, nontender mass in midline or left lower quadrant
Rectal: May reveal anal fissures, decreased tone, hard formed stool in rectal vault

Diagnostic Procedures

Consider an abdominal x-ray evaluation ($142 to $169) to rule out obstruction and look for fecal mass.

ASSESSMENT

Differential Diagnosis

Differential diagnoses include those listed in Table 66-1.

THERAPEUTIC PLAN

Phase 1: Removal of Impaction

First remove blame by explaining that the soiling is involuntary.
Initial treatment: Relieve constipation and/or impaction.
Day 1: Hypertonic phosphate enemas (3 ml/kg)
Day 2: Bisacodyl (Dulcolax) suppository ($2 to $10)
Day 3: Bisacodyl (Dulcolax) tablets, for patients 5 to 12 years old, 5 mg ($2 to $4); for patients 12 or older, 10 mg

Phase 2: Maintenance (6-12 months)

Follow an oral laxative regimen; see Chapter 44 for choices; increase dose until liquid stools occur.
Increase fiber, fruits, vegetables, and fluids in diet.
Encourage the patient to follow a regular toileting schedule (e.g., sit on toilet for 15 minutes after morning and evening meals).
Behavior modification regimen: Reward success, never punish failure.
Increase exercise.

Phase 3: Gradual Weaning

Gradually taper off laxatives as tolerated.
Maintain high fiber and fluid intake.
Monitor stool frequency.
May need to consider stool softeners (Colace 5 mg/kg/day).

Referral

Any child with suspected neurological problems should be referred to a pediatrician and/or neurologist. Any child who has experienced sexual abuse should be referred to social services, law enforcement, and mental health services.

EVALUATION/FOLLOW-UP

Follow up by telephone PRN and in 1 week.
Recheck every month until rectal vault is normal size.
Taper stool softeners once regular elimination pattern is established.

SUGGESTED READINGS

Arvin AM et al, editors: *Nelson textbook of pediatrics,* ed 15, Philadelphia, 1996, WB Saunders.

Boynton RW, Dunn ES, Stephens GR, editors: *Manual of ambulatory pediatrics,* ed 3, Philadelphia, 1994, JB Lippincott.

Chaney CA: A collaborative protocol for encopresis management in school-aged children, *J School Health* 65:360-364, 1995.

Dershewitz PA, editor: *Ambulatory pediatric care,* ed 2, Philadelphia, 1993, JB Lippincott.

Ellsworth AJ et al: *Mosby's 1998 medical drug reference,* St Louis, 1998, Mosby.

Groothuis JR et al, editors: *Current pediatric diagnosis & treatment,* ed 12, Norwalk Conn, 1995, Appleton & Lange.

Healthcare Consultants of America, Inc: *1998 Physicians fee and coding guide,* Augusta, Ga, 1998, Healthcare Consultants of America, Inc.

Loening-Baucke V: Encopresis and soiling, *Pediatr Clin North Am* 43:279-299, 1996.

Loening-Baucke V: Balloon defecation as a predictor of outcome in children with functional constipation and encopresis, *J Pediatr* 128:336-340, 1996.

Sprague JM, Lamb W, Homer D: Encopresis: a study of treatment alternatives and historical and behavioral characteristics, *Nurse Pract* 18:52-63, 1993.

Endometriosis

ICD-9-CM

Endometriosis of Uterus 617.1
Endometriosis of Pelvic Peritoneum 617.3

OVERVIEW

Definition

Endometriosis is the presence of functioning endometrial tissue outside its normal location; most frequently confined to the ovaries, uterosacral ligaments, cul-de-sac, and occasionally uterovesical peritoneum.

Incidence

The true incidence of endometriosis is unknown. In selected populations, it can range between 1% and 5%. In infertile women, the prevalence may be as high as 30%. There does not appear to be a strong racial predilection. A familial incidence has been documented.

Pathophysiology

The most widely accepted explanation focuses on the concept of retrograde flow of menstrual fluid through the fallopian tubes with implantation of viable endometrial tissue in the free pelvis. Another theory suggests that undifferentiated celomic epithelial cells remain dormant on peritoneal surface until ovaries produce enough hormones to stimulate ectopic tissue.

SUBJECTIVE DATA

History of the Present Illness

One-third of women have no symptoms.
Menstrual history: Include age at menarche, onset of dysmenorrhea, description of the pain, onset, duration, relieving factors, relationship of pain to menstrual cycle.
Obstetrical history: Number of pregnancies, outcomes, number of years attempting to become pregnant, fertility methods used.
Gynecological history: Type of birth control (past and present), history of STDs or other infections, history of gynecological surgeries.

Past Medical History

Past abdominal surgeries
Other chronic conditions

Medications

Over-the-counter medications for pain management (NSAIDs, acetaminophen)
Prescription drugs for pain management
Oral contraceptives

Family History

A woman who has an affected first-degree relative has approximately tenfold increased risk for developing endometriosis. Cervical or vaginal atresia and müllerian fusion defects with obstructed outflow are commonly associated with pelvic endometriosis; this represents another genetic or at least congenital mechanism.

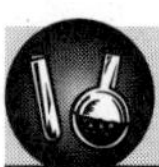

TABLE 67-1 Diagnostic Tests: Endometriosis

Test	Findings/Rationale	Cost ($)
Diagnostic laparoscopy	Allows visualization of the uterus and ovaries; confirms diagnosis of endometriosis. It may allow for treatment by ablation.	1335-1585
WBC/ESR	Rule out infection.	13-16/WBC 14-18/ESR
CA-125 assay	May be done to rule out possible ovarian cancer; also may be detected in women with endometriosis. It does not have any clinical use at this time.	62-75
Pelvic ultrasonography	May provide information in detecting and characterizing pelvic pathology if pelvic examination is limited by tenderness or obesity; however, *it is not* diagnostic.	245-295
CT or MRI	May provide presumptive evidence of endometriosis, but neither is diagnostic and would rarely be justified for an initial workup.	892-1160/CT 1560-1840/MRI

CT, Computed tomography; *ESR,* erythrocyte sedimentation rate; *MRI,* magnetic resonance imaging; *WBC,* white blood cell count.

Psychosocial History

Determine how the woman normally copes with the pain and discomfort.

Has she ever had to attend a pain clinic/program for management of pain?

Description of Most Common Symptoms

Women may be asymptomatic or may present with:

- Dysmenorrhea (66%)
- Dyspareunia (33%)
- Infertility (70%)
- Chronic pelvic pain
- Dyschezia
- Dysuria
- Low back pain (sacral pain is typical of endometriosis)
- Menstrual irregularities

The most common symptoms are pelvic pain, abnormal uterine bleeding, and infertility.

OBJECTIVE DATA

Physical Examination

A physical examination that focuses on the pelvic examination should be performed; it is best done in the immediate premenstrual period. The physical examination may be unremarkable, even in severe endometriosis.

External genitalia: Should be unremarkable

Cervix: Should be smooth, without lesions or mucopurulent discharge

Bimanual examination: May reveal tenderness in the vaginal cul-de-sac and fixed uterine retroversion with cervical motion tenderness. Tender nodules may be present in the posterior fornix or on the back of the uterus and cervix. Fixed ovarian masses are also common.

Adnexal enlargement and tenderness may indicate the presence of an endometrioma (chocolate cyst) of the ovary. These cysts may grow to 15 cm in diameter and are filled with endometrial blood and debris. Rupture of these usually painless cysts can cause an acute abdomen due to spillage of the contents of the cyst. This spillage results in further scarring and progression of the disease.

Rectovaginal examination: May demonstrate uterosacral or rectovaginal septum nodularity. Complaints of pelvic pain, dyspareunia, dysmenorrhea, abnormal bleeding, and infertility should raise suspicions.

Diagnostic Procedures

Diagnostic procedures for endometriosis are outlined in Table 67-1.

ASSESSMENT

Differential Diagnosis

Differential diagnoses include those listed in Table 67-2. Diagnosis requires direct visual and histological confirmation by either laparoscopy or laparotomy. Endometriosis is then staged based on presence, location, and quality of adhesions, endometriomas, and tubal distortion based on the stages formulated by the American Fertility Society (AFS):

Stage I—Minimal
Stage II—Mild

TABLE 67-2 Differential Diagnosis: Endometriosis

Diagnosis	Supporting Data
PID	CMT, mucopurulent discharge, abdominal pain, adnexal pain, fever; symptoms increase with menses.
Pelvic adhesions	History of previous surgeries, abdominal pain; no relationship of pain to menses.
Ovarian cysts or tumors	Women with ovarian cancer are usually older, there is no associated increase in dysmenorrhea, symptoms usually include vague GI discomforts. Surgery is required when ovaries are >5 cm in diameter to rule out malignancy.
Secondary dysmenorrhea	Abdominal pain that may not be limited to menses, depending on cause.
Uterine myomas	Increasing colicky abdominal pain, menstrual bleeding, usually in women >40. There may be bladder pressure and frequency. Examination reveals mildly tender uterus.

CMT, Cervical motion tenderness; *GI,* gastrointestinal; *PID,* pelvic inflammatory disease.

Stage III—Moderate
Stage IV—Severe

THERAPEUTIC PLAN

Not every woman with endometriosis needs therapy. Expectant management may be appropriate for the woman who is not interested in conceiving and who has little pain and mild menstrual disturbances.

Conservative therapy is more successful for moderate and severe endometriosis when fertility is desired. Usually this includes surgery to eliminate as much as possible of the endometriosis, with pregnancy planned in 12 to 15 months after the surgery.

Pharmaceutical

A number of medications can be used, but oral contraceptives or oral medroxyprogesterone acetate (Depo-Provera) are generally favored as first-line treatment (as long as fertility is not desired), since danazol and GnRH agonists are not demonstrably superior, are more expensive, and are more likely to cause side effects.

Table 67-3 outlines a pharmaceutical plan for the treatment of endometriosis.

Lifestyle/Activities

A major impact may be seen on lifestyle and activities because of pain.

Severe endometriosis may affect decisions regarding marriage partner and childbearing.

Diet

Not applicable

Patient Education

Educate family members regarding chronicity of symptoms, supportive management, and accessing appropriate networks: Endometriosis Society (800) 992-ENDO.

Patients should be encouraged to exercise (but not during painful days where increased activity may make symptoms worse).

Learn relaxation techniques.

Patients with documented endometriosis who desire pregnancy should be counseled about the relationship of endometriosis to infertility; desires and timing of childbearing should be discussed.

Recurrence of endometriosis has been reported in 30% to 50% of patients after medical therapy and in 14% to 40% of patients after conservative surgery.

Recurrence has also been reported after hysterectomy and oophorectomy, with or without estrogen replacement therapy.

Family Impact

Depending on severity of endometriosis, the family may be greatly affected, from monthly pain with menses to severe pelvic pain that interferes with activities of daily living, to drug-seeking for pain medicine to control pain and symptoms. Counseling is recommended for family on issues of infertility and pain management.

Referral

Refer the patient to an OB/GYN for laparoscopy, aggressive surgical management, or when conservative medical management is unsuccessful. A professional experienced in working with endometriosis and pelvic pain is suggested. A pain control program may be helpful.

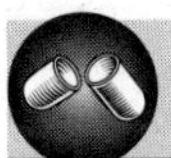

TABLE 67-3 Pharmaceutical Plan: Endometriosis

Drug	Dosage	Comments	Cost
Oral contraceptives (medium androgenic progestin formulation: 0.15 mg levonorgestrel or 0.3 mg norgestrel with 30 μg estrogen)	Use continuously without a pill-free or placebo period until the pain disappears (up to 9 mo)	Once a cyclic regimen is resumed, the pain may return. Alternatively, the patient may go without a pill-free interval for several months, then stop the continuous, active pills for 5-7 days, have withdrawal bleeding, then restart the continuous regimen for several months. If breakthrough bleeding occurs, the dose may be doubled or tripled, with the increased dose continued until the bleeding has stopped.	$14-$30/mo
Medroxyprogesterone acetate (Depo-Provera)	100 mg IM every 2 weeks for 4 doses, then 200 mg IM monthly for 4 mo	Pregnancy: X SE: Irregular bleeding, edema, weight gain, depression, insomnia, breast tenderness, alopecia, rash, acne	$37/150 mg/ml $89/400 mg/ml (2.5 ml)
Medroxyprogesterone acetate (Provera)	30 mg PO QD for 3 mo	Pregnancy: X SE: Irregular bleeding, edema, weight gain, depression, insomnia, breast tenderness	$11-$66/10 mg (100)
Other choices: Danazol (Danocrine)	Mild: 100-200 mg BID for 3-6 mo Moderate: 400 mg BID for at least 3-6 mo up to 9 mo if needed	Decreases FSH, LH Start on day 1 of menstruation if possible Pregnancy: C SE: Rash, acne, headache, decreased libido, nausea and vomiting, weight gain (virilization signs may *not* be reversible); stop drug if virilization occurs	$177/100 mg (100)
Leuprolide acetate (Lupron) (GnRH agonist)	0.5-1.0 mg SQ QD for 6 mo or 3.75-7.5 mg IM q1mo for 6 mo	Decreases estrogen to menopausal levels Pregnancy: X SE: Edema, hot flashes, decreased libido, amenorrhea, vaginal dryness	$278/1 mg/0.2 ml/SC $496/7.5 mg/vial/IM
Nafarelin (Synarel)	Nasal spray: 1 spray (200 μg) into one nostril q AM and 1 spray into other nostril q PM for 6 mo	Pregnancy: X SE: Decreased libido, vaginal dryness, increased pubic hair, flushing, depression, hot flushes, acne	2 mg/ml (10 ml) $336 for 30 day supply

FSH, Follicle-stimulating hormone; *IM,* intramuscularly; *LH,* luteinizing hormone, *SE,* side effects.

Consultation

Refer to a gynecologist if endometriosis is suspected.

Oral contraceptives would be the first choice if contraception is desired.

Follow-up

Follow up as appropriate, based on management choices.

Follow up in 2 weeks after starting medication, then every 3 months to assess effectiveness and side effects.

The patient will probably see a specialist for follow-up.

EVALUATION

Control of symptoms is the goal of therapy. Complications of endometriosis include:

Chronic pelvic pain/disruption of lifestyle
Infertility
Hysterectomy

SUGGESTED READINGS

ACOG Technical Bulletin: *Endometriosis,* No 184, 1993.

Banerjee R, Laufer M: Reproductive disorders associated with pelvic pain, *Semin Pediatr Surg* 7:52-61, 1998.

Ellsworth AJ et al: *Mosby's 1998 medical drug reference,* St Louis, 1998, Mosby.

Healthcare Consultants of America, Inc: *1998 Physicians fee and coding guide,* Augusta, Ga, 1998, Healthcare Consultants of America, Inc.

Laufer M et al: Prevalence of endometriosis in adolescent girls with chronic pelvic pain not responding to conventional therapy, *J Pediatr Adolesc Gynecol* 10:199-202, 1997.

Mishell D et al: Practice guidelines for OC selection, *Dial Contracept* 5:7-19, 1997.

Newkirk G: Endometriosis. In Johnson C, Murray J, Johnson B: *Women's health care handbook,* St Louis, 1996, Mosby.

Ryan I, Taylor R: Endometriosis and infertility: new concepts, *Obstet Gynecol Surv* 52:365-371, 1997.

Venturini P et al: Chronic pelvic pain: oral contraceptives and nonsteroidal anti-inflammatory compounds, *Cephalalgia* 17(Suppl 20):29-31, 1997.

Vercellini P: Endometriosis: what a pain it is, *Semin Reprod Endocrinol* 15:251-261, 1997.

Enuresis

ICD-9-CM

Enuresis 788.30
Nocturnal Enuresis 788.36

OVERVIEW

Definition

Enuresis is involuntary voiding after the age when control should have been established (usually 5 years old). It may be nocturnal (85%) or diurnal.

Primary enuresis: Bladder control has never been established.

Secondary enuresis: There is loss of bladder control in a child who has been consistently dry for at least 6 months,

Incidence

More common in males than females

Familial tendency

More common in large families and in the lower socioeconomic groups

Occurs in approximately:

10%-15% of 6 year olds
5% of 10 year olds
3% of 12 year olds
1% of 15 year olds

Pathophysiology

Primary Enuresis

Urinary control is a function of the central nervous system (CNS). There is delayed maturation of that portion of the CNS that permits bladder control that results in the child not sensing bladder fullness and therefore not awakening to void.

Contributing factors include:

Immature bladder with small capacity
Immature arousal from non-REM sleep
Psychological or emotional problems (e.g., new sibling, divorce)
Neurologic deficit (neurogenic bladder, spinal cord lesion)
Urologic abnormalities (urinary tract infection—UTI), vesicoureteral reflux, bifurcated bladder, tumors)
Diabetes mellitus, diabetes insipidus

Secondary Enuresis

Psychological problems
UTIs (The presence of bacteria is irritating to the bladder mucosa, producing frequency, urgency, and dysuria.)
Sexual abuse
Diabetes mellitus/diabetes insipidus

SUBJECTIVE DATA

Primary: Involuntary voiding one or more times a day, at least once a week without ever having achieved full bladder control

Secondary: Involuntary voiding one or more times a day, at least once a week after having achieved bladder control for at least 6 months

History of Present Illness

Determine onset, frequency, time frame (at what time of night does the bed wetting usually occur, is it consistent), fluid intake related to bedtime, how the parents have tried to correct the problem, how the parents and the child feel about the problem.

Depending on the age of the child, the family nurse practitioner might choose to conduct a portion of the interview with the parents and child separated.

TABLE 68-1 Differential Diagnosis: Enuresis

Diagnosis	Supporting Data
Normal developmental enuresis	Age <8 years No abnormalities on physical examination
Stress	History of stressful event such as divorce, sibling birth, death or other loss, sexual or physical abuse
Toilet training resistance	History of punitive attempts at toilet training Primary enuresis
Altered parenting	Toilet training history erratic No consistency in toileting
Urinary tract infection	Urgency, frequency, burning Urinalysis + nitrites, + blood, + leukocytes
Urinary tract anatomical abnormality	Constant wetness vs. periodic voiding, weak urinary stream, growth abnormalities, abdominal distention Abnormalities seen on KUB, VCUG, or renal ultra sound
Diabetes mellitus	Polydipsia, polyuria, polyphagia, urinalysis + sugar and ketones, blood sugar >200
Diabetes insipidus	Polydipsia, polyuria, signs and symptoms of dehydration, pale, dry skin, urine specific gravity <1.005
Seizure disorder	Awakening with bitten tongue, observations of jerking, twitching, staring episodes
Sleep apnea	Snoring, excessive fatigue and/or sleepiness during the day
Central nervous system deficit	Gait abnormalities, abnormal scoliosis examination, abnormal DTR or other parts of neurologic examination

DTR, Deep tendon reflex; *KUB,* kidneys, ureter, and bladder x-ray; *VCUG,* voiding cystourethrogram.

Past Medical History

UTI, congenital anomalies, toilet training methods (were parents demanding or punitive?)
History of sexual abuse

Family History

Enuresis, especially in father
Family history of diabetes

Psychosocial History

Ask about births, deaths, divorce, moves, school problems.

Associated Symptoms

Frequency, urgency, pain, or burning on urination
Nocturnal seizures (bitten tongue or sore muscles on awakening)

OBJECTIVE DATA

Physical Examination

Perform a complete physical and neurologic examination, usually within normal limits. Focus on constant dribbling, external anomalies of the genitalia, rectal sphincter tone, café au lait spots, abdominal masses, spinal bony defects, hairy tufts, masses and gait.

Assess for chronic urinary tract disease. Suspect if height, weight, are below the fifth percentile, and/or average BP higher than the 95th percentile for age and sex.

Diagnostic Procedures

Perform urinalysis ($14-$18) and clean voided culture ($31-$39). More invasive procedures (cystoscopy, ultrasound) are not indicated unless an abnormality is discovered on physical examination or the problem persists past age 6 years and all other diagnostic tests are negative.

ASSESSMENT

Differential diagnoses include (Table 68-1):

Normal developmental enuresis
Toilet training resistance
Altered parenting
Stress
UTI or anatomic abnormalities
Diabetes mellitus, diabetes insipidus
Seizure disorder
Sleep apnea
CNS deficit

NOTE: In the majority of cases no organic pathology can be found!

THERAPEUTIC PLAN

Involve the child in the treatment plan.

Decision to treat or not to treat must be made jointly by the child and the parents.

Treat only **children who are 8 years old** or older and who have a bladder capacity of 200 ml or greater (determined by measuring output after having the child hold voiding as long as possible).

Investigate and treat the cause if secondary enuresis.

Nonpharmaceutical

Bladder stretching exercises: Increase fluid and have child hold off voiding as long as possible.

Positively reinforce for dryness; use a gold star chart.

Education: Support and reassure; avoid punishing or embarrassing the child.

Use an "enuresis alarm"; the alarm is worn at night and is triggered by moisture. Success rate is as high as 80%. The typical course is 4 months; it must be warn until 21 consecutive nights of dryness are achieved. There is an approximate 25% relapse rate.

Pharmaceutical

Imipramine hydrochloride (Tofranil) ($2-$44) 10 to 25 mg PO hs initially. May be increased to a maximum dose of 50 mg for children under 12 years old and 75 mg for children over 12 years old. NOTE: Use imipramine hydrochloride. Imipramine pamoate may not be effective.

- Treat for 6 to 8 weeks; then taper dose over 4 to 6 weeks.
- Drug tolerance is common
- Watch for cardiac side effects (dysrhythmia, postural hypotension, anemia), as well as anticholinergic effects (dry mouth).
- **Children are more susceptible to imipramine overdose than adults. Overdose may be fatal; warn parents to store out of child's reach.**

Desmopressinacetate (DDAVP): Antidiuretic hormone ($70-$116). Use with **children age 6 years and older.**

- 20 to 40 mg intranasally
- Expensive
- Effectiveness controversial
- High relapse rate
- Helpful for short-term use (e.g., camping trips)

Referral

Refer for any anatomic abnormalities. Once UTI has been ruled out, children with chronic enuresis should have a thorough urological workup simultaneously with behavioral therapy.

EVALUATION/FOLLOW-UP

Primary enuresis

- Telephone contact in 2 weeks to check progress
- Return visit in 1 month
- Continue follow-up at 2- to 4-week intervals; phone calls and office visits may alternate

Secondary enuresis

- Individualized counseling contract
- Initial follow-up at least every 10 to 14 days
- If placed on medication, should be seen monthly
- If UTI, follow up after antibiotics are completed

SUGGESTED READINGS

Arvin AM et al, editors: *Nelson's textbook of pediatrics,* ed 15, Philadelphia, 1996, WB Saunders.

Boynton RW, Dunn ES, Stephens GR, editors: *Manual of ambulatory pediatrics,* ed 3, Philadelphia, 1994, JB Lippincott.

Dershewitz PA, editor: *Ambulatory pediatric care,* ed 2, Philadelphia, 1993, JB Lippincott.

Ellsworth AJ et al: *Mosby's 1998 medical drug reference,* St Louis, 1998, Mosby.

Groothuis JR et al, editors: *Current pediatric diagnosis and treatment,* ed 12, Norwalk, 1995, Appleton & Lange.

Healthcare Consultants of America, Inc: *1998 Physician's fee and coding guide,* Augusta, Ga, 1998, Healthcare Consultants of America, Inc.

Epididymitis

ICD-9-CM

Nonvenereal 604.90
Acute 604.99
Chlamydial 099.54
Gonorrheal 098.0
Recurrent 604.99

OVERVIEW

Definition

Epididymitis is an infectious process of the epididymis.

Incidence

There are two different etiologies, with males under 40 most susceptible for sexually transmitted disease as agent. Males age 40 and older usually have associated urinary tract infection or prostatitis. Gram-negative rods are the causative agent.

Pathophysiology

The organism travels through urethra to the ejaculatory duct, then down to the vas deferens to the epididymis.

Protective Factors Against

Condoms
Frequent sexual intercourse after age 40

Factors Increasing Susceptibility

Unprotected sex
Benign prostatic hypertrophy

SUBJECTIVE DATA

History of Present Illness

Acute swelling of epididymis and groin
Pain
Recent history of sexual activity, heavy lifting, or trauma
Urethral discharge
Dysuria

Past Medical History

Sexually transmitted disease
Mumps (may cause epididymitis)

Medications

Anticholinergics

Family History

Not significant

Psychosocial History

Long-distance bike rider (increases incidence of prostatitis)

Associated Symptoms

Fever and chills

OBJECTIVE DATA

Physical Examination

Genitalia
- Pain in scrotum radiating along spermatic cord or to flank during palpation
- Extremely tender to touch
- Erythema
- Swelling of scrotum
- Prostate may be tender
- Urethral discharge

Laboratory Tests

CBC ($13-$16): Leukocytosis and a left shift
Gram stain of urethral discharge ($15-$19): Gram-negative

Table 69-1 Differentiating Testicular Torsion and Epididymitis

	Torsion	Epididymitis
History	Previous episode common	Recent sexual activity
Pain	Sharp, sudden onset	Gradual onset
Fever	Absent	Present
Edema	Elevated testis (in order to assess this, stand at the foot of the client's bed and have the patient fold his arms over his chest)	Swollen scrotum
Urethral discharge	Absent	Possible
CBC	Normal	Elevated WBCs
Urinalysis	Normal	Bacteriuria
Testicular scan	Hypoperfused	Hyperperfused
Prehn's sign (amount of pain elicited on testis elevation)	Negative (pain increases)	Positive (pain decreases)

From Kidd P, Sturt P: *Mosby's emergency nursing reference,* St Louis, 1996, Mosby.
CBC, Complete blood count; *WBC,* white blood cell.

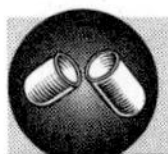

Table 69-2 Pharmaceutical Plan: Epididymitis

Drug	Dose	Comment	Cost ($)
Ceftriaxone	250 mg as single dose IM plus doxycycline	Treat sexual partner	12
Doxycycline	100 mg PO q12h ×10-21 days		6-25
Azithromycin	1 g PO as single dose for nongonococcal urethritis Use 2 g PO as single dose for gonococcal	WBCs present on smear Positive chlamydia culture	16-25
Ciprofloxacin	250-500 mg PO q12h ×21-28 days	Use for nonsexually transmitted disease, gram-negative rods	335
Ofloxacin	300 mg q12h ×10 days	Use for nonsexually transmitted disease, gram-negative rods	384
Trimethoprim/sulfamethoxazole DS (Bactrim)	160/800 mg PO q12h, ×21 to 28 days	Use for nonsexually transmitted disease, gram-negative rods	6-10

IM, Intramuscular.

diplococci (gonorrhea), white blood cells (nongonococcal, probably chlamydia)
Culture of urethral drainage ($31-$39)
Urinalysis ($15-$20): Pyuria, bacteria, hematuria

Radiographic Examinations

Scrotal ultrasound: Hyperperfusion

ASSESSMENT

The most common differential diagnosis is testicular torsion. Table 69-1 illustrates the differences between epididymitis and torsion.

THERAPEUTIC PLAN

Pharmaceutical

Pharmaceutical treatment is outlined in Table 69-2. Pain medication may be ordered for acute phase.

Lifestyle/Activities

Use condoms and limit partners.

Diet

Noncontributory

Patient Education

Elevation/support of testes relieves pain.
Use ice packs to scrotum (be sure and tell patient to use a barrier between the ice and skin) for swelling.
Bed rest is advised during the acute phase.

Family Impact

Not significant

Referral/Consultation

Consider referral to urologist for urinary tract evaluation in cases of gram-negative rod infection.

Follow-up

Repeat culture or urinalysis after antibiotic course.

EVALUATION

Delayed or inadequate treatment may decrease fertility or produce an abscess.

SUGGESTED READINGS

Denman S, Murphy P: Genitourinary infections. In Barker L, Burton J, Zieve P, editors: *Principles of ambulatory medicine*, ed 4, Baltimore; 1995, Williams & Wilkins.

Kidd P: Genitourinary conditions. In Kidd P, Sturt P, editors: *Mosby's emergency nursing reference,* St Louis, 1996, Mosby.

Presti J, Stoller M, Carroll P: Urology. In Tierney L, McPhee S, Papadakis M, editors: *Current medical diagnosis and treatment,* ed 36, Stamford, Conn, 1998, Appleton & Lange.

70 Epistaxis

ICD-9-CM

Epistaxis 784.7

OVERVIEW

Definition

Epitaxis is a nosebleed. Anterior epistaxis occurs in the anterior two thirds of the nose; posterior epistaxis occurs under the posterior half of the inferior turbinate or at the roof of the nasal cavity.

Incidence

Relatively common

Pathophysiology

The nasal septum and nasopharynx are highly vascular structures.

The nose, with its complex interior structure of folds and irregularities, warms and humidifies inspired air.

Bleeding is a result of disruption of the nasal mucosa.

Ninety percent of epitaxis in **children** are anterior nosebleeds that originate in the Kiesselbach's triangle of the anterior portion of the nares.

Anterior nosebleeds are generally considered less severe and are more easily controlled.

Posterior nosebleeds are more brisk; therefore they are considered more severe.

Posterior nosebleeds usually occur from a branch of the sphenopalatine artery.

The most common cause of epitaxis is trauma and inflammation.

Trauma includes nose picking, foreign bodies, and blunt trauma to the nose.

Inflammation can be the result of rhinitis, sneezing, blowing the nose forcibly, dryness from air that is not well humidified, and inhalant drugs and drug abuse.

Other etiologies that are far less common include nasal and sinus neoplasms, systemic diseases such as liver disease, hypertension, and blood disorders.

SUBJECTIVE DATA

History of Present Illness

Bleeding from an anterior epistaxis exits primarily from the anterior nares.

Bleeding from a posterior epistaxis presents with blood in the nasopharynx, mouth, and nares. The patients often presents sitting forward and may have difficulty breathing, swallowing, or speaking because of blood in the mouth and throat.

A foreign body in the nose presents with unilateral, foul-smelling, purulent nasal drainage with possible epistaxis.

Inquire about onset, duration, and quantity of nasal bleeding. Attempt to differentiate unilateral from bilateral nasal bleeding. Ask about trauma.

Inquire about past episodes of nasal bleeding and prior treatment.

Inquire about concurrent sinus problems, upper respiratory symptoms, and allergies.

Inquire about possible obstruction and foreign body.

Past Medical History

Inquire about blood disorders, including anemia, leukemia, clotting abnormalities, thrombocytopenia, or platelet dysfunction.

Inquire about liver disease and hypertension.

Inquire about family history of blood or bleeding disorders, including familial hereditary telangiectasia.

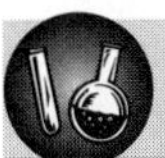

TABLE 70-1 Diagnostic Tests for Recurrent or Severe Epistaxis

Diagnostic Test	Findings/Rational	Cost ($)
Complete blood count with differential, platelets,	Evaluate significant blood loss for anemia.	13-16
PT, and PTT	Evaluate for bleeding disorder.	18-23
Computed tomographic scan (CT scan)	Evaluate for intranasal tumor.	990-1175

PT, Prothrombin time; *PTT,* partial thromboplastin time.

Medication History

Inquire about use of aspirin, nonsteroidal antiinflammatory drugs, and anticoagulation therapy.
Inquire about inhaled drugs and inhalant drug abuse.

OBJECTIVE DATA

Physical Examination

Assess blood pressure and pulse.
Note whether bleeding from one or both nares.
Attempt to visualize site of bleed by the use of a light, suction, and nasal speculum.
Assess for foreign body.

Diagnostic Procedures

Diagnostic procedures are outlined in Table 70-1.

ASSESSMENT

Anterior epistaxis
Posterior epistaxis
Recurrent epistaxis
Epistaxis secondary to systemic illness

Differential Diagnoses

Blood/coagulation disorder
Foreign body
Familial hereditary telangiectasia

THERAPEUTIC PLAN

Management of epistaxis depends on whether the bleeding is anterior or posterior.

Pharmaceutical

Vasoconstrictive drops such as Neo-Synephrine placed on a small piece of cotton and placed in the nose may also be used to control bleeding.

Antibiotics may be indicated if secondary sinusitis develops.

Nonpharmaceutical

An *anterior nosebleed* accounts for 90% of nosebleeds and should respond to the application of pressure to the anterior nasal septum. Tilt the head slightly forward. Apply pressure for 10 to 15 minutes.
Ice may be applied to the nose and lips or around the neck to promote vasoconstriction.
If the site of the bleed is easily visualized, silver nitrate cauterization may be used.
If pressure and cauterization do not control the bleeding, the nose should be packed with 1-inch Vaseline gauze strips impregnated with antibiotic ointment. The packing should remain in position for approximately 3 days.
Posterior nosebleeds account for 10% of nosebleeds and typically do not respond to cauterization and anterior packing. Posterior packing consists of passing a rubber catheter through the nose into the oropharynx and out the mouth, where a sterile gauze pack is tied to the catheter. The catheter is then withdrawn through the nose, and the pack is positioned and secured. A Foley catheter may also be used through the nose and into the oropharynx. When it is inflated and under traction, it creates hemostasis and controls the bleeding. Posterior packing should remain in place 3 to 5 days.

Patient Education

A bedside humidifier, Vaseline to the inside of the nose, and the reduction of trauma from picking or blowing the nose will help reduce recurrence of episodic, anterior nosebleeds.

Consultation/Referral

Anterior nosebleeds nonresponsive to nasal packing and posterior nosebleeds should be evaluated by a physician and/or sent to the emergency department.
Posterior nosebleeds often require hospitalization secondary

to the risk of hemorrhage or hypoxemia from the nasal packing and because of the possibility of infection.

If bleeding persists following posterior packing, surgical intervention may be indicated.

Referral may be indicated to remove a foreign body.

Referral to a otolaryngologist is indicated in cases of suspected intranasal tumors.

Referral to a hematologist is indicated in cases of blood disorders.

EVALUATION/FOLLOW-UP

Depends on the origin of the nosebleed, age of the patient, recurrence of nosebleeds, and systemic involvement

SUGGESTED READINGS

Barbarito C: Hypertension-induced epitaxis, *Am J Nurs* 98(2):48, 1998.

Dunn SA: *Primary care consultant,* St Louis, 1998, Mosby.

Friedman EM: *Ambulatory pediatric care,* Philadelphia, 1988, JB Lippincott.

Graham MV, Uphold CR: *Clinical guidelines in child health,* Gainesville, Fla, 1994, Barnarrae Books.

Healthcare Consultants of America, Inc: *1998 physicians fee and coding guide,* Augusta, Ga, 1998, Healthcare Consultants of America, Inc.

71 Failure to Thrive

ICD-9-CM

Failure to Thrive 783.4

OVERVIEW

Definition

In many ways failure to thrive (FTT) is a symptom rather than an isolated disease. In general, failure to thrive is defined as the patient's weight consistently measuring below the 3rd percentile on standardized growth charts, or a drop in weight across two major growth lines in 6 months or less. FTT is usually differentiated as organic or nonorganic.

Organic failure to thrive refers to a growth failure related to a physiological cause, whereas nonorganic failure to thrive refers to an unexplained growth failure.

Incidence

Failure to thrive occurs in **children younger than 5 years old;** the average age at diagnosis is 16 weeks. Five percent to 10% of all low-birth-weight children are identified as FTT; 3% to 5% of all pediatric hospitalizations are for evaluation of FTT. Approximately 70% of FTT cases have nonorganic causes. Box 71-1 outlines the causes of FTT.

Pathophysiology

FTT occurs when caloric intake is not sufficient to meet the metabolic needs of the child. This lack of adequate nutrition often results in developmental delays, delayed growth, decreased immune response, cognitive delays, and academic failures. Organic causes include medical conditions, such as cleft palate, which can prevent adequate caloric intake; defects in absorption, such as celiac disease; loss of calories, such as in gastroesophageal reflux; increased energy requirements, as in heart or renal disease; and prenatal causes. In nonorganic FTT there is an alteration in the parent-child relationship, resulting in difficulties in feeding and absorption.

Protective Factors Against

Parents who are identified as high-competency parents, displaying such factors as confidence in parenting skills, good interpersonal skills with their infant, and low stress are at low risk for nonorganic FTT in their infants.

Infants identified as being "adaptable," who are full-term, responsive, easy to comfort, and who feed easily are at low risk for FTT.

Factors That Increase Susceptibility

There are a number of parental stressors that predispose a child to FTT. Such parental stressors include:

- Poverty
- Little social support
- Depression or other mental health problems
- Low intelligence
- Substance abuse
- Immaturity (seen frequently in teenage parents)
- Preterm or sick newborns or those with physical deformities
- Parents who have excessive concerns about the infant's fat intake or obesity
- Abnormal feeding practices may also result in FTT

SUBJECTIVE DATA

History of Present Illness

Parents may give a history of their child vomiting frequently, having a decreased appetite, a poor suck reflex, aversive behavior (see Most Common Symptoms, p. 428) or any other trouble with feeding. It is important to elicit a comprehensive feeding history, including:

- Type of formula/food
- How often fed
- Problems with sucking, swallowing, or regurgitation

Box 71-1

Causes of Failure to Thrive

Improper Feeding (50%-90%)	Other Causes (10%-50%)
Economic: 10%-40%	Hypothyroidism
Education (lack of understanding of feeding techniques, adequate diet, etc.): 10%-40%	Cystic fibrosis
Psychological (poor parent-child interaction, emotional or maternal deprivation): 30%-40%	Subdural hematoma
Feeding intolerance: <5%	Celiac disease
	Mental retardation, unspecified
	Brain tumors
	Chronic liver disease
	Congenital heart disease
	Ulcerative colitis

From Barness L: Failure to thrive. In Hoekelman R, editor: *Primary pediatric care*, ed 2, St Louis, 1997, Mosby.

In breastfed infants the clinician needs to determine whether there are any problems with milk supply, including fat content.

Past Medical History

The clinician needs to know the child's birth weight, gestational age, and current weight, length, and head circumference.

A prenatal history is essential, including tobacco or drug use in the mother, other exposure to toxins, and the presence of HIV in the mother. The parent should be asked about any illnesses the child has had since birth and about possible lead exposure.

Sometimes parents will give a history of presumed food allergies.

The infant may have had a history of vomiting, diarrhea, lead exposure, and/or parasite exposure.

The child's stool patterns should be reviewed.

Medications

Maternal medication use or sedation during labor may contribute to FTT.

Family History

Family history is an important part of the diagnosis to help identify children with familial short stature. Heights and weights of parents, grandparents, and siblings may indicate genetic growth aberration. Other family history of malabsorption problems, such as cystic fibrosis, lactose intolerance, or other inborn errors of metabolism, may help identify organic causes for FTT. Furthermore, the childhood history of the parents may be important; parents who give a history of being poorly parented themselves are at high risk for having FTT infants.

Psychosocial History

The psychosocial aspects of the parent-child bond are probably the most important factors to consider in nonorganic FTT. The clinician needs to consider whether anything has disrupted the parent-child bond, such as maternal illness, separation of the infant from the mother, or financial stressors or other factors that impair attachment behavior.

Diet History

A diet history will be essential to determine caloric intake; a 24-hour diet recall may be helpful, but a 3- to 7-day food intake diary is usually recommended. Parents may have difficulty recording intake, in which case there may be some benefit in hospitalizing the child to record an accurate calorie count.

Description of Most Common Symptoms

Parents often describe children who have FTT as demonstrating aversive behaviors, especially in respect to eating. The infant may not suck well, may turn away from the bottle, or may spit up excessively. FTT infants usually have poor eye contact, are difficult to cuddle, or may cry or whine frequently and are difficult to comfort.

Associated Symptoms

FTT infants may have frequent diarrhea or vomiting.

OBJECTIVE DATA

Physical Examination

A complete physical examination should be done, with particular attention to:

General appearance: Measure height/length, weight, head circumference; may see a gradually declining height/length.

Head/eyes/ears/nose/throat: Assess for oral defects, thyroid enlargement, status of fontanelles (open or closed).

Cardiovascular: Listen for murmurs.

Gastrointestinal: Note whether abdomen is abnormally protuberant.

Musculoskeletal: Assess for signs of muscle wasting and other evidence of malnourishment. There may be decreased fat pads in the cheeks; the buttocks may be

TABLE 71-1 Common Findings in Infants with Inorganic Failure to Thrive

Age (months)	Findings
0-6	Prematurity
	Neonatal illness or anomaly necessitating early separation
	Feeding difficulties
	Height and weight below third percentile for age
	Unresponsiveness and withdrawal
	Watchfulness, little smiling
	Delayed socialization and vocalization
	Irregular sleep patterns
	Developmental delays
6-12	Absence of stranger anxiety
	Rumination
	No displeasure at separation
	Apathy/passivity
	Delayed milestones, such as sitting and standing
	Muscular hypotonia
12-18	Indifference to caregivers
	Small physical size
	Delayed dentition
	Little vocalization
	Little eye contact
	Intense watchfulness
	Repetitive self-stimulation behavior (rocking, head banging)

Adapted from Silva F, Needleman R: Failure to thrive: mystery, myth and method, *Contemp Pediatr* 10:114-133, 1993.

wasted and there may be poor muscle tone in the extremities.

Neurological: Assess hypotonia, gag and swallow reflexes, muscle strength, and sensation, and deep tendon reflexes.

Observe the parent/child interaction

Performing the Denver Developmental screening will help to identify developmental delays.

It will also be helpful to observe feeding of the infant whenever possible.

Table 71-1 outlines common findings in FTT.

Diagnostic Procedures

Before a diagnosis of nonorganic FTT is made, diagnostic tests are used to rule out possible organic causes for poor weight gain (Table 71-2).

ASSESSMENT

Differential Diagnosis

Chiefly the differential diagnosis must differentiate physiological or organic causes from nonorganic causes. The diagnosis is made based on poor progression on the growth chart. In FTT, the infants "fall off" the growth chart in respect to weight, with height being near normal until late in the disease and with no significant change in head circumference.

Tables 71-3 and 71-4 and Figure 71-1 outline differential diagnoses for FTT.

THERAPEUTIC PLAN

Pharmaceutical

There are no drugs indicated for FTT unless underlying disease is found.

Lifestyle/Activities

Every attempt should be made to enhance parent-child attachment.

Parents must be followed closely in the home to observe feeding behaviors and parent-child interaction and to promote bonding.

The child may need hospitalization to provide for nutritional needs.

When the child is hospitalized, the child will receive improved nutrition, but in addition, the parent needs instruction and encouragement in feeding the child and in developing parenting skills.

Diet

The diet must include adequate caloric intake to allow for "catch-up" growth.

This involves increasing the caloric intake by calculating the amount of kcal/kg/day based on the age of the child. This can be done by dividing the average caloric requirement for age by the child's percentile of median weight for age.

Caloric Needs in Children

0-6 months: 108 kcal/kg/day
6-12 months: 98 kcal/kg/day
1-3 years: 102 kcal/kg/day

Patient Education

Parents need to know how to feed without introducing extra air, how often to burp the baby, the average daily number of ounces of formula needed, and the types and amounts of

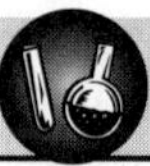

Table 71-2 Diagnostic Tests: Failure to Thrive

Test	Finding/Rationale	Cost ($)
CBC, ESR	Rule out anemia, or inflammation, hematological or collagen disorders	18-23, 16-20
Lead level	Rule out lead poisoning	41-51
Sweat-chloride screening	Rule out cystic fibrosis	16-20
Electrolytes, BUN, creatinine, U/A	Rule out renal disorders, adrenal disorders, dehydration	23-30/lyte 17-21/BUN 18-24/Cr 12-16/U/A
Growth hormone	Pituitary disease	58-74
Fasting blood glucose	Diabetes, adrenal disorders, glycogen storage disease, pituitary insufficiency or excess	16-20
Albumin	Chronic malnutrition, protein losing enteropathy	18-23
Calcium, phosphate, phosphatase	Rickets, thyroid and parathyroid insufficiency of excess	18-23/Ca; 19-24/ phosphatase;
Thyroid panel	Rule out hypothyroidism	47-61
Stool samples	Rule out cystic fibrosis	19-24/qual; 66-83/quan
TB, HIV	Rule out TB and HIV as causes for FTT	15-19/ PPD; 41-52/HIV
X-ray evaluation	Identify pulmonary disease, old fractures, and bone age (abuse) or GI problems	Varies

BUN, Blood urea nitrogen; *CBC,* complete blood cell count; *ESR*; erythrocyte sedimentation rate; *FTT,* failure to thrive; *GI,* gastrointestinal; *HIV,* human immunodeficiency virus; *PPD,* purified protein derivative; *TB,* tuberculosis; *U/A,* urinalysis.

Table 71-3 Why Isn't This Baby Growing?

Age at Onset	Diagnostic Considerations
IUGR, prematurity	Especially in symmetrical IUGR, consider prenatal infections, congenital syndromes, teratogenic exposures (anticonvulsants, alcohol)
Neonatal (0-3 mo)	Incorrect formula preparation; failed breastfeeding; neglect; poor feeding interactions; metabolic, chromosomal, or anatomical abnormality (less common); GERD; cystic fibrosis
3-6 mo	Underfeeding (possibly associated with poverty), improper formula preparation, milk protein intolerance, oral motor dysfunction, celiac disease, HIV infection, cystic fibrosis, congenital heart disease, GERD
7-12 mo	Autonomy struggles, overly fastidious parent, oral-motor dysfunction, delayed introduction of solids, intolerance of new foods
After 12 mo	Coercive feeding, highly distractible child, distracting environment, acquired illness, new psychosocial stressor (divorce, job loss, new sibling, death in the family)

Adapted from Silva F, Needleman R: Failure to thrive: mystery, myth and method, *Contemp Pediatr* 10:114, 1993; and Bauchner H: Children with special health needs. In Nelson W et al, editors: *Nelson textbook of pediatrics,* ed 15, Philadelphia, 1996, WB Saunders.
GERD, Gastroesophageal reflux disease; *HIV,* human immunodeficiency virus; *IUGR,* intrauterine growth retardation.

TABLE 71-4 Differential Diagnosis: Failure to Thrive

Diagnosis	Supporting Data
IUGR	Poor maternal weight gain, drug/alcohol ingestion during pregnancy
Malabsorption	Fatty stools, glucose-positive stools, flatulence, intestinal discomfort
Infectious disease	Giardia, parasites in stool Chronic bacteriuria
Cleft palate	Choking when eating, cyanosis when eating
GERD	Excessive vomiting, abnormal barium swallow
Dwarfism	Family history of very short stature
Inadequate calorie intake	Formula mixed wrong Frequently giving water, juice Excessive parental concerns about obesity

GERD, Gastroesophageal reflux disease; *IUGR,* intrauterine growth retardation.

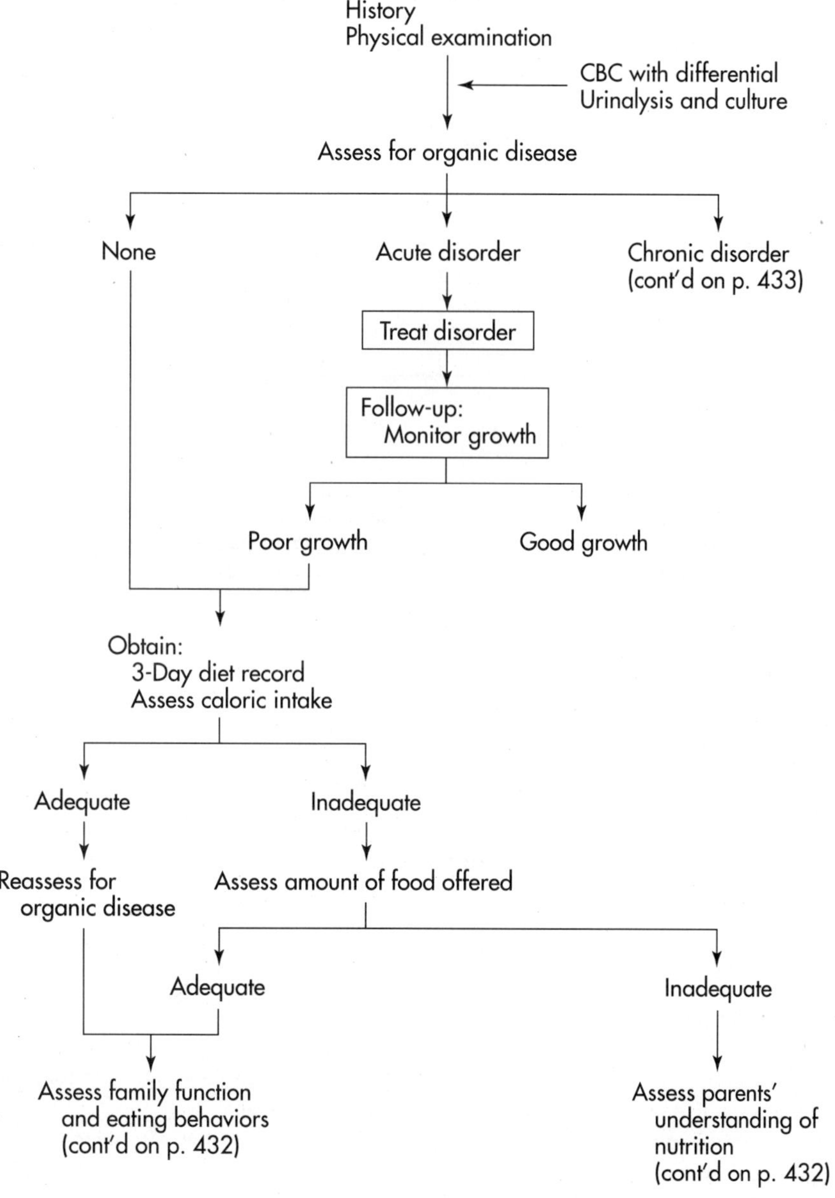

Figure 71-1 Algorithm for a patient with growth deficiency or failure to thrive. *BUN,* Blood, urea, nitrogen; *CBC,* complete blood count; *CT,* computed tomography; *GI,* gastrointestinal; *HIV,* human immunodeficiency virus; *WIC,* women, infants, children. (Adapted from Berman S: *Pediatric decision making,* ed 3, St Louis, 1998, Mosby.)

Continued

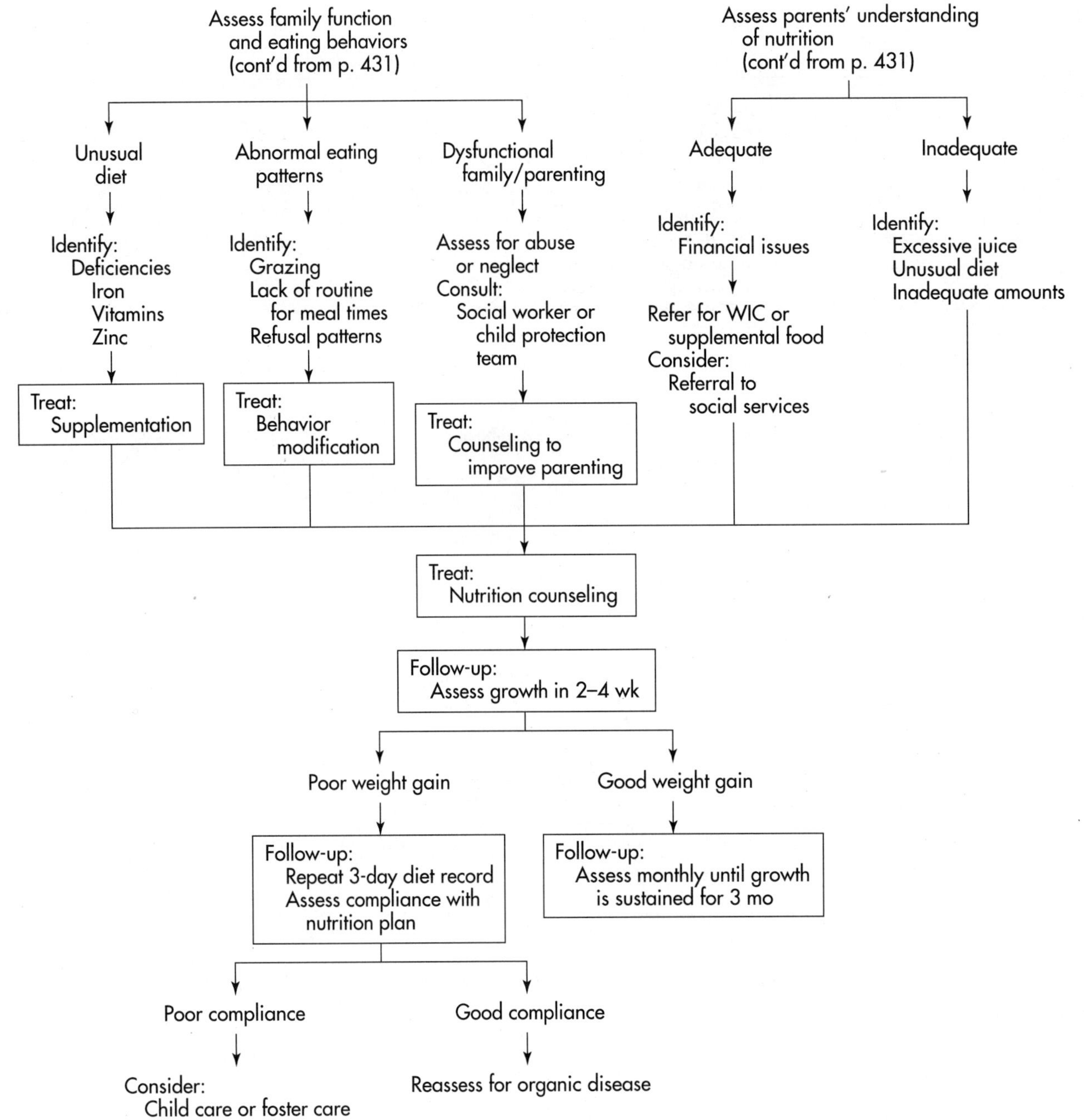

Figure 71-1, cont'd For legend see p. 431.

other food required. The parents should demonstrate how to prepare the formula they plan to use—concentrate, premixed, powder. A multiple vitamin with zinc and iron is usually recommended. Parents will need further education about how to comfort their baby, normal infant behaviors, normal child nutrition and development and the community resources available, and these facts should be reinforced at each subsequent visit.

Family Impact

FTT is a total family condition, with disruption in normal parent-child bonding; therefore the impact on the family is significant.

It is important that efforts to alter feeding behaviors and interactions with the child be directed toward all caregivers, including both parents, involved grandparents, or other extended family members, including significant others.

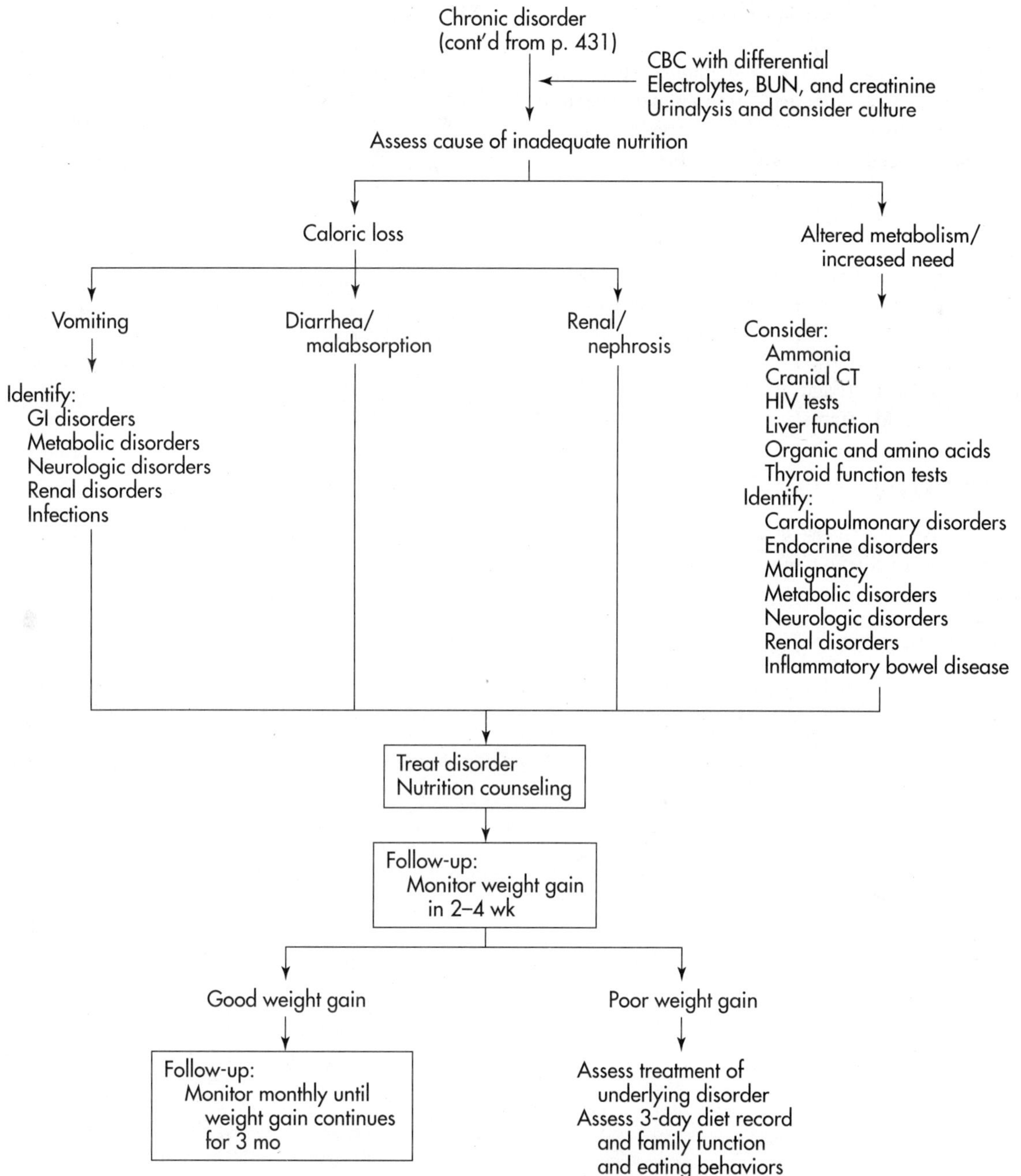

Figure 71-1, cont'd For legend see p. 431.

Furthermore, anything that can be done to strengthen family unity may play a direct role in resolution of the FTT condition.

Referral

Home health referral is frequently needed to ensure that the family has adequate resources and support to carry out the plan of care.

Referral should also be made to WIC (Women, Infants, Children) clinics and to social services to determine the financial help needed.

Referral to a nutritionist may also be helpful.

Referral to Children's Protective Services may be appropriate if FTT is due to maternal neglect.

Consultation

Children with obvious signs of malnutrition or those unresponsive to efforts to increase growth should be evaluated in conjunction with the physician regarding the need for hospitalization.

FTT in the first year of live is ominous. Most brain growth occurs in the first 6 months. Approximately one third of children with nonorganic FTT are developmentally delayed and have social and emotional problems.

Follow-up

The child with FTT must be followed frequently. Although early efforts to improve growth are often successful, the parent may not be able to sustain these efforts over time. There is a high rate of relapse in FTT. The child should be followed weekly at first and then monthly for several months until the child returns to a normal growth curve.

EVALUATION

Evaluation of the effectiveness of interventions will be based on the child's achieving normal growth and development parameters.

SUGGESTED READINGS

Burns C: *Pediatric primary care,* Philadelphia, 1996, WB Saunders.

Frank D, Silva M, Needleman R: Failure to thrive: mystery, myth and method, *Contemp Pediatr* 10:114-133, 1993.

Ellsworth A et al: *Mosby's 1998 medical drug reference,* St Louis, 1998, Mosby.

Hay W et al: *Current pediatric diagnosis and treatment,* ed 13, Norwalk Conn, 1997, Appleton & Lange.

Healthcare Consultants of America, Inc: *1998 Physicians fee and coding guide,* Augusta, Ga, 1998, Healthcare Consultants of America, Inc.

Lobo ML, Barnard KE: Failure to thrive: a parent-infant interaction perspective, *J Pediatr Nurs* 7:251-260, 1992.

Lopez R: Clinical health problem: failure to thrive, *J Am Acad Nurse Pract* 9:489-495, 1998.

Merenstein R: *Pediatric handbook,* Philadelphia, 1994, WB Saunders.

72 Fatigue

ICD-9-CM

Fatigue 300.5
Chronic Fatigue Syndrome 780.71

OVERVIEW

Definition

Fatigue can be classified as acute or chronic. Acute fatigue is normal or expected tiredness, which is intermittent and serves a protective function. Symptoms are localized, rapid in onset, and short in duration. Chronic fatigue (chronic fatigue syndrome [CFS]) is unusual and extreme tiredness with an unknown function. It has a cumulative effect and is greater than one month in duration.

Fatigue can also result from hypermetabolic causes, such as cancer, hyperthyroidism or Cushing's disease or hypometabolic diseases, such as Addison's disease or hypothyroidism.

Incidence

Incidence is unknown, but CFS is more common in females. It affects individuals of all ages and is not dependent on socioeconomic status.

Pathophysiology (CFS)

Latest research suggests the presence of low-molecular-weight 2-5A–dependent ribonuclease (Rnase) L results in inability to maintain cellular energy. Low red blood cell mass has also been associated with decreased oxygen-carrying power of the blood.

SUBJECTIVE DATA

History of Present Illness

A person with CFS will have minor but noticeable (by the patient) cognitive changes. These changes may include choosing inappropriate words and forgetfulness. Physical symptoms include joint pain, night sweats, sore throat, and swollen glands.

The description of fatigue is very important. It is unexplainable, persistent, relapsing with a definite onset, not alleviated with rest, reduces normal functioning significantly, and it is described as peripheral or muscular fatigue. Ask about duration of the symptoms; persistent fatigue lasting longer than a month needs a more comprehensive workup.

Women: In a woman of childbearing age, ask the date of her last menstrual period and her method of contraception. (Fatigue may be among the first indicators of pregnancy.) Postpartum fatigue is common for at least 6 weeks after delivery.

Children: Children often present with changes in activity level.

Past Medical History

Sleep disorders may produce fatigue. Insomnia may indicate substance abuse, and further questioning may be needed.

Repeated infections, in conjunction with sexual history (in children, a history of parental sexual and/or drug use) may suggest the need for human immunodeficiency virus testing. Acquired immunodeficiency syndrome symptoms appear, on average, 18 months after the initial infection, but dormant periods of 1.9 years may occur in children under 4 years of age. Previous treatment for hyperthyroidism may produce fatigue from hypothyroidism.

Medications

Antihypertensive agents, drugs with anticholinergic effects, antidepressants, and antihistamine drugs, pain medications, antianginal agents, and anticonvulsants, among many other medications, may cause fatigue.

Family History

A family history of chronic health problems should be elicited.
Certain anemias (e.g., sickle cell) and autoimmune diseases (e.g., lupus erythematosus) have familial tendencies.

Psychosocial History

Depression is associated with fatigue and may be triggered by loss of a job, friend, family member, or self-esteem. Psychosocial assessment should include:

- Work history
- Past or current substance abuse
- Psychiatric disorders
- Support networks
- Sexual activity and function
- Exercise/recreational activities
- Coping skills
- Relaxation techniques used
- Significant life changes

Diet History

Poor nutrition, especially inadequate protein intake, can lead to muscular fatigue with activity.

Associated Symptoms

Systemic disease will manifest other symptoms than just fatigue.
If the patient complains of shortness of breath, consider a renal, hematological, or cardiac origin.
If the patient complains of weight loss, consider infection, tumor, or hypermetabolism.
If weight gain has occurred, consider hypothyroidism and renal disease.
Bleeding may indicate a hematological or gastrointestinal origin.

OBJECTIVE DATA

Physical Examination

A complete physical examination is indicated with a chief complaint of fatigue. Particular attention should be placed on assessment of the thyroid gland, lymphatic system, heart, lungs, neurological system, and abdomen.
Baseline vital signs including weight, height, and temperature should be obtained.

Diagnostic Procedures

First level tests should include complete blood cell count (CBC), thyroid-stimulating hormone (TSH) or T_4, urinalysis, serum or urine pregnancy test (if indicated), Epstein-Barr serology, and blood glucose levels.
High-risk patients should be tested for syphilis, HIV, and tuberculosis.
If the patient is at geographical risk, a Lyme disease titer may be helpful.
If the fatigue is severe, these additional tests should be ordered: Chest x-ray evaluation, electrocardiogram, and panels for electrolytes, calcium, BUN, creatinine, and liver function.
Obtain a mammogram, Pap smear, fecal occult blood test, and sigmoidoscopy if these tests have not been performed recently and are age appropriate.
Table 72-1 outlines diagnostic tests to evaluate a complaint of fatigue.

ASSESSMENT

Differential diagnoses include anemia, thyroid dysfunction, adrenal gland dysfunction, heart or lung disease, liver disease, diabetes, tuberculosis, opportunistic infection, autoimmune disease (rheumatoid arthritis, lupus), multiple sclerosis, and myasthenia gravis (Table 72-2).

Chronic Fatigue Syndrome

Major Criteria

Fatigue lasting at least 6 months that is unrelieved with bed rest
Fatigue severe enough to reduce average daily activity by at least 50%

Minor Criteria

Mild fever or chills
Sore throat
Lymph node pain in anterior or posterior cervical or axillary nodes
Unexplained general muscle weakness
Myalgia
Prolonged fatigue (more than 24 hours) after previously tolerable levels of exercise
New generalized headaches
Migratory noninflammatory arthralgia
Sleep disturbance
Neuropsychological symptoms (photophobia, transient visual scotomata, forgetfulness, excessive irritability, confusion, difficulty thinking, inability to concentrate, depression)

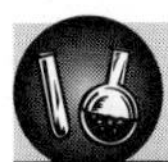

TABLE 72-1 Diagnostic Tests: Fatigue

Symptoms	Clinical Findings	Test	Cost ($)
Fatigue, palpitations, SOB	Skin: Pale skin, sclera, and mucous membranes	CBC	13-16
	Chest: Irregular heartbeat or tachycardia	Reticulocyte count	15-19
		Peripheral smear	11-14
		ECG	56-65
Fatigue, recent weight gain or loss, intolerance to temperature changes	Skin: Dry, scaly, loss of body hair or edematous extremities and face	CBC	13-16
	Eyes: Exophthalmos	TSH	56-65
	Neck: Enlarged thyroid gland with or without nodules	T_3 level	46-58
	Chest: Bradycardia or tachycardia	T_4 level	24-29
		ECG	56-65
Fatigue only, lasting >4 wk	No abnormal findings	**First-Level Tests**	
		CBC	13-16
		TSH	56-70
		U/A	14-18
		Serum or urine HCG	16-20
		Glucose level	57-72
		Epstein-Barr	N/A
		Second-Level Tests	
		T_4	24-29
		CXR	77-91
		Comprehensive metabolic panel	32-42
		ECG	56-65
		Liver profile	29-41

CBC, Complete blood cell count; *CXR*, chest x-ray evaluation; *ECG*, electrocardiogram; *HCG*, human chorionic gonadotropin; *N/A*, not available; *TSH*, thyroid-stimulating hormone; *SOB*, shortness of breath; *U/A*, urinalysis.

Physical Criteria

Documented on at least two occasions at least 1 month apart:
- Low-grade fever
- Nonexudative pharyngitis
- Palpable or tender anterior or posterior lymph nodes

THERAPEUTIC PLAN

Treatment depends on the selected diagnosis. If the patient has CFS, it is usually not possible to treat all of the patient's symptoms. Have the patient prioritize the top concerns he or she wants treated.

Pharmaceutical

For CFS, multivitamins, sleep medication, pain management, and antidepressants are frequently used. When prescribing antidepressant medications consider the following, Tricyclic antidepressants are more likely to produce fatigue but they may help with sleep. Serotonin selective reuptake inhibitors are the best choice for depression (refer to the depression chapter for dosing information). Benzodiazepines are sedating. Naproxen, Ibuprofen, and Piroxicam are the preferred NSAIDs for treating the accompanying joint pain (refer to the NSAID dosing guide in Appendix J).

Lifestyle/Activities

Regular exercise, with gradual increase in intensity based on symptoms.

Massage therapy for comfort and muscular fatigue.

Patient Education

If CFS is diagnosed, stress to patient that it is not fatal, symptoms will improve over time, and that relapses and remissions are to be expected.

Have the patient keep a diary of symptoms and bring it to the next visit. The patient should include the effect of fatigue on daily activities, sleep patterns, and diet. Fatigue should be rated on a standardized scale each day.

Fatigue can be measured using standardized scales. Commonly used scales include the Pearson Byars Fatigue Feeling Checklist, the Rhoten 10 point fatigue scale, Piper's fatigue scale, visual analog fatigue scale, and the Fatigue relief scale.

TABLE 72-2 Differential Diagnosis: Fatigue

Diagnosis	Supporting Data
Iron-deficiency and hemorrhagic anemia (refer to Chapter 11 for treatment)	CBC results RBC Children <3.8 million/mm^3 Adult men <4.7 million/mm^3 Adult women <4.2 million/mm^3 Hematocrit Children <31% Adult men <42% Adult women <37% Hemoglobin Children <11 g/dl Adult men <14 g/dl Adult women <12 g/dl
Iron-deficiency anemia	Reticulocyte count <0.5% Peripheral smear: Microcytic, hypochromic
Hemorrhagic anemia	Reticulocyte count >2% Peripheral smear: Macrocytic
Hypothyroidism (see Chapter 178 for treatment)	TSH >10 μU/ml with decreased T_4 (primary hypothyroidism) Decreased TSH with decreased T_4 indicates a pituitary disorder (secondary hypothyroidism) T_4 Adults <4.5 μg/dl Children: Varies by age; refer to laboratory indices
Hyperthyroidism CFS (see Chapter 178 for treatment)	T_4 >11.5 μg/dl To be diagnosed with CFS the patient must have the two major criteria and eight minor criteria or two major criteria, six minor criteria, and two physical criteria (see pp. 436 and 437)

CBC, Complete blood cell count; *CFS,* chronic fatigue syndrome; *RBC,* red blood cells, *TSH,* thyroid-stimulating hormone.

Referral

It may be appropriate to refer the fatigued patient to a psychiatrist or counselor for depression/substance abuse or somatization. Suicide rates are higher among CFS patients than in the normal population. Sleep testing may be indicated.

Follow-up

Schedule a return visit for 2 to 3 weeks.

EVALUATION

Suggest the patient bring a significant other to the next visit for another's appraisal of how fatigue is affecting the patient.

RESOURCES

There are two sources of information for CFS:

The American Association for CFS
c/o Harborview Medical Center
325 Ninth Ave.
Box 359780
Seattle, WA 98104
206-521-1932
debrap@u.washington.edu

Centers for Disease Control and Prevention
888-232-3228
http:www.cdc.gov/ncidod/disease/cfshome.htm

SUGGESTED READINGS

Boynton R, Dunn E, Stephans G: *Manual of ambulatory pediatrics,* Philadelphia, 1994, JB Lippincott.

Ellsworth A et al: *Mosby's 1998 medical drug reference,* St Louis, 1998, Mosby.

Farrar D, Locke S, Kantrowitz F: Chronic fatigue syndrome. 1: Etiology and pathogenesis, *Behavioral Med* 21:5-16, 1995.

Healthcare Consultants of America, Inc: *1998 Physicians fee and coding guide,* Augusta, Ga, 1998, Healthcare Consultants of America, Inc.

Kantrowitz F, Farrar D, Locke S: Chronic fatigue syndrome 2: Treatment and future research, *Behavioral Med* 21:17-24, 1995.

Kroenke K, Schultz A, Yager J: When fatigue is the major complaint, *Patient Care* 15:157-167, 1993.

Peters S: CFS: new research zeros in on physical causes, *Adv Nurse Pract* 6:71, 1998.

Ruffin M, Cohen M: Evaluation and management of fatigue, *American Family Physician* 50:625-632, 1994.

Siegel R, Melby J: Fatigue: the role of adrenal insufficiency, *Hosp Pract* 15:59-71, 1994.

73 Fever

ICD-9-CM

Fever 780.6

OVERVIEW

Description

A fever is a symptom and is considered a nonspecific response to a number of infectious and noninfectious disease processes:

The normal body temperature is considered 98.6° F orally.

There is a normal diurnal temperature variation with the body temperature being lowest in the morning and highest in the late afternoon.

There is a slight sustained rise in the body temperature following ovulation during the menstrual cycle and in the first trimester of pregnancy.

Mild elevations of body temperature can also be caused by exercise, excessive clothing, a hot bath, or hot weather.

Warm food or drink can elevate an oral temperature.

Teething can be associated with a slight temperature but does not cause fever over 101.1° F (38.4° C).

Definition

The following temperatures are defined as febrile:

Rectal or aural temperature over 100.4° F (38° C)

Oral temperature over 99.5° F (37.5° C)

Axillary temperature over 98.6° F (37° C)

Fever of unknown origin (FUO) is defined as fever over 100.9° F (38.3° C) for 3 weeks in adults and 1 week in children in which the diagnosis is not apparent after 1 week or more of studies.

See the sample flow sheet at the end of this chapter.

Classification

Low fever: Oral reading of 99° to 100.4° F (37.2° to 38° C)

Moderate fever: Oral reading of 100.5° to 104° F (38° to 40° C)

High fever: Oral reading over 104° F (40° C)

Fever over 108° F (42.2° C) causes unconsciousness, and if sustained, leads to permanent brain damage. Infectious diseases rarely cause the body temperature to exceed 106° F (41.1° C), except for central nervous system infections, when the body's ability to regulate temperature is impaired.

Incidence

Febrile illnesses during the **first 3 months of life** are uncommon, but frequently serious. Bacterial infections account for approximately 20% of these febrile illnesses, with 50% of these being serious. Viral illnesses account for 40% of febrile illnesses.

Fever in **early childhood (3 to 24 months),** on the contrary, is quite common. Twenty-six percent of sick visits to pediatricians and 55% of sick visits to hospitals are associated with fever.

Pathophysiology

Body temperature is a set point regulated by the hypothalamus.

Fever occurs when bacteria, viruses, toxins, or other agents under phagocytosis by leukocytes and cytokines are released.

Elevation in body temperature results from increased heat production by shivering or decreased heat loss by peripheral vasoconstriction.

Hyperthermia is not mediated by cytokines and occurs when body metabolic heat production or environmental heat load exceeds normal heat loss capacity or when there is impaired heat loss. Heat stroke is an example.

Infection is the most common cause of fever in both **adults and children.**

Table 73-1 Some Acute Nonbacterial Infections for Which Undifferentiated Fever May Be the First Manifestation

Infection	Transmission	Incubation Period (days)	Clinical Features
Chickenpox (varicella)	Person-to-person via respiratory secretions and direct contact; highly contagious	10-21	Malaise and fever precede or occur simultaneously with rash. Rash develops in crops as pruritic maculopapules evolving in hours to vesicles and in days to dried scabs. All stages of rash are seen in the same skin area.
German measles (rubella)	Person-to-person, via respiratory secretions and direct contact; highly contagious	14-21	1-7 day prodrome of malaise, headache, fever, mild conjunctivitis followed by maculopapular (occasionally confluent) rash which begins on forehead and spreads to trunk and extremities.
Leptospirosis (*Leptospira interrogans*)	Reservoir: Wild and domestic animals. Contact of the skin, especially if abraded, or of mucous membranes, with water, moist soil, or vegetation contaminated with urine of infected animals, as in swimming, accidental, or occupational immersion.	4-19	Fever with sudden onset, headache, chills, severe myalgia (calves and thighs), and conjunctival suffusion. Other manifestations that may be present are diphasic fever, meningitis, rash (palate exanthema), hemolytic anemia, hemorrhage into skin and mucous membranes, hepatorenal failure, jaundice, mental confusion/depression, and pulmonary involvement with or without hemoptysis.
Measles (rubeola)	Person-to-person, via respiratory secretions	9-11	3- to 4-day prodrome with fever, malaise, hacking cough, rhinitis, subsiding 1-2 days following onset of maculopapular rash spreading from face to neck to trunk to feet (by third day)
Q fever (*Rickettsia burnetti*)	Spread by airborne rickettsiae in dust contaminated by infected animals (cattle, sheep, goats) or by direct contact with infected animals or their tissue	14-26	Headache, chills, fever, anorexia, myalgias lasting 3 days to 2 weeks. Cough with rales after a few days, persisting after fever remits.
Rocky Mountain spotted fever (*Rickettsia rickettsiae*)	Bite of infected tick or contamination with tick tissues or feces	3-14	Abrupt onset of severe headache, chills, myalgia, fever; rash (second to fourth day of fever)—initially macules on wrists, ankles, palms, soles, extending in 6-12 hours to buttocks, trunk, face; becomes maculopapular by day 2 or 3 and petechial by about day 4, progressing to ecchymoses; rash may be missed on dark skin

From Barker LR, Burton JR, Ziere PD: *Ambulatory medicine,* ed 4, Baltimore, 1995, Williams & Wilkins.

The most common cause is viral but can also be bacterial, rickettsial, fungal, or parasitic (Table 73-1).

In general, **children** tend to have a greater febrile response than **adults. Elderly persons, neonates,** and those receiving medications such as nonsteroidal antiinflammatory drugs (NSAIDs) and corticosteroids may have a less marked or absent febrile response even in the presence of bacteremia.

SUBJECTIVE DATA

History of Present Illness

Ask the patient or family about the following:

Onset, duration, and pattern of fever
Was a thermometer used and by what route?
Hydration, including fluid intake, urination, vomiting, diarrhea
Level of discomfort
Immunization status, recent immunizations, or new medications
Whether family members are ill or have traveled recently
The last dose of antipyretic medication or other self-care measures
For **infants less than 2 months old,** ask about the following:
- Prematurity, maternal illnesses, including a primary herpes infection
- Maternal screenings, including group B *Streptococcus,* premature rupture of membranes
- Prolonged nursery stay with antibiotic treatment
- Ask about an infant smile, which is a useful negative predictor of meningitis

For **children,** ask about the following:
- Child's activity and whether child seems fussy or irritable, more drowsy, or not playing as usual
- Previous episodes of febrile seizures, which affect approximately 4% of children

Past Medical History

Ask about:

Current medications (Box 73-1); previous illnesses and diseases, particularly any cardiac or chronic debilitating disorders—especially immunosuppressive treatments or disorders, infections; trauma; surgery; diagnostic testing; use of anesthesia
Medication allergies

Associated Symptoms

Ask about changes in activity, appetite, chills, headache, nasal congestion, earache, sore throat, cough, abdominal pain, vomiting, diarrhea, painful urination.

OBJECTIVE DATA

Measurement of Temperature

The normal rectal or aural temperature is 0.5° C higher than a temperature measured orally, and the normal axillary temperature is correspondingly 0.5° C lower than the oral temperature.

An aural temperature is considered as accurate as a rectal temperature in **children older than 3 months of age;** rectal temperature measurement is recommended in **infants under 3 months old.**

A rectal or aural temperature is considered more reliable than an oral temperature and an oral temperature is considered more reliable than an axillary temperature.

Types of Thermometers

Glass (with mercury) thermometers are inexpensive, but they record temperature slowly and can be hard to read. The thermometer must be left in place 2 minutes for a rectal temperature, 3 minutes for an oral temperature, and 5 to 6 minutes for an axillary temperature. To ensure the accuracy of an oral reading, no food or drink should be consumed in the proceeding 10 minutes.

Digital thermometers record temperatures with a heat sensor and are powered by a battery. They measure temperature quickly, usually less than 30 seconds and display the reading on a small screen.

Tympanic thermometers are infrared devices that read the temperature of the eardrum in less than 2 seconds. Tympanic measurements are considered as accurate as a rectal reading. They require no undressing, little cooperation, and cause no discomfort.

Other types of thermometers include temperature strips, which are liquid-crystal strips that are applied to the forehead. Paper thermometers are used orally or axillary and are read by assessing the changing color dots.

Temperature-sensitive pacifiers are inaccurate. Tactile temperatures determined by touching the forehead tend to miss mild fevers.

Physical Examination

Measure temperature.
Measure vital signs, including respirations, pulse, and blood pressure.
Observe the general appearance and mental alertness of both adults and children.
Assess the following:
- Quality of the cry of an infant and ability to feed
- Anterior fontanelle of an infant
- Skin for color, rash, petechiae, purpura, dryness, turgor, capillary refill, redness, and warmth
- Nuchal rigidity
- Upper and lower respiratory involvement

Box 73-1

Drugs and Undifferentiated Fever

Hypersensitivity to a drug may result in fever. The fever may begin abruptly or may be delayed by several weeks. However, a drug taken regularly for 3 months or longer is not likely to cause fever. *Urticaria, maculopapular skin rash, and eosinophilia* are common. Chills are uncommon.

The syndrome of *serum sickness* is rare but may follow fever and present as rash, lymphadenopathy, arthritis, nephritis, and edema. The drugs most commonly implicated are barbiturates, methyldopa, penicillin, phenytoin, and sulfonamides.

A *lupuslike syndrome* is characterized by fever, arthralgias, and positive antinuclear antibody (ANA) titers. This may present following the initiation of hydralazine or procainamide.

An elevated temperature can be a result of *altered thermoregulation* which occurs because of a direct effect on the central nervous system. Common drugs are amphetamines, cocaine, or phenothiazines. Drugs with anticholinergic effects can cause decreased heat loss by diminished sweating, especially in high ambient temperatures. Monoamine oxidase inhibitors, excessive thyroid hormone, and cimetidine can elevate temperature by hypermetabolism.

A Herxheimer reaction is a fever due to the *pharmacological action of a drug* and can be seen with the use of penicillin in the treatment of syphilis. Chemotherapy is another example of fever due to the pharmacological action of a drug and is a result of rapid destruction of tumor cells.

Administration-related fever may occur after the intravenous infusion of contaminated fluids with bacterial pyrogens or as a result of phlebitis. Repeated intramuscular injections at the same site can result in an abscess which can cause fever secondary to the release of endogenous pyrogens.

Drugs That Frequently Cause Fever Due to Hypersensitivity

Allopurinol
Amphotericin B
Antihistamines
Atropine
Barbiturates
Bleomycin
Captopril
Cephalosporins
Clofibrate
Ethambutol
Heparin
Hydralazine
Ibuprofen
Iodides, including intravenous contrast media
Isoniazid
Methyldopa
Nifedipine
Nitrofurantoin
p-Aminosalicylic acid
Penicillamine
Penicillins
Phenolphthalein
Phenytoin
Procainamide
Propylthiouracil
Pyrazinamide
Quinidine
Salicylates
Streptomycin
Sulindac
Sulfonamides

Adapted from Barker LR, Burton JR, Zieve PD: *Ambulatory medicine,* ed 4, Baltimore, 1995, Williams & Wilkins, pp 296-297.

Lymphadenopathy
Swollen joints

A complete examination may be indicated (depending on the presenting complaint and age of the patient) to find a localized infection, such as otitis media, pharyngitis, sinusitis, meningitis, or pneumonia. See specific chapters for more information about individual diagnoses.

Diagnostic Procedures

Diagnostic testing depends on the age of the patient, clinical presentation, and previous medical history. In most cases, the history and physical examination will uncover the cause of the fever, which may direct any necessary testing.

However, for patients who do not have an apparent localized infection or have a localized infection but also have one or more of the following:

Are **less than 2 months of age**
Look as if they have toxic condition
Have an extremely elevated temperature
Are immunodeficient
Have an underlying chronic disease

Consider ordering the following tests:

Urinalysis ($14-$18) and culture ($29-$37)
CBC with differential ($13-$16)
Erythrocyte sedimentation rate ($16-$20)
Blood cultures ($37-$45)
Chest x-ray ($77-$91)

Cerebrospinal fluid for culture ($31-$39), cell count/differential, chemistries

Figure 73-1 summarizes the clinical approach for the care of a febrile infant.

ASSESSMENT

Infection is the most common cause of fever and can be viral, bacterial, rickettsial, fungal, or parasitic.

Other differential diagnoses include autoimmune disease,

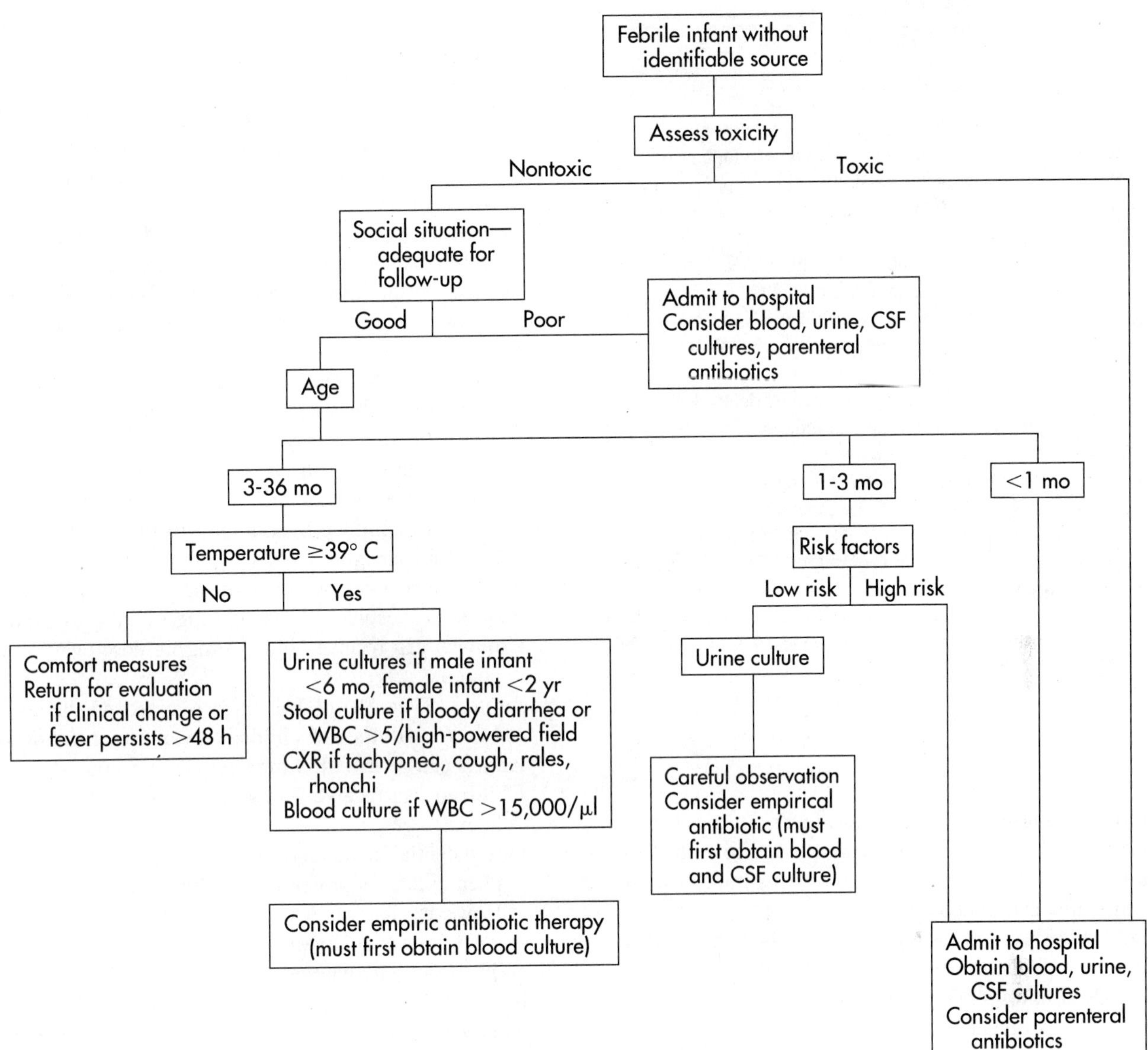

Figure 73-1 Algorithm for the treatment of a febrile infant. *CSF,* Cerebrospinal fluid; *CXR,* chest x-ray evaluation; *WBC,* white blood cell count. (From Baraff LJ et al: Practice guidelines for the management of infants and children 0 to 35 months of age with fever without source: Agency for Health Care Policy and Research, *Ann Emerg Med* 1993:22:1198.)

malignant neoplastic disease, hematological disease, cardiovascular disease, gastrointestinal disease, and endocrine disease.

Drug reactions including serum sickness, neuroleptic malignant syndrome, and malignant hyperthermia of anesthesia are diseases that cause fever as a result of chemical agents.

Central nervous system disease interferes with the thermal regulatory process and presents with fever.

A factitious fever is a fever that is faked by a patient for possible secondary gain.

THERAPEUTIC PLAN

Children and adults with fever who are disoriented, delirious, have meningismus, petechiae, or purpura should be transported to the emergency department immediately by another responsible person or by ambulance.

Children and adults who are immunodeficient or who have cardiac disease or another serious disease also need immediate evaluation, since the heart rate increases about 10 beats/min for every degree Fahrenheit. Respirations also increase.

A consultation with a physician is indicated for **any infant**

Box 73-2

Facts on Bacteremia

- The risk of associated bacteremia in infants with fever is above 50% in cases of cellulitis, adenitis, or omphalitis; 10% to 30% in cases of bacterial enteritis and pneumonia; 10% in cases with UTI; and less than 5% in cases with otitis media.
- The risk of occult bacteremia is 28% in children who appear moderately ill with an abnormal CBC. The rate of bacteremia is 13% in patients with a WBC above 15,000, compared with 2.6% in patients with a WBC between 5000 and 15,000.
- Complications of occult bacteremia include delayed-onset meningitis, periorbital or buccal cellulitis, pneumonia, epiglottitis, septic arthritis, osteomyelitis, and pericarditis.
- The risk of occult bacteremia with a temperature below 102.2° F (39° C) is 0.3%; with a temperature of 102.2° F (39° C) to 104.7° F (40.4° C) is 4%; with a temperature of 104.9° F (40.5° C) to 105.8° F (41° C) is 13%; and with a temperature over 105.8° F (41° C) is 23%.

Adapted from Berman S: *Pediatric decision making,* ed 3, St Louis, 1996, Mosby.

under 2 months of age with fever. In most cases hospitalization is necessary even if the source of the fever is identified because of the risk of dehydration, sepsis, meningitis, and pneumonia.

A **child** with fever needs immediate evaluation under the following circumstances (Hay,1995):
- The **child is under 2 months of age**
- The fever is higher than 104.2° F (40.1° C)
- The child is crying inconsolably
- The child cries when moved or touched
- The child is difficult to awaken
- The neck is stiff
- Purple spots are present on the skin
- Breathing is difficult
- The child is drooling saliva and is unable to swallow food or fluids
- A convulsion has occurred
- The child looks or acts sick

Children with fever **between the ages of 2 months and 2 years** can be treated on an outpatient basis in the presence of a localized, nonserious infection, as long as they are playful, drinking, voiding, and do not appear to have a toxic condition.

Bacteremia is more likely in a child with fever greater than 105° F (40.6° C) and should be considered even if a localized infection is found.

See Box 73-2 on bacteremia; Figure 73-2 illustrates assessment of illness in infants and children.

Pharmaceutical

Antipyretics should be considered:
- When fevers are 102° F (38.9° C) or greater
- In **children** with a history of febrile seizures
- In patients with compensated heart disease or chronic debilitating disorders, patients who become dehydrated easily, or patients who are alcoholic
- In patients who are uncomfortable and cannot rest

Considerations for not treating low to moderate fevers include the fact that antipyretics may mask the signs or symptoms of a serious disease and possibly confuse the clinical picture.

Antipyretics can be toxic in some patients.

In hyperthermic states such as thyrotoxicosis, heat stroke, and overdressing, antipyretics are ineffective. Antipyretics act by lowering the thermal set-point, and in these conditions the thermal set-point has not been changed.

In **adults and children over 2 months of age,** the drug of choice for managing fever is acetaminophen ($2 to $4), which can be given by mouth or suppository (Table 73-2).
- **Adults** can receive 325 to 650 mg every 4 to 6 hours.
- **Children** can receive 10 to 15 mg/kg/dose every 4 to 6 hours.

Ibuprofen ($3 to $9) (Table 73-3) is a second therapeutic choice for **adults** and **children over 6 months of age.**
- **Adults** can receive 400 mg every 6 to 8 hours.
- **Children** can receive 5 to 10 mg/kg/dose every 6 to 8 hours.
- One potential advantage ibuprofen has over acetaminophen is that ibuprofen has a longer duration of action. However, ibuprofen has more side effects including gastrointestinal complications.

Aspirin is an alternative choice for fever management in adults but should not be given to children or adolescents because of the possibility of developing Reye's syndrome.
- Adults can receive 325 to 650 mg every 4 to 6 hours.
- A list of medications containing aspirin can be obtained from the national Reye's Syndrome Foundation.

Patient Education

Parents may need to be instructed on the purpose of fever, the correct method to assess temperature, and when to call the health care provider. Refer to the Instruction Sheet for Parents on Managing Fever on p. 452.

If the child is younger than 3 months, a rectal temperature should be assessed.

If the child is older than 3 months, a rectal or aural temperature is appropriate.

If the child is older than 3 years, an oral temperature can be used.

An axillary temperature is an alternative if the parent is uncomfortable taking a rectal temperature or does not own an ear (aural) thermometer.

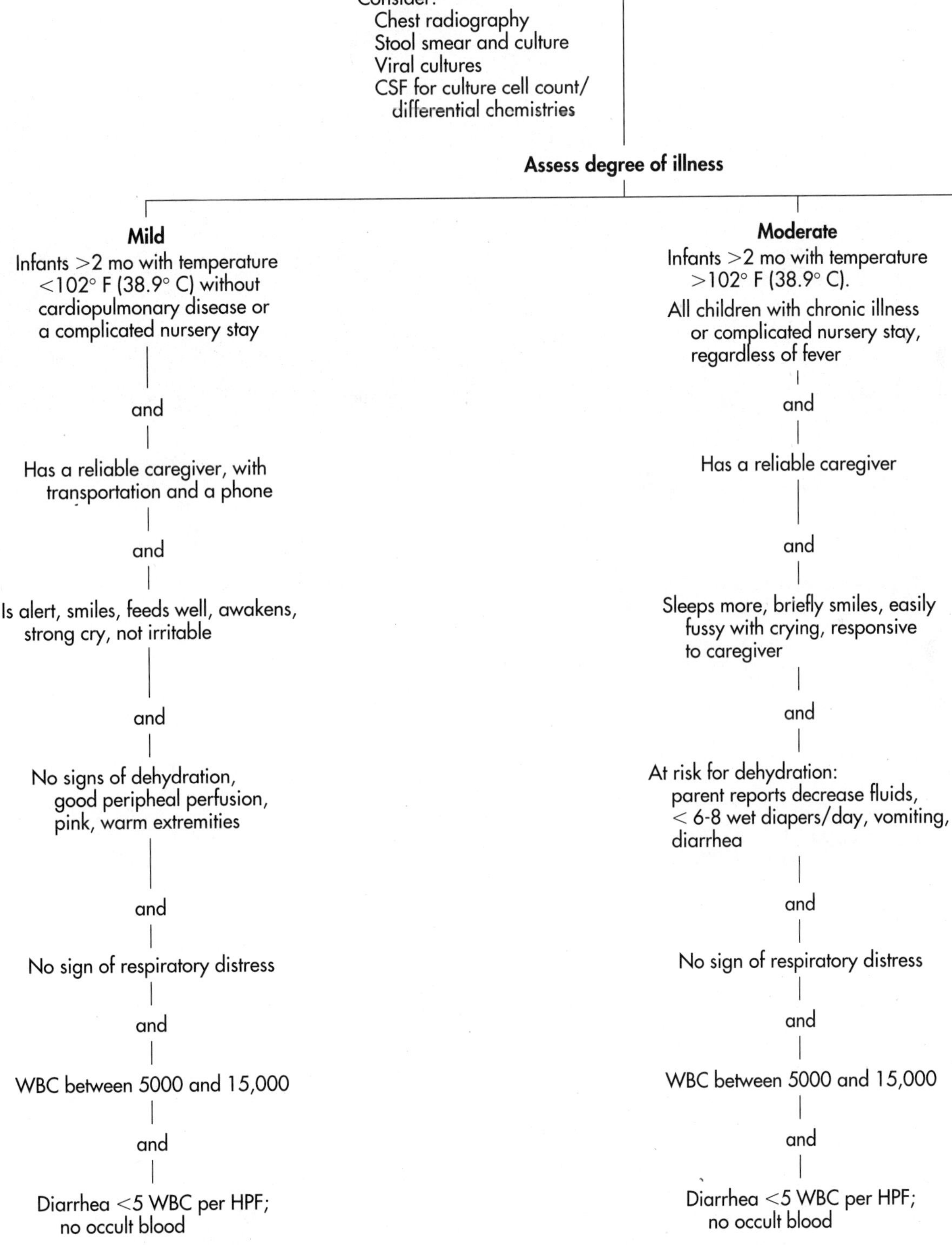

Figure 73-2 Assessing the degree of illness in infants and children with fever. *CSF,* Cerebrospinal fluid; *ESR,* erythrocyte sedimentation rate; *HPF,* high-power field; *WBC,* white blood cell count. (Adapted from Berman S: Pediatric decision making, ed 3, St Louis, 1996, Mosby.)

Continued

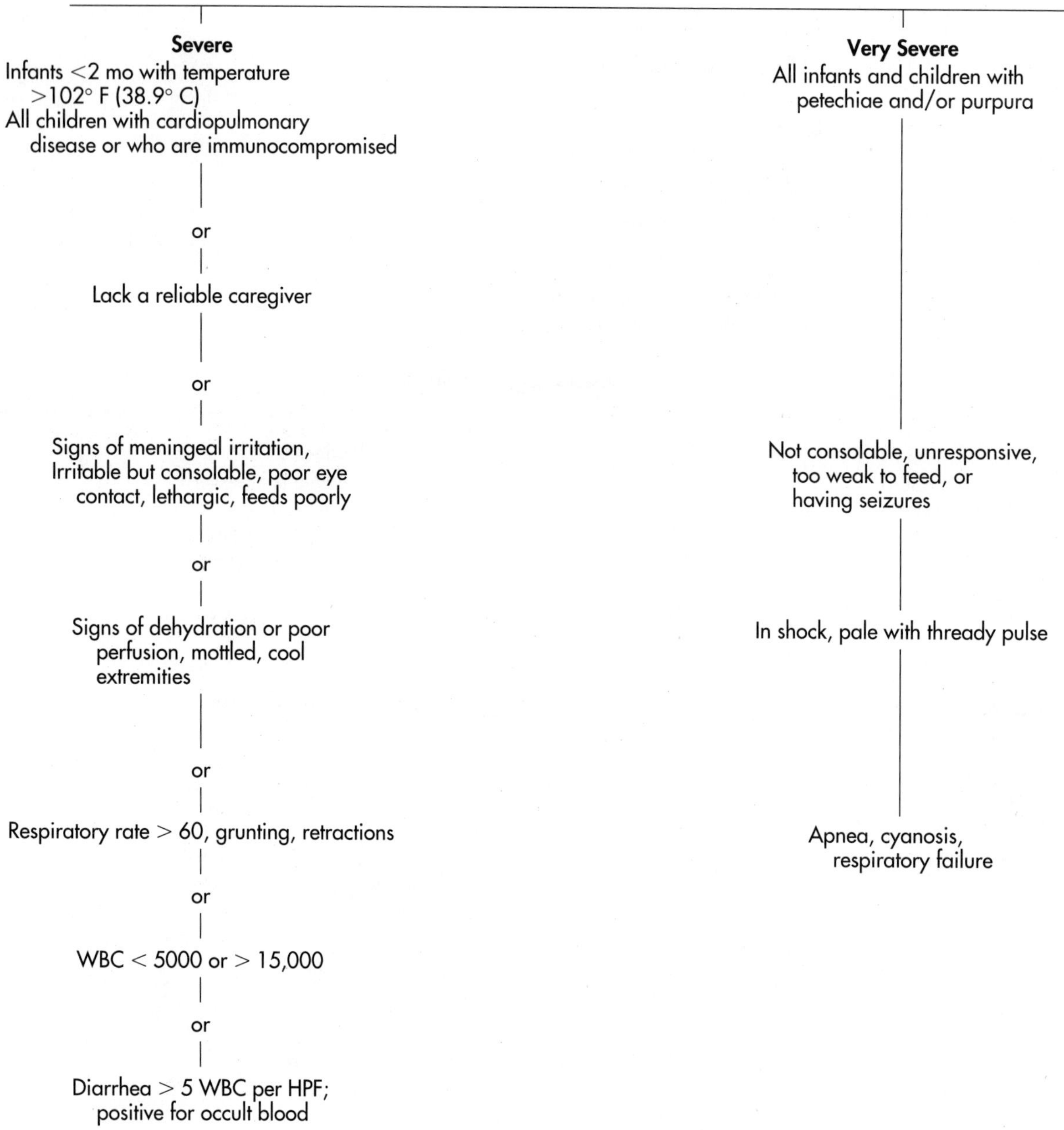

Figure 73-2, cont'd For legend see p. 445.

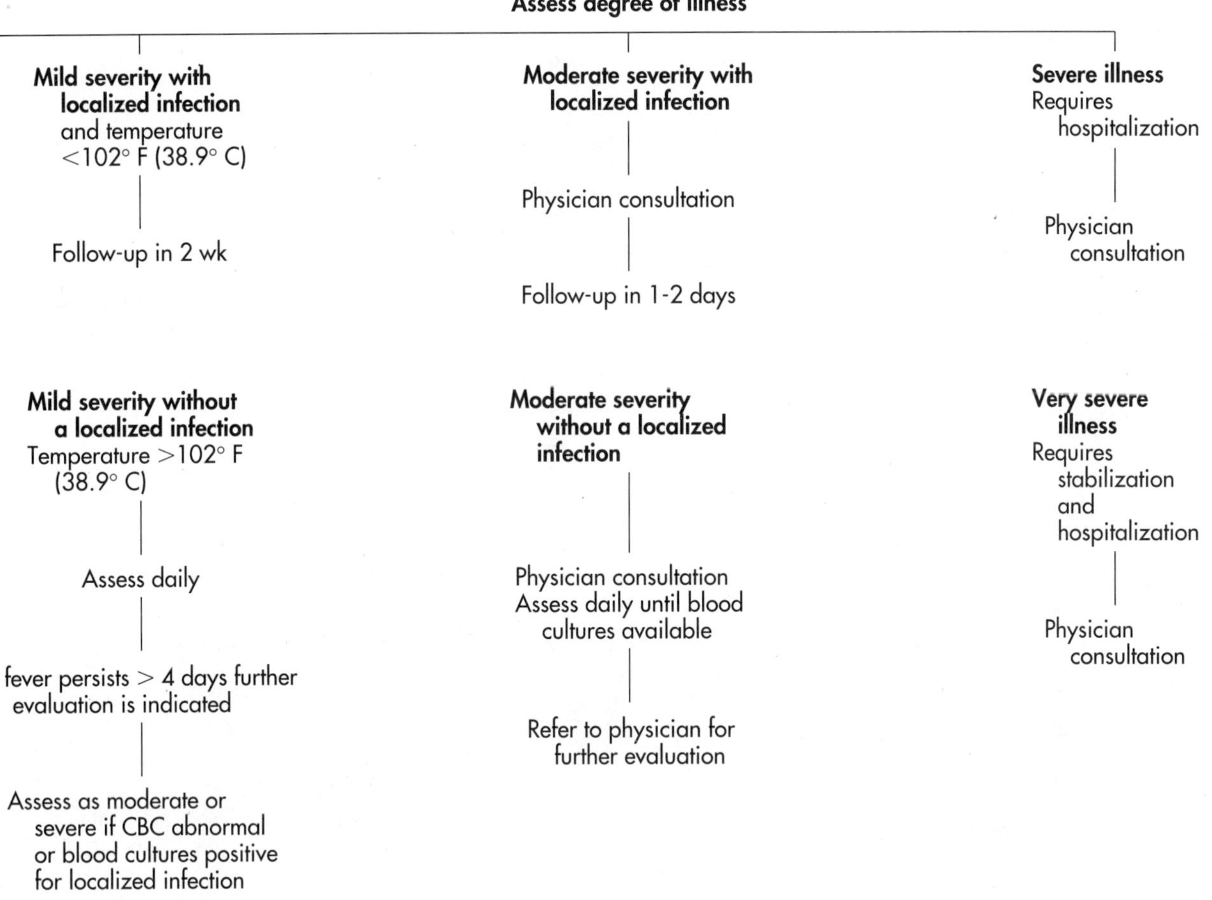

Figure 73-2, cont'd For legend see p. 445.

Teach parents to avoid the use of over-the-counter products that contain aspirin, such as Pepto-Bismol and Alka-Seltzer, when their child has a fever (Box 73-3).

Adults and parents of children should be taught when to administer antipyretics and the correct dose to avoid overdosing and underdosing. Pediatric formulations vary in their concentration. For example, elixir is 160 mg/ml whereas drops are 80 mg/0.8 ml, and chewable tablets are 80 mg each.

Hydration is important and parents should be taught to offer their children fluids every 15 to 30 minutes, depending on the child's condition. Do not withhold formula unless the child is vomiting; then Pedialyte should be substituted.

Older children and adults should also be taught to consume extra fluids when a fever is present.

Daily activities should be modified to provide for rest, light meals, and avoidance of strenuous activities.

Adults should be taught to avoid overdressing and parents should be taught not to overbundle their febrile children.

Indications for sponging with cool to lukewarm water include:

- Any fever greater than 106° F (41.1° C)
- Febrile seizures or delirium
- Patients with severe liver disease who cannot take acetaminophen
- Patients with neurologic problems in which temperature regulation mechanisms are impaired
- Environments with excessive temperatures

Ideally, acetaminophen is given 30 minutes before sponging, except in patients with liver disease. Alcohol is never used for sponging. Sponging should not cause the patient to shiver; shivering only increases body temperature.

Consultation/Referral

Consider consultation with a physician or referral for:

Any febrile infant under 2 months of age

Patients with underlying medical conditions which fever may increase risk for complications

Table 73-2 Acetaminophen Preparations

Recommended Dosage (mg)	Patient Age	Weight		Dosage Range	
		lb	kg	10 mg/kg	15 mg/kg
40	0-3 mo	6	2.7	27	41
		7	3.2	32	48
		8	3.6	36	55
		9	4.1	41	61
		10	4.5	45	68
		11	5.0	50	75
80	4-11 mo	12	5.5	55	82
		13	5.9	59	89
		14	6.4	64	95
		15	6.8	68	102
		16	7.3	73	109
		17	7.7	77	116
120	12-23 mo	18	8.2	82	123
		19	8.6	86	130
		20	9.1	91	136
		21	9.5	95	145
		22	10.0	100	150
		23	10.5	105	157
160	2-3 yr	24	10.9	109	164
		25	11.4	114	170
		26	11.8	118	177
		27	12.3	123	184
		28	12.7	127	191
		29	13.2	132	198
		30	13.6	136	205
		31	14.1	141	211
		32	14.5	145	218
		33	15.0	150	225
		34	15.5	155	232
		35	15.9	159	239
240	4-5 yr	36	16.4	164	245
		37	16.8	168	252
		38	17.3	173	259
		39	17.7	178	266
		40	18.2	182	273
		41	18.6	186	280
		42	19.1	191	286
		43	19.5	195	293
		44	20.1	201	300
		45	20.5	205	307
		46	20.9	209	314
		47	21.4	214	320

10-15 mg/kg/dose q4-6h.

Acetaminophen Preparations

Dosage for **children** is 10-15 mg/kg/dose every 4 to 6 hours.

Dosage for **adults** is 325-650 mg every 4 to 6 hours.

Children 2 months to 12 years may use:

- Infant drops and infant suspension drops, 80 mg/0.8 ml (1 dropperful).
- Children's Elixir and Suspension Liquid, 160 mg/5 ml (1 teaspoon).
- Children's chewable tablets, 80 mg.
- Junior-strength chewable tablets and swallowable caplets, 160 mg.
- Suppository 120 mg (2 grains).

Children 12 years to adult may use:

- Regular-strength tablet or caplet, 325 mg.
- Extra-strength tablets, caplets, gelcaps, or geltabs, 500 mg.
- Extended Relief Caplet, 650 mg.
- Suppository, 325 mg and 650 mg.
- Adult liquid, 500 mg/15 ml.

Contraindications include hepatic dysfunction.

Brand names include Tylenol and Tempra.

TABLE 73-2 Acetaminophen Preparations—cont'd

Recommended Dosage (mg)	Patient Age	Weight		Dosage Range	
		lb	kg	10 mg/kg	15 mg/kg
320	6-8yr	48	21.8	218	327
		49	22.3	223	334
		50	22.7	227	341
		51	23.2	232	348
		52	23.6	236	355
		53	24.1	241	361
		54	24.5	245	368
		55	25.0	250	375
		56	25.5	255	382
		57	25.9	259	389
		58	26.4	264	395
		59	26.8	268	402
400	9-10yr	60	27.3	273	409
		61	27.7	277	416
		62	28.2	282	423
		63	28.6	286	430
		64	29.1	291	436
		65	29.5	295	443
		66	30.0	300	450
		67	30.5	305	457
		68	30.9	309	464
		69	31.4	314	470
		70	31.8	318	477
		71	32.3	323	484
480	11yr	72	32.7	327	491
		73	33.2	332	498
		74	33.6	336	505
		75	34.1	341	511
		76	34.5	345	518
		77	35.0	350	525
		78	35.5	355	532
		79	35.9	359	539
		80	36.4	364	545
		81	36.8	368	552
		82	37.3	373	559
		83	37.7	377	566
		84	38.2	382	573
		85	38.6	386	580
		86	39.1	391	586
		87	39.5	395	593
		88	40.0	400	600
		89	40.5	405	607
		90	40.9	409	614
		91	41.4	414	620
		92	41.8	418	627
		93	42.3	423	634
		94	42.7	427	641
		95	43.2	432	648
640	12-14 yrs	96+	43.6	436	655

Table 73-3 Ibuprofen Preparations

Dosage for **children** is 5-10 mg/kg/dose every 6-8 hours. Maximum dose is 40 mg/kg/day.
Dosage for **adults** is 400 mg every 6-8 hours. Maximum dose is 1.2 g/day for pyrexia.
Children 6 months of age and older may use:

1. Infant oral drops, 40 mg/ml.
2. Chewable tablets, 50 mg or 100 mg.
3. Caplets 100 mg.
4. Suspension or liquid, 100 mg/5 ml.

Age	Weight (lb)	Dosage for Fever Under 102.5° F (tsp)	Dosage for Fever Over 102.5° F (tsp)
6-11 mo	13-17	¼	½
12-23 mo	18-23	½	1
2-3 yr	24-35	¾	1½
4-5 yr	36-47	1	2
6-8 yr	48-59	1¼	2½
9-10 yr	60-71	1½	3
11-12 yr	72-95	2	4
Adult	96-154	2	4

Adults may use:
Ibuprofen tablets, caplets, or gelcaps, 200 mg, 400 mg, 600 mg, or 800 mg.
Contraindications include aspirin or other nonsteroidal antiinflammatory drug allergy, peptic ulcer disease, coagulation therapy.

Brand names include Advil and Motrin

Box 73-3

Aspirin Preparations and Aspirin Combination Preparations*

The dose for adults is 325-650 mg every 4-6 hours. Maximum dosage is 4 g/day.
Adults may use:

1. Regular-strength caplets, 325 mg
2. Extra-strength caplets, 500 mg
3. Extended-strength caplets, 650 mg
4. Low-strength caplets, 81 mg

Contraindications include aspirin allergy, peptic ulcer disease, coagulation therapy, nonsteroidal antiinflammatory drug allergy, or varicella or influenza in children and teenagers, and pregnancy.

*Brand names for aspirin include Bayer and Empirin; brand names for aspirin combination products include BC Powder, Bufferin, Ecotrin, and Excedrin.

EVALUATION/FOLLOW-UP

Follow-up depends on age, diagnosis, clinical presentation, the reliability of the caregiver, and the level of support from friends and family.

For infants, young children, elderly persons, and chronically ill patients, consider a return visit within 24 hours or have telephone contact within 24 hours to reassess the patient's condition.

Instruct patients to return for further evaluation if the fever persists for more than 2 or 3 days.

REFERENCE

Hay WW: *Current pediatric diagnosis & treatment,* ed 12, Norwalk, Conn, 1995, Appleton & Lange.

RESOURCE

National Reye's Syndrome Foundation
P.O. Box 829
Bryan, Ohio 43506-0829
1-800-233-7393
email: reyessyn@mail.bright.net
Fax: 419-636-3366
http:www.bright.net/~reyessyn

SUGGESTED READINGS

Barker LR, Burton JR, Zieve PD: *Ambulatory medicine,* ed 4, New York, 1995, Williams & Wilkins.

Berman S: *Pediatric decision making,* ed 3, St Louis, 1996, Mosby.

Daaleman DO: Fever without source in infants and young children, *American Family Physician* 54(8):2503-2551, 1996. American Academy of Family Physicians, pp.

Ellsworth AJ et al: *Mosby's 1998 medical drug reference,* St Louis, 1998, Mosby.

Grimes D: *Infectious diseases,* St Louis, 1991, Mosby.

Healthcare Consultants of America, Inc: *1998 Physicians fee and coding guide,* Augusta, Ga, 1998, Healthcare Consultants of America, Inc.

Professional guide to signs & symptoms, ed 2, New York, 1996, Springhouse.

Schmitt BD: *Instructions for pediatric patients,* Philadelphia, 1992, WB Saunders.

Tierney LM, McPhee SJ, Papadakis MA: *Current medical diagnosis & treatment,* ed 35, Norwalk, Conn, 1996, Appleton & Lange.

Uphold C, Graham M: *Clinical guidelines in family practice,* Gainesville, Fla, 1994, Barmarrae Books.

Wells N et al: Does tympanic temperature measure up? *Am J Matern Child Nurs* 20:95-100, 1995.

Sample Flow Sheet for Unexplained Fever in Adults

Demographics: Name: ______________________________ Age: __________

HPI:
Onset, duration, concurrent symptoms, prior evaluation

Subjective:
History: Patients with the following illnesses or conditions are at special risk when fever is present.

1. Lymphomas, HIV, or patients receiving therapeutic doses of corticosteroids
2. Valvular heart disease, certain types congenital heart disease (ventricular septal defect, patent ductus arteriosus, coarctation of the aorta), or prosthetic heart valves or vascular grafts
3. Multiple myeloma, surgical splenectomy, or autosplenectomy secondary to sickle cell disease
4. Granulocytopenia
5. Advanced hepatic cirrhosis
6. Intravenous drug users
7. Elderly, diabetes mellitus, alcoholism

Medications: New medications, chronic medications, drug allergies, recent diagnostic testing

Immunizations: Recent immunizations, deficient immunizations

Social History: Family members with recent illness; recent travel to developing countries; employed in day care, school, or college; potential exposure to blood, body fluids; exposure to farm animals such as cattle, sheep, or goats; deer hunters; potential exposure to ticks

Objective
Vital Signs: Temp ________ BP ________ Pulse ________ Resp ________ Weight ________

Physical Examination			**Pelvic Examination**			**Laboratory Results**			
General	☐ nml	☐ abn	External	☐ nml	☐ abn	CBC	☐	PPD	☐
Skin	☐ nml	☐ abn	BUS	☐ nml	☐ abn	UA	☐	Chemistries	☐
HEENT	☐ nml	☐ abn	Vagina	☐ nml	☐ abn	ESR	☐	ASO titers	☐
Thyroid	☐ nml	☐ abn	Cervix	☐ nml	☐ abn	LFT	☐	ANA	☐
Breasts	☐ nml	☐ abn	Uterus	☐ nml	☐ abn	CXR	☐	Monospot	☐
Chest	☐ nml	☐ abn	Adnexa	☐ nml	☐ abn	Guiac	☐	HIV	☐
Heart	☐ nml	☐ abn				Blood culture	☐	RF	☐
Abdomen	☐ nml	☐ abn				________	☐	________	☐
GU	☐ nml	☐ abn				________	☐	________	☐
Extremities	☐ nml	☐ abn				________	☐	________	☐
Neurological	☐ nml	☐ abn							

Comment on abnormal findings

Differential Diagnoses of Unexplained Fever

1. Infection is the most common cause of acute unexplained fever in adults. Most episodes are self-limiting, of viral origin, and resolve without treatment.
2. Certain infections begin with fever then develop diagnostic signs or symptoms after one or several days. Examples include:
   a. Infectious mononucleosis
   b. Viral hepatitis
   c. Varicella
   d. Rubeola
   e. Rubella
   f. Recent HIV
   g. Rocky Mountain spotted fever
   h. Q fever
   i. Lyme disease
   j. Localized bacterial infections
   k. Bacteremic infections
   l. Malaria
   m. Dengue fever
   n. Scrub typhus
   o. Leptospirosis
   p. Viral hepatitis
3. Drug hypersensitivity causes a small portion of unexplained fevers
4. The most common causes of fever lasting more than 3 weeks (FUO) are as follows:
   a. Chronic infections, especially tuberculosis, subacute bacterial endocarditis, chronic osteomyelitis, cytomegalovirus infections, occult intraabdominal abscesses, urinary tract infections, and HIV infection
   b. Collagen-vascular or rheumatic diseases, especially systemic lupus erythematosus, temporal arteritis, rheumatic fever, and rheumatoid arthritis
   c. Certain neoplasms, especially lymphoma, acute leukemia, hypernephroma, hepatoma, pancreatic carcinoma, carcinoma of the lung, and malignancies involving bone
   d. Miscellaneous disorders such as granulomatous hepatitis, hyperthyroidism, drug fever, inflammatory bowel disease, sarcoidosis, thyroiditis, and recurrent pulmonary emboli

Plan

Instruction Sheet for Parents on Managing Fever

1. First of all, do not panic. **Stay calm.** Fever is the body's normal response to infections and plays an important role in fighting them.
2. Know how to take your child's temperature. There are three types of thermometers: glass mercury, digital, and an ear thermometer.
   a. A **glass mercury** thermometer is used for taking a temperature in the rectum, mouth, or under the arm. Shake down the thermometer until the mercury line is below 98.6° F (37° C). If your child is under 3 years old, check a rectal (in the bottom) temperature, which is most accurate. If your child is over 3 years old, you may check a temperature by mouth. An armpit temperature is least accurate but can be used if your child is uncooperative or if you are uncomfortable with taking a rectal temperature. Read a glass mercury thermometer by holding the thermometer horizontally and turn it back and forth until you can see the silver mercury line. Read the number. Always clean a mercury glass thermometer with rubbing alcohol after each use.
   b. A **digital** thermometer can also be used for rectal, mouth, and under the arm temperatures. They measure quickly and display the reading in numbers on a small screen. They are powered by a battery. Digital thermometers have plastic covers which are changed with each use.
   c. **Ear** thermometers are now available for use in the home. They are as accurate as a rectal temperature. Like the digital thermometer, they have small plastic covers that are changed with each use. Place the thermometer in the ear canal and pull up and back on the outside of the ear. It will measure temperature in less than 2 seconds. Ear thermometers are powered by a battery.
3. Relying on touch alone can miss mild fevers. Temperature-sensitive pacifiers are inaccurate.

Rectal Temperatures
Have your child lie on his or her stomach or side. Apply a small amount of petroleum jelly to the tip of the thermometer and insert it into the rectum about 1 inch. Keep one hand on the thermometer and one hand on your child. Leave in place 2 minutes when using a mercury glass thermometer.

Mouth Temperatures
Place the tip of the thermometer under one side of the tongue and toward the back of the mouth. Tell your child to close his or her lips and breathe through the nose. Leave in place 3 minutes when using a glass mercury thermometer. No food or drink for 10 minutes before taking the temperature.

Armpit Temperatures
Place the tip of the thermometer under a dry armpit. The shirt should be removed. Hold your child's arm next to his or her side. Leave in place 5 minutes when using a glass mercury thermometer.

See step 2c above for directions on how to take an ear temperature

4. When telling your doctor or nurse practitioner about your child's fever, do not add or subtract anything. Tell the provider how you took the temperature and the reading you got.
5. Your child has a fever if:
   a. The rectal temperature is over 100.4° F (38.0° C).
   b. The oral temperature is over 99.5° F (37.5° C).
   c. The axillary temperature is over 98.6° F (37° C).

6. Call our office ______________________ immediately if:
   Phone number
   a. Your child is less than 2 months of age.
   b. Your child's fever is over 104.2° F (40.1° C)
   c. Your child is crying inconsolably, especially when you move or touch him or her
   d. Your child is difficult to awaken, will not smile, is too weak to cry, eat, or play
   e. Your child has learned to walk, then loses the ability to stand or walk
   f. Your child's neck is stiff
   g. Your child has purple spots on the skin
   h. Your child is having difficulty breathing or has bluish lips
   i. Your child is drooling saliva and is unable to swallow food or fluids
   j. Your child cries but has no tears, has not urinated in 8 hours, his or her mouth is dry, or the soft spot on the head is sunken
   k. Your child has had a seizure
   l. If your child looks or acts sick
7. The following medications are recommended for your child when he or she has a fever: ______________________

____

8. Fluids are very important when your child has a fever. Do not withhold formula unless your child has vomiting, then give your child Pedialyte.
9. Dress your child comfortably. Do not overbundle your child.

Remember to stay calm:
Check your child's temperature.
Assess for other problems such as sore throat, ear pain, rash, diarrhea, or vomiting.
Lower your child's fever by dressing comfortably and giving acetaminophen or ibuprofen.
Monitor your child's behavior and temperature.

Adapted from the Association for the Care of Children's Health.

74 Fibromyalgia

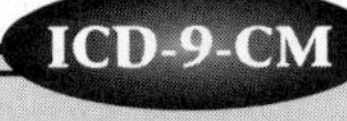

ICD-9-CM

Fibromyalgia 729.1

OVERVIEW

Definition

The American College of Rheumatology's definition of fibromyalgia includes both a 3-month history of widespread pain and pain in 11 of 18 tender points using a digital palpation force of 4 kg.

Incidence

Affects 2% of general population

In internal medicine practices, 5% to 10% of patients are seen for fibromyalgia.

In rheumatology practices, 4% to 20% of patients are seen for fibromyalgia.

Seventy-three percent to 90% are **women.**

The average age is 40 to 60, with the peak incidence between ages 45 to 55.

Pathophysiology

Although there is no clearly documented pathophysiology, there are some abnormalities that may account for the pain, poor sleep, and fatigue observed in fibromyalgia:

Sleep abnormality: Disruption of restorative delta wave stage IV (non-REM) sleep by nonrestorative alpha wave sleep.

Psychological abnormality: Emotional stressors may alter CNS serotonin, which is a chemical mediator of deep sleep and pain perception.

Activity abnormality: Pain and fatigue often result in decreased activity, which increases depression and sleep difficulties, which results in more pain and fatigue.

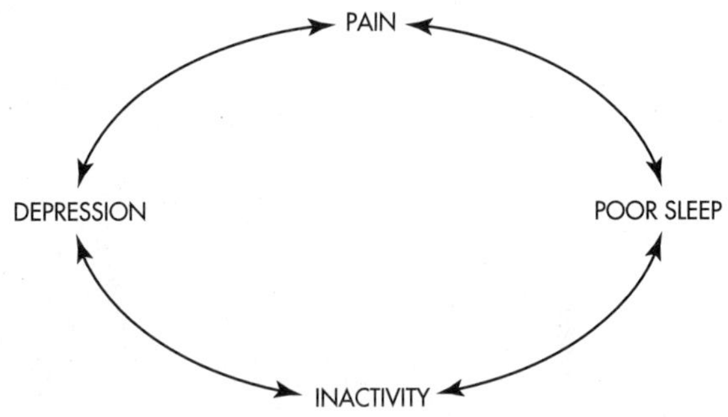

Factors That May Increase Susceptibility

Cold, humid weather

Physical/mental fatigue

Extremes of physical activity (too much/ little)

Stress

SUBJECTIVE DATA

Past Medical History

Major depression: 71% have a current or past history of depression

Rheumatological disorders: Fibromyalgia frequently complicates existing rheumatic disorders

Hypothyroidism: If not well controlled, may mimic fibromyalgia

Chronic fatigue syndrome: Similar symptoms, except fibromyalgia causes more pain

Medications

Previous relief from corticosteroids or NSAIDs (do not usually help with fibromyalgia)

Family History

Inquire about family history of rheumatologic or autoimmune disorders.

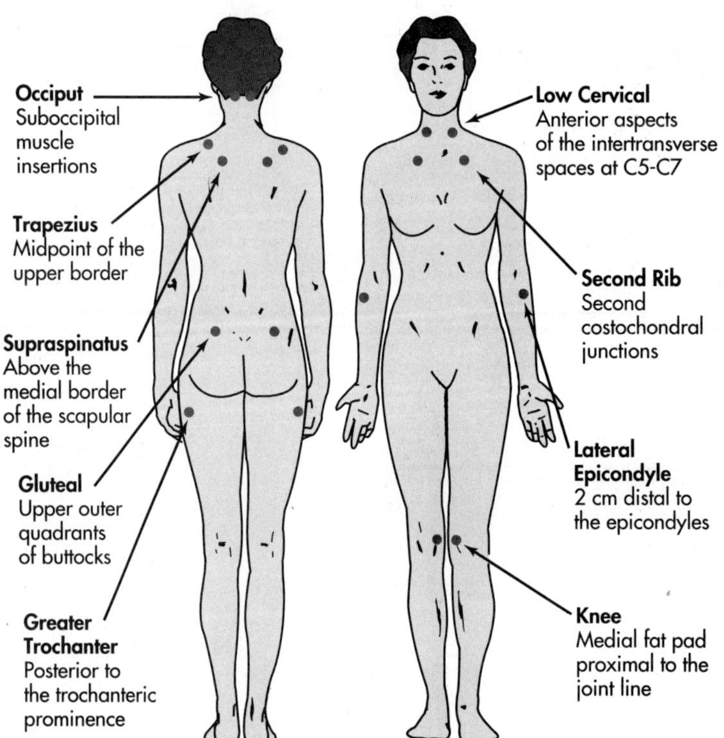

Figure 74-1 Location of specific tender points for diagnostic classification of fibromyalgia. (From Phipps W, Sands J, Marek J: *Medical-surgical nursing: concepts and clinical practice,* ed 6, St Louis, 1999, Mosby.)

Psychosocial History

Is there a functional impairment? (Patients are often unable to perform normal household and work-related tasks.)
Is there a history of depression?
Is there a history of a traumatic event preceding symptoms?

Description of Most Common Symptoms

Pain
- Widespread; must be both above and below the waist and on both right and left sides of body
- Most common areas are axial skeleton (especially cervical and low back), shoulder, pelvic girdles
- Two thirds of patients report pain on palpation all over, not just at tender points
- May result from decreased pain threshold

Sleep abnormality
Ninety percent of patients wake up tired and unrefreshed but may not be aware of a sleeping problem per se
Fatigue: 55% to 100%
Morning stiffness: 76% to 91%
Depression: 26%
Subjective sensation of swollen joints
Headache (migraine, tension)
Raynaud-like symptoms: Pallor, cyanosis, and paresthesias
Irritable bowel or bladder symptoms, or both
Paresthesias
Anxiety
Functional disability (unable to perform work or other tasks secondary to pain/fatigue)

OBJECTIVE DATA

Physical Examination

The physical examination should include manual palpation of tender points, employing a rolling motion with either the thumb or the first two fingers (using 4 kg of pressure). According to the American College of Rheumatology 1990 criteria for the classification of fibromyalgia, pain must be elicited in 11 of 18 tender sites to confirm a diagnosis of fibromyalgia (Figure 74-1):

Occiput: Bilateral, at the suboccipital muscle insertions
Low cervical: Bilateral, at the anterior aspects of the intertransverse spaces at C5 to C7
Trapezius: Bilateral, at the midpoint of the upper border
Supraspinatus: Bilateral, at origins, above the scapula spine near the medial border

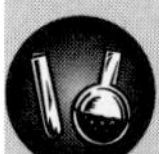

TABLE 74-1 Diagnostic Tests to Help Differentiate Fibromyalgia From Similar Disorders

Differential Diagnosis	Symptoms	Findings	Tests	Cost ($)
Chronic fatigue syndrome	Fatigue > 6 mo with no obvious cause Mild myalgias	No abnormal findings	CBC TSH Electrolytes	13-16 56-70 23-30
Polymyositis	Weakness, rash	Reproducible generalized weakness Dusky, red rash on face, neck, back, and shoulders	First-level tests ESR CPK Second-level tests EMG Muscle biopsy	 16-20 23-29 393-475 N/A
Polymyalgia rheumatica	Pain and stiffness in shoulder and pelvic girdle Age >50 Malaise	Weight loss Fever Decreased ROM, especially of shoulder	CBC ESR ANA RF	13-16 16-20 40-50 22-28
Myofascial syndrome	Pain after acute overload or chronic repetitive stress	Taut, palpable muscle band Local twitch response Trigger points: Firm palpation causes radiation outward	ESR CBC	16-20 13-16
Fibromyalgia	Widespread, aching pain Fatigue Sleep abnormality Morning stiffness	Pain elicited at 11 of 18 tender points without radiation using 4 kg of pressure	First-level tests CBC ESR Basic metabolic panel TSH Second-level tests CPK Serum protein electrophoresis ANA RF	 13-16 16-20 28-39 23-29 56-70 69-87 40-51 22-28

ANA, Antinuclear antibodies; *CBC,* complete blood cell count; *CPK,* creatine phosphokinase; *EMG,* electromyelogram; *ESR,* erythrocyte sedimentation rate; *RF,* rheumatoid factor; *ROM,* range of motion; *TSH,* thyroid-stimulating hormone.

Second rib: Bilateral, at the second costochondral junctions, just lateral to the junctions on upper surfaces

Lateral epicondyle: Bilateral, 2 cm distal to the epicondyles

Gluteal: Bilateral, in upper outer quadrants of buttocks in anterior fold of muscle

Greater trochanter: Bilateral, posterior to the trochanteric prominence

Knee: Bilateral, at the medial fat pad proximal to the joint line

Tender points must be differentiated from trigger points; pressure on trigger points causes radiating pain, which is associated with myofascial syndromes, but not with fibromyalgia.

Physical examination is otherwise negative; there should be no visible swelling or objective weakness unless this is caused by concomitant illnesses. (This is despite subjective complaints of swelling and weakness.)

Diagnostic Procedures

Fibromyalgia is a diagnosis of exclusion. All tests should be negative in the absence of concomitant disease (Table 74-1).

The initial workup should include a complete blood cell count, erythrocyte sedimentation rate, chemistries, and thyroid-stimulating hormone.

If other causes are suspected, perform a creatine phosphokinase test, serum protein electrophoresis, antinuclear antibodies, and rheumatoid factor.

Radiographs may be appropriate if pain is more localized.

ASSESSMENT

Differential diagnoses include rheumatoid arthritis, metabolic myopathies, endocrine disorders (thyroid, parathyroid, and adrenal [most common is hypothyroidism]), polymyo-

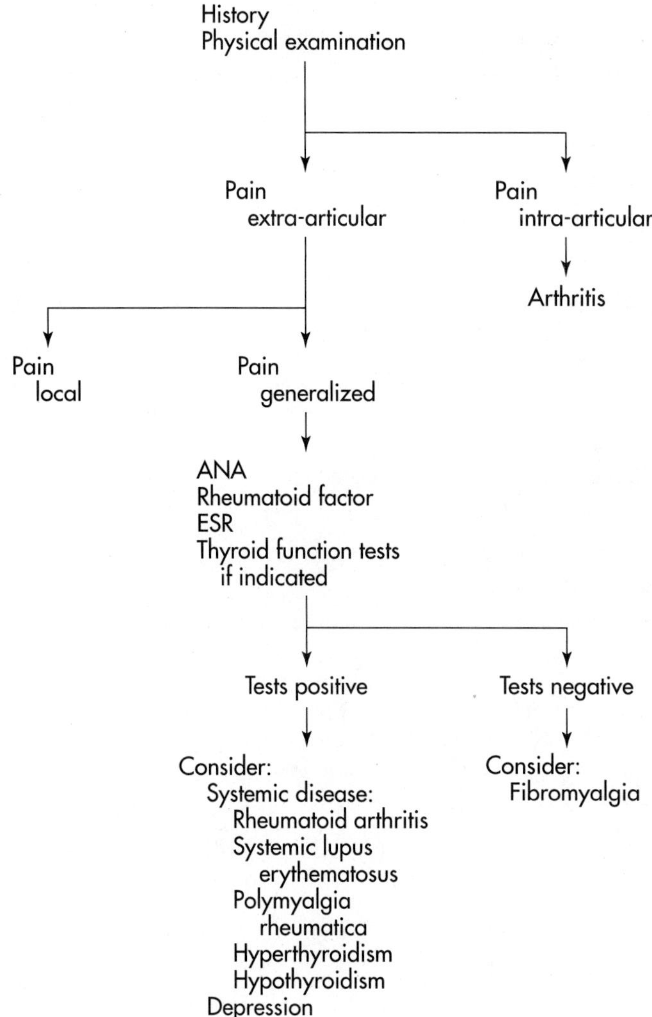

Figure 74-2 Algorithm for a patient with soft tissue pain. *ANA,* Antinuclear antibody; *ESR,* erythrocyte sedimentation rate. (Adapted from Greene HL, Johnson WP, Lemcke D: *Decision making in medicine,* ed 2, St Louis, 1998, Mosby.)

sitis, polymyalgia rheumatica, osteoarthritis, metastatic cancer, myofascial pain syndrome, ankylosing spondylitis, depression/anxiety, disc herniation, connective tissue disease, chronic fatigue syndrome.

Figure 74-2 shows an approach to the patient with fibromyalgia; Table 74-2 lists the differential diagnoses for fibromyalgia.

THERAPEUTIC PLAN

Pharmaceutical

Tricyclics help induce restful sleep and provide nonspecific analgesia for chronic pain:

Cyclobenzaprine (Flexeril) 10 to 30 mg QHS; muscle relaxer with chemical structure similar to that of tricyclic antidepressants (TCAs)

Amitriptyline (Elavil) 10 to 50 mg QHS; NOTE: Nortriptyline and desipramine are safer choices in this category

Doxepin (Sinequan) 10 to 25 mg QHS. If no relief of sleep disorder, may use with caution:

Chlorpromazine (Thorazine) 100 mg QHS

Temazepam (Restoril) 15 to 30 mg QHS (7.5 mg for elderly patients) NSAIDs and corticosteroids are not helpful.

Fluoxetine (Prozac) 20 to 40 mg QD (or another selective serotonin reuptake inhibitors [SSRI] may be used) if there is a depressive component; however, use of SSRIs with a TCA must be monitored *very* carefully. Don't combine unless the patient is under the care of a psychiatrist and TCA blood levels are monitored.

TABLE 74-2 Differential Diagnosis: Fibromyalgia

Diagnoses	Supporting Data
Chronic fatigue syndrome (CFS)	To be diagnosed with CFS, the patient must meet the criteria outlined in Chapter 72 All laboratory test results should be normal
Polymyositis	Elevated CPK ESR only minimally elevated in half of patients EMG—polyphasic potentials, fibrillations, and high frequency action potentials Muscle biopsy—necrosis of muscle fibers with inflammatory cells
Polymyalgia rheumatica	ESR >50 CBC indicative of anemia (males: H/H <42/14; females: H/H <37/12); rapid response to steroid taper
Myofascial syndrome	Trigger points—when pressure is applied, pain is referred distal to these points Quick relief of symptoms with injections of trigger points and stretching of the muscle fibers
Fibromyalgia	Pain elicited at 11 of 18 tender points using 4 kg of pressure

CBC, Complete blood cell count; *CFS*, chronic fatigue syndrome; *CPK*, creatine phosphokinase; *ESR*, erythrocyte sedimentation rate.

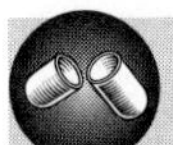

TABLE 74-3 Pharmaceutical Plan: Fibromyalgia

Medications	Precautions	Cost ($)
Cyclobenzaprine (Flexeril) 10-30 mg QHS	Use with caution in patients with urinary retention or closed-angle glaucoma; may have additive toxicity with tricyclic antidepressants	13-100
Amitriptyline (Elavil) 10-50 mg QHS	Contraindicated in pregnancy, lactation, narrow-angle glaucoma, and with MAOIs; anticholinergic side effects; use with caution if urinary retention, hyperthyroidism, hepatic or renal impairment	2-41
Doxepin (Sinequan) 10-25 mg QHS	Contraindicated in narrow-angle glaucoma, with MAOIs; use with caution if urinary retention, cardiovascular disease, hyperthyroidism or pregnancy	4-44
Chlorpromazine (Thorazine) 100 mg QHS	Contraindicated in narrow-angle glaucoma; use with caution if seizures, bone marrow depression, or liver disease are present; avoid prolonged administration	19-175
Temazepam (Restoril) 15-30 mg QHS, 7.5 mg for **elderly** patients	Use with caution in patients with anemia, hepatitis, acute narrow-angle glaucoma, or renal disease, suicidal tendencies, **children** under age 18	3-69
Nortriptyline (Aventyl) 25 mg PO QHS	Contraindicated in acute recovery phase of MI and with concurrent use of MAOIs	17-99
Desipramine (Norpramin) 25 mg PO QHS	Contraindicated in acute recovery phase of MI and with concurrent use of MAOIs	15-49
Fluoxetine (Prozac) 20-40 mg QD	Contraindicated with MAOIs; use with caution if hepatic impairment or seizure disorder	220

MAOI, Monoamine oxidase inhibitor; *MI*, myocardial infarction.

Nonpharmaceutical

Provide reassurance:

Give a name to the symptoms (the patient has probably often been told, "It's all in your head").

Relate symptoms to modifiable factors (stress, sleep, exercise)—gives the patient a sense of control over his or her body and symptoms.

Reassure the patient that fibromyalgia is not a progressive, crippling disease.

Promote exercise: Aerobic exercise for at least 30 minutes, three times per week is essential to overall management.

Refer the patient to support groups, biofeedback programs, relaxation therapy, and a hypnotherapist as appropriate.

Contact the Arthritis Foundation and Fibromyalgia Network for patient education booklets.

Emphasize that the goals are to reduce (not eliminate) pain and sleep disorders. A pharmaceutical plan is outlined in Table 74-3.

EVALUATION/FOLLOW-UP

Since there are no diagnostic tests for fibromyalgia, evaluation must be based on the patient's subjective feeling of decreased pain, fatigue, and stiffness. The examiner should also be able to either elicit fewer tender points or less tenderness at these points.

Follow monthly at first, until some improvement in symptoms is noticed. May then decrease the frequency of visits as symptoms warrant.

It is essential to emphasize the importance of ongoing aerobic exercise because it is the treatment modality that gives the most consistent positive results.

Approach must be very emotionally supportive with the philosophy of collaborating with the patient to individually tailor his or her treatment regimen. No one treatment regimen works for all fibromyalgia patients.

Consult with a physician about additional testing if there is any reason to suspect other disorders.

SUGGESTED READINGS

Bennett RM et al: A comparison of cyclobenzaprine and placebo in the management of fibrositis, *Arthritis Rheum* 31:1535-1542, 1988.

Cunningham ME: Becoming familiar with fibromyalgia, *Orthop Nurs* 15 (2), 33-36, 1996.

Ellsworth A et al: *Mosby's 1998 medical drug reference,* St Louis, 1998, Mosby.

Geel SE: The fibromyalgia syndrome: musculoskeletal pathophysiology, *Semin Arthritis Rheum* 23:347-353, 1994.

Harmon CE: Fibromyalgia: treatments worth trying, *Intern Med* 17:64-75, 1996.

Healthcare Consultants of America, Inc: *1998 Physicians fee and coding guide,* Augusta, Ga, 1998, Healthcare Consultants of America, Inc.

Hench PK: Evaluation and differential diagnosis of fibromyalgia, *Rheum Dis Clin North Am* 15:19-28, 1989.

Johnson SP: Fluoxetine and amitriptyline in the treatment of fibromyalgia, *J Family Practice* 44:128-130, 1997.

Kennedy M, Felson DT: A prospective long-term study of fibromyalgia syndrome, *Arthritis Rheum* 39:682-685, 1996.

Martin L et al: An exercise program in the treatment of fibromyalgia, *J Rheumatol* 23:1050-1053, 1996.

Multicenter Criteria Committee: The American College of Rheumatology 1990 criteria for the classification of fibromyalgia, *Arthritis Rheum* 33:160-172, 1990.

Scudds RA, McCain GA: The differential diagnosis of primary fibromyalgia syndrome (fibrositis), *Intern Med Spec* 9:83-103, 1998.

Tierny LM, McPhee SJ, Papadakis MA, editors: *Current medical diagnosis & treatment,* ed 35, Norwalk, Conn, 1996, Appleton & Lange.

Unger J: Fibromyalgia, *J Am Acad Nurse Pract* 8:27-29, 1996.

White KP, Harth M: An analytical review of 24 controlled clinical trials for fibromyalgia syndrome (FMS), *Pain* 64:211-219, 1996.

Wilke WS: Treatment of "resistant fibromyalgia," *Rheum Dis Clin North Am* 21:247-257, 1995.

Wolfe F: Fibromyalgia: the clinical syndrome, *Rheum Dis Clin North Am* 15:1-16, 1989.

75 Fifth Disease or Erythema Infectiosum

ICD-9-CM

Fifth Disease or Erythema Infectiosum 057.0

OVERVIEW

Definition

Erythema infectiosum is generally a mild illness with few or no symptoms and a characteristic rash. Fifty percent of adults have serological evidence of a previous infection. However, **pregnant women** who contract fifth disease run a 1% to 3% risk of fetal hydrops and subsequent fetal loss. Fifth disease also can result in significant anemia in patients with chronic hemolytic anemia or patients who are immunocompromised.

Pathophysiology

Factors That May Protect Against

Limited exposure to children
Previous infection

Factors That Increase Susceptibility

Children
- Less than school age

Adults
- Women
- Less than 30 years old
- Working in elementary school
- Having school age children at home
- Health care worker caring for patient in aplastic crisis induced by parvovirus B19

Patients at Risk for Complications from Fifth Disease

Pregnant patient without previous infection
Immunocompromised patient
Patient with chronic hemolytic anemia (sickle cell disease, spherocytosis, thalassemia)

Pathogen

The responsible pathogen in fifth disease is human parvovirus B19 (family Parvoviridae). The virus is a single-strand DNA that replicates in erythroid progenitor cells. The replication causes lysis of the cell with a transient anemia.

SUBJECTIVE DATA

History of Present Illness

Ask about the following:
- Current symptoms and duration of symptoms
- If any fever is present
- Presentation of rash and its relationship to any other symptoms
- Exposure to anyone else sick or who has a rash

Past Medical History

Determine whether there is any history of sickle cell disease or other chronic hemolytic anemia.
Is the patient pregnant?
Has the patient had a similar rash in the past?
Is there any history of immunocompromise?

Medications

Is the patient taking any antibiotics or other medications at this time?

Family History

Do any family members have a similar rash?
Is any family member immunocompromised or pregnant?
Does any family member have chronic hemolytic anemia?

Pyschosocial History

Has the patient been exposed to possible allergens, new foods, skin care products, detergents, clothing?
Elicit details about the patient's school attendance or occupation, as appropriate.

Description of Most Common Symptoms

Twenty percent of patients have no symptoms.
Generally, fifth disease presents with low-grade fever, sore throat, headache, and coryza.
A pruritic rash develops after the systemic symptoms resolve. The rash presents as a confluent erythematous "slapped cheek" appearance on the face. It progresses to a fine, erythematous "lacy" rash on the extremities. The rash resolves over 2 to 4 days but often recurs when the patient becomes hot, after bathing, or exposure to sunlight.
Joint pain occurs infrequently in **children.** It affects **women** more often than men. Joint pain generally resolves after 7 to 10 days but may be intermittent for months.

Complications

Chronic anemia (as opposed to transient anemia) may occur in immunocompromised patients.
Aplastic crisis is possible in patients with chronic hemolytic anemia.
Fetal hydrops and fetal death occur in 3% of pregnancies in which the mother is not immune and contracts fifth disease before 20 weeks' gestation.

OBJECTIVE DATA

Physical Examination

A problem-oriented physical examination should be conducted, with particular attention to:
- Vital signs, general appearance
- Skin: Appearance and distribution of rash
- Head/eyes/ears/nose/throat: Mucous membranes normal rather than pale

Diagnostic Procedures

No diagnostic tests are indicated for patients who do not fall in the high-risk category for complications.
Maternal serum alpha-fetoprotein (MSAFP) ($52 to $65) may be a marker for fetal aplastic crisis.

TABLE 75-1 Antibody Interpretation

IgG	IgM	Interpretation
–	–	No antibody detected
–	+	Results indicate recent infection
+	+	Results indicate recent infection
+	–	Results indicate past infection; patient is immune

Serial ultrasonography may be ordered if MSAFP is elevated to detect fetal hydrops.
Evaluation of IgG and IgM ($43 to $54) antibodies can be performed to verify infection in high-risk patients. Table 75-1 outlines interpretation of these results.

ASSESSMENT

Differential Diagnosis

Differential diagnoses (Table 75-2) include:
- Rashes: Scarlet fever, mononucleosis, rubella,* roseola, measles,* other viral exanthema, drug eruptions
- Arthralgias: Rheumatoid arthritis (juvenile or adult), Lyme disease

THERAPEUTIC PLAN

Pharmaceutical

Acetaminophen ($3 to $5) or ibuprofen ($3 to $10) for symptomatic treatment of joint pain or fever
Diphenhydramine ($2 to $16) for itching
Immunoglobulin IV in immunocompromised patients
Blood products may be necessary in severe anemia
Fetal exchange transfusion may be considered

Lifestyle/Activities

The patient is already contagious by the time the rash occurs. The infection is generally not serious, so there is no reason for the patient to stay out of day care or school.

Diet

Not applicable

Patient Education

Avoid contact with **pregnant women.**
Avoid contact with any patient with known chronic hemolytic anemia or an immunocompromised individual.

---

*Both rare because of the measles, mumps and rubella vaccine routinely given in the United States.

TABLE 75-2 Differential Diagnosis: Fifth Disease (Erythema Infectiosum)

Disease	Rash	Location	Symptoms	Timing
Scarlet fever	Flushed face and pinpoint red papules, sandpaper-like rash	Initially on face and trunk then moves to extremities	Strawberry tongue, fever, sore throat, headache	Rash and symptoms occur simultaneously
Mononucleosis	Macular/papular red, morbilliform	Trunk and upper arms; may involve face	Headache, fatigue, sore throat	Rash occurs 4-6 days after symptoms occur
Rubella	Pinpoint to 1 cm oval or round pink macules and/or papules	Begins on face and neck; spreads rapidly to trunk and extremities; rash fades in 24-48 hr	Mild fever, headache, and malaise Enlarged cervical lymph glands	Rash occurs at the height of enlarged lymph glands
Roseola	Pale pink oval macules	Begins on trunk and neck; becomes confluent	*High* fever, with few other symptoms	Rash occurs after fever resolves
Measles	Bright red to purple macules and papules; often becomes confluent	Begins behind the ears; spreads to trunk and extremities	Severe cough, fever, conjunctivitis, photophobia, and Koplik spots	Rash occurs 3-4 days after symptoms present
Fifth disease	Bright red confluent rash; pink to red confluent, lacy	Starts on face; open pattern on extremities	Mild fever, headache, sore throat, coryza	Rash occurs after systemic symptoms have resolved
Drug eruptions	Maculopapular red rash; may become confluent	Generalized; usually spares face	Possibly pruritic rash; symptoms of underlying illness	Rash begins 1-2 wk after starting medication

This is generally a benign infection for most patients.

Good hand washing technique will limit the spread of infection.

Family Impact

Very little, unless a family member has high risk factors.

Referral

Immunocompromised children

Pregnant women should contact their obstetrician regarding testing and further evaluation if they are seronegative (Figure 75-1)

Consultation

Consult a physician regarding any patient with sickle cell disease or other chronic hemolytic anemia.

Follow-up

None needed for healthy patients

Pregnant patients need to follow up with their obstetrician, depending on the results of laboratory tests and ultrasonography.

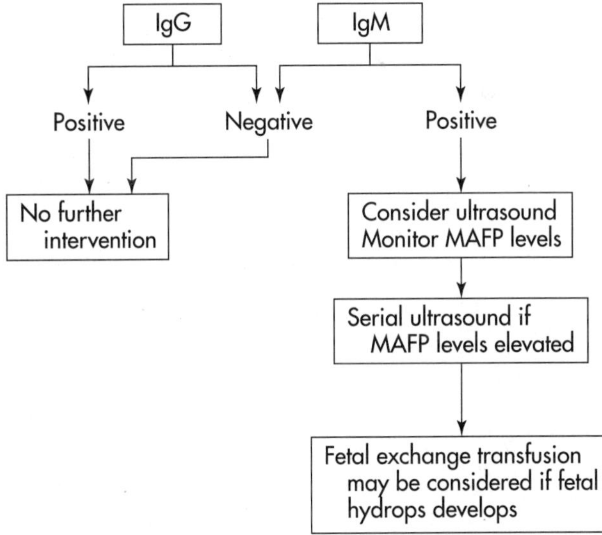

Figure 75-1 Recommendations for pregnant patients exposed to parvovirus B19. (*MAFP,* Maternal serum alpha-fetoprotein.)

EVALUATION

Complete blood count checked periodically for patients who are immunocompromised because these patients may experience chronic anemia following fifth disease.

SUGGESTED READINGS

Adler S et al: Risk of human parvovirus B19 infections among school and hospital employees during endemic periods, *J Infect Dis* 174:361-368, 1993.

Committee on Infectious Diseases, American Academy of Pediatrics: Parvovirus B19, *1997 Red Book,* 1997, pp 383-385.

Ellsworth A et al: *Mosby's 1998 medical drug reference,* St Louis, 1998, Mosby.

Finch C: Human parvovirus B19 in pregnancy, *J Obstet Gynecol Neonatal Nurs* 25:495-498, 1995.

Habif T: Exanthems and drug eruptions, *Clin Dermatol* 14:409-412, 1996.

Healthcare Consultants of America, Inc: *1998 Physicians fee and coding guide,* Augusta, Ga, 1998, Healthcare Consultants of America, Inc.

Jones M et al: Serologic diagnosis of parvovirus B19 infections, *Mayo Clin Proc* 68:1107-1108, 1993.

Kirchner J: Erythema infectiosum and other parvovirus B19 infections, *Am Family Physician* 54:335-340, 1994.

Ryan M, Leichter J: Clinical virology in children, *Am Family Physician* 54:78-84, 1994.

76 Folliculitis

ICD-9-CM

Folliculitis 704.8
Vesiculopustular Rash 782.1

OVERVIEW

Definition

Folliculitis is minor inflammation of hair follicles with or without pustules.

Incidence

More common in men who shave
More common in females who shave perineal and buttocks area

Pathophysiology

Folliculitis has multiple causes:
- Gram-negative folliculitis may occur after treatment of acne with antibiotics.
- Nonbacterial folliculitis may occur from use of oils on the skin.
- Folliculitis may be caused by occlusion.
- May occur as a response to the initiation of systemic steroids or in the tapering of a steroid dose.
- Pseudofolliculitis is caused by ingrown hairs.

Protective Factors Against

Using depilatories
Growing a beard

Factors That Increase Susceptibility

Shaving
Use of hot tubs
Public swimming pools
Use of coconut butter or oils
Tight clothing

SUBJECTIVE DATA

History of Present Illness

Itching
Burning and slight tenderness of area
Outbreak of pimples

Past Medical History

More common in patients with diabetes
Acne

Medications

Antibiotics
Corticosteroids

Family History

Noncontributory

Psychosocial History

Use of hot tubs, public swimming pools

Associated Symptoms

None

OBJECTIVE DATA

Physical Examination

Skin: Pustules of hair follicles, usually in a hairy area, neck, head, face (male), thighs
Inflammation may occur around the area with the skin becoming red and crusting (sycosis) (Figure 76-1)

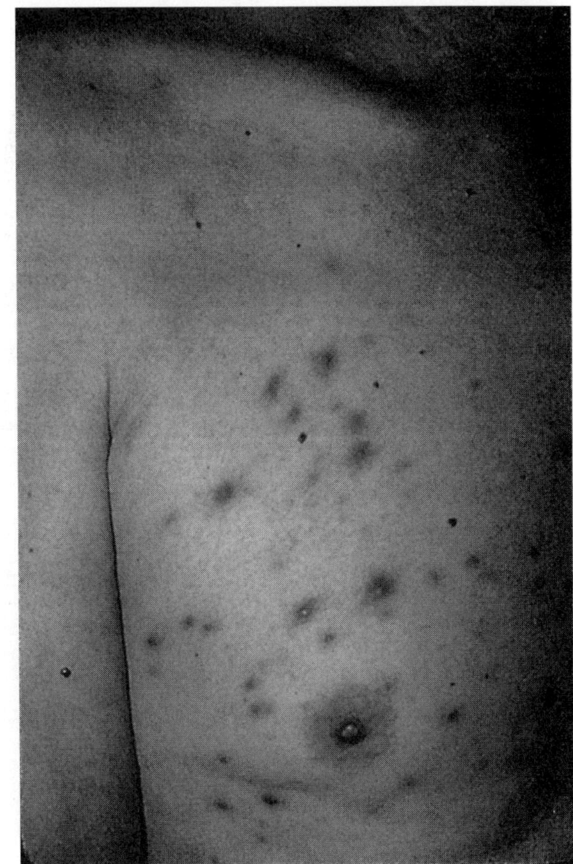

Figure 76-1 Folliculitis of trunk with erythematous papules and pustules. (Courtesy Beverly Sanders, MD. From Goldstein BG, Goldstein AO: *Practical dermatology,* ed 2, St Louis, 1997, Mosby.)

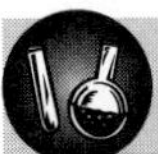

TABLE 76-1 Diagnostic Tests: Folliculitis

Diagnosis	Supporting Data
Acne	Affects mainly adolescents; includes comedones (black and white); hair is usually oily.
Miliaria	Associated with heat and humidity; found in areas of sweat gland concentration (neck, axillae, shoulders, chest); more common in infants and children; greater incidence in summer

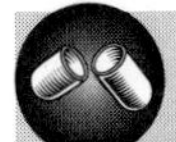

TABLE 76-2 Pharmaceutical Plan: Folliculitis

Drug	Dose	Comment	Cost
Mupirocin (Bactroban) ointment	2%, apply TID for 10 days and cover with DSD		$29/30 g
Clindamycin (Cleocin)	150-300 mg/day		$75-$120
Gentamicin Sulfate cream or ointment 0.1%	Apply to area TID-QID	May be covered with gauze DSD if desired	$4-$16
Isotretinoin	0.5 to 1 mg/kg/day PO in divided doses	Used in treatment of gram-negative folliculitis	$333-$395
3% Clioquinol and 0.5% hydrocortisone lotion or ointment	Apply to area TID or QID	Do not use in or around eyes	$2-$3
Anhydrous ethyl alcohol with 6.25% aluminum chloride	Apply TID before antibiotic ointment		

DSD, Dry sterile dressing.

Diagnostic Procedures

Gram stain ($17 to $21) and culture of pustule

ASSESSMENT

Differential Diagnosis

Differential diagnoses include those listed in Table 76-1.

THERAPEUTIC PLAN

Pharmaceutical

A pharmaceutical plan for the treatment of folliculitis is outlined in Table 76-2.

Lifestyle/Activities

Decrease hot tub use
Decrease swimming in public pools

Diet

Noncontributory

Patient Education

Cleanse areas twice daily with soap containing hexachlorophene.
Avoid minor trauma and irritants to area (cosmetics, abrasive soaps).
Be sure that hot tubs are adequately treated with chlorine.

Family Impact

None

Referral/Consultation

Refer patients with recurrent cases of folliculitis that do not respond well to antibiotics to a dermatologist.

Follow-up

Per flare-up

EVALUATION

Decrease of lesions

SUGGESTED READINGS

Berger T, Goldstein S, Odom R: Skin and appendages. In Tierney L, McPhee S, Papadakis M, editors: *Current medical diagnosis and treatment,* ed 36, Norwalk, Conn, 1998, Appleton & Lange.

Ellsworth A et al: *Mosby's 1998 medical drug reference,* St Louis, 1998, Mosby.

Healthcare Consultants of America Inc: *1998 Physicians fee and coding guide,* Augusta, Ga, 1998, Healthcare Consultants of America Inc.

Pierce N: Bacterial infections of the skin. In Barker L, Burton J, Zieve P, editors: *Principles of ambulatory medicine,* ed 4, Baltimore, 1995, Williams & Wilkins.

77 Gastroenteritis

ICD-9-CM

Gastroenteritis 558.9
Food Poisoning 005.9

OVERVIEW

Definition

Gastroenteritis is a general term for inflammation of the stomach and intestine that results in varying degrees of anorexia, nausea, vomiting, abdominal pain, and diarrhea. A number of specific illnesses are included under the category of gastroenteritis. The most common of these illnesses are viral gastroenteritis, food poisoning, and traveler's diarrhea.

Incidence

The most common cause of dehydration in **children** is vomiting and diarrhea associated with viral gastroenteritis.

Rotavirus is the most common pathogen of viral gastroenteritis in **children,** resulting in an estimated 3.7 million episodes per year in the United States.

Acute diarrhea is responsible for more than 20% of outpatient pediatric visits a year and for nearly 8 of every 100 **infant** hospitalizations.

Traveler's diarrhea is more frequently caused by bacteria and is considered the most common health problem in persons who visit developing countries; an estimated 40% to 60% of visitors to developing countries will develop diarrhea.

The incidence of food poisoning in the United States is unknown.

Pathophysiology

The vomiting and diarrhea of gastroenteritis can result from viral and bacterial infections, food poisoning, food intolerances, excessive intake of alcohol, antibiotics, parasites, altered bowel motility, and malabsorption. Gastroenteritis is predominantly caused by viral and bacterial infections that are transmitted by direct or indirect fecal-oral transmission from an infected person or by contaminated food and water.

Viral pathogens include the rotavirus, Norwalk virus, and adenovirus. Bacterial pathogens include *Salmonella* organisms, *Shigella sonnei, Campylobacter* organisms, *Escherichia coli,* and *Clostridium difficile. Giardia lamblia* is the most common intestinal parasite in the United States.

Resistance to gastroenteritis is provided by the normal bacterial flora of the intestine, the marked acidity of the stomach, and the normal motility of the gastrointestinal tract. When a person has a pathological condition or undergoes a treatment regimen, such as malnutrition or a course of antibiotics, the body's normal bacterial flora are altered, thereby increasing the individual's risk for invasion by pathogens.

Individuals who have a loss of normal gastric acidity, such as those with atrophic gastritis or those who are taking antacids and H_2-receptor antagonists, as well as those who have undergone gastric surgery, are at risk for bacterial gastroenteritis. Other factors that increase susceptibility include age and physical condition.

Pathogens that cause gastroenteritis do so by (1) secretion of an enterotoxin that causes severe inflammation and secretory diarrhea (enterotoxigenic *E. coli*); (2) invasion of the intestinal wall, which causes cellular destruction, necrosis, and possible ulceration (*Shigella* and *Campylobacter* organisms); or (3) mucosal attachment, which results in the destruction of absorptive cells in the intestinal villi (rotavirus). These pathogenic conditions reduce absorption of fluids and electrolytes and increase intestinal motility, resulting in diarrhea and potential fluid and electrolyte imbalances.

SUBJECTIVE DATA

History of Present Illness

The incubation period for gastroenteritis ranges from 12 hours to 10 days, depending on the specific organism involved.

TABLE 77-1 Assessment of Dehydration in Patients with Diarrhea

Assessment Parameter	Mild Dehydration	Moderate Dehydration	Severe Dehydration
General condition	Well, alert	Restless, irritable	Lethargic or unconscious; floppy
Eyes	Normal	Sunken	Very sunken and dry
Tears	Present	Absent	
Mouth and tongue	Moist	Dry	Very dry
Thirst	Drinks normally, not thirsty	Thirsty, drinks eagerly	Drinks poorly or not able to drink
Skin	Pinch retracts immediately	Pinch retracts slowly	Pinch retracts very slowly
Percentage of body weight loss	<5%	5%-10%	>10%
Estimated fluid deficit (ml/kg)	<50 ml/kg	50 to 100 mg/kg	>100 mg/kg

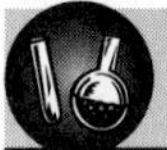

TABLE 77-2 Diagnostic Tests: Gastroenteritis

Diagnostic Test	Purpose	Cost ($)
Rectal swab/stool analysis	Evaluate for bacterial, viral, or parasitic causes	37-45
stool culture	Evaluate for blood and leukocytes	
CBC	Evaluate for bacterial response	13-16
Urinalysis	Evaluate for dehydration	14-18
Basic metabolic panel	Evaluate for electrolyte imbalances	28-39
Serology	Evaluate antibody titers	Cost varies based on organism

CBC, Complete blood count.

Gastroenteritis usually presents as nausea, vomiting, abdominal cramping or pain, and fever. Diarrhea may be present at the onset of illness or may begin the following day.

Inquire about onset of symptoms, duration, number of stools, the presence of blood, hydration, fever, vomiting, and level of discomfort.

For a **child** with symptoms consistent with gastroenteritis, ask about symptoms among classmates and day care. Determine whether other family members are ill.

For an **adult** with symptoms of gastroenteritis, ask about recent social events, recent travel, and water source.

Past Medical History

Ask the patient about his or her general health, past gastrointestinal disorders and surgeries, current medications, recent use of antibiotics, use of laxatives and antacids, and use of alcohol.

OBJECTIVE DATA

Physical Examination

A thorough physical examination should be performed, with attention to:

Height, weight, temperature, blood pressure, pulse, respirations

Hydration: Mucous membranes, skin turgor, urinary output, fontanel, tears, heart rate, level of consciousness (Table 77-1)

Abdomen: Assess for distention, hyperactive bowel sounds, diffuse tenderness, guarding, increased tympany to percussion, splenomegaly (bacterial).

Diagnostic Procedures

Diagnosis can generally be made based on history and examination (Table 77-2).

Table 77-3 Differential Diagnosis: Gastroenteritis

Agent	Age	Source	Symptoms
Viral			
Rotavirus Norwalk, adenovirus, enterovirus	Any	Food, person-to-person contact	Nausea, vomiting, fever may precede diarrhea, URI
Bacterial			
Campylobacter jejuni	Any; most common bacterial diarrhea in ages 1-5 yr	Fecal-oral, food and water, or person-to-person contact	Vomiting, fever
Salmonella	Any	Fecal-oral, animal or human source, food	Vomiting, fever, abdominal pain
Shigella	Any; peaks at 2-10 yr	Fecal-oral, rarely food	Vomiting, fever, abdominal pain
E. coli	Any; leading cause of traveler's diarrhea	Fecal-oral, food and water	Low-grade temperature, abdominal cramps, gradual onset of diarrhea
Parasitic			
Giardia lamblia	Any; peaks at 4 yr	Waterborne, seen in day care centers and communities with inadequate water treatment	Nausea, vomiting, anorexia, abdominal distention, and cramping

URI, Upper respiratory infection.

ASSESSMENT (Tables 77-3 and 77-4)

A viral pathogen is the most common cause of gastroenteritis, typically presenting with nonbloody diarrhea and no fever or a low-grade fever; it is usually self-limiting, lasting about 24 to 48 hours.

Bacterial gastroenteritis may present with bloody diarrhea and fever and can last 3 to 5 days, often requiring antibiotics to eradicate. A bacterial pathogen is the most common cause of food poisoning and traveler's diarrhea, which results in gastroenteritis.

Food poisoning often has a short incubation of 1 to 24 hours and should be suspected when groups of people who have shared a meal develop acute vomiting and diarrhea.

Traveler's diarrhea typically begins with an acute episode 3 to 5 days after arrival in a foreign location.

Protozoal infections such as *Giardia* affect travelers, as well as **children** in day care facilities.

The differential diagnosis of gastroenteritis based on cause, age, source, symptoms, stool characteristics, and treatment is outlined in Tables 77-3 and 77-4.

THERAPEUTIC PLAN

Most cases of viral gastroenteritis are self-limiting and require supportive therapy only. In the United States 95% of **children** who develop diarrhea do not need antibiotics. Oral rehydration therapy (ORT) is the most important consideration in treating mild to moderate dehydration. ORT comes in rehydrating solutions and maintenance solutions which the major difference being sodium content.

Infants and **children** are at greatest risk for dehydration because they can lose a much greater percentage of their body weight quickly.

Weight loss is the most reliable indicator of fluid loss but requires an accurate preillness weight. Often there are no physical signs of dehydration until the child is approximately 10% dehydrated. Mild dehydration is defined as a loss of 3% to 5% of total body weight; moderate dehydration is a loss of 6% to 9% of total body weight; and severe dehydration is a loss of greater than 10% of total body weight. Dehydration is further assessed by measuring urine output.

An **infant** or **child** with diarrhea and mild dehydration should be maintained on their regular diet of breast milk, formula, or table food and supplemented with ORT. For mild dehydration give 50 ml/kg per 4-hour period. Give 10 ml/kg for each loose stool. For moderate dehydration give 100 ml/kg per 4-hour period plus replacement for each loose stool.

Vomiting is not a contraindication to ORT, but the key consideration is to administer small amounts of fluids every 2 or 3 minutes. This is very labor intensive. Severe dehydration requires intravenous therapy for rehydration with normal saline solution or Ringer's lactate.

Clear liquids are not recommended. Gatorade, colas, ginger ale, apple juice, Kool-aid, popsicles, tea, Jello, and chicken soup do not contain the necessary electrolytes to correct dehydration. Foods high in fat should also be avoided. The BRAT diet (bananas, rice, applesauce, toast) has some limited benefit but should be used only on a

TABLE 77-4 Differential Diagnosis: Gastroenteritis

Diagnosis	Supporting Data
Appendicitis	Inflammation of the appendix; can present with abdominal pain which generally localizes to the RLQ; other symptoms include anorexia, nausea, vomiting, and fever
Gastritis	Generalized inflammation of the gastric mucosa; may be acute or chronic; caused by alcohol, aspirin, NSAIDs, steroids, stress or reflux; presents as anorexia, fullness, nausea, vomiting, and epigastric pain
Peptic ulcer disease	Ulcerations in the mucosal lining of the lower esophagus, stomach, or proximal small bowel; caused by increased levels of gastric acid, rapid gastric emptying genetics, stress, smoking, drugs, alcohol, and caffeine; symptoms include epigastric pain, sometimes relieved by eating, fullness, nausea, vomiting, and weight loss
Inflammatory bowel disease	Inflammation of the bowel resulting in general malaise, anorexia, fever, abdominal discomfort, and diarrhea that may be bloody
Pseudomembranous colitis	Antibiotic-associated diarrhea caused by inflammation and necrosis of the mucosal and submucosal layers of the bowel; caused by *Clostridium difficile*
Diverticulitis	Inflammation of pouchlike protrusions of the bowel wall; symptoms include LLQ abdominal pain, fever, anorexia, and nausea
Fecal impaction	Impaction may cause overflow fecal incontinence which may be mistaken for diarrhea; associated with abdominal discomfort and palpable stool in the LLQ of the abdomen or in the rectum.
Cholecystitis	Inflammation of the gallbladder; presents with RUQ pain, anorexia, nausea, and vomiting.

LLQ, Left lower quadrant; *NSAID*, nonsteroidal antiinflammatory drug; *RLQ*, right lower quadrant; *RUQ*, right upper quadrant.

TABLE 77-5 Commercially Available Oral Rehydration Solutions

Components	WHO	Pedialyte (Ross Laboratories)	Rehydralyte (Ross Laboratories)	Resol (Wyeth Laboratories)	Infalyte (Mead Johnson Laboratories)
Sodium (mEq/L)	90	45	75	50	50
Potassium (mEq/L)	20	20	20	20	25
Chloride (mEq/L)	80	35	65	50	45
Citrate (mEq/L)	30	30	30	34	30
Glucose (g/L)	20	25	25	20	30

WHO, World Health Organization.

short-term basis. Commercially Available Oral Rehydration Solutions are detailed in Table 77-5.

For adolescents and adults with acute gastroenteritis, discontinue solids for 12 hours. Fluids are important. Reintroduce solids and advance as tolerated.

Pharmaceutical

For antibacterial treatment of gastroenteritis, see Table 77-6.

Antidiarrheal medications: Used at times to shorten the course of illness and to prevent complications.

Kaolin-pectin (Kaopectate, $2 to $3): 60 ml PO every 3 to 4 hours; use not to exceed 2 days

Loperamide (Imodium, $3 to $6): 4 mg PO initial dose, then 2 mg after each loose stool to a maximum dose of 16 mg/24 hours; use is not to exceed 2 days; contraindicated in bacterial gastroenteritis

Diphenoxylate (Lomotil, $2 to $47): 5 mg PO QID

Bismuth subsalicylate (Pepto-Bismol, $2 to $35): 30 ml q30 to 60 min, not to exceed 8 doses in 2 days

NOTE: Antidiarrheal medications are contraindicated if blood is present in the stool.

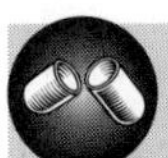

TABLE 77-6 Pharmaceutical Plan: Gastroenteritis

Pathogen	Drug/Dosage	Stool Characteristics	Cost ($)
Viral			
Rotavirus Norwalk, adenovirus, enterovirus	Predominantly symptomatic treatment, oral rehydration therapy	Large, liquid stools, variable odor, negative for blood and leukocytes	2-4 (16 oz)
Bacterial			
Campylobacter jejuni	Ciprofloxacin: 500 mg PO q12h for 5 days	Profuse bloody and watery diarrhea with mucus in streaks; positive for blood and leukocytes	290
	Azithromycin: 500 mg PO QD for 3 days		31
	Erythromycin: Children: 30-50 mg/kg/day in divided doses q6h for 7 days		11-16
	Adults: 500 mg PO BID for 5 days; take on an empty stomach		14-18
Salmonella	Ciprofloxacin: 500 mg PO BID for 3-5 days	Loose, slimy, green stool with "rotten egg" odor, positive for blood and leukocytes	290
	Trimethoprim-sulfamethoxazole: Children: 8 mg/kg trimethoprim and 40 mg/kg sulfamethoxazole per 24 hr in divided doses q12h for 14 days; Adults: DS q12h for 3-5 days		N/A
Shigella	Sames as for *Salmonella*	Watery, yellow-green, mucoid, bloody stool, no change in odor, positive for blood and leukocytes	Same as for *Salmonella*
E. coli	Same as for *Salmonella*	Green, slimy, and foul smelling stool, positive for blood and leukocytes	Same as for *Salmonella*
Parasitic			
Giardia lamblia	Metronidazole; Children: 15 mg/kg/day in divided doses q 8h for 10 days; Adults: 250 mg q8h ×5 days	Pale, bulky, greasy stool with foul odor, negative for blood and leukocytes, 30% to 60% positive for cysts	3-131

DS, Double strength.

Patient Education

Patient education handouts can be found on pp. 472 to 474.

Teach parents signs and symptoms of dehydration.

Teach parents the importance of oral rehydration and to avoid *clear liquids*.

Instruct parents to call the clinic if fluids are refused or there is continual vomiting and pain or bloody diarrhea.

Infants and **small children** may need daily weight checks.

Adults should return to the clinic if symptoms do not resolve within 3 days.

Educate patients about dietary precautions to prevent traveler's diarrhea (Box 77-1).

Consider antibiotic prophylaxis for the prevention of traveler's diarrhea if any of the following are present:

Patient has potentially reduced gastric acidity.

Patient is **elderly.**

Patient is receiving long-term histamine H_2-receptor antagonist therapy.

Patient has had gastric surgery.

Patient has a chronic illness such as diabetes, renal disease, cancer, or an immunosuppressive disorder.

Patient is taking a critically important trip or a trip that

Box 77-1

Dietary Precautions to Prevent Traveler's Diarrhea

Fluids to Avoid

Tap water, even for brushing teeth
Bottled water, unless the traveler is the one who breaks the seal
Ice made from contaminated water
Unpasteurized milk or dairy products

Fluids That Are Safe

Carbonated soft drinks
Hot drinks with boiled water
Carbonated or noncarbonated water as long as the traveler is the one who breaks the seal

Foods to Avoid

Raw fruits or vegetables, unless they can be peeled and the traveler is the one who peels them
Lettuce and other leafy vegetables
Cut-up fruit salad
Raw or rare meat and fish
Meat or shellfish that is not hot when served
All food from street vendors

From Heck JE, Cohen MB: Traveler's diarrhea, *Am Family Physician:* 48(5):793-799, 1993.

would be severely affected if the patient developed traveler's diarrhea.

Consultation/Referral

Consult/refer to collaborating physician in the following cases:

Infant younger than 3 months
Severe dehydration
Diarrhea persisting longer than 3 days in **children** and longer than 2 weeks in **adults**
Bloody diarrhea or emesis

EVALUATION/FOLLOW-UP

Follow up by telephone within 12 to 24 hours for **infants** and small **children.**

See Chapter 57 for treatment guidelines for infectious diarrhea; refer to Appendix P for typical treatment for a traveler with diarrhea.

SUGGESTED READINGS

Arvin AM et al, editors: *Nelson's textbook of pediatrics,* Philadelphia, 1996, WB Saunders.
Boyton RW, Dunn ES, Stephens GR, editors: *Manual of ambulatory pediatrics,* ed 3, Philadelphia, 1994, JB Lippincott.
Cornell S: Maintaining a fluid balance, *Adv Nurse Pract* 5:43-44, 1997.
Ellsworth A et al: *Mosby's 1998 medical drug reference,* St Louis, 1998, Mosby.
Gerchfsky M: Diarrhea, *Adv Nurse Pract* 3:12-16, 1995.
Goepp JG, Santosham M: Oral rehydration therapy. In Oski MD, McMillan JA, editors: *Principles and practice of pediatrics updates,* Philadelphia, 1993, JB Lippincott.
Dambro JR: *Griffith's five minute clinical consult,* Baltimore, 1997, Williams & Williams.
Groothuis JR et al, editors: *Current pediatric diagnosis and treatment,* ed 12, Norwalk, Conn, 1995, Appleton & Lange.
Healthcare Consultants of America, Inc: *1998 Physicians fee and coding guide,* Augusta, Ga, 1998, Healthcare Consultants of America, Inc.
Heck JE, Cohen MB: Traveler's diarrhea, *American Family Physician* 48(5):793-799, 1993.
McCargar LJ, Hotson BL, Nozza A: Fiber and nutrient intakes of chroniccare elderly patents, *J Nutr Elder* 15:13-31, 1995.
Rosenthal M: Diarrhea organisms are becoming media stars, *Infect Dis Child* 10:10-11, 1997.
Stephen TC: Outpatient management of diarrhea in infants, *PCC News* 21:1994.
Straughn A, English B: Oral rehydration therapy: a neglected treatment for pediatric diarrhea, *Matern Child Nurs* vol 6, 1996.
Uphold CR, Graham MV: *Clinical guidelines in family practice,* Gainesville, Fla, 1994, Barmarrae Books.

DIARRHEA AND VOMITING

Babies and children need fluids to live. Their bodies are made up of about 80% fluid.

Children with diarrhea lose fluids and minerals from their bodies and can become dehydrated. These fluids need to be replaced. But, most liquids such as apple juice, cola, and Gatorade have too much sugar in them, and they make diarrhea worse.

Giving babies water doesn't replace the minerals that they need and can make them very ill.

Oral Rehydration Solutions (ORS) such as Pedialyte, Ricelyte, and Rehydralyte are made to replace both the fluids and minerals that babies lose with diarrhea without making the diarrhea worse.

Children need at least twice as much fluid when they have diarrhea as they usually drink when they are healthy. To accomplish this, you should continue their regular feedings plus give them ORS frequently between meals.

The best way to get them to take all of these fluids is by giving small amounts of ORS very frequently. If you give 1 tsp to your child every minute, he or she will have taken 8 ounces in about 45 minutes.

Even if your child is vomiting, he or she can still usually take ½ to 1 tsp ORS every few minutes.

Call your doctor or clinic if your child is unable to keep down fluids, has a high fever, has blood in the stool, or begins to appear dehydrated.

SIGNS OF DEHYDRATION

A dry mouth, no drool	Drowsiness or fussiness
Thirst	Sunken looking eyes
Decreased urination (peeing)	No tears when crying

FEEDING DURING DIARRHEA

Continued feeding is an important part of treating diarrhea, so children should still be offered regular meals while they are sick.

If your child is breast- or bottle-fed, the best thing that you can do is continue to feed him or her normally.

If they eat table foods, here are some **good foods** for them to eat:

GOOD FOODS

Starchy foods such as: rice, potatoes, noodles, crackers, toast, and bananas

Cereals like: rice cereal, cream of wheat, shredded wheat, oatmeal, Cheerios, Rice Krispies, Wheaties, Kix

Soups like: soups with rice or noodles, meat and vegetables

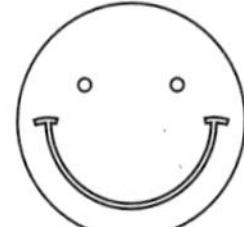

Vegetables of all kinds (without lots of butter added)

Fresh fruits, but not fruit packed in syrup

Some foods that can make diarrhea worse are foods with a lot of natural or added sugar.

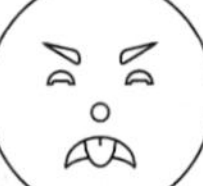

AVOID

BAD FOODS **AVOID**

Drinks such as grape juice, apple juice, orange juice, colas, ginger ale, or soft drinks (pop, soda, tonic)

Ice cream, sherbet, and popsicles

Jello or pudding

Sweetened cereals such as Sugar Smacks, Frosted Flakes, Frosted Mini Wheats, Captain Crunch, Oatmeal Swirlies

Fatty foods

 For additional information, call 410-614-2418.

COMFORT DURING DIARRHEA

Diarrhea can make children's bottoms hurt and make them irritable and cranky.

Some things that you can do to prevent and treat diaper rashes that come with diarrhea are:

Avoid using baby wipes when your child has diarrhea

Change diapers often

Wash your child's bottom with soap, rinse and pat dry

Apply Vaseline, A&D ointment or Desitin to keep the diarrhea away from your child's skin

Apply powder or corn starch to child's bottom

Diarrhea is a problem to deal with for both you and your child. Changing diapers, feeding, giving ORS, and calming a screaming child can make you cranky too. Please remember how it feels to be ill and give your child extra love when he or she is sick. If you can get someone to watch your child, take a break now and then. If you feel out of control, call the Parents' Anonymous Hotline at (800) 421-0353.

Gastroesophageal Reflux Disease

ICD-9-CM

Esophagitis 530.1
Hiatal Hernia 750.6
Heartburn 787.1
Barrett's Syndrome 530.2

OVERVIEW

Definition

Gastroesophageal reflux disease (GERD) is characterized by abnormal reflux of gastric or intestinal contents into the esophagus, resulting in esophageal inflammation.

Incidence

Adults: Sixty percent of adults in the United States experience heartburn, 10% on a daily basis.

Elderly: Elderly persons have a greater prevalence of the conditions that contribute to the development of GERD; therefore the incidence may also be increased.

Pregnant women: Seventy percent to 80% report symptoms of heartburn.

Infants: Sixty-five percent of healthy infants have physiological gastroesophageal reflux; it resolves in all but 4% by 6 months of age.

Treatment costs $2 to $3 billion annually.

Pathophysiology

Impaired antireflux mechanisms caused by increased intragastric pressure or decreased lower esophageal sphincter (LES) pressure contribute to the development and progression of GERD.

Elderly: In addition to the above, the elderly have decreased saliva production and delayed gastric emptying which contribute to reflux symptoms.

Infants and children: Physiological reflux is harmless spitting up of gastric contents. Pathological reflux is caused by abnormal relaxation of the LES unrelated to swallowing.

Factors Contributing to Reflux

Foods: High-fat diets, spicy or acidic foods, chocolate
Positions: Lying down after meals, bending over
Substances: Caffeine, cigarette smoking, or chewing tobacco
Others: Tight clothes, obesity, ascites, **pregnancy**
Infants and children: Increased risk in children with central nervous system disease and in those with a history of congenital diaphragmatic or hiatal hernia

Medications That Contribute to Reflux by Decreasing LES Pressure

Smooth muscle relaxants: Theophylline, nitrates, calcium channel blockers
Anticholinergics
Progesterone
Transdermal nicotine
Diazepam

Complications

Reflux esophagitis is caused by chronic inflammation of the esophageal wall increasing capillary permeability, edema, tissue friability, and erosion. This can lead to mild esophagitis, erosive esophagitis, or fibrotic stricture. Severe reflux is associated with an increase in risk of hemorrhage and adenocarcinoma.

SUBJECTIVE DATA

History of Present Illness

Ask about frequency, onset, progression, and duration of pain
Relationship to meals and activities
Exacerbated by specific foods, laying down, bending over
Worse at night
Relieved by antacids or non-prescription doses of H_2-receptor antagonists
Not typically exacerbated by exertion
Dysphagia, cough, weight loss, or blood loss may suggest other problems
Important to distinguish between symptoms of reflux and those of cardiac origin

Past Medical History

Ask about chronic diseases, including known cardiovascular disease
Asthma beginning in middle age without a history of allergies; asthma that occurs primarily at night (may suggest GERD-related asthma)

Medications

Over-the-counter antacids and H_2-receptor antagonists
Any other prescription, nonprescription, or herbal medications

Substances

Tobacco: Smoked or chewed
Alcohol: Amount and frequency

Diet History

High-fat diet, spicy or acidic foods, chocolate
Meal times: Relationship to pain and to bedtime

Description of Most Common Symptoms

Adults: Heartburn and regurgitation of gastric or esophageal contents into pharynx without nausea or retching
Elderly: Symptoms may be subtle; dysphagia may be the prominent symptom
Infants and children: Failure to thrive, frequent burping and regurgitation, irritability, sleep disturbance, feeding problems

Atypical Symptoms

Dysphagia (difficulty swallowing food), odynophagia (painful swallowing)
Bloating, belching, nausea, early satiety
Cough, hoarseness, exacerbation of asthma symptoms at night
Water brash: Hypersalivation produced by reflux

OBJECTIVE DATA

Physical Examination

Perform a problem-oriented physical examination, with particular attention to:
- Vital signs, height and weight, general appearance
- Lungs: Assess for adventitious sounds
- Abdomen: Bowel sounds, distention, obesity, tenderness, masses
- Rectal: Masses, tenderness, occult blood

Infants and children: Evaluate for normal growth by assessing weight, height, and head circumference
- General appearance: Hydration, activity level
- Gag and sucking reflex
- Observe being fed

Diagnostic Procedures

Adults: None indicated in patients with heartburn and regurgitation only
Infants and children: If history and physical yield normal findings, no diagnostic tests are indicated.
Patients with abnormal findings, who have initial symptoms after age 2, or who fail to respond to conservative treatment are candidates for diagnostic testing (Table 78-1 and Figure 78-1).

ASSESSMENT

Differential diagnoses are included in Table 78-2.

THERAPEUTIC PLAN

Pharmaceutical/Nonpharmaceutical

Management of GERD involves a stepped approach to care. The patient and family need to be active members of the management team.

Phase I

Institute in all adult patients.
All patients should try lifestyle changes first.
Use antacids after meals, at bedtime, and as needed.
Avoid drugs that may injure the esophageal mucosa, such as nonsteroidal antiinflammatory drugs (NSAIDs), doxycycline, quinidine.
Take all medications with a full glass of water.

Phase II

For patients who do not respond to phase I treatment, continue the above regimen and add an oral H_2 blocker.

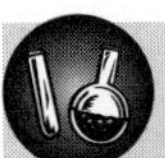

TABLE 78-1 Diagnostic Tests: Gastroesophageal Reflux Disease

Test	Findings/Rationale	Cost ($)
CBC with differential	To rule out anemias, infection	18-23
Chemistry profile	To screen for other chronic problems such as diabetes, liver disease	32-42
Barium swallow	Although the simplest and least expensive study for GERD, 40%-60% of symptomatic patients will have a normal study; useful as a screening test; can identify structural problems of the upper gastrointestinal tract and aspiration	201-240
Endoscopy	Patients with atypical symptoms or those who fail phase I treatment are candidates for endoscopic evaluation after physician consultation	544-643
Ultrasonography	To rule out pyloric stenosis in infants	361-429
GE reflux study	More specific testing for reflux	515-616
Esophagus acid reflux test	Intraluminal pH electrode for detection of reflux	340-407

CBC, Complete blood cell count; *GE*, gastroesophageal; *GERD*, gastroesophageal reflux disease; *N/A*, not available.

For GERD, a dosage higher than for other gastrointestinal conditions may be necessary (Tables 78-3 and 78-4).

Antacids can be used on an as-needed basis. Remember, magnesium-based antacids may cause diarrhea; aluminum may cause constipation. Combination products are likely to have fewer side effects.

Short-term therapy: 8 to 12 weeks

Long-term maintenance therapy with H_2 blockers, plus lifestyle modifications, is essential to prevent exacerbation of GERD. Maintenance therapy is usually half the therapeutic dose, taken at bedtime. Both omeprazole (Prilosec) and Lansoprazole (Prevacid) may be indicated in long-term treatment. There have been reports of negative long-term effects associated with the use of these drugs, such as cell hyperplasia and atrophic gastritis.

Infants and children: For infants with physiological reflux and no symptoms or signs of pathological conditions, parents can be reassured that no further treatment may be necessary. Conservative treatment measures include positioning the infant to decrease postprandial reflux. It is no longer recommended that the infant be placed in an upright, seated position; better outcomes have resulted from placing the infant in a prone position when not being held upright by the caregiver. To reduce the risk of sudden infant death syndrome, this position should be used only when monitored by the caregiver. Some infants may benefit from receiving smaller, more frequent feedings. Thickening formula with cereal has not been shown to be beneficial and may actually aggravate the condition. Infants and children with persistent or severe reflux are best managed with the assistance of a pediatric gastroenterologist.

Lifestyle/Activities

Elevate the head of the bed on 4- to 6-inch blocks.

Stop smoking.

Avoid restrictive or tight clothing or belts.

Use antacids after meals, at bedtime, and as needed.

Avoid drugs that may injure the esophageal mucosa such as NSAIDs, doxycycline, and quinidine.

Avoid drugs that may lower LES pressure, such as theophylline, anticholinergics, nitrates, calcium channel blockers, progesterone, transdermal nicotine, and diazepam.

Take all medications with a full glass of water.

Diet

Advise the patient to:

Avoid food and beverages that cause symptoms; this may include fatty, acidic, or spicy foods, chocolate, coffee, and alcohol.

Lose weight if >30% above ideal body weight.

Eat several small meals a day and do not eat within 3 hours of bedtime.

Patient Education

Discuss lifestyle changes in the previous paragraph.

Family Impact

The condition may influence the patient's ability to socialize with family, depending on symptoms.

There may be family concern about possible cancer if GERD is severe and Barrett's esophagus is present.

Referral

Refer to a physician:

Patients with dysphagia, weight loss, blood loss

Treatment failure after full course of treatment with two different medications

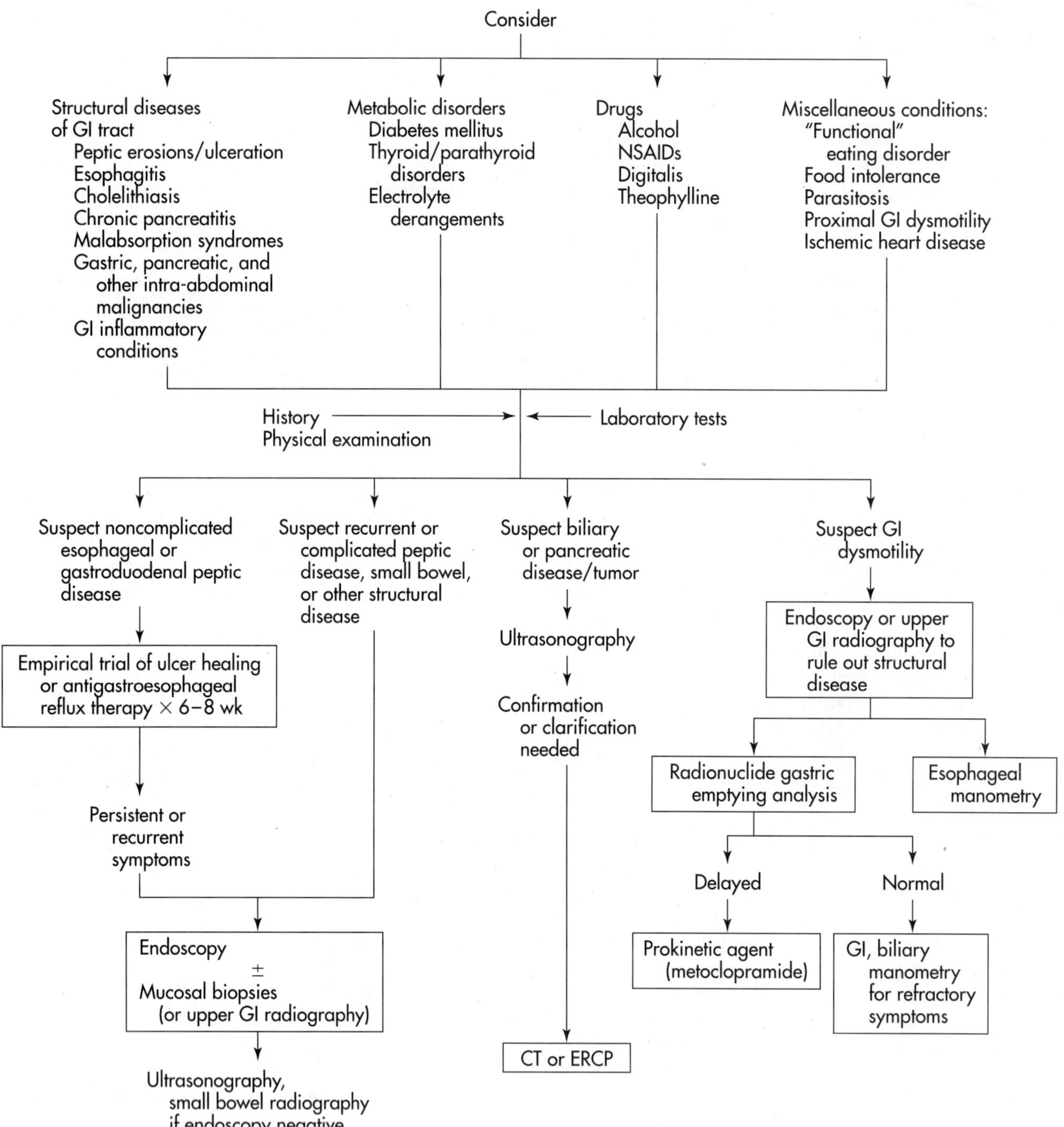

Figure 78-1 Algorithm for treatment of an **adult** patient with dyspepsia. (*CT,* Computed tomography; *ERCP,* endoscopic retrograde cholangiopancreatography; *GI,* gastrointestinal; *NSAID,* nonsteroidal antiinflammatory drug. (Adapted from Greene HL, Johnson WP, Lemcke D: *Decision making in medicine,* ed 2, St Louis, 1998, Mosby.)

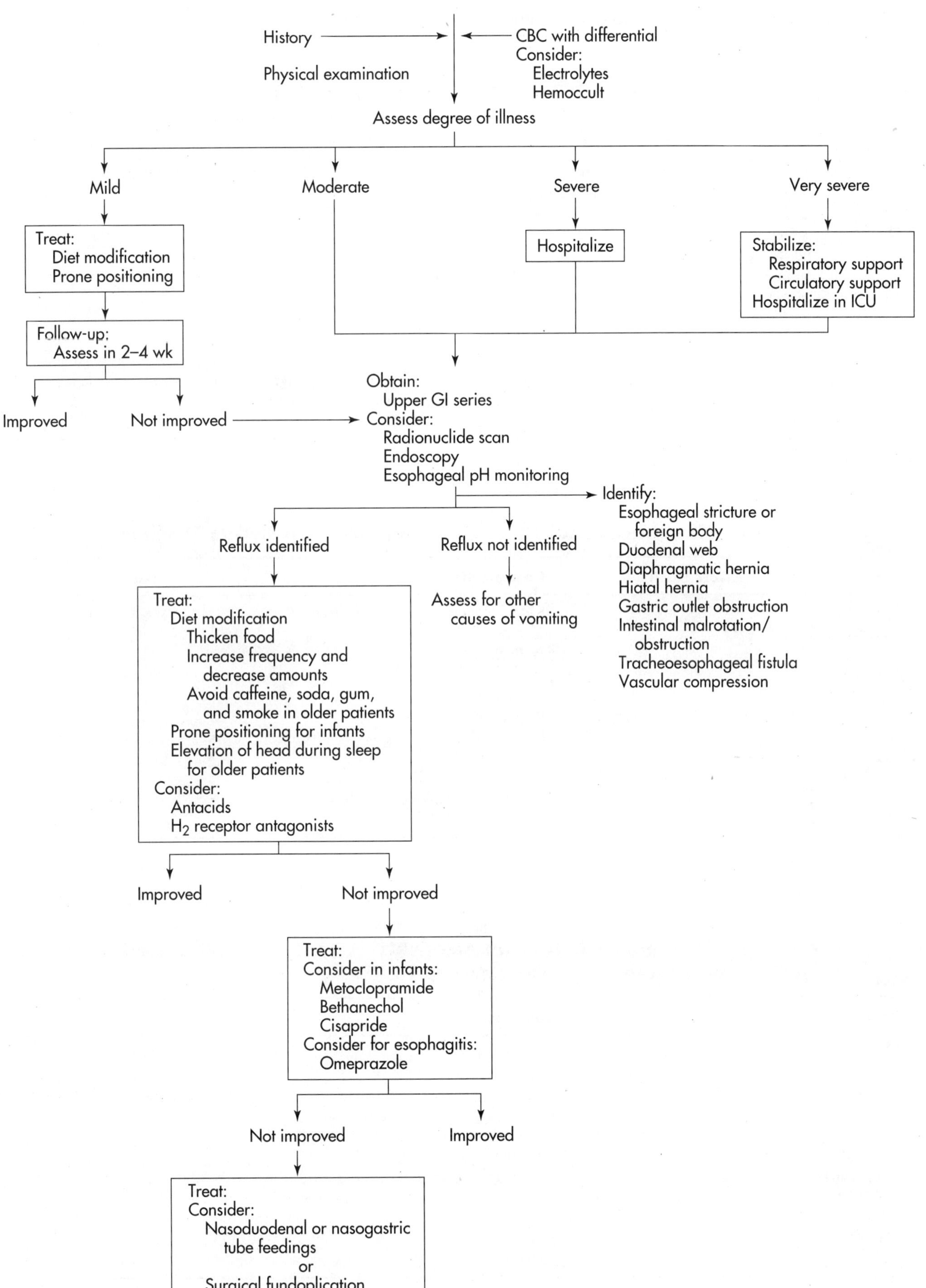

Figure 78-2 Algorithm for treatment of **pediatric** patient with gastroesophageal reflux. *GI,* Gastrointestinal; *ICU,* intensive care unit. (Adapted from Berman S: *Pediatric decision making,* ed 3, St Louis, 1996, Mosby.)

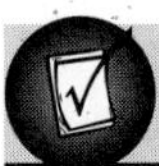

TABLE 78-2 Differential Diagnosis: Gastroesophageal Reflux

Diagnosis	Supporting Data
Cardiac chest pain	Typically unaffected by foods, position change, and antacids and aggravated by exertion
PUD	Gnawing or penetrating pain that is worse on empty stomach and may awaken patient; ulcer identified on barium swallow or endoscopic examination
Esophageal dysmotility or structural disorders	Dysphagia and regurgitation predominant features; anatomic deformities or motility abnormality on barium swallow or endoscopy
Esophageal infection (candidiasis, herpes simplex, varicella zoster, HIV, cytomegalovirus)	Immunocompromised client; odynophagia and dysphagia prominent; infection diagnosed with endoscopic brushings, biopsies, and/or cultures
Esophageal cancer	Dysphagia, odynophagia, weight loss; tumor identified on endoscopy; confirmed on tissue biopsy
Pyloric stenosis	Average age of onset is 3-4 weeks; vomiting is cardinal sign; infant continues to be hungry; weight loss, dehydration, and metabolic alkalosis can occur, caused by hypertrophy of the pyloric sphincter muscles; corrected surgically

HIV, human immunodeficiency virus; *PUD,* Peptic ulcer disease.

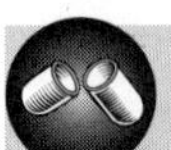

TABLE 78-3 Pharmaceutical Plan: Gastroesophageal Reflux Disease

Drug	Adult Dose*	Comments	Cost
Cimetidine (Tagamet)	800-1600 mg /day	**Elderly** more susceptible to adverse CNS reaction; decrease dose Pregnancy: B	$88-$275/800 mg (100)
Ranitidine (Zantac)	150-300 mg/day	Use cautiously with **elderly** or patients with renal or hepatic impairment Pregnancy: B	$86-$98/300 mg (30)
Famotidine (Pepcid)	40-80 mg/day	Decrease dose in severe renal impairment Pregnancy: B	$298/40 mg (100) $7/OTC: 10 mg (18)
Nizatidine (Axid)	150-300 mg/day	Decrease dose in clients with renal or hepatic impairment Pregnancy: C	$60/75 mg (30) $158/150 mg (100) $62/300 mg (30)

*Dosage for elderly may be reduced by one half.
CNS, Central nervous system.

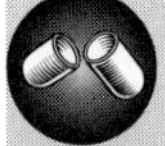

TABLE 78-4 Pharmaceutical Plan: Alternatives to H_2 Blockers, Used Alone or in Combination with H_2 Blockers for GERD

Drug	Adult Dosage	Comments	Cost
Cisapride (Propulsid)	40-80 mg/day	Fewer CNS side effects Pregnancy: C SE: Headache, diarrhea, abdominal pain; drug interaction → prolonged QT interval; check reference before prescribing	$69/10 mg (100) $122/20 mg (100) $47/Suspension: 1 mg/ml (450 ml)
Omeprazole (Prilosec)	20-40 mg/day	Use in refractory cases of GERD; treat for 8 weeks Pregnancy: C	$109/20 mg (30)
Lansoprazole (Prevacid)	15-30 mg/day	Pregnancy: C SE: Diarrhea	$325/30 mg (100)

CNS, Central nervous system; *GERD,* gastroesophageal reflux disease; *SE,* side effects.

Pregnant women with symptoms that persist despite lifestyle modifications

Patients on proton pump inhibitors

Infants and children with symptoms of pathological regurgitation

Consultation

Recurrence of symptoms after a full course of medication; a second medication is often tried for 6 to 8 weeks

Before prescribing medication for a patient more than 45 years old

EVALUATION/FOLLOW-UP

Recheck in 1 or 2 weeks to evaluate effectiveness of treatment.

If patient's condition is improving, recheck in 6 to 8 weeks or at end of first course of treatment.

Adjust follow-up based on recurring symptoms.

SUGGESTED READINGS

Barker LR, Burton JR, Zieve PD, editor: *Principles of ambulatory medicine,* ed 4, Baltimore, 1997, Williams & Wilkins.

Brady WM, Ogorek CP: Gastroesophageal reflux disease, *Postgrad Med* 100:76-89, 1996.

Clark CL, Horwitz B: Complications of gastroesophageal reflux disease, *Postgrad Med* 100:95-113, 1996.

Ellsworth A et al: *Mosby's 1998 medical drug reference,* St Louis, 1998, Mosby.

Fass R et al: Contemporary medical therapy for gastroesophageal reflux disease, *Am Family Physician* 55:205-212, 1997.

Fennerty MJ: The diagnosis and treatment of gastroesophageal reflux disease in a managed care environment: suggested disease management guidelines, *Arch Intern Med* 156:477-484, 1996.

Hart JJ: Pediatric gastroesophageal reflux, *Am Family Physician* 54:2463-2471, 1996.

Healthcare Consultants of America, Inc: *1998 Physicians fee and coding guide,* Augusta, Ga, 1998, Healthcare Consultants of America, Inc.

Hixson L: Dyspepsia. In Greene H, Johnson W, Lemcke D, editors: *Decision making in medicine,* ed 2, St Louis, 1998, Mosby.

Isselbacher KJ et al, editors: *Harrison's principles of internal medicine,* ed 13, New York, 1994, McGraw-Hill.

Jahnigen DW, Schier RW, editors: *Geriatric medicine,* ed 2, London, 1995, Blackwell.

Larsen R: Gastroesophageal reflux disease, *Postgrad Med* 101:181-187, 1997.

Uphold C, Graham M: *Clinical guidelines in family practice,* ed 2, Gainesville, Fla, 1994, Barmarrae.

Genital Warts (Human Papillomavirus)

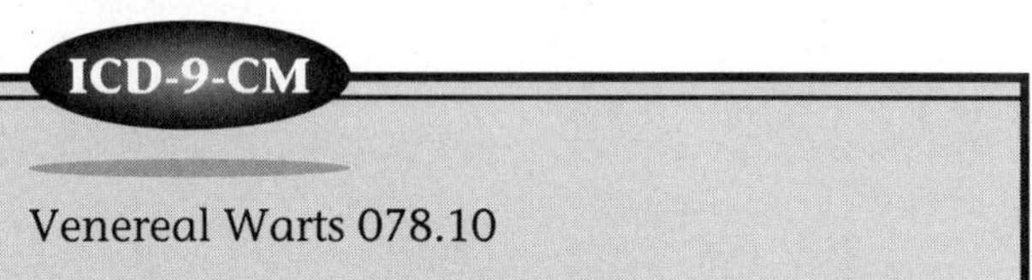

ICD-9-CM

Venereal Warts 078.10

OVERVIEW

Definition

Genital warts or condyloma acuminata is a condition characterized by pointed condylomata and is considered to be a sexually transmitted infection. It is the most common presentation of mucosal human papillomavirus (HPV) infection and the most common sexually transmitted disease (STD) in developed countries. Certain HPV infections have a major etiological role in the pathogenesis of cancer in situ and also in invasive squamous cell carcinoma of the anogenital epithelium. The virus does not always cause a lesion; subclinical infection occurs on the cervix and externally.

Incidence

Prevalence of 15% to 38% in young, sexually active **adults,** with peak incidence in persons who are between 15 and 24 years old. An increased number of cases have been reported in the past two decades; however, that number may be elevated in light of screening with Pap smears under the Bethesda Reporting System. HPV has been detected in cytologically normal cervical samples in approximately 10% of women who are seen for routine care. Approximately 25% of women with HPV will progress to high-grade squamous intraepithelial lesion (HSIL) or invasive cervical cancer.

The incubation period is 1 to 6 months but may be much longer (up to 30 years). Up to 70% regress spontaneously. The period of communicability is unknown.

Pathophysiology

HPV is a group of DNA viruses with more than 70 identified genotypes. Oncogenic HPV is associated with more severe abnormalities and more rapid progression (Table 79-1).

Factors That Increase Susceptibility

Multiple sexual partners
Lack of barrier protection
Smoking (decreases the density of Langerhans cells in the cervix)
Long-term use of oral contraceptives may increase the risk of HPV infection
Adolescents (predilection for infecting the transformation zone of the cervix)
Pregnancy (as a result of metaplasia and relative immunosuppression)
Coexistence of other STDs

SUBJECTIVE DATA

History of Present Illness

Ask about location, onset, duration, and symptoms, if any.
Ask about sexual partner or partners, any similar complaint or presentation.

Past Medical History

Previous occurrences
Any abnormal Pap smear results

Medications

Use of oral contraceptives
If there has been previous HPV treatment, what was used, how often, was the treatment completed?

Family History

Not applicable

Psychosocial History

Smoker
Sexual history, number of partners, sexual activity
Use of barrier methods of contraception

TABLE 79-1 Pathophysiology: Genital Warts

Risk for Oncogenesis	Genotypes
High	16, 18 (some place 33, 45, 56 in the high-risk category)
Intermediate	31, 33, 35, 39, 45, 51, 52, 56, 58
Low (rarely associated with cancer)	6, 11, 42, 43, 44

OBJECTIVE DATA

Physical Examination

Lymph nodes: assess for inguinal lymphadenopathy
Females: Labia, clitoris, periureteral area, perineum, cervix, vagina
Male: Frenulum, corona, glans, prepuce, shaft, scrotum
Both sexes: Perineum, perianal area, rectum, urethral meatus, urethra
Skin lesions
- Type: Pinhead papules to cauliflower-like masses; subclinical on penis, vulva, or other genital skin; may be visible only after application of acetic acid
- Color: Flesh colored, pink or red
- Palpation: Soft to the touch
- Shape: Filiform, sessile (especially on penis)
- Arrangement: May be solitary or grouped into grapelike or cauliflower-like clusters; perianal lesions may be walnut-size to apple-size

Diagnostic Procedures

Diagnostic tests are listed in Table 79-2.

ASSESSMENT

Differential Diagnosis

Differential diagnoses include those listed in Table 79-3.

TABLE 79-2 Diagnostic Tests: Genital Warts

Test	Finding/Rationale	Cost ($)
Acetowhitening	To visualize subclinical lesions, wrap the penis with a piece of gauze soaked in 5% acetic acid for 5 minutes and apply gauze to external vulvar area; use a colposcope or a 10× handheld lens; warts appear as tiny, white papules; may place acetic acid on the external genitalia; after 5 minutes, look to see whether any acetowhite changes; not recommended as a method to screen for subclinical HPV	N/A
Gonorrhea and *Chlamydia* cultures	Used to rule out other concurrent STDs	61-79/GC 39-51/Ch
RPR, VDRL	Used to rule out syphilis	18-22
Pap smear	To identify the presence of abnormal cell changes and the presence of HPV; concern about false-negative rate; consider HPV DNA typing in high-risk age group	25-31
HPV DNA typing	Consider use in adolescents; controversy exists concerning limitations and cost, but typing may be useful as adjunct to triage of patients; low-risk HPV cases could be followed via Pap smears, whereas high-risk cases could be followed by colposcopy and biopsy	61-79
Biopsy	Used for identification of abnormal cell changes	93-111

Ch, Chlamydia; *DNA,* deoxyribonucleic acid; *GC, Gonorrhea* culture; *HPV,* human papillomavirus; *RPR,* rapid plasma reagin; *STD,* sexually transmitted disease; *VDRL,* Venereal Disease Research Laboratories.

TABLE 79-3 Differential Diagnosis: Genital Warts

Diagnosis	Supporting Data
HPV	Most patients have 1-10 warts, with a surface area of 0.5-1.2 cm^2 (see the description under Physical Examination; lesions tend to be more raised than in condylomata lata)
Molluscum contagiosum	Asymptomatic clusters of white papules caused by the molluscum virus; umbilicated waxy white/gray lesions
Condylomata lata	Flat, wartlike lesions found in intertriginous areas and around the anal canal (caused by syphilis)
Lipomas, fibroma, adenomas	Round, soft, fleshy nodules
Squamous cell carcinomas	History of sun exposure, enlarging and ulcerating red nodule
Nevi	Small (<1.0 cm), circumscribed, pigmented macules or papules located in the epidermis and dermis
Seborrheic keratoses	Flesh-colored or pigmented papules or plaques with an irregular, wartlike surface and "stuck on" appearance
Psoriatic plaques	Inflammatory skin disorder ranging from isolated plaques to involvement of the whole body; well-demarcated red plaques covered with thick silvery scales, distributed over the scalp, lower back, and extensor surfaces of the extremities

THERAPEUTIC PLAN

The goal of treating visible warts is the removal of symptomatic warts. No evidence indicates that treatment of visible warts affects the development of cervical cancer. Treatment of the warts should be guided by the patient, the available resources, and the experience of the health care provider. No one method is superior. In general, warts located on moist surfaces and/or in intertriginous areas respond better to topical treatment than do warts on drier surfaces.

Complications include:

Scarring in the form of persistent hypopigmentation or hyperpigmentation with ablative therapy
Depressed or hypertrophic scars
Chronic pain syndromes (vulvodynia or hyperesthesia)

Pharmaceutical/Nonpharmaceutical

External Genital Warts

Recommended treatments are outlined in Table 79-4.

Vaginal Warts

Recommended treatments are outlined in Table 79-5.

Ureteral Meatus Warts

Recommended treatments are outlined in Table 79-6.

Anal Warts

Consider referring these patients to a surgeon for biopsy and removal. If treatment is warranted, the following approaches may be elected: cryotherapy with liquid nitrogen; TCA or BCA 80% to 90% applied to warts; or surgical removal.

Oral Warts

Cryotherapy with liquid nitrogen or surgical removal.

Management of Sex Partners

Recommendations for treatment of partners are not clear. Some researchers believe that the role of the partner in reinfection is probably minimal, and therefore treatment for the partner is not warranted. Others argue that all exposed partners should be examined and treated concurrently for visible warts.

Pregnancy

The preventive value of cesarean section regarding genital warts is unknown; thus this procedure should not be performed solely to prevent transmission of HPV.

Lifestyle/Activities

Encourage use of barrier protection

Diet

Encourage a healthy diet with adequate intake of vitamins A, C, and folate.

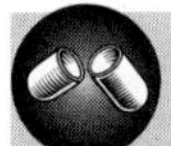

TABLE 79-4 Treatment Plan: External Genital Warts

Drug	Dosage	Comments	Cost
Patient-Applied Treatment			
Podofilox 0.5% solution or gel	Apply podofilox solution with a cotton swab, or gel with a finger, to visible warts BID for 3 days, followed by 4 days of no therapy.	May be repeated for up to 4 cycles Pregnancy: C SE: Local reactions, H/A	$52/5 mg/5 ml (3.5 ml)
Imiquimod 5% cream (Aldara)	Patients should apply cream with a finger at bedtime, three times a week (on a Monday, Wednesday, Friday schedule) for as long as 16 wk. Do not use for urethral, intravaginal, cervical, or rectal lesions.	Treatment area should be washed with mild soap and water 6-10 hr after application; many patients clear of warts by 8-10 wk or sooner Pregnancy: B SE: Local reaction, headache, flulike symptoms, myalgia	N/A
Provider-Applied Treatment			
Cryotherapy with liquid nitrogen or cryoprobe	Repeat applications every 1-2 wk.	Skill needed for best success	$70-$86/ Removal of up to 14 lesions
Podophyllin resin 10%-25% in compound tincture of benzoin (Podofilm, Podofin)	A small amount should be applied to each wart and allowed to air dry.	Some experts suggest that the preparation be thoroughly washed off 1-4 hr after application to reduce local irritation Pregnancy: X	$26-$35/25% (15 ml)
TCA or BCA 80%-90%	Apply small amount only to the warts; repeat weekly as needed. Use petrolatum jelly on surrounding skin to prevent chemical burn.	Allow to dry, at which time a white "frosting" develops; powder with talc or sodium bicarbonate (i.e., baking soda) to remove unreacted acid if an excess amount has been applied; some providers neutralize unreacted acid with liquid soap applied to the area treated; safe to use during pregnancy or with cervical HPV	$70-$86/Removal of up to 14 lesions
Surgical Removal			
By tangential scissor excision, tangential shave excision, curettage, or electrosurgery			
Alternative Treatment			
Intralesional interferon or laser surgery: interferon is painful, systemic side effects occur.			

BCA, Bichloracetic acid; *H/A,* headache; *HPV,* human papillomavirus; *N/A,* not available; *SE,* side effects; *TCA,* trichloroacetic acid.

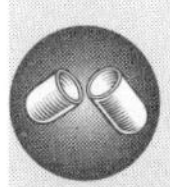

TABLE 79-5 Treatment Plan: Vaginal Warts

Treatment	Comments
Cryotherapy with liquid nitrogen	Use of a cryoprobe in the vagina is recommended.
TCA or BCA 80%-90% applied only to warts	See Cryotherapy.

BCA, Bichloracetic acid; *TCA*, trichloroacetic acid.

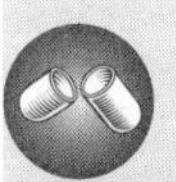

TABLE 79-6 Treatment Plan: Ureteral Meatus Warts

Treatment	Comments
Cryotherapy with liquid nitrogen	
Podophyllin 10%-25% in compound tincture of benzoin	Area must be dry before contact with normal mucosa Safety of podophyllin use during pregnancy has not been established

Patient Education

Safe sex issues

Emphasize the importance of yearly (or sooner) follow-up for cervical cancer

Family Impact

The issue of causation and blame can be a traumatic event when one partner is diagnosed with HPV. Discuss the incubation period of 2 weeks to 8 months. Being told of the relationship of HPV to carcinoma is especially frightening to the patient and family; emphasize the ability to monitor cell changes/prevention through treatment.

Referral

Cervical warts: Women with exophytic warts, high-grade squamous intraepithelial lesions must be referred to an OB/GYN.

Anogenital warts should be referred to an OB/GYN or urologist.

EVALUATION/FOLLOW-UP

After visible genital warts have cleared, a follow-up evaluation is not essential. Patients should be cautioned to watch for recurrence, most frequently encountered during the first 3 months.

RESOURCES

CDC/ STD site (includes copy of 1998 STD treatment guidelines)
http://www.cdc.gov/nchstp/dstd/breaking_news.htm

American Social Health Association
http://sunsite.unc.edu/ASHA

Ask NOAH about STDs (a site with multiple resources)
http://www.noah.cuny.edu/illness/stds/stds.html

Journal of the American Medical Association Women's Health STD site
http://www.ama-assn.org/special/std/support/support.htm

SUGGESTED READINGS

ACOG Technical Bulletin: *Genital human papillomavirus infections,* No 193, 1994.

Beutner K, Ferenczy A: Therapeutic approaches to genital warts, *Am J Med* 102:28-37, 1997.

Beutner K, Tyring S: Human papillomavirus and human disease, *Am J Med* 102:9-15, 1997.

Centers for Disease Control and Prevention: Guidelines for treatment of sexually transmitted diseases, *MMWR* 47 No RR-1:88-94, 1998.

Colletta L: Human papillomavirus in the woman with HIV: reducing risk is best strategy, *Adv Nurse Pract* 5:16-21, 1997.

Ellsworth A et al: *Mosby's 1998 medical drug reference*, St Louis, 1998, Mosby.

Foxman B, Aral S, Holmes K: Interrelationships among douching practices, risky sexual practices, and history of self-reported sexually transmitted diseases in an urban population, *Sex Transm Dis* 25:90-99, 1998.

Handsfield H: Clinical presentation and natural course of anogenital warts, *Am J Med* 102:16-20, 1997.

Hawkins JW, Roberto-Nichols DM, Stanley-Haney JL: *Condylomata acuminata: protocols for the nurse practitioner in gynecologic settings,* New York, 1995, Tiresias Press.

Healthcare Consultants of America, Inc: *1998 Physicians fee and coding guide,* Augusta, Ga, 1998, Healthcare Consultants of America, Inc.

Koutsky L: Epidemiology of genital human papillomavirus infection, *Am J Med* 102(5A): 3-8, 1997.

Reitano M: Counseling patients with genital warts, *Am J Med* 102:38-43, 1997.

Slade C: HPV and cervical cancer, *Adv Nurse Pract* 6:39-54, 1998.

80 Glaucoma

ICD-9-CM

Acute Narrow Angle Glaucoma 365.22
Open Angle 365.10
Chronic Open Angle 365.11
Glaucomatous Atrophy of Optic Disk 377.14
Narrow Angle Primary 365.20
Borderline Glaucoma 365.00

OVERVIEW

Definition

Glaucoma is a condition of the eye in which the canal of Schlemm becomes blocked, preventing the outflow of aqueous humor. As a result of the lack of outflow, the intraocular pressure increases and the optic nerve becomes cupped, leading to loss of visual field. Elevated intraocular pressure is defined as a pressure greater than 21 mm Hg. However, higher pressures leave some patients unaffected, and some persons with normal pressures develop optic nerve and visual field changes. Blockages of the canal of Schlemm can be an acute process or a chronic process. Acute glaucoma involves a narrow angle blockage and chronic glaucoma involves a wide angle of blockage.

Incidence

Glaucoma is the second most common cause for permanent blindness (after macular degeneration). There are an estimated 3 million persons in the United States who have elevated intraocular pressure. This condition occurs in as many as 15% of the **elderly** population. Glaucoma is also more common in African-Americans older than age 40 (incidence 5 times more likely than with the white population). The prevalence of glaucoma is 0.7% in persons older than age 40, 20% older than age 60.

Pathophysiology

Aqueous humor fills the posterior chamber of the eye, flows through the pupil and the anterior chamber and leaves the eye through the trabecular meshwork, a connective tissue filter at the angle between the iris and the cornea. The aqueous humor passes out of the trabecular meshwork into Schlemm's canal. The trabecular meshwork is covered by the root of the iris. Intraocular pressure is maintained by the balance between inflow and outflow of aqueous humor. Increased intraocular pressure is related to improper aqueous humor flow. Elevated intraocular pressure results in optic nerve damage. The exact mechanism of this damage is unknown, but probably relates to ischemia.

Types of Glaucoma

Primary Open-angle Glaucoma. Primary open-angle glaucoma occurs from obstruction at the microscopic level in the trabecular meshwork or from overproduction of aqueous humor. This type of glaucoma accounts for 90% of all cases of glaucoma.

Acute Closed-angle Glaucoma. Acute closed-angle glaucoma results from obstruction of the trabecular network by the iris, by a narrow angle between the anterior iris and the posterior corneal surface, small anterior chambers, or a thickened or bulging iris.

Congenital Glaucoma. Congenital glaucoma occurs rarely as a result of an autosomal-recessive gene.

Protective Factors Against

Unknown

Factors That Increase Susceptibility

Increasing age
Patients with diabetes, hypertension, or previous eye injury
Eye inflammation
Neoplasm
Neovascularization
Corticosteroid use

Closed-angle glaucoma incidence increases with pharmacological mydriatic use and with use of anticholinergics.

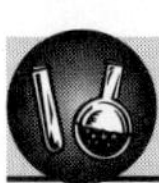

TABLE 80-1 Diagnostic Tests: Glaucoma

Test	Findings/Rationale	Cost ($)
Tonometry (intraocular pressure measurement)	Tonometry is the cardinal measurement for glaucoma. This measurement, performed in anesthetized eyes, can be done by the use of several devices. One is the Schiøtz tonometer, which sits on the eye surface and has the disadvantage of often undermeasuring intraocular pressure. Pressure can also be measured by an applanation device, or by an air-puff device used by the ophthalmologist. There is a new handheld "Tono-Pen" that easily measures intraocular pressure.	45-53
Central visual field testing	Visual fields by confrontation is a gross screening test and should be followed by a more accurate evaluation by an ophthalmologist or optometrist.	47-117
Provocative tests for glaucoma	With interpretation and without tonography; price depends on the number of isopters.	43-51

SUBJECTIVE DATA

History of Present Illness

Open-angle glaucoma is characterized by no symptoms in early stages of the disease and later slow loss of peripheral vision. Tunnel vision occurs later, and eventually there is loss of central vision.

Closed-angle glaucoma presents with unilateral symptoms and is an acute process. It presents with acute pain and pressure over one eye.

Past Medical History

Ask about:

- Past trauma to the eye
- History of intraocular surgery
- Migraine headaches
- History of chronic diseases such as hypertension, diabetes, and sarcoidosis
- History of herpes zoster and gradual onset of myopia

Medications

Steroid use may predispose an individual to open-angle glaucoma.

Closed-angle glaucoma may be precipitated in certain cases by use of antihistamines, stimulants, vasodilators, sympathomimetics, cocaine, anticholinergics (atropine for preoperative use), and clonidine.

Family History

Persons with a first-degree relative with glaucoma are five times more likely to develop glaucoma than the general population.

Psychosocial History

Closed-angle glaucoma may be precipitated by sitting in a darkened movie theater or stress leading to epinephrine excretion.

Description of Most Common Symptoms

Open-angle glaucoma
- Complaint of a mild, dull ache in the eyes
- Halos around lights

Closed-angle glaucoma
- Presents with acute unilateral eye pain and red eye

Associated Symptoms

Open-angle glaucoma is often accompanied by blurred vision.

Headache is also common.

Closed-angle glaucoma is associated with nausea, vomiting, and conjunctival infection.

Patients also report decreased visual acuity, photophobia, and halos around lights in the same way that patients with chronic glaucoma eventually present.

OBJECTIVE DATA

Physical Examination

The physical examination should include a focused examination of the eye, including:

- Visual acuity
- Pupillary response
- Accommodation
- Peripheral fields: Be alert for diminished fields of vision
- Extraocular eye movements

TABLE 80-2 Differential Diagnosis: Glaucoma

Diagnosis	Supporting Data
Open-angle glaucoma	Diminished fields of vision Funduscopic examination with an increased cup-to-disk ratio (>1:3) and a large optic cup; asymmetry of the cup between eyes and with unequal tonometry readings
Closed-angle or acute glaucoma	Rapid onset, especially in **older patients** and Asians Patient complains of severe pain and profound visual loss; diminished fields of vision Funduscopic examination with an increased cup-to-disk ratio (> 1:3) and a large optic cup Characterized by a dilated pupil that does not react to light; cornea will be cloudy; there is decreased visual acuity, and conjunctival injection Nausea and vomiting are frequently present.
Presbyopia	Natural loss of accommodation with age; inability to focus on objects at a normal reading distance, beginning around age 45
Conjunctivitis	Injected conjunctiva, exposure to others with "pink eye" Eyes matted together in AM, no pain or visual changes
Iritis/uveitis	Inflammation of iris and uveal tract (iris, ciliary body, and choroid) Unilateral pain, redness, photophobia, visual loss
Corneal abrasion	Painful with tearing, history of possible foreign body of eye Corneal abrasions seen via fluorescein stain
Red eye	Numerous conditions can cause a red eye, including keratitis, episcleritis, dry eye, blepharitis, topical drug toxicity See Chapter 155 for further delineation

Funduscopic examination: Look for cup-to-disk ratio, size of cup

Diagnostic Procedures

Diagnostic procedures include those listed in Table 80-1.

ASSESSMENT

Differential Diagnosis

Differential diagnoses include those listed in Table 80-2.

THERAPEUTIC PLAN

Treatment of acute glaucoma requires immediate lowering of eye pressure. Intravenous acetazolamide is given, followed by oral doses. Once the pressure has started to fall, pilocarpine eye drops may be started. A laser peripheral iridectomy is then performed.

Open-angle glaucoma is usually treated with medications as described next. Surgery may be required if intraocular pressure remains elevated despite medical therapy.

Pharmaceutical

The pharmaceutical plan for treatment of glaucoma is outlined in Table 80-3.

Lifestyle/Activities

Prevention is a better option than treatment. Persons should avoid eye trauma, medications that increase susceptibility, or other factors that may predispose them to development of glaucoma.

Diet

Not applicable

Patient Education

Patients older than 60 years of age who have not developed glaucoma need annual tonometry evaluation. Patients with chronic glaucoma need to be aware of signs of increasing intraocular pressure and need to schedule regular ophthalmology evaluation. Patients with chronic glaucoma also need to understand how to use eye drops; these patients should be monitored for side effects of the drugs. especially with noncardioselective beta blocker use.

Referral

Acute glaucoma is a medical emergency that requires immediate referral to an ophthalmologist for surgery. Untreated acute glaucoma will result in severe and permanent visual loss within 2 to 5 days after onset of symptoms.

TABLE 80-3 Pharmaceutical Plan: Glaucoma

Drug	Dose	Action*	Comments	Cost
Sympathomimetics				
Brimonidine 0.2% (Alphagan)	1 gt q8h	A++ B++	α_2 Antagonist Pregnancy: B SE: Oral dryness, burning, stinging, headache, blurred vision, eyelid edema	$22/0.2% (5 ml)
Apraclonidine 0.5%-1% (Iopidine)	1-2 gtt TID	A+++	Pregnancy: C SE: Dry mouth, itching, lid edema, taste aversion	$35/0.5% (5 ml); $66/(10 ml)
Epinephrine 0.1%-2% (Epifrin)	1 gt QD or BID	A+ B++	Pregnancy: C Contraindicated in narrow-angle glaucoma, soft contact lenses SE: Local irritation, blurred vision, hypertension	$28/0.5% (15 ml); $30/1% (15 ml); $32/2% (15 ml)
Dipivefrin 0.2% (Propine)	1 gt BID	A+ B++	Pregnancy: B SE: Tachycardia, hypertension, local irritation	$12-$16/0.1% (5 ml)
Beta Blockers				
Betaxolol 0.25%-0.5% (Betoptic)	1 gt bid	A+++	Pregnancy: C Contraindicated in patients with heart block, asthma SE: Fatigue, depression, bradycardia, CHF, chest pain, ocular burning, stinging, decreased corneal sensitivity	$18/0.25% (5 ml); $18/0.5% (5 ml)
Carteolol 1% (Cartrol, Ocupress)	1 gt BID	A+++	See betaxolol	$16/1% (5 ml); $29-$31/10 ml;
Levobunolol 0.25%-0.5% (Betagan)	1-2 gtt QD or BID	A+++	See betaxolol	N/A
Metipranolol 0.3% (OptiPranolol)	1 gt BID	A+++ B+	See betaxolol	N/A
Timolol (Timoptic, Betimol) .25%	1 gt BID	A+++ B+	See betaxolol	$20-$24/0.25% (10 ml); $24-$29/0.5% (10 ml)
Miotics, Direct				
Acting (Miosis)				
Acetylcholine 1%	0.5-2 ml in anterior chamber	B+++	Lasts 10 min; used for surgery	$21/1% (2 ml)
Carbachol 0.75%-3%	1-2 gtt BID or TID	B+++	Pregnancy: C SE: Blurred vision, N/V, bronchospasm; blurred vision will decrease with repeated use of drug	$18/0.75% (15 ml); $18/1.5% (15 ml)

Pilocarpine 0.25%-10% (Isoptocarpine)	1 gt BID, TID	B+++	Pregnancy: C SE: Local irritation, headache, systemic cholinergic effects	$13/0.25% (15 ml); $2-$13/0.5% (15 ml)
Pilocarpine (Ocusert-Pilo) 20 µg/hr or 40 µg/hr	1 Sustained-release insert at HS, change weekly	B+++	Pregnancy: C SE: Conjunctival irritation, ciliary spasm, H/A	$34/20 µg/hr (8); $34/40 µg/hr (8)
Miotics, Cholinesterase Inhibitors (Miosis)				
Physostigmine 0.25%-0.50% (Eserine Sulfate, Fisostin)	¼ inch of 0.25% ointment into conjunctival sac QD-TID or 1 gt 0.25%-0.5% QD-QID	B+++	Pregnancy: C SE: Seizures, hypertension, bradycardia, irregular pulse Atropine is the antidote	$12/0.25% (15 ml); $13/0.5% (15 ml); $3-$4/0.25% (3.5 g)/ointment
Demecarium 0.125%-0.25% (Humorsol)	1-2 gtt q12-84h **Children:** 1 gt q12-84h	B+++	Pregnancy: X CAUTION: In patients with recent MI, asthma, active PUD, Parkinson's disease, epilepsy	$15/0.125% (5 ml); $16/0.25% (5 ml)
Echothiophate 0.03%-0.25% (Phospholine Iodide)	1 gt BID	B+++	Pregnancy: C SE: Local irritation, headache, visual blurring, tearing	$22/0.03% (5 ml); $24/0.06% (5 ml)
Carbonic Anhydrase Inhibitors				
Acetazolamide (Diamox)	250 mg-1 g QD in divided doses	A+++	Pregnancy: C SE: Anorexia, drowsiness, confusion, malaise, depression, GI upset, tinnitus, rash, fever	$6-$45/250 mg (100)
Dichlorphenamide (Daranide)	100-200 mg initially, then 100 mg q12h Maintenance: 25-50 mg QD-TID	A+++	Pregnancy: C CAUTION: Concomitant use of corticosteroids SE: Weakness, malaise, fatigue, paresthesias of extremities, Stevens-Johnson syndrome	$50/50 mg (100)
Methazolamide (Neptazane)	25-50 mg	A+++	Pregnancy: C SE: Anorexia, malaise, depression, GI upset, paresthesias	$36-$53/25 mg (100); $51-$79/50 mg (100)
Dorzolamide 2% (Trusopt)	1 gt TID	A+++	Pregnancy: C Contraindicated: soft contact lenses SE: Burning, stinging of eyes, bitter taste, tearing, dryness, photophobia	$21/2% (5 ml)

*Mechanisms of action (each drug has the mechanism identified): *A*, decreases the rate of production of aqueous humor; *B*, increases the rate of outflow of aqueous humor from the anterior chamber of the eye; +, degree of strength.

CHF, Congestive heart failure; *COPD*, chronic obstructive pulmonary disease; *FB*, foreign body; *GI*, gastrointestinal; *gt*, drop; *gtt*, drops; H/A, headache; *MAOIs*, monoamine oxidase inhibitors; *MI*, myocardial infarction; *N/A*, not available; *N/V*, nausea and vomiting; *PUD*, peptic ulcer disease; *SE*, side effects.

Continued

TABLE 80-3 Pharmaceutical Plan: Glaucoma—cont'd

Drug	Dose	Action*	Comments	Cost
Prostaglandin Analog				
Latanoprost 0.005% (Xalatan)	1 gt QD in PM	B+++	Used when other options have failed Pregnancy: C Remove contact lenses before use; may reinsert after 15 min SE: Blurred vision, burning, stinging, conjunctival hyperemia, FB sensation	$38/0.005% (50 μg/ml)/ (2.5 ml)
Combination Drugs				
Dorzolamide hydrochloride-timolol maleate (Cosopt)	BID	As above	Combination of carbonic anhydrase inhibitor (Trusopt) and beta blocker (Timoptic); used for patients who do not respond to beta blockers alone SE: Burning, stinging of eyes	N/A
Beta blockers	May be helpful in chronic glaucoma if needed for other concomitant conditions. NOTE: Beta blockers should be used cautiously in overt heart failure, COPD/asthma, and heart block/bradycardia. Alpha adrenergic antagonists should not be used with MAOIs. Miotics should not be used with inflammation or iritis or when pupillary constriction is contraindicated.			

Consultation

The nurse practitioner should consult when there are questionable or elevated tonometry readings, eye pain without a definitive source, or an alteration in funduscopic findings.

Follow-up

Postsurgical follow-up should be done by the ophthalmologist.

In chronic glaucoma the patient should be seen every 6 to12 months for tonometry readings, but this will generally be done by the ophthalmologist or optometrist.

EVALUATION

The effectiveness of therapy will be measured by tonometry readings and failure to develop symptoms of increased intraocular pressure.

SUGGESTED READINGS

Bates B: *A guide to physical examination and history taking,* Philadelphia, 1995, JB Lippincott.

Ellsworth A et al: *Mosby's 1998 medical drug reference,* St Louis, 1998, Mosby.

Everitt DE, Avorn J: Systemic effects of medications used to treat glaucoma, *Ann Intern Med* 11:120, 1990.

Hahn M: Common eye problems in primary care, *Adv Nurse Pract* 4:3, 1996.

Healthcare Consultants of America, Inc: *1998 Physicians fee and coding guide,* Augusta, Ga, 1998, Healthcare Consultants of America, Inc.

Leske C: Risk factors for open-angle glaucoma: the Barbados Eye Study, *Arch Ophthalmol* 113:918, 1995.

Margolis KL: Physician recognition of ophthalmoscopic signs of open-angle glaucoma, *J Gen Intern Med* 4:296, 1989.

Rosenberg L: Glaucoma: early detection and therapy for prevention of vision loss, *Am Family Physician* 52:8, 1995.

Vaughan DT, Asbury T, Riordan-Eva P, editors: *General ophthalmology,* Norwalk, Conn, 1992, Appleton & Lange.

81 Gonorrhea

ICD-9-CM

Gonococcal Infections 098.0
Acute, Lower Genitourinary Tract 098.0
Unspecified Inflammatory Disease of Female Pelvic Organs and Tissue 614.9

OVERVIEW

Definition

Gonorrhea is a sexually transmitted disease caused by *Neisseria gonorrhoeae*, a gram-negative diplococcus that prefers columnar and pseudo-stratified epithelium.

Incidence

Gonorrhea occurs in about 1400 per 100,000 population, or approximately 1 million new cases each year in the United States. The condition often presents without any symptoms in the early stages (25% in men, 80% in women). The rate of gonorrhea is highest among females **15 to 19 years old.**

Pathophysiology

Gonorrheal infections are caused by gram-negative diplococci that are present in exudate and secretions on infected mucous membranes. In women the endocervical canal is the primary site of infection, and in 70% to 90% of infected women the urethra is also infected. In women who have had a hysterectomy, the urethra is the usual site of infection. Infection may also occur in the periurethral glands or Bartholin's glands. Transmission results from intimate sexual contact, and humans are the sole hosts of gonorrhea. Incubation period is generally 2 to 7 days.

Factors That Increase Susceptibility

Sexual exposure to infected individuals
No use of barrier protection
Multiple sexual partners
Infants through infected birth canal
Sexual abuse of a **child**
Autoinoculation
Intrauterine device

SUBJECTIVE DATA

History of Present Illness

Determine whether the patient has a history of previous vaginal infections, any chronic illness, sexual history (including specific practices), type of contraceptive used, most recent sexual contact, any changes in menstrual flow, and human immunodeficiency virus risks.

Women: Should be asked whether there is any dysuria, leukorrhea, labial pain and/or swelling, and any abdominal pain. If the disease is at a later stage, the patient may complain of fever, purulent vaginal discharge, abnormal menses, joint pain or swelling, and tenderness in the pelvic region.

Men: May complain of dysuria and a whitish discharge from the penis. Later this discharge may become yellow-green and he may complain of testicular pain.

Past sexual history: Ask about the number of sexual partners in the past year and if barrier methods were used. Ask about sexual orientation. Ask about any previous sexually transmitted infections and how they were treated. In women ask about the last menstrual period: date, duration, and flow.

Medications

Ask about any medications taken.

If the patient is being treated for a sexually transmitted disease (STD), what medication has been prescribed?

Family History

Not applicable

OBJECTIVE DATA

Physical Examination

Vital signs, including blood pressure and temperature

Head/eyes/ears/nose/throat: Lymph nodes should be assessed for enlargement and/or tenderness.

The throat should be assessed for tonsillar exudate, edema, and erythema if oral sex is practiced.

Women: The abdomen should be assessed for guarding, tenderness, and rebound pain. The pelvic examination should include inspection of the glands (Bartholin's and Skene's) as well as the urethra. An examination with a speculum should be done, looking at the vaginal walls for redness, discharge as well as the cervix, looking for mucopurulent discharge, cervical erythema, and friability. A bimanual examination should note any cervical motion tenderness, uterine tenderness, adnexal pain, or fullness.

Men: Assess the penis for any discharge. Check the testicles for any unusual fullness or tenderness. If anal sex is practiced, perform a rectal examination for tenderness and discharge.

Diagnostic Procedures

Diagnostic tests for gonorrhea are listed in Table 81-1.

ASSESSMENT

Differential Diagnosis

The differential diagnoses for gonorrhea are listed in Table 81-2.

THERAPEUTIC PLAN

Pharmaceutical

Table 81-3 lists recommended regimens from which to choose for the treatment of gonorrhea.

Lifestyle/Activities

Council adults that they should refrain from sexual intercourse until 7 days after completing treatment, whether a single dose treatment or a 7 to 12 day course. Also discuss the role of barrier methods to protect against sexually transmitted infections.

Diet

None

Patient Education

Counsel in a nonjudgmental, compassionate, and respectful way regarding the need for prevention: abstinence, barrier contraception.

Discuss how teens can obtain condoms, negotiate their use with partners, and use them correctly.

Family Impact

The diagnosis of an STD is a traumatic event for all involved. Encourage the patient to share this information with his or her parents or partner as appropriate and seek counseling as needed.

Referral

For sexual abuse of a **child** is suspected, the patient should be referred to a center experienced in collecting specimens, as well as for appropriate therapy. Appropriate counseling for the child and/or parent or parents is encouraged.

Follow-up

Adults: A "test of cure" is not necessary if recommended regimens have been used. If an "alternative" method has been used, a follow-up culture is recommended.

Pregnant women: A test of cure is recommended if erythromycin or amoxicillin has been used; if azithromycin is used, a follow-up test is not necessary.

Neonates and children: Follow-up cultures should be evaluated.

EVALUATION

Patients do not need to be retested for gonorrhea if they were treated using any one of the recommended regimens. If symptoms persist, they should be retested for possible reinfection.

Sex partners who have contact with a patient diagnosed with gonorrhea within the last 60 days should be treated.

The health department must be notified as specified for reportable diseases.

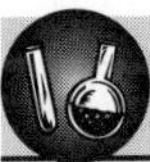

TABLE 81-1 Diagnostic Tests: Gonorrhea

Test	Finding/Rationale	Cost ($)
Microscopic examination	Wet-preparation slide may show increased WBC and decreased normal vaginal flora.	15-19
Gram stain	Identification of intracellular gram-negative diplococci provides immediate diagnosis.	15-19
Culture	Multiple laboratory tests available; sensitivity and specificity may vary. Cultures of the throat, urethra, and anus should also be considered, depending on sexual practices. Testing for chlamydia should be done at the same time. Because of the legal implications of a diagnosis of a gonorrheal infection in children beyond the neonatal period, only standard culture procedures for the isolation of *N. gonorrhoeae* should be used for children. Nonculture tests (e.g., Gram-stained smear, DNA probes, and EIA tests) should not be used alone. Specimens from the vagina, urethra, pharynx, or rectum should be streaked on selective media, and all presumptive isolates should be identified by at least two tests that involve different principles (e.g., biochemical, enzyme substrate, or serological).	Throat: 24-30 31-39/any other source (besides blood, throat, or stool); 61-79/direct probe
RPR, HIV	Any person who tests positive for a sexually transmitted infection should be offered a test for syphilis and other appropriate infections.	18-22/RPR; 8-72/HIV; 60-76/confirm Western blot test

EIA, Enzyme immunoassay; *HIV,* human immunodeficiency virus; *RPR,* rapid plasma reagin test; *WBC,* white blood cell count.

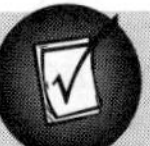

TABLE 81-2 Differential Diagnosis: Gonorrhea

Diagnosis	Supporting Data
Chlamydial infection	Considerable overlap of findings (relative to gonorrhea)
Appendicitis or ectopic pregnancy	Abdominal pain with rebound tenderness and guarding; may begin as vague abdominal pain
Cystitis	Dysuria, frequency, urgency
Men: Urethritis	Dysuria and mucoid discharge 1 week after exposure; discharge becomes purulent
Epididymitis	Acute scrotal pain, fever, dysuria, urethral discharge
Proctitis	Anorectal pain, mucopurulent or bloody discharge, tenesmus, perianal excoriation
Women: PID, cervicitis	CMT, adnexal pain, fever, abdominal pain, vaginal discharge, postcoital bleeding
Bartholinitis	Vaginal pain, erythema at Bartholin's glands
Endometriosis	Dyspareunia, dysmenorrhea, pelvic pain, premenstrual spotting, urinary urgency

CMT, Cervical motion tenderness; *PID,* pelvic inflammatory disease.

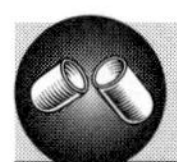

TABLE 81-3 Pharmaceutical Plan: Gonorrhea

Drug	Dose	Comments	Cost
Cefixime (Suprax) *or*	400 mg PO in a single dose	Pregnancy: B SE: Diarrhea, GI upset, rash, pruritus, headache, dizziness, superinfection	$663/400 mg (100)
Ceftriaxone *or*	125 mg IM in a single dose	Pregnancy: B SE: Local reaction, rash, diarrhea, superinfection	$12/250 mg/vial
Ciprofloxacin *or*	500 mg PO in a single dose	Pregnancy: C Not recommended in children under age 18 SE: CNS stimulation, superinfection, dizziness, rash, eosinophilia, elevated liver enzymes, photosensitivity, Stevens-Johnson syndrome, myalgia	$334/500 mg (100)
Ofloxacin *plus concurrent treatment for Chlamydia*	400 mg PO in a single dose	Contraindicated for pregnant women or for children under age 18 Pregnancy: C SE: Superinfection, rash, Stevens-Johnson syndrome, local reactions	$384/400 mg (100)
Azithromycin *or*	1000 mg (1 g) PO in a single dose	Pregnancy: B Avoid taking with antacids SE: GI upset, abdominal pain, angioedema	$16/1 g sachet
Doxycycline	100 mg PO BID for 7 days	Pregnancy: D SE: Photosensitivity, GI upset, enterocolitis, rash	$6-$123/100 mg (50)
Alternative Regimens			
Spectinomycin (Trobicin)	2 g IM in a single dose	Pregnancy: B SE: Local tenderness, urticaria, dizziness, rash, nausea, chills, fever, insomnia	$17/Spect: 400 mg/ml 2 g $7/Cefizox 500 mg $12/Cefotan 1 g/vial $11/Claforan 1 g/vial $17/Mefoxin: 2 g/vial
Ceftizoxime (Cefizox)	500 mg IM in a single dose	Pregnancy: B SE: Nausea/vomiting/diarrhea	
Cefotaxime (Claforan)	500 mg IM		
Cefotetan (Cefotan)	1 g IM		
Cefoxitin (Mefoxin)	2 g IM with probenecid 1g PO		
Uncomplicated Gonococcal Infection of the Pharynx			
Ceftriaxone *or*	125 mg IM in a single dose	See drugs listed above for comments	
Ciprofloxacin *or*	500 mg PO in a single dose		
Ofloxacin *Plus*	400 mg PO in a single dose		
Azithromycin *or*	1 g PO in a single dose		
Doxycycline	100 mg PO BID for 7 days		

Pregnant women should not be treated with quinolones or tetracyclines. They should be treated with a cephalosporin. If they are unable to tolerate a cephalosporin, they should receive a single 2 g dose of spectinomycin IM.
Children who weigh ≥45 kg should be treated with one of the regimens recommended for adults.
Children who weigh ≤45 kg should be treated with ceftriaxone 125 mg IM in a single dose.
Only parenteral cephalosporins are recommended for use in children. Ceftriaxone is approved for all gonococcal infections in children; cefotaxime is approved for gonococcal ophthalmia only. Oral cephalosporins used for treatment of gonococcal infections have not been evaluated adequately.
GI, Gastrointestinal; *IM*, intramuscularly; *SE*, side effects.

RESOURCES

American Social Health Association
http://sunsite.unc.edu/ASHA/

CDC/ STD site (includes copy of 1998 STD treatment guidelines)
http://www.cdc.gov/nchstp/dstd/breaking_news.htm

Griffith's 5-minute clinical consult: a reference for clinicians
http://www.5mcc.com

Journal of American Medical Association Women's Health STD site
http://www.ama-assn.org/special/std/support/support.htm

NOAH: Ask Noah about STDs (a site with multiple resources)
http://www.noah.cuny.edu/illness/stds/stds.html

SUGGESTED READINGS

Centers for Disease Control and Prevention: Guidelines for treatment of sexually transmitted diseases, *MMWR* 47(No RR-1):59-69, 1998.

Ellsworth A et al: *Mosby's 1998 medical drug reference,* St Louis, 1998, Mosby.

Erbelding E, Quin T: The impact of antimicrobial resistance on the treatment of sexually transmitted diseases, *Infect Dis North Am* 11:889-901, 1997.

Landers D, Sweet R: Sexually transmitted infection. In Glass RH: *Office gynecology,* ed 4, Baltimore, 1993, Williams & Wilkins.

Hawkins JW, Roberto-Nichols DM, Stanley-Haney JL: *Protocols for nurse practitioners in gynecologic settings,* ed 5, New York, 1995, Tiresias Press.

Healthcare Consultants of America, Inc: *1998 Physicians fee and coding guide,* Augusta, Ga, 1998, Healthcare Consultants of America, Inc.

Johnson CA: *Women's health care handbook,* St Louis, 1996, Mosby.

McMillan A: Sexually transmittable diseases. In Loudon N, Glasier A, Gebbie A: *Handbook of family planning and reproductive health care,* ed 3, New York, 1995, Churchill Livingstone.

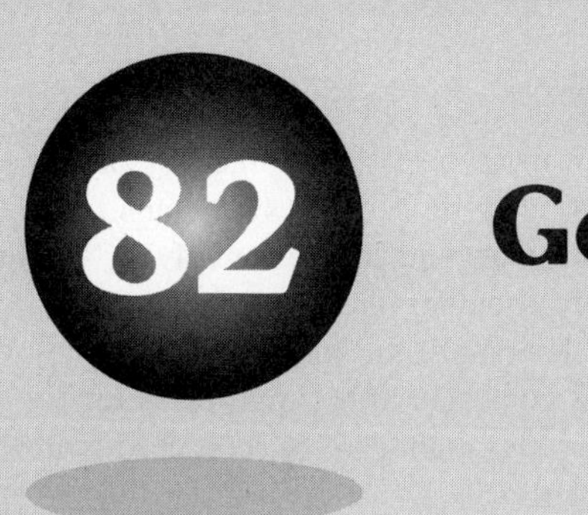

Gout

ICD-9-CM

Gout 274.9
Gouty Arthritis 274.0
Gouty Joint 274.0
Gouty Tophi 274.0
Gouty Tophi of Ear 274.81

OVERVIEW

Definition

Gout is an inflammatory arthritis caused by deposition of monosodium urate (MSU) crystals in joints as a result of an inborn error of purine metabolism and uric acid excretion.

Prevalence

An estimated 2.2 million Americans have gout. Its prevalence is 0.5% to 0.7% for men and 0.1% for women; it is rare before puberty in males and before menopause in females. It is the most common cause of inflammatory arthritis in **men over 40**.

Incidence

The incidence of gout increases as serum uric acid level rises: 0.1% of patients with serum uric acid lower than 7 mg/dl have gout, increasing to 4.5% with levels at or above 9 mg/dl. Age, obesity, and alcohol intake are factors in gout, but not to the extent that uric acid levels play. The incidence of gout is three times greater for hypertensive men taking diuretics (hyperuricemic effect) when compared with normotensive men. Other associated disorders are hyperlipidemia and diabetes.

Pathophysiology

Primary Gout

Primary gout is caused either by decreased excretion or by increased production of uric acid. Hereditary underexcretion is the most common cause of gout. After many asymptomatic years of chronic hyperuricemia (mean, 30 years), acute gout will develop in 25% of these individuals. Women are protected until menopause by estrogen, since it promotes uric acid excretion.

Secondary Gout

Secondary gout is caused by acquired conditions causing overproduction or underexcretion of uric acid.

Overproduction: Polycythemia vera, leukemia, multiple myeloma, psoriasis, hemolytic anemias, disseminated carcinoma

Underexcretion: Chronic renal insufficiency, lead poisoning, acidosis, drug ingestion (nicotinic acid, levodopa, pyrazinamide, ethambutol, cyclosporine, diuretics, low-dose salicylates).

Factors causing a rise in uric acid levels include use of diuretics, alcohol, and low-dose aspirin. Lowering of uric acid is attributed to sudden cessation of alcohol use, high-dose salicylates, or initiation of allopurinol or uricosuric drugs. Acute illness or surgery may alter uric acid levels and precipitate an attack.

Primary and Secondary Gout

Genetic factors influence the rate of uric acid clearance through the kidney.

Any sudden change in uric acid levels can precipitate symptoms of gouty arthritis.

Although not related to uric acid levels, minor trauma can trigger symptoms. Infrequently, gout may coexist with a joint infection.

Untreated chronic gout can lead to tophaceous destruction of bone and cartilage or gouty nephropathy.

SUBJECTIVE DATA

History of Present Illness

Ask about the onset, duration, and progression of symptoms.

Adults: Typically, pain is severe, generally confined to one joint of the foot or ankle in middle-aged or older men;

Children: Are not affected by gout. An acute monarthritis in a large joint in a child is more likely the result of an infectious cause.

Adolescents: Rarely have gout. If diagnosis is substantiated, a secondary cause must be ruled out.

Elderly: Older persons with gout have usually experienced at least one episode of acute arthritis, which may recur, or progress to chronic joint changes over time; elderly women may have multiple joints affected, particularly of the hands.

Past Medical History

Note history of previous attacks, including site, duration, type of treatment, and response to therapy.

History of chronic conditions (listed previously under secondary causes) may be helpful. Inquire about joint trauma, recent illness, or surgery.

Medications

Ask about history of diuretic or aspirin use.

Family History

Twelve percent of patients with gout have other family members with the condition.

Psychosocial History

Ask about ingestion of alcohol, especially beer.

Diet History

Ask about a diet high in purines such as meat, gravy, yeast products, and various vegetables such as peas, beans, spinach, and asparagus.

Description of Most Common Symptoms

Classic symptoms present with significant pain, erythema, usually of the great toe, followed by desquamation of the overlying skin. Onset of symptoms is rapid, increasing over a few hours and lasting a few days to weeks, with complete recovery. The metatarsophalangeal (MTP) joint, instep, or ankle is often the target of a first attack. MSU crystals are soluble at body temperature, and with the temperature of the great toe being lower, it predisposes the crystals to precipitate into that joint, thereby causing symptoms.

In women often more than one joint is involved, with 70% presenting with polyarticular rather than monoarticular symptoms of gout (the hands are the most common site). Chronic gout or interval gout may affect multiple joints of upper and lower extremities and can be confused with rheumatoid or osteoarthritis.

Associated Symptoms

Low-grade fever is possible; no other systemic symptoms are usually present.

OBJECTIVE DATA

Physical Examination

A physical examination should be performed with attention to weight and vital signs, temperature, and blood pressure.

Affected joints should be evaluated for redness, increased warmth, tenderness, effusion, and range of motion.

Nonpainful tophi at the Achilles tendon extensor surfaces of the forearms or, less commonly, on the helix of the ear should be noted. In early stages, tophi may appear as small, superficial yellow-white patches on the palmar and plantar surfaces of the hands and feet. Advanced tophi may ulcerate, leaving a white urate deposit on the skin surface.

Look for joint deformity, particularly of the hands and feet, and check for joint stiffness.

Diagnostic Procedures

Diagnostic tests for gout are listed in Table 82-1.

ASSESSMENT

Primary differential diagnoses include pseudogout and septic joint infection (Table 82-2).

Differential Diagnosis

Reiter's syndrome, ankylosing spondylitis, psoriatic arthritis, sarcoidosis, and gonococcal arthritis are other diseases which may present with acute monarthritis. Also consider acute rheumatic fever, cellulitis, tendinitis, bursitis, and thrombophlebitis.

THERAPEUTIC PLAN

Pharmaceutical

Pharmaceutical treatment for gout is outlined in Table 82-3.

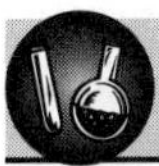

TABLE 82-1 Diagnostic Tests: Gout

Diagnostic Test	Diagnostic Value	Considerations	Cost ($)
Joint aspiration	Only confirmatory test for acute gout; find MSU crystals in phagocytes or free in tophi, seen under polarized microscope	Practitioner's technical experience with this procedure; consult with or refer to physician; use clinical judgment to omit test if symptoms classic	76-90
Serum uric acid	Limited value 20%-30% of people with acute gout have normal values	Hyperuricemia common, but acute arthritis may not be due to gout in individual with elevated uric acid	18-23
Creatinine, BUN	Will be elevated if renal insufficiency is an underlying problem	Order when uric acid elevated in young man or premenopausal woman to look for secondary cause	18-24/creatinine 17-21/BUN
24-hour urine for urate and creatinine	Order with serum uric acid and creatinine to look for secondary cause	May help determine risk for kidney stones	21-26
X-rays	Limited value in acute gout, characteristic findings in advanced gout	Helps to exclude other disorders	71-151/depends on site
CBC, ESR	Elevated with acute gout	Elevated with septic joint infection	13-16/CBC 16-20/ESR
Gram stain and culture of synovial fluid	WBC >50,000-100,000 cells/mm increases likelihood of septic joint	Aspiration limited by practitioner's experience with this procedure	15-19 31-39

BUN, Blood urea nitrogen; *CBC,* complete blood count; *ESR,* erythrocyte sedimentation rate; *WBC,* white blood count.

TABLE 82-2 Differential Diagnoses: Gout

Gout	Pseudogout	Septic Joint Infection*
More common in men over 35-40; acute and chronic arthritis	Only slightly more common in men, age over 60; acute and chronic arthritis	Age not a factor, children affected Acute arthritis
Affects MTP, ankle, instep	Generally affects the knee	Usually affects large joints, knee more common
Onset within hours	Onset occurs over days	Acute onset
Monosodium urate crystals in synovial fluid	Calcium pyrophosphate dihydrate crystals present	Purulent joint aspirate, gram-positive (*Staphylococcus aureus* common)
X-rays: acute normal; chronic asymmetrical bony erosions	X-rays of knees, wrist, symphysis-chondrocalcinosis	X-rays may show joint destruction within 10 days

MTP, Metatarsophalangeal.
*Nongonococcal

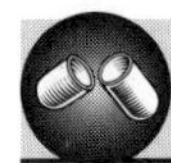

TABLE 82-3 Pharmaceutical Plan: Acute Gout

Medication/Action	Dosage	Considerations	Cost ($)
NSAIDs: First line of therapy unless contraindicated	Naprosyn 500 mg TID Indocin 25-50 mg TID-QID ×1 week, then taper over 3-5 days; (any NSAID, other than aspirin, can be used; indocin and naprosyn most studied)	Relief with Indocin achieved within 2-4 hours Avoid or use with caution in elderly with CHF or renal insufficiency In **elderly** use low-dose ranges and use drug other than indocin because of side effects Avoid NSAIDs with peptic ulcer disease, gastrointestinal bleeding, cirrhosis, or anticoagulant therapy No salicylates since they affect uric acid excretion	18-126/naprosyn; 3-89/Ibuprofen
Colchicine: Interferes with urate crystal deposition in tissues; not an analgesic, only weak antiinflammatory activity	Colchicine 0.5-1.3 mg followed by 0.50 mg-0.65 mg/hour until symptoms relieved up to a maximum of 4-8 mg	Symptoms improve by 12 hours, resolve in 2-3 days Decrease dose with renal insufficiency Diarrhea, nausea, vomiting, and abdominal discomfort are signs of toxicity and may require discontinuing the drug before relief is achieved Extremely narrow therapeutic index	4-20
Corticosteroids: Alternative antiinflammatory to NSAIDs and colchicine	Prednisone 30-50 mg/day tapered over a week Triamcinolone acetonide 60 mg IM	No advantage of parenteral over oral dosing in terms of effectiveness Intra-articular joint injections relieve symptoms without side effects of oral or parenteral therapy; before injection, do joint aspiration to rule out infection; physician consultation should be obtained	3-19/prednisone; 12/triamcinolone

CHF, Congestive heart failure; *NSAID,* nonsteroidal antiinflammatory drug.

Prevention of Recurrent Attacks

One attack of gout does not require continuous treatment with medication, but multiple attacks and/or development of tophi justify use of medication, which should be considered lifelong treatment. Options include those outlined in Table 82-4.

Asymptomatic Hyperuricemia

Treatment is generally not required for persons with uric acid levels of less than 9 or 10 mg/dl with normal renal function whose physical examinations show no tophi have developed. Consider secondary causes of hyperuricemia in these individuals and follow up annually.

Figures 82-1 and 82-2 summarize the clinical approach to the management of gout.

Patient Education

Teach the patient to avoid alcohol binges, fasting, or low-calorie diets, since these can trigger an attack; gradual weight reduction is recommended.

Generous fluid intake is important if the patient is at risk for kidney stones.

Authors differ in their opinions of the importance of a low-purine diet in reducing uric acid levels. Most agree that a low-purine diet has only modest impact on uric acid

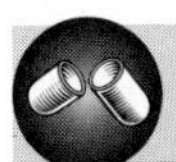

TABLE 82-4 Recurrent Attacks: Gout

Medication/Action	Drug/Dose	Considerations	Cost ($)
Colchicine	0.5-0.65 mg/day to help reduce recurrences, but doses up to 1.5-1.95 mg a day may be required	If renal insufficiency present, give 0.6 mg every other day	4-20
Uric acid–lowering drugs		Uric acid lowering–drugs can aggravate acute attack; should not be started for 2-3 weeks while taking antiinflammatory in interim Goal for these drugs is lowest dose that achieves uric acid <6 mg/dl	
Uricosuric drugs: block uric acid resorption in the proximal tubules of the kidneys	Probenecid (Benemid) 250 mg BID ×7 days, then 500 mg BID; max. 2 g;	Fairly well tolerated Requires ample fluid intake and multiple doses/day	12-35
	Sulfinpyrazone (Anturane) 50 mg BID and adjust to max. of 800 mg in divided TID-QID doses	Contraindicated in person with renal lithiasis (uric acid crystals can deposit in the kidneys and may reduce function or cause renal colic) Must have glomerular filtration rate >30-50 ml/min	12-34
Xanthine oxidase inhibitor: Decreases production of uric acid by blocking conversion of xanthine to uric acid	Allopurinol 100 mg QD starting dose; increase at weekly intervals, usual maintenance dose 300 mg per day (max. 800 mg)	Adverse effects include rash, fever, hepatitis, eosinophilia, vasculitis, and renal insufficiency	3-67

reduction, but an attempt at diet modification may prove worthwhile.

Discuss the pros and cons of treatment options, including side effects of drugs. A small percentage of patients who are taking allopurinol may develop a rash, but one fifth of patients may develop a rash when taking both allopurinol and ampicillin. A more serious but rare side effect of allopurinol is exfoliative dermatitis.

Avoid salicylates and diuretics.

Treat concomitant hypertension and diabetes mellitus.

Family Impact

The cost of medication taken long-term may have financial impact, especially for those living on a fixed income. A family member with chronic gouty arthritis may have some physical limitations affecting activities of daily living.

Consultation

Consult with a physician when joint aspiration or injection is required and the NP lacks technical expertise in these procedures.

Referral

Refer the patient to an orthopedic surgeon or rheumatologist if there is concern about a septic joint, the diagnosis is in question, or the patient's condition is unresponsive to therapy.

EVALUATION/FOLLOW-UP

Recheck within 48 hours if the patient is not responding to treatment for acute attack.

Have the patient return in 4 to 8 weeks to discuss further treatment or evaluation.

Arrange annual examination for follow-up of chronic gout.

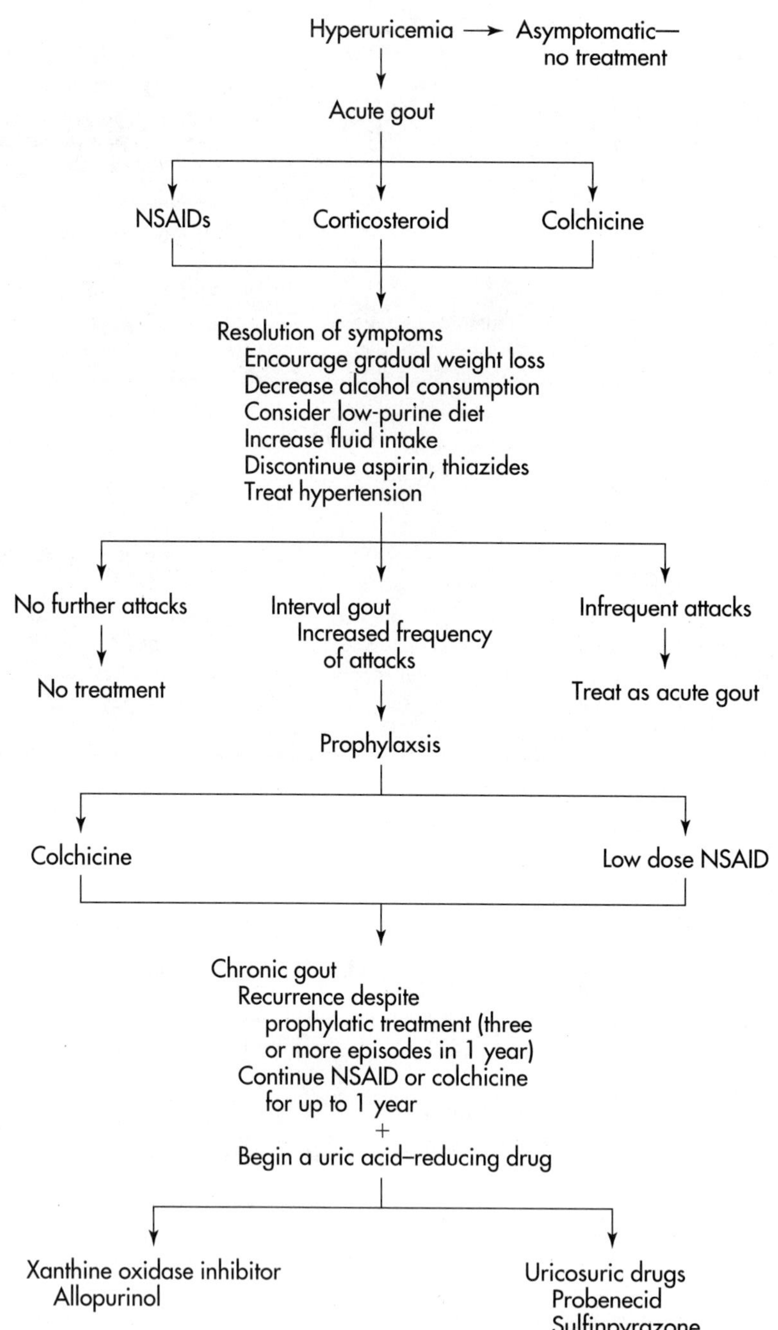

Figure 82-1 Algorithm for treatment of gout. *NSAID,* Nonsteroidal antiinflammatory drug.

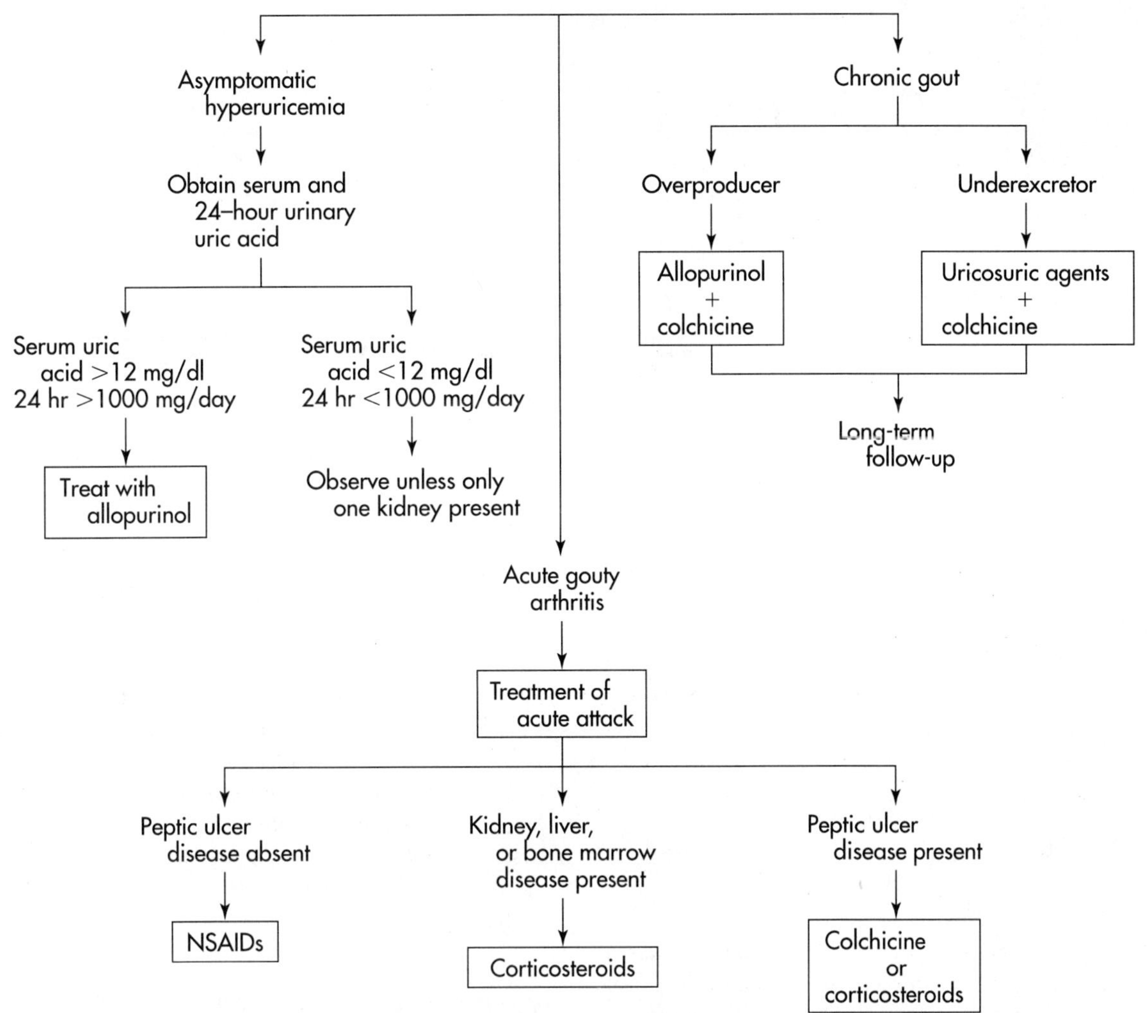

Figure 82-2 Algorithm for treatment of a patient with hyperuricemia and gout. *NSAID,* Nonsteroidal antiinflammatory drug. (Adapted from Greene HL, Johnson WP, Lemcke D: *Decision making in medicine,* ed 2, St Louis, 1998, Mosby.)

SUGGESTED READINGS

American Hospital Formulary Service: *Drug information,* Bethesda, Md, 1997, American Society of Health-Systems Pharmacists, Inc.

Ellsworth A et al: *Mosby's 1998 medical drug reference,* St Louis, 1998, Mosby.

Emmerson BT: The management of gout, *N Engl J Med* 334:445-452, 1996.

George TM, Mandell BF: Individualizing the treatment of gout, *Cleve Clin J Med* 63:150-155, 1996.

Goroll AH, May LA, Mulley AG: *Primary care medicine: office evaluation and management of the adult patient,* ed 3, Philadelphia, 1995, JB Lippincott.

Healthcare Consultants of America, Inc: *1998 Physicians fee and coding guide,* Augusta, Ga, 1998, Healthcare Consultants of America, Inc.

Hershfield MS: Gout and uric acid metabolism. In Bennett JC, Plum F, editors: *Cecil textbook of medicine,* ed 20, Philadelphia, 1996, WB Saunders.

Holland NW, Agudelo CA: Hyperuricemia and gout. In Rakel R, editor: *Conn's current therapy,* Philadelphia, 1997, WB Saunders.

Joseph J, McGrath H: Gout or 'pseudogout': how to differentiate crystal-induced arthropathies, *Geriatrics* 50:33-39, 1995.

Michet CJ et al: Common rheumatologic diseases in elderly patients, *Mayo Clin Proc* 70:1205-1213, 1995.

Towheed TE, Hochberg MC: Acute monoarthritis: a practical approach to assessment and treatment, *American Family Physician* 54:2239-2243, 1996.

Uphold CR, Graham MV: *Clinical guidelines in family practice,* Gainesville, Fla, 1994, Barmarrae Books.

Hand-Foot-and-Mouth Disease

ICD-9-CM

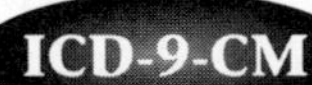

Hand-Foot-and-Mouth Disease 074.3

OVERVIEW

Definition

Hand-foot-and-mouth disease is a viral infection that causes a maculopapular rash, progressing to vesicles. The rash occurs on the extremities, usually localized to the hands and feet. This rash is generally accompanied by papules or vesicular lesions on the buccal mucosa, gums, tongue, and pharynx.

Incidence

The disease is most common in young children. In temperate climates it occurs in the summer and fall; in tropical climates it occurs throughout the year.

Pathophysiology

Protective Factors Against

Good hand washing technique
Appropriate cleansing of surfaces that have come in contact with infected secretions
Limited exposure to large number of children

Factors That Increase Susceptibility

Exposure to large groups of children, such as at day care centers
Adults who work in schools or health care settings
Poor hygiene
Crowded living conditions
Compromised immune system

Pathogens

Hand-foot-and-mouth disease is caused by organisms of the genus *Enterovirus* (nonpolio) *E.* coxsackie A16 and *Enterovirus* 71. There are 23 identified group A coxsackieviruses and four identified enteroviruses. These other enteroviruses can cause diseases that are more significant. The enteroviruses are present in the stool, saliva, and vesicular lesions of an affected patient. These viruses can survive for hours on surfaces.

SUBJECTIVE DATA

History of Present Illness

Duration of rash
Distribution of rash
Systemic symptoms such as fever or body aches

Past Medical History

Ask about frequent severe infections

Medications

Recent use of antibiotics or any other medications

Family History

Any family member ill with similar symptoms
Any family member who is immunocompromised

Psychosocial History

Current living conditions
Attending school or day care

TABLE 83-1 Differential Diagnosis: Hand-Foot-and-Mouth Disease

Disease	Rash	Location	Symptoms
Varicella	Vesicles on red base; progresses to crusts	Begins on trunk; spreads to face and extremities	Fever, headache, and malaise
Herpesvirus	Clusters of vesicles on erythematous base	Follows one or two dermatomes	Burning sensation before rash appears
Measles	Bright red to purple macules and papules	Begins behind ears; spreads to trunk and extremities	Severe cough, fever, conjunctivitis, and Koplik spots
Kawasaki's disease	Red or cracked lips, deep red maculopapular rash	Lower extremities and perineum	Fever, conjunctivitis, cervical adenopathy
Drug eruption rash	Maculopapular red rash; may become confluent	Generalized, usually spares face	Possibly pruritic rash; symptoms of underlying illness
Stevens-Johnson syndrome	Vesicles and bullous lesions	Mucous membranes of mouth, eyes and genitals	Symptoms of upper respiratory infection
Hand-foot-and-mouth	Aphthous lesions, cloudy vesicles with bright red ring	Ulcers occur in mouth; vesicles on the palms, soles; may progress up legs	Low-grade fever, sore throat, and malaise; symptoms last a few days

Description of Most Common Symptoms

Rash: Generally maculopapular, erythematous; progresses to vesicles with cloudy fluid and a red ring around the base

Mouth lesions; generally painful mouth ulcers

Fever, malaise

Approximately 10% will have abdominal pain

Associated Symptoms

Decreased oral intake due to mouth pain

OBJECTIVE DATA

Physical Examination

A problem-oriented physical examination should be conducted, with particular attention to:

- General appearance, weight, and general hydration status
- Ear/nose/throat
  - Presence of aphthous lesions anywhere in mouth or pharynx
  - Presence of saliva and patient's unwillingness to swallow
- Lymph: Presence or absence of submandibular or cervical adenopathy
- Skin: Appearance, duration, and location of rash

Diagnostic Procedures

Generally none indicated

Coxsackie group A antibodies may be evaluated in an immunocompromised patient to determine the specific virus and anticipated course of the illness

Tzanck smear may be performed to rule out other entities

CBC ($13 to $16) with differential only if diagnosis is in question or patient appears to be very ill or is immunocompromised

ASSESSMENT

Differential Diagnosis

Differential diagnoses include varicella, herpes virus, measles, Kawasaki's disease, drug eruption rash, and Stevens-Johnson syndrome; these are described in Table 83-1.

THERAPEUTIC PLAN

Pharmaceutical/Nonpharmaceutical

None curative

Acetaminophen for pain and fever

Mix diphenhydramine (Benadryl) ($2 to $16) and an antacid that contains both aluminum hydroxide and magnesium hydroxide (Maalox or Mylanta), mixed in equal parts (50% each) and apply to mouth lesions

Do not exceed 5 mg/kg/24 hr of diphenhydramine

Viscous lidocaine ($2 to $16) may be cautiously used in **adults** for mouth pain

Avoid in **children** and the **elderly** because of the risk of aspiration from elimination of gag reflex

Lifestyle/Activities

As tolerated

Diet

Soft foods

Avoid citrus, acidic or spicy foods

Maintain hydration

Patient Education

Generally self-limited infection

Rash will heal without topical treatment

Rash generally heals without scarring

Watch closely for signs of dehydration in patients who are reluctant to eat or drink (such as decreased urinary output, limited saliva, inability to cry tears)

Patient may shed the virus for weeks after symptoms resolve; however, no isolation is required in usual circumstances

Family Impact

Limited

Child required to remain out of school or day care until free of fever for 24 hours

Child may be required to remain out of day care if drooling with mouth lesions or lesions on exposed areas are oozing

Referral

Pregnant patients or a pregnant woman in contact with an infected patient may want to contact her obstetrician.

Consultation

Consider consulting with a physician for a patient with signs of dehydration or if the diagnosis is in question.

Follow-up

None needed routinely

If any question that the lesions are now infected, patient should return for a visit

EVALUATION

None

RESOURCE

Centers for Disease Control and Prevention: Hand-foot-and-mouth disease (coxsackie A) in the child care setting, *Fact sheet on childhood diseases and conditions,* updated 12/11/98, cdc.gov/ncidod/hip/abc/facts17.htm.

SUGGESTED READINGS

Committee on Infectious Diseases, American Academy of Pediatrics: *Enterovirus (nonpolio) infections,* 1997 Red Book, The Academy.

Ellsworth A et al: *Mosby's 1998 medical drug reference,* St Louis, 1998, Mosby.

Habif T: Warts, herpes simplex, and other viral infections and exanthems and drug eruptions. In Habif T: *Clinical dermatology,* St Louis, 1996, Mosby.

Healthcare Consultants of America, Inc: *1998 Physicians fee and coding guide,* Augusta, Ga, 1998, Healthcare Consultants of America, Inc.

Nelson W et al: Enteroviruses. In Nelson W et al, editors: *Nelson's textbook of pediatrics,* Philadelphia, 1996, WB Saunders.

Headache

ICD-9-CM

Headache 784.0
Migraine 346.9
Tension 307.81
Cluster 346.2

OVERVIEW

Definition

A headache is an acute or chronic, diffuse pain in different portions of the head, not confined to any nerve distribution area. Headache is usually a benign symptom and only occasionally is a manifestation of a serious illness.

Incidence

Headache is the most common complaint experienced by humans. Disabling headaches are experienced annually by at least 40% of the world population and accounts for a significant proportion of visits to health care providers and about 2.5% of visits to emergency departments. Headache affects 30% of **children** and **teens** (ages 5 to 17) and 34% of **adults** 25 to 44 years old. Ninety percent of these headaches are benign.

Headache is a frequent complaint of the **elderly**; approximately 66% of the headaches in the **elderly** are benign, 34% are secondary to systemic disease and primary intracranial lesions. Most reports indicate **women** have headaches more often than **men** (Couch, 1993; Diamond, 1992; Edmeads, 1997; and Rasmussen and Olsen, 1992).

Pathophysiology

A headache can be a symptom indicating another disease, rather than representing a disease itself. Headache can originate from activation of peripheral nociceptors in the presence of a normally functioning nervous system or as a result of injury or activation of the peripheral or central nervous system.

Headaches may arise from dysfunction, displacement, or encroachment on pain-sensitive cranial structures. Headaches can occur as a result of (1) distention, traction, or dilation of intracranial or extracranial arteries, (2) traction or displacement of large intracranial veins or their dural envelope, (3) compression, traction, or inflammation of cranial and spinal nerves, (4) spasm, inflammation, and trauma to cranial and cervical muscles, (5) meningeal irritation and raised intracranial pressure, and (6) disturbance of intracerebral serotonergic projections (Robertson and McCormack, 1998).

Classification

Headaches are broadly classified as primary (benign or idiopathic) and secondary (organic or malignant) headache disorders. Primary headaches include common tension-type (muscle-contraction) headaches, migraine headaches, and cluster headaches. These types of headaches comprise 99% of headache complaints.

Secondary headaches are caused by some underlying pathophysiology and are responsible for less than one percent of headache complaints and cerebrovascular lesions, meningeal irritation, intracranial pressure changes, arteritis, infections, and facial, cervical, systemic, or traumatic causes.

The most frequently used classification system is the 1988 four-digit system developed by the International Headache Society (IHS). The IHS system has operational diagnostic criteria for 129 different headache syndromes, divided into 13 categories. The 1988 IHS's 13 categories are provided in Box 84-1. The IHS provides diagnostic criteria for each category and subcategory.

Protective or Preventive Factors Against

No preventive measures have been clearly identified for individuals at risk for migraine and tension-type headaches.

Migraine headaches are exacerbated by lying down and relieved by standing or sitting.

Box 84-1

Major Types of Headache and Subtypes of Migraine

1. **Migraine**
1.1 Migraine without aura
1.2 Migraine with aura
1.3 Ophthalmoplegia migraine
1.4 Retinal migraine
1.5 Childhood periodic syndromes that may be precursors to or associated with migraines
1.6 Complications of migraines
1.7 Migrainous disorders not fulfilling above criteria

2. **Tension-type headache**
2.1 Episodic tension-type headache
2.2 Chronic tension-type headache
2.3 Tension type headache not fulfilling above criteria

3. **Cluster headache and chronic paroxysmal hemicrania**
3.1 Cluster headache
3.2 Chronic paroxysmal headache
3.3 Cluster headache-like disorder not fulfilling above criteria

4. **Miscellaneous headaches unassociated with structural lesion**
4.1 Idiopathic stabbing headache
4.2 External compression headache
4.3 Cold stimulus headache
4.4 Benign cough headache
4.5 Benign exertional headache
4.6 Headache associated with sexual activity

5. **Headache associated with head trauma**
5.1 Acute posttraumatic headache
5.2 Chronic posttraumatic headache

6. **Headache associated with vascular disorders**
6.1 Acute ischemic cerebrovascular disorder
6.2 Intracranial hematoma
6.3 Subarachnoid hemorrhage
6.4 Unruptured vascular malformation
6.5 Arteritis
6.6 Carotid or vertebral artery pain
6.7 Venous thrombosis
6.8 Arterial hypertension
6.9 Headaches associated with other vascular disorder

7. **Headaches associated with nonvascular intracranial disorders**
7.1 High CSF pressure
7.2 Low CSF pressure
7.3 Intracranial infection
7.4 Intracranial sarcoidosis and other noninfectious inflammatory diseases
7.5 Headache related to intrathecal injections
7.6 Intracranial neoplasm
7.7 Headache associated with other intracranial disorder

8. **Headache associated with substance or their withdrawal**
8.1 Headache induced by acute substance use or exposure
8.2 Headache induced by chronic substance use or exposure
8.3 Headache from substance withdrawal (acute use)
8.4 Headache from substance withdrawal (chronic use)
8.5 Headache associated with substance but with uncertain mechanism

9. **Headache associated with noncephalic infection**
9.1 Viral infection
9.2 Bacterial infection
9.3 Headache related to other infection

10. **Headache associated with metabolic disorder**
10.1 Hypoxia
10.2 Hypercapnia
10.3 Mixed hypoxia and hypercapnia
10.4 Hypoglycemia
10.5 Dialysis
10.6 Headache related to other metabolic abnormality

11. **Headache or facial pain associated with disorder of cranium, neck, eyes, ears, nose, sinuses, teeth, mouth, or other facial or cranial structures**
11.1 Cranial bone
11.2 Neck
11.3 Eyes
11.4 Ears
11.5 Nose and sinuses
11.6 Teeth, jaws, and related structures
11.7 Temporomandibular joint disease

12. **Cranial neuralgias, nerve trunk pain, and deafferentation pain**
12.1 Persistent pain of cranial nerve origin
12.2 Trigeminal neuralgia
12.3 Glossopharyngeal neuralgia
12.4 Nevus intermedius neuralgia
12.5 Superior laryngeal neuralgia
12.6 Occipital neuralgia
12.7 Central causes of head and facial pain other than tic douloureux
12.8 Facial pain not fulfilling criteria in groups 11 or 12

13. **Headache not classifiable**

Adapted from Dalessio DJ: Diagnosing the severe headache, *Neurology* 44 (Suppl 3): 6-11, 1994; and Dubose CD, Cutlip AC, Cutlip WD: Migraines and other headaches: an approach to diagnosis and classification, *American Family Physician* 51:1498-1504, 1995.

TABLE 84-1 Triggers or Risk Factors for Common Types of Headaches

Trigger/Risk Factors	Types of Headaches		
	Tension	**Migraine**	**Cluster**
Hormonal		Hormone replacement Menstruation Oral contraceptive therapy Pregnancy	
Exercise or exercertion		Eye strain Head injury Irregular exercise No exercise	
Environmental factors	Emotion (stressful events, anger, depression)	Bright or flashing lights Emotion (stress, anger, depression, fatigue, anxiety) Missed meals (hypoglycemia) Smoke Strong odor (perfume, paint) Too much or too little sleep Weather changes	Changes in length of daylight
Foods/ingredients		Aged cheese Alcohol Artificial sweeteners Caffeine (coffee, cola, tea) Chocolate Cultured dairy products (buttermilk, sour cream, yogurt) Fruits (avocado, bananas, citrus, figs, pineapple, raisins) Nitrates (cured meats) Sulfites Vegetables (beans, olives, onions, pickles, snow peas) Yeast	Alcohol once the cluster has started
Medications/drugs		Common drugs that cause rebound headache include: Barbiturates Opioids Ergotamine tartrate compounds Benzodiazepines Caffeine-containing analgesic preparations	Nitroglycerin once the cluster has started

Use of the following can reduce the incidence of tension-type headache:

- Glare-screens on computer terminals
- Proper ergonomics at work stations to reduce neck strain
- Good ventilation systems at work sites where personnel are exposed to chemical fumes
- Stress-reducing behaviors

No protective factors have been identified for cluster headaches.

Protective factors for secondary types of headaches include wearing seatbelts and safety helmets to prevent head injury and the use of small-cannula needles and lying down immediately after lumbar puncture (Robertson and McCormack, 1998).

Factors That Trigger Headaches

Identifying and avoiding headache risk factors and triggers can help to prevent headaches and managing them when they do occur. However, it is difficult to differentiate risk factors from prodromal symptoms in migraine (Table 84-1) (Loder, 1998).

Particularly in the **elderly,** medications may cause

Box 84-2

Medications That May Cause Headaches in Older Individuals

Cardiovascular Drugs

Vasodilators

Nitroglycerin
Isosorbide nitrate (Dilatrate-SR, Isordil, Sorbitrate)
Dipyridamole (Persantine)

Hypotensives

Reserpine
Nifedipine (Adalat, Procardia)
Atenolol (Tenormin)
Methyldopa (Aldomet)

Antiarrhythmic Agents

Quinidine
Digoxin (Lanoxicaps, Lanoxin)
Ranitidine HCl (Zantac)

Central Nervous System Drugs

Antiparkinson Agents

Levodopa (Dopar, Larodopa)
Amantadine HCl (Symadine, Symmetrel)

Sedatives

Benzodiazepines
Barbiturates
Chloral hydrate (Noctec)
(Bactrim, Cotrim, Septra)

Stimulants

Methylphenidate HCl (Ritalin)
Caffeine

Musculoskeletal Drugs

Nonsteroidal Antiinflammatory Drugs

Indomethacin (Indocin)

Analgesics

Propoxyphene (Darvon Pulvules, Dolene)
Pentazocine (Talwin)

Gastrointestinal System Drugs

Histamine$_2$ Blockers

Cimetidine (Tagamet)

Respiratory System Drugs

Bronchodilators

Aminophylline (Phyllocontin), theophylline, pseudoephedrine HCl

Immune System Drugs

Antibiotics

Trimethoprim-sulfamethoxazole

From Edmeads J: Headaches in older people, *Postgrad Med* 101:91-100, 1997.

headaches (Box 84-2). Some of the risk factors such as foods are avoidable, whereas others such as weather changes and menstrual periods are impossible to avoid.

TYPES OF HEADACHES

Primary Headaches

Migraine

Migraine Without Aura (Common Migraine)

Usually presents as a moderate to severe, throbbing, unilateral headache in the temple region or around the eye with a family history of migraine that began between 10 and 25 years of age

Higher incidence in **children** and **younger adults**

Greater occurrence in females than males in adults, but in **children** occurs with equal frequency in males and females

Peak prevalence tends to be around 40 years of age in women and 35 in men

Diagnostic Criteria for Migraine Headaches. Diagnostic criteria are as follows:

- Headache attack lasts 4 to 72 hours
- At least five attacks fulfilling two to four of the following:
  - Unilateral location
  - Pulsating quality
  - Moderate or severe intensity (inhibits or prohibits activities of daily living [ADL])
  - Exacerbated by walking stairs or similar routine physical activity
- During headache, at least one of the following occurs:
  - Nausea and/or vomiting
  - Photophobia and phonophobia
- No evidence of organic disease, or if an organic disorder is present, migraine attack not temporally related

(Cady and Farmer, 1998; Edmeads, 1997; Fettes, 1997; Heck, 1998; Lipton, Amalneik, Ferrare and Gross, 1994; and Rapoport, 1992)

Migraine with Aura (Classic Migraine)

In addition to the symptoms associated with migraine without aura, migraine with aura is characterized by typical neurological symptoms preceding the headache: visual scotomata (flashing lights), visual field defects (hemianopsia, quadrantanopsia), fortification scintillations (zigzag lines or waves), vertigo, and rarely, aural or olfactory hallucinations. Usually the symptoms of an aura cease soon after the headache starts and there is no lasting impairment.

Diagnostic Criteria for Migraine with Aura. Diagnostic criteria for migraine with aura, in addition to the criteria for migraine without aura, are listed as follows:

- At least two attacks that have at least three of the following characteristics:
- One or more fully reversible aura symptoms indicating focal cerebral, cortical, and/or brain stem dysfunction:
  - Homonymous visual disturbance
  - Unilateral paresthesias and/or numbness
  - Unilateral weakness
  - Aphasia or unclassified speech difficulty
- At least one aura symptom develops gradually over more than 4 minutes or two or more symptoms occur in succession
- No aura symptoms last more than 60 minutes; if more than one aura symptom is present, accepted duration is proportionally increased
- Headache begins before, concurrent with, or follows an aura in less than 60 minutes
- No evidence of organic disease or, if organic disorder is present, migraine attack not temporally related

Elderly: Frequency and severity of migraine diminish as one ages (Cady and Farmer, 1998; Edmeads, 1997; Fettes, 1997; Heck, 1998; Lipton, Amalneik, Ferrare and Gross, 1994; and Rapoport, 1992)

Menstrual (Hormonal) Migraine Headache

The type of migraine attack that occurs exclusively around the time of menses is called "true menstrual migraine" and affects about 14% of migraineurs. Menstrual migraines occur on a regular basis between days −2 and +3 of the menstrual cycle. Migraines that occur from days −7 to −3 of the cycle are considered premenstrual and are associated with premenstrual syndrome (PMS). Estrogen withdrawal is believed to be the trigger for the menstrual migraine (Coutin and Glasser, 1996; Fettes, 1997).

Tension-type Headache

Tension-type headache can be episodic or chronic. It is usually a bilateral, steady aching pain of mild to moderate intensity that lasts from minutes to days. The pain gradually builds with time.

This type accounts for 20% to 30% of headaches that occur more than once a month.

The female-to-male ratio is 1:1 until puberty; after puberty the ratio is 5:4.

Current theories indicate that tension-type headaches and migraine headaches occur together along a continuum, with tension headache at one end and migraine at the other.

Diagnostic Criteria for Episodic Tension-Type Headache. Diagnostic criteria are as follows:

- At least 10 previous headache episodes fulfilling the following criteria (number of days with headache less than 180 per year or less than 15 per month)
- Headache lasting from 30 minutes to 7 days
- At least two of the following pain characteristics:
  - Pressing/tightening (nonpulsating) quality
  - Mild or moderate intensity (may inhibit but does not prohibit activities)
  - Bilateral location
  - No aggravation by walking stairs or similar routine physical activity
- Both of the following:
  - No nausea or vomiting (anorexia may occur)
  - Photophobia and phonophobia are absent, or one but not the other is present
- No evidence of organic disease or organic condition present, tension headache, not temporally related

Episodic Tension-type Headache (Contraction Headache Associated With Disorder of Pericranial Muscles). This type of headache:

- Fulfills criteria for episodic tension-type headache
- Is accompanied by at least one of the following:
  - Increased tenderness of pericranial muscles demonstrated by manual palpation of pressure
  - Increased electromyelogram level of pericranial muscles at rest during physiological tests

Episodic Tension-Type Headache Not Associated With Disorder of Pericranial Muscles (Idiopathic, Essential, or Psychogenic Headache). This type of headache:

- Fulfills criteria for episodic tension-type headache
- Is accompanied by no increased tenderness of pericranial muscles

Chronic Tension-Type Headache. This type of headache is accompanied by:

- Average headache frequency 15 days per month (180 days per year) for 6 months and fulfilling the following criteria:
- At least two of the following pain characteristics:
  - Pressing/tightening quality
  - Mild or moderate severity (may inhibit but does not prohibit activities)
  - Bilateral location
  - No aggravation by walking stairs or similar physical activity
- Both of the following:
  - No vomiting

No more than one of the following: Nausea, photophobia, or phonophobia

No evidence of organic disease or, if comorbid, no temporal relation (Diamond, 1992; Heck, 1998; and Rapoport, 1992)

Cluster Headaches (Migrainous Neuralgia)

Pain begins unilaterally, usually in or around the eye or anywhere on one side of the head.

The pain quickly progresses to involve the whole side of the head and is described as a severe, boring mixture of jabs and pressure.

The pain may radiate to the teeth on one side.

The eye on the side of the pain tears and turns red and sometimes the lid droops.

Attacks of pain are associated with extracranial vasodilation, increased cerebral blood flow, and internal carotid artery changes.

Each attack lasts from 10 minutes to 3 hours.

Individuals may experience one to three attacks per day, with many of the attacks occurring at night, especially about 90 minutes after the onset of sleep.

The cluster period lasts on an average of 2 months and appears to be related to seasonal photoperiod changes (length of daylight), often occurring in the spring or fall with remission periods between clusters.

Cluster headaches account for less than 1% of headaches.

Can begin at any age and are more prevalent in **men** with a male-to-female ratio of 6-8:1.

Diagnostic Criteria for Cluster Headache. Diagnostic criteria are as follows:

At least five attacks fulfilling the following characteristics:

Severe unilateral orbital, supraorbital, and/or temporal pain lasting 15 to 180 minutes if untreated

Headache is associated with at least one of the following signs, which have to be present on the side of the pain:

- Conjunctival injection
- Lacrimation
- Nasal congestion
- Rhinorrhea
- Forehead and facial sweating
- Miosis
- Ptosis
- Eyelid edema

Frequency of attacks: From one every other day to eight per day

Episodic cluster headache: At least two periods of headache (cluster periods) lasting (untreated) from 7 days to 1 year, separated by remissions of at least 14 days

Chronic cluster headaches: Attacks occur for more than 1 year without remission or with remission lasting less than 14 days

No evidence of organic disease, or if organic disease present, cluster headache not temporally related (Diamond, 1992; Kudrow, 1991; and Heck, 1998)

Secondary Headaches

Many organic causes can produce secondary headaches of varying types,characteristics, and locations.

Cerebrovascular

Headache depends on location, type and extent of vascular lesion

Subarachnoid Hemorrhage

Approximately 98% to 100% are associated with headache

Can occur at any age; average age is about 51

Sudden onset; described as "the worst headache of my life," referred to as the "thunderclap" headache

May have a sentinel headache

Occasional family history of polycystic kidney disease or coarctation of the aorta

Nuchal rigidity occurs about 75% of the time

Neurological abnormalities common but may be absent

Computed tomographic (CT) scan can yield false-negative result (15%)

Cerebrospinal fluid bloody, electroencephalogram (EEG) may be abnormal; patient may have leukocytosis, albuminuria/glycosuria (Couch, 1993; Dalessio, 1993; Heck, 1998; and Weiss, 1993)

Intraparenchymal Hemorrhage

More than 50% of cases are associated with headache

Occurs in 3% to 10% of all strokes

Hypertension in more than 50%

Sudden onset of profound ataxia in cerebellar hemorrhage (Couch, 1993)

Ischemic Cerebrovascular Disease

Headache frequency of 17% to 54%

Headache generally mild to moderate in intensity (Couch, 1993; Edmeads, 1998)

Carotid Artery Dissection

Rare; usually occurs in young adults

Headache present in more than 80% of cases

Ipsilateral Horner's syndrome is a diagnostic clue

Approximately one third of individuals suffer infarcts (Couch, 1993)

Hypertension

Hypertension usually does not cause pain unless diastolic pressure is higher than 120 mm Hg

When headache is present, generally mild and occurs on waking but improves when patient rises (Diamond, 1992; Weiss, 1993)

Cervical Disease

Most common cause of headache beginning in middle to late life

Wide variety of cervical (neck) disease processes are involved; most common is cervical spondylosis

Pain usually has a dull, occipital, frequently asymmetrical, nonthrobbing, aching quality and associated with shoulder and low-back pain

Course is chronic and relapsing (Edmeads, 1997)

Drug Overuse (Rebound) or Withdrawal Headache

Drug overuse or withdrawal may contribute to as many as 20% of chronic headache syndromes.

Rebound Headache

Rebound headache is defined by Mathew (1997) as "the perpetuation of head pain in chronic headache sufferers that is caused by frequent and excessive use of immediate relief medication." Common terms for rebound headache are "analgesic rebound," "ergotamine rebound," and "drug-induced" headaches.

These headaches are refractory, with a daily or nearly daily frequency.

The headache varies in its severity, type, and location from time to time.

Even slight physical or intellectual effort will bring on headaches in such patients.

Headaches are accompanied by asthenia (lack or lost of strength), nausea and other GI symptoms, restlessness, anxiety, irritability, memory problems, difficulty concentrating, and depression.

Persons consuming large quantities of ergot derivatives tend to exhibit cold extremities, tachycardia, paresthesia, diminished pulses, hypertension, light-headedness, muscle pain in the extremities, weakness of the legs, and depression.

There is a drug-dependent rhythmicity of headaches. Predictable early morning (2:00 AM to 5:00 AM) headaches are frequent, particularly in patients who use large quantities of analgesics, sedatives, caffeine, or ergotamine combinations.

There is evidence of tolerance to analgesics, with patients needing increasing doses over time to obtain similar relief.

Withdrawal symptoms are observed in patients when pain medications are discontinued abruptly.

Spontaneous improvement of headache may occur simply by discontinuing medications that cause rebound.

Therapeutic efficacy of usually effective preventive medications may be compromised by ongoing consumption of immediate relief medications.

Substance-withdrawal Headache

Substance-withdrawal headache, according to Weeks (1997) "occurs (1) after use of a high daily dose of a substance for at least 3 months and (2) within hours of withdrawal." Medications that may cause withdrawal and rebound headaches include barbiturates, opioids, ergotamine tartrate compounds, benzodiazepines, and caffeine-containing analgesic preparations.

Infectious Diseases

Headache common and predominant in bacterial meningitis

Severe headache is the most frequent symptom, along with fever and nuchal rigidity in viral meningitis

Severe headache is common with acute sinusitis: A dull, nonpulsating aching headache; location depends on the sinus involved (Coutin and Glass, 1996; Dodick, 1997; Weiss, 1993)

Inflammatory Disease

Temporal Arteritis (Giant Cell Arteritis)

Usually seen in **women** (four times more often than in men) over 50 years of age Typically this is a new kind of headache for the individual

Pain tends to be focal and unvarying in location, at the temporal artery (tenderness in this area) and behind the eye

Sudden blindness may occur without warning; visual impairment occurs in a third to a half of individuals

Erythrocyte sedimentation rate (ESR) elevated with a mean of 100 mm/hr

Malaise, fever, weight loss, and jaw claudication are early symptoms; symptoms associated with polymyalgia rheumatica (Couch, 1993; Coutin and Glass, 1996; Dodick, 1997; Edmeads, 1997)

Granulomatous Angiitis

Headache common complaint (in two of three patients) in this rare, small-artery vasculitis of small vessels restricted to the central nervous system (Couch, 1993)

Neoplastic Disease

Headache associated with a brain tumor is usually deep, aching, nonthrobbing, often generalized, and intermittent; more frequent in **elderly;** however, does occur in children and young adults

Headache occasionally associated with vomiting and may be worse with exertion (e.g., coughing or straining) by increasing intracranial pressure; most severe in the morning on rising

Posterior fossa tumors frequently produce headaches

Acute hydrocephalus produces severe headache

Pseudotumor cerebri produces headache in more than 80% of individuals; is usually insidious and generalized; may be mild but can be described as "worst ever" headache; often worse in the morning or after exertion (Coutin and Glass, 1996; Diamond, 1992; Dodick, 1997; Edmeads, 1997; Heck, 1998)

Neuralgia

Postherpetic Neuralgia

Up to 50% of individuals **over 60 years of age** develop postherpetic neuralgia following shingles.

Pain is described as an intense burning pain, punctuated by stabbing exacerbations; it may persist for months to years.

V1 is the most frequently involved cranial nerve (Baumel and Eisner, 1991),

Trigeminal Neuralgia (Tic Douloureux)

Severe, disabling, lancinating (piercing, stabbing) pain in distribution of V1 or V2 cranial nerve that lasts a few seconds to minutes, interspersed with a minute or so of relief.

Pain may recur several times per day and becomes more frequent.

Exposure to environmental irritants such as wind and cold may precipitate pain (Baumel and Eisner, 1991 and Weiss, 1993).

Ophthalmological Headache

Eyestrain (Refractory Errors)

When pain (usually a dull, bilateral headache) is present, it is increased with use of eyes (e.g., with prolonged reading or computer screen viewing).

Astigmatism and refractive errors do not cause headache (Coutin and Glass, 1996).

Narrow-Angle Glaucoma

Episodic pain in and around the eye

A severe, boring ache centered in the eye (though may be diffuse on that side of the head)

Nausea and vomiting may occur

Can cause blindness if not treated (Weiss, 1993)

Optic Neuritis

Pain in or behind the eye and may be exacerbated by pressure over the eye or ocular movement (Weiss, 1993)

Tolosa Hunt Syndrome

Idiopathic granulomatous disease of the cavernous sinus or superior orbital tissue

When suspected, an ESR should be obtained

Occurs more often in **young children** (Winner, 1997)

Otalgic Headache

Headache from ear pain may originate from external canal foreign bodies, external otitis, external or middle ear neoplasia, otitis media, acoustic neuroma, and external/middle ear trauma (Weiss, 1993)

Headache Following Spinal Puncture

Occurs in 10% to 30% of individuals who receive a spinal puncture

Usually begins 15 minutes to 4 days after the procedure and lasts 4 to 8 days

Female to male ratio 2:1

Pain described as either frontal or occipital or diffuse, pounding pain or a dull ache, present when upright and relieved when lying flat (Baumel and Eisner, 1991)

Temporomandibular Joint Dysfunction

Localized facial pain, limitation of jaw motion, muscle tenderness, and joint crepitus of the temporomandibular joint

Pain in front of and behind the ear on the affected side, but may radiate over cheek and face; ear may feel full (Weiss, 1993)

Toxic and Metabolic Headaches

Toxic (Carbon Monoxide, Hypercapnia, and Acute Mountain Sickness)

A gradual intensification of headache, followed by impaired consciousness (Edmeads, 1997; Weiss, 1993)

Chinese Restaurant Syndrome

Headache caused by the ingestion of monosodium glutamate (often used in preparation of Chinese foods) by individuals who are sensitive to it

Symptoms include headache, nausea, light-headedness, and numbness and burning of head, chest, and/or arms (Edmeads, 1997; Weiss, 1993)

Chronic Hemodialysis

Individuals on chronic dialysis frequently have headaches (Weiss, 1993)

Trauma

Hematomas

Conscious individuals with epidural or acute hematomas without exception complain of headache.

Subacute or chronic subdural hematoma: Headache occurs in up to 60% of individuals; headache more severe than with that of brain tumor; suspect in individuals with headache who are alcoholic, epileptics whose seizures are not controlled, **patients over 60 years old,** or those under dialysis or anticoagulant therapy (Coutin and Glass, 1996; Dodick, 1997; Edmeads, 1997; Weiss, 1993)

Posttraumatic Headache

An immediate transient headache follows almost all head injuries.

Prevalence of chronic posttraumatic headache varies from 30% to 50%.

In addition to experiencing nonspecific headache, the patient may also have dizziness, irritability, fatigue, anxiety, insomnia, impaired concentration, and memory disturbances.

Disturbances usually last only a few months but may persist for as long as 18 months or more.

Neurological examination usually yields normal results (Coutin and Glass, 1997).

SUBJECTIVE DATA

Since headaches tend to be subjective, a focused history is the most important diagnostic tool in determining the type of headache.

Children: History in children requires input from parents. Through the history the NP must determine whether the child experiences more than one type of headache and what level of disability the headache causes. These can be estimated from specific questions, for example:

Is academic performance affected by the headaches?
How much school has the child missed because of headaches? (Winner, 1997)

Elderly: In elderly patients, headaches are more frequently associated with serious conditions or medications; therefore a history related to these areas must be obtained (Baumel and Eisner, 1990). Aspects of the history that should be obtained from a patient with complaint of headache are as described below.

History of Headache Characteristics

Number of headache types
For each type of headache the individual describes, gather the following information:
- Age at onset
- Duration (range)
  - Without treatment
  - With treatment

Figures 84-1 and 84-2 illustrate difference in history and the examination for headache based on duration.
Frequency
Location (unilateral, bilateral)
If unilateral, does it alternate sides?
Quality of pain (pulsating or constant steady ache?)
Does the pain prohibit usual daily activities?
Is the pain aggravated by mild physical activity (e.g., walking around, climbing stairs)?
Presence of associated features such as nausea, vomiting, photophobia, or phonophobia
Presence of an aura
- If yes, describe the aura
- Duration of the aura
- Relation to onset of pain

Potential Precipitating Factors

Dietary factors (e.g., tyramine and nitrite sensitivity)
Relationship to menses
Medications (e.g., oral contraceptives)
Psychosocial stressors
Other factors identified by the patient

Medications

Drugs tried for symptomatic relief of headache (both over-the-counter [OTC] and prescription medications; include highest dose reached and reason for discontinuation)
Prophylactic medications
Current medications used for the treatment of headache (include dose, length of time the drug has been taken, and effectiveness)
Medications used for reasons other than headache
Nonpharmacological therapies (e.g., biofeedback, hot or cold compresses, sleep); note their effectiveness

Pertinent Medical History

Asthma, Raynaud's syndrome
Peptic ulcer: Depression
Anxiety: Insomnia
Frequent strenuous activity (e.g., jogging, aerobics)
Fear of what headache may represent
Other

Family History

Headaches (e.g., type, frequency)

OBJECTIVE DATA

Physical Examination

A problem-oriented physical examination (PE) should be performed that includes all body systems, with emphasis on:

- Vital signs, head, neck (including lymph nodes), ears, eyes, and neurological aspects of the examination; PE usually yields normal results
- Additional components of the PE to be performed:
  - Thorax and lungs
  - Cardiovascular
  - Peripheral vascular
  - Abdomen
  - Musculoskeletal
  - Neurological
    - Cranial nerves I-XII
    - Funduscopic
    - Reflexes
  - Muscle strengths (Heck, 1998; Weiss, 1993)

Diagnostic Procedures

Most individuals with headache have normal or unrelated diagnostic findings.

Laboratory Studies

Complete blood count ($13 to $16): To rule out inflammatory and infectious conditions
WBC and differential high in meningitis: White blood count (WBC) left shift if bacterial cause
Viral syndrome: Moderately elevated WBC and lymphocytosis
When human immunodeficiency virus (HIV) is suspected, a WBC and CD_4 count should be performed ($123 to $154)
Thyroid function test to rule out hyperthyroidism ($47 or $61)
Lumbar puncture ($172 or $208) if meningitis or subarachnoid hemorrhage is suspected
Erythrocyte sedimentation rate (ESR) ($16 to $20) if temporal arteritis is suspected (a level above 80 mm/hour usually supports the diagnosis)

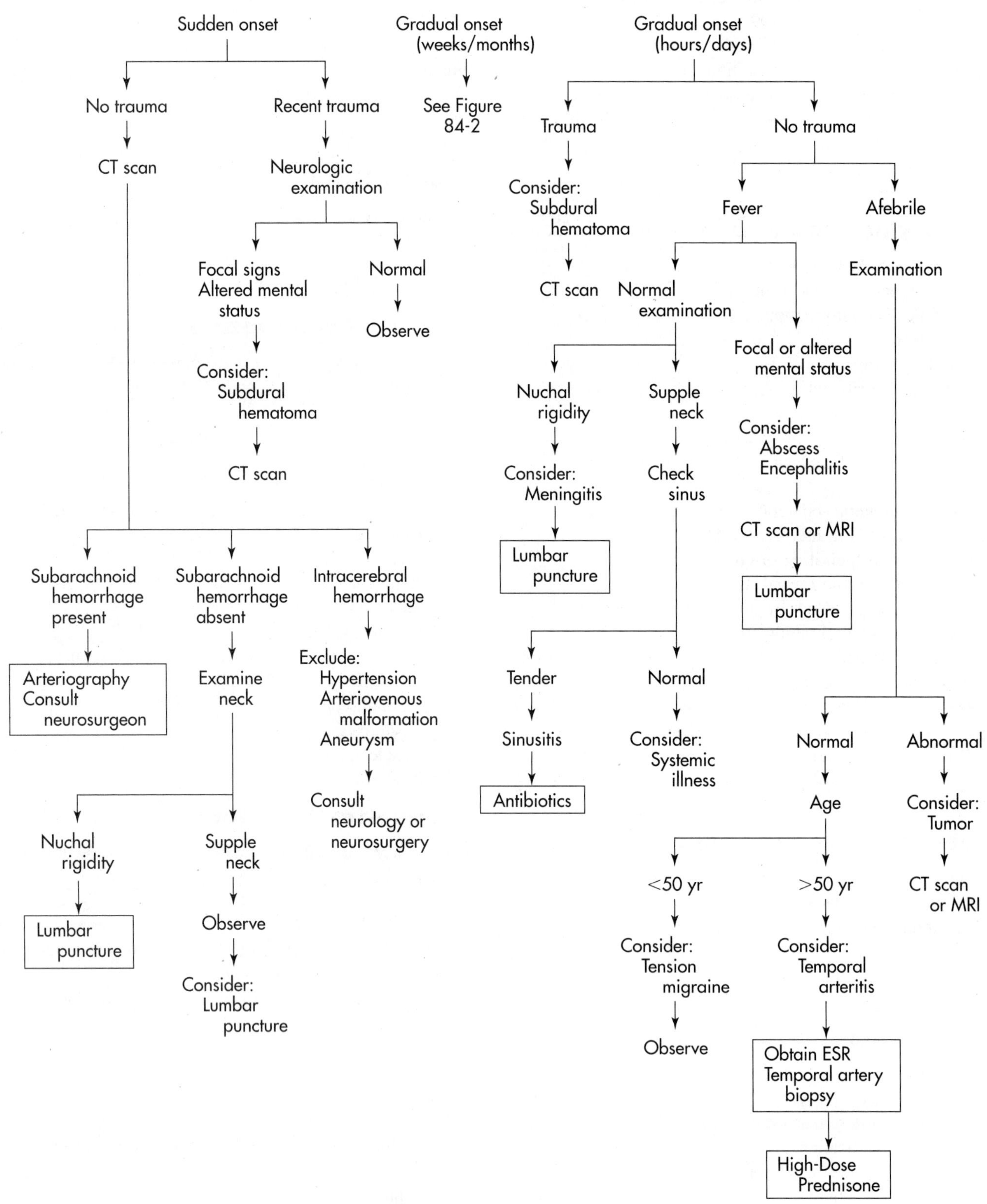

Figure 84-1 Algorithm for treatment of a patient with headache of recent onset. (Adapted from Greene HL, Johnson WP, Lemcke D: *Decision making in medicine,* ed 2, St Louis, 1998, Mosby.)

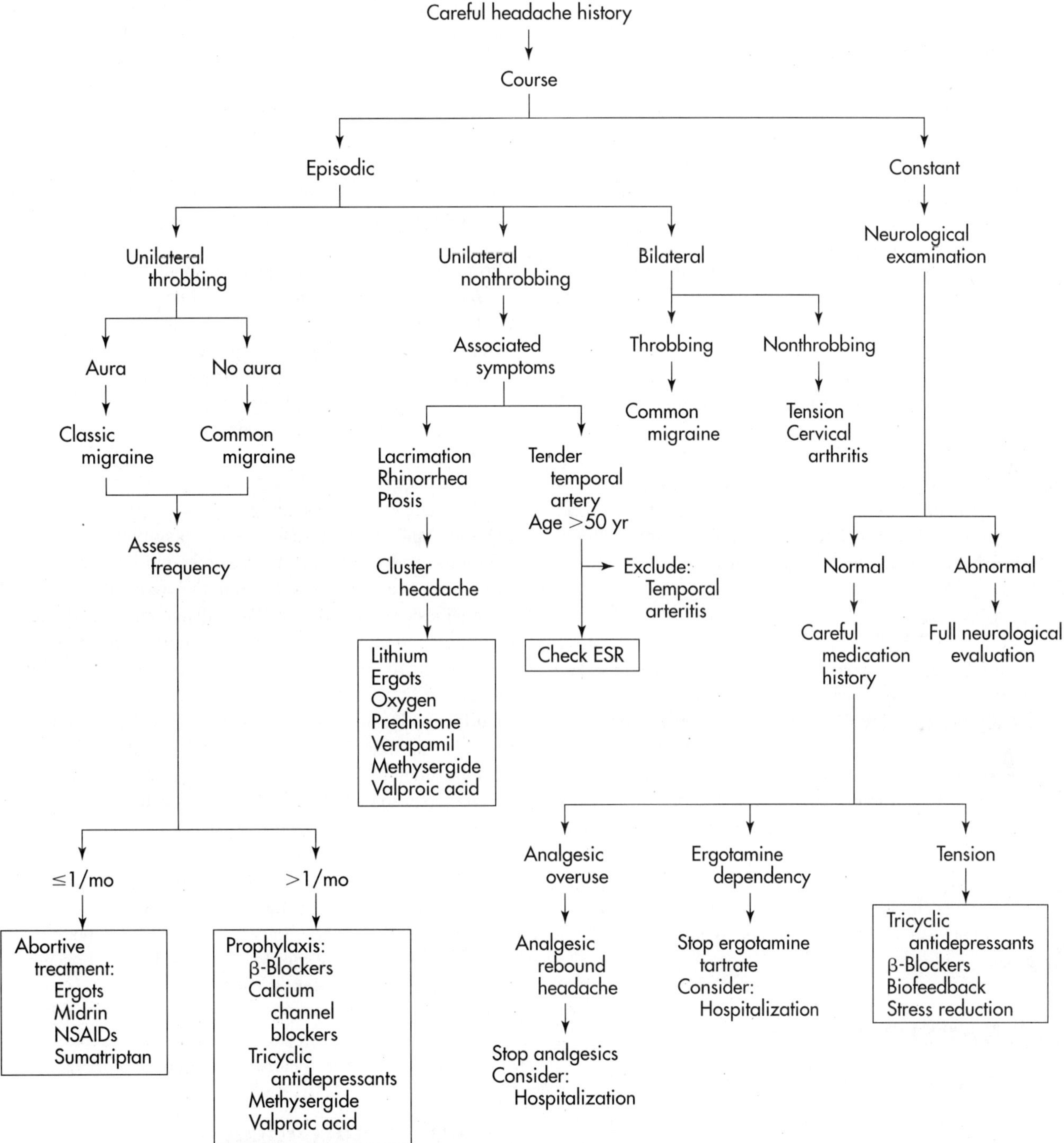

Figure 84-2 Algorithm for treatment of a patient with long-standing headache. *ESR,* Erythrocyte sedimentation rate; *NSAID,* nonsteroidal antiinflammatory drug. (Adapted from Greene HL, Johnson WP, Lemcke D: *Decision making in medicine,* ed 2, St Louis, 1998, Mosby.)

Glucose tolerance test ($45 to $57) to detect significant headache-causing metabolic abnormalities

Arterial blood gases ($78 to $98) to rule out hypoxia and/or hypercapnia (Diamond, 1992; Dodick, 1997; Heck, 1998; Weiss, 1993)

Radiological Studies

Indicated only if the patient describes an atypical headache pattern, changes in headache pattern, or recent onset of persistent headaches

Head CT scan ($990 to $1175) intracranial lesions are suspected or the patient has sinusitis that is not responsive to antibiotics

Magnetic resonance imaging (MRI) ($1781 to $2004) is preferred when posterior fossa lesions or craniospinal lesions are suspected (Coutin and Glass, 1996; Diamond, 1992; Dodick, 1997; Heck, 1998)

Other Studies

Temporal artery biopsy indicated in elderly individuals with a tender temporal artery and an elevated ESR (Coutin and Glass, 1996; Dodick, 1997; Heck, 1998)

EEG: Indicated for headaches accompanied by seizures

Lumbar puncture: When CT scan result is normal but clinical index of suspicion remains high for subarachnoid hemorrhage (Coutin and Glass, 1996)

ASSESSMENT

Differential diagnosis includes the different primary and secondary types of headaches and illnesses that are characteristically associated with a headache, which include infectious mononucleosis (Chapter 119), systemic lupus erythematosus (Chapter 110), chronic pulmonary failure with hypercapnia, Hashimoto's thyroiditis (Chapter 178), glucocorticoid withdrawal, oral contraceptives, ovulation-promoting medications, inflammatory bowel disease (Chapter 100), many of the HIV-associated illnesses (Chapter 94), and the acute blood pressure elevation that occurs in pheochromocytoma and in malignant hypertension (Chapter 96).

THERAPEUTIC PLAN

Secondary Headache Syndromes

The goal is cure, with referral for medical or surgical interventions.

Primary Headache Syndromes

The goal of treatment is pain alleviation, prevention, and the limitation of an acute episode. There is a need to limit the impact on lifestyle.

Pharmaceutical

Treatment consists of abortive (acute/symptomatic) therapy and prophylactic (preventive) therapy. Abortive therapy is used to treat symptoms once they occur or to prevent headaches after warning signs (such as an aura) have appeared. When designing an abortive (acute) treatment regimen for a patient with headache, start with OTC analgesics and gradually work up through prescription nonnarcotic analgesics, ergot drugs, and sumatriptan to narcotic analgesics (Kumar, Mathew, and Silberstein, 1995). Abortive pharmaceutical therapies with dosage and common side effects and adverse effects for migraine, tension, and cluster headaches are provided in Table 84-2.

Prophylactic (preventive) therapy should be considered for the individual who has at least one headache per week that interferes with activities of daily living.

Choice of therapy is guided by the type of headache, prior usage of typical medication, the patient's preference and needs as to route of delivery, and concurrent symptoms or problems, other medications taken, cost, and length of treatment.

Use the least potent and least addictive analgesic medication that relieves most of the pain.

Opioids and barbiturates have the potential for addiction. Caffeine and ergot contribute to rebound headaches.

Rebound headaches result from too-frequent dosing with analgesics, particularly those that contain caffeine and ergotamine; the patient needs to be weaned off these medications before proper management can be initiated; should be referred to a neurologist for evaluation.

Children: Treatment of headaches in children over 12 years old is similar to treatment in adults (may require dosage adjustments). However, treatment of headache in children younger than 12 requires modification of the adult approach (Winner, 1997).

Elderly: Elderly patients are more susceptible to cardiovascular effects of the prophylaxis headache medications. They are likely to be receiving other medications; therefore drug interactions have to be contemplated. Thus medication therapy should be initiated at low dosages and increases titrated slowly.

Prophylactic/preventive pharmaceutical therapies with dosage, common side effects, and adverse effects for migraine, tension, and cluster headaches are outlined in Table 84-3.

Nonpharmaceutical

Nonpharmaceutical strategies are an essential component of the management plan for the patient with a headache. Nonpharmacological strategies to include in the management plan are as follows:

Adequate nutrition with regular meals and adequate fluid intake

Text continued on p. 525

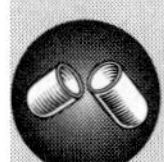

TABLE 84-2 Abortive (Acute/Symptomatic) Pharmaceutical Therapies for Common Types of Headache

Drug	Dosage	Common Side Effects or Adverse Effects	Cost ($)
Migraine Headaches			
Analgesics/NSAIDs			
Aspirin	Adult: 325 mg; 2 tabs q4-6h Children: 50-75 mg/kg/day in divided doses	Gastric intolerance, hypersensitivity reactions Contraindicated in patients with hemophilia and during pregnancy Should not be given to children during an antecedent viral infection; has been associated with Reye's syndrome	2-3
Acetaminophen	Adults: 325-500 mg QID Children: 60-120 mg, depending on age and weight	Use with caution in patients with liver disease	3-4
Naproxen sodium (Anaprox DS)	Adults: 550 mg-825 mg q12h Children: Not recommended	Hypersensitivity reactions, GI intolerance, headache, dizziness, drowsiness, vertigo, rebound headache	9-24
Ibuprofen (Motrin)	Adult: 400-800 mg, repeat PRN in 4h; should not exceed 1200 mg/day Children: 50-300 mg, depending on age and weight	Same as for naproxen	11-27
Analgesic Combinations			
Aspirin 325 mg, caffeine 40 mg, and butalbital 50 mg (Fiorinal)	Adults: 1-2 tabs or caps q4h; not to exceed 6 tabs or caps/day Children: Not recommended	Drowsiness, lightheadedness, sedation, intoxication feeling, rebound headache, GI disturbances, hypersensitivity reaction; use contraindicated during pregnancy	34-48
Acetaminophen 325 mg, caffeine 40 mg, and butalbital 50 mg (Esgic, Fioricet)	Adults: 1-2 tabs q4h; not to exceed 6 tabs/day Children: Not recommended for patients under 12 years of age	Same as for Fiorinal	6-79
Acetaminophen 325 mg and butalbital 50 mg (Phrenilin)	Adults: 1-2 tabs q4h; not to exceed 6 tabs/day Children: Not recommended for patients under 12 years of age	Drowsiness, lightheadedness, sedation, intoxication feeling, abdominal pain, rebound headache, GI disturbances, hypersensitivity reactions; use contraindicated during pregnancy	N/A
Isometheptene mucate 65 mg, acetaminophen 325 mg, and dichloralphenazone 100 mg (Midrin)	Adults: 2 caps followed by 1 cap QH until relieved; not to exceed 5 caps/12h Children: Not recommended	Hypersensitivity reaction, transient dizziness; use contraindicated in patients with glaucoma, severe renal disease, hypertension, heart disease, hepatic disease, and patients on MAO inhibitor therapy	15-39

Compiled from *1998 Physicians' desk reference,* Montvale, NJ, 1998, Medical Economics Data; Loder E: Migraine management: an overview of nonpharmacological and pharmacological interventions, *Postgrad Med* (Special Report), vol 102, 1998; Tepper SJ: Recent advances in antimigraine therapy: a clinical overview of zolmitriptan's efficacy and tolerability, *Postgrad Med* (Special Report)102:20-26, 1998; and Moore KL, Noble SL: Drug treatment of migraine, Part I. Acute therapy and drug-rebound headache, *Am Family Physician* 56:2039-2048, 1997.

AC, Before meals; *caps,* capsules; *tabs,* tablets; *MAO,* monoamine oxidase; *N/A,* not available; *NSAIDs,* nonsteroidal antiiflammatory drugs; *SL,* sublingual.

Continued

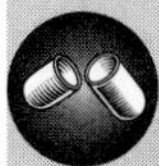

TABLE 84-2 Abortive (Acute/Symptomatic) Pharmaceutical Therapies for Common Types of Headache—cont'd

Drug	Dosage	Common Side Effects or Adverse Effects	Cost ($)
Ergot Alkaloids			
Ergotamine tartrate 1 mg and caffeine 100 mg (Ercaf, Gotamine, Wigraine) Oral	Adults: 2 tabs, followed by 1 tab q½h as needed up to 6 tabs/attack; should not exceed 10 tabs/wk Children: Not recommended	Precordial distress and pain, muscle pain in the extremities, numbness and tingling in fingers and toes, transient tachycardia or bradycardia, vomiting, nausea, weakness in the legs, diarrhea, localized edema, and hypersensitivity reactions; use contraindicated during pregnancy and in patients with peripheral vascular disease, coronary heart disease, hypertension, impaired hepatic or renal function, sepsis	N/A
Ergotamine tartrate 2 mg (Ergomar) SL	Adults: 1 tab SL, repeat q½h PRN; should not exceed 3 tabs/24h Children: Not recommended	Same as for Ercaf, Gotamine, and Wigraine (see entry above)	18
Ergotamine tartrate 2 mg and caffeine 100 mg (Cafatine, Cafergot, Migerot) Rectal	Adults: ½-1 suppository; repeat as needed after 3h Children: Not recommended	Same as for Ercaf, Gotamine, and Wigraine (see entry above)	N/A
Dihydroergotamine mesylate 1 mg (DHE 45) IM, SQ, or IV	Adult: 1 mg/1 ml IM, SQ, or IV QH to a total dose of 3 mg/3 ml Children: Not recommended	Same as for Ercaf, Gotamine, and Wigraine	N/A
Hydroxytryptamine Agonists			
Sumatriptan succinate (Imitrex) SQ	Adults: 6 mg, repeated if needed after at least 1h interval; maximum dose is two 6 mg doses/24h Children: Not recommended	Cardiovascular symptoms, chest tightness and pressure; hypersensitivity reactions, tingling, heat, flushing of face; sedation; injection-site irritation or swelling; use contraindicated in patients with ischemic heart disease, uncontrolled hypertension, hemiplegia, or basilar migraine	70-74
Sumatriptan succinate (Imitrex) Oral	Adults: 25-100 mg (maximum initial dose 100 mg), repeat as needed at 2h intervals up to 300 mg/24h Children: Not recommended	Cardiovascular symptoms, chest tightness, and pressure, hypersensitivity reactions, tingling, heat, flushing of face, atypical symptoms, sedation; contraindicated in patients with ischemic heart disease, uncontrolled hypertension	97-110
Sumatriptan succinate (Imitrex) Nasal	Adults: 5-20 mg; if needed may be repeated once after 2h; not to exceed 40 mg/day Children: Not recommended	Same as for oral forms	N/A

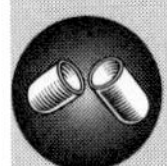

TABLE 84-2 Abortive (Acute/Symptomatic) Pharmaceutical Therapies for Common Types of Headache—cont'd

Drug	Dosage	Common Side Effects or Adverse Effects	Cost ($)
Zolmitriptan (Zomig) Oral	Adults: 1, 2.5, or 5 mg; repeat once 2h after initial dose Children: Not recommended	Nausea, dizziness, somnolence, paresthesias; use contraindicated in patients with ischemic heart disease or uncontrolled hypertension, or who have been given an ergotamine-containing medication within 24h or are on MAO medications	N/A
Narcotics/Opioids			
Acetaminophen/Codeine (various fixed dosages) Oral	Adults: 1-2 tabs q4-6h Children: Not recommended	Lightheadedness, dizziness, sedation, nausea, vomiting, hypersensitivity reactions, rebound headache; use contraindicated during pregnancy	N/A
Butorphanol nasal spray (Stadol)	Adults: 1 spray in one nostril, may repeat in 1-1½h the initial two-dose sequence may be repeated in 3-4h as needed Children: Not recommended	Somnolence, dizziness, nausea, vomiting, nasal congestion, insomnia, rebound headache, very addictive; use contraindicated during pregnancy	61
Antiemetic			
Prochlorperazine (Compazine)	Adults: 5-10 mg q4-6h Children: Not recommended for patients under 2 years of age; dosage based on weight	Drowsiness, dizziness, amenorrhea, blurred vision, hypotension, hypersensitivity reactions; use contraindicated during pregnancy	34-60
Metoclopramide (Reglan)	Adults: 10-15 mg QID, 30 min AC Children: Not recommended under 18 years of age	Restlessness, drowsiness, fatigue, insomnia, headache, confusion dizziness, mental depression with suicidal ideation; use contraindicated during pregnancy	2-71
Tension-Type Headaches			
Analgesics/NSAIDs			
Same as for migraine headache			
Analgesic Combinations			
ASA and acetaminophen-caffeine-butalbital combinations; same as for migraine headache	Adults: 1-2 tabs or caps q4h; not to exceed 6 tabs or caps/day Children: Not recommended	Drowsiness, lightheadedness, sedation, intoxication feeling, rebound headache, GI disturbances, hypersensitivity reaction; use contraindicated during pregnancy	
Isometheptene mucate 65 mg, acetaminophen 325 mg, and dichloralphenazone 100 mg (Midrin)	Adults: 1-2 caps q4h; maximum 6 caps/24h Children: Not recommended	Hypersensitivity reaction, transient dizziness; use is contraindicated in patients with glaucoma, severe renal disease, hypertension, heart disease, hepatic disease, and patients receiving MAO inhibitor therapy	34-48

Continued

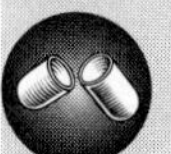

TABLE 84-2 Abortive (Acute/Symptomatic) Pharmaceutical Therapies for Common Types of Headache—cont'd

Drug	Dosage	Common Side Effects or Adverse Effects	Cost ($)
Antidepressants			
Amitriptyline (Elavil)	Adults: 10-100 mg QHS Children: Not recommended for patients under 12 years of age	Adverse effects for most systems of the body, hypersensitivity reactions; use contraindicated during pregnancy and patients on MAO inhibitor medications; start with 10 mg in elderly to reduce anticholinergic side effects	15-39
Buspirone (Buspar)	Adults: 15-60 mg QD maximum dose/day should not exceed 60 mg Children: Not recommended for patients under 18 years of age Elderly: 12.5 to 25 mg initially in elderly, titrate to effect not to exceed 200 mg	Dizziness, nausea, headache, nervousness, lightheadedness, excitement, hypersensitivity reactions; use contraindicated during pregnancy	2-19 57-100 176-181
Sertraline HCl (Zoloft)	Adults: 50-200 mg QD Children: Not recommended	Adverse effects associated with all major body systems; use contraindicated during pregnancy and patients on MAO inhibitor medications	
Muscle Relaxants			
Cyclobenzaprine (Flexeril)	Adults: 10 mg TID; should not exceed 60 mg/day Children: Not recommended for patients under 15 years of age	Drowsiness, dry mouth, dizziness, fatigue, asthenia (lack or loss of strength), nausea, constipation, dyspepsia, unpleasant taste, blurred vision, headache, nervousness, confusion, hypersensitivity reactions; use contraindicated during pregnancy, cardiac conditions, hyperthyroidism, patients on MAO inhibitor medications	N/A
Cluster Headaches			
Oxygen Therapy			
Oxygen	100% at 7 L/min per face mask during headache episode		
Ergot Alkaloids			
Ergotamine SL or Medihaler	Adults: Inhale at onset of attack, then may be repeated 3 times, 5 min apart, if needed Children: Not recommended	Precordial distress and pain, muscle pain in the extremities, numbness and tingling in fingers and toes, transient tachycardia or bradycardia, vomiting, nausea, weakness in the legs, diarrhea, localized edema, and hypersensitivity reactions; use contraindicated during pregnancy and in patients with peripheral vascular disease, coronary heart disease, hypertension, impaired hepatic or renal function, sepsis	18

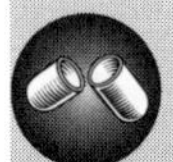

TABLE 84-2 Abortive (Acute/Symptomatic) Pharmaceutical Therapies for Common Types of Headache—cont'd

Drug	Dosage	Common Side Effects or Adverse Effects	Cost ($)
Ergotamine tartrate 1 mg and caffeine 100 mg (Ercaf, Gotamine, Wigraine) Oral	Adults: 2 tabs then q 30 min — not to exceed 6 tabs/attack	Same as for ergotamine SL	N/A
Dihydroergotamine mesylate: IM, IV	Adults: 1 ml at onset then QH, not to exceed 2 ml IV or 3 ml IM; should be reserved for emergency department use	Same as for ergotamine SL	N/A
Hydroxytryptamine Agonists			
Sumatriptan (Imitrex)	Same as for migraine headache	Same as for migraine headache	97-100
Other			
Viscous lidocaine	Adults: 4% intranasally on side of headache, 1 inhalation QH Children: Not recommended	Paresthesias, tremor, nausea, lightheadedness, hearing disturbances, slurred speech, and convulsions	7-15

N/A, Not available.

- Avoidance of trigger foods and situations
- Adequate rest: Maintain regular sleep habits
- Regular exercise
- Proper posture
- Topical heat or cold applications
- Stress-reduction techniques (work and home stresses should be discussed and reduced if possible), such as biofeedback techniques
- Individual and family counseling
- Lifestyle modifications should be implemented before considering medications

Patient Education

An important component of the management plan for a patient with a headache is providing the patient with information and counseling. Educational materials, treatment options, and available support groups can be obtained from the organizations located in the Resources section at the end of this chapter, p. 530.

The health care provider should include the following in patient education when treating a patient with a headache (Cady and Farmer, 1998; Robertson and McCormack, 1998):

- Recognition of triggers and early warning signs of headaches
- Details of pharmacotherapy, including dosage, side effects, and adverse effects, rationale for selection of medication, and cost
- Seek clinician input early when therapies do not work
- Importance of keeping a headache diary (helps both the patient and provider understand the specific nature of the headache pattern); see an example of a headache diary in Figure 84-3.
- Available resources
- Information on headaches, need for stress reduction, and dangers of drug overuse
- Validation that most headaches are genetically based and benign in nature
- Encouragement of patient's participation in treatment plan
- Importance of regular monitoring of headache treatment plan

Referral

Patients with any of the following presentations should be referred to a neurologist or a physician:

- "First or worst" headache, particularly with acute onset or abnormal neurological findings
- Headache with subacute onset that progressively worsens over days or weeks
- Headache related with fever, nausea, and vomiting that cannot be explained by a systemic disorder
- Headache associated with focal neurological findings

No obvious identifiable etiological factors for headache

EVALUATION/FOLLOW-UP

Patients with chronic headaches should be monitored regularly (monthly) to evaluate the headache diary, effectiveness of medications, compliance in taking medication, and for counseling, education, and support in maintaining treatment plan.

Text continued on p. 530

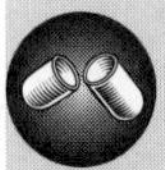

TABLE 84-3 Prophylactive (Preventive) Pharmaceutical Therapies for Common Types of Headaches

Drug	Dose	Common Side/Adverse Effects
Migraine Headache		
Beta Blockers		
Failure to respond to one beta blocker does not preclude successful use of another beta blocker in the same patient		
Atenolol (Tenormin)	Adults: 50-150 mg QD Children: Not recommended	Fatigue, hypotension, bradycardia, depression, impotence, dizziness, vertigo, nausea; use contraindicated in bradycardia, cardiogenic shock, cardiac failure, hypotension, and during pregnancy
Metoprolol (Lopressor)	Adults: 50-200 mg QD Children: Not recommended	Fatigue, hypotension, bradycardia, depression, impotence, dizziness, vertigo, nausea, headache, insomnia; use contraindicated in bradycardia, cardiogenic shock, cardiac failure, hypotension, bronchial asthma or severe COPD, hypersensitivity, and during pregnancy
Nadolol (Corgard)	Adults: 20-240 mg QD in divided doses Children: Not recommended	Same as for metoprolol
Propranolol (Inderal)	Adults: 80-240 mg QD in divided doses Children: Not recommended	Same as for metoprolol
Timolol (Blocadren)	Adults: 10-30 mg QD Children: Not recommended	Same as for metoprolol
Calcium Channel Blockers		
Most common drugs used in migraine prophylaxis		
Diltiazem (Cardizem)	Adults: 90-360 mg QD Children: Not recommended under 18 years of age	Constipation, dizziness, nausea, bradycardia, hypotension, congestive heart failure, AV heart block, edema, fatigue, hypersensitivity reactions; use contraindicated in patients with sick sinus syndrome, second or third AV heart block, atrial flutter or fibrillation, and during pregnancy
Verapamil (Calan, Isoptin); most frequently used calcium channel blocker	Adults: 120-720 mg QD Children: Not recommended	Same as for diltiazem
Tricyclic Antidepressants		
Particularly useful in patients with depression or insomnia; provides a central analgesic effect		
Amitriptyline HCl (Elavil)	Adults: 10-100 mg QD Children: Under 12 years of age not recommended	Sedation, dry mouth, weight gain, constipation, urinary retention, blurred vision; use contraindicated in patients on MAO inhibitor medication and patients with acute MI, hypersensitivity, and during pregnancy
Desipramine HCl (Norpramine)	Adults: 50-100 mg Children: Not recommended	Same as for amitriptyline

Compiled from 1998 Physicians' desk reference, Montvale, NJ, 1998, Medical Economics Data; Loder E. Migraine management: an overview of nonpharmacological and pharmacologic interventions, *Postgrad Med* (Special Report); and Noble SL, Moore KL. Drug treatment of migraine: Part II. Preventive therapy, *Am Family Physician 56*(9): 2279-2286, 1997.

COPD, Chronic obstructive pulmonary disease; *GI,* gastrointestinal.

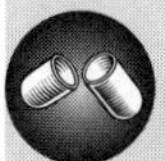

TABLE 84-3 Prophylactive (Preventive) Pharmaceutical Therapies for Common Types of Headaches—cont'd

Drug	Dosage	Common Side/Adverse Effects
Doxepine (Sinequan)	Adults: 10-200 mg QD (Maximum dose 300 mg/day) Children: Under 12 years of age not recommended	Same as for amitriptyline
Imipramine (Tofranil)	Adults: 10-150 mg QD Children: Not recommended	Same as for amitriptyline
Nortriptyline HCl (Aventyl, Pamelor)	Adults: 10-150 mg in divided doses Children: Not recommended	Same as for amitriptyline
Anticonvulsants		
Particularly useful in patients with anxiety, bipolar disorder or seizure disorders		
Divalproex sodium (Depakote)	Adults: 250-1500 mg QD; begin with 125-250 mg BID and gradually increase dosage Children: 10-15 mg/kg/day; dose should be increased 5-10 mg/kg/day/wk	Multiple adverse effects; use contraindicated in patients with hepatic disease or dysfunction, hypersensitivity, and during pregnancy
Valproic acid (Depakene)	Adults and children over 2 years of age: 15 mg/kg/day increase at 1 week intervals 5-10 mg/kg/day Children: Not recommended for children under 2 years of age	Same as for divalproex
Serotonin Antagonists		
Cyproheptadine (Periactin); drug of choice for treatment of migraine in children	Adults: 4-16 mg/day Children: Not recommended for under 2 years of age 2-6 years of age - 12 mg/day 7-14 years of age - 16 mg/day; calculated on 0.25 mg/kg/day	Multiple adverse effects; use contraindicated nursing mothers and during pregnancy
Methsergide (Sansert), approved for severe migraine that is unresponsive to other agents	Adults: 2-8 mg/day; maximum dose is 14 mg/day Children: Not recommended	Serious adverse effects; use contraindicated during pregnancy
Monoamine Oxidase Inhibitors (MAO)		
Patients must avoid tyramine-rich foods (most cheese, brewer's yeast, Chianti, canned meats, salt herring, dried fish, caviar, Italian flat beans, Chinese pea pods, broad [fava] beans, mixed Chinese vegetables, eggplant, figs, avocados, chocolate, soy sauce, and protein extracts) and sympathomimetic agents; used for refractory headaches)		
Phenelzine (Nardil)	Adults: 30-90 mg/day in divided doses Maximum dose 90 mg/day Children: Not recommended	Multiple adverse effects; use contraindicated in patients with pheochromocytoma, congestive heart failure, liver disease, or dysfunction hypersensitivity, and during pregnancy

Continued

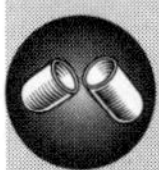

TABLE 84-3 Prophylactive (Preventive) Pharmaceutical Therapies for Common Types of Headaches—cont'd

Drug	Dosage	Common Side/Adverse Effects
Hormonal Preparation (menstrual migraine)		
Estradiol patch, start 2-3 days before expected headache (climara, Estraderm, Vivelle)	Adults: Climara; 1-22 patches over 1 wk Estraderm, Vivelle; 2-4 patches over 1 wk	
Tension-type Headaches:		
Tricyclic Antidepressants		
Amitriptyline (Elavil)	Adults: 10-150 mg QD Children: Not recommended	Same as for migraine
Nortriptyline (Aventyl, Pamelor)	Adults: 75-150 mg QD Children: Not recommended	Same as for migraine
NSAIDs		
Naproxen (Naprosyn)	Adults: 10-150 mg in divided doses Children: Not recommended	Hypersensitivity reactions, GI intolerance, headache, dizziness, drowsiness, vertigo, rebound headache
Ibuprofen (Advil, Motrin, etc.)	Adults: 250 mg BID Children: Not recommended for children under 6 months of age Children over 6 months of age: 10 mg/kg/q6-8h; max. daily dose 40 mg/kg	Same as for Naproxen
Muscle Relaxant		
Cyclobenzaprine (Flexeril)	Adults: 200 mg BID Children: Not recommended for children under 15 years of age	Drowsiness, dry mouth, dizziness; use contraindicated during pregnancy
Cluster Headaches		
Calcium Channel Blocker		
Verapamil (Calan, Isoptin)	Adults: 120 mg TID Children: Not recommended	Same as for migraine
Antidepressant		
Lithium carbonate (Lithium)	Adults: 300 mg TID Children: Not recommended for children under 12 years of age	Fine hand tremors, polyuria and mild thirst, transient and mild nausea; use contraindicated in patients with significant renal or debilitation or hydration, or sodium depletion, and during pregnancy

Date__________ Hours of sleep last night__________ Quality of sleep______________________________

Medications taken____

____

	Excellent	Very Good	Good	Fair	Poor
My health today	1	2	3	4	5

What activities did I do today (sports, work, fun exercises, other)?______________________

____

What activity did I have to eliminate because of my physical health?______________________

____

	None	Mild	Moderate	Severe
Headache rating	0	1	2	3

How long did the pain last?____

Method of relief____

Location of the pain____

Description of the pain____

Symptoms associated with headache_____________________________________

What has the weather pattern been?_____________________________________

My feelings today were:

Happy Energetic	A little uptight Nervous	Downhearted Worried or blue	Tired No energy	Hopeless Helpless
1	2	3	4	5

Things I did, ate, or drank that weren't good for me____________________________

Arguments I had____

Unexpected events that happened to me_____________________________________

Worries or fears____

Accomplishments____

Something I will do tomorrow that will be a little different______________________

Figure 84-3 Sample migraine diary for patient use. (From Cady R, Farmer K: *Headache free,* New York, 1993, Bantam. Used by permission of Bantam Books, a division of Bantam Doubleday Dell Publishing Group, Inc.)

RESOURCES

The National Headache Foundation
428 W. St James Place, 2nd Floor
Chicago, IL 60614-2750
1-800-843-2256
www.headaches.org

American Council for Headache Education
875 Kings Highway, Suite 200
Woodbury, NJ 08096-3172
1-800-255-ACHE or 609-845-0322

REFERENCES

Baumel B, Eisner LS: Diagnosis and treatment of headaches in the elderly, *Med Clin North Am* 75:661-675, 1991.

Cady RK, Farmer KU: *Headache free,* New York, 1996, Bantam.

Cady RK, Farmer KU: What patients need to know about managing migraine (Special Report), *Postgrad Med* 102:31-36, 1998.

Couch JR: Headaches to worry about, *Med Clin North Am* 77:141-167, 1993.

Coutin IB, Glass SF: Recognizing uncommon headache syndromes, *Am Family Physician* 54:2247-2252, 1996.

Dalessio DJ: Diagnosing the severe headache, *Neurology* (Suppl 3):21-30, 1994.

Diamond S: Acute headache: differential diagnosis and management of three types, *Postgrad Med* 29:21-29, 1992.

Dodick D: Headache as a symptom of ominous disease, *Postgrad Med* 101:46-64, 1997.

Edmeads J: Headache in older people, *Postgrad Med* 101:91-100, 1997.

Fettes I: Menstrual migraine, *Postgrad Med* 101:67-77, 1997.

Heck JE: Differential diagnosis of headache, *Postgrad Med* (Special Report) 102:6-12, 1998.

Kudrow L: Diagnosis and treatment of cluster headache, *Med Clin North Am* 75 (3):579-594, 1991.

Kumar KL, Mathew N, Silberstein SD: Migraine: finding the road to relief, *Patient Care* 29:90-110, 1995.

Lipton RB et al: Migraine: identifying and removing barriers to care, *Neurology* 44:563-567, 1994.

Mathew N: Rebound headache: clinical features, *Semin Head Management* 2:5-7, 1997.

Rapoport AM: The diagnosis of migraine and tension-type headache: then and now, *Neurology* 42(Suppl 2):11-15, 1992.

Rasmussen BK, Olsen J: Symptomatic and nonsymptomatic headaches in a general population, *Neurology* 42: 1225-1231, 1992.

Robertson VE, McCormack ME: Headache. In *Primary care*, Philadelphia, 1998, Lippincott-Raven Publishers.

Weeks RE: Biobehavioral considerations in the diagnosis and treatment of rebound headache, *Semin Head Manage* 2:11-13, 1997.

Weiss J: Assessment and management of the client with headaches, *Nurs Pract* 18:44-57, 1993.

Winner PK: Headaches in children: when is a complete diagnostic workup indicated? *Postgrad Med* 101:81-90, 1997.

SUGGESTED READINGS

Dubose CD, Cutlip AC, Cutlip WD: Migraines and other headaches: an approach to diagnosis and classification, *Am Family Physician* 54:1498-1504, 1995.

Ellsworth A et al: *Mosby's 1998 medical drug reference,* St Louis, 1998, Mosby.

Headache Classification Committee of the International Headache Society: Classification and diagnostic criteria for headache disorders cranial neuralgia and facial pain, *Cephalalgia* 8(Suppl 7):1-96, 1988.

Healthcare Consultants of America, Inc: *1998 Physicians fee and coding guide,* Augusta, Ga, 1998, Healthcare Consultants of America, Inc.

Loder EW: Migraine management: an overview of nonpharmacologic and pharmacologic interventions, *Postgrad Med* (Special Report) 102:13-19, 1998.

Moore KL, Noble SL: Drug treatment of migraine. Part I, Acute therapy and drug-rebound headache, *Am Family Physician* 56:2039-2048, 1997.

Noble SL, Moore KL: Drug treatment of migraine. Part II, Preventive therapy, *Am Family Physician* 56:2279-2286, 1997.

1998 Physician's desk reference, ed 52, Montvale, NJ, 1998, Medical Economics Co, Inc.

Stevens MB: Tension-type headaches, *Am Family Physician* 47:799-805, 1993.

Tepper SJ: Recent advances in antimigraine therapy: a clinical overview of zolmitriptan's efficacy and tolerability, *Postgrad Med* (Special Report) 102:1-26, 1998.

Walling AD: Cluster headache, *Am Family Physician* 47:1457-1463, 1993.

Whitney CM: New headache classification: implications for neuroscience nurses, *J Neurosci Nurs* 22:385-388, 1990.

85 Hearing Loss

ICD-9-CM

Hearing Loss 389.9
Ossicular Damage 389.03
Tympanosclerosis 385.03
Ménière's Disease 386.01
Acoustic Neuroma 225.1
Noise-Related Sensorineural Hearing Loss (SNHL) 388.12
Viral SNHL 389.18
Ototoxic SNHL 960.6
Age-Related SNHL Presbycusis 388.01

OVERVIEW

Definition

Hearing loss is a decreased ability to hear sounds. Presbycusis is the slowly progressive symmetrical loss of predominantly high-frequency hearing associated with aging.

Incidence

Hearing loss occurs in 25% to 30% of persons aged **65 and older,** and by nearly 50% of those older than 75. About 28 million Americans are affected by hearing loss, but only about 20% of people with hearing loss wear hearing aids.

Pathophysiology

Conductive hearing loss: Results from dysfunction of the middle ear, with a resulting impairment of the passage of sound vibrations to the middle ear. These are caused by obstruction (cerumen impaction), middle ear effusion, otosclerosis, and ossicular disruption. Conductive hearing loss is generally correctable.

Sensory hearing loss: Results from deterioration of the cochlea, usually as a result of the loss of hair cells from the organ of Corti. Examples of causes include noise trauma, aging, and ototoxicity. Sensory hearing loss is not correctable but may be prevented or stabilized.

Neural hearing loss: Results from lesions of the eighth cranial nerve, auditory nuclei, or auditory cortex. It is the least common cause of hearing loss. Disorders that may cause neural hearing include neuroma, multiple sclerosis, and cerebrovascular disease.

SUBJECTIVE DATA

History of Present Illness

Adults

Patient may present with complaints of difficulty hearing, or family members may identify the patient's inability to hear.

The patient may exhibit the following symptoms:

- Complains of feeling stressed or tired during conversations
- Frequently asks people to repeat themselves
- Avoids social situations
- Frequently denies having hearing problems
- Turns up TV so loudly that others complain
- Complains of nausea and vomiting, tinnitus
- Loses ability to "pop" ears
- Has a sense of fullness in ears
- Pulling at ears
- Loses equilibrium
- May complain of foreign body in the ear

Ask about involvement of one ear or both

Was the onset gradual or sudden?

Has the hearing fluctuated since the hearing loss began?

Are there associated symptoms of tinnitus, vertigo, otalgia, otorrhea, or facial weakness?

Children

Make few attempts to communicate by 12 months

Are unable to use more than 8 to 10 words at 18 months

Use two-word combinations for most of talking at age 2½
Are difficult to understand at age 3½

Past Medical History

Ask about:
- Hypertension
- Mumps
- Neurological problems
- Head trauma
- Diabetes
- Hypothyroidism
- Syphilis
- Frequent colds, congestion, allergies or ear infections as child

Medications

Ask about use of:
- High doses of aspirin
- Antibiotics: Aminoglycosides (gentamicin, streptomycin)
- Diuretics (loop: furosemide)
- Quinine

Family History

Ask about other family members with hearing loss.

Psychosocial History

Environment: Ask about occupation: Exposure to loud noises, use of protective measures, such as ear plugs
Ask about exposure to other sources of noise, such as music

OBJECTIVE DATA

Physical Examination

The physical examination should concentrate on the head and neck.

- Head/eyes/ears/nose/throat: Evaluate for an upper respiratory infection (URI)
- Ears
  - Evaluate tympanic membrane (TM), external canal
  - Complete pneumatic otoscopy: Check for TM movement
  - Tympanogram
- Neurological: Check sensation of face; note whether facial movement is symmetrical, rapid alternating movements.
- Hearing: Have patient repeat aloud words that you present in a soft whisper, normal speaking voice, or a shout. Have the opposite ear occluded, then repeat on the other side.

Children (expected response by age):
- 0-3 months: Response to noise
- 3-5 months: Child turns to sound
- 6-10 months: Child responds to name
- 10-15 months: Child imitates simple words

Weber's test: Place the tuning fork on the forehead or front teeth. Have the patient indicate where it is heard the best.
Rinne's test: The tuning fork is placed alternately on the mastoid bone and in front of the ear canal.

Diagnostic Procedures

Diagnostic tests for hearing loss are detailed in Table 85-1.

ASSESSMENT

Differential Diagnosis

Differential diagnosis includes those listed in Table 85-2.
Classification of hearing tests and types of hearing loss are detailed in Tables 85-3 and 85-4.

THERAPEUTIC PLAN

Pharmaceutical

Depends on cause of hearing loss

Lifestyle/Activities

See Patient Education

Diet

Not applicable

Patient Education

Use the following to assist with speech:
- Face people while talking
- Obtain their attention before speaking
- Use gestures
- Speak at a moderate pace
- Use adequate lighting
- Minimize background noise if possible
- Ask what can be done to facilitate the person's hearing

Use telecommunication device for the deaf (TDD) phone
Use television with words provided in written context along with speaking (closed captioned)
Hearing loss prevention:
- Wear ear plugs or ear muffs (cotton balls won't do the job)
- Keep volume low when wearing headphones

Some representative noise levels are detailed in Table 85-5.

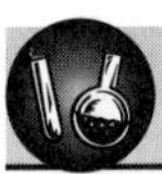

TABLE 85-1 Diagnostic Tests: Hearing Loss

Test	Finding/Rationale	Cost ($)
Audiometric studies	Hearing test conducted in soundproof room. Pure-tone thresholds in decibels (dB) are obtained over the ranges of 250-8000 Hz for both air and bone conduction. All patients with hearing loss should be referred for audiometric testing unless the cause is easily remediable (e.g., impacted cerumen). Patients can be referred directly to an audiologist. The location of an accredited audiologist can be obtained by calling the American Speech-Language Association at (800) 638-8255.	46-55
Speech discrimination testing	Evaluates the clarity of hearing. Results are reported as percentage correct.	34-41
Tympanogram	Used to detect fluid in the middle ear and to determine the mobility of the TM. An electroacoustic device is used to measure the compliance of the TM. Results are displayed in a graphic form. It is most reliable in children >6 mo.	31-37
Audiogram	Small handheld audioscopes can provide a rough indication of hearing impairment. Usually four pure tones are emitted in sequence. This test can be affected by background noise, so the examination room must be quiet.	24-29

TM, Tympanic membrane.

TABLE 85-2 Differential Diagnosis: Hearing Loss

Diagnosis	Supporting Data
Auditory brain stem	Hearing screening may be done on high-risk infants by ABR. High-risk infants include those who are premature, who received ototoxic drugs in the neonatal period, and who have a family history of hearing loss.
Conductive loss	Rinne test shows air conduction is less than bone conduction; Weber lateralizes to the involved ear. The whisper will be abnormal if >40 dB loss is present.
Cerumen impaction Ch. 62	Occlusion of the external ear canal by cerumen. Usually self-induced via attempts at cleaning.
Serous otitis media (Ch. 134)	Dull TM, hypomobile TM. Air bubbles may be seen in the middle ear, with a conductive hearing loss present.
Otosclerosis	Progressive disease with a familial tendency that affects bone surrounding the inner ear.
TM perforation	Perforation of the TM may result in decreased hearing abilities. The perforation may occur from trauma or as the result of increased pressure with otitis media. Spontaneous healing occurs in the majority of cases.
Sensorineural loss	Rinne: both AC and BC are decreased, Weber localizes to the uninvolved ear, the whisper test will be abnormal if >40 dB loss is present.
Presbycusis	Progressive, mainly high-frequency hearing loss of aging. Frequently there is a genetic predisposition. Patients complain of an inability to hear well (speech discrimination) in a noisy environment.
Noise trauma	Second most common cause of hearing loss. Sounds >85 dB are potentially damaging to the cochlea, especially with prolonged exposure. The loss typically occurs in the high frequencies (4000 Hz) and progresses to involve sounds in the normal speech frequencies. Sounds that have the potential for damage include industrial machinery, loud music, and weapons.
Ototoxicity	Hearing loss can be caused by substances that affect both the auditory and vestibular systems. Common causes include salicylates, aminoglycosides, loop diuretics, and antineoplastic agents, especially cisplatin.

TM, Tympanic membrane.

Table 85-3 Classification of Hearing Tests and Type of Hearing Loss

Classification	Rinne	Weber
Normal: Both ears	AC>BC	Midline
Conductive Loss		
Right ear	Right ear: BC>AC Left ear: AC>BC	Lateralized to right ear
Left ear	Right ear: AC>BC Left ear: BC>AC	Lateralized to left ear
Both ears	Right ear: BC>AC Left ear: BC>AC	Lateralized to poorer ear of the two
Sensorineural Loss		
Right ear	AC>BC both ears	Lateralized to left ear
Left ear	AC>BC both ears	Lateralized to right ear
Both ears	AC>BC both ears	Lateralized to better ear

AC, Air conduction; *BC,* bone conduction.

Table 85-4 Type of Hearing Loss

Category of Hearing Loss	Decibel Level (dB)
Mild hearing loss	26-40
Moderate hearing loss	41-55
Moderately severe hearing loss	56-70
Severe hearing loss	71-90
Profound hearing loss	>91

Table 85-5 Examples of Noise Levels

Noise Level (dB)	Examples
Safe Hearing Levels	
20	Whispered voice
40	Refrigerator humming
60	Normal conversation
Levels at Which Hearing Loss Can Occur	
90	Prolonged exposure to noise above 90 decibels can cause gradual hearing loss Lawn mower
100	Woodshop; no more than 15 minutes of unprotected exposure recommended
110	Chainsaw, some video arcades, headphones, stereos Regular unprotected exposure longer than 1 minute at this decibel level or higher risks permanent hearing loss
120	Loud cars, snowmobiles, rock concerts
130	Some lawn mowers, leaf blowers, power tools
140	Firecrackers
150	Gunshot or some toy guns shot from 1 foot away

Source: National Institute on Deafness and Communication Disorders, Bethesda, Md.

TABLE 85-6 Types of Hearing Aids

Device	How It Works	Cost ($)
Conventional/traditional	Amplifies sound using preprogrammed circuits.	600 and up
Programmable (analog sound processing)	Uses tiny computer chips that can be programmed to different settings, environments, background noises, types of noise; these can be reprogrammed as hearing loss changes	850-2000
Digital sound processing	Uses the latest technology with clear sound, sophisticated circuits, front and rear microphones, voice vs nonvoice sensors to make sound audible without discomfort	2000-3200

Hearing Aids

These devices can assist people with sensorineural and conductive hearing loss. Hearing aids can increase the intensity of sounds up to about 70 dB. Hearing aids can only be obtained after an evaluation by a health care provider. Medicare and most insurance companies do not pay for hearing aids. Three types of hearing aids are available, as outlined in Table 85-6.

Four basic models of hearing aids are available:

- Behind the ear: Fits in the ear and behind the ear, connected by a loop that wraps around the top of the ear.
- In the ear: Slightly smaller; fits just inside the ear and sits flush with the outer ear.
- In the canal: Fits into the ear canal and shows only slightly on the outside of the ear.
- Completely in the canal: Fits deep in the ear canal with a tiny sensor wire that protrudes from the ear.

Follow-up

If hearing loss is caused by acute disease, check for resolution in 1 to 2 weeks.

EVALUATION

Recheck hearing abilities to determine improvement.

RESOURCES

American Speech-Language-Hearing Association
10801 Rockville Pk
Rockville, MD, 20852
(800) 638-8255

National Institute on Deafness and Other Communication Disorders
Information Clearinghouse
1 Communications Ave
Bethesda, MD 20892-3456,
(800) 241-1044

Self-Help for Hard of Hearing People
7800 Wisconsin Ave
Bethesda, MD 20814
(301) 657-2248

American Academy of Otolaryngology-Head and Neck Surgery: (703) 836-4444; www.entnet.org

Better Hearing Institute 800-327-9355 or www.betterhearing.org

The Ear Foundation: www.theearfound.com

The Hearing Alliance: www.hearingalliance.com/~hearnow

National Information Center on Deafness: www.gallaudet.edu/~nicd/

Self-help for hard of hearing: www.shhh.org

SUGGESTED READINGS

Ellsworth A et al: *Mosby's 1998 medical drug reference,* St Louis, 1998, Mosby.

Healthcare Consultants of America, Inc: *1998 Physicians fee and coding guide,* Augusta, Ga, 1998, Healthcare Consultants of America, Inc.

Jackler R, Kaplan M: Ear, nose, throat. In Tierney L, McPhee S, Papadakis M, editors: *Current medical diagnosis and treatment,* Norwalk, Conn, 1998, Appleton & Lange.

Jerger J: Hearing impairment in older adults: new concepts, *J Am Geriatr Soc* 43:928, 1995.

Mitchell G: Otologic devices, *Emerg Clin North Am* 12:787, 1994.

86 Heart Murmur

ICD-9-CM

Mitral Stenosis 394.0
Endocarditis, Valve Unspecified, Unspecified Cause 424.90
Coarctation of the Aorta 747.10
Aortic Stenosis 424.1
Atrial Septal Defects 745.5
Patent Ductus Arteriosis 747.0
Mitral Valve Prolapse 424.0
Ventricular Septal Defects 745.4
Transposition of the Great Vessels 745.10
Tetralogy of Fallot 745.2

OVERVIEW

Definition

A murmur is an extra sound produced when there is turbulent blood flow into, within, or out of the heart. The characteristics of a murmur depend on the adequacy of valve function, the size of the opening, the rate of blood flow, the intensity of the myocardium, and the thickness of the chest through which the murmur must be heard.

Incidence

Data on incidence vary by type and cause of murmur.
Innocent murmurs occur in 30% to 50% of **children.**
In a **newborn** with a murmur noted within 24 hours of birth, there is a 1 in 12 risk of congenital heart disease. If a murmur is first heard when the **child** is 12 months old, there is a 1 in 50 risk of congenital heart disease.

Pathophysiology

In the past, the most common cause of murmurs was rheumatic heart disease. Other causes are now more common. Diseased valves do not open or close well. When the leaflets are thickened, the passage is narrowed so blood flow is restricted (stenosis). When the valve leaflets lose competency, the opening allows backward flow across the valve (regurgitation). Valvular disease that causes murmurs includes:

Mitral stenosis
Mitral regurgitation
Aortic stenosis
Aortic regurgitation
Tricuspid stenosis
Tricuspid regurgitation

See Appendix G for more detailed information regarding these murmurs.

Not all murmurs are the result of valvular disease. Other causes include:

High output demands that increase speed of blood flow:
Pregnancy
Thyrotoxicosis
Anemia
Structural defects (congenital or acquired) that permit blood flow through inappropriate pathways (see Chapter 41 for more detail about murmurs that affect newborns)
 Ventricular septal defect
 Atrial septal defect
Diminished strength of myocardial contraction
Altered blood flow in vessels near the heart
Innocent murmurs are commonly seen in children and adolescents because of vigorous myocardial contraction and stronger blood flow in systole and because their thinner chests make the sounds easier to hear (Seidel et al, 1995)

SUBJECTIVE DATA

History of Present Illness

In most cases patients do not present with a "murmur"; the murmur is an incidental finding during an examination. The patient may initially be seen with symptoms related to the murmur/valvular heart disease. The symptoms are usually related to the degree of heart failure and whether it is right- or left-sided heart failure.

Ask about:
- Shortness of breath (SOB)
- Exertional dyspnea
- Orthopnea
- Paroxysmal nocturnal dyspnea
- Edema
- Signs/symptoms heart failure
- Chest pain
- Fatigue
- Palpitations
- Syncope
- Hepatomegaly
- Ascites
- Dependent edema
- Leg pain or cramps

Children:
- Tires during feeding
- Cyanosis
- Knee-chest position for rest
- Naps: Longer than expected, nosebleeds, unexplained joint pain

Past Medical History

Past episodes of congestive heart failure (CHF)
History of rheumatic heart disease
Cough
Past cardiac surgery or hospitalization for cardiac workup
Chronic illness: Hypertension (HTN), diabetes mellitus (DM), bleeding disorder, hyperlipidemia, coronary artery disease (CAD), congenital heart defect (CHD)

Medications

Angiotensin-converting enzyme inhibitors
Digitalis products
Diuretics
Preprocedure penicillin
Over-the-counter medications

Family History

Ask about family history of heart disease, DM, HTN, hyperlipidemia, CHDs, sudden death (especially in young and middle-age relatives)

Psychosocial History

Ask about:
- Smoking history
- Alcohol ingestion
- Substance use/abuse
- Employment, environmental hazards, types of emotional stress
- Nutritional status
- Weight loss or gain

OBJECTIVE DATA

Physical Examination

Skin: Cyanosis, hair loss, pallor, sores
Head/eyes/ears/nose/throat: Xanthelasma
Neck: Neck vein distention, bruit
Lungs: Chest deformity, barrel chest, crackles, wheezing
Heart: Pulsations, lifts, heaves, point of maximal impulse
- Palpation: Lift, heave, PMI, thrill
- Percussion: Define the borders of the heart (limited value)
- Auscultation: Use diaphragm and bell of stethoscope in all areas:
  - Aortic area: Second intercostal space (ICS) right sternal border (RSB)
  - Pulmonic area: Second ICS LSB
  - Erbs point: Third ICS LSB
  - Tricuspid area: Fourth ICS LSB
- Identify splits, extra heart sounds, and murmurs
  - Mitral: Fifth ICS midclavicular line
- See Appendix G for specifics about grading heart murmurs

Abdominal: Hepatosplenomegaly, abdominal aorta, bruit
Extremities: Pulses

Diagnostic Procedures

Diagnostic tests are detailed in Table 86-1.

ASSESSMENT

Diastolic murmurs and murmurs associated with a thrill are always clinically significant, with underlying heart disease.

Differential Diagnosis

Table 86-2 lists differential diagnoses for heart murmur. Figures 86-1 and 86-2 outline the approach to patients with a diastolic murmur or a systolic murmur.

THERAPEUTIC PLAN

Innocent murmurs should be monitored during routine physical examinations.
In most cases the end point of valvular difficulties is heart failure.
Consider antibiotics for patients who are at high risk for bacterial endocarditis.

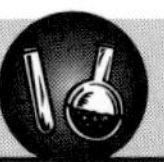

TABLE 86-1 Diagnostic Tests: Heart Murmur

Diagnostic Tests	Findings/Rationale	Cost ($)
CXR	Provides information about heart size, pulmonary circulation, pulmonary disease, and aortic abnormalities	77-91
Echocardiogram	Provides more reliable information about chamber size, hypertrophy, pericardial effusions, valvular abnormalities	675
ECG	Indicates cardiac rhythm, conduction abnormalities, and provides evidence of ventricular hypertrophy, myocardial infarction or ischemia; not recommended in follow-up, but is appropriate as baseline	56-65
Cardiac Exercise testing	Sensitivity of 60%-80% and specificity 70%-80% for CAD; not very helpful for asymptomatic patients	249-305
24 hour Holter monitoring	Most helpful for patients with symptoms consistent with arrhythmia	295-388
Thallium testing	Used commonly in conjunction with exercise testing to detect ischemia, which appears as a perfusion defect; dipyridamole (Persantine) provides similar information for patients unable to exercise	529-636

CAD, Coronary artery disease; *CXR,* chest x-ray examination; *ECG,* electrocardiogram.

TABLE 86-2 Differential Diagnosis: Heart Murmur

Diagnosis	Supporting Data	Treatment
Diastolic Murmurs		
Mitral stenosis	SOB, orthopnea, and PND seen as symptoms. Symptoms may be precipitated by onset of atrial fibrillation or pregnancy. Midsystolic or presystolic thrill at apex. Opening snap along LSB or at apex. Murmur localized at apex. Low pitched rumbling presystolic murmur. Heard best in left lateral recumbent position or after exercise. Echocardiography is the most valuable test for assessing mitral stenosis.	In most cases there is a long asymptomatic phase, followed by gradual decrease in activities. The onset of atrial fibrillation precipitates more severe symptoms. Once heart failure can no longer be controlled, surgery is indicated.
Aortic regurgitation (AR)	Usually asymptomatic until middle age; presents with left-sided failure or chest pain. Hyperactive enlarged ventricle, diastolic murmur along LSB, often blowing faint murmur. Heard best when patient is leaning forward, breath held in expiration	AR that worsens during endocarditis may warrant immediate valve replacement. Chronic AR will require valve replacement once symptoms appear.
Tricuspid stenosis	Usually caused by rheumatic fever. It should be suspected when the patient presents with symptoms of right-sided heart failure (hepatomegaly, ascites, dependent edema). Middiastolic murmur heard best along the lower LSB. S_1 is often loud; third to fifth ICS along LSB out to apex. Louder during and at peak inspiration. Echocardiography identifies the lesion, and right-side heart catheterization is diagnostic.	Tricuspid stenosis usually requires valve replacement.
Systolic Murmurs		
Mitral regurgitation (MR)	May be asymptomatic or may present with left-sided failure. Pansystolic murmur at apex, radiating into axilla or left infrascapular area, associated with S_3, blowing, high pitched, occasionally harsh or musical. Having patient do a handgrip increases the intensity of the sound.	Acute MR caused by endocarditis, MI, or ruptured chordae tendineae requires emergency surgery. Chronic MR will require surgery once left ventricular function deteriorates.
Aortic stenosis	Usually asymptomatic until middle or old age; may also have delayed or diminished carotid pulses, soft, absent, or paradoxically split S_2, prominent PMI, harsh systolic murmur (sometimes with thrill over aortic area), often radiating to neck. Best heard with patient leaning forward, holding breath in full expiration. The best diagnostic test for aortic stenosis is cardiac catheterization.	Once heart failure, angina, or syncope appears, the prognosis without surgery is poor. Surgery is indicated for all symptomatic patients.

ICS, Intercostal space; *IVDU,* intravenous drug use; *MI,* myocardial infarction; *LSB,* left sternal border; *PND,* paroxysmal nocturnal dyspnea; *SOB,* shortness of breath.

TABLE 86-2 Differential Diagnosis: Heart Murmur—cont'd

Diagnosis	Supporting Data	Treatment
Tricuspid regurgitation	This murmur may occur in situations other than disease of the valve itself. The most common is right ventricular overload caused by left ventricular overload. It also occurs with right ventricular and inferior MIs. It is a common valve problem associated with IVDU. The symptoms seen are those produced by right-sided heart failure. Atrial fibrillation is usually present. Heard best at the third to fifth ICS along LSB out to apex. Murmur becomes louder during inspiration.	Once the underlying disease is corrected, the valve problem may correct itself. If surgery is required, valve repair or a valvuloplasty is preferable to valve replacement.
Innocent murmur	Usually found in **children** or **teens** during an examination, usually grade I or II, midsystolic, without radiation, of medium pitch, blowing, brief, and accompanied by splitting of S_2. Innocent murmurs are often located in second ICS near LSB. They may not be heard in a sitting or standing position. They are heard more often with fever, exercise, or excitement.	No treatment needed.

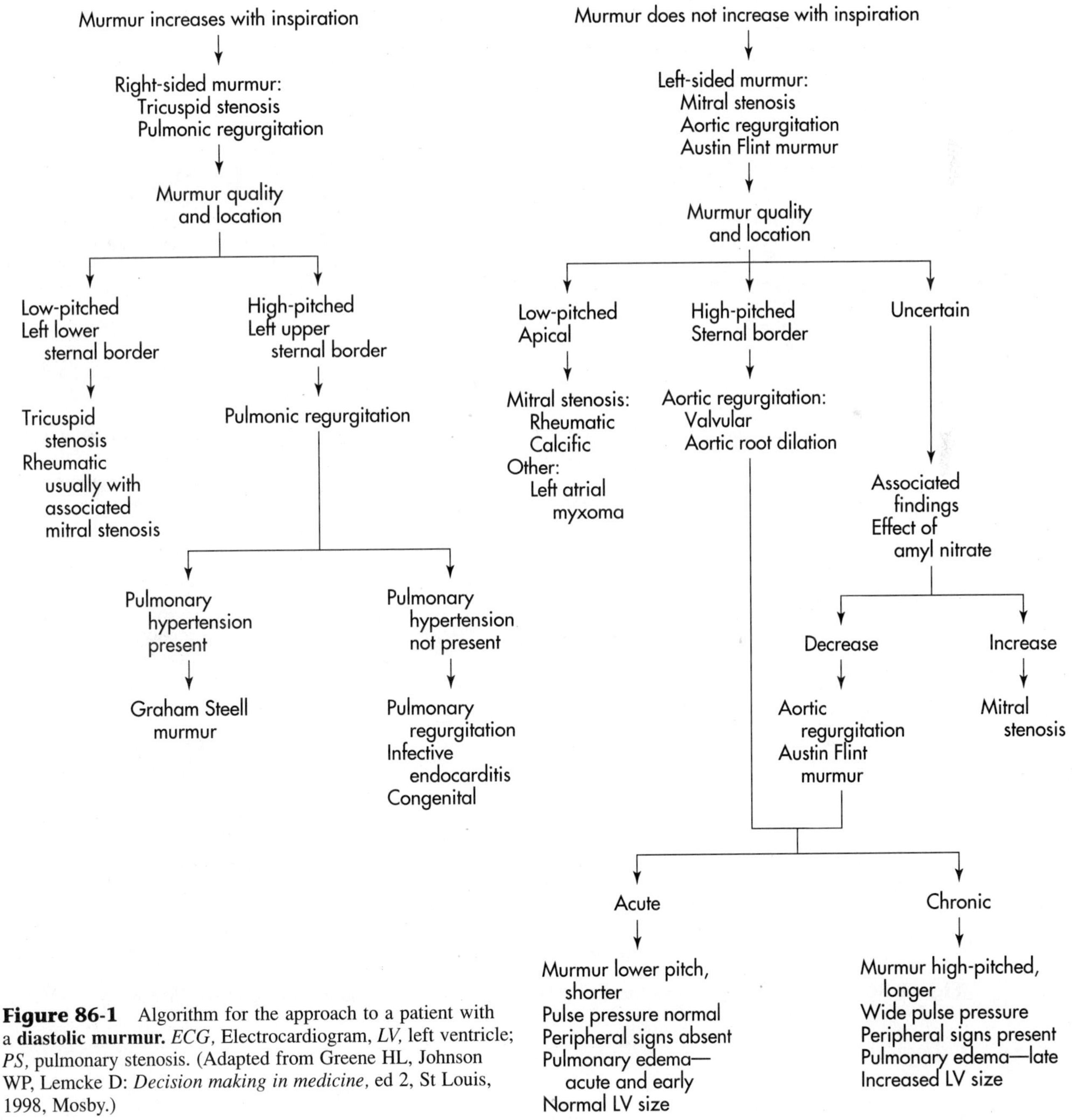

Murmur increases with inspiration
→ Right-sided murmur: Tricuspid stenosis; Pulmonic regurgitation
→ Murmur quality and location
- Low-pitched, Left lower sternal border → Tricuspid stenosis; Rheumatic usually with associated mitral stenosis
- High-pitched, Left upper sternal border → Pulmonic regurgitation
  - Pulmonary hypertension present → Graham Steell murmur
  - Pulmonary hypertension not present → Pulmonary regurgitation; Infective endocarditis; Congenital

Murmur does not increase with inspiration
→ Left-sided murmur: Mitral stenosis; Aortic regurgitation; Austin Flint murmur
→ Murmur quality and location
- Low-pitched, Apical → Mitral stenosis: Rheumatic, Calcific; Other: Left atrial myxoma
- High-pitched, Sternal border → Aortic regurgitation: Valvular, Aortic root dilation
- Uncertain → Associated findings; Effect of amyl nitrate
  - Decrease → Aortic regurgitation; Austin Flint murmur
  - Increase → Mitral stenosis

Aortic regurgitation →
- Acute → Murmur lower pitch, shorter; Pulse pressure normal; Peripheral signs absent; Pulmonary edema—acute and early; Normal LV size
- Chronic → Murmur high-pitched, longer; Wide pulse pressure; Peripheral signs present; Pulmonary edema—late; Increased LV size

Figure 86-1 Algorithm for the approach to a patient with a **diastolic murmur.** *ECG,* Electrocardiogram, *LV,* left ventricle; *PS,* pulmonary stenosis. (Adapted from Greene HL, Johnson WP, Lemcke D: *Decision making in medicine,* ed 2, St Louis, 1998, Mosby.)

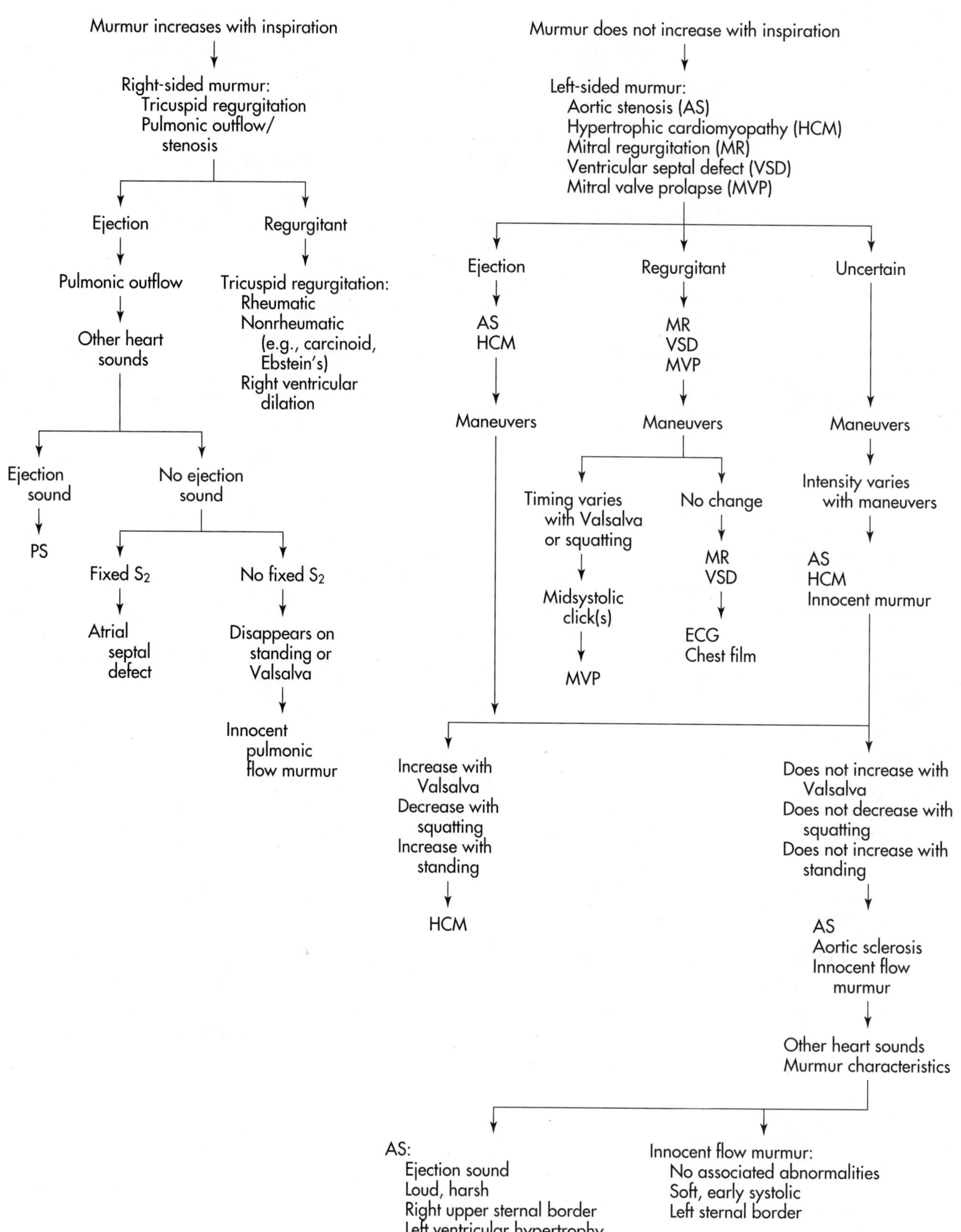

Figure 86-2 Algorithm for the approach to a patient with a **systolic murmur.** (Adapted from Greene HL, Johnson WP, Lemcke D: *Decision making in medicine,* ed 2, St Louis, 1998, Mosby.)

Pharmaceutical

Medical management with vasodilators and ACE inhibitors can reduce the severity of failure and may stabilize most patients. However, surgery (valvular repair/replacement) is usually indicated once the murmur produces symptoms. See Chapter 42 for definitive therapeutic guidelines.

Referral/Consultation

The patient should be referred to a cardiologist for diagnostic studies when a new murmur is identified or if a murmur changes or the patient becomes symptomatic.

REFERENCE

Seidel HM et al, editors: *Mosby's guide to physical examination,* St Louis, 1995, Mosby.

SUGGESTED READINGS

Ellsworth A et al: *Mosby's 1998 medical drug reference,* St Louis, 1998, Mosby.

Greene HL, Johnson WP, Lemcke D: *Decision making in medicine,* ed 2, St Louis, 1998, Mosby.

Healthcare Consultants of America, Inc: *1998 Physicians fee and coding guide,* Augusta, Ga, 1998, Healthcare Consultants of America, Inc.

Massie B, Amidon T: Heart. In Tierney L, McPhee S, Papadakis M, editors: *Current medical diagnosis and treatment,* Norwalk, Conn, 1998, Appleton & Lange.

Steward B: Clinical factors associated with calcific aortic valve disease, *J Am Coll Cardiol* 29: 630, 1997.

Warner A: Systolic and diastolic murmurs. In Greene H, Johnson W, Lemcke D, editors: *Decision making in medicine,* ed 2, St Louis, 1998, Mosby.

87 Hematuria

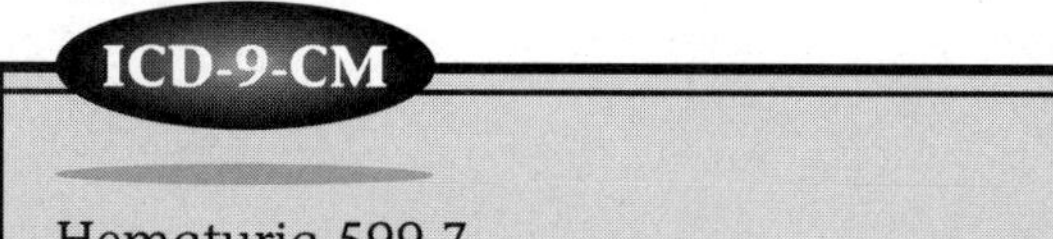

ICD-9-CM

Hematuria 599.7

OVERVIEW

Definition

Most authorities agree that three to five red blood cells (RBCs) per high-powered microscopic field (HPF) or more is the definition of clinically significant hematuria. Normal individuals excrete as many as one to three RBCs per HPF into the urine daily.

Hematuria can be a presenting complaint, an abnormality found during the evaluation of other symptoms or found on a routine urinalysis. There are three forms of hematuria: That which is caused by a disease in the genitourinary tract; innocent hematuria, present after a pelvic or prostate examination, genitourinary procedure or sometimes after vigorous exercise; and pseudohematuria, red urine without red cells. In **adults,** hematuria should be considered a sign of malignancy unless proved otherwise. In **children,** most have benign conditions that require no intervention. Time-consuming, expensive studies should be reserved for children who by history or examination are at high risk for serious renal or extrarenal disease.

Initially it is important to determine whether hematuria does in fact exist. False-positive indicators of hematuria can occur when dipsticks react to hemoglobin or myoglobin, or the condition may be pigmenturia, caused by any of a variety of foods and drugs. A microscopic examination must be done to confirm the presence of RBCs.

Incidence

Asymptomatic microscopic hematuria in a young patient carries a lower risk of a concomitant finding of significant genitourinary tract disease; there is a higher risk in patients with macroscopic hematuria, particularly in older males. One percent to 5% of **children** and **adults** show evidence of microhematuria on routine urinalysis; fewer than 2% of these patients have a serious and treatable urinary tract disease.

SUBJECTIVE DATA

History of Present Illness

The description of the hematuria may suggest a cause: Blood clots and bright-red urine are more likely to have a urological source; dark-, cola-, or tea-colored urine suggests glomerulonephritis, hepatitis, or subacute bacterial endocarditis.

Initial hematuria, the presence of blood at the beginning of the urinary stream that clears during the stream, is more likely caused by urethral bleeding; terminal hematuria, the presence of blood at the end of the stream, points to bleeding from the prostate gland or bladder neck.

Total hematuria, the presence of blood throughout the urinary stream, implies a bladder or upper tract source.

Gross, painless hematuria throughout voiding may be indicative of neoplasm.

Recent trauma may indicate possible renal, ureteral, or urethral injury.

Past Medical History

A history of pharyngitis 2 weeks before the development of cola-colored hematuria is classic for poststreptococcal glomerulonephritis.

Upper respiratory infections other than strep sore throat can also cause glomerulonephritis.

A prior history of nephritis may indicate chronic nephritis as the cause of hematuria.

A history of stone disease or malignancy should be investigated.

Diabetes mellitus or sickle cell trait or disease should be explored.

A hematological history is important as well as systemic illnesses such as lupus, polycythemia vera, or rheumatic fever.

Determine whether the patient has a history of a bleeding disorder.

Last menstrual period.

Medications

Anticoagulants: Papillary necrosis, bleeding resulting from high international normalized ratio (INR)

Antibiotics: Interstitial nephritis

Salicylates

Methenamine preparations

Sulfonamides have been implicated in hematuria, and can cause discoloration of urine

Estrogen-containing birth control pills have been known to cause a loin-pain hematuria syndrome, a disorder predominantly of young women

Drugs such as phenazopyridine and rifampin darken urine in such a way that it can be mistaken for hematuria

Analgesic abuse can cause papillary necrosis

Cyclophosphamide may produce hemorrhagic cystitis

Family History

A family history of hematuria, renal insufficiency, hearing loss, or cystic renal disease should be elicited.

In blacks and some persons of Mediterranean origin question about sickle-cell trait and sickle-cell disease.

Hearing deficit: Alport syndrome

Microscopic hematuria: IgA nephropathy, benign familial hematuria, hypercalciuria

Renal insufficiency or failure: Polycystic kidney disease

Sickle cell disease/trait: Sickle cell nephropathy

Psychosocial History

Question about strenuous exercise or long-distance running.

Smoking is a major risk factor for transitional cell carcinoma.

Occupational exposure to aromatic amines, dyes, or benzidine is also a major risk factor for a neoplasm.

Diet History

Ascertain whether the diet includes large quantities of beets, rhubarb, berries, or paprika. These contain dyes that can darken the urine.

Amount of water, colas, teas, coffee consumed daily.

Associated Symptoms

Accompanying symptoms can be nonspecific.

Suprapubic pain, urgency and frequency as well as dysuria often occur with urinary tract infections (UTIs), but bladder carcinoma can also produce the same symptoms.

Nephrolithiasis can present as painless hematuria or flank pain radiating to the abdomen and groin.

Renal artery emboli can also cause flank pain and hematuria.

Arthralgias, especially when accompanied by fever and rash may suggest a systemic illness such as a vasculitis or an infection such as endocarditis.

OBJECTIVE DATA

Physical Examination

The physical examination should emphasize signs of systemic disease, as well as signs of medical renal disease.

Vital signs: Baseline measurements should include blood pressure (lying and standing), weight, and temperature. Height and weight of children should be plotted on standardized growth charts.

Table 87-1 identifies important areas of the physical examination, along with possible findings and conditions that may cause them.

Diagnostic Procedures

The appropriate workup depends on whether the patient has macroscopic hematuria or asymptomatic hematuria, on the age and gender of the patient, and on the clinical presentation.

Clues from the history and physical examination should direct the laboratory follow-up. The most prominent etiological possibilities include neoplasms, nephrolithiasis, infections, and intrinsic renal disease, especially glomerulonephritis. The first step is a repeat urinalysis. Table 87-2 summarizes the diagnostic procedures for hematuria. Figure 87-1 outlines the approach to the patient with hematuria.

ASSESSMENT

Differential Diagnosis

The most common illnesses found in **children** include those shown in Table 87-3. In **adults,** the sources of bleeding are outlined in Table 87-4.

THERAPEUTIC PLAN

Treatment depends on the selected diagnosis.

Hematuria with pyuria: Bacterial cultures should be obtained and infections treated appropriately.

Acute uncomplicated UTIs can be effectively treated, before the infecting organism is identified, with oral trimethoprim-sulfamethoxazole.

Table 87-1 Physical Examination: Hematuria

Assessment	PE Findings	Conditions
BP	Hypertension	Renal parenchymal disease
Skin	Rash, purpura, petechiae, pallor	Lupus, polycythemia vera, strep infection, vasculitis
HEENT	Lymphadenopathy, pharyngitis	Poststreptococcal glomerulonephritis
Heart	Friction rub, murmur	Bacterial endocarditis, rheumatic fever
Lungs	Crackles	Volume overload
Abdomen	Organomegaly (one or more kidneys, liver, spleen), CVAT or suprapubic tenderness	Flank mass (hydronephrosis, polycystic kidney, Wilms' tumor), polycystic kidneys, volume overload, infection
Prostate examination	Enlargement, nodules	BPH, carcinoma
External genitalia/pelvic	Bleeding from urethral, vaginal or other lesions, signs of inflammation, trauma, presence of FB	Infection, menstruation, tumor, trauma
Extremities	Peripheral edema	Glomerular disease
Musculoskeletal	Joint pain, soft tissue swelling	Connective tissue disease, rheumatic fever

BP, Blood pressure; *BPH,* benign prostatic hypertrophy; *CVAT,* costovertebral angle tenderness; *FB,* foreign body; *HEENT,* head, eyes, ears, nose, throat; *PE,* physical examination.

Hematuria with proteinuria, RBC casts, or dysmorphic red blood cells: Immunological studies should be performed and a renal biopsy considered. Consultation with a nephrologist indicated.

Hematuria as a result of urolithiasis: Strain urine, increase fluid intake to ten 10-ounce glasses of fluid a day.

Pyuria without bacteriuria: Most frequently occurs with chlamydial infections or coliform infections of low colony count; may occur with tuberculosis of the urinary tract or an interstitial nephritis such as analgesic nephropathy. Treat appropriately.

Persistent gross hematuria: A urologist should always be consulted.

Pharmaceutical

Treatment depends on the selected diagnosis.

Lifestyle/Activities

Activity and lifestyle modifications are determined by the diagnosis.

Women experiencing postcoital cystitis, for example, should void just before and immediately following sexual intercourse.

Use of a diaphragm for birth control is not recommended.

Showers versus baths are advised.

Use of scented perfumes, powders, and sprays in the genital area is discouraged.

Referral

Appropriate referrals for the patient with hematuria may include a nephrologist, urologist, or immunologist. **Gross painless hematuria in an adult is always an indication for urological consultation.**

Referral to a urologist is recommended for **children** who have persistent UTIs involving the same organism, for all boys with UTIs, for boys and girls in whom pyelonephritis is suspected and for girls who have two or more infections in 6 months.

Follow-up

Follow-up is determined by the identified cause of hematuria. In the female with a complicated UTI, a follow-up urinalysis is important after treatment to ensure resolution of the hematuria. A completely normal result to a repeat study in a healthy young person requires no further investigation other than a follow-up urinalysis in 1 or 2 months. However, in an **older patient,** whose risk of malignancy is much greater, RBCs greater than 3 to 5 RBCs per high-power field should be taken seriously even if the repeat urinalysis is clear. Urinary tract malignancies can present in this manner.

EVALUATION

In patients with negative results to their evaluations, repeat evaluations are necessary to avoid a missed malignancy. Urinary cytology can be repeated in 3 to 6 months, and

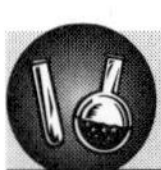

TABLE 87-2 Diagnostic Tests: Hematuria

Test	Findings/Rationale	Cost ($)
U/A with microscopic examination	First-level test for basic screening: Presence of pyuria and bacteriuria suggests infectious cause such as cystitis, pyelonephritis, or prostatitis; pyuria without bacteriuria frequently occurs with chlamydial infections, TB of urinary tract, or interstitial nephritis, such as analgesic nephropathy Proteinuria, RBC casts, and dysmorphic RBCs indicate intrinsic renal disease, particularly glomerulonephritis	14-18
PT, PTT, bleeding time	To rule out bleeding disorder	18-23/PT 23-29/PTT 19-24/bleeding
Urine cultures	To rule out bacterial growth: Infection	31-39
Urine cytology	To identify bladder neoplasm (three voided samples are recommended to maximize sensitivity)	121-144
Serum creatinine/ BUN	First-level test to indicate renal function	17-21/BUN 18-24/creat
PPD and urine AFB cultures	Tests for patient with sterile pyuria to rule out tuberculosis of the urinary tract	15-19/ PPD 18-24/AFB
Hemoglobin electrophoresis	Test for patient at risk for sickle hemoglobinopathies	41-51
Throat culture and ASO titers	Test for patient with a history of URI symptoms to rule out streptococcal infections	24-30/throat culture 29-37/ASO
LDH	Test when renal emboli suspected	20-25
Serum complements and ANA	Test for patient with evidence of systemic disease	42-52/ANA 47-59
24-Hour urine collection/eval	To detect hypercalciuria (**children** only); hypercalciuria is a common cause for hematuria in **children**	24-30
24-Hour urine collection/eval	To quantify proteinuria, calcium, uric acid; heavy proteinuria is associated with glomerular lesions	21-26
IVP	First-level test to identify most stones, some bladder lesions, obstructions, intrinsic ureteral lesions	280-333
Renal ultrasonography	Can detect renal masses not found on IVP and determine whether a lesion is fluid-filled or solid; alternative for those allergic to IVP dye or at high risk for contrast nephropathy; role unclear, sensitivity may be lower than other tests	347-416
Cystoscopy	Visualizes the bladder and urinary outlet tract for bleeding	447-540
Renal angiography	Reserved for evaluation of possible renal trauma, suspicious renal masses and possible arteriovenous malformations	268-325

AFB, Acid-fast bacillus, *ANA,* antinuclear antibody; *ASO,* antistreptolysin O; *BUN,* blood urea nitrogen; *IVP,* intravenous pyelogram; *LDH,* lactic acid dehydrogenase; *PPD,* purified protein derivative of tuberculin; *PT,* prothrombin time; *PTT,* partial thromboplastin time; *RBC,* red blood cells.

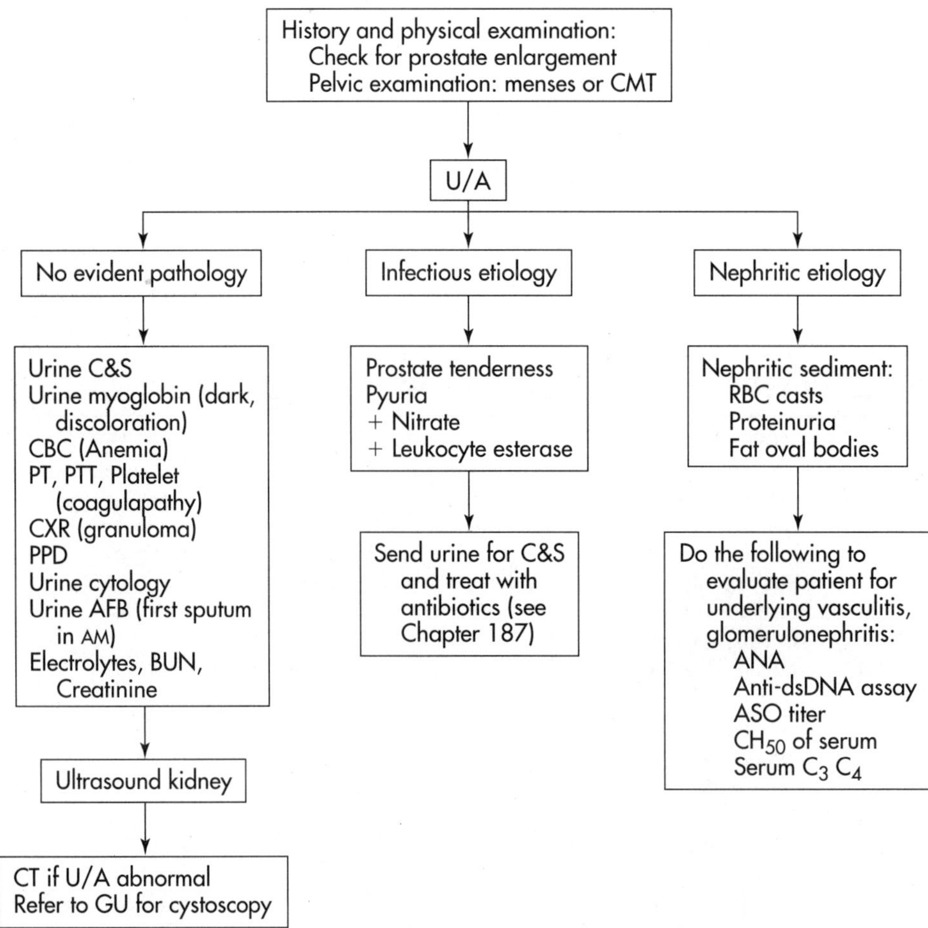

Figure 87-1 Algorithm for the approach to a patient with hematuria. *AFB,* Acid-fast bacillus; *ANA,* antinuclear antibody; *ASO,* antistreptolysin O; *BUN,* blood urea nitrogen; *C&S,* culture and sensitivity; *CBC,* complete blood cell count; *CMT,* cervical motion tenderness; *CXR,* chest x-ray examination; *PPD,* purified protein derivative of tuberculin; *PT,* prothrombin time; *PTT,* partial thromboplastin time; *RBC,* red blood cells; *U/A,* urinalysis; *UTI,* urinary tract infection.

TABLE 87-3 Differential Diagnosis: Hematuria in Children

Diagnosis	Supporting Data
Glomerulonephritis	Inflammation of glomeruli, hematuria, proteinuria, RBC casts in urine, edema, oliguria, hypertension, flank pain, and increased BUN and creatinine.
UTI	Symptoms of cystitis include dysuria, urgency, frequency, and suprapubic abdominal pain. Symptoms of pyelonephritis include fever, vomiting, irritability, CVAT, flank pain, and dysuria. Urine dipstick reveals positive result for leukocytes and nitrites. A positive urine culture is also found.
Alport's syndrome	Progressive hereditary nephritis: Glomerulonephritis, sensorineural deafness, ocular abnormalities. Symptoms include hematuria, proteinuria, and progressive renal insufficiency. Hearing deficit is for higher sounds and may not become evident until teenage years. Males are more severely affected than females. Definitive diagnosis requires a renal biopsy.
Benign familial hematuria	Seen in children and young adults as persistent microscopic hematuria, with or without proteinuria. If proteinuria occurs, it rarely results in nephrotic syndrome. Definitive diagnosis requires renal biopsy. This condition is nonprogressive and benign and requires no treatment.
Idiopathic hypercalciuria	Hypercalciuria is present in approximately 3% of healthy children. It has no relationship to ↑ dietary intake of calcium. It is caused by excessive GI absorption of calcium or a renal leak of calcium as a result of ↓ tubular reabsorption. Identified by a screening random urine comparing calcium to creatinine ratio. If ratio >0.22, a 24-hour urine collection should be done.
Miscellaneous	Strenuous exercise, blunt trauma, a bleeding disorder, sickle-cell trait or disease can all cause hematuria. Exercise, trauma, and bleeding disorder should be evident from history. Testing should be conducted for sickle cell trait or anemia if suspected.

BUN, Blood urea nitrogen; *CVAT,* costovertebral angle tenderness; *GI,* gastrointestinal; *RBC,* red blood cells; *UTI,* urinary tract infection.

TABLE 87-4 Sources of Bleeding in Adults with Hematuria

Source	Location	Percent
Upper tract source	Kidneys, ureters	10
	Stone disease	42
	Medical renal disease: medullary sponge kidney, glomerulonephritis	19
	Renal cell carcinoma	10
	Transitional cell carcinoma of ureter or renal pelvis	7
Lower tract source	Transitional cell carcinoma of bladder (in absence of infection)	Unknown
	Males: BPH most common cause	

BPH, Benign prostatic hypertrophy.

cystoscopy and upper tract imaging may be repeated in 1 year. **Children** with repeated UTIs should be evaluated for the possibility of sexual abuse.

SUGGESTED READINGS

Fang L: Evaluation of the patient with hematuria. In Goroll A, May L, Mulley A, editors: *Primary care medicine: office evaluation and management of the adult patient,* ed 3, Philadelphia, 1995, JB Lippincott.

Hassay K: Effective management of urinary discomfort *Nurse Pract* 20(2):36-46, 1995.

Healthcare Consultants of America, Inc: *1998 Physicians fee and coding guide,* Augusta, Ga, 1998, Healthcare Consultants of America, Inc.

Leiner S: Recurrent urinary tract infection in otherwise healthy adult women, *Nurse Pract* 20:48-56, 1995.

McCarthy J: Outpatient evaluation of hematuria: locating the source of bleeding, *Postgrad Med* 101:125-131, 1997.

Presti J, Stoller M, Carroll P: Evaluation of hematuria. In Tierney L, McPhee S, Papadakis M, editors: *1998 Current medical diagnosis and treatment,* ed 37, Norwalk, Conn, 1997, Appleton & Lange.

Portale A et al: Kidneys and electrolytes. In Rudolph A, Kamei R, editors: *Rudolph's fundamentals of pediatrics,* ed 2, Norwalk, Conn, 1998, Appleton & Lange.

Spector D: Hematuria. In Barker L, Burton J, Zieve P, editors: *Principles of ambulatory medicine,* ed 4, Baltimore, 1995, Williams & Wilkins.

Sutton J: Evaluation of hematuria in adults, *JAMA* 263:2475-2480, 1990.

Hemorrhoids

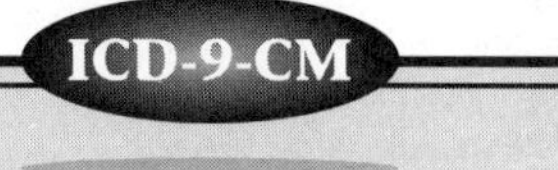

ICD-9-CM

Hemorrhoids 455.6

OVERVIEW

Definition

Hemorrhoids are varicosities of the lower rectum or anus. Internal hemorrhoids occur above the internal sphincter. External hemorrhoids occur outside the external sphincter.

Incidence

Most common in adults

Pathophysiology

The veins of the hemorrhoidal plexus dilate secondary to prolapse and entrapment by the internal sphincter.

Contributing factors to prolapse include constipation, straining while defecating or lifting, prolonged sitting, pregnancy, episiotomy, obesity, loss of muscle tone as a result of aging, hypertension, anal infection, and anal intercourse.

SUBJECTIVE DATA

History of Present Illness

Ask the patient about:

Onset and duration of pain, itching, burning, and bleeding.

Prolapse and protrusion requiring manual replacement.

Constipation, straining, lifting, prolonged sitting.

Concurrent medical conditions such as pregnancy and hypertension.

Concurrent anal infection and/or recent anal intercourse.

Self-help measures and response to treatment.

Past Medical History

Inquire about history of anal surgery or episiotomy.

OBJECTIVE DATA

Physical Examination

Position a male patient in a side-lying position or ask him to stand and rest his body across the examining table. A female patient can be positioned in a side-lying or lithotomy position. A child can be positioned in a side-lying position.

Assess the rectum and anus for large, dilated veins noting any inflammation, ulcers, excoriations, or bleeding. Assess rectal muscle tone.

External hemorrhoids usually present as a soft, painless mass just outside the anus.

Internal hemorrhoids may or may not be visualized by an external exam. They may be palpated on internal digital exam with a gloved, lubricated finger.

A thrombosed hemorrhoid may present as a firm, bluish, painful mass.

Diagnostic Procedures

Diagnostic procedures are summarized in Table 88-1.

ASSESSMENT

External hemorrhoids

Internal hemorrhoids

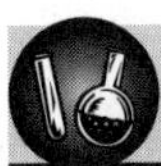

TABLE 88-1 Diagnostic Tests: Hemorrhoids

Test	Findings/Rationale	Cost ($)
Hemoglobin and hematocrit	Assess for anemia with significant rectal bleeding.	13-16/CBC
Proctosigmoidoscopy	Assess for internal hemorrhoids, rectosigmoid cancer, strictures, polyps, and inflammatory bowel disease	149-182
Barium enema	Assess for colorectal lesions (polyps, cancer), diverticulosis, strictures, fistulas and sinus tracts, and inflammatory bowel disease	394-471

Differential Diagnosis

Anal tags
Polyps
Carcinoma
Pruritus ani

THERAPEUTIC PLAN

Pharmaceutical

Many products are available because of their anesthetic, astringent, or protective factors (Table 88-2).

Stool softeners may also be considered: Docusate sodium (Colace) $2 to $23

- **Adults:** 50 to 200 mg PO QD
- **Children** under 3 years old: 10 to 40 mg PO QD
- **Children** 3 to 6 years old: 60 mg PO QD
- **Children** 6 to12 years old: 40 to 120 mg PO QD

Diet

The patient will need:

- A high-fiber diet
- To increase fluid intake
- A psyllium product (Metamucil) QD

Patient Education

Educate patient about causes, contributing factors, and treatments.

Most hemorrhoids respond to conservative treatment therapies.

Lifestyle Modifications

The patient should be encouraged to:

- Lose weight
- Practice proper lifting techniques
- Prevent constipation
- Bowel training

The patient should be encouraged to avoid:

- Prolonged sitting
- Straining
- Anal intercourse

Anal hygiene measures include:

Cleansing with mild unscented soap and water after each bowel movement

Using unscented, uncolored soft toilet tissue, blotting area without rubbing

Pain Management

Ice packs or sitz baths BID or TID for 15 minutes
Witch hazel/glycerin pads (Tucks)

Consultation/Referral

Consult with a physician and/or refer to a surgeon for non-reducible, thrombosed, ulcerated, or strangulated hemorrhoids. Rubber band ligation, thermal technique, cryosurgery, and surgical resection have all been used to treat hemorrhoids.

Complete hemorrhoidectomy may be indicated for severe hemorrhoids or complications from hemorrhoids.

Complications

Thrombosis
Ulceration
Fissure
Strangulation
Secondary infection
Prolapse
Secondary anemia
Incontinence

EVALUATION/FOLLOW-UP

Follow-up depends on the severity, history of recurrence, response to treatment, and concurrent medical problems.

TABLE 88-2 Products for Treatment of Hemorrhoids

Product Manufacturer/ Supplier	Dosage Form	Anesthetic	Vasoconstrictor‡	Astringent	Protectant	Other Ingredients
Americaine Hemorrhoidal Heritage Consumer	Ointment	Benzocaine, 20%				Benzethonium chloride, 0.1%, polyethylene glycol 300, polyethylene glycol 3350
Anusol Warner-Lambert Consumer	Ointment	Pramoxine HCl, 1%		Zinc oxide, 12.5%	Mineral oil, cocoa butter, kaolin, peruvian balsam	Benzyl benzoate, dibasic calcium phosphate, glyceryl monooleate, glyceryl monostearate, polyethylene wax
Anusol Warner-Lambert Consumer	Suppository	Benzyl alcohol			Topical starch, 51%	Tocopheryl acetate, hydrogenated vegetable oil
Balneol Solvay Ph'cals	Lotion				Mineral oil, lanolin oil	Propylene glycol, glyceryl stearate/ PEG-100 stearate, PEG-40 stearate, laureth-4, PEG-4 dilaurate, sodium acetate, carbomer 934, triethanolamine, methylparaben, dioctyl sodium sulfosuccinate, fragrance, acetic acid
Calmol 4 Mentholatum	Suppository			Zinc oxide, 10%	Cocoa butter, 80%	Glyceryl stearate, methylparaben, propylparaben, bismuth subgallate
Fleet Medicated C. B. Fleet	Pad			Witch hazel, 50%	Glycerin, 10%	Methylparaben, water, aloe vera gel, benzethonium chloride
Fleet Pain-Relief C. B. Fleet	Pad	Pramoxine HCl, 1%			Glycerin, 12%	Water, sodium citrate, octoxynol-9, citric acid, sodium benzoate, disodium EDTA, cetylpyridinium chloride, eucalyptol, menthol
Hemorid for Women Consumer Health Care/Pfizer	Suppository		Phenylephrine HCl, 0.25%	Zinc oxide, 231 mg	Hard fat, 88.25%	Aloe
Hemorid for Women Consumer Health Care/Pfizer	Cream	Pramoxine HCl, 1%	Phenylephrine HCl, 0.25%		Petrolatum, 30%, mineral oil, 20%	Water, stearyl alcohol, cetyl alcohol, methylparaben, propylparaben, polysorbate 80, aloe vera gel
Hemorid for Women Consumer Health Care/Pfizer	Ointment	Pramoxine HCl, 1%	Phenylephrine HCl, 0.25%		Petrolatum, 82.15%, mineral oil, 12.5%	Aloe, white wax
Lanacane Creme Combe	Cream	Benzocaine, 6%		Zinc oxide	Glycerin	Benzethonium chloride, 0.1%, aloe, chlorothymol, dioctyl sodium sulfosuccinate, ethoxydiglycol, fragrance, glyceryl stearate SE, isopropyl alcohol, methylparaben, propylparaben, sodium borate, stearic acid, sulfated castor oil, triethanolamine, water, zinc oxide, pyrithione zinc

Lanacane Maximum Strength Combe	Cream	Benzocaine, 20%			Dimethicone, mineral oil	Benzethonium chloride, 0.2%, acetylated lanolin alcohol, aloe, cetyl acetate, cetyl alcohol, fragrance, glycerin, glyceryl stearate, isopropyl myristate, methylparaben, PEG-100 stearate, propylparaben, sorbitan stearate, stearamidopropyl PG-dimonium chloride phosphate, water, pyrithione zinc
Lanex* Carma Labs	Ointment	Menthol			Petrolatum, lanolin, cocoa butter	Spermaceti, beeswax, paraffin
Medicone Merz Consumer	Suppository		Phenylephrine HCl, 0.25%		Hard fat, 88.7%	Corn starch, methylparaben, propylparaben
Medicone Merz Consumer	Ointment	Benzocaine, 20%			Light mineral oil, white petrolatum	
Nupercainal Novartis Consumer	Ointment	Dibucaine, 1%			Lanolin, white petrolatum, light mineral oil	Acetone, sodium bisulfite, purified water
Nupercainal Novartis Consumer	Suppository			Zinc oxide, 0.25 g	Cocoa butter, 2.1 g	Acetone sodium bisulfite, bismuth subgallate
Pazo Bristol-Myers Products	Ointment	Camphor, 2%	Ephedrine sulfate, 0.2%	Zinc oxide, 5%	Lanolin, petrolatum	
Peterson's Ointment Lee Ph'cals	Ointment	Phenol, camphor		Zinc oxide, tannic acid		
Preparation H Whitehall-Robins Healthcare†	Ointment		Phenylephrine HCl, 0.25%		Petrolatum, 71.9%, mineral oil, 14%, shark liver oil, 3%, lanolin, glycerin	Benzoic acid, methylparaben, propylparaben, red thyme oil, water, Tenox GT-2, Tenox 4B, FALBA
Preparation H† Whitehall-Robins Healthcare	Cream		Phenylephrine HCl, 0.250%		Petrolatum, 18%, glycerin, 12%, shark liver oil, 3%, lanolin	BHA, carboxymethyl cellulose, cetyl alcohol, citric acid, disodium edetate, methylparaben, propylparaben, sodium benzoate, sodium lauryl sulfate, stearyl alcohol, water, tegacid, Arlacel 186, Tenox GT-2, Tenox 2, medical antifoam emulsion, Rhodigel

Adapted from Hemorrhoidal Product Table, *Nonprescription products: formulations and features '98-99*, pp 189-192.

*New listing.

†Manufacturer/supplier did not confirm information for this edition. Product listing is reprinted from the '97-98 edition.

‡Patients who are taking monoamine oxidase inhibitors or who have diabetes, hyperthyroidism, hypertension, cardiovascular disease, or difficulty in urination due to prostate enlargement should not use products containing a vasoconstrictor without first consulting a physician.

Continued

Table 88-2 Products for Treatment of Hemorrhoids—cont'd

Product Manufacturer/ Supplier	Dosage Form	Anesthetic	Vasoconstrictor‡	Astringent	Protectant	Other Ingredients
Preparation H† Whitehall-Robins Healthcare	Suppository		Phenylephrine HCl, 0.25%		Cocoa butter, 79%, shark liver oil, 3%	Methylparaben, propylparaben, corn starch
Procto Foam Non-Steroid Schwarz Pharma	Foam	Pramoxine HCl, 1%				Cetyl alcohol, glyceryl monostearate, PEG-100 stearate blend, methylparaben, polyoxyethylene 23 lauryl ether, polyoxyl 40 stearate, propylene glycol, propylparaben, purified water, trolamine, isobutane, propane
Rectacaine Reese Ph'cal	Suppository		Phenylephrine HCl, 0.25%		Hard fat, 88.7%	Corn starch, methylparaben, propylparaben
Rectacaine Reese Ph'cal	Ointment				Petrolatum, 71.9%, mineral oil, 14%, shark liver oil, 3%, glycerin	Beeswax, benzoic acid, BHA, corn oil, lanolin alcohol, methylparaben, paraffin, propylparaben, thyme oil, tocopherol, water
Tronolane Ross Products/Abbott Labs	Suppository			Zinc oxide, 5%	Hard fat, 95%	
Tronolane Ross Products/Abbott Labs	Cream	Pramoxine HCl, 1%		Zinc oxide	Glycerin	Beeswax, cetyl alcohol, cetyl esters wax, methylparaben, propylparaben, sodium lauryl sulfate, purified water
Tronothane Hydrochloride Abbott Labs	Cream	Pramoxine HCl, 1%			Glycerin	Cetyl alcohol, cetyl esters wax, sodium lauryl sulfate, methylparaben, propylparaben
Tucks Warner-Lambert Consumer	Pad			Witch hazel, 50%	Glycerin	Alcohol, propylene glycol, sodium citrate, diazolidinyl urea, citric acid, methylparaben, propylparaben, water
Tucks Clear Warner-Lambert Consumer	Gel	Benzyl alcohol		Witch hazel, 50%	Glycerin, 10%	Carbomer 974P, disodium edetate, propylene glycol, sodium hydroxide, water
Vaseline Pure Petroleum Jelly Chesebrough-Pond's	Ointment				White petrolatum, 100%	
Witch Hazel Hemorrhoidal Pads Dickinson Brands	Pad			Distilled witch hazel, 50%	Glycerin, 10%	Purified water, benzethonium chloride, methylparaben, aloe vera gel

Adapted from Hemorrhoidal Product Table, *Nonprescription products: formulations and features '98-99*, pp 189-192. © 1998 by American Pharmaceutical Association. Reprinted with permission.

SUGGESTED READINGS

Bates B: *A guide to physical examination and history taking,* ed 5, Philadelphia, 1991, JB Lippincott.

Doughty DB: *Gastrointestinal disorders,* St Louis, 1993, Mosby.

Dunn SA: *Primary care consultant,* St Louis, 1998, Mosby.

Ellsworth A et al: *Mosby's 1998 medical drug reference,* St Louis, 1998, Mosby.

Healthcare Consultants of America, Inc: *1998 Physicians fee and coding guide,* Augusta, Ga, 1998, Healthcare Consultants of America, Inc.

Tierney LM, McPhee SJ, Papadakis MA: *Medical diagnosis & treatment,* ed 35, Norwalk, Conn, 1996, Appleton & Lange.

Hepatitis

ICD-9-CM

Hepatitis 573.3
Alcoholic Hepatitis 571.1
Chronic Hepatitis 571.40
Viral Hepatitis: Type A Without Coma 070.1
Viral Hepatitis: Type B 070.30
Chronic Hepatitis: Type B Without HDV Without Coma 070.32
Hepatitis: Type C Without Coma 070.51
Chronic Hepatitis: Type C Without Coma 070.54
Hepatitis: Type D 070.52
Hepatitis: Type E 070.53

OVERVIEW

Definition

Hepatitis is a general term denoting inflammation of the liver, which can be caused by viral/bacterial sources or from chemical damage. Some viral infections (Epstein-Barr, mononucleosis, cytomegalovirus) can systemically inflame the liver; however, in this chapter we will focus on those hepatotropic viruses that primarily cause hepatitis. The following designations have been established for hepatitis-causing viruses: A, B, C, D, E, and G.

Incidence

Incidence depends on exposure to situations predisposing one to the virus. **Hepatitis A** (HAV) is found in infected water and food and is common in crowded situations such as low income housing, schools, dormitories. Clinical manifestations of a hepatitis A infection may be silent, especially in **children.**

Hepatitis B (HBV) is common in individuals exposed to needle punctures and/or blood products and those engaged in frequent, unprotected sexual intercourse. Intravenous drug users and homosexual men have the highest incidence. Health care workers who are not vaccinated for hepatitis B have an incidence of 15% to 30%. When a **pregnant woman** has HBV, a cesarean section is performed to protect the infant. Chronic HBV occurs in more than 90% of **neonates** infected with HBV at birth. About 10% of other populations are subject to a chronic HBV disease state. Each year more than 100,000 people contract HBV; approximately 90% to 95% will recover in 6 months and not contract HBV again (Hepatitis Foundation International online). The prevalence of chronic hepatitis B in the United States is 3.9 million cases.

Hepatitis C (HCV) is the leading cause of posttransfusion hepatitis; therefore individuals who receive repeated blood transfusions will have a higher incidence. Hepatitis C is also seen in individuals who are exposed to blood, such as health care workers, or those whose habits expose them to trauma resulting in exposure to blood, such as homosexual men. It accounts for 20% of hepatitis cases; almost 4 million Americans are inflicted with hepatitis C. Chronic liver disease occurs in approximately 75% to 80% of individuals with hepatitis C, approximately 1.25 million cases. At least 20% of patients with chronic hepatitis C develop cirrhosis, increasing their risk for hepatocellular carcinoma.

Hepatitis D occurs only in conjunction with hepatitis B, with the same routes of transmission. Hepatitis D virus presents in one of two modes: similar in severity to the co-existing HBV or as a superinfection in an individual who has chronic HBV. The superinfection carries a more severe prognosis and often results in fulminant hepatitis or severe chronic hepatitis that proceeds to cirrhosis.

Hepatitis E viral infection is more commonly seen in India, Asia, Africa, and Central America but is rare in the United States. It is usually a mild, self-limiting disease in patients over 15 years old. Hepatitis E infection occurs after water supplies have been contaminated, such as during monsoon season. Cases imported into the United States have occurred. There is no carrier state with hepatitis E; HEV does not progress to chronic liver disease. In **pregnant women** it presents with a considerable (10% to 20%) mortality rate.

TABLE 89-1 Pathophysiological Mechanisms of Hepatitis

Type of Hepatitis	Route of Transmission	Incubation Period
A	Fecal-oral	2-6 wk
B	Blood and body fluids	6 wk-6 mo
C	Blood and body fluids (inefficient mode of transmission)	5-10 wk
D	Blood and body fluids; coexists only with hepatitis B*	
E	Fecal-oral	2-9 wk
G	Percutaneous	Not yet determined

*Concurrent infection results in a more virulent manifestation than hepatitis B alone.

Hepatitis G is transmitted percutaneously. Its clinical significance is not yet clear. Hepatitis G may result in mild elevations of serum aminotransferase levels (ALT and AST usually below 300 IU/L during acute phase); however, chronic carriers may have normal values. Diagnostic tests for hepatitis G are not yet commercially available.

Pathophysiology

The liver performs numerous metabolic and regulatory functions, and decreased function is the source of the presenting symptoms in hepatitis. Complete regeneration can take place, even when 70% of the liver is destroyed. Cirrhosis results from necrosis of the hepatic cells, leading to fibrosis of hepatic tissue, eventual loss of hepatic architecture, and ultimately loss of hepatic function.

The pathophysiology of hepatitis is summarized in Table 89-1.

Factors That Increase Susceptibility

High-risk groups for hepatitis are listed in Box 89-1.

Box 89-1

Groups at High Risk for Hepatitis

Hepatitis A: Day care centers, mentally challenged individuals in institutions, and person who travel to foreign countries.

Hepatitis B: Intravenous drug users who share needles; homosexual men; individuals undergoing hemodialysis; hemophiliacs; health care personnel, such as nurses, laboratory staff, surgeons, and personnel performing hemodialysis; and sexually promiscuous persons.

Hepatitis C: Individuals receiving frequent blood transfusions, homosexual men, intravenous drug users (most common mode of transmission—60% to 90%), and hospital personnel.

Hepatitis D: Since hepatitis B has to be present for hepatitis D to survive, the high-risk groups are the same as hepatitis B.

Hepatitis E: Individuals living in areas such as those mentioned in hepatitis A.

Hepatitis G: Individuals exposed to percutaneous sticks from needles infected with the virus.

SUBJECTIVE DATA

Past Medical History

The patient may remember the exposure to the viral agent, but past medical history may also be inconclusive in identifying how and where the individual may have encountered the exposure.

Psychosocial History

Significant for sexual practices, recreational use of drugs, and/or other habits or occupations that place the individual at risk for hepatitis viral infections.

For hepatitis A, it is important to determine whether the patient's other contacts have exhibited symptoms of the same illness. With food contamination, events such as weddings or other gatherings, and use of a school cafeteria or any other common source should be identified.

Description of Most Common Symptoms

NOTE: The subjective symptoms presented here will be ambiguous in nature and related to an alteration in the normal function of the liver.

Hepatitis A: Signs and symptoms will appear at the end of prodromal period; these include fatigue, weakness, and mild gastrointestinal disturbances. A striking aversion to cigarettes may occur. Some may have joint pain, fever, hepatomegaly, lymphadenopathy, and jaundice.

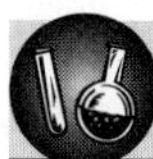

Table 89-2 Diagnostic Tests: Hepatitis

Tests	Findings/Rationale	Cost ($)
Hemoccult	Presence of occult blood loss should be evaluated via a stool specimen, optimally with voluntary evacuation, since there is a percentage of false positives with a specimen from a digital rectal examination	13-17
Monospot	Rule out mononucleosis.	20-25
Thyroid screen	Rule out hypothyroidism.	47-61 (panel)
Electrolytes, renal and liver function tests	Important to assess hepatic function AST is maximally elevated in the acute phase (>1000), then tapers off. AST and ALT levels do not always correlate with the degree of liver damage. Total and direct bilirubin will be elevated. Jaundice is usually detectable with a total bilirubin level above 2 mg/dl; does not reflect the severity of the illness.	23-30/elec; 29-41/LFT; 28-39/basic metabolic panel; 32-42/comprehensive metabolic panel
HIV	Rule out HIV.	41-52
Liver biopsy	Determines extent of the disease; not usually performed until disease is believed to be chronic, as defined by clinical history of unresolved symptoms with AST/ALT elevations of 6 months or longer. Does not provide useful prognostic value in the acute phase of hepatitis. Essential before interferon therapy is started.	1030-1101
CBC with differential	Anemia, possible infection. Lymphocytosis >10% atypical cells characteristic for Epstein-Barr. Leukopenia is common with hepatitis A.	18-23
CXR	Can be delayed until the serology test results are known; however, if H&P indicates cytomegaloviral infection, a CXR would be useful. If CMV infection present, the CXR may demonstrate bilateral, diffuse white infiltrates.	77-91

ALT, Alanine aminotransferase; *AST,* aspartate aminotransferase; *CBC,* complete blood cell count; *CMV,* cytomegalovirus; *CXR,* chest x-ray evaluation; *H&P,* history and physical examination; *HIV,* human immunodeficiency virus; *LFT,* liver function tests.

Hepatitis B: General malaise, joint swelling, rash pruritus, hepatomegaly, and gastrointestinal symptoms. Jaundice presents with more nausea and vomiting.

Hepatitis C: Acute illness with fever, chills, malaise, and nausea and vomiting.

Assess for weight loss, presence of cough, dyspnea, and a history of yeast infections; all of these would be significant to rule out human immunodeficiency virus (HIV). History of menorrhagia in women and constipation in both genders may indicate hypothyroidism.

OBJECTIVE DATA

Physical Examination

Skin: Jaundice, rashes (mononucleosis), dryness (hypothyroidism), or spider angiomata.

Neurological: Altered mental status (thyroid disorders)

Head/eyes/ears/nose/throat: Fever, pharyngitis, or cervical lymphadenopathy (mononucleosis); oral lesions (HIV); size of thyroid gland

Abdominal: Imperative to assess liver size and/or tenderness, splenomegaly, and/or presence of ascites; constipation (hypothyroidism)

Diagnostic Procedures

Diagnostic procedures for hepatitis are summarized in Table 89-2.

Hepatitis screening will determine which viral infection is responsible for the illness and stage of the infection. Information to keep in mind related to the different serum markers are outlined in Table 89-3 and Figure 89-1; Table 89-4 summarizes interpretation of laboratory values of tests for hepatitis B.

ASSESSMENT

Differential Diagnosis

The differential diagnoses for hepatitis include those found in Table 89-5.

TABLE 89-3 Hepatitis Screening Tests

Type of Hepatitis	Test	Interpretation	Comments	Cost ($)
A	IgM*–anti-HAV	Acute or recent infection	IgM–anti-HAV assay is diagnostic for hepatitis A infection. It is usually detectable at the time of clinical presentation and persists for several months.	50
	IgG-anti-HAV	Recovery	Indicates HAV is gone.	
B	See more explicit testing for HBV below; HBsAb should be included in all routine prenatal profiles		Anti-HBc can persist for 3-6 months or more (indefinitely). The core antigen itself (HBcAg) does not appear freely in the serum, so the antibody (anti-HBc) level is what is measured.	42-53/HBcAB, IgG, IgM; 42-53/surface antibody; 37-47/surface antigen
C	Anti-HCV	Acute, chronic, or recovered	RIBA is the most sensitive indicator for HCV, which is HCV RNA. HCV RNA is identified within a few days of exposure to HCV and is present well before any anti-HCV antibodies are discovered.	51-64
D	HDAg and Anti-HDV IgM	Acute infection		51-65
	Anti-HDV IgG	Previous infection		
E	Tests not available			
G	Antigen direct probe			61-79
	Hepatitis panel includes hepatitis B surface antigen, surface antibody, core antibody, hepatitis A antibody, hepatitis C antibody			108-151

RIBA, Recombinant immunoblot assay.
*Way to remember what IgM/IgG means: *M,* miserable (acute infection); *G,* gone (infection resolved).

THERAPEUTIC PLAN

The therapeutic plan will be to follow the liver enzyme levels and closely observe symptoms. Figure 89-2 summarizes treatment for a patient who has been exposed to hepatitis.

Pharmaceutical

Pharmaceutical measures are discussed under each type of hepatitis as appropriate.

Hepatitis A

HAV infection commonly requires no treatment. If an epidemic of HAV is noted in the community from a common source of food or water contamination, close contacts should be offered passive immunity with serum immunoglobulin (Gamastan, Gammar) 0.02 ml/kg IM. This vaccine is safe and inexpensive ($24 to $30). Usually causal contacts such as co-workers do not need to be vaccinated.

Individuals expecting to be exposed to HAV (travelers, institutional workers, daycare employees, military personnel, etc.) should receive an inactivated HAV vaccine (Havrix). **Children** 2 to 18 years old would receive two 360 enzyme-linked immunosorbent assay (ELISA) unit (0.5 ml) IM injections given 1 month apart. **Adults** receive one dose at 1440 ELISA units ($55 to $76). Both populations should receive a booster injection in 6 months.

Hepatitis B

Treatment of the acute stage of HBV consists of observation of liver enzymes and hepatitis markers to identify individuals who may benefit from interferon therapy. Approximately 90% to 95% of acute infection will spontaneously resolve. Consult with a physician regarding initiation of therapy with

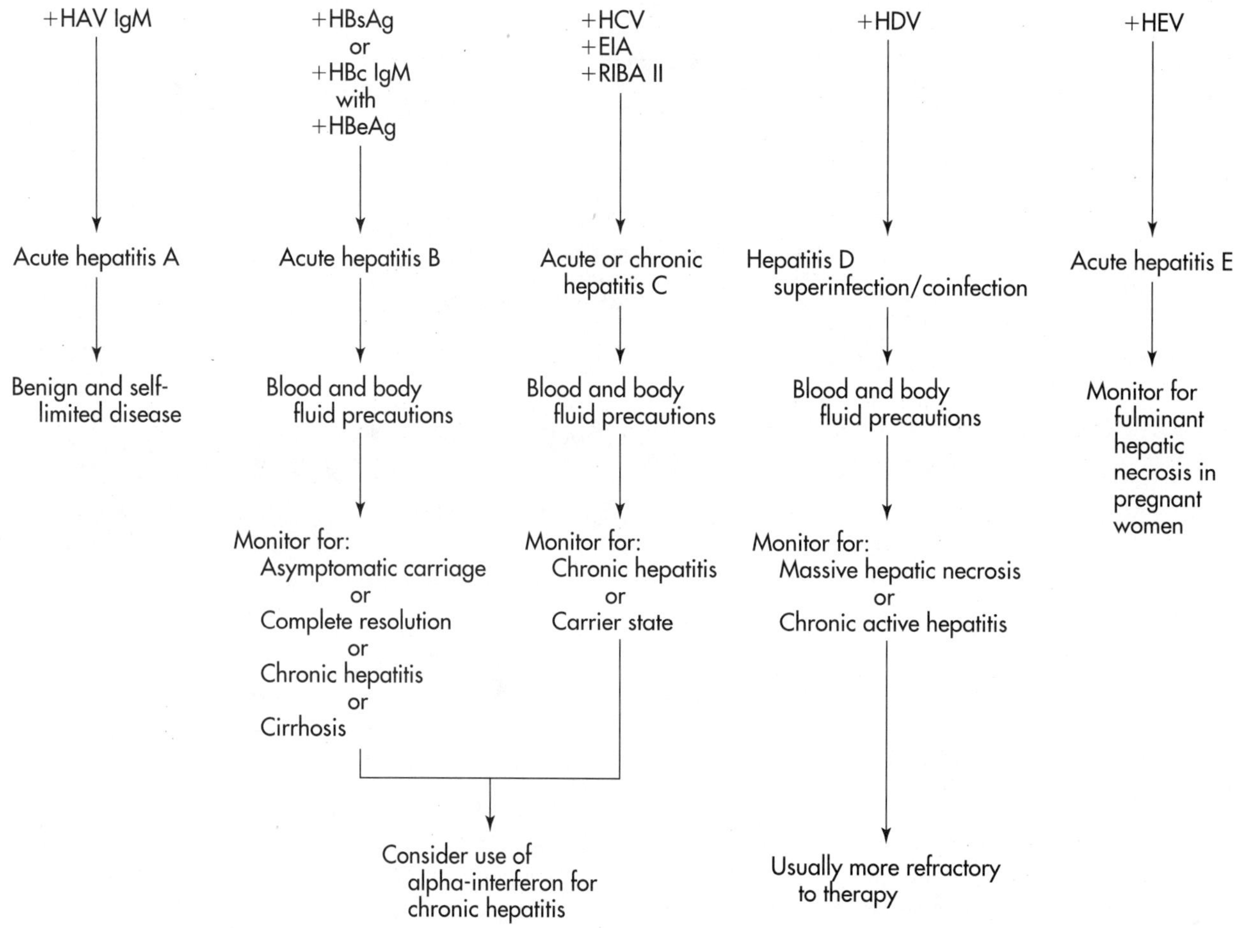

Figure 89-1 Algorithm for treatment of a patient with viral serology that indicates an acute hepatitis infection. (Adapted from Grodzin CJ, Schwartz SC, Bone RC: *Diagnostic strategies for internal medicine,* St Louis, 1996, Mosby.)

TABLE 89-4 Interpretation of Laboratory Results of Tests for Hepatitis B

HBsAG	Anti HB	Anti HBC	IgM	Interpretation
Pos	Neg	Neg	Neg	HBsAg is the first evidence of HBV infection. It appears before any biochemical evidence presents itself, heralding liver disease, and persists throughout the clinical illness. Presence of HBsAg implies infectivity. Early acute HBV infection.
Pos	Neg	Pos	Pos	Indicates acute HBV infection.
Pos	Neg	Pos	Neg	Indicates chronic HBV infection.
Neg	Neg	Pos	Pos/neg	Indicates early convalescence from HBV.
Neg	Pos	Pos	Neg	Anti-HBs indicates recovery from HBV infection, and along with the disappearance of HBsAg levels, denotes recovery and protection from recurrent HBV infection. Recovery/immunity to HBV.
Neg	Pos	Neg	Neg	Indicates immunity to HBV infection.

TABLE 89-5 Differential Diagnosis: Hepatitis

Diagnosis	Supporting Data
Anemia	Fatigue, weakness, shortness of breath, beefy red sore tongue with pernicious anemia, nausea, vomiting, anorexia, weight loss, diarrhea, constipation, pale oral mucosa, headaches, lightheadedness, generalized pallor, ecchymosis, petechiae, signs/symptoms of an opportunistic infection
CMV	Fatigue, myalgia, headache, nonproductive cough, watery diarrhea, fever, tachypnea, shortness of breath, cyanosis, jaundice, spider angiomas, splenomegaly, hepatomegaly
Epstein-Barr viral infection	Pharyngitis that may be severe, cervical lymphadenopathy, fever, splenomegaly, rash, atypical lymphocytosis, elevated hepatocellular enzymes and lactic dehydrogenase, malaise, headache, chills, nausea, palatal petechiae
Chronic fatigue syndrome	Major criterion: Prolonged. overwhelming fatigue that is unresolved with rest for at least 6 months Minor criteria: Mild fever, painful anterior or posterior cervical or axillary nodes, unexplained generalized muscular weakness, migratory arthralgia without joint swelling or redness, myalgia, cognitive dysfunction, nonexudative pharyngitis
Acquired hypothyroidism	Energy loss, fatigue, forgetfulness, sensitivity to cold, unexplained weight gain, constipation, anorexia, decreased libido, joint stiffness, muscle cramping, thick dry tongue, hoarseness, slowed speech, dry flaky skin, periorbital edema, drooping upper eyelids, dry sparse hair pattern, thick brittle nails with visible transverse and longitudinal grooves, intention tremor, nystagmus, weak pulse, bradycardia, absent or decreased bowel sounds, hypotension
Depression	Predominantly sad mood, loss of interest and/or pleasure in activities that were previously pleasurable, irritability, apathy, suicidal ideation/attempts, increased or decreased appetite, sleep disturbances, decreased libido, constipation, or diarrhea

alpha-interferon, a cytokine that is currently the only approved antiviral agent used to eradicate viral replication and end chronic hepatitis infection (Table 89-6). Refer the patient to a gastroenterologist.

Cytokines are proteins synthesized by cells in response to certain and various invasions (including viral) that lead to biochemical changes. Interferon binds to specific cellular receptors, resulting in at least two dozen proteins that promote viral resistance. Approximately 50% of patients treated with alpha-interferon will respond; however, about 25% to 30% of those patients will relapse, leaving 25% to 30% who sustain a prolonged response (Liaw et al, 1997).

Factors that improve interferon therapy response are low HBV-DNA levels, high serum alanine aminotransferase (ALT), short-term infection, and active inflammation on liver biopsy (Davis, 1997). If these factors do not exist, a tapering course of prednisone over 6 weeks may increase response rates. This approach should be undertaken cautiously, since corticosteroid withdrawal can lead to hepatic failure in these individuals (Davis, 1997).

Side effects of interferon are flulike symptoms, especially at the initiation of treatment; these tend to decrease with continued therapy. The flulike symptoms can be minimized by being well hydrated and administering the dose at bedtime. Acetaminophen 30 minutes before the interferon dose may also help.

Prophylaxis for HBV can be achieved by both passive (high-titered anti-HBs immunoglobulin [HBIg]) and active immunization (HBV vaccine: Recombivax HB, Engerix-B). Prophylactic treatment before exposure consists of three deltoid IM injections of HBV vaccine (initial injection, then in 1 month and 6 months; $33 to $90, depending on age). Dosage depends on the formulation of the vaccine. Immunocompromised individuals should receive a higher dose.

Prophylaxis for unvaccinated individuals exposed to HBV should be with both HBIg and HBV vaccine. Adult dosage of HBIg is 0.06 ml/kg IM followed by a complete course of HBV vaccine. Another dose of HBIg can be given 1 month later. This is the same protocol used for **infants** born to HbsAg-positive mothers or the mothers' sexual contacts.

When the previously vaccinated individual is exposed to HbsAg-positive blood or body fluids, serum anti-HBs titers should be obtained. If the antibody level is less than 10 million IU/ml, the individual should be treated with the same regimen as for an unvaccinated person.

Hepatitis C

Therapy for HCV includes interferon. A liver biopsy should be performed before the therapy is initiated. Interferon should be considered for all patients with persistently elevated ALT levels, anti-HCV in serum, and histological evidence of chronic, uncompensated hepatitis.

The regimen consists of alpha-interferon 3 million U SQ three times weekly for 6 to 12 months. The patient's CBC, ALT, thyroid-stimulating hormone (TSH) levels, and HCV RNA should be monitored. Patients in whom a course of interferon fails should be given another course for 12 months. Clinical trials evaluating interferon and ribavirin

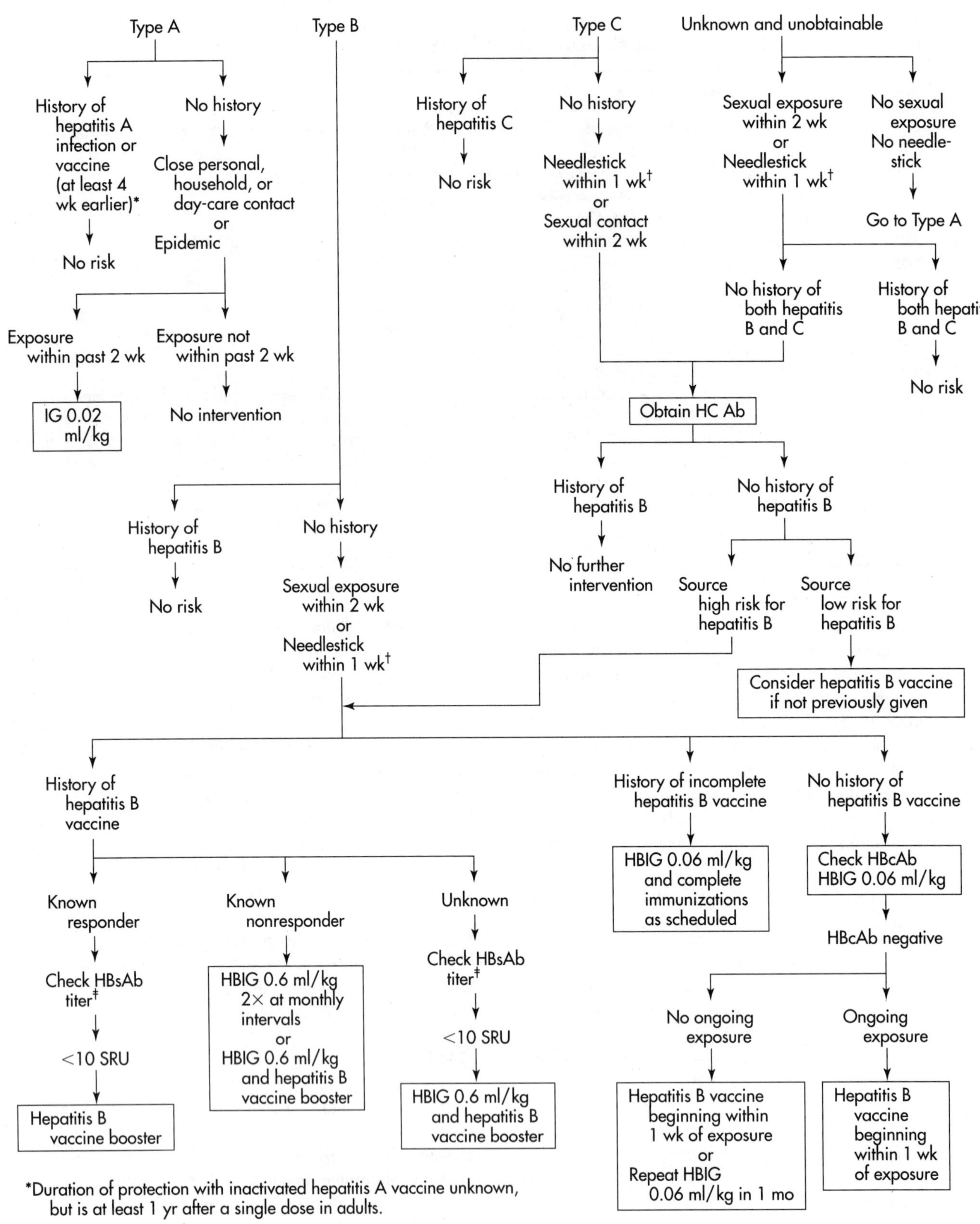

*Duration of protection with inactivated hepatitis A vaccine unknown, but is at least 1 yr after a single dose in adults.

†Treat permucosal exposure to blood similarly to a needlestick.

‡If not known to be >10 SRU in the last 24 mo.

Figure 89-2 Algorithm for treatment of a patient who has been exposed to hepatitis. (Adapted from Greene HL, Johnson WP, Lemcke D: *Decision making in medicine,* ed 2, St Louis, 1998, Mosby.)

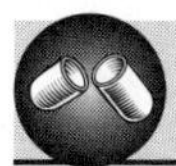

TABLE 89-6 Pharmaceutical Plan: HBV Treatment with Alpha-Interferon

Drug	Dose	Comment	Cost ($)
Alpha-interferon	Most common alpha-interferon regimen consists of 16-wk course of 5 million U self-administered SQ daily. Some studies show equal effectiveness with 10 million U three times per week, but the side effects may be more severe. In Europe a regimen of 5 million units three times a week is used, showing similar effectiveness; however, this regimen has not been approved in the United States (Davis, 1997).	Pregnancy: C Avoid breastfeeding SE: Dizziness, confusion, numbness, seizures, coma, edema, hypotension, rash, dry skin, flulike symptoms, myalgias, fatigue	53/Alpha-2b, 5 million U/vial

(Virazole) therapy are currently under way and have shown some benefit.

HCV exposure prophylaxis of serum immunoglobulin is used but has no proven effectiveness. One regimen is two IM injections of 0.06 ml/kg of HBIg within the first 2 weeks of exposure.

Hepatitis D

HDV always occurs with HBV infection and the only effective treatment for chronic infection is high doses of interferon over 9 months to 1 year.

Patient Education

Hepatitis A

- Transmitted via fecal-oral route.
- Usually a 6-week course of illness with a high recovery rate.
- *No* carrier state; *no* chronic state.
- Detectable serum IgG–anti-HAV confirms HAV immunity. Preventive measures include hand washing. Pooled human immune serum globulin (ISG 0.02 mg/kg IM) effective only when administered within 2 weeks of exposure.
- Fulminant hepatitis A is infrequent; however, when it does occur, it has a 50% mortality rate.

Hepatitis B

- Detectable in blood, breast milk, saliva, tears, nasal secretions, menstrual fluid, urine, semen, and in bloodsucking insects that have bitten infected individuals.
- Appears in blood as a virion called the Dane particle.
- HBV may occasionally exist in a quiescent nonhepatotoxic state (chronic carrier state).
- HBeAg (hepatitis B e antigen) is present when the liver is making large quantities of HBcAg during viral replication. When HBeAg is present for more than 3 to 4 months, a chronic HBV state is likely. HBeAg is used to manage a patient in the chronic state and signifies ongoing viral replication and liver damage. Anti-HBeAg is associated with resolution of the infection.
- Chronic HBV exists when transaminases remain elevated for 6 months or more. It may be transient and spontaneously resolve. Occasionally it progresses to an active ongoing hepatocellular necrosis (chronic active hepatitis) and eventually cirrhosis, with a dramatic increased risk of hepatoma.
- HBV is responsible for almost 80% of the primary cases of hepatocellular carcinoma (hepatoma) worldwide.
- Icteric phase lasts 2 to 6 weeks, peaks in 14 days with a variable period of disappearance.
- Prompt administration of anti-HBs (HBIg) and HBV vaccine to **neonates** is highly effective in prevention of vertical transmission of HBV. This protocol is also recommended for treatment of accidental needlesticks or splashes.

Hepatitis C

- Seroconversion may not occur for as long as 6 months.
- Half of the individuals acquiring posttransfusion HCV will develop chronic hepatitis with potential for cirrhosis.

Hepatitis D (Delta)

- HDV causes infection only when it coexists with HBV.
- Clinically important because it is associated with a higher rate of fulminant hepatitis and a high fatality rate. There is also a substantially higher risk of developing chronic hepatitis B liver disease.
- Hepatitis D viral superinfection usually correlates to a more severe and rapid progression of HBV infection.
- Serum anti-HDV proteins are diagnostic for HDV infection.

Family Impact

The family impact of any infectious disease is worrisome. and the patient may be guilt-ridden if the disease is inadvertently passed on to loved ones. Support is needed throughout the course of the workup, diagnosis, and treatment.

Safe sexual practices should be reviewed, since hepatitis is sexually transmitted. Condom use should be encouraged, although sexual partners of patients infected with hepatitis C seem to have a low transmission rate.

Fatigue is a common symptom of hepatitis, and the patient should be educated about appropriate behavioral management. Assist the patient in assessing the home and work situation to identify where energy can be conserved. Give the patient "permission" to ask for assistance and to take needed rest breaks.

Referral

If liver function test results remain elevated or progressively elevate, the patient should be referred to a gastroenterologist for a possible liver biopsy to assess the extent of hepatic damage. Interferon therapy is usually managed by gastroenterologists or infectious disease specialists.

EVALUATION/FOLLOW-UP

Follow-up should be on a monthly basis to assess disease progression. If the patient presents with an increase in severity of symptoms, the follow-up will be more frequent. Blood work should be performed every 2 months, or more frequently if the symptoms worsen.

RESOURCES

American Liver Foundation
1425 Pompton Ave
Cedar Grove, NJ 07009-1000
800-GO-LIVER or 888 4 HEP ABC
www.liverfoundation.org

Hepatitis/Liver Disease Hotline
800-223-0179 for printed material
and reference to the nearest support group
(The local health department is a good resource as well)

The Hep C Connection
1741 Gaylord St.
Denver, CO 80206
303-393-1202
Hepatitis C hotline: 800-522-HEPC
www.hepc-connection.org

Hepatitis C Foundation
1502 Russett Dr.
Warminster, PA 18974
215-672-2606
www.hepcfoundation.org

Hepatitis Foundation International
30 Sunrise Terrace
Cedar Grove, NJ 07009-1423
800-891-0707
www.hepfi.org

Everson GT and Weinberg, H
Living with Hepatitis C: A survivor's guide
New York, NY Hatherleigh Press, 1998
800-906-1234

REFERENCES

Davis GL, Lau JY: Factors predictive of a beneficial response to therapy of hepatitis C, *Hepatology* 26(suppl 1):122S-127S, 1995.

Liaw Y et al: Response of patients with dual hepatitis B virus and C virus infection to interferon therapy, *J Interferon Cytokine Res* 17:449-452, 1997.

SUGGESTED READINGS

Ellsworth A et al: *Mosby's 1998 medical drug reference,* St Louis, 1998, Mosby.

Friedman LS: Liver biliary tract and pancreas. In Tierney L, McPhee S, Papadakis M, editors: *Current medical diagnosis & treatment,* Norwalk, Conn, 1997, Appleton & Lange.

Gluckman S, DiNubile M: Hepatitis exposure. In Greene H, Johnson W, Maricic M, editors: *Decision making in medicine,* ed 2, St Louis, 1998, Mosby.

Groer M, Shekleton M: Disorders of digestions absorption excretion and metabolism. In Groer M, Shekleton M, editors: *Basic pathophysiology: a conceptual approach,* St Louis, 1979, Mosby.

Hayden F: Antimicrobial agents: antiviral agents. In Hardman J, Limbird L, editors: *Goodman & Gillman's the pharmacological basis of therapeutics,* ed 9, New York, 1996, McGraw-Hill.

Healthcare Consultants of America, Inc: *1998 Physicians fee and coding guide,* Augusta, Ga, 1998, Healthcare Consultants of America, Inc.

Norris J: Infection. In McMahon E, Ambrose M, Deutsch D, editors: *Diseases,* Springhouse, Pa, 1993, Springhouse.

Ohno H et al: Human hepatitis B virus enhancer 1 is responsive to human interleukin-6, *J Med Virol* 52:413-418, 1997.

Saab S, Martin P: Hepatitis C: a practical approach to diagnosis and management, *Family Pract Recert* 20:21-43, 1998.

Sechopoulos P, Jensen D: Case 3. In Grodzin C, Schwartz S, Bone R, editors: *Diagnostic strategies for internal medicine,* St Louis, 1996, Mosby.

Shulman S: Viral hepatitis. In Shulman S, Phair J, Sommers H, editors: *The biologic and clinical basis of infectious diseases,* Philadelphia, 1992, WB Saunders.

Uphold C, Graham M: *Clinical guidelines in family practice,* ed 2, Gainesville, Fla, 1994, Barmarrae.

Zeldis JB, Friedman LS: Acute and chronic viral hepatitis. In Rakel RE, editor: *1997 Conn's current therapy,* Philadelphia, 1997, WB Saunders.

90 Hernia

ICD-9-CM

Hernia, Abdominal 553.20
Hernia, Inguinal 550.9
Hernia, Umbilical 553.1
Hernia, Femoral 553.0

OVERVIEW

Definition

A hernia is the result of an abnormal opening or weakness of the abdominal musculature that allows protrusion of the abdominal viscera.

Types of hernias include inguinal, femoral, umbilical, incisional, and epigastric. Hernias are classified as reducible, nonreducible or incarcerated, and strangulated.

Incidence

Inguinal hernias are responsible for 99% of all groin hernias in **children under 3** years old.

Inguinal hernias occur more commonly in boys.

There is a 1% prevalence rate of inguinal hernias among full-term **infants.**

There is a 13% to 30% prevalence rate of inguinal hernias among **premature infants.**

One third of inguinal hernias are diagnosed before the patient is 6 months old.

A unilateral inguinal hernia is more likely to develop on the right side; 10% to 15% of **infants and children** will have bilateral hernias.

Umbilical hernias are very common and are considered a normal variant of development.

Umbilical hernias occur more commonly in **black children,** with a prevalence rate of 40% to 60%, whereas **white children** have a rate of 4%.

Most umbilical hernias close spontaneously, and by 1 year of age the prevalence rate drops to 12% for **black children** and 2% for **white children**.

Umbilical hernias occur with equal frequency in boys and girls.

Femoral hernias occur most commonly in **women** and are very rare in **children.**

Pathophysiology

Hernia is a congenital defect that results from conditions that cause increased intraabdominal pressure, such as chronic coughing, obesity, pregnancy, chronic constipation with straining, and heavy lifting.

SUBJECTIVE DATA

History of Present Illness

Ask about:

- Onset and duration of symptoms
- Presence of a bulge, swelling, or lump in the abdomen, umbilicus, groin, scrotum
- Softness and reducibility
- Pain, nausea, vomiting, abdominal cramping
- Whether swelling is constant or intermittent

Past Medical History

Ask about:

- Past surgery in the area or presence of a scar
- Underlying medical conditions

OBJECTIVE DATA

Physical Examination

Abdomen: Assess bowel sounds. Assess for lymphadenopathy. Inspect for protruding subcutaneous mass. Ask patient to lift head. Assess for tenderness and reducibility.

Assess for scars. Palpate femoral pulses. Assess for tenderness and mass. NOTE: *A strangulated hernia will present as discolored and painful. Do not reduce.*

Genitourinary

Males: Assess scrotum and testes for lymphadenopathy. Transilluminate the scrotum if a mass is present. Assess for inguinal hernia by invaginating the scrotum and advancing the finger into the inguinal canal. Ask the patient to cough or bear down. Assess for a bulge on the tip or along the side of the finger.

Females: Attempt to locate the inguinal ring between the inguinal ligament and os pubis. Place a hand over the inguinal ring and ask the patient to bear down.

Diagnostic Procedures

Abdominal ultrasonography ($351 to $419) may be indicated if there is uncertainty about the nature of the abdominal mass.

ASSESSMENT

Inguinal hernias may or may not be visible. When visible, the hernia may present as a soft swelling in the groin or scrotum. Inguinal hernias are difficult to identify in females. An inguinal mass and a hydrocele in an infant is most likely an inguinal hernia.

Femoral hernias present with pain and swelling over femoral canal. The swelling or mass is more medial and higher in the proximal thigh. The pulse can be palpated.

Umbilical, incisional, and epigastric hernias are diagnosed by the location of the bulge or mass.

Differential Diagnosis

Differential diagnoses are listed in Table 90-1.

TABLE 90-1 Differential Diagnosis: Hernia

Diagnosis	Supporting Data
Hydrocele	A collection of fluid between the two layers of the tunica vaginalis in the scrotum; swelling progresses throughout the day, resolving at night; hydroceles usually resolve spontaneously
Varicocele	Results from the dilation of veins in the spermatic cord in the scrotum; rare before puberty
Epididymitis	Inflammation of the epididymis, usually caused by infection
Testicular tumor	May present as a slow-growing, painless mass that is firm and free of fixation; the tumor usually displaces the testicle
Lymph node	Enlarged and sometimes painful lymph nodes can easily be palpated in the inguinal area of children and adults; may be indicative of an infection
Lipoma	Fatty tumor

THERAPEUTIC PLAN

Inguinal hernias, including femoral hernias in patients of all ages, should be surgically repaired. The timing depends on the presence of complications.

Umbilical hernias often resolve spontaneously and do not impose a significant risk of incarceration or strangulation. Surgical repair is often cosmetic.

Complications

The risk of incarceration of an inguinal hernia is greatest in children under 1 year old.

Incarcerated hernias may cause pain, nausea, and vomiting.

Ninety-five percent of incarcerated hernias can be reduced.

Strangulated hernias are a surgical emergency because of the risk of vascular compromise. Pain and discoloration may be present.

Patient Education

Discuss exacerbating and alleviating factors with the patient.

Discuss signs and symptoms of incarceration and strangulation.

The patient may need preoperative and postoperative instructions.

Lifestyle modifications may include no heavy lifting.

Educate parents about umbilical hernias as a normal variant.

Consultation/Referral

Refer the patient to a surgeon.

EVALUATION/FOLLOW-UP

Inguinal hernias will require postoperative follow-up.

Umbilical hernias can be monitored for problems.

SUGGESTED READINGS

Dershewitz RA: *Ambulatory pediatric care,* Philadelphia, 1998, JB Lippincott.

Dunn SA: *Primary care consultant,* St Louis, 1998, Mosby.

Healthcare Consultants of America, Inc: *1998 Physicians fee and coding guide,* Augusta, Ga, 1998, Healthcare Consultants of America, Inc.

Hoekelman RA: *Primary pediatric care,* ed 2, St Louis, 1992, Mosby.

Hoekelman, RA: *Primary pediatric care,* ed 3, St Louis, 1997, Mosby.

Herpes Simplex/ Genital Herpes

ICD-9-CM

Eczema Herpeticum 054.0
Neonatal Herpes Simplex 771.2
Herpes Labialis 054.9
Genital Herpes 054.1
Herpes Simplex with Ophthalmic Complications 054.40

OVERVIEW

Definition

Herpes simplex is a series of cutaneous infections with herpes simplex virus; HSV-1 is usually associated with oral infections, and HSV-2 with genital infections. Nongenital herpes simplex virus infection, whether primary or recurrent, is characterized by grouped vesicles arising on an erythematous base on keratinized skin or mucous membranes.

Incidence

Herpes simplex is most commonly seen in **young adults** (genitalis), and gingivostomatitis in **children.** The incubation period is 2 to 20 days. Four out of five people harbor HSV-1; one in six has HSV-2.

PATHOPHYSIOLOGY

Transmission is usually skin to skin, skin to mucosa, or mucosa to skin contact. Increased HSV-1 transmission is associated with crowded living conditions. After the virus invades the host, it is able to enter sensory nerve terminals, move up to sensory sacral ganglia that supply skin and mucosa of infected site, and remain in latent state without apparent cell damage. Various triggers, often unknown to the particular individual, cause virus to become reactivated to replicate viral components.

Factors that Increase Susceptibility

Skin/mucosa irradiation
Altered hormonal states (menstruation, pregnancy)
Fever
Upper respiratory infection
Altered immune system (human immunodeficiency virus, malignancy, transplantation, chemotherapy, systemic corticosteroids, irradiation, immunosuppressive drugs)

SUBJECTIVE DATA

History of Present Illness

Primary Episode

Any or all of the following may be present:

- Pain and itching, localized to area of outbreak
- Ulcerative lesions
- Fever
- Headache, stiff neck
- Mild photophobia
- Malaise
- Constipation
- May be asymptomatic
- Dysuria
- Urethral/vaginal discharge
- Inguinal adenopathy
- Myalgia
- Pharyngitis
- Urinary retention
- Backache

Recurrent Episodes

Itching
Prodromal tingling or shooting pains (often 1 to 2 days before outbreak)
Urethral or vaginal discharge
Small, painful vesicles
Erythema
Dysuria

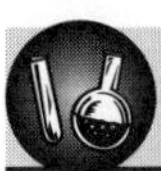

TABLE 91-1 Diagnostic Tests: Herpes Simplex

Diagnostic Test	Finding/Rationale	Cost ($)
Tzanck smear	Unroof the vesicle using either the blunt edge of a scalpel (No. 21) or a cytobrush Transfer specimen to glass slide and fix immediately using Cytospray Positive smear shows characteristic multinucleated giant cells Sensitivity of Tzanck smear is 85%-95%, with 95% specificity	24-30
Pap smear	Specimen taken from mucous membranes Sensitivity is only 60%-70%, with 95% specificity	25-31
Culture	(Confirmatory test of choice) Unroof vesicle or sample from ulcer if all lesions are open Rub base of lesion vigorously (but gently— THIS HURTS!) with cotton or Dacron-tipped swab Place the swab immediately into transport media and follow guidelines for transport and storage (some need to be placed on ice, others refrigerated) Virus detected in 90% of vesicles, 70% of ulcers, and 25% of crusted lesions Results are usually available in 3 days, but most laboratories wait 7 days before determining culture to be negative	61-75
Herpes simplex antigen by direct fluorescent antibody technique	Newer test—may replace culture in future	39-51; 61-79/ direct probe; 98-126/amplified probe

Tender lymph nodes
Less systemic symptoms

Additional Information

Ask about location, onset, duration, and appearance of the lesion(s)
Ask if burning or pareretheses present before eruption
Ask about associated symptoms of fever, myalgia, malaise
Ask about previous occurrences
Ask about exposure to infected person(s), including oral sores, especially if patient participates in oral sex
With recurrent outbreaks ask about recent exposure to reactivating factors: physical trauma, exposure to sunlight/tanning beds, stress, menses

OBJECTIVE DATA

Physical Examination

A problem oriented physical should be considered, with special attention paid to the following types of episodes.

Primary Episode

Vital signs, including temperature and blood pressure
Examination of the mouth for fissures, lesions
Examination of the external genitalia: Erythema is often noted, followed by grouped, often umbilicated vesicles, which may evolve into pustules. They may become eroded and turn into ulcers.
Male: lesions present on penis, buttocks, thighs, urethral discharge
Female: lesions present on labia, fourchette, cervix, buttocks, thigh (examination may be painful, with speculum examination impossible)
Groin: inguinal adenopathy
Abdomen: bladder distention secondary to urinary retention may be present; more common in women

Recurrent Episodes

Perform a physical examination as for a primary episode; clinical symptoms are less severe. Distribution is often less severe.

Diagnostic Procedures

Diagnostic procedures include those found in Table 91-1.

Whom to Test

Patients with genital herpes suspected on clinical grounds
Pregnant women with lesions; lesions present at term may indicate a need for C-section to prevent transmission to the infant

TABLE 91-2 Differential Diagnosis: Herpes Simplex

Diagnosis	Supporting Data
Syphilis	Clean, painless ulcer with a hard base
Chancroid	The combination of a painful ulcer and tender inguinal lymphadenopathy suggests a diagnosis of chancroid.
Lymphogranuloma venereum	An initial ulcerative or vesicular lesion develops, often unnoticed. There is lymph node enlargement, softening and suppuration with draining sinuses, and a positive groove sign.
Granuloma inguinale	These painless, progressive, ulcerative lesions without regional lymphadenopathy are uncommon in United States. The lesions are vascular and bleed easily on contact.
Impetigo	Vesicles rupture, with release of honey-colored discharge/crust formation, and are painful.

ASSESSMENT

Differential diagnoses include those found in Table 91-2.

THERAPEUTIC PLAN

Pharmaceutical

Initial Clinical Episode of Genital Herpes (HSV-2)

Recommended Regimens. The regimens listed in Table 91-3 have the best results if started as soon as possible following outbreak of symptoms; they are found to be most helpful if started within 48 hours.

Recurrent Episodes of Genital Herpes

For patients with obvious prodromes or easily recognized lesions, initiation of medication will suppress viral shedding and hasten healing (Table 91-4).

Suppressive Therapy

Suppressive therapy reduces the frequency of genital herpes by ≥75% among patients who have frequent recurrences (i.e., 6 or more recurrences a year). Safety and efficacy have been documented among patients receiving daily therapy with acyclovir for as long as 6 years and with valacyclovir and famciclovir for 1 year (Table 91-5). After 1 year of suppressive therapy, discontinuation of therapy should be discussed with the patient to assess the patient's psychological adjustment to genital herpes and rate of recurrent episodes, as the frequency of recurrence decreases over time.

Management of Sex Partner(s)

Symptomatic patients should be evaluated for HSV-2. Asymptomatic partners of newly diagnosed patients with HSV-2 should be questioned concerning histories of typical and atypical lesions, and they should be encouraged to examine themselves for lesions in the future and seek medical care promptly if lesions should occur.

Pregnancy

The safety of systemic acyclovir and valacyclovir therapy in pregnant women has not been established. So far, this registry does not show evidence of increased risk of birth defects after acyclovir treatment, although the sample size is too small to reach reliable conclusions.

The first clinical outbreak of herpes in pregnancy may be treated with oral acyclovir. Investigations suggest that acyclovir treatment near term may reduce the rate of C-sections among women with frequently recurring outbreaks or newly acquired infection. However, routine administration of acyclovir to pregnant women is not recommended at this time.

At the onset of labor, all women should be examined and carefully questioned regarding whether they have symptoms of genital herpes. Infants of women who do not have symptoms or signs of genital herpes infection or signs of its prodrome may be delivered vaginally.

Lifestyle/Activities

Warn about transmittability of lesions by direct contact
Encourage use of barrier contraceptives; safer sex
Urge avoidance of stress

Diet

Not applicable

Patient Education

Patients should be told about the natural history of the disease, with emphasis on the potential for recurrent episodes, asymptomatic viral shedding, and sexual transmission.

Patients should be advised to refrain from sexual activity when lesions or prodromal symptoms are present.

The use of condoms with new or uninfected partners should be encouraged.

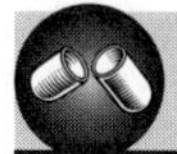

TABLE 91-3 Initial Treatment of Genital Herpes

Drug	Dose	Comments	Cost
Acyclovir (Zovirax) *or*	400 mg PO TID for 7-10 days *or* 200 mg PO 5× day for 7-10 days **Children:** (2-12 yrs) 20 mg/kg (up to 800 mg/dose) for 5 days	Not recommended <2 years of age (however, no unusual toxicity or pediatrics specific problems have been observed in studies done in children using doses of up to 3000 mg/m^2/d or 80 mg/kg/d) Pregnancy: C—register pregnant patients with registry 800-722-9292, x 8465 SE: N/V, H/A, CNS disturbances (esp. elderly), vertigo, rash, malaise, fatigue	\$98/200 mg (100); \$189/400 mg (100); \$84/susp: 200 mg/5 ml (480 ml)
Famciclovir (Famvir) *or*	125 mg PO TID for 7-10 days or some sources recommend 500 mg TID for 7 days; if creatinine clearance ≥60 ml/min, give 500 mg q8h; if between 40 and 59 ml/min, give 500 mg q12h; if between 20 and 39, give 500 mg q24h	Not recommended in children Pregnancy: B—register pregnant patients with registry [800-366-8900, x 5231] SE: H/A, fatigue, GI upset	\$29/125 mg (10); \$116/500 mg (21)
Valacyclovir (Valtrex)	1 g PO BID/TID for 7 days; if creatinine clearance ≥50 ml/min, give 1 g q8h; if between 30 and 49 ml/min, give 1 g q12h; if between 10 and 29 ml/min, give 1 g q24h	Not recommended for children Pregnancy: B—register pregnant patients with registry 800-722-9292, x 39437 SE: H/A, dizziness, GI upset, abdominal pain	\$282/500 mg (100)

CNS, Central nervous system; *GI*, gastrointestinal; *H/A*, headache; *N/V*, nausea and vomiting; *SE*, side effects.
NOTE: Treatment may be extended if healing is incomplete after 10 days of therapy.

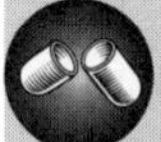

TABLE 91-4 Recommended Regimens for Treatment of Recurrent Genital Herpes

Drug	Dose	Comments	Cost
Acyclovir (Zovirax) *or*	400 mg PO TID for 5 days *or* Acyclovir 200 mg PO 5× day for 5 days *or* Acyclovir 800 mg PO BID for 5 days	See Table 91-3	See Table 91-3
Famciclovir (Famvir) *or*	125 mg PO BID for 5 days	See Table 91-3	See Table 91-3
Valacyclovir (Valtrex)	500 mg PO BID for 5 days	See Table 91-3	See Table 91-3

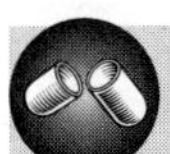

TABLE 91-5 Recommended Regimens for Daily Suppressive Therapy

Drug	Dose	Comments	Cost
Acyclovir	400 mg PO BID	See Table 91-3	See Table 91-3
Famciclovir	250 mg PO BID	See Table 91-3	See Table 91-3
Valacyclovir	250 mg PO BID *or* 500 mg PO QD *or* 1 g PO QD	500-mg QD dose appears less effective than other valacyclovir dosing regimens	See Table 91-3

Viral shedding may occur during asymptomatic periods, more so in patients who have had genital herpes <1 year.

Patients having their first outbreak of genital herpes should be advised that:

- Episodic antiviral therapy during recurrent episodes might shorten the duration of the lesions.
- Suppressive therapy can ameliorate or prevent recurrent outbreaks.

Patients should be made aware of the side effects of antiviral therapy.

Xylocaine gel may be used topically three to four times a day for comfort. (Do not use around the urethra.)

Avoidance of immunocompromised patients

Family Impact

Herpes can be very devastating to the patient since it is never cured and the potential for relapse is common. Warn patients about cross transmittal between oral and genital lesions. Encourage good hand washing.

Referral/Consultation

Refer to dermatologist if disseminated herpes.

Refer to OB/GYN if unable to urinate due to painful lesions. (Voiding in a tub of hot water may help with painful lesions.)

EVALUATION/FOLLOW-UP

Follow-up lesions every week until lesions healed.

RESOURCES

Wellcome DIALOG
Burroughs Wellcome Co. Booklet
1-800-843-8889

The Herpes Resource Center
1-800-230-6039

Healthy Imagination: An audiotape for relaxation, guided imagery, and positive affirmations
Available through ASHA or by writing Insight Images
187 Calle Magdalena
Suite 210
Encinitas, CA 92024

SUGGESTED READINGS

Brown Z et al: The acquisition of herpes simplex virus during pregnancy, *N Engl J Med* 337(8):509-515, 1997.

Cassidy L et al: Are reported stress and coping style associated with frequent recurrence of genital herpes? *Genitourinary Med* 73(4):263-266,1997.

Centers for Disease Control and Prevention: Guidelines for treatment of sexually transmitted diseases, *MMWR* 47(RR-1):59-69, 1998.

Ellsworth A et al: *Mosby's 1998 medical drug reference,* St. Louis, 1998, Mosby.

Fleming D et al: Herpes simplex virus type 2 in the US, 1976-1994, *N Engl J Med* 337(16):1105-1111, 1997.

Harvard Health Watch: *Genital herpes,* September, Boston, 1997, Harvard Health Watch.

Hawkins JW, Roberto-Nichols DM, Stanley-Haney JL: *Herpes protocols for nurse practitioners in gynecologic settings,* ed 5, New York, 1995, Tiresias Press.

Healthcare Consultants of America, Inc.: *1998 Physicians fee and coding guide*, Augusta, Ga, 1998, Healthcare Consultants of America, Inc.

Green J, Koesis A: Psychological factors in recurrent genital herpes, *Genitourinary Med* 73(4):253-258, 1997.

Johnson C: *Women's health care handbook,* St Louis, 1996, Mosby.

McMillan A: *Sexually transmittable diseases: handbook of family planning and reproductive health,* ed 3, New York, 1995, Churchill Livingstone.

Solomon A, Smith S: (1997). Understanding herpes simplex virus: diagnosis, transmission, and management, *Female Patient* 22:37-43, 1997.

Herpes Zoster (Shingles)

ICD-9-CM

Herpes Zoster 053.9
Herpes Zoster without Ophthalmology Complications 053.2
(Site-specific Codes Preferred by Medicare)

OVERVIEW

Definition

Herpes zoster is an acute dermatomal infection associated with reactivation of varicella zoster virus, which usually occurs in three stages: prodrome, active, and chronic.

Incidence

More than 66% are >**50 years,** 5% of cases are in **children <15 years of age.**
It occurs in 10% to 20% of the population at some time, in males and females equally.

Pathophysiology

Reactiviation of the varicella-zoster virus that has been dormant in a dorsal root ganglion
Transmitted by airborne route
Approximately one third as contagious as varicella (susceptible contacts can contract varicella via airborne route)

Factors That Increase Susceptibility

Altered immune system (human immunodeficiency virus [HIV] [8× incidence], malignancy, transplantation, chemotherapy, systemic corticosteroids, irradiation, immunosuppressive drugs, age >55)

SUBJECTIVE DATA

History of Present Illness

Prodrome

Headache, malaise, fever occur in 5% of patients.

Tenderness, neuritic pain or paresthesia (itching, burning or tingling) in the involved dermatome precedes skin eruption by 3 to 5 days, but it can have a range of 1 to 14 days.

Pain is described as stabbing, pricking, boring, penetrating, or shooting. Allodynia (heightened sensitivity to mild stimuli) may be reported.

Active Vesiculation

Red swollen plaques appear.
Vesicles arise from erythematous base, usually in clusters, along dermatome pattern (unilateral).
Crust forms after vesicles rupture (falls off in 2 to 3 weeks).
Headache, malaise, and fever may also be present.

Additional Information

Ask about location, onset, duration, and appearance of the lesion(s).
Ask if burning, itching, or pareretheses were present before eruption.
Ask about associated symptoms of fever, myalgia, malaise.
Ask about previous occurrences.

Past Medical History

Ask about immunosuppressed states: HIV, immunosuppression, chemotherapy, radiotherapy, lymphoproliferative disorders, carcinoma

Medications

Ask about steroids, chemotherapy, immunosuppressive drugs.

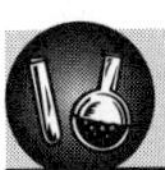

TABLE 92-1 Diagnostic Tests: Herpes Zoster

Diagnostic Test	Finding/Rationale	Cost ($)
Tzanck smear	Unroof the vesicle using either the blunt edge of a scalpel (No. 21) or a cytobrush. Transfer specimen to glass slide and fix immediately, using Cytospray. Positive smear shows characteristic multinucleated giant cells. Sensitivity of Tzanck smear is 85% to 95% with 95% specificity.	24-30
Culture	Confirmatory test of choice. Unroof vesicle or sample from ulcer if all lesions are open. Rub base of lesion vigorously (but gently— THIS HURTS!) with cotton or Dacron-tipped swab. Place the swab immediately into transport media and follow guidelines for transport and storage (some need to be placed on ice, others refrigerated). Virus is detected in 90% of vesicles, 70% of ulcers, and 25% of crusted lesions. Results are usually available in 3 days, but most laboratories wait 7 days before determining culture to be negative.	61-75

Family History

Ask if family members have had chicken pox.

Psychosocial History

Ask about HIV risk factors
Ask about chronic alcohol ingestion or intravenous drug use

OBJECTIVE DATA

Physical Examination

A problem-oriented physical examination should be considered, with special attention paid to:

Vital signs, including temperature and blood pressure
Skin: Erythematous base with grouped clear vesicles, sometime hemorrhagic
  Follows dermatome
  Sites of predilection:
    Thoracic: 50%
    Trigeminal nerve: 10% to 20%
    Lumbosacral/cervical: 10% to 20%
Lymph: Regional lymph nodes often enlarged and tender
Eye: Nasociliary involvement of trigeminal nerve: one third of cases
  Be alert for vesicles on side and tip of the nose.
  Do visual acuity.

Diagnostic Procedures

Diagnostic procedures include those found in Table 92-1.

ASSESSMENT

Differential diagnoses include those found in Table 92-2.

TABLE 92-2 Differential Diagnosis: Herpes Zoster

Diagnosis	Supporting Data
Herpes simplex	Grouped umbilicated vesicles, followed by ulceration; skin lesions may be accompanied by headache, malaise, myalgia
Contact dermatitis	Well demarcated plaques of erythema and edema, with vesicles; often linear arrangement of vesicles
Conjunctivitis (if eye involved)	Injected conjunctiva, itching of eye, matting of eye in AM
Impetigo	Vesicles that rupture, with release of honey-colored discharge/crust formation, painful

THERAPEUTIC PLAN

Goals
Minimizing pain
Reducing viral shedding
Speed crusting of lesions
Preventing or reducing postherpetic neuralgia (PHN)

Pharmaceutical

Table 92-3 contains the pharmaceutical plan for herpes zoster.

Lifestyle/Activities

Application of moist dressings (Burow's solution) to the involved dermatome is soothing and helps decrease pain. Apply for 30 minutes several times a day.

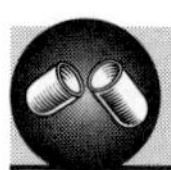

TABLE 92-3 Pharmaceutical Plan: Herpes Zoster

Drug	Dose	Comments	Cost
Acyclovir (Zovirax)	800 mg PO 5× for 7-10 days; should be given IV for ophthalmic zoster or immunocompromised host	Decreases pain and hastens healing if given within 48 hr of onset of rash Not recommended in **children** <2 (however, no unusual toxicity or pediatric specific problems have been observed in studies done in children using doses of up to 3000 g/m²/day or 80 mg/kg/day) Pregnancy: C—register pregnant patients with registry 800-722-9292, x8465 SE: N/V, H/A, CNS disturbances (esp. **elderly**), vertigo, rash, malaise, fatigue	$989/200 mg (100); $189/400 mg (100); $84/susp: 200 mg/5 ml (480 ml)
Famciclovir (Famvir)	500 mg po q 8h for 7days; if creatinine clearance ≥60 ml/min, give 500 mg q8h; if between 40 and 59 ml/min, give 500 mg q2h; if between 20 and 39, give 500 mg q24h	Not recommended in **children** Pregnancy: B—register pregnant patients with registry [800-366-8900, x 5231]) SE: H/A, fatigue, GI upset	$29/125 mg (10); $116/500 mg (21)
Valacyclovir (Valtrex)	1 g PO TID for 7 days; if creatinine clearance ≥50 ml/min, give 1 g q8h; if between 30 and 49 ml/min, give 1 g q12h; if between 10 and 29 ml/min, give 1 g q24h	Not recommended for children Pregnancy: B—register pregnant patients with registry 800-722-9292, x39437 SE: H/A, dizziness, GI upset, abdominal pain	$282/500 mg (100)

Pain management: early control of pain is indicated since lesions can be very painful.
Oral corticosteroids (prednisone) improve quality of life issues (decreased acute pain, improved sleep, and return to normal activity) when given with antiviral agent. Prednisone 30 mg BID days 1 to 7, 15 mg BID days 8 to 14, and 7.5 mg days 15 to 21 recommended in some patients >50 years of age (Kost RG, Straus S: Postherpetic neuralgia: pathogenesis, treatment, and prevention, *N Engl J Med* 335:32-42, 1996).
IV, Intravenously; *CNS,* central nervous system; *GI,* gastrointestinal; *H/A,* headache; *N/V,* nausea and vomiting; *SE,* side effects.

Diet

Not applicable

Patient Education

Isolate patient from neonates, pregnant women, people who have not had chicken pox, and immunosuppressed patients, since the active lesions are potentially infectious, although spread of infection is rare.

Emphasize prevention via varicella immunization for those who have not had chicken pox.

Family Impact

Herpes zoster can be very painful and debilitating, especially to the **elderly** and immunocompromised. Encourage thorough hand washing.

Referral/Consultation

Refer to dermatologist if disseminated herpes or more than two dermatomes.

Involvement of ophthalmic branch of trigeminal nerves requires immediate consultation with ophthalmologist. Ophthalmic steroids will be used, as well as mydriatics.

Follow-up

Follow up lesions every week until lesions healed (in immunocompetent host: 2 to 3 weeks).

EVALUATION

Complications of trigeminal nerve involvement include uveitis, keratitis, conjunctivitis, retinitis, optic neuritis, and glaucoma.

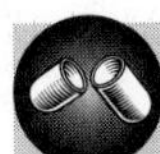

TABLE 92-4 Treatment of Postherpetic Neuralgia

Drug	Dose	Comment	Cost
Capsaicin 0.75% (Zostrix)	Cream applied to affected area 3-4× daily Do not apply to open or abraded areas	Helps decrease pain impulses in PHN Good hand washing after application Pregnancy: N/A SE: Burning sensation, local irritation, contact dermatitis	N/A

N/A, Not available; *SE,* side effects.

PHN is associated with nerve inflammation, infection, and scarring (Table 92-4). Risk of PHN is >40% in those over 60 years of age and also with ophthalmic zoster.

Recurrent zoster can occur in immunocompromised individuals.

SUGGESTED READINGS

Baron R, Haendler G, Schulte H: Afferent large fiber polyneuropathy predicts the development of postherpetic neuralgia, *Pain* 73(2):231-238, 1998.

Biorgen S: Clinical snapshot of herpes zoster, *Am J Nurs* 98(2):46-47, 1998.

Bowsher D: Management of postherpetic neuralgia, *Postgrad Med* 73(864):623-629, 1997.

Chasuk R: Treatment for postherpetic neuralgia, *J Family Practice* 45(3):203-204, 1997.

Chiarello S: Tumescent infiltration of corticosteroids, lidocaine, and epinephrine into dermatomes of acute herpetic pain of post herpetic neuralgia, *Arch Dermatol* 134(3):279-281, 1998.

Ellsworth A et al: *Mosby's 1998 medical drug reference,* St. Louis, 1998, Mosby.

Healthcare Consultants of America, Inc: *1998 Physicians fee and coding guide*, Augusta, Ga, 1998, Healthcare Consultants of America, Inc.

Millerchip S: Postherpetic neuralgia, *Professional Nurs* 13(5):310-313, 1998.

Reifsnider E: Common adult infectious skin conditions, *Nurse Pract* 22(11):17-20, 1997.

Straus S: Shingles: sorrows, salves, and solutions, *JAMA* 269:1836, 1993.

93 Hirsutism

ICD-9-CM

Hirsutism 704.1

OVERVIEW

Definition

Hirsutism is the growth of excessive terminal hair in androgen-dependent areas of a woman's body such as the upper lip, chin, chest, inner thighs, back, and abdomen.

Incidence

Hirsutism is a common clinical condition affecting about 5% of women in the United States. The most common causes are polycystic ovary syndrome (PCOS) (78%) and idiopathic hirsutism (15%).

Pathophysiology

Hair follicles are present over the entire surface of the skin, except for the lips, palms of the hands, and soles of the feet. Most of the hair covering the body is vellus hair, which is fine and lightly pigmented. At the onset of puberty and in response to the increase in androgen production in both sexes, vellus hair in the axillae, lower pubic triangle, arms, and lower legs is replaced by terminal hair, which is coarser and more pigmented. Androgen-sensitive areas include the lip, chin, sideburns, chest, upper pubic triangle, and intergluteal region. Normally the terminal hair growth in these areas is limited to adult men. Under the influence of increased androgen production and/or an increase in the sensitivity of the hair follicle to normal androgen concentrations, women may develop terminal hair growth in the normally male distribution. This may be accompanied by other androgenic skin disorders such as alopecia, seborrhea, or acne. *Once established, the androgen pattern of hair growth persists even when androgens are withdrawn.*

The predominant circulating androgens are testosterone and dihydrotestosterone (DHT). Testosterone is converted to DHT in the skin and the hair follicle by 5 alpha-reductase. DHT is a more potent androgen than testosterone and is believed to be the androgen principally responsible for hair growth, especially on the face. Up to 50% of circulating androgens are secreted from the ovaries and adrenals. The remainder are produced by the conversion of androstenedione (the major C19 steroid produced by the ovaries but also produced by the adrenals) and dehydroepiandrosterone (DHEA, the major adrenal androgen) in peripheral tissues. Most circulating androgens are bound to sex hormone–binding globulin (SHBG) and albumin. That which is unbound, free testosterone, is the most biologically active. SHBG is decreased, and the free testosterone level is increased by elevated levels of testosterone, insulin, and obesity. SHBG is increased, and the free testosterone level is decreased by elevated levels of estrogen or thyroid hormone.

Causes of Hirsutism

Can be classified as ovarian, adrenal/genetic, drug-related, or idiopathic (Table 93-1).

SUBJECTIVE DATA

History of Present Illness

Onset, progression: Slow from puberty, possibly PCOS or late-onset congenital adrenal hypoplasia (CAH); rapid onset, possibly androgen-secreting tumor

Symptoms of Androgen Excess

Acne, oily skin

Signs of Androgen Excess

Clitoromegaly, temporal balding, change in voice; change in body habitus (loss of female body contour); increase in

TABLE 93-1 Classification and Causes of Hirsutism

Body System	Causes of Hirsutism
Ovarian	Polycystic ovary syndrome* Neoplasms Sertoli-Leydig cell tumors Hilar cell tumors Lipoid cell tumors Adrenal rest tumors
Adrenal/genetic	Congenital adrenal hyperplasia 21-hydroxylase deficiency 11α-hydroxylase deficiency 3α-hydroxysteroid dehydrogenase deficiency Cushing's syndrome Neoplasms Adrenal carcinoma Adrenal adenoma
Drugs (proprietary name)	Cyclosporine (Sandimmune) Danazol (Danocrine) Phenytoin (Dilantin) Glucocorticoids Minoxidil (Loniten) Diazoxide (Hyperstat) Penicillamine Hexachlorobenzene Oral contraceptives with 19-nortestosterone Anabolic steroids
Idiopathic	

*Most common causes of hirsutism.

muscle mass, especially in the upper shoulder girdle; increased libido

Signs and Symptoms of Thyroid Dysfunction

Intolerance for heat/cold, tremors, tachycardia, fatigue, dry skin, coarse or silky hair

Galactorrhea

Menses/Fertility

Menarche age

Menorrhagia, oligomenorrhea, or amenorrhea

Infertility

Medications

Drug history (see Table 93-1)

Family History

Ethnic factors: Hair follicle numbers: Mediterranean > Nordic > Oriental; hair pattern in family

Psychosocial History

Psychosocial impact, regardless of degree of hirsutism

OBJECTIVE DATA

Observation

Pay particular attention to hair growth in androgen-responsive areas (face, chest, breasts, abdomen, lower back, arms, and legs)

Ferriman & Gallway score: Interpret in relation to ethnic background of patient; usually a score ≥8 signifies hirsutism (Figure 93-1)

Acne, oily skin

General Physical Examination

Pay particular attention to:

Thyroid

Thorough abdominal examination

Pelvic Examination

Clitoromegaly: Shaft diameter >1 cm measured transversely at the base of the clitoris *or* a clitoral index >35 mm (the product of the largest sagittal and transverse dimensions of the glans clitoris)

Palpable tumors: Note that androgen-secreting ovarian neoplasms may be small (1 to 2 cm) and patients with hirsutism may be obese, making the physical examination either unsatisfactory or inadequate

Physical Signs of Other Syndromes

Acanthosis nigricans: Hyperpigmented, thickened verrucous skin changes around the neck, axilla, or intertriginous areas; presence suggests insulin resistance, particularly for thin women; may be a sign of occult malignancy, but is frequently seen in simple obesity

Hyperprolactinemia: Galactorrhea, amenorrhea, and hypertension

Cushing's: Central obesity, muscle weakness and/or wasting, abdominal striae, suboccipital fat pad, bruisability, amenorrhea, symptoms of diabetes, hypertension, and psychosis

Diagnostic Procedures

NOTE: *Check your local laboratory for normal values.* Laboratory tests are best obtained during follicular phase or just after a withdrawal bleed (Tables 93-2 and 93-3).

If rapid virilization, abdominal or pelvic mass, and/or high laboratory values as defined in Tables 93-2 and 93-3 are present, evaluate for an adrenal/ovarian tumor: Ultrasound ($347-$416), computed tomography scan ($347-

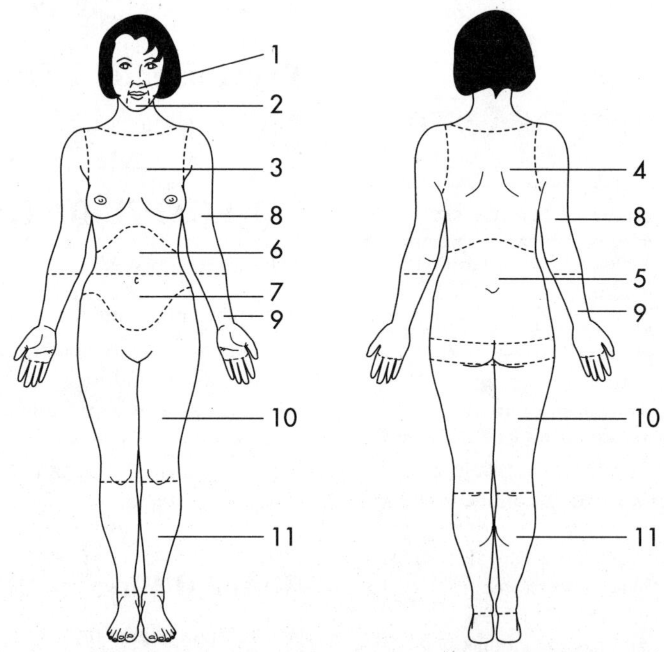

(Grade 0 at all sites indicates absence of terminal hair.)

Site	Grade	Definition
1. Upper Lip	1	A few hairs at outer margin.
	2	A small moustache at outer margin.
	3	A moustache extending halfway from outer margin.
	4	A moustache extending to mid-line.
2. Chin	1	A few scattered hairs.
	2	Scattered hairs with small concentrations.
	3 & 4	Complete cover, light and heavy.
3. Chest	1	Circumareolar hairs.
	2	With mid-line hair in addition.
	3	Fusion of these areas, with three-quarter cover.
	4	Complete cover.
4. Upper back	1	A few scattered hairs.
	2	Rather more, still scattered.
	3 & 4	Complete cover, light and heavy.
5. Lower back	1	A sacral tuft of hair.
	2	With some lateral extension.
	3	Three-quarter cover.
	4	Complete cover.
6. Upper abdomen	1	A few mid-line hairs.
	2	Rather more, still mid-line.
	3 & 4	Half and full cover.
7. Lower abdomen	1	A few mid-line hairs.
	2	A mid-line streak of hair.
	3	A mid-line band of hair.
	4	An inverted V-shaped growth.
8. Arm	1	Sparse growth affecting not more than a quarter of the limb surface.
	2	More than this; cover still incomplete.
	3 & 4	Complete cover, light and heavy.
9. Forearm	1, 2, 3, 4	Complete cover of dorsal surface; 2 grades of light and 2 of heavy growth.
10. Thigh	1, 2, 3, 4	As for arm.
11. Leg	1, 2, 3, 4	As for arm.

NOTE: Scores in each area are added. Total score of ≥8 indicates hirsutism.

Figure 93-1 Ferriman and Gallway Score. (From Ferriman D, Gallway JD, Clinical assessment of a body hair growth in women, *J Clin Endocrinol Metabol* 21:1440, 1961.©The Endocrine Society.)

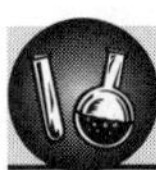

TABLE 93-2 Initial Diagnostic Tests: Hirsutism

Diagnostic Test	Findings/Rationale	Cost ($)
Total Testosterone	Normal range: 20-80 ng/dl Values >200 ng/dl require further testing for androgen producing tumor (Speroff et al, 1994)	83-103
DHEA-S	Upper limit of normal: 350 æg/dl Values >700 æg/dl is a marker for abnormal adrenal function and strongly suggest a tumor (Speroff et al, 1994)	81-102
17-hydroxyprogesterone*	Baseline level: <200 ng/dl Levels from 200 ng/dl-800 ng/dl require ACTH testing Levels >800 ng/dl are diagnostic of 21-hydroxylase deficiency (CAH) (Speroff, Glass, and Kase, 1994)	87-107

ACTH, Adrenocorticotropic hormone; *CAH,* congenital adrenal hyperplasia; *DHEA,* dehydroepiandrosterone.
*Some experts do not believe this to be an initial diagnostic test.

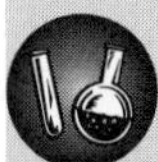

TABLE 93-3 Additional Tests Obtained Based on History and/or Physical Examination

Diagnostic Test	Findings/Rationale	Cost ($)
Prolactin	Normal: <25 ng/ml (NOTE: Girls 13-15 years of age have three times the adult levels) Increased in: 10%-25% of women with galactorrhea and normal menses; 10%-15% of women with amenorrhea without galactorrhea; 75% of women with both galactorrhea and amenorrhea/oligomenorrhea with ↑ prolactin; 20% have hypothyroid, do TSH	70-89
TSH	Enlarged thyroid, signs and/or symptoms of thyroid dysfunction	56-70
Fasting glucose: insulin ratio *or* 2- or 3-hour GTT with glucose and insulin levels	Lack of normal postprandial increase in blood glucose, ↑ insulin levels (fasting glucose to fasting insulin ratio <3 for significant hyperinsulinemia) If glucose : insulin ratio is <5, use troglitazone (Rezulin) or metformin (Glucophage) in treatment	16-20/glucose; 40-51/insulin; 45-67/GTT
24-hour urinary cortisol	Suspect Cushing's syndrome (least common final diagnoses)	57-73
LH/FSH ratio	Diagnosis and management of infertility Differential diagnosis of gonadal disorders	61-76/LH; 62-78/FSH

FSH, Follicle-stimulating hormone; *LH,* luteinizing hormone; *TSH,* thyroid-stimulating hormone.

$416), magnetic resonance imaging ($1560-$1840), and/or ovarian/adrenal catheterization (not available)

ASSESSMENT

Causes of hirsutism and associated findings are listed in Tables 93-4 and 93-5.

THERAPEUTIC PLAN

Pharmaceutical

Hirsutism is slow to respond to treatment due to the hair growth cycle. Caution the patient that hormonal suppression will be necessary for at least 6 months before she will notice a decrease in hair growth. Electrolysis is not recommended until hormonal suppression has been used for at least 6 months. The combination of hormonal suppression and electrolysis is the most complete and effective treatment of hirsutism. After 1 to 2 years of treatment, the patient can stop the medication and watch for a return of ovulatory cycles. If the patient remains anovulatory, hirsutism could recur eventually, but testosterone suppression continues for 6 months to 2 years after discontinuation of the medication. When a patient's symptoms are particularly resistant, combination therapy may be used (Tables 93-6 and 93-7).

Treat insulin resistance if:
  Fasting glucose : insulin ratio is less than 5.

TABLE 93-4 Mechanism of Hirsutism

Cause of Hirsutism	Mechanism
Hirsutism without Virilization	
Polycystic ovary syndrome	Ovarian androgen overproduction
Idiopathic	Increased peripheral conversion of androgens
Late-onset congenital adrenal hyperplasia	Adrenal androgen overproduction
Cushing's syndrome (ACTH-induced)	Adrenal androgen overproduction
Insulin resistance/obesity	Ovarian androgen overproduction
Iatrogenic (medication-induced)	Varies ranging from direct androgenic activity to nonandrogenic effects
Hirsutism with Virilization	
Ovarian hyperthecosis	Autonomous ovarian androgen production
Ovarian neoplasms	Autonomous ovarian androgen production
Adrenal neoplasms, especially adrenal carcinoma	Autonomous adrenal androgen production

From Nussbaum S: Evaluation of hirsutism. In Goroll A, May L, Mulley A, editors: *Primary care medicine*, ed 3, Philadelphia, 1995, JB Lippincott.

TABLE 93-5 Associated Findings: Hirsutism

Cause	Associated Findings
Hirsutism without Virilization	
PCOS (75%)	Perimenarchial onset
	Irregular menses, oligomenorrhea, and/or amenorrhea
	Anovulation/infertility
	+/- Hypertension
	+/- ↑ Testosterone
	Normal DHEA-S
	Normal 17-hydroxyprogesterone
	+/- Hyperglycemia
	+/- ↑ Insulin levels
	+/- Obesity
	LH/FSH ratio >3
	+/- Lipid abnormalities
	+/- Ultrasound reveals polycystic ovaries
Idiopathic (15%)	Diagnosis of exclusion
Late-onset CAH (3%)	↑ DHEA-S (<2 times normal→suspect CAH; >2 times normal→suspect adrenal tumor)
	↑ Testosterone
	+/- Regular menses
	REFER
Cushing's syndrome (ACTH-induced) (Ch. 48)	Truncal obesity
	Fat in cheeks and behind neck
	Thin skin
	Purple abdominal striae
	Hypertension
	Acne
	Facial plethora
	Muscle weakness
	+/- Virilization (late sign)
	+ Dexamethasone suppression test
	Excessive cortisone secretion (↑ 24-hour free cortisol excretion and ↑ late evening plasma cortisol level
	REFER
	REFER

ACTH, Adrenocorticotropic hormone; *CAH,* congenital adrenal hyperplasia; *DHEA,* dehydroepiandrosterone; *PCOS,* polycystic ovary syndrome.

TABLE 93-5 Associated Findings: Hirsutism—cont'd

Cause	Associated Findings
Insulin resistance/obesity	See PCOS Android obesity Acanthosis nigricans Lipid abnormalities Hypertension +/- Hyperglycemia Lack of normal postprandial increase in blood glucose ↑ Insulin levels (fasting glucose to fasting insulin ratio <3 for significant hyperinsulinemia)
Hyperprolactinemia	Galactorrhea ↑ Prolactin levels Other manifestations of this disease are more prominent than hirsutism
Iatrogenic (medication-induced)	See medication list
Hirsutism with Virilization	
Ovarian hyperthecosis	Hyperplasia of the androgen-secreting thecal cells Same clinical manifestations as PCOS, but more severe Acanthosis nigricans Insulin resistance
Ovarian neoplasms	Rapid onset of hirsutism Recent onset of menstrual irregularity Testosterone >200 ng/dl
Adrenal neoplasms, especially adrenal carcinoma	Rapid onset of hirsutism Recent onset of menstrual irregularity Testosterone >200 ng/dl DHEA-S >700 æg/dl

There is a strong family history of diabetes and the patient is obese or has irregular cycles or hirsutism.

There is evidence that hyperinsulinemia has adverse health effects in general (Table 93-8).

Lifestyle/Activities

Cosmetic measures
- Shaving
- Bleaching with hydrogen peroxide
- Chemical depilatories
- Plucking
- Waxing
- Electrolysis

Stress management: Stress can contribute to androgen excess

Diet

Diet modification and weight loss, especially for those who are insulin resistant

Patient Education

Treatment may last for months; noticeable improvement may not come for 6 months.

Infertility can be a problem. Ovulation induction may be necessary.

If excessive virilization has occurred, voice and hair follicle changes are not reversible.

Consultation

Consult with gynecologist and/or endocrinologist.

Follow-up

See specific medications for follow-up instructions.

Other than specific recommendations above, at least recheck in 2 months; other follow-up depends on their goals and your program.

EVALUATION

Oligomenorrhea and obesity (often seen in PCOS) have an increased risk of endometrial cancer.

Hirsute women tend to have higher blood pressures and lower low-density lipoprotein cholesterol levels.

Android obesity with a high waist-to-hip ratio, increased insulin resistance, and coronary artery disease is common.

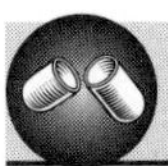

TABLE 93-6 Pharmaceutical Plan: Suppression of Androgen Overproduction

Drug	Dose	Comments	Cost
Oral contraceptives	1 tab per day on 28-day packet	Formulations with desogestrel, gestodene, or norgestimate (examples: Desogen, Ortho-Cept, Ortho-Cyclen) ↑ SHBG and ↓ free testosterone levels	~$28/mo
Medroxyprogesterone acetate	Choose one: 150 mg IM q3 months 30 mg PO/day (Speroff et al, 1994) 10 mg PO/day for 10 days cycling every 1-2 months (Marantides, 1997)	Not applicable for children Contraindicated: Undiagnosed vaginal bleeding, breast cancer, hepatic dysfunction Pregnancy: X SE: Irregular bleeding, edema, weight gain, depression, insomnia, breast tenderness, acne, hirsutism, alopecia	$37/150 mg/ml, 1-ml vial
GnRH agonists Leuprolide (Lupron)	Leuprolide 3.75 mg monthly, with add back estrogen and progesterone either in an OC or 0.625 conjugated estrogens or 1 mg estradiol combined with 2.5 mg medroxyprogesterone acetate or 0.35 mg norethindrone	Suppresses the pituitary; reserved for the severe case of ovarian hyper-androgynism (significant hyperthecosis) and hyperinsulinism Pregnancy: X SE: Pain, acne, rash, syncope, GI upset, emotional liability, vaginal discharge	$398/3.75-mg vial
Dexamethasone (Decadron)	Given nightly in a dose of 0.5 mg (equals 5-7.5 mg of prednisone); if cortisol secretion is suppressed (morning plasma cortisol <2 æg/dl), reduce dose	For women who have adrenal enzyme deficiency; if there are only moderate elevations of DHEA-S, this is not indicated Pregnancy: C SE: HPA axis suppression, masks infection, glaucoma, cataracts, hypokalemia, hypocalcemia, hypernatremia, osteoporosis, carbohydrate intolerance	$12-$52/0.5 mg (100)

GI, Gastrointestinal; *OC*, oral contraceptive; *DHEA*, dehydroepiandrosterone; *HPA*, hypothalamic-pituitary-adrenal; *SE*, side effects; *SHBG*, sex hormone–binding globulin.

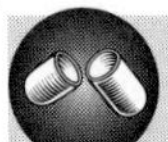

TABLE 93-7 Pharmaceutical Plan: Drugs That Block the Effect of Androgens

Drug	Dose	Comments	Cost
Spironolactone (Aldactone)	50-250 mg daily (usually 100-200 mg daily); start at 25-50 mg and increase dose, depending on patient response	Use when OCs are unacceptable or in addition to OCs. If the patient is anovulatory, use a progestational agent to avoid endometrial hyperplasia. For acne, a cream of 2%-5% spironolactone has been used. *Ovulation can occur while on this medication, and teratogenic effects on a fetus could occur.* Therefore effective contraception is important. Monitor BP and K+ on initiation, at 2 weeks, and after each dose change. Monitor K+ regularly on high doses. SE: Hyperkalemia, GI upset, H/A, impotence, hirsutism, voice deepening, menstrual changes	$71/50 mg (100); $119/100 mg (100)

BP, Blood pressure; *GI*, gastrointestinal; *H/A*, headache; *OC*, oral contraceptive; *SE*, side effects.

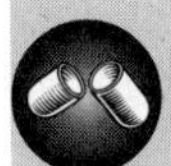

TABLE 93-7 Pharmaceutical Plan: Drugs That Block the Effect of Androgens—cont'd

Drug	Dose	Comments	Cost
Flutamide (Eulexin)	250 mg BID or TID	Nonsteroidal antiandrogen. It inhibits hair growth and has few side effects. *Make sure patient is using effective contraception because of teratogenic effects on fetus.* Pregnancy: D SE: Hot flashes, loss of libido, GI upset, rash	$269/125 mg (180)
Cyproterone acetate (Androcur)	Used in combination with estrogen; administer on days 5-15 of the menstrual cycle in doses of 25-100 mg daily with 20-35 μg ethinylo-estradiaol on days 5-26; transdermal estrogen can be used	Progestational agent. Adverse lipoprotein profile. OC + spironolactone is as effective as cyproterone. *Make sure patient is using effective contraception because of teratogenic effects on fetus.*	Not available in United States
Finasteride (Proscar)	5 mg daily	5 alpha-reductase inhibitor. *Make sure patient is using effective contraception because of teratogenic effects on fetus.* SE: Decreased libido, hepatic dysfunction	$195/5 mg (100)

TABLE 93-8 Treatment of Insulin Resistance

Drug	Dose	Comments	Cost
Metformin (Glucophage)	Start with ½ tab at dinner for 1 week; then ½ tab breakfast and dinner for a week; then, 1 tab with dinner for a week; then 1 tab BID. Warn about diarrhea/ nausea, cut back if a problem; check glucose:insulin after 1 month on full dose; work up to 850 mg BID; increase to 1000 mg BID as necessary	20% won't tolerate this due to GI side effects, but most respond and regulate cycles within 3 months. *Make sure patient is using effective contraception because of teratogenic effects on the fetus.* At the very least, chart basal body temperature at home, and if temp remains elevated for 16 days, stop medication. Pregnancy: B Confirm normal renal function before initiating. Interactions with: Cimetidine, digoxin, quinidine, ranitidine, triamterene, phenytoin, nicotinic acid, calcium channel blockers SE: Metallic taste, lactic acidosis (avoid with renal insufficiency)	$46/500 mg (100); $79/850 mg (100)

ALT, Alanine aminotransferase; *d/c,* decrease; *LFT,* liver function tests; *SE,* side effects.

Continued

TABLE 93-8 Treatment of Insulin Resistance—cont'd

Drug	Dose	Comments	Cost
Troglitazone (Rezulin)	400 mg daily; may increase to 600 mg in 1 month; if no response after 1 month of 600 mg, discontinue drug	There is a real problem with liver toxicity; LFTs monthly for 8 months, then q2mo for rest of year. See drug warning update and current manufacturer recommendations for LFT testing. Do not start on drug if ALT levels are elevated >1.5× normal. If ALT levels >1.5 — 2× normal during therapy, retest weekly until levels return to normal or rise about 3× normal (d/c drug). Take with food. (Interferes with CYP3A4) Pregnancy: B SE: Asthenia, dizziness, nausea, back pain	\$104/200 mg (30); \$160/400 mg (30)

Medical treatment of hirsutism may not address all the health care issues; each issue should be treated individually.

REFERENCES

Marantides D: Management of polycystic ovary syndrome, *Nurse Pract* 22(12):34, 36-38, 40-41, 1997.

Speroff L, Glass RH, Kase N: *Clinical gynecologic endocrinology and infertility*, ed 5, Baltimore, 1994, Williams & Wilkins.

SUGGESTED READINGS

Adashi E: Insulin and related peptides in hyperandrogenism, *Clin Obstet Gynecol* 34(4):872-882, 1991.

Aiman J: Virilizing ovarian tumors, *Clin Obstet Gynecol* 34(4): 835-847, 1991.

Barnes R: Adrenal dysfunction and hirsutism, *Clin Obstet Gynecol* 34(4): 827-834, 1991.

Bates GW, Cornwell C: Iatrogenic causes of hirsutism, *Clin Obstet Gynecol* 34(4):848-851, 1991.

Conn J, Jacobs H: The clinical management of hirsutism, *Eur J Endocrinol* 136(4):339-348, 1997.

Delaney M: Hirsutism. In Carr P, Freund K, Somani S, editors: *The medical care of women*, Philadelphia, 1995, WB Saunders.

Ellsworth A et al: *Mosby's 1998 medical drug reference*, St Louis, 1998, Mosby.

Ferriman D, Gallway JD: Clinical assessment of body hair growth in women, *J Clin Endocrinol Metabol* 21:1440, 1961.

HealthCare Consultants of America: *1998 physicians fee and coding guide*, Augusta, Ga, 1998, HealthCare Consultants of America, Inc.

Kalve E, Klein J: Evaluation of women with hirsutism, *Am Family Physician* 54(1):117-124, 1996.

Kessel B, Liu, J: Clinical and laboratory evaluation of hirsutism, *Clin Obstet Gynecol* 34(4):805-816, 1991.

Lobo R: Hirsutism in polycystic ovary syndrome: current concepts, *Clin Obstet Gynecol* 34(4):817-826, 1991.

Lovely L: Personal communication via e-mail, March 23, 1998.

Monroe S, Andreyko J: Hirsutism. In Glass R, editor: *Office gynecology*, ed 4, Baltimore, 1993, Williams & Wilkins.

Nussbaum S: Evaluation of hirsutism. In Goroll A, May L, Mulley A, editors: *Primary care medicine*, ed 3, Philadelphia, 1995, JB Lippincott.

Prelevic G: Insulin resistance in polycystic ovary syndrome, *Curr Opin Obstet Gynecol* 9(3):193-201, 1997.

Sakiyama R: Approach to patients with hirsutism, *West J Med* 165(6):386-391, 1996.

Schriock EA, Schriock ED: Treatment of hirsutism, *Clin Obstet Gynecol* 34(4):852-863, 1991.

Star W: Hirsutism. In Star W, Lommel L, Shannon M, editors: *Women's primary health care: protocols for practice*, Washington, DC, 1995, American Nurses Association Publishing.

Watson R, Bouknight R, Alguire P: Hirsutism: evaluation and management, *J Gen International Med* 10(5):283-292, 1995.

Wild R: Lipid metabolism and hyperandrogenism, *Clin Obstet Gynecol* 34(4):864-871, 1991.

94 HIV/AIDS

ICD-9-CM

Human Immunodeficiency Infection 042

OVERVIEW

Definitions

HIV-1: Human immunodeficiency virus type 1

The retrovirus recognized as the agent that induces AIDS

HIV-2: Human immunodeficiency virus type 2

A virus closely related to but less virulent than HIV-1 and epidemic only in West Africa

AIDS: Acquired immunodeficiency syndrome

A transmissible retroviral disease caused by infection with HIV and manifested by depression of cell-mediated immunity, CD4 count less than 200. The outcome of this process is an increase in opportunistic infections initiated by bacterial, fungal, protozoan, and viral pathogens.

Incidence

From 1981 to 1996 a total of 573,800 persons ages ≥13 years with AIDS were reported to the Centers for Disease Control and Prevention (CDC) by state and local health departments. As of June 1996, the estimated prevalence of AIDS was 223,000 U.S. residents ages ≥13 years. Prevalence represents not only the rate of new AIDS cases but also the duration of illness for those presently diagnosed with AIDS. This increase of AIDS prevalence reflects declines in AIDS deaths and stable AIDS incidence (Table 94-1).

AIDS Indicator Conditions

HIV+ persons with CD4 cell counts <200 or a CD4 <14%
Candidiasis of bronchi, trachea, or lungs
Candidiasis of esophagus
Cervical cancer, invasive
Coccidioidomycosis, disseminated or extra pulmonary
Cryptococcosis, extra pulmonary
Cryptosporidiosis, chronic intestinal (>1-month duration)
Cytomegalovirus disease (other than liver, spleen, or nodes)
Cytomegalovirus retinitis (with loss of vision)
Encephalopathy, HIV-related
Herpes simplex: chronic ulcer(s) (>1-month duration); or bronchitis, pneumonitis, or esophagitis
Histoplasmosis, disseminated or extra pulmonary
Isosporiasis, chronic intestinal (>1-month duration)
Kaposi's sarcoma
Lymphoma, Burkitt's (or equivalent term)
Lymphoma, immunoblastic (or equivalent term)
Lymphoma, primary, of brain
Mycobacterium avium complex or *M. kansasii,* disseminated or extra pulmonary
Mycobacterium tuberculosis, any site (pulmonary or extra pulmonary)
Mycobacterium, other species or unidentified species, disseminated or extra pulmonary
Pneumocystis carinii pneumonia
Pneumonia, recurrent
Progressive multifocal leukoencephalopathy
Salmonella septicemia, recurrent
Toxoplasmosis of brain
Wasting syndrome due to HIV

Pathophysiology

The major target for HIV is the CD4 T lymphocyte; macrophages and monocytes may also be infected. The virus attaches to the CD4 cell, enters the cytoplasm, and uncoats. Using the viral enzyme reverse transcriptase, a DNA copy of the viral RNA genome is transcribed and duplicated. This new DNA integrates into the DNA of the host cell. This process generates viral buds that separate from the host cell, thereby initiating viral replication.

HIV is transmitted by sexual exposure and intravenous drug use (IDU), through blood and blood products, and from mother to fetus. Within 2 to 6 weeks following exposure and

TABLE 94-1 1993 Revised Classification System for HIV Infection and Expanded AIDS Surveillance Case Definition for Adolescents and Adults

	Clinical Categories		
CD4 + T-cell categories	(A) Asymptomatic, Acute (primary) HIV, or PGL	(B) Symptomatic, not (A) or (C) conditions	(C) AIDS Indicator Conditions
(1) >500	A1	B1	C1
(2) 200-499	A2	B2	C2
<200 AIDS-indicator T-cell count	A3	B3	C3

From Centers for Disease Control and Prevention: 1993 revised classification system for HIV infection and expanded surveillance case definition for AIDS among adolescents and adults, *MMWR* 44(RR-7):1-19, 1992.
PGL, Persistent generalized lymphadenopathy.
Shaded cells indicate AIDS.

lasting approximately 1 to 2 weeks, there will be symptoms indicative of acute retroviral conversion for approximately 50% to 70% of those exposed. These symptoms are characteristic of infectious mononucleosis or "flulike" in character and include fever, arthralgias, myalgias, and fatigue. Physical examination may reveal a diffuse erythematous rash and generalized adenopathy. This clinical presentation coincides with high levels of viral replication, which are measured by HIV RNA and the presence of p24 antigen. CD4 cells drop dramatically, and CD8 cells generally rise in response to the virus. Seroconversion generally takes 6 to 12 weeks following transmission. The levels of HIV RNA are sharply reduced, and CD4 returns to higher levels but generally not to preinfection levels. This is followed by a prolonged stage of asymptomatic clinical latency. During this stage there is a large viral reservoir actively replicating in the lymphoid tissues. As this clinical latency continues and disease progresses, the framework of the lymph tissue disintegrates, accounting for the rise of viral burden detectable in the plasma. Immunologic damage increases, and opportunistic infections develop unabated. The rate of disease progression is outlined in Figure 94-1.

Risk Categories for HIV Infection

Persons who have sexually transmitted diseases
High-risk categories
- IDU, gay and bisexual men, hemophiliacs, regular sexual partners of persons in these categories

Lower-risk categories
- Prostitutes and persons who received blood or artificial insemination during 1978 to 1985
- Persons who consider themselves at risk or request testing
- Women at risk who are of childbearing age
- Persons living in high prevalence communities or born in high prevalence countries
- All pregnant women
- Patients with clinical or laboratory findings suggestive of HIV infection
- Patients with active tuberculosis
- Recipient and source of blood or body fluid exposures
- Health care workers who perform exposure-prone invasive procedures
- Hospital admissions for patients ages 15 to 45 years in facilities where the seroprevalence is ≥1% or AIDS case rates are ≥1/1000 discharges
- Donors of blood, semen, and organs (this is the only category in which testing is mandatory in all states)

SUBJECTIVE DATA

Past Medical History

Fatigue
Malaise
Fevers without cause that are ≥100° F
Night sweats
Swollen or painful lymph nodes.
Unexplained loss of ≥10% body weight
Loss of appetite
Cough, SOB, chest tightness, orthopnea, tachypnea, or history of tuberculosis or PPD testing
Oral thrush/candidiasis
Changes in central nervous system function, including headaches, changes in mental status, stiff neck, seizures, and cognitive, motor, and behavioral changes
Skin rashes, lesions, bruises

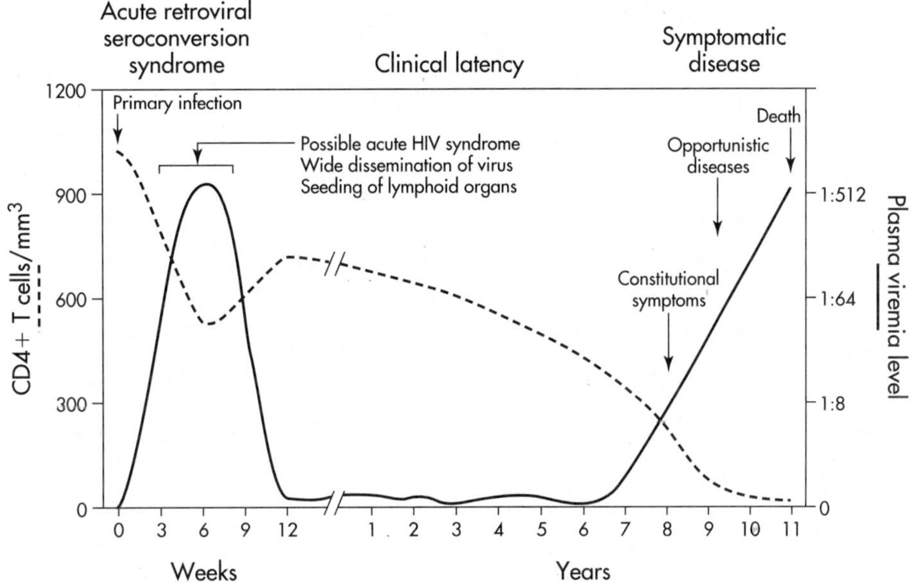

Figure 94-1 The typical course of HIV infection without therapy. (From Barlett JA: *Care and management of patients with HIV infection*, Durham, NC, 1996, Glaxo Wellcome. Reproduced with permission.)

Herpes zoster/shingles
Allergies (e.g., foods, pets, environment)
Sexually transmitted infections: Gonorrhea, chlamydia, syphilis, condylomata, hepatitis, herpes simplex
Sexual preference and safe sex practices
Female patients: Pregnancy history, pap smear history, vaginal infections, and contraceptive use
Children: Pregnancy history, including drug exposure, labor and delivery history, gestational age at birth and weight, growth patterns, feeding patterns, developmental milestones, and history of illnesses
Substance use/abuse, illicit or prescribed
Smoking
Assess ongoing high-risk behavior exposures that may place the patient at risk for opportunistic infections or HIV transmission to others.
Access the patient's perception and knowledge about HIV infection. Had the patient ever known anyone infected with HIV? Has he or she ever taken care of anyone with HIV infection or AIDS?

Medications

Medication history: Prescribed, over-the-counter, and herbs, vitamins, and other non-traditional therapies

Family History

Cardiopulmonary
Diabetes
Gastrointestinal
Cancer
Depression
Suicide
Substance abuse
Is the patient's family aware of the diagnosis? If not, will they be informed?
Prior family experience with HIV infection

Psychological History

Signs and symptoms of depression
Suicide ideation
Prior psychologic or psychiatric care
Support network of family and friends
Present employment status and medical/dental benefits

OBJECTIVE DATA

Physical Examination

A physical examination should be performed that includes the areas identified in Table 94-2.

Diagnostic Procedures

Diagnostic procedures are included in Table 94-3.

ASSESSMENT

The range of diagnoses are numerous and varied, depending on patient history and physical examination (Figure 94-2).

Table 94-2 Physical Examination of Clients with HIV/AIDS

Areas	Symptoms/Findings	Differential Diagnoses
Mouth	Whitish coating on tongue, gums, roof of mouth	Oral candidiasis
	Fine lines or ridges on sides of tongue	Hairy leukoplakia
	Purple spots or lesions	Kaposi's sarcoma
	Bleeding gums	ITP
	Lesions	Herpes simplex, aphthous ulcers
Eyes	Cotton-wool spots, exudate plus hemorrhage	Cytomegalovirus retinitis
Neck	Swollen, painful lymph nodes	Lymphadenopathy
	Nuchal rigidity	Cryptococcosis
Lungs	Auscultation for extraneous sounds (rales, wheezes, rhonchi)	PCP *Pneumococcus* *Mycobacterium tuberculosis*
	Cough	Bacterial pneumonia
Abdomen	Abnormal tenderness	ITP
	Enlarged liver/spleen	Hepatitis Cirrhosis Cancers
Genitourinary/rectal	Warts	Venereal warts
	Whitish coating of membranes	Candidal infection
	Ulcers/lesions	Herpes simplex Syphilis
Skin (entire body examination)	Purple lesions	Kaposi's sarcoma
	Vesicular lesions	Herpes simplex or zoster
	Bruising	ITP
	Dry, flaking skin	Seborrheic dermatitis
	Rashes	Drug reactions Syphilis Disseminated disease
	Warts/papules	Molluscum/HPV
Neurologic	Memory loss	Cryptococcosis
	Personality changes	Toxoplasmosis
	Decreased cognitive function	Central nervous system lesions
	Decreased or increased reflexes	HIV dementia
	Neuropathies	Progressive multifocal leukoencephalopathy
Gynecologic	Yeast/white discharge	Vaginal candidiasis STD
	Papular lesions	Condylomata acuminatum
	Vesicles	Herpes Syphilis

HPV, Human papillomavirus; *ITP,* idiopathic thrombocytopenic purpura; *PCP, Pneumocystis carinii* pneumonia; *STD,* sexually transmitted disease.

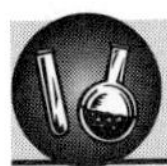

TABLE 94-3 Diagnostic Tests: HIV/AIDS

Diagnostic Test	Findings/Rationale	Cost ($)
HIV Serology	Test results are reported as negative, positive, or indeterminate. A positive HIV serology requires both a positive ELISA and the confirmatory, positive Western blot. If the test result is questionable based on patient history, repeat testing is warranted.	41-52/Elisa; 60-76/Western Blot
CD4 Count	Results direct initiation and use of prophylaxis of antiretrovirals, treatment for opportunistic infections, and diagnostic tests. Collected initially and repeated every 3-6 months.	123-151
CBC	Initially, repeat q3-6 months	18-23
HIV RNA	Used primarily for disease staging and monitoring response to antiretroviral therapies. Frequency of testing should coincide with CD4 screening.	165
VDRL or RPR	Initially and yearly, if sexually active	18-22
Chemistry panel	Initially and when warranted based on disease status or adverse drug reaction	32-42
Hepatitis panel	The choice of diagnostic test is determined by patient history. Hepatitis B immunization status can be determined.	108-151
PPD	Initially and yearly. Should be repeated in nonreactors who are suspected of having or having been exposed to TB. Induration ≥5 mm is considered positive.	15-19
CXR	When clinically warranted	77-91
PAP smear	Initially and repeat every 6-12 months, based on patient immune status	25-31
Toxoplasmosis serology	Initially and when severely immunocompromised (CD4 ≤100)	46-57

CBC, Complete blood count; *CXR,* chest x-ray; *PPD,* purified protein derivative; *RNA,* ribonucleic acid; *RPR,* rapid plasma reagin; *VDRL,* Venereal Disease Research Laboratories.

Most Common Presentations

Persistent generalized lymphadenopathy
Cytopenias: Anemia, leukopenia, thrombocytopenia
Pulmonary symptoms suggesting *Pneumocystis carinii* pneumonia (PCP)
Kaposi's sarcoma
Candidiasis: Vaginal, esophageal, oral
Constitutional symptoms: Weight loss, night sweats, fatigue, chronic fever and/or chronic diarrhea for 30 days
Bacterial infections, primarily pulmonary
Tuberculosis
Sexually transmitted infections
Neurological syndromes
HIV-associated dementia: Difficulty concentrating, memory loss, and mental slowing
Peripheral syndrome: Pain and paresthesia of the feet

THERAPEUTIC PLAN

Pharmaceutical

Antiretroviral medication decisions are made in collaboration with a physician. Medication selection is based on clinical presentation of the patient and laboratory data. Recommendations are rapidly changing on the basis of new research. *Therefore, all recommendations must be periodically reviewed and modified due to ongoing new pharmaceutical approaches* (Table 94-4).

Indications to Treat

Initiation of antiretroviral therapy is based on disease progression risk. CD4 ≤500/mm is no longer the sole criteria for drug initiation; HIV RNA copies per milliliter along with CD4 and a symptomatic patient are the three cornerstones to drug therapy. When HIV RNA ≥5000 to 10,000 copies per milliliter and the CD4 count and clinical status indicate disease progression, begin drug therapy. Viral burden is becoming the dominant criteria for drug initiation or pharmaceutical change, regardless of the CD4 and clinical picture. It is presently recommended to begin antiretroviral therapy with HIV RNA 5000 copies per milliliter and to maintain that level or reduce viral load to an undetectable level. This reduces the relative risk of opportunistic infections.

AZT continues to be the sole drug recommended by the U.S. Public Health Service *only* for the prevention of perinatal HIV transmission. Pregnancy carries a 15% to 35% risk of HIV infection for the infant. This can be reduced by two thirds with the use of AZT. HIV is transmitted through breast milk. Therefore counsel patients of this danger and advise bottle feeding (Table 94-5).

Psychosocial

Determine the interest and need for psychological counseling for the patient and those close to him or her. Depression and/or suicide risk must be assessed.

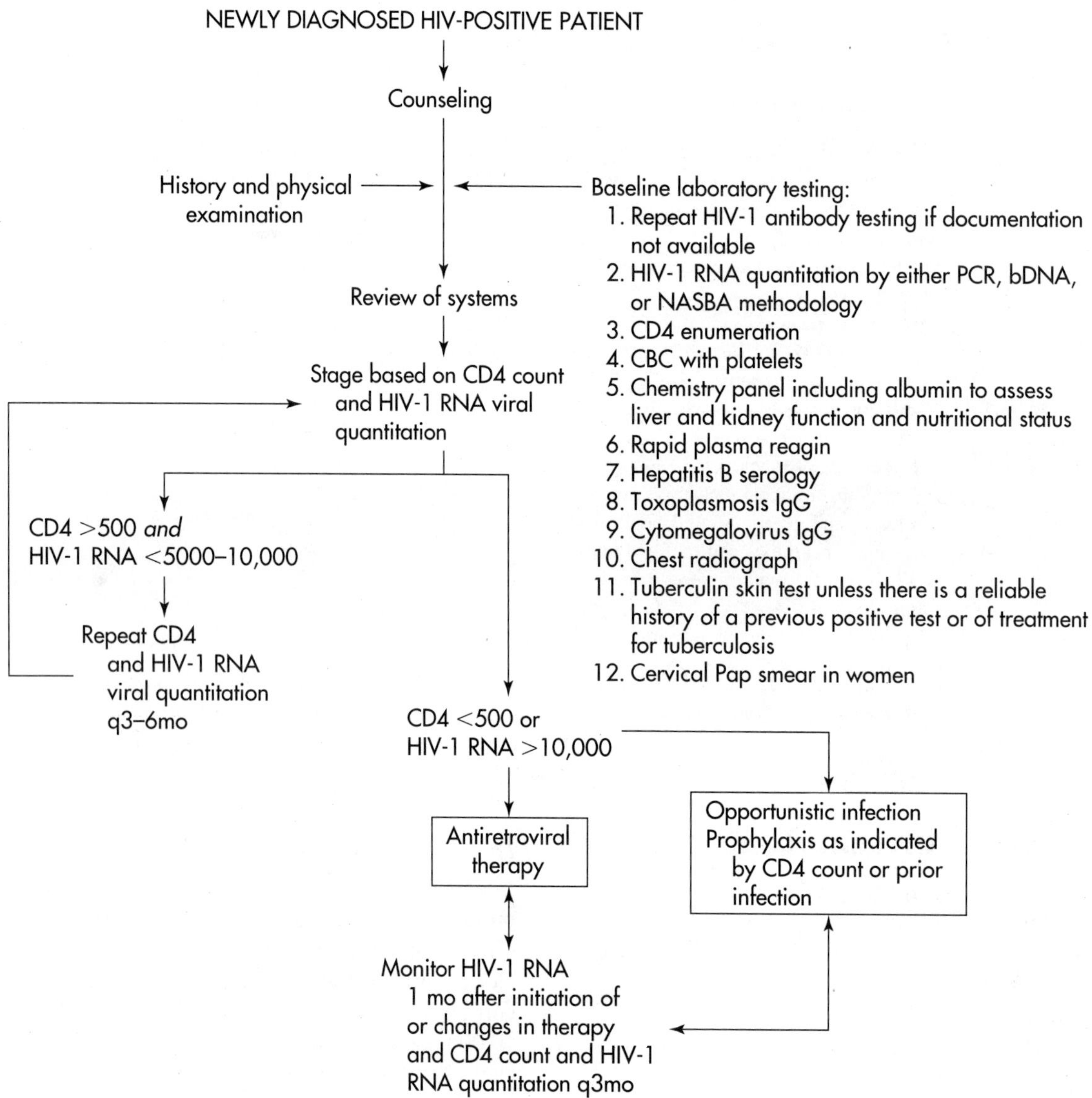

Figure 94-2 Algorithm for client newly diagnosed HIV-positive. (From Greene HL, Johnson WP, Lemcke D: *Decision making in medicine*, ed 2, St Louis, 1998, Mosby.)

Review the natural history of HIV infection and course of disease.

Assess patient's involvement and level of desire to participate in health care decisions.

With the patient's cooperation, or anonymously with local health department assistance, notify sexual and needle-sharing partners of risk status. Primary care providers, specialist MDs, and dentists involved in care should be informed.

Diet

The role of nutrition must not be undervalued by the medical team, patient, and caregivers. The patient's cultural or religious interests must be incorporated into dietary planning.

The health care team should include the expertise of a nutritionist.

Be prepared for patient questions regarding vitamin and/or mineral supplementation.

Food supplements of high caloric replacement are valuable dietary additions.

Patient Education

Review lifestyle behaviors associated with disease prevention: smoking, alcohol and other substance abuse; exercise; and safe sex practices.

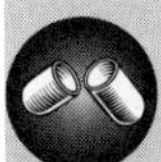

TABLE 94-4 Combination Drug Therapy: Select a Protease Inhibitor to Be Administered With One of the Nucleoside Analogs

Drug	Dose	Comments	Cost
Protease Inhibitor:			
Saquinavir (Invirase; new formulation: Fortovase)	600 mg TID with meals	Pregnancy: B Indinavir (C) GI intolerance	$573/200 mg (270)
Indinavir (Crixivan)	800 mg TID between meals	Nephrolithiasis ↑ Indirect bilirubin	$338/200 mg (270)
Ritonavir (Norvir)	600 mg BID with meals	Gastrointestinal intolerance Peripheral paraesthesia ↑ Transaminase levels	$146/100 mg (100)
Nucleoside Analog:			
Zidovudine (Retrovir) {AZT}	100 mg 3-5× daily	Pregnancy: C Gastrointestinal intolerance/headache/malaise	$155/100 mg (100)
Didanosine (Videx) (ddI)	≥60 kg 200 mg BID ≤60 kg 125 mg BID	Peripheral neuropathy/ pancreatitis	$89/100 mg (60)
Zalcitabine (Hivid) (ddC)	0.75 mg TID	Peripheral neuropathy	$230/0.750 mg (100)
Stavudine (Zerit) (d4T)	40 mg BID	Peripheral neuropathy	$233/40 mg (60)
Lamivudine (Epivir) (3TC)	150 mg BID	GI intolerance/headache	$230/150 mg (60)
Select a Protease Inhibitor From Above List to Give with 3TC and AZT:			
3TC AZT	See above	Side effects of combined drug therapy are additive; see above	See costs above

Bartlett JG: *The Johns Hopkins Hospital guide to medical care of patients with HIV infection*, Baltimore, 1996, Williams & Wilkins.

Household pets are a concern because they may carry microbes that cause diarrhea. If a pet develops diarrhea, veterinary care should be sought for the pet. Litter boxes should be cleaned daily, and pets should be kept indoors. Do not feed them raw meat. Wash hands frequently and thoroughly.

Food preparation: Avoid raw eggs, undercooked poultry, seafood, and meat. Wash produce. Keep raw meat utensils washed and counter tops and cutting boards washed and clean.

Travel: Avoid contaminated food and water. Review immunization needs for travel.

Occupational risks: Major occupational settings that pose risks for HIV-infected individuals are health care settings, day care settings, and animal shelters.

TABLE 94-5 Pregnant Women Perinatal Transmission Prevention: U.S. Public Health Service Recommendation

Drug	Dosage
Prenatal AZT	100 mg 5× daily initiated at 14-34 weeks' gestation
Labor/delivery AZT	IV infusion 2 mg/kg for 1 hour followed by 1 mg/kg/hr till delivery
Neonatal AZT	Syrup: 2 mg/kg q6h; initiate within 8-12 h after birth for 6 weeks

From Barlett JA: *Care and management of patients with HIV infection*, Durham, NC, 1996, Glaxo Wellcome, Inc.

Family Impact

The inclusion of family and friends into the care of patients diagnosed with HIV/AIDS is at the direction of the patient. Once the family is included, the health care team must be prepared to address the emotional and informational needs of the patient and family. Do not overlook the opportunities to educate family and friends so that they are well-informed caregivers.

Consultation/Referral

Prevention of Opportunistic Diseases

Tuberculosis

HIV/AIDS has substantially increased the prevalence of tuberculosis in the United States as well as isoniazid (INH) and rifampin-resistant strains. Tuberculosis also represents a significant health threat to those who live and work in crowded facilities and communities.

Indications

Purified protein derivative (PPD) ≥5 mm

Prior positive PPD without INH prophylaxis

High-risk exposure

Treatment

INH and pyridoxine (vitamin B_6) for 12 months

Beware of INH/hepatitis risk; perform liver function tests at 1 and 3 months after initiating INH

PCP

PCP is the major AIDS-defining diagnosis and the major identifiable cause of death in patients with AIDS.

Indications

Prior PCP

CD4 ≤200

Thrush

Treatment: Alternative regimens

TMP-SMX: 1 regular-strength tablet PO/day or 1 double-strength tablet PO three times weekly

Dapsone 50 mg PO BID or 100 mg daily

Adverse reactions reported with TMP-SMX are rash, fever, nausea/vomiting, neutropenia, and hepatitis

Toxoplasmosis

Toxoplasma gondii is a protozoan organism. It is ubiquitous in nature. Cats are the primary host and reservoir. Symptoms for immunocompromised patients include headache, confusion, fever, lethargy, and seizures.

Indications

CD4 ≤100

Positive *T. gondii* serology

Treatment

TMP-SMX DS: 1 or 2 tablets daily (precise dose has not been decided; consult)

Mycobacterium avium complex (MAC)

MAC refers to a group of atypical mycobacteria of which *M. avium* and *Mycobacterium intracellulare* are the most important. They are widely isolated from the soil and water and are a threat to those who are immunocompromised.

Indication

CD4 ≤75

Treatment

Clarithromycin 500 mg PO BID

Azithromycin 1250 mg PO once weekly

Rifabutin 300 mg PO daily

Follow-up

Patient returns 2 weeks after initial visit to discuss laboratory results. The plan of care, including initiation of medications, will be reviewed with the patient at that time, allowing for patient involvement and questions.

The frequency of follow-up visits is based on patient status, medication stability, and routine laboratory review. Three- to 6-month intervals are most common for the healthy, established patient.

Pap: 2× in first year, annually thereafter except if:

History of HPV

Previous Pap with SIL

Symptomatic HIV infection

Dental: 2×/year

Multiple medications/schedules are very challenging and confusing for your patients. Review this issue with each patient visit.

Immunizations

Pneumovax: Initially and consider boosters q5-7 years

Influenza: Annually

Tetanus: Every 10 years

HBV: Series of three

Periodically review the patient's financial status. Assist or refer to social services when needed.

EVALUATION

No single subspecialty deals effectively with the care of HIV-infected individuals and their families. Expand your collaborative relationships with the health team and caregiving community.

Addiction, homelessness, and mental illness preclude effective patient care. Address these issues first.

Drug regimens are changing often and quickly. Consult with infectious disease specialist and/or treatment center.

Gaining experience and knowledge in the management of HIV/AIDS involves acquiring information from specialists and interacting effectively with consultants. Your experience with HIV/AIDS is a factor in your patient's survival.

RESOURCES

National AIDS Hotline (800) 342-2437

This number has everything a state hotline has, including trained counselors, and is open 24 hours a day. If you need referrals to local agencies or services, your state hotline number may have more up-to-date information.

National AIDS Clearinghouse (800) 458-5231

This number gives you access to the full range of the CDC's published information. You can get referrals to AIDS service organizations and services, order publications, get information about AIDS in the workplace, find out about the latest clinical trails, or use automated service to get information by fax. You can also order a free catalogue of HIV/AIDS education and prevention materials.

National Institutes of Health
AIDS Clinical Trails Information Service (800) Trials-A
This number provides up-to-date information on clinical trails that evaluate experimental drugs and other therapies for adult and children at all stages of HIV infection.

National Lesbian and Gay Health Association (202) 939-7880

National Minority AIDS Council (202) 483-6622

National Women's Health Network (202) 347-1140

National Hemophilia AIDS Foundation (800) 424-2634

Positively Aware (Bimonthly publication)
1258 West Belmont Ave.
Chicago, IL 60657-3292
(312) 404-8726.

GMHC Treatment Issues
The Gay Men's Health Crisis Newsletter of Experimental AIDS Therapies
129 W. 20th St.
New York, NY 10011
An excellent publication for not only gay men, but for all individuals infected with HIV

SUGGESTED READINGS

Abdullah G: AIDS therapy: hitting a moving target, *Patient Care* 31(12):43-70, 1997.

Barlett JA: *Care and management of patients with HIV infection*, Durham, NC, 1996, Glaxo Wellcome.

Bartlett JG: *The Johns Hopkins Hospital guide to medical care of patients with HIV infection*, Baltimore, 1996, Williams & Wilkins.

Carpenter CCJ et al: Antiretroviral therapy for HIV infection, *JAMA*, 276(2):146-154, 1996.

Centers for Disease Control and Prevention: 1993 revised classification system for HIV infection and expanded surveillance case definition for AIDS among adolescents and adults, *MMWR* 44(RR-7):1-19, 1992.

Centers for Disease Control and Prevention: USPHS/IDSA guidelines for the prevention of opportunistic infections in persons infected with Human Immunodeficiency Virus: a summary, *MMWR* 44(RR-8):1-34, 1995.

Centers for Disease Control and Prevention: Update: trends in AIDS incidence, deaths, and prevalence—United States, 1996, *MMWR* 46(RR-8):165-173, 1996.

Ellsworth AJ et al: *Mosby's 1998 medical drug reference*, St Louis, 1998, Mosby.

Healthcare Consultants of America, Inc.: *1998 physicians fee and coding guide*, Augusta, Ga, 1998, Healthcare Consultants of America, Inc.

Kitahata MM et al: Physicians' experience with the acquired immunodeficiency syndrome as a factor in patients' survival, *N Engl J Med* 334(11):701-705, 1997.

Saag MS et al: HIV viral load markers in clinical practice, *Nature Med* 2(6):625-629, 1996.

Weiner RH: HIV: an update for primary care physicians, *Emerg Med* 29(1):52-62, 1997.

Hyperlipidemia (Hyperlipoproteinemia)

ICD-9-CM

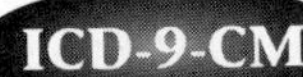

Hyperlipidemia 272.4

OVERVIEW

Definition

Hyperlipidemia is an excessive accumulation of one or more of the lipoproteins in the blood. Primary lipidemia is an hereditary or spontaneous genetic disorder of metabolism. Secondary hyperlipidemia is hyperlipidemia caused by disease (e.g., diabetes mellitus, renal disease).

Incidence

Patients with established coronary heart disease (CHD) have a 5 to 7 times greater risk of a myocardial infarction (MI) than those without CHD (NIH, 1997).

Pathophysiology

Hyperlipidemia results from excessive production, defective removal, or both.

Protective Factors Against

Exercise
Estrogen

Factors that Increase Susceptibility to Coronary Artery Disease with Increased Cholesterol

History of coronary artery disease (CAD) such as MI or angina
At least two of following:
Male ≥45 years, Women ≥55 years
+Family history of CAD (MI, sudden death of parent/sibling <55 years in a male or <65 years of age in a female)
Cigarette smoking
Hypertension
Low high-density lipoprotein (HDL) cholesterol (<35 mg/dl)
HDL >60 mg/dl
Diabetes mellitus
History of CVA or peripheral vascular disease
Obesity (>30% over desirable weight)
Increased total cholesterol and low-density lipoprotein (LDL) cholesterol in men <35 years of age and premenopausal women

Causes of Elevated Triglycerides

Diabetes mellitus
Obesity
Ethanol consumption
Oral contraceptives
Renal disorders (Frishman and Mahmood, 1995).

SUBJECTIVE DATA

Past Medical History

Previous history of a lipid disorder
Presence of conditions associated with lipid abnormalities: Diabetes mellitus, renal disease, hypothyroidism

Medications

Recent use of antibiotics, any other medications
Use of oral contraceptives

Family History

Ask about family history of lipid abnormalities, premature CAD.

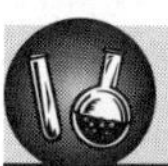

TABLE 95-1 Diagnostic Tests: Hyperlipidemia

Diagnostic Test	Findings/Rationale	Cost ($)
Lipid Panel	Fasting lipid profiles should include total cholesterol, HDL, LDL, and triglycerides measurements. Screening cholesterol can be performed in a nonfasting state. Triglycerides are the most affected by recent high fat intake. If an LDL is not measured, use the following equation to calculate: LDL = Total cholesterol – HDL cholesterol – (Triglycerides/5) **Normal Cholesterol** Adult: Total cholesterol measurement <200 is desirable HDL cholesterol measurement >35 and <60 is desirable LDL cholesterol measurement: High LDL: 160 mg/dl or greater Borderline LDL: 130-159 mg/dl Children: Infant <1 mo: 45-100 mg/dl 2 mo-12 mo: 65-175 mg/dl >12 mo: Same as adult **Normal Triglyceride** Adult: If serum is clear, triglyceride is generally <165 mg/dl. Triglycerides >1000 mg/dl can be seen when a primary lipid disorder is increased by alcohol or fat intake or by medications such as corticosteroids or estrogens. Children: 10-121 mg/dl	49-62

HDL, High-density lipoprotein; *LDL,* low-density lipoprotein.

Diet History

Ask about increased ingestion of caffeine or carbonated drinks.

Alcohol consumption

24-hour diet recall; intake of fats: saturated, unsaturated

Description of Most Common Symptoms

Usually no specific symptoms are identified.

Associated Symptoms

None

OBJECTIVE DATA

Physical Examination

A problem-oriented physical should be conducted, with particular attention to:

Vital signs and weight, general appearance

Usually no specific physical findings are noted

Xanthomas may be detected in severe lipid disorders

Diagnostic Procedures

Diagnostic procedures include those found in Table 95-1.

National Cholesterol Education Program (NCEP) guidelines: without a family history of premature CAD or familial hyperlipidemia, routine screening is not necessary in **children.**

If triglycerides are elevated, further testing should be done to evaluate whether it is the result of underlying pathology (e.g., diabetes mellitus, hypothyroidism [Frishman and Mahmood, 1995]).

ASSESSMENT

Various lipoprotein disorders are presented in Table 95-2.

THERAPEUTIC PLAN

Clinical trials (LRC-CPPT, Helsinki Heart Study) have clearly demonstrated a relationship between high cholesterol and CAD. Reduction of cholesterol levels reduces the incidence of cardiac events (4S, CARE WOSCOPS). The National Cholesterol Education Project (NCEP) has recommended guidelines for the diagnosis and management of high cholesterol levels.

TABLE 95-2 Differential Diagnosis of Hyperlipidemia

Lipoprotein Disorder	Defect	Cholesterol	Triglyceride	Comments
Familial hypercholesterolemia (FH)	Decreased LDL receptors	300-600 but may be higher; LDL high	normal	Incidence is 1/500 and responsible for 3%-6% of premature MIs. Men with FH have a 50% likelihood of MI by age 50 and women by age 60. Presents with xanthelasma and accelerated atherosclerosis. Can be detected in childhood. Consider hypothyroidism, nephrotic syndrome and hepatic obstruction.
Familial combined hyperlipidemia	Overproduction of VLDL by the liver	250-600; LDL high	200-600	1%-2% of population have this disorder accelerated atherosclerosis associated with diabetes or obesity. Both cholesterol and triglyceride may be elevated at different times and in different family members.
Familial hypertriglyceridemia	Hepatic overproduction or defective lipolysis of VLDL triglycerides	Normal	200-5000	Xanthomas. Elevated triglycerides may cause pancreatitis. Consider nephrotic syndrome, hypothyroidism, alcoholism, oral contraceptives. Low risk for atherosclerosis.
Hyperchylomicronemia	Lipolytic defect for chylomicrons	Increased	1000-10,000 chylomicrons	Rare, autosomal-recessive condition. Symptoms include xanthomas, lipemia retinalis, recurrent abdominal pain, hepatosplenomegaly pancreatitis. Onset in infancy or childhood. Aggravated by high fat intake, diabetes, and alcohol. Low risk for atherosclerosis.
Mixed hypertriglyceridemia		300-1000	500->10,000; chylomicrons high	Symptoms include recurrent abdominal pain, hepatosplenomegaly, xanthomas, glucose intolerance. Symptoms begin in adult life. Aggravated by high fat and alcohol intake and diabetes. Nil to low risk for atherosclerosis.
Dysbetalipoproteinemia	Accumulation of remnantlike lipoproteins called beta VLDLs	200-500	200-500	Palmar xanthomas are typical with yellow discolorations; other xanthomas common. Aggravated by alcohol and estrogen. Increased risk of atherosclerosis and premature atherosclerosis of coronaries, carotids, and abdominal aorta. Cholesterol/triglyceride ratio in VLDL exceeds 0.3.

Adapted from Nicoll D et al: *Pocket guide to diagnostic tests,* ed 2, Stamford, Conn, 1997, Appleton Lange; Cressman M. In Matzen R, Lang R, editors: *Clinical preventive medicine*, St. Louis, 1993, Mosby; and Grundy S: Disorders of lipids and lipoproteins. In Stein J, editor: *Internal medicine,* ed 5, St Louis, 1998, Mosby.

LDL, Low-density lipoprotein; *VLDL,* very low–density lipoprotein.

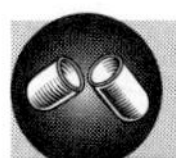

TABLE 95-3 Pharmaceutical Plan: HMG CoA Reductase Inhibitors

Drug	Initial Dose	Maximum Dose	Cost ($)
Atorvastatin (Lipitor)	10 mg/day	80 mg/day	$164/10 mg (90); $254/20 mg (90); $306/40 mg (90);
Cerivistatin (Baycol)	0.3 mg/day	0.3 mg/day	N/A
Fluvastatin (Lescol)	20-40 mg/day q HS	80 mg/day	$115/20 mg (100); $128/40 mg (100)
Lovastatin (Mevacor)	20 mg/day with meals	80 mg/day with meals	$125/20 mg (60); $225/40 mg (60)
Pravastatin (Pravachol)	10-20 mg/day q HS	40 mg/day	$169/10 mg (100); $170/20 mg (90); $288/40 mg (90)
Simvastatin (Zocor)	5-10 mg/day every evening	40 mg/day	$107/5 mg (60); $113/10 mg (60); $204/20 mg (60); $206/40 mg (60)

From National Institutes of Health, National Heart, Lung, and Blood Institute, National Cholesterol Education Program: *Cholesterol lowering in the patient with coronary heart disease* (Publication No. 97-3794), Washington, DC, 1997, NIH; and Woodhead G: The management of cholesterol in coronary heart disease risk reduction, *Nurse Pract: Am J Primary Health Care* 21(9):45-53, 1996.
N/A, available.

Pharmaceutical

Initiate pharmaceutical therapy when:
- LDL cholesterol >190 mg/dl without CHD and fewer than two risk factors
- LDL cholesterol >160 mg/dl without CHD and two or more risk factors
- LDL cholesterol >130 mg/dl in known CHD

Goal LDL levels:
- <100 mg/dl in known CHD
- <130 mg/dl without CHD, two or more risk factors
- <160 mg/dl without CHD, fewer than two risk factors (NCEP, 1997)

Types of Pharmaceutical Intervention

HMG CoA Reductase Inhibitors. Table 95-3 contains the pharmaceutical plan for HMG CoA reductase inhibitors.
- Produce greatest LDL lowering
- Inhibit cholesterol synthesis
- Usually given in a single dose in the evening to maximize LDL reduction
- Pregnancy: X
- Side effects: Gastrointestinal (GI) complaints, myopathies, elevated transaminases
- Repeat lipid and transaminases values 4 to 8 weeks after beginning drug, and at 3 months and as indicated thereafter
- Decrease LDL, total cholesterol, increase HDL, decrease triglycerides

Nicotinic Acid. Table 95-4 contains the pharmaceutical plan for nicotinic acid

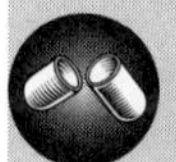

TABLE 95-4 Pharmaceutical Plan: Nicotinic Acid

Drug	Initial Dose	Maximum Dose	Cost
Niacin	125 mg BID and titrate up	1.5-3 g day	$4-$6/SR: 125 mg (100); $1-$3/100 mg (100); $2-$64/500 mg (100)

- Water-soluble B vitamin that affects lipids and lipoproteins
- Decreases LDL and triglycerides, increases HDL (20% to 25%)
- Especially useful in those with elevated LDL, elevated triglycerides, and low HDL
- Pregnancy: A
- Side effects: Flushing, GI complaints, hepatotoxicity, gout, and hyperglycemia
- Flushing can be reduced by taking niacin with a meal or after a meal and with aspirin; tolerance often develops
- Use with caution in those with associated conditions of type 2 diabetes or gout

Bile Acid Sequestrants (Resins). Table 95-5 contains the pharmaceutical plan for bile acid sequestrants.
- Bind with bile acids in the intestine

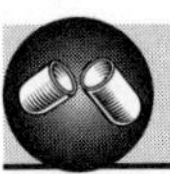

TABLE 95-5 Pharmaceutical Plan: Bile Acid Sequestrants

Drug	Initial Dose	Maximum Dose	Cost
Cholestyramine (Questran)	4 g BID	24 g day (BID-TID dosing)	$83/4 g (60)
Colestipol (Colestid)	5 g BID	30 g day (BID-QID dosing)	$110/5 g (90)

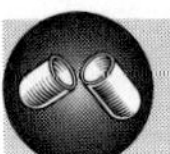

TABLE 95-6 Pharmaceutical Plan: Fibric Acids

Drug	Initial Dose	Maximum Dose	Cost
Gemfibrozil (Lopid)	600 mg BID before meals	1200 mg day	$41-$66/600 mg (60)

- Enhance LDL receptor activity
- Lower LDL, increase HDL (3% to 5%), may increase triglycerides
- Safe to use in combination with statins
- Pregnancy: C
- Side effects: Mainly GI complaints
- Administer within 1 hour of eating
- Interfere with absorption of certain medications: warfarin, digoxin, beta-blockers, thiazide diuretics; oral medications should be taken 1 to 2 hours before or 4 to 6 hours after administration of bile acid sequestrants

Fibric Acids. Table 95-6 contains the pharmaceutical plan for fibric acids.

- Effective in triglyceride lowering
- Not recommended by the Food and Drug Administration as single drug therapy for patients with CHD
- Reduce LDL (10% to 15%), increase HDL (10% to 15%)
- Pregnancy: B
- Side effects: Mainly GI complaints, may aggravate gallstones
- Increases the anticoagulant effect of warfarin (Coumadin), ↑ pro-time/international normalized ratio (PT/INR)

Lifestyle/Activities

Exercise/physical activity

Diet

Primary Prevention

- NCEP recommendation for the general public is equivalent to a STEP I Diet
- Saturated fat intake: 8% to 10% total calories, 30% or less of calories from total fat, and cholesterol <300 mg/day
- STEP II Diet: Instituted if STEP I diet ineffective and in all CAD patients
  - Saturated fat intake <7% of calories and cholesterol to <200 mg/day
  - Registered dietitian or qualified nutritionist helpful in educating on STEP II diet (NCEP 1993).
  - Goal is permanent change in eating habits
- INITIATE diet management
  - In all patients with CAD and LDL >100 mg/dl
  - LDL cholesterol >160 in those without CHD and fewer than two risk factors
  - LDL cholesterol >130 mg/dl in those without CHD and two or more risk factors

Patient Education

- Weight management/maintenance
- Medication compliance
- Importance of office and laboratory follow-up if taking cholesterol medications

Family Impact

Rule out familial hyperlipidemia

Referral

- Refer to registered dietitian if necessary
  - Children
  - Familial hyperlipidemia (refer to lipid specialist)
  - Pregnant women

EVALUATION/FOLLOW-UP

Secondary Prevention: For patients 20 to 70 years of age a measurement of cholesterol should be performed every 5 years unless otherwise indicated.

REFERENCES

Frishman WH, Mahmood SF: Lipid disorders. In Crawford M, editor: *Current diagnosis and treatment of cardiology*, Norwalk, Conn, 1995, Appleton and Lange.

National Institutes of Health, National Heart, Lung, and Blood Institute, National Cholesterol Education Program: *Cholesterol lowering in the patient with coronary heart disease* (Publication No. 97-3794), Washington, DC, 1997, NIH.

SUGGESTED READINGS

National Cholesterol Education Program Expert Panel: *Second report of the expert panel on detection, evaluation, and treatment of high blood cholesterol in adults (Adult Treatment Panel II)* (NIH Publication No. 93-3095), Washington, DC, 1993, U.S. Department of Health and Human Services, Public Health Service, National Institutes of Health, National Heart, Lung, and Blood Institute.

Woodhead G: The management of cholesterol in coronary heart disease risk reduction, *Nurse Pract: Am J Primary Health Care* 21(9):45-53, 1996.

96 Hypertension

ICD-9-CM

Hypertension, Unspecified 401.9
Hypertension, Accelerated 401

OVERVIEW

Definition

Primary (essential) hypertension is an elevation of blood pressure (BP) of more than 140 mm Hg systolic and more than 90 mm Hg diastolic on the average of two or more readings taken at each of two or more visits. Hypertension can be classified into stages, depending on the blood pressure measurement. Hypertension classifications are detailed in Table 96-1.

Urgent hypertension refers to an elevated diastolic blood pressure (DBP) between 120 and 160 mm Hg without symptoms or acute retinopathy.

Severe, accelerated, or malignant hypertension is an elevation of the diastolic blood pressure (DBP) of more than 120 mm Hg with evidence of target organ damage (TOD), such as retinal hemorrhages, exudates, or papilledema, left ventricular hypertrophy or dysfunction, and renal or cerebrovascular injury.

Isolated systolic hypertension (ISH) is a persistent elevated systolic blood pressure (SBP) of more than 160 mm Hg with a diastolic blood pressure (DBP) less than 90 mm Hg.

Hypertensive crisis is a severe elevation of the diastolic BP of more than 120 to 130 mm Hg and is considered an emergency in the presence of acute or ongoing target organ damage, that is, rapid or progressive deterioration of the central nervous system, myocardial, hematological, or renal function.

Pregnancy-induced hypertension (PIH) is an elevated systolic BP 33 mg Hg above and/or diastolic BP 15 mg Hg above normal BP before 20 weeks' gestation.

"White-coat" hypertension is defined as an elevated systolic or diastolic BP that occurs in the office setting (presumably resulting from the patient's response to the presence of medical staff), but normal blood pressure during usual activities outside the office setting.

Secondary hypertension is caused by another underlying pathological condition. The causes of secondary hypertension include:

- Aortic coarctation
- Chronic alcohol use
- Cushing's syndrome
- Oral contraceptives
- Pheochromocytoma
- Polycystic kidney disease
- Pregnancy
- Renovascular disease

Incidence and Susceptibility

Approximately 50 million Americans have elevated BP that requires monitoring or drug therapy. The prevalence increases with age, is greater for blacks than for whites, and occurs more frequently in the less educated, lower socioeconomic populations. Blacks have higher rates of stage 3 hypertension (HTN) with an increased mortality resulting from stroke, heart disease, and end-stage renal disease. There is a higher incidence in **children** who exhibit other risk factors for cardiovascular disease or have hypertensive parents. **PIH** occurs in approximately 7% of all pregnancies. Isolated systolic hypertension (ISH) is seen primarily in **elderly** persons (more than 60 years old), with 4 million people estimated to have ISH.

Factors That Increase Susceptibility

Risk factors that compound the risk for developing HTN include dyslipidemia, cigarette smoking, diabetes mellitus, being older than 60 years of age, and sex (men and postmenopausal women). There is also a strong correlation between a family history of HTN and/or stroke and the development of HTN; this may be the result of genetics, shared environment, or common lifestyle habits.

TABLE 96-1 Classifications of Hypertension

Category	Systolic*	Diastolic*
>Optimal	<120	<80
Normal	<130	<85
High normal	130-139	85-89
Hypertension		
Stage 1	140-159 or	90-99
Stage 2	160-179 or	100-109
Stage 3	≥180 or	≥110

From the Joint National Committee on Detection, Evaluation and Treatment of High Blood Pressure: *The sixth report of the Joint National Committee on Detection, Evaluation and Treatment of High Blood Pressure,* Bethesda, Md, 1997, National Institutes of Health, US Department of Health and Human Services.

*Not taking antihypertensive drugs and not acutely ill. When systolic and diastolic BP fall into different categories, the higher category should be used to classify the individual's BP status. Isolated systolic HTN is defined as systolic BP 140 mm Hg or greater, and diastolic BP less than 90 mm Hg and staged appropriately. Based on the average of two or more readings taken at each of two or more visits after an initial screening.

Boxes 96-1 and 96-2 detail cardiovascular risk factors and target organ damage.

Hypertension in Children and Adolescents

Children and adolescents with a persistently elevated BP that is higher than 95% of children of the same age and sex are at risk for developing the same complications as adults with HTN. Secondary HTN is more common in **children** than in adults. The incidence of secondary HTN is greatest in infancy and late childhood (Table 96-2).

Pathophysiology

Hypertension results from an increase in the total peripheral resistance caused by arteriolar constriction. The regulation of arteriolar constriction is controlled by hemodynamic, neural, renal, and humoral factors. Hemodynamic factors include volume/pressure receptors and chemoreceptors found in the periphery. These receptors provide autoregulation to changes within the system.

The central and autonomic nervous systems regulate BP through the stimulation of alpha- and beta-receptors on the arterioles and venules. The kidneys also provide a humoral response to maintain BP in the presence of decreased blood flow to the kidneys, which results in the release of renin and its subsequent vasoconstrictors, angiotensin and aldosterone. Other humoral mechanisms that regulate BP include the natriuretic hormone and hyperinsulinemia.

Box 96-1

Components of Cardiovascular Risk Stratification in Patients with Hypertension

Major Risk Factors

Smoking
Dyslipidemia
Diabetes mellitus
Age: Older than 60 years
Sex: Men and postmenopausal women
Family history of cardiovascular disease in women younger than 65 years or men younger than 55 years

Box 96-2

Target Organ Damage Related to Hypertension

Heart disease: Left ventricular hypertrophy
Angina or myocardial infarction
Heart failure
Stroke or transient ischemic attack
Nephropathy
Peripheral arterial disease
Retinopathy

From the Joint National Committee on Detection, Evaluation and Treatment of High Blood Pressure: *The sixth report of the Joint National Committee on Detection, Evaluation and Treatment of High Blood Pressure,* Bethesda, Md, 1997, National Institutes of Health, US Department of Health and Human Services.

SUBJECTIVE DATA

History of Present Illness

Symptoms may include blurred vision, chest pain, claudication, dizziness, dyspnea, fatigue, flushing, headaches, hematuria, muscle cramps, palpitations, tingling or cold extremities, or weakness, usually resulting from end-organ damage or the underlying primary disorder. Patients with early primary HTN are usually asymptomatic.

History-taking should include questions about the duration of symptoms, aggravating/relieving factors, and last menstrual period.

Past Medical History

Patients may report a history of:

Cardiovascular disease: Angina, myocardial infarction (MI), heart failure
Cerebrovascular disease: Transient ischemic attack (TIA), cerebrovascular accident (CVA), or seizures

TABLE 96-2 Hypertension in Children and Adolescents

Age	Girls: 50th Percentile for Height (BP)	Girls: 75th Percentile for Height (BP)	Boys: 50th Percentile for Height (BP)	Boys: 75th Percentile for Height (BP)
1	104/58	105/59	102/57	104/58
6	111/73	112/73	114/74	115/75
12	123/80	124/81	123/81	125/82
17	129/84	130/85	136/87	138/88

From the Joint National Committee on Detection, Evaluation and Treatment of High Blood Pressure: *The sixth report of the Joint National Committee on Detection, Evaluation and Treatment of High Blood Pressure,* Bethesda, Md, 1997, National Institutes of Health, US Department of Health and Human Services.

Renal disease: Renal artery stenosis, pheochromocytoma, polycystic kidney disease, Cushing's syndrome
Diabetes mellitus
Dyslipidemia
Gout
Toxemia of pregnancy

Medication History

History-taking should include information on all recent and currently prescribed and over-the-counter medications. Contraceptives, steroids, nonsteroidal antiinflammatory drugs (NSAIDs), nasal decongestants, cold remedies, appetite suppressants, sodium bicarbonate products (antacids), licorice, tricyclic antidepressants, MAO inhibitors, cyclosporine, and erythropoietin can increase and/or interfere with blood pressure therapy.

Family History

Ask about anyone in the family with a history of:

Diabetes mellitus
Dyslipidemia
Hyperparathyroidism
Hypertension
Peripheral vascular disease
Premature coronary artery disease (CAD) (in persons younger than 50 years old)
Renal disease
Stroke, TIA, or seizures
Thyroid disorders

Psychosocial History

History-taking should include information on smoking and alcohol use, diet (especially sodium, cholesterol, and fat intake), employment and family status, educational level, and leisure-time activities.

Information regarding use of illegal drugs (such as cocaine) must also be obtained, since these drugs may contribute to or cause elevated BP.

OBJECTIVE DATA

Physical Examination

A complete physical examination should be conducted to assess for end-target organ damage.

Blood pressure evaluation
Two or more BP readings at least 2 minutes apart, with the patient in the supine or seated position and after standing for 2 minutes.
The initial readings should be taken after 5 minutes of rest.
The patient should not have drunk coffee or smoked cigarettes within 30 minutes of the evaluation.
Check BP in both arms on at least one occasion to verify that the results are equivalent.
The appropriate cuff size should have the bladder encircle at least 80% of the arm above the antecubital space.
Height and Weight
Head: Funduscopic examination for arteriolar narrowing, nicking, hemorrhages, exudates, and papilledema
Neck: Examination for carotid bruits, distended veins, or thyromegaly
Heart: Examination for increased rate, size, precordial heave, clicks, murmurs, arrhythmias, and S_3 or S_4 heart sounds
Abdomen: Examination for bruits, enlarged kidneys, masses, or abnormal aortic pulsations
Extremities: Examination for decreased or absent peripheral arterial pulsations, bruits, or edema

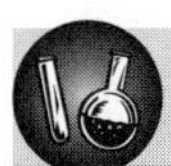

Table 96-3 Diagnostic Tests: Hypertension

Test	Findings/Rationale	Cost ($)
Urinalysis	Identify proteinuria	15-20
CBC	Provide baseline data, identify anemia	18-23
Blood glucose	Rule out diabetes mellitus	15-20
Multiphasic blood chemistry (potassium, calcium, creatinine, uric acid, cholesterol, triglycerides, magnesium)	Provide baseline data Identify comorbid conditions: Dyslipidemia	72-105/general health panel (includes basic metabolic, thyroid, CBC)
12-Lead ECG	Provide baseline data about heart function and rule out LVH and cardiomegaly	56-65
May also consider: Glycosylated hemoglobin	Identify the presence of diabetes and control over last 3 mo	34-43
TSH	Identify thyroid disorders that can affect BP readings	47-61/included in general health panel or thyroid panel
Echocardiography	Provide more specific data regarding heart	675

BP, Blood pressure; *CBC,* complete blood cell count; *LVH,* left ventricular hypertrophy; *TSH,* thyroid-stimulating hormone.

Table 96-4 Additional Diagnostic Tests and Differential Diagnoses

Symptoms	Differential Diagnosis	Diagnostic Tests	Cost ($)
Paroxysmal HTN, headache, palpitations, pallor, perspiration	Pheochromocytoma	24-hour urine collection/ assessment for protein and VMA	54-67/VMA 21-26/albumin
Abdominal bruit lateralizing to renal area or heard during diastole	Renovascular disease	Renal angiography Renal US	703-843 259-319
Abdominal or flank masses	Polycystic kidney	Renal US	259-319
Delayed or absent femoral artery pulses and decreased BP in lower extremities	Aortic coarctation	CXR MRI Echocardiogram	77-91/chest 1552-1839/MRI 675/echo
Truncal obesity with purple striae	Cushing's syndrome	24-hour urine collection/ assessment for free cortisol	57-73

BP, Blood pressure; *CXR,* chest x-ray evaluation; *HTN,* hypertension; *MRI,* magnetic resonance imaging; *US,* ultrasonography; *VMA,* vanilmandelic acid.

Neurological assessment: Examination for deep tendon reflexes, gait, cranial nerves

Diagnostic Procedures

Laboratory testing may be used to assess cardiovascular risk factors as well as evaluating end-organ function. Tests may include those listed in Table 96-3. Additional diagnostic procedures may be indicated to identify the cause of secondary HTN (Table 96-4).

ASSESSMENT

Differential Diagnosis

The differential diagnosis should focus on distinguishing true primary HTN from pseudohypertension resulting from a faulty BP reading and secondary HTN. Suspect an underlying pathological basis for secondary HTN when:

Drug therapy is ineffective in a compliant patient

Elevated BP occurs in individuals under 25 years old or

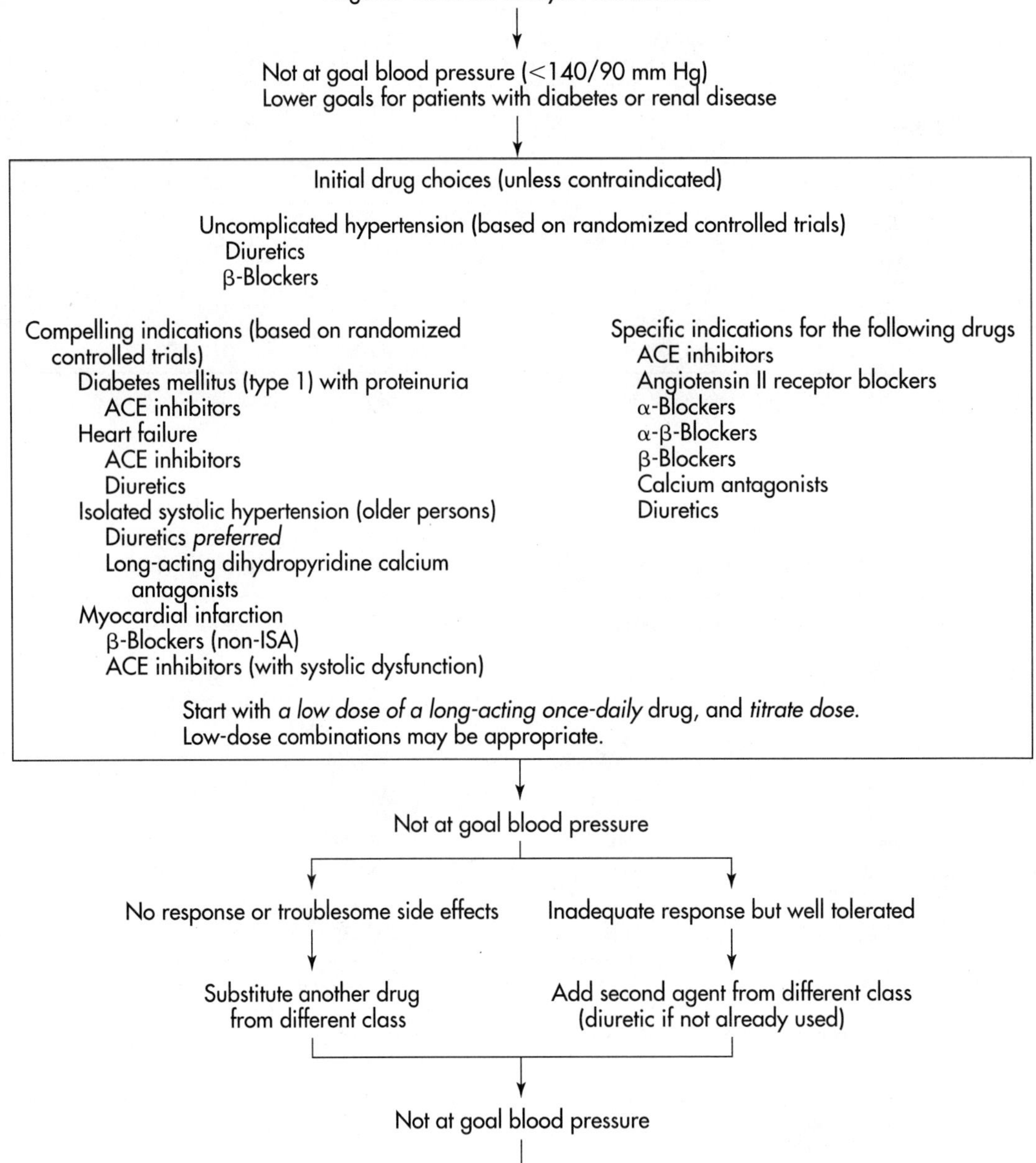

Figure 96-1 Algorithm for the treatment of hypertension. *ACE,* Angiotensin-converting enzyme; *ISA,* intrinsic sympathomimetic activity. (From the Joint National Committee on Detection, Evaluation and Treatment of High Blood Pressure: *The sixth report of the Joint National Committee on Detection, Evaluation and Treatment of High Blood Pressure,* Bethesda, Md, 1997, National Institutes of Health, US Department of Health and Human Services.)

TABLE 96-5 Risk Stratification and Treatment

BP Stages	Risk Group A No Risk Factors; No TOD/CCD	Risk Group B At Least One Risk Factor, Not Including DM; No TOD/CCD	Risk Group C TOD/CCD and/or Diabetes, With or Without Other Risk Factors
High normal (130-139/85-89)	Lifestyle modification	Lifestyle modification	Drug therapy*
Stage 1 (140-159/90-99)	Lifestyle modification (up to 12 mo)	Lifestyle modification† (up to 6 mo)	Drug therapy
Stages 2 and 3 (≥160/≥100)	Drug therapy	Drug therapy	Drug therapy

From the Joint National Committee on Detection, Evaluation and Treatment of High Blood Pressure: *The sixth report of the Joint National Committee on Detection, Evaluation and Treatment of High Blood Pressure,* Bethesda, Md, 1997, National Institutes of Health, US Department of Health and Human Services.
*For those with heart failure, renal insufficiency, or diabetes.
†For patients with multiple risk factors, clinicians should consider drugs as initial therapy plus lifestyle modifications. Lifestyle modification should be adjunctive therapy for all patients recommended for pharmacological therapy.
A patient with diabetes and a BP of 142/94 mm Hg plus LVH should be classified as having Stage 1 HTN with TOD and with another major risk factor (diabetes). This patient would be categorized as stage 1, risk group C, and recommended for immediate initiation of pharmacological treatment.
TOD/CCD, Target organ damage/clinical cardiovascular disease.

over 60 years old in the absence of a family history of hypertension

Associated symptoms occur, such as edema, abnormal pulses or heart sounds, hirsutism, striae, palpitations, perspiration, and dizziness

THERAPEUTIC PLAN

Pharmaceutical

The decision to begin drug therapy should be based on the degree of HTN, the presence of target organ damage, and the presence of clinical cardiovascular disease and other risk factors (Figure 96-1). Table 96-5 identifies treatment strategies for those at risk.

The drug of choice, based on age, need, and comorbid disease, should be initiated at a low dose and titrated upward to provide 24-hour coverage. Ideally, long-acting, once-daily dosing may be preferred because of better compliance and coverage. Twice-daily dosing may provide similar benefits at a lower cost (Tables 96-6 and 96-7).

Combination therapy may provide fewer side effects than would higher doses of a single agent (Table 96-8). If no other indications are evident to initiate a particular agent, drug therapy should begin with a diuretic or beta-blocker, because these have been shown to reduce mortality and morbidity. For patients with comorbid conditions, specific agents may be indicated or contraindicated (Table 96-9).

Drug Interactions

Specific antihypertensive agents may interact with other medications or foods (Table 96-10).

Special Considerations

Special considerations in the treatment of patients with HTN are outlined in Table 96-11, and Table 96-12 reviews the use of antihypertensive drugs in pregnant patients.

Lifestyle Modifications

Lose weight if overweight.

Limit alcohol intake to less than 1 ounce of ethanol per day (24 oz. beer, 8 oz. wine, or 2 oz. 100-proof whiskey).

Exercise aerobically on a regular basis.

Reduce sodium intake to less than 2.3 g of sodium or less than 6 g of sodium chloride.

Maintain adequate dietary intake of potassium, calcium, and magnesium.

Stop smoking and decrease dietary saturated fat and cholesterol. Reducing fat intake will decrease caloric intake for weight control.

Diet

Dietary modification is an essential strategy in the control and prevention of HTN. The diet should be high in fruits,

Text continued on p. 612

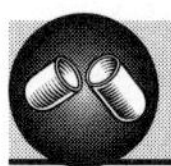

TABLE 96-6 Pharmaceutical Plan: Diuretic Therapy for Hypertension

Drug	Dose	Comments	Cost
Potassium Sparing		Monitor potassium levels for hyperkalemia	
Spironolactone (Aldactone)	25-200 mg/day in 4-5 divided doses **Children:** 1-3/kg/day in divided doses	Take with meals or milk Pregnancy: D SE: Diarrhea, vomiting, rash, pruritus, hyperkalemia	\$5-\$39/25 mg (100) \$71/50 mg (100) \$119/100 mg (100)
Triamterene (Dyrenium)	25-100 mg /day Max 300 mg/day **Children:** 2-4 mg/kg/day	Not recommended for use in children Pregnancy: D SE: Diarrhea, nausea, fatigue, weakness, hyperkalemia	\$32-\$34/50 mg (100) \$34/100 mg (100)
Amiloride (Midamor)	5-10 mg QD Max: 20 mg/day	Pregnancy: B SE: Headache, orthostatic hypotension, nausea, diarrhea, anorexia, hyperkalemia	\$26-\$46/5 mg (100)
Thiazide Type			
Chlorothiazide (Diuril)	250-500 mg QD/BID	Pregnancy: B SE: Adverse lipid values, photosensitivity, hypokalemia, hyponatremia	N/A
Hydrochlorothiazide (e.g., HCTZ, Esidrix)	12.5-50 mg QD	Pregnancy: B SE: Adverse lipid values, photosensitivity, hypokalemia, hyponatremia	\$2-\$13/25 mg (100) \$2-\$21/50 mg (100)
Metolazone (Zaroxolyn)	5 mg QD Max 20 mg/day	Pregnancy: B SE: Hypokalemia, hyponatremia, hyperglycemia, hyperuricemia, gout, blurred vision	\$53/2.5 mg (100) \$59/5 mg (100) \$68/10 mg (100)
Other			
Indapamide (Lozol)	2.5 mg QD; after 1 week may increase to 5 mg/day	Pregnancy: B SE: Hypokalemia, hyponatremia, hyperglycemia, hyperuricemia, gout, blurred vision	\$65/1.25 mg (100) \$66-\$85/2.5 mg (100)
Loop Diuretics			
Bumetanide (Bumex)	0.5-1 mg IV/IM 0.5-2 mg PO (1 mg Bumex ≅ 40 mg furosemide)	Pregnancy: C SE: Muscle cramps, headache, ototoxicity, electrolyte imbalance, hyperuricemia	\$37-\$45/1 mg (100) \$63-\$72/2 mg (100)
Ethacrynic acid (Edecrin)	0.5 -1 mg/kg up to 50 mg IV 25-100 mg PO QD/BID **Children:** 25 mg QD	Use in infants not recommended Pregnancy: B SE: Fluid/electrolyte imbalance, ototoxicity, deafness, vertigo, tinnitus, GI upset, headache, rash	\$20/IV: 50 mg/vial \$30/25 mg (100) \$43/50 mg (100)
Furosemide (Lasix)	1 mg/kg up to 20-40 mg IV 20-80 mg QD/BID **Children:** PO: 2 mg/kg/day as single dose	Pregnancy: C SE: Photosensitivity, xanthopsia, vertigo, paresthesia, jaundice, tinnitus, hypokalemia	\$2-\$16/20 mg (100) \$3-\$22/40 mg (100) \$6-\$37/80 mg (100)

GI, Gastrointestinal; *HCTZ,* hydrochlorothiazide; *SE,* side effects.

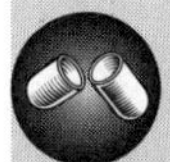

TABLE 96-6 Pharmaceutical Plan: Diuretic Therapy for Hypertension—cont'd

Drug	Dose	Comments	Cost
Torsemide (Demadex)	5-20 mg IV/PO QD	Pregnancy: B Interactions with amphotericin B, anticoagulants, hypokalemia-causing medications, lithium, salicylates (high-dose) SE: Constipation, dizziness, GI upset, headache	$53/5 mg (100) $49/10 mg (100) $53/20 mg (100) $216/100 mg (100)
Combination Diuretics			
Triamterene, HCTZ (Dyazide)	1-2 caps QD	Pregnancy: C SE: Drowsiness, muscle cramps, weakness, headache, GI upset, dry mouth, impotence, urine discoloration	N/A
Spironolactone + HCTZ (Aldactazide)	Used for maintenance: 4 tabs in single or divided doses	Pregnancy: Not recommended SE: Hyperkalemia, gynecomastia, headache, menstrual changes, photosensitivity, GI disturbances	N/A

GI, Gastrointestinal.

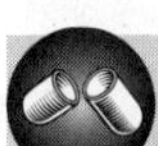

TABLE 96-7 Pharmaceutical Plan: Adrenergic Inhibitors for Hypertension

Drug	Dose	Comments	Cost
Peripheral Agents			
Guanadrel sulfate (Hylorel)	10-75 mg BID	Pregnancy: B SE: Postural hypotension, diarrhea, fatigue, headache, drowsiness, peripheral edema, nocturia, urinary frequency	$72/10 mg (100)
Guanethidine monosulfate (Ismelin)	10-150 mg QD	Pregnancy: C SE: Postural hypotension, diarrhea, dizziness, bradycardia, weakness, inhibition of ejaculation	$50/10 mg (100)
Reserpine (Serpasil) (also acts centrally)	0.05-0.25 QD	Pregnancy: C SE: Nasal congestion, sedation, depression, activation of peptic ulcer, drowsiness	$3-$6/0.1 mg (100)

From the Joint National Committee on Detection, Evaluation and Treatment of High Blood Pressure: *The sixth report of the Joint National Committee on Detection, Evaluation and Treatment of High Blood Pressure,* Bethesda, Md, 1997, National Institutes of Health, US Department of Health and Human Services.

CBC, Complete blood count; *CD,* combination drug; *LFT,* liver function test; *N/V,* nausea and vomiting; *SE,* side effects; *SR,* slow release. *Continued*

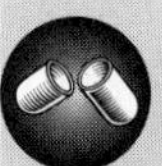

Table 96-7 Pharmaceutical Plan: Adrenergic Inhibitors for Hypertension—cont'd

Drug	Dose	Comments	Cost
Central Alpha-Agonists			
Clonidine HCl (Catapres)	0.2-1.2 mg BID/TID Max 2.4 mg/day	Give first dose at HS to avoid sedation; do not discontinue abruptly Pregnancy: C SE: Drowsiness, dizziness, sedation, nightmares, dry mouth, constipation, anorexia	\$2-\$56/0.1 mg (100)
Methyldopa (Aldomet)	250 mg BID-TID, increase q 2 days as needed Max 3 g/day	Pregnancy: C SE: Sedation, headache, dizziness, decreased libido Monitor CBC, LFTs periodically	\$6-\$27/125 mg (100) \$7-\$34/250 mg (100)
Alpha-Blockers			
Doxazosin mesylate (Cardura)	1 mg QD, increasing to 16 mg if needed; usual range 4-16 mg	Take first dose at HS to avoid orthostatic symptoms Pregnancy: C SE: Dizziness, headache	\$89/1 mg (100)
Prazosin hydrochloride (Minipress)	1 mg BID/TID, increase up to 6-15 mg in divided doses	See doxazosin mesylate	\$6-\$48/1 mg (100)
Terazosin hydrochloride (Hytrin)	1 mg at HS, increase PRN; usual dose 1-5 mg QD Max 20 mg/day	See doxazosin mesylate	\$135/All forms (100)
Beta-Blockers			
Acebutolol (Sectral)	400 mg QD, usual dose 400-800 mg	Pregnancy: B SE: Fatigue, dizziness, headache, impotence, bronchospasm, may mask insulin induced hypoglycemia, decreased exercise tolerance, hypertriglyceridemia	\$121/400 mg (100)
Atenolol (Tenormin)	25 mg QD, increasing to q 1-2 wk to	Pregnancy: C SE: See acebutolol	\$9-\$88/25 mg (100)
Betaxolol (Kerlone)	10 mg QD increased to 20 mg after 7-14 days	Pregnancy: C SE: See acebutolol	\$72/10 mg (100) \$108/20 mg (100)
Bisoprolol (Zebeta)	2.5-5.0 QD, max dose 20 mg QD	Pregnancy: C SE: See acebutolol	\$27/5 mg, 10 mg (30)
Carteolol HCl (Cartrol)	2.5-10 mg QD	Pregnancy: C SE: See acebutolol	\$99/2.5 mg, 5 mg (100)
Metoprolol tartrate (Lopressor)	100 mg/day, max 450 mg/day	Pregnancy: B SE: See acebutolol	\$11-\$57/50 mg (100) \$16-\$82/100 mg (100)
Metoprolol succinate (Toprol-X)	SR 50-100 mg QD, max 400 mg/day		\$67/SR: 100 mg (100)
Nadolol (Corgard)	40 mg QD, increase q 3-7 days, maintenance 40-320	Pregnancy: C SE: See acebutolol	\$85-\$105/40 mg (100) \$116-\$144/80 mg (100)

From the Joint National Committee on Detection, Evaluation and Treatment of High Blood Pressure: *The sixth report of the Joint National Committee on Detection, Evaluation and Treatment of High Blood Pressure,* Bethesda, Md, 1997, National Institutes of Health, US Department of Health and Human Services.

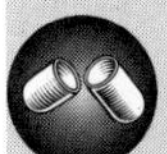

TABLE 96-7 Pharmaceutical Plan: Adrenergic Inhibitors for Hypertension—cont'd

Drug	Dose	Comments	Cost
Penbutolol sulfate (Levatol)	10-20 mg QD	Pregnancy: C SE: See acebutolol	N/A
Pindolol (Visken)	5 mg BID, max 60 mg/day	Pregnancy: B SE: See acebutolol	$23-$80/5 mg (100)
Propranolol HCl (Inderal, Inderal LA)	40 mg BID. Usual range 120-240/day Max/day 640 mg LA 80 mg QD Max 120-160 mg	Pregnancy: C SE: See acebutolol	$2-$60/40 mg (100) $3-$82/80 mg (100) $73-$96/LA: 80 mg (100) $90-$133/120 mg (100)
Timolol maleate (Blocadren)	10 mg BID initially, then 20-40 mg/day in divided doses	Pregnancy C SE: See acebutolol	$26-$57/10 mg (100) $54-$97/20 mg (100)
Combination Alpha- and Beta-Blocker			
Carvedilol (Coreg)	6.25-50 mg BID	Pregnancy: C SE: See acebutolol Contraindicated in significant hepatic dysfunction, CHF class IV, severe bradycardia Do not discontinue abruptly; taper over several weeks Take with food Response less in black patients	N/A
Labetalol (Normodyne, Trandate)	100 mg BID initially, may increase q 2-3 day, max 2.4 g/day	Pregnancy: C SE: See acebutolol Many drug interactions; check drug book before prescribing	$44-$47/100 mg (100) $63-$66/200 mg (100) $84-$87/300 mg (100)
Direct Vasodilators			
Hydralazine (Apresoline)	10 mg QID, increase by 10-25 mg/day to max of 300 mg/day	Pregnancy: C SE: Dizziness, tremors, headache, anxiety, anorexia, N/V/day Take with meals Monitor CBC, ANA titer during therapy	$2-$21/10 mg (100) $2-$29/25 mg (100) $4-$62/50 mg (100)
Calcium Antagonists/Nondihydropyridines			
Diltiazem (Cardizem SR, CD, Dilacor XR)	SR 60-120 mg BID, increase q 2 wk Max 350 mg/day	Pregnancy: C SE: Dizziness, headache, conduction arrhythmias, edema, nausea, gingival hyperplasia Drug interactions: check prior to RX	$71-$92/SR 60 mg (100) $81-$105/90 mg (100)
Mibefradil (Posicor)	50-100 mg QD	See diltiazem	N/A
Verapamil (Covera, Calan)	80 mg TID or 240 mg SR Max dose 480 mg		$52-$119/SR: 180 mg (100) $54-$136/240 mg (100) $5-$48/80 mg (100)

Continued

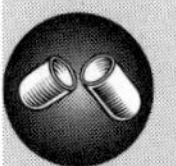

Table 96-7 Pharmaceutical Plan: Adrenergic Inhibitors for Hypertension—cont'd

Drug	Dose	Comments	Cost
Dihydropyridines			
Amlodipine (Norvasc)	5 mg QD, increase up to 10 mg QD	Pregnancy: C SE: Dysrhythmia, peripheral edema, flushing, gingival hypertrophy, flushing, headache	$103/5 mg (100) $178/10 mg (100)
Felodipine (Plendil)	5 mg QD, usual range 5-10 mg Max 20 mg/day	See amlodipine	$90/2.5 mg, 5 mg (100) $161/10 mg (100)
Isradipine (DynaCirc)	2.5 mg BID, increase in 2- to 4-wk intervals; max 10 mg BID	See amlodipine	$52-$56/2.5 mg (100) $82/5 mg (100)
Nicardipine (Cardene SR)	SR 30 mg BID, may increase to 60 mg BID	See amlodipine	$40/30 mg (60) $63/45 mg (60)
Nifedipine (Procardia XL, Adalat)	10 mg PO TID; usual range 10-20 mg TID XL 30-60 mg; titrate to 120 mg max	See amlodipine	$11-$53/10 mg (100) $17-$95/20 mg (100) $90-$120/SR: 30 mg (100) $151-$207/60 mg (100)
Nisoldipine (Sular)	20 mg QD increase by 10 mg/wk Max 60 mg/day	See amlodipine	$82/10, 20, 30, 40 mg (100)
ACE Inhibitors			
Benazepril (Lotensin)	10 mg QD, increase PRN to 20-40 mg/day	Pregnancy: C first trimester; D second and third trimesters SE: Cough, headache, dizziness, fatigue, decreased libido	$64/10, 20, 40 mg (100)
Captopril (Capoten)	12.5 mg BID/TID; usual range 25-150 mg BID/TID Max 450 mg /day	See benazepril	$63-$67/12.5 (100) $68-$73/25 mg (100) $116-$124/50 mg (100) $155-$165/100 mg (100)
Enalapril (Vasotec)	2.5-5 mg QD, usual dose 20-40 mg	See benazepril	$72/2.5 mg (100) $91/5 mg (100) $136/20 mg (100)
Fosinopril (Monopril)	10 mg QD, then 20-40 mg divided BID or QD Max 80 mg/day	See benazepril	$71/10 mg (100) $76/20 mg (100) $22/40 mg (30)
Lisinopril (Prinivil, Zestril)	10 mg QD, usual dose 20-40 mg/day	See benazepril	$81/10 mg (100) $87/20 mg (100) $127/40 mg (100)
Moexipril (Univasc)	7.5 mg PO 1 hr AC QD, usual dose 7.5-30 mg	See benazepril	$40/7.5, 15 mg (100)
Quinapril (Accupril)	10 mg QD, adjust dose q 2 wk, max 80 mg/day divided QD or BID	See benazepril	$91/5 mg, 10 mg, 20 mg (100)
Ramipril (Altace)	2.5 mg QD, adjust dose q 2 wk, usual range 2.5-20 mg/day in QD or BID doses	See benazepril	$69/2.5 mg (100) $74/5 mg (100) $86/10 mg (100)
Trandolapril (Mavik)	1 mg QD (nonblack patients) or 2 mg QD (black patients), increase q 1 wk Max dose 8 mg/day	See benazepril	$63/1 mg, 2 mg, 4 mg (100)

From the Joint National Committee on Detection, Evaluation and Treatment of High Blood Pressure: *The sixth report of the Joint National Committee on Detection, Evaluation and Treatment of High Blood Pressure,* Bethesda, Md, 1997, National Institutes of Health, US Department of Health and Human Services.

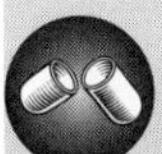

TABLE 96-7 Pharmaceutical Plan: Adrenergic Inhibitors for Hypertension—cont'd

Drug	Dose	Comments	Cost
Angiotensin II Receptor Blockers			
Losartan (Cozaar)	25-50 mg QD	Pregnancy: C first trimester; D second and third trimesters SE: Angioedema (rare), dizziness, insomnia, nasal congestion; increased BUN, creatinine	$110/All forms (100)
Valsartan (Diovan)	80-320 mg QD		$114/80 mg, 160 mg (100)
Irbesartan (Avapro)	150-300 mg QD		Not available

TABLE 96-8 Combination Drugs for Hypertension

Drug	Trade Name
β-adrenergic blockers and diuretics	
Atenolol, 50 or 100 mg/chlorthalidone, 25 mg	Tenoretic
Bisoprolol fumarate, 2.5, 5, or 10 mg/hydrochlorothiazide, 6.25 mg	Ziac*
Metoprolol tartrate, 50 or 100 mg/hydrochlorothiazide, 25 or 50 mg	Lopressor HCT
Nadolol, 40 or 80 mg/bendroflumethiazide, 5 mg	Corzide
Propranolol hydrochloride, 40 or 80 mg/hydrochlorothiazide, 25 mg	Inderide
Propranolol hydrochloride (extended release), 80, 120, or 160 mg/hydrochlorothiazide, 50 mg	Inderide LA
Timolol maleate, 10 mg/hydrochlorothiazide, 25 mg	Timolide
Angiotensin-converting enzyme (ACE) inhibitors and diuretics	
Benazepril hydrochloride, 5, 10, or 20 mg/hydrochlorothiazide, 6.25, 12.5 or 25 mg	Lotensin HCT
Captopril, 25 or 50 mg/hydrochlorothiazide, 15 or 25 mg	Capozide*
Enalapril maleate, 5 or 10 mg/hydrochlorothiazide, 12.5 or 25 mg	Vaseretic
Lisinopril, 10 or 20 mg/hydrochlorothiazide, 12.5 or 25 mg	Prinzide, Zestoretic
Angiotensin II receptor antagonists and diuretics	
Losartan potassium, 50 mg/hydrochlorothiazide, 12.5 mg	Hyzaar
Calcium antagonists and ACE inhibitors	
Amlodipine besylate, 2.5 or 5 mg/benazepril hydrochloride, 10 or 20 mg	Lotrel
Diltiazem hydrochloride, 180 mg/enalapril maleate, 5 mg	Teczem
Verapamil hydrochloride (extended release), 180 or 240 mg/trandolapril, 1, 2, or 4 mg	Tarka
Felodipine, 5 mg/enalapril maleate, 5 mg	Lexxel
Other combinations	
Triamterene, 37.5, 50, or 75 mg/hydrochlorothiazide, 25 or 50 mg	Dyazide, Maxide
Spironolactone, 25 or 50 mg/hydrochlorothiazide, 25 or 50 mg	Aldactazide
Amiloride hydrochloride, 5 mg/hydrochlorothiazide, 50 mg	Moduretic
Guanethidine monosulfate, 10 mg/hydrochlorothiazide, 25 mg	Esimil
Hydralazine hydrochloride, 25, 50, or 100 mg/hydrochlorothiazide, 25 or 50 mg	Apresazide
Methyldopa, 250 or 500 mg/hydrochlorothiazide, 15, 25, 30, or 50 mg	Aldoril
Reserpine, 0.125 mg/hydrochlorothiazide, 25 or 50 mg	Hydropres
Reserpine, 0.10 mg/hydralazine hydrochloride, 25 mg/hydrochlorothiazide, 15 mg	Ser-Ap-Es
Clonidine hydrochloride, 0.1, 0.2, or 0.3 mg/chlorthalidone, 15 mg	Combipres
Methyldopa, 250 mg/chlorothiazide, 150 or 250 mg	Aldochlor
Reserpine, 0.125 or 0.25 mg/chlorthalidone, 25 or 50 mg	Demi-Regroton
Reserpine, 0.125 or 0.25 mg/chlorothiazide, 250 or 500 mg	Diupres
Prazosin hydrochloride, 1, 2, or 5 mg/polythiazide, 0.5 mg	Minizide

*Approved for initial therapy.

TABLE 96-9 Considerations for Individualizing Antihypertensive Drug Therapy

Indication	Drug Therapy
Compelling Indications Unless Contraindicated	
Diabetes mellitus (type 1) with proteinuria	ACE I
Heart failure	ACE I, diuretics
Isolated systolic hypertension (older patients)	Diuretics (preferred), CA (long-acting DHP)
Myocardial infarction	β-blockers (non-ISA), ACE I (with systolic dysfunction)
May Have Favorable Effects on Comorbid Conditions*	
Angina	β-blockers, CA
Atrial tachycardia and fibrillation	β-blockers, CA (non-DHP)
Cyclosporine-induced hypertension (caution with the dose of cyclosporine)	CA
Diabetes mellitus (types 1 and 2) with proteinuria	ACE I (preferred), CA
Diabetes mellitus (type 2)	Low-dose diuretics
Dyslipidemia	α-Blockers
Essential tremor	β-Blockers (non-CS)
Heart failure	Carvedilol, losartan potassium
Hyperthyroidism	β-Blockers
Migraine	β-Blockers (non-CS), CA (non-DHP)
Myocardial infarction	Diltiazem hydrochloride, verapamil hydrochloride
Osteoporosis	Thiazides
Preoperative hypertension	β-Blockers
Prostatism (BPH)	α-Blockers
Renal insufficiency (caution in renovascular hypertension and creatinine level ≥265.2 μmol/L [≥3 mg/dL])	ACE I
May Have Unfavorable Effects on Comorbid Conditions*†	
Bronchospastic disease	β-Blockers‡
Depression	β-Blockers, central α-agonists, reserpine‡
Diabetes mellitus (types 1 and 2)	β-Blockers, high-dose diuretics
Dyslipidemia	β-Blockers (non-ISA), diuretics (high-dose)
Gout	Diuretics
Second- or third-degree heart block	β-Blockers,‡ CA (non DHP)‡
Heart failure	β-Blockers (except carvedilol), CA (except amlodipine besylate; felodipine)
Liver disease	Labetalol hydrochloride, methyldopa‡
Peripheral vascular disease	β-Blockers
Pregnancy	ACE I,‡ angiotensin II receptor blockers‡
Renal insufficiency	Potassium-sparing agents
Renovascular disease	ACE I, angiotensin II receptor blockers

From the Joint National Committee on Detection, Evaluation and Treatment of High Blood Pressure: *The sixth report of the Joint National Committee on Detection, Evaluation and Treatment of High Blood Pressure,* Bethesda, Md, 1997, National Institutes of Health, US Department of Health and Human Services.

ACE I, angiotensin-converting enzyme inhibitors; *BPH,* benign prostatic hyperplasia; *CA,* calcium antagonists; *DHP,* dihydropyridine; *ISA,* intrinsic sympathomimetic activity; *MI,* myocardial infarction; *non-CS,* noncardioselective.

*Conditions and drugs are listed in alphabetical order.

†These drugs may be used with special monitoring unless contraindicated.

‡Contraindicated.

TABLE 96-10 Selected Drug Interactions with Antihypertensive Therapy

Class of Agent	Increase Efficacy	Decrease Efficacy	Effect on Other Drugs
Diuretics	Diuretics that act at different sites in the nephron (e.g., furosemide + thiazides)	Resin-binding agents NSAIDs Corticosteroids	Diuretics raise serum lithium levels Potassium-sparing agents may exacerbate hyperkalemia due to ACE inhibitors
β-Blockers	Cimetidine (hepatically metabolized β-blockers) Quinidine (hepatically metabolized β-blockers) Food (hepatically metabolized β-blockers)	NSAIDs Withdrawal of clonidine Agents that induce hepatic enzymes, including rifampin and phenobarbital	Propranolol hydrochloride induces hepatic enzymes to increase clearance of drugs with similar metabolic pathways β-Blockers may mask and prolong insulin-induced hypoglycemia Heart block may occur with nondihydropyridine calcium antagonists Sympathomimetics cause unopposed α-adrenoceptor-mediated vasoconstriction β-Blockers increase angina-inducing potential of cocaine
ACE inhibitors	Chlorpromazine or clozapine	NSAIDs Antacids Food decreases absorption (moexipril)	ACE inhibitors may raise serum lithium levels ACE inhibitors may exacerbate hyperkalemic effect of potassium-sparing diuretics
Calcium antagonists	Grapefruit juice (some dihydropyridines) Cimetidine or ranitidine (hepatically metabolized calcium antagonists)	Agents that induce hepatic enzymes, including rifampin and phenobarbital NSAIDs	Cyclosporine levels increase* with diltiazem hydrochloride, verapamil hydrochloride, mibefradil dihydrochloride, or nicardipine hydrochloride (but not felodipine, isradipine, or nifedipine) Nondihydropyridines increase levels of other drugs metabolized by the same heptic enzyme system, including digoxin, quinidine, sulfonylureas, and theophylline Verapamil hydrochloride may lower serum lithium levels
α-Blockers			Prazosin hydrochloride may decrease clearance of verapamil hydrochloride
Central α_2-agonists and peripheral neuronal blockers		Tricyclic antidepressants (and probably phenothiazines) Monoamine oxidase inhibitors Sympathomimetics or phenothiazines antagonize guanethidine monosulfate or guanadrel sulfate Iron salts may reduce methyldopa absorption	Methyldopa may increase serum lithium levels Severity of clonidine hydrochloride withdrawal may be increased by β-blockers Many agents used in anesthesia are potentiated by clonidine hydrochloride

From the Joint National Committee on Detection, Evaluation and Treatment of High Blood Pressure: *The sixth report of the Joint National Committee on Detection, Evaluation and Treatment of High Blood Pressure,* Bethesda, Md, 1997, National Institutes of Health, US Department of Health and Human Services.

*This is a clinically and economically beneficial drug-drug interaction because it both retards progression of accelerated atherosclerosis in heart transplant recipients and reduces the required daily dose of cyclosporine.

ACE, Angiotensin-converting enzyme; *NSAIDs,* nonsteroidal anti-inflammatory drugs.

TABLE 96-11 Special Considerations in Treating Patients with Hypertension

Characteristic	Recommendation
Demographics	Black patients tend to respond better to diuretics and calcium antagonists than to beta-blockers or ACE inhibitors; no differences have been found in treatment responses regarding sex or age groups.
Elderly	This group responds to all classes of drugs.
Quality of life	Undesirable side effects of drug therapy may worsen quality of life and play a role in noncompliance.
Economic constraints	Drug therapy, routine laboratory tests, follow-up office visits, and time off from work should be considered in selecting therapy
Patients with comorbid disease	Chose medications that may help treat coexisting disease.
Children	Lifestyle modifications should be initiated first and drug therapy begun for higher levels of BP or unsuccessful response to lifestyle modifications. Choice of drugs for children is similar to adults, but at smaller doses. ACE and angiotensin II blockers should be avoided in pregnant or sexually active young women or in combination with anabolic steroids. The underlying cause, severity, and potential complications should determine intensity and type of therapy required. Children with insulin-dependent diabetes mellitus and primary renal disease should be treated with drug therapy to slow disease progression.

ACE, Angiotensin-converting enzymes; *BP,* blood pressure.

TABLE 96-12 Use of Antihypertensive Drugs in Pregnant Patients

Suggested Drug	Comments
Central alpha-agonists	Methyldopa (Aldomet) is the drug of choice.
Beta-blockers	Atenolol and metoprolol appear to be safe in late pregnancy (Pregnancy C). Labetalol HCl also appears to be effective.
Calcium antagonists	Potential synergism with magnesium sulfate may lead to precipitous hypotension.
ACE inhibitors, angiotensin II receptor blockers	Fetal abnormalities, including death, can be caused, and these drugs should not be used in pregnant patients.
Diuretics	Diuretics are recommended for chronic hypertension if prescribed before pregnancy or if patients appear salt sensitive. Their use is not recommended in patients with preeclampsia.
Direct vasodilators	Hydralazine hydrochloride is the parenteral drug of choice, based on its long history of safety and efficacy.

From the Joint National Committee on Detection, Evaluation and Treatment of High Blood Pressure: *The sixth report of the Joint National Committee on Detection, Evaluation and Treatment of High Blood Pressure,* Bethesda, Md, 1997, National Institutes of Health, US Department of Health and Human Services.

vegetables, low-fat dairy foods, and reduced in amounts of saturated and total fats. Also, sodium should be reduced and the amount of calcium and magnesium should be increased. However, no data exist to recommend mineral supplements.

Patient Education

Education for patient and family should include:

- Lifestyle modification
- Actions and side effects of medications
- Self-measurement of BP
- Necessity for compliance when asymptomatic

Family Impact

The long-term impact of complications caused by uncontrolled HTN include irreversible TOD and premature death. Certainly, the financial, emotional, and physical strain of serious cardiovascular, cerebrovascular, and renal disease caused by HTN will impact family dynamics.

TABLE 96-13 Recommendations for Follow-up Based on Initial Blood Pressure Measurements in Adults*

Systolic	Diastolic	Follow-up Recommended†
<130	<85	Recheck in 2 years
130-139	85-89	Recheck in 1 year
140-159	90-99	Confirm within 2 months; provide advance advice about lifestyle modifications
160-179	100-109	Evaluate or refer to source of care within 1 month
≥180	≥110	Evaluate or refer to source of care immediately or within 1 week, depending on clinical situation

From the Joint National Committee on Detection, Evaluation and Treatment of High Blood Pressure: *The sixth report of the Joint National Committee on Detection, Evaluation and Treatment of High Blood Pressure,* Bethesda, Md, 1997, National Institutes of Health, US Department of Health and Human Services.

*If systolic and diastolic categories are different, follow recommendations for shorter follow-up.

†Modify the scheduling of follow-up according to reliable information about past blood pressure, other cardiovascular risk factors, or TOD.

Family members also need to know their family's cardiovascular history, and that having a family member with HTN also increases their risk of also having HTN. Stress the importance of family members exercising, watching their diet, and having their BP checked periodically.

Referral

Referral is indicated for patients with:

- Stage 3 HTN (or hypertensive emergencies)
- Presence of TOD
- HTN unresponsive to therapy
- Suspected secondary HTN

Consultation

Consider consultation with MD for patients with:

- Stage 2 HTN unresponsive to therapy
- Sudden onset HTN in previously controlled, compliant patients

EVALUATION/FOLLOW-UP

Once the patient's condition is stabilized, follow-up for hypertensive patients should be at 3- to 6-month intervals. Normotensive patients should be evaluated every 1 or 2 years. Table 96-13 identifies recommendations for follow-up based on initial BP measurements in adults.

SUGGESTED READINGS

Calhoun D, Oprаril S: Treatment of hypertensive crisis, *N Engl J Med* 323:1177-1182, 1990.

Dipiro J et al: *Pharmacotherapy: a pathophysiologic approach,* Norwalk, Conn, 1997, Appleton & Lange.

Ellsworth A et al: *Mosby's 1998 medical drug reference,* St Louis, 1998, Mosby.

Healthcare Consultants of America, Inc: *1998 Physicians fee and coding guide,* Augusta, Ga, 1998, Healthcare Consultants of America, Inc.

Hurst JW: Hypertension. In *Atlas of the heart,* New York, 1988, JB Lippincott.

Joint National Committee on Detection, Evaluation and Treatment of High Blood Pressure: *The sixth report of the Joint National Committee on Detection, Evaluation and Treatment of High Blood Pressure,* Bethesda, Md, 1997, National Institutes of Health, US Department of Health and Human Services.

Kannam J, Levy D: Isolated systolic hypertension in the elderly, *Hosp Practice* 28(9)57-61, 1993.

National High Blood Pressure Education Program Working Group on HTN Control in Children and Adolescents: Update on the 1987 task force report on high blood pressure in children and adolescents: a working group report form the National High Blood Pressure Education Program, *Pediatrics* 98:649-658, 1996.

Task Force on Blood Pressure Control in Children: Report of the second task force on blood pressure control in children, *Pediatrics* 79:1-25, 1987.

US Public Health Service, US Department of Health and Human Services: Put prevention into practice, *Nurse Pract* 9:27-31, 1997.

97 Impetigo

ICD-9-CM

Vesiculopustular Rash 782.1

OVERVIEW

Definition

Impetigo is a contagious infection of the skin.

Incidence

Impetigo is the most common skin infection seen in **children.**

Pathophysiology

There are two forms: Streptococcal, which produces crusted lesions, and staphylococcal, which produces bullae. The incubation period is up to 3 days. Impetigo is communicable up to 48 hours after treatment is initiated.

Protective Factors Against Impetigo

Good hygiene

Factors That Increase Susceptibility to Impetigo

Poor hygiene
Overcrowding

SUBJECTIVE DATA

History of Present Illness

Sores
Pruritus
Minor trauma (insect bites, scratches)

Past Medical History

Recent chickenpox, scabies, insect bites

Medications

None significant

Family History

Determine whether another member in the home has recently had impetigo.

Psychosocial History

Living conditions

Associated Symptoms

Fever

OBJECTIVE DATA

Physical Examination

Skin: Most often involves face, nose, perioral, and exposed areas. Lesions begin as macules, then evolve into vesicles, finally becoming pustular. There may be a mixture of lesions. Usually there is a clear vesicle on an erythematous base. Bullae with clear fluid progressing to cloudy fluid may be present (Figures 97-1 and 97-2).
Undress the patient and check entire body for lesions.
Lymph nodes: Check for regional adenopathy.

Diagnostic Procedures

Laboratory tests are usually not necessary; diagnosis is made on clinical grounds.
If there is doubt, a Gram stain ($17 to $21) and culture of the drainage can be performed.

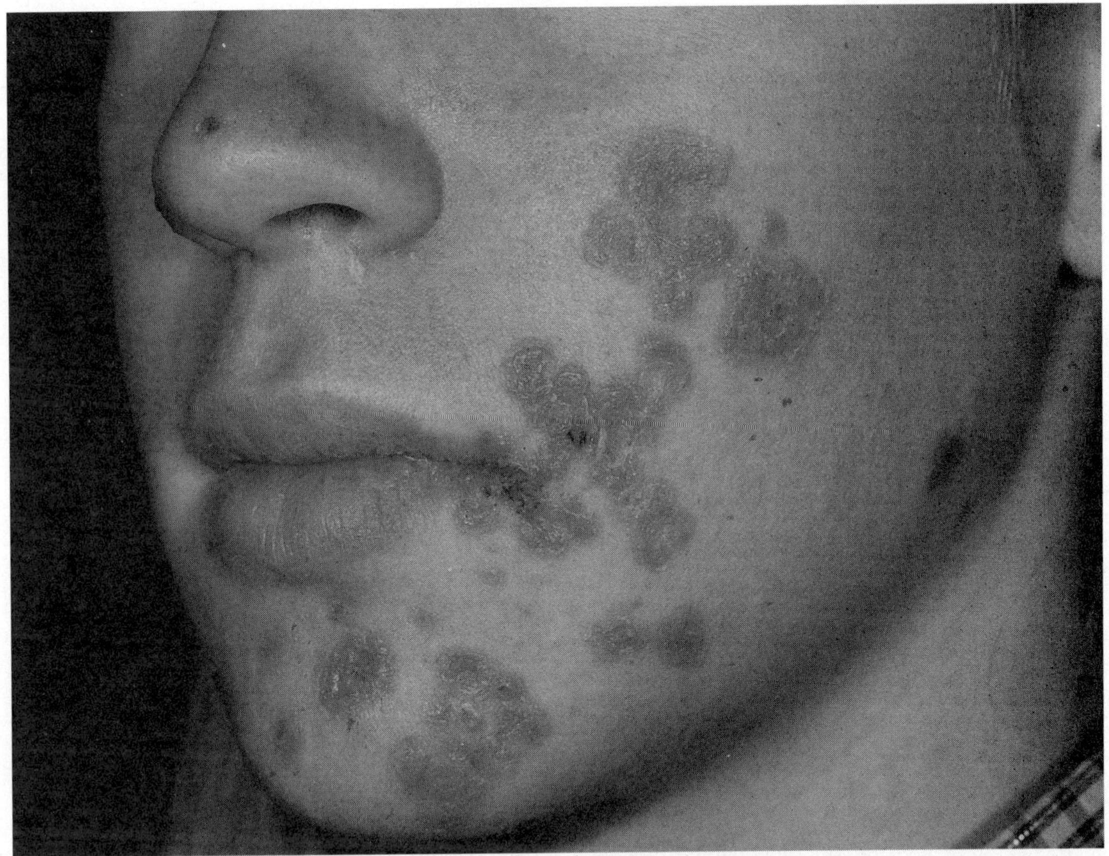

Figure 97-1 Impetigo. A thick, honey-yellow adherent crust covers the entire eroded surface. (From Habif T: *Clinical dermatology,* ed 2, St Louis, 1996, Mosby.)

ASSESSMENT

Differential Diagnosis

Differential diagnoses include those listed in Table 97-1.

THERAPEUTIC PLAN

Pharmaceutical

A pharmaceutical plan for treatment of impetigo is outlined in Table 97-2.

Lifestyle/Activities

Remove crusts by gentle washing with warm water and antibacterial soap.
Wash linen and towels separately.
Trim fingernails to minimize scratching.

Diet

Noncontributory.

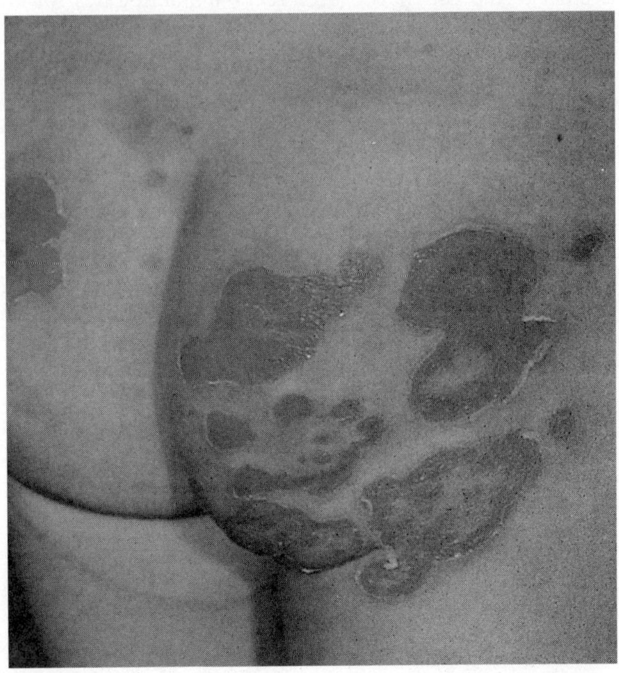

Figure 97-1 Bullous impetigo. Huge lesions with a glistening, eroded base and a collarette of moist scale. (From Habif T: *Clinical dermatology,* ed 2, St Louis, 1996, Mosby.)

TABLE 97-1 Differential Diagnosis: Impetigo

Diagnosis	Supporting Data
Herpes simplex	Usually history of recurrences; grouped vesicles, or discrete erosions
Contact dermatitis	Erythema and edema; history of exposure to suspected irritant; location suggests cause; asymmetrical distribution with linear lesions
Ecthyma	Deeper form of impetigo with ulceration and scarring

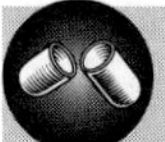

TABLE 97-2 Pharmaceutical Plan: Impetigo

Drug	Dose	Comment	Cost
Mupirocin ointment	2% (dispense as 15 g) Use TID for 10 days	Use only for very small lesion/area; consider oral antibiotics	$29/30 g
Dicloxacillin	250 mg QID 12.5-25 mg/kg/day in four divided doses for 10 days		$20-$94 $16/Oral solution
Cephalexin	50 mg/kg/day for 10 days		$15-$130
Erythromycin	250 mg QID or 30-50 mg/kg/day in four divided doses for 10 days		$14-$20

Patient Education

Teach that if left untreated or not adequately treated, impetigo could progress to systemic infection with serious complications.

The child should not return to school until the lesions are clear or the patient has been receiving antibiotics for 48 hours.

Teach that change in urine color and output should be noted and the health care provider called.

Warn about possible renal problems in rare cases.

Family Impact

Check other family members for lesions.

Referral/Consultation

Refer the patient to a physician if: There are symptoms of acute glomerulonephritis (see Chapter 156).

There is no improvement after 4 days.

Bullae appear in a newborn or infant.

Follow-up

By phone in 24 hours, particularly if topical treatment was used

EVALUATION

Fewer lesions and less vesicles

Normal results on urinalysis

SUGGESTED READINGS

Berger T, Goldstein S, Odom R: Skin and appendages. In Tierney L, McPhee S, Papadakis M, editors: *Current medical diagnosis and treatment,* ed 36, Norwalk, Conn, 1998, Appleton & Lange.

Boynton R, Dunn E, Stephens G: *Manual of ambulatory pediatrics,* ed 4, Philadelphia, 1998, JB Lippincott.

Ellsworth A et al: *Mosby's 1998 medical drug reference,* St Louis, 1998, Mosby.

Healthcare Consultants of America, Inc: *1998 Physicians fee and coding guide,* Augusta, Ga, 1998, Healthcare Consultants of America, Inc.

Pierce N: Bacterial infections of the skin. In Barker L, Burton J, Zieve P, editors: *Principles of ambulatory medicine,* ed 4, Baltimore, 1995, Williams & Wilkins.

98 Impotence

ICD-9-CM

Impotence 302.72

OVERVIEW

Definition

Impotence or erectile dysfunction is the inability to achieve and maintain an erection of the penis with sufficient rigidity (tumescence) to allow for sexual intercourse. The condition may be chronic, occasional, or situational.

Incidence

It is estimated that 10 to 30 million men are affected by impotence.

Most men experience occasional impotence from fatigue or tension.

Only 5% of affected men seek professional help for impotence.

Impotence can affect any male after puberty.

Impotence is age related, affecting 25% of men older than 60 years of age.

Chronic impotence can affect younger men as well as older men.

Treatment can restore sexual function in approximately 95% of cases.

Eighty-five percent of cases of chronic impotence result from physical causes (although many cases have coinciding psychological factors).

Pathophysiology

Vascular problems: Arteriosclerosis, hypertension (Chapter 96), coronary artery disease, peripheral arterial insufficiency, chronic renal insufficiency, or renal failure (Chapter 156)

Endocrine disorders: Diabetes mellitus (Chapter 55), thyroid disease (Chapter 178), adrenal disorders, hyperprolactinemia, hypogonadism, pituitary disorders

Neurological disorders: Brain or spinal cord injuries, Alzheimer's disease (Chapter 9), Parkinson's disease (Chapter 139), multiple sclerosis (Chapter 120), epilepsy

Psychological disorders: Affective, psychotic, and personality disorders

Prescription and over-the-counter medications: Antihypertensive agents; cardiac drugs; diuretics; psychoactive medications, including antidepressants, tranquilizers, and sedatives; anticholinergic agents; antiparkinson's drugs; indomethacin; metronidazole

Oncological radiation treatments

Prostate, bladder, rectum, and colon surgery

Alcohol, cigarettes, illegal drugs, and substance abuse

Penile deformities and prostate infections

Congenital syndromes

SUBJECTIVE DATA

History of Present Illness

Ask the patient about:

- Onset and duration of symptoms, including libido, the ability to achieve and maintain an erection, orgasm, ejaculation, and satisfaction with sex life
- Current sexual relationships and past sexual experiences and behaviors

Concurrent medical conditions, including endocrine disorders, vascular problems, neurological problems, and psychiatric problems
Smoking, alcohol, and substance abuse

Medication History

Ask the patient about all current prescription and over-the-counter medications taken; many of these can cause erectile dysfunction (Box 98-1).

Past Medical History

Ask about past genitourinary surgeries.
Ask about sexual development and secondary sex characteristics.

OBJECTIVE DATA

Physical Examination

As part of the physical examination, assess the following:
Vital signs, including blood pressure
Body habitus and secondary sex characteristics
Presence of gynecomastia
Abdomen and inguinal area for scars from past genitourinary surgeries
Genitourinary area: Penis, scrotum, testes
Prostate and anal sphincter tone
Femoral and lower extremity pulses
Neurological examination of perianal sensation and lower extremities

Diagnostic Procedures

Diagnostic procedures for impotence include those listed in Table 98-1.

ASSESSMENT

Differential Diagnosis

Differential diagnoses for male sexual disfunction are listed in Table 98-2.

THERAPEUTIC PLAN

Pharmaceutical

Androgen deficiency can be treated with testosterone injections, 200 mg IM q 2 to 3 weeks ($13 to $59). Prostatic cancer should be excluded by a screening PSA and ultrasonography.

Sildenafil (Viagra) ($17 to $23) 50 mg PO 1 hour before sexual intercourse. (May be taken 30 minutes to 4 hours before intercourse.) Dose may be adjusted to the maximum dose of 100 mg per day or decreased to 25 mg per day. *Viagra is contraindicated in patients who take concurrent organic nitrates and should not be prescribed to any patient who may have access to nitrates in any form, at an time, for any reason.* Success rate is 66%. Side effects are headache and flushing. If the patient is taking a cytochrome P-450 isoenzyme 3A4 inhibitor (see Appendix D for a list of these drugs) (e.g., cimetidine, erythromycin, ketoconazole, and mibefradil) use a smaller dosage, since clearance of sildenafil is decreased.

Intraurethral alprostadil (MUSE) penile suppository. Side effects are penile pain and hypotension. Efficacy is inconsistent.

Vacuum constrictive devices are appropriate for patients with venous disorders of the penis. The device draws the penis into an erect state by inducing a vacuum within a cylinder. Once an adequate erection is achieved, a constrictive rubber band is placed around the proximal

Box 98-1

Drugs That Cause Erectile Dysfunction

Antihypertensive Medications
Beta-blockers
Thiazide diuretics
Spironolactone
Methyldopa
Reserpine
Clonidine
Guanethidine
Calcium-channel blocking agents

Central Nervous System Medications
Monoamine oxidase inhibitors
Opioids
Phenothiazine antipsychotic agents
Tricyclic antidepressant agents
Haloperidol
Selective serotonin reuptake inhibitors

Endocrine System Medications
Estrogens
Antiandrogens
Gonadotropin antagonists

Miscellaneous
Cimetidine
Metoclopramide
Fibric acid derivatives
Disopyramide
Nicotine
Sympathomimetic agents (epinephrine, phenylephrine, pseudoephedrine)

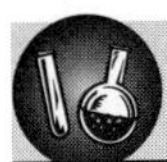

TABLE 98-1 Diagnostic Tests: Impotence

Test	Findings/Rationale	Cost ($)
Urinalysis	Assess for infection	14-18
Complete blood count	Assess for anemia, infection	13-16
Serum creatinine	Assess renal function	18-23
Albumin		18-23
Blood urea nitrogen		17-21
Lipid profile	Assess for hyperlipidemia	49-62
Fasting blood	Assess for diabetes	16-20
Thyroid profile, thyroid-stimulating hormone	Assess for thyroid disease	47-61
Testosterone level	Assess for appropriate testosterone level	80-101
Follicle-stimulating hormone, luteinizing hormone, prolactin	Assess for hypothalamus-pituitary-gonadal hormonal axis function	70-89
Prostate-specific antigen	Screen for prostate cancer	64-81
Penile Doppler ultrasound	Evaluate abnormal penile blood flow	137-198
Penile angiography	Detailed evaluation of arterial vasculature	N/A
Nocturnal penile tumescence	Evaluate psychogenic versus organic erectile dysfunction	161-214
Dynamic infusion cavernosography	Evaluate neuropathic versus vascular impotence, assesses arterial inflow abnormalities, venous leaks	223-272
Sacral evoked testing	Evaluate for neuropathy of pelvic region	N/A

N/A, Not available.

TABLE 98-2 Differential Diagnosis: Impotence

Diagnosis	Supporting Data
Loss of libido	May indicate an androgen deficiency secondary to hypothalamic, pituitary, or testicular disease. Serum testosterone and gonadotropin levels should be assessed.
Loss of erections	May result from arterial, venous, neurogenic, or psychogenic causes. Can be secondary to the use of many medications. Occasional impotence despite nocturnal or early morning erections indicate a probable psychogenic cause. A gradual loss of erections over time suggests an organic cause.
Loss of emission	Retrograde ejaculation may occur as a result of surgery, medications, or diabetes. May be secondary to an androgen deficiency.
Loss of orgasm	Usually psychogenic if libido and erection are intact.
Premature ejaculation	Usually anxiety related.

See pathophysiology for the many causes of impotence.

end of the penis to prevent loss of erection. The cylinder is then removed before intercourse.

Injection therapy consists of the direct injection of vasoactive substances into the penis. A tuberculin syringe is used and the injection site is the base and lateral aspect of the penis. Complications include dizziness, hypotension, nausea, pain, fibrosis, infection, and priapism.

Underlying medical conditions such as diabetes, thyroid disease, coronary heart disease, and/or renal disease should be treated.

Surgical

Penile prostheses may be directly implanted into the corporal body of the penis. The protheses vary and may be rigid, malleable, hinged, or inflatable. Sensation, ejaculation, and orgasm generally are not altered. A penile implant is irreversible and is often considered a procedure of last resort.

Patients with arterial disorders or venous occlusions may be candidates for vascular reconstruction.

Patient Education

Impotence is not necessarily a part of aging.

Spouses and/or sexual partners should be included in the treatment plan.

Smoking and alcohol cessation should be recommended.

Complications

Infertility

Social isolation and poor self-esteem

Dysfunctional sexual/intimate relationships

Consultation/Referral

Consultation with a physician, psychiatrist, urologist, plastic surgeon, vascular surgeon, endocrinologist, or neurologist may be indicated, depending on the cause of impotence.

Sex therapy and/or psychotherapy may be indicated for psychogenic impotence and/or dysfunctional intimate relationships.

EVALUATION/FOLLOW-UP

Depends on cause, severity, and patient motivation.

RESOURCES

Impotence Institute of America
Impotents Anonymous (IA)
8201 Corporate Drive, Suite 320
Landover, MD 20785-2229
(800) 669-1603

SUGGESTED READINGS

Dunn SA: *Primary care consultant,* St Louis, 1998, Mosby.

Ellsworth A et al: *Mosby's 1998 medical drug reference,* St Louis, 1998, Mosby.

Gerchufsky M: Impotence: the problem men don't talk about, *Adv Nurse Pract* 3:13-16, 1995.

Gray M: *Genitourinary disorders,* St Louis, 1992, Mosby.

Healthcare Consultants of America, Inc: *1998 Physicians fee and coding guide,* Augusta, Ga, 1998, Healthcare Consultants of America, Inc.

Tierney L, McPhee, S, Papadakis, M: *Current medical diagnosis and treatment,* ed 35, Norwalk, Conn, 1996, Appleton & Lange.

Infertility

ICD-9-CM

Infertility, Male 606.9
Infertility, Female 628.9

OVERVIEW

Definition

Infertility is the inability to achieve fertilization and pregnancy after 1 full year of unprotected intercourse. Sterility is the inability to reproduce, whereas infertility implies a decrease in the ability to conceive in a certain time frame while the potential for conception remains a possibility.

Primary infertility is defined as having no history of a pregnancy; secondary infertility is defined as having a prior pregnancy regardless of the outcome.

Incidence

It is estimated at least 14%—1 of every 7 married couples of reproductive years—and an unknown number of unmarried couples and singles will experience difficulty in conceiving during a given time of 1 year.

One to two percent of couples are involuntarily sterile.

Infertility is experienced as a life crisis by most couples and feelings of frustration, anger, depression, grief, guilt, and anxiety are common.

Only 51% of couples with primary infertility and 22% of couples with secondary infertility will actually seek treatment.

Factors Affecting Fertility

Many persons voluntarily delay marriage and childbearing in favor of establishing careers. This may precipitate an age-related decline in fertility, especially in women.

Women 35 to 40 years old demonstrate a decline in fertility, with a sharp decline evident in most women in their forties.

In some cases the choice of prior contraception may lead to infertility, as with the use of some intrauterine devices (IUDs).

An increased number of sexual partners leads to greater potential for exposure to sexually transmitted diseases, which may lead to complications that cause infertility.

Because of a general increase in knowledge regarding infertility and conception in the American culture, many couples today are simply less willing to accept childlessness and are increasingly aware of available services and options for resolving infertility.

Physiology of Conception

For pregnancy to occur, the following physiological conditions and events must be present and functioning appropriately.

The woman must ovulate for pregnancy to happen.

The man must have sufficient motile sperm in the ejaculate that is deposited at the cervix in the vagina.

Sperm should be in the fallopian tubes within seconds.

The fallopian tubes must be patent and of normal anatomy for fertilization to take place.

The endometrium must be sufficiently developed to allow for implantation.

The uterus should be free of anatomical defects and the pelvis should be free of conditions that could interfere with conception.

Pathophysiology

The pathophysiology of infertility can be divided into female factors, male factors, and couple factors.

Female factors account for 40% of infertility cases. The most common factors are ovulation disorders, tubal disease, and endometriosis (Box 99-1).

Male factors account for another 40% of infertility cases.

Box 99-1

Female Factor Causes of Infertility

Ovulatory

Central Defects

Chronic hyperandrogenemic anovulation
Hyperprolactinemia (drug, tumor, empty sella)
Hypothalamic insufficiency
Pituitary insufficiency (trauma, tumor, congenital)

Peripheral Defects

Gonadal dysgenesis
Premature ovarian failure
Ovarian tumor
Ovarian resistance

Metabolic Disease

Thyroid disease
Liver disease
Renal disease
Obesity
Androgen excess, adrenal, or neoplastic

Pelvic

Infection

Appendicitis
Pelvic inflammatory disease
Uterine adhesions (Asherman's syndrome)

Endometriosis

Structural Abnormalities

DES exposure
Failure of normal fusion of the reproductive tract
Myoma

Cervical

Congenital

DES exposure
Müllerian duct abnormality

Acquired

Surgical treatment
Infection

Adapted from Martin MC: Infertility. In DeCherney AH, Pernoll ML, editors: *Current obstetric & gynecology diagnosis & treatment,* Stamford, Conn, 1994, Appleton & Lange.

DES, Diethylstilbestrol.

Men's fertility is much more susceptible to environmental factors than that of women. For instance, spermatogenesis can be affected by such environmental factors as drug use (Box 99-2) and scrotal temperatures. In addition, congenital anomalies, undescended testes, varicoceles, infections, and pituitary and hypothalamic disorders also lead to male factor infertility (Box 99-3).

Couple factor infertility accounts for approximately 20% of infertility cases. Coital timing and frequency, sperm-cervical mucus interaction, sperm penetration, and antisperm antibodies are possible couple factors.

In 5% to 10% of cases, the cause of infertility is undetermined.

SUBJECTIVE DATA

History of Present Illness

Both partners in a relationship contribute to infertility; therefore both partners should be evaluated, even if the source of the problem seems apparent. To evaluate only one partner is inappropriate because of the high incidence of multiple problems. Ideally, the initial assessment begins with an extended fertility history of both individuals. The couple's ages, previous pregnancies, and length of time attempting conception are important factors to be noted as well as the frequency of intercourse, use of lubricants

Box 99-2

Drugs and Toxins Implicated in Male Infertility

Germ Cell Depletion

Chemotherapeutic agents
Radiotherapy

Testicular Toxin

Alcohol

Pituitary Suppression

Alcohol

Impaired Spermatogenesis

Alcohol
Nitrofurantoin
Sulfa drugs

Decreased Libido/Impotence

Narcotics
Minor tranquilizers
Clofibrate
Estrogens
Cyproterone

Source: the American College of Obstetrics and Gynecology: Male infertility, *ACOG Technical Bulletin* No 142, June 1990.

Box 99-3

Male Factor Causes of Infertility

Endocrine Disorders

Hypothalamic disorders (Kallmann's syndrome)
Pituitary failure (tumor, radiation, surgery)
Hyperprolactinemia (drug, tumor)
Exogenous androgens
Thyroid disorders
Adrenal hyperplasia

Abnormal Spermatogenesis

Chromosomal abnormalities
Mumps orchitis
Cryptorchidism
Chemical or radiation exposure
Varicocele

Abnormal Motility

Absent cilia (Kartagener's syndrome)
Varicocele
Antibody formation

Sexual Dysfunction

Retrograde ejaculation
Impotence
Decreased libido

Anatomical Disorders

Congenital absence of vas deferens
Obstruction of vas deferens
Congenital abnormalities of ejaculatory system

Adapted from Martin MC: Infertility. In DeCherney AH, Pernoll ML, editors: *Current obstetric & gynecology diagnosis & treatment,* Stamford, Conn, 1994, Appleton & Lange

(which can be spermicidal), anorgasmia, impotence, and dyspareunia.

Medical History for Male Factor Infertility

Diethystilbestrol (DES) exposure in utero
Congenital abnormalities, including hypospadias, undescended testis
Prior paternity
Frequency of intercourse
Previous surgery, including testicular, prostate, or hernia repair
Retrograde ejaculation
Varicocele
Previous infections and treatments, including sexually transmitted diseases (STDs), postpubertal mumps
Drugs and medications, including genital radiation, chemotherapy, and anabolic steroids
Excessive exposure to heat (hot tubs, saunas), toxic chemicals, pesticides
General health (diet, medications, exercise, review of systems)
Use of nicotine, alcohol, or illegal substances such as marijuana and other street drugs

Medical History for Female Factor Infertility

DES exposure in utero
History of sexual development, including onset menses
Menstrual cycle characteristics (length, duration, molimina), last menstrual period
Contraceptive history, including use of IUD
Prior pregnancies and outcome, including history of ectopic pregnancy or abortion
Previous surgeries especially pelvic surgery, including ruptured appendix, adnexal/ovarian mass or cyst
Prior infections including STDs, pelvic inflammatory disease (PID)
Leiomyomas
Endometriosis
Obesity or eating disorders
History of cervicitis, abnormal Pap smears, cone biopsy, cautery, obstetric trauma
Thyroid disease
Hirsutism, galactorrhea, hot flushes, severe psychological stress
General health (diet, weight stability, medications, exercise)
Use of nicotine, alcohol, and illegal substances such as marijuana and other street drugs

OBJECTIVE DATA

Physical Examination

A complete physical examination should be performed, with attention to the following:

Height, weight, and vital signs
Overall body habitus and appropriate hair distribution for both males and females
Thyroid gland should be palpated for evidence of enlargement or nodules
Breast development in females and the presence of gynecomastia in men
The skin of the abdomen should be inspected for scars, particularly in the inguinal area, that may indicate prior genital surgery

Physical examination of the male should include careful evaluation of the genitalia, assessing for testicular descent, size, and consistency, the presence and consistency of the epididymis and vas deferens, and the possible presence of a varicocele or penile anomalies or lesions

Physical examination of the female should include an external examination of the genitalia with careful observation for signs of infection, lesions, or anomalies of the clitoris, labia, Skene's and Bartholin's glands, vulva, and perineum; bimanual examination may reveal pelvic tenderness, pelvic mass, uterosacral nodularity, decreased mobility, or enlarged/irregular uterine contour

Diagnostic Procedures

The more common infertility factors can be evaluated by the following tests: a semen analysis, documentation of ovulation, a postcoital test, and evaluation of tubal patency. A semen analysis should be collected after 2 to 3 days (but no more than 7 days) of abstinence; the semen is collected in a clean, sterile container and must be sent immediately to the laboratory so that it can be evaluated within 1 hour of ejaculation.

Normal Semen Parameters

Liquefaction	30 minutes
Sperm count	20 to 250 million/ml
Motility	Greater than 50%
Volume	2 to 5 ml
Morphology	Greater than 50% to 60%
Normal pH	7.2 to 7.8

If abnormalities are identified, additional semen analysis should be performed 2 weeks after the initial analysis. If abnormalities persist, the patient should be referred to urologist for further evaluation.

Basic methods to assess ovulation include basal body temperature, serum progesterone, and endometrial biopsy.

A pattern of regular menses (every 26 to 36 days) is presumptive of ovulation. Many clinicians use basal body temperature charting to document ovulation. There is a slight rise in the basal body temperature at the time of ovulation which is sustained until the onset of menses. Temperature is assessed daily and the pattern of the temperature is assessed monthly. Ovulation can only be documented in retrospect in this manner.

Serum progesterone levels can be measured 7 days after estimated ovulation. Values greater than 15 ng/ml are consistent with normal ovulation; levels less than 5 ng/ml may indicate anovulation. Intermediate values may indicate a luteal phase defect. Serum progesterone levels can vary, because they are released in a pulsating fashion, which may affect clinical interpretation.

An endometrial biopsy detects ovulation through sampling of the endometrial lining of the uterus, which builds in response to ovulation.

The postcoital test evaluates sperm-cervical interaction. Cervical mucus is removed from the endocervical canal 2 to 8 hours after coitus and its quantity, clarity, pH, and spinnbarkeit are assessed. The findings of 5 to 10 progressively motile sperm per high-powered field in clear, acellular mucus with a spinnbarkeit of greater than 8 cm generally excludes a cervical factor.

Tubal patency can be evaluated by a hysterosalpingogram. This procedure involves taking fluoroscopic x-ray films as a contrast medium flows through the uterus and the fallopian tubes, facilitating visualization of these structures.

Tables 99-1 through 99-3 and Figures 99-1 through 99-3 outline procedures and considerations for assessing infertility in men and women.

ASSESSMENT

See the causes of infertility for differential diagnoses.

THERAPEUTIC PLAN

Patient Education

Many couples need basic information on reproductive physiology, including time of ovulation and the impact of coital frequency (see the basal body temperature record on pp. 633 and 634). Sixty percent of normal, healthy couples will conceive by 6 months; 90% will conceive by 12 months; and 95% will conceive by 24 months after beginning unprotected sex. Intercourse once a week over a 6-month period will result in a 16% chance of pregnancy. Increased coital frequency of four times per week around the time of ovulation will increase the chance of pregnancy to 83%.

An infertility evaluation is generally initiated after 1 year of attempting pregnancy, unless maternal age is a factor. In 5% to 10% of couples, completion of the basic workup will not reveal any abnormalities, and their infertility may be unexplained.

Lifestyle Modifications

Health care providers should advise all patients on the importance of a healthy diet, multivitamins and zinc, and exercise.

Smoking cessation should be recommended and alcohol moderation should be stressed.

Potential environmental hazards or toxins should be identified and eliminated if possible.

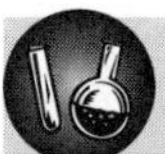

Table 99-1 Diagnostic Tests: Male Infertility

Test	Indications	Side Effects	Cost ($)/Risk
Complete PE, including GU	Assessment of testicular size, descent, and consistency; presence and consistency of the epididymis and vas deferens; rule out presence of a varicocele, penile anomalies, lesions, or infection	None	Cost of an office visit/ no risk
Cultures for gonorrhea and chlamydia	Rule out STDs; recurrent STDs can cause scarring and blockage of the reproductive tract	Mild discomfort	37-45/gon; 49-62/chlam/no risk
Semen analysis	Confirm presence of viable sperm	None	N/A/no risk
Serum FSH, LH	Low FSH and LH may indicate hypothalamic or pituitary dysfunction; elevated FSH and LH may indicate testicular failure	Discomfort from venipuncture	315-495/minimal risk
Serum testosterone	May indicate a problem of hormone production at the level of the testes	Discomfort from venipuncture	80-101/minimal risk
Serum prolactin	Elevated prolactin may indicate a pituitary adenoma	Discomfort from venipuncture	70-89/minimal risk
Sperm antibodies	Can result from a vasectomy and recurrent STDs	Discomfort from venipuncture	N/A/minimal risk
Sperm penetration assay	Evaluates the functional ability of sperm to penetrate hamster eggs	None	N/A/minimal risk
Testicular biopsy	Evaluates testicular failure versus an obstruction	Local discomfort	N/A/ risk of surgical procedure
Microsurgery	Correction of an obstruction or varicocele Reversal of a vasectomy Exploration of an anomaly	Local discomfort, risk of an infection	N/A/risk of surgical procedure

FSH, Follicle-stimulating hormone; *GU,* genitourinary; *LH,* luteinizing hormone; *N/A,* not available; *PE,* physical examination; *STD,* sexually transmitted disease.

Organization of Diagnostic Testing

Testing can be organized according to the women's menstrual cycle. If she has regular periods, then ovulation is presumed.

Basal body temperature charting documents ovulation and is maintained throughout the cycle.

A semen analysis can be done at any time.

Hysterosalpingography is performed after menstruation but before ovulation.

A postcoital test is performed at midcycle around the time of ovulation.

An endometrial biopsy is completed 1 or 2 days before the expected menses.

Couples should be given an explanation of each test, including risks, benefits, and costs. The couple should be allowed to decide testing intervals, and the testing should be organized in an efficient and logical sequence to minimize stress and cost.

A woman with irregular periods or no periods secondary to anovulation will require ovulation induction before a postcoital test or endometrial biopsy can be performed.

However, a semen analysis and hysterosalpingography should be performed before initiating ovulation induction medications.

A diagnostic laparoscopy is performed to assess whether pelvic adhesions or endometriosis are present in the pelvis. The laparoscopy should not be completed before the other testing unless the woman is experiencing severe pelvic pain or ovulation induction is being considered.

A current semen analysis should be documented to rule out male factor infertility before any surgical procedure is conducted on the man or woman to evaluate infertility.

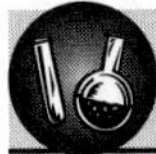

TABLE 99-2 Diagnostic Tests: Female Infertility

Test	Indications	Side Effects	Cost ($)/Risk
Complete PE, including GU	Assessment of external genitalia for infection, lesions, and anomalies; bimanual examination may reveal pelvic tenderness, pelvic mass, uterosacral nodularity, decreased uterine mobility, or enlarged/irregular uterine contour	None	Cost of office visit/no risk
Pap smear	Evaluation for cervical dysplasia and cervical cancer	Mild discomfort, occasional spotting	53-65/minimal risk
Cultures for gonorrhea and chlamydia	Assess for STDs Recurrent STDs can cause scarring and blockage of the reproductive tract	Mild discomfort	37-51/gon/minimal risk 49-62/chlam
Wet preparation	Assess for presence of *Trichomonas* or candidal organisms, leukocytes Assess pH	None	19-23/minimal cost and risk
Basal body temperature charting	Documentation of ovulation	None	N/A/no risk
LH kits	Documentation of ovulation Available over-the-counter	None	N/A/no risk
Serum progesterone levels	Documentation of ovulation	Discomfort of venipuncture	59-73/minimal risk
Endometrial biopsy	Evaluation of the endometrial lining, which builds in response to ovulation and increased progesterone levels	Uterine cramping, spotting	142-170/risk of perforation and/or infection of uterus
Serum FSH, LH, TSH, prolactin	Evaluation of hypo-thalamic, pituitary, or thyroid dysfunction; elevated LH to FSH ratio with hirsutism, obesity, and amenorrhea is consistent with polycystic ovarian disease Elevated FSH and LH levels is consistent with ovarian failure Low FSH and LH levels are consistent with anovulation Elevated prolactin levels may be indicative of a pituitary adenoma Elevated TSH is consistent with hypothyroidism	Discomfort from venipuncture	315-495/FSH, LH/minimal risk 56-70/TSH 70-89/prolactin
Cervical mucus antisperm antibodies	Can be found in both serum and cervical mucus Can impair sperm-egg interaction	Mild discomfort from venipuncture and examination	N/A/minimal risk

FSH, Follicle-stimulating hormone; *GU,* genitourinary; *LH,* luteinizing hormone; *N/A,* not available; *PE,* physical examination; *STD,* sexually transmitted disease; *TSH,* thyroid-stimulating hormone.

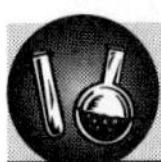

TABLE 99-2 Diagnostic Tests: Female Infertility—cont'd

Test	Indications	Side Effects	Cost ($)/Risk
Hystero-salpingogram	Evaluates tubal patency by use of x-ray evaluation and contrast medium, allowing for visualization of the uterus and fallopian tubes as the dye flows through these structures	Uterine cramping, bleeding, nausea, and dizziness	181-216/moderate risk, including uterine perforation and allergic reaction
Hysteroscopy	Evaluates inside uterine cavity for presence of uterine septum, polyps, and adhesions Particularly valuable for lysis of adhesions with Asherman's syndrome, a condition in which there is internal scarring of uterus	Moderate discomfort from procedure; vagal stimulation from cervical manipulation can cause mild bradycardia, hypertension, and diaphoresis	N/A/moderate risk
Diagnostic laparoscopy	Evaluates the size, shape, surface, color, consistency, and mobility of the uterus, tubes, and ovaries Operative work includes lysis of adhesions, vaporization of endometriosis, correction of anatomical defect, remove portion of damaged tube or ectopic pregnancy	Moderate abdominal discomfort, nausea and vomiting from anesthesia and bowel manipulation, sore throat from endotracheal intubation, possible shoulder pain from insufflation of carbon dioxide	1186-1398/moderate risk

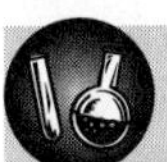

TABLE 99-3 Diagnostic Tests: Couples Infertility

Test	Indications	Side Effects	Cost/Risk
Postcoital test	Evaluates sperm-cervical interaction Timing is imperative; 48-72 hr when the cervical mucus is receptive—otherwise it serves as barrier	None	N/A/minimal risk

N/A, Not available.

Pharmaceutical

A pharmaceutical plan for treating infertility is outlined in Table 99-4.

Support Groups

Support groups for infertile couples are helpful in alleviating feelings of isolation and provide a supportive environment in which they may identify with other couples who are experiencing the same problem.

Alternative Therapies

Artificial insemination involves the collection of semen by masturbation and placing it into the cervix or directly into the uterus, thus bypassing the cervix, when there is a problem with cervical mucus production. This procedure is also performed when there is poor motility and a low sperm count.

Therapeutic donor insemination is indicated in cases with severely low sperm count or no sperm, sex-linked genetic diseases, and severe male antisperm antibodies. Many

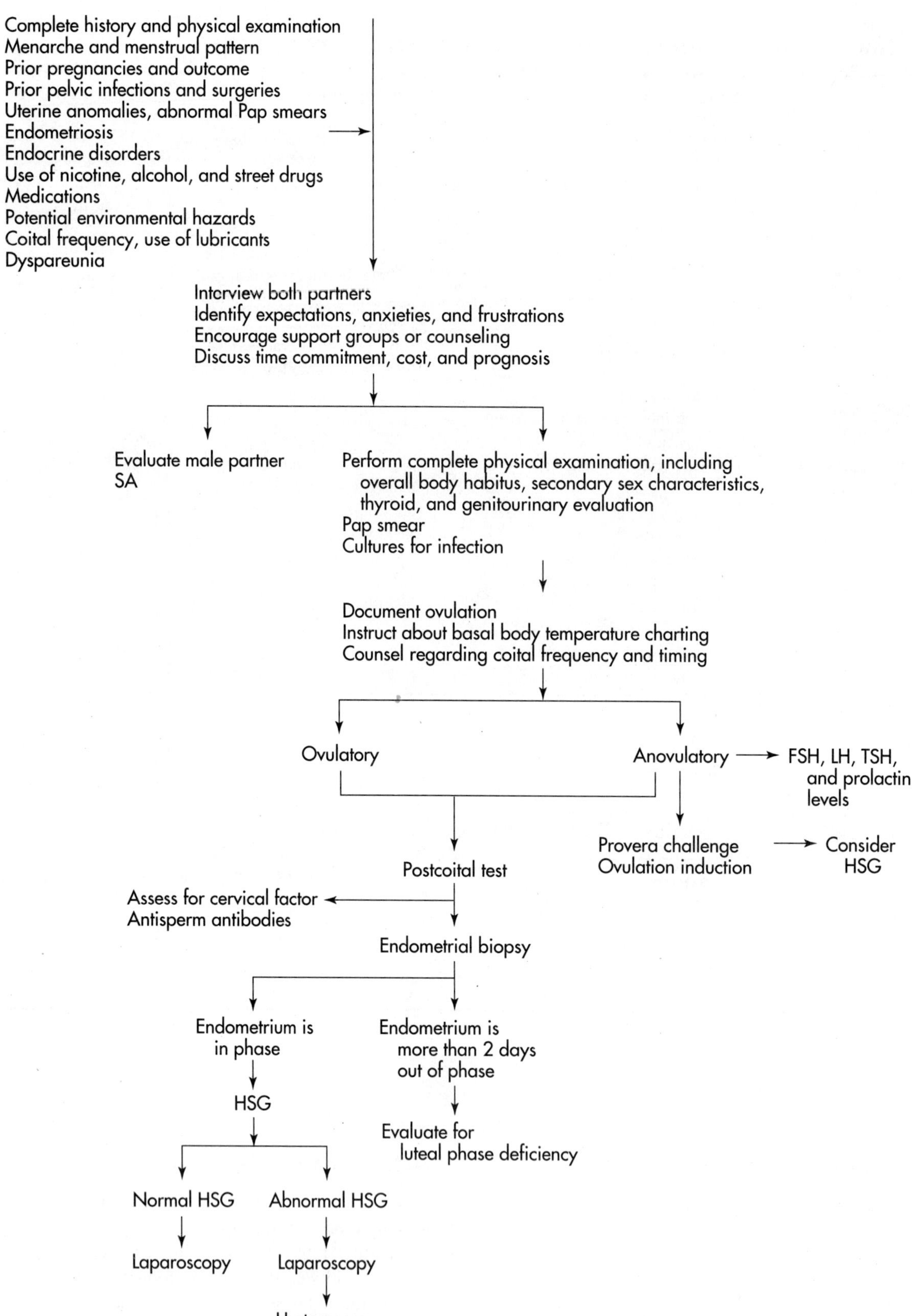

Figure 99-1 Algorithm for the treatment of female infertility. *FSH,* Follicle-stimulating hormone; *HSG,* hysterosalpingogram; *LH,* luteinizing hormone; *SA,* semen analysis; *TSH,* thyroid-stimulating hormone.

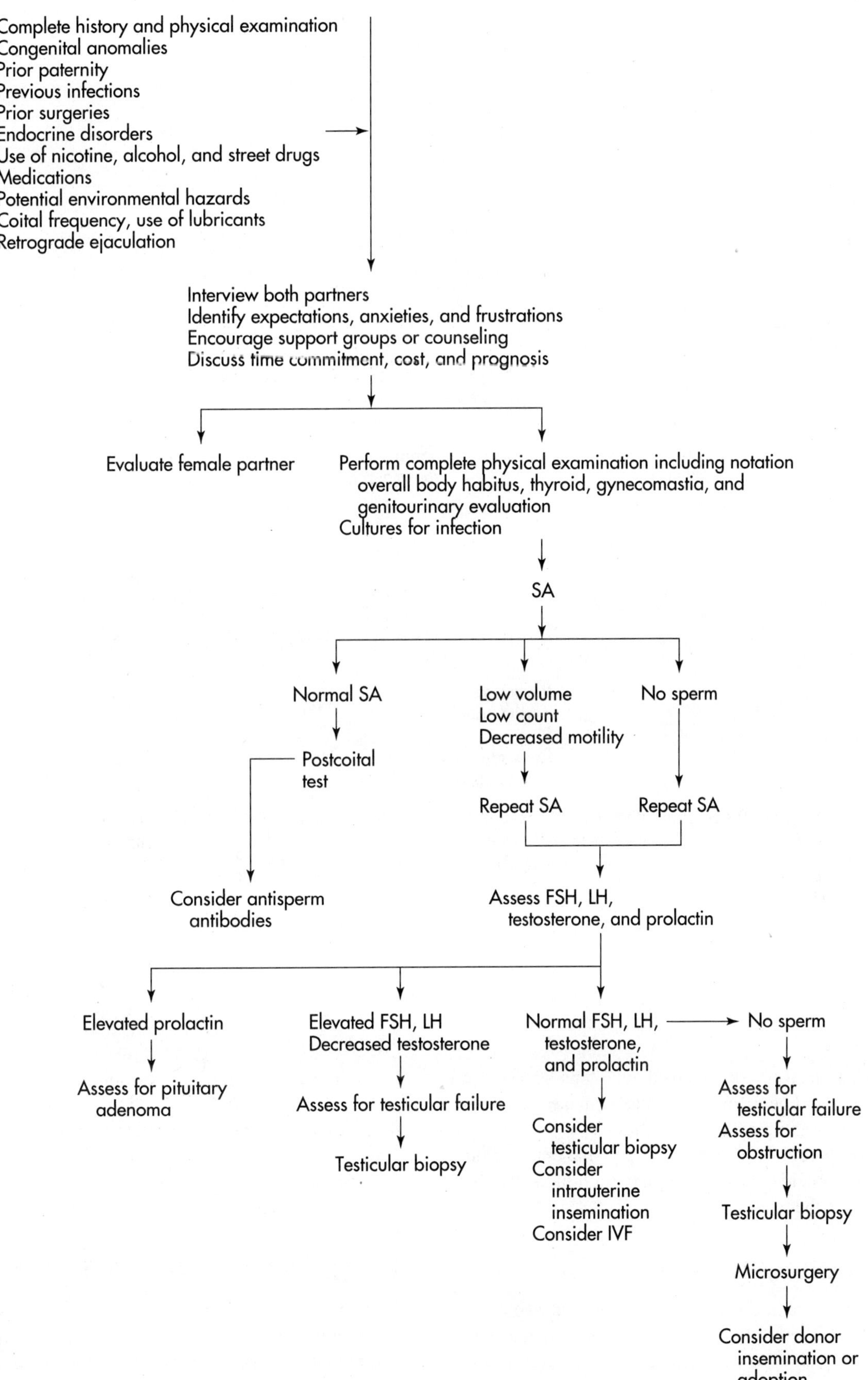

Figure 99-2 Algorithm for the treatment of male infertility. *FSH,* Follicle-stimulating hormone; *IVF,* in vitro fertilization; *LH,* luteinizing hormone; *SA,* semen analysis.

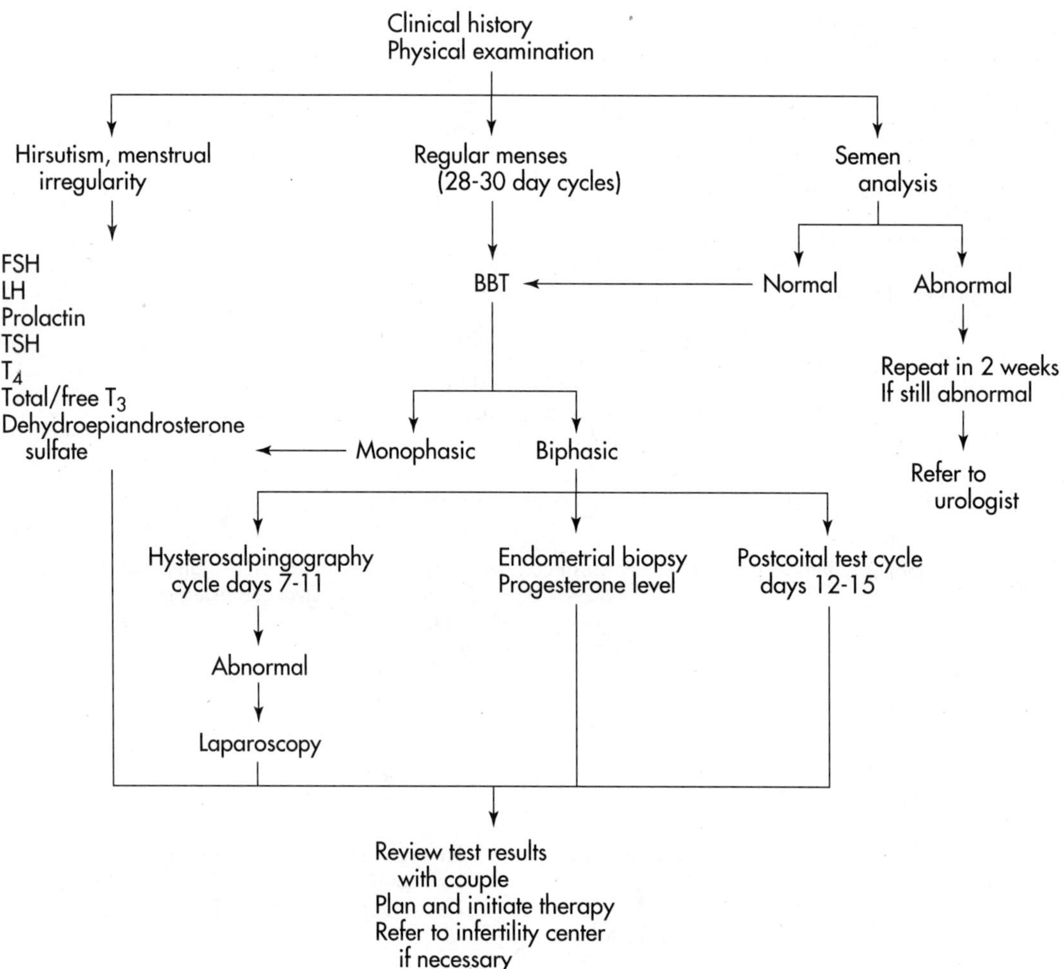

Figure 99-3 Algorithm for the treatment of an infertile couple. *BBT,* Basal body temperature; *FSH,* follicle-stimulating hormone; *LH,* luteinizing hormone; *TSH,* thyroid-stimulating hormone. (Adapted from Greene HL, Johnson WP, Lemcke MJ: *Decision making in medicine,* ed 2, St Louis, 1993, Mosby.)

psychological factors are involved with this choice, and counseling should be recommended to evaluate the ethical, religious, legal, and medical ramifications.

Adoption should be considered as a viable option. Some couples may decide that not having a child is the best alternative for them.

Consultation/Referral

Referral to a reproductive endocrinologist would be appropriate for consideration of the use of the latest reproductive technologies, such as in vitro fertilization, embryo transfer, gamete intrafallopian transfer, zygote intrafallopian transfer, intracytoplasmic sperm injection, and preembryo cryopreservation techniques. However, these reproductive technologies are not appropriate for all couples or for all problems of infertility, because the ethical considerations are tremendous, and the emotional and financial stressors are considerable during these procedures.

EVALUATION/FOLLOW-UP

Most infertility evaluations can be completed within 12 to 18 months if the health care provider is both organized and committed and the couple is both reliable and kept well informed.

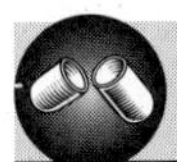

TABLE 99-4 Pharmaceutical Plan: Infertility

Drug	Indication	Mechanism of Action	Dose	Cost ($)/Side Effects
Clomiphene citrate (Clomid, Serophene)	Ovulation induction: treatment of luteal phase deficiency	Thought to bind to estrogen receptors in the pituitary, blocking them from detecting estrogen. Causes hypothalamus to release GnRH, stimulating the release of FSH and LH.	50 mg/day for 5 days; starting fifth day on of cycle, may increase to 200 mg/day; ovulation is expected about day 14 from the start of the clomiphene therapy	163-218/Hot flushes, headache, ovarian enlargement, nausea, visual disturbances, multiple gestation
Once ovulation has occurred at a specific dose, there is no advantage in increasing the dose. Also, once ovulation is established, the PCT and EMB should be performed on all women because the antiestrogenic properties of clomiphene citrate can have adverse effects on cervical mucus and endometrial development.				
Human menopausal gonadotrophins (MMG, Pergonal)	Ovulation induction	Direct stimulation of ovarian follicle	IM injections dosage variable Pergonal LH FSH in 0.75:0.75 ratio plus HCG	57-125 /Ovarian enlargement, hyperstimulation, multiple births, local irritation at injection site
Purified FSH (Metrodin)	Treatment of polycystic ovarian disease	Direct action on ovarian follicle	75 U plus HCG	N/A/Ovarian enlargement, hyperstimulation, multiple births, local irritation at injection site
HCG (Profasi)	Ovulation induction	Acts directly on ovarian follicle to stimulate meiosis and rupture of follicle	2000-10,000 U IM following last day of menotropins/ gonadotrophins or 5-9 days after last dose of clomiphene	N/A
Danocrine (Danazol)	Treatment of endometriosis; combination of estrogen, progestin, and androgen suppresses ovarian activity	Initially 400 mg BID decreasing to 100-200 mg BID for 3-9 mo	Mild hirsutism, acne edema, weight gain, elevation of liver enzymes	118-300
Progesterone (Progestoral)	Treatment of luteal phase deficiency	Direct stimulation of the endometrium	Vaginal suppositories 25-50 mg BID or 50 mg QHS, rectal suppositories q12h Progesterone capsules 100 mg by mouth TID	35-45/Breast tenderness, local irritation, headaches
GnRH agonists (Synarel, Lupron)	Treatment of endometriosis	Suppression of LH/ FSH and ovarian functions	Synarel: 200 µg intranasally BID for 6 mo Lupron:Depot 3.75 mg IM q 28 days for 6 mo	400-500/Nasal irritation, nosebleeds with Synarel, hot flashes, vaginal dryness, headache, mild bone loss, myalgia with both Synarel and Lupron

From Fogel CI, Woods NF: *Women's health care,* Thousand Oaks, Calif, 1995, Sage Publications.

EMB, Endometrial biopsy; *FSH,* follicle-stimulating hormone; *GnRH,* gonadotropin-releasing hormone; *HCG,* human chorionic gonadotropin; *LH,* luteinizing hormone; *N/A,* not available; *PCT,* postcoital test; *TSH,* thyroid-stimulating hormone.

RESOURCES

March of Dimes
Birth Defects Foundation
National Office
1275 Mamaroneck Avenue
White Plains, NY 10605

Toll-free number (888) 663-4637
Web site http://www.modimes.org
E-mail resourcecenter@modimes.org

SUGGESTED READINGS

Cefalo RC, Moos MK: *Preconceptional health promotion: a practical guide,* Rockville, Md 1988, Aspen Publication.

Martin MC: Infertility. In DeCherney AH, Pernoll ML, editors: *Current obstetric & gynecology diagnosis & treatment,* Stamford, Conn, 1994, Appleton & Lange.

Ellsworth A et al: *Mosby's 1998 medical drug reference,* St Louis, 1998, Mosby.

Fogel CI, Woods NF: *Women's health care,* Thousand Oaks, Calif, 1995, Sage Publications.

Friedman EA, Borton M, Chapin DS: *Gynecological decision-making,* ed 2, Philadelphia, 1988, BC Decker.

Gray M: *Genitourinary disorders,* St Louis, 1992, Mosby.

Hankins JW, Roberto DM, Stanley-Haney JL: *Protocols for nurse practitioners in gynecologic settings,* ed 4, New York, 1993, Tiresias Press.

Healthcare Consultants of America, Inc: *1998 Physicians fee and coding guide,* Augusta, Ga, 1998, Healthcare Consultants of America, Inc.

Infertility. *ACOG Technical Bulletin* No 125, Feb 1989.

Loriaux TC: Male infertility: a challenge for primary health care providers, *Nurse Pract* 16:38-45, 1991.

Male infertility. *ACOG Technical Bulletin* No 142, June 1990.

Medical induction of ovulation. *ACOG Technical Bulletin* No 120, Sept 1998.

Moss WM: *Contraceptive surgery for men and women,* ed 2, Durant, Okla, 1991, Essential Medical Informations Systems, Inc.

New reproductive technologies. *ACOG Technical Bulletin* No 140, March 1990.

Wilson B: The effects of drugs on male sexual function and fertility, *Nurse Pract* 16:12-22, 1991.

INSTRUCTIONS FOR KEEPING
TEMPERATURE RECORDS

1. Insert date at top of column in space provided for date of month.
2. Each morning, upon awakening, but before you get out of bed, place your thermometer under your tongue for at least two minutes. Do this every morning, even during menstruation. Be sure not to eat, drink, or smoke before taking your temperature.
3. Accurately record temperature reading on the graph by placing a dot in the proper location (see example below). Indicate days of coitus (intercourse) by placing a downpointing arrow (↓) in the space provided.
4. The first day of menstrual flow is considered to be the start of a cycle. Indicate each day of flow by blocking the square indicated (■) on the graph, starting at the extreme left under the first day of your cycle.
5. Any obvious reasons for temperature variation, such as colds, infection, insomnia, indigestion, etc., should be noted on the graph above the reading for the day.
6. Ovulation may be accompanied, in some women, by a twinge of pain in the lower abdomen. If you notice this, indicate the day it occurred on the graph.
7. Start a new cycle on the next graph.

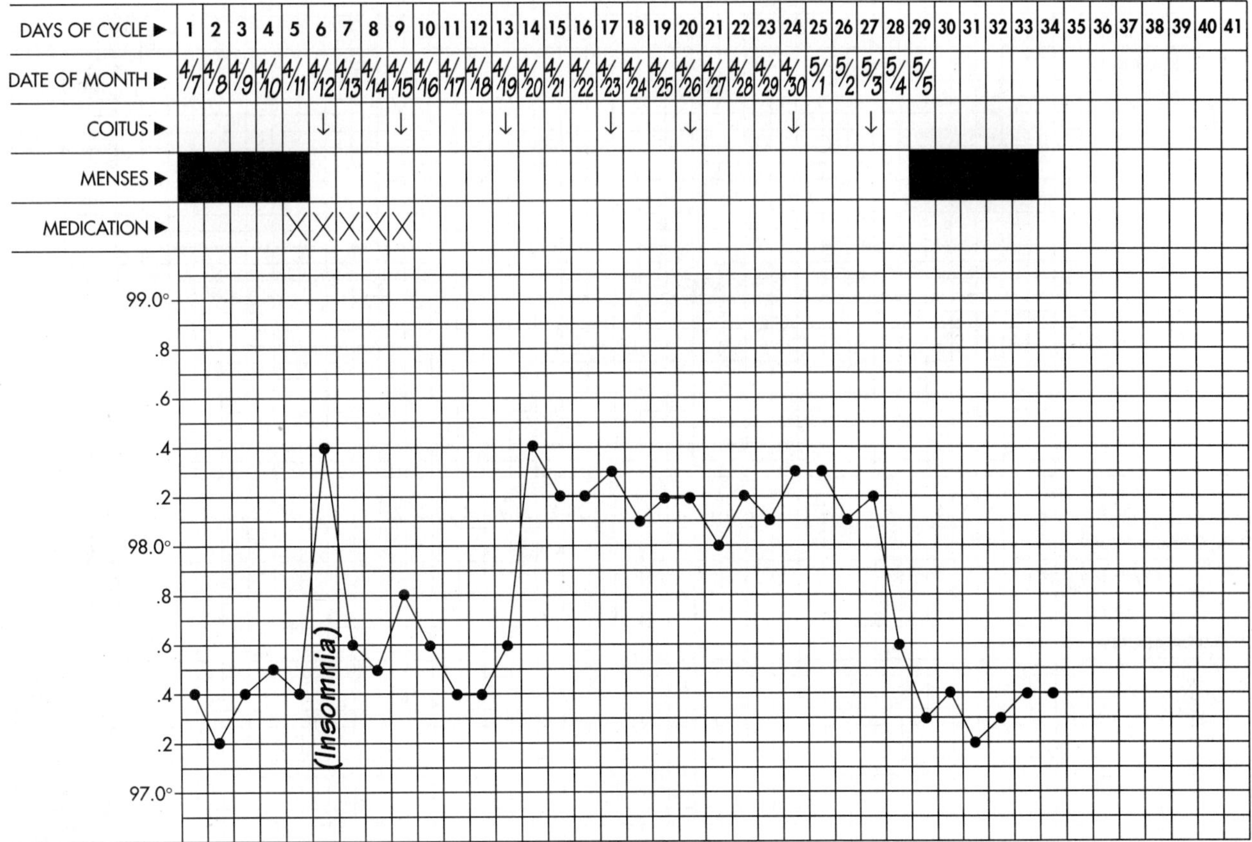

BASAL BODY TEMPERATURE RECORD
See instructions at front of chart.

NAME: ____________________

AGE: ____________________

↓ COITUS

■ MENSES

DAYS OF CYCLE ▶	1	2	3	4	5	6	7	8	9	10	11	12	13	14	15	16	17	18	19	20	21	22	23	24	25	26	27	28	29	30	31	32	33	34	35	36	37	38	39	40	41
DATE OF MONTH ▶																																									
COITUS ▶																																									
MENSES ▶																																									
MEDICATION ▶																																									
99.0°																																									
.8																																									
.6																																									
.4																																									
.2																																									
98.0°																																									
.8																																									
.6																																									
.4																																									
.2																																									
97.0°																																									

DAYS OF CYCLE ▶	1	2	3	4	5	6	7	8	9	10	11	12	13	14	15	16	17	18	19	20	21	22	23	24	25	26	27	28	29	30	31	32	33	34	35	36	37	38	39	40	41
DATE OF MONTH ▶																																									
COITUS ▶																																									
MENSES ▶																																									
MEDICATION ▶																																									
99.0°																																									
.8																																									
.6																																									
.4																																									
.2																																									
98.0°																																									
.8																																									
.6																																									
.4																																									
.2																																									
97.0°																																									

DAYS OF CYCLE ▶	1	2	3	4	5	6	7	8	9	10	11	12	13	14	15	16	17	18	19	20	21	22	23	24	25	26	27	28	29	30	31	32	33	34	35	36	37	38	39	40	41
DATE OF MONTH ▶																																									
COITUS ▶																																									
MENSES ▶																																									
MEDICATION ▶																																									
99.0°																																									
.8																																									
.6																																									
.4																																									
.2																																									
98.0°																																									
.8																																									
.6																																									
.4																																									
.2																																									
97.0°																																									

Inflammatory Bowel Disease

ICD 9 CM

Inflammatory Bowel Disease 558.9
Crohn's Disease 555.9
Ulcerative Colitis 556.0

OVERVIEW

Definition

Inflammatory bowel disease (IBD) in general refers to any chronic, inflammatory condition of the small and/or large bowel. Specifically, the two most common types of inflammatory bowel disease are ulcerative colitis and Crohn's disease. These two entities share many features secondary to bowel inflammation such as diarrhea, pain, fever, and blood loss, but differ in terms of distribution of disease, histological findings, incidence and type of extra-intestinal symptoms, response to medications and surgery, and prognosis.

Incidence

Ulcerative colitis occurs at a rate of 5 per 100,000 per year.

The incidence of Crohn's disease has increased dramatically since first described in 1932 from 20 to 70 per 100,000 per year.

The most common age of onset is **15 to 40 years.**

It is three to five times more common among European or North American Jews.

It has an **equal to slightly higher rate among females** to males.

It has a familial tendency.

Pathophysiology

The cause of IBD is unknown.

Research has focused on many variables, including autoimmune factors, genetic factors, infectious agents, food allergies, collagen disorders, and psychosocial factors.

Ulcerative colitis affects only the colon. It usually extends upward from the rectum.

Inflammation affects only the mucosal and submucosal layers, presenting as continuous lining involvement.

Crohn's disease can occur anywhere in the gastrointestinal tract from the mouth to the anus.

Inflammation has transmural involvement, which is a predisposing factor to fistula formation, and presents as healthy tissue interspersed with areas of affected tissue.

SUBJECTIVE DATA

History of Present Illness

The most prominent clinical features of ulcerative colitis are rectal bleeding and diarrhea. Severity ranges from intermittent bleeding, mild diarrhea with no systemic involvement, to severe disease characterized by marked diarrhea, bleeding severe enough to cause anemia, abdominal cramping, tenderness, anorexia, and weight loss.

Associated systemic manifestations of ulcerative colitis include skin lesions, eye lesions, arthritis, and liver disease.

Early manifestations of Crohn's disease are often vague and episodic and may go unrecognized for years. These initial manifestations include general malaise, anorexia, fever, mild abdominal discomfort, and diarrhea. As the disease progresses, so do the most consistent symptoms—abdominal pain and diarrhea.

Rectal bleeding may occur but is not as common as with ulcerative colitis. Advanced disease may result in obstruction, abscess formation, and fistula development (Box 100-1).

Perianal disease is common with Crohn's disease and may present as an edematous skin tag, a wide, painless fissure, an abscess, an anal ulcer, or anal stenosis.

Nutritional deficiencies are common in Crohn's disease secondary to malabsorption and stricture formation.

Associated systemic manifestations of Crohn's disease include joint problems, skin lesions, ocular disorders, and aphthous ulcers of the mouth.

Box 100-1

Symptoms of Advanced Crohn's Disease

Obstructive Symptoms	Abscess Formation	Fistula Development
Colicky abdominal pain	Fever	May or may not produce signs or symptoms, depending on organ involvement, such as between the bowel, skin, bladder, or vagina
Obstipation	Leukocytosis	
Abdominal distention	Pain	
Nausea	Tender abdominal mass	
Vomiting	Guarding	

Other systemic disorders associated with Crohn's disease include kidney stones, gallstones, osteoporosis, liver disorders, vascular problems, and psychiatric disorders.

Children and adolescents may experience growth retardation and/or delayed sexual development.

Past Medical History

Ask about past episodes of diarrhea and abdominal pain and its course.

Ask about autoimmune disorders, food allergies/intolerances, collagen disorders, and gastrointestinal disorders.

Ask about a family history of inflammatory bowel disease.

Determine the patient's ethnic origin.

Medication History

Ask about all prescription and over-the-counter medications, and herbal remedies currently being taken. Ask about antidiarrheal medications.

Psychosocial History

Ask about psychosocial stressors and methods of coping.

Ask about past psychiatric disorders and treatments.

OBJECTIVE

Physical Examination

A physical examination should be performed, with attention to the following:

- Vital signs, height, weight
- Abdomen: Assess bowel sounds, pain, guarding, rebound, masses, distention.
- Rectum: Assess tone, integrity, abscess, masses, guaiac for occult blood.
- A complete physical examination is often indicated to rule out extraintestinal involvement.

Diagnostic Procedures

Diagnostic tests for IBD are listed in Table 100-1.

ASSESSMENT

Differential Diagnosis

Table 100-2 distinguishes ulcerative colitis from Crohn's disease; Table 100-3 lists differential diagnoses for IBD.

Complications

Complications of IBD are found in Box 100-2.

THERAPEUTIC PLAN

Pharmaceutical

The goal of medical treatment is to decrease inflammation or suppress the immune system's response. Antibiotics and antidiarrheal medications are sometimes indicated in certain situations.

Sulfasalazine (Azulfidine) ($11 to $23) is a combination salicylate/sulfonamide and is the most commonly prescribed maintenance medication for both ulcerative colitis and Crohn's disease.

Children (more than 2 years old)

- Initial dose: 40 to 60 mg/kg/day in 3 to 6 doses.
- Maintenance dosage: 30 mg/kg/day in 4 divided doses.

Adults

- Initial dose: 1 to 2 g /day; increase to 3 to 4 g/day in divided doses after meals until clinical symptoms are controlled.
- Maintenance dosage: 2 g/day, to a maximum dose of 4 g/day.

Initiate sulfasalazine therapy with corticosteroids, since it may take 2 weeks to achieve therapeutic results.

Olsalazine (Dipentum) ($62) is an alternative to sulfasalazine therapy for adults; it is administered 500 mg PO BID

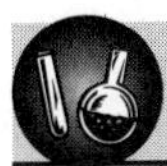

TABLE 100-1 Diagnostic Tests: Inflammatory Bowel Disease

Test	Findings/Rationale	Cost ($)
CBC	Evaluate for anemia, infection	13-16
Stool for guaiac	Evaluate for occult blood	N/A
Stool for culture and sensitivity	Evaluate for bacterial infection	37-45
Serum albumin and total protein	Decreased with advanced disease and malnutrition	18-23 22-27
Vitamin B_{12} levels	Decreased with distal ileitis or distal ileal resection	53-67
Liver function studies	Evaluate for liver disease	29-41
Folic acid levels	Levels may be reduced	49-62
X-ray (flat plate) evaluation of the abdomen	Rule out dilation and/or obstruction	142-169
Barium studies and upper GI (barium enema is contraindicated in acute ulcerative colitis)	Evaluate for mucosal irregularities, ulcers, fissures, cobblestoning, skip lesions, stenosis, stricture, areas of diffuse narrowing, pseudodiverticula, pseudopolyps, sinus tracts, fistula formation, colonic shortening	275-328
Endoscopy (colonoscopy is contraindicated in the presence of acute ulcerative colitis because of the risk of perforation; however, sigmoidoscopy can be performed)	Evaluate mucosal irregularities, ulcers, fissures, cobblestoning, skip areas, fistulas, rectal sparing, shortening of the colon, pseudopolyps	799-956 254-302
Biopsy	Diagnosis and to rule out malignancy; aid in differentiating ulcerative colitis from Crohn's disease	N/A
CT scan of abdomen	Evaluate mesenteric abnormalities, thickening of the bowel wall; abscess and fistula formation	807-956

Adapted from Doughty DB, Jackson DB: *Gastrointestinal diseases,* St Louis, 1993, Mosby.
CBC, Complete blood cell count; *CT,* computed tomography; *GI,* gastrointestinal; *N/A,* not available.

with meals. Olsalazine is **not recommended for use in children.**

Corticosteroids ($14 to $20) are used during acute exacerbations to suppress inflammation. They can be administered orally, intravenously, intramuscularly, or rectally. Administration should be of short duration because of the potential for serious side effects; they should be tapered slowly.

Prednisone 0.25 to 0.75 mg/kg/day for moderate to severe disease symptoms. Side effects include adrenal suppression; bone thinning; weakened resistance to infection; affective mood changes; impaired glucose tolerance; cushingoid appearance, including moonface; hirsutism; acne; and growth retardation in children.

Hydrocortisone enemas (Cortenema) and rectal foam (Cortifoam) are used to alleviate symptoms of the lower colon and anogenital area.

Mesalamine (Rowasa) ($60) enemas or suppositories are used for proctitis and proctosigmoiditis.

The use of immunosuppressive agents such as mercaptopurine (6-MP) has been controversial but is thought to have limited steroid-sparing utility and allows for reduction in steroid dosage or problems with withdrawal.

Metronidazole (Flagyl) ($7) is an antiinfective agent limited to use for fistulas or perianal involvement in Crohn's disease.

Antidiarrheal agents include psyllium products for bulking effect with watery diarrhea: Diphenoxylate (Lomotil) ($7 to $13), loperamide (Imodium) ($3 to $5), codeine and cholestyramine (Questran) for diarrhea related to malabsorption of bile salts. (Use of codeine or loperamide is generally contraindicated in IBD, except when there is a definite diagnosis of Crohn's disease that does not involve the large intestine.)

Surgical

Surgery is frequently indicated for patients with ulcerative colitis to relieve strictures, but also in emergency situations when the disease is unresponsive to medical measures, has intractable bleeding, or an unresponsive megacolon has developed.

TABLE 100-2 Distinguishing Ulcerative Colitis from Crohn's Disease

Means of Assessment	Ulcerative Colitis	Crohn's Disease
Symptoms		
Abdominal pain	Unusual	Usual
Hemorrhage	Usual	Unusual
Fistula formation	Very unusual	Not rare
Anal changes	Unusual	Usual
Palpable intestinal mass	Never	Often
Involvement of rectum	Almost always	Not so often
Scope		
Rectoscopy	No normal mucous membrane	Quite normal, or islands of normal mucous membrane
X-ray Evaluation		
Spreading	Continuous	Discontinuous
Strictures	No	Often
Mucosal appearance	Granulomatous, superficial ulcerations	Deep, undetermined ulcerated fissures
Shortened, arched colon	Often	No
Evaluation by Pathology		
Mucosa	Largely lacking, superficial ulcerations	Discrete ulcerations, fissures, cobblestone appearance
Connective tissue	Increased, the intestine generally somewhat constricted, no strictures, less length	Normal amount of connective tissue, normal or dilated intestine between stricturing parts
Fistula	None	Often
Involved terminal ileum	Never	Often
Inflammation	Mucosa and submucosa	All layers
Lymph nodes	Reactive, hyperplasia	Sarcoid, conglomerate

Adapted from Cooke DM: Inflammatory bowel disease: primary health care management of ulcerative colitis and Crohn's disease, *Nurse Pract* 16:27-39, 1991.

TABLE 100-3 Differential Diagnosis: Inflammatory Bowel Disease

Diagnosis	Supporting Data
Irritable bowel syndrome (IBS)	Functional disorder of bowel motility resulting in abdominal pain, bloating, diarrhea alternating with constipation
Peptic ulcer disease	Ulcerations in the mucosal lining of the esophagus, stomach, or small intestine; abdominal pain may be relieved by eating or may awaken individual at night
Gastroenteritis	Inflammation of the stomach and intestines, caused by viral or bacterial infections; presents as anorexia, nausea, vomiting, abdominal pain, and diarrhea
Pseudomembranous enterocolitis	Antibiotic-associated diarrhea characterized by inflammation and necrosis of the mucosal and submucosal layers of the bowel wall; results from an infection by *Clostridium difficile*
Diverticulitis	Inflammation of pouchlike protrusions caused by herniations of the mucosal and submucosal layers of the colon wall; symptoms include fever, LLQ abdominal pain, anorexia, and nausea
Cholecystitis	Inflammation of the gallbladder, associated with gallstones; symptoms include RUQ pain, anorexia, nausea, and vomiting; pain may radiate to scapula
Pancreatitis	Inflammation of the pancreas, associated with excessive alcohol intake; presents with abdominal pain, nausea, and vomiting
Peritonitis	Inflammation of the peritoneum resulting from infection, trauma, obstruction, ischemia, or may occur postoperatively; abdominal pain, fever, abdominal rigidity, nausea, vomiting, and distention are common

LLQ, Left lower quadrant; *RUQ*, right upper quadrant.

Box 100-2

Complications of Ulcerative Colitis and Crohn's Disease

Ulcerative Colitis

Massive bleeding
Toxic megacolon*
Perforation
Adenocarcinoma
Extraintestinal manifestations, including
- Skin lesions: Erythema nodosum, pyoderma gangrenosum
- Eye lesions: Uveitis, conjunctivitis, episcleritis
- Joint abnormalities: Migratory arthritis, ankylosing spondylitis
- Liver disease: Fatty liver, sclerosing cholangitis, chronic hepatitis, bile duct cancer

Crohn's Disease

Abscess formation
Intestinal obstruction
Perianal disease
Malnutrition
Growth retardation

Adapted from Doughty DB, Jackson DB: *Gastrointestinal diseases,* St Louis, 1993, Mosby.

*Toxic megacolon is a rare but serious complication of ulcerative colitis occurring in approximately 5% of patients, with an average mortality rate of 25%. Mucosal inflammation spreads to the submucosal, muscular, and serosal layers of the colon, paralyzing the smooth muscle, which allows the colon to dilate. The colon then loses the barrier function of the epithelium, permitting the uptake of bacterial toxins and antigens. Clinical manifestations include severe abdominal distention, abdominal pain, fever, chills, leukocytosis with a left shift, anorexia, nausea, vomiting, and bloody diarrhea. The risks of perforation and peritonitis add to the high mortality rate.

Typically the procedure used is a proctocolectomy with ileostomy. This procedure is considered curative for ulcerative colitis.

Surgical interventions can be therapeutic in Crohn's disease as well, but there is a significant recurrence rate. Indications for surgery include intestinal obstruction, abscess formation with toxicity, fistula of the bladder or vagina, and colon failure with intractable bleeding and diarrhea. Typically the procedure used is resection of the diseased bowel, with reanastomosis. (Recurrence is common at the site of reanastomosis.)

Diet

No single diet causes or corrects IBD.

IBD is frequently accompanied by a lactose deficiency.

A low-fiber, low-residue diet is often recommended.

Bolus obstructions can result from nuts, popcorn, tough meat, raw fruit, corn, coleslaw, and uncooked vegetables.

IBD patients are at risk for protein deficiencies, and a diet high in calories (2500 to 3000 cal/day) and in protein (120 to 150 g/day) is advisable.

A deficiency of fat-soluble vitamins A, D, E, and K can occur.

Vitamin B_{12} deficiencies and iron deficiencies can occur; vitamin B_{12} injections should be considered. Most patients are not able to tolerate oral iron preparations, and parenteral and/or periodic infusions should be considered. Concurrent administration of oral iron supplements and sulfasalazine can result in decreased levels of sulfasalazine.

Total parenteral nutrition is used in cases of intensive flare-up, significant malnutrition, or in preparation for surgery to allow the bowel to rest.

Cancer Screening

Ulcerative colitis is a risk factor for colorectal cancer. The risk with Crohn's disease for colorectal cancer is slightly less than that with ulcerative colitis, but it is still higher than in the general population.

Malignancies tend to occur in the affected portion of the bowel.

Rectal bleeding is a common and often very obvious presenting symptom.

Colonoscopy should be performed every 2 years for anyone who has had a diagnosis of ulcerative colitis for more than 5 to 10 years. An upper gastrointestinal and small bowel series should also be considered for patients with Crohn's disease. A biopsy should be performed of any suspicious areas to assess for dysplastic changes.

Family Planning and Sexuality

IBD is not a contraindication to pregnancy.

Conception can be delayed by malnutrition and/or steroid therapy.

If conception occurs during remission, the pregnancy may go to full term without complications.

There is an increased risk of miscarriage if conception occurs during an active phase of the disease.

There is no increased risk of birth defects from the use of sulfasalazine or corticosteroids.

Sulfasalazine and steroid therapy may diminish sperm counts.

A male with a total proctocolectomy is at risk for impotence.

Individuals may feel a diminished sexual desire because of an altered body image or from an underlying depression from long-standing illness or steroid use.

Referral/Consultation

Refer the following patients to an internist or gastroenterologist: A newly diagnosed patient, a patient with uncontrollable symptoms, a patient with acute exacerbation of symptoms, or a patient needing screening for colorectal cancer.

Refer patients for psychosocial evaluation and counseling as indicated.

Refer patients for nutritional counseling as indicated.

Refer patients for support and self-help groups as indicated.

EVALUATION/FOLLOW-UP

Most patients will follow a cyclic course of remission and flare-up.

The overall mortality rate for ulcerative colitis is between 12% and 15% because of the risk for serious complications such as hemorrhage, perforation, and toxic megacolon.

An estimated 50% to 65% of Crohn's patients will undergo surgery at some point in their life for intestinal resection or colectomy.

The overall prognosis remains modest with Crohn's disease, unlike ulcerative colitis, which can be cured by a colectomy.

RESOURCES

Crohn's and Colitis Foundation of America (CCFA)
386 Park Avenue South
New York, NY 10016-7374
(212) 685-3440
(800) 343-3637

United Ostomy Association (UOA)
19772 MacArthur Blvd. #200
Irvine, CA 92612
(714) 660-8624
(800) 826-0826

SUGGESTED READINGS

Cooke DM: Inflammatory bowel disease: primary health care management of ulcerative colitis and Crohn's disease, *Nurse Pract* 16(8):27-39, 1991.

Doughty BD, Jackson DB: *Gastrointestinal disorders,* St Louis, 1993, Mosby.

Hay WH et al: *Current pediatric diagnosis & treatment,* ed 12, Norwalk, Conn, 1995, Appleton & Lange.

Healthcare Consultants of America, Inc: *1998 Physicians fee and coding guide,* Augusta, Ga, 1998 Healthcare Consultants of America, Inc.

101 Influenza

ICD-9-CM

Influenza 478.1

OVERVIEW

Definition

Influenza is an acute, febrile, viral illness associated with upper and lower respiratory involvement.

Incidence

Influenza occurs worldwide in pandemics, epidemics, localized outbreaks, and sporadic cases.

Outbreaks peak in the winter months in temperate climates.

Influenza affects healthy **children** at a rate of 10% to 40% annually, with a hospitalization rate of 1%.

The risk of complications from lower respiratory tract infection ranges from 0.2% to 25%.

Neonates with influenza have a higher morbidity rate from sepsis, apnea, and lower respiratory tract disease.

Children who have sickle cell disease, bronchopulmonary dysplasia, asthma, cystic fibrosis, malignancies, diabetes, or chronic renal failure have a higher rate of complications from influenza secondary to bronchitis and pneumonia.

Pathophysiology

Influenza viruses are orthomyxoviruses.

There are three types of viruses: type A, B, and C, each with many strains.

Types A and B produce clinically indistinguishable infections; whereas type C is usually a minor illness.

Transmitted by direct contact person to person, large droplet infection, or by articles contaminated by nasopharyngeal secretions.

The virus penetrates the surface of upper respiratory tract mucosal cells, producing lysis and destruction of the ciliated epithelium.

The viscosity of the mucosa decreases thus facilitating the spread of the virus to the lower respiratory tract.

Inflammation and necrosis of the bronchiolar and alveolar epithelium result, filling the alveoli with an exudate containing leukocytes, erythrocytes, and hyaline membrane.

Influenza resembles many other febrile illnesses, but it is always accompanied by a cough.

Influenza is highly contagious and can spread rapidly among **children** and **adolescents** in schools and colleges, especially among those living in dormitories or residential facilities or members of athletic teams.

Transmission to other family members is also common.

Influenza is most infectious in the 24 hours before the onset of symptoms and during the period of peak symptoms.

Viral shedding in the nasal secretions usually ceases within 7 days of the onset of illness.

The incubation period is 1 to 3 days.

SUBJECTIVE DATA

History of Present Illness

Ask about sudden onset of fever, chills, rigor, headache, malaise, diffuse myalgia, and a dry cough.

Inquire about progression of respiratory symptoms, which may include sore throat, rhinitis, nasal congestion, a prominent cough, and substernal soreness. Malaise may progress to prostration.

Inquire about associated symptoms of conjunctivitis, abdominal pain, and nausea and vomiting.

Influenza is usually self-limiting, with acute symptoms

lasting 2 to 7 days, followed by a convalescent period of about a week.

Confirm the age of the patient. **Infants, young children,** and the **elderly** are at greatest risk for complications. **Pregnant women** are also at risk for complications.

Past Medical History

Ask about general health and any underlying medical problems specifically a history of cardiac disease including rheumatic heart disease; pulmonary disease including asthma; diabetes; renal disease; malignancies; and HIV/AIDS.

Influenza can alter the metabolism of certain medications such as theophylline, which can result in toxicity from elevated serum concentrations.

OBJECTIVE DATA

Physical Examination

Perform a physical examination, with general observation and special attention to the following:

- Vital signs, especially temperature and respiration
- Upper and lower respiratory assessment: Pharyngeal injection, flushed face, anterior cervical adenopathy, and conjunctival redness are common signs
- Assess for lower respiratory involvement, including crackles and rhonchi

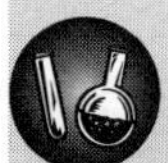

TABLE 101-1 Diagnostic Tests: Influenza

Test	Findings/Rationale	Cost ($)
Viral culture	Nasopharyngeal swabs, if they are to be used, should be obtained within the first 72 hours of illness, since the quantity of virus shed decreases rapidly	58-72
Serological testing	Diagnosis is made retrospectively by significant change in antibody titer between acute and convalescent sera	51-64
CBC	Leukopenia is common; conversely, ↑ WBC may indicate a secondary bacterial infection; Hgb and Hct may be elevated	13-16
Urinalysis	Proteinuria may be present	14-18

CBC, Complete blood cell count; *Hct,* hematocrit; *Hgb,* hemoglobin; *WBC,* white blood cell count.

Diagnostic Procedures

Diagnostic procedures are outlined in Table 101-1.

ASSESSMENT

Influenza resembles many other mild febrile illnesses and can be difficult to diagnose unless there is an epidemic.

Complications of Influenza

Sinusitis
Otitis media
Bronchitis
Pneumonia (especially influenza type A)
Reye's syndrome (especially influenza type B)

THERAPEUTIC PLAN

Pharmaceutical

Amantadine and rimantadine (Table 101-2) are FDA approved for prophylaxis against influenza A infections in **adults.** Only amantadine is approved for the treatment in **children.**

Antiviral prophylactic therapy, if indicated, should be initiated within 48 hours of onset of symptoms and continued for 2 to 5 days or for 24 to 48 hours after the patient becomes asymptomatic.

Amantadine and rimantadine are not effective against influenza B and are not approved for **infants** less than a year of age. Dosage should be reduced in the **elderly** and in patients with significant renal insufficiency. Elderly patients are more likely to have CNS and GI side effects. Amantadine is classified as pregnancy category C. Rimantadine is recommended in patients with renal failure. Rimantadine is also available in syrup form (50 mg/ml). Dosage adjustments are based on creatinine clearance (Table 101-3).

Antipyretics such as acetaminophen are recommended. **Children and adolescents** should not receive salicylates because of the risk of Reye's syndrome.

Antitussives may help reduce cough.

Antibiotics may be indicated for secondary bacterial infections.

Aerosolized ribavirin with oxygen for 12 to 18 hours a day over 3 to 7 days has been associated with a modest shortening of clinical symptoms.

TABLE 101-2 Recommended Doses for Amantadine and Rimantadine

Use	Ages 1-9*	Ages 10-65*	Age 65 and older
Treatment†	5 mg/kg/day; max dose 150 mg/day, in 1 or 2 divided doses	Weight <40 kg: 5 mg/kg/day in 1 or 2 divided doses Weight >40 kg: 200 mg/day in 1 or 2 divided doses	100 mg/day; dosage reduced in patients with impaired renal function
Prophylaxis	100 mg/day for children weighing >20 kg and adults	100 mg BID	100 mg QD

*Only amantadine is approved for treatment in children.
†Initiate within 48 hours of onset of symptoms; continue for 2 to 5 days.

TABLE 101-3 Amantadine and Rimantadine Dosage Adjustments Based on Creatinine Clearance

Creatinine Clearance (ml/min)/(ml/sec)	Dose
>50/0.83	Usual adult and adolescent dose
30-50/0.50-0.83	200 mg the first day, then 100 mg once a day
15-29/0.25-0.48	200 mg the first day, then 100 mg every other day
<15/0.25	200 mg once every 7 days
Hemodialysis patients	200 mg once every 7 days

TABLE 101-4 Influenza Vaccination Schedule

Age	Vaccine	Dose	No. of Doses
6-35 mo	Split virus	0.25 ml IM	1-2*
3-8 yr	Split virus	0.5 ml IM	1-2*
9-12 yr	Split virus	0.5 ml IM	1
>12 yr	Whole virus	0.5 ml IM	1

*Infants and children receiving influenza vaccine for the first time should receive two doses administered 1 month a part.

Patient Education

Encourage fluids and rest.

Instruct the patient about medications and the natural course of the illness.

Instruct the patient to return to the clinic if fever persists for more than 4 days or if the cough becomes productive. (Along with an elevated white count, this could indicate a bacterial infection.)

Prevention

Influenza vaccine provides partial immunity (about 85% efficacy) for a few months to 1 year (Table 101-4). The composition is changed periodically and is based on prevalent strains of the preceding year.

Annual vaccination with the trivalent influenza virus vaccine 0.5 ml intramuscularly is recommended each October or November for persons **65 years of age** and older, **children and adolescents** who are receiving aspirin therapy, nursing home residents, and persons with chronic lung or heart disease or other debilitating illnesses, including immunosuppressive disorders, diabetes, renal disease, and sickle cell anemia.

Immunization of **adults** who are in contact with **children** at high risk may be an important means of protection for these children. This includes health care workers and family members. Conversely, **children** who are members of households with high-risk adults should be vaccinated for the same reasons.

Split-virus vaccines are recommended for **children** under 13 years of age.

Influenza vaccine is strongly recommended for all **pregnant women** who are in their second and third trimester during the influenza season. Immunization is considered safe at any stage of **pregnancy.**

Administration of the vaccine is contraindicated in patients with hypersensitivity to chicken or egg protein.

Side effects include local erythema, induration, and tenderness. Myalgias and fever are rare but possible.

Consultation/Referral

Referral may be necessary for high-risk patients or those with complications.

EVALUATION/FOLLOW-UP

Closely monitor **infants, children, elderly persons,** and patients with chronic diseases.

Report influenza to local health department.

SUGGESTED READINGS

American Academy of Pediatrics: Influenza. In Peter G, editor: *1997 Red book: Report of the Committee on Infectious Diseases,* ed 24, Elk Grove Village, Ill, 1997, The Academy.

Ellsworth A et al: *Mosby's 1998 medical drug reference,* St Louis, 1998, Mosby.

Healthcare Consultants of America, Inc: *1998 Physicians fee and coding guide,* Augusta, Ga, 1998, Healthcare Consultants of America, Inc.

Tierney LM, McPhee SJ, Papadakis MA: *Current medical diagnosis & treatment,* ed 36, Norwalk, Conn, 1997, Appleton & Lange.

Wilson SF, Thompson JM: *Respiratory disorders,* St Louis, 1990, Mosby.

Irritable Bowel Syndrome

ICD-9-CM

Irritable Bowel Syndrome 564.1

OVERVIEW

Definition

Irritable bowel syndrome (IBS) is a functional disturbance of intestinal motility characterized by abdominal pain, sometimes with rectal pain; change in bowel habit, usually constipation and/or constipation alternating with diarrhea; bloating; and flatulence. There is a high correlation with emotional factors as well as intolerance to certain foods. IBS often becomes chronic, with symptoms among individuals, but typically remains constant in presentation for a particular person. IBS has been referred to as mucous colitis, spastic bowel, or spastic colitis.

Incidence

It is estimated 9% to 20% of the **adult** population are affected by IBS.

The incidence among **children** and **adolescents** is unknown, but it is thought to be relatively uncommon or possibly underdiagnosed.

Symptoms typically appear in **late adolescence** and **early adulthood.**

More common in women then in men.

Initial presentation is rarely seen in an **individual over 50 years of age.**

IBS demonstrates a familial pattern.

IBS accounts for 50% of the referrals to gastroenterologists because of concern for organic disease.

Pathophysiology

A functional bowel disorder is a chronic or recurrent gastrointestinal disorder that is not explained by organic causes. IBS is the most common of these disorders. There are several theories regarding the pathophysiology of IBS, including:

Altered bowel motility accounting for the diarrhea and constipation,

Increased sensitivity of the gut and response of the intestines to distention accounting for the abdominal pain and bloating,

The effect of other associated factors, including psychosocial stressors, psychologic dysfunction, food intolerances, abuse, and menstruation.

SUBJECTIVE DATA

History of Present Illness

IBS is consistent with continuous or recurrent symptoms for at least 3 months.

Assess for abdominal pain or cramps and inquire about location, intensity, radiation, aggravating factors, alleviating factors specifically defecation, and pain at night.

NOTE: Awakening in the morning with abdominal pain is significantly different from awakening from abdominal pain at night and should be differentiated by the clinician. Pain that wakes an individual from sleep is more likely to have an organic cause.

The left lower quadrant is the most frequent site of abdominal pain in IBS.

Diarrhea or constipation, or alternating between both, is likely to be present (note amount, frequency, and consistency of stool). Assess for painless diarrhea.

Bloating and distention, often flatulence, especially after meals, is common.

Mucus in stool; no blood in stool.

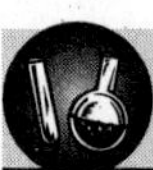

TABLE 102-1 Diagnostic Tests: Irritable Bowel Syndrome

Test	Rationale/Findings	Cost ($)
CBC with sedimentation rate	Rule out anemia, infection, and inflammatory causes	13-16 16-20
Comprehensive metabolic panel	Rule out diabetes, abnormal liver function; an elevated magnesium level may indicate diuretic or laxative abuse	32-42
Stool guaiac	Rule out occult blood	N/A
Stool ova and parasite	Rule out ova and parasites	23-28
Stool culture	Rule out bacterial infection	37-45
U/A	Assess hydration and rule out concurrent urinary tract infection	14-18
Abdominal x-ray evaluation (flat-plate and upright films)	Rule out obstruction	142-169
Barium enema	Rule out organic causes such as diverticulitis, inflammatory bowel disease, or malignancy	275-328
Abdominal sonography or flexible sigmoidoscopy	Rule out organic causes	254-302
Colonoscopy	Rule out organic causes	799-956
Lactose hydrogen breath test	Rule out lactose intolerance	N/A

CBC, Complete blood cell count; *N/A,* not available; *U/A,* urinalysis.

Past Medical History

Patient may have sought numerous providers because of unrelieved symptoms or lack of cure.

Note any previous episodes with a similar clinical course.

Note any chronic disease, food, or drug allergies.

Inquire about a family history of IBS or other gastrointestinal disorders.

Ask about past sexual or domestic abuse (increased stress).

Psychosocial History

Ask about the patient's stress level and how it is managed.

Inquire about past or present counseling.

Medications

Note all medications currently being taken (prescription, over-the-counter, vitamins, and herbal therapies), including use of laxatives or enemas.

Associated Symptoms

Assess changes in appetite or weight. Weight loss is not associated with IBS.

Assess for aggravating dietary factors such as dairy products, grains, citrus fruit, and sugar-free products that contain sorbitol. Assess for caffeine and alcohol intake.

Assess for psychosocial stressors.

Assess for psychiatric illness such as depression, anxiety, somatization, cancer phobia, and physical and sexual abuse.

Inquire about last menstrual period and relationship to symptoms.

Assess for fever.

Assess for urinary frequency.

Assess for recent travel or camping (or any possible exposure to contaminated water).

Children

Assess growth parameters. Any child who does not follow his or her weight and height curves may be experiencing malabsorption.

School-age children may present and describe abdominal pain but may be less likely to describe change in bowel habit.

Assess a school-age child for whether or not he or she will use the bathroom at school. Many children will hold stool and urine at school because of lack of privacy and time constraints.

OBJECTIVE DATA

Physical Examination

A physical examination should be performed with attention to the following:

Vital signs, height, weight

Abdomen: Assess for bowel sounds, distention, pain, and organomegaly

Rectum: Assess for tenderness, masses, stool for occult blood

TABLE 102-2 Differential Diagnosis: Irritable Bowel Syndrome

Diagnosis	Supporting Data
Inflammatory bowel disease (IBD) (ulcerative colitis, Crohn's disease)	Characterized by frequent bloody diarrhea, severe abdominal pain, nausea, fever, chills, weakness, anorexia, weight loss; cause unknown
Lactose intolerance	Deficiency in the enzyme lactase, which leads to an inability to digest lactose and results in bloating, gas, nausea, diarrhea, and abdominal cramps
Diverticulosis/diverticulitis	Pouchlike herniations through the wall of the colon that can cause crampy pain, fever, and leukocytosis during periods of inflammation
Colorectal cancer	Characterized by melena, a change in bowel habits, and the passage of blood; caused by a neoplasm in the colon or rectum
Obstruction	Obstruction of the small bowel may cause severe pain, vomiting of fecal material, dehydration, and a drop in blood pressure
	Obstruction of the colon causes less severe pain, marked abdominal distention, and constipation
	The most common cause is mechanical obstruction from adhesions, impacted feces, tumor of the bowel, hernia, intussusception, volvulus, or strictures from inflammatory bowel disease
Peptic ulcer disease	Loss of the mucous membrane of the stomach or duodenum; characterized by gnawing epigastric pain that is worse at night
	Caused by an excessive secretion of gastric acid, inadequate protection of the mucous membrane, stress, heredity, and certain drugs
Infectious diarrhea	Results from bacterial, viral, or parasitic infections
Gallstones and biliary pain	Gallstones in the gallbladder may cause abdominal pain, nausea, vomiting, eructation, flatulence, and intolerance to certain foods
Gastroesophageal reflux	Backflow of stomach contents into the esophagus as a result of incompetence of the lower esophageal sphincter, causing burning pain
Diabetic autonomic neuropathy	May present as diarrhea
Psychiatric disorders	Anxiety, depression, and somatoform disorders may present with gastrointestinal complaints

Diagnostic Procedures

The patient's history is the cornerstone of the diagnosis of IBS. The clinician should consider the possibility of organic causes of symptoms while balancing the risk and expense of testing (Table 102-1).

ASSESSMENT

Diagnostic considerations for IBS include the following:

Persistent or recurrent abdominal pain or discomfort for a period of at least 3 months

Pain relieved by defecation or associated with a change in the frequency or consistency of stool

Change in bowel habit in terms of altered stool frequency, altered stool form (hard stool or loose stool), altered stool passage (straining or sensation of urgency, or a feeling of incomplete evacuation)

Passage of mucus

Bloating or a feeling of abdominal distention

The diagnosis is made by careful history-taking and the absence of clinical findings. Differential diagnoses for irritable bowel syndrome include those listed in Table 102-2.

THERAPEUTIC PLAN

Pharmaceutical

No single agent has been proven effective.

Bulk-forming agents such as psyllium (Metamucil): 1 rounded tablespoon in juice BID to TID (helps with constipation and diarrhea).

Loperamide ($3 to $6) (Imodium) 4 mg PO initially, then 2 mg after each unformed stool, for a maximum total daily dose of 16 mg; or diphenoxylate ($6 to $47) (Lomotil) 2.5 to 5.0 mg PO after each unformed stool. Both of these agents can cause rebound constipation.

Antispasmodics and anticholinergics such as dicyclomine ($3 to $35) (Bentyl) 10 to 20 mg BID or hyoscyamine ($11 to $37) (Levsin) 0.125-0.25 mg PO TID to QID are used with meals for postprandial cramping.

Lactaid 1 to 3 caplets with meals for lactose intolerance.

Relieve bloating and flatulence with simethicone (Mylicon) 80 mg with meals and at bedtime.

Paroxetine ($57 to $64) (Paxil) 20 mg each morning is a good choice for a depressed patient with constipation, since it has some anticholinergic action. Use fluoxetine ($215 to $220) (Prozac) 20 mg each morning or sertraline ($176 to $181) (Zoloft) as a second-line drug, since both of these agents can produce GI problems, including constipation. As a last resort (**except do not use in the elderly**), consider the anticholinergic agent amitriptyline ($3 to $69) (Elavil) 50 to 100 mg at bedtime for a depressed patient with diarrhea.

Lubricants such as mineral oil have been used for constipation.

Lifestyle/Activities

Encourage the patient to walk 20 to 45 minutes at least four or five times a week.

Diet

Encourage the patient to do the following:

Maintain a food diary to help identify exacerbating foods.

Increase fluid intake (water) to 2000 ml/day.

Increase fiber intake to 25 to 35 g/day.

Avoid large meals.

Avoid spicy and fatty foods.

Monitor caffeine intake.

Avoid lactose, fructose, and sorbitol in foods such as milk products, citrus fruits, and juices, and sugar-free candy and gum if they increase symptoms.

Patient Education

Define constipation, diarrhea, and "normal" bowel habits for the patient.

Inform the patient that IBS is a chronic disorder with real symptoms, and it is not considered a precursor to cancer, colitis, or altered life expectancy.

Review lifestyle modifications, including increasing fluids, fiber, and exercise (see the patient handout on p. 649)

Encourage bowel training by instructing the patient to sit on the toilet after meals to take advantage of the normal urge to defecate after eating caused by the gastrocolic reflex.

Validate the patient's feelings and frustrations.

Stress management and biofeedback may help.

Heat to the abdomen helps trapped gas escape and allows the colon to decompress. (Heat is contraindicated if inflammation is suspected, as with appendicitis or diverticulitis.)

Children may sit in a warm tub of water.

Consultation/Referral

For uncontrolled IBS or symptoms consistent with organic disease, consider referring the patient to an internist or a gastroenterologist.

For psychopathology (anxiety, depression, posttraumatic stress disorder from abuse), refer the patient for evaluation and counseling.

Nutritional counseling and self-help and support groups may be beneficial.

EVALUATION/FOLLOW-UP

Schedule an initial follow-up in 1 to 2 weeks to assess improvement.

Every 1 to 3 months, adjust follow-up on the basis of recurring signs and symptoms.

Twenty-five percent of those diagnosed with IBS will ultimately have a permanent remission.

SUGGESTED READINGS

Bonis P, Norton R: The challenge of irritable bowel syndrome, *Am Family Physician* 53:1229-1239, 1996.

Carlson E: Irritable bowel syndrome, *Nurse Pract* 23:82-91, 1998.

Cerda J, Drossman D, Scherl E: Effective compassionate management of IBS, *Patient Care* 30:131-142, 1996.

Dalton CB, Drossman DA: Diagnosis and treatment of irritable bowel syndrome, *Am Family Physician* 55:875-880, 1997.

Ellsworth A et al: *Mosby's 1998 medical drug reference,* St Louis, 1998, Mosby.

Goroll A, May L, Mulley A, editors: *Primary care medicine: office evaluation and management of the adult patient,* Philadelphia, 1995, JB Lippincott.

Hancock L, Selig P: Irritable bowel disease. In Youngkin E, Davis M, editors: *Women's health: a primary care clinical guide,* Norwalk, Conn, 1994, Appleton & Lange.

Healthcare Consultants of America, Inc: *1998 Physicians fee and coding guide,* Augusta, Ga, 1998, Healthcare Consultants of America, Inc.

Hurst JW: *Medicine for the practicing physician,* Norwalk Conn, 1996, Appleton & Lange

Isselbacher KJ et al: *Harrison's principles of internal medicine,* ed 13, New York, 1994, McGraw-Hill.

Johnson TR, Apgar B: Irritable bowel syndrome, *Female Patient* 20:48-58, 1995.

Lonergan E, editor: *Textbook of family practice,* ed 5, Philadelphia, 1995, WB Saunders.

McWade LJ: Irritable bowel syndrome: diagnosis and management in school-aged children and adolescents, *J Pediatr Health Care* 6:82-83, 1992.

Rakel R, editor: *Textbook of family practice,* ed 5, Philadelphia, 1995, WB Saunders.

Uphold C, Graham M: *Clinical guidelines in family practice,* ed 2, Gainesville Fla, 1994, Barmarrae.

Irritable Bowel Syndrome

What is irritable bowel syndrome?

Irritable bowel syndrome has been called many names over the years, including nervous colon, spastic colon, nervous colitis, mucous colitis. It is quite common, affecting 9% to 20% of the adult population. It seems to affect women more than men. It often starts in the late teens to early adult years.

What causes irritable bowel syndrome?

The exact cause is unknown. The symptoms are a result of the intestinal tract moving too slowly or too fast. Abdominal pain, bloating, gas, and changes in bowel movements such as diarrhea and constipation are common.

Will irritable bowel syndrome hurt me?

Irritable bowel syndrome is uncomfortable, but it does not lead to cancer, diverticulitis, colitis, or decreased life expectancy.

What makes irritable bowel syndrome worse?

Irritable bowel syndrome seems to be made worse by certain foods and by stress.

Foods that commonly cause IBS

Milk	Citrus	Onions	Cheese	Chocolate
Potatoes	Butter	Coffee/tea	Barley/rye	Yogurt
Yeast	Oats	Eggs	Alcohol	Corn
Nuts	Fruit	Wheat		

How is irritable bowel syndrome treated?

It is important to change your eating habits. Adding both fiber and water to your diet helps the diarrhea and constipation. Try to drink 8 to 10 glasses of water a day. Avoid excess caffeine and alcohol. Fiber can be found in beans, vegetables, fruits, cereals, and breads. Exercise is very important. Walking 20 to 45 minutes several days a week has been very helpful to many people. Avoid using laxatives because your body can become dependent on them. Sometimes medicine is used to help symptoms, but that depends on each patient. Setting aside time each day to sit on the toilet after a meal will help keep your bowels more regular. Not everyone has a bowel movement every day, but the stool should be soft and pass easily. Find ways to reduce stress.

Kawasaki's Disease

ICD-9-CM

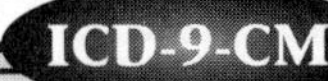

Kawasaki Syndrome 446.1

OVERVIEW

Definition

Kawasaki's disease is also known as mucocutaneous lymph node syndrome and infantile polyarteritis. It is a febrile illness with an acute onset from inflammation of the arteries, particularly the coronary arteries.

Incidence

Boys are affected greater than girls (1.5:1). In the United States, incidence is greatest between 18 and 24 months. The highest risk is among Asian boys. Kawasaki's disease is the leading cause of acquired heart disease in children in the United States.

Pathophysiology

The cause is unknown, but it is believed to be associated with the dust mite. It is a type III hypersensitivity reaction with depositing of immune complexes. These complexes increase blood viscosity and produce aneurysm formation. May also be caused by a superantigen secreted by *Staphylococcus aureus.*

The disease has four stages:

- Stage I (11 days): Signs and symptoms are fever, conjunctivitis, irritability, rash, cervical lymphadenopathy, elevated erythrocyte sedimentation rate
- Stage II (10 to 14 days long, second and third week of illness): Cardiac complications, fever, irritability, desquamation of fingers and toes
- Stage III (6 to 10 weeks): Conjunctivitis and aneurysms of peripheral vessels
- Stage IV (duration unknown): Coronary complications in adulthood, thrombosis, myocardial infarction, dysrhythmias, congestive heart failure

Protective Factors Against

Avoiding recently shampooed rugs

Factors That Increase Susceptibility

Living by bodies of water

SUBJECTIVE DATA

History of Present Illness

Rash
Fever greater than 5 days' duration unresponsive to antibiotics
Diarrhea in infants
Irritability
Cough
Joint pain
Conjunctivitis

Past Medical History

Recent respiratory illness
Recent streptococcal infection

Medications

Recent antibiotics but no change in fever

Family History

Not usually significant

Psychosocial History

Recent exposure to dust and dust mites

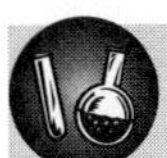

TABLE 103-1 Diagnostic Test: Kawasaki Disease

Test	Findings/Rationale	Cost ($)
CBC	Leukocytosis with a shift to the left (neutrophils with immature forms); thrombocytosis, anemia	13-16
U/A	Proteinuria, sterile pyuria	14-18
ESR	Elevated	16-20
C-reactive protein	Positive	26-32
Liver enzymes	Elevated	29-41
CXR	Pulmonary infiltrates and cardiomegaly may be present	72-91
ECG	Dysrhythmia	56-65
Echocardiogram	Mitral insufficiency, aneurysms, pericardial effusion	675

CBC, Complete blood cell count; *CXR*, chest x-ray evaluation; *ECG*, electrocardiogram; *ESR*, erythrocyte sedimentation rate; *U/A*, urinalysis.

Associated Symptoms

Arthralgia

Erythema and induration at recent Bacille Calmette-Guérin inoculation site

OBJECTIVE DATA

Physical Examination

A physical examination should be performed, with attention to the following:

General appearance: Irritability in infants, vital signs to rule out fever

Head/eyes/ears/nose/throat:

Ear: Tympanic membrane may be pink, poor light reflex, concomitant otitis media

Eye: Bilateral tearing without exudate, injection of conjunctiva

Lymphadenopathy: Usually anterior cervical chain is enlarged

Throat: Enlarged, erythematous tonsils without exudate may be present

Mouth: Strawberry tongue, dry, erythematous, cracked lips

Integument:

Indurative edema or erythema of the soles and palms

Desquamation of hands and feet beginning in the fingertips

Nonvesicular diffuse, polymorphous rash mostly on the trunk

Cardiac: May hear murmur of mitral valve regurgitation or friction rub

Diagnostic Procedures

Diagnostic tests for Kawasaki's disease are listed in Table 103-1.

TABLE 103-2 Differential Diagnosis: Kawasaki's Disease

Diagnosis	Supporting Data
Scarlet fever	Lymphadenopathy, nausea and vomiting, headache, positive result to a screening test for streptococcal organisms, sore throat, papular rash on neck progressing to trunk and extremities, flushed face
Measles	Cough, coryza, conjunctivitis, Koplik's spots (small, bluish-gray papules on a red base) in the mouth, rash starts on face then progresses to trunk, fine brownish desquamation may occur

ASSESSMENT

Differential Diagnosis

Differential diagnoses are listed in Table 103-2.

THERAPEUTIC PLAN

Pharmaceutical

Hospitalization is required for administration of intravenous gamma globulin and the monitoring of the child's cardiac condition. Pharmaceutical treatment is outlined in Table 103-3.

Dipyridamole and warfarin therapy may be initiated if the child develops coronary artery aneurysm. This medication is usually dosed by the pediatric cardiologist. Corticosteroid use is contraindicated and has been associated with aneurysm formation.

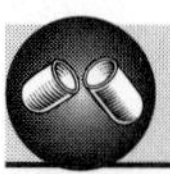

TABLE 103-3 Pharmaceutical Plan: Kawasaki's Disease

Drug	Dose	Comments	Cost ($)
Acute Phase			
Aspirin	80 to 100 mg/kg/day in four divided doses	Discontinue if child develops varicella or flu to prevent Reye's syndrome	9-37/ECA
Subacute/Convalescent Phase			
Aspirin	3 to 5 mg/kg/day in a single dose	Discontinue if child develops varicella or flu to prevent Reye's syndrome	9-37/ECA

ECA, Enteric-coated aspirin.

Lifestyle/Activities

Depending on the degree of cardiac involvement, activity may be limited.

Diet

Noncontributory

Patient Education

Parents should be taught that administration of live virus vaccines (measles, mumps, and rubella) should be delayed 5 months after administration of intravenous gamma globulin.

Parents should be taught that coronary artery damage may not manifest itself until adulthood, therefore echocardiograms are repeated throughout adolescence.

Family Impact

Parents may have anxiety regarding prognosis and probability of acute cardiac death.

Consultation/Referral

Patients suspected of having Kawasaki disease should be evaluated by a pediatric cardiologist and followed by this specialist if cardiac complications are present.

Follow-up

Patients should be followed throughout all four stages: initially in 1 week, then in 1 month, then in 6 months, and annually.

EVALUATION

Beware of the development of aneurysms in unusual places such as the hepatic, axillary, and brachial arteries. Arteriography may need to be performed for detection.

SUGGESTED READINGS

Ellsworth A et al: *Mosby's 1998 medical drug reference,* St Louis, 1998, Mosby.

Fredriksen M: An infant with persistent fever, *Clin Rev* 8:129-136, 1998.

Healthcare Consultants of America, Inc: *1998 Physicians fee and coding guide,* Augusta, Ga, 1998, Healthcare Consultants of America, Inc.

Rubin B, Cotton D: Kawasaki disease: a dangerous acute childhood illness, *Nurse Pract* 23:34-48, 1998.

104 Lead Poisoning (Plumbism)

ICD-9-CM

Lead Poisoning 984.9

OVERVIEW

Definition

As defined by the Centers for Disease Control* (CDC) in 1991, lead poisoning is characterized by a blood lead level greater than or equal to 10 µg/dl.

Incidence

Adults: Lead poisoning in an adult is a rare occurrence, usually a result of occupational exposure in an unsafe work site. More than 3 million workers in the United States are potentially exposed to lead in the workplace.

Children: Children 6 to 36 months old are at the highest risk for lead poisoning, although lead poisoning can be a hazard until children are approximately 6 years of age. National estimates from 1988 to 1991 showed that approximately 1.7 million children in the United States had blood lead levels of more than 10 µg/dl. It is difficult to estimate the costs associated with lead poisoning. Studies have demonstrated that screening is cost effective.

Pathophysiology

Lead is primarily orally ingested and enters the bloodstream via the stomach. Children absorb approximately 50% of the lead they ingest, compared with adults, who absorb only 10%. Lead is a protean poison; it causes cellular disturbance in most body tissues and organs. It interferes with heme synthesis, causing an anemia that mimics iron-deficiency anemia. The major concern in lead poisoning in young children is the effect on the developing nervous system. Lead is thought to interfere with the development of nerve pathways. Lead is also substituted for calcium in the bone matrix. The lead that accumulates in the bone provides a source for remobilization and continued toxicity after exposure ceases.

Complications of Lead Poisoning

Chronic anemia, mild to severe in nature, results from lead interference in the heme synthesis pathway. Lead's interference with brain development can cause complications as minor as no identifiable problem to as severe as mental retardation or seizure. Severe lead poisoning can cause coma and death. Complications of lead intoxication include learning disabilities, behavior disorders, sleep disorders, developmental delay, poor appetite, nausea, and vomiting.

Primary Sources of Lead Exposure

Lead paint is the most common source. It is ingested in the form of paint chips or, more frequently, lead paint dust. Most homes built before 1950 were painted with lead-based paint. Lead was not banned from paint until 1978. Lead-painted surfaces that are in poor repair offer the greatest risk.

Drinking water offers a minor risk. Elevated lead levels are usually found in old homes with lead-soldered pipes.

Soil with lead paint dust and/or leaded gasoline contamination (from car exhaust) can be a risk factor.

Occupations and hobbies can be a source of exposure. Children are generally exposed by playing by or living next to contaminated work sites or by contaminated clothing.

Airborne lead from car exhaust is a minor source of exposure.

Ceramics and lead crystal can be a source. There is an increased risk in products purchased outside the United States.

Folk remedies have been a minor source of exposure (e.g., Mexican: azarcon; Asian: chuifong tokuwan; Middle Eastern: alkohl).

---

*Now called the Centers for Disease Control and Prevention.

Factors Contributing to Lead Poisoning

Age <6 years old
Exposure to lead hazard
Low blood hemoglobin, hematocrit, and iron
Pica behaviors
Poor diet
Presence of developmental delay (as a result of prolonged hand/mouth behaviors)
Poor hand washing

SUBJECTIVE DATA

History of Present Illness

Ask the patient (in children, ask the patient's parents) about:
- The presence or absence of clinical symptoms, including fatigue, irritability, distractibility, inability to concentrate, unusual sleep patterns, poor appetite, nausea, vomiting, coordination problems; most children with lead poisoning will be asymptomatic
- The child's developmental history with attention to language development, and ability to concentrate
- Mouthing activities, including pica behaviors, use of a bottle, pacifier or thumb sucking
- Nutritional status

Past Medical History

Ask the patient (in children, ask the patient's parents) about:
- Past blood lead levels
- History of anemia
- History of developmental delay
- History of gastrointestinal, hematological, renal, reproductive and neurological disorders

Medications

Vitamins or any prescription or nonprescription drugs the child is taking

Family History

Family history of lead poisoning

Environmental History

Age and condition of child's primary residence (or residences)
Living near an active lead smelter, battery recycling plant, or other industry likely to release lead
Occupation (plumber, pipe fitter, auto repair person, printer, battery manufacturing, pottery workers, rubber industry, jewelers, welders, and so on) and hobby interests of adults in the household

Diet History

Iron and calcium intake
Infant formula: Amount and type
Meal frequency
Amount of fat in diet; a high-fat diet is associated with increased lead absorption

Description of Most Common Symptoms

Most infants and children present with no overt symptomatology.
The most common symptoms are loss of appetite, nausea, vomiting, and irritability.
Behavioral symptoms are often not realized until treatment reverses the effects of lead poisoning.

OBJECTIVE DATA

Physical Examination

A complete physical examination should be performed; it can often be done at a scheduled well child visit.

- Vital signs
- Growth parameters, including height, weight, head circumference; should be plotted on growth charts
- General appearance
- Particular attention should be paid to the neurological examination; psychosocial skills, cognition, language, and behavior should all be observed

Diagnostic Procedures

Diagnostic procedures include those found in Table 104-1. Many offices use a home assessment risk questionnaire to help identify children at risk for lead poisoning. This is acceptable, but it must be used consistently. The CDC recommends that all children should have a blood lead level evaluation done by 12 months of age. Children at high risk should be screened at 6 months.

ASSESSMENT

Differential Diagnosis

Differential diagnoses for lead poisoning are listed in Table 104-2.

THERAPEUTIC PLAN

The plan of care is based on the patient's blood lead level. Care should be based on the risk classification developed by the CDC in 1991 (Table 104-3).

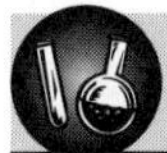

TABLE 104-1 Diagnostic Tests: Lead Poisoning

Test	Finding/Rationale	Cost ($)
Blood lead level	A venous sample with a lead level of ≥10 μg/dl is considered confirmation of lead poisoning. A finger stick sample must be confirmed with a venous sample because of the risk of contamination in the finger stick sample. A venous sample is the most cost-effective approach.	20 (varies)
Abdominal x-ray or CXR	Used to identify lead particles in abdomen and lines of increased density in metaphyseal plate of long bones.	41-57
Hemoglobin	To assess for anemia; often part of a routine visit.	11-14
U/A, serum creatinine	To detect renal dysfunction.	15-20/U/A 18-24/creat
Zinc protoporphyrin or free erythrocyte protoporphyrin level	Reflects the toxic effect of lead on the erythrocyte enzyme ferrochelatase. Zinc protoporphyrin levels begin to rise in adults when the blood level >30-40 μg/dl. It is only of ancillary value in evaluating occupational lead exposure.	34-43

CXR, Chest x-ray examination; *U/A,* urinalysis.

TABLE 104-2 Differential Diagnosis: Lead Poisoning

Diagnosis	Supporting Data
Attention deficit disorder	Impulsivity, decreased ability to concentrate, hyperactivity, decreased ability to restrain behavior, easily bored with repetitive tasks, inability to stop and think about consequences before acting, excessive movements
Learning disability	Patient's demonstrated achievement on standardized tests in reading, math, or written expression substantially below the expected scores for age, schooling, and intelligence
Developmental delay	A spectrum of disorders characterized by deficits in cognitive, social, and emotional functioning
Iron deficiency anemia	Fatigue, irritability, difficulty concentrating
CNS tumor	Headache, irritability, difficulty concentrating, vomiting
Metabolic disorder	Seizures, coma, irritability, weight loss

CNS, Central nervous system.

Pharmaceutical

A pharmaceutical plan for lead poisoning is outlined in Tables 104-4 and 104-5.

A lead level and complete blood count with differential liver function studies and renal panel should be done at the end of therapy.

Be aware that lead levels may rebound as a result of the body's attempt to equilibrate. Lead will be freed from the bone and will enter the circulation. Repeat chelation test as often necessary.

Testing of blood lead levels (by venous sample only) should be performed monthly.

At a lead level >70 μg/dl the health department will intervene to ensure that the child is living in lead-safe housing (see Table 104-6).

Lifestyle/Activities

Lead poisoning is best prevented. Primary prevention would include:

Engineering controls: Isolation via containers, ventilation, substitution of less-hazardous materials

Personal protective equipment: Respirator use

Work practices: Housekeeping to remove lead dust accumulation

Personal hygiene and periodic inspections

Education of Parents

Discuss lead hazard and health implications.

Assess homes for peeling or chipping paint. Look closely at

TABLE 104-3 CDC Risk Classifications

Class	Blood Lead	Intervention
Class I	<9 μg/dl	Assess risk factors at all well-child visits until the patient is 3 years old. A 6-month-old child who is at high risk because of housing or family history of lead poisoning should have a lead level checked every 6 months until he or she is 3 years old.
Class IIa	10-14 μg/dl	Rescreen every 6 months using only venous obtained samples. Assess risk factors for lead hazard sources. Provide dietary education; increase iron-containing foods. Increase foods containing calcium. Low-fat diet to reduce absorption and retention of lead. Consider starting multivitamins with iron. Provide education regarding protecting child from lead hazards: Home cleaning Hand washing education Decreasing hand to mouth behaviors
Class IIb	15-19 μg/dl	Rescreen every 3 months with a venous sample. Assess risk factors for lead hazards. Provide above-mentioned education regarding diet, environment, and health behaviors. Some states require home evaluation by the health department at this level. Be aware of local regulations.
Class III	20-44 μg/dl	Complete medical assessment with referral to lead poisoning program if available. Identify and eliminate lead hazards. Refer to the local healthy department for environmental evaluation. Provide education regarding diet, environment, and health behaviors. Rescreen monthly.
Class IV	Blood lead 45-69 μg/dl	Immediate retest with a venous sample. Begin oral chelation therapy with succimer.

TABLE 104-4 Pharmaceutical Plan: Lead Poisoning

Drug	Dose	Comments	Cost
Succimer (Chemet)	350 mg/m^2 or 10 mg/ml q8h for 5 days, then reduced to 350 mg/m^2 or 10 mg/ml q12h for 14 days	Not recommended for children <1 year old FDA approved for children only Pregnancy: C SE: GI upset, elevated AST, ALT, rash, pain, cramps, flulike symptoms, dizziness, drowsiness; succimer is a capsule in sprinkle formulation; it can be opened and mixed with food; has a strong sulfurlike odor	$318/100 mg (100)

ALT, Alanine aminotransferase; *AST,* aspartate aminotransferase; *FDA,* Food and Drug Administration; *GI,* gastrointestinal; *SE,* side effects.

TABLE 104-5 Succimer Pediatric Dosing

Weight	Dose (mg) q8h for 5 Days then q12h for 14 Days	Number of Capsules
18-35 lb (8-15 kg)	100	1
36-55 lb (16-23 kg)	200	2
56-75 lb (24-34 kg)	300	3
76-100 lb (35-44 kg)	400	4
>100 lb (>45 kg)	500	5

TABLE 104-6 Therapeutic Approach for Class V Lead Poisoning

Class	Blood Lead	Intervention
Class V	>70 μg/dl	The child should be admitted to the hospital for intravenous chelation therapy with $CaNa_2$ EDTA. EDTA may be given in combination with intramuscular BAL.

BAL, British anti-Lewisite; *EDTA,* ethylenediaminetetraacetic acid.

windows, the opening and closing can increase lead dust. Children are drawn to windows out of curiosity.

Floors and window sills should be cleaned with a wet mop or sponge. An effective cleaning agent is trisodium phosphate, which is available in hardware stores.

Lead paint removal should only be done by a qualified contractor; removing the paint improperly can increase the lead hazard.

Iron and calcium deficiencies increase the absorption of lead.

Diet counseling is important.

Children with elevated lead levels or lead hazards in their homes should not use a pacifier and should be weaned from the bottle by 12 months of age.

Hands should be washed after play and before eating.

Discourage hand/mouth behaviors such as thumbsucking and nail biting.

Referral

Refer to MD:

- All patients with blood lead levels >44 μg/dl by venous sample confirmation
- Any child with any elevated lead level that is symptomatic

Consultation

Blood lead level of 20 to 44 μg/dl.

Consult with appropriate health professional for treatment of language, behavior and attention disorders, and developmental delay.

A case of occupational lead poisoning should be reported to the health department. 27 states require reporting of elevated lead levels under the Adult Blood Lead Epidemiology and Surveillance program administered by NIOSH.

EVALUATION/FOLLOW-UP

Follow-up will be based on the classification of the lead poisoning.

RESOURCES

Code of federal regulations
http://law.house.gov/cfr.htm

Duke University Occupational and Environmental Medicine
http://152.2.65.120/oem

CDC home page
http://www.cdc.gov

OSHA regulations
http://www.osha.gov

EPA home page
http://epa.gov/

NIOSH homepage
http://www.cdc.gov/niosh/homepage.html

Envirolink
http://www.envirolink.org

SUGGESTED READINGS

American Academy of Pediatrics Committee on Drugs: Treatment guidelines for lead exposure in children, *Pediatrics* 96:155-160, 1995.

Baker RC, editor: *Handbook of pediatric primary care,* Boston, 1996, Little Brown & Co.

Brody D, Pirkle JL, Kramer RA: Blood lead levels in the US population: phase I of the third national health and nutrition examination survey, *JAMA* 272:277-283, 1994.

Centers for Disease Control and Prevention: *Preventing lead poisoning in young children,* Atlanta, Ga, 1991, CDC.

Ellsworth A et al: *Mosby's 1998 medical drug reference,* St Louis, 1998, Mosby.

Healthcare Consultants of America, Inc: *1998 Physicians fee and coding guide,* Augusta, Ga, 1998, Healthcare Consultants of America, Inc.

Kimbrough RD, LeVois M, Webb DR: Management of children with slightly elevated blood lead levels, *Pediatrics* 93:188-191, 1994.

Sargent JD: The role of nutrition in the prevention of lead poisoning in children, *Pediatr Ann* 23:636-642, 1994.

Staudinger K, Roth V: Occupational lead poisoning, *Am Family Physician* 57:719-728, 1998.

Leukemia

ICD-9-CM

Acute Lymphocytic Leukemia (ALL) 204.0
Chronic Lymphocytic Leukemia (CLL) 204.1
Hairy Cell Leukemia 202.4
Acute Nonlymphocytic Leukemia (ANLL), Acute Myelocytic Leukemia (AML), or Acute Granulocytic Leukemia (AGL) 205.0
Chronic Myelocytic Leukemia (CML) or Chronic Granulocytic Leukemia (CGL) in Adults 205.1
Lymphoid Leukemia 204.9

OVERVIEW

Definition

Leukemia is a proliferation of immature white blood cells (WBCs) originating in the bone marrow.

Pathophysiology

The overproliferation of immature WBCs in the bone marrow can completely replace the normal bone marrow precursors leading to a decrease in red blood cells (RBCs), platelets, and granulocytes. Leukemic cells may also proliferate in other reticuloendothelial tissues and in other extramedullary sites such as the central nervous system, testes, bones, or skin (Lampkin, 1997). It is theorized that the cause is ecogenetic in basis—a genetic transformation of the progenitor (stem) cell that occurs in response to environmental agents.

Risk Factors

Genetic Predisposition

The presence of Diamond-Blackfan anemia carries an increased risk of AML
Patients with Down's syndrome (trisomy 21) have a 10 to 20 times higher incidence of leukemia
The presence of Bloom's syndrome and Fanconi's anemia leads to an increased risk of AML
Ataxia/telangiectasia
Identical twins carry a 25% increased risk of ALL
Nontwin siblings of a patient with ALL also carry an increased risk of ALL
History of fetal loss
Advanced maternal age

Possible Environmental Factors

Ionizing radiation
Chronic chemical exposure (e.g., to benzene)
Previous malignancy treated with alkylating agents
Exposure to electromagnetic fields
Exposure to herbicides and pesticides
Maternal use of alcohol, contraceptives, diethylstilbestrol (DES), or cigarettes

Viral Infections

HTLV-I: Linked to adult T-cell leukemia lymphoma
HTLV-II: Linked to hairy cell leukemia
HTLV-III: Linked to Kaposi's sarcoma
Epstein-Barr virus (EBV): Associated with L_3 subtype of ALL

Immunodeficiency

Long-term use of immunosuppressive drugs
Wiskott-Aldrich syndrome

Congenital hypogammaglobulinemia
Ataxia/telangiectasia

Types and Incidence

The incidence of all types of leukemia is approximately 13/100,000 per year. In general, males are affected more often than females and whites more than blacks.

Acute Lymphocytic Leukemia

Abnormal proliferation of immature lymphocytes in the bone marrow
Affects approximately 4/100,000 **children** each year
Approximately 3500 new cases each year in the United States
Peak incidence is in children 3 to 5 years old
Males affected more than females (1.3:1)
Accounts for 75% to 80% of all childhood leukemias

Acute Myelogenous Leukemia

Abnormal proliferation of immature myeloid stem cells in the bone marrow
Ratio of AML to ALL is 1:4
Accounts for 15% to 25% of **childhood** leukemias
10% of the cases of childhood AML occur in **infants** under 2 years old
Incidence is relatively constant from birth through adolescence

Chronic Lymphocytic Leukemia

A persistent absolute lymphocytosis for 3 months or longer
The most common type of leukemia in the United States
Males affected more than females (2 to 3:1)
75% of patients are **60 years old** or older

Chronic Myelogenous Leukemia

Abnormal proliferation of differentiating myeloid cells in blood and bone marrow

Juvenile Chronic Myelogenous Leukemia

Accounts for 1% to 5% of all childhood leukemias
If it is seen in children, it almost always is seen in those under 2 years of age
Relatively rapid course
Cytogenetic marker: Philadelphia (Ph^1) chromosome

Adult Chronic Myelogenous Leukemia

Median age of onset is 45 years
Natural course of disease: Progresses from chronic to accelerated, then to the blast phase

Leukemia in Pregnancy

Occurs in fewer than 1/100,000 pregnancies annually
Limited studies done
Two large studies (Caligiuri and Mayer, 1993):
  Seventy-two cases of leukemia from 1975 to 1988
  Types/incidence:
    AML: 61%
    ALL: 28%
    CML: 7%

SUBJECTIVE DATA

History of Presenting Signs and Symptoms

Acute leukemias: Symptoms present 1 to 2 weeks before diagnosis
Chronic leukemias: Symptoms chronic and less obvious
ALL and AML: Most common presenting symptoms include pallor, bleeding, fever, and pain
Bone marrow infiltration and failure cause these signs and symptoms
CML: Most cases are diagnosed during the chronic phase. Symptoms at diagnosis may include splenomegaly, hepatomegaly, fever, night sweats, pallor, weight loss, bone pain, and lymphadenopathy. If hyperleukocytosis is present, complications include focal or diffuse neurological findings, respiratory distress, metabolic disturbances, or priapism.
Juvenile CML: Usually affects children 2 years old or younger. Symptoms include cutaneous lesions (eczema, xanthomata, and café-au-lait spots), generalized lymphadenopathy, marked splenomegaly, hepatomegaly, and hemorrhagic problems. A facial rash (erythematous, maculopapular, or desquamative) is common and may have been present for months before diagnosis. Also, respiratory symptoms including cough, expiratory wheezing, and tachypnea may be present.
CLL: Most cases are diagnosed during chronic phase. Symptoms at diagnosis include malaise, increased fatigability, generalized lymphadenopathy, and splenomegaly. As the disease progresses, symptoms of anemia, granulocytopenia, thrombocytopenia, and hypogammaglobulinemia may develop.

Past Medical History

Recent history of viral illness
History of prior illnesses, surgery
Genetic abnormalities
Exposure to HTLV-I virus
Allergies

Medications

Exposure to cytotoxic drugs, benzene, chloramphenicol
Medications, including home remedies, nonprescription drugs, vitamin/mineral supplements, and borrowed medicine

Family History

Family history of cancer

Psychosocial History

Tobacco, alcohol and/or drug use
Immunizations and screening tests
Home situation and significant others, including family and friends

Description of Most Common and Associated Symptoms

Anemia: Present in most cases at diagnosis. Symptoms include malaise, weakness, dyspnea, irritability, fatigue, anorexia, pallor, and heart murmur.
Thrombocytopenia: Present in 75% cases of childhood leukemia. Symptoms include petechiae, easy bruising, epistaxis, menorrhagia, gastrointestinal and intracranial hemorrhage, and hematuria.
Neutropenia: Fever at diagnosis is present in 60% cases of childhood leukemia. Other symptoms include persistent infections, abscesses.
Central nervous system involvement: Present in fewer than 10% cases. Symptoms include headache, vomiting, and visual disturbances.
Bone pain: Present in approximately 23% of cases at diagnosis. Pain is from the overproliferation of leukemia cells within the bone marrow space, and possibly from bony destruction by leukemic infiltration.
Gastrointestinal symptoms: Caused by proliferation of leukemic cells in the abdominal viscera, liver, and spleen. Symptoms include anorexia, weight loss, abdominal pain, and hepatosplenomegaly.
Generalized lymphadenopathy: Common at diagnosis; results from infiltration by leukemic cells.
Genitourinary symptoms: In males, testicular ALL can present with a painless, firm, unilateral, or bilateral enlargement; some degree of discoloration may be present.

OBJECTIVE DATA

Physical Examination

Perform a complete physical examination, with increased attention to:

Vital signs
Weight
Signs/symptoms of infection
General appearance
Skin: Excessive bruising, petechiae, pallor, rashes, infections, leukemia cutis: leukemic skin infiltration associated mostly with AML
Lymph system: Check neck, axillae, supraclavicular and infraclavicular, epitrochlear, and inguinal regions for nodal enlargement
Head/eyes/ears/nose/throat: Fundi—papilledema
Chest: Murmurs from anemia; wheezing and decreased breath sounds from a possible mediastinal mass
Abdomen: Hepatosplenomegaly
Genitourinary: Male: check testes for unilateral or bilateral firm, painless enlargement with or without some degree of scrotal discoloration

Diagnostic Procedures

Diagnostic procedures are listed in Table 105-1.

Prognostic Factors

Initial WBC evaluation: High risk if WBCs higher than 50,000
Age at diagnosis: Poor prognosis if patient is younger than 2 years old or older than 10 years old
Hemoglobin level: Poorer prognosis when low
Platelet count: Poorer prognosis when low
Race: Blacks have poorer prognosis
Presence of mediastinal mass, organomegaly, or lymphadenopathy: More tumor burden requiring more intense chemotherapy

ASSESSMENT

The bone marrow test is the definitive diagnostic test for leukemia.
Differential diagnoses include those listed in Table 105-2.
Children: Most likely diagnosis is ALL, then AML
Adults: Most likely diagnosis CML or CLL
Pregnant women: Most likely AML, then ALL, and least often CML

THERAPEUTIC PLAN

Refer the patient to a physician if the complete blood count (CBC), differential, history, and physical examination are highly indicative of leukemia. The goal of treatment is to eradicate leukemic blast cells so normal cells can regrow.

Pharmeceutical

ALL

Treatment consists of combination chemotherapy, often following specific multicenter protocols. Cranial-spinal radiation is used if there is central nervous system (CNS) involvement. The length of the treatment would be 2 years plus a few months for girls and 3 years plus a few months for boys.

Chemotherapy includes:

Prednisone/dexamethasone
Vincristine
Asparaginase
Methotrexate

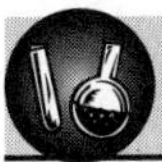

TABLE 105-1 Diagnostic Tests: Leukemia

Test	Findings/Rationale	Cost ($)
CBC with differential	WBC >50,000 in 20% of patients with ALL Initial WBC level is single most important predictor of prognosis Low absolute neutrophil count is present Hemoglobin <10 g/dl Thrombocytopenia (platelets <100,000) present in 75% of cases at diagnosis May or may not see blast cells on differential; bone marrow may be "packed" before one can see blasts on a peripheral smear	18-23
Bone marrow	Definitive diagnostic test Bone marrow aspiration shows 25% blasts: Cytogenetics, immunophenotyping, and special stains are done to differentiate type of leukemia	401-499
Lumbar puncture	Lumbar puncture to rule out CNS involvement	172-208
CXR	To check for mediastinal mass	77-91
Serum immunoglobulin levels quantitative	Low in 30% of ALL patients at diagnosis	69-87/IgG 140/IgG subclasses
Uric acid	Increased serum uric acid levels can lead to uric acid nephropathy and renal failure	18-23
Liver function tests	Results can be elevated if there is liver involvement	29-41
Calcium/phosphorus	May see ↑ calcium and ↓ phosphorus	18-23/ca 18/phos
Blood culture tests if patient is febrile	To rule out bacteremia/sepsis, identify bacteria, and treat with sensitive antibiotics	37-45

CBC, Complete blood cell count; *CNS*, central nervous system; *CXR*, chest x-ray evaluation; *WBC*, white blood cells.

TABLE 105-2 Differential Diagnosis: Leukemia

Diagnoses	Supporting Data
Aplastic anemia	No abnormal blasts in peripheral blood
Marrow infiltration with solid tumor	Often there is other lymph node enlargement; CBC is usually normal; no circulating blasts
Autoimmune pancytopenia	Similar to aplastic anemia; approximately a third of cases of aplastic anemia are caused by autoimmune factors; no abnormal blasts in peripheral blood
Immune thrombocytopenia	Isolated ↓ in platelets, bruises
Severe megaloblastic anemia	MCV ↑, normal platelets, ↓ Hgb (MCV in ALL usually near normal or low)
Overwhelming infection	Signs and symptoms of infection appear before CBC changes
Rheumatoid arthritis	Often normal CBC with joint swelling and pain
Marrow suppression as a result of drugs, toxins, or infections	Negative history of exposures of patient/parents

CBC, Complete blood cell count; *Hgb*, hemoglobin; *MCV*, mean corpuscular volume.

6-Mercaptopurine
Thioguanine
Cytoxan
Ara-C (cytosine arabinoside)
Doxorubicin

AML

Treatment consists of very intense combination chemotherapy. The duration of treatment is shorter than for ALL. Cranial-spinal radiation is indicated if there is CNS involvement. Bone marrow transplant (BMT) may be undertaken if a complete match can be found. Most of the treatment is performed in the hospital. Chemotherapy consists of intense doses of:

Idarubicin
Ara-C (cytosine arabinoside)
Etoposide (VP-16)
6-Thioguanine
Dexamethasone
Daunomycin

CML

Juvenile CML is generally resistant to therapy. Median survival length is less than 9 months from diagnosis. BMT is the only possible curative treatment.

For adult CML the goal of treatment is to provide symptomatic relief by lowering the WBC count and reducing liver and spleen size. Hydroxyurea or busulfan, given as single agents, can be used to regulate leukocytosis. BMT is the only possible curative treatment.

Hydroxyurea 1 to 3 g/day PO as a single dose on an empty stomach
Busulfan (Myleran) 4 to 8 mg/day PO (initial doses often 0.1 mg/kg/day)
Alpha-interferon

CLL

Stable, asymptomatic patients with or without lymphadenopathy and/or splenomegaly do not require treatment.

Symptomatic patients (those with weight loss, malaise, anemia, thrombocytopenia) are treated with alkylating agents (chlorambucil or cyclophosphamide in standard doses), with or without corticosteroids.

Leukemia in Pregnancy

AML or ALL requires immediate and aggressive treatment with combination chemotherapy.

If AML or ALL is diagnosed in the first trimester, the prognosis is very poor for both mother and child.

If AML or ALL is diagnosed and treated in the second or third trimester, there is a 75% chance of remission and only a 1.5% incidence of congenital anomalies.

CML has a slow, indolent course.

Lifestyle/Activities

No intramuscular injections
No rectal temperature-taking or use of suppositories
No tampons
Use a soft toothbrush or toothettes for oral care

Diet

Not applicable

Patient Education

The patient and family must become fully informed about the disease, the diagnosis, and the treatment plan.

The patient and family can be taught about expected and toxic side effects of chemotherapy.

Supportive care and guidelines for lifestyle and activities modifications must be clear to the family and primary care provider.

Family Impact

The impact of having a loved one diagnosed with leukemia is devastating. Assisting the family in finding support systems and resources is important. Most oncology centers are well versed in resources for patients and families.

Referral/Consultation

The patient should be referred to a hematologist/oncologist in a timely manner to avoid complications from delay.

Follow-up

The communication between the hematologist/oncologist and primary care provider must be clear, concise, and current.

Supportive Care Guidelines

If there is central line access, provide antibiotic prophylaxis before dental work is done.

If the patient is febrile, always check CBC with differential immediately to rule out a fever from neutropenia.

Hold all immunizations during treatment. Immunizations can be resumed 6 months to 1 year after treatment.

Avoid use of live virus vaccines (MMR, oral polio).

Siblings of patients need to avoid live virus vaccines also.

Varicella zoster immunoglobulin (VZIG) must be given within 72 to 96 hours of exposure to varicella in nonimmune children.

Trimethoprim-sulfamethoxazole (Bactrim) 5 mg/kg/day for 3 days/week can be prescribed for prophylaxis to prevent the development of *Pneumocystis carinii* pneumonia.

Monthly use of intravenous or aerosolized pentamidine is recommended if the patient is allergic to Bactrim.

Empirical use of broad-spectrum antibiotics for fever and neutropenia is recommended.

EVALUATION

The overall cure rate for pediatric cancers is reaching 75%. By the year 2000, it is estimated that 1 in 900 individuals aged 20 to 29 years will be a survivor of childhood cancer. Many pediatric oncology centers have developed clinics specifically designed to provide comprehensive evaluation of childhood cancer survivors.

Box 105-1

Five-Plus Evaluation: Leukemia

Central Nervous System

Risk factors: Cranial (XRT) radiation therapy, CNS relapse, intrathecal drugs

Neuropsychology evaluation: All patients less than 8 years old when irradiated, PRN for school or behavior problems

Endocrine evaluation: T_4, TSH; LH, FSH, testosterone/estrogen if puberty is delayed

Growth: Growth curve, growth velocity; bone age, growth hormone testing, somatomedin C, IGF-BP3, if abnormal

Dental examination, ophthalmological examination, audiogram based on s/p cranial XRT

Gonadal Function

Risk factors: Cranial spinal XRT, testicular relapse s/p XRT, TBI, Cytoxan >7.5 g/m^2 total dose

Endocrine: Growth curve, growth velocity, FSH, LH, testosterone/estrogen, semen analysis

Liver

Risk factors: Chemotherapy, transfusions

Liver function tests annually

If LFT abnormal, or there has been a history of abnormal LFTs, or multiple transfusions have been necessary, obtain hepatitis studies (A,B,C)

Kidneys

Risk factors: Cytoxan, antibiotic therapy

Urinalysis, BUN, creatinine annually

Hematology

CBC annually

Others

If methotrexate was given for more than 3 years: CXR, pulmonary function tests

Cytoxan ≥5 g/m^2 total dosage: Urinalysis, urine cytology, BUN, creatinine annually.

Anthracycline total dose >250 mg/m^2 or any dose with thoracic XRT: ECG, Echo, GXT, for 5 years from diagnosis; repeat every 2 to 3 years if normal; if abnormal, every year.

Risk for second malignancies: Early: ANLL, CML, NHL, brain tumors; late: carcinomas (thyroid, skin, liver, breast)

From Children's Hospital Medical Center, Cincinnati, Ohio. Reprinted with special thanks to Cynthia DeLaat, MD, and Judy Correll, RN, CPNP.

BUN, Blood urea nitrogen; *CXR,* chest x-ray evaluation; *ECG,* electrocardiogram; *Echo,* echocardiogram; *FSH,* follicle-stimulating hormone; *LFT,* liver function test; *LH,* luteinizing hormone; *s/p,* status post; T_4, thyroxine; *TBI,* total body irradiation; *TSH,* thyroid-stimulating hormone; *XRT,* external radiation therapy.

Children's Hospital Medical Center in Cincinnati, Ohio, has a long-term clinic, the ATP 5+ Clinic, where the issues outlined in Box 105-1 are evaluated on a regular basis.

RESOURCES

American Cancer Society
www.cancer.org

Granny Barb and Art's Leukemia Links
www.acor.org/leukemia/frame.html

Leukemia Society of America, Inc.
800 Second Avenue
New York, NY 10016
(212) 573-8484
1-800-4LSA
www.leukemia.org

National Cancer Institute
Cancer Information Service
Building 31, Room 10A18
Bethesda, MD 20892
(800) 4-CANCER (800-422-6237)

REFERENCES

Caligiuri MA, Mayer RJ: Pregnancy and leukemia, *Semin Oncol* 16:338-396, 1993.

Lampkin B: Acute lymphoblastic leukemia. In Arceci RJ, editor: *Hematology/oncology/stem cell transplant handbook,* ed 2, Cincinnati, 1997, Hematology/Oncology Division of the Children's Hospital Medical Center.

SUGGESTED READINGS

Altman AJ et al: The prevention of infection. In Ablin AR, editor: *Supportive care of children with cancer,* Baltimore, 1993, The Johns Hopkins University Press.

Antonelli NM et al: Cancer in pregnancy: a review of the literature, Part II, *Obstet Gynecol Surv* 51:135-142, 1996.

Baer MR: Management of unusual presentations of acute leukemia. In Bloomfield CD, Herzig GP, editors: *Hematology/oncology clinic of North America: management of acute leukemia,* Philadelphia, 1993, WB Saunders.

Bates B: *Physical examination and history taking,* ed 2, Philadelphia, 1995, JB Lippincott.

Bennetts GA: Immunization of patients with malignant disease. In Ablin AR, editor: *Supportive care of children with cancer,* Baltimore, 1993, The John Hopkins University Press.

Cohen DG: Leukemia in children and adolescents—acute lymphocytic leukemia. In Foley GV, Fochtman D, Mooney KH, editors: *Nursing care of the child with cancer,* ed 2, Philadelphia, 1993, WB Saunders.

Healthcare Consultants of America, Inc: *1998 Physicians fee and coding guide,* Augusta, Ga, 1998, Healthcare Consultants of America, Inc.

Panzarella C et al: *Pediatric oncology nursing study guide,* Skokie, Ill, 1993, Association of Pediatric Oncology Nurses.

Reynoso EE et al: Acute leukemia during pregnancy: the Toronto Leukemia Study Group experience with long-term follow-up of children exposed in utero to chemotherapeutic agents, *J Clin Oncol* 5:1098-1106, 1987.

Salerno M: Hematological and oncological disorders. In Millonig VL, editor: *Adult nurse practitioner certification review guide,* ed 2, Potomac, Md, 1994, Health Leadership Associated, Inc.

Sambrano J: Chronic myelogenous leukemia. In Arceci RJ, editor: *Hematology/oncology/stem cell transplant handbook,* ed 2, Cincinnati, 1997, Hematology/Oncology Division of the Children's Hospital Medical Center.

Skidmore-Roth L: *Mosby's nursing drug reference,* St Louis, 1999, Mosby.

Tierney J: Hematological/oncological/immunological disorders. In Millonig VL, editor: *Adult nurse practitioner certification review guide,* ed 2, Potomac, Md 1994, Health Leadership Associated, Inc.

Waterburg L, Zieve PD: Selected illnesses affecting lymphocytes: mononucleosis, chronic lymphocytic leukemia, and the undiagnosed patient with lymphadenopathy. In Barker LR, Burton JR, Zieve PD, editors: *Principles of ambulatory medicine,* ed 4, Baltimore, 1995, Williams & Wilkins.

Wiley FM: Leukemia in children and adolescents—acute myelogenous leukemia. In Foley GV, Foctman D, Mooney KH, editors: *Nursing care of the child with cancer,* ed 2, Philadelphia, 1993, WB Saunders.

106 Lice (Pediculosis)

ICD 9-CM

Pediculosis Capitis 132.0
Pediculosis Pubis 132.2
Pediculosis Corporis 132.1

OVERVIEW

Definition

Lice is infestation of the skin or hair by the species of blood-sucking lice capable of living as external parasites on the human host. There are three types of lice that inhabit the human host:

Pediculosis humanus corporis is the body louse; it infests the body but actually emerges from lining or seams of infested clothing, upholstery, or bedding to bite the human host.

Pediculosis capitis is the head louse; it infests the scalp and head hair. This louse is clear in color when hatched but becomes red-brown after feeding. It is the size of a sesame seed.

Phthirus pubis is the crab louse; it infests the genital region (sometimes referred to as pediculosis pubis). It may also affect hair of axilla, chest, abdomen, thighs, facial hair, and eyelashes. This is one of the most common sexually transmitted diseases.

Incidence

6 to 12 million cases annually in the United States; **50% to 75% of cases <12 years old;** can be epidemic in day care, kindergartens, summer camps, and schools; 1:4 elementary school age contact annually; nearly 80% of school districts have at least one outbreak during the school year

Occurs in all ages, races, and socioeconomic groups and in all geographic regions; can occur in any season but is most common August through November

Pediculosis Capitis

Occurs most commonly in **5 to 12 year olds,** more in girls; may spread to other family members; occurs <1% in blacks secondary to structure of their hair shaft; acquired through personal contact

Pediculosis Corporis

Occurs most commonly in crowded living conditions, situations of poverty, and where laundering is limited, such as in the homeless population

Phthirus Pubis

Highly contagious (1 contact >90% acquired); occurs during intimate personal and/or sexual contact; can occur in **children** as a result of sexual abuse; most commonly occurs in females 15 to 19 and males >20 years of age

Pathophysiology

Lice are ectoparasites that, when spread from direct or fomite contact, pierce the skin to feed. When they bite, they infuse saliva to prevent clotting and probe for a vessel. The louse lays 100 to 300 eggs (nits) during a lifetime. Nits attach to the hair shaft by a cementlike structure and are difficult to remove. Lice cannot live off the human host for more than 24 to 48 hours. It is the saliva of the louse that creates symptoms—itching may not begin for 4 weeks when sensitivity to saliva occurs. Lice live up to 30 days, and the females lay up to 100 eggs. Nits are protected by a cocoonlike state and are stuck to the hair shaft.

In the United States, lice do not transmit pathogens; however, in other regions of the world they may carry disease. The greatest harm from lice in the United States is likely the misguided use of highly caustic substances in an attempt to kill lice.

Protective Factors Against

Lifestyle behaviors and situations that do not provide exposure

Being of African-American descent (In Africa, the reverse is true since lice have adapted to infest curly hair. Straight-haired Europeans or Americans in Africa are protected from infestations.)

NOTE: Clean hair and good hygiene do not prevent infestation with lice.

Factors That Increase Susceptibility

Pediculosis Capitis

Childhood, especially with enrollment in day care, school, or camp

Family member with infestation

Sharing hair combs, brushes, hair decorations, and other objects that touch the head where lice are present

Pediculosis Corporis

Homelessness

Poor hygiene

Infrequent laundering

Infrequent change of clothing

Close contact in crowded situations with individuals who are lice infested

Sharing clothing or bedding that is contaminated

Phthirus Pubis

Sexual contact with individual infected with pubic lice

SUBJECTIVE DATA

History of Present Illness

Ask about known exposure

Ask about duration of symptoms (itching may not be noted for 4 weeks)

Usual complaint: Intense itching, often worse at night. (With pediculosis capitis [head lice], itching at occipital hairline and behind ears is most common.)

Children: Presence of pubic lice is indicative of sexual abuse; investigate this possibility

Past Medical History

Last menstrual period, contraception used

Allergies

If postpartum woman, ask if she is breastfeeding

Medications

Current prescription and over-the-counter drug use

Family History

Ask about infestation in family member

Psychosocial History

Pediculosis Capitis

Ask if child enrolled in day care, kindergarten, school, or camp.

Ask about sharing clothing, hair brushes/combs, barrettes, and other personal items; participation in sports where equipment is shared; participation in theater where wigs and borrowed clothes are shared.

Pediculosis Corporis

Inquire about living arrangements. Is the environment crowded? Is the patient homeless? Can he or she bathe, shampoo, and launder clothing as needed? Are pillows, bedding, and clothing shared?

Ask if clothing is purchased from yard sales and thrift shops and not laundered before use.

Ask if clothes found on the street or in lost/found are worn.

Phthirus Pubis

Ask about multiple sexual partners.

Associated Symptoms

Children with head lice may have sleeplessness, irritability, or difficulty concentrating in school because of itching.

OBJECTIVE DATA

Physical Examination

Strong lighting and a magnifying lens facilitate identification of lice and nits. Examiner should always wear gloves when examining for lice.

Visualize hair shaft of all body and head hair for evidence of lice. (Lice are size of sesame seed—3 to 4 mm—and gray-brown; they move quickly away from light and hide.)

Identify nits in hair. (Nits are tear-drop shaped, 0.8 mm and cream colored; empty ova shells are white and attached near base hair shaft at scalp or pubic area.) Hair may appear "peppered" with nits, although there are usually not >12 active at any time. If nits are >1 inch from scalp, the lice have probably already hatched.

Observe skin for pinpoint red bites and/or black specks of lice feces. These may be impossible to visualize, and they are not necessary for diagnosis.

Note presence of pinpoint blood spots on underclothes.

Check back of neck and postauricular areas for erythema.

Palpate for cervical lymphadenopathy, which may occur with secondary infections associated with head lice.

Check for other sexually transmitted diseases, which may co-exist with pediculosis pubis.

Observe for secondary bacterial infection of skin.

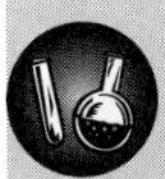

TABLE 106-1 Diagnostic Procedures: Lice

Diagnostic Test	Findings/Rationale	Cost ($)
Microscopic evaluation	A louse may be removed for examination under a microscope for confirmation, if desired. Mineral oil applied to the slide facilitates visualization.	15-18
Wood's lamp	Lice fluoresce. This is normally not necessary for diagnosis.	Not available

Diagnostic Procedures

Diagnostic procedures include those found in Table 106-1.

ASSESSMENT

Confirm type of lice infestation: capitis, corporis, or pubis.

Pediculosis Capitis

Rule out hair artifacts (spray, gel), dandruff, seborrhea, psoriasis, impetigo, eczematous dermatitis, tinea capitis.

Pediculosis Corporis

Rule out contact dermatitis, lichen simplex chronicus, eczematous dermatitis.

Pediculosis Pubis

Rule out eczema, seborrheic dermatitis, tinea cruris, folliculitis, molluscum contagiosum; rule out other concurrent sexually transmitted diseases (Table 106-2).

THERAPEUTIC PLAN

Pharmaceutical

Pediculicides are required to kill lice and nits. Most are contraindicated in **children** <2 and in **pregnant** and **lactating women.** During use, the patient's eyes should be covered and shut (Table 106-3).

Mechanical Removal of Nits

More certain and safer than pharmaceutical products but time consuming. Good lighting, a magnifying glass, and tweezers are advised.

Nit Removal

Nits must be mechanically removed. There are commercial preparations, such as Step 2 or Clear, that assist in nit removal. A 50/50 white vinegar/water solution may also be used to loosen nits. There is recent anecdotal support for use of olive oil for this purpose (never machine oil, which may be harmful). A nit comb (metal ones work better) is used to remove all nits from the hair shafts. This can be a time-consuming process. Nit combs may be purchased over the counter at the pharmacy. Recently, the National Pediculosis Association (NPA, http://www.headlice.org) has introduced the trademarked special nit comb, the LiceMeister, which is receiving strong anecdotal support from parent-users. It has a strong plastic handle and 1½-inch metal teeth that comb through hair with less pulling and discomfort. This comb is nonbreakable and reusable. It can be used with wet, dry, or damp hair. It appears to be especially valuable if one lives alone and must check his or her own hair. The LiceMeister is available at 1-888-542-3634 for $14.95 + shipping.

It is easier to remove nits by back-combing the hair. The comb may be cleaned with water frequently. Lice may be removed with fingers or tweezers.

To treat lice-infested eyelashes, apply petrolatum to lashes BID for 10 days. Lice either suffocate or slide off the slick lashes.

Lifestyle/Activities

Since transmission occurs from person to person, educate children and parents about mode of transmission and preventive measures such as not sharing combs, brushes, hair decorations, hats, scarves, helmets, headphones, bedding, or sleeping bags. Coats and hats should be hung separately, not touching those of others. Sleeping mats should be individually labeled and kept separately in plastic bags, not stacked. *All family members need to be examined and treated at the same time.*

Diet

None

Patient Education

Reassure that pediculosis is curable, does not cause long-term effects, and is a common problem in all socioeconomic groups.

TABLE 106-2 Differential Diagnosis: Lice

Diagnosis	Supporting Data
Hair Artifacts (spray, gel)	History recent use of hair products Combs out easily Shampoos out without difficulty
Dandruff	Irregular white flakes Easily removed
Seborrhea	Gradual onset Face, scalp, body folds: yellow to red, often greasy lesions with white dry scales and sticky crusts
Lichen simplex chronicus	Areas within easy reach of fingers Excoriation and thickening of skin without other specific findings Most common in middle-aged women and those under extreme stress
Psoriasis	Knees, elbows, scalp: Pustules possible Erythematous papulosquamous lesions
Tinea capitis	Scalp Grayish scaling Round areas with broken hairs obvious Wood's light fluoresces yellow-green; KOH testing: spores and hyphae
Contact dermatitis	Exposed area or one previously sensitized Edema and redness or darkening Weeping vesicles or bullae
Tinea cruris	Groin, pubis, thighs Warm, humid environment Tight clothing Large, scaling, demarcated plaques Possible central clearing Papules and pustules may be present at margins Wood's light fluoresces red; KOH testing: Spores and hyphae
Impetigo	Small vesicles that gradually enlarge with red halo and central honey-colored crusts Common in children
Folliculitis	Small, red, domed pustules over hair follicles; hair may or may not be broken
Molluscum contagiosum	Genital, trunk, neck: Usually nonpruritic Pearly white papules or nodules, mostly round or ovoid with classic umbilicated top, located in clusters
Eczematous dermatitis	Dorsa of hands and feet, ears, skin creases Dry, thick, scaly excoriation

Teach how to disinfect the personal articles of the infested individual and to clean the environment, reinforcing that lice do not jump or fly but spread through crawling (Box 106-1).

Advise parents to inform school authorities of infested children and keep children out of school until treated.

Reinforce the importance of mechanical removal of lice and nits from infested hair. Hair should be separated into multiple sections while each part of the scalp is exposed, examined, and methodically treated. Nits are removed with a nit comb. (A different comb should be used for each infested person and cleaned frequently during the removal process.)

Family Impact

It is important to assess the patient/parent/family perception of the problem of lice since there are many misconceptions about infestation. Clarification is essential. Lice infestations are stigmatizing to the family because of the myth about poor hygiene causing lice. Children may be ridiculed by peers, leading to poor self-image. They may miss enough schoolwork to jeopardize learning.

Referral

Referral to an MD is necessary for:

- Treatment failures
- Lice in eyelashes that persist despite treatment
- Co-existing dermatologic conditions

Consultation

If pediculosis pubis is identified in a child, appropriate authorities should be notified of potential child sexual abuse.

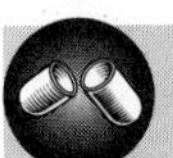

TABLE 106-3 Pharmaceutical Plan: Lice

Type Pediculicide	Availability	Instructions/Comments	Cost
Pyrethrins with Piperonyl Butoxide 0.3% (A200, RID, Triple X) Natural botanical pesticide	Over-the-counter	Pregnancy: C Apply on dry hair. Leave shampoo on ×10 min. Rinse. May need reapplication in 7-10 days. Usually drug of choice in pregnancy—consult MD. **Pyrethrins and Permethrin should not be used by those allergic to ragweed or chrysanthemums.**	\$6/60 ml
Permethrin 1% cream rinse (Nix)*	Over-the-counter (5% is prescription)	Apply after shampooing hair. Leave on ×10 min. Rinse thoroughly. Do not shampoo again for 24 hours. Reapplication is not usually necessary. **Pyrethrins and Permethrin should not be used by those allergic to ragweed or chrysanthemums.** Pregnancy: B Do not use in children <2 mos.	\$18/60 g
Lindane (Kwell)† 1% lotion 1% cream 1% shampoo	Prescription	Shampoo and leave ×4 min. Repeat in 1 week. Do not use on acutely inflamed skin. Use with caution: Can cause neurotoxicity and seizures, especially in children. DO NOT SWALLOW.	\$3-\$11/60 ml
Co-trimoxazole (Bactrim)	Double strength 1 BID ×3 days	One single, unrandomized, unblinded trial reported this treatment was effective for lice. A second therapy 10 days later may be necessary to kill emerging nymphs before they reproduce (Beckwith, 1998).	7-74/DS 400 smx/ 50 TMP (100)

*Considered drug of choice because of 97% to 99% cure rate and minimal side effects.

†Strong pesticides have an increased potential for absorption and systemic side effects. Nurse practitioners would be well advised to document prior treatment failures and the potential for side effects, especially if medication is used inappropriately. Despite the side effects, does not appear as effective as over-the-counter drugs.

Box 106-1

Lice Disinfection

Machine wash all washable clothing and bedding used within last 48 hours, using hot water and detergent (water should be >125° Fahrenheit and washed for a minimum of 20 minutes).

Dry clothing and bedding as possible on high heat in a clothes dryer at least 20 minutes.

Dry-clean clothing and personal items that cannot be washed. Upholstered furniture, pillows, and stuffed animals may be ironed with hot iron.

Soak personal hair products such as hair brushes, combs, and barrettes in 2% Lysol or Pediculicide for 1 hour.

Clean other objects that have been in contact with infested hair in last 48 hours, such as curlers, headphones, earpieces of glasses, helmets, car seats, with Lysol 2% or Pediculicide.

Place other items that have been exposed to infestation in plastic bag and keep closed for 2 weeks; lice will die.

Vacuum mattresses, rugs, upholstered furniture, and stuffed animals regularly.

Remind patients/parents not to use insecticides or chemicals (such as kerosene, gasoline, or pet shampoos) not meant to be used on humans.

Hair cuts and head shaving are last resort measures.

Recommend that all family members and close contacts should be examined for presence of infestation and treated at the same time as the identified patient.

American Head Lice Information Center, http://headliceinfo.com

Consultation should be sought for treatment of **children** under 2 years of age and **pregnant** and **lactating women.**

Follow-up

During lice season, the parent should check the child's hair every 3 days. Once treated for lice, the individual should be reexamined, at least by a family member, several days after treatment. Reapplication of Pediculicide is often necessary 7 to 10 days after the initial treatment. In the case of pediculosis pubis, all sexual contacts for the past month should receive treatment.

EVALUATION

Successful outcome is resolution of lice infestation without relapse and family empowered by education to minimize or prevent future exposure.

RESOURCE

National Pediculosis Association (NPA), Box 149 Newton, MA 02161. Tel: (617) 449-6487; http://headlice.org

REFERENCE

Beckwith C: *Head lice: new and improved?* Pharmacist's letter (Document No. 140507), Stockton, Calif, April 22, 1998, Therapeutic Research Center.

SUGGESTED READINGS

A modern scourge: parents scratch their heads over lice, *Consumer Reports,* February 1998, pp 62-63.

Copeland L: *The lice-buster book*, New York, 1995, Warner Books.

Crain EF, Gershel JC: *Clinical manual of emergency pediatrics*, New York, 1997, McGraw-Hill.

Fenstermacher K, Hudson BT: *Practice guidelines for family nurse practitioners*, Philadelphia, 1997, WB Saunders.

Fitzpatrick TB et al: *Color atlas and synopsis of clinical dermatology*, New York, 1992, McGraw-Hill.

Forsman KE: Pediculosis and scabies: what to look for in patients who are crawling with clues, *Postgrad Med* 98(6):89-100, 1995.

Havens CS, Sullivan ND, Tilton P: *Manual of outpatient gynecology*, Boston, 1996, Little, Brown.

Hawkins JW, Roberto-Nichols DM, Stanl-Haney JL: *Protocols for nurse practitioners*, New York, 1995, The Tiresias Press.

Lichtman R, Papera S: *Gynecology—well woman care*, Norwalk, Conn, 1990, Appleton & Lange.

Mengel MB, Schwiebert LP: *Ambulatory medicine: the primary care of families*, Stamford, Conn, 1996, Appleton & Lange.

Millonig VL: Back to school signals "head lice season," *J Am Acad Nurse Pract* 3(3):136-137, 1991.

Pigott KG: Lice and scabies, *Lippincott's Primary Care Pract* 1(1):93-96, 1997.

Pigott KG: Lice and scabies treatment, *Lippincott's Primary Care Pract* 2(1):109-110, 1997.

Reifsnider E: Common adult infectious skin conditions, *Nurse Pract* 22(11):17-33, 1997.

Sokoloff F: Identification and management of pediculosis, *Nurse Pract* 19(3):62-64, 1994.

Star WL, Lommel LL, Shannon MT: *Women's primary health care: protocols for practice*, Washington, DC, 1995, American Nurses Publishing.

Uphold CR, Graham MV: *Clinical guidelines in family practice*, Gainesville, Fla, 1994, Barmarrae Books.

Wong D: *Nursing care of infants and children*, ed 5, St Louis, 1995, Mosby.

Youngkin EO, Davis MS: *Women's health—a primary care clinical guide*, Norwalk, Conn, 1994, Appleton & Lange.

Lower Back Pain

Lumbosacral Strain and Herniated Nucleus Pulposus

ICD-9-CM

Intervertebral Disk Disorder 722
Lumbago 724.0
Due to Intervertebral Disk Displacement, Lumbar, or Lumbosacral Area 722.10
Backache, Unspecified 724.5

OVERVIEW

Definition

Lumbosacral Strain

Lumbosacral strain (LBS) is defined as stretching or tearing of muscles, tendons, ligaments, or fascia of the lumbosacral area secondary to trauma or mechanical injury. Acute lower back pain is defined as symptoms of less than 3 months' duration.

Herniated Nucleus Pulposus (HNP)

Herniated nucleus pulposus (HNP) is the rupture of an intervertebral disc with herniation of nucleus pulposus into the spinal canal. Sciatica refers to pain and paresthesias extending down the leg in a dermatomal pattern; the most common cause is HNP at L_{4-5} and L_5S_1.

Incidence

Low back problems affect virtually everyone at some point in life; 50% of working adults are affected every year, and 15% to 20% seek health care. For persons younger than 45 years of age, low back problems are the most common cause of disability. Low back pain is more common between 20 to 40 years of age than at any other age and costs approximately $30 billion per year in direct and indirect costs. Only about 10% of patients with low back pain experience HNP.

Children

Strains of the ligaments/muscles of the back are unusual in **children,** unless they occur as a result of trauma, infection, inflammation, or malignancies.

Pathophysiology

Etiology of lumbosacral strain unclear; herniation occurs with tears in annulus fibroses, which allows contents of pulposus to protrude.

Protective Factors Against LBS and HNP

Proper body mechanics
Appropriate weight maintenance
Conditioned state

Factors that Increase Susceptibility to LBS and HNP

Overweight
Mechanical disorders (e.g., scoliosis, kyphosis)
Nonmechanical disorders (e.g., ankylosing spondylitis, prostate cancer, pelvic and renal disease)
Occupational strain
Leg length differences
Poor posture
Poor body mechanics with lifting

SUBJECTIVE DATA

History of Present Illness

Inquire regarding duration of symptoms and any known trauma.
Children: Inquire regarding trauma, infection, inflammation, malignancy.
Adults/elderly: Ask about occupation, leisure/hobby activities, underlying physical conditions.

Past Medical History

Inquire about:

Prior history of back pain or other painful conditions, treatment measures, compliance, outcome

Use of alcohol, tobacco products

Last normal monthly period, considering pelvic inflammatory disease and ectopic pregnancy as possible causes of lower back pain; rule out pregnancy before initiating any radiologic tests

History of weight loss, systemic disease, malignancy

Prior history affective disorder(s)

Medications

Recent use of acetaminophen, nonsteroidal antiinflammatory drugs (NSAIDs) or other over-the-counter preparations with responses

Other current medications

Family History

Inquire about family history of back problems, treatment, outcome(s), malignancies.

Psychosocial History

Children

Inquire about caregiver(s), usual level of activity.

Adults/Elderly

Inquire about stresses in work place/job satisfaction, leisure activities, financial resources, support systems, internal/external locus of control, self-rating of health, total work loss (due to back pain) in past 12 months.

Diet History

Inquire as to overall nutrition pattern, with emphasis on weight reduction, if needed, and a balanced diet.

Description of Most Common Symptoms

Lumbosacral Strain

Must identify a mechanism of injury, if known

Pain that has increased over time and accompanied by stiffness

Pain located primarily in back, but may radiate to buttock(s) or thigh(s); pain increased with movement and relieved with rest

Muscle spasms in lower back

Elderly: Symptoms less severe

Herniated Nucleus Pulposus

Radicular pain (shooting, electrical) below the knee

Paresthesia or numbness along sensory distribution of nerve root

Elderly: The nucleus pulposus is more fibrotic, making the incidence and/or symptoms much less common

Associated Symptoms

Sleep disturbance, life stressors, weakness, hypesthesia, weight loss, fever, malaise, presence of genitourinary symptoms: dysuria, vaginal discharge, prostatism, night sweats

OBJECTIVE DATA

Physical Examination

The physical examination should be conducted with attention to vital signs, weight, general appearance, and systems other than musculoskeletal to rule out mechanical, systemic, or psychosocial causes for back pain. The examination should be conducted in a systematic head-to-toe fashion, incorporating standing, sitting, and lying positions of the patient for the examination.

Gait

Walking to examination room, as well as removing shoes, and getting on examination table, noting flexion or other difficulties performing these functions

Children: Note activity level

Standing

Note patient undressed with back exposed

Note posture in bare feet

Walk on heels (L_{4-5}) and toes (S_{1-2}); unable to perform this if nerve root irritation

Back: Examine spinal column from front, back, and side; note any scoliosis and abnormalities of expected S curvature; lumbar lordosis may be seen in acute LBS

Note level of shoulder tips, scapular ranges, iliac crests, gluteal folds, popliteal creases should be equal; in LBS, unequal levels may be present

Perform spinal range of motion (ROM)(flexion, extension, lateral bending, rotation); severe guarding may support a diagnosis of fracture, spinal infection, or tumor

Palpate paravertebral muscles for spasm and/or tenderness; may be seen in acute LBS

Sitting

Lungs: Check for signs of pleural effusion or consolidation.

Heart: Note rate, rhythm, and any signs of recent cardiac event (rub, effusion).

Extremities/neurological: Check deep tendon reflexes (DTRs) of knees (L_4) and Achilles (S_1), Babinski. Observe for bilaterally equal responses. If unequal responses, consider nerve root irritation. Test strength, vibratory, and proprioceptive sensation bilaterally (should be equal). Weakness in dorsiflexion of ankle or great toe (L_{4-5}) suggests nerve root dysfunction (Figure 107-1).

Light touch sensation of medial (L_4), dorsal (L_5), and lateral (S_1) aspects of foot.

Perform sitting straight-leg raise (SLR) (sitting knee extension) (Figure 107-2). Knee should extend without radiation of pain below knee; this is also one way to check for malingering behavior, as results should equal those of SLR performed in lying position.

Check for ankle and toe (L_5) dorsiflexion strength bilaterally; they should be equal.

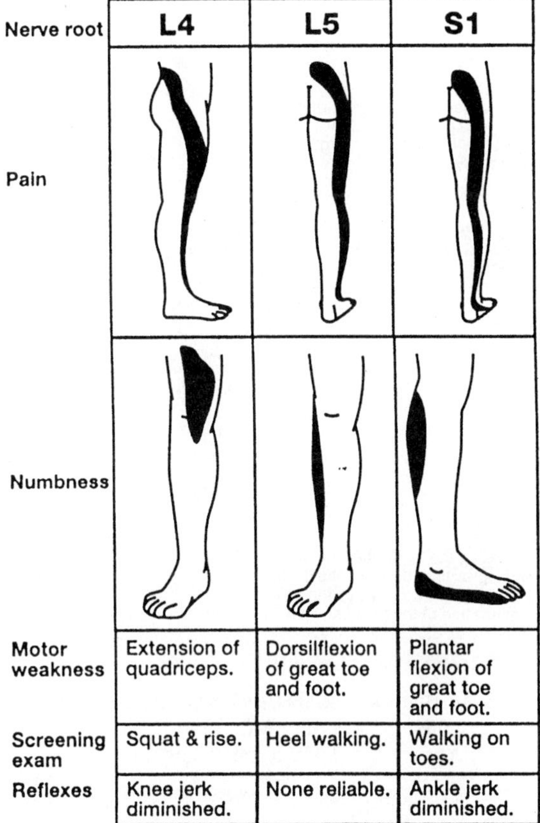

Nerve root	L4	L5	S1
Pain			
Numbness			
Motor weakness	Extension of quadriceps.	Dorsiflexion of great toe and foot.	Plantar flexion of great toe and foot.
Screening exam	Squat & rise.	Heel walking.	Walking on toes.
Reflexes	Knee jerk diminished.	None reliable.	Ankle jerk diminished.

Figure 107-1 Testing for lumbar nerve root compromise. (From Bigos BS et al: Acute low back problems in adults. In *Clinical practice guideline, quick reference guide*, Number 14 [AHCPR Pub. No. 95-0643], Rockville, Md, 1994, U.S. Department of Health and Human Services, Public Health Service, Agency for Health Care Policy and Research.)

Supine

Abdomen: Check for tenderness of peptic ulcer disease and/or bruits/enlargement of dissecting aortic aneurysm.

Extremities: *F*lexion, *Ab*duction, *E*xternal *R*otation (FABER or Patrick test) of hips; decreased ROM may indicate hip or sacroiliac joint problem

Neurological: Standard SLR (Figure 107-3); normally the hip can be flexed to 80 degrees without pain, except in thigh. A positive test is one that elicits (shooting, sharp, electrical) pain that radiates below the knee on the affected side at 30-degree flexion or less.

Crossed SLR: SLR of *un*affected leg; a positive test is when the SLR of the unaffected leg causes radicular pain in the affected leg to be reproduced.

Sensory assessment of buttocks and perineum to rule out saddle anesthesia of cauda equina syndrome (compression of nerves at $L_{4\text{-}5}$ level, which needs emergency surgical decompression).

Indicators for Pelvic Examination

Reports of abdominal pain, dyspareunia, vaginal discharge

Rest of examination unequivocal

Indicators for Rectal Examination

Men over the age of 50

Rest of examination equivocal

Specialized Examination Techniques for Malingering Behavior

"Pain behaviors" of distress such as amplified grimacing, distorted gait or posture, or rubbing of painful body parts may cloud the picture. Interpreting inconsistencies or pain behaviors as malingering may not be useful because they could be viewed as a plea for help. The goal is to

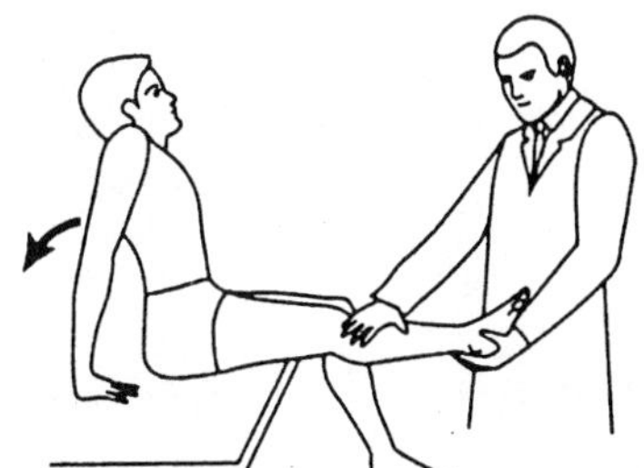

Figure 107-2 Instructions for sitting knee extension test. (From Bigos BS et al: Acute low back problems in adults. In *Clinical practice guideline, quick reference guide*, Number 14 [AHCPR Pub. No. 95-0643], Rockville, Md, 1994, U.S. Department of Health and Human Services, Public Health Service, Agency for Health Care Policy and Research.)

(1) Ask the patient to lie as straight as possible on a table in the supine position.

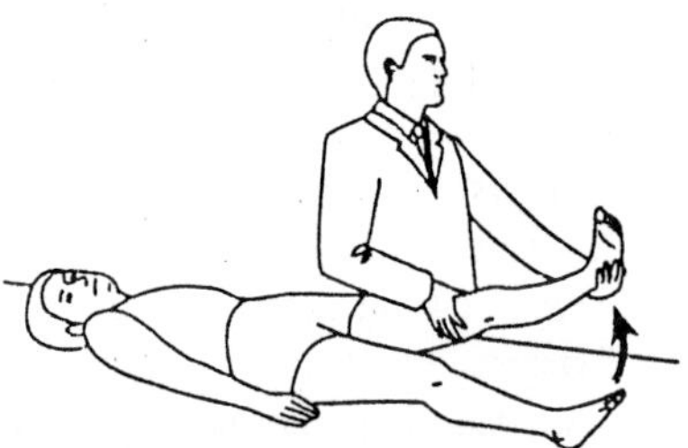

(2) With one hand placed above the knee of the leg being examined, exert enough firm pressure to keep the knee fully extended. Ask the patient to relax.

(3) With the other hand cupped under the heel, slowly raise the straight limb. Tell the patient, "If this bothers you, let me know, and I will stop."

4) Monitor for any movement of the pelvis before complaints are elicited. True sciatic tension should elicit complaints before the hamstrings are stretched enough to move the pelvis.

(5) Estimate the degree of leg elevation that elicits complaint from the patient. Then determine the most distal area of discomfort: back, hip, thigh, knee, or below the knee.

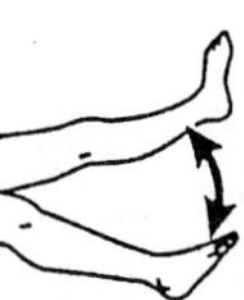

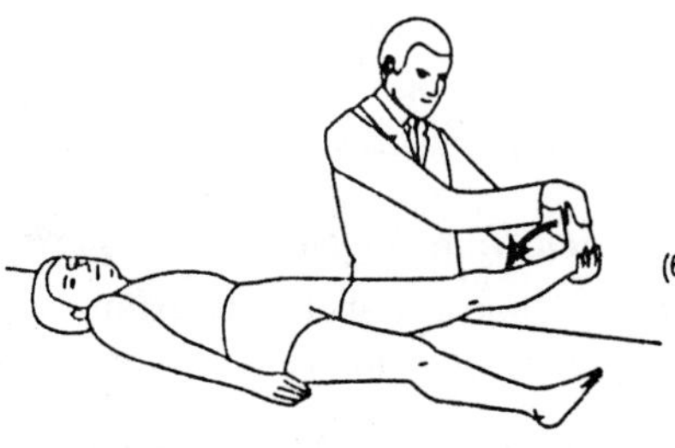

(6) While holding the leg at the limit of straight leg raising, dorsiflex the ankle. Note whether this aggravates the pain. Internal rotation of the limb can also increase the tension on the sciatic nerve roots.

Figure 107-3 Instructions for the straight leg raising test. (From Bigos BS et al: *Clinical practice guideline, quick reference guide,* Number 14 [AHCPR Pub. No. 95-0643], Rockville, Md, 1994, U.S. Department of Health and Human Services, Public Health Service, Agency for Health Care Policy and Research.)

facilitate recovery and avoid the development of chronic low back disability.

However, there may be times when malingering behavior must be ruled out. The following tests may be used in these cases:

Waddell signs: A standardized group of nonorganic physical signs

Tenderness: Which is nonanatomical or superficial

Simulation: Simulate movement without actually performing it

Axial loading: Pressure to top of head should not produce pain

Distraction: Examine SLR in sitting and supine position and compare results

Regionalization: Inappropriate location of pain from normal neuro anatomy

Overreaction: Disproportionate verbalization, facial expression, or tremor

Others:

Magnuson's test: Mark areas that were tender when palpated; return to the marked areas later in the examination to see if pain can be reproduced. With malingering behavior, those marked areas are not likely to reproduce pain.

Hoover's test: Put examiner's hands under both heels. (Patient can be standing, sitting, or lying.) Ask patient to raise affected leg. If the pain is real, the heel on the other leg will push into the examiner's hands.

Diagnostic Procedures

X-rays or laboratory testing are generally not necessary at the initial visit unless there is history of trauma or suspicion of systemic or structural changes (Table 107-1).

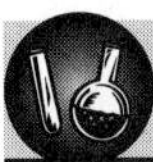

TABLE 107-1 Primary Differential Diagnosis: Lower Back Pain

Symptoms	Findings	Diagnostic Tests
Acute LBS		
Pain with movement and relieved with rest, minimal pain initially and increasing over time, stiffness, radiation to buttocks/thigh, negative GU signs	Painful gait, lumbar lordosis, asymmetry, muscle spasm or tenderness, DTRs normoreactive, negative SLR/crossed SLR	None
HNP		
Radicular pain below knee, numbness or paresthesia, sleep disturbance, difficulty getting comfortable, pain w/defecation, negative GU signs	Unable to walk on heels and/or toes, unequal DTRs, decreased strength/vibratory sensation/proprioception unilaterally, + SLR/crossed SLR	Consultation/referral with collaborating physician about MRI

DTR, Deep tendon reflex; *GU,* genitourinary; *HPN,* herniated nucleus pulposus; *LBS,* lumbosacral strain; *MRI,* magnetic resonance imaging; *SLR,* straight-leg raising.

TABLE 107-2 Secondary Differential Diagnosis: Lower Back Pain

Diagnoses	Supporting Data
Pelvic inflammatory disease (PID)	Cervical/vaginal discharge Lower abdominal pain Cervical motion tenderness Laboratory evidence w/*Neisseria gonorrhea* or *Chlamydia trachomatis*
Prostate tumor	Prostatic induration on prostate exam Elevation of PSA Asymptomatic
Prostate infection	If acute: Fever, irritative voiding signs, perineal or suprapubic pain, exquisite tenderness on examination, + urine culture If chronic: Irritative voiding signs, perineal or suprapubic discomfort (may be dull and poorly localized), + expressed prostatic secretions (EPS)/culture
Malingering behavior	Inconsistencies with history and examination, overexaggeration of signs, conflicting examination results, + Waddell signs
Spinal cord disease	Back pain (may precede neurological signs) Back pain aggravated by lying down, bearing weight, sneezing/coughing Progressive weakness, recent weight change Sensory loss, usually in lower extremities Late findings include bowel/bladder dysfunction Back pain may be local, root, or both
Osteoporosis	Back pain may be asymptomatic or severe Spontaneous fractures Demineralization, especially of spine, hip, pelvis
Osteoarthritis	Morning stiffness <30 minutes Pain relieved by rest Minimal articular inflammation X-ray findings (narrowed joint space, osteophytes, bony cysts, lipping of marginal bone)

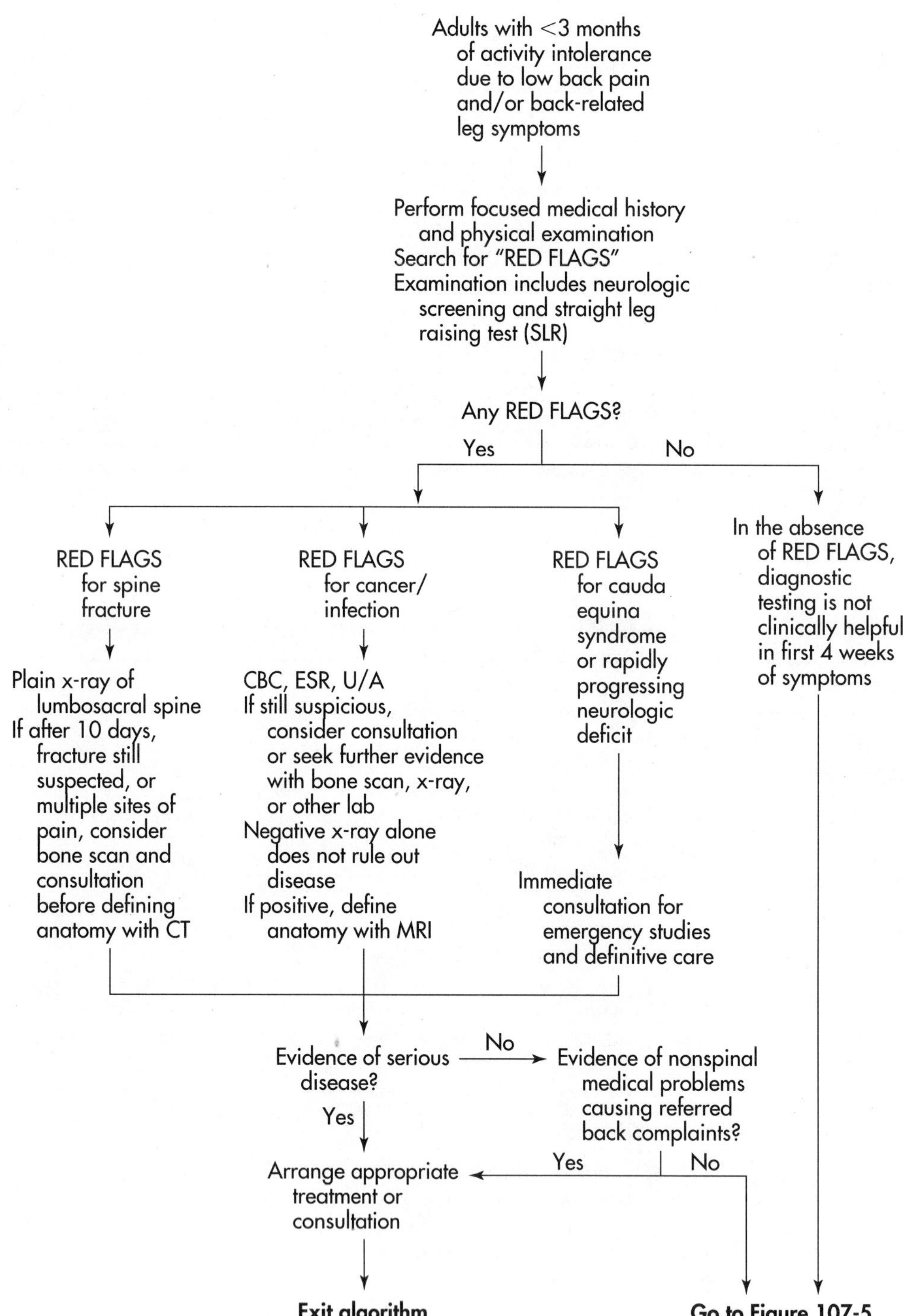

Figure 107-4 Initial evaluation of acute low back problem. *CBC,* Complete blood count; *ESR,* erythrocyte sedimentation rate; *U/A,* urinalysis. (From Bigos BS et al: *Clinical practice guideline, quick reference guide*, Number 14 [AHCPR Pub. No. 95-0643], Rockville, Md, 1994, U.S. Department of Health and Human Services, Public Health Service, Agency for Health Care Policy and Research.)

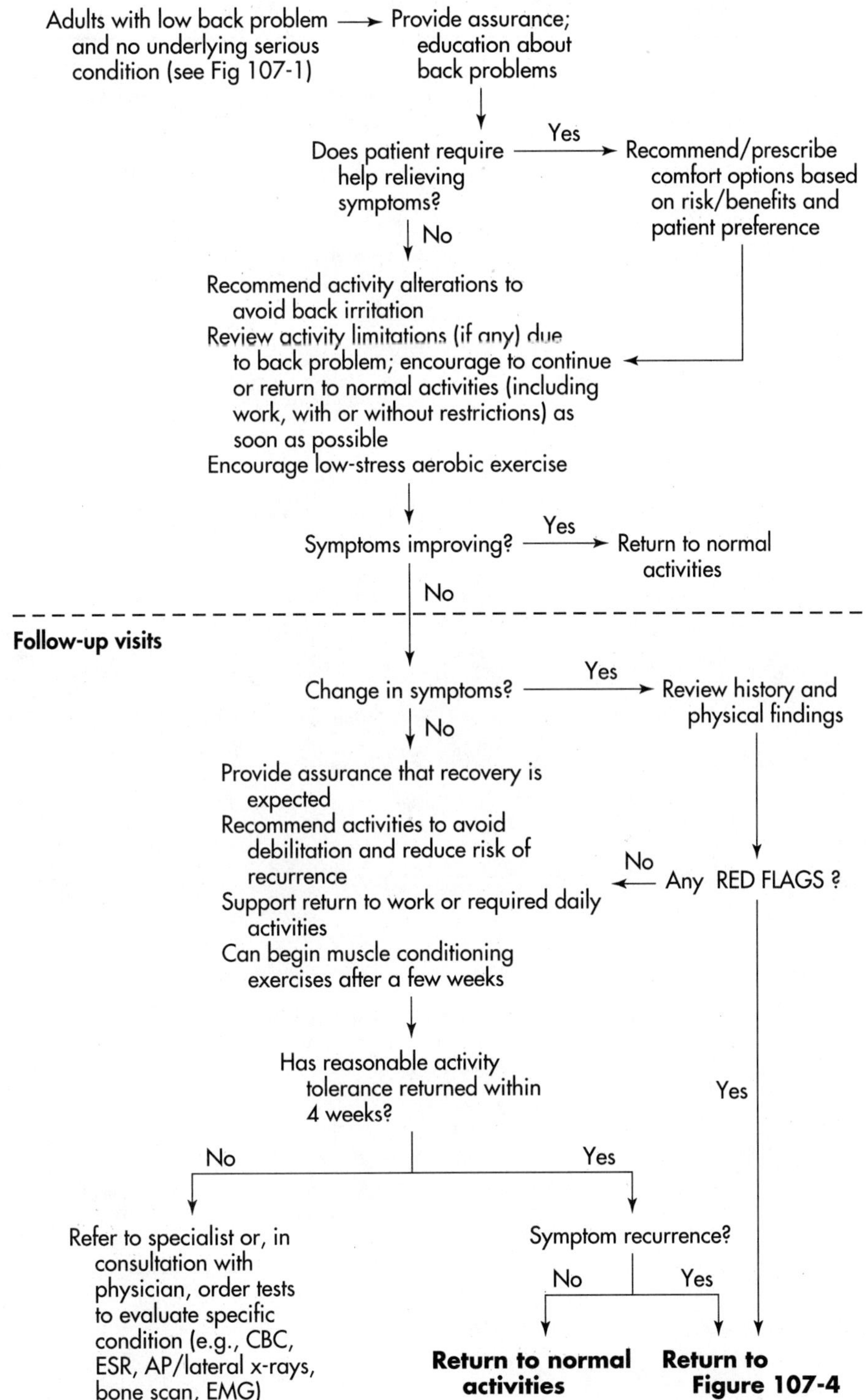

Figure 107-5 Treatment of low back problem on initial and follow-up visits. *AP,* Anteroposterior; *CBC,* complete blood count; *EMG,* electromyelogram; *ESR,* erythrocyte sedimentation rate. (From Bigos BS et al: *Clinical practice guideline, quick reference guide,* Number 14 [AHCPR Pub. No. 95-0643], Rockville, Md, 1994, U.S. Department of Health and Human Services, Public Health Service, Agency for Health Care Policy and Research.)

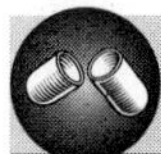

TABLE 107-3 Nonsteroidal Antiinflammatory Drugs

Drug/Pregnancy Classification	Adult Dose	Children	Cost ($)	Maximum Daily Dose
Proprionic Acid Derivatives				
Ibuprofen (Motrin, Advil, Nuprin) **Pregnancy: B**	600-800 mg TID to QID	Not recommended	4-107	
Naproxen (Naprosyn, Anaprox) **Pregnancy: B**	500 mg BID	Not recommended	18-26	1000 mg/day
Fenoprofen (Fenopron)	600 mg TID	Not recommended	19-63	2400 mg/day
Ketoprofen (Orudis) **Not recommended in pregnancy**	150-300 mg in divided doses TID or QID	Not recommended	80-114	300 mg/day
Flurbiprofen (Ansaid) **Pregnancy: B**	100 mg BID to TID	Not recommended	106-125	300 mg/day
Oxaprozin (Daypro) **Pregnancy: C**	600-1200 mg/day	Not recommended	121	1200 mg/day
Oxicams				
Piroxicam (Feldene) **Not recommended in pregnancy**	10-20 mg/day	Not recommended	14-257	20 mg/day
Acetic Acid Derivatives				
Indomethacin (Indocin) **Not recommended pregnancy or in elderly**	50 mg TID to QID	Not recommended	3-89	150-200 mg/day
Sulindac (Clinoril) **Not recommended in pregnancy**	150-200 mg BID	Not recommended	26-120	400 mg/day
Tolmetin (Tolectin) **Pregnancy: C**	400 mg TID to QID		26-92	2000 mg/day
Diclofenac (Voltaren) **Pregnancy: B**	50 mg BID to TID	Not recommended	84-108	150 mg/day
Etodolac (Lodine) **Pregnancy: C**	200-400 mg/TID	Not recommended	113-128	1200 mg/day
Nabumetone (Relafen) **Pregnancy: C**	1000-2000 mg/day	Not recommended	102-123	2000 mg/day

Continued

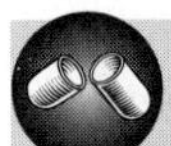

TABLE 107-3 Nonsteroidal Antiinflammatory Drugs—cont'd

Drug/Pregnancy Classification	Adult Dose	Children	Cost ($)	Maximum Daily Dose
Fenamates				
Meclofenamate (Meclomen)	50-100 mg TID to QID		16-76	400 mg/day (Use for short periods)
Mefenamic acid (Ponstel)	250 mg	Under 14: Not recommended	96	
Pregnancy: C				
Pyrazoles				
Ketorolac (Toradol)	10 mg q4-6h	Not recommended	122	Use ONLY for short periods
Pregnancy: C				
Contraindicated in patients with renal failure or at risk for renal failure. Do not use concomitantly with other nonsteroidal antiinflammatory drug				

ASSESSMENT

Differential diagnoses include: pelvic inflammatory disease, prostate tumor/infection, aortic aneurysm, abdominal tumor, uterine/fibroids, vertebral fracture, possible cauda equina syndrome, malingering behavior, renal colic, bladder infection, malignancy, spinal cord disease, pyelonephritis, osteoporosis, osteoarthritis, spinal stenosis, peptic ulcer disease, bursitis. This list is not all inclusive but should remind the NP to consider discogenic causes, malignancies, vascular lesions, infections, intraabdominal or pelvic causes, neurologic complications, congenital, trauma, and metabolic bone diseases as possible causes of lower back pain (Table 107-2). **Children: Because pain due to sprains of ligaments and muscles is unusual in children,** inflammation, infections, tremors, and trauma must be considered.

THERAPEUTIC PLAN

See Figures 107-4 and 107-5.

Pharmaceutical

Nonprescription drugs such as acetaminophen, aspirin, or NSAIDs (ibuprofen, naproxen, ketoprofen) provide relief for most persons. If an NSAID from one class is not tolerated or does not provide relief, another NSAID within the same or different class may be prescribed.

Muscle relaxants do not appear to be more effective than NSAIDs and should be reserved for those whom NSAIDs do not help or those in whom NSAIDs are contraindicated. If muscle relaxants are used, they should be limited to a course of 1 to 2 weeks; they should be avoided or used in reduced dosages in **older patients** who are at risk of falling.

Opiates are *not* necessary in the management of acute lumbosacral strain; if they are used for more severe pain, they should be taken for a short period of time only. Poor patient tolerance, drowsiness, clouded judgment, decreased reaction time, and the potential for misuse (dependence) may occur (Table 107-3).

Lifestyle/Activities

Proper body mechanics
Continuation of daily activities is preferred
When to return to work: A goal is to return to light work in 4 to 7 days and to normal duty within 1 to 2 weeks
Discussion of ergonomic issues involved in work, home, or leisure activities and ways to remedy any problems identified
Sleeping facilitated by lying on either side with knees flexed; if on back, pillows under knees and small pillow under lower back

Diet

None

Patient Education

Aerobic conditioning exercises (walking, swimming, stationary biking, light jogging) may be recommended to avoid debilitation. If a person was sedentary before this event, walking is preferred; if more active, light jogging is permitted.

Exercises may increase the pain, but patient must work through pain unless intolerable.

Back braces/belts, transcutaneous electrical nerve stimulation, shoe lifts (unless leg length discrepancy), biofeedback, and traction have not been shown to be beneficial.

Adjunct therapies such as ultrasound and massage have no effect on outcome but provide symptomatic relief and may be used for 3 weeks or less.

Chiropractic manipulation, if used in the first month, has been found to be safe and effective.

Bed rest is reserved for patients with rare severe leg pain and should not exceed 2 to 4 days. Other patients should maintain physical activity.

If patient must stand, he or she should rest one foot on low stool to relieve pressure on back and every 5 to 15 minutes switch the foot resting on the stool.

Men should lift no more than 20 pounds if pain is severe, 60 pounds if mild; women should lift no more than 20 pounds if pain is severe and no more than 35 pounds if pain is mild.

Patient should sit no longer than 20 minutes if back pain is severe; if no back pain, up to no longer than 50 minutes without getting up and walking around 5 to 10 minutes.

Local application of ice may help initially in decreasing edema and/or pain; after 2 to 3 days either ice or heat may be applied.

Explore community resources available (exercise programs, swimming pools, physical therapists, walking trails).

One of the most important aspects of patient education involves *prevention.* Education regarding proper body mechanics in lifting, weight loss (if needed), and overall muscular conditioning should be stressed.

Family Impact

Time lost from work with lost wages can temporarily affect every member of the family. If a family is noninsured or underinsured, the financial consequences can be great.

Disability or the development of a chronic pain syndrome can affect every member of the family for an indefinite period of time. If one member of the family exhibits behaviors of a sick individual, the entire family's functioning is impaired.

Briefly assess family, support systems, difficulty getting/taking medications, transportation/financial resources.

Referral

Children: Because strains of the back are uncommon in children and may be related to trauma, malignancies, infections, or inflammation, many children will require referral to a neurologist or pediatrician.

Adults: Refer to orthopedist, neurologist, internist, or vascular surgeon as appropriate those in whom HNP, fractures, malignancies, aortic aneurysms, cauda equina syndrome, spinal cord disease, renal colic are suspected.

Consultation

Consider consulting with MD on any patient in whom you suspect infection, malingering, prior treatment failures, or current treatment failure.

Follow-up

Most episodes of acute lumbosacral strain will resolve spontaneously within 4 weeks

May schedule return visit in 2 weeks with instructions to call/return if questions or no improvement

EVALUATION

If recovery does not go as expected, attempt to build a trusting relationship, emphasizing self-care and minimizing chance of chronic pain.

SUGGESTED READINGS

Barker LR, Burton JR, Zieve PD, editors: *Principles of ambulatory medicine*, Baltimore, 1995, Williams & Wilkins.

Bigos BS et al: Acute low back problems in adults. In *Clinical practice guideline, quick reference guide*, Number 14 (AHCPR Pub. No. 95-0643), Rockville, Md, 1994, U.S. Department of Health and Human Services, Public Health Service, Agency for Health Care Policy and Research.

Deen HG: Concise review for primary care physicians, *Mayo Clin Proc* 71:283-287, 1996.

Gillette RD: Behavioral factors in the management of back pain, *Am Family Physician* 53:1313-1318, 1996a.

Gillette RD: A practical approach to the patient with back pain, *Am Family Physician* 53:670-676, 1996b.

Gorroll AH, May LA, Mulley AG, editors: *Primary care management*, Washington, DC, 1995, American Psychological Association.

McIntosh E: Low back pain in adults, *Adv Nurse Practitioner* August 1997, pp 17-25.

Tierney LM, McPhee SJ, Papadakis MA, editors: *Current medical diagnosis and treatment,* Stamford, Conn, 1996, Appleton & Lange.

Weinstock MB, Neides DM, editors: *The resident's guide to ambulatory care*, Columbus, 1996, Anadem Publishing.

Lower Extremity Pain and Limp in Children

ICD-9-CM

Growing Pains in Children 781.9
Legg-Calvé-Perthes Disease 732.1
Osgood-Schlatter Disease 732.4
Benign Hypermotility Syndrome 728.5
Chondromalacia, Knee 717.7

OVERVIEW

Definition

Limb pain is defined as subjective discomfort localized in the soft tissues, bones, or joints. It has both acute and chronic definitions, with chronic being limb pain of >6 months. A limp is considered the inability to walk with a normal gait due to pain.

Incidence

Limb pain is the third most common childhood complaint (although no numbers are available to indicate how frequent) after abdominal pain and headache. Approximately 15% of school-age children are affected by growing pains. Legg-Calvé-Perthes disease usually occurs between the ages of 5 and 7 years, whereas in adolescents slipped femoral epiphyses and patellar problems are common.

Pathophysiology

Dependent on the cause; growing pains are nonarticular limb pains usually associated with physical activity

SUBJECTIVE DATA

History of Present Illness

Ask about:

- Timing: Onset, time of day pain noted; at night versus during school test
- Frequency and duration
- History of trauma: Falling/injury
- Location: Unilateral versus bilateral
- Effect of pain on activities of daily living
- Aggravation or relieving factors: influence of rest and nonsteroidal antiinflammatory drugs (NSAIDs) on decreasing pain
- Precipitating factors:
  - Other illness
  - Drug exposure
  - Immunization
  - Travel
  - Tick exposure

Past Medical History

Ask about previous leg injuries or surgery

Ask about previous systemic diseases: leukemia, juvenile rheumatoid arthritis, systemic lupus erythematosus, inflammatory bowel disease

Medications

Ask about use of analgesics or NSAIDs

Family History

Ask about history of arthritis or rheumatic disease.

Psychosocial History

School performance, preceding stressful events

A suspicion of child abuse should be considered if the degree of injury is out of proportion to the history or is recurrent

Diet History

Nutritional intake

TABLE 108-1 Associated Symptoms: Lower Extremity Pain

Associated Symptoms	Suggested Diagnosis to Consider
Fever	Infection, SLE, JRA, leukemia
Photosensitivity or malar rash	SLE, dermatomyositis, parvovirus
Raynaud phenomenon	SLE, scleroderma
Oral ulcers	SLE, IBD
Abdominal pain	HSP, SLE
Dysphagia	SLE, dermatomyositis, scleroderma
Eye inflammation	JRA, Reiter syndrome, IBD, spondyloarthritis
Weight loss, poor linear growth, fatigue	Chronic inflammatory illness or malignancy

HSP, Henoch-Schönlein purpura; *IBD,* inflammatory bowel disease; *JRA,* juvenile rheumatoid arthritis; *SLE,* systemic lupus erythematosus.

Associated Symptoms

Associated symptoms are found in Table 108-1.

OBJECTIVE DATA

Physical Examination

A complete physical examination is warranted to identify whether the cause of limb pain is systemic or local.

- General: Overall impression; chronically ill appearing, loss of weight
- Skin: Rash
- Head/eyes/ears/nose/throat: Lymphadenopathy of the eye, inflammation, ulcers of the mouth
- Lungs/cardiovascular: Provide baseline data
- Abdominal: Hepatosplenomegaly
- Extremities
  - Assess gait
  - Look for swelling and deformity
  - Check for symmetry, leg length, and muscle wasting
  - Palpate extremities for tenderness (osteomyelitis or fracture)
  - Active and passive range of motion
  - Muscle strength
  - Deep tendon reflexes

Diagnostic Procedures

Diagnostic procedures are determined by the history and physical examination (Table 108-2). If the pain is intermittent and does not affect daily function and the physical examination is normal, no diagnostic testing may be indicated.

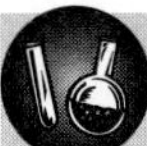

TABLE 108-2 Diagnostic Procedures: Lower Extremity Pain and Limp

Diagnostic Test	Findings/Rationale	Cost ($)
ESR	Indicates inflammation, helpful to distinguish arthritis from arthralgia	16-20
CBC	Presence of occult malignant disease (leukemia, anemia, ITP), osteoarticular infection, and inflammatory joint disease	18-23
U/A, blood chemistry	If systemic disease is present, will identify renal or hepatic dysfunction	15-20/U/A; 32-42/chem
ANA, RF	ANA is not specific for rheumatic disease; RF, although positive in up to 80% of adults with RA, is not as specific or sensitive for children	42-52/ANA; 22-28/RF
X-rays of hips, pelvis, lower extremity; CXR	Appropriate if orthopedic conditions are suspected: trauma, tumor, avascular necrosis, and slipped capital femoral epiphysis; comparison should always be done to the "normal" extremity; CXR provides a screening tool for multisystem diseases	112-134/hip; 127-151/pelvis
Bone scan	Useful in distinguishing between arthritis and occult malignant disease; the results are positive in osteomyelitis before there are x-ray changes	Varies
Ultrasound	Useful to evaluate soft tissues and documentation of fluid	Varies

ANA, Antinuclear antibody; *CBC,* complete blood count; *CXR,* chest x-ray; *ESR,* erythrocyte sedimentation rate; *ITP,* idiopathic thrombocytopenic purpura; *RA,* rheumatoid arthritis; *RF,* rheumatoid factor; *U/A,* urinalysis.

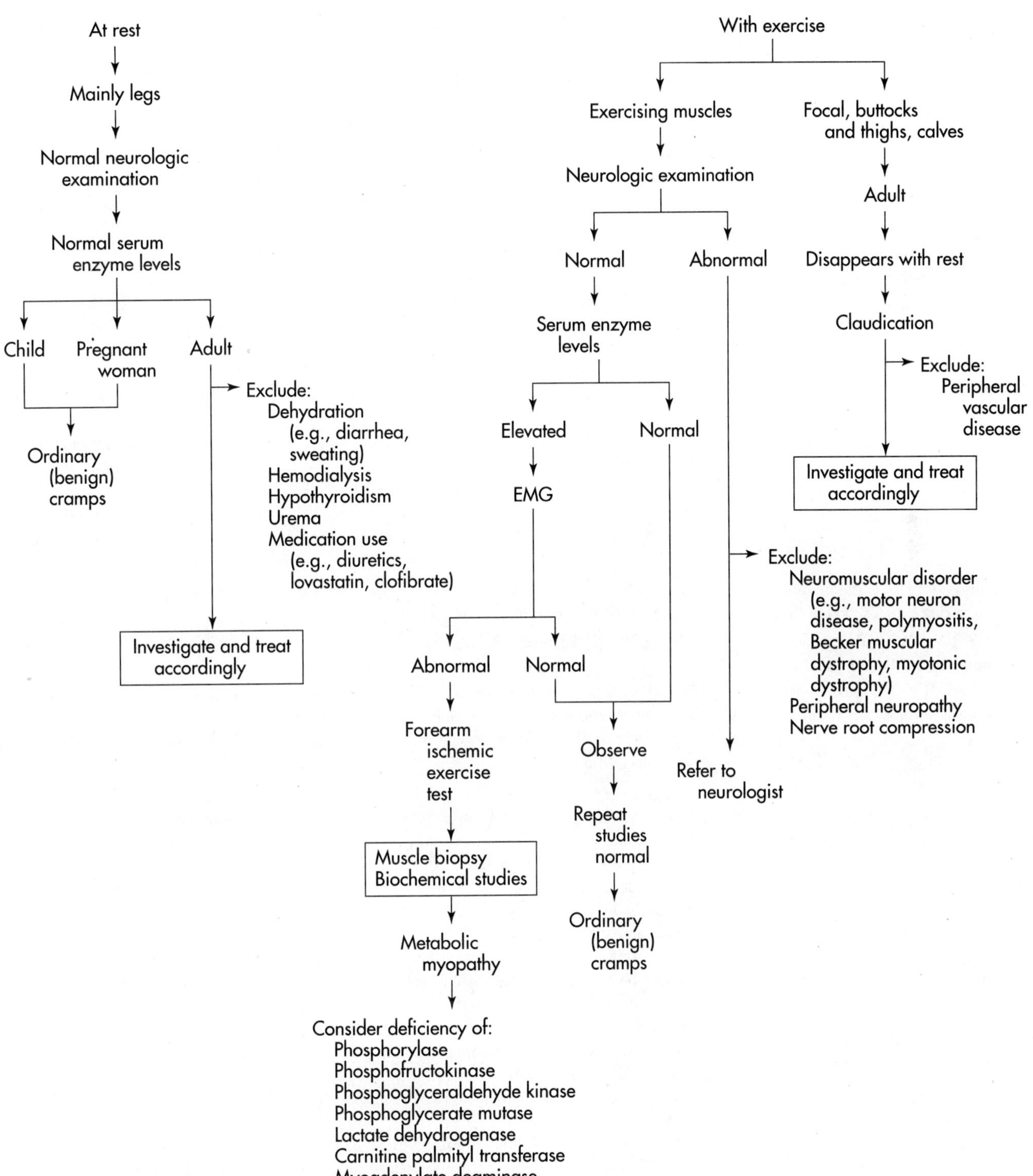

Figure 108-1 Algorithm for patient with muscle cramps and aches. (Adapted from Greene HL, Johnson WP, Lemcke D: *Decision making in medicine*, ed 2, St Louis, 1998, Mosby.)

TABLE 108-3 Differential Diagnosis: Lower Extremity Pain and Limp in Children

Diagnosis	Supporting Data
Trauma	
Contusions, sprains, strains, fractures, overuse syndromes (Ch. 123, 125, 127)	History of trauma identified, pain usually occurs after physical activity; children are most likely to sustain fractures since their tissues are more flexible; usually able to localize the pain to a specific spot; pain increases with more activity and is decreased with rest; usually unilateral; when due to mild trauma, the pain or limp should disappear in 2-3 weeks
Structural	
SCFE, Osgood-Schlatters, benign hypermotility syndrome, chondromalacia, Legg-Calvé Perthes	Hypermotility: pain increases after physical activity, more common in girls and especially in children who excel in gymnastics and ballet; pain occurs at the end of the day; pain, unlike growing pains, is localized to the joints and does not interrupt sleep; pigamentous laxity is also present SCFE: Insidious onset of limping and pain that increases in severity; pain may localize to the knee, thigh, or groin; flexion of the hip produces marked outward rotation and reproduces symptoms Schlatter's: Swelling and pain over the tibial tubercle, usually bilateral; more common in active boys; knee x-rays show fragmentation of the tibial tubercle and soft tissue swelling Chondromalacia: Pain climbing stairs and riding a bike Legg-Calvé Perthes: Is a disturbance of the epiphyseal ossification usually associated with a limp and pain referred to the medial aspect of the knee
Infection	
Cellulitis (Ch. 31), osteomyelitis, Lyme disease (Ch. 111), septic arthritis	Fever, erythema, sudden onset, child may appear toxic, usually able to localize area of pain to specific location, ↑WBC, ↑ESR Lyme: Flulike illness preceding joint pain
Hematological/Oncological	
Leukemia (Ch. 105), sickle-cell disease, primary bone tumors	Pain that wakens child from sleep is seen in both primary bone tumors and those that infiltrate the bone (leukemia); pain that interferes with ADLS should be investigated vigorously; unilateral pain is seen in primary bone tumors, ↑WBC with leukemia, ↓platelets with ITP
Rheumatic Disease	
JRA (Ch. 115), SLE (Ch. 110), vasculitis (HSP, Kawasaki's [Ch. 103])	Arthritis: Raynaud's phenomenon may be present; fever, eye inflammation, morning stiffness and evening pain after prolonged use, persistent pain, no history of injury, joint swelling, tenderness to palpation; reduced ROM, ↑WBC, ↑ANA, ~RF; HSP; polyarthritis, typical rash, abdominal colic; usually follows an URI Kawasaki's: Rash, fever, conjunctival erythema without discharge, LA, desquamation of palms and soles SLE: Young female with rash and joint pain
Growing pains	Pain may be severe enough to wake from sleep, relatively transient pains, worse late in day and at night, history of increased physical activity, poorly localized pains involving thighs, knees, shins, and ankles, usually outside joints; physical examination is normal, as are diagnostic tests; never unilateral pains and does not cause a limp; symptom-free periods; in older children the pains resemble cramps, or restless legs; no associated signs of erythema, decreased ROM or local tenderness
Osgood-Schlatter (Ch. 131)	Pain over tibial tuberosity
IBD (Ch. 102)	Lack of linear growth, anemia, increased ESR may appear prior to GI symptoms
Psychogenic causes	Should be considered if has a chronic history of pain for years; multiple physical examinations and laboratory results within normal limits; poor school attendance; patient tends to see multiple specialists and undergo treatments without improvement

ADL, Activities of daily living; *ANA*, antinuclear antibody; *ESR*, erythrocyte sedimentation rate; *GI*, gastrointestinal; *HSP*, Henoch-Schönlein purpura; *IBD*, inflammatory bowel disease; *ITP*, idiopathic thrombocytopenic purpura; *JRA*, juvenile rheumatoid arthritis; *LA*, lymphadenopathy; *ROM*, range of motion; *SCFE*, slipped capital femoral epiphysis; *SLE*, systemic lupus erythematosus; *URI*, upper respiratory disease; *WBC*, white blood count.

ASSESSMENT

Most serious causes of limb pain or limp are unilateral. Limping is a common complaint among children: it is never normal. The causes are many, ranging from ill-fitting shoes to a sprained ankle to the earliest manifestation of a malignant tumor (Figure 108-1).

Common causes of limb pain in children are found in Table 108-3.

THERAPEUTIC PLAN

Depends on cause of limb pain

Osgood-Schlatter: See Chapter 131

Growing pains: Growing pains may be treated with leg massage and analgesics (limit use to 5 days)

Lifestyle/Activities

Once growing pains are diagnosed, parents may want to monitor excessive physical activity.

A warm bath may help prevent/relieve some of the symptoms.

Tights or other supportive hose may help.

Application of warmth seems to help growing pains.

Diet

Not applicable

Patient Education

Demonstrate how to massage child's lower extremities.

Family Impact

Having a child wake in the late evening or at night with leg pain can be disconcerting for parents. Reassure them that massage, warmth, and analgesics should help decrease the discomfort. Reassure them that transient growing pains are not a sign of underlying pathology.

Referral

Refer any child suspected having a systemic illness to a pediatrician.

Refer any child with continued limp to an orthopedist.

Consultation

Consult with collaborating physician about antibiotics/need for hospitalization if cellulitis is suspected.

EVALUATION

Pain that is unilateral with no history of trauma and that causes limping should be investigated thoroughly. Pain that increases in frequency, duration, and intensity should be evaluated carefully to rule out inflammatory joint disease or occult malignancy.

SUGGESTED READINGS

Abu A, Russell G: Recurrent limb pain in schoolchildren, *Arch Dis Child* 74:336, 1996.

Eichenfield A: Rheumatic diseases. In Rudolph A, Kamei R, editors: *Rudolph's fundamentals of pediatrics,* ed 2, Stamford, Conn., 1998, Appleton & Lange.

Stern L: Muscle cramps and aches. In Greene HL, Johnson WP, Lemcke D: *Decision making in medicine*, ed 2, St Louis, 1998, Mosby.

Healthcare Consultants of America, Inc: *1998 physicians fee and coding guide,* Augusta, Ga, 1998, Healthcare Consultants of America, Inc.

Lower Extremity Ulcers*

ICD-9-CM

Lower Extremity Ulcers 707.1
Insufficiency, Venous (Peripheral) 459.8
 Arterial (Peripheral) 443.9
Ulcer, Stasis (Leg) (Venous) 454.0
Neuropathy, Peripheral (Nerve) 356.9
 In Diabetes Mellitus 250.6

OVERVIEW

Definition

Venous insufficiency is a disturbance in the forward flow of blood in the lower extremities that may progress to increased hydrostatic pressure, venous hypertension, and ultimately dermal ulceration. It presents as partial thickness skin loss ulcer.

Arterial insufficiency is an inadequate arterial perfusion to an extremity or location. Ulceration associated with arterial insufficiency results in full-thickness skin loss.

Peripheral neuropathy is altered nerve function in the lower extremities; it may involve diminished or absent sensation to touch, pain, or temperature; absence of sweating; foot deformities; and altered gait/weight bearing. Ulceration associated with peripheral neuropathy may present as partial thickness, but commonly as a full-thickness skin loss.

Incidence

Venous Insufficiency

One percent (1%) of the general population and 3.5% of **individuals over the age of 65** are afflicted with venous ulcers of the lower extremities. The rate of recurrence is 29 to 59%. **Among the elderly, women are affected three times more often than men.**

Arterial Insufficiency

Of all vascular lower extremity ulcers, only about 10% are due entirely to arterial insufficiency and ischemia. Another 10% to 20% are due to a combination of venous and arterial disease.

Peripheral Neuropathy

Symmetric polyneuropathy is most common in patients with diabetes. It is estimated that 15% of diabetic patients will develop a lower extremity ulcer; 50% to 70% of all patients undergoing amputations have diabetes.

Pathophysiology

Venous Insufficiency

Valvular incompetence; obstruction of deep venous system; congenital absence or malformation of valves of the venous system; regurgitation from deep to superficial venous system

Contributing factors: Malnutrition, hypoalbuminemia, immobility, and trauma

Arterial Insufficiency

Arteriosclerosis is a thickening and decreased elasticity of the arterial walls; atherosclerosis develops as a result of the accumulation of plaque, lipids, fibrin, platelets, and other cellular debris into and along the wall of the artery; the dynamics of arterial blood flow are affected by atherosclerotic plaque

Contributing factors: Smoking, diabetes mellitus, hyperlipidemia, hypertension

Peripheral Neuropathy

Cause unknown, but is probably multifactorial; ischemic injury to sensory, autonomic, and motor nerves and hyperglycemia have been implicated

Contributing factors: Diabetes, smoking, advanced age, Hansen's disease, and spinal cord lesion

---

*The authors would like to thank Jane Wurtzel, BSN, RN, CETN, ET Nurse at the Milwaukee VA Medical Center, Milwaukee, Wis.; and Dr. Scott Pruitt, Department of Surgery, Duke University Medical Center, Durham, N.C. for their assistance in writing this chapter.

SUBJECTIVE DATA

History of Present Illness

Venous insufficiency: Event that precipitated ulcer; length of time ulcer present; type of treatments used; pain
Arterial insufficiency: Event that precipitated ulcer; length of time ulcer present; type of treatments used; pain
Peripheral neuropathy: Event that precipitated ulcer; length of time ulcer present; type of treatments used; pain; footwear

Past Medical History

Venous insufficiency: Previous deep venous thrombosis and varicosities, reduced mobility, obesity, vascular ulcers, phlebitis, trauma, congestive heart failure (CHF), orthopedic procedures, pain reduced by elevation, nutritional deficits
Arterial insufficiency: Diabetes, previous vascular procedures/surgery, smoking; anemia, sickle cell disease, arthritis, increased pain with activity and/or elevation, intermittent claudication, hypertension, hyperlipidemia
Peripheral neuropathy: Diabetes, spinal cord injury, Hansen's disease, paresthesia of extremities

Medications

All currently used prescriptive and over-the-counter (OTC) medications such as immunosuppressants, corticosteroids, growth factors, NSAIDs, pentoxifylline (Trental), vasoconstrictive agents, anticoagulants, analgesics, caffeine, and nicotine

Family History

History of diabetes, arterial insufficiency, cardiac disease, obesity, lower extremity ulcers

Psychosocial History

Consider cognitive functioning, hygiene, access to health care, adequate footwear and prosthetic devices, difficulty maintaining employment, support of family and/or significant other(s), smoking, manual dexterity, visual acuity, patient's ability and/or motivation to adhere to prescribed medical regimen, patient's goal for therapy, financial resources

Description of Most Common Symptoms

Venous insufficiency: Minimal pain
Arterial insufficiency: Painful ulcer; intermittent claudication; resting, positional, nocturnal pain; decreased response to analgesics
Peripheral neuropathy: Diminished sensation, usually painless

OBJECTIVE DATA

Physical Examination

A problem-oriented physical examination should be conducted with particular attention to the following conditions.

Venous Insufficiency

Located on medial aspect of lower leg, superior to medial malleolus
Skin appears ruddy with surrounding erythema and/or brown staining
Shallow wound with irregular wound margins
Moderate to heavy exudate
Edema
Possible cellulitis
Peripheral pulses present/palpable
Normal capillary refill, less than 3 seconds

Arterial Insufficiency

Located on toe tips or web spaces, phalangeal heads around lateral malleolus, areas exposed to pressure or repetitive trauma
Extremity is pale on elevation
Dependent rubor
Skin taut, thin, dry; hair loss lower extremities
Atrophy of subcutaneous tissue
Thickened toenails
Deep, pale wound bed
Wound margins symmetrical, punched out in appearance
Edema variable
Skin temperature decreased
Granulation tissue rarely present
Infection frequent
Possible necrosis, eschar, and gangrene
Peripheral pulses absent or diminished
Capillary refill delayed more than 3 seconds

Peripheral Neuropathy

Located on plantar aspect of foot, metatarsals, heels, altered pressure points or callus formation; color normal with trophic skin changes
Depth variable
Wound margins well defined
Exudate variable
Edema
Cellulitis or underlying osteomyelitis common
Skin temperature warm
Possible granulation tissue
Infection frequent
Necrotic tissue variable
Peripheral pulses palpable/present

Capillary refill normal

Motor Neuropathy

Diminished reflexes

Orthopedic deformities such as hammer toes, malformation of the great toe

Altered gait

Sensory Neuropathy

Diminished sensitivity to touch

Reduced response to pin prick/monofilament testing

Autonomic Neuropathy

Xerosis, fissures common

Charcot's foot (degenerative changes involving cartilage and bone in the foot, whereas hypertrophic changes occur at the joint edges, resulting in an irregular deformity with instability at the joint), pathologic fractures

Diagnostic Procedures

Noninvasive Studies

1. Palpate peripheral pulses: Begin distally with dorsalis pedis and posterior tibial pulses and progress proximally until a pulse can be palpated.
2. Ankle-brachial index (ABI) indicated for arterial and mixed etiology ulcers. Procedure can be done either in the vascular laboratory or by individuals. Equipment: Blood pressure cuff, Doppler, gel (may substitute K-Y Jelly or Surgilube)
   a. Lay patient flat.
   b. Place blood pressure (BP) cuff around arm.
   c. Apply gel to antecubital fossa.
   d. Hold Doppler at a 45-degree angle and place over brachial pulse.
   e. Inflate BP cuff until Doppler sound disappears and slowly deflate cuff until sound returns. This is the BRACHIAL SYSTOLIC PRESSURE.
   f. Record this reading.
   g. Using fingers or Doppler probe, locate dorsalis pedis or posterior tibial pulses.
   h. Apply BP cuff around the leg just above the ankle.
   i. Apply gel and locate dorsalis pedis or posterior tibial pulses using Doppler probe.
   j. Inflate BP cuff until Doppler sound disappears. Slowly deflate cuff until the sound returns. This is the ANKLE SYSTOLIC PRESSURE.
   k. Record pressure reading.

   To calculate the ABI, divide the ankle pressure reading by the brachial pressure reading.

$$\text{ABI} = \frac{\text{Ankle Systolic Pressure}}{\text{Brachial Systolic Pressure}}$$

   General range for ABI findings
   1-1.1—Normal
   <0.9—Indicates presence of occlusive disease
   <0.8—Indicates intermittent claudication
   0.75—Loss of palpable pulse
   <0.5—Rest pain or threatened loss of limb
3. Toe pressures: Procedure is the same as ABI, only the blood pressure cuff is placed on great toe. May be indicated in some patients, especially patients with diabetes and those with atherosclerosis because of calcified arteries in the calf.
4. Other tests such as ultrasonic Doppler waveforms ($257 to $300), pulse volume recording (PVR), and transcutaneous oxygen tension may be considered.

Invasive Studies

Invasive studies such as venograms and arteriograms should be performed only after the decision has been made to surgically approach the problem by either interventional radiology or surgical reconstruction.

Laboratory Studies

Serum glucose ($16 to $20)

Cholesterol ($17 to $21)

Triglyceride levels ($19 to $24)

Serum albumin ($18 to $23)

Prothrombin time/partial thromboplastin time ($18 to $23)

Radiological Studies

Plain film of the extremity if osteomyelitis is suspected

Bone scan, Indium-labeled leukocyte scan, or magnetic resonance imaging may be recommended if plain film negative and osteomyelitis is still suspected.

ASSESSMENT

Differential diagnosis to include:

Bilateral edema: Edema of legs secondary to CHF; nephrotic syndrome, cirrhosis, acute and chronic thrombophlebitis, cellulitis, lymphedema, salt retaining drugs, constricting garments, and dependency; other diagnoses include rheumatoid arthritis, carcinomas, sickle cell anemia, fungal infection, trauma, bullous diabeticorum

Unilateral edema: Lymphedema secondary to obstruction, cellulitis, compartmental syndrome, thrombophlebitis

THERAPEUTIC PLAN

Pharmaceutical/Nonpharmaceutical

Drugs

Drug therapy used in lower extremity ulcers is found in Table 109-1.

Wound Care

The goal of topical wound care for the patient with a lower extremity ulcer is to promote a favorable environment by removing/preventing impediments (e.g., necrosis, infection, excessive or pooled exudate).

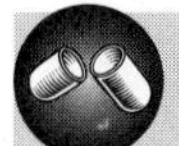

TABLE 109-1 Pharmaceutical Plan: Lower Extremity Ulcers

Drug	Dose	Category	Cost ($)	Indications
Oral Antibiotics				
Cephalexin (Keflex)	500 mg QID	Cephalosporin	31-253	Staphylococci
Dicloxacillin (Dynapen)	250-500 mg QID	Penicillin	19-94	Staphylococci
Clindamycin (Cleocin)	150-450 mg q6h	Lincomycin derivative	75-232	Aerobic and anaerobic streptococci
Amoxicillin and clavulanate (Augmentin)	500 mg q8h 500 mg q12h 875 mg q12h	Penicillin, broad-spectrum	82-86	Staphylococci, *Escherichia coli, Klebsiella,* streptococci
Ciprofloxacin (Cipro)	500-750 mg q12h	Quinolone	335-572	Staphylococci, streptococci, *Pseudomonas*
Vasodilator/Antiplatelet Agents				
Pentoxifylline (Trental)	400 mg TID-QID	Blood viscosity reducing agent	57	Arterial insufficiency, intermittent claudication
Enteric-coated aspirin	325 mg daily	Nonnarcotic analgesic	9-33	Alters platelet function
Dipyridamole (Persantine)	25-74 mg TID	Coronary vasodilator	3-55	Alters platelet function/antiplatelet agent, questionable efficacy
Neuropathic Analgesics				
Amitriptyline (Elavil)	10-25 mg QHS	Tricyclic antidepressant	2-41	Neuropathic pain
Gabapentin (Neurontin)	300 mg QHS × 1 day 300 mg BID × 1 day 300 mg TID, then adjust dosage	Anticonvulsant/ miscellaneous	90	Neuropathic pain
Carbamazepine (Tegretol)	100 mg BID with food; gradually increase in increments of 100 mg BID as needed	Anticonvulsant/ miscellaneous	16-21	Neuropathic pain (Draw levels and CBC q3-6 months to monitor for toxic levels and neutropenia.)
Parenteral Antibiotics				
Nafcillin (Nafcil/Unipen)	2 g q4h	Penicillin	6-11	Group A streptococci, *Staphylococcus aureus*
Cefazolin (Kefzol/Ancef)	1 g q6-8h	Cephalosporin	2-7	Staphylococci

NOTE: Patient response to drug therapy is individualized.

Venous Insufficiency

Compression therapy: Short stretchy bandages, therapeutic support stockings (TED hose are not therapeutic; they provide only 8 to 12 mm Hg compression; therapeutic stockings provide 25 to 35 mm Hg compression [moderate compression]; some patients are unable to tolerate 25 to 35 mm Hg compression and must begin with stockings providing 18 to 25 mm Hg compression [mild compression]), Unna's boot, four-layer wrap, mechanical pump; *compression therapy contraindicated in patients with an ABI less than 0.8 mm HG*

Topical therapy
- Wound cleansing with saline or noncytotoxic commercial cleanser
- Necrotic tissue
  - Remove necrotic tissue: Conservative sharp debridement (mechanical); enzymatic debriding agents (chemical)
  - Dressings that maintain moist wound surface (autolysis)
- Nonnecrotic tissue
  - Moist wound healing (transparent dressings, hydro-

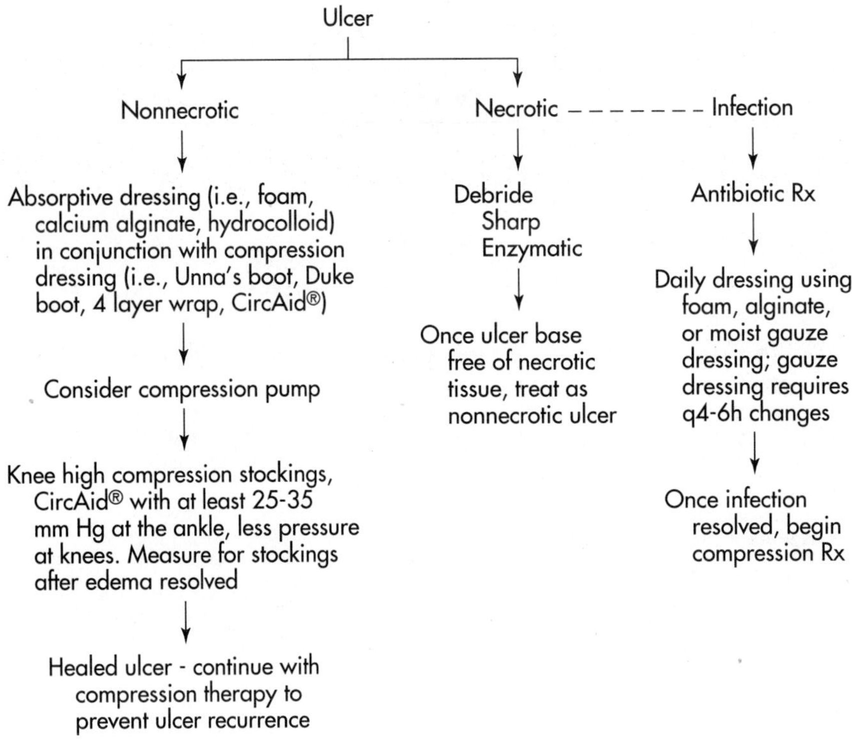

Figure 109-1 Wound care algorithm for venous insufficiency ulcers.

gels, collagen, hydrocolloid, calcium alginates, Unna's boot); protect surrounding skin to avoid maceration (e.g., ointments, protective skin sealants, or absorptive dressing)

Complications: Infection, osteomyelitis, chronic ulcer

NOTE: If signs and symptoms of wound infection appear or wound fails to respond to treatment within 2 to 4 weeks, consider culture and sensitivity with Gram stain and/or punch biopsy and antibiotic therapy. If wound fails to heal or pain increases, refer for vascular work-up (Figure 109-1).

Arterial Insufficiency

Wound cleansing with saline or noncytotoxic commercial cleanser

Necrotic tissue

- Debridement may be contraindicated in arterial wounds; consult with vascular surgeon and/or emergency technician (ET)/wound ostomy continence (WOC) nurse and follow their recommendations.

Nonnecrotic wound: *Topical dressings require judicious use in ischemic ulcers*

- Peripheral pulses present
  - Hydrogels, collagens, calcium alginates may be used
  - Occlusive dressings (hydrogel wafer, transparent dressings, and foam dressings) *may be used with caution*
- Absent peripheral pulses
  - Occlusive dressings contraindicated
  - Protect surrounding skin
  - Avoid topical therapy that may cause fragile epidermis to macerate
  - Consider antibiotic therapy when signs/symptoms of infection are present. NOTE: Clinical manifestations of infection may be subtle due to reduced blood flow.

Complications: Infection, gangrene (may result in amputation), osteomyelitis (may result in amputation) (Figure 109-2).

Peripheral Neuropathy

Nonweight bearing on affected area

Wound cleansing with saline or noncytotoxic commercial cleanser

Necrotic tissue

- Surgical consult for conservative sharp debridement
- Enzymatic agents
- Autolysis using transparent dressing, or other moisture-retentive dressings

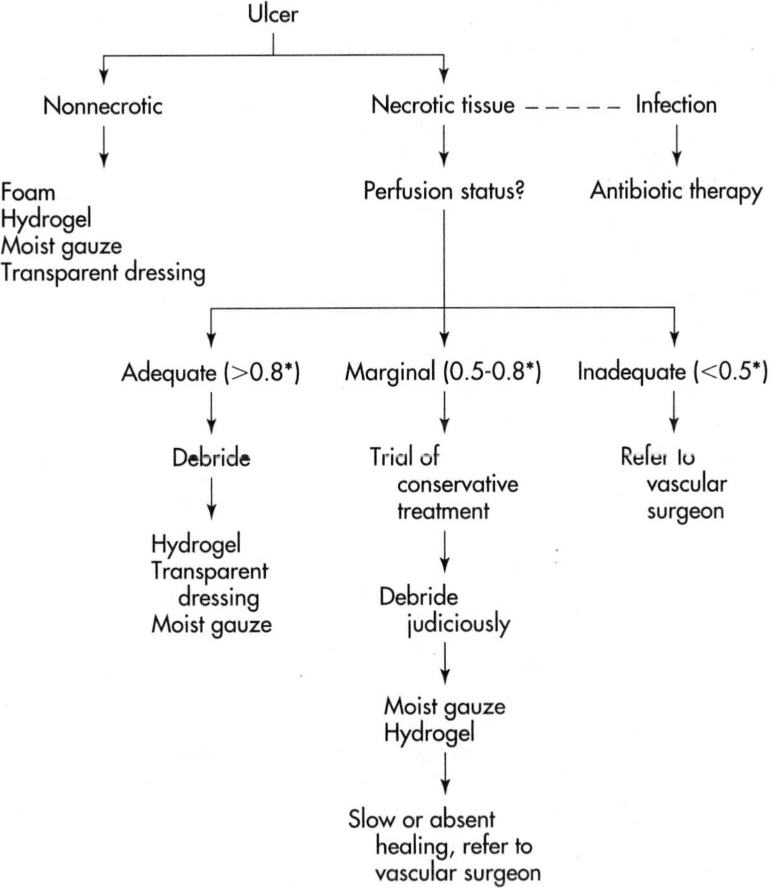

Figure 109-2 Wound care algorithm for arterial insufficiency ulcers.

Nonnecrotic wound with crater formation or pooled exudate
  Absorptive dressing (e.g., calcium alginate, foam, moist gauze)
Shallow ulcers with minimal drainage
  Transparent dressing, hydrogel, or moist gauze
  Protect surrounding skin: Solvent may be used to protect fragile skin when removing adhesives; friction may increase size of wound if maceration present; sealants or ointments may be used to prevent maceration of surrounding skin

Complications: Infection, gangrene (may result in amputation), osteomyelitis (may result in amputation) (Figure 109-3).

NOTE: See wound care product information in Table 109-2 and Box 109-1.

Lifestyle/Activities

Venous Insufficiency

Keep legs higher than heart
Discourage sitting with acute angulation and/or legs crossed
Discourage standing for prolonged periods
Ambulate to tolerance
Discourage constrictive clothing
Correctly fit and apply vascular support devices (e.g., zinc oxide impregnated support dressings, pressure gradient stockings, elastic wraps, sequential compression devices)
Provide pressure reduction for heels and other bony prominences
Implement measures to keep surrounding skin clean and pliable
Adequate nutrition
Comply with prescribed medications

Arterial Insufficiency

Maintain legs in a neutral or dependent position
Avoid crossing legs
Avoid exposure to cold
Avoid smoking
Prevent thermal, mechanical, and chemical trauma; prevent moisture between toes
Avoid friction

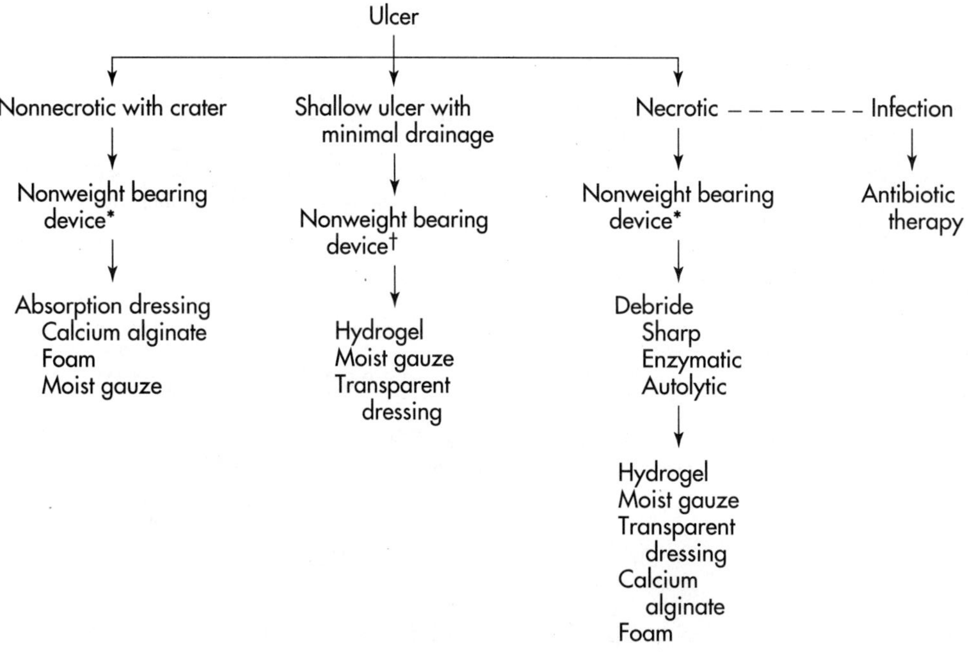

Figure 109-3 Wound care algorithm for peripheral neuropathy ulcers.
*Nonweight-bearing device (i.e., orthotics, special shoe); refer to orthotist or prosthetics.
†Nonweight-bearing device (i.e., orthotics, special shoe, contact casting); referral may vary, depending on available resources; consider wound ostomy continence, enterostomal continence nurse, orthotist, rehabilitation medicine, orthopedist.

Routine professional foot care for toenails, corns, calluses
Use of proper, well-fitting footwear
Avoid constrictive clothing
Keep surrounding skin clean and pliable
Pressure reduction for heels and other bony prominences
Ambulate to tolerance

Peripheral Neuropathy

Maintain legs in a neutral or dependent position
Avoid exposure to cold
Avoid constrictive garments
Prevent thermal, mechanical, and chemical trauma; prevent moisture between toes
File calluses to prevent thickening and cracking
Avoid friction
Routine professional foot care for toenails, corns, and calluses
Use of proper footwear
Daily inspection of feet
Avoid self-treatment of corns and calluses
Provide pressure reduction for heels and other bony prominences
Implement measures to keep surrounding skin clean and pliable; moisturize after bathing and as necessary with a nonirritating agent such as petrolatum or xipamide with water (e.g., Eucerin or Absorbase cream)
Avoid fragrance or other sensitizing agents

Diet

It is important to maintain weight control, positive nitrogen balance, and glucose control. Nutritional needs should be based on the patient's underlying medical problems. If ulcer is present, consider supplementing the diet with vitamin C, 500 mg BID, and zinc, 15 to 20 mg daily, to promote wound healing. Dietary recommendations should be practical to promote compliance.

Patient Education

Venous Insufficiency

No smoking
Adequate nutrition: Low salt, maintain/attain ideal body weight
Skin care: Avoid trauma (mechanical, chemical, thermal)
Maintain clean, well lubricated skin
Optimize venous return: Elevate legs above heart
Discourage sitting with legs crossed
Discourage standing for prolonged periods
Comply with prescribed medications
Compression therapy

Arterial Insufficiency

No smoking
Compliance with medications
Diabetes control

TABLE 109-2 Options in Lower Extremity Wound Management

Category/ Trade Name	Manufacturer	Description	Indications	Applications	Advantages	Disadvantages
Absorptive Wound Fillers						
Bard Absorption Dressing Multidex Calcium alginates	Bard Home Health Div. DeRoyal See separate category	Hydrophilic dressings which absorb exudate, dead cells, and bacteria	Exudating wounds Non-tunneling deep wounds Infected wounds Partial or full-thickness wounds	Irrigate with saline or commercial non-cytotoxic cleanser Change daily Secondary dressing	Absorbs exudate Moist environment Nonocclusive Odor reduction Comfortable Inert Cleanses debris Many distributed in unit dose packs Pain reduction	Difficult to apply May increase wound pH May sting when applied Needs secondary dressing Application techniques vary
Calcium Alginates						
Kaltostat Restore CalciCare Sorbsan	ConvaTec Hollister Dow B. Hickam	A hydrophilic nonwoven dressing or calcium sodium alginate fibers Alginates are processed from brown seaweed into pad or twisted fiber form. Exudate transforms fibers to gel at wound interface	Light to heavily exudating wounds Moist wound environment Autolysis Partial or full thickness wounds	Irrigate with saline or commercial non-cytotoxic cleanser Change daily or with frequency of compression dressing Cover with appropriate dressing to promote moist wound environment	Absorptive Decreases pain Nonocclusive Moist wound environment Conformable Easy, trauma-free removal May use in infected or non-infected wounds Permeable to gases Reduces wound pain Nonirritating to wound Accelerates wound healing time to clean up wound Less frequent dressing changes Aids in control of minor bleeding	Requires secondary dressing Characteristic odor May desiccate peri-wound skin May promote hypergranulation tissue Permeable to fluids and bacteria

NOTE: There are many wound care products on the market. This list represents only a small sampling of available products under each category. You may want to consult with a wound ostomy continence/enterostomal therapy nurse or sales representative for other options.

Continued

TABLE 109-2 Options in Lower Extremity Wound Management—cont'd

Category/ Trade Name	Manufacturer	Description	Indications	Applications	Advantages	Disadvantages
Compression Dressings						
Coban (use with Unna's boot) CircAid Profore Unna's boot	3-M Coloplast/Sween Smith & Nephew/United Biersdorf	Elastic stockings or bandages applied to the lower extremities	Venous insufficiency	Irrigate with saline or commercial non-cytotoxic cleanser Change Q3-7 days PRN exudate May require use of protective cream/ointment to prevent contact dermatitis (do not apply to ulcer)	Promotes venous blood return Prevents blood pooling Decreases edema	Arterial ulcers Ulcers with mixed arterial-venous etiology ABI <0.8 Contact dermatitis may develop due to zinc oxide impregnated wraps
Enzymatic Debriding Agents						
Santyl Accuzyme	Knoll Pharmaceuticals Health Point Medical	Debriders digest necrotic tissue by differing methods	Dermal ulcers, partial or full-thickness wounds	Irrigate with saline or commercial non-cytotoxic cleanser	Daily application Nonsurgical method of debridement Does not harm healthy tissue (these 2 products only) Provides moist environment	Secondary dressing May require cross-hatching of eschar
Foams						
Allevyn LYOfoam PolyMem	Smith & Nephew/United ConvaTec Ferris Manufacturing	Absorbs exudate May be non-adherent or have adhesive backing	Management of exudating cutaneous wounds Infected or non-infected wounds	Irrigate with saline or commercial non-cytotoxic cleanser	Daily application Non-occlusive May use under compression dressing	May require secondary dressing

Gauze	Numerous	Nonocclusive fiber dressing with loose, open weave	Minimal-heavy exudating wounds Infected wounds Debridement	Irrigate with saline or commercial non-cytotoxic cleanser Change q6-8h	Readily available Deep wound packing May use with infected wounds or with topical agents Non-occlusive Comfortable	Wound bed may desiccate Non-selective wound debridement May cause bleeding/ pain on removal Secondary dressing required Frequent dressing changes Dressing may "shed"
Hydrocolloids Comfeel Duoderm CGF Restore Tegasorb	Coloplast/Sween ConvaTec Hollister 3-M	A wafer dressing composed of hydrophilic particles in an adhesive form covered by a water resistant film or foam	Clean, granular wounds Minimal to moderate exudating wounds Venous ulcers in conjunction with Unna's boot Partial thickness wounds Full-thickness wounds without tunneling or undermining Noninfected wounds only Autolysis	Irrigate with saline or commercial non-cytotoxic cleanser Change q3-7 days	Forms moist gel wound bed Impermeable to fluids/bacteria Conformable Good thermal insulation	For noninfected wounds only Contraindicated for arterial/neuropathic Impermeable to gases May leave residue on skin
Amorphous Hydrogels Carrasorb Carrasyn Gel IntraSite gel Restore Hydrogel Solosite	Carrington laboratories Carrington Laboratories Smith & Nephew/ United Hollister Smith & Nephew/ United	Gel composed of 94% water to 96% glycerin	Partial thickness or full thickness wounds Arterial and neuropathic ulcers	Irrigate with saline or commercial non-cytotoxic cleanser Cover with gauze/ transparent dressing to prevent dehydration of gel	Forms moist wound Conformable Manages exudate by swelling Autolysis	May dehydrate Minimal to moderate absorption Requires secondary dressing May require BID-TID dressing changes if appropriate secondary dressing not used

Continued

Table 109-2 Options in Lower Extremity Wound Management—cont'd

Category/ Trade Name	Manufacturer	Description	Indications	Applications	Advantages	Disadvantages
Skin Sealants						
AllKare protective Barrier Wipes Skin Gel Protective Wipes Skin Prep Sween Prep	ConvaTec Hollister Smith & Nephew/United Coloplast/Sween	Vapor-permeable film, nonwater soluble	Prevents epidermal stripping caused when adhesive products	Irrigate with saline or commercial non-cytotoxic cleanser Apply, allow to dry before placing adhesive on skin	Protects skin from epidermal stripping when adhesives are removed	Burns if applied to denuded skin Must apply prior to each application of adhesive
Transparent Dressings						
Opsite Tegaderm	Smith & Nephew/United 3-M	A semi-occlusive, translucent dressing with partial or continuous adhesive composed of polyurethane or copolymer thin film	Partial-thickness wounds Clean, granular wounds Minimally exudating wounds Peripheral neuropathy ulcers Cover dressing for hydrogels, alginates, enzymatic debriding agents	Irrigate with saline or commercial non-cytotoxic cleanser Change q3-7 days Requires at least 24 hr wear time for effective use Apply skin sealant to periwound skin before applying	Semi-occlusive Gas permeable Easy inspection of wound Protection Impermeable to fluids/bacteria Comfortable Self-adherent Pain reduction Moist environment Resists shear	For noninfected wounds only Not absorptive May cause peri-trauma on removal Maceration may occur with large amounts of exudate
Cell Proliferation						
Becaplermin (Regranex) Pregnancy: C	Ortho-McNeil	A recombinant human platelet-derived growth factor in a topical gel	Lower extremity, diabetic neuropathic ulcer in conjunction with other ulcer care practices. DO not use in children <16 years.	Each square inch of ulcer surface requires ⅔ inch length of gel (cm^2 of ulcer requires 0.25 cm)	Very few side effects	Cover with saline-moistened dressing Leave in place 12h Remove and rinse with saline to remove residue Cover with plain, moist dressing Wound and SQ tissue must have adequate blood supply Complex dosing (Box 109-1)

> **Box 109-1**
>
> ### Calculations for Regranex Gel Dosing
>
> Measure the greatest length and greatest width of the ulcer.
> Calculate the length of gel that should be squeezed from the 15-g tube using the following formulas:
>
> **Inches**
>
> Length × Width × 0.6
> For example, if the ulcer measures 1 inch by 2 inches, a 1¼-inch length of gel should be used [1 × 2 × 0.6 = 1.2].
> Each square inch of ulcer surface will require approximately ⅔-inch length of gel.
>
> **Centimeters**
>
> Length × Width ÷ 4
> For example, if the ulcer measures 4 cm by 2 cm, a 2-cm length of gel should be used ([4 × 2] ÷ 4 = 2).
> Each square centimeter of ulcer surface will require approximately a 0.25-cm length of gel.

From Regranex package insert, December 1997, Ortho-McNeil Pharmaceutical, Raritan, New Jersey.

Neutral or dependent position for legs (depends on pain tolerance)
Avoid leg crossing
Avoid exposure to cold, friction
Avoid constrictive clothing
Avoid moisture between toes
Avoid going barefoot
Routine professional foot care for toenails, corns, calluses
Use of well-fitting footwear
Pressure reduction for heels and other bony prominences

Peripheral Neuropathy

No smoking
Compliance with medications
Control diabetes
Avoid exposure to cold
Avoid friction
Avoid moisture between toes
Avoid going barefoot
Routine professional foot care for toenails, corns, calluses
Use of well-fitting footwear
Pressure reduction for heels and other bony prominences
Avoid use of external use of heat (heating pad, hot water bottle, hydrotherapy)
Daily foot care which includes skin inspection, wash and dry well, especially between toes, keep skin moisturized, clean socks
Avoid use of over-the-counter medications for corns and calluses
Avoid temperature extremes
Request referral for orthotic footwear if altered gait or orthopedic deformity occurs

Family Impact

Economic: Cost of initial treatment; loss of wages and productivity; disability frequently experienced; cost of recurrent treatment
Family dynamics: Increased responsibility for caregiver; possible altered emotional status (e.g., depression, anxiety, dependency)

Referrals

WOC/ET nurse: Refer for wound care or debridement, depending on comfort level of nurse practitioner
Social worker: Refer depending on patient's psychosocial situation
Home health: Refer if assistance needed for wound care
Vascular surgeon: Refer if ABI <0.5, pain increases, or ulcer fails to respond within 2 to 4 weeks
Dietitian
Podiatrist
Orthotist
Endocrinologist
Other referrals as indicated

Consultation

If nurse practitioner does not have admitting privileges to local hospital, consult primary care physician if patient exhibits signs of cellulitis not responding to oral antibiotics and requires parenteral antibiotics or sudden loss of pulse with cyanosis of lower extremity. Symptoms of cellulitis that may require parenteral antibiotics and hospitalization may be edema of lower extremity with nonlocalized erythema; patient may or may not be febrile.

EVALUATION/FOLLOW-UP

NOTE: Each patient's follow-up should be individualized.

Venous insufficiency: Every 4 to 7 days for the first 2 weeks if compression dressing becomes saturated, because decrease in edema will require more frequent dressing changes; then, if followed by home health or family member instructed to change dressing weekly and PRN for dressing saturation, every 3 to 4 weeks; if not followed by home health or family member changing dressing, then weekly and PRN for dressing changes.
Arterial insufficiency: Weekly for the first 2 weeks, then every 4 weeks and PRN for change in status of affected lower extremity.

Peripheral neuropathy: Weekly for 4 to 6 weeks; then every 2 to 3 weeks and PRN for change in status of affected lower extremity.

SUGGESTED READINGS

Ackerman Z et al: Skin zinc concentrations in patient with varicose ulcers, *Int J Dermatol* 29(5):360-362, 1990.

Alguire PC, Mathes BM: Chronic venous insufficiency and venous ulceration, *J Gen Intern Med* 12(6):374-382, 1997.

Arnold TE et al: Prospective multicenter study of managing lower extremity venous ulcers, *Ann Vasc Surg* 8(4):356-362, 1994.

Barr DM: The Unna's boot as a treatment for venous ulcers, *Nurse Pract* 21(7):55-56, 61-64, 71-72, 1996.

Black SB: Venous stasis ulcers: a review, *Ostomy Wound Management* 41(8):20-22, 24-26, 28-30, 1995.

Cheatle TR, Scurr JH, Smith PD: Drug treatment of chronic venous insufficiency and venous ulceration: a review, *J Royal Soc Med* 84(6):354-358, 1991.

Clinical fact sheet: Arterial insufficiency, Costa Mesa, Calif., 1996, Wound Ostomy Continence Nurses Society.

Clinical fact sheet: Quick assessment of leg ulcers, Costa Mesa, Calif., 1996, Wound Ostomy Continence Nurses Society.

Clinical fact sheet: Peripheral neuropathy, Costa Mesa, Calif., 1996, Wound Ostomy Continence Nurses Society.

Clinical fact sheet: Venous insufficiency (stasis), Costa Mesa, Calif., 1996, Wound Ostomy Continence Nurses Society.

DePalma RG: Venous ulceration: a cross-over study from nonoperative to operative treatment, *J Vasc Surg* 24(5):788-792, 1996.

Erickson CA et al: Healing of venous ulcers in an ambulatory care program: the roles of chronic venous insufficiency and patient compliance, *J Vasc Surg* 22(5):629-636, 1995.

Ellsworth AJ et al: *Mosby's 1998 medical drug reference*, St Louis, 1998, Mosby.

Falanga V, Eaglestein WH: *Leg and foot ulcers*, London, 1995, Martin Dunitz Ltd.

Hafner J et al: Management of venous leg ulcers, *VASA* 25(2):161-167, 1996.

Harris AH, Brown-Etris M, Troyer-Caudle J: Managing vascular leg ulcers. Part I: assessment, *Am J Nurs* 96(1):38-43, 1996.

Hess CT: *Nurses clinical guide: wound care*, Springhouse, Penn., 1995, Springhouse Corp.

Holloway GA: Arterial ulcers: assessment and diagnosis, *Ostomy Wound Management* 42(3):50-51, 1996.

Hume M, Basmajian A: Venous ulcers, the nurse and the care budget, *J Vasc Nurs* 11(1):23-24, 1993.

Karp DL, Fahey VA: Chronic venous disease. In Fahey VA, editor: *Vascular nursing*, Philadelphia, 1994, WB Saunders.

Kenkre JE et al: A randomized controlled trial of electromagnetic therapy in the primary care management of venous leg ulcerations, *Family Practice* 13(3):235-241, 1996.

Kowallek DL, DePalma RG: Venous ulceration: active approaches to treatment, *J Vasc Nurs* 15(2):50-57, 1997.

Lagua R, Claudio V: *Nutrition and diet therapy reference dictionary,* ed 4, Florence, Ky, 1996, International Thomas Publishing.

Levin ME, O'Neal LW, Bowkin JH: *The diabetic foot*, ed 5, St Louis, 1993, Mosby.

Marculescu GL et al: *Standards of care: patient with dermal wounds: lower extremity ulcers*, Costa Mesa, Calif., 1993, Wound Ostomy Continence Nurses Society.

Maune J, Giordano J: Experience with open-heeled Unna boot application technique, *J Vasc Nurs* 15(2):63-72, 1997.

Mayberry JC et al: Nonoperative treatment of venous stasis ulcer. In Bergan JJ, Yao JS, editors: *Venous disorders*, Philadelphia, 1991, WB Saunders.

Moffat C: The Charing Cross approach to venous ulcers, *Nurs Stand* 5(12):6-9, 1990.

Morison M, Moffatt C: *A color guide to the assessment and management of leg ulcers*, ed 2, St Louis, 1994, Mosby.

Nelzen O, Bergquist D, Lindhagen A: Long-term prognosis for patient with chronic leg ulcers: a prospective cohort study, *Eur J Vasc Endovasc Surg* 13(5):500-508, 1997.

Richard LE: Compression therapy and venous ulceration: another point of view, *J Wound Ostomy Continence Nurs* 24(3):180, 1997.

Sanford JP et al: *The Sanford guide to antimicrobial therapy*, Kansas City, Mo, 1997, Hoechst Marion Roussel.

Sieggreen MY, Maklebust J: Managing leg ulcers, *Nursing* 26(12):41-46, 1996.

Sieggreen MY et al: Commentaries on venous leg ulcers diagnostic and treatment draft guidelines, *Adv Wound Care* 9(4):18-26, 1996.

Smith PD: The microcirculation in venous hypertension, *Cardiovasc Res* 32(4):789-795, 1996.

Stacey MC et al: The influence of dressings on venous ulcer healing—a randomized trial, *Eur J Vasc Endovasc Surg* 13(2):174-179, 1997.

Stacey MC: Clinical trials in the treatment of chronic venous ulcerations. In Negus D, Jantet G, Coleridge-Smith PC, editors: *Phlebotomy '95*, Berlin, 1995, Springer-Verlag.

Zink M, Rouseau P, Holloway GA Jr.: Lower extremity ulcers. In Bryant RA, editor: *Acute and chronic wounds: nursing management*, St Louis, 1992, Mosby.

Lupus (Systemic Lupus Erythematosus)

ICD-9-CM

Systemic Lupus Erythematosus 710.0
Discoid Lupus Erythematosus 695.4

OVERVIEW

Definition

Systemic lupus erythematosus (SLE) is a chronic, autoimmune disease that causes inflammation of various parts of the body, especially the skin, joints, blood, and kidneys. SLE is highly variable in its nature, with periods of exacerbation and remission.

There are three types of LE: discoid, systemic, and drug-induced. Discoid LE is limited to the skin. Systemic LE generally is more severe than discoid; it affects almost any organ or system of the body. Drug-induced LE is similar to systemic SLE. It may first appear as a rash, but any organ or system may be involved.

Incidence

1,400,000 to 2,000,000 (1994)

Occurs most frequently in females ages 15 to 45

Adult females 10 to 15 times more frequent than in adult males

60% of cases females in late 20s or older

Childhood onset more severe; 3/100,000 children

Increased incidence in African, Native American, Asian descent

Pathophysiology

Autoimmune disorder with environmental and genetic factors

Environmental factors: Infection, antibiotics, ultraviolet light, extreme stress, drugs

Genetic factors: No known gene causes illness; 10% have close relative with disease; **5% of children born to individuals with SLE develop illness**

Hormonal factors may be implicated in the disease; **cyclic increase in symptoms associated with menstrual periods and/or during pregnancy suggests that hormones may be involved**

SUBJECTIVE DATA

No characteristic clinical pattern; may be acute or insidious; characterized by recurrent seasonal remissions and exacerbations, especially during spring and summer.

Requires careful history with focus both on systemic and on single organ symptoms (Table 110-1)

Migratory nonerosive *polyarthralgia/arthritis:* Prolonged morning stiffness in multiple joints, less stiffness after using joints, spine not involved

Constitutional symptoms: Malaise, *fever,* anorexia, *weight loss*

Multi-system involvement: *Fatigue, rash, anemia,* diffuse adenopathy, alopecia, oral and nasal ulcers, pleuritic chest pain, Raynaud's phenomenon, dry eyes and mouth, abdominal pain, nausea, vomiting, diarrhea, constipation, irregular menstruation or amenorrhea, headaches, irritability, depression, renal dysfunction, urinary frequency, dysuria, bladder spasms, urinary tract infection

Typical presentation: **Young woman** with symmetric polyarthritis or arthralgia, facial rash (butterfly rash), fever, fatigue, and weight loss

Past Medical History

Recent viral infection, hormonal abnormality, ultraviolet radiation; seizures, visual disturbances

Medications

Drugs that may induce SLE are *hydralazine, procainamide,*

penicillin, isonicotinic acid hydrazide, chlorpromazine, phenytoin, and quinidine.

Family History

SLE, autoimmune disorders

OBJECTIVE DATA

Physical Examination

Assess temperature for fever and blood pressure for hypertension

Integumentary: Pallor, signs of bleeding, including petechiae and bruising; erythema forming a butterfly pattern on cheeks and nose, lesions and necrosis on fingertips, toes, elbows; hairline for hair loss

TABLE 110-1 Frequency of Lupus Symptoms

Percent	Symptom
95	Arthralgia
90	Fever >100° F
90	Arthritis
81	Fatigue
74	Rashes
71	Anemia
50	Kidney involvement
45	Chest pain on deep breathing (pleurisy)
42	Butterfly-shaped rash across cheeks and nose
30	Photosensitivity
27	Hair loss
17	Raynaud's phenomenon
15	Seizures
12	Mouth/nose ulcers

From the Lupus Foundation of America, 1996.

Musculoskeletal: Inspect extremities and joints for signs of arthritis, lymphadenopathy, peripheral neuropathy; range of motion, and joint discomfort

Cardiovascular/respiratory: Auscultate lungs and heart to determine presence of pleural or pericardial friction rub

Abdomen: Palpate spleen and liver for tenderness, splenomegaly, or hepatomegaly

Psychosocial: Determine level of anxiety, fear, depression

Diagnostic Procedures

There is no definitive laboratory test to diagnose SLE. Commonly used tests include:

- Complete blood count, rheumatoid arthritis factor, erythrocyte sedimentation rate, Venereal Disease Research Laboratories
- Antinuclear antibody: High titer confirms lupus; low titer confirms autoimmune disease (i.e., RA)
- Anti-DNA or anti-dsDNA: 40% to 75% with SLE
- Anti-Sm: 20% to 25% with SLE; for false-positive serologic test for syphilis
- Anti-nRNP (antinuclear ribonucleoprotein): 40% with SLE
- Anti-Ro: 40% with SLE
- Antiphospholipid antibodies: 30% with SLE
- <Serum C3, C4; 50% to 70%
- LE cell prep: Determine presence of cell that has ingested swollen antibody-coated nucleus of another cell; used less frequently than ANA, which is more sensitive for SLE
- Urinalysis: Cellular casts predictive of early SLE renal disease; 20% to 30% (Table 110-2)

ASSESSMENT

SLE is difficult to diagnose because many symptoms mimic those of other illnesses. Diagnosis is made by careful review

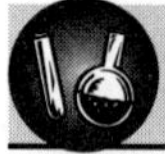

TABLE 110-2 Diagnostic Tests

Symptoms	Findings	Cost ($)
Fatigue, fever, weight loss, migratory arthritis, headaches, alopecia, depression, seizures, anemia, rash, photosensitivity, oral ulcers, Raynaud's syndrome, dyspnea (4 of 11 criteria)	Joint swelling and tenderness, discoid lesions, reducible joint abnormalities, hypertension, adenopathy	13-16/CBC 22-28/RF 18-22/VDRL 16-20/ESR 14-18/Urinalysis 49-51/ANA
	+ANA	54-71 each/anti-SM, anti-nRNP, anti-Ro; 47-59/serum C3, C4

ANA, Antinuclear antibody; *CBC*, complete blood count; *ESR*, erythrocyte sedimentation rate; *RF*, rheumatoid factor; *VDRL*, Venereal Disease Research Laboratories.

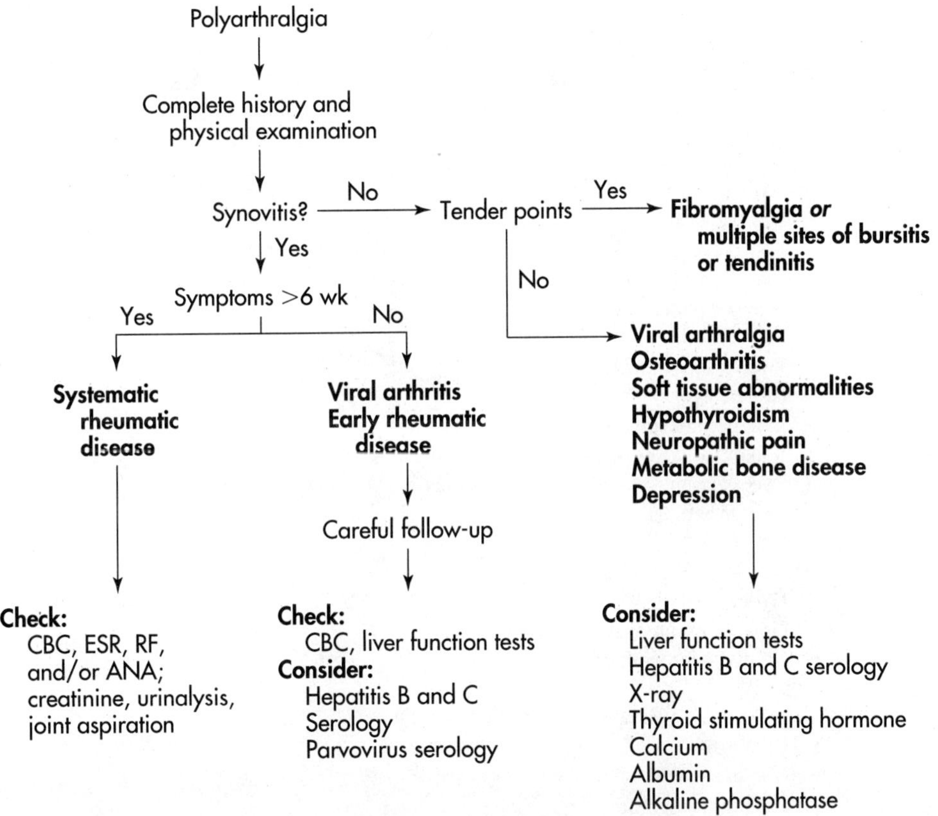

Figure 110-1 Differential diagnosis algorithm for systemic lupus erythematosus. *ANA*, Antinuclear antibodies; *CBC*, complete blood count; *ESR*, erythrocyte sedimentation rate; *RF*, rheumatoid factor. (From American College of Rheumatology Ad Hoc Committee on Clinical Guidelines: Guidelines for the initial evaluation of the adult patient with acute musculoskeletal symptoms, *Arthritis Rheum* 39[1]:1-8, 1996.)

of the entire medical history, current symptoms, and analysis of laboratory tests (Figure 110-1).

At some point in the disease history, an individual should have 4 or more of the 11 criteria in Table 110-3 to be diagnosed with systemic lupus erythematosus (American College of Rheumatology Ad Hoc Committee on Clinical Guidelines, 1996).

THERAPEUTIC PLAN

Goals:

- Reduce inflammation
- Suppress abnormalities of immune system responsible for tissue inflammation
- Avoid or decrease severity of flare-ups

Pharmaceutical/Nonpharmaceutical

Pharmaceutical/nonpharmaceutical interventions can be found in Tables 110-4 and 110-5 and Boxes 110-1 and 110-2.

Patient Education

Encourage regular exercise to maintain full range of motion and prevent contractures.

During exacerbations, rest is indicated.

Apply heat packs to relieve joint pain and stiffness.

Use warmth and protect hands from injury if Raynaud's disease is also present.

Maintain rest and balanced diet; no evidence of selective diets influencing course of disease.

Eat cool, bland foods if sore mouth.

Avoidance of infection (meticulous mouth care, hand washing, avoiding crowds and people with known infection).

Avoid ultraviolet light; wear protective clothing, sunscreen.

Avoid precipitating factors: Fatigue, allergy shots (immunotherapy), infection, stress, surgery, drugs, exposure to ultraviolet light, food (parsley, figs, celery) and drugs (tetracycline) that augment effect of ultraviolet light.

Signs and symptoms of exacerbation (flare): Increased pain, increased fatigue, fever, abdominal pain, SOB, headache, dizziness, blurred vision, recurring nose

TABLE 110-3 The Eleven Criteria Used for the Diagnosis of Lupus

Criteria	Definition
Malar rash	Rash over the cheeks
	Discoid rash
	Red raised patches
Photosensitivity	Sun exposure causes or intensifies skin rash
Oral ulcers	Nose or mouth
	Often painless
Arthritis	Two or more peripheral joints
	Nonerosive
Serositis	Inflamed mucous membrane
Pleuritis or pericarditis	Inflammation of pleura or pericardium
Renal disorder	Excessive protein in urine (>0.5 g/day or 3+ on test sticks)
	And/or cellular casts
Neurologic	Headaches
	Aseptic meningitis
	Hydrocephalus
	Organic brain syndromes
	Cranial neuropathies
	CVA
	Movement disorders
	Psychosis
Seizures	Convulsions in absence of drugs or metabolic disturbances
Hematologic	Hemolytic anemia
	Leukopenia (WBC <4000 cells per cubic millimeter) on two or more occasions
	Lymphopenia (<1500 lymphocytes per cubic millimeter) on two or more occasions
	Thrombocytopenia (<100,000 platelets per cubic millimeter)
Immunologic	Positive LE prep test
	Positive anti-DNA test
	Positive anti-Sm test
	False-positive syphilis test (VDRL)
	Positive ANA

Source: American Rheumatism Association: *Eleven Criteria for SLE,* 1996.
ANA, Antinuclear antibody; *CVA,* cerebrovascular attack; *DNA,* deoxyribonucleic acid; *VDRL,* Venereal Disease Research Laboratories; *WBC,* white blood count.

Box 110-1

Pediatric Pharmaceutical Recommendations

- Long-term hydroxychloroquine potentially efficacious
- Methotrexate promising
- Aggressive antihypertensive therapy (e.g., hydralazine hydrochloride [Apresoline] PO 0.75-7.5 mg/kg/day to max of 200 mg/day)
- Do not over treat with corticosteroids or immunosuppressive agents
- Cyclophosphamide should be reserved for severe life threatening disease (vasculitis, CNS disease, thrombocytopenia)

Box 110-2

Promising Pharmaceutical Interventions

- Dehydroepiandrosterone (DHEA)
- Thalidomide
- 2-Chlorodeoxyadenosine
- Bromocriptine
- Tamoxifen

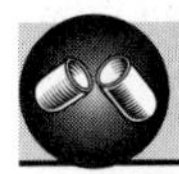

TABLE 110-4 Pharmaceutical Treatment

Drug	Dose	Cost ($)	Comments
Nonsteroidal Anti-inflammatory Drug (NSAID)			
Nabumetone (Relafen)	**Adults:** Initially 1 g/day BID; max 2 g/day Pregnancy: C	102-123	Most common treatment; avoid ibuprofen (Motrin), sulindac (Clinoril), tolmetin (Tolectin); they can be associated with aseptic meningitis
Anti-malarials			
Chloroquine (Aralen) Hydroxychloroquine (Plaquenil)	Chlor: 250 mg/day Hydroxy: 200 mg BID Pregnancy: C NOTE: Chloroquine and hydroxychloroquine are regarded as unsafe during pregnancy	8-18/chlor 104-116/hydroxy	Retinopathy leading to retinal degeneration dose-related; baseline ophthalmologic examination q3-6 mo
Corticosteroids			
Prednisone (Deltasone)	**Adults:** Initially 5-6 mg/day, divided in 1-4 doses **Child:** 0.14-2 mg/kg/day or 4-60 mg/m^2/day, divided in 4 doses Pregnancy: C	8-32	Used when other treatments fail and joints remain swollen and painful; reserved for major organ involvement; beneficial long-term prognosis in SLE nephritis
Cytotoxic Drugs			
Azathioprine (Inuran)	**Adult and Child:** 1-2 mg/kg/day in divided doses; maintenance dosage ½ starting dose Pregnancy: D	118	Reduce inflammation, suppress immune system; may take 6-8 wk to see affect; corticosteroid sparing (decreases amount of corticosteroid needed); use contraceptive measures during treatment and 12 wk after completion

TABLE 110-5 Prevention of Exacerbation (Flares)

Risk	Measure
Photosensitivity	Avoidance of (excessive) sun exposure Application of sun screen (SPF 30)
Muscle weakness, fatigue	Regular exercise; minimum 30 minutes, 3 times per week
Infection	Immunizations (*allergy immunotherapy* contraindicated—may cause flares) Avoid people with colds or infections
Stress	Support groups Counseling Talking with friends, family, primary provider
General health hazards	Smoking cessation Reduce alcohol intake Maintain prescribed medication schedule Regular medical check-ups

bleeds, puffy eyelids, hemoptysis, increasing swelling of feet and legs.

Referral

Consultation or referral to rheumatologist or clinical immunologist:

Severe constitutional symptoms (e.g., disabling fatigue, fever, weight loss)

Vasculitis, involvement of lungs, heart, kidneys, or nervous system

Undiagnosed after initial evaluation (tests inconclusive)

EVALUATION/FOLLOW-UP

Treatment based on specific needs and symptoms. Ongoing supervision is essential to proper treatment as the course of lupus may vary significantly.

Individuals receiving hydroxychloroquine should have an eye exam prior to starting therapy and every 6 months thereafter.

RESOURCE

Lupus Foundation of American
1300 Piccard Dr. Suite 200
Rockville, MD 20850-4303
800-558-0121

Lupus Network Canada
http://www.lupusnet.ucalgary.CA

REFERENCE

American College of Rheumatology Ad Hoc Committee on Clinical Guidelines: Guidelines for the initial evaluation of the adult patient with acute musculoskeletal symptoms, *Arthritis Rheum,* 39(1):1-8, 1996.

SUGGESTED READINGS

Crofts P, D'Cruz D: Systemic lupus erythematosus part 2: the role of the nurse, *Nurs Standard* 11(44):40-44, 1997.

Davis JC, Tassiulas IO, Boumpas DT: Lupus nephritis, *Curr Opin Rheumatol* 8:415-423, 1996.

Gare BA: Epidemiology of rheumatic disease in children, *Curr Opin Rheumatol* 8:449-454, 1996.

Gladman DD: Prognosis and treatment of systemic lupus erythematosus, *Curr Opin Rheumatol* 8:430-437, 1996.

Johnson AE et al: Undiagnosed systemic lupus erythematosus in the community, *Lancet* 347:367-369, 1996.

Khamashta MA, Hughes GRV: Pregnancy in systemic lupus erythematosus, *Curr Opin Rheumatol* 8:424-429, 1996.

Lahita RG: *What is lupus?* Rockville, Md, 1996, Lupus Foundation of America, Inc.

Shmerling RH: *Learning the signs of lupus flare-ups,* Lupus Foundation of America newsletter article library, 1996, pp 93-117.

Silverman E:. What's new in the treatment of pediatric SLE? *J Rheumatol* 23:1657-1660, 1996.

Strand V: Approaches to the management of systemic lupus erythematosus, *Curr Opin Rheumatol* 9:410-420, 1997.

West SG: Lupus and the central nervous system, *Curr Opin Rheumatol* 8:408-414, 1996.

van Vollenhoven RF, Engleman EG, McGuire JL: Dehydroepiandrosterone in systemic lupus erythematosus: results of a double-blind, placebo-controlled, randomized clinical trial, *Arthritis Rheum* 38(12):1826-1831, 1995.

Lyme Disease

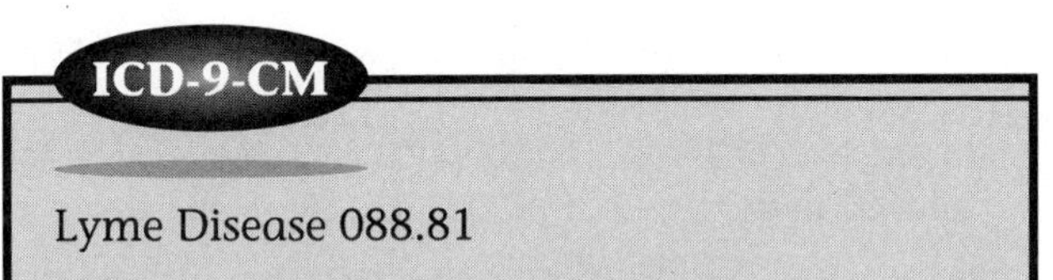

ICD-9-CM

Lyme Disease 088.81

OVERVIEW

Definition

Infection caused by *Borrelia burgdorferi*, a spirochete; most common arthropod-borne disease in the United States. It is transmitted by prolonged attachment of 2 days or more by an infected tick.

Incidence

Highest incidence in northeast, upper Midwest, and northern California; however, cases have been reported in all 50 states.

Prevalence associated with increased deer population in endemic areas. Most infections occur between the months of May through August in most of the United States, January through May in the Pacific Northwest.

Protective Factors Against

None

Factors that Increase Susceptibility

Exposure to tick-infested areas, particularly during May through August

Common Pathogens

Ixodes dammini (deer tick) in Northeast and Midwest
I. pacifica in Far West
I. ricinus in Europe
Incubation period: 2 to 36 days, median 9 days

SUBJECTIVE DATA

History of Present Illness

Ask about duration of symptoms
Ask about possible exposure to tick bites, such as recent camping trip, hiking, or working in yard
Ask about occupation (e.g., farming, logging, landscaping)
Ask patient to describe duration, characteristics of any skin lesions
Question about recent occurrence of headache, fatigue, fever, myalgias
Less then 50% of patients with Lyme disease recall a preceding tick bite

Past Medical History

Any history of arthritis, systemic lupus erythematosus, or recent viral syndrome
Previous history of Lyme disease and/or treatment
Previous history of lyme vaccine

Medications

Current and recent medication therapy to rule out any recent infections, such as syphilis, or the existence of any chronic problem, such as arthritis or systemic lupus erythematosus, which patient may not have included in past medical history

Family History

Ask about any other family members with similar symptoms
Ask about family history of rheumatoid arthritis

Diet History

Ask about recent ingestion of inadequately cooked meat, or possibly contaminated water to rule out tularemia

Description of Most Common Symptoms

Malaise, fatigue, headache, fever, chills, stiff neck, muscle and joint pain, lymphadenopathy, backache, anorexia, nausea and vomiting, abdominal pain, and erythema migrans, a skin lesion at the site of tick bite that begins as a red bull's eye with central clearing and enlarges over days to weeks. Lesions over 5 cm in diameter are most specific for diagnosis of Lyme disease (Figure 111-1).
Erythema migrans does not occur in all cases; in some patients, arthritis is the first and only sign.

OBJECTIVE DATA

Physical Examination

Carefully inspect skin for lesions
Palpate for lymphadenopathy
Perform a thorough cardiac examination for secondary carditis, which occurs in 6% to 10% of untreated cases, manifested by atrioventricular conduction abnormalities and left ventricular dysfunction (shifted PMI, presence of S3, S4).
Inspect joints (particularly knee, shoulder, hip, elbow, and ankle) for swelling, tenderness, or erythema.
Perform neurological examination; 10% to 20% of untreated cases result in neurological complications, including meningitis (headache and neck pain), encephalitis (sleep disturbances, poor memory, irritability, dementia), and cranial neuropathies (Bell's palsy, decreased sensation, weakness, loss of reflexes).

Diagnostic Procedures

Indirect fluorescent antibody: Very nonspecific, poor diagnostic tool
Enzyme-linked immunosorbent assay (ELISA) ($43-$53): Usual method (high occurrence of false-positive results with: viral infections, systemic lupus erythematosus, rheumatoid arthritis)
Western blot assay ($81-$103): Confirmatory, helps identify false positive ELISA results
ELISA and Western blot identify 50% of early Lyme disease and 100% of patients with later complications of carditis, neuritis, and arthritis

ASSESSMENT

Differential diagnoses include:
Syphilis, rheumatoid arthritis, meningitis/encephalitis, *viral syndrome*
Systemic lupus erythematosus, Rocky Mountain spotted fever, tularemia, Bell's palsy (Table 111-1)

THERAPEUTIC PLAN

Pharmaceutical

Adults (including **nonpregnant, nonlactating females,** and **children over 8 years**)
Doxycycline 100 mg BID ×10 to 21 days or,
Tetracycline 250 to 500 mg QID ×10 to 21 days, or
Erythromycin 250 mg QID ×10 to 21 days for patients allergic to penicillin (PCN) or tetracycline
Amoxicillin 250 to 500 mg TID ×10 to 21 days is **preferred treatment for pregnant or lactating women and for children under the age of 8 years**
Child dose: 25 to 50 mg/kg/day in divided doses, maximum dose 1 to 2 g/day
Erythromycin 30 mg/kg/day divided into q6h dosing for **children under age 8 who are allergic to PCN**
Consult physician about treatment of patients with cardiac or neurologic manifestations; intravenous therapy of PCN 20 million U/day, or ceftriaxone 2 g/day for 14 days is recommended
Doxycycline BID or amoxicillin TID ×30 days is effective for patients with arthritis
Nonsteroidal antiinflammatory drugs may be used as an analgesic (see Table 111-2)

Patient Education

Lyme disease vaccine is now available and should be given to individuals who either live in a community with a high incidence of Lyme disease or by virtue of their work and lifestyle have high exposure to tick-infested area. Individuals with previous uncomplicated Lyme disease who are at continued high risk should be considered to receive the vaccine. This vaccine is approved for individuals ages 15 to 70. Three injections are given over a 1-year period. **It is not recommended during pregnancy.**

Avoid exposure to ticks by wearing light-colored clothes so ticks are easily detected.
Wear long pants tucked into socks and long-sleeved shirt tucked in at waist.
Use insect repellent (DEET) safe for all ages; read precautions on container.
Avoid tick-infested areas during May through August.
Keep area around house and yard free of brush and tall grass.
Inspect entire body following potential exposure.
Use tweezers to remove attached tick.

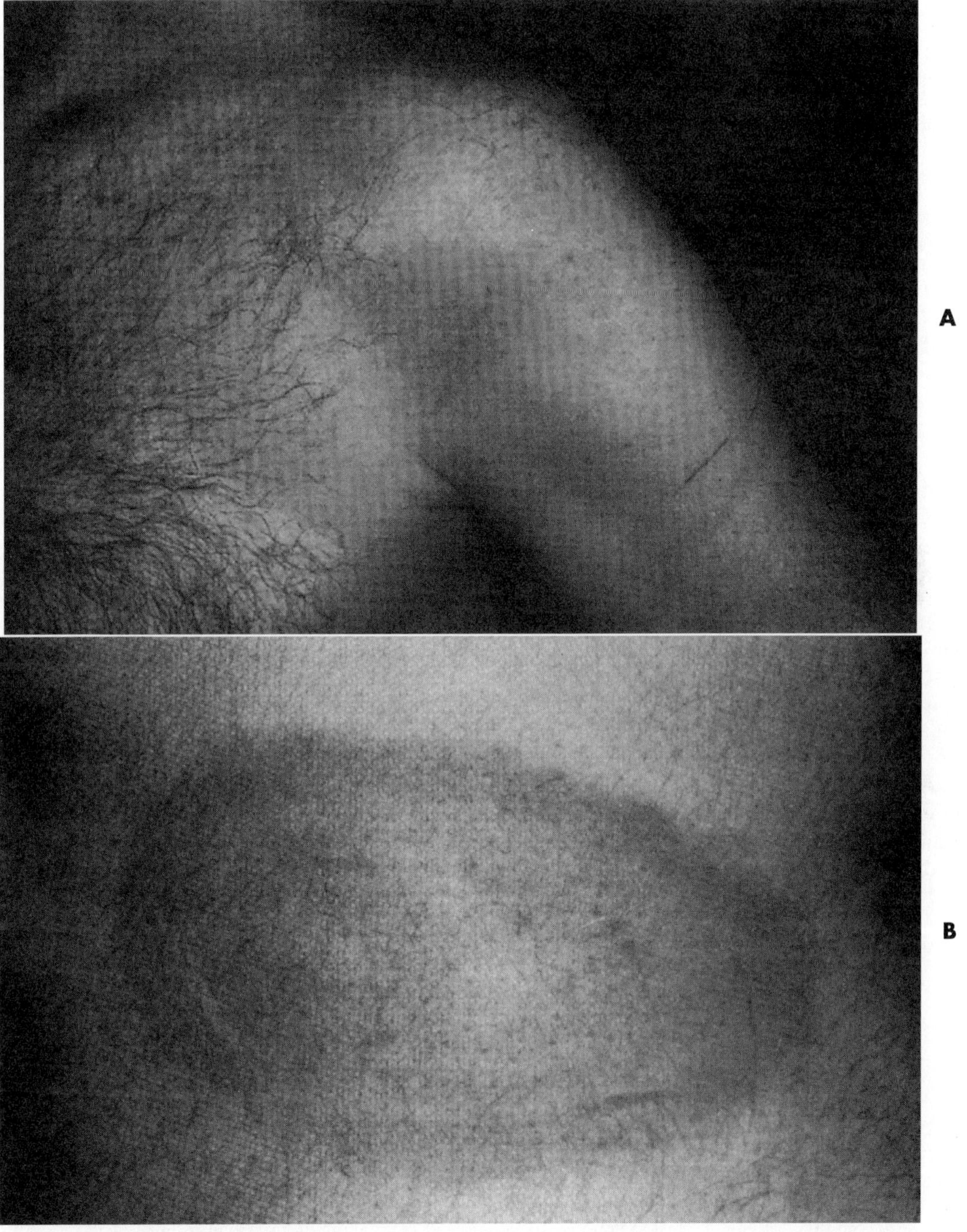

Figure 111-1 **A,** Lyme borreliosis, erythema migrans. A very large annular lesion is seen on the shoulder. The pen line marks the border of the previous day, the lesion having expanded by 1 cm in 24 hours. **B,** Lyme borreliosis, erythema migrans. Solitary annual lesion on the lateral thigh occurring at the site of an asymptomatic tick bite. (From Fitzpatrick T et al: *Color atlas and synopsis of clinical dermatology*, ed 2, New York, 1992, McGraw-Hill.)

TABLE 111-1 Differential Diagnosis: Lyme Disease

Diagnosis	Supporting Data
Syphilis	Chancre, nonpruritic rash (maculopapular) to trunk, palms, and soles *Cerebrospinal fluid:* Increased mononuclear cells and protein, decreased glucose Diagnostic test: Venereal Disease Research Laboratory ($18-$22); rapid plasma reagin ($42-$54) more sensitive, or fluorescent treponemal antibody absorption test
Rheumatoid arthritis	Joint swelling, particularly proximal interphalangeal, metacarpophalangeal joints and wrist, *synovial cysts* **Labs:** *Complete blood count* ($13-$16), hematocrit 30%-34%, hemoglobin may be decreased, normocytic normochromic, white blood count normal, erythrocyte sedimentation rate elevated
Viral syndrome	Abrupt onset, fever (as high as 106° F), malaise, headache, *clear nasal discharge, cough*
Systemic lupus erythematous	Photosensitivity, oral ulcers, persistent proteinuria, seizures

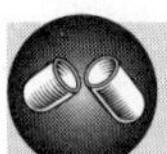

TABLE 111-2 Pharmaceutical Treatment Plan

Drug	Adult Dose	Child Dose	Cost ($)
Medications Indicated for Adults, Including Nonpregnant and Nonlactating Females and Children >8 Years			
Doxycycline	100 mg BID ×10-21 days	Not indicated for small children	60-123
Tetracycline	250-500 mg QID ×10-21 days	Not indicated for small children	4-10
Erythromycin (for patients allergic to penicillin or tetracycline)	250 mg QID ×10-21 days	30 mg/kg/day in divided doses q6h for **children under 8 who are allergic to penicillin**	14-16
Amoxicillin (preferred treatment for **pregnant or lactating women and for children under the age of 8 years)**	250-500 mg TID ×10-21 days	25-50 mg/kg/day in divided doses; max dose 1-2 g/day	8-27

TABLE 111-3 Complications of Lyme Disease

Complications	Findings
Palpitations with AV conduction abnormalities presence of S3, S4	Lyme carditis
Headache, nausea, vomiting, fatigue, depressed consciousness, impaired concentration, neck pain	Lyme meningitis (present in 80% of those with neurologic problems associated with Lyme disease) Diagnostic test: Cerebrospinal fluid may have mild to moderate mononuclear pleocytosis (<500) with elevated protein and normal glucose concentrations
Sixth nerve palsy, facial (Bell's) palsy	Facial nerve paralysis
Sleep disturbances, poor memory, irritability, dementia	Lyme encephalitis
Diffuse arthralgia, synovial fluid with WBC counts >25,000 cells/mm^3, arthritis manifested in knees, shoulder, hip, ankle, elbow	Lyme arthritis

Most ticks removed are not infected with *B. burgdorferi;* therefore prophylactic antimicrobial therapy is not recommended.

No data exist to document resistance to reinfection following treatment.

Reinfection vs. recurrence in endemic regions is difficult to distinguish.

Referral

Patients with cardiac or neurologic manifestations should be referred to physician.

Follow-up by cardiologist or neurologist may be indicated (Table 111-3).

EVALUATION/FOLLOW-UP

Follow-up evaluation at end of treatment (2 to 3 weeks) is adequate for uncomplicated cases. Patients with more severe symptoms such as cardiac or neurologic manifestations should be seen more frequently.

SUGGESTED READINGS

Angelov L: Unusual features in the epidemiology of Lyme borreliosis, *Eur J Epidemiol* 12(l):9-11, 1996.

Bartlett CR, Brown JW: New and emerging pathogens, part 2: Tick, tick, tick, tick, boom! The explosion of tick borne diseases, *Med Lab Observ* 28(3):44-52, 1996.

Deltombe T, et al: Lyme borreliosis neuropathy: a case report, *Am J Phys Med Rehabil* 75(4):314-316, 1996.

Ellsworth AJ, et al: *Mosby's 1988 medical drug reference,* St Louis, 1998, Mosby.

Fitzpatrick TB, et al: *Color atlas and synopsis of clinical dermatology,* ed 15, New York, 1994, McGraw-Hill.

Halperin JJ: Neuroborreliosis, *Am J Med* 98(4A):52S-56S, 1995.

Healthcare Consultants of America, Inc: *1998 Physicians fee and coding guide*, Augusta, Ga., 1998, Healthcare Consultants of America, Inc.

Herman L, Robinson TT, Birrer RB: Lyme disease: ready cure, but a challenging diagnosis, *J Am Acad Physician Assistants* 9(10):39-40, 43-44, 47-48, 1996.

Masters EJ: Erythema migrans: rash as key to early diagnosis of Lyme disease, *Postgrad Med* 94(1):133-134, 137-138, 1993.

Newland JA: Nurse practitioner extra: primary care protocol, Lyme disease, *Am J Nurs* 95(7):16, 1995.

Schneiderman H: What's your diagnosis? erythema migrans of Lyme disease, *Consultant* 35(5):677-678, 680, 1995.

Steere AC: Musculoskeletal manifestations of Lyme disease, *Am J Med* 98(4A):44S-48S, 1995.

Verdon ME, Sigal LH: Recognition and management of Lyme disease, *Am Family Physician* 56(2):427-436, 439-440, 1997.

Ziska MH, Donta ST, Demarest FC: Physician preferences in the diagnosis and treatment of Lyme disease in the United States, *Infection* 24(2):182-186, 1996.

Lymphadenopathy

ICD-9-CM

General Lymphadenopathy 785.6
Due to Toxoplasmosis 130.7
Lymphadenitis 289.3
Infectional Lymphadenitis 683

OVERVIEW

Definition

Painless lymph node >10 mm in size (except epitrochlear >5 mm and inguinal >15 mm)
Adenitis is inflammation of lymph node, usually caused by *Staphylococcus* or *Streptococcus*
Cat scratch fever will also cause enlarged lymph nodes
Enlarged lymph nodes are common with viral infections in **children**
Systemic illnesses such as mononucleosis, acquired immunodeficiency syndrome, or Kawasaki disease can cause generalized lymphadenopathy (LA)

Incidence

The annual incidence of LA is 0.5% in the primary care setting
Children frequently have palpable, firm, freely movable and nontender lymph nodes (referred to as "shotty" lymph nodes)

Pathophysiology

Lymph tissue serves to provide an appropriate environment for maturation of lymphoid cells, to provide a filtration system for antigens, and to act as the center of both humoral and cellular immunity. Lymph nodes serve as secondary lymphoid organs, providing filtration of antigens and presented to lymphocytes as part of the immune response. There are more than 500 lymph nodes in the body, ranging in size from less than 1 mm to 2 cm in diameter. Lymph node enlargement confined to one lymph node group or involving contiguous regions is termed regional LA. Generalized LA refers to enlargement of at least two or more noncontiguous lymph node groups.

LA is a symptom. Enlargement of lymph nodes may be broadly classified into infectious, neoplastic, inflammatory, and miscellaneous. The extent of the response and enlargement depends on the nature, virulence, and degree of stimulus; the ability of the host to react; and the site of entry.

Factors that Increase Risk

Autoimmune disease
Immunodeficiency

SUBJECTIVE DATA

History of Present Illness

When was lymph node enlargement noted?
Is it recurrent?
Are lymph nodes painless or tender?
Have the lymph nodes changed in size over time?

Past Medical History

Ask about recent infections, illnesses, or trauma, which may cause enlarged lymph nodes
Ask about exposure to someone who has been ill
Recent dental work
Ask about unusual exposure to animals (toxoplasmosis, cat scratch fever, rat bite fever, anthrax, erysipeloid and

ticks), ingestion of unpasteurized milk or travel to exotic lands such as Third World countries, China, South America

History of blood product use or transfusion

Ask about high risk factors for human immunodeficiency virus:

- Gays/bisexuals or their partners
- Intravenous drug abusers or their partners
- History of frequent sexually transmitted diseases
- Multiple partners
- Prostitutes
- Newborns of infected women
- Those receiving blood transfusions

Medications

Anticonvulsants (especially phenytoin and mephenytoin) can cause LA

Medication associated with systemic allergic response (skin rash, fever, hepatosplenomegaly and eosinophilia)

Family History

Ask about family history of lymphoma or other malignancies

Ask about autoimmune diseases

Psychosocial History

Risk:

- Veterinarians
- Laboratory workers
- Farmers
- Fishermen
- Butchers
- Exposure to silicone

Associated Symptoms

Ask about systemic symptoms:

- Night sweats
- Pruritus, generalized or local
- Weight loss
- Anorexia
- Fever
- Fatigue
- Arthralgias
- Morning stiffness
- Malaise
- Dry eyes
- Dry mouth
- Skin rash
- Sore throat
- Cough
- Pain involved in lymph node after alcohol

OBJECTIVE DATA

Physical Examination

Because there is wide range of causes of LA and the systemic nature of the diseases associated with it, a complete physical will be needed.

- Vital signs/general appearance
- Skin: Rash (syphilis, childhood exanthems, systemic lupus erythematosus, sarcoidosis)
- Head, eyes, ears, nose, and throat:
  - Exophthalmos, thyroid enlargement, hairy leukoplakia or candidiasis, petechial eruption at the junction of the soft and hard palate
- Lymph: Usually only consider nodes in three regions:
  - Cervicofacial
  - Axillary
  - Inguinal
  - Use the three middle fingers to inspect and palpate the lymph node characteristics on both sides of the body:
    - Location
    - Size, in centimeters
    - Tenderness or other inflammatory signs present: Erythema, warmth
    - Degree of fixation
    - Texture: Hard, soft or firm
- It is particularly important not to miss supraclavicular nodes. It may be necessary to have the patient perform the Valsalva maneuver to make these nodes more easily palpable.
- Cardiovascular: Heart murmur or symptoms of subacute bacterial endocarditis
- Abdominal: Check for hepatosplenomegaly
- Joints: Evidence of arthritis
- Any lymph node >1 cm is considered to be enlarged, although in the supraclavicular area a palpable lymph node that is less than 1 cm is often a significant finding.

Diagnostic Procedures

Diagnostic procedures include those found in Table 112-1.

ASSESSMENT

Differential diagnoses include those found in Tables 112-2 to 112-4 and Fig. 112-1.

THERAPEUTIC PLAN

Pharmaceutical

Dependent on cause of LA

Lifestyle/Activities

Dependent on cause of LA

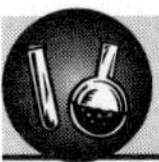

Table 112-1 Diagnostic Tests: Lymphadenopathy

Diagnostic Test	Findings/Rationale	Cost ($)
CBC, peripheral smear, ESR	Give clues to lymphocytosis seen in EBV, CMV, or other infection; anemia of chronic disease; or ↑ ESR seen in systemic illness	18-23/CBC; 54-68/smear; 16-18/ESR
Blood chemistry	↑ Liver enzymes seen in EBV, CMV, toxoplasmosis, or leptospirosis	32-42/metabolic panel
Throat culture, monospot, PPD, HIV, VDRL, rheumatoid factor, ACE level, ANA	May be helpful, depending on history and physical examination and above initial laboratory work-up	24-30
Blood cultures and serology for EBV, CMV, toxoplasmosis, leptospirosis, brucellosis	May be needed in special circumstances	37-45
CXR or CT	Used to determine the extent of the LA involving the central groups rather than to evaluate its etiology; mediastinal LA in young people is suggestive for malignancy; in sarcoidosis bilateral hilar adenopathy may be found; calcification of lymph nodes on CXR implies TB or histoplasmosis; abdominal CT is the preferred method for retroperitoneal LA	77-91/CXR; 947-1126/CT
Lymphangiography	More specific for neoplastic disease	1255-1504
Lymph node biopsy	Usually necessary to diagnose serious disease; excisional lymph node biopsy is the gold standard	416-494

ACE, Angiotensin-converting enzyme; *ANA,* antinuclear antibody; *CBC,* complete blood count; *CMV,* cytomegalovirus; *CT,* computed tomography; *CXR,* chest x-ray; *EBV,* Epstein-Barr virus; *ESR,* erythrocyte sedimentation rate; *HIV,* human immunodeficiency virus; *PPD,* purified protein derivative; *TB,* tuberculosis; *VDRL,* Venereal Disease Research Laboratories.

Table 112-2 Differential Diagnosis: Lymphadenopathy

Diagnoses	Supporting Data
Lymphoma (Ch. 113)	Firm rubbery, irregular, hard nodes; some tenderness may be seen in Hodgkin's with firmer nodes than non-Hodgkin's lymphoma
Mononucleosis (Ch. 119)	Sore throat, fever, dysphagia, lymphadenopathy, especially posterior cervical, anorexia, headache, abdominal pain; 50% or more lymphocytes and 10% or more atypical lymphocytes, positive monospot
HIV/AIDS (Ch. 94)	Fatigue, malaise, fevers without cause, night sweats, swollen or painful lymph nodes, weight loss, anorexia, cough, shortness of breath, thrush, skin rashes
Sarcoidosis	Malaise, fever, or bilateral hilar and paratracheal lymphadenopathy on chest x-ray
Lymphadenitis	Tender lymph node, overlying erythema, with or without being fluctuant; the involved node is superinfected; most common pathogens: *Staphylococcus pyogenes* and *S. aureus;* treat with first-generation cephalosporin or an antistaphylococcal penicillin and warm soaks
Cat scratch disease (reactive lymph node)	History of scratch by cat at involved area, primary lesion; infected, scabbed ulcer or papule, with symptoms of generalized infection 3 weeks later (fever, malaise, headache) and tender, enlarged regional lymph nodes; organism: *Bartonella henselae,* a gram-negative rod; disease is self-limiting, although the node may remain enlarged for several months

TABLE 112-3 Differential Diagnosis Based on Lymph Node Involvement

Diagnostic Assessment	Area	Supporting Data
Head and neck	Occipital nodes	Drain the scalp and back of the head. They ↑ in response to lice, ringworm, folliculitis.
	Preauricular nodes	Drain anterior pinnae, external auditory meatus, temporal scalp, lateral eyelids, and palpebral conjunctivae. They ↑ in response to squamous cell carcinoma, erysipelas, herpes zoster, conjunctival infections.
	Postauricular nodes	Drain external auditory meatus, posterior pinnae, temporal scalp. They ↑ in size with external otitis, scalp conditions, rubella.
	Submental, submandibular	Drain the medial angle of the eye, tongue, lips, and cheeks. They ↑ with dental infections, oral cancer, oral lesions.
	Superior deep cervical nodes	Drain palatine tonsils and tongue. ↑ Seen with pharyngeal or tonsillar infections.
	Inferior deep cervical nodes	Drainage from nodes of entire head and neck, along with some from arm and thorax. Because of their wide drainage, infectious and neoplastic processes must be considered when enlargement of these nodes is seen.
	Supraclavicular	Receive some drainage from abdominal organs, so if increase is seen (usually on left), abdominal neoplasia should be suspected.
	Superficial cervical nodes	Drain from pinnae of ear and the parotid gland. Any disorder involving these organs will cause nodes to enlarge. These nodes are also involved in lymphoma.
Axillary	Anterior nodes	Drain the mammary glands and the anterior chest
	Posterior nodes	Posterior chest and upper extremity
	Lateral nodes	Drain the upper extremity
	Central and apical	Receive drainage from other axillary nodes
		Consider upper extremity lesions and breast cancer
Epitrochlear	Drainage from the ulnar ½ of hand	Enlargement seen with many infectious diseases
Inguinal	Superficial Chain: Drains upper abdominal wall, genital area, gluteal, and the medial lower extremity; deep chain: Drains posterior and lateral foot, popliteal nodes, the superficial inguinal nodes.	Enlargement is seen with extremity lesions, and sexually transmitted diseases.
Generalized	Higher incidence of generalized LA is seen in **children** and **teens** due to the increased amount and greater responsiveness; thus LA is less likely to represent serious disease.	

TABLE 112-4 Differential Diagnosis by System

Symptoms	Diagnoses to Consider
LA, with prolonged fever, conjunctivitis, mucous membrane erythema and rash	Kawasaki disease
Rash + LA	Measles, varicella, or rubella
Exudative pharyngitis + LA	EBV, CMV, adenovirus, or *S. pyogenes*
Hepatosplenomegaly	EBV, CMV, HIV, or malignant neoplasm

CMV, Cytomegalovirus; *EBV,* Epstein-Barr virus; *HIV,* human immunodeficiency virus.

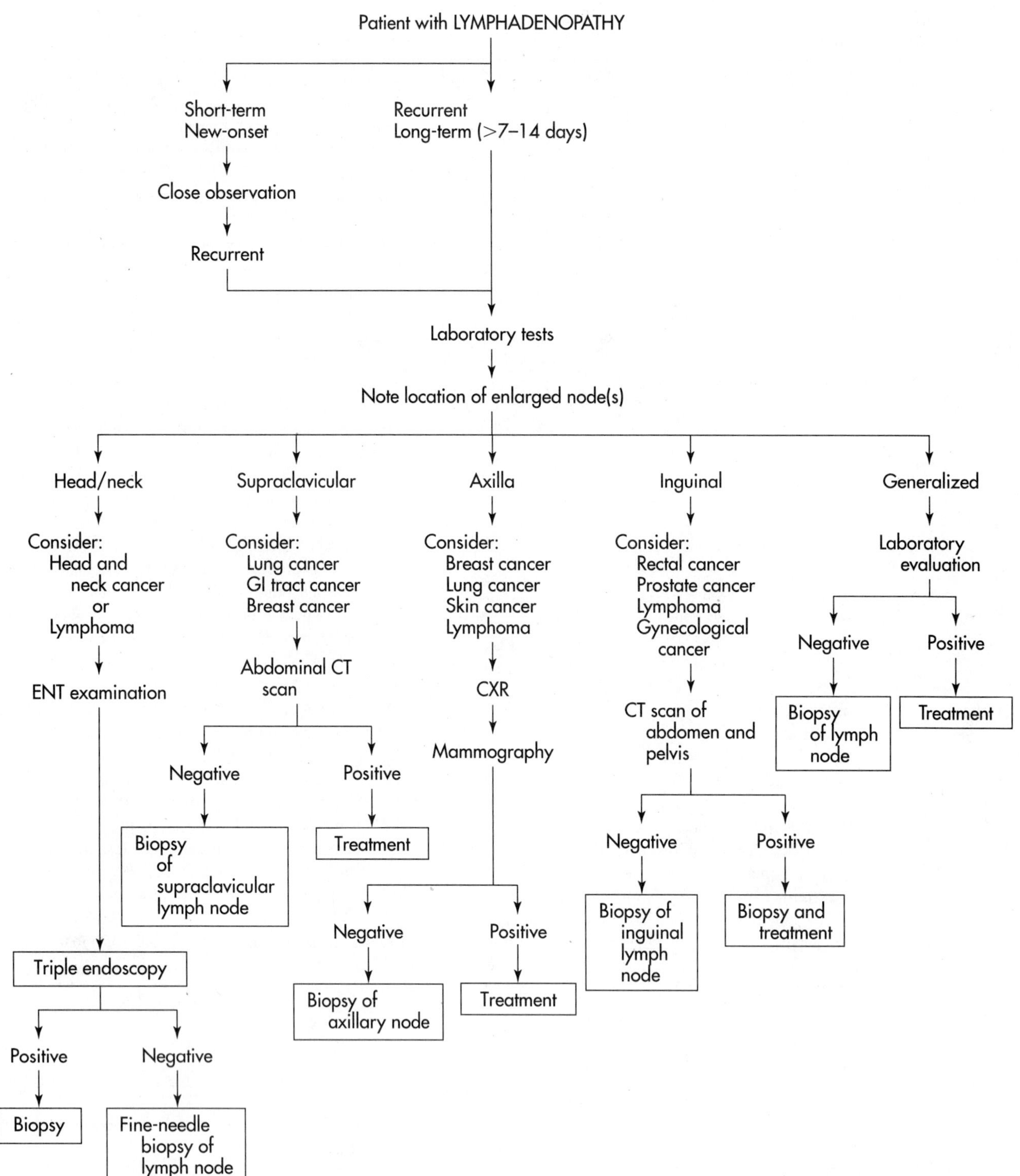

Figure 112-1 Algorithm for patient with lymphadenopathy. *CT,* Computed tomography; *CXR,* chest x-ray; *ENT;* ear, nose, and throat; *GI,* gastrointestinal. (Adapted from Greene HL, Johnson WP, Lemcke D: *Decision making in medicine*, ed 2, St Louis, 1998, Mosby.)

Diet

Not applicable

Patient Education

Explain how and why lymph nodes work
Explain how in **children** lymph nodes are easily felt and even seen
Describe the watchful waiting period of an enlarged lymph node in **children** and **teens**, and why more aggressive follow-up is needed for adults

Referral/Consultation

Refer anyone in whom diagnosis is unclear or if aggressive follow-up is needed to general surgeon for lymph node biopsy.

Follow-up

In **young children and teens,** it is reasonable to observe a lymph node for 1 to 4 weeks, measuring the lymph node carefully. Lymph node biopsy should be considered if the node has:

- Increased in size after 2 weeks
- Remained the same for 4 to 6 weeks
- Is persistently abnormal for 8 to 12 weeks

Risk factors for more serious disease in **children and teens** include:

- Abnormal chest x-ray
- Lymph node enlargement >2 cm
- Night sweats
- Weight loss
- Anemia
- Presence of supraclavicular nodes
- Fixed and matted nodes

Risk factors for **adults** include:

Work-up similar to above, except risk of serious disease is more likely.
Risk factors for serious disease in adults are:

- Age >40
- Weight loss
- Presence of supraclavicular LA

EVALUATION

Resolution of the lymph node or referral for biopsy

SUGGESTED READINGS

Getz M, Graziano F: Lymphadenopathy. In Taylor R, editor: *Difficult diagnosis 2*, Philadelphia, 1992, WB Saunders.

Gonzalalez-Osete G, Modiano M: Lymphadenopathy. In Greene H, Johnson W, Lemcke D, editors: *Decision making in medicine*, ed 2, St Louis, 1998, Mosby.

Healthcare Consultants of America, Inc.: *1998 Physicians fee and coding guide*, Augusta, Ga., 1998, Healthcare Consultants of America, Inc.

LaRow J, Wehbe P, Pasual A: Cat scratch disease in a child with unique MRI findings, *Arch Pediatr Adolesc Med* 152(4):394-396, 1997.

Schwartz S, Fried W: Case 6. In Grodin C, Schwartz S, Bone R, editors: *Diagnostic strategies for internal medicine*, St Louis, 1996, Mosby.

113 Lymphoma

ICD-9-CM

Lymphoma 202
Hodgkin's Lymphoma 201.9

OVERVIEW

Definition

Lymphoma is a malignant disease of the lymphoid tissue that can be classified as Hodgkin's or non-Hodgkin's lymphoma. It is usually a painless, unilateral, enlarging, firm, neck mass (70% present in neck), in upper third of neck.

Non-Hodgkin's lymphoma is a malignant disease of the lymphoid tissue with no Reed-Sternberg cells present.

Incidence

Hodgkin's lymphoma: 3.5/100,000; approximately 7500 per year in the United States; males more than females; bimodal distribution: one peak between **ages 20 and 29,** and a second one **over age 50;** non-Hodgkin's lymphoma has an incidence of 9/100,000

Children

- 0 to 6 years: One of top four malignancies
- 6 to 12 years: Hodgkin's one of top two malignancies
- >12 years: Hodgkin's most frequent malignancy of head/neck

Pathophysiology

Malignant transformation of an uncertain progenitor cell to the Reed-Sternberg cell; disease spreads to lymphoid tissue and eventually to nonlymphoid tissue; in Hodgkin's the spread is usually to contiguous areas of lymph nodes, with vascular invasion late in the course of the disease

Risk Factors

Autoimmune disease
Immunodeficiency
Onset <1 month of age

SUBJECTIVE DATA

History of Present Illness

Painless, enlarged lymph nodes

Past Medical History

Ask about:

- Recent infections that may cause enlarged lymph nodes or exposure to someone who is ill
- Unusual exposure to animals, ingestion of unpasteurized milk, travel to exotic lands such as Third World countries, China, and South America
- History of blood product usage
- High risk factors for human immunodeficiency virus

Medications

None significant

Family History

Ask about family history of lymphoma or other malignancies.

Associated Symptoms

Fever
Night sweats
Weight loss
Fatigue
Anorexia
Generalized pruritus (Hodgkin's)
Pain in involved node after alcohol ingestion (Hodgkin's)

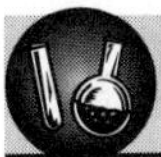

TABLE 113-1 Diagnostic Procedures: Lymphoma

Test	Findings	Cost ($)
CBC with diff	Usually normal, but may see a leukemic phase	18-23
Chemistry: liver, renal function tests	LDH helpful in evaluating the extent of the disease and aggressiveness of the tumor; increased LDH indicates more widespread disease	32-42/ metabolic panel
ESR	May indicate an inflammatory process	16-20
CXR	May show a mediastinal mass in lymphoblastic lymphoma	77-91
CT or MRI scan of abdomen and pelvis	Assists with staging	807-956/CT: Ab; 892-1160/pelvis; 1515-1790/MRI: ab; 1560-1840/pelvis
Lymph node biopsy	Hodgkin's: Reed-Sternberg cells; supraclavicular nodes usually have the highest yield	416-494/ superficial biopsy
Lumbar puncture	Indicated in high-risk morphology for non-Hodgkin's lymphoma	174-208
Lymphangiogram	More specific for neoplastic disease; can detect abnormal lymph architecture even before the nodes are enlarged	1255-1504
Bone marrow biopsy	Usually necessary to diagnose serious disease	401-499

CBC, Complete blood count; *CT,* computed tomography; *CXR,* chest x-ray; *ESR,* erythrocyte sedimentation rate; *LDH,* lactate dehydrogenase; *MRI,* magnetic resonance imaging.

TABLE 113-2 Differential Diagnosis: Lymphoma

Diagnoses	Supporting Data
Mononucleosis	Sore throat, fever, dysphagia, lymphadenopathy, especially posterior cervical, anorexia, headache, abdominal pain
Acquired immunodeficiency syndrome	Fatigue, malaise, fevers without cause, night sweats, swollen or painful lymph nodes, weight loss, anorexia, cough, shortness of breath, thrush, skin rashes
Sarcoidosis	Malaise, fever, or bilateral hilar and paratracheal lymphadenopathy on CXR
Cat scratch disease (reactive lymph node)	History of scratch by cat at involved area; primary lesion: infected, scabbed ulcer or papule, with symptoms of generalized infection 3 weeks later (fever, malaise, headache) and tender, enlarged regional lymph nodes

OBJECTIVE DATA

Physical Examination

A problem-oriented physical examination should be conducted, with particular attention to:

Vital signs and weight, general appearance, growth parameters in children

Lymph: Check neck, axilla, groin for enlarged nodes; evaluate for size, shape, consistency, location, fixation, and duration/rate of change (See Chapter 112 for more details about enlarged lymph nodes.)

Abdomen: Liver/spleen enlargement

Diagnostic Procedures

Diagnostic procedures include those found in Table 113-1.

ASSESSMENT

Differential diagnoses include other lymphomas, mononucleosis, sarcoidosis, acquired immunodeficiency syndrome, autoimmune disease, and cat scratch disease (Tables 113-2 and 113-3).

See Figure 112-1.

THERAPEUTIC PLAN

Indolent non-Hodgkin's lymphomas are usually not curable and are treated with palliative therapy. Patients with intermediate or high-grade lymphomas are treated with curative intent, usually with combination chemotherapy.

Hodgkin's disease: Patients with localized disease are treated with radiation therapy. Patients with disseminated disease are treated with aggressive combination chemotherapy.

TABLE 113-3 Staging

Hodgkin's	Survival Rate
Stage I: Single node group	90% 5 years
Stage II: Two or more groups on same side of diaphragm	90% 5 years
Stage III: Node groups on both sides of diaphragm	75% 10 years
Stage IV: Dissemination involving nonlymphatic organs	66% 10 years
Subclassification A: asymptomatic B: symptomatic	Better prognosis

Pharmaceutical

Combination chemotherapy

Nonpharmaceutical

Subtotal or total nodal irradiation

Patient Education

Effect of therapy on gonads; consider sperm banking
Risk of secondary malignancies

Referral

All patients should be referred to a surgeon for excisional biopsy, and if malignant to an oncologist.

RESOURCES

Lymphoma Research Foundation, Canada
www.lymphoma.ca/

Oncolink
www.oncolink.com

National Cancer Institute
Cancer Net, 1-800-422-6237
www.graylab.ac.uk/cancerweb not well

SUGGESTED READINGS

Barker L, Burton J, Zieve P: *Principles of ambulatory medicine*, ed 4, Baltimore, 1995, Williams & Wilkins.

Dershewitz R: *Ambulatory pediatric care*, Philadelphia, 1993, JB Lippincott.

Healthcare Consultants of America, Inc.: *1998 physicians fee and coding guide*, Augusta, Ga., 1998, Healthcare Consultants of America, Inc.

Ramsey P, Larson E: *Medical therapeutics*, ed 2, Philadelphia, 1993, WB Saunders.

Linker C: Blood. In Tierney L, McPhee S, Papadakis M, editors: *Current medical diagnosis and treatment*, ed 37, Stamford, Conn, 1998, Appleton & Lange.

Schwartz A: Patterns of exercise and fatigue on physical activities of cancer survivors, *Oncol Nurs Forum* 25(3):485-491, 1997.

Warmkessel J: Caring for patients with non-Hodgkin's lymphoma, *Nursing* 27(6):48-49, 1997.

114 Meniere's Disease

ICD-9-CM

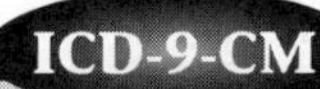

Meniere's Disease 386.0

OVERVIEW

Definition

Meniere's disease (MD) is an idiopathic disease characterized by hearing loss, tinnitus, and episodic vertigo. The hearing loss is fluctuating, usually low frequency, sensorineural, and associated with tinnitus. The vertigo is a spontaneously occurring sensation of movement that is accompanied by unsteadiness and lasts from minutes to hours, frequently accompanied by nausea and vomiting (Slattery and Fayad, 1997).

Incidence

It primarily affects Caucasians, with a prevalence of approximately 1/1000 of population. The disease occurs in **children,** but the peak onset is between **20 and 50** years of age. 85% of people have only one ear affected.

Pathophysiology

The principal underlying pathology is endolymphatic hydrops. There are a number of theories regarding the development of MD; it is probably a multifactorial process. The factors include:

Structural abnormalities of the temporal bone

Immunological: Immune complex deposition has been found in the endolymphatic sac

Viral: Possible role of neurotropic viruses

Vascular: Association between migraines and MD suggests a vascular pathogenesis

Metabolic: Exposure of the hair cells with chronic loss of hair cell motility

SUBJECTIVE DATA

History of Present Illness

One of the early symptoms is vertigo. This is usually described as a sensation of motion when there is no motion or an exaggerated sense of motion in response to a bodily movement associated with nausea and vomiting. The episode is often preceded by an aura of fullness or pressure in the ear lasting from 20 minutes to several hours. Between attacks the hearing is normal.

Hearing loss fluctuates and is finally lost, affecting lower pitches first.

Patients may present with complaints of difficulty hearing, or family members may identify an inability of the patient to hear.

Complains of nausea and vomiting, tinnitus

Loss of ability to "pop" ears

Sense of fullness in ears

Pulling at ears

Loss of equilibrium

May complain of foreign body in the ear

Ask about involvement of one ear or both

Was the onset gradual or sudden?

Has the hearing fluctuated since the hearing loss began?

Are there associated symptoms of tinnitus, vertigo, otalgia, otorrhea, or facial weakness?

Past Medical History

Ask about:

- Hypertension
- Mumps
- Neurological problems
- Head trauma
- Diabetes

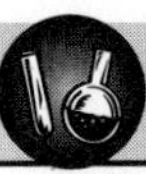

TABLE 114-1 Diagnostic Procedures: Meniere's Disease

Diagnostic Test	Finding/Rationale	Cost ($)
Rapid plasma reagin	Should be done to rule out syphilis, a known cause of Meniere's disease.	18-22
Audiometric studies	Hearing test conducted in soundproof room. Pure-tone thresholds in decibels (dB) are obtained over the ranges of 250-8000 Hz for both air and bone conduction. All patients with hearing loss should be referred for audiometric testing unless the cause is easily remedied (impacted cerumen). Patients can be referred directly to an audiologist. The location of an accredited audiologist can be obtained by calling the American Speech-Language Association at 1-800-638-8255.	119-159 (comprehensive examination)
Speech discrimination testing	Evaluates the clarity of hearing. Results are reported as percentage correct.	88-104
Tympanogram	Used to detect fluid in the middle ear and to determine the mobility of the tympanic membrane (TM). An electro-acoustic device is used to measure the compliance of the TM. Results are displayed in a graphic form. It is most reliable in children >6 mos.	31-37
Audiogram	Small hand-held auriscopes can provide a rough indication of hearing impairment. Usually four pure tones are emitted in sequence. This test can be affected by background noise, so the examination room must be quiet.	24-29
Glycerol dehydration test	Measures the audiometric response to an oral dose of glycerol. Improvement in scores for hearing low-frequency and discriminating speech is diagnostic as there is no other condition in which this change is observed.	Not available
Caloric testing	Reveals loss or impairment of nystagmus induced with cold substance in involved ear.	38-45 each ear
Electrocochleography	Presents with a highly characteristic waveform of MD, although the results may be negative in the early and late stages of the disease.	141-169
Electronystagmography	Objective recording of the nystagmus induced by head and body movements. It helps to quantify the degree of vestibular dysfunction.	142-171

Hypothyroidism
Syphilis
Migraine

Medications

Ask about use of:
- Aspirin (high dose)
- Antibiotics: Aminoglycosides (gentamicin, streptomycin)
- Diuretics (loop-furosemide)
- Quinine

Family History

Ask about a family history of hearing loss.
Ask about a familial disposition to Meniere's disease.

Psychosocial History

Ask about occupation: exposure to loud noises, use of protective measures, ear plug.
Ask about exposure to other sources of noise, loud music.

OBJECTIVE DATA

Physical Examination

The examination should concentrate on the head and neck.

- Head, eyes, ears, nose, and throat: Evaluate for an upper respiratory infection
- Ear: Evaluate tympanic membrane (TM), external canal
  - Complete pneumatic otoscopy; check for TM movement
  - Tympanogram
- Neurological: Check sensation of face, note if facial movement is symmetrical, random alternating movements
  - Do Romberg test
  - Evaluate gait
  - Check for nystagmus: Nylen-Barany maneuver (limited use when the patient is able to visually fixate)
  - Fukuda test (patient walks in place with eyes closed) can detect subtle defects; a + response is when the patient rotates toward the diseased labyrinth

Table 114-2 Differential Diagnosis: Meniere's Disease

Diagnosis	Supporting Data
Conductive loss	Rinne shows air conduction <bone conduction; Weber lateralizes to the involved ear; the whisper will be abnormal if >40 dB loss is present
Cerumen impaction	Occlusion of the external ear canal by cerumen; usually self-induced via attempts at cleaning
Serous otitis media	Dull tympanic membrane (TM), hypomobile TM; air bubbles may be seen in the middle ear, with a conductive hearing loss present
Acoustic neuroma	Hearing loss, vertigo, nausea and vomiting, deterioration of speech discrimination
Otosclerosis	Progressive disease with a familial tendency that affects bone surrounding the inner ear
TM perforation	Perforation of the TM may result in decreased hearing abilities; the perforation may occur from trauma or as the result of increased pressure with otitis media; spontaneous healing occurs in the majority of cases
Sensory-neural loss	Rinne, both AC and BC are decreased; Weber localizes to the uninvolved ear; the whisper test will be abnormal if >40 dB loss is present
Presbycusis	Progressive, mainly high-frequency hearing loss of aging; frequently with genetic predisposition; patients complain of an inability to hear well (speech discrimination) in a noisy environment
Noise trauma	Second most common cause of hearing loss; sounds >85 dB are potentially damaging to the cochlea, especially with prolonged exposure; the loss typically occurs in the high frequencies (4000 Hz) and progresses to involve sounds in the normal speech frequencies; sounds that have the potential for damage: industrial machinery, loud music, and weapons
Ototoxicity	Hearing loss can be caused by substances that affect both the auditory and vestibular systems; common causes: salicylates, aminoglycosides, loop diuretics and antineoplastic agents, especially cisplatin

Hearing: Have patient repeat aloud words presented in a soft whisper, normal speaking voice, or shout. Have the opposite ear occluded, then repeat on other side.
Children: Expected hearing findings by age:
- 0-3 mos: response to noise
- 3-5 mos: child turns to sound
- 6-10 mos: child responds to name
- 10-15 mos: child imitates simple words

Weber: Place the tuning fork on the forehead or front teeth. Have the patient indicate where it is heard the best.

Rinne: The tuning fork is placed alternately on the mastoid bone and in front of the ear canal.

Diagnostic Procedures

Diagnostic procedures include those outlined in Table 114-1.

ASSESSMENT

Differential diagnoses include those found in Table 114-2. Hearing loss classifications and categories are listed in Tables 114-3 and 114-4.

Table 114-3 Classification of Hearing Test and Types of Hearing Loss

Classification	Rinne	Weber
Normal: both ears	AC > BC	Midline
Conductive loss	Rt ear: BC > AC	Lateralized to right ear
Right ear	Lt. Ear AC > BC	
Left ear	Rt. Ear: AC > BC	Lateralized to left ear
	Lt. Ear: BC > AC	
Both ears	Rt. Ear: BC > AC	Lateralized to poorer ear of the two
	Lt. Ear: BC > AC	
Sensorineural loss	AC > BC both ears	Lateralized to left ear
Right ear		
Left ear	AC > BC both ears	Lateralized to right ear
Both ears	AC > BC both ears	Lateralized to better ear

AC, Air conduction; *BC*, bone conduction.

TABLE 114-4 Categories of Hearing Loss

Category of Hearing Loss	dB level
Mild hearing loss	26-40 dB
Moderate hearing loss	41-55 dB
Moderately severe hearing loss	56-70 dB
Severe hearing loss	71-90 dB
Profound hearing loss	>91 dB

THERAPEUTIC PLAN

Treatment is currently empirical. No treatment has modified the clinical course and prevented the progressive hearing loss.

The vertigo eventually disappears in about 70% of patients. Nonsurgical treatment is considered effective in about 80% of patients.

Pharmaceutical

Acute attack: Aim is to sedate the vestibulo-brain stem, use only for 2 weeks and gradually wean (Table 114-5).

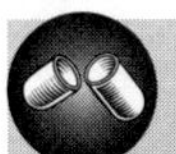

TABLE 114-5 Pharmaceutical Plan: Acute Attacks

Drug	Dose	Comments	Cost
Prochlorperazine (Compazine)	5-10 mg 3-4×/d or 15-30 mg spansule q AM or 10 mg spansule q12h (sustained release)	Considered antidopaminergic agent Pregnancy: C SE: Drowsiness, lowered seizure threshold, amenorrhea, photosensitivity, extrapyramidal reactions	$34-$60/5 mg (100); $52-$89/10 mg (100); $25/supp: 2.5 mg (12); $28/5 mg (12)
Promethazine (Phenergan)	25 mg PO q6h Children: 12.5-25 mg Supp: 12.5, 25, 50 mg	Antihistamine, anticholinergic Pregnancy: C SE: Sedation, sleepiness, dry mouth, lowered seizure threshold	$7-$18/12.5 mg (100); $3-$33/25 mg (100)
Diazepam (Valium)	2-5 mg PO TID/QID	Vestibular suppressant; recommended as drug of choice for acute vertigo; many people with vertigo, particularly elderly, respond well to decreased dose and frequency. Pregnancy: D SE: Dizziness, drowsiness, dry mouth, orthostatic hypotension	$2-$66/5 (100); $2-$109/10 mg (100)
Glycopyrrolate (Robinul)	1-2 mg PO QD/BID	Anticholinergic when combined with diazepam is very helpful in controlling inner ear symptoms of nausea and vomiting Pregnancy: B SE: Dry mouth, distorted visual acuity, or increase symptoms of BPH. Contraindications: Glaucoma, symptomatic BPH	$18/1 mg (100); $28/2 mg (100)
Dimenhydrinate (Dramamine)	50-100 mg TID/QID	Recommended for refractory cases Pregnancy: B SE: Drowsiness, blurring of vision, dry mouth, constipation	$2-$6/50 mg (100); $4/liq: 12.5 mg/4 ml (120 ml)
Meclizine (Antivert)	25 mg PO TID QID	Used for vertigo; slower onset and longer duration of action than most other antihistamines; recommended for refractory cases Pregnancy: B SE: Drowsiness, fatigue, dry mouth, blurred vision	$3-$49/25 mg (100)

BPH, Benign prostatic hypertrophy; *SE,* side effects.

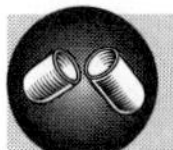

TABLE 114-6 Pharmaceutical Plan: Maintenance

Drug	Dose	Comments	Cost
Furosemide (Lasix)	20-80 mg QD	K supplementation will be needed Pregnancy: C SE: GI upset, electrolyte imbalance, rash, photosensitivity	\$2-\$16/20 mg (100); \$3-\$22/40 mg (100); \$6-\$37/80 mg (100)
Amiloride (Midamor)	5 mg QD	K-sparing diuretic Pregnancy: B SE: Headache, gastrointestinal upset, hyperkalemia, muscle cramps, dizziness, impotence	\$26-\$46/5 mg (100)
Hydrochlorothiazide*	12.5-50 mg QD	K supplementation is usually needed Pregnancy: B SE: Electrolyte disorders, orthostatic hypotension, GI disturbances	\$2-\$13/25 mg (100); \$4-\$38/50 mg (100)
HCTZ and triamterene (Dyazide)*	1 tablet QD	Provides diuretic action with need for K supplementation Pregnancy: D (B according to manufacturer)	\$32-\$34/50 mg (100)
Betahistine (Serc)	8 mg TID	Clinical studies have revealed this histamine analogue helpful in improving hearing loss, vertigo, and tinnitus in the short term (not available in United States) Betahistine with or without diuretic is the recommended maintenance Be aware of future developments regarding this drug	Not available
Nimodipine (Nimotop)	30 mg BID	Used for patients who have failed diuretic therapy (use in refractory cases) Pregnancy: C SE: GI upset	\$526/30 mg (100)
Eriodictyol glycoside (lemon bioflavonoid extract)	2 mg capsule TID for a trial period of 6 months	May act as a blocking agent for histidine decarboxylase	Not available

GI, Gastrointestinal; *SE*, side effects.
*Preferred initial maintenance therapy.

Maintenance

Aim is to attempt to modify the endolymphatic hydrops itself by lowering endolymphatic pressure. Long-term maintenance therapy is usually not recommended due to the fluctuant nature of the disease. Maintenance therapy usually includes diet modifications combined with pharmacologic interventions (Table 114-6).

Ablative Therapy

Ablative therapy involves the use of aminoglycosides to control vertigo via vestibulotoxic effects. Partial ablation of the labyrinth is recommended to control the severity of ataxia and perhaps stabilize hearing. Administration of low doses of intramuscular streptomycin is the treatment of choice (1 g 5 days/week until ablation occurs). Ablation is demonstrated via absence of ice water caloric test. Ablation should be done by an ear, nose, and throat specialist.

Lifestyle/Activities

Bed rest may reduce the severity of vertigo in an acute attack. In chronic vertigo exercise is one of the most important therapies. It enhances the ability of the central nervous system to compensate for labyrinth dysfunction. The patient should begin body conditioning exercises after the nausea and vomiting has resolved and continue until vertigo occurs.

Specific exercises to promote adaptation of the vestibular system may be prescribed by the otolaryngologist.

Diet

Low-salt diet (<2 g sodium daily): A strict low-sodium diet with a daily allowance of 1500 mg of sodium/day is advised. A more practical approach of avoiding excessively salty foods and not adding table salt to foods is probably a more realistic expectation.

Restriction of caffeine, nicotine, and alcohol is also suggested.

Patient Education

Completely explain the disorder, indicating the expected course of the disease and medications.

Discuss the need to live with unpredictable illness.

Referral/Consultation

A variety of options for medical and surgical treatment are available if the patient is referred to an otolaryngologist. Medical options include intratympanic aminoglycosides to control vertigo. Surgical options include procedures that are not destructive to hearing: endolymphatic sac surgery (effective in approximately 80% to control vertigo), vestibular nerve section (effective in 90% to 95% to control vertigo; however, the surgery is major in that the posterior cranial fossa is opened), sacculotomy, cryosurgical treatment, and insertion of tympanostomy tubes. Other surgeries destroy any remaining hearing: labyrinthectomy, cochleosacculotomy, and vestibulocochlear neurectomy. Cochlear implantation is an option; end-stage Meniere's disease is a recognized indication for implantation.

Follow-up

Usually done by otolaryngologist

EVALUATION

Improvement in vertigo with preserved hearing ability is the goal.

Resources

The Meniere's Network: www.meniere2.htm

The Ear Foundation: www.theearfound.com

REFERENCE

Slattery W, Fayad J: Medical treatment of Meniere's disease, *Otolaryngol Clin North Am* 30(6):1027-1037, 1997.

SUGGESTED READINGS

Arts H, Kileny P, Telian S: Diagnostic testing for endolymphatic hydrops, *Otolaryngol Clin North Am* 30(6):987-1005, 1997.

Clendaniel R, Tucci D: Vestibular rehabilitation strategies in Meniere's disease, *Otolaryngol Clin North Am* 30(6):1145-1158, 1997.

Derebery M: The role of allergy in Meniere's disease, *Otolaryngol Clin North Am* 30(6):1007-1016, 1997.

Ellsworth AJ et al: *Mosby's 1998 medical drug reference*, St Louis, 1998, Mosby.

Gibson W, Arenberg I: Pathophysiologic theories in the etiology of Meniere's disease, *Otolaryngol Clin North Am* 30(6):961-967, 1997.

Grant I, Welling D: The treatment of hearing loss in Meniere's disease, *Otolaryngol Clin North Am* 30(6):1123-1144, 1997.

Healthcare Consultants of America, Inc: *1998 Physicians fee and coding guide*, Augusta, Ga., 1998, Healthcare Consultants of America, Inc.

Quaranta A, Marini F, Sallustio V: Long-term outcome of Meniere's disease: endolymphatic mastoid shunt versus natural history, *Audio Neurootolaryngol* 3(1):54-60, 1998.

Rodgers G, Telischi F: Meniere's disease in children, *Otolaryngol Clin North Am* 30(6):1101-1104, 1997.

Saeed S: Fortnightly review: diagnosis and treatment of Meniere's disease, *Br Med J* 316(7128):368-372, 1998.

Silverstein H et al: Dexamethasone inner ear perfusion for the treatment of Meniere's disease: a prospective, randomized, double-blind, crossover trial, *Am J Otolaryngol* 19(2):196-201, 1998.

115 Meningitis

ICD-9-CM

Bacterial Meningitis 320
Unspecified Viral Meningitis 047.9
Meningococcemia 036.2
Meningococcemia Meningitis 036.0

OVERVIEW

Definition

Meningitis is an inflammation of the meninges of the brain caused directly or indirectly by an infectious agent, either bacterial or viral.

Etiology and Incidence

Meningitis is usually the result of hematogenous spread of organisms secondary to an infection at another site (e.g., otitis media and pneumonia). It is less commonly caused by the direct introduction of pathogens following head trauma (e.g., paranasal sinus fracture) or neurosurgery. Meningitis occurs most often in the **very young** and **elderly** and/or debilitated persons.

Bacterial Meningitis

See Table 115-1 for the incidence and pathogens of meningitis.

Aseptic Meningitis

Nonbacterial meningitis is usually viral, accounts for two thirds of all central nervous system (CNS) infections, and is generally less severe than bacterial meningitis. Enteroviruses are the most common agent in **children under 1 year** and account for about 80% of aseptic meningitis at all ages. Other agents include fungi and spirochetes.

Pathophysiology

Organisms that have entered the meningeal space multiply and spread throughout the cerebral spinal fluid. Infection may also affect nearby cranial nerves or contribute to parenchyma abscesses. A fibrous exudate, which accompanies the inflammatory response, may impede cerebrospinal fluid (CSF) flow: accumulation can block the narrow Sylvian duct leading to the hydrocephalus. Inflammatory swelling may exert pressure on the hypopituitary gland, stimulating excess secretion of antidiuretic hormone and secondary cerebral edema. Bulging fontanels (infants) and nuchal rigidity and opisthotonus from meningeal irritation (older children and adults) may occur as disease progresses.

Factors that Increase Susceptibility

Individuals who:

- Have sickle cell anemia, diabetes, alcoholism
- Had a basilar skull fracture
- Have an indwelling CSF shunting device
- Are debilitated and/or institutionalized
- Have had contact with others who have meningitis

SUBJECTIVE DATA

History of Present Illness

Bacterial and aseptic meningitis present similarly—there is no reliable symptom that readily distinguishes one from the other.

TABLE 115-1 Bacterial Meningitis Incidence and Pathogens

	Neonates	Older Infants/ Children	Adults	Postsurgical/ Post-traumatic
Incidence	100 per 100,000 live births	90% before age 6 After 1 mo, 50 per 100,000 6-8 mos, 80 per 100,000	Extremely rare	
Pathogen	Group B *Streptococcus*, *Streptococcus pneumoniae*, gram-negative enteric	*Haemophilus influenzae B*,* *Neisseria meningitidis*, *S. pneumoniae*	*Listeria monocytogenes* *S. pneumoniae* *N. meningitidis*	*S. aureus*, gram-negative bacilli

*The introduction of the *H. influenzae B* vaccine has dramatically reduced the incidence of *H. influenzae* meningitis.

Neonates

Onset usually acute; hypothermia, hypotonia, weak or abnormal cry, apnea, and seizures

Young Infants

Onset is generally acute with nonspecific symptoms of temperature instability or hypothermia, irritability, lethargy, poor feeding, unusual cry, jitters, and/or hypotonia

Older Infants, Children, and Adults

Onset is usually acute, although it is sometimes subacute. A prodromal febrile illness rapidly progresses to vague complaints of irritability, listlessness, or general malaise; older children and adults may complain of photophobia, myalgia, headaches and stiff neck, and vomiting. Seizures may also occur.

Past Medical History

Inquire about:

Recent infections (especially ear and respiratory, or partially treated meningitis).

Facial or cranial injuries and/or surgery

Immunization status

Associated Symptoms

A diffuse macular, maculopapular, or purpuric rash may occur, depending on the type of infection. Abdominal pain and diarrhea may also be present if the offending agent is an enterovirus.

OBJECTIVE DATA

Physical Examination

Physical examination should focus on:

Vital signs: Temperature, heart rate, and blood pressure may help to identify septicemic shock.

General appearance: Pay particular note to mental status.

Skin: Inspect/palpate for presence of a rash, petechiae/ purpura (fever with purpura is associated with meningococcal infections, even though the patient may not appear acutely ill at the time).

Head: Inspect/palpate for bulging/enlarged fontanels in infants; a marked increase in head circumference may also be present.

Eyes: Inspect for papilledema (this is a late symptom and, if present early, usually indicates the presence of a space-occupying lesion).

Ear, nose, and throat: Inspect for sources of inflammation/infection, palpate for lymphadenopathy (oropharyngeal vesicles suggest enterovirus).

Cardiovascular: Assess capillary refill and peripheral pulses, and turgor.

Neurological: Assess cranial nerves, muscle strength/ tone, motor coordination and sensory status, reflexes, and meningeal irritation (Kernig and Brudzinski signs).

Kernig: When the patient is supine with hip and knee flexed toward abdomen, extension of knee elicits pain.

Brudzinski: When child is supine, passive flexion of the neck elicits flexion of the knees and hips.

Other: Symptoms of tachycardia, delayed capillary refill, hypotension, and oliguria may accompany septicemic shock.

Diagnostic Procedures

Diagnostic procedures include those in Table 115-2.

Cerebrospinal Fluid Analysis

CSF analysis is outlined in Table 115-3.

ASSESSMENT

Differential diagnoses: Other infectious processes may also present with fever, myalgia, headache, and general malaise (Reye's syndrome, CNS disturbances) (Table 115-4).

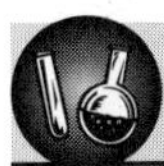

TABLE 115-2 Diagnostic Procedures: Meningitis

Diagnostic Test	Finding/Rationale	Cost ($)
CBC with differential count	Indicates the presence of infection by increased WBCs and shift to left	18-23
Cultures: blood and CSF	Should be obtained when meningitis is suspected. Results may be positive in up to 90% of *Haemophilus influenzae* and 80% of pneumococcal meningitis. Meningitis cannot be ruled out if cultures are negative. Aseptic meningitis should be considered. Antibiotic treatment of mother may influence the results in newborn.	37-45
Gram stain CSF	Provides invaluable information that aids in selecting antibiotic treatment.	15-19
Latex agglutination	Helpful in the setting of prior antibiotic therapy that may interfere with culture results.	N/A
CT/MRI	Rule out space-occupying lesions.	990-1175/CT 1781-2004/MRI
CXR	Rules out pneumonia as cause of sepsis.	77-91
Lumbar puncture (LP)	Although aseptic meningitis is generally benign and self-limiting, there is no reliable symptom that readily distinguishes it from bacterial. **(A lumbar puncture in the presence of a space-occupying lesion can cause brain stem herniation and should not be performed if papilledema is present.)** LP should be performed in any infant in which sepsis is suspected (goal is LP within 30 minutes and then begin empiric therapy).	174-208

CBC, Complete blood count; *CT,* computed tomography; *CXR,* chest x-ray; *MRI,* magnetic resonance imaging; *N/A,* not available.

TABLE 115-3 Cerebrospinal Fluid Analysis

	Neonate Normal	>1 mo Normal	Bacterial	Aseptic
Appearance	Clear	Clear	Turbid	Clear
White Blood Cells	<30	<10	>500	<500
Organisms	Absent	Absent	+ Gram stain	Negative Gram stain
Protein	<90 mg/dl	<40 mg/dl	>100 mg/dl	<100 mg/dl
Glucose	70-80 mg/dl	50-60 mg/dl	Elevated	Decreased

TABLE 115-4 Differential Diagnosis: Meningitis

Diagnosis	Supporting Data
Bacterial meningitis	Usually acutely ill, increased WBCs, low CSF glucose, increased CSF protein
Aseptic (viral) meningitis	Insidious onset, mildly elevated WBCs, low to normal glucose, normal to mildly elevated protein
Reye's syndrome	Irritability, fever, seizures, coma
CNS-occupying lesion: mass, infection	Headache, vision change, diplopia, nausea, tinnitus, lethargy, progressing to stupor as intracranial pressure increases

CNS, Central nervous system; *CSF,* cerebrospinal fluid; *WBC,* white blood cell.

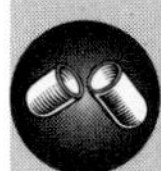

TABLE 115-5 Bacterial Pathogens in Meningitis and Empiric Therapy by Age Group*

Age Group	Likely Organisms	Empiric Therapy (Drug of Choice in Bold)
Neonate	Group B and D *Streptococcus, Escherichia coli,* and other Gram organisms, *Listeria monocytogenes*	Ampicillin + gentamicin *or* **ampicillin (50 mg/kg IV q8h) + cefotaxime (100 mg/kg q12h IV)**
1-3 mos	Group B *Streptococcus* (late onset), *Streptococcus pneumoniae,* and rarely, *L. monocytogenes*	Vancomycin with either **ampicillin + gentamicin** *or* **ampicillin** (50-100 mg/kg IV q8h) + **cefotaxime** (150 mg/kg IV q12h) or **ceftriaxone + dexamethasone** 0.4 mg/kg q12h × 2 days or 0.15 mg/kg q6h × 4 days; **first dose 15-20 min before first dose of antibiotic;** chloramphenicol, rancomycin, + dexamethosone is alternate therapy
3 mos-7 yr	*S. pneumoniae, H. influenza,* and *Neisseria meningitidis*	**Cefotaxime** (150 mg/kg IV q12h) or **ceftriaxone** (75 mg/kg initial dose, then 100 mg/kg/day q12h) (vancomycin is used for ceftriaxone-resistant *S. pneumoniae*) + dexamethasone first dose 15-20 min before first dose of antibiotic. 0.4 mg/kg q12h × 2 days or 0.15 mg/kg q6h × 4 days
7-50	*S. pneumoniae, N. meningitidis, Listeria,* and occasionally, *Haemophilus influenzae*	Cefotaxime (2 g q4h IV) or ceftriaxone (2 g q12h IV) + dexamethasone before first dose of antibiotic 0.4 mg q12h IV ×2 days + ampicillin 50 mg/kg q6h IV
>50	*S. pneumoniae* most common; rare *H. influenzae, Listeria, Pseudomonas aeruginosa, N. meningitidis*	Ampicillin 50 mg/kg q6h IV + cefotaxime or ceftriaxone + dexamethasone (doses as above)

*Empiric use of vancomycin must be customized, depending on the incidence of *S. pneumoniae* resistance to penicillin and cephalosporins in the community.

THERAPEUTIC PLAN

Immediate medical consultation/referral, hospitalization, and prompt initiation of broad-spectrum antibiotics are warranted. CSF analysis is preferred before the initiation of antibiotic therapy. However, there is a direct relationship between early treatment and positive outcomes in bacterial meningitis, and therapy should not be postponed for CSF analysis if the patient appears ill and/or is deteriorating rapidly.

Pharmaceutical

Antibiotic treatment is empiric based on the age of the patient, history, and the likely causative organisms (Table 115-5).

Lifestyle/Activities

Not applicable due to seriousness of illness

Diet

Not applicable

Patient Education

Discuss the seriousness of the illness and the need for aggressive/supportive care.

Discuss the availability of a vaccine that is effective for most strains of meningococcus. A single dose of 0.5 ml is given by SQ injection. The vaccine is helpful in controlling outbreaks in adults and children >2 but is poorly immunogenic in children <2. Unfortunately, this is the group most at risk for contracting the disease.

Family Impact

The Centers for Disease and Control and Prevention (CDC) recommends prophylactic antibiotics to patient's close contacts. Close contacts are defined as "those residing with the index case or spending 4 or more hours with the index case for 5 of 7 days before the onset of illness" (CDC, 1997). Those at risk for infection would then include household members, classmates, day care or preschool workers. The prophylaxis should be administered as soon as possible after the patient's diagnosis, preferably within 24 hours. The risk of contracting meningococcal disease is approximately 4/1000 for those who have had close contact

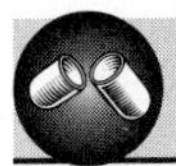

TABLE 115-6 Prophylactic Antibiotic Therapy

Drug	Dose	Comment	Cost
Rifampin (Rifadin, Rimactane)	Children <1 mo: 5 mg/kg q12h × 2 days Children >1 month: 10 mg/kg q12h × 2 days Adults: 600 mg q12h × 2 days	Pregnancy: C SE: Flu syndrome, headache, drowsiness, mental confusion, rash, pruritus; use backup method of contraception; body fluids may be colored orange and may discolor contacts, do not wear during treatment	$149/gel cap:150 mg (100); $161-$211/300 mg (100) Available as suspension
Ciprofloxacin (Cipro)	Adults: 500-mg dose	Pregnancy: C SE: Nausea, vomiting, and diarrhea; do not take within 2 hrs of antacids; multiple drug interactions; check reference before prescribing	$334/500 mg (100)
Ceftriaxone (Rocephin)	Children <15 yrs 125 mg IM Adult: 250 mg IM can be diluted in 2.1 ml of 1% lidocaine to reduce pain at injection site	Pregnancy: B Drug of choice during pregnancy SE: Pain at injection site, rash, urticaria, nausea, vomiting, and diarrhea	250 mg/vial $12

SE, Side effects.

with a known patient. This risk is minimized by prophylaxis (Table 115-6).

Referral/Consultation

Meningococcal disease is a medical emergency because of its rapid progression and poor outcomes. It is imperative to consult if you are suspicious of this disease. The goal in most Emergency Departments is to have the first dose of antibiotic given within an hour of arrival due to the seriousness of this illness. It may be appropriate to administer the initial dose of antibiotics without delay. *Do not postpone the patient's transfer to a tertiary setting to administer the medication.*

EVALUATION/FOLLOW-UP

Observe for neurological and developmental sequelae. Refer for multidisciplinary evaluation and treatment if necessary.

REFERENCE

Centers for Disease Control and Prevention: Control and prevention of meningococcal disease and control and prevention of serogroup C meningococcal disease: evaluation and management, *MMWR* 46(RR-5): 1-21, 1997.

SUGGESTED READINGS

American Academy of Pediatrics: Committee on Infectious Diseases: *The red book report of the committee on infectious diseases*, ed 23, New York, 1994, the Academy.

Booy R, Kroll J: Bacterial meningitis and meningococcal infection, *Curr Opin Pediatr* 10(1):13-18, 1998.

Ellsworth AJ et al: *Mosby's 1998 drug reference*, St Louis, 1998, Mosby.

Griffin DE: Central nervous system infections. In Stobo J et al, editors: *The principles and practice of medicine,* ed 23, Stamford, Conn., 1996, Appleton & Lange.

Hay W, et al: *Current pediatric diagnosis and treatment*, ed 13, Stamford, Conn., 1997, Appleton & Lange.

Healthcare Consultants of America, Inc.: *1998 Physicians fee and coding guide*, Augusta, Ga., 1998, Healthcare Consultants of America, Inc.

Herf C, et al: Meningococcal disease: recognition, treatment and prevention, *Nurse Pract* 23(8):30-46, 1998.

Lau A, et al: Infectious diseases. In Rudolph A, Kamei R, editors: *Rudolph's fundmentals of pediatrics*, ed 2, Stamford, Conn, 1998, Appleton & Lange.

McCrone E, Venna N, Bergethon P: Infections of the nervous system. In Noble J et al, editors: *Textbook of primary care medicine*, ed 2, St Louis, 1996, Mosby.

Meadow W, Lanton J: A proactive data based determination of the standard of care in pediatrics, *Pediatrics* 101(4Part I):E6, 1998.

Phillips C, Simor A: Bacterial meningitis in children and adults: changes in community acquired disease may affect patient care, *Postgrad Med* 103(3):102-104, 1998.

Powell K: Meningitis. In Hoekelman R et al, editors: *Primary pediatric care*, ed 3, St Louis, 1997, Mosby.

Schuckat A, et al: Bacterial meningitis in the U.S. in 1995, *N Engl J Med* 337(14):970-976, 1997.

Sommers M, Johnson S, editors: *Davis's manual of nursing therapeutics for diseases and disorders*, Philadelphia, 1997, FA Davis.

Menopause

ICD-9-CM

Premenopausal Menorrhagia 627.0
Menopausal or Female Climacteric States 627.2
State Associated with Artificial Menopause 627.4

OVERVIEW

Definition

Menopause is the permanent cessation of menstruation following the decline of ovarian estrogen production.

Perimenopause is the period extending from immediately before to after menopause (generally 45 to 55 years of age). For most women, the transition lasts approximately 4 years. This period is marked by altered ovarian function.

Incidence

Menopause that occurs in a woman less than 30 years of age is premature; between 30 and 40 is considered early (and autoimmune disorders should be ruled out). The average age of menopause is 51.4 years.

Physiology

The major source (90%) of estradiol before menopause is the ovarian follicle. General atresia of ovarian follicles begins at puberty, increasing after age 35, leading to a decline in ovarian production of estrogen and progesterone.

Estrogen normally participates in a negative feedback system; thus with decreased estrogen, gonadotropin hormones are no longer inhibited, so increased levels of FSH and LH are secreted. FSH and LH never return to premenopausal levels. Ovarian testosterone levels are maintained at or about the levels before menopause.

Surgical menopause occurs when the uterus is removed, which causes an abrupt end of menstruation and/or when ovaries are surgically removed, which brings about an abrupt end to both ovulation and menstruation.

SUBJECTIVE DATA

History

Ask date of last menstrual period (LMP). Was it normal for her (length, duration, flow)? Menses are often more frequent or less frequent, with either more than normal flow or less, and of longer or shorter duration. Menstrual flooding often occurs at the beginning of flow. Menses may also be irregular; skipping months at a time is common. Determine the length of time without a period.

She may also complain of:

- Hot flush (vasomotor reaction): Sensation of heat, mostly about head, neck, and upper torso, with increased skin temperature and arterial vasodilation
- Dyspareunia related to vaginal dryness
- Night sweats
- Dry skin or hair
- Joint stiffness

Ask about:

- Urinary changes; in particular question about incontinence, with cough, sneeze, laughing, sexual intercourse
- Headache
- Irritability
- Insomnia
- Depression
- Loss of sense of well being

Past Medical History

Gynecologic history: Surgery (including hysterectomy), endometriosis, infertility, last Pap smear, any breast problems, date of last mammogram, any sexually transmitted diseases

Obstetrical history: Pregnancies, abortions, stillbirths

Any history of fractures, deep vein thrombosis, history of breast cancer

Medications

Ask about:
- Contraceptive use past and present
- Any over-the-counter treatments to relieve symptoms, including herbal remedies and vitamins
- Douches
- Calcium

Family History

Age mother, siblings became menopausal
Any history of thyroid disorder, polycystic ovarian disease, diabetes, osteoporosis, Alzheimer's disease, obesity, mental illness, heart disease
Diethylstilbestrol exposure
Cancer: If positive for breast or ovarian cancers, at what age were they diagnosed?

Psychosocial History

Alterations in sleep pattern
Sexual history: Dysfunction, unresponsiveness, recent changes
Ask about:
- Fatigue, mood swings, irritability
- History of substance use/abuse: Alcohol, tobacco, drugs
- Physical activity, hobbies
- Abuse or family violence
- Marital status, work, family dynamics
- Diet history

OBJECTIVE DATA

Physical Examination

A complete physical examination is warranted:

- Vital signs, including blood pressure, pulse, temperature, height (baseline for osteoporosis assessment), and weight
- Head, Eyes, Ears, Nose, and Throat: Especially important with smokers, pay attention to oral cavity, condition of teeth and gums
- Neck: Assess thyroid, adenopathy
- Heart: Rate, rhythm, murmur, edema, peripheral pulses
- Lungs
- Breasts: Assess density of the tissue, nipples may become smaller and flatter, assess for dimpling, puckering, retractions, axillary lymph nodes
- Abdomen: Shape, masses, bowel sounds, areas of tenderness, assess abdomen size in relation to spine; is it becoming larger because lower spine is curving inward?
- Musculoskeletal: Assess for arthritic changes, joint mobility, lordosis, scoliosis
- Neuro: Assess cranial nerves, reflexes, muscle strength, and symmetry
- Skin: Assess integrity, smoothness, unusual lesions (NOTE: 20% of melanomas start in the perigenital areas)
- Pelvic examination
  - External genitalia: Look for atrophy of the vulva, decreased subcutaneous tissue, decreased labia majora and minora; skin may become thinner with loss of pubic hair; dystrophies and pruritus are common. Assess the urethra and clitoris for atrophy
  - Vagina: Becomes shorter and narrower, with some loss of rugae (primary cause of dyspareunia complaints)
  - Cervix becomes pale and shrinks, endocervix becomes atrophic; os may become stenotic; also look for polyps as a cause of abnormal bleeding
  - Pelvic floor: Assess for cystocele, rectocele, prolapse. Also have patient cough to assess for stress incontinence
  - Bimanual: Uterus may become smaller; adnexa are often nonpalpable
  - Rectal examination: Assess for polyps, hemorrhoids, sphincter tone, hemoccult

NOTE: If a patient is posthysterectomy, do not assume that the cervix was removed; older hysterectomies were often done leaving the cervix intact, which may be a cause of bleeding

Diagnostic Procedures

Diagnostic procedures include those found in Table 116-1.

ASSESSMENT

Differential diagnoses include those found in Table 116-2.

THERAPEUTIC PLAN

Pharmaceutical: Hormone Replacement Therapy (HRT)

Definitions

Estrogen Replacement Therapy (ERT): Refers to administration of estrogen alone (used in women who do not have a uterus)
Hormone Replacement Therapy (HRT): Administration of estrogen and a progestin in menopause for a women with an intact uterus

Effect of Unopposed Estrogen on the Uterus

Stimulates endometrial cell biosynthesis:
- Proliferative endometrium may progress to cyclic or adenomatous hyperplasia.
- Adenomatous hyperplasia has a 25% chance of progressing to atypical adenomatous hyperplasia (premalignant) and adenocarcinoma.

TABLE 116-1 Diagnostic Procedures: Menopause

Diagnostic Test	Finding/Rationale	Cost ($)
Pap smear	Recommended as part of annual examination, every 3 yrs >65 if past three examinations have been within normal limits, or every 3 yrs if s/p hysterectomy	25-31
Endometrial biopsy	If menstrual irregularities occur (may consider a transvaginal ultrasound instead; if endometrial stripe is >4 mm, proceed to do a endometrial biopsy).	142-170
Mammogram	Yearly after 40; check insurance coverage; some companies cover only every other year	99-125
Cholesterol	Recommended as part of baseline data, repeat every 5 yrs	17-21
Blood sugar	Recommended as part of baseline data	16-20
TSH, T4	Rule out thyroid dysfunction	86-109/panel
Prolactin	Elevated prolactin levels may cause amenorrhea	70-89
HCG	Rule out pregnancy with secondary amenorrhea	28-35/qual
FSH	May or may not be helpful; consider using it to determine ovarian function in a woman who had her uterus removed but ovaries were left in place; if patient has been on oral contraceptive pills to regulate bleeding, check FSH on days 6 or 7 of placebo pill.	62-78
FOB	Part of annual examination for women after 40	13-17

FOB, Fecal occult blood; *FSH,* follicle-stimulating hormone; *HCG,* human chorionic gonadotropin; *s/p,* status post; *TSH,* thyroid-stimulating hormone.

TABLE 116-2 Differential Diagnosis: Menopause

Diagnosis	Supporting Data
Pregnancy	Secondary amenorrhea, breast tenderness, fatigue, nausea, weight gain
Thyroid disease	Weight gain, fatigue or nervousness, intolerance to heat, palpitations, irritability
Diabetes	Fatigue, polyuria, polydipsia, polyphagia
Hyperprolactinemia	Elevated prolactin level, amenorrhea, may be associated with galactorrhea

Adenocarcinoma of endometrium after estrogen use is generally low stage, low grade, and associated with fewer cases of myometrial invasion.

Progesterone counteracts this effect.

Contraindications to and Precautions to Be Taken With HRT

Unexplained vaginal bleeding
Chronic impaired liver disease
Carcinoma of the breast
Active liver disease
Recent vascular thrombosis (with or without emboli)
Endometrial cancer

Relative Contraindications to HRT

Seizure disorder
Uncontrolled hypertension
Uterine leiomyomas
Familial hyperlipidemia
Migraine headaches
Thrombophlebitis
Endometriosis
Gallbladder disease

Effects of Oral Hormone Replacement Therapy on the Body

HRT and Breast Cancer. Whether or not HRT increases the risk of breast cancer is still controversial. The risks and benefits must be evaluated on an individual basis, based on a woman's family and personal history.

HRT and Lipids

Estrogens

Low-density lipoproteins: Serum level decreases; the more elevated the level is before therapy, the more dramatic the decrease

High-density lipoproteins (HDLs): Serum level increases, although it takes 3 months of therapy to increase levels

Triglycerides: Serum level increases slightly

Progestins

Greatest effect on HDL

May blunt negative effect of estrogen on triglycerides

HRT and the Heart

Estrogens

Increase in endothelial prostacyclin, which is a powerful inhibitor of platelet aggregation

Direct vasodilating effect on coronary arteries
Some positive effect mediated through alterations in lipid profile
Progestins
Animal studies suggest vasodilating effect of estrogen is independent of progestin type and dosage

HRT and Bones. Several studies have shown that estrogen therapy can arrest bone loss and reduce the incidence of bone fractures, even if treatment is begun later in life.

HRT and Genitourinary Systems

Estrogens are effective in ameliorating atrophy of the vaginal epithelium and associated systems.
Clinical studies indicate that estrogens are effective in relieving some urinary tract symptoms.
Estrogen receptors have been identified in the urethra, and an increase in the number of superficial cells of the urethral epithelium have been reported with estrogen replacement.
Estrogens have a beneficial effect on reducing the symptoms of urgency, nocturia, and frequency in some women, as well as a positive effect on complaints of dyspareunia secondary to vaginal atrophy.

HRT and the Skin. Estrogen replacement has been shown to increase the thickness and collagen content of the skin.

HRT and Other Body Systems

Newer studies are pointing towards a positive effect of HRT on risks of colon cancer and Alzheimer's disease.
Several randomized, double-blind, cross-over, placebo-controlled drug trials have shown improvement in both cognitive and affective end-points with estrogen use in areas including memory, insomnia, anxiety, and irritability.
Postmenopausal osteoporosis affects jaw bones and may be a factor in tooth loss. Studies have indicated that estrogen may aid in tooth retention.

Options for HRT

Continuous Combined HRT

Conjugated estrogens, 0.625 mg/day, and medroxyprogesterone acetate (MDA), 2.5 mg/day or 5 mg/day
Goal is amenorrhea
Advantages: No withdrawal bleeding; easy to follow regimen; lower dose of progestin may increase tolerance
Disadvantages: Erratic bleeding at start of therapy
Regular or irregular vaginal bleeding is major reason for patients stopping HRT
May result in some withdrawal bleeding for the first 6 months
Restrict biopsies during that period
Endometrial biopsy if bleeding persists thereafter
If no pathology is found:
Increase medroxyprogesterone acetate to 5 mg/day
Decrease conjugated estrogen to 0.3 mg/day (this dose is not approved for prevention of osteoporosis, so pay special attention to lifestyle changes)
Prempro combines conjugated estrogens 0.625 mg and MDA 2.5 mg in a single tablet
Prempro 5 combines conjugated estrogens 0.625 mg and MDA 5 mg in a single tablet. It may be worth considering this initial treatment for the first 6 months to decrease the risk of breakthrough bleeding.

Cyclic Sequential HRT

Conjugated estrogens 0.625 mg on calendar days 1 to 25 plus MDA 10 mg on days 16 to 25
Possible estrogen withdrawal symptoms when off hormones
Endometrial biopsy is indicated if vaginal bleeding occurs on calendar days that patient is on therapy
Advantages: Most widely studied in the United States, predictable bleeding
Disadvantages: Cyclic withdrawal bleeding, progestin may be difficult to tolerate

Continuous Sequential HRT

Conjugated estrogens 0.625 mg/day plus MDA 10 mg for first 2 weeks each month
No estrogen withdrawal symptoms
No endometrial hyperplasia with 2 weeks of progestins
80% to 90% have withdrawal bleeding
Endometrial biopsy if bleeding occurs before the 10th day of the month
If no pathology, increase progestin (dosage or number of days of therapy) or continue current therapy
Advantages: Easy to follow regimen, therapy is never discontinued, may be easier to assess abnormal bleeding
Disadvantages: Cyclic withdrawal bleeding, progestin may be difficult to tolerate
Premphase combines conjugated estrogens 0.625 and MDA 5 mg in a single tablet for the second half of a 4-week cycle of a continuous sequential regimen of HRT

Cyclic Combined HRT

Both conjugated estrogens 0.625 mg and MDA 2.5 mg on calendar days 1 to 25 with break for the remainder of the month
Often results in bleeding for 3 to 6 months
Predictable bleeding pattern
Bleeding usually lasts 1 to 2 days and is scant
Ultimately, amenorrhea is expected
Fewer progesterone side effects than with continuous combined therapy
or
Both conjugated estrogens 0.625 mg and MDA 2.5 mg daily, Monday through Friday
Ultimately amenorrhea expected
Fewer hormonal side effects

Low-Dose Estrogens

Conjugated estrogen 0.3 mg
As effective as 0.625 mg in maintaining bone mass but only if given with 1500 mg elemental calcium/day

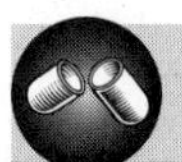

TABLE 116-3 Oral Estrogen Products for Postmenopausal Women

Generic Name Brand Name/ Manufacturer	Hot Flashes*	Prevention of Osteoporosis	Urogenital Atrophy*	Cost
Conjugated Equine Estrogens				
Premarin/Wyeth Ayerst	1.25 mg/day	0.625 mg/day	0.3-1.25 mg/day or more	$28/0.625 (100); $54/1.25 mg (100)
Micronized Estradiol				
Estrace/Bristol-Myers/Squibb	1-2 mg/day	0.5 mg/day	1-2 mg/day	$33/1 mg (100); $48/2 mg (100)
Estropipate (Piperazine Estrone Sulfate)				
Ogen/Pharmacia-Upjohn Ortho-Est/Ortho	0.625-5 mg/day	0.625 mg/day	0.625-5 mg/day	$35-$53/0.625 mg (100); $47-$74/1.25 mg (100); $100-$129/2.5 mg (100)
Esterified Estrogens				
Estratabs/Solvay Menest/Smith Kline Beecham	0.3-1.25 mg/day	Not FDA-labeled for this indication	0.3-1.25 mg/day	$12-$21/0.3 mg (100); $18-$29/0.625 mg (100); $29-$40/1.25 mg (100)
Ethinyl Estradiol				
Estinyl/Schering	0.02-0.05 mg/day	Not FDA-labeled for this indication	Not FDA-labeled for this indication	$30/0.02 mg (100); $51/0.05 mg (100); $104/0.5 mg (100)

FDA, Food and Drug Administration.
*Most manufacturers recommend titration to minimal effective dose.
Estrogen dosage equivalents: conjugated equine estrogens 0.625 mg = micronized estradiol 1 mg = estropipate 0.625 mg = transdermal estradiol 0.05 mg = esterified estrogens 0.625 mg.

Effect on prevention of coronary heart disease is not known

Transdermal Estrogen

Transdermal 17B-estradiol 0.05 mg every 3½ days (or weekly if using Climara) plus MDA 2.5 mg for the first 2 weeks each month

Direct delivery to bloodstream, bypassing first pass effect of liver metabolism

Skin rash occurs in 15% of patients

More expensive than oral preparations

Special considerations:

- Cigarette smokers may require higher doses of estrogens
- Consider in patients with migraine headaches who do not tolerate oral estrogens
- Consider in patients with elevated triglycerides >300 mg/dl
- Consider in patients with cholelithiasis, transdermal preparations do not alter the composition of bile
- Consider in patients taking oral estrogens who experience increasing symptoms of fibrocystic breast disease
- Consider in patients with history of thromboembolic disease; no demonstrable changes in clotting factors

Estrogen with Androgen

Esterified estrogens 1.25 g and methyltestosterone 2.5 g (Estratest) PO QD

Esterified estrogens 0.625 g and methyltestosterone 1.25 g (Estratest HS) PO QD

Indicated for women complaining of decreased libido

Also indicated for postmenopausal women with low body weight, poor musculature/coordination, or osteoporosis

It is contraindicated for women with seborrhea/acne or a history of polycystic ovarian disease

The effects attributed to testosterone were demonstrated only in women with testosterone levels below the normal range or 20 to 60 ng/dl

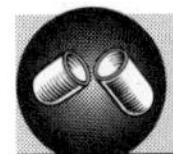

TABLE 116-4 Transdermal Estradiol Products

Brand Manufacturer	Patch Design	Dosage Strengths	Hot Flashes	Osteoporosis Prevention	Urogenital Atrophy	Cost
Alora/Procter & Gamble	Matrix	0.05 mg/day; 0.075 mg/day; 0.1 mg/day	0.05 mg/day patch twice weekly	Not FDA-approved for this indication	0.05 mg/day patch twice weekly	N/A
Climara/ Berlex	Matrix	0.05 mg/day; 0.1 mg/day	0.05 mg/day patch once weekly	Not FDA-labeled for this indication	0.05 mg/day patch once weekly	$57/0.05 mg/day (24); $55/0.1 mg/day (24)
Estraderm/ Ciba-Geigy	Reservoir	0.05 mg/day; 0.1 mg/day	0.05 mg/day patch twice weekly	0.05 mg/day patch twice weekly	0.05 mg/day patch twice weekly	Same as Berlex
FemPatch/ Parke-Davis	Matrix	0.025 mg/day	0.025 mg/day patch once weekly	Not FDA-labeled for this indication	0.025 mg/day patch once weekly	Same as Berlex
Vivelle/ Ciba-Geigy	Matrix	0.0375 mg/day; 0.05 mg/day 0.075 mg/day 0.1 mg/day	0.05 mg/day patch twice weekly	Not FDA-labeled for this indication	0.05 mg/day patch twice weekly	Same as Berlex

FDA, Food and Drug Administration; *N/A*, not applicable.

Selective Estrogen Receptor Modulators (SERMs)

SERMs are mixed estrogen agonists/antagonists: Selective ability to act like estrogen in the bone and cardiovascular tissue while blocking estrogen effects on breast and uterus

Raloxifene hydrochloride (Evista) 60 mg daily (60 mg [30] $59)
- Used only after menopause to prevent osteoporosis, although its effect on fractures is not known
- Does not prevent hot flushes (in fact, may increase them)
- There is no documented increase in risk of either breast or uterine cancers; in fact, early studies show that raloxifene may prevent breast cancer in women at higher risk
- There is no withdrawal bleeding
- There is no breast tenderness
- Contraindicated in patients with liver disease or history of thromboembolic disease and during pregnancy (Category X)
- Early studies show a moderate positive effect on lipids; (see Tables 116-3 to 116-7)

Patient Education

Warn patient taking HRT of the following side effects and the need to contact her health care provider should they occur:
- **A** = Abdominal pain
- **C** = Chest pain
- **H** = Headaches that are unusual
- **E** = Eye problems
- **S** = Severe leg pain

Remind patients of the importance of regular examinations, including Pap smears and mammography.

Encourage women to seek follow-up if they have unexplained/abnormal uterine bleeding.

Teach patients breast and vulvar self-examinations.

Some women choose not to take replacement hormones during or after menopause. Others have contraindications to HRT. The self-help tips in Box 116-1 should be explained to patients.

Perimenopausal women need to be informed that pregnancy is still a possibility until menopause actually occurs. Contraception needs to be discussed.

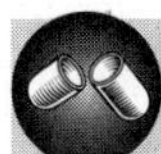

TABLE 116-5 Intravaginal Estrogen Products

Generic Name Brand Name/ Manufacturer	Dosage for Urogenital Atrophy	Strength	Cost ($)
Conjugated Estrogens			
Premarin/Wyeth Ayerst	½-2 g/day; use cyclically	0.625 mg/g, 45-g tube	29-32
Micronized Estradiol			
Estrace/Bristol-Myers Squibb	2-4 g/day for 1-2 weeks, then gradually cut dose by half for a similar period; may use 1 g one to three times a week for maintenance therapy	0.1 mg/g, 42.5-g tube	26
Micronized Estradiol			
Estring/Pharmacia-Upjohn	Vaginal ring inserted into the vagina for up to 90 days	0.0075 mg/day	26
Estropipate			
Ogen/Pharmacia-Upjohn	2-4 g/day; use cyclically	1.5 mg/g, 45-g tube	39
Dienestrol			
Ortho Dienestrol/ Ortho Pharmaceuticals	1-2 applicators/day for 1-2 weeks, then gradually cut dose by half for a similar period; may use 1 applicator 1 to 3 times/week for maintenance therapy	0.01%, 78-g tube	23; 24 with applicator

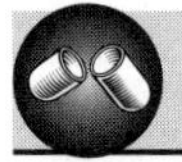

TABLE 116-6 Oral Progesterone Products for Postmenopausal Women

Drug	Dose	Comments	Cost
Medroxyprogesterone (Provera, Cycrin)	2.5-5 mg based on regimen chosen	Precaution: Pregnancy SE: Thromboembolic events, edema, depression, insomnia, nausea, somnolence, breast tenderness, acne, hirsutism alopecia	$29-$35/2.5 mg (100); $44-$53/5 mg (100)

SE, Side effects.

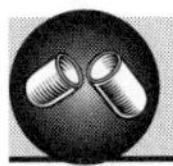

TABLE 116-7 Combined Estrogen and Progesterone Products

Drug	Dose	Comments	Cost ($)
Estrogen 0.625 mg and medroxyprogesterone 5 mg (Premphase)	Take estrogen 1 tablet QD for 14 days; then take estrogen + medroxyprogesterone (combined tablet) 1 tablet QD for 14 days	Examination and Pap recommended yearly while taking product Pregnancy: X SE: Nausea and vomiting, breast tenderness, breakthrough bleeding, intolerance to contact lenses, depression, increased size of uterine fibroids	46
Estrogen 0.625 mg and medroxyprogesterone 2.5 mg (Prempro) and estrogen 0.625 mg and medroxyprogesterone 5 mg	Take 1 tablet QD; if break-through bleeding, can increase to tablet that contains medroxyprogesterone 5 mg	Examination and Pap recommended while taking product Pregnancy: X SE: Nausea and vomiting, breast tenderness, breakthrough bleeding, intolerance to contact lenses, depression, increased size of uterine fibroids	50

SE, Side effects.

Box 116-1

Patient Education: Menopause

To Prevent Osteoporosis

Take 1500 mg of calcium daily along with 400 to 800 IU of vitamin E.
Do weight-bearing exercises regularly (brisk walking, jogging, bicycling).
Avoid alcohol, caffeine, and carbonated sodas, all of which are high in phosphate and increase bone loss.
Decrease protein intake; too much protein depletes bones of calcium.
Eat whole grains, fruits, and leafy green vegetables.
Consider adding soy to your diet.
Consider a multivitamin.

To Prevent Heart Disease

Exercise regularly.
Eat a low-fat diet (no more than 2 g of fat per 100 calories).
Practice stress reduction exercises.
Monitor blood pressure, cholesterol, and triglycerides.
Consider taking a low-dose (80 mg) aspirin a day.

To Reduce Hot Flushes/Flashes

Take vitamin E and maintain a diet high in vegetables.
Consider adding Evening Primrose Oil to your vitamin regimen (if you are at risk for breast cancer, substitute Black Current Oil); both are available at health food stores.
Add B complex vitamins.
Clonidine 0.05 to 0.15 PO QD. Watch for significant rebound effect (including hypertension if discontinued suddenly).
Methyldopa 250-500 mg PO BID.
Medroxyprogesterone 20 mg PO QD.
Megestrol acetate 20 mg PO QD.
Be aware that hot drinks, alcohol, spicy foods, stress, and heat may all trigger hot flushes and make them worse.

To Treat Diminished Libido

Consider adding dehydroepiandrosterone: preliminary studies show incremental increases in testosterone.
Vitamin C 500 mg PO QD-QID.
B Complex vitamins.
Tryptophan.
Methyltestosterone 2.5 mg PO QD; monitor carefully for androgen excess that may be irreversible; check liver function test and lipids q3 months.

Hormone Replacement Side Effects

Gastrointestional symptoms, usually nausea, may respond to a switch to a lower estrogen or to a transdermal patch.
Progesterones are associated with bloating, cramping, irritability, breast tenderness, insomnia, depression, hirsutism, hair loss, PMS symptoms, changes in libido, and acne. Decreasing the daily progesterone dose or taking it on alternate days may help alleviate symptoms.
Estrogen side effects are associated with breast changes (tenderness, enlargement), nausea and vomiting, breakthrough bleeding, weight gain, PMS symptoms, edema, leiomyomata enlargement.

Referral/Consultation

Sex therapist for prolonged sexual dysfunction
Counseling: Stresses of the middle years, depression

Follow-up

Annual examination: Pap smear, breast examination, pelvic examination
Mammogram

SUGGESTED READINGS

ACOG: Health maintenance for perimenopausal women, *ACOG Technical Bulletin* No. 210, 1995.

1997 Drug Topics Red Book, Facts and Comparisons, Montvale, NJ, 1997, Medical Economics.

Ellsworth A et al: *Mosby's 1998 medical drug reference*, St Louis, 1998, Mosby.

Healthcare Consultants of America, Inc: *1998 Physicians fee and coding guide*, Augusta, Ga., 1998, Healthcare Consultants of America, Inc.

Gallagher JC, et al: Why HRT makes sense, *Patient Care* 30(13):66-92, 1996.

Gambrell RD: Overcoming the side effects of hormone replacement therapy, *Women's Health Primary Care* 1(2):160-171, 1998.

Goldzieher JW: Postmenopausal androgen therapy, *Female Patient* 22(4):10-13, 1997.

Harvard Women's Health Watch: *Testosterone and HRT*, Cambridge, Mass, 1996, Harvard Press.

Hawkins JW, Roberto-Nichols DM, Stanley-Haney JL: *Protocols for nurse practitioners in gynecologic settings*, ed 5, New York, 1995, Tiresias Press.

Johnson S: Menopause and hormone replacement therapy, *Med Clin North Am* 82(2):297-320, 1998.

Kaplan H, Abisla M: In transition: empowering your menopausal patients, *Adv Nurse Pract* 5(6):28-33, 1997.

Norwitz ER: Managing the menopause without estrogen, *Female Patient* 22(2):42-59, 1997.

Paganini-Hill A: Long-term risks and benefits of estrogen replacement therapy, *Adv Nurse Pract* 4(3):22-25, 1996.

Scanlon C: Estrogen replacement: are the benefits worth the risks? *Hosp Pract* 32(4):67-69, 1997.

Scharbo-Dehaan M: Management strategies for hormonal replacement therapy, *Nurse Pract* 19(12):47-56, 1994.

117 Mitral Valve Prolapse

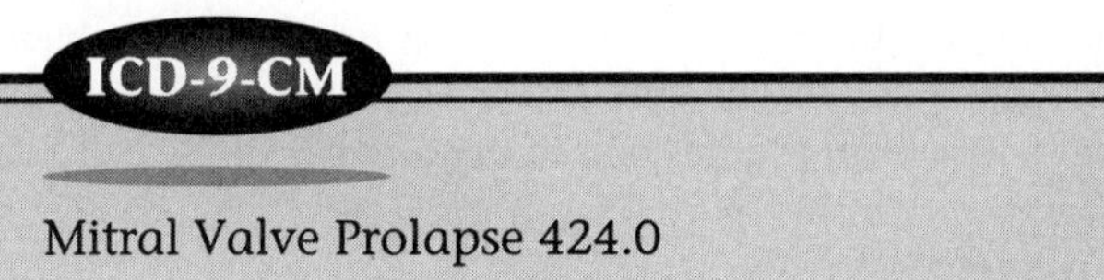

ICD-9-CM

Mitral Valve Prolapse 424.0

OVERVIEW

Definition

Anatomic mitral valve prolapse (MVP) is an abnormality of the mitral valve leaflet(s), the supporting chords, or both in which the mitral valve leaflet(s) prolapses back into the left atrium during ventricular systole.

Mitral valve prolapse syndrome (MVPS) is anatomic MVP in association with one or more of the following symptoms: fatigue, palpitations, mood swings, atypical chest pains, lightheadedness, migraine headaches, exercise intolerance, shortness of breath, anxiety or panic attacks, and dizziness associated with postural changes. The term MVPS refers to the occurrence or coexistence of symptoms unexplainable on the basis of the valvular abnormality.

Incidence

The reported prevalence of MVP varies from 5% to more than 15%. According to the Framingham Heart Study, 7.6% of women and 2.5% of men have MVP. The true incidence of MVPS is unknown. The prevalence of MVP increases with age; MVP is rare under the age of 10 years.

Pathophysiology

Symptoms are believed to be the result of anxiety disorders or various forms of neuroendocrine or autonomic dysfunction. Metabolic changes associated with MVPS include:

High serum and urine catecholamines
Catecholamine regulation abnormality
Hyperresponsiveness to adrenergic stimulation
Parasympathetic abnormality
Baroreflex modulation abnormality
Renin-aldosterone regulation abnormality
Decreased intravascular volume
Decreased standing ventricular diastolic volume
Atrial natriuretic peptide secretion abnormality

In addition, magnesium deficiency may also play a role in MVPS symptoms.

Complications

Relatively infrequent complications of MVP include infective endocarditis, severe mitral regurgitation, sudden cardiac death, potentially dangerous arrhythmias, and cerebral ischemia. Patients at a higher risk of sudden death include: advanced age, male gender, history of recurrent syncope, history of sustained supraventricular arrhythmias, complex ventricular arrhythmias, family history of cardiac sudden death, presence of a holosystolic murmur, and left ventricular or left atrial enlargement.

SUBJECTIVE DATA

History of Present Illness

When analyzing the patient's symptoms, pay particular attention to aggravating and alleviating factors (see Box 117-1).

Medications

Ask about the use of over-the-counter medications that contain epinephrine, ephedrine, phenylpropanolamine, pseudoephedrine, or caffeine. (Examples: Actifed, Anacin, Benadryl, Chlor-Trimeton, Congestac, Excedrin, Sudafed, and Vanquish.)

Inquire about patient knowledge of antibiotic prophylaxis.

Family History

MVP may be inherited: therefore, ask about family history of MVP. Family members with a suspicion of MVP should undergo a physical examination and an echocardiogram.

Box 117-1

Factors Associated with Increased Intensity or Frequency of MVPS Symptoms

Emotional stress
Excessive fatigue
Unaccustomed physical activity
Anxiety or nervousness
Caffeine
Medicines with stimulants
Sweets
Being in a hot, dry environment
Dehydration
Flu, cold, or other illnesses
Lack of sleep
Alcohol
Smoking
Skipping meals
Rushing around
Lying on the left or right side
Menses
Menopause

Reprinted with permission from *Taking Control* questionnaire, 1995, The MVP Program of Cincinnati. ©K. A. Scordo.

Psychosocial History

Lifestyle Changes

Obtain information about lifestyle changes that have occurred within a few years of the onset of symptoms. MVPS symptoms often occur after a major stressor or accumulation of stressors such as illness, a job change, death, or divorce.

Diet

Ask about intake of foods and substances that contain caffeine, tyramine, nitrites, and phosphates. Caffeine can worsen MVPS symptoms such as chest pain and palpitations, whereas tyramine and nitrites can provoke migraine headaches (Box 117-2). Nitrites are found in cured or processed meats, ham, bacon, sausage, and hot dogs. Phosphates—found in many sodas—reduce magnesium absorption.

Also, ask about the patient's intake of concentrated sugars such as those found in candy bars, pastries, and doughnuts.

Description of Most Common Symptoms

Chest pain, chest tightness—usually atypical of that of angina pectoris
Palpitations, extra heartbeats, heart pounding, fluttering, or racing
Lightheadedness, dizziness, or forceful heartbeat, mainly associated with positional changes
Shortness of breath—with or without exertion
Fatigue
Exercise intolerance
Anxiety or panic attacks
Mood swings
Migraine headaches

Associated Symptoms

Other commonly reported symptoms include insomnia, chronic cold hands and feet, gastrointestinal disturbance, inability to concentrate or a feeling of fogginess, numbness and/or tingling of the arms and/or legs, difficulty swallowing, and a feeling of a lump in the throat.

Adolescents

Although young adults may complain of similar symptoms, common complaints are palpitations, chest pain, and shortness of breath.

Elderly

Exertional dyspnea, particularly in males over 50, may be related to the progression of mitral insufficiency, and not to the syndrome of MVP.

OBJECTIVE DATA

Physical Examination

A complete physical examination should be done, with particular attention to:

General: Low body weight, low blood pressure (B/P)
Orthostatic B/P: Frequently see ↑ of heart rate up to 140 beats/min going from lying to standing position
Head/eyes/ears/nose/throat: High arched palate
Musculoskeletal: Scoliosis, hyperextensible joints, a straight back, and an arm span greater than height
Heart:
Auscultation: The auscultatory hallmark of MVPS is a mid-to-late systolic click, loudest at the apex, with or without a mid-to-late systolic murmur. Listen for changes in the timing of the click and murmur with positional changes. With standing, the click and murmur occur earlier in systole. The murmur may become holosystolic. Prompt squatting from a standing position causes the click and murmur to occur later in systole. Also, note changes in heart rate. Standing from a sitting or lying position is frequently associated with an acceleration in heart rate, whereas prompt squatting is associated with a slowing of the heart rate. Because these changes are related to changes in left ventricular volume, they may be difficult to appreciate in patients who take beta-blockers.

Box 117-2

Foods and Substances That Contain Caffeine, Tyramine, and Phosphate*

Caffeine (mg)*	Tyramine† (10-25 mg)	Phosphate (mg)‡
AuBonPain (9 oz) (171)	Red wine (Chianti, burgundy, sherry, vermouth)	Dr. Pepper (44)
Dunkin' Doughnut Coffee (8 oz) (104)	Broad beans and pods (lima beans, fava beans, lentils, snow peas and soy beans)	Diet Dr. Pepper (44)
Coffee Beanery (8 oz) (82)	Aged cheese	Coca-Cola Classic (41)
Starbucks (6 oz) (81)	Smoked fish or meat	Cherry Coca-Cola (37)
Coffee Brewed (8 oz) (88)	Pickled herring and salted dry fish	TAB (30)
Coffee Instant (8 oz) (71)	Dry and fermented sausage (bologna, corned beef, pepperoni and salami)	Mr. Pibb (29)
McDonald's (6 oz) (60)	Sauerkraut	Caffeine-free diet Coke (18)
Mountain Dew (12 oz) (54)	Brewer's yeast, yeast vitamin supplements	Diet Cherry Coca-Cola (18)
Mello Yellow (12 oz) (53)	Overripened avocados	Welch's Sparkling Grape Soda (34)
TAB (12 oz) (47)		Sprite (0)
Coca-Cola (12 oz) (45)		Diet Sprite (0)
Shasta cola (12 oz) (44)		Minute Maid Orange (0)
Mr. Pibb (12 oz) (41)		Mello Yello (trace)
Tea Brewed (6 oz) (41)		Fresca (trace)
Dr. Pepper (12 oz) (40)		7Up and Diet 7Up (only as present in water)
Pepsi Cola (12 oz) (38)		
Chocolate Milk (8 oz) (8)		
Cake, chocolate 1/18th of 9" (14)		
Candy, chocolate (1 oz) (8)		

Source:

*Caffeine labeling: Council on Scientific Affairs. *JAMA*, 252, Aug. 10, 1984; Tufts University *Diet Nutri Lett* 12:(5), July 1994.

†Anon: Foods interacting with MAOI inhibitors. *Med Lett Drug Ther* 1989;31:11-12; McCabe, B: Dietary tyramine and other pressor amines in MAOI regimes: a review, *J Am Diet Assoc* 86:1059-1064, 1986.

‡Consumer Information Center, The Coca-Cola company 1/94; consumer affairs, Dr. Pepper/Seven-Up Corporation 4/94.

MVPS is a dynamic syndrome, and auscultatory features may vary from one examination to another. Therefore multiple examinations under different conditions may be needed.

Children

Auscultatory findings in children with MVP are similar to those described in adults.

Diagnostic Procedures

Diagnostic procedures are outlined in Table 117-1.

ASSESSMENT

Many symptoms associated with MVPS are nonspecific and are present in a variety of other clinical conditions. Differential diagnoses are listed in Table 117-2.

THERAPEUTIC PLAN

Pharmaceutical

Traditionally, beta-blockers are used to treat associated MVPS symptoms. However, there is no evidence that supports their efficacy. In addition, these medications do not guarantee symptom control and are not without side effects. Many patients with MVPS are young and wish to avoid medication. Therefore encourage the use of nonpharmacological interventions. Reserve beta-blockers for patients with frequent migraine headaches and for patients with rapid resting heart rates who are highly symptomatic. As patients adopt nonpharmacological measures, beta-blockers can be discontinued. Tenormin (atenolol) 25 to 50 mg at bedtime is effective. Table 117-3 contains a pharmaceutical plan for MVPS.

Antibiotic Prophylaxis

MVP with valvar regurgitation and/or thickened leaflets is considered a moderate-risk factor for the development of bacterial endocarditis, whereas MVP without valvar regurgitation is considered a negligible-risk factor. Recommended antibiotic prophylaxis for dental, oral, respiratory tract, or esophageal procedures is found in Tables 117-4 and 117-5.

For patients who currently take an antibiotic normally used for endocarditis prophylaxis, select a drug from a different class rather than increase the dose of the current antibiotic. When possible, have the patient delay the procedure 9 to 14 days after completion of the antibiotic.

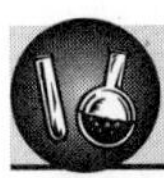

TABLE 117-1 Diagnostic Procedures: Mitral Valve Prolapse

Diagnostic Test	Finding/Rationale	Cost ($)
Echocardiogram	A two-dimensional echocardiogram is used to confirm the diagnosis. Also, the echo is useful to assess mitral leaflet thickness, associated tricuspid and aortic valve prolapse, wall thickness and wall motion, and chamber size. Doppler ultrasound determines the degree of mitral regurgitation—an important factor that determines the risk of complications. Look for billowing of the mitral leaflets in the parasternal long-axis view and thickened, redundant, floppy mitral leaflets.	675
Electrocardiogram	Although not specific for the diagnosis of MVPS, nonspecific ST-segment and T-wave changes, particularly in the inferior leads (II, III, and aVf) may be noted. These changes may normalize with exercise or with the administration of beta-blockers.	55-65
Graded exercise stress testing	Because of the frequent occurrence of false-positive stress test in women with MVPS, obtain a stress echocardiogram or nuclear exercise study to rule out chest pain of ischemic origin.	249-305
Holter monitoring or event monitor recording	For patients who complain of daily palpitations, a 24-hour Holter monitor may be required to assess for the presence of arrhythmias. For patients who have episodic palpitations, an event monitor may be required. Often sinus tachycardia is reported during complaints of "heart palpitations."	295-388
Additional tests	In patients suspected of magnesium deficiency, obtain an RBCmg (atomic absorption spectroscopy). (Because only 1% of magnesium is present in the serum and interstitial body fluids, avoid standard serum magnesium testing.) To determine the presence and degree of dysautonomia, noninvasive cardiovascular reflex tests may be required.	Not available

TABLE 117-2 Differential Diagnosis: Mitral Valve Prolapse

Diagnosis	Supporting Data
Esophagitis	Odynophagia and dysphagia
Hypoglycemia	Autonomic symptoms: Sweating, palpitations, anxiety and tremulousness
Fibromyalgia	Fatigue, sleep disorders, chronic headaches, more frequent in women, trigger points
Anxiety disorder	Apprehension, worry, headaches, tachycardia, epigastric pain, chest pain, dyspnea, smothering feelings, dizziness, (alarm response)
Chronic fatigue syndrome	Symptoms for >6 mos, impaired memory, sore throat, tender cervical lymph nodes, headaches, joint pain, unrefreshing sleep, muscle pain

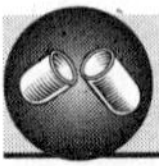

TABLE 117-3 Pharmaceutical Plan: Mitral Valve Prolapse

Drug	Dose	Comments	Cost
Atenolol (Tenormin)	25-50 mg QHS	Pregnancy: C SE: Fatigue, dizziness, lethargy, nausea, impotence, conduction arrhythmias	$9-$88/25 (100) $5-$90/50 (100)

SE: Side effects.

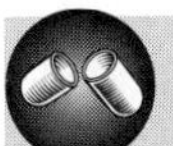

TABLE 117-4 Antibiotic Prophylaxis: Adults

Drug	Dose	Comments	Cost
Amoxicillin	2 g PO 1 hour before the procedure	Pregnancy: B SE: Nausea, vomiting, diarrhea; rash; anaphylaxis	\$17-\$49/500 mg (100)
Clindamycin	600 mg PO 1 hour before the procedure	For patients allergic to penicillin Pregnancy: B SE: Pseudomembranous colitis, nausea and vomiting, abdominal pain, leukopenia	\$231/300 mg (100)
Cephalexin	2 g 1 hour before the procedure	For patients allergic to penicillin Pregnancy: B SE: Pseudomembranous colitis, diarrhea	\$31-\$253/500 mg (100)
Azithromycin or clarithromycin	500 mg 1 hour before the procedure	For patients allergic to penicillin Pregnancy: B (azi); C (clar) SE: Nausea, vomiting, and diarrhea	\$31/250 mg (6)/eryth; \$185/500 mg (60)/clar

SE: Side effects.

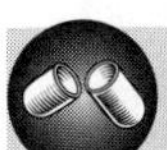

TABLE 117-5 Antibiotic Prophylaxis: Children

Drug	Dose	Comments	Cost
Amoxicillin	50 mg/kg orally 1 hour before procedure	See Table 117-4	See Table 117-4
Clindamycin	20 mg/kg orally	Penicillin (PCN) allergy See Table 117-4	See Table 117-4
Azithromycin or clarithromycin	15 mg/kg orally	PCN allergy See Table 117-4	

Lifestyle/Activities

Exercise: Encourage regular cardiovascular exercise. Include information about the mode, intensity, duration, frequency, and progression of physical activity. For effective symptom control, exercise should be performed for 45 to 60 minutes 3 days a week. Prescribe exercise that uses large muscle groups and is rhythmic and aerobic in nature, such as rowing, brisk walking, and stationary bicycling.

Diet

Caffeine: Avoid foods and beverages that contain caffeine.

Simple carbohydrates: Avoid concentrated sugars, especially those found in candy bars, pastries, and doughnuts. If patients have a craving for a sweet treat, instruct them to eat a well-balanced meal first.

Amines, nitrites, and tyramine: Teach migraine sufferers to avoid foods and beverages that contain amines, nitrites, and tyramine.

Crash or fad diets: Because many MVPS patients are sensitive to volume depletion, have them avoid crash diets. The initial rapid weight loss associated with crash diets is largely due to water and sodium loss and can worsen MVPS symptoms.

Fluid and sodium intake: Encourage patients to drink a minimum of eight 8-ounce glasses of water a day and, unless otherwise contraindicated, not to restrict their sodium intake. Choose snacks such as pretzels and tomato juice.

Magnesium: Encourage a diet rich in magnesium. Good sources of magnesium include nuts, shellfish, legumes, cereal grains, green leafy vegetables, apples, apricots, brown rice, lima beans, peaches, wheat, and whole grains.

Patient Education

Avoid catecholamine and cAMP stimulation: Teach patients to avoid medications with epinephrine, phenylpropanolamine, pseudoephedrine, or ephedrine. Caution patients to carefully read medication labels. For patients who require antihistamines, prescribe astemizole (Hismanal) or loratadine (Claritin). These medications have little or

SYMPTOM CHECK LIST

Name________________________ Week #____________ Week ending ____/____/____

Please place a number next to the symptom that best indicates the frequency that you experienced this symptom during the **past week:**

5 - All of the time

4 - Most of the time

3 - A good bit of the time

2 - Some of the time

1 - A little of the time

0 - None of the time

Symptom	Frequency
Chest pain and/or chest discomfort	
Arm pain and/or arm discomfort	
Palpitations/extra beats/ skipped beats/heart pounding	
Shortness of breath	
Fatigue	
Headache	
Anxious (Feeling nervous or frightened)	
Mood swings	
Dizziness and/or lightheadedness	
Passing out spells (Losing consciousness)	
Muscle cramps	

Please discuss other symptom(s) you experienced this past week. Use the reverse side of this paper.

This week:

I saw my physician ___Yes ___No. If yes, was this a routine visit? ___Yes ___No. If no, please explain.

I missed ___ days from work. I went to the emergency room for treatment. ___Yes ___No. If yes, what symptom(s) prompted you to go to the emergency room?

Figure 117-1 Mitral valve prolapse symptom check list. (Copyright 1988 Kristine A. Scordo, Dayton, Ohio. Reproduced with permission.)

no central or autonomic nervous system effects. In addition, encourage smoking cessation and minimal to no alcohol consumption. Both of these substances can worsen MVPS symptoms.

Feet up: Many patients who experience chest pain find relief by lying down and leaning their legs against a wall. Have them take in slow, deep breaths through the nose. An alternative position is to sit crossed-legged (Indian style) and lean forward. Symptom relief may be related to changes in left-ventricular end-diastolic volume.

Locomotion: Teach patients who have episodes of palpitations without lightheadedness to perform an activity that will increase their heart rate when they first notice the extrasystoles. In addition to refocusing their attention on the activity, the extrasystoles are either suppressed or overridden with an increased heart rate.

Pursed-lip breathing: Teach patients with shortness of breath—or the inability to take in a deep breath—to use pursed-lip breathing. Have them breathe in through their nose then slowly breathe out through pursed lips. Have them repeat this until they are able to take full, deep breaths.

Reassurance: Reassure patients that the prognosis for MVPS is excellent and rarely requires valve replacement.

Stress reduction techniques: Techniques such as mindful hatha-yoga help to alleviate MVPS symptoms.

Support groups: Many patients with MVPS find that participation in a support group is helpful. When they share, they learn from one another and gain insight into their problems.

Family Impact

MVPS is a family affair—symptoms affect children and spouses. When appropriate, include spouses and children in support groups and during formal or informal MVPS education.

Referral

Refer patients with mitral insufficiency or symptoms of congestive heart failure to a cardiologist.

Consultation

Refer for counseling patients whose anxiety and/or panic attacks are not controlled by the use of nonpharmacological measures. Persistent MVPS symptoms after use of nonpharmacological interventions are usually a manifestation of an underlying psychological problem.

Follow-up

Yearly physical examination and echocardiogram
Children: Similar follow-up as for adults

EVALUATION

Figure 117-1 depicts a simple way to objectively measure patients' progress. Have them complete this questionnaire weekly and graph their results.

RESOURCES

The MVP Program of Cincinnati
10525 Montgomery Road
Cincinnati, OH 45242
(513) 745-9911

National Society for MVP and Dysautonomia
c/o Baptist Health Foundation
PO Box 83060
Birmingham, AL 35283-0605
www.mvprolapse.com/index.html

For mitral valve literature; lists multiple printed resources:
www.mvprolapse.com/lit.htm

SUGGESTED READINGS

Boudoulas H: Mitral valve prolapse: etiology, clinical presentation and neuroendocrine function, *J Heart Valve Dis* 1:175-188, 1992.

Boudoulas J: Mitral valve prolapse: serious or not? *Hosp Med* 1:43-62, 1992.

Boudoulas H, Wooley C: Mitral valve prolapse: clinical presentation and diagnostic evaluation. In Boudoulas H, Wooley C, editors: *Mitral valve prolapse and the mitral valve prolapse syndrome*, New York, 1988, Futura Publishing.

Dajani A et al: Prevention of bacterial endocarditis: recommendations by the American Heart Association, *JAMA* 277(22):1794-1801, 1997.

Galland L, Baker S, McLellan R: Magnesium deficiency in the pathogenesis of mitral valve prolapse, *Magnesium* 5:165-174, 1986.

Fernandes J et al: Therapeutic effect of a magnesium salt in patients suffering from mitral valvular prolapse and latent tetany, *Magnesium* 4:283-290, 1985.

Feigenbaum H: *Echocardiography*, ed 5, Philadelphia, 1994, Lea & Febiger.

Frances U, Collet F, Luccioni R: Long-term follow-up of mitral valve prolapse and latent tetany: preliminary data, *Magnesium* 5:175-181, 1986.

Levy D, Savage, D: Prevalence and clinical features of mitral valve prolapse, *Am Heart J* 113:1281-1290, 1987.

Rokicki W, Krzystolik-Ladzinska J, Goc B: Clinical characteristics of primary mitral valve prolapse syndrome in children, *Acta Cardiol* L:147-153, 1995.

Savage D et al: Mitral valve prolapse in the general population. I. Epidemiologic features: the Framingham Study, *Am Heart J* 106:571-576, 1983.

Scordo K: Mitral valve prolapse syndrome: interventions for symptom control, *Dimensions Crit Care Nurs* 17(4):177-186, 1998.

Scordo K: Factors associated with participation in an mitral valve prolapse support group, unpublished raw data, 1998.

Scordo K: Mitral valve prolapse syndrome: nonpharmacologic management, *Crit Care Nurs Clin North Am* 9:555-564, 1997.

Scordo K: *Taking control: living with the mitral valve prolapse syndrome*, ed 2, Dayton, Ohio, 1996, Kardinal Publishing.

Scordo K: Mitral valve prolapse syndrome: women as second class citizens, *Capsules Comments Crit Care Nurs* 2:1-6, 1994.

Scordo K: The effects of aerobic exercise on symptomatic women with mitral valve prolapse, *Am J Cardiol* 76:863-868, 1991.

Zuppiroli A et al: Natural history of mitral valve prolapse, *Am J Cardiol* 75:1028-1032, 1995.

118 Molluscum Contagiosum

ICD-9-CM

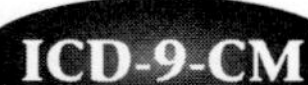

Molluscum Contagiosum 078.0

OVERVIEW

Definition

Molluscum contagiosum is a benign epidermal neoplasm.

Incidence

Common in infants, young children, **immunocompromised persons, sexually active adolescents**

Pathophysiology

Caused by pox virus, which causes the epidermis to proliferate and form papules

Protective Factors Against

Intact immune system
Condoms

Factors that Increase Susceptibility

Chronic illness
Unprotected sex

SUBJECTIVE DATA

History of Present Illness

Usually insidious onset
Single skin-colored lesion noticed

Past Medical History

Previous sexually transmitted diseases
Human immunodeficiency virus infection
Substance abuse

Medications

Noncontributory

Family History

Not usually significant

Associated Symptoms

None

OBJECTIVE DATA

Physical Examination

Skin: Begin as skin-colored lesions progressing to discrete pearly white or yellowish lesions that are umbilicated dome-shaped papules (Figure 118-1)
2 to 5 mm diameter
May have multiple papules
Center is filled with a cheesy substance
Common locations are trunk, face, arms, genitalia
If on genitalia in child, consider sexual abuse

Diagnostic Procedures

Not necessary
Microscopic examination of scraping will show basophilic epidermal cells

ASSESSMENT

Differential diagnosis is outlined in Table 118-1.

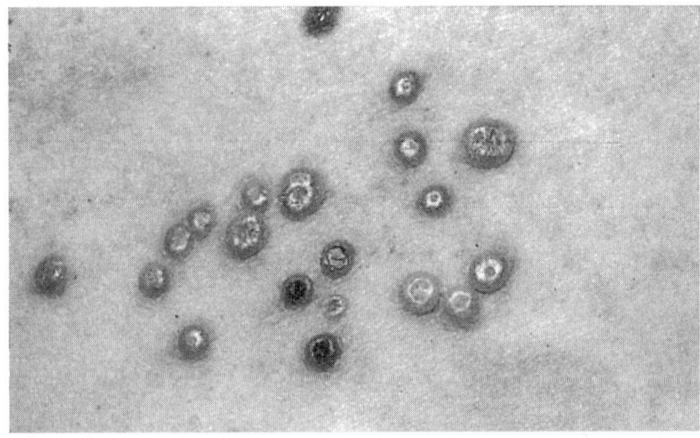

Figure 118-1 Molluscum contagiosum, showing typical discrete smooth umbilicated grouped lesions. (From Cox NH, Lawrence CM: *Diagnostic problems in dermatology*, St Louis, 1998, Mosby.)

TABLE 118-1 Differential Diagnosis: Molluscum Contagiosum

Diagnosis	Supporting Data
Acne	More common in adolescents; hair may be oily; includes comedones, both black and white
Wart	Flat lesion with pinpoint depression; more common in females ages 12 to 16

TABLE 118-2 Pharmaceutical Plan: Molluscum Contagiosum

Drug	Dose	Comment	Cost ($)
Trichloroacetic acid	30% apply to base of each lesion	Avoid surrounding skin	Not available
Salicylic acid cream 25%-60% ointment 25%-60% 5% gel	Apply thin layer to lesion q3-5d, cover, apply to skin once QD		3-16
1%-2% Lotion	Apply to area QD up to TID		
5%-27% Solution	Apply QD up to BID		
Tretinoin gel (Retin A)	0.01% apply to lesions QD	Keep away from eye, nares, mouth, avoid exposure to ultraviolet light, may worsen acne, use in child over age 12	21
Aldara cream (Imiquimod)	5% apply 3× week leave on for 6-10 hours; wash with soap and water; limit use to 16 weeks	Not recommended in under 18 years of age	108

THERAPEUTIC PLAN

Pharmaceutical

Pharmaceutical plan is outlined in Table 118-2.

Surgical

Remove each lesion with sharp curette, electrosurgery, or cryotherapy (apply liquid nitrogen to lesion).

Lifestyle/Activities

Safe sex

Diet

Noncontributory

Patient Education

Teach that lesions will usually subside without treatment in 6 to 9 months, but may last for years
Removal may produce scarring
Teach signs and symptoms of secondary infection from touching lesions
Teach contact with lesion can spread to another person

Family Impact

Prevent contact with infected family member

Referral/Consultation

Refer to dermatologist multiple lesions unresponsive to treatment

Follow-up

Recheck in 1 week

EVALUATION

Decrease in number of lesions
No secondary infection

SUGGESTED READINGS

Berger T, Goldstein S, Odom R: Skin and appendages. In Tierney L, McPhee S, Papadakis M, editors: *Current medical diagnosis and treatment*, ed 36, Stamford, Conn., 1998, Appleton and Lange.
Boynton R, Dunn E, Stephens G: *Manual of ambulatory pediatrics*, ed 4, Philadelphia, 1998, JB Lippincott.
Ellsworth AJ, et al: *Mosby's 1998 medical drug reference*, St Louis, 1998, Mosby.
Pierce, N: Bacterial infections of the skin. In Barker L, Burton J, Zieve P, editors: *Principles of ambulatory medicine*, ed 4, Baltimore, 1995, Williams & Wilkins.

119 Mononucleosis (Mono)

ICD-9-CM

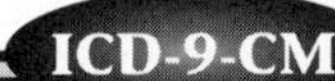

Infectious Mononucleosis 075

OVERVIEW

Definition

Mononucleosis (mono) refers to the presence of an abnormally high number of mononuclear leukocytes in the body.

Incidence

Approximately 12% to 30% of the total cases of mono occur among university students and military cadets. By adulthood, most individuals have had at least one infection with the Epstein Barr virus (EBV). Mono most often occurs in **adolescents** from higher socioeconomic groups and college students. The peak incidence occurs in boys from 16 to 18 and in girls 14 to 16. It is rare in children under 5 years, but the infection occurs early in life among lower socioeconomic groups and in developing countries.

Pathophysiology

Mono results from a viral syndrome caused by the EBV. The virus is introduced when the host comes in close contact with another individual who is shedding EBV in the oropharynx. Mono is commonly known as the "kissing disease" because of the close contact needed for transmission. The virus replicates in epithelial cells of the pharynx and salivary glands. A localized inflammatory response produces the pharyngeal exudate. The virus is then carried via the lymphatics to the lymph nodes. Local and generalized lymphadenopathy develops. Mono has an incubation period of 30 to 50 days.

SUBJECTIVE DATA

History of Present Illness

Past Medical History

Exposure to person with mono, history of upper respiratory infection in past
History of recent strep throat
Last menstrual period for female
Allergies

Medications

Recent use of antibiotics, any other medications

Family History

Ask about other family members who may be sick.

Psychosocial History

Smoking history
Ability to perform normal activities, extent to which fatigue has interfered with work or school expectations
Assess ability to cope with interference with normal activities

Diet History

Ask about the type of diet the patient usually eats

Description of Most Common Symptoms

Fever/fatigue for 1 week
Sore throat (patient may describe it as the worst patient has ever had)
Dysphagia
Swelling of lymph nodes, especially posterior cervical lymph nodes
Between 10% and 50% have atypical presentations: rash nonspecific, gastrointestinal complaints

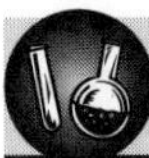

TABLE 119-1 Diagnostic Procedures: Mononucleosis

Diagnostic Test	Finding/Rationale	Cost ($)
CBC, with differential	WBC >10,000—20,000 Lymphocytes over 50% with numerous atypical lymphocytes/monocytes	18-23
Monospot	+ after 7-10 days	20-25
Strep screen	20% of patients have concurrent strep with mono	19-24
Liver function tests	May see mild elevation with mono	29-41

CBC, Complete blood count; *WBC,* white blood count.

TABLE 119-2 Differential Diagnosis: Mononucleosis

Diagnosis	Supporting Data
Strep pharyngitis	Pharyngitis, fever, malaise, + strep screen
Measles	Cough, coryza and conjunctivitis, Koplik spots
Viral exanthems	Rash and fever
Viral hepatitis	Jaundice, fever, fatigue
CMV	Fatigue, malaise, pharyngitis (CMV is a member of herpes family and can cause mononucleosis; nearly identical clinical and laboratory features of CMV with mono, except CMV does not cause exudative pharyngitis or extensive LA)
HIV	Sero-conversion to HIV+ may produce similar symptoms: Fatigue, pharyngitis
Chronic fatigue syndrome	Profound, debilitating fatigue; fatigue exacerbated by physical exertion, and not alleviated by rest; also may see low-grade fever, sore throat, myalgia, sleep disturbances, short-term memory deficits

CMV, Cytomegalovirus; *HIV,* human immunodeficiency virus; *LA,* lymphadenopathy.

Associated Symptoms

Anorexia
Headache
Abdominal pain
Jaundice (rare)

OBJECTIVE DATA

Physical Examination

A problem-oriented physical should be conducted, with particular attention to:

Vital signs, weight, general appearance
Skin: Maculopapular rash
Head, eyes, ears, nose, and throat: Assess for erythema of pharynx and exudate.
Petechiae at the junction of hard/soft palate occurs in 25%.
Facial edema, especially eyelid edema, is rarely encountered in young adults and is suggestive of mono.
Lymph: Cervical and epitrochlear. Significant lymphadenopathy is almost always present; if not, question diagnosis.
Abdominal
  Hepatomegaly (50%)
  Splenomegaly (75%)
  Children: Assess for dehydration and activity level.

Diagnostic Procedures

Diagnostic procedures are outlined in Table 119-1.

ASSESSMENT

Differential diagnoses are outlined in Table 119-2.

THERAPEUTIC PLAN

Pharmaceutical

Symptomatic treatment only
  Acetaminophen for fever and pain relief
  If antibiotics needed for concomitant strep throat, avoid ampicillin or amoxicillin since they cause a rash in 80% of patients treated

Nonpharmaceutical

Bed rest for fatigue
Maintenance of adequate fluid intake

Anesthetic lozenges for pain relief
Salt water gargles

Diet

Soft diet

Patient Education

Teach the patient to avoid splenic rupture by avoiding minor trauma, heavy lifting, overexertion, and contact sports for 1 to 2 months (rupture usually occurs between 4th and 21st day of illness).
Teach the patient strategies to avoid constipation because it can cause increased pressure on the spleen.
Reassure that the illness is self-limiting and isolation is unnecessary.
Reassure that the EBV is not responsible for chronic fatigue syndrome.

Referral

Marked splenomegaly
Respiratory compromise
Excessively enlarged tonsils and difficulty swallowing
Jaundice
Hyperbilirubinemia

Follow-up

Report abdominal pain and upper quadrant pain radiating to the shoulder promptly.
If the patient experiences shortness of breath or inability to swallow, emergency services should be accessed immediately.
Assess splenomegaly weekly until it no longer persists.

EVALUATION

Antibodies may remain + in blood for up to a year after the illness

SUGGESTED READINGS

Boynton R, Dunn E, Stephens G: *Manual of ambulatory pediatrics*, ed 4, Philadelphia, 1998, Lippincott.
Ellsworth A et al: *Mosby's 1998 medical drug reference*, St Louis, 1998, Mosby.
Healthcare Consultants of America, Inc: *1998 Physicians fee and coding guide*, Augusta, Ga., 1998, Healthcare Consultants of America, Inc.
Hickey S, Strasburger V: What every pediatrician should know about infectious mononucleosis in adolescents, *Pediatr Clin North Am* 11(6):1541-1556, 1997.
Robinson D: Mononucleosis. In Sommers M, Johnson S, editors: *Davis's manual of nursing therapeutics for diseases and disorders*, Philadelphia, 1996, FA Davis.
Wohl D, Isaacson J: Airway obstruction in children with infectious mononucleosis, *Ear Nose Throat J* 74:630-633, 1995.

Multiple Sclerosis

ICD-9-CM

Multiple Sclerosis 340.0

OVERVIEW

Definition

Multiple sclerosis (MS) is a chronic inflammatory demyelinating disease of the central nervous system (CNS) associated with periods of disability (relapsing/flares) alternating with periods of recovery (remission), which often results in progressive neurologic disability. MS may affect all parts of the CNS and produces a multiplicity of symptoms.

There are two phases of disease:

1. Exacerbating-remitting (average one attack per year); after several years, most individuals enter
2. Chronic-progressive phase (50% within 10 years; 60% within 15 years)

Incidence

250,000 to 350,000 Americans, with increasing incidence both nationally and worldwide

30/100,000 prevalence in high risk areas: northern Europe, United States, Canada, southern Australia, New Zealand

Low prevalence around equator

Most common neurologic disease in individuals under 40 years of age; average age 30; **diagnosed as young as 10 years of age; can occur as late as 60 to 70 years of age**

Women: Two to three times rate of men

Factors associated with adverse outcome:

- Older age at onset
- Male
- Cerebellar involvement
- Persisting deficits in brain stem
- Higher frequency of attacks in first 2 years after onset
- High levels of disability
- Short first interattack interval (accelerated deterioration)

Pathophysiology

Etiology unknown; autoimmune disease

Theories of four possible causes:

- Genetics: Presence of genes that code for certain histocompatibility leukocyte antigen genes
- Environmental factors: Documented occurrences of clusters and epidemics reinforce this hypothesis; however, no identified environmental factor
- Immunologic factors: Decreased suppressor T-lymphocytes; excess immunoglobulin; high levels of IgG secreted; loss of suppressor cell inducers
- Viruses: Most widely accepted causal agent; exposure in adolescence, which triggers autoimmune response penetrating blood-brain barrier and causing structural lesions in the CNS

Hormonal factors may be implicated in the disease. Cyclic increase in symptoms associated with menstrual periods, during climacteric, and/or pregnancy suggest hormones may be involved

SUBJECTIVE DATA

History of Present Illness

No characteristic clinical pattern; symptoms extremely variable

Requires careful history with focus on the *temporal profile* of the neurologic deficit, which usually starts unilaterally or focally and eventually becomes bilateral and progressive

Family History

Ask about family history of multiple sclerosis or other autoimmune diseases.

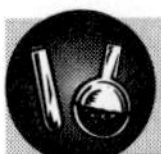

TABLE 120-1 Diagnostic Procedures: Multiple Sclerosis

Symptoms	Findings	Diagnostic Tests	Costs ($)
Most Common			
Decrease in color perception, dull ache behind eye, tingling, numbness, feeling of tightness (as if body part is wrapped in cast), paresthesias, fluctuating weakness of limbs, urgency, intermittent pain, depression	Asymmetrical weakness, sensory loss, pale optic disks, nystagmus, (+) Babinski, spastic gait, ataxia, diminished visual acuity	MRI (good evidence of MS) CSF (not specific for MS; adjunct to support diagnosis) Evoked potential (not specific for MS; may detect abnormalities not clinically evident)	1781-2004 172-208/LP
Less Common			
Facial weakness, hearing loss, trigeminal neuralgia, euphoria, confusion	Hyporeflexia, writhing facial muscles afferent pupillary defect, deafness, muscle atrophy, dementia		
Uncommon			
Aphasia, apraxia	Aphasia, apraxia		

CSF, Cerebrospinal fluid; *LP,* lumbar puncture; *MRI,* magnetic resonance imaging.

Description of Most Common Symptoms

Fatigue, limb weakness, paresthesia, aching pain, double vision, monocular impairment of vision, slurred speech, urgency, constipation, imbalance, impotence, depression, temperature lability

Associated Symptoms

Facial weakness, hearing loss, trigeminal neuralgia, euphoria, confusion, nystagmus

Uncommon Symptoms

Severe apraxia or aphasia, extrapyramidal movement disorders, seizures, perineal pains, hypersomnolence

OBJECTIVE DATA

Physical Examination

Neurological examination
- Most common signs: Asymmetrical weakness, sensory loss, pale optic disks, nystagmus, (+) Babinski, spastic gait, ataxia, diminished visual acuity
- Less common signs: Hyporeflexia, writhing facial muscles, afferent pupillary defect, deafness, muscle atrophy, significant dementia
- Uncommon signs: Aphasia, apraxia

Diagnostic Procedures

The diagnosis of MS should remain primarily clinical since confirmatory tests are nonspecific; however, the following tests in Table 120-1 may increase diagnostic sensitivity and should be evaluated in the clinical context.
- MRI: Gold standard; multiple (two to three) white matter lesions clinically definitive (Table 120-2)
- Cerebrospinal fluid: Cell count less than 40 WBCs; protein under 100 mg/dl; oligoclonal immunoglobulin bands (+); IgG index above 0.70
- Evoked potential (visual, auditory, somatosensory, motor) studies: Identify subclinical areas of disease

ASSESSMENT

Multiple sclerosis is difficult to diagnose because many symptoms mimic those of other diseases. Diagnosis is generally made by means of observation of the temporal clinical course, in conjunction with a neurologic examination and laboratory tests.

Differential diagnoses include the following (refer to Table 120-3).
- *Systemic lupus erythematosus*
- *Myalgia encephalomyelitis/chronic fatigue syndrome*
- Lyme disease
- CNS lesions/tumors
- *Acquired immunodeficiency syndrome*
- Seizure disorder
- *Peripheral neuropathy*

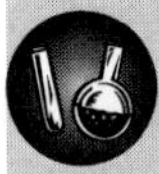

TABLE 120-2 Influence of Positive MRI/CSF Oligoclonal Bands on Diagnosis of Multiple Sclerosis

History (No. of Attacks)	Clinical Evidence	MRI/Oligoclonal Bands	Diagnosis
Two	Two lesions	Clinical diagnosis	Clinically definite MS
Two	Two lesions	+MRI	Clinically definite MS
		–MRI	Clinically probable MS
Two	One lesion	+Oligoclonal bands	Lab supported definite MS
		–Oligoclonal bands	Clinically probable MS
One	One lesion	+MRI* +Oligoclonal bands	Laboratory-supported definite MS
		+MRI* -Oligoclonal bands	Clinically probable MS
One	One lesion	–MRI +Oligoclonal bands	Not diagnostic
One	One lesion	–MRI –Oligoclonal bands	Not diagnostic

CSF, Cerebrospinal fluid; *MRI,* magnetic resonance imaging.
*New lesions developing on follow-up MRI; single MRI not diagnostic (Ford and Johnson, 1995).

TABLE 120-3 Differential Diagnosis: Multiple Sclerosis

Diagnoses	Supporting Data
Multiple sclerosis	Episodic focal neurologic symptoms dependent on locations of demyelinating lesions MRI: Demonstrates the widespread multifocal areas of demyelination CSF: Up to 50 mononuclear cells/mm^3 (higher levels should raise suspicion of other diseases); protein up to 80 mg/dl; glucose normal; oligoclonal bands of IgG (occurs in 80% of cases); visual-auditory-somatosensory-evoked potential helps detect asymptomatic involvement of the appropriate systems
Systemic lupus erythematosus	Episodic symptoms, including fatigue, fever, weight loss, migratory myalgias, migratory arthralgias, arthritis, rash, depression, headaches, seizures +MRI +ANA Anti-dsDNA Low C3 High ESR
Chronic fatigue syndrome	Fatigue, migratory myalgias, migratory arthralgias, migratory painful paresthesias, memory and cognitive disturbances, dizziness, sensation of dysequilibrium, sleep disturbance, anhedonia Diagnosis is one of exclusion

ANA, Antinuclear antibody; *CSF,* cerebrospinal fluid; *MRI,* magnetic resonance imaging.

THERAPEUTIC PLAN

Pharmaceutical

Goals
- Treat acute exacerbations (Tables 120-4 and 120-5)
- Manage chronic symptoms (Table 120-6)
- Delay progression of disease (Table 120-7)

Under study (most promising, fewer exacerbations):
- Cladribine 2CD-A, reduces the number of new or active lesions by programming lymphocyte cell death; plasma exchange has met with mixed results

Patient Education

Health promotion/maintenance: Physical therapy, exercise, group therapy, individual counseling
Safety issues in the home related to leg spasticity, decreased visual acuity, changes in balance
Provide information about illness; treatment is palliative, and course is unpredictable
Provide current research on MS, medications, side effects
Provide family planning services; **pregnancy not contraindicated; exacerbations found in postpartum period**

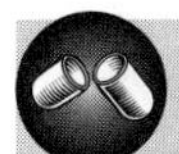

TABLE 120-4 Treatment Recommendations: Multiple Sclerosis

Syndrome	Cost/Treatment
Mild relapse of relapsing-remitting	None
Moderate-severe relapse of relapsing-remitting	$17-$30/IVMP (intravenously administered methylprednisolone) 500 mg QD ×5 days
Recent accelerated deterioration in progressive disease	IVMP 500 mg QD ×5 days
Sustained deterioration in severe progressive refractory to IVMP	$220-$404/Oral low-dose methotrexate

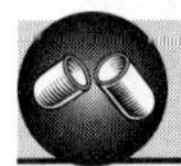

TABLE 120-5 Acute Exacerbations

Drug	Dosage	Comments
Intravenously administered methylprednisolone (IVMP)	500 mg QD ×5 days	
IV dexamethasone $5-$30	8 mg ×7 days, 4 mg ×4 days, 2 mg ×3 days	Efficacy comparable to IVMP

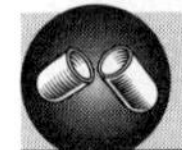

TABLE 120-6 Chronic Symptoms

Symptom	Drug Cost/ Generic (Trade)	Dose	Comments
Spasticity	$11-$52/baclofen (Lioresal)	Adult: PO 15-25 mg TID	Drug of choice; may increase weakness of spastic limbs; abrupt withdrawal may cause hallucinations Pregnancy: C
	$2-$43/diazepam (Valium)	Adult: PO 2-10 mg BID-QID Child >6 mo: PO 1-2.5 mg TID-QID	Causes sedation and dependency; avoid abrupt withdrawal Pregnancy: D
	$135/tizanidine (Zanaflex)	Adult: 4 mg PO @ hs increase by ½ tablet (2 mg) q3 days, not to exceed 36 mg/day (12 mg TID)	Decreased hypotension, give with food, decreased dosage needed with OC due to 50% decreased clearance of drug
	$72/dantrolene (Dantrium)	Adult: PO 25-50 mg/day; max 400 mg/day ×1 wk Child: PO 1 mg/kg/day in divided doses BID-TID; max 100 mg QID	Negative effect on strength; monitor for hepatic toxicity at least q3 months Pregnancy: C
Fatigue	$19-$85/amantadine (Symmetrel)	Adult: PO 100 mg/BID; max 400 mg/day	Ankle edema; nervousness, sleep disturbances; blurred vision Pregnancy: C
Depression	$176-$181/sertraline $215-$220/fluoxetine $184-$189/fluvoxamine $57-$65/paroxetine	Adult: PO 25-200 mg QD PO 10-80 mg/day PO 25-300 mg/day PO 10-50 mg/day	First line for depression; contraindicated in those with hypersensitivity to it and those taking monoamine oxidase inhibitors Pregnancy: B

BUN, Blood urea nitrogen; *GI,* gastrointestinal; *Hct,* hematocrit; *Hgb,* hemoglobin; *NSAID,* nonsteroidal antiinflammatory drug; *OC,* oral contraceptives; *RBC,* red blood cells; *U/A,* urinalysis.

Continued

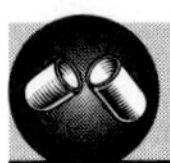

TABLE 120-6 Chronic Symptoms—cont'd

Symptom	Drug Cost/ Generic (Trade)	Dose	Comments
Bladder Dysfunction	$18-$50/oxybutynin (Ditropan)	Adult: PO 5 mg BID-TID Child >5 y/o: PO 5 mg BID; max 5 mg TID	Decreases frequency; may produce dry mouth, accommodation disturbances, tachycardia, mental confusion secondary to anticholinergic side effects of Ditropan Pregnancy: C
	$6-$48/prazosin (Minipress)	Adult: PO 0.5 mg/day to most effective tolerated dose	Decreases outflow obstruction; monitor blood urea nitrogen (BUN), uric acid; may cause hypotension, syncope, fatigue Pregnancy: C
	$70/desmopressin (DDAVP)	Adult: Intranasal 0.1-0.4 mg QD in divided doses; SC 0.2-0.4 mg QD in divided doses Child 3 mo-12 y/o: intranasal 0.05-0.3 mg QD in divided doses	Decreases nocturia: may cause nasal irritation, headache, lethargy Pregnancy: B
Ataxia Tremors	$57-$73/clonazepam (Klonopin)	Adult: PO 0.5 mg/day TID; max dose 20 mg/day Child <10 y/o: PO 0.01-0.03 mg/kg/day q8h; max dose .05 mg/kg/day	Sedative, muscle relaxing effects limiting factors Pregnancy: C
	$10-$39/carbamazepine (Tegretol)	Adult: PO 200 mg BID; max dose 1200 mg/day	UA, creatinine, BUN q 3 mo; RBC, Hct, Hgb, reticulocyte counts q wk for 4 wk then q mo; ophthalmic examination before, during, and after treatment; severe skin reaction may occur Pregnancy: C
	$1-$14/isoniazid (INH)	Adult: PO 5 mg/kg/day Child: PO 10 mg/kg/day	Hepatitis and bone marrow suppression have occurred; avoid use in hepatic or renal disease; vitamin B_6 supplements 25 mg QD recommended Pregnancy: C
	Beta-blockers and/or $14-$16/Valproic acid (Depakene)		Generally disappointing results
Pain	NSAIDs		Contraindicated in patients with asthma, renal, hepatic or ulcer disease, GI bleeding is potential side effect from chronic NSAID administration Pregnancy: B
	$2-$19/amitriptyline (Elavil)	Adult: 15-75 mg/day	Caution in patients with cardiac, hepatic, renal disease, extreme caution in elderly secondary to severe anti-cholinergic effects Pregnancy: C

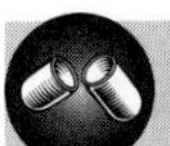

TABLE 120-7 Drugs Used to Reduce Rate of Relapse, Slow Progression

Drug	Dose	Comments	Cost ($)
Azathioprine (Imuran)	*Adult:* PO 1-3 mg/kg/day	Reduces frequency of relapses, modestly retards progression; commonly induces anemia, gastrointestinal complaints, reactivation of latent viral infection; monitor RBC, transaminase levels monthly Pregnancy: D	$118
Cyclophosphamide (Cytoxan)	*Adult:* PO/IV 750 mg/m^2 q mo	Systemic toxic effects may outweigh benefits Pregnancy: D	152-280
Cyclosporine (Sandimmune)	*Adult, Child:* PO/IV 15 mg/kg/day initially; 5-10 mg/kg/day maintenance IV 5-6 mg/kg/day	Reduces progression to wheelchair-confined status; does not affect number of lesions. Risk of renal toxicity and hypertension outweigh modest benefits Pregnancy: C	42-168
Methotrexate (MTX)	*Adult:* PO/IM/IV 7.5 mg q wk	Reduces progressive disability; monitor RBC, transaminase levels, BUN monthly; patients should avoid pregnancy, alcohol, ASA, trimethoprim-sulfamethoxazole, anticoagulants Pregnancy: X	220-404
Interferon beta (Betaseron)	*Adult:* SC 0.25 mg QOD *Child:* Safety and efficacy not established	Influences rate of exacerbation and progressive disability; discontinue use with pregnancy, skin necrosis, severe depression, lack of compliance, and continued frequent exacerbations Pregnancy: C	72
Glatiramer acetate (Copaxone)	SC 20 mg QD	Lowers relapse rate in patients who become resistant to interferon Beta treatment	23-37
Interferon beta-1a (Avonex)	*Adult:* SC/IM 30 µg weekly *Child:* Safety and efficacy not established	Use cautiously with chronic progressive MS, suicidal tendencies or mental disorders, cardiac disease, seizures Pregnancy: C	710

ASA, Aspirin *BUN,* blood urea nitrogen; *RBC,* red blood count.

Encourage avoiding excessive fatigue; maintaining well-balanced diet; there is no evidence that specific diets affect the course of the disease

Referral

MS is a multifaceted disease, often requiring care from neurologists, urologists, physical therapists, home health, and psychologists. Management of acute exacerbations, hospitalizations, and chronic symptoms should be coordinated by neurologist.

Positive finding on neurological examination requires referral to neurologist.

Pregnancy requires referral to obstetrician.

Bladder dysfunction requires referral to urologist.

Spasticity requires referral to physical therapist.

The primary care provider is in an ideal position to care for patient by coordinating services, offering emotional support, managing episodic illness.

EVALUATION/FOLLOW-UP

Annual laboratory tests: Complete blood count, chemistry profile, urinalysis, screening tests, influenza vaccinations along with thorough examinations to assess client's condition

Episodic illness: Increased risk of sinusitis; pseudoexacerbations caused by fever and infection

Interferon beta-1b may cause depression of white blood cells and elevation of liver function tests. Follow monthly for 3 months, then every 3 months.

RESOURCE

National Multiple Sclerosis Society
733 Third Ave.
New York, NY 10017
1-800-344-4867
info@NMSS.org

REFERENCE

Ford HL, Johnson MH: Telling your patient he/she has multiple sclerosis, *Postgrad Med J* 71(838):449-452, 1995.

SUGGESTED READINGS

Brod SA, Lindsey JW, Wolinsky JS: Multiple sclerosis: clinical presentation, diagnosis and treatment, *Am Family Phys* 54(4):1309-1311, 1996.

Collard RC, Koehler RPM, Mattson DH: Frequency and significance of antinuclear antibodies in multiple sclerosis, *Neurology* 49:857-861, 1997.

Hogencamp WE, Rodriguez M, Weinshenker BG: The epidemiology of multiple sclerosis, *Mayo Clin Proc* 72:871-878, 1997.

Hunter SF, et al: Rational clinical immunotherapy for multiple sclerosis, *Mayo Clin Proc* 72:765-780, 1997.

Kaufman MD: Multiple sclerosis. In *Saunders manual of medical practice*, Philadelphia, 1996, WB Saunders.

Palacce J, Rothwell P: New treatments and azathioprine in multiple sclerosis, *Lancet* 350:261, 1997.

Pender MP: Recent advances in the understanding, diagnosis and management of multiple sclerosis, *N Zealand J Med* 26:157-161, 1996.

Poser CM: The epidemiology of multiple sclerosis: a general overview, *Ann Neurol* 36(S2):S180-193, 1994.

Rudick R et al: Management of multiple sclerosis, *N Engl J Med* 337:1604-1611, 1997.

Swain SE: Multiple sclerosis: primary health care implications, *Nurse Pract* 21(7):40-54, 1996.

Thompson AJ: Multiple sclerosis: symptomatic treatment, *J Neurol* 243:559-565, 1996.

van Oosten BW, et al: Multiple sclerosis therapy: a practical guide, *Drugs* 49(2):200-212, 1995.

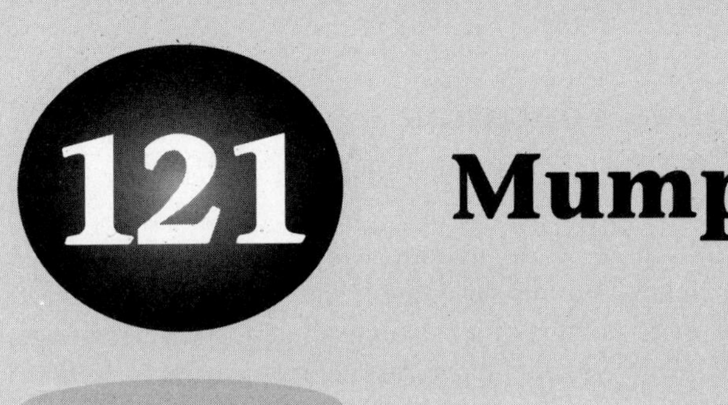

121 Mumps

ICD-9-CM

Mumps Without Mention of Complication 072.9

OVERVIEW

Definition

Mumps is an acute, systemic disease caused by a paramyxovirus. It is characterized by swelling of the salivary glands but can involve multiple organs and may be moderately debilitating.

Incidence

Mumps outbreaks occur in late winter and spring. It has a 16- to 18-day incubation period and is contagious for 1 or 2 days before and 3 to 7 days after swelling is noted.

Pathophysiology

Administration of the mumps vaccine or contracting the illness confers lifelong immunity. Serological studies show that more than 85% of unimmunized adults have had a mumps infection.

Mumps is spread by direct contact and respiratory routes. Humans are the only known natural hosts.

SUBJECTIVE DATA

History of Present Illness

Patient has had 1 or 2 days of fever, headache, malaise, and swelling of one or more salivary glands.

Past Medical History

Ask about the patient's immunization history, recent exposure to mumps or other infections, and any known allergies.

Medications

Determine whether the patient is currently taking any medications.

Family History

Ask about any recent illness of household members and the immunization status of family members.

Description of Most Common Symptoms

Parotitis
Aseptic meningitis (usually without sequelae)
Orchitis (usually unilateral) occurs in 20% to 30% of postpubertal males

Associated Symptoms

Encephalitis and pancreatitis are rare. Oophoritis occurs in 5% of postpubertal females.

OBJECTIVE DATA

Physical Examination

Head/eyes/ears/nose/throat: Observe the parotid gland: Swelling and pain will be present on palpation at the angle of mandible; the swelling pushes the earlobe up and outward.

Stensen's duct: Swelling, redness, and yellow drainage without pus will be present. The submandibular and sublingual gland will be swollen.

Genitals: Observe for orchitis, epididymitis, or oophoritis.

TABLE 121-1 Differential Diagnosis: Mumps

Diagnosis	Supporting Data
Cervical adenitis	Angle of jaw may be observed but earlobe not displaced; Stensen's duct normal
Bacterial parotitis	Pus in Stensen's duct; systemic toxicity

Diagnostic Procedures

The diagnosis is made on clinical grounds. Serological tests can confirm the diagnosis, since mumps is now a rare infection. The virus can be isolated from saliva, blood, urine, and cerebrospinal fluid during the acute phase of the disease. Skin tests are unreliable.

ASSESSMENT

Differential Diagnosis

Differential diagnoses for mumps include those listed in Table 121-1.

THERAPEUTIC PLAN

Pharmaceutical

None

Lifestyle/Activities

Supportive care is appropriate. Scrotal support can be provided for orchitis.

Diet

As tolerated.

Encourage fluids.

Sour foods cause pain because they stimulate salivary flow, and swallowing is painful.

Patient Education

The **child** should not attend school or day care for 9 days after the onset of swelling.

Immunization with mumps vaccine should be given routinely as a measles/mumps/rubella (MMR) vaccine at 12 to 15 months of age and again at 4 to 6 years of age.

Mild fever without upper respiratory symptoms is not a contraindication to vaccination.

Mumps can occur in highly vaccinated populations, including individuals who have had mumps immunization.

Permanent sequelae (such as sterility) or death is uncommon.

Family Impact

The need for child care during the period of communicability may pose a problem for working parents.

Referral/Consultation

Women who become pregnant within 3 months after receiving mumps vaccine or who are infected during the first trimester of pregnancy should be referred to an OB/GYN.

Unimmunized children with severe egg allergies should be referred to an allergist for immunization.

Follow-up

Aseptic meningitis occurs in 50% of cases.

EVALUATION

Rare complications include arthritis, renal involvement, thyroiditis, mastitis, pancreatitis, and hearing impairment.

SUGGESTED READINGS

American Academy of Pediatrics: Mumps. In Peter G, editor: *1997 Red book: report of the committee on infectious disease,* ed 24, Elk Grove Village, Ill, 1997, The Academy.

American Public Health Association: *Control of communicable diseases manual,* ed 16, Washington, DC, 1995, The Association.

Ellsworth A et al: *Mosby's 1998 medical drug reference,* St Louis, 1998, Mosby.

Healthcare Consultants of America, Inc: *1998 Physicians fee and coding guide,* Augusta, Ga, 1998, Healthcare Consultants of America, Inc.

122 Muscular Dystrophy

ICD-9-CM

Congenital Muscular Dystrophies 359.0
Duchenne's Muscular Dystrophy 359.1
Becker's Muscular Dystrophy 359.1
Myotonic Dystrophy 359.2

OVERVIEW

Definition

Muscular dystrophy (MD) is a genetically determined (X-linked recessive) disease that features progressive muscle fiber degeneration in the absence of other nervous system abnormalities. There are approximately eight types of MD. The most common are Duchenne's (Duchenne type) muscular dystrophy (DMD) and Becker's (Becker type) (BMD). In Duchenne type, the disease usually develops before age 5. Becker type is similar to Duchenne type but has a milder course (average age at onset, 11 years). Weakness may present later in life, and ambulation is preserved into the third decade.

Incidence

Duchenne MD has an incidence of 1:4000 **children.**

Pathophysiology

Duchenne-Becker is an X-linked disease resulting in complete (Duchenne) or partial (Becker) loss-of-function mutations in the dystrophin gene product. It is theorized that dystrophin maintains the integrity of the muscle cell wall. Where it is deficient, there is an influx of calcium, a breakdown of the calcium complex, and an excess of free radicals. These lead eventually to irreversible destruction of the muscle cells (Lissauer and Clayden, 1997).

SUBJECTIVE DATA

History of Present Illness

Ask the patient or family about:
- Muscle weakness
- Difficulty walking on toes and climbing stairs (patient goes up one by one)
- Waddling gait
- Frequent falls
- Any swallowing problems
- Leg pain, which may be an early component
- Whether developmental milestones were normal until the child began walking

Past Medical History

Ask the patient or family about:
- Frequent respiratory infections
- History of falls
- Inability to keep up with running and sports

Medications

Noncontributory

Family History

Muscle diseases

Psychosocial History

School performance
Sports abilities

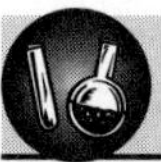

TABLE 122-1 Diagnostic Tests: Muscular Dystrophy

Test	Finding/Rationale	Cost ($)
CPK	Elevated CPK levels, which decrease over time Marked ↑ in Duchenne's, moderate ↑ in Becker's May be affected by multiple drugs and disorders	23-39
Muscle biopsy	Degeneration of muscle fibers with progressive fibrosis (fiber-splitting, necrosis, regeneration with interspersed fibrosis)	194-235/superficial 354-470/deep
EMG	Recommended for myotonic dystrophy	393-475
Dystrophin level	Low to absent in muscle biopsy specimens	N/A
CT of brain	Reveals gyrus abnormalities and cerebral hypodensity	990-1175
Genetic testing	Identify female carriers via DNA analysis	385-695

CPK, Creatine phosphokinase; *CT,* computed tomography; *DNA,* deoxyribonucleic acid; *EMG,* electromyelogram; *N/A,* not available.

OBJECTIVE DATA

Physical Examination

Most patients will present with concerns about weakness and frequent falls. The purpose of the examination is to evaluate the extent of muscle weakness and to suspect MD. A complete physical examination should be completed, with particular attention to:

- Head/eyes/ears/nose/throat: Facial weakness; high forehead with receding hairline
- Respiratory: Respiratory effort
- Cardiovascular: Cardiac conduction defects, arrhythmias
- Musculoskeletal: Gait (look for a waddling gait)
  - Weakness in proximal muscles
  - Gowers' sign: Sign of generalized muscle weakness: Patient maneuvers to a position supported by both arms and legs, pushes off the floor to rest hands on knees, then pushes himself upright.
  - Pseudohypertrophy of the calves and deltoids (feel large and firm), exaggerated biceps
  - Decreased strength: Inability to do push-ups
  - Winging of scapula
  - Contractions of Achilles tendons
- Neurological: Intelligence may be decreased

Diagnostic Procedures

Diagnostic procedures for muscular dystrophy are listed in Table 122-1.

ASSESSMENT

Differential Diagnosis

Differential diagnoses include those listed in Table 122-2 and Figure 122-1.

THERAPEUTIC PLAN

Treatment consists of supportive care in most cases.

Pharmaceutical

Prednisone 0.15 to 0.75 mg/kg/day may be helpful in improving muscle strength in boys. This should be prescribed by a neurologist/orthopedist/specialist who is coordinating the patient's care.

Lifestyle/Activities

Depend on level of muscular disability.

Stretching exercises and night splints may play a role in the treatment plan.

Exercise will help the patient maintain muscle power and mobility and will delay the onset of scoliosis.

Walking can be prolonged with use of orthoses.

Diet

Depends on level of muscular disability

Monitor nutritional status

Patient Education

Use of a good sitting posture helps minimize the risk of scoliosis.

Referral/Consultation

Discuss any concerns over developmental delays with the physician. Refer any child with suspected muscle weakness for more specialized testing.

Recommend that the patient see a perinatologist and receive genetic counseling if there is a positive family history of the disease.

TABLE 122-2 Differential Diagnosis: Muscular Dystrophy

Diagnosis	Supporting Data
Myasthenia gravis	Hypotonia and weakness, weak cry, and feeding difficulties that respond to anticholinesterase therapy; positive family history
Congenital myotonic dystrophy	Disease of early childhood, an autosomal-dominant inherited disease; symptoms include difficulty swallowing and varying degrees of respiratory difficulty
Spinal muscular atrophy syndromes	Caused by degeneration of the nuclei of the motor cranial nerves and anterior horn cells; weakness is the primary symptom seen, with floppiness and poor head and extremity control; decreased deep tendon reflex

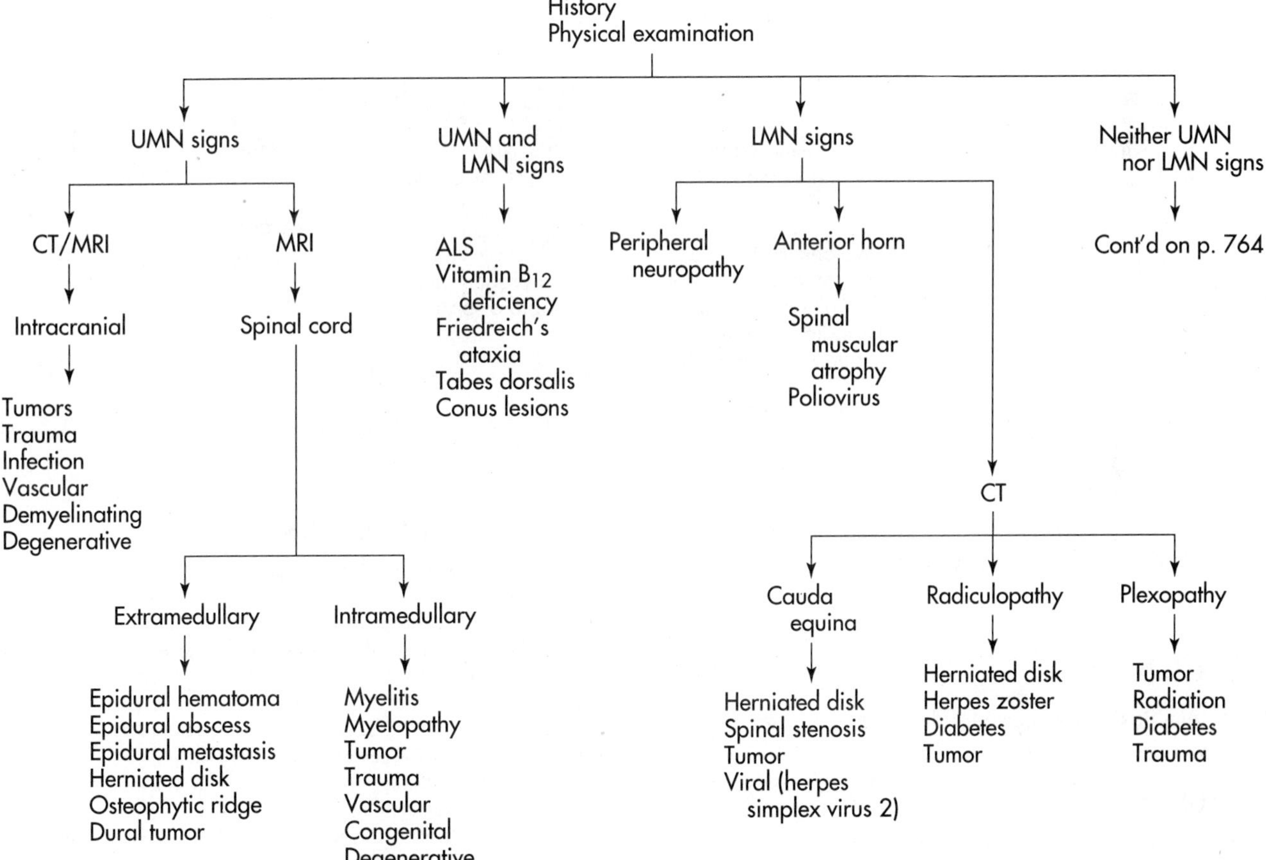

Figure 122-1 Algorithm for treatment of a patient with weakness. *ALS,* Amyotrophic lateral sclerosis; *CK,* creatine kinase; *LMN,* lower motor neuron; *TFTs,* thyroid function tests; *UMN,* upper motor neuron. (From Greene HL, Johnson WP, Lemcke D: *Decision making in medicine,* ed 2, St Louis, 1998, Mosby.)

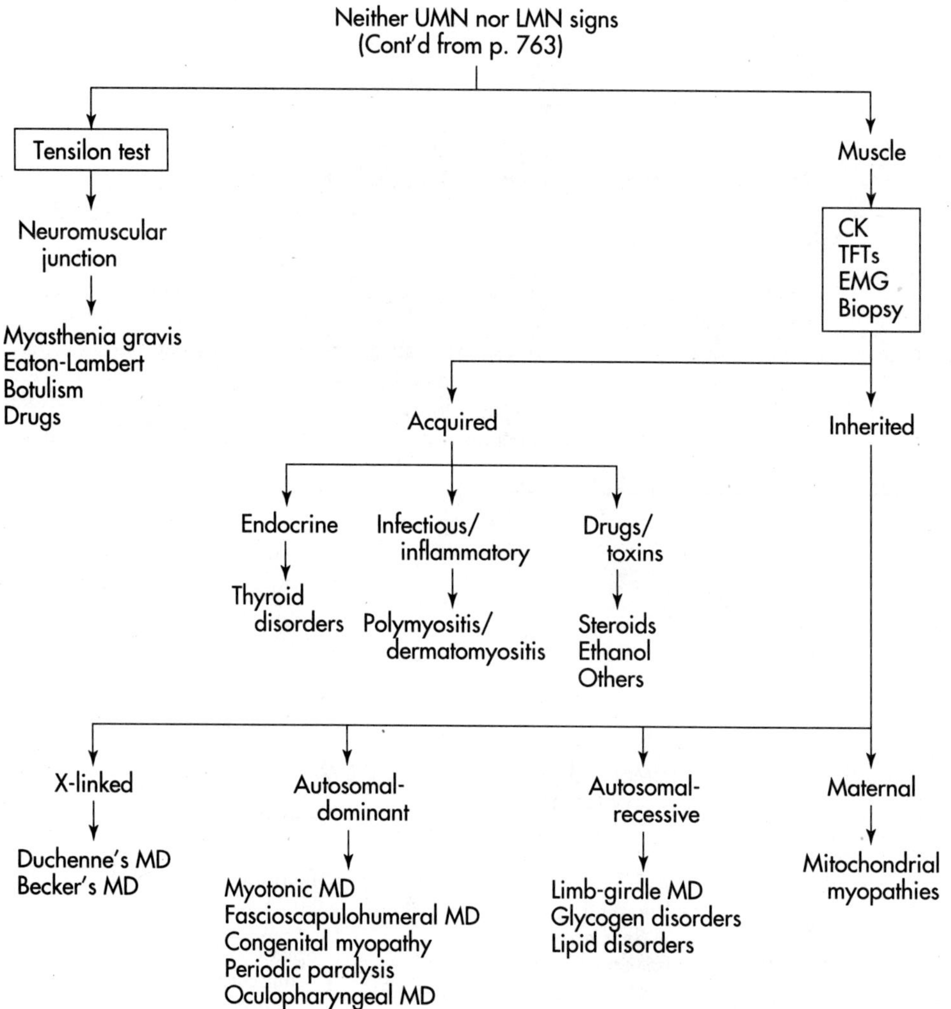

Figure 122-1, cont'd For legend see p. 763.

Recommend family counseling; prevention is accomplished through identification of whether the mother is a carrier of the implicated gene.

EVALUATION

Timely diagnosis of a muscular disorder is important. Outcome depends on the level of muscular disability.

RESOURCES

Parent self-help groups for information and support
Muscular Dystrophy Association: www.mdausa.org

REFERENCE

Lissauer T, Clayden G: *Illustrated textbook of pediatrics,* St Louis, 1997, Mosby.

SUGGESTED READINGS

Dubowitz V: *Muscle disorders in childhood,* Philadelphia, 1995, WB Saunders.

Eggers S, Zatz M: How the magnitude of clinical severity and recurrence risk affects reproductive decisions in adult males with different forms of progressive muscular dystrophy, *J Med Ethics* 35:189-195, 1998.

Eggers S, Zatz M: Social adjustment in adult males affected with progressive muscular dystrophy, *Am J Med Genetics* 81:4-12, 1998.

Ferriero D, Weiss W: The nervous system. In Rudolph A, Kamei R, editors: *Rudolph's fundamentals of pediatrics,* ed 2, Norwalk, Conn, 1998, Appleton & Lange.

Healthcare Consultants of America, Inc: *1998 Physicians fee and coding guide,* Augusta, Ga, 1998, Healthcare Consultants of America, Inc.

Rankin L: Weakness. In Greene H, Johnson W, Lemcke D, editors: *Decision making in medicine,* ed 2, St Louis, 1998, Mosby.

VanderKooi A et al: Limb girdle muscular dystrophy: pathology and immunohistochemical re-evaluation, *Muscle Nerve* 21:584-590, 1998.

Voit T: Congenital muscular dystrophy: 1997 update, *Brain Devel* 20:65-74, 1998.

123 Musculoskeletal Injuries: Ankle

ICD-9-CM

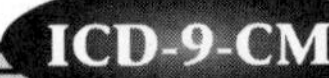

Sprains and Strains 848.9

OVERVIEW

Definitions

A sprain is an injury to one of the ligamentous structures of the body. A fracture is a loss in continuity in the substance of the bone.

Anatomy

The ankle joint is composed of three bones: The distal fibula (lateral malleolus), the distal tibia (medial malleolus), and the talus. These bones are held together medially by the deltoid ligament and laterally by three ligaments: The anterior talofibular ligament, the calcaneofibular ligament, and the posterior talofibular ligament (Figures 123-1 and 123-2). The distal tibia and fibula are connected together by the tibiofibular ligament and the syndesmosis.

Pathophysiology

Sprain

Ligaments, which connect bones together, can sustain injuries. Ligamentous injuries are classified as grade I, grade II, or grade III, depending on the extent of injury. A completely torn ligament is classified as a grade III sprain, whereas a mildly stretched ligament is classified as a grade I sprain. Ankle sprains may occur as a result of an inversion, eversion or rotation of the ankle. Inversion injuries are the most common with the foot turning inward at the ankle such as occurs with basketball injuries. Less common eversion injuries occur when a wrestler tries to get a wider stance. Tibiofibular injuries may occur with a forced rotation of the ankle.

Fracture

Ankle fractures also occur as a result of inversion or eversion injuries to the ankle. The fracture may be a small avulsion fracture of the fibula or tibia caused by the attachments of ligaments being sheered off as a result of force applied to the ligaments. Additionally, the actual force acting on the ankle may fracture the distal fibula, tibia, or both. If the supporting structures about the ankle are also disrupted along with the fracture, then the talus may dislocate out of the mortise. Also proximal fibular fractures may occur as a result of force displaced with severe ankle fractures and dislocations.

Common Injuries

Ankle sprains are most commonly caused by inversion of the ankle, resulting in injury to one or more of the lateral ankle ligaments—the anterior talofibular, the calcaneofibular, and the posterior talofibular. Eversion ankle injuries commonly involve the deltoid ligament of the medial ankle.

Ankle fractures involve the medial malleolus, the lateral malleolus, or both.

SUBJECTIVE DATA

History of Present Illness

Ask about:

- Exact mechanism of injury; timing of injury
- Description/location of pain
- Radiation, quality, timing, severity, aggravation/relief
- Previous treatment

Past Medical History

Previous injuries, especially ankle trauma; surgical history; exercise history

Any allergies

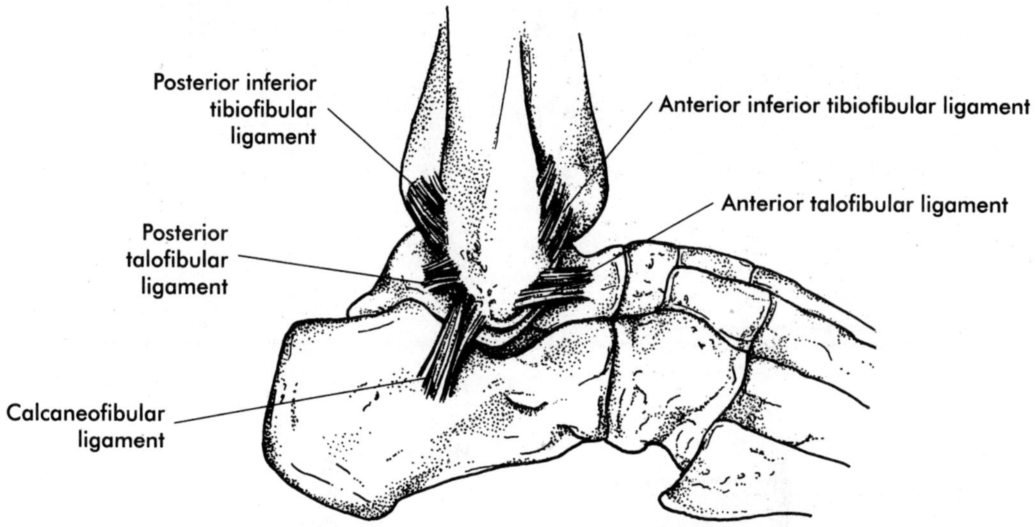

Figure 123-1 Lateral ligaments of the ankle. The composite of ligaments of the syndesmosis and the four ligaments of the ankle joint. (From Baxter DE: *The foot and ankle in sport,* St Louis, 1995, Mosby.)

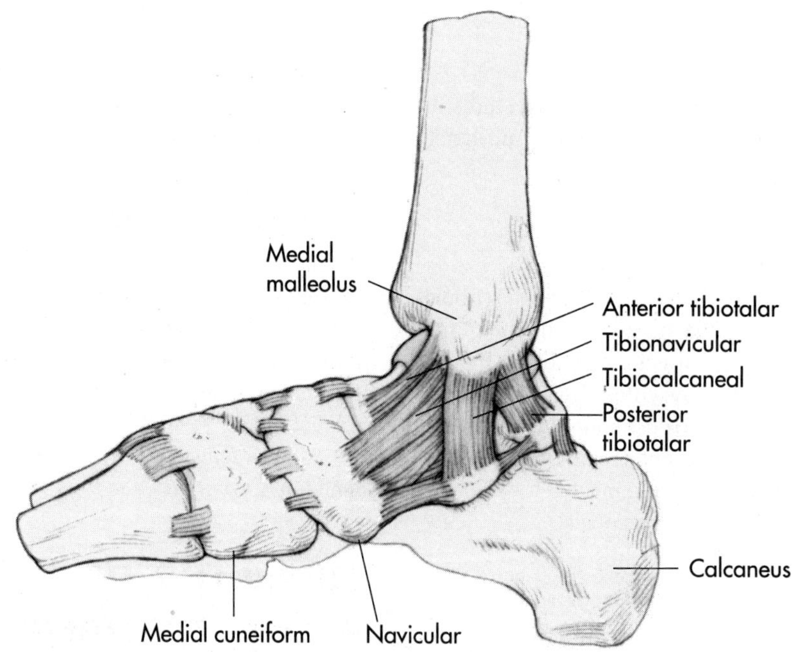

Figure 123-2 The deltoid ligament, which attaches the medial malleolus of the tibia to several underlying bones. It consists of anterior tibiotalar, tibionavicular, tibiocalcaneal, and posterior tibiotalar portions. (From Mathers LH et al: *Clinical anatomy principles,* St Louis, 1995, Mosby.)

Medications

Recent or present use of pain medications, nonsteroidal antiinflammatory drugs (NSAIDs), other medications

Family History

Orthopedic problems

Psychosocial History

Ask the patient about:

Occupational—job description
Smoking, alcohol intake
Conditioning history (e.g., aerobic training such as running, strength training such as weight lifting)

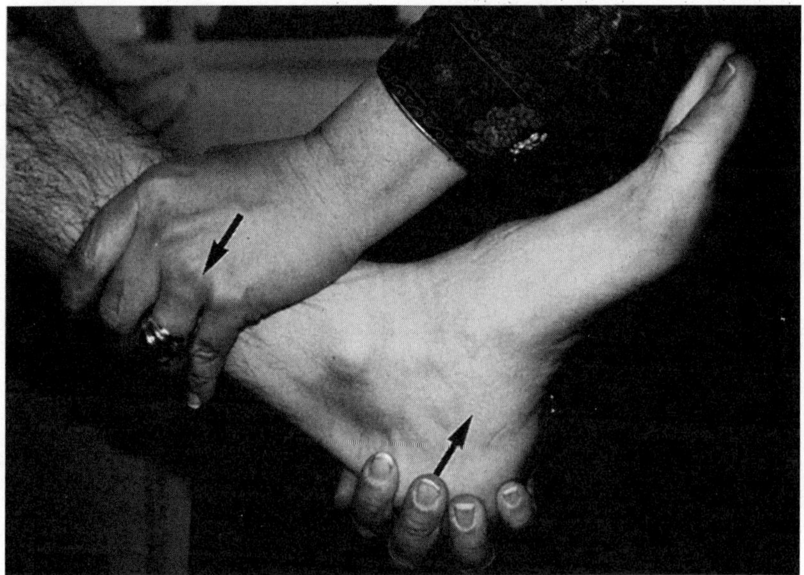

Figure 123-3 The anterior drawer test. One of the examiner's hands grasps the distal tibia, while the other hand grasps the patient's heel and attempts to displace the foot anteriorly. (From Scuderi GR, McCann PD, Bruno PJ: *Sports medicine: principles of primary care,* St Louis, 1997, Mosby.)

Pertinent History of Common Ankle Injuries

Ankle sprains usually result from an inversion injury in which the lateral ligaments of the ankle are damaged. Eversion injuries, although less common, do occur as do injuries to the tibiofibular ligament. Ankle fractures may occur as a result of inversion or eversion injuries.

Associated Symptoms

Swelling, deformity, masses, paralysis, gait changes

OBJECTIVE DATA

Physical Examination

A problem-oriented physical examination should be conducted, with particular attention to:

Vital signs: Should be relatively normal with common nonlife-threatening injuries.

General: Note gait, patient response to pain, and how the patient is holding the injured extremity.

The musculoskeletal examination should include observation for swelling and effusion, palpation of adjacent and actual areas of injury, evaluation of range of motion (ROM), and physical testing to diagnose a specific condition.

Inspect the ankle while the patient is bearing weight.

Check for malleolar pain or bone tenderness on the posterior edge or tip of lateral or medial malleolus.

ROM: Point to the ceiling, point to the floor.

Bend the sole of the foot first away and then toward other foot (inversion/eversion).

Abduct and adduct the foot.

Neurovascular assessment should be performed distal to the injury. Check pulses, sensation, and capillary refill.

Specific Physical Findings of Common Ankle Injuries

Ankle sprains include mild to severe swelling over the area involved and mild to severe pain over the lateral ligaments and lateral malleolus. Inversion ankle sprains are often difficult to differentiate from distal fibular avulsion fractures, since both present with similar physical findings. Assessment includes palpation of the distal tibia, fibula, all ankle ligaments, and the fifth metatarsal base. Joint laxity reveals a positive anterior drawer sign (Figure 123-3), indicating a significant ligament injury. Palpate the proximal fibula with all severe ankle injuries to assess for proximal fracture.

Diagnostic Procedures

Diagnostic procedures for ankle injuries are outlined in Table 123-1.

Radiographic Findings of Common Ankle Injuries

Ankle sprains usually reveal normal findings on film, with soft tissue swelling present, but they can include avulsion fractures of the distal fibula or tibia. Ankle fractures may reveal malleolar fractures of the tibia or fibula or bimalleolar

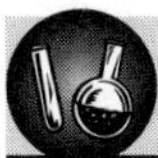

TABLE 123-1 Diagnostic Tests: Ankle Injury

Tests	Findings/Rationale	Cost ($)
Ankle x-ray evaluation	Consider when significant pain, swelling, effusion, or contusion is present. Consider use of Ottawa ankle rules for determining who needs to have x-ray evaluation. Obtain x-ray if the following are present: Pain in malleolar zone Bone tenderness on the posterior edge or tip of lateral or medial malleolus Unable to bear weight, both immediately and in the emergency department For ankle injuries always obtain anteroposterior, lateral, oblique, and mortise-view films. Also consider x-ray evaluation of the foot if the fifth metatarsal base is tender. Comparison views of the opposite normal extremity may be helpful if the injury involves a growth plate in a child.	108-129

TABLE 123-2 Differential Diagnosis: Ankle Injuries

Diagnosis	Supporting Data
Bursitis	Limitation of movement caused by swelling, pain on movement, point tenderness; site is erythematous and warm. The most common site for the ankle is the Achilles bursa.
Gout (Ch. 82)	Increased uric acid production; red, hot; swollen joint, exquisite pain, limited range of motion, tophi, low-grade fever; more common in men >40 years old.
Osteoarthritis (Ch. 15)	Articular deterioration and bony overgrowth of the joint surface. Pain is the most common symptom, occurring with motion and activity, relieved by rest. Findings on physical examination include crepitus, swelling, restriction of movement, and joint enlargement. X-ray evaluation reveals joint space narrowing, spur formation, sclerosis, and subchondral cyst formation.
Rheumatoid arthritis	Multiple joints involved. Females most commonly affected. Usually subacute in onset, often symmetrical. Morning stiffness >1 hr; joint involvement with redness, swelling, heat, and stiffness. X-ray evaluation reveals soft tissue swelling, joint space narrowing, erosion, and deformity.
Tendinitis (Ch. 175)	Microscopic tears of the involved muscles with inflammation. Joints have normal range of motion, no swelling, and appear normal on x-ray evaluation.

fracture of both the tibia and fibula. Trimalleolar fractures reveal a bimalleolar fracture, as well as a fracture of the posterior tibial malleolus.

ASSESSMENT

Differential Diagnosis

Differential diagnoses include those listed in Tables 122-2 and 122-3.

THERAPEUTIC PLAN

RICE

The RICE formula for treatment of an injury stands for rest, ice, compression, and elevation:

Rest any injured part of the musculoskeletal system. Rest time varies according to the seriousness of the injury.

Ice all musculoskeletal injuries to attempt to control swelling. Continue ice application as long as swelling exists. Ice can be applied for 15 minutes at a time.

Compression controls edema and provides comfort and/or support. Compression can be accomplished with ace wraps, neoprene braces, custom made splints, and commercially made splints (e.g., "air cast")

Elevate all injured extremities.

Joint Protection/Immobilization

The injured joint should be protected by applying a splint, allowing for postinjury swelling. Never apply a circumferential cast to an acutely injured extremity. Use crutches for lower extremity injuries. Many splints are commercially made and easy to apply. Custom-made splinting material includes plaster and Fiberglass. Immobilization will also assist in pain control.

TABLE 123-3 Physical Findings in Ankle Sprains by Grade

Symptoms	Grade I	Grade II	Grade III
Tendon	No tear	Partial tear	Complete tear
Loss of functional ability	Minimal	Some	Great
Pain	Minimal	Moderate	Severe
Edema	Minimal	Moderate	Severe
Bruising	Usually not/limited	Frequently	Yes
Weight bearing	No problem	Usually a problem	Almost always unable to bear weight

Adapted from Wexler W: The injured ankle, *Am Family Physician* 57:476, 1998.

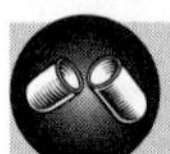

TABLE 123-4 Pharmaceutical Plan: NSAIDs

Drug	Dosage	Comments	Cost
Naproxen (Naprosyn)	250-500 BID	NSAIDs are indicated for MS injury. NSAIDs inhibit prostaglandin synthesis, which decreases pain. *Do not* prescribe to patients with peptic ulcer disease, allergy to NSAIDs /ASA, renal dysfunction, or pregnant women. Pregnancy: B (D if used near term; etodolac: C)	\$12-\$80/250 mg (100); \$18-\$126/500 mg (100); \$100/SR 500 mg (75)
Ibuprofen (Motrin)	200-800 mg QID Maximum: 3.2 g/day		\$3-\$9/200 mg (100); \$4-\$80/600 mg (100)
Etodolac (Lodine)	200-400 mg q6-8h		\$114/200 mg (100); \$128/300 mg (100); \$132/400 mg (100)

Splints for Particular Injuries

Bimalleolar splint: Ankle sprains

Posterior splint for lower extremity: Ankle sprains, Jones fracture, foot fractures, fractures of the lateral or medial malleolus

Posterior splint with stirrups: Provides additional support by decreasing inversion and eversion of the foot at the ankle; indicated for severe ankle sprains, malleolus fractures, foot fractures

Pharmaceutical

Antiinflammatory drugs and muscle relaxants are the drugs of choice for musculoskeletal injury (Tables 123-4 and 123-5).

See Appendix J for more detailed prescribing of NSAIDs.

Myorelaxants are indicated for pain related to muscle spasm and prescribed for short periods of time with fractures (3 to 5 days).

Narcotic analgesics are indicated only for fractures with severe pain and should be given for only several days.

Patient Education

RICE: Emphasize the importance of rest, ice application, use of splints/ace wraps, and elevation. All of these measures will tend to decrease swelling and help to control pain.

Pathophysiology: Explain the pathophysiology of the injury and expected outcomes.

Cast/splint care: Give detailed information, including bathing instructions, removal and reapplication if indicated, and observation for signs of neurovascular compromise.

Medications: Include potential medication side effects and instructions for administration. The patient should take NSAIDs with food to avoid abdominal discomfort. Muscle relaxants/narcotic analgesics may cause drowsiness; the patient should not operate machinery or work above ground level.

Referral

Immediately refer the patient to an orthopedic surgeon for the following fractures: long bone, displaced, intraarticular, and all fractures with neurovascular compromise. Also refer the patient for ankle injuries with significant instability or mortise widening.

Within 3 to 5 days of injury the patient should be seen by an orthopedic surgeon for simple nondisplaced fractures and for grade II or III ankle sprains after appropriate splinting and patient education.

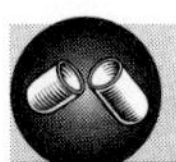

TABLE 123-5 Pharmaceutical Plan: Muscle Relaxants

Drug	Dose	Comments	Cost
Cyclobenzaprine (Flexeril)	10 mg TID	Pregnancy: B SE: Drowsiness, confusion, constipation, dry mouth, blurred vision, urinary retention	\$13-\$100/10 mg (100)
Chlorzoxazone (Parafon Forte)	250-750 mg TID-QID	Pregnancy: C SE: Dizziness, drowsiness, nausea, hepatotoxicity	\$5-\$58/250 mg (100); \$16-\$104/500 mg (100)
Orphenadrine citrate (Norflex)	100 mg BID	Pregnancy; C SE: Tachycardia, transient dizziness, urinary retention, ↑ IOP, blurred vision, dry mouth	\$127/100 mg (100)
Methocarbamol (Robaxin)	1000-1500 mg QID ×23 days; then 750 mg TID	Pregnancy: C SE: Drowsiness, GI upset, blurred vision, headache, hypotension	\$6-\$49/500 mg (100); \$8-\$72/750 mg (100)
Carisoprodol (Soma)	350 mg TID/QID	Pregnancy C SE: Dizziness, drowsiness, nausea, epigastric distress, tachycardia	\$7-\$179/350 mg (100)

IOP, Intraocular pressure; *GI,* gastrointestinal; *SE,* side effects.

Refer to an orthopedic surgeon: All patients with minor ankle sprains that do not respond to conservative management.

EVALUATION/FOLLOW-UP

Recheck all minor ankle sprains in 1 week.

Begin rehabilitation for minor ankle sprains as soon as possible to prevent contractures and loss of conditioning.

Patient should continue to take NSAIDs with food.

SUGGESTED READINGS

Alonso J: Ankle fractures. In Masear V, editor: *Primary care orthopedics,* Philadelphia, 1996, WB Saunders.

Anderson B: *Office orthopedics for primary care,* Philadelphia, 1995, WB Saunders.

Balano K: Anti-inflammatory drugs and myorelaxants: pharmacology and clinical use in musculoskeletal disease, *Primary Care* 23:329-334, 1996.

Chorley JN et al: Management of ankle sprains, *Pediatr Ann* 26:56-64, 1997.

Connolly J: Acute ankle sprains: getting and keeping patients back up on their feet, *Consultant* 36:1631-1639, 1996.

Dichristina D. Fractures and ligamentous injuries of the ankle. In Masear V, editor: *Primary care orthopedics,* Philadelphia, 1996, WB Saunders.

Ellsworth A et al: *Mosby's 1998 medical drug reference,* St Louis, 1998, Mosby.

Healthcare Consultants of America, Inc: *1998 Physicians fee and coding guide,* Augusta, Ga, 1998, Healthcare Consultants of America, Inc.

Wexler R: The injured ankle, *Am Family Physician* 57:474-482, 1998.

Musculoskeletal Injuries: Elbow

ICD-9-CM

Sprains and Strains 848.9
Tendinitis 762.90

OVERVIEW

Definitions

A sprain is an injury to one of the ligamentous structures of the body. A dislocation is a disruption of the relationship between the humerus and ulna. (A loss of relationship can also occur between the radius and ulna.) A fracture is a loss in continuity in the substance of the bone.

Anatomy

The elbow is a hinge joint, permitting motion of the humerus and ulna on one plane. The elbow forms the articulation of the humerus, radius, and ulna. It consists of a single synovial cavity, with the radius and ulna protecting the joint (Figures 124-1 and 124-2). Four ligaments are important in evaluating elbow injuries (Figure 124-3). The radial head is held in place by the annular ligament, and the radial collateral ligament. In addition, the ulnar collateral ligament and anterior capsule add stability to the joint. These structures can be severely damaged with fracture or dislocation of the joint (Magnusson, 1992).

Pathophysiology

Common Injuries/Fractures

Nursemaid's elbow: Subluxation of the annular ligament around the radial neck at the elbow. Nursemaid's elbow is the result of longitudinal traction on the hand with the elbow extended and the forearm in a pronated position, as in pulling a child up by the arm.

Dislocation of the elbow: Dislocation of the elbow requires considerable energy, so 30% to 40% of all dislocations also have associated fractures. The most common dislocation is posteriorly. The mechanism of injury is a fall on an outstretched hand, most commonly seen in adults.

Factures of the head and neck of the radius: Occurs as a result of a fall on an outstretched hand.

Fractures of the distal humerus: A supracondylar fracture is commonly seen in children under 15 years old and, rarely, in persons over 20 years old. The strength of the collateral ligament and joint capsule are greater than that of bone. This is opposite in adults, and a posterior elbow dislocation is sustained instead. The result is anterior displacement of the distal fragment of the humerus, endangering the brachial artery and median nerve.

Epicondylar fracture: Most common in children; often involves the apophyses.

Olecranon fracture: Usually occurs from a direct blow or fall on an outstretched hand.

Factors Associated with Increased Risk of Injury

Poor physical conditioning
Failure to warm up muscles adequately
Intensity of competition
Collision and contact sports participation
Rapid growth
Overuse of joints (Seidel et al, 1995)
Nursemaid's elbow: Pulling child up by one wrist or hand
Occurs in children between 1 and 3 years old; rare after age 6

SUBJECTIVE DATA

History of the Present Illness

Exact mechanism of injury
Timing of injury
Description/location of pain, radiation, quality, timing, severity
Aggravating/relieving factors

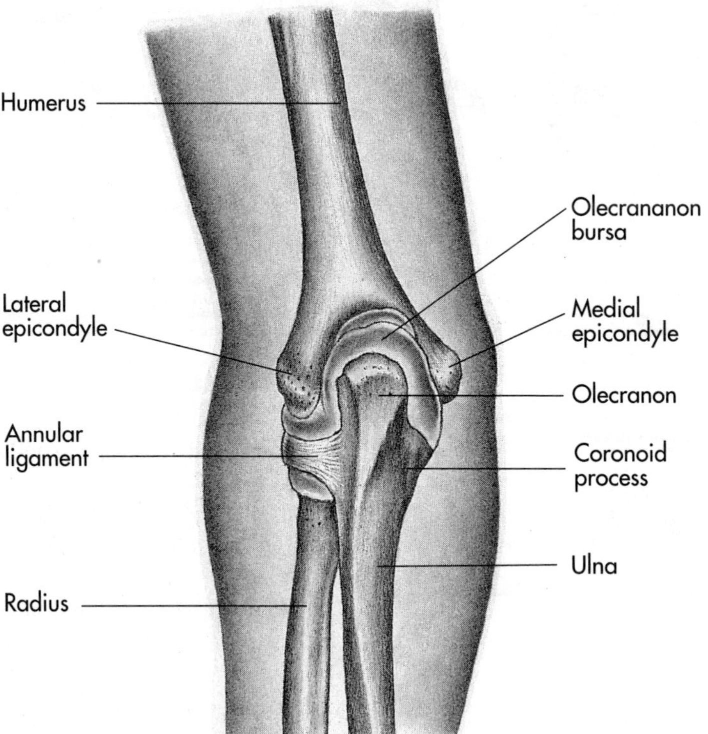

Figure 124-1 Structures of the left elbow joint; posterior view. (From Seidel HM et al: *Mosby's guide to physical examination,* ed 4, St Louis, 1999, Mosby.)

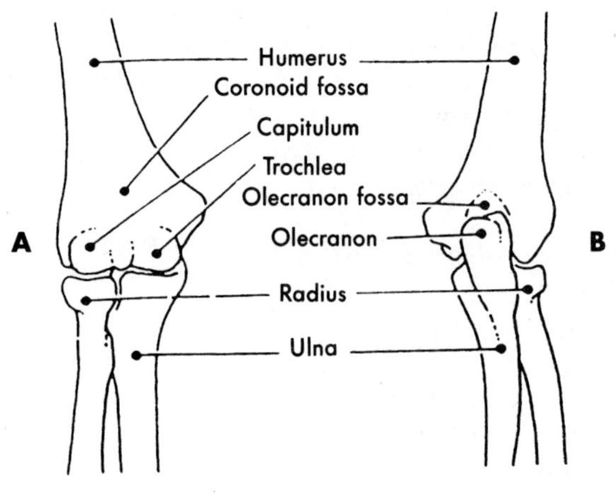

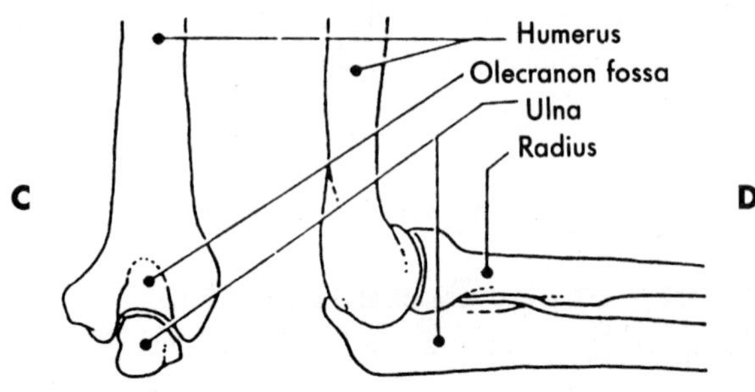

Figure 124-2 Bony anatomy of the distal humerus and elbow region. **A,** Anterior view; **B,** posterior view; **C,** posterior view, 90 degrees flexion; **D,** lateral view; right elbow is shown. (From Connolly JF: *DePalma's management of fractures and dislocations,* Philadelphia, 1981, WB Saunders.)

Previous treatment
Any joint complaints: Stiffness, limitation of motion, pain with motion, joint locking, or giving way
Effects of activity on joint should also be noted

Past Medical History

Previous injuries, surgical history, exercise history, chronic illness, osteoporosis, skeletal deformities

Medications

Recent or present use of pain medications, nonsteroidal antiinflammatory drugs (NSAIDs), other medications

Family History

Family history of orthopedic problems

Psychosocial History

Occupational job description
Lifting history
Smoking, alcohol intake
Conditioning history

Allergies

Any allergies

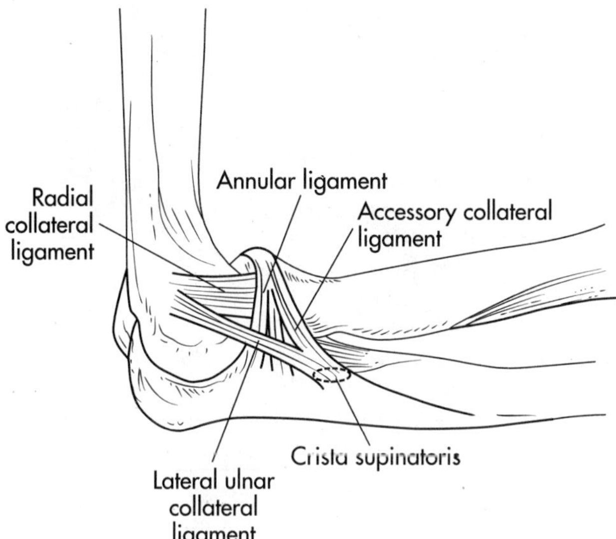

Figure 124-3 Lateral view of the lateral collateral and annular ligaments of the elbow. (From Nicholas JA, Hershman EB: *Upper extremity in sports medicine,* ed 2, St Louis, 1995, Mosby.)

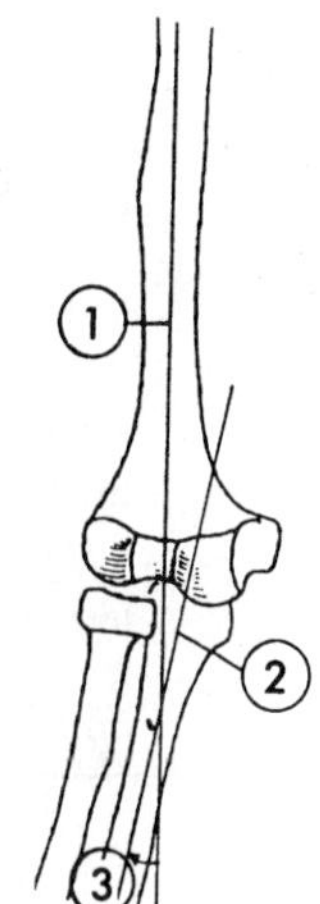

Figure 124-4 Carrying angle *(3)* is formed by intersection of lines drawn parallel to the long axis of humerous *(1)* and ulna *(2)*. (From Ramamarti CP: *Orthopaedics in primary care,* Baltimore, 1979, Williams & Wilkins.)

Pertinent History of Common Elbow Injuries

Nursemaid's elbow: No obvious history of injury noted; child typically stops using his or her elbow and avoids motion of arm because of pain

Dislocation of the elbow: Patient or caregiver may describe a fall on an outstretched hand, with pain and decreased range of motion (ROM)

Fractures of the head and neck of the radius: Characterized by tenderness of elbow, local swelling and pain

Fracture distal radius: In a supracondylar fracture, patient will complain of localized tenderness and swelling

Olecranon fracture: Patient presents with elbow in flexion, and there is diffuse tenderness

Associated Symptoms

Swelling, deformity, masses, paralysis

OBJECTIVE DATA

Physical Examination

A problem-oriented physical examination should be performed, with particular attention to:

- Vital signs: Should be relatively normal with common, nonlife-threatening injuries
- General: Note patient response to pain, gait, and how the patient is holding the injured extremity
- Musculoskeletal: Observe for swelling and effusion, palpation of adjacent and actual areas of injury, evaluate ROM, and special physical testing to diagnose a specific condition

Elbow: Inspect elbow in flexed and extended positions for contour

Palpate the extensor surface of the ulna, olecranon, and the medial and lateral epicondyles of the humerus.

ROM

- Bend and straighten the elbow.
- With elbow bent at 90 degrees, rotate the hand from palm side up to palm side down.
- Apply force while patient flexes and extends the elbow.
- Determine the carrying angle; this is helpful in assessing subtle supracondylar fractures. The carrying angle is formed by the intersection of lines drawn parallel to long axis of humerus and ulna. This angle is normally up to 12 degrees; asymmetrical carrying angles of greater than 12 degrees are often associated with fracture (Figure 124-4).

Neurovascular: Assess distal to the injury. Check pulses, sensation, and capillary refill. Radial nerve function should be evaluated by assessing wrist and finger extension. The sensory component should be tested in the web space between the thumb and index finger. Check for median nerve function by checking the flexion and abduction of the thumb and index finger. The sensory component is tested over the palmar aspects of the thumb to the radial half of the ring finger. The ulnar nerve should be tested by having the patient pinch a piece of paper between the fingers and thumb and assessing the patient's ability to hold onto the paper as the examiner pulls outward.

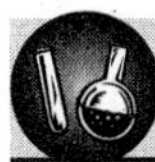

TABLE 124-1 Diagnotic Tests: Elbow Injuries

Test	Findings/Rationale	Cost ($)
X-ray evaluation	Consider x-ray evaluation with significant pain, swelling, effusion, or contusion. Routine views should include anterior-posterior and lateral views. Consideration should include an oblique view for certain injuries. Anteroposterior and oblique views are taken with the elbow extended. Lateral views are taken with the elbow at 90 degrees. Special attention should be paid to the radial head and the fat pads; doing so reduces the risk of missing fractures. Injuries that produce intraarticular hemorrhage cause distention of the synovium and displace the fat pad out of the fossa so it is seen on lateral views. With a posterior fat pad sign, >90% of patients have an intraarticular injury. The anterior fat pad can also be altered and resembles a boat's sail when viewed on x-ray films.	102-122

Specific Physical Findings of Common Injuries of Elbow

Nursemaid's elbow: Resistance to supination and tenderness on direct palpation of the head of the radius

Dislocation of the elbow: Obvious deformity with posterior dislocation of the elbow with the elbow held in flexion; prominent olecranon

Fractures of the head and neck of the radius: Characterized by tenderness of elbow, local swelling and pain on passive rotation of the forearm; joint effusion frequently present

Fracture of the distal humerus (supracondylar fracture): **Children** present with the forearm supported by the other arm and the elbow flexed at 90 degrees; prominence of the olecranon usually present

Olecranon: Tenderness and pain over the olecranon, palpable separation at the fracture site, and inability to extend the elbow against force; ulnar nerve function is vulnerable and should be evaluated by checking sensation over the palmar aspect of the fifth digit and hypothenar eminence

Diagnostic Procedures

Diagnostic procedures are outlined in Table 124-1.

Radiographic Findings of Common Elbow Injuries

Nursemaid's elbow: Subluxation of the annular ligament around radial neck at the elbow may be seen on x-ray evaluation, or the films may appear normal; x-ray evaluation not routinely done unless there is swelling or deformity

Dislocation of the elbow: Obvious deformity with posterior dislocation of the elbow

Fractures of the head and neck of the radius: May include everything from a disruption of the usual gradual sweep of the radial head to an obvious comminuted or displaced fracture

Fracture of distal radius: In a supracondylar fracture the distal fragment is often displaced on the lateral view

Olecranon fracture: X-ray film of the olecranon is usually diagnostic in the lateral view: fracture is demonstrated, and the amount of displacement in the 90 degree flexion position displacement more than 2 mm is an indication for surgery

ASSESSMENT

Differential Diagnosis

Differential diagnoses include sprain, strain, fracture, tendinitis, osteoarthritis, rheumatoid arthritis, cellulitis, gout, gonococcal arthritis, tumors, degenerative changes, congenital disorders, overuse syndromes, and infections (Table 124-2).

THERAPEUTIC PLAN

The RICE formula for treatment of an injury stands for rest, ice, compression, and elevation.

Rest any injured part of the musculoskeletal system. Rest time varies according to the seriousness of the injury.

Ice all musculoskeletal injuries in an attempt to control swelling. Continue ice application as long as swelling exists. Ice can be applied for 15 minutes at a time.

Compression controls edema and provides comfort and/or support. Compression can be accomplished with Ace wraps, neoprene braces, custom-made splints, and commercially made splints.

Elevate all injured extremities. Upper extremities should be elevated with a sling.

TABLE 124-2 Differential Diagnosis: Elbow Injuries

Diagnosis	Supporting Data
Bursitis	Limitation of movement caused by swelling, pain on movement, point tenderness; site erythematous and warm. The most common site is the olecranon.
Gout (Ch. 82)	Increased uric acid production: Red, hot; swollen joint, exquisite pain, limited range of motion, tophi, low-grade fever, more common in men >40 years old.
Osteoarthritis (Ch. 15)	Articular deterioration and bony overgrowth of the joint surface. Pain is the most common symptom, occurring with motion and activity, relieved by rest. Physical findings include crepitus, swelling, restriction of movement, joint enlargement. X-ray evaluation reveals joint space narrowing, spur formation, sclerosis, and subchondral cyst formation.
Rheumatoid arthritis	Multiple joints involved. Females most commonly affected. Usually subacute in onset, often symmetrical. Morning stiffness >1 hour, joint involvement with redness, swelling, heat, and stiffness. X-ray evaluation reveals soft tissue swelling, joint space narrowing, erosion, and deformity.
Tendinitis (Ch. 175)	Microscopic tears of the involved muscles with inflammation. Joints have normal range of motion, no swelling, and appears normal on x-ray films.

Specific Treatments for Elbow Injuries

Nursemaid's elbow: Reduction is easily accomplished by supinating and flexing the forearm while applying manual pressure over the radial head. The pain is immediately relieved. A sling should be worn for 5 to 7 days after the episode (Figure 124-5).

Dislocation of the elbow: Reduction should be performed as soon as possible. It can be accomplished by gentle, steady traction on the wrist with countertraction on the shoulder. After reduction the elbow is immobilized in a splint for 3 weeks. Displaced or comminuted fractures in adults are treated by early surgery.

Fractures of the head and neck of the radius: Undisplaced fractures in adults and children are treated conservatively. A splint and sling are applied with elbow flexed at 90 degrees for 1 to 2 weeks. The sling is continued for 2 more weeks.

Fracture of distal radius: About one third of fractures are not displaced and require only splinting and follow-up. The other two thirds have a distal segment displaced. Reduction of the fragment should be prompt.

Olecranon fracture: The undisplaced fracture is treated for 2 more weeks, followed by sling and range-of-motion exercises. Displaced fractures require open reduction and internal fixation to restore bony alignment and repair the triceps insertion.

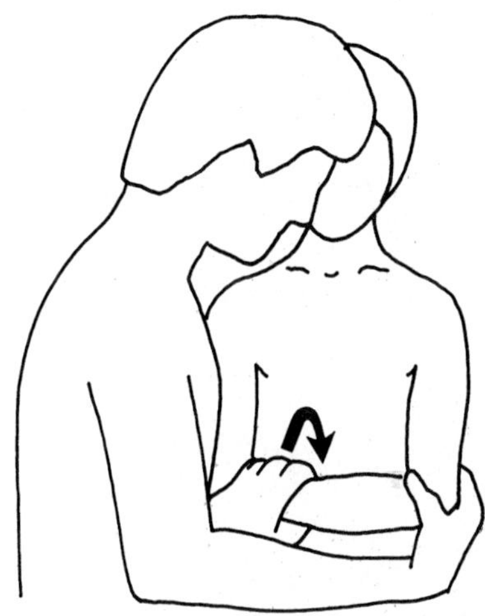

Figure 124-5 Reduction of a "pulled elbow." (From Mercier LR: *Practical orthopedics,* ed 4, St Louis, 1996, Mosby.)

Joint Protection and Immobilization

The injured joint should be protected by applying a splint; allow for postinjury swelling. Never apply a circumferential cast to an acutely injured extremity. Many splints are commercially made and easy to apply. Custom-made splinting material includes plaster and fiberglass. Immobilization will also assist in easing pain in the injured part.

Splints for Particular Injuries

Nursemaid's elbow: Sling

Dislocation of elbow: Molded posterior plaster splint with elbow at 90 degrees

Fracture of the head and neck of the radius: Light posterior splint with elbow flexed at 90 degrees

Olecranon fracture: Molded posterior plaster splint

Dislocation: Posterior splint with the elbow in as much flexion as circulation will allow; elbow suspended in a sling

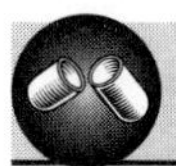

TABLE 124-3 Pharmaceutical Plan: NSAIDS

Drug	Dosage	Comments	Cost
Naproxen (Naprosyn)	250-500 BID	NSAIDs are indicated for MS injury. NSAIDs inhibit prostaglandin synthesis, which decreases pain *Do not* prescribe to patients with peptic ulcer disease, allergy to NSAIDs/ASA, renal dysfunction, or pregnant women. Pregnancy: B (D if used near term; etodolac: C)	\$12-\$80/250 mg (100); \$18-\$126/500 mg (100); \$100/SR 500 mg (75)
Ibuprofen (Motrin)	200-800 mg QID Maximum: 3.2 g/day		\$3-\$9/200 mg (100); \$4-\$80/600 mg (100)
Etodolac (Lodine)	200-400 mg q6-8h Pregnancy: C		\$114/200 mg (100); \$128/300 mg (100); \$132/400 mg (100)

ASA, Aspirin; *NSAID*, nonsteroidal antiinflammatory drug.

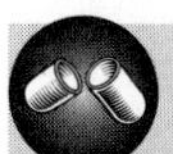

TABLE 124-4 Pharmaceutical Plan: Muscle Relaxants

Drug	Dose	Comments	Cost
Cyclobenzaprine (Flexeril)	10 mg TID	Pregnancy: B SE: Drowsiness, confusion, constipation, dry mouth, blurred vision, urinary retention	\$13-\$100/10 mg (100)
Chlorzoxazone (Parafon Forte)	250-750 mg TID-QID	Pregnancy: C SE: Dizziness, drowsiness, nausea, hepatotoxicity	\$5-\$58/250 mg (100); \$16-\$104/500 mg (100)
Orphenadrine citrate (Norflex)	100 mg BID	Pregnancy: C SE: Tachycardia, transient dizziness, urinary retention, ↑ IOP, blurred vision, dry mouth	\$127/100 mg (100)
Carisoprodol (Soma)	350 mg TID/QID	Pregnancy: C SE: Dizziness, drowsiness, nausea, epigastric distress, tachycardia	\$7-\$179/350 mg (100)
Methocarbamol (Robaxin)	1.5 g QID (two 750 mg tabs)	Pregnancy: C SE: Drowsiness, GI upset, blurred vision, headache, hypotension	\$6-\$49/500 mg (100) \$8-\$72/750 mg (100)

IOP, Intraocular pressure; *GI*, gastrointestinal; *SE*, side effects.

Pharmaceutical

NSAIDs and muscle relaxants are the drugs of choice for musculoskeletal injury (Tables 124-3 and 124-4). See Appendix J for more detail on prescribing NSAIDs.

Myorelaxants are indicated for pain related to muscle spasm and prescribed for short periods of time (3 to 5 days) when a fracture is present.

Narcotic analgesics are indicated only for fractures with severe pain and should be given for only a few days.

Patient Education

RICE: Emphasize the importance of rest, application of ice, use of splints/Ace wraps, and elevation to decrease swelling and help to control pain.

Pathophysiology: Explain pathophysiology of the injury and expected outcomes.

Cast/splint care: Give detailed information concerning care, including bathing instructions, removing and reapplying if indicated, and observing for signs of neurovascular compromise (especially important in cases of elbow dislocation—watch carefully for the first 36 hours for vascular impairment).

Medications: Include instructions for administration and potential side effects. Instruct the patient to take NSAIDs with food to avoid abdominal discomfort. Muscle relaxants and narcotic analgesics may cause drowsiness; the patient should not operate machinery or work above ground level.

Discuss the mechanism of nursemaid's elbow. Encourage caregivers to avoid lifting the child by one arm.

Referral/Consultation

Patients with the following should be referred immediately to an orthopedic surgeon: long-bone fractures, displaced fractures, intraarticular fractures, and all fractures with neurovascular compromise, dislocations of the elbow, and condylar fractures.

Patients should be referred to an orthopedic surgeon to be seen in 3 to 5 days for simple, nondisplaced fractures after appropriate splinting and patient education.

EVALUATION/FOLLOW-UP

Recheck all minor injuries/sprains in 1 week. For patients whose injury is not showing improvement, consider referral to an orthopedic surgeon.

Begin rehabilitation for minor injuries/sprains as soon as possible to prevent contractures and loss of conditioning.

Advise the patient to continue NSAIDs with food.

REFERENCES

Magnusson A: Humerus and elbow. In Rosen P, Barkin R, editors: *Emergency medicine: concepts and clinical practice,* ed 3, St Louis, 1992, Mosby.

Seidel HM et al: *Mosby's guide to physical examination,* ed 4, St Louis, 1995, Mosby.

SUGGESTED READINGS

Anderson B: *Office orthopedics for primary care,* Philadelphia, 1995, WB Saunders.

Balano K: Anti-inflammatory drugs and myorelaxants: pharmacology and clinical use in musculoskeletal disease, *Primary Care* 23:329-334, 1996.

DaSilva M et al, editors: Pediatric throwing injuries about the elbow, *Am J Orthoped* 27:90-96, 1998.

Ellsworth A et al: *Mosby's 1998 medical drug reference,* St Louis, 1998, Mosby.

Healthcare Consultants of America, Inc: *1998 Physicians fee and coding guide,* Augusta, Ga, 1998, Healthcare Consultants of America, Inc.

Irshad F, Gregory R: Reliability of fat pad sign in radial head/neck fractures of the elbow, *Injury* 28:433-435, 1997.

Kalding C, Whitehead C: Musculoskeletal injuries in adolescence, *Primary Care* 25:211-223, 1998.

Masear V, editor: *Primary care orthopedics,* Philadelphia, 1996, WB Saunders.

Mercier L: *Practical orthopedics,* ed 4, St Louis, 1995, Mosby.

Rettig A: Elbow, forearm and wrist injuries in athletes, *Sports Med* 25:115-130, 1998.

Shearman C, Med B, El-Khoury G: Pitfalls in radiologic evaluation of extremity trauma. Part I. The upper extremity, *Am Family Physician* 57:995-1002, 1998.

Skaggs S, Pershad J: Pediatric elbow trauma, *Pediatr Emerg Care* 13:425-434, 1997.

Musculoskeletal Injuries: Foot

ICD-9-CM

Sprains and Strains 848.9

OVERVIEW

Definitions

A sprain is an injury to one of the ligamentous structures of the body. A dislocation is the complete separation of the contact between two bones in a joint, often caused by pressure or force pushing the bone out of joint. A fracture is a loss in continuity in the substance of the bone.

Anatomy

The foot has 26 bones, including the tarsal bones, the metatarsals, and the phalanges. The forefoot includes the phalanges and the metatarsals. The midfoot includes the three cuneiform bones, the cuboid, and the navicular bone. The hindfoot includes the talus and calcaneus (Figure 125-1). After soft tissue injuries, fractures and dislocations of the foot are the second most common injuries sustained. The talus and the calcaneus are most often involved. Injuries of the foot are uncommon in **children,** because their feet are very resilient.

Incidence

Fractures of the foot in a **child** result from severe direct trauma, such as fall from heights or a car accident. Children have almost twice as many foot soft tissue injuries as adults.

Pathophysiology

Talus fracture: Fractures of the talus are relatively rare because of the well-secured location of the talus in the ankle joint. Men with this injury outnumber women 3 to 1, men being more prone to violent injury. The talus is the second most frequently injured tarsal bone; the most common site is the superior lateral dome of the talus. Fractures usually result from falls on the heel or forefoot. The mechanism of injury is acute hyperextension of the midfoot (if the forefoot strikes a rung on the ladder during a fall), occurring with falls from heights or car accidents.

Calcaneal fracture: The os calcis is the largest bone of the foot, transferring body weight to the ground, and serves as the attachment for the Achilles tendon. The os calcis is fractured more often than any other tarsal bone, accounting for 1% to 2% of all fractures. Tarsal fractures are uncommon in **children** and are usually less significant because of the elasticity of supportive structures in children. Calcaneal fractures usually result from a fall from a height or a vertical compressive load in both adults. The compression fracture seen in adults is not seen in children because their bones are more compact. Calcaneal fractures usually peak in people between the 30 and 50 years of age, with a peak incidence at age 45. Men are affected five times more often than women. An acute contusion of the heel pad can occur following a hard landing on the heel. The injury usually heals spontaneously.

Forefoot Injuries

The most common stress fracture of the lower extremity most often involves the third metatarsal. Stress fractures of the feet of **children** due to jumping are common because of the increased porosity of the bones.

Fifth metatarsal fracture: Among the most common fractures of all injuries of the foot. The mechanism of injury includes inversion stress on the forefoot, which produces an avulsion of the styloid process at the base of the fifth metatarsal; a lateral blow to the base of the fifth metatarsal may also produce a fracture.

Phalangeal fracture: Most phalangeal fractures are caused by direct stubbing or trauma to the toes, usually at night in an unlit area. There is rarely a significant displacement.

Achilles tendon rupture: Second most frequently ruptured tendon; the diagnosis is frequently missed. The patient can have a partial tear and still have minimal pain with reasonable strength.

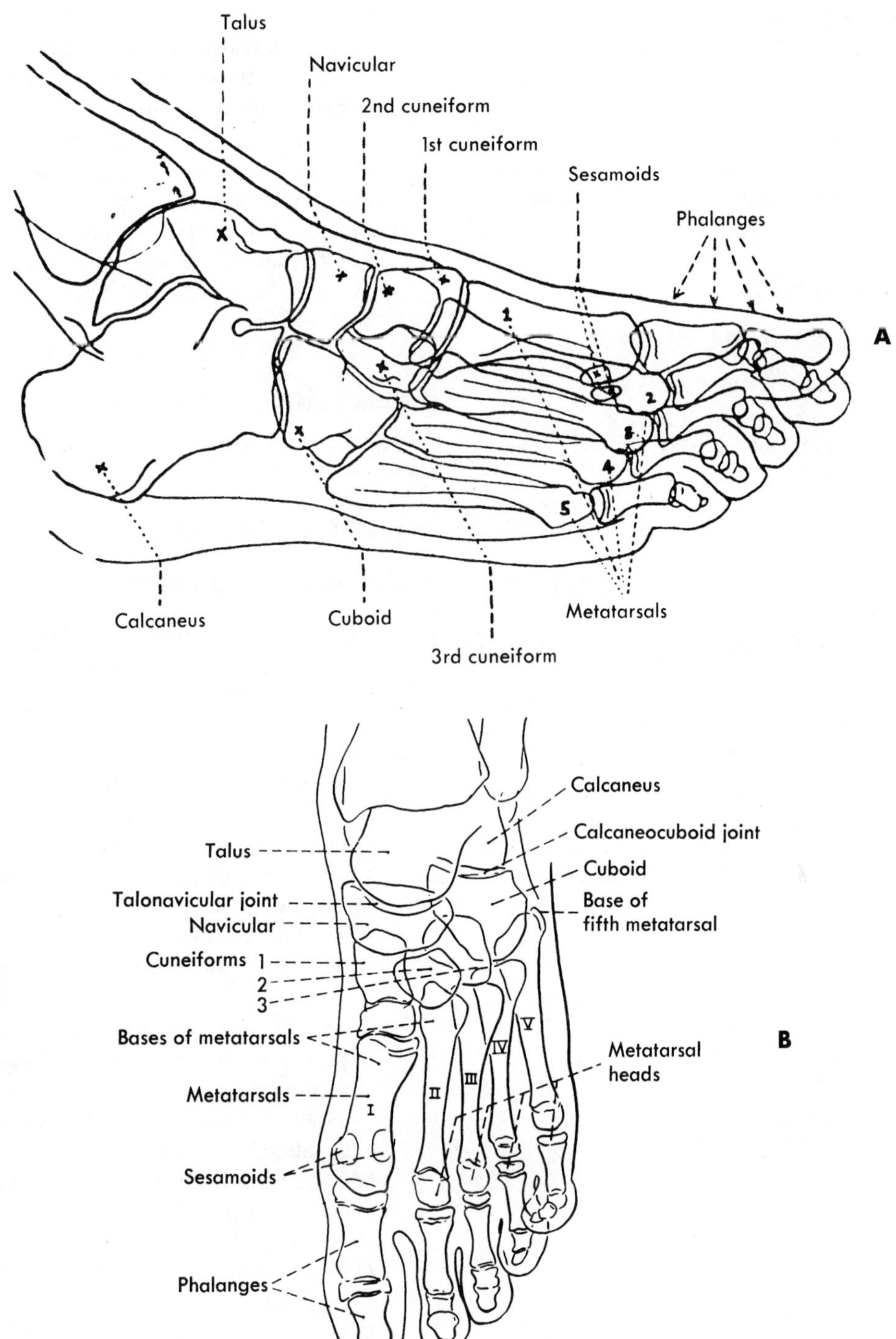

Figure 125-1 Anatomical structure of the foot. **A,** Oblique view; **B,** anteroposterior view. (From Mann RA: *Surgery of the foot,* ed 6, St Louis, 1993, Mosby.)

Factors Associated with Increased Risk of Injury

Osteoporosis
Poor physical conditioning
Failure to warm up muscles adequately
Intensity of competition
Collision and contact sports participation
Rapid growth
Overuse of joints (Seidel et al, 1995)
Feet with a long second metatarsal or a short first metatarsal (increased stress placed on the second metatarsal)

SUBJECTIVE DATA

History of the Present Illness

Exact mechanism of injury; timing of injury; size and weight of the object causing the injury; description and location of pain, radiation, quality, timing, severity, aggravation/relief; previous treatment.

Joint complaints: Stiffness, limitation of motion, pain with motion, joint locking or giving way. The effects of activity on joint should also be noted.

Past Medical History

Previous injuries; surgical history; exercise history, chronic illness, osteoporosis, skeletal deformities

Medications

Recent or present use of pain medications, nonsteroidal antiinflammatory drugs (NSAIDs), other medications

Family History

Orthopedic problems

Psychosocial History

Occupational job description
Lifting history
Smoking, alcohol intake
Conditioning

Allergies

Any allergies

Pertinent History of Common Foot Injuries

Talus fracture: Patient complains of ankle pain and swelling of the normal ankle contours.

Calcaneal fracture: Patient complains of swelling, bruising, and pain of the rearfoot and pain on both lateral and medial aspects of the calcaneus.

Forefoot injuries: Injuries usually occur from a direct blow, especially with fractures of the second, third, or fourth metatarsals. Usually there is no history of direct trauma, but of just the metatarsals beginning to hurt. In fifth metatarsal fractures the patient complains of pain at the base of the metatarsal.

Phalangeal fracture: Patient complains of pain and swelling in the involved toes. A history of stubbing or direct trauma to a blunt object will be given.

Achilles tendon rupture: Patient will give a history of a "pop" at the back of the heel and report that it felt like being kicked in the heel.

Associated Symptoms

Swelling, deformity, masses, paralysis, gait changes

OBJECTIVE DATA

Physical Examination

As with any injury sustained from a fall from a height, injuries of the lower extremity (26%) and lumbar spine (10%) should be investigated. A problem-oriented physical examination should be performed, with particular attention to:

Vital signs: Should be relatively normal with common, nonlife-threatening injuries.
General: Note patient response to pain, gait, and how the patient is holding the injured extremity.
Musculoskeletal: Observe for swelling and effusion, palpation of adjacent and actual areas of injury, assess range of motion (ROM), and perform special physical testing to diagnose a specific condition.
Inspect the feet while the patient is bearing weight.
Expect smooth and rounded malleolar prominences, prominent heels, and metatarsophalangeal (MTP) joints. Calluses or corns indicate chronic pressure or irritation.
Observe the contour of the feet and the position, size, and number of toes. The feet should be in alignment with the tibia.
Expect the foot to have a longitudinal arch, although the foot may flatten with weight bearing,
Palpate the Achilles tendon and the anterior surface of the ankle. Using thumb and fingers, compress the forefoot and each MTP joint.
ROM
- Point the foot toward the ceiling and floor.
- Bend the foot at the ankle, turn sole of foot toward and then away from the other foot (inversion, eversion).

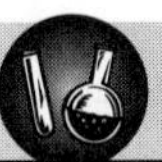

TABLE 125-1 Diagnostic Tests: Foot Injuries

Test	Findings/Rationale	Cost ($)
X-ray evaluation	Consider x-ray evaluation when significant pain, swelling, effusion, or contusion is present. Comparison views of the opposite normal extremity may be helpful if the injury involves a growth plate in a **child.** Anteroposterior and lateral views should be obtained. If possible, an oblique view of the talus should also be taken, because it will help delineate the surrounding joints of the foot and the full extent of injury. Axial views are needed to help identify calcaneal fractures.	109-129
Bone scan	A bone scan may help to diagnose a stress fracture of the foot, but it is an expensive procedure and is usually not necessary.	274-366

Bend and straighten the toes.

Neurovascular: Assess the area distal to the injury. Check pulses, sensation, and capillary refill.

Specific Physical Findings of Common Foot Injuries

Talus fracture: Tenderness over the superolateral talar dome may indicate a fracture in this area. Swelling or displacement of the talus will alter the normal ankle contours.

Calcaneal fracture: Tenderness over the medial and lateral aspects of the calcaneus. Edema and ecchymosis that extends over the sole of the foot may be seen with a calcaneal fracture. Subtalar joint motion and weight bearing will be painful.

Forefoot fracture: Soft tissue swelling, which may be extensive if the foot is not elevated. There will be localized tenderness over the involved site.

Phalangeal fracture: No signs of inflammation, but ecchymosis and tenderness are evident when the joint is palpated.

Achilles tendon rupture: A patient with a complete tear of the Achilles tendon will have an abnormal result to the Thompson test (patient lying prone, a hard squeeze of the calf should produce a plantar flexion of the foot). With a complete tear, there is no plantar flexion. The patient with a partial tear has a normal result to a Thompson test but usually has a palpable defect.

Diagnostic Procedures

Diagnostic procedures are outlined in Table 125-1.

Radiographic Findings of Common Foot Injuries

Talus fracture: Seen best on lateral and oblique views.

Calcaneal fracture: The relationship of the posterior facet of the subtalar joint to the posterior and anterior aspects of the calcaneus should be calculated. This relationship (called Bohler's angle) is normally between 20 and 40 degrees. Reduction of this angle indicates a possible calcaneal fracture.

Forefoot fracture: Anteroposterior (AP), lateral, and oblique views should be obtained. The superimposition of the metatarsal shafts can be visualized. Dorsal angulation at the fracture site may occur. In stress fractures, the initial x-ray evaluation results may be normal, and callus formation may not be visible for 2 to 4 weeks.

Phalangeal fracture: X-ray films usually provide no diagnostic information. However, x-ray evaluation should be ordered for index and great toe injuries, including AP and oblique views.

ASSESSMENT

Differential Diagnosis

Differential diagnoses include sprain, strain, fracture, tendonitis, osteoarthritis, rheumatoid arthritis, cellulitis, gout, gonococcal arthritis, tumors, degenerative changes, congenital disorders, overuse syndromes, and infections (Table 125-2 and Figure 125-2).

THERAPEUTIC PLAN

The RICE formula for treatment of an injury stands for rest, ice, compression, and elevation:

Rest any injured part of the musculoskeletal system. Rest time varies according to the seriousness of the injury.

Ice all musculoskeletal injuries in an attempt to control swelling. Continue ice application as long as swelling exists. Ice can be applied for 15 minutes at a time.

Compression controls edema and provides comfort and/or support. Compression can be accomplished with ace wraps, neoprene braces, custom-made splints, and commercially made splints.

Elevate injured extremity.

TABLE 125-2 Differential Diagnosis: Foot Injuries

Diagnosis	Supporting Data
Bursitis	Limitation of movement caused by swelling, pain on movement, point tenderness; site erythematous and warm. The bursa in the foot that may be involved is the subcalcaneal bursa.
Gout (Ch. 82)	Increased uric acid production: Red, hot; swollen joint, exquisite pain, limited range of motion, tophi, low-grade fever, more common in men >40 years old. The great toe is the most common site.
Osteoarthritis (Ch. 15)	Articular deterioration and bony overgrowth of the joint surface. Pain is the most common symptom, occurring with motion and activity, relieved by rest. Physical findings include crepitus, swelling, restriction of movement, joint enlargement. X-ray evaluation reveals joint space narrowing, spur formation, sclerosis, and subchondral cyst formation.
Rheumatoid arthritis	Multiple joints involved. Females most commonly affected. Usually subacute in onset, often symmetrical. Morning stiffness >1 hour, joint involvement with redness, swelling, heat, and stiffness. X-ray evaluation reveals soft tissue swelling, joint space narrowing, erosion, and deformity.
Tendinitis (Ch. 175)	Microscopic tears of the involved muscles with inflammation. Joints have normal range of motion, no swelling, and appear normal on x-ray films.
Plantar fasciitis	An overuse syndrome; inflammation of the plantar fascia. This occurs from the repetitive stretching of the plantar fascia. It tends to occur more in people whose feet pronate excessively or in runners who have not stretched adequately. The patient complains of pain along the arch or heel. The pain is often intense enough to cause the patient to limp or walk on the lateral surface of the foot. Examination reveals tenderness to firm, deep palpation of the medial edge of the fascia or at the origin on the anterior surface of the calcaneus. X-ray evaluation does not contribute to the diagnosis. Treatment includes administration of NSAIDs, rest, cold application, or injection into the subcalcaneal bursa with Marcaine.

Specific Treatments for Foot Injuries

Talus fracture: Any injury with significant displacement should be reduced as soon as possible. Fractures of the body of the talus that are not displaced need to be immobilized for 6 to 8 weeks.

Calcaneal fracture: Admission to the hospital is usually required for best management of this fracture, especially if comminuted or compressed.

Forefoot fracture: Initial conservative treatment of metatarsal shaft fractures should be a short leg splint, nonweight bearing. A semirigid splint for 4 to 6 weeks is adequate for a fifth metatarsal fracture if the bone is not markedly displaced.

Phalangeal fracture: Toes should be splinted for support by buddy taping to the adjacent toes. Markedly angulated fractures may require reduction.

Achilles tendon rupture: Surgery is the treatment of choice. Results are best if the surgery is done at an early stage, although delayed primary repair is an option. Conservative treatment with a cast is also an option, but there is a higher rerupture rate and the patient usually has decreased strength.

Joint Protection and Immobilization

The injured joint should be protected by applying a splint; be sure to allow for postinjury swelling. *Never apply a circumferential cast to an acutely injured extremity.* Use crutches for lower extremity injuries. Many splints are commercially made and easy to apply. Custom-made splinting material includes plaster and fiberglass. Immobilization will also assist in pain control.

Pharmaceutical

Antiinflammatory drugs and muscle relaxants are the drugs of choice for musculoskeletal injury (Tables 125-3 and 125-4). See Appendix J for more detailed prescribing information. Myorelaxants are indicated for fracture pain related to muscle spasm and prescribed for short periods of time (3 to 5 days). Narcotic analgesics are indicated only for fractures with severe pain and should be given for only several days.

Patient Education

RICE: Emphasize the importance of rest, ice application, use of splints/Ace wraps, and elevation. All of these measures will tend to decrease swelling and help to control pain.

Pathophysiology: Explain the pathophysiology of the injury and expected outcomes.

Cast/splint care: Give detailed information, including bathing instructions, as well as removal/application of cast if indicated, and observation for signs of neurovascular compromise.

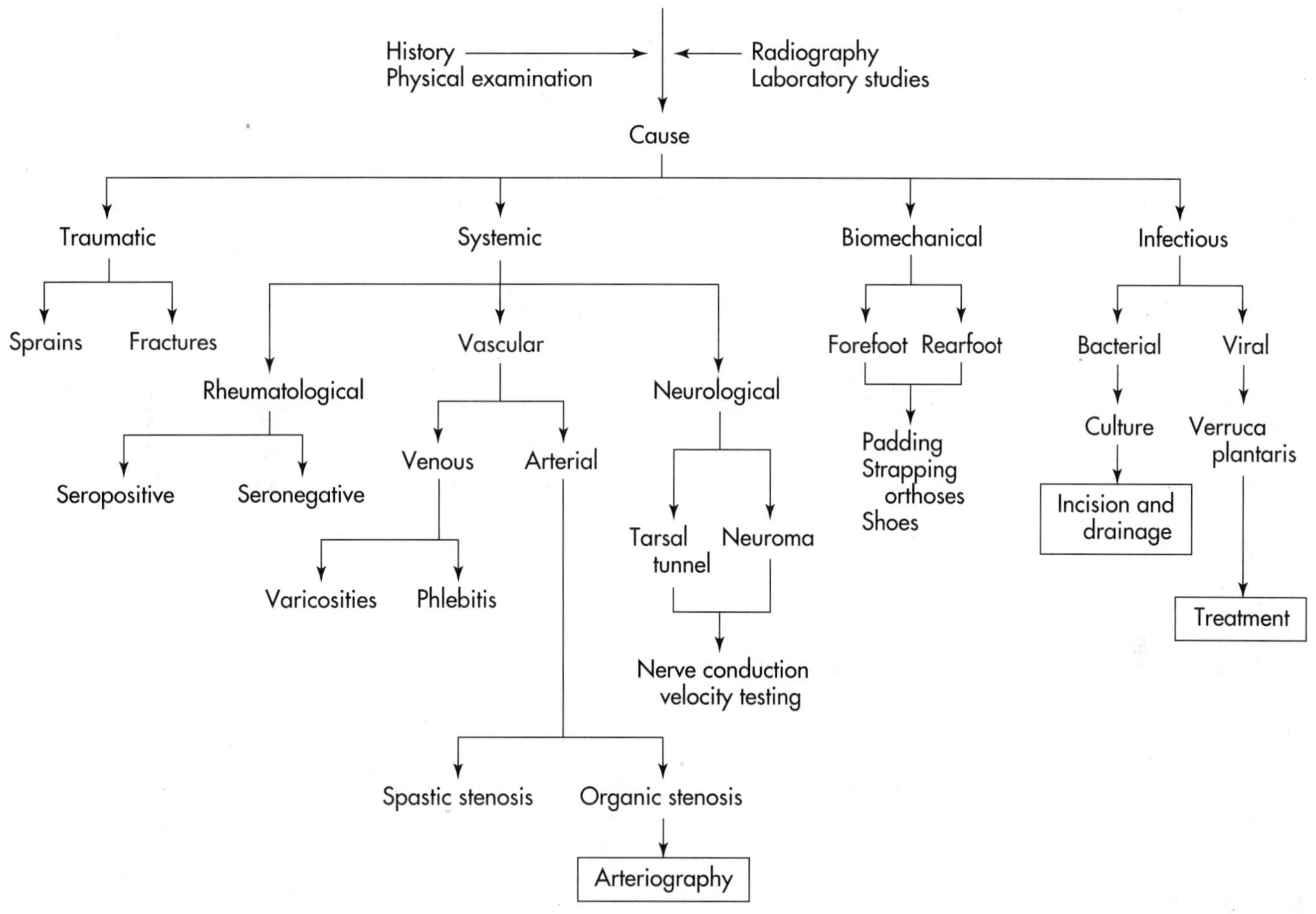

Figure 125-2 Algorithm for treatment of the patient with foot pain. (Adapted from Greene HL, Johnson WP, Lemcke D: *Decision making in medicine,* ed 2, St Louis, 1998, Mosby.)

Table 125-3 Pharmaceutical Plan: NSAIDs

Drug	Dosage	Comments	Cost
Naproxen (Naprosyn)	250-500 BID	NSAIDs are indicated for musculoskeletal injury. NSAIDs inhibit prostaglandin synthesis which decreases pain	\$12-\$80/250 mg (100); \$18-\$126/500 mg (100); \$100/SR 500 mg (75)
Ibuprofen (Motrin)	200-800 QID Maximum: 3.2 g/day	*Do not* prescribe to patients with peptic ulcer disease, allergy to NSAIDs/ASA, renal dysfunction, or pregnant women.	\$3-\$9/200 mg (100); \$4-\$80/600 mg (100)
Etodolac (Lodine)	200-400 mg q6-8h	Pregnancy: B (D if used near term; etodolac: C)	\$114/200 mg (100); \$128/300 mg (100); \$132/400 mg (100)

Adapted from Wexler W: The injured ankle, *Am Family Physician* 57:476, 1998.
ASA, Aspirin; *NSAID,* nonsteroidal antiinflammatory drug.

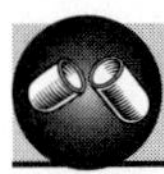

TABLE 125-4 Pharmaceutical Plan: Muscle Relaxants

Drug	Dose	Comments	Cost
Cyclobenzaprine (Flexeril)	10 mg TID	Pregnancy: B SE: Drowsiness, confusion, constipation, dry mouth, blurred vision, urinary retention	$13-$100/10 mg (100)
Chlorzoxazone (Parafon Forte)	250-750 mg TID-QID	Pregnancy: C SE: Dizziness, drowsiness, nausea, hepatotoxicity	$5-$58/250 mg (100); $16-$104/500 mg (100)
Orphenadrine citrate (Norflex)	100 mg BID	Pregnancy: C SE: Tachycardia, transient dizziness, urinary retention, ↑ IOP, blurred vision, dry mouth	$127/100 mg (100)
Carisoprodol (Soma)	350 mg TID/QID	Pregnancy: C SE: Dizziness, drowsiness, nausea, epigastric distress, tachycardia	$7-$179/350 mg (100)
Methocarbamol (Robaxin)	1.5 g QID (two 750 mg tabs)	Pregnancy: C SE: Drowsiness, GI upset, blurred vision, headache, hypotension	$6-$49/500 mg (100); $8-$72/750 mg (100)

IOP, Intraocular pressure; *GI,* gastrointestinal; *SE,* side effects.

Medications: Include instructions for administration as well as potential medication side effects. Instruct the patient to take NSAIDs with food to avoid abdominal discomfort.

Muscle relaxants/narcotic analgesics may cause drowsiness; the patient should not operate machinery or work above ground level.

Referral

Immediately refer the patient to an orthopedic surgeon for long bone fractures, displaced fractures, intraarticular fractures of the calcaneus, fractures/dislocations, Achilles tendon rupture, and all fractures with neurovascular compromise.

Refer the patient to an orthopedic surgeon to be seen in 3 to 5 days for simple and nondisplaced fractures after appropriate splinting and patient education.

EVALUATION/FOLLOW-UP

Recheck all minor sprains in 1 week. For patients whose injury is not showing improvement, consider referral to an orthopedic surgeon.

Continue NSAIDs with food.

REFERENCE

Seidel HM et al: *Mosby's guide to physical examination,* ed 4, St Louis, 1995, Mosby.

SUGGESTED READINGS

Anderson B: *Office orthopedics for primary care,* Philadelphia, 1995, WB Saunders.

Balano K: Anti-inflammatory drugs and myorelaxants: pharmacology and clinical use in musculoskeletal disease, *Primary Care* 23:329-334, 1996.

Ballas M, Tytko J, Mannarino F: Commonly missed orthopedic problems, *Am Family Physician* 57:267-274, 1998.

Ellsworth A et al: *Mosby's 1998 medical drug reference,* St Louis, 1998, Mosby.

Healthcare Consultants of America, Inc: *1998 Physicians fee and coding guide,* Augusta, Ga, 1998, Healthcare Consultants of America, Inc.

Mann RA: *Surgery of the foot,* ed 6, St Louis, 1993, Mosby.

Mercier L: *Practical orthopedics,* ed 4, St Louis, 1995, Mosby.

Rosen P, Barkin R, editors: *Emergency medicine: concepts and clinical practice,* ed 3, St Louis, 1995, Mosby.

Snyder M: Foot pain. In Greene H, Johnson W, Lemcke D, editors: *Decision making in medicine,* ed 2, St Louis, 1998, Mosby.

Musculoskeletal Injuries: Hand

ICD-9-CM

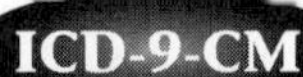

Sprains and Strains 848.9

OVERVIEW

Definitions

A sprain is an injury to one of the ligamentous structures of the body. A fracture is a loss in continuity in the substance of the bone.

Anatomy

The hand consists of five metacarpals and five phalanges with an intricate pulley system in association extensor and flexor tendons (Figures 126-1 and 126-2).

Pathophysiology

Common Injuries of the Hand

Gamekeeper's thumb or skier's thumb is caused by a forced hyperabduction of the thumb. This common injury to the ulnar collateral ligament of the metacarpophalangeal (MCP) joint of the thumb is easily missed and can result in significant disability if not managed properly (Figure 126-3).

Boxer's fracture (fifth metacarpal fracture) is usually caused by a forceful punch with a closed hand. This is the most common metacarpal fracture and usually results in distal fifth metacarpal fracture with angulation of the distal fragment (Figure 126-4).

Common Injuries of the Fingers

Mallet finger is a flexion deformity of the distal interphalangeal (DIP) joint of the finger that occurs with a forced flexion of the distal phalanx. The extensor tendon as it attaches to the distal phalanx is ruptured, or the dorsal base of the distal phalanx, which serves as the insertion site for the extensor tendon, fractures (Figure 126-5). Distal phalanx fractures are very common and are frequently associated with a crush injury.

SUBJECTIVE DATA

History of the Present Illness

Exact mechanism of injury
Timing of injury
Description/location of pain
Radiation, quality, timing, severity
Aggravation/relief
Previous treatment

Past Medical History

Previous injuries
Surgical history
Exercise history

Medications

Recent or present use of pain medications, nonsteroidal anti-inflammatory drugs (NSAIDs), other medications

Family History

Family history of orthopedic problems, arthritis

Psychosocial History

Occupational job description
Smoking, alcohol intake
Conditioning history

Allergies

Any allergies

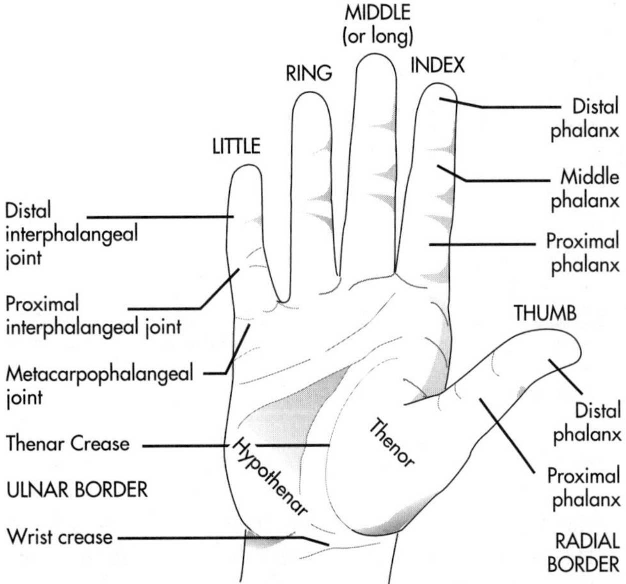

Figure 126-1 Volar view of the hand, showing anatomical terminology useful in describing the hand. (From Kidd PS, Sturt PL: *Mosby's emergency nursing reference,* St Louis, 1996, Mosby.)

Pertinent History of Common Hand Injuries

Hand: A patient with gamekeeper's/skier's thumb will relate a history of forced hyperabduction of the thumb, such as when skiers fall while holding onto ski poles. Boxer's fracture is associated with a forceful punch with a closed fist.

Fingers: Mallet finger, also called baseball finger, is usually caused by a jamming injury of the finger or a forced flexion of the distal phalanx. This commonly occurs with a jamming injury. Distal phalanx fractures are frequently associated with crush injuries.

Associated Symptoms

Swelling, deformity, masses, paralysis

OBJECTIVE DATA

Physical Examination

A problem-oriented physical examination should be performed, with particular attention to:

Vital signs: Should be relatively normal with common, nonlife-threatening injuries.

General: Note patient response to pain and how the patient is holding the injured extremity.

Musculoskeletal: Observe for swelling and effusion, palpate adjacent and actual areas of injury, evaluate range of motion (ROM), and perform physical tests to diagnose a specific condition.

Inspect the dorsal and palmar aspects of the hands, noting contour, position, shape, number, and completeness of digits, as well as bilateral symmetry.

Palpate each joint in the wrist and hand.

Evaluate ROM by having the patient do the following:

Bend fingers forward at the metacarpophalangeal (MCP) joint, then stretch joints up and back at the knuckle.

Touch the thumb to each finger; make a fist (Figure 126-6).

Spread the fingers apart and then touch them together.

Bend the wrist up and down. Expect flexion of 90 degrees and hyperextension of 70 degrees.

With palm side down, turn hand right and left.

Neurovascular: Assess the hand distal to the injury. Check pulses, sensation, and capillary refill.

Specific Physical Findings of Common Hand Injuries

Hand: Gamekeeper's or skier's thumb presents with pain of the ulnar aspect of the MCP joint of the thumb and with possible abnormal opening of the MCP joint with stress when compared with the opposite thumb (see Figure 126-3). There may be ecchymosis and swelling over the joint. Boxer's fractures present with swelling along the dorsal-lateral surface of the hand, and pain is elicited when the fifth metacarpal is palpated. Commonly there is a malrotation of the involved digit.

Fingers: Mallet finger presents with a flexion deformity of the distal phalanx and inability to actively extend the DIP joint.

Distal phalanx fractures: Often associated with crush injuries and therefore may present with lacerations, contusions, and subungual hematoma.

Diagnostic Procedures

A diagnostic procedure for an injury of the hand is outlined in Table 126-1.

Radiographic Findings of Common Hand Injuries

Hand: X-ray evaluation of *gamekeeper's thumb* usually yields normal findings, but occasionally an avulsion fracture of the ulnar aspect of the distal thumb metacarpal will be found. *Boxer's fractures* reveal a fracture of the fifth metacarpal, which frequently is medially angulated.

Fingers: *Mallet finger* injury may reveal a normal film or an avulsion fracture of the proximal dorsal surface of the distal phalanx at the extensor tendon insertion site. *Finger fractures* may show crush injuries to the distal phalanx; transverse or spiral fractures of the phalanges may also be present.

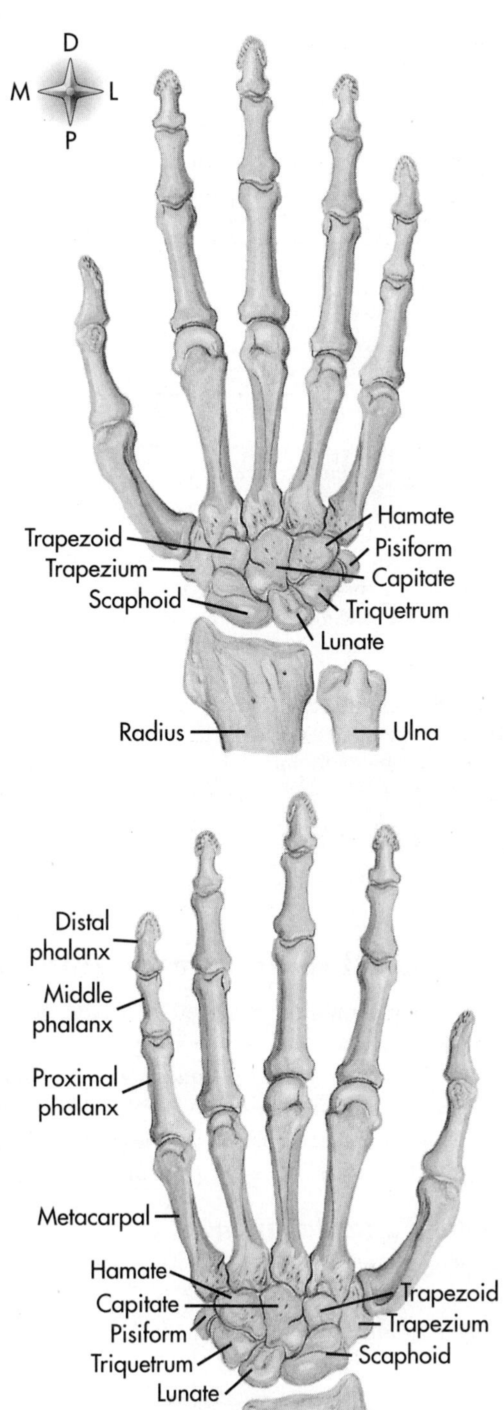

Figure 126-2 Dorsal view of the bones of the right hand and wrist. (From Thibodeau GA, Patton KT: *Anatomy and physiology,* ed 4, St Louis, 1999, Mosby.)

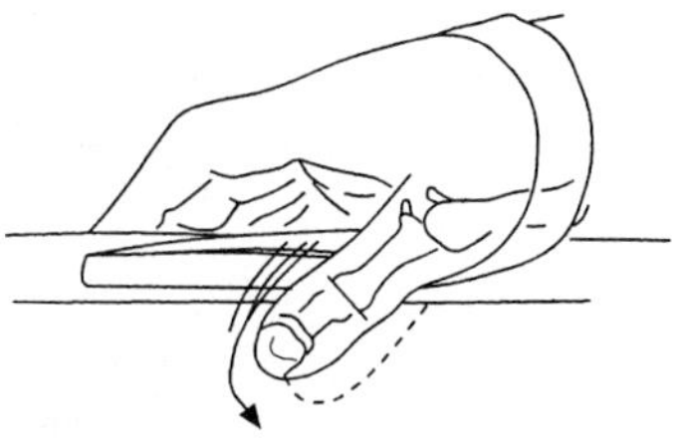

Figure 126-3 Gamekeeper's or skier's thumb. Ulnar collateral ligament sprain, tear, or avulsion. (From Hartley A: *Practical joint assessment, upper quadrant,* St Louis, 1995, Mosby.)

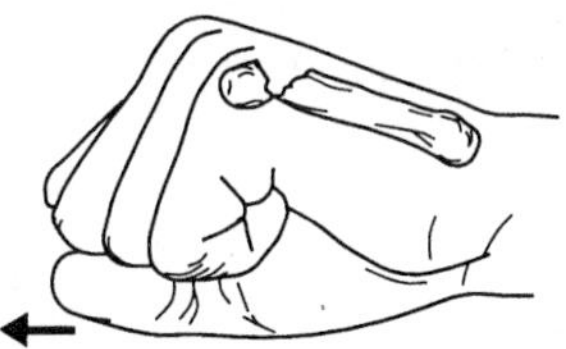

Figure 126-4 Boxer's fracture, a fracture of the neck of the fifth metacarpal. (From Hartley A: *Practical joint assessment, upper quadrant,* St Louis, 1995, Mosby.)

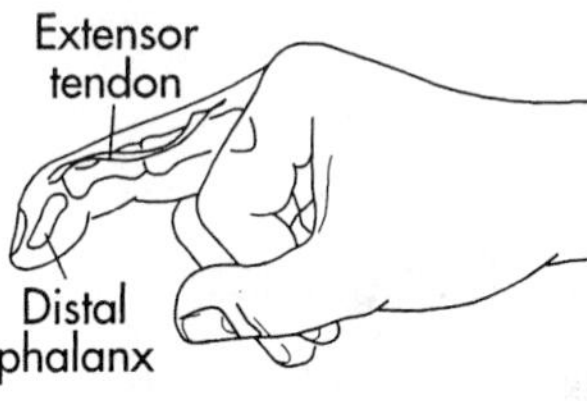

Figure 126-5 Mallet finger. (From Hartely A: *Practical joint assessment, upper quadrant,* St Louis, 1995, Mosby.)

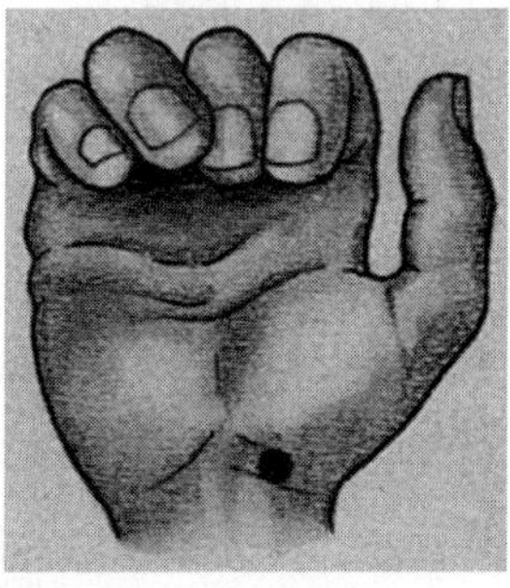

Figure 126-6 Normally, the axes of the flexed fingers point to the navicular *(dot)*. A fracture with rotation will cause the fingers to overlap when a fist is made. The resultant functional disability may be great. (From Mercier LR: *Practical orthopedics,* ed 4, St Louis, 1996, Mosby.)

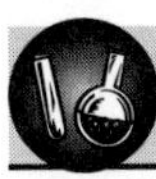

TABLE 126-1 Diagnostic Tests: Hand Injuries

Test	Findings/Rationale	Cost ($)
Hand/finger x-ray evaluation	Consider when there is significant pain, swelling, deformity, or contusion. Comparison views of the opposite normal extremity may be helpful if the injury involves a growth plate in a **child.**	100-110/hand 76-90/finger

TABLE 126-2 Differential Diagnosis

Diagnosis	Supporting Data
Bursitis (Ch. 82)	Limitation of movement caused by swelling, pain on movement, point tenderness; site is erythematous and warm.
Gout	Increased uric acid production: red, hot; swollen joint, exquisite pain, limited ROM, tophi, low-grade fever, more common in men >40 years old.
Osteoarthritis (Ch. 15)	Articular deterioration and bony overgrowth of the joint surface. Pain is the most common symptom, occurring with motion and activity, relieved by rest. Physical findings include crepitus, swelling, restriction of movement, joint enlargement. X-ray evaluation reveals joint space narrowing, spur formation, sclerosis, and subchondral cyst formation.
Rheumatoid arthritis	Multiple joints involved. Women most commonly affected. Usually subacute in onset, often symmetric. Morning stiffness >1 hr, joint involvement with redness, swelling, heat, and stiffness. X-ray evaluation reveals soft tissue swelling, joint space narrowing, erosion, and deformity.
Tendinitis (Ch. 175)	Microscopic tears of the involved muscles with inflammation. Joints have normal ROM, no swelling, and appear normal on x-ray evaluation.

ROM, Range of motion.

ASSESSMENT

Differential Diagnosis

Differential diagnoses include sprain, strain, fracture, tendonitis, osteoarthritis, rheumatoid arthritis, cellulitis, gout, gonococcal arthritis, tumors, degenerative changes, congenital disorders, overuse syndromes, and infections. The most common diagnoses are presented in Table 126-2.

THERAPEUTIC PLAN

RICE

The RICE formula for treatment of an injury stands for rest, ice, compression, and elevation:

Rest any injured part of the musculoskeletal system. Rest time varies according to the seriousness of the injury.

Ice all musculoskeletal injuries to attempt to control swelling. Continue ice application as long as swelling exists. Ice can be applied for 15 minutes at a time.

Compression controls edema and provides comfort and/or support. Compression can be accomplished with Ace wraps, neoprene braces, custom-made splints, and commercially made splints (e.g., finger splints).

Elevate all injured extremities.

Joint Protection and Immobilization

The injured joint should be protected by applying a splint; allow for postinjury swelling. Never apply a circumferential cast to an acutely injured extremity. Many splints are commercially made and easy to apply. Custom-made splinting material includes plaster and fiberglass. Immobilization will also assist in easing pain in the injured part.

Splints for Particular Injuries

Thumb spica: Gamekeeper's thumb, scaphoid fracture
Ulnar gutter: Boxer's fracture
Metal finger splint: Finger sprain, finger fracture
Stax splint: Mallet finger

Pharmaceutical

NSAID and muscle relaxants are the drugs of choice for musculoskeletal injury (Tables 126-3 and 126-4). See Appendix J for more detail on prescribing NSAIDs.

Myorelaxants are indicated for pain related to fractures secondary to muscle spasm and prescribed for short periods of time (3 to 5 days). It is presently not necessary for most hand injuries.

Narcotic analgesics are indicated only for fractures with severe pain and should be given for only a few days.

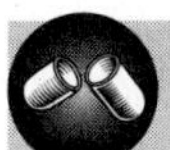

Table 126-3 Pharmaceutical Plan: Hand Injuries

Drug	Dosage	Comments	Cost
Naproxen (Naprosyn)	250-500 BID	NSAIDs are indicated for musculoskeletal injury; they inhibit prostaglandin synthesis, which decreases pain. *Do not* prescribe to those with peptic ulcer disease, allergy to NSAIDs/ASA, or renal dysfunction or to pregnant women. Pregnancy: B (D if used near term; etodolac: C)	$12-$18/250 mg (100); $18-$126/500 mg (100); $100/SR 500 mg (75)
Ibuprofen (Motrin)	200-800 mg QID; maximum 3.2 g/day		$3-$9/200 mg (100); $4-$80/600 mg (100)
Etodolac (Lodine)	200-400 mg q6-8h		$114/200 mg (100); $128/300 mg (100); $132/400 mg (100);

ASA, Aspirin; *NSAID,* nonsteroidal antiinflammatory drug.

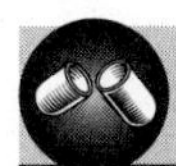

Table 126-4 Pharmaceutical Plan: Muscle Relaxants

Drug	Dose	Comments	Cost
Cyclobenzaprine (Flexeril)	10 mg TID	Pregnancy: B SE: Drowsiness, confusion, constipation, dry mouth, blurred vision, urinary retention	$13-$100/10 mg (100)
Chlorzoxazone (Parafon Forte)	250-750 mg TID-QID	Pregnancy: C SE: Dizziness, drowsiness, nausea, hepatotoxicity	$5-$58/250 mg (100); $16-$104/500 mg (100)
Orphenadrine citrate (Norflex)	100 mg BID	Pregnancy: C SE: Tachycardia, transient dizziness, urinary retention, ↑ IOP, blurred vision, dry mouth	$127/100 mg (100)
Methocarbamol (Robaxin)	1000-1500 mg QID	Pregnancy: C SE: Drowsiness, GI upset, blurred vision, headache, hypotension	$6-$49/500 mg (100); $8-$72/750 mg (100)
Carisoprodol (Soma)	350 mg TID/QID	Pregnancy: C SE: Dizziness, drowsiness, nausea, epigastric distress, tachycardia	$7-$179/350 mg (100)

IOP, Intraocular pressure; *GI,* gastrointestinal; *SE,* side effects.

Patient Education

RICE: Emphasize the importance of rest, application of ice, use of splints/Ace wraps, and elevation to decrease swelling and help to control pain.

Pathophysiology: Explain pathophysiology of the injury and expected outcomes.

Cast/splint care: Give detailed information concerning splint care, including bathing instructions, removing and reapplying it if indicated, and observing for signs of neurovascular compromise.

Medications: Include instructions for administration and potential side effects. Instruct the patient to take NSAIDs with food to avoid abdominal discomfort. Narcotic analgesics may cause drowsiness; the patient should not operate machinery or work above ground level.

Referral

Patients with the following should be referred immediately to an orthopedic surgeon: displaced fractures, intraarticular fractures, and all fractures with neurovascular compromise.

Patients should be referred to an orthopedic surgeon to be seen in 3 to 5 days for simple, nondisplaced fractures after appropriate splinting and patient education.

Suspected gamekeeper's thumb always needs referral to an orthopedic or hand surgeon.

EVALUATION/FOLLOW-UP

Recheck all minor injuries/sprains in 1 week. For patients whose injury is not showing improvement, consider referral to an orthopedic surgeon.

Begin rehabilitation for minor injuries/sprains as soon as possible to prevent contractures and loss of conditioning.

Continue NSAIDs with food.

SUGGESTED READINGS

Anderson B: *Office orthopedics for primary care,* Philadelphia, 1995, WB Saunders.

Balano K: Anti-inflammatory drugs and myorelaxants: pharmacology and clinical use in musculoskeletal disease, *Primary Care* 23:329-334, 1996.

Ballas MT et al: Commonly missed orthopedic problems, *Am Family Physician* 57:267-274, 1998.

Bonatz E: Bones and soft tissue injuries to the hands. In Maeser V, editor: *Primary care orthopedics,* Philadelphia, 1996, WB Saunders.

Dvorkin M: *Office orthopedics,* Norwalk, Conn, 1993, Appleton & Lange.

Eiff MP et al: *Fracture management for primary care,* Philadelphia, 1998, WB Saunders.

Ellsworth A et al: *Mosby's 1998 medical drug reference,* St Louis, 1998, Mosby.

Healthcare Consultants of America, Inc: *1998 Physicians fee and coding guide,* Augusta, Ga, 1998, Healthcare Consultants of America, Inc.

Lillegard WA: Common upper extremity injuries, *Arch Family Med* 5:159-168, 1996.

Martin R: Initial assessment and management of common fractures, *Primary Care* 23:405-409, 1996.

Savage PL: Casting and splinting techniques. In Maeser V, editor: *Primary care orthopedics,* Philadelphia, 1996, WB Saunders.

Snider RK: *Essentials of musculoskeletal care,* Rosemont, Ill, 1997, American Academy of Orthopedic Surgeons.

Torburn L: Principles of rehabilitation, *Primary Care* 23:335-343, 1996.

Musculoskeletal Injuries: Knee

ICD-9-CM

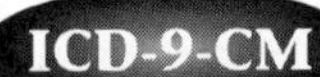

Sprains and Strains 848.9

OVERVIEW

Definitions

A sprain is an injury to one of the ligamentous structures of the body. A fracture is a loss in continuity in the substance of the bone.

Anatomy

The knee joint includes four bones: the distal femur, the patella, the proximal fibula, and the proximal tibia. Soft, pliable cartilage, the medial and lateral menisci, lie within the tibiofemoral joint and function to reduce stress and act as a cushion between the femur and tibia. Intraarticular ligaments called the anterior cruciate ligament (ACL) and posterior cruciate ligament (PCL) stabilize the knee in an anterior and posterior fashion. The extraarticular ligaments, the medial collateral ligament (MCL) and the lateral collateral ligament (LCL), maintain varus and valgus stability of the knee. The extensor mechanism of the knee is maintained by the quadriceps ligament, the patella, and the patellar tendon (Figure 127-1).

Pathophysiology

Fracture

Factures are classified as either open or closed. Open fractures are exposed to the external environment and are highly prone to serious infection. Description of a fracture includes anatomical location as well as degree of displacement, rotation, translation, or shortening. Fractures into the joint are called intraarticular fractures. Fracture patterns are described as transverse, oblique, spiral, comminuted, or greenstick. Salter-Harris classification is commonly used to describe growth plate fractures in **children.**

Sprain

Ligaments, which connect bones together, can sustain injuries. Ligamentous injuries are classified as grade I, grade II, or grade III, depending on the extent of injury. A completely torn ligament is classified as a grade III sprain, whereas a mildly stretched ligament is classified as a grade I sprain.

Specific Knee Injuries

Meniscus: Meniscal injuries usually result from a tear to either the lateral or medial meniscus secondary to some type of physical activity.

Ligament: ACLs, PCLs, MCLs, and LCLs are commonly injured while one is engaging in athletic activities. Tibial plateau fractures are generally associated with high-impact injuries to the knee.

SUBJECTIVE DATA

History of the Present Illness

Ask the patient about:
- Exact mechanism of injury
- Timing of injury
- Description/location, radiation, quality, timing, and severity of pain
- Measures that aggravate/relieve pain
- Previous treatment

Past Medical History

Ask the patient about:
- Previous injuries, surgeries
- Exercise history

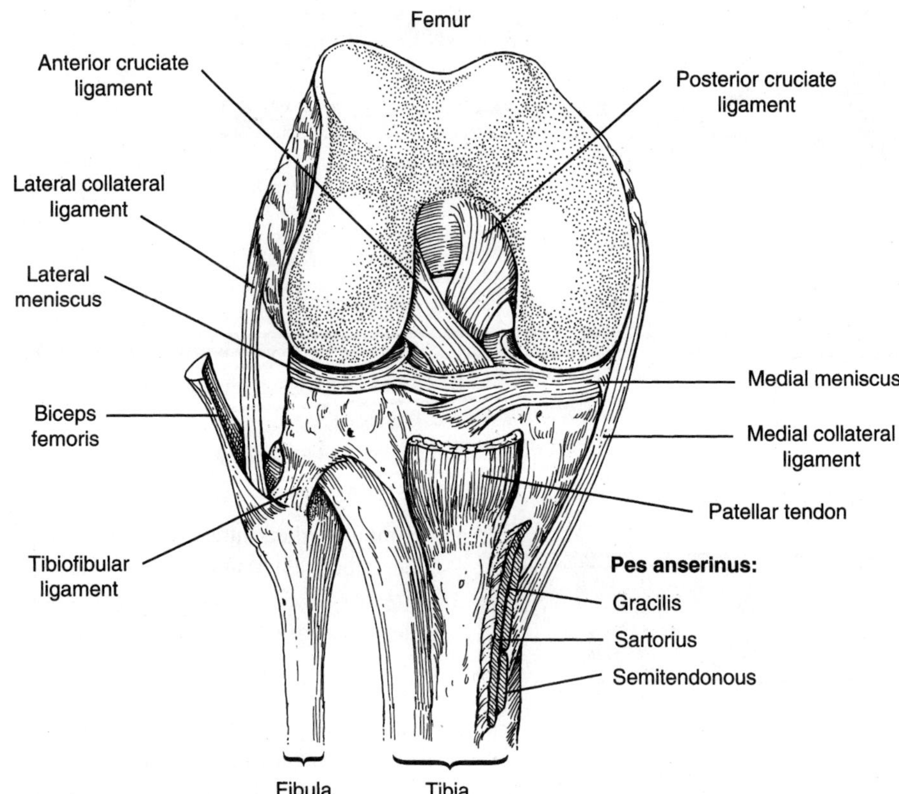

Figure 127-1 Anterior view of the knee. (From Scuderi GR, McCann PD, Bruno PJ: *Sports medicine: principles of primary care,* St Louis, 1997, Mosby.)

Family History

Orthopedic problems

Psychosocial History

Occupational job description
Smoking, alcohol intake
Conditioning history

Allergies

Any allergies

Pertinent History of Common Knee Injuries and Fractures

Meniscus injuries occur in all age groups and are frequently associated with athletic activity in which a hyperextension, hyperflexion, or rotational injury occurs.

Collateral ligament injuries occur as a result of varus or valgus stress to the knee.

ACL injuries occur with twisting motion, a quick stop, or a hyperextension. *ACL injuries* are also associated with an audible pop.

PCL injuries are associated with a direct blow to the anterior portion of the tibia.

Tibial plateau fractures are associated with high-impact varus or valgus stress and axial compression. Tibial plateau fractures are also commonly seen in postmenopausal women with osteoporosis.

Associated Symptoms

Swelling, deformity, masses, paralysis, gait changes

OBJECTIVE DATA

Physical Examination

A problem-oriented physical examination should be performed, with particular attention to:

Vital signs: Should be relatively normal with common nonlife-threatening injuries.

General: Note the patient's gait, response to pain, and how the patient is holding the injured extremity.

Musculoskeletal: Observe for swelling and effusion, palpate adjacent and actual areas of injury, evaluate range of motion (ROM), and perform physical testing to diagnose a specific condition (Table 127-1).

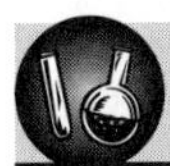

TABLE 127-1 Diagnostic Tests: Knee Injuries

Diagnosis	Mechanism of Injury/History	Physical Findings	Special Tests
Meniscal injuries	Associated with hypertension, hyperflexion, or rotation of the knee	Mild swelling and joint line tenderness	Positive result to McMurray test (see Figure 127-2)
Anterior cruciate ligament injury	Twisting motion, a quick stop, or hyperextension of the knee; associated with an audible pop	Frequently associated with an effusion and anterior drawer sign	Positive result to Lachman's test (see Figure 127-6)
Posterior cruciate ligament injury	Associated with direct force to the anterior tibia.	Minimal swelling and + drawer sign	Positive sag sign of Godfrey (see Figure 127-7)
Medial collateral ligament injury	Associated with force to the lateral knee with resultant valgus stress.	Mild swelling, joint line pain, +/– joint effusion, pain or laxity with valgus stress	Valgus stress maneuvers +
Lateral collateral ligament injury	Associated with force to the medial side of the knee with resultant varus stress	Mild swelling, joint line tenderness, pain and/or laxity with varus stress; effusion may or may not be present	Varus stress maneuvers yield positive response (pain)
Tibial plateau fractures	Associated with high-energy valgus or varus force to the knee or fall from a height with axial force to the proximal tibia; may be seen in **elderly** patients rather than meniscus or ligamentous injuries	Inability to bear weight, painfully swollen, common effusion and hemarthrosis; associated with soft tissue injuries; can lead to acute compartment syndrome	

Inspect the knees in both flexed and extended positions, noting the major landmarks: Tibial tuberosity, medial and lateral tibial condyles, medial and lateral epicondyles of the femur, adductor tubercle of the femur, and the patella. Inspect the knee for its natural concavities on the anterior aspect, on each side, and above the patella.

Palpate the popliteal space, noting any swelling or tenderness. Then palpate the tibiofemoral joint space, identifying the patella, the suprapatellar pouch, and the infrapatellar fat pad. The joint should feel firm and smooth, without tenderness, bogginess or crepitus.

ROM

Bend each knee; expect 130 degrees of flexion.

Straighten leg; expect full extension and up to 15 degrees of hyperextension.

Neurovascular: Assess the area distal to the knee injury. Check pulses, sensation, and capillary refill.

Specific Physical Findings of Common Knee Injuries

Meniscus injuries present with mild swelling, joint line tenderness, and a positive result to the McMurray's test (Figure 127-2).

MCL injuries are associated with joint line pain, mild swelling, +/– joint effusion, pain and/or laxity with valgus stress (Figure 127-3).

LCL injuries include joint line pain and pain and/or laxity with varus stress (Figure 127-4); swelling or effusion may or may not be present.

ACL injuries frequently include a joint effusion with a positive anterior drawer sign or positive result to a Lachman's test (Figures 127-5 and 127-6).

PCL injuries are associated with minimal swelling, but positive posterior drawer sign or a positive sag sign of Godfrey (Figure 127-7).

Tibial plateau fractures are associated with a painful, swollen knee and inability to bear weight. An effusion is common and associated soft tissue injuries frequently coexist.

Diagnostic Procedures

Diagnostic procedures are outlined in Table 127-2.

Radiographic Findings of Common Injuries

Soft tissue injuries: ACL, MCL, PCL, LCL, and meniscus injuries usually yield normal films, with the exception of a

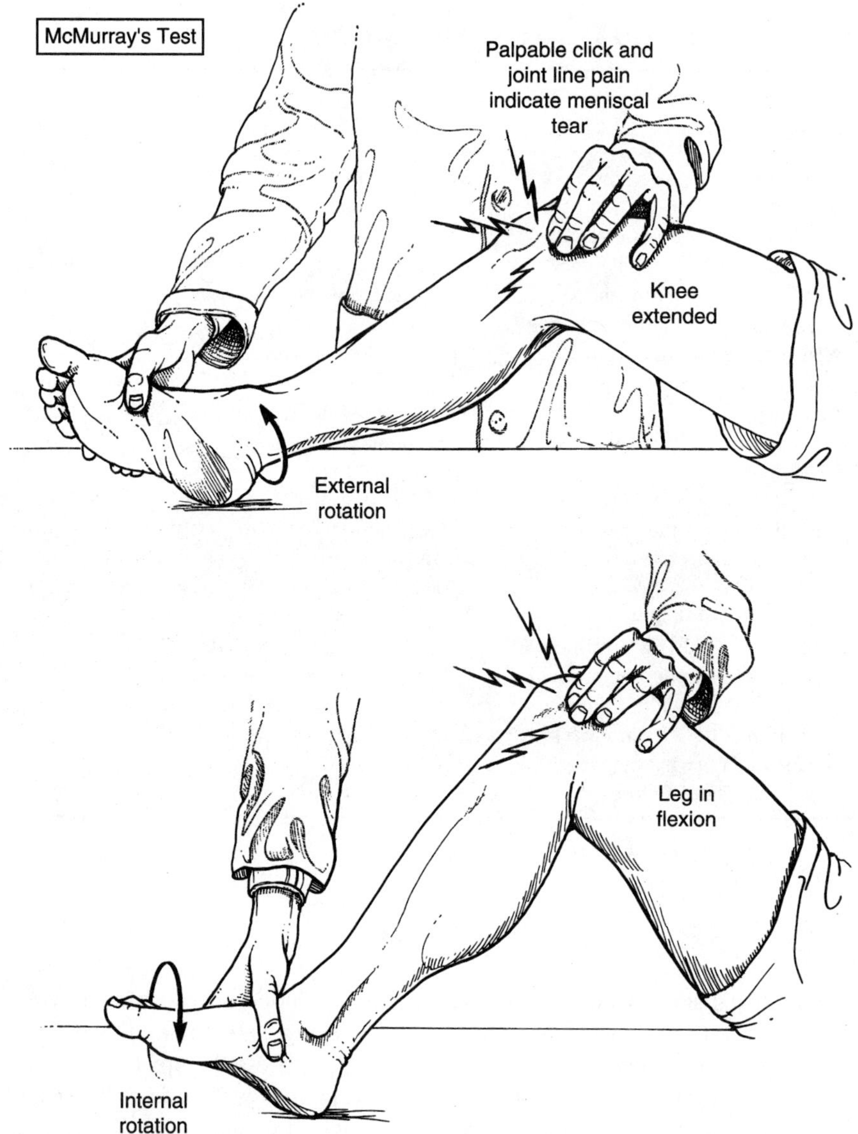

Figure 127-2 McMurray's test. The leg in flexion is moved from valgus, external rotation, to varus, internal rotation. Alternatively, the knee can be extended during the maneuver. A meniscal tear is suspected with a palpable click or joint line pain. (From Scuderi GR, McCann PD, Bruno PJ: *Sports medicine: principles of primary care,* St Louis, 1997, Mosby.)

visible joint effusion or soft tissue swelling. Occasionally a ligament rupture will reveal a small avulsion fracture. Tibial plateau fractures may exist on either the lateral or the medial plateau, or both.

ASSESSMENT

Differential Diagnosis

Differential diagnoses include sprain, strain, fracture, tendonitis, osteoarthritis, rheumatoid arthritis, cellulitis, gout, gonococcal arthritis, tumors, degenerative changes, congenital disorders, overuse syndromes, and infections. The most common diagnoses are listed in Table 127-3.

THERAPEUTIC PLAN

RICE

The RICE formula for treatment of an injury stands for rest, ice, compression, and elevation:

Rest any injured part of the musculoskeletal system. Rest time varies according to the seriousness of the injury.

Ice all musculoskeletal injuries to attempt to control

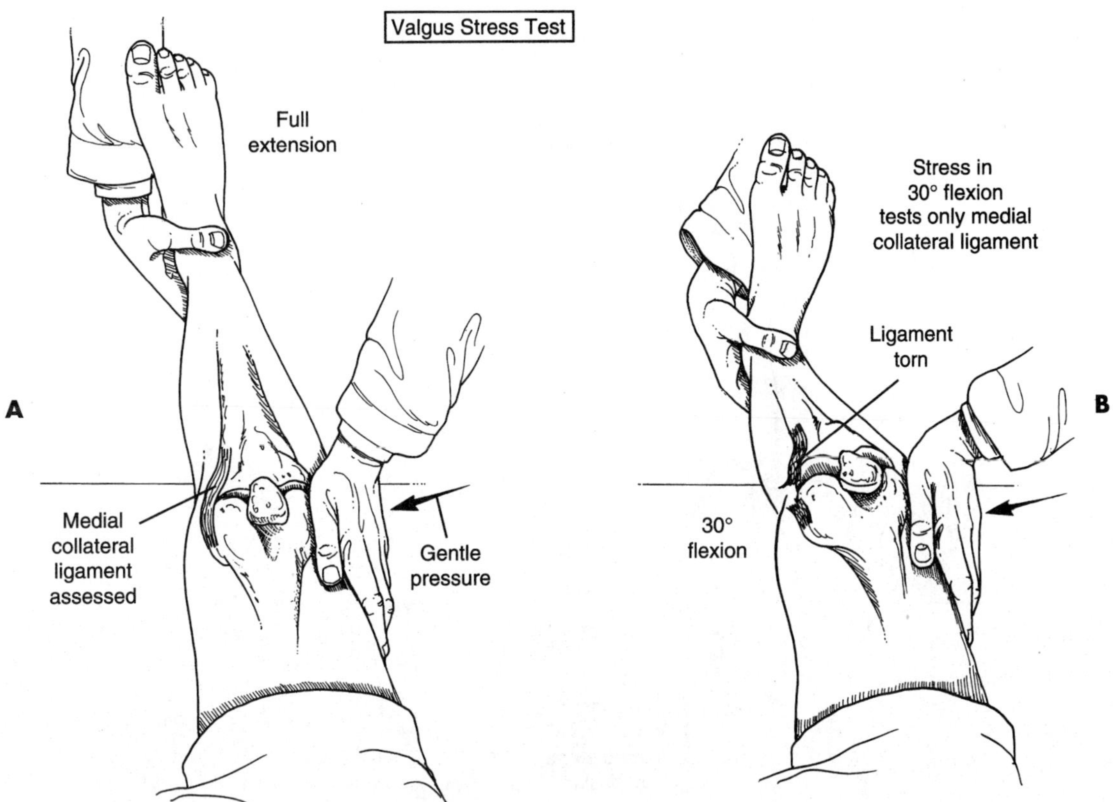

Figure 127-3 The valgus stress test is performed **A,** at full extension to assess secondary restraints and **B,** at 30 degrees of flexion to assess the medial collateral ligament. (From Scuderi GR, McCann PD, Bruno PJ: *Sports medicine: principles of primary care,* St Louis, 1997, Mosby.)

swelling. Continue ice application as long as swelling exists. Ice can be applied for 15 minutes at a time.

Compression controls edema and provides comfort and/or support. Compression can be accomplished with Ace wraps, neoprene braces, custom made splints, and commercially made splints (e.g., "air cast").

Elevate all injured extremities.

Joint Protection/Immobilization (Knee Immobilizer, Bulky Jones Wrap)

The injured joint should be protected with application of a splint, which should allow for postinjury swelling. Commercially available knee immobilizers apply compression and immobilize the knee in full extension. If a commercial knee brace is not available, the knee can be adequately immobilized in full extension with a bulky wrap of Kerlex rolls and Ace wraps. Crutches should be used for knee injuries.

Pharmaceutical

NSAIDs and muscle relaxants are the drugs of choice for musculoskeletal injury (Tables 127-4 and 127-5).

Myorelaxants are indicated for pain of fractures related to muscle spasm and are prescribed for short periods of time (3 to 5 days).

Narcotic analgesics are indicated for fractures and severe pain and should be given for only a few days.

See Appendix J for more detailed prescription information for NSAIDs.

Patient Education

RICE: Emphasize the importance of rest, application of ice, use of splints/Ace wraps, and elevation to decrease swelling and help to control pain.

Pathophysiology: Explain pathophysiology of the injury and expected outcomes.

Cast/splint care: Give detailed information concerning splint care, including bathing instructions, removing and reapplying it if indicated, and observing for signs of neurovascular compromise.

Medications: Include instructions for administration and potential side effects. Instruct the patient to take NSAIDs with food to avoid abdominal discomfort. Narcotic analgesics may cause drowsiness; the patient should not operate machinery or work above ground level.

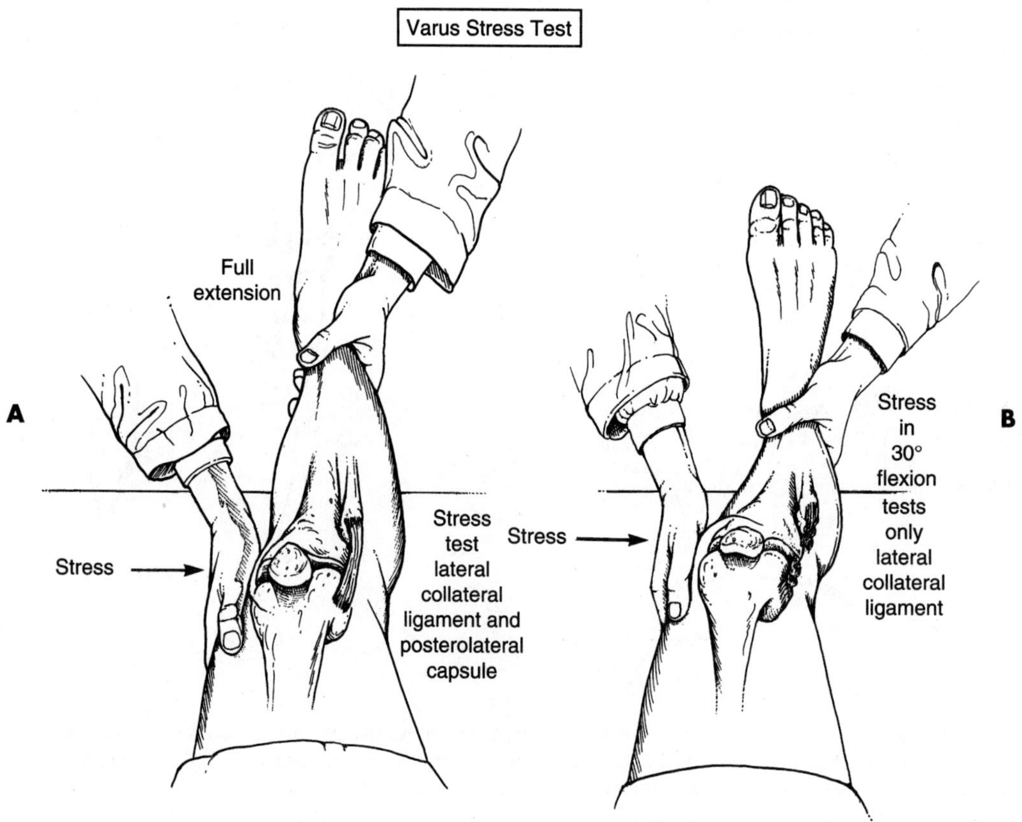

Figure 127-4 The varus stress test is performed **A,** at full extension to assess secondary restraints and **B,** at 30 degrees of flexion to assess the lateral collateral ligament. (From Scuderi GR, McCann PD, Bruno PJ: *Sports medicine: principles of primary care,* St Louis, 1997, Mosby.)

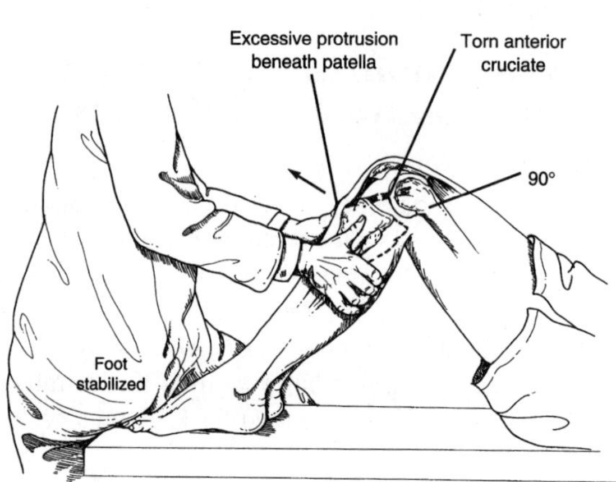

Figure 127-5 The anterior drawer test is performed at 90 degrees of flexion with an anteriorly directed force applied to the proximal tibia. (From Scuderi GR, McCann PD, Bruno PJ: *Sports medicine: principles of primary care,* St Louis, 1997, Mosby.)

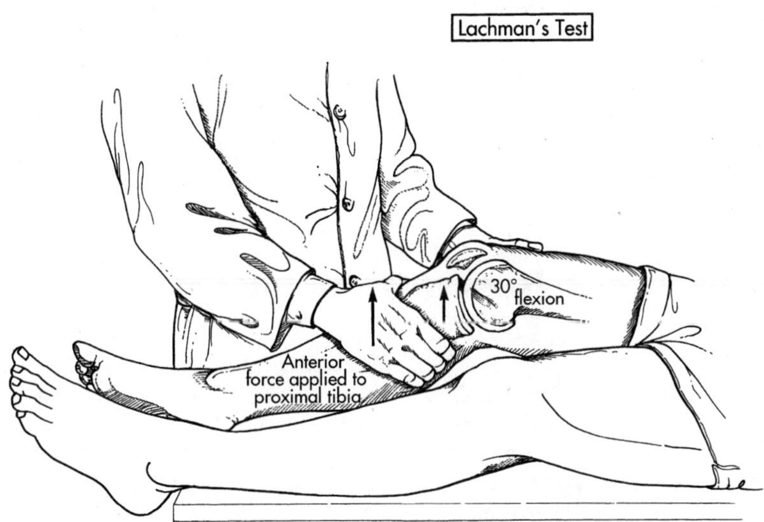

Figure 127-6 The Lachman test is performed at 30 degrees of flexion with an anteriorly directed force applied to the proximal tibia while the opposite hand stabilizes the thigh. (From Scuderi GR, McCann PD, Bruno PJ: *Sports medicine: principles of primary care,* St Louis, 1997, Mosby.)

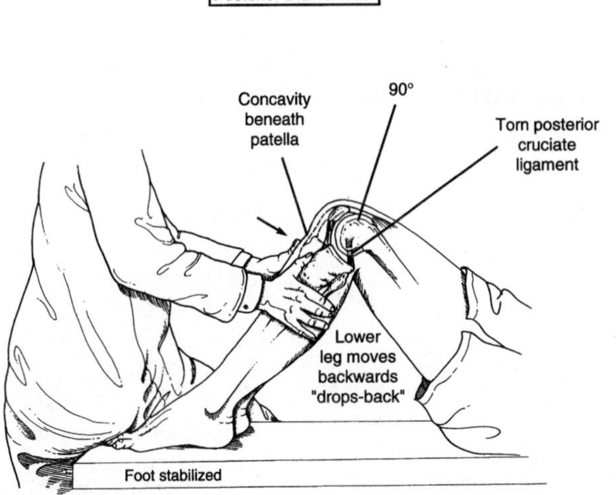

Figure 127-7 Posterior cruciate ligament deficiency results in a posterior sag (Godfrey's sign) in the resting position, which can be appreciated at 90 degrees of flexion by comparing the contour of the anterior knee with that of the opposite side. Further posteriorly directed force produces the posterior drawer test to assess the extent of laxity. (From Scuderi GR, McCann PD, Bruno PJ: *Sports medicine: principles of primary care,* St Louis, 1997, Mosby.)

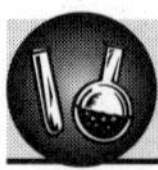

TABLE 127-2 Diagnostic Tests: Knee Injuries

Test	Finding/Rationale	Cost ($)
X-ray evaluation	Obtain when there is significant pain, swelling, effusion, contusion, or high-impact injury. Always obtain multiple views: Anteroposterior, lateral, and oblique. Obtain a sunrise view of the patella if trauma occurred directly to the patella.	113-132

TABLE 127-3 Differential Diagnosis: Knee Injuries

Diagnosis	Supporting Data
Bursitis	Limitation of movement caused by swelling, pain on movement, point tenderness; site is erythematous and warm. The most common site is the prepatellar bursae in the knee.
Gonococcal arthritis	Suspect in young adult who presents with an edematous, erythematous knee with no history of trauma.
Gout (Ch. 82)	Increased uric acid production: Red, hot; swollen joint, exquisite pain, limited range of motion, tophi, low-grade fever, more common in men >40 years old.
Osteoarthritis (Ch. 15)	Articular deterioration and bony overgrowth of the joint surface. Pain is the most common symptom, occurring with motion and activity, relieved by rest. Physical findings include crepitus, swelling, restriction of movement, joint enlargement. X-ray evaluation reveals joint space narrowing, spur formation, sclerosis, and subchondral cyst formation.
Rheumatoid arthritis	Multiple joints involved. Women most commonly affected. Usually subacute in onset, often symmetric. Morning stiffness >1 hr, joint involvement with redness, swelling, heat, and stiffness. X-ray evaluation reveals soft tissue swelling, joint space narrowing, erosion, and deformity.
Tendinitis (Ch. 175)	Microscopic tears of the involved muscles with inflammation. Joints have normal range of motion, no swelling, and appear normal on x-ray evaluation.

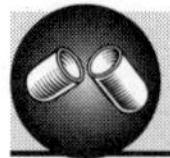

TABLE 127-4 Pharmaceutical Plan: Knee Injuries

Drug	Dosage	Comments	Cost
Naproxen (Naprosyn)	250-500 BID	NSAIDs are indicated for musculoskeletal injury; they inhibit prostaglandin synthesis, which decreases pain. *Do not* prescribe to those with peptic ulcer disease, allergy to NSAIDs/ASA, or renal dysfunction or to pregnant women. Pregnancy: B (D if used near term; etodolac: C)	\$12-\$80/250 mg (100); \$18-\$126/500 mg (100); \$100/SR 500 mg (75)
Ibuprofen (Motrin)	200-800 mg QID; maximum 3.2 g/day		\$3-\$9/200 mg (100); \$4-\$80/600 mg (100)
Etodolac (Lodine)	200-400 mg q6-8h		\$114/200 mg (100); \$128/300 mg (100): \$132/400 mg (100)

ASA, Aspirin; *NSAID*, nonsteroidal antiinflammatory drug.

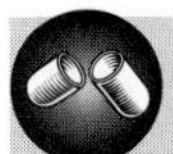

TABLE 127-5 Pharmaceutical Plan: Muscle Relaxants

Drug	Dose	Comments	Cost
Cyclobenzaprine (Flexeril)	10 mg TID	Pregnancy: B SE: Drowsiness, confusion, constipation, dry mouth, blurred vision, urinary retention	\$13-\$100/10 mg (100)
Chlorzoxazone (Parafon Forte)	250-750 mg TID-QID	Pregnancy: C SE: Dizziness, drowsiness, nausea, hepatotoxicity	\$5-\$58/250 mg (100); \$16-\$104/500 mg (100)
Orphenadrine citrate (Norflex)	100 mg BID	Pregnancy: C SE: Tachycardia, transient dizziness, urinary retention, ↑ IOP, blurred vision, dry mouth	\$127/100 mg (100)
Methocarbamol (Robaxin)	1000-1500 mg QID	Pregnancy: C SE: Drowsiness, GI upset, blurred vision, headache, hypotension	\$6-\$49/500 mg (100); \$8-\$72/750 mg (100)
Carisoprodol (Soma)	350 mg TID/QID	Pregnancy: C SE: Dizziness, drowsiness, nausea, epigastric distress, tachycardia	\$7-\$179/350 mg (100)

IOP, Intraocular pressure; *GI,* gastrointestinal, *SE,* side effects.

Referral

Patients with the following should be referred immediately to an orthopedic surgeon: displaced fractures, intra-articular fractures, and all fractures with neurovascular compromise.

Patients should be referred to an orthopedic surgeon to be seen in 3 to 5 days for simple, nondisplaced fractures, and grade II and III sprains after appropriate splinting and patient education.

EVALUATION/FOLLOW-UP

Recheck all minor injuries/sprains in 1 week. For patients whose injury is not showing improvement, consider referral to an orthopedic surgeon.

Begin rehabilitation for minor injuries/sprains as soon as possible to prevent contractures and loss of conditioning.

Continue NSAIDs with food.

Refer to an orthopedic surgeon any injury that does not respond to conservative care.

SUGGESTED READINGS

Anderson B: *Office orthopedics for primary care,* Philadelphia, 1995, WB Saunders.

Balano K: Anti-inflammatory drugs and myorelaxants: pharmacology and clinical use in musculoskeletal disease, *Primary Care* 23:329-334, 1996.

Budoff JE et al: Knee problems: diagnostic tests for injuries, *Consultant* 37:915-930, 1997.

Dvorkin ML: *Office orthopedics,* Norwalk, Conn, 1993, Appleton & Lange.

Eiff MP: *Fracture management for primary care,* Philadelphia, 1998, WB Saunders.

Ellsworth A et al: *Mosby's 1998 medical drug reference,* St Louis, 1998, Mosby.

Garth W, Fagan K: Knee injuries in sports. In Masear V, editor: *Primary care orthopedics,* Philadelphia, 1996, WB Saunders.

Healthcare Consultants of America, Inc: *1998 Physicians fee and coding guide,* Augusta, Ga, 1998, Healthcare Consultants of America, Inc.

Koutures CG et al: The acutely injured knee, *Pediatr Ann* 26:50-55, 1997.

Martin R: Initial assessment and management of common fractures, *Primary Care* 23:405-409, 1996.

Meislin R: Managing collateral ligament tears of the knee, *Phys Sports Med* 24:67-80, 1996.

Swenson EJ: Diagnosing and managing meniscal injuries in athletes, *J Musculoskeletal Med* 12(5):35-45, 1995.

Torburn L: Principles of rehabilitation, *Primary Care* 23:335-343, 1996.

Musculoskeletal Injuries: Shoulder

ICD-9-CM

Sprains and Strains 848.9
Other Bursitis 727.3
Tendinitis 762.90
Rotator Cuff Tear 840.4

OVERVIEW

Definitions

Shoulder injuries are common, because the shoulder has the widest range of motion (ROM) of any joint, thus predisposing it to instability and injury. Eight percent to 13% of all athletic injuries involve the shoulder, and shoulder dislocations account for more than 50% of all major joint locations seen in the emergency department. Traumatic injuries are common in football and ice hockey.

Children are vulnerable to the same injuries as adults; however, the strength of the joint capsule and its ligament is two to five times greater than that of the epiphyseal plate. *Therefore, an injury that produces a sprain or dislocation in an adult often causes a fracture through the growth plate of a child.*

A sprain is an injury of one of the ligamentous structures of the body. A dislocation is the complete separation of the contact between two bones in a joint, often caused by pressure or force pushing the bone out of joint. A fracture is a loss in continuity in the substance of the bone.

Anatomy

Shoulder: The shoulder is a ball-and-socket joint that permits movement of the humerus on many axes. It consists of three bones (the clavicle, humerus, and scapula) and three joints:

The glenohumeral joint forms the articulation of the humerus and the glenoid fossa of the scapula. The acromion and coracoid processes and the ligaments between them form the capsule surrounding and protecting the joint.

The acromioclavicular (AC) joint forms the articulation between the acromion process and the clavicle.

The sternoclavicular joint forms the articulation between the manubrium and the clavicle. All three joints comprise the shoulder girdle (Figure 128-1).

The rotator cuff plays an essential role in the movement of the shoulder. It consists of four muscles that originate on the scapula and insert on the humeral head:

Supraspinatus (most commonly injured)
Infraspinatus
Teres minor
Subscapularis

Pathophysiology

Fracture of Clavicle

The clavicle is typically injured by a fall against the shoulder or on an outstretched hand. The clavicular fracture accounts for 5% of all fractures and is the most commonly fractured bone during **childhood.** Fractures of the clavicle are classified into three types:

Proximal third: Results from a blow to the chest (relatively rare, 5%)

Middle third: Accounts for 80% of all injuries; results from an indirect force applied to the lateral aspect of the shoulder

Distal third: Results from a direct blow to the top of the shoulder (15% of injuries)

Glenohumeral Dislocation

This joint is the most frequently dislocated joint in the body. The lack of body stability along with a wider range of motion (ROM) predisposes this joint to dislocation. There are two distinct incidence peaks—the first in men **20 to 30 years old** and the second in women **61 to 80 years old.** Dislocations are most commonly anterior and result from a fall on the externally rotated abducted arm. This forces the humerus out of the glenoid cavity into its anterior position. Posterior dislocations are less common and may result from a force directed against the internally rotated arm. Many posterior dislocations may occur during a seizure in patients with convulsive disorders.

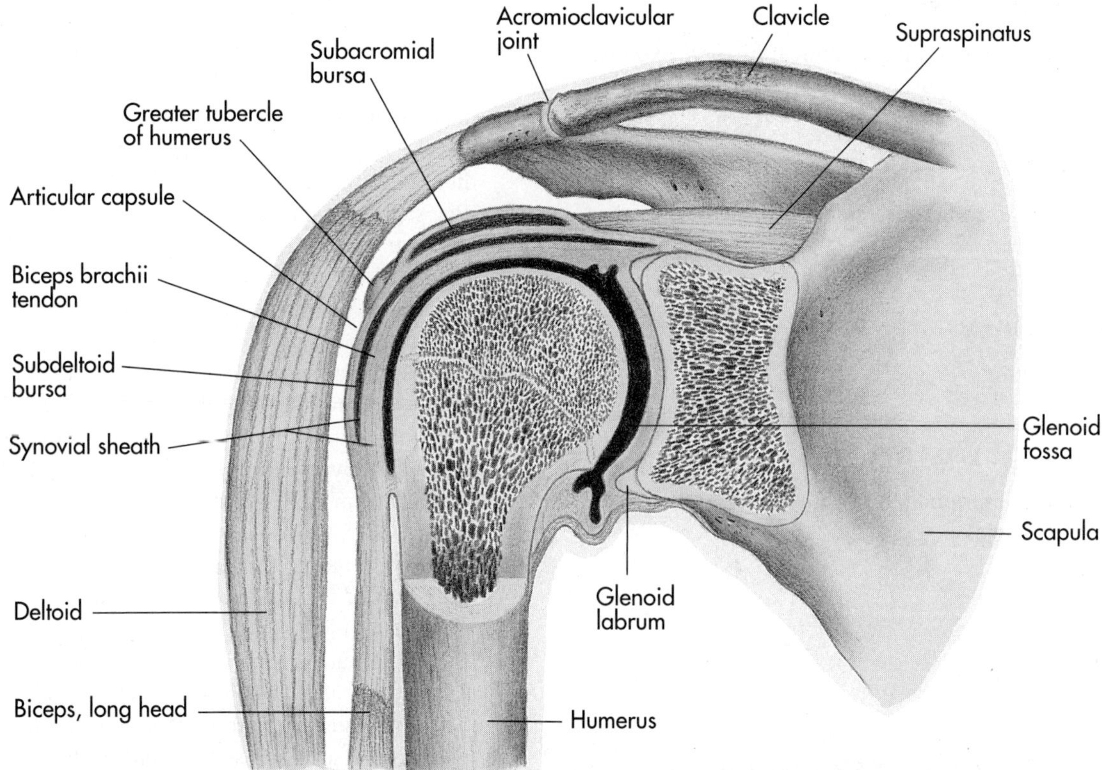

Figure 128-1 Structures of glenohumeral and acromioclavicular joints. (From Seidel HM et al: *Mosby's guide to physical examination,* ed 4, St Louis, 1999, Mosby.)

Acromioclavicular Separation

A separation of the AC junction usually occurs as a result of a fall on the shoulder or from a direct blow to the top of the shoulder with the arm in adduction. The acromion is driven away from the clavicle. An AC separation can be graded I through V based on the degree of damage sustained by the acromioclavicular and coracoclavicular ligaments. Grades I and II are sometimes known as incomplete separation, and grades III through V are called complete. These most commonly occur in males and account for 12% of all dislocations around the shoulder girdle. Most injuries occur in contact sports.

Fracture of the Proximal Humerus

Fractures of the proximal humerus account for 4% to 5% of all fractures. They occur primarily in **older persons** in whom the structural changes associated with osteoporosis weaken the proximal humerus. The mechanism of injury involves a fall on an outstretched, abducted arm. In older patients the humerus tends to fracture, whereas in younger patients it tends to dislocate.

Factors Associated with Increased Risk of Injury

Poor physical conditioning
Failure to warm up muscles adequately before exercise
Intensity of competition
Collision and participation in contact sports
Rapid growth
Overuse of joints (Seidel et al, 1995)

SUBJECTIVE DATA

History of the Present Illness

Exact mechanism of injury
Timing of injury
Description/location, radiation, quality, timing, and severity of pain
What exacerbates/relieves pain
Previous treatment
Any joint complaints: Stiffness, limitation of motion, pain with motion, joint locking or giving way
Effects of activity on joint should be determined; specifically ask about pain at night that awakens patient

The history of shoulder problems usually involves some combination of pain, stiffness, instability, and weakness. (Significant shoulder weakness is usually associated with a rotator cuff tear or an underlying nerve lesion.)

Associated Symptoms

Swelling, deformity, masses, paralysis, gait changes

Past Medical History

Previous injuries or dislocations; surgical history; exercise history, chronic illness, osteoporosis, skeletal deformities

Medications

Recent or present use of pain medications, NSAIDs, other medications

Family History

Orthopedic problems

Psychosocial History

Occupational job description with lifting history
Smoking, alcohol intake
Conditioning history

Allergy

Any allergies

Pertinent History of Common Shoulder Injuries

Shoulder dislocation: Patient will describe a fall onto his or her arm and will complain of severe pain with movement. The arm is held in slight abduction and external rotation by the opposite extremity.

AC separation: Patient will describe a fall on the shoulder or a blow to the top of the shoulder. Tenderness and swelling is present over the AC joint.

Fractured clavicle: Patient will complain of pain in the clavicle, with tenderness and swelling at site, holding the affected extremity close to the body.

Proximal humerus fracture: Patient will describe a fall on an outstretched arm. The affected arm is held close to the body, and all movements are restricted by pain.

OBJECTIVE DATA

Physical Examination

A problem-oriented physical examination should be conducted, with particular attention to:

Vital signs: Should be relatively normal with common nonlife-threatening injuries.

General: Note gait, patient response to pain, and how the patient is holding the injured extremity.

Musculoskeletal: Observe for swelling and effusion, palpate adjacent and actual areas of injury, evaluate ROM, and perform physical tests to diagnose a specific condition.

Shoulder: Inspect the contour of the shoulders, shoulder girdle, clavicles, and scapulae for symmetry of size and contour. Note any obvious deformity, ecchymosis, laceration, swelling, or hematoma. Palpate the sternoclavicular and acromioclavicular joints, clavicle, scapulae, coracoid process, greater trochanter of the humerus, biceps groove, and shoulder muscles. Start at the sternoclavicular joint and move laterally to the clavicle to the acromioclavicular joint, followed by palpation of the scapula, glenohumeral joint, and humerus. The presence of any point tenderness, crepitus, swelling, or deformity should be noted.

ROM: Both active and passive ROM should be evaluated. Active ROM is best evaluated in the sitting position, which eliminates contributions of the lumbar spine and lower extremity joints. Passive ROM is best evaluated in the supine position. The degrees of abduction, forward flexion, extension, and internal and external rotation should be recorded and compared with that of the unaffected extremity:

Shrug shoulders.
Raise both arms forward and over the head.
Extend and stretch both arms behind back.
Lift arms laterally and straight over head.
Swing each arm across the front of the body.
Place both arms behind the hips, elbows out.
Place both arms behind the head, elbows out.

Check cranial nerve (CN) XI by having the patient shrug his or her shoulders against your downward pressure.

Impingement test: Elevate patient's arm with one hand while preventing scapular motion with the other hand. Grimacing suggests impingement.

Crossover test: Place hand on opposite shoulder. Examiner pushes down on elbow while patient resists. Pain indicates acromioclavicular joint pathology.

Neurovascular: Assess the region distal to the injury. Check pulses, sensation, and capillary refill.

Specific Physical Findings of Common Shoulder Injuries

Dislocation: The acromion is more prominent than usual; there is an absence of normal fullness of the humeral head beneath the deltoid and acromion process. Little ROM is possible without severe pain. Anteriorly, the arm is held externally rotated, the anterior shoulder is full, and internal rotation is painful. The patient leans away from the shoulder and cannot adduct or internally rotate the shoulder.

AC separation: The patient should be examined in a sitting or standing position, because the supine position can mask joint instability. Type I injuries may have mild tenderness and swelling over the joint margin. There is no joint deformity, and a full ROM is possible. Type II injuries produce moderate pain, whereas type III injuries are associated with severe pain and the arm is adducted

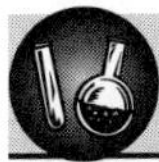

TABLE 128-1 Diagnostic Tests: Shoulder Injuries

Test	Findings/Rationale	Cost ($)
X-ray evaluation	Consider when there is significant pain, swelling, effusion, or contusion. Comparison views of the opposite normal extremity may be helpful if the injury involves a growth plate in a **child.** Views should include AP, transscapular, and axillary lateral.	shoulder: 109-128; clavicle: 95-112
Arthrography	90% Sensitive for rotator cuff tears, but invasive and requires dye.	273-324
Magnetic resonance imaging (MRI) of shoulder	Noninvasive, 84%-100% accuracy when combined with clinical findings. Rare for impingement syndrome, since MRI is expensive. Refer to orthopedist, who will decide which text is most appropriate.	1468-1741
AC joint with and without weights	AC views use less intensity to better view the injury. Complete dislocations may be differentiated from incomplete dislocations by an AP view taken while the patient has a 10-kg weight hanging from both wrists (not holding). Widening will be present on the affected side if complete dislocation has occurred. These views are expensive and painful so are generally not done.	113-134

AC, Acromioclavicular; *AP,* anteroposterior.

close to the body. The shoulder hangs down and the clavicle rides high, producing an obvious deformity.

Fracture of the clavicle: With a midclavicular fracture, the shoulder is slumped downward, forward, and inward. The proximal fragment of the clavicle is displaced upward. Crepitus and a palpable deformity may be present.

Fracture of the proximal humerus: Tenderness, deformity, hematoma, or crepitus may be present over the fracture site.

Diagnostic Procedures

Diagnostic procedures are outlined in Table 128-1.

Radiographic Findings With Common Shoulder Injuries

AC separation: Widening between the coracoid process and the clavicle will be present.

Fracture of the clavicle: X-ray films reveal the separation of the clavicle, showing the greenstick fracture common in **children.** Most fractures are nondisplaced.

Fracture of the proximal humerus: X-ray films show that most fractures are nondisplaced (80% to 85%).

Glenohumeral dislocation: X-ray films show a dislocation. Fractures may be present in up to 50% of all cases. The most common situation is a compression fracture of the posterolateral aspect of the humeral head. The defect is best viewed on an internal rotation view of the glenohumeral joint.

ASSESSMENT

Differential Diagnosis

Differential diagnoses include sprain, strain, fracture, tendinitis, osteoarthritis, rheumatoid arthritis, cellulitis, gout, gonococcal arthritis, tumors, degenerative changes, congenital disorders, overuse syndromes, and infections (Figure 128-2). The most common diagnoses are presented in Table 128-2.

THERAPEUTIC PLAN

RICE

The RICE formula for treatment of an injury stands for rest, ice, compression, and elevation:

- **R**est any injured part of the musculoskeletal system. Rest time varies according to the seriousness of the injury.
- **I**ce all musculoskeletal injuries to attempt to control swelling. Continue ice application as long as swelling exists. Ice can be applied for 15 minutes at a time.
- **C**ompression controls edema and provides comfort and/or support. Compression is difficult with the shoulder.
- **E**levate all injured extremities.

Shoulder dislocation: The dislocation should be reduced as soon as possible. It is usually reducible if good muscular relaxation is obtained. Gentle, straight traction on the arm

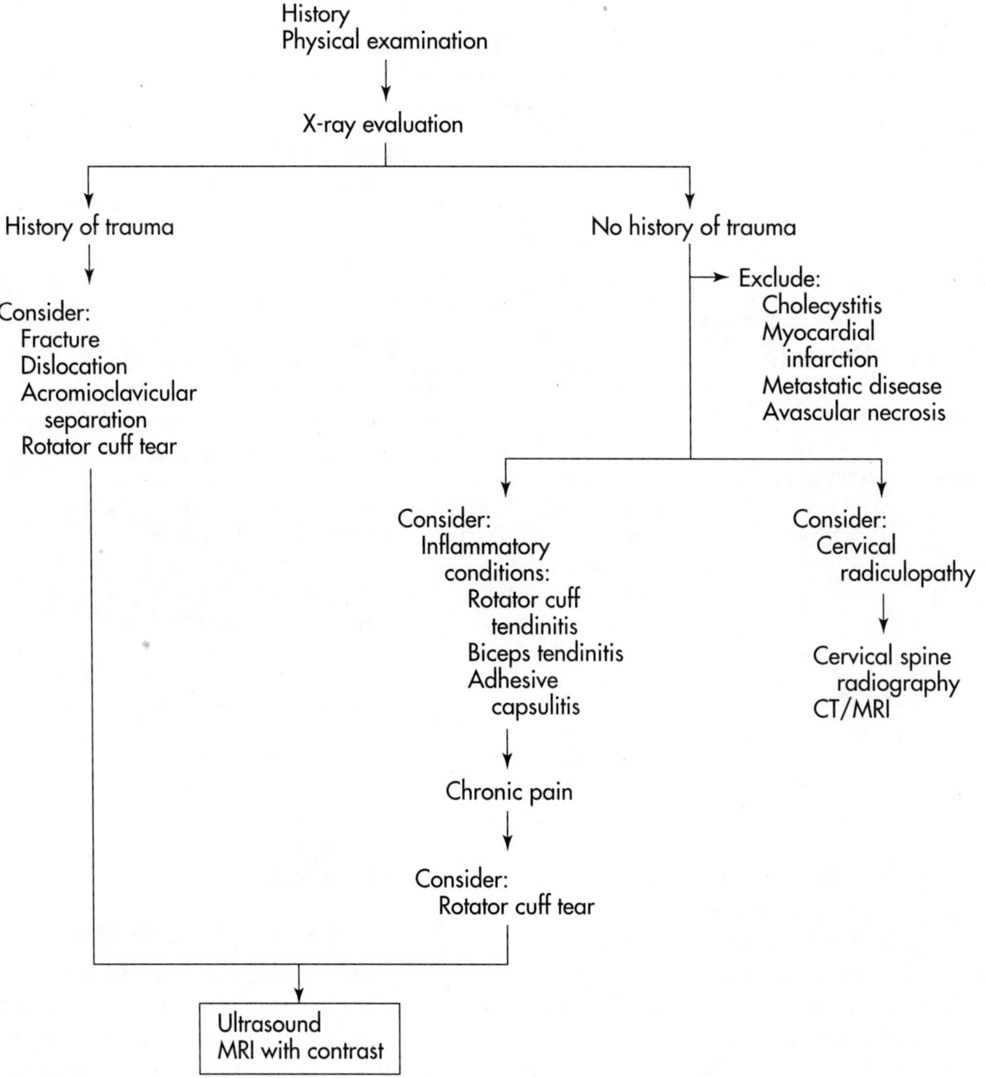

Figure 128-2 Algorithm for treatment of a patient with shoulder pain. (Adapted from Greene HL, Johnson WP, Lemcke D: *Decision making in medicine,* ed 2, St Louis, 1998, Mosby.)

is usually sufficient to reduce both anterior and posterior dislocations. Rehabilitation exercises are helpful.

AC separation: Reduction by manual pressure is performed, but reduction is difficult to maintain. A sling is used to minimize pain, and active ROM exercises are begun as soon as possible.

Fracture of the clavicle: Reduce by manipulating both shoulders upward, outward, and backward to reestablish the length of the clavicle. Midclavicular fractures are treated with a clavicular splint, a sling, or a sling and swathe.

Proximal humerus: Initial treatment consists of applying a sling and swathe. As soon as clinical union has occurred, functional exercises can be initiated.

Joint Protection/Immobilization

Splints for Particular Injuries

Shoulder dislocation: Sling or sling and swathe used for 1 to 2 weeks after reduction

Fracture of the clavicle: Figure-of-eight or clavicle strap (which holds shoulders upward, outward, and backward); worn for 4 to 5 weeks for a **child,** 5 to 6 weeks for an adult. The addition of a sling may be helpful.

Fracture of the proximal humerus: Sling and swathe

Pharmaceutical

Nonsteroidal antiinflammatory drugs (NSAIDs) and muscle relaxants are the drugs of choice for treatment of a

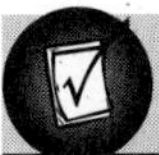

TABLE 128-2 Differential Diagnosis: Shoulder Injuries

Diagnosis	Supporting Data
Bursitis	Limitation of movement caused by swelling, pain on movement, point tenderness; site is erythematous and warm. The most common site is the subdeltoid
Gout (Ch. 82)	Increased uric acid production: red, hot; swollen joint, exquisite pain, limited range of motion, tophi, low-grade fever, more common in men >40 years old.
Osteoarthritis (Ch. 15)	Articular deterioration and bony overgrowth of the joint surface. Pain is the most common symptom, occurring with motion and activity, relieved by rest. Physical findings include crepitus, swelling, restriction of movement, joint enlargement. X-ray evaluation reveals joint space narrowing, spur formation, sclerosis, and subchondral cyst formation. Common finding in acromioclavicular joint. Crossover maneuver is painful.
Rheumatoid arthritis	Multiple joints involved. Women most commonly affected. Usually subacute in onset, often symmetric. Morning stiffness >1 hr, joint involvement with redness, swelling, heat, and stiffness. X-ray evaluation reveals soft tissue swelling, joint space narrowing, erosion, and deformity.
Tendinitis (Ch. 175)	Microscopic tears of the involved muscles with inflammation. Joints have normal range of motion, no swelling, and appear normal on x-ray evaluation. Biceps tendinitis is often secondary to impingement syndrome. Tenderness at the bicipital groove and pain with abduction.
Impingement syndrome	Tendinitis resulting from impingement due to overuse, acute injury, excessive overhead use, or anatomic abnormalities. Stage I: Acute injury; mild activity-related pain but no weakness or decrease in range of motion. Heals with conservative treatment; Most common <25 y/o. Stage II: Seen predominantly in 25-40 y/o. More chronic initiation, with thickening of subacromial bursae and supraspinatus tendinitis. Major symptoms are pain at night and interference with activities of daily living. Complains of popping or clicking. Painful range of motion. Positive Neer's sign. Stage III: Full or partial tear of the rotator cuff tendons. Usually seen in patients >40. Complains of weakness, stiffness, pain at night. Impaired range of motion, weakness of rotator cuff muscles.

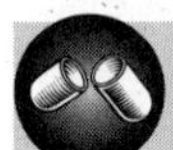

TABLE 128-3 Pharmaceutical Plan: NSAIDs

Drug	Dosage	Comments	Cost
Naproxen (Naprosyn)	250-500 BID	NSAIDs are indicated for MS injury. NSAIDs inhibit prostaglandin synthesis which decreases pain *Do not* prescribe to patients with	$12-$80/250 mg (100); $18-$126/500 mg (100); $100/SR 500 mg (75)
Ibuprofen (Motrin)	200-800 mg QID Maximum: 3.2 g/day	peptic ulcer disease, allergy to NSAIDs/ASA, renal dysfunction, or pregnant women	$3-$9/200 mg (100); $4-$80/600 mg (100)
Etodolac (Lodine)	200-400 mg q6-8h	Pregnancy: B (D if used near term; etodolac: C)	$114/200 mg (100); $128/300 mg (100); $132/400 mg (100)

ASA, Aspirin; *NSAID*, nonsteroidal antiinflammatory drug.

musculoskeletal injury (Tables 128-3 and 128-4). Myorelaxants are indicated for pain related to fracture and secondary muscle spasm and are prescribed for short periods of time (3 to 5 days). See Appendix J for more detailed prescription information for NSAIDs.

Narcotic analgesics are indicated only for fractures with severe pain and should be given for only a few days.

Patient Education

RICE: Emphasize the importance of rest and ice application to shoulder. The use of an Ace wrap can help hold the ice in place. All of these measures will tend to decrease swelling and help to control pain.

Pathophysiology: Explain the pathophysiology of the injury and expected outcomes.

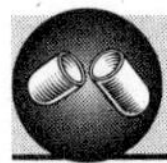

Table 128-4 Pharmaceutical Plan: Muscle Relaxants

Drug	Dose	Comments	Cost
Cyclobenzaprine (Flexeril)	10 mg TID	Pregnancy: B SE: Drowsiness, confusion, constipation, dry mouth, blurred vision, urinary retention	\$13-\$100/10 mg (100)
Chlorzoxazone (Parafon Forte)	250-750 mg TID-QID	Pregnancy: C SE: Dizziness, drowsiness, nausea, hepatotoxicity	\$5-\$58/250 mg (100); \$16-\$104/500 mg (100)
Orphenadrine citrate (Norflex)	100 mg BID	Pregnancy: C SE: Tachycardia, transient dizziness, urinary retention, ↑ IOP, blurred vision, dry mouth	\$127/100 mg (100)
Carisoprodol (Soma)	350 mg TID/QID	Pregnancy: C SE: Dizziness, drowsiness, nausea, epigastric distress, tachycardia	\$7-\$179/350 mg (100)
Methocarbamol (Robaxin)	1.5 g QID (two 750 mg tabs)	Pregnancy C SE: Drowsiness, GI upset, blurred vision, headache, hypotension	\$6-\$49/500 mg (100); \$8-\$72/750 mg (100)

IOP, Intraocular pressure; *GI,* gastrointestinal; *SE,* side effects.

Sling: Slings may be helpful to decrease pain. Caution is needed with older patients or patients with diabetes, since the shoulder can become frozen if it is not moved.

Medications: Include potential medication side effects and instructions for administration. Instruct the patient to take NSAIDs with food to avoid abdominal discomfort.

Muscle relaxants/narcotic analgesics may cause drowsiness; the patient should not operate machinery or work above ground level.

Tell the patient that primary dislocations of the shoulder in patients younger than 30 years old have a high rate of recurrence, often with little trauma. Recurrent dislocations may require corrective surgery.

Referral/Consultation

Patients with the following should be referred immediately to an orthopedic surgeon: long-bone fractures, displaced fractures, intraarticular fractures, and all fractures with neurovascular compromise.

Patients should be referred to an orthopedic surgeon to be seen in 3 to 5 days for simple, nondisplaced fractures after appropriate splinting and patient education.

EVALUATION/FOLLOW-UP

Recheck all minor injuries/sprains in 1 week. For patients whose injury is not showing improvement, consider referral to an orthopedic surgeon.

Begin rehabilitation for minor injuries/sprains as soon as possible to prevent contractures and loss of conditioning. Gentle stretching (bend forward, lean over chair/stool, swing arm in pendulum fashion) for 3 to 5 minutes five to ten times a day is very effective in maintaining shoulder motion.

Advise the patient to continue NSAIDs with food.

The most common complication seen with proximal humerus fractures is a frozen shoulder. This can be prevented with an early rehabilitation program. Patients who have diabetes are at increased risk for this complication.

REFERENCE

Seidel HM et al: *Mosby's guide to physical examination,* ed 4, St Louis, 1995, Mosby.

SUGGESTED READINGS

Anderson B: *Office orthopedics for primary care,* Philadelphia, 1995, WB Saunders.

Balano K: Anti-inflammatory drugs and myorelaxants: pharmacology and clinical use in musculoskeletal disease, *Primary Care* 23:329-334, 1996.

Daya M: Shoulder. In Rosen P, Barkin R, editors: *Emergency medicine: concepts and clinical practice,* ed 3, St Louis, 1992, Mosby.

Ellsworth A et al: *Mosby's 1998 medical drug reference,* St Louis, 1998, Mosby.

Healthcare Consultants of America, Inc: *1998 Physicians fee and coding guide,* Augusta, Ga, 1998, Healthcare Consultants of America, Inc.

Lemos L: The evaluation and treatment of injured acromioclavicular joints in the athlete, *Am J Sports Med* 26:137-144, 1998.

Lyon R, Street C: Pediatric sports injury: when to refer or x-ray, *Pediatr Clin North Am* 45:221-244, 1998.

Mercier L: *Practical orthopedics,* ed 4, St Louis, 1995, Mosby.

Shearman C, Med B, El-Khoury G: Pitfalls in the radiologic evaluation of extremity trauma: Part I. The upper extremity, *Am Family Physician* 57:995-1002, 1998.

Musculoskeletal Injuries: Wrist

ICD-9-CM

Strains and Sprains 848.9
Tendinitis 762.90

OVERVIEW

Definitions

A sprain is an injury to one of the ligamentous structures of the body. A dislocation is the complete separation of the contact between two bones in a joint, often caused by pressure or force pushing the bone out of joint. A fracture is a loss in continuity in the substance of the bone.

Anatomy

The wrist is composed of the distal radius, distal ulna, and the eight carpal bones, along with their attaching ligaments (Figure 129-1).

Pathophysiology

Wrist fractures commonly occur as a result of a fall on an outstretched hand. Fracture of the distal radius is common among **elderly** persons because of osteoporotic bone changes. Carpal bones can be fractured and or dislocated. The most common ligamentous injury of the wrist is the scapholunate ligament, which helps maintain position of the carpal bones and therefore injury leads to instability of the wrist.

Common Wrist Injuries

A Colles fracture is a fracture of the distal radius and is the most common type of **adult** wrist fracture. The distal radius fragment is displaced dorsally. Smith's fracture of the distal radius with a volar displaced fragment is less common. A scaphoid fracture (also called a navicular fracture) is the most common carpal bone fracture because of its anatomical location, in which it spans both rows of carpal bones.

SUBJECTIVE DATA

History of the Present Illness

Exact mechanism of injury
Timing of injury
Description/location, radiation, quality, timing, and severity of pain
Factors that exacerbate/relieve pain; such as movement, medication, immobilization
Previous treatment

Past Medical History

Previous injuries and surgeries
Exercise history

Medications

Recent or present use of pain medications, nonsteroidal antiinflammatory drugs (NSAIDs), other medications

Family History

Orthopedic problems

Psychosocial History

Occupational job description
Smoking, alcohol intake
Conditioning history

Allergies

Any allergies

Pertinent History of Common Wrist Injuries

Colles fracture is associated with a fall on an outstretched hand.

Scaphoid fractures are usually seen in **young adults** who have sustained a fall on an outstretched hand.

Associated Symptoms

Swelling, deformity, masses, paralysis

OBJECTIVE DATA

Physical Examination

A problem-oriented physical examination should be conducted with particular attention to:

Vital signs: Should be relatively normal with common nonlife-threatening injuries.

General: Note patient's gait, response to pain, and how the patient is holding the injured extremity.

Musculoskeletal: Observe for swelling and effusion, palpate adjacent and actual areas of injury, evaluate range of motion (ROM), and perform physical testing to diagnose a specific condition.

Inspect the dorsal and palmar aspects of the hands, noting contour, position, shape, number, and completeness of digits.

Palpate each joint in the wrist and hand.

Examine ROM:

- Bend fingers forward at the metacarpophalangeal (MCP) joint, then stretch joints up and back at the knuckle.
- Touch the thumb to each finger; make a fist.
- Spread the fingers apart and then touch them together.
- Bend the wrist up and down. Expect flexion of 90 degrees and hyperextension of 70 degrees.
- With palm side down, turn the hand right and left.

Neurovascular assessment should be performed distal to the injury. Check pulses, sensation, and capillary refill.

Specific Physical Findings of Common Wrist Injuries

Colles fracture presents with the classic "dinner fork" appearance, with considerable pain and resistance to ROM on palpation. Concomitant median nerve injury commonly occurs with a Colles fracture. Numbness and tingling of the thumb, index, long, and radial half of the ring fingers should be noted.

Scaphoid fractures present with a painful wrist, localized to the anatomical snuffbox. Elicitation of pain when this

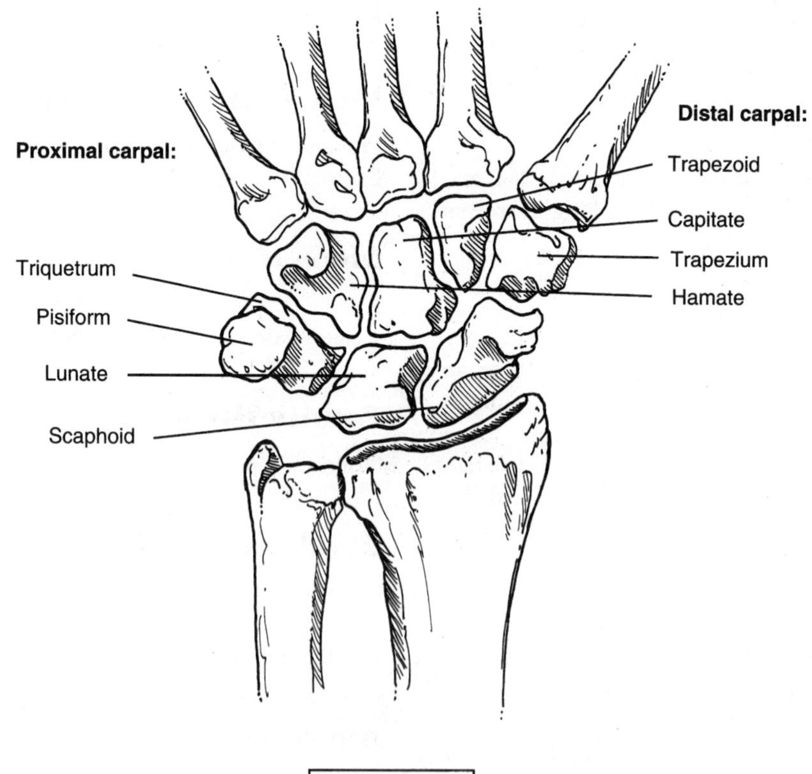

Figure 129-1 Wrist bones. The carpal bones consist of the proximal row (scaphoid, lunate, and triquetrum), the distal row (trapezium, trapezoid, capitate, and hamate), and the pisiform. (From Scuderi GR, McCann PD, Bruno PJ: *Sports medicine: principles of primary care,* St Louis, 1997, Mosby.)

area is palpated is reason to consider a scaphoid fracture, even when x-ray films appear normal (Figure 129-2).

Diagnostic Procedures

Diagnostic procedures are outlined in Table 129-1.

Radiographic Findings with Wrist Injuries

Colles fractures reveal a fractured distal radius with a dorsally displaced distal fragment. Smith's fracture reveals a fractured distal radius with a volar displaced fragment.

Scaphoid fractures typically do not show up on initial x-ray films but may be evident on follow-up films 7 to 10 days after the injury.

ASSESSMENT

Differential Diagnosis

Differential diagnoses include sprain, strain, fracture, tendinitis, osteoarthritis, rheumatoid arthritis, cellulitis, gout, gonococcal arthritis, tumors, degenerative changes, congenital disorders, overuse syndromes, and infections. The most common diagnoses are listed in Table 129-2.

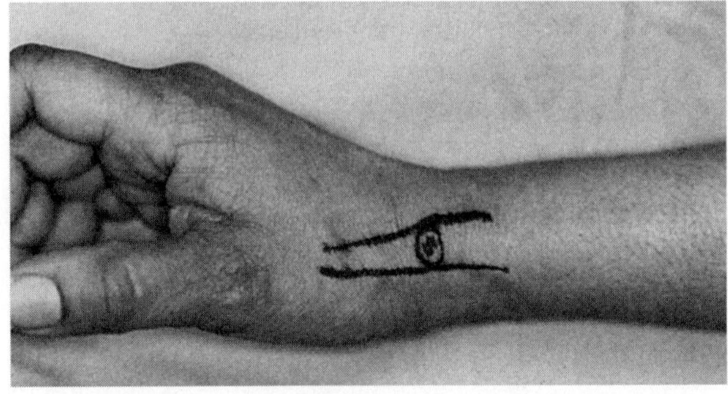

Figure 129-2 The "anatomic snuffbox" is easily viewed in this wrist. The dorsal boundary is the extensor pollicis longus, and the extensor pollicis brevis and abductor pollicis longus provide the palmar boundary. The proximal boundary is the radial styloid (not demarcated). The scaphoid *(S)* can be palpated in this region. (From Scuderi GR, McCann PD, Bruno PJ: *Sports medicine: principles of primary care,* St Louis, 1997, Mosby.)

THERAPEUTIC PLAN

The RICE formula for treatment of an injury stands for rest, ice, compression, and elevation:

Rest any injured part of the musculoskeletal system. Rest time varies according to the seriousness of the injury.

Ice all wrist injuries to attempt to control swelling. Continue ice application as long as swelling exists. Ice can be applied for 15 minutes at a time.

Compression controls edema and provides comfort and/or support. Compression can be accomplished with Ace wraps, custom-made splints, and commercially made splints. Any injury with snuffbox tenderness requires a thumb spica splint.

Elevate all injured extremities. Upper extremities should be elevated with a sling.

Joint Protection and Immobilization

The injured joint should be protected by applying a splint, allowing for postinjury swelling. Never apply a circumferential cast to an acutely injured extremity. Many splints are commercially made and easy to apply. Custom-made splinting material includes plaster and fiberglass. Immobilization will also assist in easing pain in the injured part.

Splints for Particular Wrist Injuries

Volar cock-up: Wrist sprains, Colles fractures

Sugar tong upper extremity: Colles fracture, forearm fractures

Thumb spica: Scaphoid fractures; all wrist injuries with snuffbox tenderness

Pharmaceutical

NSAIDs and muscle relaxants are the drugs of choice for treatment of a musculoskeletal injury (Tables 129-3 and 129-4).

Myorelaxants are indicated for pain related to muscle spasm and are prescribed for short periods of time (3 to 5 days). See the Appendix for more detailed prescription information for NSAIDs.

Narcotic analgesics are indicated only for fractures with severe pain and should be given for only a few days.

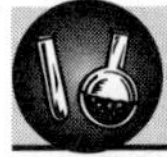

TABLE 129-1 Diagnostic Tests: Wrist Injuries

Tests	Findings/Rationale	Cost ($)
Wrist x-ray evaluation	Consider with significant pain, swelling, deformity, contusion or snuffbox tenderness. Always obtain multiple views and with snuffbox tenderness obtain additional navicular or scaphoid views of the wrist. Comparison views of the opposite normal extremity may be helpful if the injury involves a growth plate in a **child.**	102-121

TABLE 129-2 Differential Diagnosis: Shoulder Injuries

Diagnosis	Supporting Data
Bursitis	Limitation of movement caused by swelling, pain on movement, point tenderness; site is erythematous and warm. The most common site are is the olecranon.
Gout (Ch. 82)	Increased uric acid production: red, hot; swollen joint, exquisite pain, limited range of motion, tophi, low-grade fever, more common in men >40 years old.
Osteoarthritis (Ch. 15)	Articular deterioration and bony overgrowth of the joint surface. Pain is the most common symptom, occurring with motion and activity, relieved by rest. Physical findings include crepitus, swelling, restriction of movement, joint enlargement. X-ray evaluation reveals joint space narrowing, spur formation, sclerosis, and subchondral cyst formation.
Rheumatoid arthritis	Multiple joints involved. Women most commonly affected. Usually subacute in onset, often symmetric. Morning stiffness >1 hr, joint involvement with redness, swelling, heat, and stiffness. X-ray evaluation reveals soft tissue swelling, joint space narrowing, erosion, and deformity.
Tendinitis (Ch. 175)	Microscopic tears of the involved muscles with inflammation. Joints have normal range of motion, no swelling, and appear normal on x-ray evaluation.

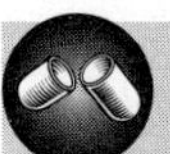

TABLE 129-3 Pharmaceutical Plan: NSAIDs

Drug	Dosage	Comments	Cost
Naproxen (Naprosyn)	250-500 BID	NSAIDs are indicated for MS injury. NSAIDs inhibit prostaglandin synthesis which decreases pain	$12-$80/250 mg (100); $18-$126/500 mg (100); $100/SR 500 mg (75)
Ibuprofen (Motrin)	200-800 mg QID Maximum: 3.2 g/day	*Do not* prescribe to patients with peptic ulcer disease, allergy to NSAIDs/ ASA, renal dysfunction, or pregnant women.	$3-$9/200 mg (100); $4-$80/600 mg (100)
Etodolac (Lodine)	200-400 mg q6-8h	Pregnancy: B (D if used near term; etodolac: C)	$114/200 mg (100); $128/300 mg (100); $132/400 mg (100)

ASA, Aspirin; *NSAID,* nonsteroidal antiinflammatory drug.

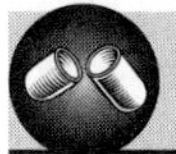

TABLE 129-4 Pharmaceutical Plan: Muscle Relaxants

Drug	Dose	Comments	Cost
Cyclobenzaprine (Flexeril)	10 mg TID	Pregnancy: B SE: Drowsiness, confusion, constipation, dry mouth, blurred vision, urinary retention	$13-$100/10 mg (100)
Chlorzoxazone (Parafon Forte)	250-750 mg TID-QID	Pregnancy: C SE: Dizziness, drowsiness, nausea, hepatotoxicity	$5-$58/250 mg (100); $16-$104/500 mg (100)
Orphenadrine citrate (Norflex)	100 mg BID	Pregnancy: C SE: Tachycardia, transient dizziness, urinary retention, ↑ IOP, blurred vision, dry mouth	$127/100 mg (100)
Carisoprodol (Soma)	350 mg TID/QID	Pregnancy: C SE: Dizziness, drowsiness, nausea, epigastric distress, tachycardia	$7-$179/350 mg (100)
Methocarbamol (Robaxin)	1.5 g QID (two 750 mg tabs)	Pregnancy: C SE: Drowsiness, GI upset, blurred vision, headache, hypotension	$6-$49/500 mg (100); $8-$72/750 mg (100)

IOP, Intraocular pressure; *GI,* gastrointestinal; *SE,* side effects.

Patient Education

RICE: Emphasize the importance of rest, ice application, use of splints/Ace wraps and elevation. All of these measures will tend to decrease swelling and help to control pain.

Pathophysiology: Explain the pathophysiology of the injury and expected outcomes.

Cast/splint care: Give detailed information concerning splint care including bathing instructions, removal and reapplication if indicated, and observation for signs of neurovascular compromise.

Medications: Include potential medication side effects and instructions for administration. Instruct the patient to take NSAIDs with food to avoid abdominal discomfort.

Muscle relaxants/narcotic analgesics may cause drowsiness; the patient should not operate machinery or work above ground level.

Referral/Consultation

Patients with the following should be referred immediately to an orthopedic surgeon: long-bone fractures, displaced fractures, intraarticular fractures, and all fractures with neurovascular compromise, dislocations of the elbow, and condylar fractures.

Most Colles and Smith's fractures require immediate referral due to bone fragment displacement, need for reduction and common neurovascular compromise.

Refer all patients with scaphoid fracture, even if nondisplaced, to an orthopedist. These fractures have a poor blood supply and nonunion is fairly common.

Patients should be referred to an orthopedic surgeon to be seen in 3 to 5 days for simple, nondisplaced fractures after appropriate splinting and patient education.

EVALUATION/FOLLOW-UP

Recheck all minor injuries/sprains in 1 week. For patients whose injury is not showing improvement, consider referral to an orthopedic surgeon.

Begin rehabilitation for minor injuries/sprains as soon as possible to prevent contractures and loss of conditioning.

Advise the patient to continue NSAIDs with food.

Refer the patient to an orthopedic surgeon if the injury does not respond to conservative care.

SUGGESTED READINGS

Anderson B: *Office orthopedics for primary care,* Philadelphia, 1995, WB Saunders.

Balano K: Anti-inflammatory drugs and myorelaxants: pharmacology and clinical use in musculoskeletal disease, *Primary Care* 23:329-334, 1996.

Ballas MT: Commonly missed orthopedic problems, *Am Family Physician* 57:267-274, 1998.

Dvorkin M: *Office orthopedics,* Norwalk, Conn, 1993, Appleton & Lange.

Eiff MP et al: *Fracture management for primary care,* Philadelphia, 1998, WB Saunders.

Ellsworth A et al: *Mosby's 1998 medical drug reference,* St Louis, 1998, Mosby.

Healthcare Consultants of America, Inc: *1998 Physicians fee and coding guide,* Augusta, Ga, 1998, Healthcare Consultants of America, Inc.

Lillegard WA: Common upper extremity injuries, *Arch Family Med* 5:159-168, 1996.

Savage PL: Casting and splinting techniques. In Maeser V: *Primary care orthopedics,* Philadelphia, 1996, WB Saunders.

Torburn L: Principles of rehabilitation, *Primary Care* 23:335-343, 1996.

Myocardial Infarction

ICD-9-CM

Acute Myocardial Infarction of Anterolateral Wall 410.0
Acute Myocardial Infarction, Unspecified Site 410.9

OVERVIEW

Definition

A myocardial infarction (MI) results when there is a lack of oxygen to the myocardium over a prolonged period of time that leads to necrosis of heart muscle.

Incidence

Each year in the United States, 900,000 persons suffer an MI. Approximately 225,000 of these individuals die, most as a result of arrhythmia. Mortality is greatest within the first 2 hours of the onset of symptoms. On average, women who have an MI are 10 years older than men who have an MI. However, by the time men and women are age 75, the incidence of coronary disease in women exceeds that in men (Douglas, 1993; Ryan et al, 1996).

Pathophysiology

The coronary arteries develop atherosclerotic changes with superimposed thrombi. These plaques cause a narrowing of the lumen of the arteries, and the development of thrombi further narrows the vessel. This may eventually lead to occlusion of the artery, thus causing ischemia to a particular area. If this ischemia is prolonged, infarction of muscle occurs (Pasternak, 1992). Myocardial infarction is rare during pregnancy. However, the greatest mortality occurs with MI late in pregnancy.

Precipitating Risk Factors

Cigarette use
Hyperlipidemia/hypercholesterolemia
Hypertension
Family history of premature coronary artery disease (CAD)
Obesity
Diabetes mellitus
Postmenopausal woman not receiving estrogen replacement therapy (ERT)

SUBJECTIVE DATA

Past Medical History

Assess presence of risk factors for coronary artery disease:

- Family history of premature CAD
- Age >65 in women
- Age >45 in men
- Previous history of atherosclerotic heart disease, diabetes, and hypertension
- Recent surgical procedure that may have resulted in a large blood loss

Medications

Previous and current medications
Medication allergies

Psychosocial History

Assess recent recreational drug use (cocaine can cause coronary spasm)

Description of Most Common Symptoms

Assess pain characteristics (usually occurs at rest; of longer duration than angina, and usually unrelieved by rest and/or nitroglycerin).

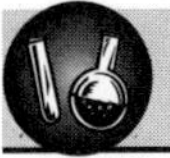

TABLE 130-1 Diagnostic Tests: Myocardial Infarction

Tests	Findings/Rationale	Cost ($)
ECG	ST-T changes, ST segment elevation with T wave inversions; Q wave development within 24-48 hr; Q wave absent in NQWMI (non–Q wave MI; nontransmural)	56-65
Cardiac enzymes	CPK-MB current standard	23-29/total;
	Are elevated in first 6-8 hr, peak within 24 hr, resolve within 72 hr	43-55/iso
Troponin I and troponin T	Markers for acute myocardial infarction; increased serum levels occur early after muscle damage	34-46/quant
	Troponin I present for up to 7 days after infarct; troponin T may be present for 10-14 days	
LDH (lactic dehydrogenase)	Elevation detectable 12 hr after chest pain, and peaks within 24-49 hr (Ryan et al, 1996)	20-25
Echocardiography	Assess LV wall motion abnormalities and valvular structures	675
CBC, electrolytes, PT/PTT	Rule out ischemia resulting from anemia	18-23/CBC;
	Elevated WBCs not abnormal in acute MI; check electrolytes—may contribute to ventricular arrhythmias if abnormal potassium	23-30/elect; 22-27/PT;
	Rule out elevated PT/PTT, which may indicate liver problem	23-29/PTT
CXR	Pulmonary venous congestion	77-91

CBC, Complete blood cell count; *CPK-MB,* creatine phosphokinase (with M and B isoenzyme subunits); *CXR,* chest x-ray examination; *ECG,* electrocardiogram; *PT,* prothrombin time; *PTT,* partial thromboplastin time; *WBCs,* white blood cells.

Pain can be described as a retrosternal ache, heaviness, or tightness, with radiation to jaw, neck, left arm, or through to the back. There may be an associated shortness of breath, nausea and vomiting, or diaphoresis.

MI may present with acute onset of dyspnea, congestive heart failure, or confusion in the absence of chest discomfort. This can be seen in persons with diabetes and **elderly persons.**

Atypical presentations may occur (Pasternak, 1992):
- Congestive heart failure
- Atypical location of pain (left arm or jaw pain only)
- Mental status changes secondary to decrease in cardiac output resulting in decreased cerebral perfusion from associated cerebral arteriosclerosis (**elderly** patients may present with confusion)
- Syncope
- Indigestion-like presentation

OBJECTIVE DATA

Physical Examination

A thorough physical examination should be performed, with particular attention to:

General appearance: Anxious, restlessness; Levine's sign (fist clenched against chest); diaphoresis, pallor.

Vital signs: Heart rate may vary from bradycardia to tachycardia; premature ventricular contractions common. Blood pressure may vary from hypotensive to hypertensive. The patient may develop a fever within 24 to 48 hours after the onset of MI because of tissue necrosis. The respiratory rate may be tachypneic.

Neck: The jugular venous pressure (volume overload) will be elevated.

Chest: Note the presence of rales, indicating left ventricular (LV) dysfunction.

Cardiac: An S_4 gallop is frequently present; this indicates decreased LV compliance. An S_3 gallop indicates LV dysfunction. Murmurs are commonly audible.
- New systolic murmurs are important and may indicate:
  - Mitral regurgitation
  - Ventricular septal defect

Pericardial friction rubs most commonly occur during the second or third day after the MI (Jaffe, 1995; Pasternak, 1992).

Diagnostic Procedures

Diagnostic procedures are outlined in Table 130-1.

ASSESSMENT

An MI can be confirmed if two of the following criteria are present (Jaffe, 1995):
- Prolonged ischemic-type chest discomfort
- ECG changes consistent with ischemia
- Elevated cardiac enzymes

Differential Diagnosis

Differential diagnoses are listed in Table 130-2.

TABLE 130-2 Differential Diagnosis: Myocardial Infarction

Differential Diagnosis	Symptoms	Diagnostic Procedure	Cost ($)
Pericarditis	Pleuritic pain, relieved with sitting and leaning forward; with or without rub	Echocardiography to rule out tamponade	675
Pulmonary embolus	Sudden-onset SOB, chest pain, hemoptysis	V/Q scan, ECG; inferior ST elevation	890-1060/VQ; 56-65/ECG
Aortic dissection	ST elevation or depression, NSST-T changes, abrupt onset severe chest pain, SOB	CT chest, MRI, or TEE	947-1126/CT; 1475-1860/MRI; 878-1035/TEE
Gallbladder disease	Nausea, vomiting, RUQ or epigastric pain, RUQ tenderness	Ultrasound GB	358
Pancreatitis	Elevated lipase/amylase, midepigastric pain	Serum amylase and lipase, CT scan of abdomen	24-30/amylase; 18-35/lipase; 953-1120/CT

CT, Computed tomography; *GB,* gallbladder; *NSSTT,* nonspecific ST-T (wave segment changes on electroencephalogram); *RUQ,* right upper quadrant; *SOB,* shortness of breath; *TEE,* transesophageal echocardiography.

THERAPEUTIC PLAN

Refer the patient to a physician if an MI is suspected—immediate intervention decreases mortality. Most of the therapeutic plan will be determined by the cardiologist and/or cardiology nurse practitioner.

Acute Intervention

Hospitalize immediately
Administer oxygen in initial course
Continuously monitor by electrocardiography; monitor and treat arrhythmias as appropriate
Bed rest for 24 hours and as condition warrants
Pharmacological intervention
- Thrombolytic medications should be used at the physician's discretion if there are no contraindications.
- Aspirin 325 mg may be used if there are no contraindications or allergies; aspirin has been proven to reduce mortality in long-term use.
- Heparin IV can be administered by standard or weight-adjusted protocol.
- Angiotensin-converting enzyme (ACE) inhibitors are given within the first 24 hours if the patient's blood pressure is stable and thrombolytic therapy has been completed. ACE inhibitors help prevent adverse remodeling and may improve longevity (see Chapter 96 for specific information about ACE inhibitors).
- Nitrates: Nitroglycerin SL provides vasodilation; *avoid long-acting nitrates in the early course of an MI.* Intravenous nitroglycerin is the preparation of choice in acute MI (Ryan et al, 1996). Give nitroglycerin 5 μg/min IV; increase slowly.
- Beta-blockers: Decrease myocardial oxygen demand, reduce morbidity and mortality during an evolving infarction (metoprolol 5 mg intravenously ×3, 2 minutes apart, followed by oral administration of 50 mg every 6 hours, starting 15 minutes after last intravenous dose).
- Analgesia: Morphine sulfate 2 to 6 mg intravenously every 2 to 4 hours as needed for pain.

Long-Term Pharmaceutical Care

Long-acting nitrates: May be started before the patient is discharged or as an outpatient if necessary for recurrent angina.
Isosorbide dinitrate (ISDN) half-life = 40 to 90 minutes; isosorbide-5-mononitrate (ISMN) half-life = 4 to 5 hours.
Table 130-3 outlines MI treatment with long-acting nitrates.

Long-Term Use of Beta-Blockers

Unless contraindicated because of hypotension, bradycardia, heart block (second or third degree), severe chronic obstructive pulmonary disease, or other conditions, beta-blockers should be started during hospitalization for an acute MI. Secondary prevention/long-term use: Titrate to tolerance in long-term use; reduces long-term mortality by decreasing incidence of sudden and nonsudden cardiac death (Ryan et al, 1996).

Table 130-4 outlines the pharmaceutical plan for treatment of MI using beta blockers.

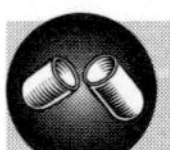

TABLE 130-3 Pharmaceutical Plan: Long-Acting Nitrates

Drug	Dosage	Maximum Dose	Cost
Isosorbide dinitrate (Isordil titradose)	Initial: 10 mg TID Maximum: 40 mg TID	Pregnancy C SE: Headache, flushing, dizziness, weakness, orthostatic hypotension	$30/10 mg (100)
Isosorbide mononitrate (ISMN)	10 mg BID Initial: 30 mg QD (Imdur) Maximum: 120 mg QD	Pregnancy: B SE: Orthostatic hypotension, headache, dizziness, caution with calcium channel blockers	$51/10 mg (100); $54-$76/20 mg (100)

SE, Side effects.

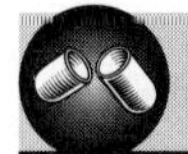

TABLE 130-4 Pharmaceutical Plan: Beta Blockers

Drug	Dosage	Comments	Cost
Atenolol (Tenormin)	25 mg QD-100 mg QD	Pregnancy: D SE: Fatigue, bradycardia, depression, sexual dysfunction, nightmares, heart failure	$9-$88/25 mg (100); $5-$90/50 mg (100)
Metoprolol (Lopressor)	25 mg BID-100 mg BID	Pregnancy: C SE: Fatigue, bradycardia, depression, sexual dysfunction, nightmares, heart failure	$11-$57/50 mg (100); $11-$82/100 mg (100)
Propranolol (Inderal)	10 mg TID-80 mg TID	Pregnancy: C SE: Fatigue, bradycardia, depression, sexual dysfunction, nightmares, heart failure	$1-$33/10 mg (100); $2-$35/20 mg (100); $2-$60/40 mg (100); $3-$82/80 mg (100)

SE, Side effects.

Calcium Channel Blockers

No evidence exists that use of calcium channel blockers leads to a reduction in mortality after acute MI. Calcium channel blockers should *not* be used in acute MIs unless beta-blockers are contraindicated or ineffective, and only if there is evidence of continued ischemia or atrial-fibrillation with a rapid ventricular rate and absence of LV dysfunction, congestive heart failure, or atrioventricular block (Ryan et al, 1996).

Calcium channel blockers can be used in patients whose angina or hypertension is not adequately controlled with other medications. If beta-blockers are not tolerated, calcium channel blockers, which slow the heart rate, may be appropriate as an alternative if there is preserved LV function (Ryan et al, 1996).

Complications

Cardiogenic shock
Cardiac arrest
Arrhythmias
Congestive heart failure
Postinfarction angina
Pericarditis
Dressler's syndrome (post MI syndrome)

Lifestyle/Activities

Discuss with the patient:
- Lifestyle and risk factor modification
- Smoking cessation
- Activity limitations

Diet

Low-fat/low-cholesterol diet: Consult with a dietitian if necessary, especially when associated medical conditions are present (renal failure, diabetes mellitus).

Patient Education

Importance of medication compliance: Include side effects, mechanism of action, benefits
Disease process and long-term implications and treatment

Lifestyle changes: Modification of risk factors: smoking, low-fat diet, exercise, stress reduction

Family Impact

Economic impact if patient is the breadwinner
Emotional lability and depression common after MI
Family member support is imperative

Referral

A patient with an acute MI should be referred to a physician.

Consultation

If the patient has an increase in recurrent chest pain/angina after an infarct, he or she should be referred to a physician.

Follow-up

Prescribe exercise stress testing to assess functional capacity; assess efficacy of the current treatment plan; risk stratification.

Consider cardiac rehabilitation program if appropriate.

Follow-up with healthcare provider within 1 to 2 weeks after discharge and then as indicated.

Evaluation of lipid profile should be performed as appropriate.

EVALUATION

Evaluate for recurrent chest pain or discomfort; reevaluate lifestyle changes (e.g., exercise, diet, return to work, daily activities); 10% to 15% of patients will have a recurrence of MI within 1 year.

REFERENCES

Douglas P: *Cardiovascular health and disease in women,* Philadelphia, 1993, WB Saunders.

Jaffe A: Acute myocardial infarction. In Crawford M: *Current diagnosis and treatment in cardiology,* Norwalk, Conn, 1995, Appleton & Lange.

Pasternak R, Braunwald E, Sobel B: Acute myocardial infarction. In Braunwald E: *Heart disease: a textbook of cardiovascular medicine,* Philadelphia, 1992, WB Saunders.

Ryan TJ et al: ACC/AHA guidelines for the management of patients with acute myocardial infarction: a report of the American College of Cardiology/American Heart Association Task Force on Practice Guidelines (Committee on Management of Acute Myocardial Infarction), *J Am Coll Cardiol* 28:1328-1428, 1996.

SUGGESTED READINGS

Arnstein P, Buselli E, Rankin S: Women and heart attacks: prevention diagnosis and care, *Nurse Pract* 21:57-69, 1996.

Crawford M: Approach to cardiac disease diagnosis. In Crawford M: *Current diagnosis and treatment in cardiology,* Norwalk, Conn, 1995, Appleton & Lange.

Ellsworth A et al: *Mosby's 1998 medical drug reference,* St Louis, 1998, Mosby.

Healthcare Consultants of America, Inc: *1998 Physicians fee and coding guide,* Augusta, Ga, 1998, Healthcare Consultants of America, Inc.

Reiss C, Eisenberg P: Ischemic heart disease. In Woodley M, Whelan A, editors: *The Washington manual,* Boston, 1992, Little Brown & Co.

Osgood-Schlatter Disease

ICD-9-CM

Juvenile Osteochondrosis of Lower Extremity, Excluding Foot 732.4

OVERVIEW

Definition

Osgood-Schlatter disease is a condition that involves inflammation and pain over the tibial tuberosity. It is also referred to as epiphysitis or apophysitis of the knee.

Incidence

Osgood-Schlatter disease is most common in athletic adolescents or preadolescents. It is very common in **children, ages 10-14,** who are participating in sports on a regular basis. It is more common in males than females.

Pathophysiology

The condition results when tendinitis of the anterior patellar tendon occurs. The patella is embedded in this tendon, and recurrent strain of this tendon results in associated osteochondrosis of the tibial tubercle. In its mildest state, there is avascular necrosis in the region of the tibial tubercle, and hypertrophic cartilage forms in the distal tendon itself in an attempt to repair the injury. On occasion, ossicles have been found that are separate from the tubercle. Severe cases of Osgood-Schlatter disease may result in an epiphyseal separation of the tibial tubercle.

Protective Factors Against

Stretching before exercise may be beneficial in that it may limit excessive strain of a tight tendon. Delayed or limited athletic participation until later in adolescence may allow for a longer period of growth and development of tendons, ligaments, and the quadriceps muscles and may help reduce stress of the patellar tendon.

Factors That Increase Susceptibility

As mentioned previously, excessive athletic endeavors, particularly at a young age, increase susceptibility. Furthermore, those activities requiring excessive running, jumping, lateral movement of the knees, and contraction of the quadriceps often contribute to the development of Osgood-Schlatter disease.

SUBJECTIVE DATA

History of Present Illness

Osgood-Schlatter presents as a gradually increasing pain and swelling over the tibial tubercle. Pain occurs during or immediately after activity or after direct trauma to the area. Pain decreases with cessation of the activity. Sudden pain may indicate that there is a pathologic fracture through an area of ischemic necrosis.

Past Medical History

Noncontributory

Medications

Nonsteroidal antiinflammatory drugs (NSAIDs) are recommended by some providers; others believe that NSAIDs have no specific benefit over other analgesics, any of which should be used to effectively manage pain.

Family History

No specific correlation between family members has been shown.

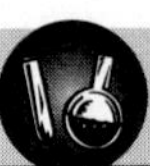

TABLE 131-1 Diagnostic Procedures: Osgood-Schlatter Disease

Diagnostic Test	Finding/Rationale	Cost ($)
X-ray of tibia/fibula	X-ray will confirm the enlargement of the tibial tubercle. The examiner should be alert for the presence of ossicles, necrosis, or fracture.	105-126

Psychosocial History

The patient may give a history of increasing athletic participation, trying out for a team, or increasing mileage (in runners).

Descriptions of Most Common Symptoms

Pain and swelling over the tibial tuberosity are the cardinal symptoms.

Associated Symptoms

Nighttime leg cramps may occur.

OBJECTIVE DATA

Physical Examination

Examination of the knee should include range of motion, testing for varus/valgus pain, McMurray's and drawer tests.

Tenderness of the tibial tuberosity is present. Mild inflammation may be visible. After long-standing disease, the tibial tuberosity will be prominent.

Diagnostic Procedures

Diagnostic procedures include those found in Table 131-1.

ASSESSMENT

Differential diagnoses include those found in Table 131-2.

THERAPEUTIC PLAN

Pharmaceutical

Pharmaceutical treatment is outlined in Table 131-3.

Lifestyle/Activities

Rest and avoiding activity that causes repetitive contraction of the quadriceps, or deep knee bending may be helpful.

Strengthening surrounding muscles, particularly the quadriceps has been found to be beneficial in some cases. (This can be done by simple lifting exercises that involve placing 1-pound objects such as canned vegetables or dried beans in each of two tube socks tied together and draped across the ankle. The athlete will gradually increase repetitions of extension of the lower legs.)

Recurrent conditions, or those resulting in severe pain, may require a rest period of 6 to 8 weeks.

Diet

No dietary changes will affect the course of this condition.

Patient Education

Rest

- Ice after sports
- Compression with a knee immobilizer (in severe cases) may help
- Stretching before exercise may also be beneficial

Family Impact

Overall family impact is not generally significant, but adolescents in pain or unable to participate in desired athletic activities may disrupt family harmony.

Referral

Casting per an orthopedist may be indicated in very severe cases to allow for full rest.

Surgery has been shown to provide relief for patients with ossicle development, but this step is rarely indicated unless long-term conservative therapy is not successful.

Consultation

The clinician should consult an orthopedist if there is a fracture or the probability of occult fracture (sudden onset of acute pain).

Also consult for conditions unresponsive to standard therapy.

Follow-up

See the patient in the office 1 to 2 weeks after the initial presentation to monitor symptoms and effectiveness of therapy.

TABLE 131-2 Differential Diagnosis: Osgood-Schlatter Disease

Diagnosis	Supporting Data
Avascular necrosis of the tibial tubercle	Fracture, agranulation, or procallus formation on x-ray
Growing pains	Pain more generalized, no localization or tenderness of tibial tuberosity
Hip abnormalities	Diffuse pain over distal femur, no localization over tibial tuberosity
Chondromalacia patellae	Seen in young adults, especially women; no history of recent trauma; pain occurs in peripatellar area with exertion such as stair-climbing or as deep aching in the knees; pain usually recurrent; patella may seem to face medially; tenderness of patella or medial aspect of knee on compression of the patella in the medial femoral groove; x-ray is unremarkable

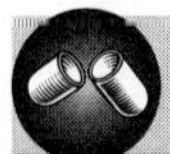

TABLE 131-3 Pharmaceutical Treatment: Osgood-Schlatter Disease

Drug	Dose	Comments	Cost
NSAIDs		See Appendix J for detailed information about NSAIDs	
Tylenol with Codeine No. 3 (30 mg codeine) 325 mg of Tylenol	1 tab q 4h PRN for pain	Pregnancy: C SE: Dizziness, drowsiness Risk of habituation, constipation, nausea and vomiting	Codeine only: $21/15 mg (100); $36-$42/30 mg (100)

Further follow-up is indicated for acute exacerbation of symptoms or significant changes in symptomatology.

EVALUATION

The clinician should work with the patient to help determine the degree of stress/athletic participation that may be undertaken without significant pain. Patients need to understand how to minimize stress (stretching, supporting muscle strengthening exercises), how to prevent pain (postparticipation icing of the tubercle), and how to treat pain (usually NSAIDs).

SUGGESTED READINGS

Burns C: *Pediatric primary care*, Philadelphia, 1996, WB Saunders.

Ellsworth A, et al: *Mosby's 1998 medical drug reference,* St Louis, 1998, Mosby.

Fox J: *Primary health care of children*, St Louis, 1997, Mosby.

Healthcare Consultants of America, Inc.: *1998 Physicians fee and coding guide*, Augusta, Ga, 1998, Healthcare Consultants of America, Inc.

McCance K: *Pathophysiology*, St Louis, 1998, Mosby.

Polin R: *Pediatric secrets*, St Louis, 1995, Mosby.

Osteoporosis

ICD-9-CM

Postmenopausal Osteoporosis 733.01

OVERVIEW

Definition

Osteoporosis is a systemic skeletal disease characterized by low bone mass and micro architectural deterioration of bone tissue, leading to enhanced bone fragility and consequent increase in fracture risk.

Incidence

Fifty percent of postmenopausal white women experience an osteoporotic fracture (only one in eight men in a comparable age group). Lifetime risk of hip fracture for a 50-year-old woman is 15%; the risk doubles every 10 years. $14 billion is spent annually on treatment. Hip fractures increase mortality, compromise functional ability, and increase risk for nursing home admission. Vertebral fractures account for more than 5 million restricted activity days in women aged 45 and older; they cause a loss of height, deform the spinal column, and lead to decreasing lung function.

Pathophysiology

Normally osteoclasts remove damaged bone from micro fractures that are caused by everyday stresses; osteoclasts then attract osteoblasts that replace bone matrix. Bone is lost if osteoclasts create a cavity of excessive depth or if osteoblasts incompletely fill a cavity. *Trabecular bone, the interior meshwork of the bone, is more susceptible to fracture and has a greater turnover rate than the exterior cortical bone.* Sites with a high proportion of trabecular bone such as the *spine, pelvis, distal radius and proximal femur are generally the first to have osteoporotic changes and fractures.*

The strength of bone in later life depends on (1) the peak strength of bone attained in early adulthood and (2) hormone deficiency-related bone loss. Normal levels of vitamin D, parathyroid hormone, calcitonin, thyroid hormone, and phosphorus are necessary for healthy bone metabolism.

Risk Factors for Osteoporosis

Risk factors are outlined in Box 132-1.

Protective Factors Against

Black race; obesity; early menarche; continuous estrogen replacement therapy (ERT) immediately after menopause; regular, varied, weight-bearing exercise 2 to 3 times weekly; diet rich in calcium with sufficient vitamin D; adequate vitamin K and mineral intake, thiazide diuretics

SUBJECTIVE DATA

History of Present Illness

Often asymptomatic

Ask about scoliosis, loss of 1.5 inches or more than maximum self-reported height, abdominal protuberance and change in fit of clothes, acute pain with sudden onset localized to specific vertebrae with local tenderness, chronic pain in paraspinal muscles that is localized to lumbar area, falls and/or inability to bear weight on a leg, constipation

Past Medical History

Ask about history of fractures, scoliosis, menstrual history, age of menarche, any form of ovarian function loss

Box 132-1

Modifiable and Nonmodifiable Risk Factors for Osteoporosis

Nonmodifiable	Modifiable
Advancing age	Low calcium intake
Postmenopausal status	Sedentary lifestyle
White or Asian race	Cigarette smoking
Female gender	>2 cups caffeine/day lifetime
Family history	Low weight for height
Light skin	Estrogen deficiency
Thin, small body frame	Glucocorticoid, phenytoin use
Scoliosis	Excessive thyroid hormones
Multiple myeloma, Cushing's	Excessive alcohol, sodium, protein intake

Long term use of Depo-Medrol may result in secondary osteoporosis

Box 132-2

How to Estimate Calcium Intake

Identify the daily servings of foods that provide substantial calcium (Table 132-1).

Use Table 132-1 to calculate total milligrams of calcium or add 300 mg calcium.

Add 200 mg calcium for women and 300 mg for men (from other foods).

If patient is taking a vitamin or mineral supplement, add milligrams calcium received.

Calculate the total 24-hour calcium intake from the previous steps.

Compare the total with recommended optimal calcium intake (see Table 132-2).

including late menarche, athletic amenorrhea, amenorrhea secondary to anorexia nervosa, bulimia and/or poor nutritional habits, hyperprolactinemia, gonadotropin-releasing hormone agonist therapy, premature or surgical menopause, irregular menses and/or oligomenorrhea, chronic illness, thyroid disorders, malignancies such as multiple myeloma, endocrinopathies such as hypogonadism if male, seizures.

Medications

Ask about current and past medications; chronic drug therapy, especially with anticonvulsants; cyclosporine, heparin, methotrexate, or corticosteroids; if menopausal, ask about ERT.

Diet History

Review over the lifetime for anything affecting nutrition such as bulimia; anorexia; gastrectomy; intestinal bypass; malabsorption syndrome; chronic renal failure; a diet high in protein, caffeine, sodium, and phosphate and/or low in calcium.

Obtain a 24-hr diet history and use Box 132-2 to estimate calcium intake.

Family History

Ask about family history of osteoporosis, particularly maternal hip fracture.

Psychosocial/Lifestyle History

Children and adolescents: Ask about current and lifetime physical activity patterns, including types of exercise and recreational sports; participation in weight-bearing sports; nicotine use, caffeine and alcohol intake; general nutritional habits, particularly calcium intake; and inadequate or excessive exercise and/or nutritional habits.

Adults: Ask about current and lifetime physical activity patterns and nutritional habits. Calculate years of cigarette smoking. Evaluate for alcohol use more than two drinks per day and caffeine intake equal to two cups of coffee or more. Calculate calcium intake as discussed under diet history.

Older adults/elderly: Ask postmenopausal women about ERT. If they have taken estrogen, ask what dosage, date started, pattern of use, on ERT. Ask about risk factors for falls in older women (Box 132-3).

Older men: Assess for osteoporosis in men after the seventh decade, especially if they have a history of alcoholism, corticosteroid therapy, chronic debilitating disease, endocrine abnormalities especially hypogonadism, malignancy, or gastrectomy.

Pregnant and nursing mothers: Obtain a 24-hour diet history and evaluate to see if these persons are meeting the increased calcium requirements (see Table 132-2).

Description of Most Common Symptoms

Symptoms may not be present. Common subtle symptoms are height loss, kyphosis (dowager's hump), protuberant abdomen, abdominal discomfort, negatively changed body image, difficulty fitting clothes, and back pain. Vertebral fracture may present with gradual, acute or chronic, or referred pain to the back, neck, shoulders, or arms.

Associated Symptoms

Depression and anxiety may accompany fractures and chronic pain; fear of fracture with self-imposed limitation of physical and social activity; limited mobility and independence; decreased self-esteem; caregiver burden

TABLE 132-1 Calcium Content of Selected Foods

Dairy Foods*	Calcium Content (mg)	Nondairy Foods*	Calcium Content (mg)
Skim milk	300	Calcium-fortified orange juice	300
Whole milk	290	Oysters raw 13-19	226
Yogurt (plain, low-fat)	415	Salmon, canned, 3 oz	167
Frozen yogurt (fruit)	240	Sardines, canned with bones	372
Swiss cheese, 1 oz	270	Collard greens, cooked	357
Cheddar, mozzarella cheese, 1 oz	205	Turnip greens, cooked	252
Part-skim ricotta cheese, 4 oz	335	Broccoli, cooked	100
Vanilla ice cream	176	Soybeans, cooked	131
Cottage cheese (low-fat) 4 oz	78	Tofu, 4 oz	108
		Almonds, 1 oz	75

Adapted from Tresolini CP, Gold DT, Lee LS: *Working with patients to prevent, treat, and manage osteoporosis: a curriculum guide for the health professions*, San Francisco, 1996, National Fund for Medical Education.
*1 cup unless otherwise specified.

TABLE 132-2 Optimal Calcium Requirement Recommended by the National Institutes of Health Consensus Panel

Age Group	Optimal Daily Intake of Calcium (mg)
Infant	
Birth-6 mo	400
6 mo-1 yr	600
Children	
1-5 yr	800
6-10 yr	800-1200
Adolescents/young adults	
11-24 yr	1200-1500
Men	
25-65	1000
Over 65 yr	1500
Women	
25-50	1000
Over 50 (postmenopausal)	
On estrogens	1000
Not on estrogens	1500
Over 65 yr	1500
Pregnant and nursing	1200-1500

Modified from NIH Consensus Conference: Optimal calcium intake, *JAMA* 272:1943, 1994.

OBJECTIVE DATA

Physical Examination

Do a complete history and physical examination to rule out other pathology.

Observe for visible deformity of the spine and palpate for tenderness.

Box 132-3

Risk Factors for Falls in Older Women

- Poor vision (reduced depth perception and contrast sensitivity)
- Poor muscle strength, evidenced by difficulty rising from a chair using arms
- On feet <4 hours/day, no walking exercise
- Postural hypotension
- Use of medications that may affect balance
- Concurrent medical problems
- Environmental hazards

Record height and compare with self-reported maximum height.

Diagnostic Procedures

Laboratory

Obtain laboratory data to rule out other pathology and to identify secondary causes of osteoporosis. Complete blood count ($13 to $16), sedimentation rate ($16 to $20), serum calcium ($18 to $23), phosphorus ($47 to $61), alkaline phosphatase ($19 to $24), proteins and creatinine levels ($18 to $24), liver function tests ($29 to $41), thyroid function tests ($47 to $61), urine calcium ($24 to $30), and glucose and protein ($28 to $39) are normal in uncomplicated osteoporosis. The alkaline phosphatase may be elevated following a fracture. In the presence of a low bone mass, abnormalities suggest secondary osteoporosis.

Biochemical markers have been approved for monitoring the effect of osteoporosis treatment, but it is not known if they can help predict fracture risk. Serum markers of bone breakdown include deoxypyridinoline, pyridinoline, phenazopyridine collagen cross-links; serum markers of

TABLE 132-3 Techniques for Measuring Bone Mass

Method	Body Site	Procedure Duration (min)	Approximate Medicare Reimbursement ($)
Dual-energy x-ray absorptiometry (DXA)	Spine or hip	15	130
Peripheral dual-energy x-ray absorptiometry (pDXA)	Forearm, phalanges	10 2	70 70
Single-energy x-ray absorptiometry (SXA)	Heel or forearm	10	70
Radiographic absorptiometry (RA)	Phalanges	5	40
Quantitative computed tomography (QCT)	Spine	30	120
Peripheral quantitative computed tomography (pQCT)	Forearm	15	70

Adapted from Siris ES, Schussheim DH: Osteoporosis: assessing your patient's risk: early identification can prevent later complications, *Women's Health Primary Care* 1(1):99-106, 1998.

bone formation are alkaline phosphatase, osteocalcin, and procollagen-1 extension peptides. Consult with physician to evaluate use of these in selected patients.

Radiographic

Bone densitometry measures the average density of bone mineral in the region scanned. It is the best available measure of bone strength. Use densitometry to:

Establish a diagnosis of osteoporosis (compare bone mass density [BMD] with young normal T-score value)

Predict future fracture risk (compare BMD to young adult values to estimate actual fracture risk and compare BMD to age-matched Z-score to estimate risk compared with others of same age)

Monitor changes in BMD due to medical problems or therapeutic intervention (compare new value, in density units, to previous measurement)

The National Osteoporosis Foundation Clinical Guidelines recommends determining BMD in estrogen-deficient women:

When vertebral abnormality is seen in radiography

On initiation of glucocorticosteroid therapy

In primary hyperparathyroidism

Consider screening all women at age 65 and all women between 50 and 65 who have more than one risk factor.

Dual-energy x-ray absorptiometry (DXA) is the gold standard for measuring BMD. However, ultrasound has recently been approved by the FDA, and other smaller, less costly techniques are rapidly becoming available. Table 132-3 contrasts current techniques for bone assessment.

ASSESSMENT

Differential Diagnoses

Table 132-4 identifies *normal, osteopenia, osteoporosis,* and *severe osteoporosis* on the basis of bone densitometry.

Menopause-related bone loss (type I) is associated with high bone turnover and osteoclastic overactivity. Greatest loss in vertebral bodies and long bones (vertebral and Colles fracture).

Age-related bone loss (type II) caused by impaired bone formation and osteoclastic underactivity. Greatest bone loss is in cancellous and cortical bone (hip fracture).

Secondary Osteoporosis (Box 132-4) is caused by endocrinopathies, drugs, medical conditions, and genetic abnormalities.

THERAPEUTIC PLAN

Health Promotion

General Teaching Plan

Prevention in the best treatment!

The goal is maintenance of bone mass through life without fractures.

Begin patient education in childhood and continue throughout life. Include the family unit. Tailor the plan to individual needs.

Emphasize good nutrition and adequate calcium intake throughout the lifespan.

Teach the importance of a healthy lifestyle.

Assist with smoking cessation.

TABLE 132-4 World Health Organization Classification System for Osteoporosis

Results*	Diagnosis
Within 1 standard deviation (SD) of young adult mean	Normal
Between 1 and 2.5 SD below mean, repeat in 2 years	Low bone mass (osteopenia)
Greater than 2.5 SD below mean	Osteoporosis
Greater than 2.5 SD below mean and one or more fragility fractures exist	Severe osteoporosis

From World Health Organization: Assessment of fracture risk and its application to screening for postmenopausal osteoporosis, *WHO Study Group technical report* series 843, Geneva, 1994, WHO.

*Results can be affected by positioning of the body in the DXA scan, presence of current or old fractures, arthritis, extraneous calcifications.

Box 132-4

Causes of Secondary Osteoporosis

Endocrinopathies

Hypercortisolism
Hyperthyroidism
Hyperparathyroidism
Hypogonadism
Hyperprolactemia

Drugs

Corticosteroids
L-thyroxin
Heparin
Barbiturates
Phenytoin
Methotrexate
Alcohol
Aluminum-containing antacids
Tobacco
Isoniazid

Other Conditions

Immobilization
Diabetes mellitus
Chronic renal failure
Hepatic disease
Scurvy
Chronic obstructive lung disease
Rheumatoid arthritis
Osteomalacia
Systemic mastocytosis
Malabsorption

Genetic Conditions

Marfan's syndrome
Osteogenesis imperfecta
Klinefelter's syndrome
Turner's syndrome
Ehlers-Danlos syndrome
Homocystinuria

Teach patients to develop an exercise plan that allows for gradual buildup of muscle strength and endurance. Avoid excessive exercise.

Participate in regular, diverse, weight-bearing exercise (Box 132-5) two or three times weekly.

Treadmills, stair climbers, tennis, low impact aerobics are also desirable exercises.

Exercise

General: Exercise is site specific. If exercise ceases, bone mass will be lost. Bones must be overloaded if exercise is to be effective. (Box 132-5 lists weight-bearing activities.) In patients whose activity level is reduced, nonweight-bearing exercises may be sufficient to improve bone density.

Box 132-5

Weight-bearing Exercises

Walking
Jogging
Basketball
Soccer
Hiking
Aerobic dancing
Gymnastics
Stair climbing
Skiing
Dancing

Children: Teach that peak bone mass is achieved by the late teens. Weight-bearing and resistive exercises are necessary for development and maintenance of bone mass. Instruct that bicycling and swimming do not develop bone mass. Encourage development of muscle strength and posture and participation in a variety of sports and recreational activities. Basketball, soccer, and tennis are good bone-building sports

Adolescents: Continue to promote a physically active lifestyle. Promote muscle strengthening and weight-bearing exercises. Teach women to avoid excessive exercise and/or reduction in body fat that may result in amenorrhea (e.g., distance running). Continue to encourage good posture and body mechanics.

Adults: Encourage a moderate, regular exercise regimen that includes strength training for 20 to 30 minutes two or three times per week and/or weight-bearing exercise for 30 to 45 minutes three or four times per week. Ensure strength and flexibility of muscles.

Elderly (without osteoporosis): Promote continuance of moderate exercise of resistance training and weight-bearing exercise. Assess fall risk by physical examination and balance and mobility testing and correct deficiencies.

Fall Prevention

Elderly: Assess for visual acuity and refer as necessary; assess medications for effect on central nervous system such as balance, drowsiness, and confusion (antihistamines, opioid analgesics). Assess medications for their ability to affect sight (blurred vision, e.g., tricyclic

Box 132-6

Home Modification to Improve Safety

Remove throw rugs and make certain that carpet edges are securely fastened to the floor.
Reduce clutter, especially in traffic area.
Increase wattage of lighting in hallways, bathrooms, kitchens, stairwells, and entrances to home.
Use night lights near bed, in hallways, and in bathrooms to improve night safety.
Install safety handrails in shower, tub, and around toilet.
Provide nonskid surfaces for bathrooms and shower stalls.
Have sand or salt available to spread on porches, stairs, and sidewalks for use in snowy or icy weather.
Use a portable phone for safety and security.

antidepressants). Assess medications for their ability to cause orthostatic hypotension (e.g., antihypertensives).
Encourage development of muscular strength and flexibility.
Teach patients to avoid reaching but if necessary, use a safety step stool (with wide steps, friction surface, and hand rails). Instruct on proper lifting techniques.
Use a cane or walker to increase stability if needed.
Wear supportive, cushioned, low-heeled shoes. Avoid scuffs and high heels.
Teach patient to avoid rushing to answer a phone or door.
Instruct patients on measures to increase home safety (Box 132-6).

Nutrition

All ages: Teach and encourage good nutritional practices throughout the lifespan.

Calcium Supplementation

A quick route to estimate calcium supplementation is contained in Box 132-7.
For an individualized estimation of calcium supplementation, use the process described under diet history to determine the current calcium intake. Subtract this amount from the recommended daily requirements.

Prescribing Guidelines and Teaching Points

Take calcium on a consistent basis.
Only elemental calcium is absorbed; if the label does not state the type of calcium, assume that "Calcium" is referring to elemental calcium.
Calcium carbonate ($3 to $9) contains 40% of elemental calcium, the highest proportion of all types of calcium, and it is the least expensive.
If taken with food, there is little difference in absorption rates between the different types of calcium; if taken on an empty stomach, calcium citrate is best absorbed. Calcium citrate does not require gastric acid for absorption. If achlorhydria exists, take calcium citrate. Calcium citrate is best absorbed at a higher stomach pH. Elderly patients have higher stomach pH and may also be taking antacids and histamine blockers (e.g., Zantac, Axid, and Tagamet or omeprazole) further raising their stomach pH. Therefore calcium citrate may be the best supplement. Calcium supplements are best absorbed if taken in smaller amounts multiple times per day.

Box 132-7

Quick Route Estimation of Calcium Supplementation

If daily requirement is:
1000 mg, supplement with 500 mg
1500 mg, supplement with 1000 mg

Some research indicates calcium supplements are best absorbed if taken HS.
Take 500 mg calcium per dose. If 1000 mg is needed, take 500 mg BID.
Do not exceed 2000 mg calcium per day unless prescribed.
Chewable tablets are a good alternative for persons who have trouble swallowing pills. Tums or generic alternatives are good sources of calcium carbonate.
There is variability in absorption rates for calcium tablets. To evaluate if a calcium tablet will be absorbed adequately, place a tablet in white vinegar and stir every 5 minutes for 30 minutes. The supplement should be 75% dissolved. This test can be bypassed with chewable forms of calcium where solubility is not an issue.
After an illness that results in bed rest, boost calcium intake to 2000 mg for a period about 7 times as long as the patient spent in bed.
Add a multivitamin with 400 IU vitamin D to ensure adequate calcium absorption. Use vitamin D_3 for those confined indoors.
Avoid calcium supplements derived from dolomite, oyster shells, and bone meal. These may contain higher levels of lead than other supplements.
If taken at the same time, calcium interferes with iron absorption. This may be a problem with persons who ingest low levels of iron. Take calcium HS or at other times that are between meals to avoid this complication.
Calcium supplements may have an adverse effect on phosphorus, zinc, and magnesium when these substances are ingested in inadequate amounts.
Milk-alkali syndrome (hypercalcemia, metabolic alkalosis, and renal failure) may result from concurrent ingestion of high amounts of calcium (2000 mg or more) and alkali when there is concurrent use of thiazide diuretics, pre-existing renal failure, or dehydration.
Calcium intakes exceeding recommendations may result in renal calculi.
Use thiazides with caution to avoid milk-alkali syndrome.

Hormone Replacement Therapy (ERT)

Estrogen

Counsel perimenopausal and postmenopausal women about estrogen replacement therapy; it is never too late; but immediate replacement is preferable.

Discuss benefits: Prevents bone loss and osteoporotic fractures; protects from coronary artery disease; elevates high-density lipoprotein levels; relieves menopausal/genitourinary symptoms.

Discuss risks and side effects: Intermittent bleeding, breast tenderness, abdominal fullness and weight gain, hypertension, thrombosis, migraine headaches, and endometrial hyperplasia (if progesterone is not administered).

Contraindicated in women with breast cancer. Consult with physician regarding potential use of tamoxifen and raloxifene.

Prescribe (if acceptable to the patient):

Conjugated estrogens ($28-$33) 0.3 mg or 0.625 mg, *or*

Estradiol ($27 to $55) 0.5 or 1 mg, *or*

Estrone sulfate 0.625, *or*

Estradiol transdermally (Estraderm) as skin patches changed 2 × weekly and provide 0.05 to 0.1 mg of hormone daily

All of the above estrogen forms appear to be effective; more information is available about conjugated estrogens

If the uterus is present, add progesterone to the regime to decrease the risk of endometrial cancer; if a hysterectomy has been performed, this is not necessary

Do breast examinations, mammogram, pelvic examinations and Pap smear before initiating ERT to rule out malignancy or other contraindication

ERT prescriptive regimens

Estrogen, days 1 to 25 of each calendar month, followed by 5 to10 mg medroxyprogesterone acetate on days 14 to 25 (omit day 26 to end of month), *or*

Estrogen continuously, progesterone days 1 to 14; may result in irregular spotting; increase progesterone dose temporarily to achieve amenorrhea sooner, *or*

Estrogen along with 2.5 mg medroxyprogesterone acetate daily every day; advise the patient that this regime may cause some initial spotting but will stop in a few months

Omit medroxyprogesterone if the uterus is not present

Nonestrogen Receptor Modulator

Raloxifene hydrochloride (Evista) ($59 for 30)

A selective estrogen receptor modulator that has estrogen-like effects on bone and on lipid metabolism but lacks estrogen-like effects on the uterus and breast. This drug is for females at risk of osteoporosis who are not actively experiencing menopausal symptoms. The effect on reduction of fractures has not been established.

Give 60-mg tablet daily without regard to time of day or meals.

Do not give concurrently with estrogen or cholesterol lowering medicine. Give calcium supplements and vitamin D if the diet is inadequate. Give only after menopause. Contraindicated in patients with a history of thrombosis/phlebitis.

Obtain a baseline measure of bone density before pharmacologic therapy. Measure bone density every 2 years to evaluate effects of pharmacologic treatment for osteoporosis.

Secondary and Tertiary Care

Consult with physician for diagnosis and follow-up of osteopenia and/or suspected fractures, in the presence of secondary causes, in complicated cases, and when patients are unable to comply with prescribed regime. Plan will depend on patient problems (e.g., care of patient with fracture, physical therapy for soft tissue trauma).

Pharmacological Therapies

Biphosphonates

Alendronate (Fosamax) (Biphosphonate) ($174-$438)

Decreases bone resorption and prevents bone loss

Binds to hydroxyapatite and specifically inhibits the activity of osteoclasts; inhibits osteoclastic resorption

First-line: 1000 times more potent as osteoclast inhibitor than etidronate. Does not cause osteomalacia or inhibit mineralization of bone.

For the treatment of *postmenopausal* osteoporosis, give 10 mg per day with at least 6 oz plain water ½ hour before the first food or beverage of the day. To avoid esophagitis, instruct the patient to wait at least 30 minutes in an upright position before eating or drinking anything else. Wait 30 minutes after taking the medication before taking any other medication. For *prevention* of osteoporosis (e.g., in patients receiving long-term glucocorticoid therapy), give 5 mg/day.

Consider prescribing supplemental calcium and vitamin D if their diet is inadequate.

Do not give to patients with esophageal strictures. Give with caution to patients who have a history of hiatal hernia, dysphagia, gastritis, or peptic ulcers.

Etidronate (Didronel) ($109-$218)

Less effective but less expensive than alendronate when given cyclically in 400-mg doses daily for 2 weeks every 3 months

May reduce osteoporosis when given prophylactically to patients receiving long-term doses of glucocorticoid.

Calcitonin-Salmon (Miacalcin)

Suppresses osteoclast activity and bone resorption

Has an analgesic effect on osteoporotic fracture pain and is usually reserved for those with severe osteoporotic fractures and vertebral fractures

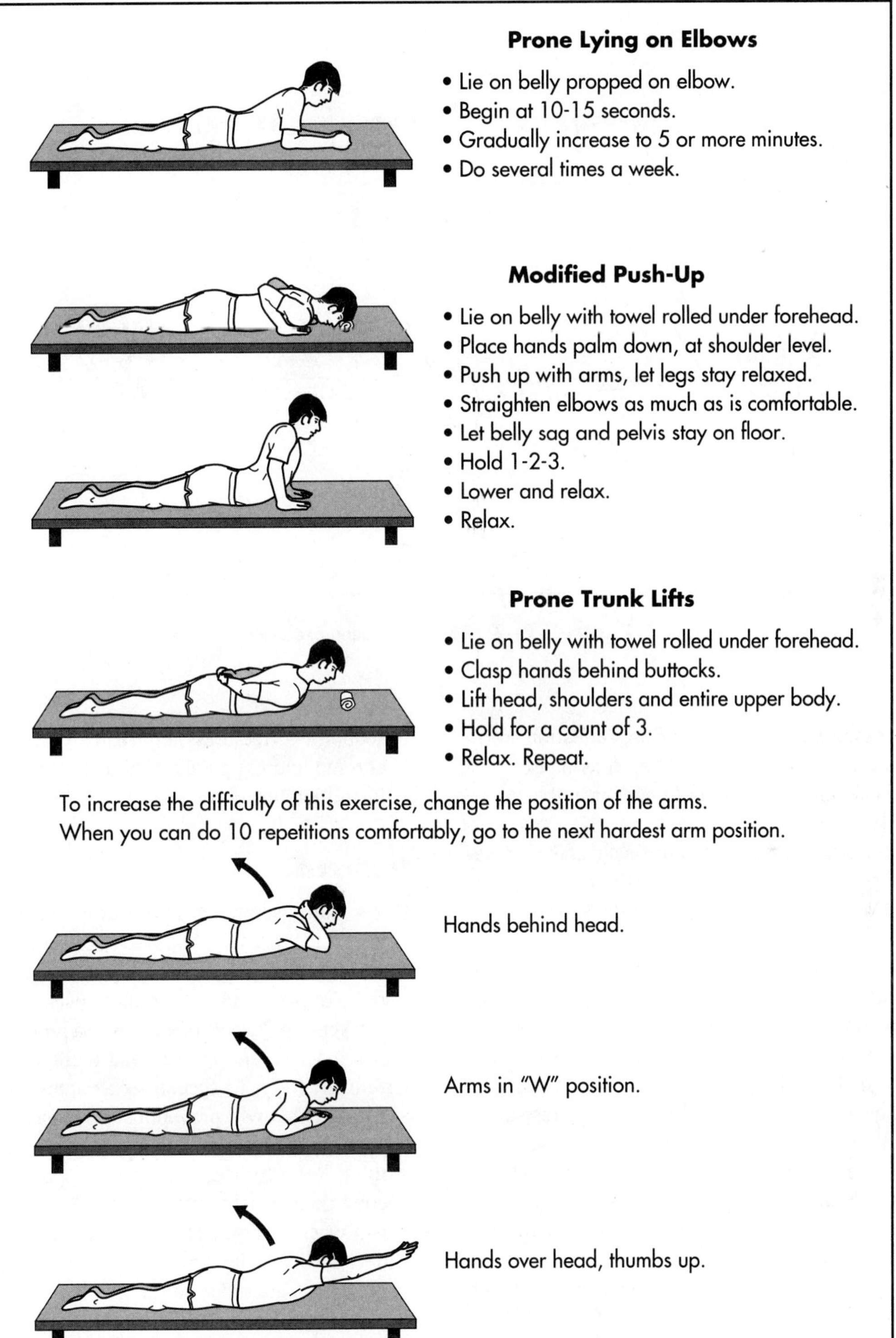

Figure 132-1 Exercises to prevent/minimize kyphotic deformity.

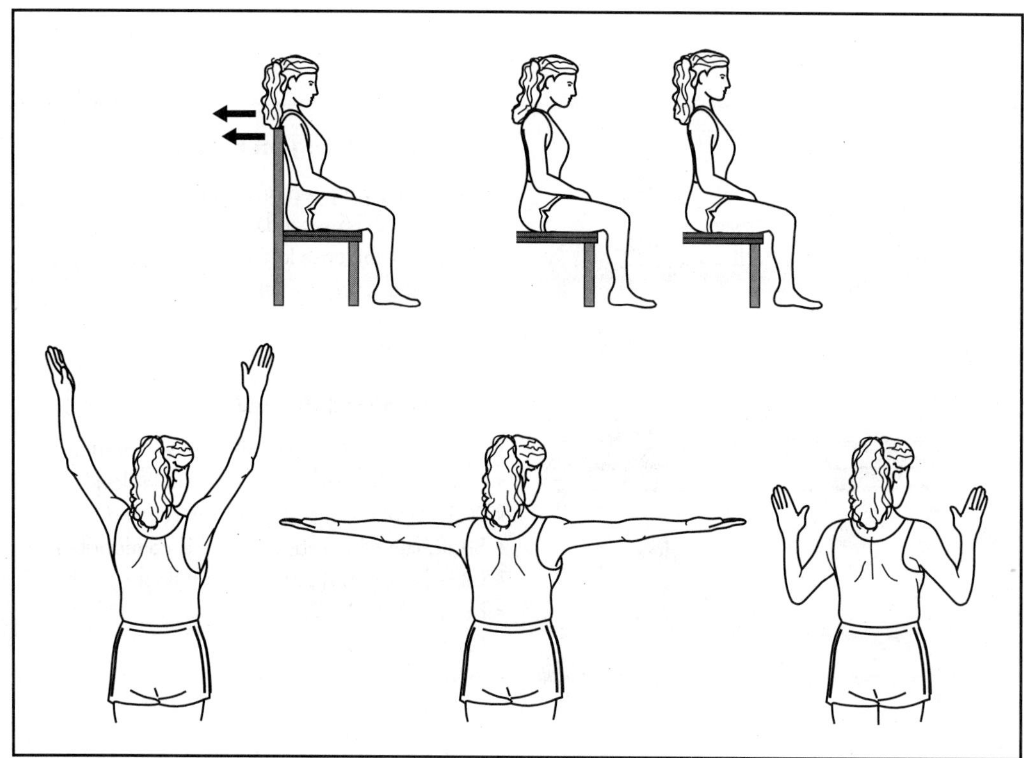

Figure 132-2 Spinal extension exercises.

Available as nasal spray and injection; injection form expensive and has more side effects such as nausea

Take adequate calcium and vitamin D concurrently

Sodium Fluoride

Use is controversial. Consult with physician and pharmacist. High doses are required. Bone density may increase, but the bone formed is more brittle ($9 to $13)

Exercise

Individuals with established osteoporosis: Consult with physician before initiating exercise program. General guidelines: If initiating exercise, start walking as much as possible for daily activity and an endurance walking program three or four times per week. Use resistance training cautiously to avoid overload to the skeleton. If already exercising, promote continuance of moderate exercise regimen of weight-bearing exercise. Continue or begin exercises to prevent/minimize kyphotic deformity (Figure 132-1). Encourage spinal extension exercises (Figure 132-2) and teach good body mechanics. Teach patients to avoid spinal flexion exercises (Figure 132-3). Reassess for fall risk and intervene appropriately.

Family Impact

Facilitate healthy lifestyle in all family members to prevent osteoporosis.

Osteoporotic fractures may lead to loss of independence, chronic pain, caregiver burden, financial burden, and institutionalization

Referral

Use a multidisciplinary approach in preventing and managing osteoporosis. A variety of professionals may be helpful, including primary care physicians, geriatricians, radiologists, and endocrinologists, as well as social workers, physical therapists, radiologists, nutritionists, pharmacists, and recreational therapists.

Children: Refer to specialists as appropriate to facilitate a lifestyle that will prevent osteoporosis and/or for medical conditions that may cause osteoporosis.

Adults: Refer for fractures and as appropriate for secondary conditions causing osteoporosis (e.g., to AA for alcoholism or endocrinologist for hypogonadism).

Elderly: Older adults may benefit from persons specialized in care of the older adult.

Consultation

Consult with physician when osteopenia and/or osteoporosis present, before initiating medications to treat osteoporosis, before initiating exercises following fracture, and for secondary causes of osteoporosis as appropriate

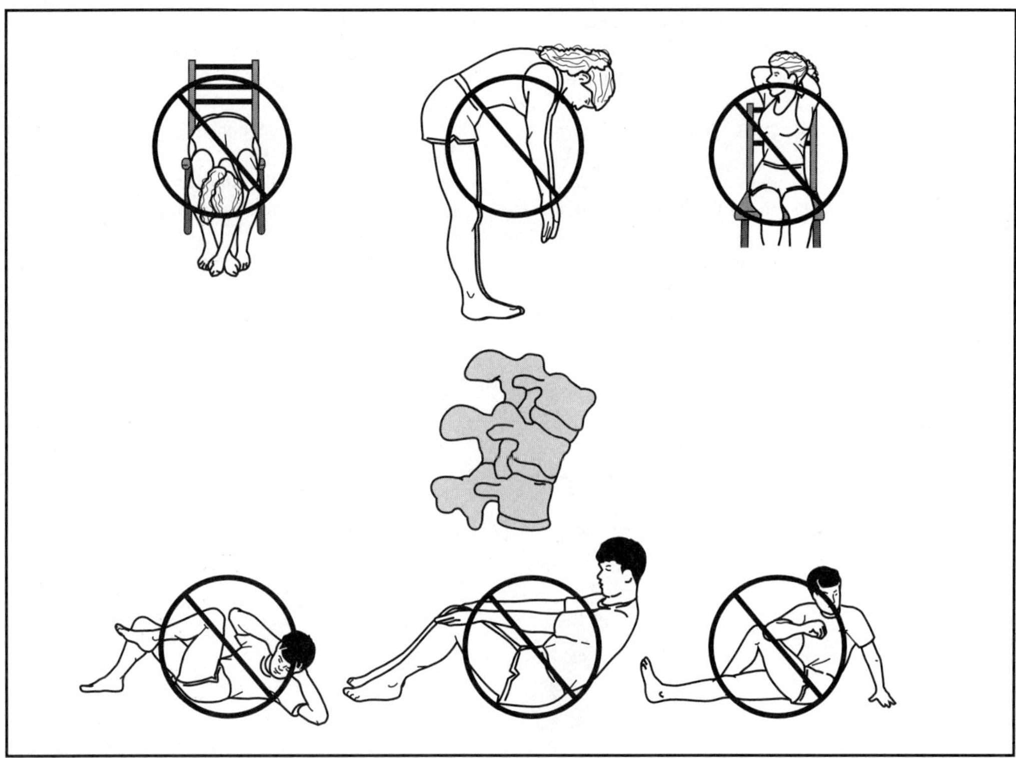

Figure 132-3 Spinal flexion exercises to be avoided.

Box 132-8

National Osteoporosis Foundation Recommendations Regarding Bone Mass Screening

Bone mass measurements should be obtained in estrogen-deficit women as part of the consideration for the use of hormone replacement or the need for other treatment modalities.

For women whose bone mass is one standard deviation (SD) below the mean peak bone mass, hormone replacement or some other form of treatment should be recommended.

Women with bone mass one SD above the mean require no intervention.

Women with bone mass within one SD of the mean should be followed with repeat measurements at 1-to 5-year intervals, depending on the initial value.

Follow-up

Box 132-8 lists the National Osteoporosis Foundation recommendations regarding bone mass screening. Follow-up of patients with confirmed osteoporosis will depend on the individual situation.

EVALUATION

Prevention is the optimal outcome. Resolution of osteoporosis, decrease in advancement of osteoporosis, and/or prevention of complications such as fracture, pain, and excess disability are other desirable outcomes.

SUGGESTED READINGS

Abramowicz M: New drugs for osteoporosis, *Med Lett* 38(965):1-3, 1996.

Abrams W, Berkow R, editors: *The Merck manual of geriatrics*, Whitehouse Station, NJ, 1995, Merck & Co.

Barrett-Connor C, Chang J, Edelstein S: Coffee-associated osteoporosis offset by daily milk consumption, *JAMA* 271:280-283, 1994.

Birge SJ: Osteoporosis and hip fracture. In Kaiser TE, editor: *Clinics in geriatric medicine: care of the older woman,* ed 9, Philadelphia, 1993, WB Saunders.

Deal CL: Osteoporosis: prevention diagnosis and management, *Am J Med* 102 (suppl 1A):35S-36S, 38S-39S, 1997.

Ellsworth A, et al: *Mosby's 1998 medical drug reference,* St Louis, 1998, Mosby.

Healthcare Consultants of America, Inc: *1998 Physicians fee and coding guide*, Augusta, Ga, 1998, Healthcare Consultants of America, Inc.

Janis LW: Prevention of osteoporosis. In Rubin R, et al: *Medicine: a primary care approach*, Philadelphia, 1996, WB Saunders.

Jibrin J: Calcium supplements made simple, *Prevention* March: 81-85, 156, 1997.

Kanis J, et al: The diagnosis of osteoporosis, *J Bone Min Res* 8:1137-1141, 1994.

Kessenich CR: Update on pharmacologic therapies for osteoporosis, *Nurse Pract* 21(8):19-24, 1996.

Kessinich CR: The pathophysiology of osteoporotic vertebral fractures, *Rehab Nurs* 22(4):192-195, 1997.

Kirk JK, Spangler JG: Alendronate: a biphosphonate for treatment of osteoporosis, *Am Family Physician* 54(6):2053-2060, 1996.

Kupecz D: Alendronate for the treatment of osteoporosis, *Nurse Pract* 21(1):86-89, 1996.

Lindsay R: *Osteoporosis: a guide to diagnosis prevention and treatment*, New York, 1992, Raven Press.

Lindsay R, Marcus R, Recker R: Osteoporosis: what's new in prevention and treatment, *Patient Care* August 1996, pp 24-31, 35-36, 38, 44, 46, 49, 53.

Lufkin E, Zilkoski M: Diagnosis and management of osteoporosis, *Am Family Physician Monograph* 1:3-17, 1996.

McGee C: Secondary amenorrhea leading to osteoporosis: incidence and prevention, *Nurse Pract* 22(5):38, 41-42, 44-45, 48, 51-52, 57-58, 63, 1997.

Moussa J, Elias Y, Libanati C: Osteoporosis: prevention and treatment in the primary care setting, *Primary Care Rep* 3(1):1-8, 1997.

National Osteoporosis Foundation: Bone densitometry and its use in the diagnosis of osteoporosis, *Osteoporosis Clinical Updates* 1(3):1-3, 1996.

National Osteoporosis Foundation: *Boning up on osteoporosis: a guide to prevention and treatment,* Washington, DC, 1991, The Foundation.

NIH Consensus Conference: Optimal calcium intake, *JAMA* 272(24):1942-1947, 1994.

Notelovitz M: Osteoporosis in postmenopausal women: pathophysiology prevention and management, *Clin Ger* 2:1-13, 1994.

Riggs A, editor: The prevention and treatment of osteoporosis, *New Engl J Med* 327:620-627, 1992.

Siris ES, Schussheim DH: Osteoporosis: assessing your patient's risk: early identification can prevent later complications, *Women's Health Primary Care* 1(1):99-106, 1998.

Svitil K: Boning up: Important news about osteoporosis-particularly if you have arthritis, *Arthr Today* November-December: 37-41, 1997.

Tierney LM, McPhee SJ, Papadakis MA, editors: *Current medical diagnosis and treatment,* Stamford, Conn, 1998, Appleton & Lange.

Uphold C, Graham M: *Clinical guidelines in family practice*, Gainesville, Fla, 1994, Barmarrae Books.

Whiting SJ, Wood R, Kim K: Pharmacology update: calcium supplementation, *J Am Acad Nurse Pract* 9(4):187-192, 1997.

World Health Organization: Assessment of fracture risk and its application to screening for postmenopausal osteoporosis, *WHO Study Group technical report* series 843, Geneva, 1994, WHO.

133 Otitis Externa

ICD-9-CM

Infective Otitis Externa, Unspecified 380.10

OVERVIEW

Definition

Infection of the external auditory canal, known as swimmer's ear

Incidence

Affects all ages, occurs following swimming, aggressive cleaning of the canal, or trauma

Pathophysiology

Trauma, excessive dryness or wetness can cause a change in the pH of the ear canal from acid to alkaline, making the external canal susceptible to superinfection. Organisms that cause external otitis include:

Staphylococcus aureus
Pseudomonas
Streptococcus
Pneumococcus
Candida
Aspergillus

Protective Factors Against

Avoiding excessive trauma when cleaning ears
Use of prophylactic ear solutions after frequent bathing/swimming
Acid pH
Intact epithelial lining

Factors That Increase Susceptibility

Trauma to ear canal from aggressive cleaning
Excessive dryness of ear canal
Excessive moisture in ear canal
Frequent swimming/showering
High humidity
Underlying dermatitis

SUBJECTIVE DATA

History of Present Illness

Otalgia
Ear discharge
Tenderness when ear is moved

Past Medical History

Past episodes of external otitis, hearing loss
Use of hearing aids
Use of steroids

Medications

Use of steroids
Preventive medicines used

Family History

Not usually significant

Psychosocial History

Frequent swimming or bathing

Associated Symptoms

Fever (uncommon)
Nausea

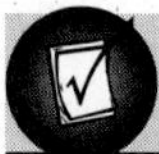

TABLE 133-1 Differential Diagnosis: Otitis Externa

Diagnoses	Supporting Data
Acute otitis media	Typically rapid onset, TM is erythematous, injected, and opaque. An effusion develops in the middle ear, causing poor TM mobility. Frequently a fever is present, and the TM may be bulging. Purulent discharge may be seen if the TM perforates.
Malignant otitis externa	Persistent external otitis in the patient with diabetes or who is immunocompromised may result in osteomyelitis of the skull base. It is usually caused by *Pseudomonas*. The patient presents with persistent foul aural discharge, granulations of the ear, and deep otalgia.
Furuncle	Discrete pustule with surrounding erythema visualized in canal.

TM, Tympanic membrane.

OBJECTIVE DATA

Physical Examination

General appearance, including vital signs
Head/eyes/ears/nose/throat:
- Ear:
  - Tenderness with pinna movement or pressure on tragus
  - Ear canal is erythematous, edematous, and inflamed with moist debris
  - Tympanic membrane (TM) is usually normal, good mobility
  - If canal grossly swollen, TM may not be visible
  - Pinna may be swollen and inflamed
- Neck
  - Preauricular, postauricular cervical nodes may be enlarged on affected side

Diagnostic Procedures

None

ASSESSMENT

Differential diagnoses include those found in Table 133-1.

THERAPEUTIC PLAN

Pharmaceutical

Pharmaceutical treatment can be found in Table 133-2.

For symptomatic pain relief, use acetaminophen, ibuprofen, or codeine.

Extreme swelling of external canal may necessitate the placement of a wick to facilitate contact of otic drops with canal. Both otic drops and systemic antibiotic may be needed.

Lifestyle/Activities

Ear must be kept dry
- No swimming
- No shampooing without protection
- No showers
- Do not use cotton: it will retain moisture

Diet

Noncontributory

Patient Education

Instillation of drops:
- Lie on side, pull affected auricle back and up; then instill drops without allowing dropper to touch ear; remain in position for at least 5 minutes

Ear canal should be kept dry for 7 days

Acetic acid 2% (vinegar) (or ½ acetic acid 2%, ½ alcohol) can also be used to prevent recurrence

Instill 2 drops BID and after contact with water

Prevention
- Avoidance of precipitating factors
- Prophylaxis with topical solutions
- Solutions containing alcohol or preparations with boric or acetic acid have been used

Family Impact

Inability to participate in family water activities during acute phase

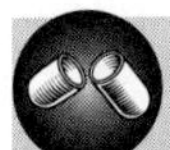

TABLE 133-2 Pharmaceutical Plan: Otitis Externa

Drug	Dose	Comments	Cost
Polymyxin, neomycin, hydrocortisone and propylene glycol (Cortisporin Otic); Corticosporin TC	Adults: 4 gtts in affected ear TID or QID × 7 days Child: 3 gtts TID or QID	Antibiotic and steroid to decrease inflammation; TC adds surfactant to cut through cerumen Max. 10 days Caution: perforated TM, chronic otitis media, asthma Pregnancy: C	$32/10 ml; TC: $40/10 ml
Amoxicillin with clavulanate (Augmentin)	45 mg/kg/day q12h	External otitis with fever, cellulitis of pinna or tender postauricular adenopathy should be treated with systemic antibiotics.	$27/125 mg/5 ml (150 ml); $52/250 mg/5 ml (150 ml); $58/250 mg (30); $82/500 mg (30)
Clarithromycin (Biaxin)	15 mg/kg/day	For patients allergic to penicillin Pregnancy: C SE: Nausea, vomiting, diarrhea	$26/125 mg/5 ml (100 ml); $49/250 mg/5 ml (100); $185/250 mg, 500 mg (60)
Otic Domeboro (acetic acid) or Vosol Otic solution	5 gtts in each ear after water exposure	Prophylactic use during swimming season or ↑ bathing (serve as drying agents) Change pH in ear canal to acidic Antifungal and antibacterial agents	$3-$33/2% (15 ml)
Ciprofloxacin (Cipro)	N/A	Pregnancy: C SE: irritation burning on instillation	N/A
Ofloxacin (Floxin)	1-12 y/o: 5 gtts BID >12 y/o: 10 gtts BID × 10 days	See ciprofaxin	N/A

N/A, Not available; *SE,* side effects; *TM,* tympanic membrane.

Need to institute preventive measures and be alert to beginning symptoms

Referral/Consultation

Refer to collaborating physician or otolaryngologist if:

Symptoms worse after 24 hours
No response to treatment in 48 to 72 hours
Foreign body in ear that is not removable
Hearing loss

Follow-up

Reevaluate ear if no improvement in 1 week.

EVALUATION

Reevaluate and discuss need for preventive measures.

SUGGESTED READINGS

Bojab D, Bruderly T, Abdulrazzak Y: Otitis externa, *Otolaryngol Clin North Am* 29(5):761-782, 1996.

Boyton R, Dunn E, Stephens G: *Manual of ambulatory pediatrics,* ed 4, Philadelphia, 1998, JB Lippincott.

Brook I, Frazie E, Thompson D: Aerobic and anaerobic microbiology of external otitis, *Clin Infect Dis* 15:955, 1992.

Clark W, et al: Microbiology of otitis externa, *Otolaryngol Head Neck Surg* 116(1):23-25, 1997.

Eden A, Fireman P, Stook S: Managing acute otitis: a fresh look at a familiar problem, *Contemp Pediatr* 13(3):64-93, 1996.

Ellsworth A et al: *Mosby's 1998 medical drug reference,* St Louis, 1998, Mosby.

Healthcare Consultants of America, Inc: *1998 physicians fee and coding guide*, Augusta, Ga, 1998, Healthcare Consultants of America, Inc.

Jackler R, Kaplan M: Ear nose throat. In Tierney L, McPhee S, Papadakis M, editors: *1998 current medical diagnosis and treatment*, ed 37, Stamford Conn, 1998, Appleton & Lange.

Mirza N: Otitis externa: management in the primary care office, *Postgrad Med* 99(5):153-154, 1996.

Russell J et al: What causes acute otitis externa? *J Laryngol Otolaryngol* 107:898, 1993.

Sundstrom J et al: Pseudomonas aeruginosa in otitis externa: a particular variety of the bacteria? *Arch Otolaryngol Head Neck Surg* 122(8):833-836, 1996.

134 Otitis Media

ICD-9-CM

Acute OM 382.0
Acute Suppurative OM 381

OVERVIEW

Definition

Otitis media (OM) is inflammation of the middle ear. Acute OM (AOM) is defined as the presence of fluid in the middle ear associated with signs or symptoms of acute local or systemic illness. OM with effusion (OME) is defined as the presence of fluid in the middle ear in the absence of signs or symptoms of acute infection.

Incidence

OM is second only to upper respiratory infection (URI) for largest number of office visits for children. Peak incidence is **3 to 36 months;** it is least frequent in the 4- to 6-year age group. At least 93% of children have one incident by age 7. Boys have higher incidence than girls.

Pathophysiology

OM typically follows an URI. The most accepted theory is that the eustachian tubes become blocked from chronic negative pressure. This leads to formulation of fluid or effusions in the middle ear. This fluid becomes infected (Table 134-1) and inflamed, causing bulging of the tympanic membrane (TM).

Protective Factors Against

Breastfeeding

Factors That Increase Susceptibility

Day care
Exposure to smoke
Bottle fed
Anatomical anomalies of the mid-face
Eskimo, Latino, or Native American race
Sibling or parent with OM
Allergies such as atopic dermatitis or asthma

Factors Associated with Increased Risk of Recurrence

Young age at first ear infection
Male gender
Positive family history of recurrent ear infections
Participation in day care
Exposure to cigarette smoke
Native American or Eskimo ancestry
Individuals with Down syndrome or cleft palate

SUBJECTIVE DATA

History of Present Illness

Preceded by URI: Rhinorrhea, cough, low grade fever
Describe ear pain, pulling on ear, discomfort
Decreased ability to hear
Home measures tried

Past Medical History

Past history of ear infections, insertion of myringotomy tubes
Allergies

Table 134-1 Common Organisms

Commonly Identified Organisms	Beta Lactamase–Producing
Streptococcus pneumonia (31%)	None
H. influenza (22%)	20%-40%
Moraxella catarrhalis (7%)	90%
Viruses (17%)	

Hearing abilities
Bottle/breast fed
Takes a bottle to bed
Craniofacial abnormalities

Medications

Past antibiotics used for ear infections, response
Allergies to antibiotics

Family History

Family history of ear infections
Family history of allergies, atopic dermatitis, asthma
Parents/family members who smoke in house

Psychosocial History

Attends day care
Frequent absences from school due to URI/OM

Diet

History of food allergies

Descriptions of Most Common Symptoms

Otalgia: Worse at night
Otorrhea: Signifies rupture of TM
Hearing loss
Fever
Tinnitus
Pulling or rubbing at ears
Adults: Pain most prominent sign
Elderly: May not exhibit fever

Associated Symptoms

Restless or diminished sleep
Diarrhea/vomiting

OBJECTIVE DATA

Physical Examination

General appearance/vital signs, weight
Head/eyes/ears, nose/throat
- Determine sinus tenderness
- Determine nasal erythema, bogginess from allergies
- Determine pharynx erythema, edema

Ear
- Check for external ear pain
- TM
  - Assess for position, color, translucency, and mobility of TM:
  - Check for erythema, bulging, infection
  - Absent landmarks
  - Diminished or absent light reflex, dullness
  - Presence of bubbles or air fluid levels
  - Check mobility using pneumoscope
  - Assess for mastoid tenderness

Neck: Palpate for enlarged/tender lymph nodes
Respiratory: Auscultate for adventitious breath sounds
Abdomen: Bowel sounds, tenderness

Diagnostic Procedures

Diagnostic procedures include those found in Table 134-2.

ASSESSMENT

Differential diagnoses include those found in Table 134-3. Episodes of OM should be classified as acute OM or OM with effusion.

THERAPEUTIC PLAN

Treatment depends on the correct diagnosis of OM. OM should be classified as AOM or OME. AOM requires documentation of middle ear effusion and signs or symptoms of acute local or systemic illness. Treatment of OME is only warranted if effusions persist >3 mos. It is expected that OME will follow an episode of AOM, lasting up to 3 months. Prophylaxis should be reserved for recurrent AOM, defined as >3 distinct and well-documented episodes/6 months or >4 episodes/12 months.

Approximately 80% of children with OM will have clinical resolution by 7 to 14 days without antibiotics, compared to 95% of those treated with antibiotics (Table 134-4).

Pharmaceutical

Those more at risk for treatment failure include those with:
- Perforation of TM
- Underlying medical conditions

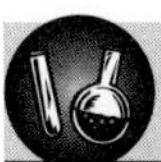

TABLE 134-2 Diagnostic Procedures: Otitis Media

Diagnostic Test	Finding/Rationale	Cost ($)
Tympanogram	Can be helpful when used as adjunct to physical examination; not helpful in child <6 or 7 months old due to flexibility of their ear canals; tympanometry: decreased compliance in AOM or OME, and + pressure in AOM, with + or – pressure in OME	31-37
Acoustic reflectometry	New diagnostic option uses sonar technology; device works best if child is not crying; use instrument first before attempting to visualize TM	N/A
CBC	Usually not done in most instances; may be done when patient looks toxic	18-23
Ear drainage culture	Not routinely done—usually treated empirically; tympanocentesis may be considered for nonresponse to treatment or recurrent infections	31-39
Sinus films	May be considered in recurrent cases	146-173
Audiometry	Usually done after repeated OM when there is concern about hearing loss	24-29

AOM, Acute otitis media; *CBC,* complete blood count; *N/A,* not available; *OM,* otitis media; *OME,* otitis media with effusion; *TM,* tympanic membrane.

TABLE 134-3 Differential Diagnosis: Otitis Media

Diagnoses	Supporting Data
Acute otitis media (AOM)	Typically rapid onset, tympanic membrane (TM) is erythematous, injected and opaque. An effusion develops in the middle ear, causing poor TM mobility with both positive and negative insufflation. Frequently a fever is present, and the TM may be bulging. Purulent discharge may be seen if the TM perforates. High likelihood of bacterial infection. Antibiotics indicated.
Subacute OM	Defined as OM that lasts 4-8 weeks. The TM remains dull or with erythematous appearance. The drum may bulge slightly, retract, or return to normal position. Mobility is decreased due to effusion.
OM with effusion (OME)/ serous OM	OM >12 wks. TM usually in retracted position. Effusion becomes thick and mucoid. Effusion may be clear or dark. Air bubbles signify a likely indication that the effusion will resolve. Negative otalgia, TM dull to clear. Decreased TM mobility only with positive pressure insufflation. No fever. Low likelihood of bacterial infection. Antibiotics not indicated.
External OM	Inflammation of external ear canal, frequently with exudate visible in canal. Pain with movement of pinna or turning head. Inflammation may involve TM.
Hyperemia of TM	The TM becomes reddened with crying or high temperature. TM has normal mobility, and landmarks are visible.

Recurrent or chronic OM
Children younger than 15 months to 2 years

Antibiotic prophylaxis: Consider to prevent recurrent OM. Use is controversial. May want to use during fall, winter, and spring when child has experienced three episodes of AOM in the prior 6 months or 4 episodes in past 12 months (Table 134-5).

Lifestyle/Activities

Smoking cessation
Avoidance of secondhand smoke
Eliminate or decrease pacifier use
Consider influenza vaccine as a means to decrease AOM episodes
Consider pneumococcus vaccine in children >2

Diet

No modifications needed

Patient Education

Prevention
Encourage breastfeeding
Reduce exposure to second-hand smoke
Use family day care settings if possible
Feed in an upright position

Discuss need for completion of antibiotics/resistance
Assist as needed with smoking cessation
Encourage parents not to put child to bed with bottle
Side effects of medications such as upset stomach, diarrhea, allergy reactions

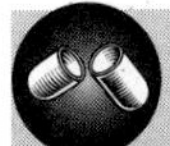

TABLE 134-4 Pharmaceutical Treatment: Otitis Media

Drug	Dose	Comments	Cost
First Line			
Amoxicillin	**Adults:** 500 mg TID × 7 days **Children:** 40 mg/kg/day divided q8h × 10 days; recent reports of 60-80 mg/kg/day	Not effective if high beta-lactam community Pregnancy: B SE: N/V, rash, diarrhea, Stevens-Johnson syndrome	\$3-\$5/125 mg/5 ml (150); \$4-\$8/250 mg/5 ml (150); \$9/125 mg (60); \$23-\$26/250 mg (100)
Erythromycin	**Adults:** 500 mg BID **Children:** 50 mg/kg/day divided q6-8h	Pregnancy: B SE: N/V, diarrhea, abdominal pain	\$11-\$16/200 mg/5 ml (200 ml); \$22/400 mg/5 ml (200); \$18-\$40/500 mg (100)
TMP/SMX (Bactrim)	**Adults:** 1 Double strength (DS) tab BID **Children:** 8 mg/kg/day TMP divided q12h	Pregnancy: C SE: H/A, insomnia, leukopenia, hemolytic anemia, Stevens-Johnson syndrome	\$27-\$43/200 mg SMX/40 mg TMP/5 ml (480 ml); \$7-\$79/400 mg SMX/80 TMP (100); \$9-\$121/800 mg SMX/160 mg TMP (DS) (100)
Second Line			
Amoxicillin with clavulanate (Augmentin)	**Adults:** 500 mg q12h **Children:** Base dosage on amox component: <12 wks: 30/mg/kg q12h >12 wks: 45 mg/kg/day q12h >40 kg: As adult If suspect penicillin-resistant, ↑ dose to 80 mg/kg/day	Pregnancy: B SE: GI upset, rash, urticaria, vaginitis, superinfection, anaphylaxis	\$27/125 mg/31.25 mg/5 ml (150 ml); \$52/250 mg/62.5 mg/5 ml (150 ml); \$58/250 mg/125 mg (30); \$82/500 mg/150 mg (30); \$86/875 mg/125 mg (30)
Cefuroxime (Ceftin)	**Adult:** 250-500 BID × 10 days **Child:** 3 mos-12 yrs: 30 mg/kg/day divided q12h	Pregnancy: B SE: Diarrhea, GI upset, bitter taste, vaginitis, hypersensitivity	\$29/125 mg/5 ml (100 ml); \$35/125 mg (20); \$94/250 mg (30); \$119/400 mg (30)
Loracarbef (Lorabid)	**Adults:** 200 mg q12h × 10 days **Children:** >6 mos: 30 mg/kg/day q12h × 10 days	Pregnancy: B SE: GI upset, rash, H/A, somnolence, dizziness, superinfection	\$24-\$34/100 mg/5 ml (100 ml); \$37/200 mg/5 ml (100 ml); \$94/200 mg (30); \$119/400 mg (30)
Cefprozil (Cefzil)	**Adults:** 250-500 mg q12h ×10 days **Children:** 6 mos-12 yrs: 30 mg/kg/day divided q12h × 10 days	Pregnancy: B SE: Diarrhea, N/V, abdominal pain, dizziness, superinfection	\$27/125 mg/5 ml (100 ml); \$50/250 mg/5 ml (100); \$317-\$356/250 mg (100); \$612-\$672/500 mg (100)
Clindamycin (Cleocin)	**Adults:** 150-300 mg q6h ×10 days **Children:** 20-30 mg/kg/d divided q4h doses	Pregnancy: Caution SE: Pseudomembranous colitis, diarrhea, GI upset, N/V, jaundice, superinfection	
Ceftriaxone (Rocephin)	**Children:** 50 mg/kg in one dose	Pregnancy: B, used when compliance is an issue SE: Local reactions, rash, diarrhea, anaphylaxis, superinfection	\$12/250 mg/vial
Ofloxacin (Floxin Otic)	1-12 y/o: 5 gtts BID × 10 days >12 y/o: 10 gtts BID × 14 days	Used for AOM with PE tubes and chronic suppurative OM in adults with perforated TM Pregnancy: C SE: Local reactions, dizziness, earache	Not available

The traditional duration is 10 days; recent literature suggests 5 days may suffice (Pichichero ME, Cohen R: Shortened course of antibiotic therapy for acute otitis media, sinusitis and tonsillopharyngitis, *Pediatr Infect Dis J* 16[7]:680-695, 1997). Indicators for short-course therapy: no performation in TM, no chronic AOM, no craniofacial abnormalities; no immunocompromise; age >2 years.
GI, Gastrointestinal; *H/A*, headache; *N/V*, nausea and vomiting; *SE*, side effects.

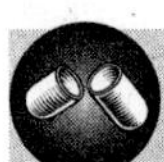

TABLE 134-5 Antibiotic Prophylaxis

Drug	Dose	Comments	Cost
Amoxicillin	20 mg/kg/day	See Table 134-4	See Table 134-3
Sulfisoxazole (Gantrisin)	50 mg/kg/day (>2 mos)	Pregnancy: C SE: Blood dyscrasias, Stevens-Johnson syndrome	$12/500 mg/5 ml (120 ml)

SE, Side effects.

Encourage to have child's ears rechecked after treatment if nonverbal or still having symptoms
Reassure parents that episodes of OM diminish with time as the eustachian tube lengthens
Avoid fluids entering the ear if perforated eardrum is present

Family Impact

Concern about child with painful episodes and potential for hearing/speech impairment

Referral

Refer to ear, nose, and throat specialist for possible tube insertion:
- Six episodes by 6 years of age
- Five episodes in 1 year
- Three episodes in 6 months
- Effusion present after 3 months with no resolution
- Decreased hearing

Consultation

Consult concerning no response to antibiotic in 24 hours
Infants <3 mos

Follow-up

Recheck child in 24 hours if appears toxic or extremely irritable; return in 10 to 14 days for recheck of erythema, effusion and mobility. Recheck in 4 to 6 weeks for OME resolution.
Treatment failure should be considered if symptoms persist despite good compliance with initial therapy.
A change in antibiotic therapy should be considered in these patients.

EVALUATION

Pain and fever should improve in 48 to 72 hours
Consider prophylaxis treatment if:
- Three episodes in 6 months or 4 in year
- Continue during peak occurrence of URI
- Recheck every month while getting prophylaxis

SUGGESTED READINGS

Boyton R, Dunn E, Stephens G: *Manual of ambulatory pediatrics,* Philadelphia, 1998, JB Lippincott.

Calandra L: Otitis media with effusion, *Adv Nurse Pract* 6(2):22, 67-70, 1998.

Dowell S et al: Otitis media-principles of judicious use of antimicrobial agents, *Pediatrics* 101(1):165-171, 1998.

Ellsworth A et al: *Mosby's 1998 medical drug reference,* St Louis, 1998, Mosby.

Healthcare Consultants of America, Inc: *1998 physicians fee and coding guide,* Augusta, Ga, 1998, Healthcare Consultants of America, Inc.

Smith C: Managing otitis media: present methods, future directions, *Am J Nurse Pract* 2(2):27-31, 1998.

Ovarian Cysts/Masses

ICD-9-CM

Benign Neoplasm of Ovary 220
Malignant Neoplasm of Ovary, Primary Site 183.0

OVERVIEW

Definition

Ovarian cysts are nonneoplastic adnexal masses. Most ovarian cysts are functional or physiological in nature—normal transient variations in the physiologic enlargement of the ovary related to a disproportionate increase in ovarian hormones.

Incidence

Most women have functional ovarian cysts that never cause problems or come to medical attention unless found on coincident pelvic examination. They are one of most common causes of adnexal mass and tenderness in **women of childbearing age.** Generally they do not occur before puberty or after menopause. They account for as much as 4% of pelvic pain.

Pathophysiology

There are three types of functional physiological ovarian cysts: follicle cysts, corpus luteum cysts, and theca lutein cysts. The other most common ovarian cysts are dermoid cysts, endometriomas, and mucinous cystadenomas—all benign adnexal masses.

Functional Ovarian Cysts

Table 135-1 lists the characteristics of functional ovarian cysts.

Follicle Cysts

Most common of ovarian cysts; physiological structures resulting from faulty resorption of fluid from incompletely developed ovarian follicles; usually asymptomatic, disappearing spontaneously within <60 days; may be associated with abnormally long or short intermenstrual interval, thus causing irregular periods

Corpus Luteum Cysts

Less common; transient structure seen only in ovulating women; result from failure of corpus luteum to degenerate after ovulation, so often coincide with ovulation or early pregnancy; more likely to be clinically significant; cause local pain and tenderness on examination; most resorb spontaneously; some rupture (2%); some persist, causing ovarian enlargement, pain, and menstrual irregularity

Theca Lutein Cysts

Least common functional ovarian cysts; may occur independently or in normal pregnancy but usually associated with trophoblastic tumors (hydatid moles) and gonadotropin or clomiphene (Clomid) simulation; commonly bilateral; disappear after ovarian stimulation withdrawn

Other Common Benign Ovarian Cysts

Although less common than functional cysts, these benign ovarian masses occur more commonly than others.

Endometriomas

Also known as "chocolate cysts" because they contain old blood, these occur during reproductive age. They are caused when cyclic menstrual blood in the endometrial tissue implants on the ovaries or elsewhere, causing cyclic pain and dysmenorrhea. Rarely are they asymptomatic. When endometriomas exceed 2 cm, surgery is generally necessary.

Dermoid Cysts (Cystic Teratomas)

These cysts are germ cell tumors; greater than 99% are benign. Common in **children** and **adolescents,** they grow large and cause pressure on other organs before symptoms occur. The cysts are composed of hair, sebaceous material, and sometimes teeth or other calcifications. They are diagnosed by ultrasonography. Surgical removal is generally required.

Mucinous Cystadenomas

These cysts are rare before puberty; 40% occur after

TABLE 135-1 Characteristics of Functional Ovarian Cysts

Characteristic	Follicle Cyst	Corpus Luteum Cyst	Theca Lutein Cyst
Size	Microscopic to 8 cm	3 cm or >	25-30 cm
Occurrence in menstrual cycle	First half	Second half at ovulation	Second half
Associated menstrual irregularity	Normal or delayed menstrual period	Scanty flow followed by delayed menstrual period with menses, may have prolonged flow	Secondary amenorrhea
Potential complications	Rare Usually resorb	May rupture May cause torsion	May rupture May cause torsion May involve problems of trophoblastic growth

menopause. They are composed of epithelium and thick, sticky fluid, may become huge and are prone to torsion.

Polycystic Ovary (PCO) or Stein Leventhal Syndrome

PCO is associated with multiple inactive ovarian cysts. The cause is androgen excess and anovulation. It affects **15- to 30-year-olds;** causes infertility. In addition to bilateral PCOs, patient has small breasts, large clitoris, obesity, secondary amenorrhea, enlarged muscle mass, acne, and oily skin. Fifty percent have hirsutism with male pattern distribution. These are all symptoms associated with virilization. Symptoms of this syndrome become more apparent with each postmenarchal year. A follicle-stimulating/luteinizing hormone (LH) ratio can help diagnose this disorder; instead of the usual 2:1 ratio, in PCO syndrome the LH level is increased several times the normal level.

With adnexal mass, the practitioner must always suspect cancer until proven otherwise.

Ovarian Cancer

Potentially lethal malignancy of ovarian tissue; asymptomatic in early stages. Cause unknown. In 75% of cases, malignancy has spread before symptoms occur. Sometimes vague (GI) symptoms (anorexia, early satiety, dyspepsia, bloating, and increased belching) 6 months or less before disease is discovered. Irregular mass, adhered to surrounding tissue; firm nodules are frequently noted in the cul de sac or along the uterosacral ligaments. Tumors of germ cell origin usually occur in women under age 30, whereas those of epithelial origin occur after age 30. Cancer of the ovary is rare under age 20 but increases steadily thereafter. Approximately 1.6% of women develop ovarian cancer during their lifetimes. The average age at diagnosis is about 50.

Five to ten percent of cases of ovarian cancer are hereditary and associated with BRCA 1 and BRCA 2 genes, located on the 17th and 13th chromosomes, respectively. With this genetic make-up, the overall lifetime risk of breast cancer is 80%; the lifetime risk of ovarian cancer is 60%.

Protective Factors Against Ovarian Cysts

Factors that suppress ovarian activity
Use of oral contraceptives and pregnancy

Protective Factors Against Ovarian Cancer

Oral contraceptive use
Multiparity
Breastfeeding
Early first pregnancy
Bilateral tubal ligation

Factors That Increase Susceptibility to Ovarian Cysts

Being of childbearing age

Factors That Increase Susceptibility to Ovarian Cancer

Increased ovulation
Nulliparity
Infertility
Irradiation of pelvis
Endometriosis
Late childbearing
Family history of breast or ovarian cancer, especially first degree relatives
Personal history of breast, colorectal, or endometrial cancer
Menarche >14 years old
Menopause <45 years old
Talc use on perineum
High fat diet
Fertility drug use (possible)

SUBJECTIVE DATA

History of Present Illness

Functional Ovarian Cyst

May present with complaints of vague local pressure, heaviness, and aching or cramping in affected side, sometimes aggravated by sexual intercourse, menstruation, or defecation. Menstrual irregularities are common. Some functional ovarian cysts are asymptomatic and discovered during routine bimanual pelvic examination.

Ask:

- About type, location, and extent of pain
- About duration of symptoms
- About associated symptoms and association of symptoms with the menstrual cycle
- What helps or makes the pain worse
- How the symptoms have affected her life thus far

Suspicion of Torsion or Rupture

Ask:

- About last menstrual period (LMP): Usually occurs 14 to 60 days after last period
- About general aching followed by sudden severe abdominal pain
- About weakness, syncope, dizziness that may occur with sudden blood loss
- What activity preceded sudden pain: Often will report exercise, trauma, or sexual intercourse immediately preceding
- About nausea and vomiting and whether it preceded or followed the pain

Ovarian Cancer

Ask about:

- Increasing abdominal girth, vague GI complaints (dyspepsia, anorexia, early satiety, increased bloating and belching), weight change
- Presence of risk factors

Past Medical History

Suspected Functional Cysts

Ask about menstrual history: Age at menarche or menopause, LMP

Ask about obstetrical history. Ask about sexual history, dyspareunia, use of contraception, especially oral contraceptive pills (OCPs), exposure to sexually transmitted disease. Determine high risk behaviors that might cause pelvic inflammatory disease (PID), confusing the diagnosis. Ask about chronic illnesses, injuries, surgeries, and allergies.

Medications

Note use of OCPs. Ask about use of analgesia for discomfort. Ask about use of medications for indigestion, nausea, and constipation. Ask about use of anticoagulants.

Family History

Ask about first-degree relatives who have had cancer, especially breast, endometrial, or ovarian. Ask about female relatives with a history of ovarian cysts

Psychosocial History

Ask about smoking, alcohol, and other drug use. Inquire about sexually risky behavior, including multiple sexual partners. Ask how pelvic aching affects lifestyle, including sexual relationship.

Diet History

Determine if high-fat diet places her at risk for ovarian cancer.

OBJECTIVE DATA

Physical Examination

Perform a problem-oriented physical examination, with special attention to general appearance, vital signs, abdominal and pelvic examination, and systems that reflect virilization.

Check weight and height.

Note abdominal girth, presence of ascites and fluid wave.

Check bowel sounds and palpate for general tenderness, guarding, rebound and other peritoneal signs, and organomegaly.

Check for hirsutism and note hair distribution pattern—male vs female. Note temporal baldness, skin changes, including acne (see Chapter 93).

In preteen girls, note Tanner's staging.

Examine the breasts and check for nipple discharge.

Perform pelvic examination gently to avoid inadvertent rupture of ovarian cyst. Note size of clitoris (>10 mm = virilization; 2 to 4 mm = normal). Note size, contour, and position of uterus. Note cervical motion tenderness and presence of cervical and/or vaginal discharge, performing wet preparations or cultures as needed. Assess adnexa for tenderness and presence of mass or enlarged ovary.

Perform rectovaginal examination to confirm size of adnexal mass and locate in relation to uterus. Note tender nodularity posterior cul de sac and along uterosacral ligaments.

If patient presents with history of sudden severe abdominal pain, note position on examination table. With ruptured cyst, patient will usually lie quietly with knees drawn up toward abdomen as movement increases pain. Assess for acute abdomen—pain, guarding, rigidity, rebound, and other peritoneal signs.

Diagnostic Procedures

The diagnostic procedures in Table 135-2 may be ordered to confirm or rule out ovarian cysts versus other differential diagnoses.

ASSESSMENT

Differential diagnoses of adnexal masses include functional ovarian cyst, benign ovarian tumor, endometrioma, tuboovarian abscess, GI illness like diverticulum or

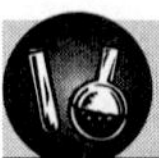

TABLE 135-2 Diagnostic Procedures: Ovarian Cysts

Diagnostic Tests	Finding/Rationale	Cost ($)
Serum hCG	To rule out intrauterine or ectopic pregnancy when patient presents with acute abdomen/possible ruptured ovarian cyst	28-35/qual 51-65/quan
Culdocentesis	To check for intraperitoneal bleeding or infection by tapping cul de sac of Douglas; performed by MD	122-146
CBC, including WBC and differential	To determine presence of infectious process to evaluate fluid and red cell volume and presence of anemia secondary to blood loss	18-23
FSH, LH, 17 ketosteroids	Rule out polycystic ovary syndrome	62-78/FSH; 61-76/LH; 50-63/17
LPA	Ovarian cancer activating factor: LPA is a lipid normally produced in certain hematopoietic cells and is found in serum; about 90% of patients with stage 1 ovarian cancer and 100% of stages 2-4 have elevated LPA levels; test is more sensitive than Ca 125 but is not currently in widespread use; watch for more details as more data are available	
Pelvic or transvaginal ultrasonography	To differentiate between cyst and solid mass and aids in determining which should be followed and which referred	347-416/pelvis; 369-439/transvag
CA 125 Radioimmunoassay	Tumor sensitive antigen for patients at high risk for ovarian cancer; >35 U/ml is found in 60%-80% of those with ovarian cancer but is also found in 1% of healthy women	62-78
Laparoscopy	May be necessary for diagnosis	1186-1398

CBC; Complete blood count; *FSH,* follicle-stimulating hormone; *hCG,* human chorionic gonadotropin; *LH,* luteinizing hormone; *LPA,* lysophosphatidic acid.

cancer, ovarian cancer, uterine fibroid, ectopic pregnancy (Table 135-3).

When patient presents with findings suggestive of ruptured cyst, rule out ruptured ectopic pregnancy, appendicitis, acute salpingitis, tuboovarian abscess/PID.

THERAPEUTIC PLAN

Management of Ovarian Cysts

Management of ovarian cysts is summarized in Table 135-4.

Pharmaceutical

Use of OCPs may aid resolution in 80% of functional cysts within 2 months. (See family planning for more details on OCPs.) If a theca lutein cyst is suspected, any drug being used to stimulate ovarian activity should be discontinued immediately.

Lifestyle/Activities

Teach what to expect if torsion or hemorrhage occurs; reassure that these are rare complications, but prepare patient to notify caregiver or go directly to the Emergency Department. Advise about lifestyle changes that decrease risk of ovarian cancer.

Diet

None

Patient Education

Discuss possible cause and course of functional cysts. Identify factors that protect against or increase risk for ovarian cyst and ovarian cancer.

Family Impact

Anxiety related to a mass and the possibility of malignancy. Confirmation of a diagnosis of cancer is associated with inherent fears of pain, mutilation, and death. Family members must deal with painful emotions and possible loss of a loved one.

Complications of ovarian cysts such as rupture or torsion involve emergency situations that create anxiety for family.

A diagnosis of PCO disease, associated with an uncertain childbearing future, may evoke strong feelings.

Table 135-3 Differential Diagnosis: Ovarian Cysts

Diagnosis*	Supporting Data
Benign ovarian tumor	
Dermoid cyst (cystic teratoma)	May be asymptomatic
	Mass anterior to uterus which displaces uterus backward
	Ultrasonography + calcifications
Mucinous cystadenoma	Reproductive age and postmenopausal women
	Enlarged abdomen (if large) weight gain
	Pressure symptoms (if large)
	+ Ultrasonography
	Palpable adnexal mass—smooth and irregular contour
	Reproductive age
	Cyclic pain and dysmenorrhea—occurs 1-2 days before menses
Endometrioma	Palpable adnexal mass—typically immobile
	+ Ultrasonography
Tuboovarian abscess/salpingitis	Sexually active female—high-risk sexual behavior
	Fever/chills
	++ White blood count
	+ Cervical discharge
	Cervical motion tenderness
	DNA probe: + Chlamydia, gonorrhea
	Diffuse, thickened, tender adnexa
	Pelvic pain—increasing with urination secondary to pressure change
	Possible purulent drainage on culdocentesis
	Guarding, + peritoneal signs possible
Ovarian cancer	Postmenopausal women most commonly
	Palpable adnexal mass—firm, irregular
	Immobile
	Vague gastrointestinal complaints in previous weeks
	+ Ultrasonography
	Increased Ca 125
Uterine fibroids	Palpable irregularly contoured uterus
	Firm, nontender
	Fairly mobile uterus
Pelvic adhesions	History of pelvic inflammatory disease or abdominal surgery
	Uterus fixed position
Ectopic pregnancy	Reproductive age
	Late menses followed by irregular bleeding
	Abdominal pain on affected side
	Normal or slightly enlarged uterus (approx 6-wk size possible)
	Small, tender adnexal mass on affected side—2-3 cm
	Soft swelling immediately lateral to fundus
	+ Beta hCG—does not double in 48 hours as with IUP; >3000 IUP evident on vaginal ultrasound—> 6000 IUP evident on pelvic ultrasound
	Serum progesterone <8 mg/ml (80% accurate)
	Physical findings of early pregnancy
	Nonclotting bloody aspirate on culdocentesis
Ruptured cyst	Pelvic pain
	Tenderness on pelvic examination
	+ Ultrasonography
	Serous, serosanguinous, or clear fluid aspirate on culdocentesis
Appendicitis	Fever
	++ White blood count
	Periumbilical, then right lower quadrant tenderness at McBurney's point
	Right lower quadrant pain
	+ Rebound and peritoneal signs
	Guarding
	Decreased bowel sounds
	Nausea and vomiting

*Because of symptoms associated with adnexal masses causing pressure on the bladder or gastrointestinal tract, genitourinary or gastrointestinal disorders must often be considered in a list of differential diagnoses and ruled out or confirmed by appropriate diagnostic tests.
N/A, Not available; *IUP,* intrauterine pregnancy.

TABLE 135-4 Management of Ovarian Cysts

Age	Plan
Prepuberty	Mass <5 cm, cystic, asymptomatic; watch ×1-2 months, repeating ultrasound to evaluate size Enlarging: Refer for surgery Persistent after 2 months: Refer Mass, solid or 8 cm or >: Refer for surgery
Reproductive age	<5 cm, asymptomatic: Watch 1-2 cycles Unchanged on reexamination: OCPs 1-2 months Persistent: Continue evaluation on OCPs or refer Enlarging: Refer
>40 years old or postmenopausal	Consider cancer until proven otherwise; refer cystic or solid

OCP, Oral contraceptive pills.

Referral

Refer to OB/GYN:

- Cysts >8 cm or persisting 2 cycles (large cysts are more subject to torsion and hemorrhage); if suspect lesion is not functional cyst; in postmenopausal patient (if cyst <5 cm and patient does not have other risk factors, observe; recheck at 6 weeks, 3 months, and 6 months)
- If there is any increase in size of mass
- Any **child** who is prepubertal with an adnexal mass
- Any **older woman** who is postmenopausal with an enlarged ovary
- For emergent care in event of rupture or torsion symptoms
- Patients with PCO syndrome: For initial diagnosis and early management; but, depending on setting, may be co-managed by the primary care provider

Consultation

When uncertainty occurs about diagnosis or management of adnexal masses

Follow-up

Most functional cysts resolve in 8 weeks either spontaneously or with the aid of OCPs. Patients on OCPs should be followed for untoward effects. Women with a history of functional ovarian cysts should continue to have annual clinical examinations. Cysts sometime recur.

If an adnexal mass occurs during pregnancy, ectopic must be ruled out. A fetal sac of intrauterine pregnancy should be seen with an human chorionic gonadotropin level of 6500 IU on pelvic ultrasound or 2000 IU with transvaginal ultrasound. *Physician management is warranted.*

Patients with PCO should have an annual examination to reevaluate the appropriateness of oral contraception and to determine the desire for childbearing, which would require ovulation induction. Because of their anovulatory status without treatment, they need to be followed carefully for endometrial cancer related to prolonged unopposed endogenous estrogen.

Follow-up for ovarian cancer depends on patient situation. It is usually done by a physician and oncology team. Because of its insidious nature, most ovarian cancer has spread before diagnosis. Despite aggressive treatment, 5-year survival is 30% or less.

EVALUATION

Successful outcome is resolution of ovarian cyst without complications. In the event of a malignant adnexal mass, a successful outcome involves early diagnosis while cancer is in situ, aggressive treatment, and long-term survival.

SUGGESTED READINGS

Andolf E: Ultrasound screening in women at risk for ovarian cancer, *Clin Obstet Gynecol* 36(2):423-431, 1993.

Barber HK, Creasman WT, Knapp RC: A rational approach to ovarian masses, *Patient Care* 27:50-67, 74, 1993.

Benson RC, Pernoll ML: *Handbook of obstetrics and gynecology*, New York, 1994, McGraw-Hill.

Bodurka DC et al: Gynecologic cancer: what to watch for, when to refer, *Patient Care* 31(19):15-18, 27-28, 35-42, 1997.

Bowman MA et al: Who are you screening for cancer and when? *Patient Care* 30:54-76, 83-87, 1996.

Carlson KJ et al: *Primary care of women*, St Louis, 1995, Mosby.

Carlson KJ, Skates SJ, Singer DE: Screening for ovarian cancer, *Ann Intern Med* 121:124-132, 1994.

Gallup DG: An update on the diagnosis and treatment of common malignant ovarian tumors, *J Med Assoc Ga* 86:181-185, 1997.

Gallup DG, Talledo OE: Management of the adnexal mass in the 1990s, *Southern Med J* 90(10):972-980, 1997.

Haering WA: Evaluation strategies for functional benign ovarian cysts, *J Am Acad Physician Assistants* 1:201-210, 1988.

Havens CS, Sullivan ND, Tilton P: *Manual of outpatient gynecology*, Boston, 1996, Little Brown.

Healthcare Consultants of America, Inc: *1998 physicians fee and coding guide*, Augusta, Ga, 1998, Healthcare Consultants of America, Inc.

Igoe BA: Symptoms attributed to ovarian cancer by women with the disease, *Nurse Pract* 22(7):122, 127-144, 1997.

Lemcke DP et al: *Primary care of women*, Norwalk, Conn, 1995, Appleton & Lange.

Lichtman R, Papera S: *Gynecology well woman care*, Norwalk, Conn, 1990, Appleton & Lange.

Mann WJ: Diagnosis and management of epithelial cancer of the ovary, *Am Family Physician* 49(3):613-618, 1994.

Mengel MB, Schwiebert P, editors: *Ambulatory medicine: the primary care of families*, Stamford, Conn, 1996, Appleton & Lange.

Star WL, Lommel LL, Shannon MT: *Women's primary care: protocols for practice*, Washington DC, 1995, American Nurses Publishing.

Youngkin EO, Davis MS: *Women's health: a primary care clinical guide*, Norwalk, Conn, 1994, Appleton & Lange.

136 Overweight and Obesity

ICD-9-CM

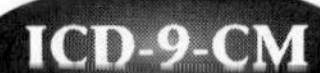

Obesity 278.0

OVERVIEW

Definition

Overweight is defined as a body mass index (BMI) of 25 to 29.9 kg/m. *Obesity* is identified when BMI is >30 kg/m^2. A BMI of 30 is about 30 pounds over weight. Overweight and obesity are not mutually exclusive, since obese persons are also overweight.

Incidence

54.9% of U.S. adults >20 are overweight.

Obesity is higher in certain ethnic populations, particularly in women.

44% of African-American women >20 are overweight.

39% of Hispanic women >20 are overweight.

25% to 30% in prepubertal **children** and 18% to 25% of **adolescents** are obese.

56% of Hispanic **children** and 41% of African-American **children** are overweight compared to 28% of Caucasian **children** (Hellmich, 1992). Obesity (BMI >85th percentile) is 29% among Navajo **children** and 40% among Pueblo Indians (Davis, Gomez, and Lambert, 1993).

Pathophysiology

Obesity is a significant and independent predictor of coronary heart disease (CHD) morbidity and mortality; even mild to moderate weight gain has significant influence in the morbidity and mortality this is caused by chronic illness (Kannel, 1990; Willett, Manson, and Stampfer, 1995).

Obesity is negatively related to high-density lipoprotein (HDL)2 and HDL3 cholesterol and positively correlated with plasma total cholesterol, low-density lipoprotein (LDL) cholesterol, and triglyceride levels (Grundy et al, 1997; Kris-Etherton, 1990). The prevalence of diabetes, hypertension, and hyperlipidemia is three times higher in overweight adults. Obesity also increases the risk of certain types of cancer: colon, rectum, prostate, gallbladder, breast, cervix, endometrium, ovary, and biliary tract.

The location of body fat depots, rather than body weight, is associated with type II diabetes mellitus and CHD, elevated concentrations of very low–density lipoproteins (VLDL), LDL, apoprotein (APO) B-100, insulin resistance. and hypertension (Bjorntorp, 1990; 1992).

Central (abdominal) fat distribution "apple" has been shown to be related to elevated blood glucose, plasma insulin, VLDL-cholesterol and triglycerides, and low concentrations of HDL cholesterol (Kaplan, 1989).

Protective Factors Against

Prevention of overweight and obesity is the most successful method of long-term health.

Risk/Susceptibility

Risk of Binge Dieting

Weight loss efforts are not without risk. The weight loss produced by dietary restriction is a result of the loss of both fat and lean body tissue (fat-free mass, FFM). This contributes to the dilemma of weight cycling when the individual gains weight while eating less.

Binge eaters account for 40% of obese participants in weight control programs (Delvin, Walsh, and Spitzer, 1992; Hakala, 1994). About half of obese individuals in treatment have nonpurging bulimia: they binge eat two to three times a week, have feelings of lack of control over eating behavior, and have significant concern with body weight and shape (Foreyt and Goodrick, 1991).

Some obese individuals have food dependence, similar to substance dependence.

Risk of Obesity in Children

Parental obesity: Overweight parents increase risk of overweight child

Excessive weight of siblings: Assess sibling weight

Mother's preference for a chubby baby: Assess cultural

values regarding weight gain for infant, appearance of a "chubby" baby

BMI >95th percentile: Identifies child in need of treatment

BMI >85th percentile with psychosocial problems: Identifies child in need of treatment

High infant birth weight: Assess infant's birth weight, mother's weight gain during pregnancy

SUBJECTIVE DATA

History of Present Illness

Adults/Elderly

Determine length of overweight and obesity (e.g., Has the patient been overweight since childhood? Was the weight gain related to pregnancy? Menopause? Retirement? Stressful life change event such as a move or job change?)

Children

Determine the emotional impact of overweight and obesity on the child. Frequently children engage in inappropriate weight loss efforts in secret.

Determine their perceptions of themselves: fat, slim, or just right.

Past Medical History

Is there a history of heart disease, diabetes, angina, hypertension, hyperlipidemia, pancreatic disorders, musculoskeletal disorders?

Determine if the obesity has limited mobility and physical endurance.

Medications

Use of over-the-counter medications, medications used for weight loss, sleep assistance, prescription medications

Family History

Family history of diabetes, CHD, hypertension, angina, hyperlipidemia, overweight/obesity

Psychosocial History

Is there a history of addictive behaviors, substance abuse, emotional disorders, psychiatric treatment?

Determine if the patient has had economic, social, and job discrimination related to obesity.

Lifestyle Assessment

Adults and Children

Dietary recall, pattern of weight loss/gain, bingeing, purging, amount and frequency of physical activity, length of time engaging in physical activity (both chronology and duration)

Parental/Child Knowledge and Values

Assess the child/family for the following:

Parental knowledge of nutrition, including balance of fat, protein and carbohydrates

Duration of breastfeeding/early introduction of solid foods: Assess time of breast/bottle cessation, introduction of solid foods

Using food as reward, comfort measure: Assess parental interpretation of infant cues; use of food/feeding as comfort measure

Family Lifestyle

Assess the family situation for the following:

Lower socioeconomic status: Assess food choices/ resources for shopping and nutritional choices

Mother's marital status (single parent): Assess mother's social support sources

Several caretakers in childbearing: Assess feeding choices for caregivers

Assess snack food choices/ foods available for nutrition in the home

Physical inactivity: Assess number of hours of TV/videos watched; amount, frequency, and duration of child's physical activity

Description of Most Common Symptoms

Determine the body image and self-esteem of the obese patient.

Some ethnic groups do not necessarily equate overweight and obesity with being unattractive.

Associated Symptoms

Determine associated symptoms the patient may be experiencing, such as hyperglycemia, gastrointestinal disturbances, musculoskeletal disorders, activity intolerance

OBJECTIVE DATA

Physical Examination

A thorough examination, including vital signs, should be conducted to determine the extent of overweight/obesity and the concurrent conditions that occur (Tables 136-1 and 136-2).

Diagnostic Procedures

Diagnostic procedures include those found in Table 136-3.

TABLE 136-1 Physical Examination: Adults

Test	Findings/Rationale
Body mass index (BMI)	The Body Mass Index (BMI) is an expression of body weight relative to height. BMI is calculated as weight (in kilograms) divided by the square of height (m^2). Use of BMI is limited for reflecting body fat because it does not distinguish fat weight from nonfat weight. A BMI equal to or greater than 27.8 and 27.3 (kg/m^2) for males and females, respectively, has been equated with obesity. Individuals with high BMI should be further examined for fat distribution and health risks associated with overweight and obesity, such as blood lipids.
Weight-to-height ratio	Determines an individual's relative weight to height.
Fat distribution	Measuring where fat is deposited on the body is an important dimension of the assessment of body fat because of its relationship to morbidity and mortality outcomes. Waist-to-hip ratio (WHR) is the simplest method for determining regional fat and describes the anatomical distribution of fat tissue on the waist and hips. The waist circumference is measured at the narrowest spot between the ribs and hips or, when a narrow point is not evident, the midpoint between the lowest rib and the iliac crest. The hip circumference is measured at the widest circumference over the great trochanters. The WHR is calculated by dividing the waist measurement by the hip measurement. A WHR greater than 1 in men and 0.9 in women is associated with substantial increase in risk for hypertension, stroke, and diabetes.

TABLE 136-2 Physical Examination: Children

Test	Findings/Rationale
Weight-for-age methods	Although widely used, weight-for-age percentiles are inadequate to assess overweight because the contributions of stature and lean tissue are not taken into account (Himes and Dietz, 1994). Another method considers weight relative to the weight-for-age percentile that corresponds to the stature-for-age percentile. However the percentiles of weight-for-stature are more narrow than those of weight-for-age, resulting in overestimation of the target weight (Himes and Dietz, 1994).
BMI	Using the BMI, the child is classified as overweight when the index is equal to or exceeds the 85th percentile. The percentiles are age and gender specific: for example, in children ages 12 to 14, the 85th percentile for boys is >23, for girls >23.4; for 15- to 17-year-old males >24.3, for girls >24.8 (Harlan, 1993). In adolescents, the BMI is significantly associated with subcutaneous and total body fatness and is highly specific for individuals with the greatest amount of body fat, making it a useful approach for measurement of fatness in this age group (Himes and Dietz, 1994). It is important to note that specific cutoff points of the BMI that are associated with morbidity and mortality in children and adolescents have not been adequately established.
Skinfold measurements	Some investigators advocate the use of anthropometric (skinfold) measurements as a particularly practical approach for field measurement in children and adolescents (Lohman, 1992). Using this technique, special calipers grasp a skinfold which is held between the tester's thumb and fingers to provide a measurement in millimeters for a double fold of skin and subcutaneous fat (Lohman, 1984).

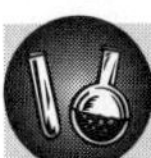

Table 136-3 Diagnostic Procedures: Obesity/Overweight

Diagnostic Test	Findings/Rationale	Cost ($)
Total cholesterol	Helps determine the patient's overall cardiovascular risk status	49-62/lipid panel
HDL	See cholesterol	
LDL	See cholesterol	
VLDL	See cholesterol	
TSH	Screening for other obesity associated diseases	47-61/thyroid panel
FPG	Determines risk for diabetes/hyperglycemia	15-20

FPG, Fasting plasma glucose; *HDL,* high-density lipoprotein; *LDL,* low-density lipoprotein; *TSH,* thyroid-stimulating hormone; *VLDL,* very low–density lipoprotein.

Table 136-4 Differential Diagnosis: Obesity/Overweight

Diagnosis	Supporting Data	Diagnostic Tests
Hypothyroid (Ch. 178)	Fatigue, weight gain	Thyroid-stimulating hormone
Noninsulin-dependent diabetes mellitus (Ch. 55)	Weight gain, fatigue	Fasting blood sugar

ASSESSMENT

Adult/Elderly

A BMI equal to or greater than 27.8 and 27.3 (kg/m^2) for males and females, respectively, has been equated with obesity (NIH Consensus Development Conference Statement, 1993) (Table 136-4).

A waist-to-hip ratio greater than 1 in men and 0.9 in women is associated with substantial increase in risk for hypertension, stroke, and diabetes.

Child

Using the BMI, the child is classified as overweight when the index is equal to or exceeds the 85th percentile. The definition of obesity in children using triceps skinfold measurement is thickness greater than or equal to 85th percentile and weight for height, age, and sex greater than or equal to the 85th percentile. The 85th percentile corresponds roughly to 120% of ideal body weight and is the accepted definition of obesity in children (NIH Consensus Development Conference Statement, 1993).

THERAPEUTIC PLAN

A treatment algorithm is found in Figure 136-1.

Pharmaceutical

Drugs may be used as part of a comprehensive weight loss program, including dietary and physical activity for patients with BMI >30 with no concomitant obesity-related risk factors or diseases, and for patients with BMI >27 with concomitant obesity-related risk factors (hypertension, dyslipidemia, CHD, type 2 diabetes, and sleep apnea). Weight loss drugs should never be used without lifestyle modifications. Continual assessment of drug therapy for efficacy and safety is necessary (Table 136-5).

Lifestyle/Activities

Exercise

Physical activity is particularly important in aiding and sustaining weight loss through increased total energy expenditure, preservation of lean body mass, and changes in metabolism (King and Tribble, 1991).

Obese people carry much more weight around than their lean counterparts and expend more calories when they expend energy. If weight is lost and activity levels remain the same, caloric intake needs to be further reduced to compensate for both the reduced resting metabolic rate and the reduced nonresting energy expenditure (Pi-Sunyer, 1991).

The energy equation of energy intake and expenditure needs to be a major consideration in weight loss efforts. It is the combination of exercise and caloric restriction that contributes to success of weight loss and maintenance (Avila and Hovell, 1994; Blair, 1993; Foreyt and Goodrick, 1991; Ballor and Poehlman, 1994).

Exercise is most advantageous in weight loss because it maintains the RME and the TEF. In addition, exercise produces a favorable effect on plasma lipids and carbohydrate metabolism (Calles-Escandon and Horton, 1992). It is not only the amount of exercise but the intensity of the exercise that may be important in weight loss.

Children

The goal of weight reduction in children is to achieve sustained weight loss of fat tissue without affecting BMI or

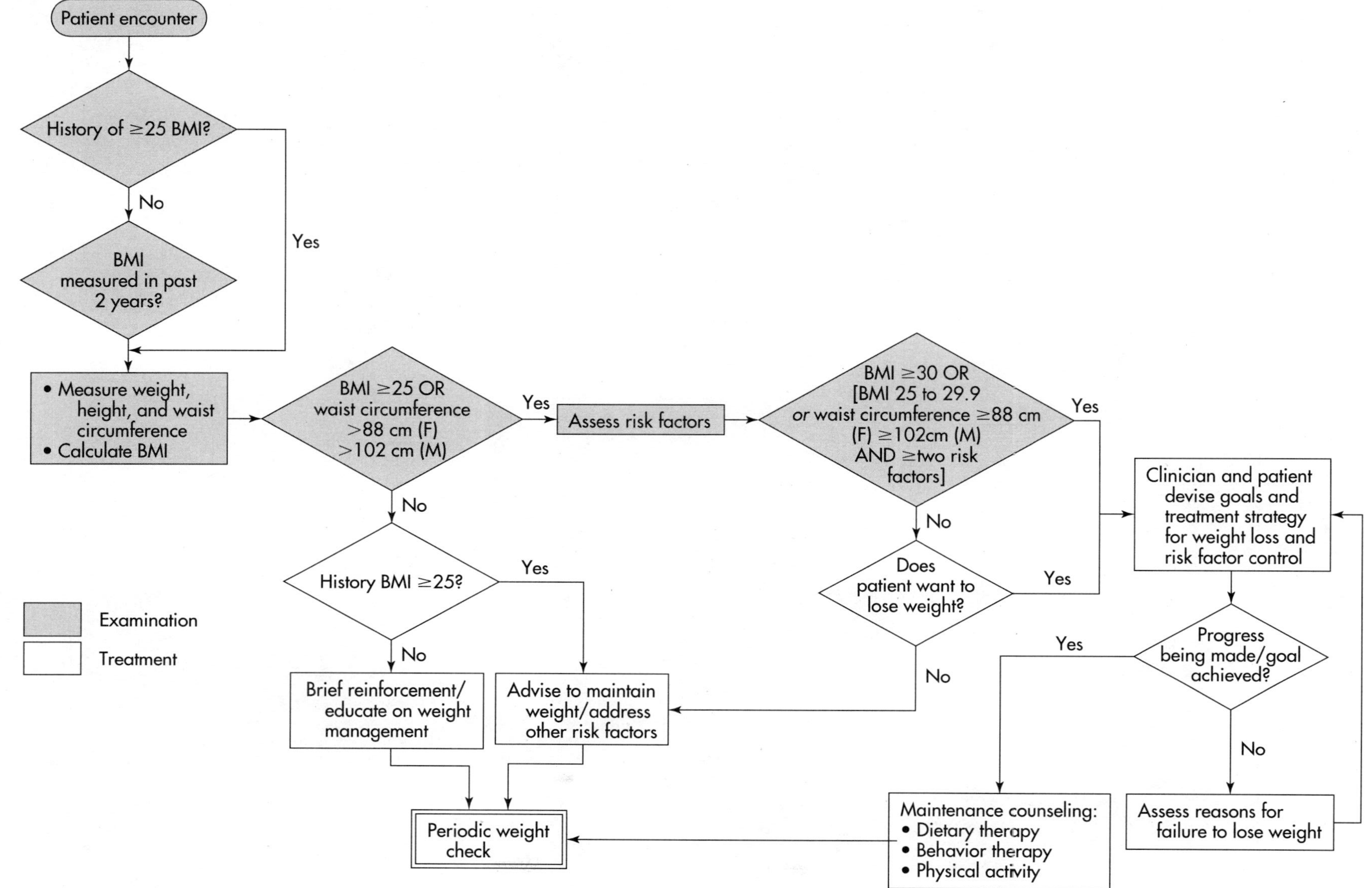

Figure 136-1 Treatment algorithm for obesity and overweight. This algorithm applies only to the assessment for overweight and obesity and subsequent decisions based on that assessment. It does not reflect any initial overall assessment for other conditions and diseases that the provider may wish to do. *BMI*, Body mass index. (From National Institutes of Health: *Clinical guidelines on the identification, evaluation, and treatment of overweight and obesity in adults*, Rockville, Md, 1998, NIH.)

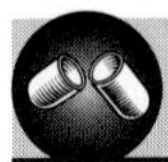

TABLE 136-5 Pharmaceutical Treatment: Obesity and Overweight

Agent	Drugs	Dose	Adverse Effects	Cost
Anorexigenic Agents				
Reduction of Energy Intake				
Those that affect the catecholaminergic system	Benzphetamine (Didrex) CS III	25-50 mg	Pregnancy: Didrex (X), Tenuate (B) SE: HTN, potential for abuse, CNS overstimulation, dry mouth	Didrex N/A $5-39/Tenuate: 25 mg (100); $46-$97/SR: 75, 100 mg (100)
	Diethylpropion hydrochloride (Tenuate) CS IV	25 mg TID		
	Phendimetrazine (Bontril, Metra, Adipex [ER])	35 mg BID/TID 1 hr AC ER: 105 mg QD, 30-60 min before AM meal		
	Phenylpropanolamine hydrochloride (e.g., Dexatrim; OTC)	25 mg TID 30 min AC or ER: 50-75 mg QD midmorning with glass H_2O	Pregnancy: Not recommended SE: Dry mouth, anticholinergic effect, insomnia	$12/ER: 75 mg (60); $2/25 mg (100)
Those That Affect the Serotonergic System				
Sibutramine (Meridia): Centrally acting appetite depressant that inhibits reuptake of serotonin, norepinephrine, and dopamine	Meridia	10 mg QD (may be ↑ to 15 mg QD if wt loss of 4 lb occurs in 4 wks)	Pregnancy: C SE: Dry mouth, anorexia, insomnia, and constipation, HTN	$60/10 mg (15)
Phentermine (Ionamin)	Ionamin	15-30 mg before breakfast or 10-14 hr before HS		$4/15 mg (100); $4-$99/30 mg (100)
Experimental Agents				
Reduction of absorption of nutrients; inhibits pancreatic and gastric lipase; blocks action of enzymes or block absorption of nutrients from GI tract	Orlistat	Clinical trials ongoing; recently approved for use	Fat-soluble vitamins may require replacement because of partial malabsorption; ↑ gas, ↑ bowel movements	N/A
Increase energy expenditure Ephedrine, and beta-adrenoceptor agonist increase metabolic rate through changes in the sympathetic nervous system or uncoupling oxidative phosphorylation	BRL-26830A (experimental)	None approved by FDA for weight loss		N/A

CNS, Central nervous system; *CS,* controlled substance; *FDA,* Food and Drug Administration; *GI,* gastrointestinal; *HTN,* hypertension; *N/A,* not available; *SE,* side effects.

linear growth. There is no generally accepted standard for the effective treatment of obesity in children. Interventions may address either prevention of overweight or treatment of the problem.

The focus of most weight reduction interventions and research has been on coupling physical activity and moderate caloric restriction during the growth period.

The main methods of treatment of childhood obesity are modification of diet, exercise, diet and exercise together, and child-oriented or family-based behavior modification programs.

The interventions include parent education in behavioral and problem-solving techniques and mothers' attendance at weight loss classes.

Exercise is an important adjunct to weight loss and subsequent reduction of unfavorable lipoproteins in children.

Behavioral modification such as recognition of stimuli related to eating, behavioral substitution, goal setting and self-monitoring with contracts are techniques that have been successful. Program interventions such as "Shapedown" focuses on the child's cognitive behavioral and affective elements of weight management.

Rather than using restrictive diets, emphasize healthy eating habits, exercise behavior, and communication skills in both prevention and reduction efforts. Efforts should be made to assist the child to normalize, not restrict, food; to increase physical activity; and to gain a feeling of empowerment.

Diet

Adults

Dietary restriction is the most commonly used strategy for weight loss and maintenance and includes primarily two levels of calorie restriction.

The low-calorie diet (LCD) is 1000 to 1500 calories (12 to 15 Kcal/kg body weight). The very low–calorie diet (VLCD) is about 800 calories (6 to 19 Kcal/kg body weight). Weight loss using VLCD averages 1.5 to 2.5 kg/week; after 12 to 16 weeks the average loss is 20 kg. The use of VLCD has been associated with adverse complications, but it is generally safe when used under proper supervision in moderate and severely obese patients.

VLCD produces rapid short-term weight loss, with about half of patients gaining more than half of their lost weight after 1 year (Holden, Darga, and Olson, 1992; Kern, Trozzolino, and Wolfe, 1994).

Other strategies of dietary restriction include changes in dietary proportions of fat, protein, and carbohydrates (e.g., 30% of total caloric intake as fats).

Children

Dietary restrictions in infants, young children, and even adolescents are unsafe and may retard both physical and mental growth and development. Moderate dietary nutrition coupled with exercise will not contribute to a decrease in linear growth.

Weight reduction therapy should be focused primarily on those children and adolescents who have obesity-related morbidity. These include those with a BMI greater than the 95th percentile or those with a BMI greater than the 85th percentile who perceive their adiposity to be a significant psychosocial problem.

Finally, identify "problem" foods such as cookies and chips, which are habitual. Encourage the reduced consumption of "problem" foods, rather than worry about the occasional pizza or ice cream treat.

Enlist parental assistance to plan and structure healthy meals and snacks.

Patient Education

Behavior modification is the most widely recognized and studied approach to weight loss; management includes behavior modification elements.

Programs using behavior approaches involve the systematic examination of factors preceding and following the target behavior (eating). The core of behavioral approaches is self-monitoring (Foreyt and Goodrick, 1993a).

Stimulus control is based on the concept of controlling the environment and modifying cues that lead to inappropriate eating or exercise (Foreyt and Goodrick, 1993b). For example, altering behavior topology, such as the speed at which one eats, has been successful (Foreyt and Goodrick, 1993b).

Contracts that focus on increasing healthy behaviors associated with weight loss are used with contingency management when the individual receives a reward for appropriate behavior (Foreyt and Goodrick, 1993a). Their weight loss methods include alterations in cognitive-behavioral patterns. Thinking patterns that are reframed away from self-rejection and toward self-acceptance have been effective in therapy for binge eating (Foreyt and Goodrick, 1993a).

Family Impact

The family role in weight loss efforts cannot be overemphasized. Esteem support is demonstrated by such things as verbal reinforcement, using behavioral techniques along with the participant, and attendance at meetings with the participant.

Informational support includes assistance with monitoring the participant's weight loss activities and prompting appropriate eating behavior. Instrumental support includes refraining from criticism of the participant's progress (Black, Gleser, and Kooyers, 1990).

Family involvement in childhood weight management is important. In long-term management of obesity in children, successful programs include those with parents as active participants, family support to encourage behavior changes, and family motivational structures.

Referral/Consultation

Morbidly obese individuals—particularly those with accompanying risks such as hypertension and co-morbid chronicity such as noninsulin-dependent diabetes mellitus—should be referred to specialists.

Follow-up

It is necessary to encourage the weight loss efforts beyond 20 weeks and provide frequent support to the patient in his or her weight management attempts (Perri et al, 1989).

EVALUATION

Recognize that treatment for obesity is generally unsuccessful. The majority of weight loss attempts are self-directed and are usually the most successful at long-term success: 72% of people who had maintained a significant weight loss had done so on their own, whereas 20% had enrolled in commercial programs, 3% used diet pills, and 5% enrolled in a medical-based program (Foreyt and Goodrick, 1993a).

Identify your own personal experiences and beliefs about body image, attractiveness, and benefits of weight loss.

The goal of weight loss should be to prevent the associated risks factors related to end-stage organ damage.

RESOURCES

Overeaters Anonymous, 1-505-891-2664.
TOPS (Take Off Pounds Sensibly), 1-800-932-8677.

REFERENCES

Avila P, Hovell MF: Physical activity training for weight loss in Latinas: a controlled study, *Int J Obesity-Related Metabol Disorders* 18(7):476-482, 1994.

Ballor DL, Poehlman ET: Exercise-training enhances fat-free mass preservation during diet-induced weight loss: a meta-analytical finding, *Int J Obesity* 18:35-40, 1994.

Bjorntorp P: "Portal" adipose tissue as a generator of risk factors for cardiovascular disease and diabetes, *Arteriosclerosis* 10(4):493-496, 1990.

Bjorntorp P: Regional obesity. In Bjorntorp P, Brodoff BN, editors: *Obesity*, Philadelphia, 1992, JB Lippincott.

Black DR, Gleser LJ, Kooyers KJ: A meta-analytic evaluation of couples weight-loss programs, *Health Psych* 9(3):330-347, 1990.

Blair SN: Evidence for success of exercise in weight loss and control, *Ann Intern Med* 119(7 part 2):702-706, 1993.

Calles-Escandon J, Horton ES: The thermogenic role of exercise in the treatment of morbid obesity: a critical evaluation, *Am J Clin Nutr* 55(2 Suppl):533S-537S, 1992.

Davis S, Gomez Y, Lambert L: Primary prevention of obesity in American Indians, *Ann NY Acad Sci* 699:167-180, 1993.

Delvin MJ, Walsh BT, Spitzer RL: Is there another binge eating disorder? A review of the literature on overeating in the absence of bulimia nervosa, *Int J Eating Disorders* 11:333-337, 1992.

Foreyt JP, Goodrick GK: Factors common to successful therapy for the obese patient, *Med Sci Sports Exercise* 23(3):292-297, 1991.

Foreyt JP, Goodrick GK: Evidence for success of behavior modification in weight loss and control, *Ann Intern Med* 119(7 part 2):698-701, 1993a.

Foreyt JP, Goodrick GK: Weight management without dieting, *Nutrition Today* 28(2):4-9, 1993b.

Grundy SM et al: Guide to primary prevention of cardiovascular disease: a statement for healthcare professionals from the Task Force on Risk Reduction American Heart Association Science Advisory and Coordinating Committee, *Circulation* 95:2329-2331, 1997.

Hakala P: Weight reduction programs at a rehabilitation center and a health center based on group counseling and individual support: short- and long-term follow-up study, *Int J Obesity-Related Metabol Disorders* 18(7):483-489, 1994.

Harlan WR: Epidemiology of childhood obesity, *Ann NY Acad Sci* 699:1-5, 1993.

Himes JH, Dietz WH: Guidelines for overweight in adolescent preventive services: recommendations from an expert committee, *Am J Clin Nutrition* 9:307-316, 1994.

Holden JH et al: Long-term follow-up of patients attending a combination very-low calorie diet and behaviour therapy weight loss programme, *Int J Obesity-Related Metabol Disorders* 16(8):605-613, 1992.

Kannel WB: CHD risk factors: a Framingham study update, *Hosp Pract* 25(7):119-130, 1990.

Kaplan NM: The deadly quartet: upper body obesity glucose intolerance, hypertriglyceridemia and hypertension, *Arch Intern Med* 149:1514-1520, 1989.

Kern PA, Trozzolino L, Wolfe G: Combined use of behavioral models and very low calorie diets in weight loss and maintenance, *Am J Med Sci* 307(5):325-328, 1994.

King AC, Tribble DL: The role of exercise in weight reduction in nonathletes, *Sports Med* 11(5):331-349, 1991.

Kris-Etherton PM: *Cardiovascular disease: nutrition for prevention and treatment,* Chicago, 1990, American Dietetic Association.

Lohman TG: Advances in body composition assessment, *Curr Iss Exercise Science Service* (monograph 3), Champaign Ill, 1992, Human Kinetics.

Lohman TG, Pollock ML, Slaughter MJ: Methodological factors and the prediction of body fat in female athletes, *Med Sci Sports Exercise* 16:92-96, 1984.

National Institutes of Health Consensus Development Conference Statement: Health implications of obesity, *Ann Intern Med* 103(6):1073-1077, 1993.

Pi-Sunyer FX: Obesity: determinants and therapeutic initiatives, *Nutrition* 7:292-294, 1991.

Willett WC, Manson JE, Stampfer MJ: Weight change and coronary heart disease in women, *JAMA* 273:461-465, 1995.

SUGGESTED READINGS

Ellsworth A et al: *Mosby's 1998 medical drug reference*, St Louis, 1998, Mosby.

Healthcare Consultants of America, Inc.: *1998 Physicians fee and coding guide*, Augusta, Ga, 1998, Healthcare Consultants of America, Inc.

House T: Obesity in women: examining today's issues, *Adv Nurse Pract* 5(11):55-59, 1997.

McArdle WD, Katch FI, Katch VL: *Exercise physiology: energy nutrition and human performance*, Philadelphia, 1991, Lea & Febiger.

National Institutes of Health: *Clinical guidelines on the identification, evaluation, and treatment of overweight and obesity in adults,* Rockville, Md, 1998, NIH.

Perri MG, Nezu AM, Patti ET : Effect of length of treatment on weight loss, *J Consult Clin Psychol* 57(3):450-452, 1989.

White JH: The process of embarking on a weight control program, *Health Care Women Int* 5:77-91, 1984.

Palpitations/ Arrhythmias

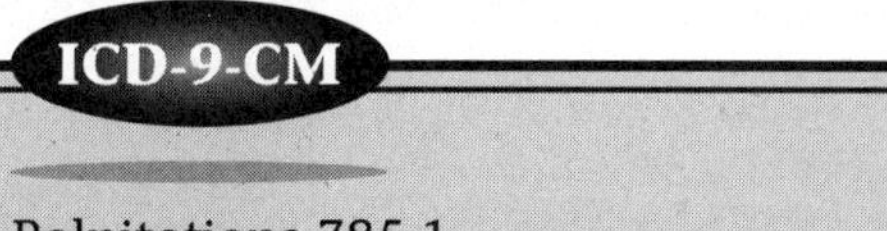

ICD-9-CM

Palpitations 785.1

OVERVIEW

Definition

Palpitations are abnormalities of cardiac rhythm. They are described as skipped beats, extra beats, or racing heart. Most of these abnormalities do not represent serious arrhythmias; however, serious arrhythmias may present with mild symptoms initially. Awareness of the heartbeat can also reflect increased stroke volume in noncardiac conditions (exercise, thyrotoxicosis, anemia, anxiety). Increased perception of the heartbeat may also be due to cardiac abnormalities that increase stroke volume (valvular disease or bradycardia) or to a cardiac arrhythmia itself.

If there is a sufficient decrease in arterial pressure or cardiac output, symptoms will develop (especially in an upright position) such as impaired cerebral blood flow, dizziness, blurring of vision, or loss of consciousness.

Incidence

Complaints of rhythm abnormalities are very common. Tachycardia is more common than bradycardia in **children.** The new onset of premature beats is often due to conditions such as digoxin toxicity, drug ingestions, hypoxia, hypokalemia, acidosis, or underlying cardiac disease.

In adults the following percentages might be expected in terms of causation of arrhythmias:

Cardiac	43%
Psychiatric	31%
Unclear	16% (Weber and Kapoor, 1996)

Pathophysiology

Depends on the arrhythmia present

SUBJECTIVE DATA

History of Present Illness

Ask about:

- Onset of abnormal rhythm, how often they occur, regular or irregular rhythm (have patient tap out rate/rhythm)
- How palpitations stop: do they settle down gradually or do they stop suddenly?
- Complaints of chest pain or lightheadedness
- Association of arrhythmia with exercise or position
- Previous episodes of arrhythmia
- Activities preceding onset of arrhythmia

Associated Symptoms

Shortness of breath
Nausea and vomiting, diaphoresis

Past Medical History

Coronary artery disease, hypertension, angina, previous myocardial infarction or cardiac surgery (angioplasty or coronary artery bypass graft)
Past episodes of syncope
Ever told he or she had a heart murmur
Hyperthyroidism
Anemia
Anxiety

Medications

Digoxin
Over-the-counter decongestants
Street drugs: Cocaine, amphetamines

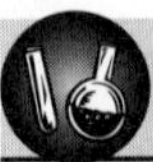

TABLE 137-1 Diagnostic Procedures: Palpitations/Arrhythmias

Diagnostic Tests	Findings/Rationale	Cost ($)
12-lead ECG	Always should be obtained. Documenting the rhythm can be difficult, since the symptoms may be infrequent. A sinus arrhythmia is a normal finding in children. A normal ECG is frequently found. Evaluate for delta waves characteristic of an accessory pathway (Wolff-Parkinson-White syndrome).	56-65
24-hour Holter monitor	If the arrhythmia is frequent (every day or every few days), a Holter monitor for 24 hours is indicated. If the episodes occur less frequently, the Holter record is likely to be normal.	295-388
Event recorder (30-day)	For infrequent episodes of arrhythmia. The patient carries an event monitor, places it on the chest when an episode occurs, recording the rhythm. This allows capture of infrequent events.	541-659
Treadmill testing	This may be an option if the arrhythmia occurs with exercise or to determine the severity of the arrhythmia in light of sports participation.	249-305/stress test

TABLE 137-2 Differential Diagnosis: Palpitations/Arrhythmias

Diagnosis	Supporting Data
Premature contractions	Episodes that are fleeting, occurring at rest. The patient is more aware of the compensatory pause than the premature beat.
Paroxysmal tachycardia	Palpitations that start with sudden onset, last several seconds to minutes, and end abruptly may be seen with paroxysmal tachycardia.
Anxiety (Ch. 13)	Slow onset and slowly resolving episodes are more consistent with anxiety.
SVT/paroxysmal SVT or (PSVT)	c/o palpitations, chest pain, shortness of breath, a sense that the heart is racing. Most common in children. Most patients do not have underlying heart disease. Typically the episode occurs at rest, but it may occur with exertion. Rate is usually above 100, with regular rate. Causes of SVT include metabolic demand: pregnancy, thyroid, fever; impaired stroke volume—valvular or myocardial disease; increase in sympathetic tone— anxiety or excitement. The common arrhythmias included in SVT are: atrial tachycardia (rate 100-200), atrial flutter (rate 220-360), atrial fibrillation (most common of all sustained arrhythmias; present in 3%-4% in people >70) and paroxysmal SVT.
Wolff-Parkinson-White syndrome	The ventricle is excited through an accessory pathway. This produces a characteristic ECG pattern with a short PR interval and a slurred QRS complex (the delta wave).
Ventricular tachycardia	When three or more ectopic beats arise from lower than the bundle of His, the arrhythmia is termed ventricular. The range is 130-200 beats/min. Ventricular tachycardia is usually associated with organic heart disease.

ECG, Electrocardiogram; *SVT,* supraventricular tachycardia.

Caffeine
Cardiac rate-altering drugs: Beta blockers, nondihydropyridine calcium channel blockers

Family History

Structural heart disease
Sudden death

Psychosocial History

Amount of caffeine intake
Ethanol history
Smoking history

OBJECTIVE DATA

Physical Examination

A complete screening examination should be done, with particular attention to the heart. In most cases the examination is unremarkable.

General: Overall appearance
Cardiovascular: Rate, rhythm, presence of murmurs, extra heart sounds
Extremities: Edema, pulses

Diagnostic Procedures

Diagnostic procedures are outlined in Table 137-1.

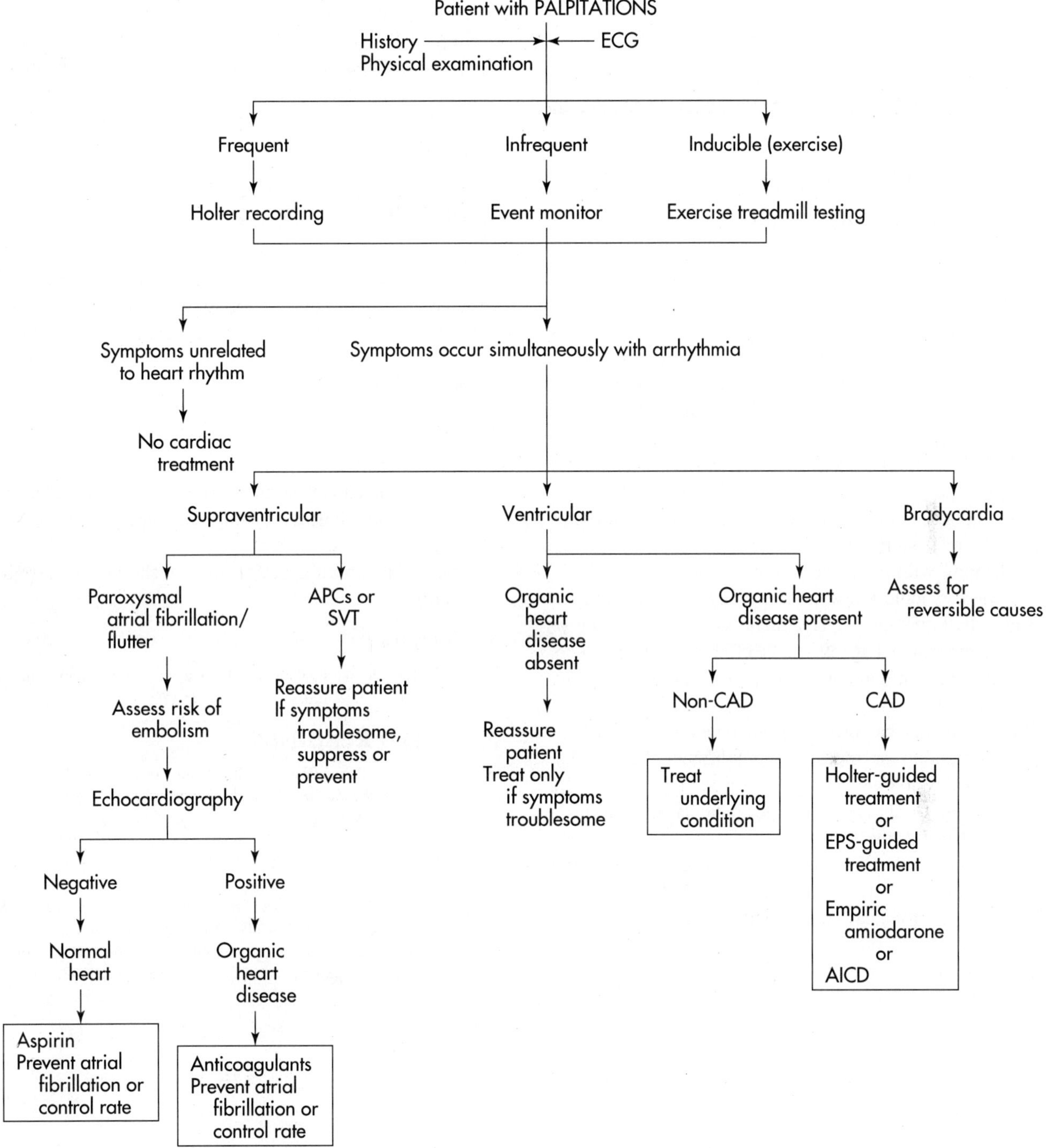

Figure 137-1 Algorithm for patient with palpitations. *AICD,* Automatic implantable cardioverter-defibrillator; *APC,* atrial premature contraction; *CAD,* coronary artery disease; *ECG,* electrocardiogram; *EPS,* electrophysiologic study; *SVT,* supraventricular tachycardia. (Adapted from Greene HL, Johnson WP, Lemcke D: *Decision making in medicine*, ed 2, St Louis, 1998, Mosby.)

ASSESSMENT

Descriptions of the palpitations should provide some indication of what might be causing the rapid beating of the heart (Table 137-2, Figure 137-1).

THERAPEUTIC PLAN

Pharmaceutical/Nonpharmaceutical

Treatment depends on the cause of the arrhythmia and how symptomatic the patient is.

Supraventricular Tachycardia in Children and Adolescents

There are three options for supraventricular tachycardia (SVT):

No therapy: Adolescents with rare, self-limiting SVT, a structurally normal heart and no evidence of Wolff-Parkinson-White syndrome may not require any treatment. The patient should be taught about vagal maneuvers:

In infants, do not do carotid massage or apply orbital pressure.

Rectal stimulation (by taking rectal temperature) frequently is effective.

Gagging with nasogastric tube is also effective.

Patients should know when to seek medical help.

Antiarrhythmic agents: Treatment with beta-blocking or calcium channel agents can be effective. Beta blockers can cause fatigue, which is unacceptable to many adolescents.

Radiofrequency catheter ablation: When medications are unacceptable or there is breakthrough tachycardia, electrophysiologic testing is considered. This is the treatment of choice in younger patients, since it has a high success rate.

In patients with SVT localized to the atrium (atrial fibrillation or flutter), consideration should be given to inciting factors: caffeine, hyperthyroid, or alcohol use. Correction of these factors is usually sufficient to control the arrhythmia. In patients >70 with atrial fibrillation and underlying heart disease that is not controllable, anticoagulation therapy may be considered if there are no contraindications. The issue of absolute need for anticoagulation with atrial fibrillation is currently under investigation.

In patients with paroxysmal SVT, since there is a chance of syncope, pharmacologic therapy is directed to altering conduction properties of the atrioventricular (AV) node and sinus tract. Drugs that are effective include digoxin or beta blockers.

Lifestyle/Activities

Palpitations are a common complaint in adolescents. For most adolescents a particular cause may not be found. Emphasize the importance of avoiding caffeine or other stimulants and obtaining adequate sleep, sufficient fluids, and routine exercise.

Referral

Serious abnormalities such as AV block, symptomatic SVT, or ventricular tachycardia warrant immediate referral to a cardiologist/hospital, using the emergency transport system.

A patient with a prolonged QT interval should be referred to a cardiologist.

REFERENCE

Weber B, Kapoor W: Evaluation and outcomes of patients with palpitations, *Am J Med* 100:138, 1996.

SELECTED READINGS

Brook M, Moore P, Van Hare G: Circulation. In Rudolph A, Kamei R, editors: *Rudolph's fundamentals of pediatrics*, ed 2, Stamford, Conn, 1998, Appleton & Lange.

Brugada P: Investigation of palpitations, *Lancet* 341:1254, 1993.

Ellsworth A et al: *Mosby's 1998 medical drug reference*, St Louis, 1998, Mosby.

Healthcare Consultants of America, Inc.: *1998 physicians fee and coding guide*, Augusta, Ga, 1998, Healthcare Consultants of America, Inc.

Kern K, Fenster P: Palpitations. In Greene H, Johnson W, Lemcke D, editors: *Decision making in medicine*, ed 2, St Louis, 1998, Mosby.

Pancreatitis

ICD-9-CM

Acute Pancreatitis 577.0
Chronic Pancreatitis 577.1

OVERVIEW

Definition

Pancreatitis is an inflammation of the pancreas caused by a variety of mechanisms: alcohol abuse, cholelithiasis, trauma, or drugs.

Incidence

Unknown

Pathophysiology

Pancreatitis can be caused by many conditions. Regardless of cause, the end result is the same: liberation of pancreatic enzymes into the tissues of the pancreas. In the mildest form of pancreatitis, edema results, but no changes in the structure or function of the pancreas occur. In severe pancreatitis, repeated attacks occur, leading to loss of tissue and acinar units so patients develop pancreatic insufficiency with steatorrhea or diabetes. In the most severe form, tissue destruction occurs, leading to involvement of the blood vessels and hemorrhage pancreatitis. The mortality rate of hemorrhage pancreatitis ranges from 50% to 85%.

Precipitating Factors

Alcohol ingestion
Cholelithiasis
Medications
Pancreatic cancer
Abdominal trauma/surgery
Ulcer with pancreatic involvement
Viral infections
Metabolic hypercalcemia, hypertriglycemia

SUBJECTIVE DATA

History of Present Illness

Symptoms range from mild epigastric pain to sudden intense abdominal pain with shock and cyanosis. Patients will present with:

- Complaints of abdominal pain, usually worse with walking and lying down, better with sitting and leaning forward. The pain may radiate to the back
- Nausea and vomiting
- Epigastric pain

Ask about:

- Abdominal trauma
- Previous episodes of pancreatitis or gallbladder attacks in the past
- A heavy meal immediately preceding the attack
- Bowel movements (BMs), episodes of diarrhea, last BM

Past Medical History

Ask about:

- Episodes of gastritis
  - History of diabetes or glucose intolerance
  - Cholecystitis/cholelithiasis
  - Peptic ulcer disease
  - Hyperlipidemia

Medications

Ask about use of sulfonamides, thiazides, furosemide, tetracycline, valproic acid.

Family History

Ask about family history of:

- Alcohol abuse/dependence
- Pancreatitis

Psychosocial History

Ask about alcohol ingestion; use CAGE questionnaire (see Chapter 171).
Ask about tobacco use.

OBJECTIVE DATA

Physical Examination

The extent of the physical examination will depend on the acuteness of the patient's symptoms. The main focus of the examination will be the abdomen, but a more complete examination may be warranted, depending on the patient's complaints.

Vital signs: May see fever of 38.4° to 39° C, tachycardia, hypotension
General: Observe for jaundice
Lungs
Cardiovascular
Abdominal
Bowel sounds (may be absent), peristaltic waves, distention
Inspection: Look for Cullen's sign (discoloration around umbilicus) or Grey Turner's sign (flank discoloration)
Percussion
Palpation: Assess for tenderness, especially in the upper abdomen (usually without guarding, rigidity or rebound); masses; Murphy's sign; liver size and tenderness
Rectal: Check for abdominal tenderness, rectal tenderness, occult blood

Diagnostic Procedures

Diagnostic procedures are outlined in Table 138-1.

ASSESSMENT

Differential diagnoses are outlined in Table 138-2.

THERAPEUTIC PLAN

Pharmaceutical/Nonpharmaceutical

Depends on the extent of the pancreatitis and the presence of infection
The treatment of acute pancreatitis is supportive. Patients with the following signs should be admitted to the intensive care unit:
White blood count (WBC) >16,000
Serum glucose >200 mg/dl
Tachycardia >130
Low urine output
Decreasing serum calcium
Respiratory distress

General measures for acute pancreatitis
P = Pain control, meperidine
A = Arrest shock, intravenous fluids
N = Nasogastric tube for vomiting
C = Calcium monitoring
R = Renal evaluation
E = Ensure pulmonary function
A = Antibiotics
S = Surgery or special procedures in selected cases (Dambro, 1998, p. 768)

Chronic pancreatitis:
Pain control, alcohol abstinence
Pancreatic enzyme supplements for maldigestion
Diabetes mellitus: Insulin

Lifestyle/Activities

Alcohol cessation

Diet

Oral intake should be withheld since it stimulates release of pancreatic enzymes and therefore continued tissue damage during the acute phase. No fluid or food should be given until the patient is pain free and has bowel sounds.
A low-fat diet should be followed in chronic pancreatitis.
Small meals high in protein are recommended for chronic pancreatitis.

Patient Education

The importance of alcohol abstinence should be stressed.

Referral

A surgeon/internal medicine physician should be consulted in all cases of severe acute pancreatitis during the workup phase to make sure that, if the cause is surgically correctable, exploration is done quickly.

Follow-up

Dependent on symptoms
Follow-up of amylase level—if it remains elevated, should do ultrasound for pseudocyst.

EVALUATION

In most patients acute pancreatitis is a mild disease that resolves spontaneously in a few days.
The severity of pancreatitis can be determined by using Ranson's criteria. When three or more of the following are present, a more severe course can be predicted:
Age >55
WBC >16,000

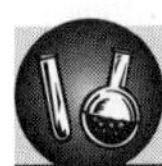

TABLE 138-1 Diagnostic Procedures: Pancreatitis

Diagnostic Test	Findings/Rationale	Cost ($)
Serum amylase	The most specific aid in the diagnosis of pancreatitis, often only transiently elevated, and may return to normal in 48-72 hours; as many as 20% of patients with pancreatitis have a normal or borderline amylase; elevations of 1000U/dl are almost always caused by pancreatitis or obstruction of the pancreatic duct; morphine can mildly elevate an amylase level	24-30
Lipase, ALT, AST, alk phosphatase	Lipase elevated in pancreatitis; ALT and AST elevated when associated with alcoholic hepatitis or choledocholithiasis, mild elevations of alkaline phosphatase	28-35/lipase; 18-24/alk; 29-41/LFT
CT/US	An enlarged pancreas on either a CT scan or ultrasound increases the likelihood that the pancreas is the cause of the acute abdominal pain; best in diagnosing late complications, especially pseudocysts or abscess	952-1120/CT; 351-419/US
Bilirubin	Mildly elevated bilirubin is seen with pancreatitis (about 20% of patients)	23-30
Glucose	May be increased in severe pancreatitis	16-20
Calcium	May be mildly decreased in pancreatitis; in severe pancreatitis, the calcium level may be very low, low enough to cause tetany; a decrease in serum calcium correlates well with the severity of the disease	18-23
CBC	↑ WBCs will be seen in acute pancreatitis	18-23
FOB	Check for GI or rectal bleeding	13-17

ALT, Alanine aminotransferase; *AST,* aspartate aminotransferase; *CBC,* complete blood count; *CT,* computed tomography; *FOB,* fecal occult blood; *GI,* gastrointestinal; *LFT,* liver function test; *US,* ultrasound; *WBC,* white blood count.

TABLE 138-2 Differential Diagnosis: Pancreatitis

Diagnosis	Supporting Data
Cholelithiasis	RUQ abdominal pain, jaundice, epigastric tenderness, + Murphy's sign; in chronic cholecystitis, pain may be present after meals, heartburn; US: gallstones
PUD/perforation	Severe abdominal pain, patient appears toxic, abdominal guarding and rigidity
Intestinal obstruction	Abdominal pain, distention and vomiting are hallmark symptoms. Obstipation (inability to pass gas or stool) may also be present. Bowel sounds may be absent, high pitched, or weak, depending on the location of the bowel obstruction.
IBS/IBD	LLQ abdominal pain, constipation, diarrhea
Chronic pancreatitis	90% caused by alcohol abuse, increased amylase; as the pancreatitis goes on, pancreatic function decreases. Fat malabsorption occurs, calcification may be seen on plain abdominal film in 20% of patients. Diabetes mellitus may also be present. Abdomen: CT shows characteristic changes: dilated ducts, pseudocysts, and enlargement of the pancreas
Carcinoma of the pancreas	Pain is the most common presenting symptom. Complains of dull ache in the epigastrium with radiation depending on the location of the tumor. Patient also complains of constipation and crampy lower abdominal pain. Initial diagnosis frequently is IBS. Jaundice may be seen only with tumor of head of pancreas. CT scan and endoscopy examination via ERCP will show tumor.

CT, Computed tomography; *ERCP,* endoscopic retrograde cholangiopancreatography; *IBD,* infectious bowel disease; *IBS,* irritable bowel syndrome; *LLQ,* left lower quadrant; *PUD,* peptic ulcer disease; *RUQ,* right upper quadrant; *US,* ultrasound.

Blood glucose >200 mg/dl
Base deficit >4 mEq/L
Aspartate aminotransferase >250 U/L
Lactate dehydrogenase >350 U/L

RESOURCES

Pancreatitis Partners, www.ddc.musc.edu/partners.htm

National Digestive Diseases Information Clearinghouse, Box NDDIC, Bethesda, MD; 301-468-6344.

REFERENCE

Dambro M: *Griffith's 5 minute clinical consult*, Baltimore, 1998, Williams & Wilkins.

SUGGESTED READINGS

Ellsworth A et al: *Mosby's 1998 medical drug reference*, St Louis, 1998, Mosby.

Friedman L: Liver, biliary tract and pancreas. In Tierney L, McPhee S, Papadakis M, editors: *Current medical diagnosis and treatment*, Stamford, Conn, 1998, Appleton & Lange.

Healthcare Consultants of America, Inc.: *1998 Physicians fee and coding guide*, Augusta, Ga, 1998, Healthcare Consultants of America, Inc.

Skaife P, Kingsnorth A: Acute pancreatitis: assessment and management, *Postgrad Med* 72:277, 1996.

139 Parkinson's Disease

ICD-9-CM

Paralysis Agitans (Parkinson's Disease) 332.0

OVERVIEW

Definition

Parkinson's disease (PD) is a chronic, progressive neurodegenerative disorder of movement and posture.

There are four categories:

- Idiopathic parkinsonism
  - Parkinson's disease (most common)
- Symptomatic parkinsonism
  - Drug-induced
  - Hypoxia
  - Infectious
  - Trauma
  - Tumor
  - Cerebrovascular accident
  - Metabolic
- Parkinson-plus syndromes
- Heredodegenerative diseases

Incidence

PD is the fourth most common neurodegenerative disease. It affects nearly 1% of the population **≥65 years of age.** PD usually appears between the ages of 50 and 75, and the incidence increases with age. The mean age of onset is 57 years, and by 70 years of age is six times that of the general population. Male 3: female 2.

Etiology

Unknown; current theories include environmental toxins, genetic predisposition, and infectious disease

Pathophysiology

There is a loss of cells in the substantia nigra of the basal ganglia of the brain that produce dopamine. (Dopamine is a neurotransmitter essential for control of voluntary movement.) There is a resultant increase in acetylcholine pathway activity. Dopamine concentration is decreased by 80% before symptoms of PD appear.

SUBJECTIVE DATA

History of Present Illness

The signs of PD are gradual and frequently overlooked by the patient, family, and health provider and/or attributed to the aging process. The most prominent indicators of PD are:

- Resting tremor: Initial complaint in 70% of patients; characteristically disappears with action, and reappears when posture is resumed; commonly seen in the lips, chin, and tongue; also tremor in the hand may increase with the purposeful activity of walking; the more recognizable sign is the "pill-rolling" action of the thumb and forefinger
- Bradykinesia: Abnormal slow movements are observed in a number of activities such as:
  - Difficulty initiating movement
  - Reduction in spontaneous facial expression
  - Decreased blinking
  - Slurred speech and lower-pitched, less audible voice
- Rigidity: Resistance to passive limb movement, producing the ratchet type motion called cogwheeling; stiffness also evident in the neck, wrists, shoulders, and trunk
- Postural instability: Decreased postural reflexes create a need for the patient with PD to stoop forward, which generates difficulty walking; to prevent falling, the patient will exhibit festination or an involuntary posture of hurried, short steps attempting to catch up to his or her center of gravity

Behavioral and personality changes such as fearfulness, anxiety, and passivity are frequently identified by the patient or the family. Mental impairment is not associated with PD but rather a slowing of thought processes, bradyphrenia, which is simply an inability to move quickly through mental sets.

Autonomic dysfunction presents with increased constipation, bladder dysfunction, impotence, and orthostatic hypotension.

Two forms of restlessness are observed with PD: akathisia, which is a general restlessness; and restless leg syndrome, which occurs generally at night and often interferes with sleep.

Micrographia: Small handwriting is a significant finding of PD. When writing a paragraph, the letters may initially be legible and of normal size, but will deteriorate as the writing continues.

Past Medical History

Medication history suggesting drug-induced symptoms:
- Reglan
- Neuroleptic type medication (Haldol)
- Antiemetics
- Antihypertensives

Occupational and environmental exposure history (e.g., carbon monoxide, manganese, or cyanide)

Onset and progression of symptoms

Family History

Family history of essential tremor

Psychosocial History

What is the patient's satisfaction with activities of daily living?

Has the daily living environment been assessed for safety?

Are there social networks of friends and family?

How have activities of recreation or employment been affected?

Diet History

Has there been any demonstration of dysphagia or difficulty swallowing?

OBJECTIVE DATA

Physical Examination

Vital signs focusing on orthostatic blood pressure

Observe posture and gait

Cranial nerves
- Sense of smell frequently decreased
- Blink reflex reduced
- Abnormal extraocular movement

Motor and extrapyramidal symptoms: Rigidity, hand and foot posturing

Sensory evaluation for peripheral neuropathies

Reflexes are difficult to examine but may be hyperactive

Diagnostic Procedures

Diagnostic procedures are outlined in Table 139-1.

ASSESSMENT

Differential diagnoses are outlined in Table 139-2 and Figures 139-1 and 139-2.

THERAPEUTIC PLAN

Pharmaceutical

Pharmaceutical treatment is outlined in Table 139-3.

Patients <60: Start solo therapy with selegiline as initial management.

Lifestyle/Activities

Exercise helps maintain and strengthen overall muscle tone and aids in reducing depression.

Home and work environment may need to be evaluated by the patient or family for safety and function.

Diet

Carbidopa/levodopa should be taken 30 to 60 minutes before meals to avoid reduced absorption of drug by the interference of dietary protein. If clinically significant drug response fluctuations occur, a reduced protein diet should be presented to the patient and family by a nutritionist, respecting cultural and religious dietary interests.

Advise the patient to avoid megadoses of vitamin B_6 (50 to 100 mg or ≥) which may reduce the activity of carbidopa and increase the side effects of levodopa. A daily vitamin containing lower doses of vitamin B_6 poses no risk.

Patient Education

PD is a progressive disease. This should be discussed with patient and family.

Educate the patient about the possibility of recurrent bronchitis and pneumonia secondary to dysphagia and silent aspirations.

Home safety must be stressed to avoid accidents contributing to hip fractures as the patient ages and/or becomes increasingly symptomatic.

Discuss with the patient symptoms of bradykinesia and the impact on social relationships.

Educate the patient about the symptoms of depression and the strong association to PD.

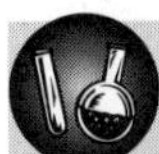

TABLE 139-1 Diagnostic Procedures: Parkinson's Disease

Diagnostic Test	Findings/Rationale	Cost ($)
CBC, UA, chemistry	Baseline laboratory data	18-23/CBC; 15-20/UA; 32-43/chem
Liver function tests	Done along with serum copper if Wilson's disease is suspected	29-41
Serum copper	Done if Wilson's disease is suspected	45-58
CT or MRI	Should be considered for patients with unilateral Parkinsonism, atypical symptoms, or poor drug treatment response; MRI can rule out mass lesions, infarctions, or normal pressure hydrocephalus; although it is expensive, MRI is the preferred test because it can demonstrate brain stem atrophy	990-1175/CT; 1781-2004/MRI
Schwab and England ADL Scale or Unified Parkinson Disease Rating Scale	May help establish the initial diagnosis	N/A
Low-dose trial of levodopa/carbidopa	Cost-conscious clinicians might recommend a low-dose levodopa to replace the missing dopamine and confirm diagnosis; levodopa is always given with carbidopa to limit peripheral side effects	N/A

ADL, Activities of daily living; *CBC,* complete blood count; *CT,* computed tomography; *MRI,* magnetic resonance imaging; *N/A,* not available; *UA,* urinalysis.

TABLE 139-2 Differential Diagnosis: Parkinson's Disease

Diagnoses	Supporting Data
Essential tremor	Is absent at rest Worsens with voluntary movement Frequently affects the head, rarely the legs Also may see a voice tremor
Drug-induced parkinsonism	Medication history includes: Reglan Tigan, Compazine Reserpine
Atypical parkinsonism	Unilateral presentation Atypical presentation Poor medication response
Wilson's disease	Hepatolenticular degeneration characterized by excessive deposits of copper in the liver and brain; neurological symptoms are related to basal ganglia dysfunction: rigidity or parkinsonian tremor; pathognomonic sign: Kayser-Fletcher ring (brownish ring around cornea)
Neurodegenerative diseases (e.g., progressive supranuclear palsy, striatonigral degeneration)	Often diagnosed initially as PD, but show little or no response over time and a rapid progression of the disease

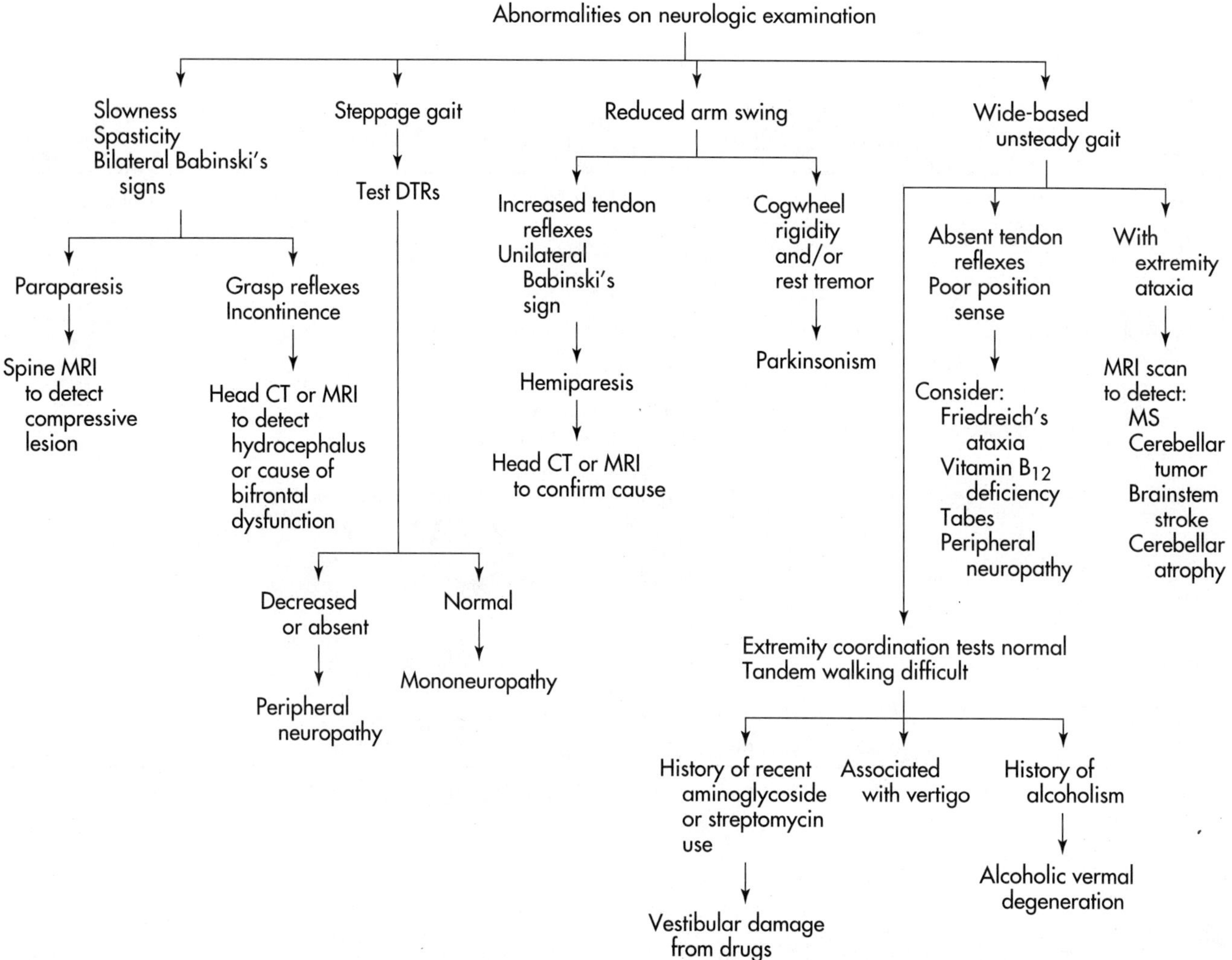

Figure 139-1 Algorithm for patient with gait disturbance (orthopedic disease excluded). *CT,* Computed tomography; *DTR,* deep tendon reflex; *MRI,* magnetic resonance imaging; *MS,* multiple sclerosis. (Adapted from Greene HL, Johnson WP, Lemcke D: *Decision making in medicine*, ed 2, St Louis, 1998, Mosby.)

Review medication use and potential side effects at each patient visit.

Family Impact

Educate the family about PD symptoms, medications and their side effects, and disease progression.

Families may find themselves in need of support groups offering respite from daily care. Identify appropriate community groups.

Referral/Consultation

Identify a neurologist to initially confirm the diagnosis and establish a treatment plan.

Seek specialist consultation every 6 to 12 months to ensure appropriateness of treatment plan and reassure patient of health care team commitment.

Physical, speech, and occupation therapy will be valuable.

Surgical interventions for PD are controversial. The pursuit of this type of symptom reduction should be presented by the neurologist.

EVALUATION/FOLLOW-UP

Follow-up is determined by the medical and psychosocial status of the patient and the medication needs and response throughout the course of the illness.

Discuss activities of daily living and patient satisfaction with level of function.

Compare the frequency and timing of PD symptoms with medication schedule. An increase in symptoms or unusual presentation may reflect reduced compliance, reduced drug effectiveness, or dietary interferences.

Stay alert to the symptoms of depression and the value of antidepressants and also to anxiety disorders.

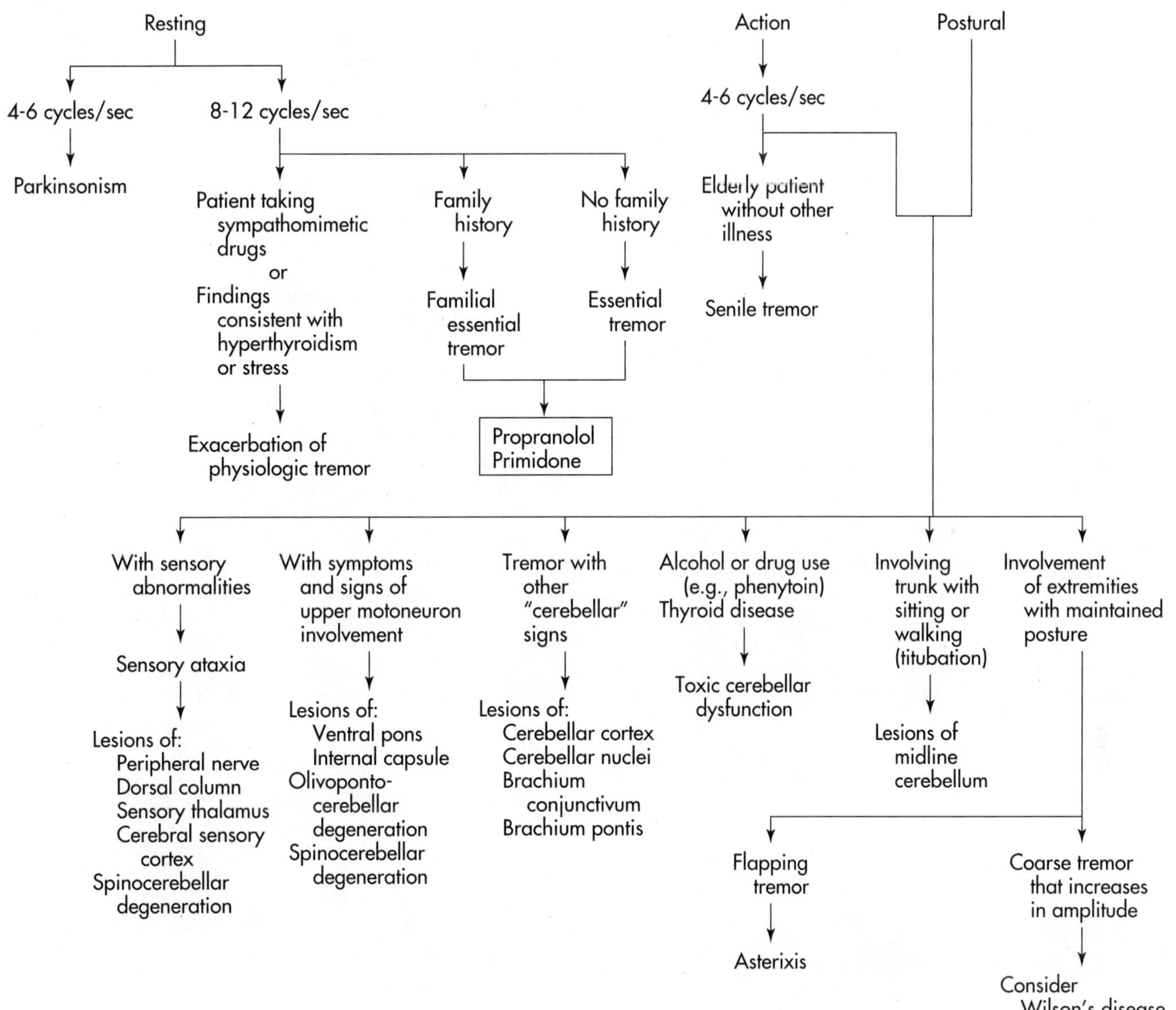

Figure 139-2 Algorithm for patient with tremor. (Adapted from Greene HL, Johnson WP, Lemcke D: *Decision making in medicine*, ed 2, St Louis, 1998, Mosby.)

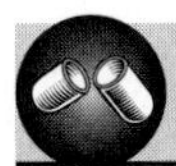

Table 139-3 Pharmaceutical Plan: Parkinson's Disease

Drug	Adult Dose	Comments	Cost
Amantadine (Symmetrel)	100 mg BID	Low rate of side effects; can be started at full dose without upward titration, but many patients have no response and/or drug loses effectiveness over a few months; caution in **elderly** Pregnancy: C SE: Lightheadedness, insomnia, nausea, dizziness, mottling of legs, dependent edema, confusion Excreted by kidney: Caution with impaired renal function	\$19-\$85/10 mg (100); \$40-\$72/syrup: 50 mg/ 5 ml (480 ml)
Anticholinergics			
Benztropine (Cogentin) Trihexyphenidyl (Artane)	0.5-2 mg TID 2-5 mg TID	Not tolerated well by **elderly** Use not encouraged by movement specialists Pregnancy: C SE: Dry mouth, constipation, blurred vision, urinary retention, ↑ heart rate, gastrointestinal disturbances	\$2-\$18/0.5 mg (100); \$3-\$25/1 mg (100); \$20-\$33/2 mg/5 ml (480 ml); \$5-\$22/2 mg (100)
Carbidopa (25 mg) plus levodopa (100 mg) = Sinemet Gold standard of treatment: Begin drug when disability interferes with life/ activities of daily living	CR: 1 tablet BID, not less than 6 hr apart or 25 mg/100 mg TID Also can give generic version: 1 tab TID or QID Give on empty stomach/take with 4 oz water or other nondairy liquid	Significant improvement in bradykinesia, rigidity, and some improvement in tremor; patients with mild PD often become symptom free; more disabled patients experience less dramatic improvements; after 5-8 years of drug, the majority of patients have drug response fluctuations and an on-off syndrome marked by rapid switches between mobility and immobility; slow-release forms provide a longer half-life and lower peak plasma level of levodopa, which may reduce drug-induced fluctuations Pregnancy: C SE: Dyskinesia, nausea, mental changes, fatigue, numbness, headache, weakness, orthostatic hypotension, dry mouth, dysphagia	\$29-\$66/10 mg/ 100 mg (10); \$62/SR: 25 mg/ 100 mg (100); \$129/50 mg/ 200 mg (100)

CR, Continuous release; *N/A,* not available; *SE,* side effects.

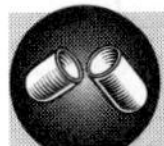

TABLE 139-3 Pharmaceutical Plan: Parkinson's Disease—cont'd

Drug	Adult Dose	Comments	Cost
Dopamine Agonists			
Pergolide (Permax)	0.05 mg QD × 1-2 days; gradually increase by 0.1 or 0.15 mg/day q third day; max. 5 mg	Adjunct therapy to Sinemet to ↓ symptoms; often prescribed early in diagnosis to postpone use of carbidopa/levodopa or in conjunction with carbidopa/levodopa to increase symptom relief Pregnancy: B SE: Hypotension, psychosis, hallucinations, paranoia, dyskinesia, somnolence, insomnia, nausea and vomiting, dizziness, fatigue, visual hallucinations	$15/0.05 mg (30); $106/0.25 mg (100)
Ropinirole (Requip)	2-4 mg BID	Pregnancy: D SE: Drowsiness, somnolence, euphoria, postural hypotension, bradycardia	N/A
Pramipexole (Mirapex)	0.125 mg, 0.25 mg, 1 mg, or 1.5 mg tablets	Pregnancy: D SE: Somnolence, nausea, hallucinations Can be used alone or in combination with levodopa Used to treat all stages of PD	N/A
Cabergoline (Dostinex)	0.25 mg twice/week; dose may be increased by 0.25 mg 2 ×/wk up to max of 1 mg twice/wk	Pregnancy: Unknown SE: Headache, dizziness, nausea, fatigue	$168/0.5 mg (8)
Bromocriptine (Parlodel)	1.25 mg BID with meals; increase q2-4 wks by 2.5 mg/day; max: 100 mg/day	Pregnancy: D SE: Headache, dizziness, nausea and vomiting, anorexia, orthostatic hypotension	$108-$158/ 2.5 mg (100)
Selegiline (Elderpryl)	5 mg at AM and noon	Monoamine oxidase B inhibitor; expensive drug. May provide neuroprotective affects and delay, temporarily, the use of levodopa. and slow progression of disease Pregnancy: C SE: Nausea and vomiting, hallucinations, confusion, dyskinesia, constipation **Never should take meperidine (Demerol)**	$130/5 mg (60)
Tolcapone (Tasmar) and Entacapone		Catechol-*o*-methyltransferase (COMT) inhibitors: When COMT activity is blocked, dopamine is retained in the brain for a longer period of time; results in reduced doses of levodopa needed	N/A

RESOURCES

American Parkinson's Disease Association, (800) 223-2732.
Parkinson's Disease Foundation, (800) 457-6676.
Parkinson's Referral Line, (888) 400-2732. (Developed by American Parkinson Disease Assoc. and SmithKline Beecham)
Internet resource: http://neuro-www.mgh.harvard.edu/forum

SUGGESTED READINGS

Aminoff MJ, Burns RS, Silverstein PM: Update on Parkinson's Disease, *Patient Care* May 30, 1997, pp 12-25.

Barker LR, Burton JR, Zieve PD: *Principles of ambulatory medicine,* ed 4, Baltimore, 1995, Williams and Wilkins.

Calne DB: Diagnosis and treatment of Parkinson's disease, *Hosp Pract* 30(1):83-89, 1995.

Calne S: Examining causes and care of idiopathic parkinsonism, *Nurs Times* 90(16):38-40, 1994.

Ellsworth A et al: *Mosby's 1998 medical drug reference*, St Louis, 1998, Mosby.

Healthcare Consultants of America, Inc: *1998 Physicians fee and coding guide*, Augusta, Ga, 1998, Healthcare Consultants of America, Inc.

Imke S: Parkinson's: a medical management update, *Adv Nurse Pract* 6(1):25-28, 1998.

Kieburtz K, Shoulson I, McDermott M: Safety and efficacy of pramipexole in early Parkinson disease, *JAMA* 278:125-130, 1997.

Montgomery E: Tremor. In Greene H, Johnson W, Lemcke D, editors: *Decision making in medicine,* ed 2, St Louis, 1998, Mosby.

Professional Development: Parkinson's disease, Part I, vol 92, no 1, Jan 3, 1996.

Sweeney PJ: Parkinson's disease: managing symptoms and preserving function, *Geriatrics* 50(9):24-31, 1995.

Tapper VJ: Pathophysiology, assessment, and treatment of Parkinson's disease, *Nurse Pract* 22(7):76-95, 1997.

Uphold CR, Graham MV: *Clinical guidelines in family practice,* Gainesville, Fla, 1994, Barmarrae Books.

Watts R: The role of dopamine agonists in early Parkinson's disease, *Neurology* 46(2):S34-S57, 1996.

Pelvic Inflammatory Disease

ICD-9-CM

Inflammatory Disease of Female Pelvic Organs and Tissue 614.9

OVERVIEW

Definition

Pelvic inflammatory disease (PID) is an acute, chronic, or subacute inflammation caused by infection of the upper genital track, including the uterus, fallopian tubes, or ovaries. It usually refers to salpingitis.

Incidence

One million cases occur in the United States annually (Chin, 1996). Of this number, **one third are under the age of 19 years** (Kottmann, 1995).

Pathophysiology

Protective Factors Against

Sexual abstinence
Use of barrier contraception, oral contraceptives, or progestin-only contraceptives

Factors That Increase Susceptibility

General debilitation
Vaginal or cervical infection
Intrauterine device (IUD) use
Invasive procedures (including abortion)
Substance abuse (Kendig, 1995)
Age younger than 25 years
Multiple sexual partners
History of PID
Menstruation
Douching
Smoking (MacKay, Soper, and Sweet, 1997)

Common Pathogens

Most often bacterial, although it can be fungal or parasitic
Ascending *Chlamydia trachomatis* (chlamydia) (20%) or *Neisseria gonorrhea* (gonorrhea) (10% to 16%). Less often it may be caused by *Mycoplasma hominis, Ureaplasma urealyticum, Bacteroides, Peptostreptococcus, Escherichia coli, Haemophilus influenza*, and *Streptococcus agalactiae* (CDC, 1993).

SUBJECTIVE DATA

History of Present Illness

Ask about an unusual vaginal discharge; if the patient has had a noticeable discharge, a vaginal infection may have ascended
Ask about number of sexual partners during lifetime and about recent new partner(s)
Ask about menstrual pattern and last normal menstrual period (symptoms usually begin during or immediately following menses)
Ask about bleeding or pain with intercourse or spotting between periods; often these PID symptoms are overlooked (MacKay, Soper, and Sweet, 1997)
Ask about contraceptive method (especially IUD)

Past Medical History

Ask about history of PID
Ask about history of sexually transmitted diseases (STDs)
Ask about history of invasive procedures
Allergies

Medications

Need for use of pain medication

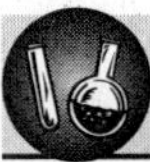

TABLE 140-1 Diagnostic Procedures: Pelvic Inflammatory Disease

Diagnostic Test	Findings/Rationale	Cost ($)
Vaginal discharge wet mount	Identification of increased number of WBCs and to rule out bacterial vaginosis	15-19
Gram stain of cervical discharge	Identification of organism	15-19
GC/chlamydia cultures (or gen probe)	Identification of most common causative organism	49-62
Urine human chorionic gonadotropin	r/o pregnancy	17-23
Complete blood count	Identify elevated WBCs indicating infection	18-23
C-reactive protein	May be elevated in PID	26-32
Erythrocyte sedimentation rate	May be elevated in PID	16-20
Ultrasound	Determine tubo-ovarian abscess if adnexal fullness detected	327-416

PID, Pelvic inflammatory disease; *WBC*, white blood cells.

Family History

No relationship has been established

Psychosocial History

Diet: Ask about history of nutritional deficiency
Substance use: Ask about frequency of use of recreational drugs or alcohol

Description of Most Common Symptoms

Often symptoms are subtle, or the woman may be asymptomatic.
Other symptoms may include increased vaginal discharge; anorexia; constant, dull, bilateral, lower abdominal pain; irregular bleeding; pain with intercourse; urinary urgency.
Severe PID symptoms include fever, nausea and vomiting, severe pelvic or abdominal pain, and significant vaginal bleeding.

Associated Symptoms

Symptoms of a urinary tract infection
Women with history of PID may develop chronic pelvic pain

OBJECTIVE DATA

Physical Examination

A problem-oriented physical should be conducted, with particular attention to:

- General appearance; slow or shuffled gait
- Vital signs
  - Fever >38.3° C (101° F); severe PID if >39° C (102.2° F)
- Abdominal
  - Tender with possible guarding; normal bowel sounds
- Pelvic
  - Cervical motion tenderness
  - Tenderness in uterus and adnexa on bimanual examination
  - Purulent discharge at cervical os
  - Adnexal fullness or mass
- Rectal
  - No masses, no fecal occult blood

Diagnostic Procedures

Diagnostic procedures are outlined in Table 140-1.

ASSESSMENT

Differential diagnoses include appendicitis, cholecystitis, perforated ulcer, pancreatitis, pregnancy (particularly ectopic), peritonitis, mild PID vs. severe PID (Table 140-2, Figure 140-1).

THERAPEUTIC PLAN

Pharmaceutical

Therapy must provide broad-spectrum coverage of likely organism. Coverage should include *N. gonorrhoeae, C. trachomatis*, anaerobes, gram-negative facultative bacteria, and streptococci.
Outpatient antibiotic therapy is appropriate for mild PID (temperature <38° C, white blood count <11,000, minimal evidence of peritonitis, active bowel sounds, able to tolerate oral nourishment.) Treatment regimens are based on CDC (1998) guidelines.
Partner treatment is necessary for success of plan (Table 140-3).

TABLE 140-2 Differential Diagnosis: PID

Diagnosis	Supporting Data
Appendicitis	Anorexia, periumbilical pain or right lower quadrant abdominal pain followed by nausea and vomiting; possibly rebound tenderness; involuntary guarding with examination
Cholecystitis	Steady, aching epigastric or right upper quadrant abdominal pain; nausea and vomiting; indigestion; flatulence
Gastroenteritis	Sharp pain and vomiting occurring simultaneously; diarrhea; anorexia
Cystitis	Pain or burning with urination; low abdominal pain; bladder tenderness; cramping
Peritonitis	Severe, constant, colicky epigastric pain; restlessness; vomiting; increased total serum amylase
Pregnancy (esp. ectopic)	Sudden, sharp pain in lower abdomen; adnexal mass; missed menses; possible vaginal bleeding; shoulder pain
Pelvic inflammatory disease	Abdominal tenderness; adnexal tenderness; cervical motion tenderness
Mild	Dull abdominal pain; pain with intercourse; urinary urgency; irregular bleeding; possible mucopurulent discharge from cervix; fever >38° C (100.4° F)
Severe	Nausea and vomiting; severe abdominal or pelvic pain; significant bleeding; fever >39° C (102.2° F)

Lifestyle/Activities

Use of condoms with sexual intercourse

Contact surveillance through health department: any partner who had sexual contact within the last 60 days should be treated because of the risk of reinfection and urethral gonococcal or chlamydial infection in sex partner

Partners should be treated empirically for both gonorrhea and chlamydia

Bed rest if possible until acute symptoms resolve

Diet

Healthy diet improves general health and increases chance of recovery from infection.

Patient Education

Partner treatment is necessary to prevent spread or recurrence; abstinence until both partners complete entire course of treatment is necessary.

Both partners need to take all of medication.

If left untreated, infertility or ectopic pregnancy may result secondary to scarring and obstruction of the genital tract, especially the fallopian tubes.

Family Impact

The discovery of an STD can be disruptive to a relationship. Offer to assist the woman in discussing the diagnosis and treatment regimen with her partner.

Referral

Moderate to severe PID requires aggressive therapy and probable hospitalization

Refer to/consult with MD any cases with the following:

- Moderate to severe adnexal and uterine pain
- Fever >39° C (102.2° F)
- Guarding
- Adolescent
- Any person where compliance with treatment is an issue
- Rebound tenderness
- Positive human chorionic gonadotropin (pregnant)
- Presence of IUD
- Failure of outpatient therapy
- Inability to rule out appendicitis or ectopic pregnancy
- Tubo-ovarian abscess on ultrasound
- Severe illness, nausea and vomiting or high fever
- Immunodeficient (human immunodeficiency virus, taking immunosuppressive therapy, or has another disease)

Consultation

Consider consulting with MD on any patient in whom you are unsure of the severity of the PID or in whom symptoms are vague, making diagnosis difficult.

Follow-up

Reevaluation of the patient's condition/progress should be done within 24 to 48 hours after treatment is begun. She should call or return if symptoms return or do not resolve.

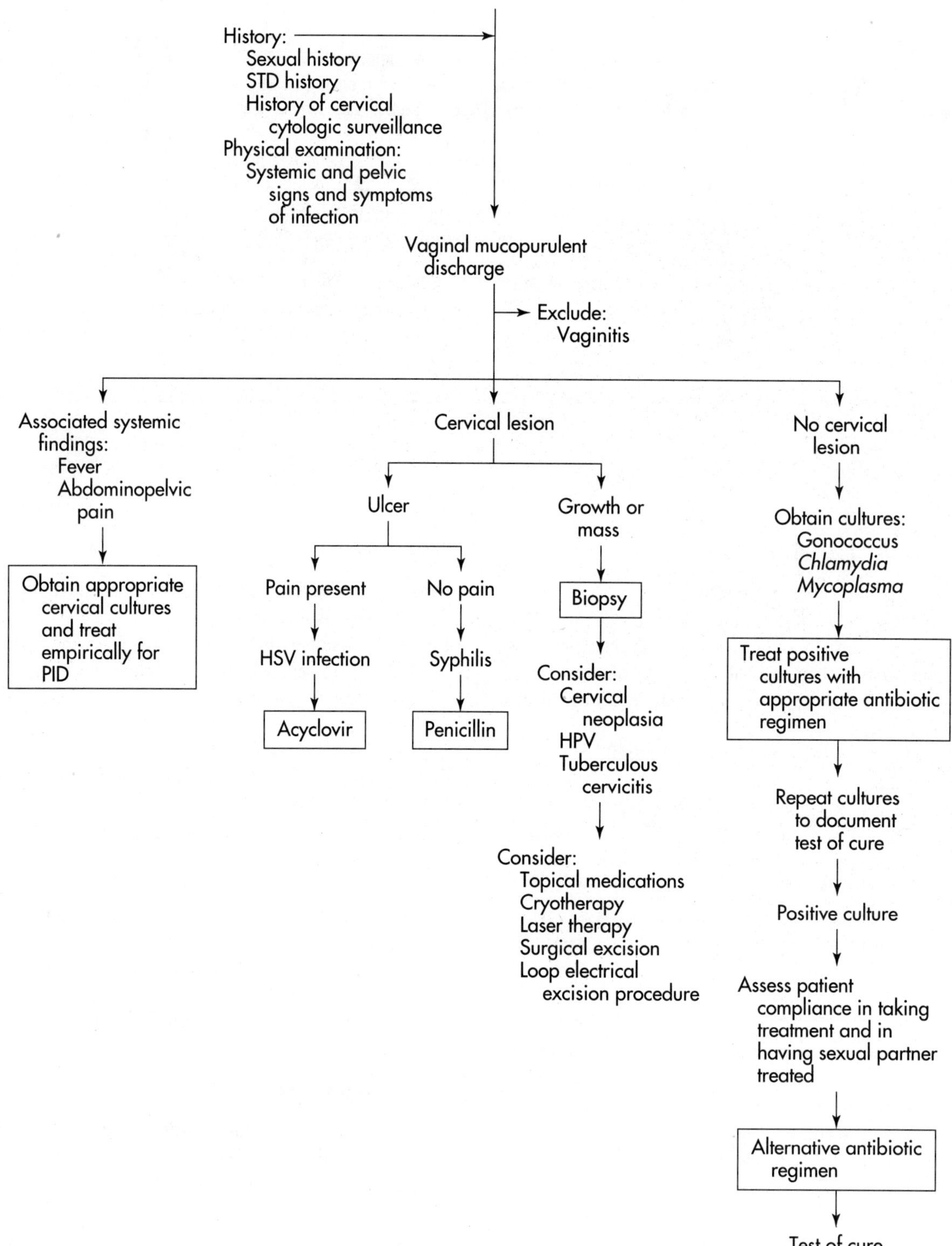

Figure 140-1 Algorithm for patient with cervicitis. *HPV,* Human papilloma virus; *HSV,* herpes simplex virus; *PID,* pelvic inflammatory disease; *STD,* sexually transmitted disease. (Adapted from Greene HL, Johnson WP, Lemcke D: *Decision making in medicine*, ed 2, St Louis, 1998, Mosby.)

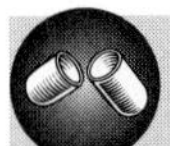

TABLE 140-3 Treatment Regimens for Outpatient Treatment of PID

Drug	Dose	Comment	Cost
Ofloxacin (Floxin) + metronidazole (Flagyl)	400 mg BID ×14 days 500 mg BID ×14 days	Ofloxacin covers gonorrhea and chlamydia; it does not provide anaerobe coverage which is why metronidazole is added Pregnancy: Oflox: C SE: Nausea, pseudomembranous colitis Interaction with antacids. Take on empty stomach Pregnancy: Met: B SE: Nausea and vomiting, metallic taste, dry mouth, Antabuse reaction	$384/oflox: 400 mg (100); $7-$238/met: 500 mg (100)
or			
Ceftriaxone (Rocephin) + doxycycline (Vibramycin)	250 mg IM ×1 dose + 100 mg BID ×14 days	The optimal choice of cephalosporin is unclear; cefoxitin has better anaerobic coverage, ceftriaxone has better coverage against gonorrhea and chlamydia; other third-generation cephalosporins would work (ceftizoxime or cefotaxime); no data available on oral cephalosporin for PID Pregnancy: Ceftriaxone: B SE: Rash, painful injection site Pregnancy: Doxy: D SE: Nausea, vomiting, diarrhea, photosensitivity, interactions with antacids, iron, carbamazepine; take with food Pregnancy: Probenecid: B SE: Anorexia, nausea, vomiting; drug interactions: check before Rx	$12/250 mg (vial); $6-$123/doxy: 100 mg (50)
or			
Cefoxitin sodium + probenecid (Benemid) + doxycycline	2 g IM 1 g PO single dose 100 mg BID ×14 days	As for ceftriaxone and doxycycline	$12-$35/prob: 500 mg (100)
or			
Trovafloxacin (Trovan)	200 mg QD ×10-14 days	Good activity against anaerobes (comparable to metronidazole); can also be given intravenously Pregnancy: Not recommended SE: Dizziness (take at bedtime or with food to decrease), nausea, vomiting, diarrhea, headache Interactions: Aluminum/magnesium, iron vitamin preparations, and sucralfate decrease absorption of Trovan	N/A
Azithromycin	2 g PO	Covers chlamydia and gonorrhea Pregnancy: B	N/A

N/A, Not available; *SE*, side effects.

Patient must return for a test of cure (TOC) 2 weeks after initial diagnosis and initiation of treatment. (Some experts recommend doing TOC in 4 to 6 weeks after therapy.)

EVALUATION

Successful outcome is resolution of symptoms and negative TOC.

At each annual visit, careful assessment of any signs or symptoms of a vaginitis or STD should be performed.

REFERENCES

Centers for Disease Control and Prevention: Guidelines for treatment of sexually transmitted diseases, *MMWR* 47(RR-1):1-118, 1998.

Chin V: Pelvic inflammatory disease. In Havens CS, Sullivan ND, Tilton P, editors: *Manual of outpatient gynecology*, Boston, 1996, Little, Brown.

Kendig S: Women at risk for infection: the woman who is chemically dependent, *JOGNN* 24(8):776-781, 1995.

Kottmann LM: Pelvic inflammatory disease: clinical overview, *JOGNN* 24(8):759-767, 1995.

MacKay T, Soper D, Sweet RL: PID: suspect more, treat more, hospitalize less, *Patient Care* 31(12)109-129, 1997.

SUGGESTED READINGS

Ellsworth A et al: *Mosby's 1998 medical drug reference*, St Louis, 1998, Mosby.

Healthcare Consultants of America, Inc: *1998 physicians fee and coding guide*, Augusta, Ga, 1998, Healthcare Consultants of America, Inc.

Pelvic Pain

ICD-9-CM

Pelvic Pain 625.9

OVERVIEW

Definitions

Acute pelvic pain is sudden onset of severe lower abdominal pain assessed to be gynecological in nature. Chronic pelvic pain is pain in any region of the pelvis that has lasted 6 months or longer, is unresponsive to treatment of symptoms, and is severe enough to affect a woman's daily functioning and relationships. *Pain is an illness itself.* Dysmenorrhea is painful menstruation; either primary, in which there is no detectable pathological condition of the pelvic region, or secondary, in which pelvic pathology is present (see Chapter 60).

Incidence

Chronic pelvic pain accounts for up to 10% of outpatient gynecological consultations, approximately 20% of laparoscopies, and 12% of hysterectomies in the United States. It is estimated that dysmenorrhea affects more than 50% of menstruating women; about 10% are incapacitated for 1 to 3 days each month. Dysmenorrhea is the greatest single cause of absenteeism from school and work among young women, with estimates of more than 140 million working hours lost annually. The clinician must first determine whether the pain is acute and life-threatening, subacute but progressive and serious, chronic, or self-limited.

ACUTE PELVIC PAIN

Pathophysiology

Acute pain may arise from a number of causes, including:

- Infections resulting in pelvic inflammatory disease (PID)
- Ovarian pathology (ovarian cysts, Mittelschmerz, adnexal torsion)
- Ruptured pelvic abscess
- Extrauterine pregnancy *(must be ruled out in all patients with acute pelvic pain)*
- Uterine perforation
- Uterine leiomyomata
- Bladder pathology
- Postsurgical pain
- Secondary to resolved pelvic pathology
- Urethral pathology
- Secondary to pregnancy, regardless of outcome
- Primary or secondary as a focal site of stress

SUBJECTIVE DATA

History of the Present Illness

Ask the patient:

- Duration of symptoms
- Onset of pain
- Remissions and exacerbations
- Describe pain: Sharp, dull, penetrating, aching?
- Location of pain: Does it stay in one place or is it throughout the abdomen?

When does the pain occur? Does it wake the patient up?
Does a particular thing trigger the pain (e.g., eating, urinating, defecating, sexual intercourse)?
Does anything relieve the pain?
Any weight gain or loss?
Diarrhea, blood in stools or urine?
Any increase in vaginal discharge, vaginal bleeding?
Elicit responses concerning the timing in relation to menses, changes in the character of menses (PID typically occurs within the first week of the menstrual cycle; endometriosis just before and during menses, and ovarian cyst problems generally occur midcycle)

Past Medical History

Ask the patient about:
Date of last menstrual period
Form of birth control (tubal ligation increases risk of ectopic pregnancy; intrauterine device [IUD] increases the risk of ectopic pregnancies and may increase the risk of PID)
Use of barrier methods of birth control
Sexual history: Exposure to sexually transmitted diseases (STDs)
Onset and frequency of sexual activity
Number and sex of partners; does partner have other partners? Does partner have signs of infection?
Pain with intercourse?

Medications

Oral contraceptives
Over-the-counter analgesics

Obstetrical History

Note the number of pregnancies, term births, abortions (spontaneous or induced), problems with any pregnancies, history of infertility, infertility treatments.

Surgical History

Pelvic surgery in the past 12 to 24 months
Any diagnostic pelvic workups, such as laparoscopy, endometrial biopsy, colonoscopy, endometrial biopsy

Psychosocial History

Unusual stressors at the time pain began?
History of sexual trauma?
Life changes, such as moving, new job, new relationship, end of relationship?
Trips to the emergency department for similar pain?

Diet History

Document high caffeine intake, foods high in lactose, spicy foods.

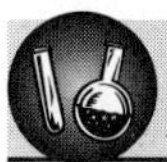

TABLE 141-1 Diagnostic Tests: Pelvic Pain

Test	Findings/Rationale	Cost ($)
Human chorionic gonadotropin	HCG is still detectable 9-35 days after a spontaneous abortion and 16-60 days after an induced abortion	28-35/qual 51-65/quan
CBC	Leukocytosis suggests an inflammatory response; normal WBC level occurs in 56% of patients with acute PID and 37% with acute appendicitis	18-23
ESR	Nonspecific sign of inflammation	16-20
U/A, urine culture	Pyuria indicates a UTI or an inflamed appendix in a posterior position, or contamination of urine by purulent vaginal discharge	15-20/U/A 31-39/culture
Cultures for gonorrhea, chlamydia	Rule out causative organisms for infection, PID	49-62/Chl 61-70/GC (probe)
Wet prep	Look for WBCs, clue cells, trichomonads, hyphae	15-18
Stool guaiac	Look for GI bleeding as source of pain	13-17
Ultrasound pelvis	Useful to distinguish uterine from extrauterine pregnancy, diagnosing appendicitis, luteal cysts, PID, spontaneous abortion; be sure to check blood flow to both ovaries to rule out torsion	347-416
Flat/upright abdominal x-ray evaluation	If concerned about a renal stone or free air under the diaphragm	142-169
Other specific x-ray evaluations	Radiological studies such as barium enema, IVP, CT scan as indicated by findings	Varies

CBC, Complete blood cell count; *CT*, computed tomography; *ESR*, erythrocyte sedimentation rate; *GI*, gastrointestinal; *HCG*, human chorionic gonadotropin; *IVP*, intravenous pyelography; *PID*, pelvic inflammatory disease; *U/A*, urinalysis; *WBC*, white blood cells.

Description of Most Common Symptoms

The patient may present with a sudden onset of symptoms, chills, fever, nausea, vomiting, diarrhea or constipation, increased vaginal discharge, acute cramping. The patient may relate either continuous or intermittent episodes of urinary frequency and urgency, menstrual pain, and missed menses.

OBJECTIVE DATA

Physical Examination

A complete physical examination should be performed, with special attention to:

- Vital signs
  - Blood pressure, pulse (tachycardia and hypotension may be signs of sepsis or dehydration), temperature (may be associated with PID or appendicitis), and respirations
- Abdominal examination
  - Bowel sounds normal, hyperactive, hypoactive, absent
  - Any bruits, generalized or localized tenderness, guarding, rebound tenderness, old scars from previous surgeries, distention
  - Use percussion to evaluate whether liver, spleen, and/or bladder is enlarged; any pain elicited with light touch; deep palpation, any organomegaly or masses
- Pelvic examination
  - Complete vaginal and vulvar examination, cervix (dilation, tissue at the os, lesions, cervical motion tenderness), discharge (mucopurulent, frothy, malodorous)
- Bimanual
  - Adnexal pain (unilateral or bilateral), masses (present in 70% to 98% of adnexal torsion), uterine size, and tenderness
  - Rectal examination: Pain or tenderness, masses, melena; fecal occult testing; flank tenderness, suprapubic tenderness
- Elicit psoas sign; perform obturator maneuver

Diagnostic Procedures

Diagnostic procedures for pelvic pain are outlined in Table 141-1.

ASSESSMENT

Differential Diagnosis

Differential diagnosis include:

- Pregnancy-related disorders: Ectopic pregnancy, abortion (spontaneous, septic, threatened, or complete), intrauterine pregnancy with bleeding of the corpus luteum
- Gynecological disorders: PID, endometriosis, ovarian cyst hemorrhage or rupture, adnexal torsion, Mittelschmerz, uterine leiomyomata degeneration or torsion, primary dysmenorrhea, tumor
- Nonreproductive tract disorders
  - Gastrointestinal (GI): Appendicitis, irritable bowel syndrome (IBS), mesenteric adenitis, diverticulitis
  - Urinary tract: Urinary tract infection, renal calculus

Table 141-2 outlines differential diagnoses for acute pelvic pain.

THERAPEUTIC PLAN (for nonpregnant patients with a negative pregnancy test)

Pharmaceutical

Antibiotics if indicated for PID (see Chapter 140), UTI (see Chapter 187)

Treatment for primary dysmenorrhea (see Chapter 60)

Patient Education

Teaching and comfort measures for mittelschmerz

Treatment and teaching for IBS (see Chapter 102)

Complications

Generalized sepsis, hemorrhage, perforation of bowel, rupture of abscess, ruptured ectopic pregnancy, shock, bowel obstruction, interference with activities of daily living with mittelschmerz, dysmenorrhea, IBS

Family Impact

It can be frightening to family members when a loved one is in pain. To a sexual partner it may be frustrating and frightening when sexual intercourse causes pain.

Referral

Refer the patient to MD:

- For suspected ectopic pregnancy (will need an ultrasound), appendicitis, ovarian pathology, abscess, complications of uterine leiomyomata, suspected pelvic adhesions, suspected bowel or other tumors
- For hospitalization if symptoms worsen or return after treatment or if there is no response to treatment

EVALUATION/FOLLOW-UP

For nonreferred patients:

- Reevaluate the patient's condition in 48 hours as warranted by clinical findings.

TABLE 141-2 Differential Diagnosis: Pelvic Pain

Diagnosis	Supporting Data
PID (see Chapter 140)	Acute PID is the leading diagnostic consideration in patients with acute pelvic pain unrelated to pregnancy. The pain, usually bilateral, but may be unilateral in 10% Diagnostic criteria for PID: All of the following must be present and no other causes for the illness is found Lower abdominal tenderness Adnexal tenderness and Cervical motion tenderness Additional criteria to support a diagnosis of PID include: Oral temperature >101° F Abnormal cervical or vaginal discharge Elevated ESR Elevated C-reactive protein Laboratory documentation of gonorrhea or chlamydia
Acute appendicitis (see Chapter 14)	Leukocytosis, periumbilical pain that migrates to the RLQ, slightly ↑ temperature, nausea, vomiting, anorexia, rebound tenderness
Adnexal torsion	Usually unilateral pain, but may be bilateral; pain is intense and progressive, with a tense, tender adnexal mass Often antecedent history of repetitive, transitory pain Pelvic U/S confirms the diagnosis
Ruptured or hemorrhagic cyst of the corpus luteum	Usually causes bilateral pain, but may be unilateral U/S aids in the diagnosis
Endometriosis (see Chapter 67)	Causes deep chronic or recurrent pain, but may occasionally cause acute pelvic pain Usually a history of infertility, dysmenorrhea, and deep dyspareunia; pelvic examination reveals fixed uterine displacement and tender uterosacral and cul-de-sac nodularity Definitive diagnosis requires laparoscopy

ESR, Erythrocyte sedimentation rate; *PID*, pelvic inflammatory disease; *RLQ*, right lower quadrant; *U/S*, ultrasonography.

Repeat bimanual and/or abdominal examination in 1 week and review status.

Seek an immediate clinical consultation if symptoms become worse.

Follow-up as appropriate for specific conditions such as PID and primary dysmenorrhea.

CHRONIC PELVIC PAIN

Incidence

Fifty percent of cases are enigmatic, 25% are secondary to endometriosis, and 25% are related to other pathological conditions, including subacute and chronic salpingitis.

SUBJECTIVE DATA

History of Present Illness

The patient may present with chronic pain with or without menstrual exacerbation, dysmenorrhea, dyspareunia, dyschezia, nausea, vomiting and/or diarrhea associated with the pain, or chronic constipation and chronic intermittent cramping.

Ask the patient about:
- Symptoms of chronic bowel disease, any previous diagnosis for such and results of treatments
- Symptoms of chronic urinary tract anomaly, kidney disease
- Location of pain, duration, exacerbation, and what precedes onset of pain
- Description of pain: Sharp, dull, aching cramping; intermittent or continuous?
- Pain: What relieves it?
- Weight gain or loss
- Symptoms that accompany pain

Past Medical History

Sexual history: Include history of STDs, how long with current partner, sexual responsiveness, dyspareunia: how often, how long, relieved by changes in positions, contraceptive history, including IUD

Gynecological history: Age at menarche, dysmenorrhea, characteristics of menses (flow, duration, regularity)

Surgical history

Medical history: Specific for urinary and GI complaints

Pelvic surgery: Laparoscopy, laparotomy, tubal ligation, hysterectomy, repair of cystocele, urethrocele, appendectomy, myomatectomy, cervical cone biopsy, loop electrosurgical excision of cervix
Pregnancy history: Ectopic pregnancies, infertility treatments

Medications

Oral contraceptives
Pain medication and how often
Antidepressants

Psychosocial History

Diet
Exercise
Life stressors
Major life changes
History of abuse, assault, and incest
Age over 30 and nulligravida

OBJECTIVE DATA

Physical Examination

A complete physical examination should be performed, with special attention to:

Vital signs: Blood pressure, pulse
Abdominal: Bowel sounds (hypoactive or hyperactive, sluggish, absent, bruits, sites of acute, dull pain elicited on superficial or deep palpation, any guarding, rebound tenderness, scars, distention, asymmetry, organomegaly, masses)
Pelvic: Observe external genitalia for edema, areas of trauma, cervix for lesions, discharge, unusual odor, color
Bimanual: Check cervix for cervical motion tenderness, uterus for tenderness, masses, shape, size, consistency, adnexal for shape, size, tenderness, masses, tender nodules through the posterior fornix and along the uterosacral ligaments during rectovaginal examination
Rectal: Pain, tenderness, masses, melena, rectovaginal masses, fistulas, adhesions
Elicit psoas sign; perform obturator maneuver

Diagnostic Procedures

See Table 141-1 for diagnosis of pelvic pain.

ASSESSMENT

Differential Diagnosis

Differential diagnoses include:

Consider possible causes listed under acute pelvic pain
GI pathology, including pancreatitis, bowel obstruction, ulcers, GERD, cholecystitis, cholelithiasis, biliary colic, diverticulitis, ileitis, carcinoma, irritable bowel syndrome, ulcerative colitis, hepatitis, urinary calculus
Endometriosis is diagnosed only by laparoscopy, not by clinical diagnosis alone
Psychogenic causes related to post-traumatic stress disorder, stress
Enigmatic pain
Pelvic congestion syndrome in women who do not have orgasmic relief (pelvic congestion syndrome following precipitous delivery often includes varicosities of the uterine ligaments)
Somatization disorders
Musculoskeletal origin

THERAPEUTIC PLAN (nonpregnant women with no other cause of pelvic pain)

Endometriosis

See Chapter 67.

Functional Ovarian Cysts

These fluid-filled cavities occur commonly in reproductive-age women, do not represent a pathological process, and usually disappear spontaneously. They have no clinical significance unless they cause significant pain, are large enough to rupture, or cause torsion (in which case surgical intervention is necessary). All *monophasic* oral contraceptive pills reduce the incidence of functional cysts; the most success has been reported with those containing 35 μg of estrogen. These should be considered in women who have a history of recurrent, clinically significant cyst formation (see Chapter 135).

Irritable Bowel Syndrome

IBS is a functional GI disorder attributed to intestinal origin, associated with symptoms of pain and altered defecation and/or symptoms of bloating and distention. Pain with IBS is often attributed to bowel hyperactivity. Management of IBS includes increased fiber in the diet, prescribing anticholinergics (e.g., Bentyl 10 to 20 mg QID), and lorazepam (Elavil) 25 to 50 mg QHS; may increase to 75 to 150 mg QHS if needed. Amitriptyline has some anesthetic qualities for the colon. Psychosocial management as indicated; dietary and exercise instruction as appropriate (see Chapter 102).

Lifestyle/Activity Modification for All Pelvic Pain

Lifestyle changes to reduce stress
Diet: Limit consumption of refined sugars (cookies, cakes, jelly, honey), salt intake to 3 g or less a day

Limit intake of alcohol and nicotine
Avoid caffeine (including chocolate, coffee, tea, soft drinks)
Increase intake of complex carbohydrates (fresh fruits, vegetables, whole grains, pasta, rice, potatoes)
Consume moderate amounts of protein and fats (decrease animal fats and increase vegetable oils)
Exercise three times a week for 30 to 40 minutes each time
Sexual intercourse/masturbation (orgasm releases oxytocin)

Referral

Refer the patient:

For laproscopic examination
For pelvic venography
For psychological support
As indicated by history and physical examination findings
For pain control

SUGGESTED READINGS

Apgar B: *Women's health care handbook,* St Louis, 1996, Mosby.
Ellsworth A et al: *Mosby's 1998 medical drug reference,* St Louis, 1998, Mosby.
Hawkins J, Roberto-Nichols D, Stanley-Haney JL: *Protocols for nurse practitioners in gynecological settings,* New York, 1995, Tiresias Press.
Healthcare Consultants of America, Inc: *1998 Physicians fee and coding guide,* Augusta, Ga, 1998, Healthcare Consultants of America, Inc.
Jamieson D, Steege J: The association of sexual abuse with pelvic pain complaints in a primary care population, *Am J Obstet Gynecol* 177:1408-1412, 1997.
Mishell D et al: Practice guidelines for OC selection, *Dial Contracept* 5:7-19, 1997.
Steege J: Office assessment of chronic pelvic pain, *Clin Obstet Gynecol* 40:554-563, 1997.
Vourakis C: Substance abuse concerns in the treatment of pain, *Nurs Clin North Am* 33:47-60, 1998.

Peptic Ulcer Disease

ICD-9-CM

Peptic Ulcer Disease 533. 9
Duodenal Ulcer 532.9
Gastric Ulcer 531.9

OVERVIEW

Definition

An ulcer, a sore, or lesion that forms in the lining of the stomach or duodenum where acid and pepsin are present.

A *duodenal ulcer* affects the proximal part of the small intestine. These ulcers follow a chronic course characterized by remissions and exacerbations.

A gastric ulcer affects the stomach mucosa.

Incidence

Approximately 20 million Americans develop at least one ulcer during their lifetime. Ulcers are rare in **teenagers** and even more uncommon in **children.** In **young children,** ulcers of the stomach and duodenum are typically secondary to systemic illnesses or drugs. In **older children** and **adolescents,** duodenal ulcers have a relapsing course that is increasingly thought to be related to co-existing, chronic, active antral gastritis and *Helicobacter pylori* infection. Duodenal ulcers usually occur for the first time between ages 30 and 50, more frequently in men than women. Approximately 80% of all ulcers are duodenal, and 20% are gastric. Approximately 5% of all gastric ulcers are malignant. Each year ulcers affect about 4 million people, more than 40,000 people have surgery because of persistent symptoms or problems from ulcers, and about 6,000 people die of ulcer-related complications.

Pathophysiology

Peptic ulcer disease (PUD) occurs when the mucosal barrier is impaired or overwhelmed by aggressive factors such as acid or pepsin. By definition, ulcers extend through the muscularis mucosae and are >5 mm. The role of stress in the development of PUD is uncertain. Three major causes of PUD are recognized: nonsteroidal antiinflammatory drugs (NSAIDs), chronic *H. pylori* infection, and acid hypersecretory states such as Zollinger-Ellison syndrome.

Protective Factors Against

Stomach's natural defenses
- Mucus production: Lubricant-like coating that shields stomach tissues
- Bicarbonate production: Neutralizes and breaks down digestive fluids
- Good blood supply: Increases cell renewal and repair

Factors That Increase Susceptibility

Bacterial virulence
Physiological stress: Surgical procedures, severe trauma, burns, shock
Medications: Corticosteroids, NSAIDs (increases risk of gastric ulcers 40-fold)
Gender/age: **Male age 30 to 50, female** >60 years of age
Familial predisposition
Physiological incompetence: Bile reflux from incompetent pyloric sphincter, delayed or abnormal gastric emptying
Children: See Box 142-1

Box 142-1

Factors That Increase Susceptibility to PUD in Children

Primary Factors That Increase Susceptibility

Association with bile acid and reflux
Association with *H. pylori*

Secondary Factors That Increase Susceptibility

Stress
- Major systemic illness
- Burns
- Head trauma

Excess acid
- G-cell hyperplasia (pseudo-Zollinger Ellison syndrome)
- Mastocytosis

Drugs
- NSAIDs
- Corticosteroids
- Corrosives

Gastroduodenal Crohn's disease
Cystic fibrosis
Sickle cell disease
Juvenile-onset diabetes mellitus

Common Pathogens

Helicobacter pylori

SUBJECTIVE DATA

History of Present Illness

Obtain a clear statement of the chief complaint.

Ask about the manifestation of pain; note the location, intensity, and whether or not the pain radiates or is relieved/aggravated by food.

Explore gastrointestinal (GI) symptoms of nausea, vomiting, change in bowel habits, dysphagia, weight loss/gain, change in appetite.

Ask about other symptoms such as history of testicular atrophy, gynecomastia, and alopecia (may be indicative of hepatic cirrhosis).

Blood type: Type O has been associated with the adherence of *H. pylori*.

Allergies

Elderly: Ask about excessive belching, bloating, flatulence, nausea/vomiting, diarrhea, rectal bleeding, number of bowel movements/day, dietary history.

Past Medical History

Ask about:
- Previous episodes of PUD
- Any other chronic illnesses, especially ones that might be treated with NSAIDs
- Rheumatoid arthritis

Medications

NSAIDs, especially aspirin and higher doses of other NSAIDs
- During first 3 months of NSAID therapy
- Increased age
- Concomitant steroid therapy

Family History

Ask about family history of polyps, GI cancers, alcohol consumption, smoking, and psychological disorders

Psychosocial History

Elderly: Consider losses/role changes in the past year; may need to ask about death of loved ones, retirement, changes in living situations

Diet History

Ask about the consumption of alcohol, caffeine, foods that increase or relieve the symptoms, and patterns of consumption and elimination

Ask the patient to record diet for 3 days—this will give a more accurate pattern

Description of Most Common Symptoms

Up to 20% may be asymptomatic (silent ulcers)

Duodenal Ulcer

Intermittent epigastric pain—gnawing/burning (present in 80% to 90% of patients), heartburn; pain often occurs between meals and in the early hours of the morning, may awaken nights; nausea and vomiting (N/V) (significant N/V is uncommon and suggests gastric outlet syndrome or gastric malignancy), loss of appetite; fatigue/weakness; tarry stools; dyspepsia

Gastric Ulcer

Pain often aggravated or triggered by food: weight loss common

Elderly: May be asymptomatic until disease has advanced (GI bleeding, pancreatitis)

Associated Symptoms

Chest pain, diarrhea

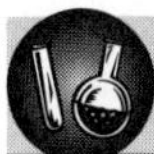

TABLE 142-1 Diagnostic Procedures: Peptic Ulcer Disease

Diagnostic Test	Findings/Rationale	Cost ($)
H. pylori	All patients with new or recurring ulcers should be tested for *H. pylori* if they are in a high risk category	72-91
Upper GI series	Will detect 90% of peptic ulcers	293-350
Hemoglobin/hematocrit	To check for anemia	11-14
Albumin/renal panel	Useful if signs of nutritional deficiency is present	18-23/alb; 28-39/renal
Endoscopy	Becoming the test of choice because it is more sensitive; ulcers can be diagnosed photographically and tissue taken for biopsy at time of procedure; indicate if clinical symptoms persist despite negative barium studies- rule out malignancy of gastric ulcers; locate bleeding site in those with diagnosed or suspected blood loss	870-1025 (including control of bleeding and biopsy)

GI, Gastrointestinal.

OBJECTIVE DATA

Physical Examination

A problem-oriented physical should be conducted, with particular attention to:

Vitals signs and weight, general appearance, hydration status, including turgor and orthostatic changes
Cardiovascular: Rule out cardiac insufficiency
Abdomen: Complete examination, especially note areas of tenderness, bruits, hums, or rubs; note size of organs, costovertebral angle tenderness; mild localized epigastric tenderness to deep palpation may be present
Genital/rectal: Examine external genitalia for atrophy, digital rectal examination

Diagnostic Procedures

Diagnostic procedures are outlined in Table 142-1.

ASSESSMENT

Differential diagnoses include those found in Table 142-2.

THERAPEUTIC PLAN

The goals of treatment are to relieve the pain, aid healing, prevent recurrence, and prevent complications.

Pharmaceutical

There are a variety of regimens used for eradication of *H. pylori*. There is not any one "right" regimen. Table 142-3 shows the most common regimens used today. TID regimens should be taken with meals, and QID regimens should be taken with meals and at HS. Table 142-4 shows side effects of the drugs.

Children

In children with primary ulcers, long-term maintenance therapy with an H_2 blocker is an option that might be considered to reduce the high rate of ulcer recurrence. However, consideration must also be given to cost and compliance with long-term acid suppression. Eradication of *H. pylori* if identified is appropriate for children.

Children with secondary ulcers are usually at low risk for recurrence once the underlying illness has been resolved.

Lifestyle/Activities

Smoking cessation
Discontinue the use of NSAIDs
Discontinue/decrease the consumption of alcohol and caffeine
Stress management

Diet

No specific diet; avoid irritating foods
Decrease caffeine

Patient Education

Disease process, expected outcomes and possible complications
Stress reduction
Stop smoking
Medications, especially NSAIDs

TABLE 142-2 Differential Diagnosis: Peptic Ulcer Disease

Diagnosis	Supporting Data
Peptic ulcer disease	Previous history of disease treated with antacids; antisecretory agents; epigastric pain relieved by eating or taking antacids; positive *H. pylori*
Gastric cancer	Early gastric cancer rarely gives rise to symptoms; the most common presenting symptoms are epigastric pain that mimics peptic ulcer pain (relieved by food and antacids), weight loss, and acute or chronic bleeding; anorexia, nausea, and vomiting may also occur
Angina	ECG normal resting; ST/T segment changes during stress; serial cardiac enzymes elevated; pain described as squeezing, heaviness, viselike, or crushing over the midsternum
Cholecystitis	RUQ pain with nausea and occasional vomiting after meals; may radiate to the back; dark urine, stool lighter in color; direct bilirubin, alkaline phosphatase elevated, SGOT LDH slightly elevated, US of gallbladder reveals stones
Pancreatitis	Abdominal pain, nausea, vomiting often precipitated by a large meal and/or alcohol; epigastric pain may become generalized or radiate to the back with some relief noted with flexion of the trunk; pancreatitis pain may localize to the RUQ

ECG, Electrocardiogram; *LDH,* lactate dehydrogenase; *RUQ,* right upper quadrant; *SGOT,* serum glutamic oxaloacetic transaminase; *US,* ultrasound.

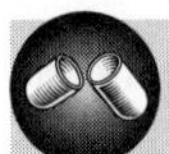

TABLE 142-3 Pharmaceutical Plan: Peptic Ulcer Disease

Drug	Dose	Comments	Efficacy	Cost
Bismuth (Pepto-Bismol) Metronidazole (Flagyl) Tetracycline Omeprazole (Prilosec)	2 tablets QID 250 mg TID/QID 500 mg TID 20 mg BID	Duration of regimen: 1-2 weeks; omeprazole should be continued up to 4 weeks	94%-98%	\$2-\$4/bismuth: 262 mg (30); \$3-\$131/met: 200 mg (100); \$6-\$19/tet: 500 mg (100); \$109/omep: 20 mg (30)
Bismuth Metronidazole Tetracycline (Helidac includes above medications) + H_2 blocker (dose depends on drug selected)	2 tablets QID 250 TID/QID 500 mg QID	Duration: 1-2 weeks; H_2 blocker may be continued for 4-6 weeks; not recommended for children; give with full glass of water; avoid alcohol during treatment; may antagonize OCP; photosensitivity	77%-82%	See individual drugs above Cost depends on drug selected
Bismuth Metronidazole Amoxicillin	2 tablets QID 250 TID 500 mg TID/QID	Duration: 1-2 weeks	1 wk: 75%-81% 2 wk: 80%-94%	\$17-\$49/amox, 500 mg (100), plus cost of bismuth and metronidazole
Bismuth Clarithromycin (Biaxin) Tetracycline	2 tablets QID 500 mg TID 500 mg QID	Duration: 1-2 weeks	>90%	\$185/clar, 500 mg (100), plus cost of bismuth and tetracycline
Bismuth Clarithromycin Amoxicillin	2 tablets QID 500 mg TID 500 mg QID	Duration: 1-2 weeks	>90%	See individual drugs above
Bismuth Clarithromycin Omeprazole	2 tablets QID 500 mg BID 20 mg BID	Duration: 8 days	80%	See individual drugs above

Adapted from Prescribers Letter: Efficacy of peptic ulcer treatment (Document No. 130804), *Prescribers Letter*, Stockton, Calif, 1998, Therapeutic Research Center.

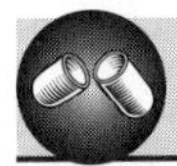

Table 142-3 Pharmaceutical Plan: Peptic Ulcer Disease—cont'd

Drug	Dose	Comments	Efficacy	Cost
Metronidazole Omeprazole Clarithromycin	500 mg BID 20 mg BID 500 mg BID	Duration: 1-2 weeks	87%-91%	See individual drugs
Amoxicillin Omeprazole Clarithromycin	1 g BID 20 mg BID 500 mg BID	Duration: 1-2 weeks	80%-95%	See individual drugs
Amoxicillin Omeprazole Metronidazole	1 g BID 20 mg BID 500 mg BID	Duration: 1-2 weeks	77%-86%	See individual drugs
Amoxicillin Omeprazole	500 mg TID 40 mg QD	Duration: 2 weeks	54%-79%	See individual drugs
Amoxicillin Clarithromycin	500 mg TID 500 mg TID	Duration: 2 weeks	>90%	See individual drugs
Amoxicillin Metronidazole	750 mg TID 500 mg TID	Duration: 2 weeks	>85%	See individual drugs
Clarithromycin Omeprazole	500 mg TID 40 mg QD	Duration: 2 weeks Decrease clarithromycin dose if creatinine clearance is <30 ml/min; not recommended for children	64%-83%	See individual drugs
Clarithromycin Ranitidine bismuth citrate (Tritec)	500 mg TID 400 mg BID	Duration: 2 weeks	74%-84%	Tritec: Not available
Clarithromycin Amoxicillin Lansoprazole (Prevacid)	500 mg BID 1 g BID 30 mg BID	Duration: 2 weeks; not recommended for children	86%-92%	$325/lanso plus cost of amoxicillin and clarithromycin: 30 mg (100)

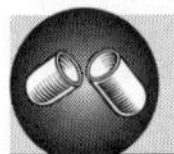

Table 142-4 Side Effects

Drugs	Pregnancy/Side Effect Profile
Bismuth	Pregnancy: Not recommended; do not give to children during varicella or influenza; not recommended for use with children <3 SE: Darkened tongue and stool
Metronidazole	Pregnancy: B SE: Seizures, peripheral neuropathy, GI upset, metallic taste, constipation, dysuria
Clarithromycin	Pregnancy: C SE: GI upset, abnormal taste, headache
Amoxicillin	Pregnancy: B SE: Diarrhea, headache, urticaria, superinfection
Tetracycline	Pregnancy: D SE: superinfection, photosensitivity, GI upset, enterocolitis, rash
Omeprazole	Pregnancy: C SE: Headache, diarrhea, dizziness, rash, constipation, cough
Lansoprazole	Pregnancy: B SE: Diarrhea, abdominal pain, nausea
Ranitidine bismuth citrate (Tritec)	Pregnancy: C SE: Taste disturbances, diarrhea, headache, nausea and vomiting
Bismuth, metronidazole tetracycline (Helidec)	Pregnancy: D SE: Nausea/diarrhea, abdominal pain, darkening of tongue, constipation, insomnia
Ranitidine	Pregnancy: B SE: Headache, GI upset, jaundice, rash, CNS disturbances, arthralgia, myalgia

CNS, Central nervous system; *GI,* gastrointestinal; *SE,* side effects.

Referral/Consultation

Persons who fail to respond to treatment
Significant weight loss
Symptoms of peritonitis (abdominal rigidity, rebound tenderness, fever)
Suspected gastric ulcers

Follow-up

Follow-up in 2 to 4 weeks of initial visit and 6 to 8 weeks thereafter until stable

EVALUATION

Consider rechecking *H. pylori* status if dyspepsia continues, since its presence may be a weak predictor of persistent infection.

REFERENCE

Prescribers Letter: Efficacy of peptic ulcer treatment (Document No. 130804), *Prescribers Letter*, Stockton, Calif, 1998, Therapeutic Research Center.

SUGGESTED READINGS

Ament ME: Peptic ulcer disease in children: diagnosis, treatment and the implication of *H. pylori* (guest editor). *Gastroenterol Clin North Am* 23(4):707-725, 1994.

Aronson B: Update on peptic ulcer drugs, *Am J Nurs* 98(1):41-46, 1998.

Cave DR, Hoffman JS: Management of *Helicobacter pylori* infection in ulcer disease, *Hosp Pract* 31(1):63-75, 1996.

Cerda JJ et al: Peptic ulcer disease: now you can cure, *Patient Care* 29(20):101-117, 1995.

Cornell S: New treatments for peptic ulcer disease, *Adv Nurs Pract* 5(3):57-59, 1997.

Cryer B, Feldman M: Treatment and prevention of NSAID-induced ulcers, *Fed Pract* Dec:22-37, 1995.

Damianos AJ, McGarrity TJ: Treatment strategies for *H. pylori* infection, *Am Family Physician* 57:2765-2774, 1997.

Dohil R, Israel D, Hassal E: Effective 2-week therapy for *Helicobacter pylori* disease in children, *Am J Gastroenterol* 92(2):244-247, 1997.

Ellsworth A et al: *Mosby's 1998 medical drug reference*, St Louis, 1998, Mosby.

Healthcare Consultants of America, Inc: *1998 physicians fee and coding guide*, Augusta, Ga, 1998, Healthcare Consultants of America, Inc.

Heslin JM: Peptic ulcer disease: making a case against the prime suspect, *Nurs 97* Jan:34-40, 1997.

Johnson DA: New dimensions in *Helicobacter pylori* infection, *Emerg Med* Feb:74-85, 1996.

Jones N, Sherman P: *Helicobacter pylori* infection in children, *Curr Opin Pediatr* 10(1):19-23, 1998.

Kato S et al: Omeprazole-based dual and triple regimens for *Helicobacter pylori* eradication in children, *Pediatrics* 100(1):E3, 1997.

Lewis JH: Peptic ulcer disease: update on management in the *H. pylori* era, *Consultant* Jan:91-94, 1995.

McColl K et al: Assessment of symptomatic response as predictor of *Helicobacter pylori* status following eradication therapy in patients with ulcer, *Gut* 42(5):618-622, 1998.

National Institutes of Health: *Stomach and duodenal ulcers* (NIH publication No 95-38), Bethesda, Md, 1995, National Digestive Diseases Information Clearing House.

Rowland M, Drumm B: Clinical significant of *Helicobacter* infection in children, *Br Med Bulletin* 54(1):95-103, 1998.

Peripheral Neuropathy

ICD-9-CM

Neuropathy, Neuropathic 355.9
Alcoholic Neuropathy 357.5
Peripheral Neuropathy 356.9
Peripheral Neuropathy Due to Diabetes 250.6
Charcot-Marie-Tooth 365.1

OVERVIEW

Definition

Peripheral neuropathy is the inability to perceive sensation, specifically in the extremities. Often the patient complains of tingling, burning or other abnormal sensations.

Incidence

Peripheral neuropathy is a common feature of many systemic diseases. There are numerous causes for neuropathy, although the most common causes in the developed countries are diabetes (58% of persons with diabetes have neuropathy) and alcoholism. An etiology is not determined in 13% to 22%, whereas in up to 42% a familial neuropathy is found. Alcoholic neuropathy is believed to be the second most common cause of neuropathy.

Pathophysiology

Large myelinated axons include motor axons and the sensory axons, which are responsible for vibration, proprioception, and light touch. The axons responsible for light touch, pain, and temperature are within small myelinated fibers. Small unmyelinated axons are also involved in sensory conduction and transmit pain and temperature. Both types of small fibers are affected by neuropathies and are called small fiber neuropathies.

Once injured, the nerve has limited ways to respond to injury. Damage can occur at the level of the axon, motor neuron, or dorsal root ganglion (frequently with incomplete recovery) or at the level of the myelin sheath.

SUBJECTIVE DATA

History of Present Illness

Describe the onset of the neuropathy; acute vs. gradual
Is there lack of sensation or motor movements or both?
Description of pain: Burning, lightning like, aching, feeling of tightness, or paresthesias
Hyperesthesia (e.g., sheets rubbing over feet)
Feelings of numbness or reduced sensation
Muscle wasting or weakness: Tripping, loss of grip strength
Muscle cramping or twitching
Difficulty climbing stairs, getting out of a chair, lifting, and swallowing, and dysarthria
Exposure to tick bite (Lyme disease)
Symptoms preceded by infective illness, inoculations, or surgery

Past Medical History

Systemic diseases associated with neuropathy: Diabetes, hypothyroidism, pernicious anemia

Medications

Many medications can cause a peripheral neuropathy, usually a distal symmetric axonal sensorimotor neuropathy. Box 143-1 identifies drugs that cause neuropathy and the location of nerve damage.
Ask about vitamin usage.

Family History

Presence of hammer toes, high arches, weak ankles, gait abnormalities, or muscular dystrophy (which might suggest long-standing or hereditary neuropathy) (Charcot-Marie-Tooth disease or porphyria [motor symptoms occur first, weakness is often marked proximally and in upper limbs])

Box 143-1

Drugs That Cause Neuropathy

Axonal Damage	Demyelinating
Vincristine	Amiodarone
Interferon	Chloroquine
Phenytoin	Suramin
Amitriptyline	Gold
Colchicine	
Pyridoxine	**Neuropathy**
Lithium	Thalidomide
Dapsone	Cisplatin
Cimetidine	Pyridoxine
Nitrous oxide	
Hydralazine	

Psychosocial History

Ask about:
- Human immunodeficiency virus risk factors
- Foreign travel (leprosy)
- Alcohol ingestion
- Smoking

Diet History

24-hour diet recall
Vitamin use (especially B_6)

OBJECTIVE DATA

Physical Examination

A complete physical examination is warranted due to the complexities of some diagnoses.

General: Overall appearance, evidence of chronic disease or weight loss, orthostatics
  Check for lymphadenopathy
Skin: Lesions, transverse lines in nail beds
Head/eyes/ears/nose/throat: Fundus (optic pallor: leukodystrophy or B_6 deficiency)
Lung: Peak expiratory flow rate and respiratory rate (Guillain-Barré)
Abdominal: Hepatomegaly or splenomegaly
Neurological: Cranial nerve examination: identify distal vs. proximal involvement
  Motor: Evaluate for fasciculations or cramps or loss of muscle bulk
  Tone: Normal or reduced
  Pattern of weakness: Symmetric vs. asymmetric
    Distal or proximal; upper vs. lower extremities
    Confined to a particular nerve or root level
  Sensation: Light touch, pain, vibration, temperature, position sense, two-point discrimination
  Romberg
  Deep tendon reflexes
Muscular: Look for trophic changes: loss of hair in affected areas or ulceration
  Look for loss of muscle bulk
Cardiovascular: Peripheral pulses and edema

Diagnostic Procedures

Diagnostic procedures are outlined in Table 143-1.

The workup for peripheral neuropathy can be very extensive, so a focused clinical evaluation can significantly narrow the differential diagnosis.

The most important question to ask: Does the patient actually have a peripheral neuropathy? Symptoms of generalized weakness may mimic peripheral neuropathy and should be ruled out before proceeding with extensive testing.

ASSESSMENT

Five keys to differential diagnosis are:
- Age at onset
- Rate of progression
- Motor vs. sensory vs. autonomic involvement
- Distal vs. proximal vs. global
- Associated neurologic or systemic diseases

See Tables 143-2 and 143-3 and Figure 143-1.

THERAPEUTIC PLAN

It is important to identify and treat peripheral neuropathies since they are frequently a symptom of a systemic illness, they can be slowed or cured, and they have a direct impact on the patient's quality of life. Rigid glucose control in diabetic patients will help decrease symptoms. Physical therapy to stretch and massage can be helpful in the relief of muscle cramping and leg aches. Electrical stimulation also has been found to be helpful with burning and tingling.

Surgical treatment includes the implantation of spinal electrodes and decompression of the posterior tibial nerves. Only patients with prolonged incapacitating pain should be considered for surgical treatment (Figure 143-2).

Pharmaceutical

Pharmaceutical treatment is outlined in Table 143-4.

Lifestyle/Activities

Caution should be used when wearing new shoes: Assess for improper fit.

Minor cuts and infections should be followed aggressively.

Avoid hot soaks.

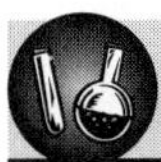

TABLE 143-1 Diagnostic Procedures: Peripheral Neuropathy

Diagnostic Test	Findings/Rationale	Cost ($)
FBG, HgbA1C	Rule out diabetes and control of glucose	16-20/FPG; 34-43/Hgb
Renal and liver panels, U/A	Screening baselines	32-42/comprehensive metabolic panel 15-20/U/A
Vitamin B_{12}	Done if patient presents with distal symmetric sensorimotor neuropathy	53-67
TSH	Rule out hypothyroidism	86-109/thyroid panel + TSH; 56-70/TSH
ESR, CBC	Check for inflammation	18-23/CBC 16-20/ESR
Nylon monofilament test (Semmes-Weinstein monofilament)	The test is abnormal when the patient cannot sense the touch of the monofilament when it is pressed against the foot with just enough pressure to bend the filament; indicates loss of protective threshold; see Chapter 55 for complete description of how to do test	N/A
Biothesiometer and Neurometer	Biothesiometer establishes vibration perception threshold; Neurometer monitors current perception threshold	N/A
EMG, nerve conduction studies	Most useful initial laboratory studies for peripheral neuropathy; can confirm presence of a neuropathy and provide information as to the type of fibers involved, pathophysiology (axonal vs. demyelination) and a symmetric vs. asymmetric or multifocal pattern	393-475
LP, CXR, ECG, FVC	Should be done if acute progressive neuropathy suspected; LP is useful in evaluating myelopathies and polyradiculopathies	172-208/LP 77-91/CXR 56-65/ECG 96-117/spirometry
Autonomic studies	Include determination of HR variation with standing/tilting, B/P variation to sustained hand grip and a measure of sympathetic skin response; these tests can provide objective evidence of autonomic insufficiency and a measure of small fiber function	134-167
CSF evaluation	Provides information related to myelopathies and polyradiculopathies; elevated protein with less than 5 WBCs is present in acquired inflammatory neuropathy (Guillain-Barré)	74-92
Nerve biopsy	Useful only in very specific cases to diagnose vasculitis, leprosy, amyloid neuropathy, and sarcoidosis	477-562
Doppler studies	Rule out vascular disease	257-300

B/P, blood pressure; *CBC,* complete blood count; *CSF,* cerebrospinal fluid; *CXR,* chest x-ray; *ECG,* electrocardiogram; *EMG,* electromyelogram; *ESR,* erythrocyte sedimentation rate; *FBG,* fasting blood glucose; *HR,* heart rate; *FVC,* forced vital capacity; *LP,* lumbar puncture; *N/A,* not available; *TSH,* thyroid-stimulating hormone; *U/A,* urinalysis; *WBC,* white blood cell.

TABLE 143-2 Differential Diagnosis: Peripheral Neuropathy Based on Symptom

Symptom/Presentation	Examination Findings	Diagnosis
Focal or mono neuropathies	Sensory loss in specific nerve distributions	Common compressive neuropathies: Carpal tunnel, ulnar neuropathy, peroneal neuropathy, or neoplastic infiltration or compression
Multifocal neuropathies	All nerves of the body are affected, with the longest axons being most vulnerable; axons degenerate most distal to proximal	Diabetes Vasculitis Sarcoidosis Leprosy Acquired immunodeficiency syndrome (AIDS)
Generalized motor weakness	Usually proximal in predominantly motor neuropathies	Motor neuron disease, disorders of neuromuscular junction, and myopathy
Distal symmetric sensorimotor polyneuropathies (DSSP)	Depressed deep tendon reflexes or diminished vibration sense in the legs may be initial symptoms in diabetes Alcoholism: Distal neuropathy accompanied by painful cramps, muscle tenderness, and painful paresthesias, > legs than arms AIDS: Variety of neuropathies; tendon reflexes lost at ankle, even when still present in knees and arms	Most common neuropathy seen; diabetes, hypothyroid, alcoholism (made worse by nutritional deficiencies), vitamin B_{12} deficiency, thiamine deficiency, connective tissue diseases, amyloidosis, AIDS, Lyme disease, toxic neuropathies (hexacarbons, ethylene oxide, carbon monoxide, glue sniffing, gold, mercury, thallium)
Proximal sensory neuropathies	May see cranial nerve abnormalities	Relatively rare, porphyria
Predominantly motor neuropathies	Distal: Weakness, tripping on toes, loss of grip strength, muscle cramps, restless legs Proximal: Difficulty in climbing stairs, getting out of a chair, lifting, swallowing	Usually proximal and includes acquired inflammatory neuropathies such as Guillain-Barré, diabetes, arsenic poisoning, lymphoma, diphtheria, hypothyroidism
Cranial nerve involvement	Lyme: Meningitis, cranial neuropathy	Diabetes, Guillain-Barré, human immunodeficiency virus, Lyme, diphtheria
Neuropathies involving upper limbs	G-B: sometimes follows infective illness; weakness begins in legs, spreading to a variable degree but usually involving the arms and one or both sides of the face; the muscles of respiration may be affected	Guillain-Barré, diabetes, porphyria, vitamin B_{12} deficiency, lead neuropathy
Small fiber neuropathies	Burning pain, lancinating pain, aching or uncomfortable paresthesia	Leprosy, diabetes, alcoholic neuropathy, amyloidosis, AIDS, hereditary

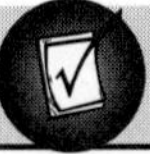

TABLE 143-3 Differential Diagnosis Based on Onset

Onset	Diagnoses/Conditions to Consider
Neuropathies with abrupt/rapid onset	Ischemic neuropathies, polyarteritis nodosa, rheumatoid arthritis, diabetes, nerve compression, penetrating wounds, thermal injury, Guillain-Barré syndrome, toxins, tick paralysis, porphyria
Subacute onset	Many toxins, drugs, nutritional neuropathies, uremic neuropathy, vasculitis, amyloid, malignancy, infection
Chronic onset	Diabetic neuropathy, chronic inflammatory neuropathies, lead toxicity, dysproteinemia, myeloma

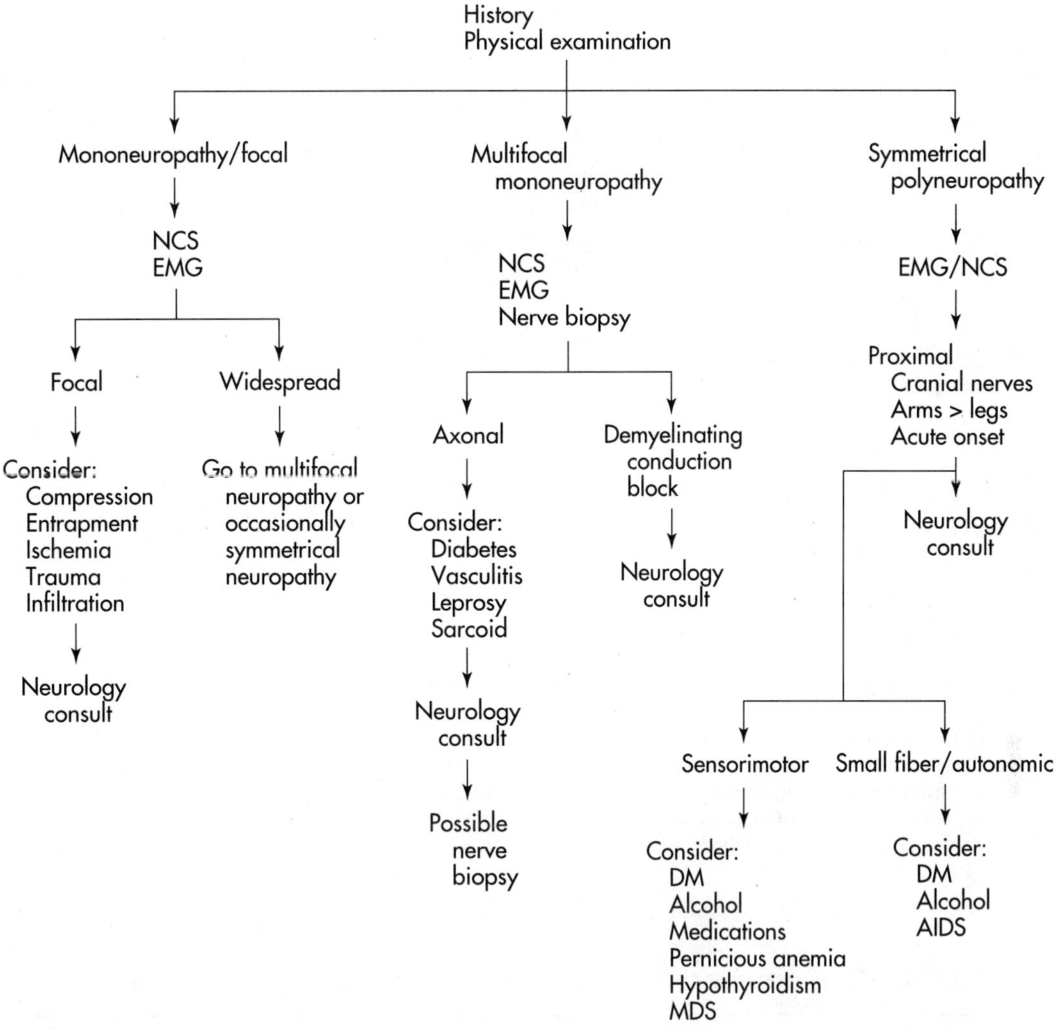

Figure 143-1 Algorithm for patient with peripheral neuropathy. *AIDS,* Acquired immunodeficiency syndrome; *DM,* diabetes mellitus; *EMG,* electromyelogram; *NCS,* nerve conduction studies. (Modified from Tolander L: Peripheral neuropathy. In Greene H, Johnson W, Lemcke D, editors: *Decision making in medicine*, ed 2, St. Louis, 1998, Mosby; and Poncelet A: An algorithm for the evaluation of peripheral neuropathy, *Am Family Physician* 57[4]:755-764, 1998.)

Avoid heating pads.

Avoid use of H_2O_2, iodine, povidone iodine (Betadine), and astringents such as witch hazel.

Clean minor cuts with soap, and apply topical antibiotic.

Diet

Encourage a well-balanced diet to counteract any nutritional deficiencies.

Patient Education

Daily foot inspection

Gentle washing with soap and water followed by application of moisturizers (helps to maintain healthy skin that can better resist breakdown and infection)

Reinforce that, even with adequate preventive care, many patients develop ulcers. Since neuropathy is present, the ulcers will be painless.

Family Impact

The risk of lower extremity amputation is a real concern when the patient has decreased sensation. For diabetic patients, amputation occurs up to 45 times more frequently than patients who do not have diabetes.

Referral

See Figure 143-1 for suggested referral strategies.

Refer to neurologist any patient with motor neuropathies that are progressing

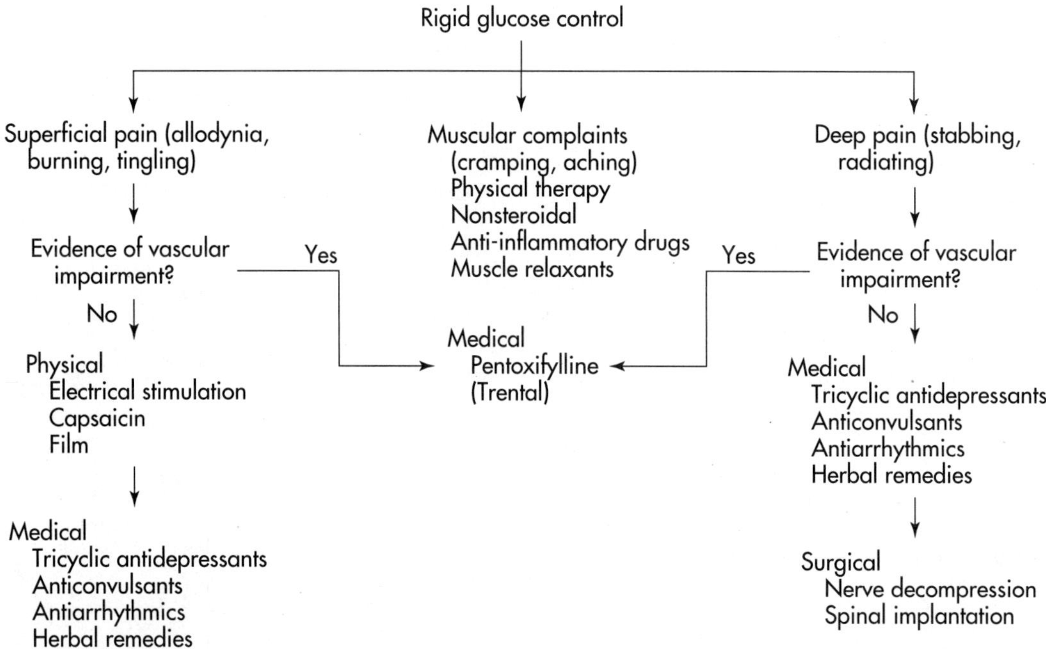

Figure 143-2 Management of painful diabetic neuropathy. This treatment algorithm builds on a foundation of optimum glucose management and focuses on the nature and location of pain. Superficial pain should be addressed with physical modalities. If physical modalities are ineffective, oral medication may be prescribed. Muscular complaints usually respond to physical therapy and muscle relaxants. Pain arising from vascular compromise may respond to pentoxifylline. Deep complaints in patients without significant vascular compromise can be addressed through medical or surgical means. (From Page J, Chen R: Management of painful diabetic neuropathy, *J Am Podiatr Med Assoc* 87[8]:370-379, 1997.)

TABLE 143-4 Pharmaceutical Treatment: Peripheral Neuropathy

Drug	Dose	Comments	Cost
Analgesics			
Ibuprofen Sulindac	600 mg QID 200 mg BID	Use NSAIDs with caution in diabetes mellitus due to risk of nephrotoxicity; short-term therapy only Pregnancy: B (D if used near term) SE: GI upset, GI bleeding, tinnitus	$3-$9/ibupro: 200 mg (100); $4-$80/600 mg (100)
Tricyclic Antidepressants			
Amitriptyline (Elavil)	10-25 mg HS, may increase to 150 mg/day; (chronic pain dose usually at lower end of range)	Decrease ability to reuptake norepinephrine and serotonin Pregnancy: D SE: Anticholinergic responses: dry mouth, tiredness, headache, constipation, urinary retention, insomnia, palpitations, increased sweating; desipramine has fewer anticholinergic effects due to more selective action	$3-$69/50 mg (100); $4-$91/100 mg (100)

CBC, Complete blood count; *GI*, gastrointestinal; *LFT*, liver function test; *NSAID*, nonsteroidal antiinflammatory drug; *SE*, side effects.

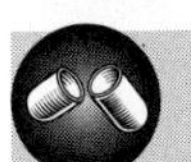

Table 143-4 Pharmaceutical Treatment: Peripheral Neuropathy—cont'd

Drug	Dose	Comments	Cost
Nortriptyline (Pamelor)	25 mg HS, increase in 3- to 5-day increments to 75-150 mg/day	Pregnancy: C SE: See amitriptyline	\$17-\$99/25 mg (100); \$21-\$178/50 mg (100)
Imipramine (Tofranil)	75-100 mg HS	Pregnancy: C SE: See amitriptyline	\$2-\$26/25 mg (100); \$3-\$74/50 mg (100)
Desipramine (Norpramin)	25 mg QD, increase by 25 mg/day q3-5 days to 100-200 mg/day (geriatric >150 mg not recommended)	Pregnancy: C SE: See amitriptyline	\$10-\$59/25 mg (100); \$15-\$112/50 mg (100)
Trazodone (Desyrel)	50 mg TID; max 400 mg/day	Pregnancy: C SE: See amitriptyline	\$5-\$139/50 mg (100); \$12-\$243/100 mg (100)
Anticonvulsants			
Gabapentin (Neurontin)	300 mg on day 1, 300 mg BID on day 2 and 300 mg TID on day 3	Pregnancy: C SE: Somnolence, dizziness, ataxia, fatigue, nystagmus, tremor, impotence Monitor CBC, LFTs	\$90/300 mg (100)
Carbamazepine (Tegretol)	100 mg BID; may increase 100 mg q12h until pain subsides; max 1.2 g/day; maintenance 200-400 mg BID	Second-line therapy Pregnancy: C SE: Ataxia, drowsiness, nausea, constipation, diarrhea, thrombocytopenia, agranulocytosis, aplastic anemia	\$16-\$21/100 mg (100); \$10-\$39/200 mg (100)
Local Anesthetics			
Mexiletine (Mexitil)	200 mg q8h; max 1200 mg/day	Pregnancy: C SE: Tremor, lightheadedness, coordination difficulties, dizziness, gastrointestinal upset, heartburn	\$82-\$98/200 mg (200); \$95-\$112/250 mg (100)
Hemorheologic Agents			
Pentoxifylline (Trental)	400 mg TID with meals (can ↓ to 400 mg BID if SE occur)	Used for intermittent claudication; found to improve arterial supply in diabetes mellitus patients Pregnancy: C SE: Dizziness, headache, tremor, anxiety, confusion, GI upset	\$56/400 mg (100)
Topical Counter-Irritants			
Capsaicin 0.75% (Zostrix)	Cream applied to painful areas QID; use only what can be rubbed into area	Reduce conduction in type C fibers, making them less sensitive to stimuli; do not inhale or breathe drug; wash hands after application Pregnancy: N/A SE: Burning, stinging or warm sensation at site, coughing, sneezing	N/A
Potential Future Agents			
Iloprost Tolrestat	N/A	Iloprost: A stable prostacyclin analog Tolrestat: Aldose reductase inhibitor (currently in trials for diabetic retinopathy)	N/A
Herbal Remedies			
Evening primrose	Contains active ingredient of gamma–linolenic acid. Possibly helpful since persons with diabetes have impaired metabolism of linoleic acid to linolenic acid.		
Borage oil			

TABLE 143-5 Follow-up for Peripheral Neuropathy

Degree of Foot Problem	Symptom	Treatment
No pathology	Normal monofilament test; no evidence of peripheral arterial occlusive disease; no history of ulcer	Daily foot examination Foot examination by provider 2-3×/yr
Neuropathy	Abnormal monofilament	As for No pathology plus protective footwear
Neuropathy with deformity	Abnormal monofilament	As for No pathology plus referral for custom shoe or surgery to correct deformity
History of ulcer	No evidence of vascular disease	As for No pathology plus more frequent visits to evaluate feet
Ulcer	No evidence of vascular disease, no infection	Debridement of ulcer/dressings referral
Charcot's joint	Confirmed by x-ray	Increased monitoring, referral
Infected ulcer	No evidence of vascular disease	Referral
Evidence of vascular disease	Abnormal vascular studies	Referral

Modified from Armstrong D, Lavery L: Diabetic foot ulcers: prevention, diagnosis and classification, *Am Family Physician* 57(6):1330, 1998.

Consultation

Any neuropathies that do not clearly indicate a diagnosis should be discussed with collaborating physician.

Follow-up

Follow-up is determined by the degree of pathology. Although the classification system was developed for use with diabetic foot pathology, it seems appropriate for patients with peripheral neuropathy (Table 143-5).

EVALUATION

Any foot ulcer needs aggressive follow-up. Debridement is needed to remove necrotic tissue and surrounding callus. Referral to a foot specialist is suggested to determine involvement of underlying structures such as tendon, joint capsule, or bone.

SUGGESTED READINGS

Armstrong D, Lavery L: Diabetic foot ulcers: prevention, diagnosis and classification, *Am Family Physician* 57(6):1325-1334. 1998.

Ellsworth A et al: *Mosby's 1998 medical drug reference*, St Louis, 1998, Mosby.

Emanuele N, Emanuele M: Diabetic neuropathy: therapies for peripheral and autonomic symptoms, *Geriatrics* 52(4):40-49, 1997.

Healthcare Consultants of America, Inc: *1998 physicians fee and coding guide*, Augusta, Ga, 1998, Healthcare Consultants of America, Inc.

Page J, Chen R: Management of painful diabetic neuropathy, *J Am Podiatr Med Assoc* 87(8):370-379, 1997.

Poncelet A: An algorithm for the evaluation of peripheral neuropathy, *Am Family Physician* 57(4):755-764, 1998.

Tolander L: Peripheral neuropathy. In Greene H, Johnson W, Lemcke D, editors: *Decision making in medicine,* ed 2, St Louis, 1998, Mosby.

Pertussis

Whooping Cough, Bordetella *pertussis*

ICD-9-CM

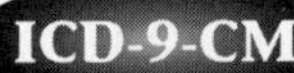

Whooping Cough 033.9
Vaccination Against V03.6

OVERVIEW

Definition

Pertussis is an acute bacterial disease involving the respiratory tract. Whooping cough syndrome may also be caused by *Bordetella parapertussis, Mycoplasma pneumoniae, Chlamydia trachomatis, C. pneumonia, B. bronchiseptica,* and certain adenoviruses.

Incidence

Humans are the only known hosts. Incubation period is 6 to 20 days. It is communicable for 3 weeks after the onset of paroxysmal stage in untreated patients and for 5 days after the onset of treatment.

Affects females more than males. **Infants 1 to 2 months old** are highly susceptible. Highest rates in **children <5 years of age.** Adults may be an important reservoir of infection in children. Adults may not have a typical presentation.

Outbreaks occur periodically. There has been a marked decline in incidence and mortality rates over the past 40 years in communities with active immunization programs. Incidence rates have increased in communities where immunization rates have fallen, but immunizing against pertussis or having the disease does not convey lifelong immunity.

Pathophysiology

Spread by respiratory secretions. Most severe in first year of life. Prolonged immunity after first attack. Second attack rarely occurs.

Protective Factors Against

DTaP (acellular preparations) immunizations at 2, 4, and 6 months of age. Boosters at 12 to 15 months and at school entry. No immunization after 7 years of age since the disease is relatively mild in older persons.

SUBJECTIVE DATA

History of Present Illness

Mild upper respiratory symptoms that progress to severe paroxysms of cough. Fever is absent or minimal. Symptoms wane gradually with 6 to 10 weeks' duration.

Past Medical History

Immunization history, previous infection, recent exposure

Medications

Current medications

Family History

Illness among family members

Psychosocial History

School/day care exposures

Description of Most Common Symptoms

The symptoms last about 6 weeks and are divided into three stages:

Catarrhal stage: Insidious onset, lacrimation, sneezing, coryza, anorexia, malaise, and hacking night cough

Paroxysmal stage: Often with a characteristic respiratory whoop, followed by vomiting; in infants <6 months, symptoms may be atypical; apnea is a common man-

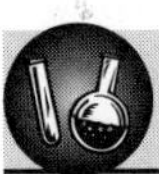

Table 144-1 Diagnostic Procedures: Pertussis

Diagnostic Test	Findings/Rationale	Cost ($)
Nasopharyngeal culture	To try to confirm organism; negative cultures are common, especially late in the course of the disease; a special medium (Bordet-Gengou agar) must be requested	31-39
Complete blood count	White blood count is usually 15,000-20,000, 60%-80% are lymphocytes	27-34

Table 144-2 Differential Diagnosis: Pertussis

Diagnoses	Supporting Data
Bacterial tracheitis	Respiratory stridor, high fever, copious purulent secretions; follows streptococcal, staphylococcal or *Haemophilus influenzae* type B infection
Congenital subglottic stenosis	Presents as prolonged or recurrent episodes of croup
Croup	Child wakens at night with barking cough, hoarseness, inspiratory stridor, and possible respiratory distress; usually afebrile; episodes are mild to moderate and resolve quickly when exposed to humidity

ifestation, and the whoop is often absent; a cough lasting >2 weeks in an adult is suggestive of pertussis

Convalescent stage: Begins 4 weeks after onset with a decrease in frequency and severity of cough

Associated Symptoms

Pneumonia, seizures, and encephalopathy

OBJECTIVE DATA

Physical Examination

Observe respirations, nasal congestion, auscultate chest

Diagnostic Procedures

Diagnostic procedures are outlined in Table 144-1.

ASSESSMENT

Differential diagnoses include: Bacterial tracheitis, congenital subglottic stenosis, and croup (Table 144-2)

THERAPEUTIC PLAN

Pharmaceutical

Pharmaceutical treatment is outlined in Table 144-3.

Lifestyle/Activities

Supportive care

Students and school staff should not attend school until 5 days of antibiotic treatment

Diet

As tolerated, encourage fluid intake

Patient Education

Discuss need for immunization, possible adverse events after pertussis vaccine, and antipyretic prophylaxis after administration of diphtheria-tetanus-pertussis (DTP) immunization. Booster doses of pertussis not recommended for patients >6 y/o unless to control outbreaks.

Family Impact

Immunization and treatment of family members

Referral

Immediate referral with hospitalization of infants <6 mo

Consultation

All other cases

Follow-up

Report to local health authority

14-day course of erythromycin ethyl succinate for household and close contacts, regardless of immunization status

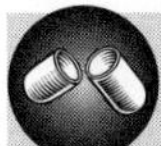

TABLE 144-3 Pharmaceutical Treatment: Pertussis

Drug	Dose	Comments	Cost
Erythromycin ethyl succinate (EES) *or*	800 mg q12h ×14 days (max 4 g/day) Children: 10-12.5 mg/kg/d q6h ×14 days	Drug of choice Pregnancy: B SE: N/V/D, abdominal cramping, anorexia Many drug interactions: check before Rx	\$14-\$16/250 mg (100); \$26-\$154/500 mg (100); \$13-\$27/susp: 200 mg/5 ml (480 ml); \$22-\$49/400 mg/5 ml (480 ml); \$20/chewable: 200 mg (40)
Clarithromycin (Biaxin)	250 mg BID for 7-14 days Children: 7.5 mg BID, max 500 mg BID	Pregnancy: C SE: N/V/D	\$26/125 mg/5 ml (100 ml); \$49/250 mg/5 ml (100 ml); \$185/250, 500 mg (60)

N/V/D, Nausea, vomiting, and diarrhea; *SE,* side effects.

EVALUATION

Pneumonia is the most common cause of death.

SUGGESTED READINGS

American Academy of Pediatrics: Pertussis. In Peter G, editor: *1997 red book: report of the Committee on Infectious Disease*, ed 24, Elk Grove Village, Ill, 1997, American Academy of Pediatrics.

American Public Health Association: *1995 control of communicable diseases manual*, ed 16, Washington DC, 1995, the Association.

Ellsworth A et al: *Mosby's 1998 medical drug reference*, St Louis, 1998, Mosby.

Healthcare Consultants of America, Inc: *1998 physicians fee and coding guide*, Augusta, Ga, 1998, Healthcare Consultants of America, Inc.

Uphold C, Graham M: *Clinical guidelines in family practice*, ed 2, Gainesville, Fla, 1994, Barmarrae Books.

Pityriasis

ICD-9-CM

Pityriasis Rosea 696.3

OVERVIEW

Definition

Pityriasis rosea: Exanthematous, maculopapular red scaling eruption that occurs largely on the trunk

Incidence

Pityriasis is mainly a disorder of fair-skinned whites, and is uncommon in those with Mediterranean heritage. It is common in **ages 10 to 35,** occurring more in the spring and fall in temperate climates. It accounts for approximately 2% of outpatient dermatologic visits. M=F.

Pathophysiology

Unknown cause
Perhaps a viral or autoimmune disorder

Protective Factors Against

None

Factors That Increase Susceptibility

Climate
Fair complexion

SUBJECTIVE DATA

History of Present Illness

Development of skin lesion, usually on trunk; then 1 to 2 weeks later a generalized secondary eruption occurs

Complaints of itching:
- Absent (25%)
- Mild (50%)
- Severe (25%)

Treatments tried and results

Past Medical History

Noncontributory

Medications

Recent use of corticosteroids

Family History

Less than 5% affected give positive family history

Psychosocial History

Ask about stressful situations

Associated Symptoms

Fever and malaise is rare

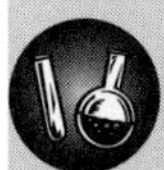

TABLE 145-1 Diagnostic Procedures: Pityriasis

Diagnostic Test	Findings/Rationale	Cost ($)
Potassium hydroxide wet mount	Rule out tinea corporis	15-19
Rapid plasma reagin	Rule out syphilis	18-22
Lyme titer	If suspicious of Lyme disease	34-42

TABLE 145-2 Differential Diagnosis: Pityriasis

Diagnosis	Supporting Data
Drug eruption	Consider if captopril or barbiturates, whole body involvement
Secondary syphilis	Maculopapular rash, especially on palms and soles, also occurs on face, scattered discrete lesions, positive serology
Lyme disease	Systemic symptoms initially; solitary annular lesion with distinct red border and partially clearing center; may develop secondary lesions: smaller, lack central induration; exposure to *Borrelia burgdorferi* via tick bite
Tinea corporis	Small, scaling, sharply marginated lesions; peripheral enlargement and central clearing, annular configuration; single lesions, with occasional scattered multiple lesions
Guttate psoriasis	Lesions that occur rapidly, frequently after streptococcal pharyngitis; more frequent in young adults; no marginal collarette

OBJECTIVE DATA

Physical Examination

A problem-oriented approach, with particular attention to:
- Height, weight, general appearance
- Skin: General skin lesions: type, shape, arrangement, distribution
  - Hair/nail involvement
  - Discrete erythematous fine scaling lesions scattered in a characteristic pattern: the long axes of the lesions following the lines of cleavage in a "Christmas Tree" distribution. Usually confined to the trunk and proximal aspects of arms and legs
  - Rarely involves face; color dull pink or tawny
  - "Herald Patch": 2- to 6-cm patch that precedes the rash by days to weeks; oval, slightly raised patch, bright red, with fine collarette scale at periphery

Diagnostic Procedures

Diagnostic procedures are outlined in Table 145-1.

ASSESSMENT

Differential diagnoses include those found in Table 145-2.

THERAPEUTIC PLAN

Pharmaceutical

Pharmaceutical treatment is outlined in Table 145-3.

Lifestyle/Activities

Symptomatic treatment
Colloidal bath
Lukewarm oatmeal bath
Ultraviolet B phototherapy or natural sunlight exposure for itching (works best if in first week of rash)

Diet

Not applicable

Patient Education

Reassure patient that he or she does not have a "blood disease" and is not contagious
Usually spontaneous remission in 6 to 12 weeks
Recurrence is uncommon, but does occur
Hot water may exacerbate rash
Strenuous activity may aggravate rash

Referral

Refer to dermatologist:

If no improvement in expected time frame
If rash persists for >6 weeks, a skin biopsy is needed to rule out parapsoriasis

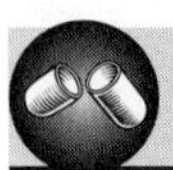

TABLE 145-3 Pharmaceutical Plan: Pityriasis

Drug	Dose	Comments	Cost
Diphenhydramine (Benadryl) Elixir: 12.5 mg/5 ml	25-50 mg q6h Children: 5 mg/kg/day	Competes with H_1 receptor sites Pregnancy: B (should not be used in first trimester) SE: Causes drowsiness	$2-$15/12.5 mg/5 ml (480 ml); $2-$22/25 mg (100); $2-$24/50 mg (100)
Topical corticosteroid (See Appendix R for more details)	Apply sparingly to affected areas BID daily	May be used if pruritus bothersome Pregnancy: C	$4-$27/(60 g)

SE, Side effects.

EVALUATION/FOLLOW-UP

Return for reevaluation if lesions last 6 weeks.

SUGGESTED READINGS

Dunn S: *Primary care consultant*, St Louis, 1998, Mosby.

Ellsworth A et al: *Mosby's 1998 medical drug reference*, St Louis, 1998, Mosby.

Fitzpatrick T et al: *Color atlas and synopsis of clinical dermatology*, ed 3, New York, 1997, McGraw Hill.

Habif F: *Clinical dermatology: a color guide to diagnosis and therapy*, ed 3, St Louis, 1996, Mosby.

Healthcare Consultants of America, Inc: *1998 physicians fee and coding guide*, Augusta, Ga, 1998, Healthcare Consultants of America, Inc.

Horio T: Skin diseases that improve by exposure to sunlight, *Clin Dermatol* 16(1):59-65, 1998.

Pomeranz A, Fairley J: Pityriasis, *Pediatr Clin North Am* 45(1):49-63, 1998.

Wyndham M: Pityriasis, *Practitioner* 241(1575):358, 1997.

Pneumonia

ICD-9-CM

Pneumonia 486.0
Mycoplasma 483.0
Bacterial 482.9
Viral 480.9

OVERVIEW

Definition

Pneumonia is an inflammatory process of the parenchyma of the lung (bronchioles and the alveolar spaces) that is caused by infection.

Classification

Community-acquired
Hospital-acquired (nosocomial)

Incidence

Pneumonia is the most common cause of death due to an infectious disease.
Pneumonia is the sixth overall cause of death in the United States and the fourth leading cause of death among the **elderly.**
Pneumonia occurs most often during the winter months and early spring.
One to two percent of hospitalized patients develop pneumonia, with a mortality rate of 30% even with adequate antimicrobial therapy.

Pathophysiology

Aspirated oropharynegeal secretions
Inhalation of infected droplets
Lymphohematogenous spread from another site
Direct introduction of organisms from a diagnostic or treatment procedure or trauma

Protective Factors Against

Cough and gag reflexes to protect against gross aspiration.
Mucociliary lining of the tracheobronchial tree.
Immune response: leukocytes and phagocytosis.

Factors That Increase Susceptibility

Altered upper respiratory tract flora: Predisposition to more virulent organisms as a result of recent antibiotic therapy, recent hospitalization, diabetes, or alcoholism
Altered immune status: Diabetes, acquired immunodeficiency syndrome (AIDS), alcoholism, malignancy, chemotherapy, uremia, sickle cell disease
Impaired cough and gag reflex: Increased risk of aspiration with altered mental status, alcohol or drug intoxication, anesthetics, cerebrovascular accident, seizure
Impaired function of natural defense mechanisms: Mucociliary clearance damaged by smoking, inhaled environmental pollutants, chronic obstructive pulmonary disease (COPD), congestive heart failure (CHF), alcohol, viral infection
Mechanical bypass of normal defense: Tracheal intubation, chest tube
Underlying lung pathology: Pulmonary embolus or contusion, foreign body, atelectasis
Chest wall pain: Postoperative pain, chest trauma, myopathy

Common Pathogens

Streptococcus pneumoniae is by far the most common cause of bacterial pneumonia accounting for 90% of cases.
Staphylococcus aureus and *Haemophilus influenzae* type B may also cause bacterial pneumonia.
Influenza A is the most common cause of viral pneumonia in older **children, adolescents,** and **adults.**

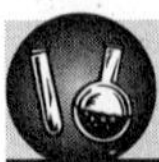

TABLE 146-1 Diagnostic Procedures: Pneumonia

Diagnostic Test/Cost	Findings/Rationale
Chest x-ray ($77-$91)	Bacterial pneumonia presents with lobar or segmental consolidation, abscess, pneumatocele, or pleural fluid; mycoplasmal and viral pneumonia will present with interstitial infiltrates with possible hyperexpansion but no consolidation; fungal, mycobacterial, staphylococcal pneumonia present with patchy distribution of granulomas with possible necrosis and cavity development
Pulse oximetry	Determines oxygen saturation; less than 90% indicates need for supplemental oxygen therapy
Complete blood count ($13-$16)	Assess for leukocytosis, which may or may not be present with bacterial pneumonia and neutrophilia, which may be present with mycoplasmal or viral pneumonia
Blood culture ($31-$39)	Bacteremia is present in 10%-25% of cases and is associated with high fever
Sputum cultures ($31-$39)	Assess organism identification; adequate sampling imperative and may be hampered by dehydration and weak cough; can be obtained by bronchoscopy or transtracheal aspiration
Acid fast stains and culture	Assess for tuberculosis
Arterial blood gases	Pao_2 <80 mm Hg indicates hypoxemia; used to determine severity of the illness
Immunofluorescent staining and enzyme-linked immunosorbent assay	Rapid viral diagnostic techniques for respiratory syncitial virus; both tests are done on nasopharyngeal secretions and may identify cases that may benefit from early ribavirin treatment
Diagnostic thoracentesis	Assess pleural fluid for culture and fluid analysis
Serum specimens for cold agglutinins	Present in about 50% of cases caused by viral or mycoplasmal infections
Bacterial antigen detection tests	Assess for *S. pneumoniae* and *H. influenzae*

Respiratory syncytial virus (RSV) is the most common cause of pneumonia in **infants.**

Mycoplasma pneumoniae is common in **school-age children** and **young adults.**

Other pathogens that cause pneumonia in **infancy** include *Chlamydia,* group B streptococcus, parainfluenza viruses, and *Bordetella pertussis.*

Aspiration pneumonia may be caused by *S. aureus, Escherichia coli, Klebsiella pneumoniae, Pseudomonas aeruginosa, Proteus,* and *Enterbacter.*

The most common pathogens in **people 65 and older** are *S. pneumoniae, H. influenza,* and other gram-negative bacilli. Other possible pathogens include *M. catarrhalis, Legionella* species, *Mycobacterium tuberculosis,* and endemic fungi.

SUBJECTIVE DATA

History of Present Illness

Typically pneumonia presents with an abrupt onset of fever, chills, and productive cough, but it can have an atypical presentation with an insidious onset and dry cough.

Inquire about onset and duration of symptoms.

Inquire about associated symptoms, including difficulty breathing, shortness of breath, wheezing, retractions, nasal flaring, difficulty sleeping, difficulty speaking or weak cry, difficulty eating, rhinorrhea, earache, sore throat, hoarseness.

Inquire about possibility of aspiration and/or foreign body.

Inquire about systemic symptoms, including fever, chills, rash, malaise, muscle aches, vomiting, and seizures.

Inquire about self-help measures and other family members who might be ill.

Inquire about recent hospitalizations, antibiotics, or treatments.

Inquire about smoking and the possibility of alcohol or drug use/abuse.

Past Medical History

For **children** inquire about underlying disease such as reactive airway disease, bronchopulmonary dysplasia, cystic fibrosis, tracheomalacia, congenital heart disease, sickle cell disease, seizures, and human immunodeficiency virus (HIV)/AIDS. Inquire about medications.

For **adults** inquire about underlying disease such as COPD, diabetes, chronic renal failure, CHF, liver disease, cancer, and HIV/AIDS. Inquire about medications.

Inquire about immunization status for both **children** and **adults.**

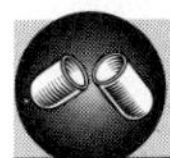

TABLE 146-2 Pharmaceutical Therapy for Empiric Outpatient Treatment

Drug	Dose	Comments	Cost ($)
Erythromycin	20 mg/kg/day divided into q12h doses	0-7 days old	11-16/eryth
Erythromycin/sulfisoxasole (Pediazole)	40 mg/kg/day (erythromycin) PO divided into q6h doses × 10 days	>2 months old Alternatives include trimethoprim/sulfamethoxazole (TMP/SMZ)	Not available
Amoxicillin	60-80 mg/kg/day divided into three doses × 10 days	Alternatives include Pediazole, TMP/SMZ, Ceclor, Suprax, or Augmentin	3-8

OBJECTIVE DATA

Physical Examination

Assess vital signs for temperature elevation, tachypnea, tachycardia, hypotension, hypertension.

Observe for pallor or cyanosis, dyspnea, pursed lips, grunting, or nasal flaring.

Inspect the chest for retractions and use of accessory muscles, increased anteroposterior diameter.

Dullness to percussion may indicate lobar consolidation.

Ascultate the chest, assessing for asymmetry and equal inspirations/expirations.

Assess for crackles/rales, wheezing, bronchial breath sounds, increased vocal fremitus, bronchophony, egophony, and whispered pectoriloquy.

Infants with a respiratory rate >60 breaths/minute and **children** less than 3 years old with a respiratory rate >40 breaths/minute with chest retractions are sensitive and specific indications of lower respiratory tract infection.

Diagnostic Procedures

Diagnostic procedures are outlined in Table 146-1.

ASSESSMENT

When the presenting features are fever and cough consider one of the following:

Lower respiratory tract infection such as pneumonia and bronchitis
(In **children,** bronchiolitis is more common than bronchitis)
Pulmonary embolus (fever, usually low grade)
Septic pulmonary cough

When the presenting features is dyspnea in a **younger patient** consider one of the following:

Pulmonary embolus
Pneumonia
Pneumothorax
Reactive airway disease/asthma
Costochondritis/pleuritis

When the presenting feature is dyspnea in an **older adult** consider one of the following:

Acute myocardial infarction
Pulmonary embolism
CHF
Exacerbation of COPD
Pneumonia
Pulmonary abscess
Rib fracture

THERAPEUTIC PLAN

Pharmaceutical

Pharmaceutical treatment is outlined in Tables 146-2 and 146-3.

Consider administering procaine penicillin IM or ceftriaxone (Rocephin) IM to ensure initial compliance and avoid problems related to vomiting.

Severely ill **infants, children** and **elderly** should be hospitalized and treated with intravenous antibiotic therapy.

Indications for hospitalization are moderate to severe respiratory distress, including respiratory rate >70 per minute, marked retractions, cyanosis, grunting, oxygen saturation less than 88% to 90%, systemic toxicity, dehydration, or mental status change.

Infants and **children** at greatest risk of deterioration include those with sickle cell disease, malnutrition, or immunodeficiency; those who are taking immunosuppressive drugs; those with cardiac or pulmonary disease; and those who are premature.

Infants and **children** whose families have no communication or means of transportation should be considered high risk.

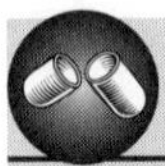

TABLE 146-3 Dosing for Older Patients

For young adult, otherwise healthy	Erythromycin 500 mg QID × 7-10 days	Alternatives include doxycycline, azithromycin, clarithromycin, and dirithromycin
Adult >60 years old, or co-morbidity	Trimethoprim/sulfamethoxazole (Bactrim DS) one tablet BID × 7-10 days, plus erythromycin or doxycycline	Alternatives include azithromycin, clarithromycin, oral second or parenteral third-generation cephalosporin, amoxicillin-clavulanate (Augmentin), plus erythromycin or doxycycline
Suspected aspiration	Clindamycin ($45-$231) (Cleocin) 150-300 mg q6h × 10 days; take with a full glass of water	Amoxicillin-clavulanate

Box 146-1

Indications for Hospitalization for an Adult With Community-Acquired Pneumonia

Age >65 years
Unstable vital signs (heart rate >140 beats/min, systolic blood pressure <90 mm Hg respiratory rate >30/min).
Altered mental status
Hypoxemia (PO_2 < 60 mm Hg)
Severe underlying disease (chronic obstructive pulmonary disease, diabetes mellitus, liver disease, heart failure, renal failure)
Immunocompromised (HIV infection, cancer, corticosteroid use)
Complication from pneumonia (extrapulmonary infection, meningitis, cavitation, multilobar involvement, sepsis, abscess, empyema, pleural effusion)
Severe electrolyte, hematologic, or metabolic abnormality (sodium <130 mEq/L, hematocrit <30%, absolute neutrophil count <1000/mm^3, serum creatinine >2.5 mg/dl).
Failure to respond to outpatient treatment within 48 to 72 hours

From King DE, Pippin HJ: Community-acquired pneumonia in adults: initial antibiotic therapy, *Am Family Physician* 56(2):544-549, 1997.

H. influenzae is a common pathogen in smokers and should be treated with a macrolide.

Most antibiotics should be prescribed for 10 to 14 days, except azithromycin, which is given for 5 days because of its long half-life and significant pulmonary penetration.

Azithromycin should not be used if bacteremia is suspected because it does not yield appreciable serum levels.

If *Pseudomonas aeruginosa* is suspected, use a cephalosporin such as ceftazidime or cefepime.

Fluoroquinolones are not recommended for empiric monotherapy for community-acquired pneumonia.

Hospitalization should be considered with any of the indicators in Box 146-1.

Patient Education

Stress the importance of rest, fluids, nutrition, antibiotics, and antipyretics.

Teach deep-breathing and cough techniques.

Report to health care provider any change in color or characteristics of sputum, decreased activity tolerance, persistent fever, or increased chest pain or no overall improvement.

Encourage smoking cessation if appropriate.

Recommend influenza and pneumococcal vaccines as appropriate.

Consultation/Referral

Consultation with a physician is indicated for severe respiratory distress or in the presence of co-morbidity.

Consult when referring for inpatient hospitalization.

EVALUATION/FOLLOW-UP

Assess for response to treatment and improvement within 48 to 72 hours.

SUGGESTED READINGS

Ashbourne J, Downey P: Pneumonia. In Rosen P, editor, *Emergency medicine: concepts and clinical practice,* St Louis, 1993, Mosby.

Berman S: *Pediatric decision making,* ed 2, Philadelphia, 1991, BC Decker.

Ellsworth AJ et al: *Mosby's medical drug reference.* St Louis, 1998, Mosby.

French M: Pneumonia in the elderly, *Adv Nurse Pract* 3(5):40-44, 1995.

Grimes D: *Infectious diseases,* St Louis, 1991, Mosby.

Guidelines for the Initial Management of Adults With Community-Acquired Pneumonia: Diagnosis, assessment of severity, and initial antimicrobial therapy, *Am Rev Respir Dis* 148:1418-1426, 1993.

Healthcare Consultants of America, Inc: 1998 physicians fee and coding guide, Augusta, Ga, 1998, Healthcare Consultants of America, Inc.

King DE, Pippin HJ: Community-acquired pneumonia in adults: initial antibiotic therapy, *Am Family Physician* 56(2):544-549, 1997.

Staufler J: Ling. In Tierney L Jr, McPhee S, Papadakis M, editors, *Current medical diagnosis & treatment,* Norwalk, Conn, 1996, Appleton & Lange.

Wilson SF, Thompson JM: *Respiratory disorders,* St Louis, 1990, Mosby.

Postabortion Care

ICD-9-CM

Legal Abortion (Under Medical Supervision) 635.9
Gynecological Examination V72.3
Family Planning Advice V25.09

OVERVIEW

Definition

Postabortion care consists of a scheduled examination 2 to 4 weeks after a therapeutic or elective abortion to assess the patient's physical and emotional status, with identification of any unexpected events or complications

Incidence

The risk of serious complications as a result of an abortion during the first 12 gestational weeks for women of all ages is about 1 to 2/100,000. The more advanced the pregnancy, the more likely that complications will occur. In 1994, an estimated 1.4 million abortions took place. Every year, 3/100 women ages 15 to 44 have an abortion.

Pathophysiology

First-trimester abortion: Dilation of the cervix and removal of the products of conception by suction curettage (D&C). *Laminaria digitata* may be used to soften the cervix and reduce the need for forcible dilation. *Laminaria* are seaweed that absorb water, swell, and gently open the cervix.

Second-trimester abortion: Dilation of the cervix and extraction of the fetus and placenta with ring forceps and a large curette (D&E). Another method is to use prostaglandin preparations to stimulate uterine contractions. The placenta is often retained after the fetus is expelled and must be removed surgically. Progesterone antagonists (RU-486—not available in the United States), which block progesterone receptor sites in the decidua, induce bleeding in pregnant women within a few days. These drugs also sensitize the uterus to prostaglandins, which are given after the antagonists.

SUBJECTIVE DATA

History of Present Condition

Ask about date of procedure, type of abortion (D&C, D&E)
Last menstrual period
Any bleeding following the procedure, and when
Pain associated with bleeding, any clots, fever
If antibiotics were given, was the full course completed?
Has there been any sexual intercourse since the procedure?
Any use of tampons or douching since the procedure?
Any complaints of constipation or diarrhea since the procedure?
Amount of physical activity since the procedure
Method of birth control
Family/partner support
How does the woman/partner feel about the procedure?
Any questions about the procedure?
Obtain operative report, cultures done at the time of procedure

Possible Complaints

Fever, body aches, chills
Severe pain/cramping
Heavy bleeding (more than one pad an hour) or clots
Abdominal pain: Onset, duration, location
Nausea and/or vomiting
Foul vaginal discharge
Dizziness or vertigo

Past Medical History

History of previous pelvic inflammatory disease or sexually transmitted diseases, especially chlamydia and gonorrhea
Ask about previous episodes of bacterial vaginosis and treatment

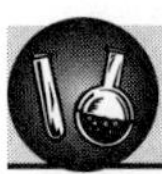

TABLE 147-1 Diagnostic Procedures: Postabortion

Diagnostic Test	Finding/Rationale	Cost ($)
Urine HCG	A highly sensitive urine pregnancy test to rule out retained products of conception, missed abortion	17-23
Pap smear	Consider a Pap smear if patient wants birth control and will be seen in your office and it has been >1 yr since last one	25-31
Genital cultures	If cultures not done before procedure, consider doing tests for chlamydia and gonorrhea	61-79
Wet prep	Check for clue cells, white blood cells, and trichimoniasis	15-19
U/A	Assess for UTI	15-20
CBC with differential and ESR	Rule out infection if complications are present	18-23
Transvaginal ultrasound	Identify possible products of conception or inflammation	369-439

CBC, Complete blood count; *ESR,* erythrocyte sedimentation rate; *HCG,* human chorionic gonadotropin; *U/A,* urinalysis; *UTI,* urinary tract infection.

Medications

Current medications if any

OBJECTIVE DATA

Physical Examination

A problem-focused examination should be performed, with special attention to:

Vital signs, including blood pressure, temperature, respirations, and pulse
Head/eyes/ears/nose/throat: Look for sign of upper respiratory infection, otitis, pharyngitis
Lymph nodes: Look for lymphadenopathy, tenderness
Heart: Murmurs, irregular rhythms
Lungs: Breath sounds, adventitious sounds
Abdominal: Bowel sounds, masses, guarding, organomegaly, rebound tenderness, referred pain, suprapubic tenderness, bladder distention
Pelvic examination: Use sterile speculum if <1 week since procedure
Cervix: Is os closed, any signs of trauma or purulent discharge or tissue?
    Assess for bleeding, and site of bleeding
Bimanual: Check size of uterus, consistency, any cervical motion tenderness, fullness
    Check for adnexal masses, tenderness
Rectovaginal examination: Assess for tenderness, hard stool, or bleeding

Consider a complete examination if patient is going to continue to be seen in your office on a regular basis.

Diagnostic Procedures

Diagnostic procedures are outlined in Table 147-1.

ASSESSMENT

Differential diagnoses are outlined in Table 147-2.

THERAPEUTIC PLAN

Review birth control options including risks, benefits, and side effects. Help to determine the best method for her and her partner (see Chapter 198).
Review history for contraindications for contraceptive choices.
If patient started on oral contraceptive pills (OCPs) since the procedure, evaluate any side effects.
Continue the method if no contraindications or if patient desires.

Pharmaceutical

As indicated by symptoms and findings on examination
Medications may include:
    Antibiotics (usually coverage of chlamydia, gonorrhea, and bacterial vaginosis) but will depend on cultures (see Chapters 35, 81, and 192)
    Nonsteroidal antiinflammatory drugs
    Stool softener
    Ergotrate

Diet

Not applicable

Patient Education

Emphasize the need for follow-up.
Encourage patient to call if she is unhappy with birth control or method and wants to stop it.
Have patient return to office if her menses do not begin in 3 to 4 weeks.
Discuss with patient that abortion is not a satisfactory

TABLE 147-2 Differential Diagnosis: Postabortion

Diagnosis	Supporting Data
Postabortion examination, no complications	No bleeding or uterine tenderness, decreasing size of uterus, no fever, os closed, no discharge, no CMT
Retained products of conception	Continued and excessive vaginal bleeding Enlarged, soft uterus
Missed abortion	Positive pregnancy test, positive confirmation by ultrasound
Uterine infection (endometritis)	Fever, uterine or pelvic tenderness, lochia with foul odor, abdominal pain
Delayed involution	Continued bloody discharge, uterus soft and boggy; involution usually takes place within 1 month, and menstruation begins 4-6 weeks after the abortion
PID (Ch. 140)	CMT, fever, adnexal tenderness, abdominal pain
UTI (Ch. 187)	Suprapubic tenderness, dysuria, frequency, ~CVAT
Uterine perforation	Abdominal pain, abdominal guarding, abdominal rigidity, hypotension
Systemic illness	URI, gastroenteritis

CMT, Cervical motion tenderness; *CVAT,* costovertebral angle tenderness; *PID,* pelvic inflammatory disease; *UTI,* urinary tract infection.

method of birth control: encourage her to be proactive and prevent the pregnancy before it occurs.

Discuss the signs and symptoms of depression and let patient know that many women may experience various feelings, including depression and guilt, following an abortion.

Family Impact

An abortion, whether elective or therapeutic, is a traumatic event for all involved. In some cases the woman's family may not be aware that it occurred. Encourage her to share this information with parents or partner as appropriate and seek counseling as needed.

Referral

Social Service or counseling referral if patient is having problems with unresolved issues.

If pregnancy test is positive, continue OCPs if the patient wishes, and refer her back to center that provided abortion services to be evaluated. Serial quantitative human chorionic gonadotropins (HCGs) may be indicated if a missed abortion is suspected. Explain that the HCG may be elevated for a short time after abortion and may need to be repeated several times and followed to a value less than 5 to ensure a return to a prepregnancy state. A referral to an OB/GYN is indicated if a missed abortion is suspected.

EVALUATION/FOLLOW-UP

Yearly examination for health maintenance and contraception.

There may be a small rise in the risk of breast cancer related to a history of induced abortion among young women of reproductive age. These are preliminary results, but they warrant close breast follow-up in women who have had the procedure.

Monitor patient closely for signs and symptoms of depression. It may be worthwhile to have her return in 1 to 3 months after the procedure to screen for depression.

Complications of abortion include:
- Sepsis
- Hemorrhage
- Uterine perforation

RESOURCE

www.agi-usa.org/pubs/fb_abortion2/fb_abort2.html

SUGGESTED READINGS

Daling J et al: Risk of breast cancer among white women following induced abortions, *Am J Epidemiol* 144(4):373-380, 1996.

Ellsworth A et al: *Mosby's 1998 medical drug reference*, St Louis, 1998, Mosby.

Healthcare Consultants of America, Inc: *1998 physicians fee and coding guide*, Augusta, Ga, 1998, Healthcare Consultants of America, Inc.

Levallois P, Rioux J: Prophylactic antibiotics for suction curettage abortion: results of a clinical controlled trial, *Am J Obstet Gynecol* 158(1):100-105, 1988.

Mattox J: *Core textbook of obstetrics and gynecology*, St Louis, 1998, Mosby.

Penney G: Preventing infective sequelae of abortion, *Human Reprod* 12(11 suppl):107-112, 1997.

Sawaya G et al: Antibiotics at the time of induced abortion: the case for universal prophylaxis based on a meta-analysis, *Obstet Gynecol* 87 (5 Pt 2):884-890, 1996.

Stevenson M, Radcliffe K: Preventing pelvic infection after abortion, *Int J STD AIDS* 6(5):305-312, 1995.

Pregnancy Problems: Early and Late Bleeding

ICD-9-CM

Placenta Previa without Hemorrhage 641.0
Hemorrhage from Placenta Previa 641.1
Placenta Abruptio 641.2
Placenta Detachment (Partial) (Premature) (with Hemorrhage) 641.1
Spontaneous Abortion 634.9
Threatened Abortion 640.0
Premature Labor 644.2

OVERVIEW

Definition

Threatened abortion is a pregnancy in which a live fetus is present, the cervix is closed, and bleeding occurs with or without cramping. Loss is possible. No tissue is passed.

Inevitable abortion is a pregnancy in which spontaneous loss is almost certain to occur.

Missed abortion is an early pregnancy loss in which the fetus has died but spontaneous abortion has not occurred.

Incomplete abortion is an early loss of pregnancy in which only a portion of the products of conception is passed, leaving some tissue retained.

Ectopic pregnancy is a pregnancy developing outside the uterine cavity, usually in a fallopian tube. Generally it becomes evident at 12- to 16-weeks' gestation.

Implantation bleeding is vaginal spotting that occurs at the time of trophoblast implantation. It is not a threat to the pregnancy. It occurs at 27 to 35 days after the last normal menstrual period.

Hydatidiform mole is an abnormal development of the placenta with the presence of grapelike vesicles and the absence of a fetus.

Abruptio placenta is the premature separation of the placenta from the uterine wall before delivery of the fetus. It may be complete or partial. Bleeding may or may not be visible (Figure 148-1).

Placenta previa is the implantation of the placenta located low on the uterine wall. Types are determined by whether the placenta is near or over the internal cervical os (Figure 148-2).

Incidence

First-trimester Bleeding

Bleeding in the first trimester occurs usually at the 9th to the 12th week of gestation, and 10% to 15% of these pregnancies will end in abortion. Although the cause is often unknown, most often spontaneous abortion is due to a defect, either chromosomal or developmental (Hayashi and Castillo, 1993). Ectopic pregnancy is the leading cause of first-trimester maternal mortality (Guyette, 1997). All but threatened abortion can lead to infection.

Ectopic pregnancies can cause life-threatening hemorrhage as well, whereas abortions usually do not. Most of the blood loss from such hemorrhages is maternal, although some fetal blood loss is possible as well.

Second-trimester Bleeding

Bleeding in the second trimester is the hallmark of a hydatidiform mole. Incidence is the highest in Oriental women living in Asia (up to 1/200 pregnancies) and lowest in Caucasian women of Western European/U.S. origins (1/2000).

Third-trimester Bleeding

Serious hemorrhages occur in 2% to 3% of all pregnancies and are usually due to either abruptio placenta or placenta previa. Placenta previa in one form or another occurs in 1 in 200 births. Thirty percent of third trimester cases of hemorrhages are due to placental abruption (Pernoll, 1994).

Pathophysiology

Factors that Increase Susceptibility

Early (9 to 20 weeks)
- Infections (e.g., urinary tract infection, STDs)
- Anatomic abnormalities of the uterus
- Systemic disorders (such as lupus)

Abruptio placentae (premature separation)

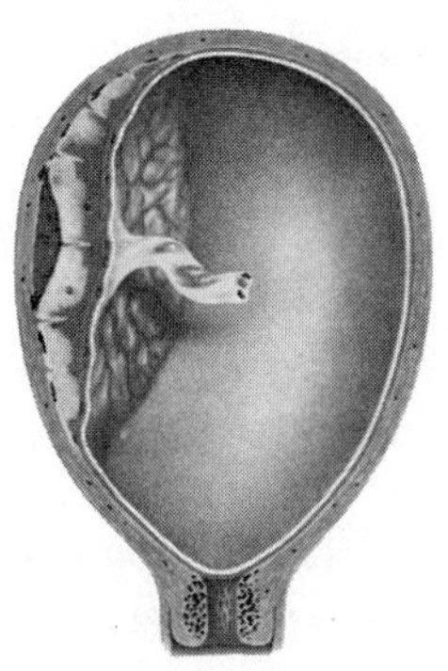

Partial separation (concealed hemorrhage)

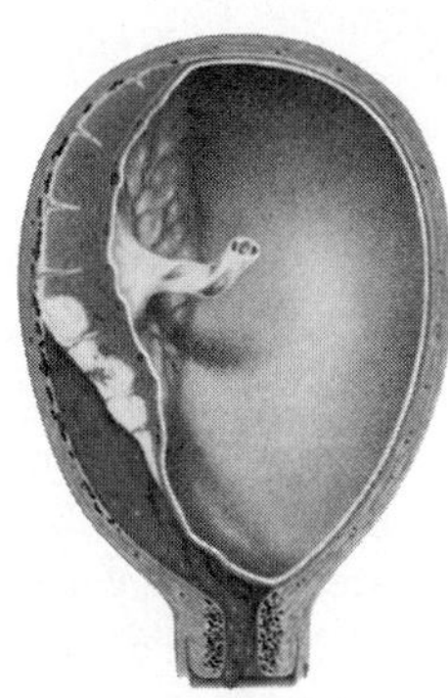

Partial separation (apparent hemorrhage)

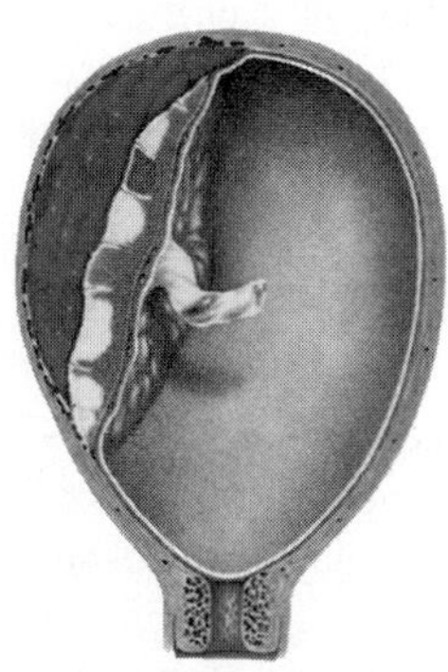

Complete separation (concealed hemorrhage)

Figure 148-1 Abruptio placentae. Premature separation of normally implanted placenta. (From Poole JH: Maternal hemorrhagic disorders. In Lowdermilk DL, Perry SE, Bobak IM, editors: *Maternity and women's health care*, St Louis, 1997, Mosby.)

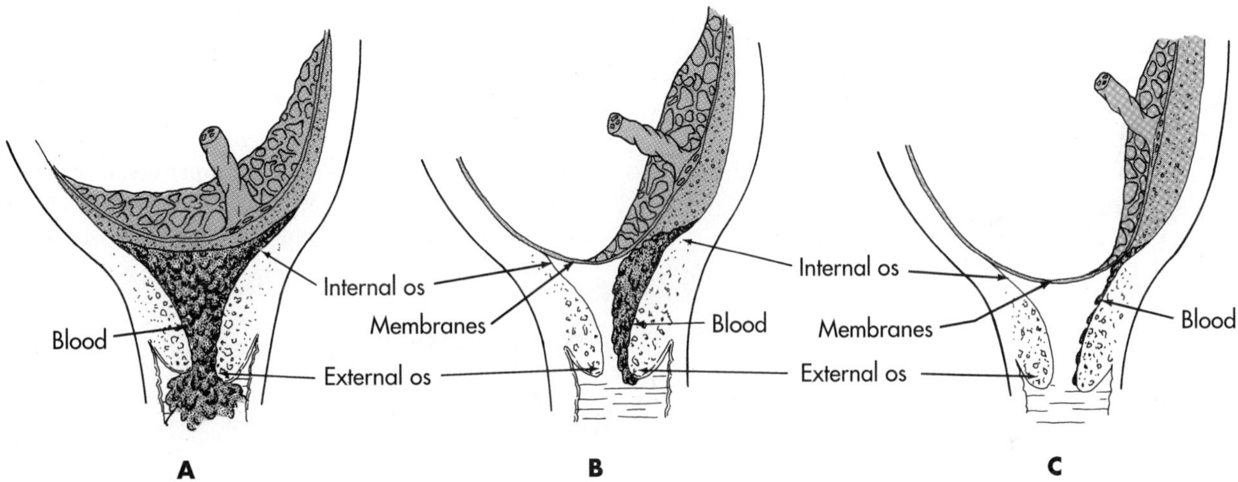

Figure 148-2 Types of placenta previa after onset of labor. **A,** Complete, or total. **B,** Incomplete, or partial. **C,** Marginal, or low lying. (From Poole JH: Maternal hemorrhagic disorders. In Lowdermilk DL, Perry SE, Bobak IM, editors: *Maternity and women's health care*, St Louis, 1997, Mosby.)

- Immunologic factors
- Genetic causes
- Hormonal abnormalities
- Incompetent cervix
- Poor nutrition
- Intrauterine device use or endometriosis (ectopic)

Late (20 weeks to term)

- Abruption: Multiple pregnancy or hydramnios
  - Uterine leiomyomas
  - Trauma
  - Short umbilical cord
- Previa
  - Multiple pregnancy
  - Anything causing scarring or uterine wall (e.g., cesarean scar, pelvic inflammatory disease [PID], or endometritis)

Factors Common to Both Previa and Abruptio

Maternal age >35
Hypertension
Diabetes
Substance use (smoking, alcohol, cocaine)
Lack of prenatal care

SUBJECTIVE DATA

History of Present Illness

Determine estimated date of delivery.

Data collection is based somewhat on length of gestation when the bleeding occurred.

Ask how much she is bleeding.

How many pads is she soaking per hour? What color is

the bleeding? The characteristics of bleeding can help differentiate the cause of bleeding in early pregnancy (see Table 148-3). Has it occurred before? Bear in mind that bleeding from placenta previa can cease and resume.

Determine her age.

Ask where she had prenatal care if she is not a regular patient.

Ask if she has any pain.

If so, what type of pain? Does it radiate? Bear in mind that internal hemorrhage will sometimes cause referred shoulder pain. Ask about duration.

Have her describe her activities for the last 24 hours. The bleeding may be extrauterine if it occurred with intercourse, did not increase with activity, or was not associated with cramping; or if the patient had experienced an abnormal vaginal discharge before the bleeding began. Extrauterine bleeding can be caused by cervical polyps or malignancies, vaginal trauma or varices, cervicitis, or hemorrhoids.

Explore any possibility of trauma to the abdomen.

Ask if she has had any burning on urination or other symptoms of cystitis.

Determine if she has any allergies.

Past Medical History

Ask about:

History of infertility, endometriosis, STIs, PID, or ectopic pregnancy

Past pregnancies (e.g., number, complications, types of deliveries, lengths of gestations)

Systemic diseases, diabetes, and hypertension

Contraceptive use

Medications

Any medications (prescription or over-the-counter) in the first trimester

Family History

Ask about:

Any genetic or familial diseases

Diethylstilbestrol exposure

Psychosocial History

Frequency of use of recreational drugs, alcohol, or tobacco

Diet History

Ask about diet and prenatal vitamins.

OBJECTIVE DATA

Physical Examination

Vital signs (remember that tachycardia will occur before hypotension with hemorrhage)

Abdominal

Check for abdominal tenderness, boardlike abdomen, and presence or absence of Cullen's sign (bluish ring around umbilicus that signifies internal abdominal bleeding)

Check fetal heart tones (presence and rate)

Perineal: Visual check of external vaginal bleeding

With Early Pregnancy Bleeding

Perform speculum examination to determine status of cervix (open or closed) and the presence of vaginal bleeding, polyps, tissue, or vaginal discharge for culture or wet mount.

Perform a bimanual examination to determine the size of the uterus, the presence of adnexal mass, or cervical motion tenderness.

With Late Pregnancy Bleeding

DO NOT PERFORM A VAGINAL EXAMINATION. Vaginal examination can lead to further hemorrhage in the case of placenta previa. Measure fundal height and mark with indelible pen; if intrauterine bleeding is present, the fundal height will rise.

Diagnostic Procedures

Diagnostic procedures are outlined in Table 148-1. See also Figure 148-3.

ASSESSMENT

Differential diagnoses are determined by timing of the bleeding.

Early: Type of spontaneous abortion, ectopic, hydatidiform mole, implantation bleeding, or extrauterine bleeding (Table 148-2)

Late: The challenge in third-trimester bleeding is to differentiate between placenta previa and abruptio placenta (Table 148-3). Placenta previa usually involves painless bleeding, whereas abruptio is usually accompanied by pain. Extrauterine bleeding may also be a cause of late pregnancy bleeding.

THERAPEUTIC PLAN

Any episode of bleeding for a pregnant patient should be taken seriously and evaluated. Risk to the fetus and the mother may be significantly high.

If assessment reveals complete abortion, the patient may return home. Schedule a return visit for 2 weeks.

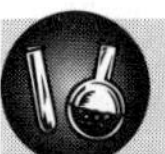

TABLE 148-1 Diagnostic Procedures: Bleeding in Pregnancy

Diagnostic Test	Findings/Rationale	Cost ($)
Blood type, Rh	Indicated since blood transfusion may be required; Rhogam may be necessary for Rh-negative women	16-21
Hemoglobin and hematocrit	Indicated to determine extent of blood loss	11-14
Serum human chorionic gonadotropin (HCG) level	Beta HCG should double every 2 days for the first 10 weeks of gestation (Guyette, 1997); levels will be abnormally low with ectopic pregnancy; abnormally high levels may indicate hydatidiform mole; decreasing levels are consistent with a spontaneous abortion	51-65 (quant)
Serum progesterone level	Level below 5 ng/dl indicates nonviable pregnancy (Guyette, 1997)	59-73
Ultrasound	Invaluable no matter what the timing or cause of bleeding; determines the presence of a viable fetus and the status and location of the placenta	352-419

Any other types of abortion, hydatidiform mole, or suspicion of ectopic require immediate referral. If contents of the uterus are not expelled within 1 month after fetal death, coagulopathy may occur.

Most threatened abortions will occur, regardless of any intervention. The treatment is bed rest and no sexual activity. The mother may feel that she is doing everything she can by remaining on bed rest; therefore she should be encouraged to do so (Guyette, 1997). She should be monitored with weekly visits to assess the status of the fetus and check for infection.

Ectopic pregnancy is an emergency situation since hemorrhage from a ruptured ectopic can be catastrophic and life-threatening.

Most types of extrauterine bleeding can be treated under protocols for pregnancy; however, cervical polyps should be removed by a physician (Guyette, 1997).

Patients with suspected placenta previa or abruptio must be referred immediately to a physician on an emergency basis.

Pharmaceutical

Medications are not used to attempt to stop an early pregnancy loss. Iron supplements may be used based on hemoglobin results. Give RhoGam if RH negative.

Lifestyle/Activities

If a patient goes home on bed rest, the entire family will be affected. Be sure to assess her level of support (both physical and emotional)

Diet

A diet high in iron will assist in maintaining adequate stores for the woman and the pregnancy.

Patient Education

If she is on bed rest, be sure she knows to maintain adequate hydration and understands the importance of high fiber.

If possible, include the partner in education sessions. If a reason for the bleeding can be identified, the couple will probably want to know how to prevent it from happening again—with this pregnancy or the next. This may be particularly difficult to discuss (as in the case of an STD); however, honest explanations offer the most complete and useful information. Often the cause cannot be identified, and this fact should be shared with the couple as well.

If the patient did not seek prenatal care, reasons for this should be discussed, and possibilities should be explored.

Family Impact

The patient who is bleeding during pregnancy is often frightened and concerned for her own well-being and that of her baby. With bleeding, loss of the fetus becomes a real possibility. Loss may occur even with the best of care. It is important to remember that grief is very real, even in early pregnancy loss. A nonjudgmental attitude is very important—even if the woman had no prenatal care. Ambivalence is a normal maternal emotional response early in pregnancy, and the mother may feel guilt if the pregnancy is lost in the midst of this ambivalence. The entire family may be affected by grief, and this possibility should be recognized and discussed.

Referral

Most cases of bleeding during pregnancy should be immediately referred to an MD or to the Emergency Department. Late pregnancy bleeding is an emergency situation if the bleeding is not extrauterine. Ectopic pregnancy is also an emergency.

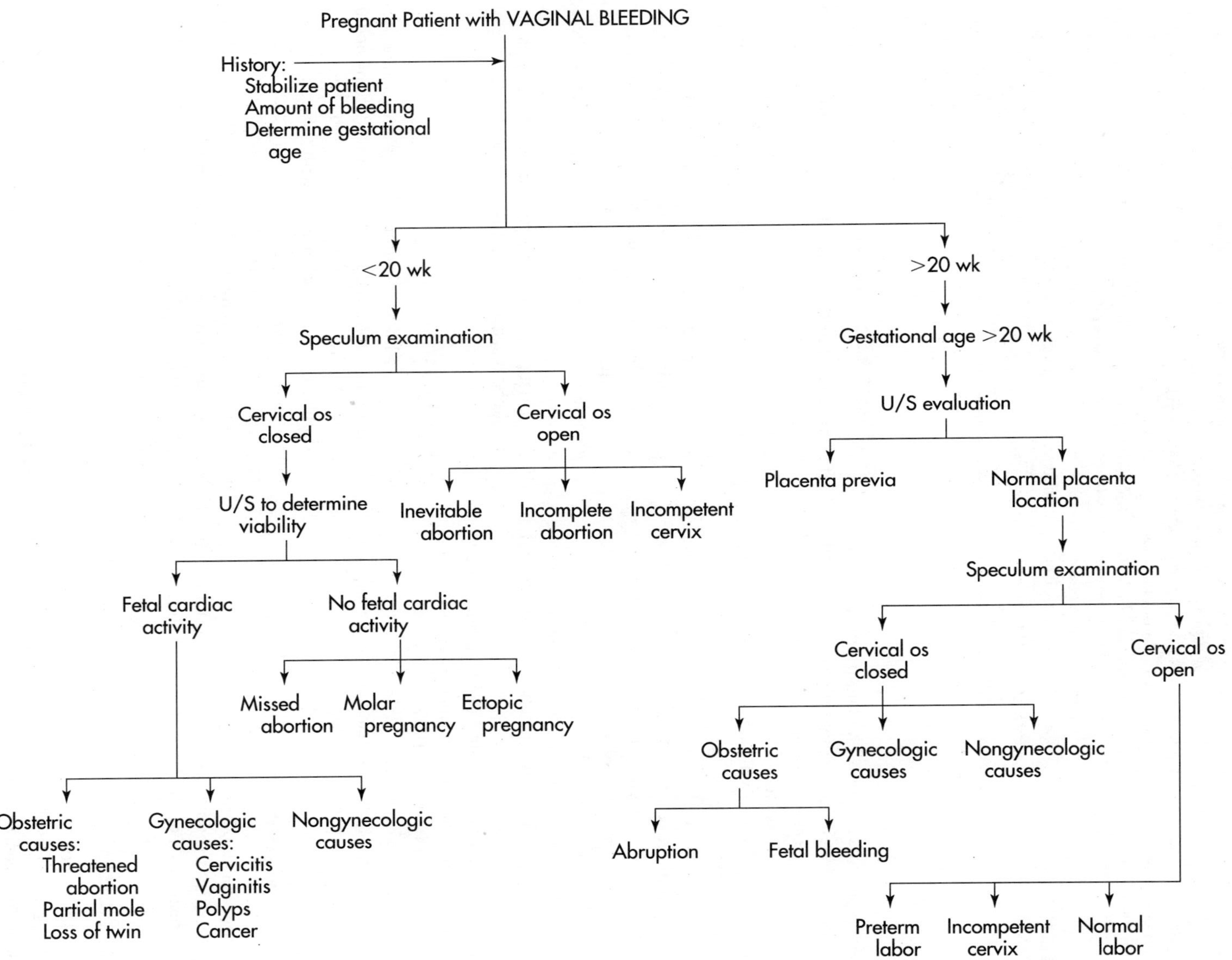

Figure 148-3 Algorithm for pregnant client with vaginal bleeding. *U/S*, Ultrasound. (Adapted from Greene H, Johnson W, Lemcke D, editors: *Decision making in medicine*, ed 2, St. Louis, 1998, Mosby.)

TABLE 148-2 Differentiation of Types of Abortions

Type of Abortion	Description
Complete	Bleeding and cramping present; complete expulsion of the products of conception; uterus firmly contracted
Incomplete	Bleeding, cramping, pelvic pressure; some passage of tissue; cervix open; uterus smaller than expected size
Missed	Spotting without cramping or passage of tissue; cervix closed; uterus smaller than expected size
Threatened	Spotting or slight bleeding; cervix closed; no tissue passed; size of uterus consistent with dates
Inevitable	Moderate bright red bleeding; products of conception at cervical os; uterine size consistent with dates
Hydatidiform Mole	Brownish spotting to heavy bleeding; passage of grape-like vesicles; uterus large for dates Increased suspicion with very young or older women (10× more common in women >45)
Ectopic	Nonspecific symptoms; spotting, cramping, or unilateral pelvic pain present; may feel tearing sensation and shoulder pain if rupturing; adnexal mass or fullness present; severe nausea and vomiting

TABLE 148-3 Comparison of Placenta Previa and Abruptio Placenta

Symptom	Previa	Abruptio
Bleeding	Minimal to severe, usually after 28th week; first episode may occur during sleep; may have repeated episodes that tend to be more severe than the first	Absent to moderate
Pain	None	Moderate to severe back or abdominal
Shock	Present with severe bleeding	Signs of shock may be disproportionate to amount of visible bleeding
Uterus	Nontender	Tender and rigid

Early pregnancy bleeding associated with spontaneous abortion usually does not involve life-threatening hemorrhage; however most cases should be referred because surgical intervention (D&C) may be required.

Patients who experience a pregnancy loss should be offered counseling or the contact number for a support group such as Resolve Through Sharing (Kowalski, 1991).

Consultation

Consider consulting with MD if you are unsure about whether a patient has expelled all the products of conception in a spontaneous abortion or in the case of threatened abortion.

Follow-up

All patients with a hydatidiform mole should be followed closely by an MD because choriocarcinoma occurs in 0.5% to 9.5% of these patients (Hayashi and Castillo, 1993). They are monitored with beta human chorionic gonadotropin levels for 24 months. They should use a reliable form of birth control for that time.

EVALUATION

Patients should be evaluated physically and emotionally on return visit.

If loss of early pregnancy occurs, the patient should make an appointment for 2 weeks following the loss. During the interim, she should report any signs of infection. A thorough pelvic examination should be performed on the next visit.

Patients who experienced bleeding late in pregnancy should be followed as with any postpartum patient after loss or delivery.

REFERENCES

Guyette L: Bleeding in pregnancy: deciphering this danger sign, *Adv Nurse Pract* 5(9):34-40, 1997.

Hayashi RH, Castillo MS: Bleeding in pregnancy. In Knuppel RA, Drukker JD, editors: *High-risk pregnancy: a team approach,* Philadelphia, 1993, WB Saunders.

Pernoll ML: Third-trimester hemorrhage. In DeCherney AH, Pernoll ML, editors: *Current obstetric and gynecologic diagnosis and treatment,* ed 8, Norwalk, Conn, 1994, Appleton & Lange.

SUGGESTED READINGS

Ellsworth A et al: *Mosby's 1998 medical drug reference*, St Louis, 1998, Mosby.

Greene H, Johnson W, Lemcke D, editors: *Decision making in medicine*, ed 2, St Louis, 1998, Mosby.

Kowalski K: No happy ending: pregnancy loss and bereavement, *NAACOG Clin Iss Perinatal Womens Health Nurs* 2(3) 368-380, 1991.

Healthcare Consultants of America, Inc: *1998 physicians fee and coding guide*, Augusta, Ga, 1998, Healthcare Consultants of America, Inc.

Poole JH: Maternal hemorrhagic disorders. In Lowdermilk DL, Perry SE, Bobak IM, editors: *Maternity and women's health care*, St Louis, 1997, Mosby.

Pregnancy Problems: Hypertension in Pregnancy

Pregnancy-induced Hypertension (PIH), Preeclampsia, Toxemia

ICD-9-CM

Preeclampsia, Mild 642.4
Preeclampsia, Severe 642.5

OVERVIEW

Definitions

Preeclampsia

Preeclampsia is a condition of pregnancy characterized by the presence of edema, hypertension, and proteinuria after the 20th week of gestation.

Eclampsia

Eclampsia is the occurrence of seizures in the patient with preeclampsia.

Chronic Hypertension

Chronic hypertension is hypertension that is present in the pregnant patient before conception or before the 20th week of gestation or 42 days postpartum.

Incidence

In the United States, 6% of women develop preeclampsia during their first pregnancy (Mabie and Sibai, 1994). There is a 15% incidence among women of lower socioeconomic status (Knuppel and Drukker, 1993).

Pathophysiology

Protective Factors Against

Unknown; perhaps diet adequate in protein, vitamins, calcium, and magnesium throughout pregnancy

Factors That Increase Susceptibility

Primigravity
Maternal age <18 or >35
Mother or sister with history of PIH
Diabetes
Preeclampsia with a previous pregnancy
Low socioeconomic status
Multiple gestation
Large fetus
Hydatidiform mole
Chronic hypertension
Residence in western or southern United States (Sibai et al., 1995)

Etiology

The cause of preeclampsia is unknown. It is a multisystem disease characterized by vasospasm, resulting in hypertension and decreased blood flow to all organs, including the placenta. The vasospasm causes a fluid shift from intravascular space into the intervascular space, resulting in hypovolemia and increased hematocrit. The cure is delivery of the placenta.

NOTE: When assessing and treating any pregnant patient, the practitioner must bear in mind that two patients are involved, the mother and the fetus.

SUBJECTIVE DATA

History of Present Illness

At every prenatal visit ask about edema of the hands and face upon arising in the morning. This nondependent edema is especially a warning sign if accompanied by hypertension and proteinuria.

Ask about changes in vision, epigastric pain or nausea, or headaches. Visual changes are caused by the cerebral effects of preeclampsia. Ask about dizziness, drowsiness, or confusion. These are warning signs and should be followed up.

Determine gravida and parity.

Determine any previous complications of this pregnancy.

Determine estimated date of delivery.

Ask about prenatal care.

Ask if she is feeling fetal movement.

Past Medical History

Ask about:

- Any complications of previous pregnancies
- A history of hypertension
- Allergies to medications
- Renal or hepatic disease
- Diabetes

Medications

Ask about use of aspirin, prenatal vitamins, calcium, or other vitamin or mineral intake.

Family History

Ask about any history of hypertension in the family, particularly history of PIH for a mother or a sister.

Diet History

Ask about nutritional status both before and during pregnancy, particularly intake of protein, calcium, magnesium, and vitamins.

Description of Most Common Symptoms

Edema of the hands and face on arising in the morning

Visual changes such as blurred vision, seeing flashes of light, blind spots

Headaches

Diplopia

Dizziness

Drowsiness

Nausea and vomiting

Associated Symptoms

Oliguria, confusion, hyperreflexia, epigastric pain, decreased fetal movement

OBJECTIVE DATA

Physical Examination

A complete prenatal assessment should be performed, with particular attention to:

Blood pressure

Because of its damaging effects, hypertension is the most important finding in the diagnosis of preeclampsia. The blood pressure should be taken with the patient seated with her supported arm extended and elevated to the level of her heart. Be sure to use the appropriate-sized cuff.

Blood pressure readings should be compared with prepregnant or first-trimester readings obtained as a baseline (if available). Bear in mind that an increase in diastolic pressure of 15 mm Hg over baseline or an increase in systolic of 30 mm Hg over baseline is ominous—*even if the blood pressure is not 140/90*.

In addition, the mean arterial pressure (MAP) should be calculated by the following formula:

$$\text{MAP} = \frac{(\text{SP} - \text{DP})}{\text{DP} + [3]}$$

A MAP of 105 or greater represents or an increase in MAP of 20 mm Hg represents hypertension (ACOG, 1992).

If a blood pressure elevation is found, the patient must remain in the clinic or return for a repeat blood pressure check 6 hours later (Mabie & Sibai, 1994). *Never take lightly an elevated blood pressure in a pregnant woman.*

PIH can be superimposed on chronic hypertension. Prognosis for the mother and fetus in this case is worse than with either condition alone (Mabie & Sibai, 1994).

Edema: Note location and severity. Dependent edema is a common finding in pregnancy. Weight gain in excess of 2 lbs per week or sudden weight gain over 1 to 2 days is cause for concern (Mabie & Sibai, 1994).

Fetal status: Fetal heart tones (FHTs) should be taken.

Diagnostic Procedures

Although the development of preeclampsia is relatively unpredictable for most women, certain predictive tests show promise (Table 149-1).

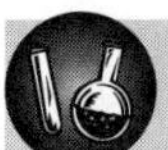

TABLE 149-1 Diagnostic Procedures: Preeclampsia

Diagnostic Test	Finding/Rationale	Cost ($)
Uric acid* concentration	One of the most sensitive indicators; in normal pregnancy, serum urate concentration <4.5 mg/100 ml.	18-23
Creatinine*	Serum creatinine levels >0.8 mg/100 ml should be considered suspicious.	18-24
Serial Hgb and HCT	Since one of the features of preeclampsia is failure of plasma volume expansion, a rising Hgb or HCT is a feature of developing disease.	11-14 repeated
Serial platelet	Platelet consumption is a common feature of preeclampsia, so serial platelet counts are useful in diagnosis and assessing the progression of disease.	14-18 repeated
MAP	A MAP of 85 during the second trimester may be predictive of hypertension during the third trimester (O'Brien, 1992).	N/A
Roll-over test	Some clinicians find the roll-over test useful in women with predisposing factors. It is performed between 28 and 32 weeks' gestation (Knuppel & Drukker, 1993). It is a screening test, and preeclampsia should not be ruled out based on negative results of this test alone. Steps of the procedure are found in Box 149-1.	N/A
Doppler flow velocimetry	Doppler flow velocimetry is being used to monitor blood flow velocity through the uterine artery and the umbilical artery at 22-24 weeks' gestation (Liberati et al., 1997). A systolic/diastolic ratio >3 is abnormal.	524-536
Proteinuria	This is the last sign of preeclampsia to develop and indicates fetal jeopardy. Obtain a clean-catch specimen and complete a reading by dipstick. A reading of 1+ is significant. If proteinuria is present, patient should remain in or return to the clinic for another reading 6 hours later.	15-20
24-Hour urine for proteinuria	Quantifies proteinuria.	21-26

*Lower values than upper limit of normal for nonpregnant women. READINGS WILL NOT APPEAR AS ABNORMAL ON LABORATORY RESULTS.
Hct, Hematocrit; *Hgb,* hemoglobin; *N/A,* not available.

ASSESSMENT

Differential diagnoses include transient hypertension, PIH, chronic hypertension, PIH superimposed on chronic hypertension (Table 149-2).

Box 149-1

Steps of the Roll-over Test

Step 1: Measure the patient's blood pressure in the left lateral position.
Step 2: Leaving the cuff in place, roll the patient to the supine position.
Step 3: Immediately retake the blood pressure. Have the patient remain supine.*
Step 4: Retake the blood pressure in 5 minutes.

Results

Positive increase of ≥20 mm Hg at the 5-minute reading
Negative increase of <20 mm Hg at the 5-minute reading

*A wedge may be placed under the patient's right hip to prevent vena cava syndrome.

THERAPEUTIC PLAN

Pharmaceutical

Nurse practitioners will be involved with the care of mild preeclamptics only. Mild preeclamptics receive no medication except prenatal vitamins.

One baby aspirin per day may prevent PIH in women with risk factors. This preventive measure should not be instituted without an MD consult because aspirin has been associated with premature closure of the ductus arteriosus (Mabie & Sibai, 1994).

Patient Education

After referral to the MD if the patient is placed on home care for mild preeclampsia, the nurse practitioner is uniquely qualified to educate and monitor her.

Bed rest in left lateral position; up only for eating and bathroom
Dipstick urine for protein; report 1+ reading
Be sure she knows how to read the dipstick
Nutrition: No added salt, but no need to avoid sodium

TABLE 149-2 Differential Diagnosis: Hypertension in Pregnancy

Diagnoses	Supporting Data
Transient hypertension	Single occurrence of blood pressure elevation after 20 weeks' gestation or within 24 hours postpartum; no nondependent edema or proteinuria
PIH	Hypertension occurring after 20 weeks' gestation with no history of hypertension; usually occurs with edema and proteinuria
Chronic hypertension	Hypertension present before 20 weeks, gestation without non-dependent edema or proteinuria
PIH superimposed on chronic hypertension	Hypertension present before 20 weeks' compounded by signs of PIH after 20 weeks' gestation
HELLP syndrome	A syndrome consisting of the following: hemolysis, elevated liver (enzymes), low platelets

altogether; include foods high in fiber, 60 to 70 g of protein, 1200 mg calcium, 8 to 10 glasses of water per day (Palmer, 1997)

Fetal status: Fetal kick counts should be done after a meal for 1 hour every day; patient should report any decrease in fetal movement immediately

Daily weight: Weigh in same clothes at same time every day

Scheduled appointments: Keeping appointments is important to allow her to remain at home and still monitor her status and that of the fetus

It is important to explain that the course of this disease is unpredictable; patient may be able to avoid hospitalization or she may not; management is aimed at preventing the worsening of the condition; she needs to understand that even if she feels better, she is not cured until delivery has occurred

Family Impact

Bed rest is difficult. It is important that the patient have support persons to provide transportation, prepare meals, and care for the house and other children.

Referral

The detection of hypertension in pregnancy calls for immediate referral to an MD (OB/GYN).

Consultation

A dietitian should be called to assist the patient with meal planning at home.

A social service consult may be needed if the patient cannot afford help in the home or does not have family support.

Follow-up

All patients should be followed closely until 6 weeks postpartum or until chronic hypertension is brought under control postpartum.

EVALUATION

A return to baseline blood pressure or control of chronic hypertension signifies resolution. Blood pressure should be monitored until it remains within acceptable range.

REFERENCES

American College of Obstetricians and Gynecologists: Invasive hemodynamic monitoring in obstetrics and gynecology, *Int J Gynaecol Obstet* 42(2):199-205, 1993.

Knuppel RA, Drukker JE: Hypertension in pregnancy. In Knuppel, RA, Drukker JE, editors: *High-risk pregnancy: a team approach,* ed 2, Philadelphia, 1993, WB Saunders.

Liberati M et al: Uterine artery Doppler velocimetry in pregnant women with lateral placentas, *J Perinatal Med* 25(2):133-138, 1997.

Mabie WC, Sibai BM: Hypertensive states of pregnancy. In DeCherney AH, Pernoll ML, editors: *Current obstetrics and gynecologic diagnosis and treatment,* Norwalk, 1994, Appleton & Lange.

O'Brien WF: The prediction of preeclampsia, *Clin Obstet Gynecol* 35:351-364, 1992.

Palmer DG: Hypertensive disorders in pregnancy. In Lowdermillk DL, Perry SE, Bobak IM, editors: *Maternity and women's health care,* ed 6, St Louis, 1997, Mosby.

Sibai BM et al: Risk factors for preeclampsia in healthy nulliparous women: a prospective multicenter study, *Am J Obstet Gynecol* 172:642-648, 1995.

SUGGESTED READINGS

Ellsworth A et al: *Mosby's 1998 Medical drug reference,* St. Louis, 1998, Mosby.

Healthcare Consultants of America, Inc: *1998 Physicians fee and coding guide,* Augusta, Ga, 1998, Healthcare Consultants of America, Inc.

150 Premenstrual Syndrome

ICD-9-CM

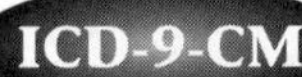

Premenstrual Syndrome 525.4

OVERVIEW

Definition

Premenstrual syndrome (PMS) is defined as periodic recurrence of a combination of annoying, unpleasant, often distressing physical, psychological, and behavioral symptoms that occur in the second half (premenstrual or luteal phase) of the menstrual cycle and persist not more than 4 days after the onset of menses. When present, symptoms interfere with the woman's activities of daily life, work, and relationships. The hallmark feature is presence of a minimum 7-day symptom-free interval in the first ½ of the cycle.

Incidence

Recurring premenstrual symptoms are almost universal among women who ovulate. For 20% to 40%, symptoms are severe enough to disrupt life and require medical intervention; 5% suffer debilitating symptoms.

Peak incidence: 26 to 35 years old. May occur from age 20 to 50. Rare in teens. Does not occur before puberty or after menopause.

Pathophysiology

The exact cause is unknown. Numerous causative theories have been proposed, including various hormonal imbalances, exaggerated response to prostaglandin, various nutritional imbalances, fluid retention, disorders in endorphin levels, and abnormal serotonin levels.

Pathophysiology likely involves three interrelated factors: (1) abnormal levels of CNS neurotransmitters; (2) ovulation as a precipitating event; and (3) individual perceptions and interpretations of and reactions to PMS symptoms.

Protective Factors Against

Being of prepuberty age
Postmenopausal state, whether surgical, medically induced, or natural
Anovulatory state
Pregnancy
Regular exercise

Factors That Increase Susceptibility

Being of reproductive age
Ovulatory cycles
Increased parity
Stressful lifestyle, especially in preceding year
Dysfunctional family of origin
Associated factors: History of depression (including that postpartum) and/or history of migraines

SUBJECTIVE DATA

More than 100 PMS symptoms have been reported. Clusters of complaints are characteristic; if a woman presents with an isolated premenstrual complaint, a different diagnosis must be considered. Box 150-1 presents a list of common complaints.

History of Present Illness

Symptoms are best assessed with a daily symptom diary, calendar, or checklist for a minimum of two cycles. Retrospective recall is less accurate, with a tendency to overestimate.

Several preprinted checklists are available (Moo's Menstrual Distress, Vargyas' Premenstrual Syndrome Symptomatology), but an open-ended diary using a point scale (0 = none; 1 = mild; 2 = moderate; 3 = severe/extreme) works equally well.

Having the woman list and prioritize the most bothersome symptoms allows an optimal management plan.

Self-diagnosis is common. If this is the case, ask the patient what made her draw the conclusion that she is experiencing PMS.

Box 150-1

Most Common Complaints

Most Common Physical Complaints*	Most Common Psychological/Behavioral Complaints*
Bloating/weight gain	Irritability
Breast tenderness	Depression
Headache	Emotional liability
Skin changes, including acne	Tension and anxiety; "keyed up"; "on edge"
Pelvic pain	Aggressiveness
Change in bowel habits	Social withdrawal
Fatigue; marked lack of energy	Accident proneness/poor coordination
Joint pain	Loss of control; feeling overwhelmed
Insomnia	Change in sexual desire/libido
Change in appetite	Decrease interest in usual activities
Hot flashes	Difficulty concentrating

*The character of complaints is less important than timing pattern: Are they worse premenstrually with absence of symptoms or improvement after menses?

Ask when she first experienced these physical, psychological, and/or behavioral symptoms.
Ask how symptoms vary throughout the menstrual cycle.

Past Medical History

Ask about:
- History of chronic illness, noting any effects of PMS on the illness
- Lupus, fibrocystic disease, thyroid disease, and chronic fatigue syndrome, which may mimic PMS
- History of psychiatric illness, hospitalization, drug treatment, psychotherapy
- Previous surgery
- Drug and/or other allergies
- Conduct detailed menstrual history: menarche, LMP, dysmenorrhea, frequency, duration, flow
- Obstetrical history
- Postpartum depression

Note current and past contraceptive use and any relationship to symptoms

Medications

Note current use of prescription or over-the-counter (OTC) medications, including those for menstrual-related symptoms. (Some OTC drugs for relief of premenstrual symptoms contain caffeine, which can exacerbate PMS.)

Family History

Ask about:
- First-degree relatives with PMS
- Family history of psychiatric illness

Psychosocial History

Ask about a typical day and stress level. Determine how this varies throughout the menstrual cycle.
Ask how symptoms affect work or school, leisure, and relationships.
Ask about use of alcohol, tobacco, or street drugs.
Determine how significant others have responded to diagnosis, if applicable. (Remember that PMS diagnosis is controversial and sometimes discounted by others, including health care professionals. For some, diagnosis is stigmatizing. For those reasons, the syndrome should be validated and treated seriously by the nurse practitioner.)

Diet History

Ask about food cravings
Use dietary recall to determine fat, refined sugar, sodium, and caffeine intake, especially on days of PMS symptoms

OBJECTIVE DATA

Physical Examination

There are no characteristic physical findings associated with PMS.
Problem-oriented physical examination should be performed, with attention to symptom-related clusters, vital signs, weight and presence of edema, skin, heart, thyroid, breasts, abdomen, and pelvis.

Diagnostic Procedures

There is no single test diagnostic for PMS since no physiologic or biochemical factors are consistently altered. Laboratory tests may be ordered on the basis of individual symptoms or to rule out organic causes of symptoms or additional problems.

ASSESSMENT

PMS is a diagnosis of exclusion. History and physical examination must be directed to answering two questions: (1) Does she ovulate? (2) Do these complaints suggest some other disorder that explains the entire clinical picture or exacerbates PMS?

Differential diagnoses include chronic illness with exacerbation related to menstrual cycle, acute illness with coincidental occurrence during luteal phase of menstrual cycle, psychiatric illness; marital discord, social or family distress, chemical abuse, and sexual abuse.

THERAPEUTIC PLAN

Pharmaceutical

No drug has been approved by Food and Drug Administration for treatment of PMS. Medications may be ordered to relieve target symptoms when self-help strategies are not successful. Table 150-1 describes pharmaceutical treatment.

Suppression of ovulation prevents PMS. Oral contraceptives (OCPs) may be used for this purpose, particularly in women needing contraception. Other hormones used for ovulation suppression are reserved for nonresponsive cases and implemented in consultation with a physician. Table 150-2 contains a list of these OCPs.

Other drugs used for PMS on basis of anecdotal reports from patients; randomized clinical trials are lacking or conflicting:

- Pyriodoxine (vitamin B_6): 50 mg/day during luteal phase. CAUTION: >100 mg/day may cause peripheral neuropathy.
- Vitamin E: 400 IU/day luteal phase
- Magnesium: 100 to 250 mg/day luteal phase, increase water intake.
- Evening primrose oil (gamma linoleic acid): 500 mg TID luteal phase
- Calcium 100 mg luteal phase

Lifestyle/Activities

Teach record keeping system with menstrual-symptom diary, checklist, or calendar. Being actively involved in management is sometimes therapeutic. (See patient handout on p. 924.)

Help see predictable timing of symptoms to enable planning for stress reduction and scheduling difficult situations at work or in personal life for symptom-free intervals as much as possible. (This decreases patient's sense of vulnerability and increases her sense of control.)

Recommend regular aerobic exercise like walking, running, swimming, biking; encourage exercise she is likely to do regularly.

Role play, asserting needs and dealing with difficult situations.

Diet

Suggest these dietary changes especially during premenstrual phase:

- Frequent small meals low calorie, high complex carbohydrates, low fat, low refined sugar, minimal sodium
- Low caffeine intake
- Limited alcohol intake
- Multivitamin daily

Patient Education

PMS is treated symptomatically.

Encourage use of self-help strategies in managing the target symptoms of PMS (Table 150-3).

Discourage placing blame for all negative circumstances on PMS to avoid perpetual victim role.

Educate about illness and the relationship with menstrual cycle.

Family Impact

For the 7 to 14 days each month that the woman experiences PMS symptoms, the impact on home maintenance, marital interaction, and parenting may be quite negative and disruptive. Conversation with the partner or other family members can provide opportunities for education and for gaining insight into the level of understanding and family support available.

Referral

PMS support groups

Marriage or family therapy as needed

Assertiveness training, as needed

Psychotherapy, if indicated

Consultation

Lack of responsiveness to therapy

Need for ovulation suppression beyond OCPs

Follow-up

Most women with PMS require treatment for at least 2 years. With self-help strategies and NSAID therapy, follow up for three cycles then annually.

EVALUATION

Several different regimens may be necessary before optimal treatment is identified. The treatment regimen should be evaluated throughout three cycles before being modified unless it obviously exacerbates symptoms or is otherwise not tolerated.

RESOURCES

Drjamesmd.hypermart.net

Patient education handout: http://omni.AC.UK/UMLS/detail/C0033046.html

His and her PMS calendar: www.coolpress.com

www.pms.com

Link to multiple sites: www.pmsing-woman.com/pms.html

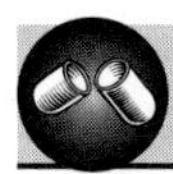

TABLE 150-1 Symptomatic Treatment for Premenstrual Syndrome

Target Symptoms	Drug of Choice	Dose	Clinical Implications	Cost
Anxiety/ irritability	Alprazolam (Xanax)	0.25 mg PO q6h to q8h during luteal phase	Pregnancy: D Dependence with continued use Caution with CYP450 inhibitors SE: CNS depression, drowsiness, headache, ataxia, withdrawal seizures	$5-$66/0.25 mg (100); $6-$80/0.5 mg (100); $57/5 mg (100); $100/10 mg (100)
Breast tenderness (mastalgia)	Danazol	200 mg/day initially; then 100 mg/day with clinical response × 2 mo; convert to luteal phase regimen 100 mg/day day 14-28 after 4 months	Only drug FDA approved Androgenic SE: Hirsutism, weight gain, acne, menstrual irregularities, headaches, and nausea	$177/100 mg (100)
	Bromocriptine (Parlodel)	2.5 mg PO QD during luteal phase	Tabs may be given vaginally if PO dose causes nausea SE: Hypotension, headache, syncope	$108-$158/ 2.5 mg (100)
	Tamoxifen (Nolvadex)	10-20 mg QD	Pregnancy: D SE: Hot flashes, vaginal discharge, irregular menses, GI upset	$85-$90/10 mg (60)
Depression/ mood liability	Buspirone (BuSpar) or	5 mg PO q12h luteal or continuous	Pregnancy: B May need to increase dose to 40-60 mg/day SE: Dizziness, nausea, headache, dream disturbance, tinnitus, sore throat, nasal congestion	$57/5 mg (100); $100/10 mg (100)
	Fluoxetine (Prozac)	20-40 mg PO QD in AM	Pregnancy: B CYP450 interactions SE: CNS stimulation, insomnia, somnolence, anorexia, decreased libido	
Fluid Retention/ weight gain	Spironolactone (Aldactone)	50-100 mg QD luteal phase	Potassium-sparing mild diuretic; lower risk of rebound edema Also may relieve mastalgia	$5-$39/25 mg (100); $71/50 mg (100); $119/100 mg (100)
Headache, joint pain	Ibuprofen or Naproxen (Naprosyn)	300-800 mg PO QID PRN 250-500 mg PO q12h PRN	Caution: GI side effects Pregnancy: B (D third trimester)	$3-$9/200 mg (100)

Consultation with MD concerning these drugs is appropriate
CNS, Central nervous system; *FDA*, Food and Drug Administration; *GI*, gastrointestinal; *SE*, side effects.

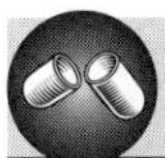

TABLE 150-2 Oral Contraceptives for Premenstrual Syndrome

Drug	Dose	Comments	Cost ($)
Low-dose estrogen: Transdermal estradiol plus cyclic progesterone to induce withdrawal (i.e., Norlutate 5 mg for 7-10 days each month)	0.2 mg daily day 26 of cycle through menstrual flow (7 days total) Use two 0.1-mg patches simultaneously	Does not interfere with menses; minimal side effects; progestin minimizes risk Pregnancy: X SE: Increased risk of endometrial cancer or hyperplasia, fluid retention, BTB, increased size of uterine fibroids	14-40/pack
Luprolide (Lupron) GnRH agonist	3.75 mg IM monthly	Causes hypoestrogen state with inherent risk of CHD and osteoporosis; 6-month maximum use Pregnancy: X SE: Hot flashes, vaginitis, depression, decreased libido, gastrointestinal upset	Not available
Danazol (synthetic steroid with androgenic activity)	200-400 mg QD luteal phase or continuous	Causes adverse effects on lipids; monitor lipid profile Pregnancy: X SE: See Table 150-1	See Table 150-1

BTB, Breakthrough bleeding; *CHD,* coronary heart disease; *IM,* intramuscularly; *SE,* side effects.

TABLE 150-3 Self-help Strategies

Target Symptom	Self-Help Measures
Anxiety/irritability	Stress reduction Yoga Paced breathing/relaxation exercises/guided imagery Frequent aerobic exercise
Breast tenderness	Supportive brassiere Reduced caffeine Reduced sodium intake
Depression	Exercise Alteration of circadian rhythm —bright light exposure in evening —decrease sleep early luteal phase
Sleep disruption	Regular pattern of sleep Avoiding stimulants (diet or activity) before bedtime Warm milk Warm bath If insomnia occurs, get out of bed until feels sleepy

SUGGESTED READINGS

Altshuler LL, Hendrick V, Parry B: Pharmacological management of premenstrual disorder, *Harvard Rev Psychiatry* 2(5):233-245, 1995.

Carter J, Verhoef MJ: Efficacy of self-help and alternative treatment of premenstrual syndrome, *Women's Health Institute* 4(3):130-136, 1994.

Chuong CJ, Pearsall-Otey LR, Rosenfeld BL: A practical guide to relieving PMS, *Contemp Nurse Pract* 1:31-37, 1995.

DeCherney AH, Pernoll ML: *Current obstetric and gynecologic diagnosis and treatment*, Norwalk, Conn, 1994, Appleton & Lange.

Endicott J, Johnson SR, Keye WR: Helping the patient with PM, *Patient Care* 24(3)44-48, 55-58, 63, 66-68, 75, 82, 1990.

Hawkins JW, Roberto EM, Stanley-Haney JL: *Protocols for nurse practitioners in gynecologic setting,* New York, 1994, Tiresias.

Hendrick V, Altshuler LL, Burt VK: Course of psychiatric disorders across the menstrual cycle, *Harvard Rev Psychiatry* 4(4):200-207, 1996.

Palmer DG: Hypertensive disorders in pregnancy. In Lowdermillk DL, Perry SE, Bobak IM, editors: *Maternity and women's health care,* ed 6, St Louis, 1997, Mosby.

Hsia LS, Long MH: Premenstrual syndrome: current concepts in diagnosis and management, *J Nurse Midwifery* 35(6):351-353, 1990.

Johnson SR: Clinician's approach to the diagnosis and management of premenstrual syndrome, *Clin Obstet Gyncol* 35(3):637-657, 1992.

Lemke DP et al: *Primary care of women,* Norwalk, Conn, 1995, Appleton & Lange.

Lindow KB: (1991). Premenstrual syndrome: family impact and nursing implications. *J Obstet Gynecol Neonatal Nurs* 20(2):135-138, 1991.

Mastrangelo R: Taming the beast known as PMS, *Adv Nurse Pract* 2:11-14, 1994.

Rubinow DR, Schmidt PJ: The treatment of premenstrual syndrome: forward into the past, *N Engl J Med* 332(23):1574-1575, 1995.

Smith, RP: *Gynecology in primary care,* Baltimore, 1997, Williams & Wilkins.

Star WL, Lommel LL, Shannon MT: *Women's primary health care: protocols for practice,* Washington, DC, 1995, American Nurses Publishing.

Taylor DL: Evaluating therapeutic change in symptom severity at the level of individual women experiencing severe PMS, *Image: J Nurs Scholarship,* 26(1):25-33, 1994.

Youngkin EQ, Davis MS: *Women's health: a primary care clinical guide,* Norwalk, Conn, 1994, Appleton & Lange.

Premenstrual Syndrome Record
of

____
Woman's Name

Instructions: Record information for each day of your menstrual cycle for 3 cycles to help in the diagnosis of premenstrual syndrome (PMS).

Rating Scale: 0 No symptoms today
1 Mild symptoms that do not interfere with daily activities or relationships
2 Moderate symptoms that somewhat interfere with daily activities/relationships
3 Severe symptoms that interfere a lot with daily activities/relationships

Day of cycle	1*	2	3	4	5	6	7	8	9	10	11	12	13	14	15	16	17	18	19	20	21	22	23	24	25	26	27	28	29	30	31	32	33
Date																																	
Most Bothersome Symptoms																																	

*First Day of Menstrual Period

Prostate Problems

ICD-9-CM

Prostatitis 601.9
Benign Prostatic Hyperplasia 236.5
Prostate Cancer 185

OVERVIEW

Definition

Acute bacterial prostatitis is an infection usually caused by gram-negative rods and, less commonly, gram-positive organisms such as enterococcus. The signs and symptoms include fever, irritative voiding symptoms (frequency, nocturia, urgency), perineal or suprapubic pain, exquisitely tender prostate on physical examination, and positive culture.

Chronic bacterial prostatitis is an infectious process that may evolve from acute bacterial prostatitis, but not always. Gram-negative rods are the most common etiologic agent, and only one gram-negative rod, enterococcus, is associated with chronic infection.

Benign prostatic hypertrophy or *hyperplasia (BPH)* is defined as urinary outflow obstruction with decreased force/caliber of urinary stream, nocturia, sensation of incomplete emptying, hesitancy, frequency, urgency, and high post-void residual.

Prostate cancer is a malignant neoplasm of the prostate gland.

Incidence

Prostatitis is the most important cause of urinary tract infections in men. Both acute and chronic prostatitis can occur in men of any age, but is not seen in children.

Benign prostatic hypertrophy affects **one in every four men by age 80** in the United States. Symptoms are unusual before age 50. Symptomatology is reported in nearly half of the men 50 to 64 years old in the general population.

Prostate cancer has overtaken lung and colon cancers to be the most common cancer in males, comprising 21% of all newly discovered cancers in males. The lifetime probability that a man will have prostate cancer is between 6% to 9%, but the probability of death from prostate cancer is approximately 2%.

Pathophysiology

Prostatitis is most likely caused by ascending urethral infection, reflux of infected urine, extension of rectal infection, or hematogenous spread.

The causes of benign prostatic hypertrophy are not fully understood; the disorder is associated with two factors: male sex and increasing age. The etiology of age-related hyperplasia is unknown, although is thought to be related to androgenic changes at the cellular level. The earliest changes of BPH occur in the periurethral glands, with nodular hyperplasia. As these nodules grow and coalesce over the years, true prostatic tissue is compressed outward. As the gland enlarges, urethral resistance to urine flow increases, and muscular hypertrophy of the bladder ensues.

Prostate cancer incidence increases with age, and African-Americans have a threefold higher incidence; however, there is no clear cut etiologic relationship to environment, socioeconomic status, fertility, or endogenous androgen level. Regional differences do exist and may reflect unknown environmental factors or variation in detection methods.

Protective Factors Against

Prostatitis
Children/adolescents
Benign prostatic hypertrophy
Young age
Prostate cancer
White/Asian
Young age

Factors that Increase Susceptibility

Prostatitis
Advancing age
Prior history of prostatitis
Benign prostatic hypertrophy
Advancing age
Prostate cancer
Black
Advancing age

Common Pathogens

Gram-negative rods such as *Escherichia coli* are the most common; others are *Klebsiella* or *Pseudomonas*

A gram-positive rod, enterococcus, is often associated with chronic infection

SUBJECTIVE DATA

History of Present Illness/Most Common Symptoms

Acute Bacterial Prostatitis

Symptoms occur acutely; if symptoms are not acute, must consider alternate diagnosis. Symptoms include fever, urgency, nocturia, perineal, or suprapubic pain. May also experience low back pain and fatigue.

Elderly: May be asymptomatic.

Chronic Bacterial Prostatitis

Symptoms occur less acutely or after episode of acute bacterial prostatitis. Symptoms include fever, nocturia, frequency, perineal, or suprapubic pain, which is often dull and poorly localized.

Elderly: May be asymptomatic.

Benign Prostatic Hypertrophy

Symptoms may occur over a number of years. Symptoms include decreased force and caliber of stream, nocturia, feeling of incomplete emptying, hesitancy, and dribbling.

Elderly: Symptoms may be more pronounced.

Prostate Cancer

Symptoms may occur over a period of months until noticeable. Symptoms include hesitancy, frequency, nocturia, decreased force and caliber of stream, urge incontinence.

Elderly: Symptoms are more likely to be present.

Past Medical History

Ask about history of previous episode(s) of prostatitis, family history for prostatic disease(s), medication history, sexual history (sexually transmitted disease [STD]), delayed sexual drive, early cessation of sexuality, smoking, high-fat diet.

Medications

Use of decongestants, antidepressants, antihypertensives, anticholinergics.

Family History

Ask about family history of prostate/urinary diseases.

Psychosocial History

In considering prostate cancer especially, ask about multiple sexual partners and multiple STDs.

Diet History

Ask about the amount of fat in the diet.

Associated Symptoms

With acute bacterial prostatitis, may have occasional hematuria, penile tip pain, pain with bowel movements.

With chronic prostatitis, may also experience hematospermia or painful ejaculation.

With prostate cancer, 20% of men may present with symptoms of metastatic cancer such as spinal/bone pain and gross hematuria.

OBJECTIVE DATA

Physical Examination

A problem oriented approach should be conducted, paying particular attention to:

Vital signs, weight, general appearance, hydration. Given the wide variety of presentations in patients with BPH, a complete physical examination may be necessary.

Abdomen: Check for distended bladder, abdominal pain.

Musculoskeletal: Check for pain in back with range of motion or palpation.

Genital/rectal: Perform examination of external genitalia. Assess for prostate tenderness, enlargement, or nodules.

Diagnostic Procedures

Based on presentation of symptoms and/or age

Elderly: May choose to be more aggressive in testing because of increased risk for both BPH and prostate cancer

For diagnostic procedures, see Table 151-1 and Figures 151-1 to 151-3.

Acute/Chronic Bacterial Prostatitis

First line: Segmented urine cultures (urines representing urethral, bladder, and postprostatic massage)

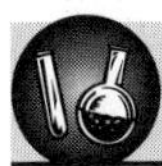

TABLE 151-1 Diagnostic Procedures: Prostate

Symptoms	Findings	Diagnostic Tests	Costs ($)
Acute Bacterial Prostatitis			
Acute onset fever, urgency, nocturia, frequency	Fever, perineal, suprapubic, or sacral pain, warm and tender prostate	Segmented urine cultures Complete blood count; expressed prostatic excretions	31-39 13-16
Chronic Bacterial Prostatitis			
Above symptoms occur less acutely or recurrently or after episode of acute bacterial prostatitis	Poorly localized perineal, scrotal, or lower back pain, enlarged prostate with varying degrees of tenderness, bogginess, and asymmetry	Same as for acute bacterial prostatitis	Same as acute bacterial prostatitis
Benign Prostatic Hypertrophy			
Dribbling, nocturia, urgency hesitancy, feeling of incomplete emptying bladder	Focal or uniformly enlarged and nontender prostate, residual urine >100 ml, examination of abdomen may reveal distended bladder	Urinalysis Post-void residual	14-18
Prostate Cancer			
Hesitancy, frequency, nocturia, decreased force and caliber of stream, urge incontinence; perhaps gross hematuria	Indurated prostate Elevated PSA	DRE PSA Basic metabolic panel Acid phosphatase	64-81 28-39 30-38

DRE, Digital rectal examination; *PSA,* prostate specific antigen.

Second line: Complete blood count

Third line: Expressed prostatic secretions (obtained as a result of prostatic massage and usually obtained by specialist due to chance of bacteremia)

BPH

First line: Digital rectal examination (DRE)

Second line: Urinalysis

Third line: Post-void residual/urinalysis by catheterization

Prostate Cancer

First line: DRE, Prostate-specific antigen

Second line: Renal functions, acid phosphatase

Third line: Post-void urine residual/urinalysis by catheterization

ASSESSMENT

Differential diagnoses include *nonbacterial prostatitis, prostatodynia (myalgia of pelvic floor), STD, urethral stricture,* acquired or congenital bladder neck contracture, *chronic urethritis, pyelonephritis, acute diverticulitis* (Table 151-2).

THERAPEUTIC PLAN

Pharmaceutical

The choice of antibiotic therapy for acute and/or chronic prostatitis is the same; however, chronic prostatitis is treated for at least 12 weeks in contrast to the 14 to 30 days for acute prostatitis. Therapy for BPH includes consideration of antiandrogens and alpha-adrenergic antagonists. Treatment for prostate cancer for nurse practitioners includes immediate referral (Table 151-3).

Nonpharmacological treatment for BPH can include herbal therapy: saw palmetto, 80 mg BID for 8 weeks (up to 160 mg of the lipophilic [fat-soluble] extract BID); vitamin B_6 (500-1000 mg/QD); zinc (50-100 mg/QD). If zinc is taken for more than a month, copper (1 to 2 mg/QD) should be added as zinc depletes the body's stores of copper.

Lifestyle/Activities

Acute and/or chronic bacterial prostatitis can cause men to feel fatigued and acutely ill. Should seek early intervention.

BPH symptoms may cause men to feel as if they cannot

Text continued on p. 933

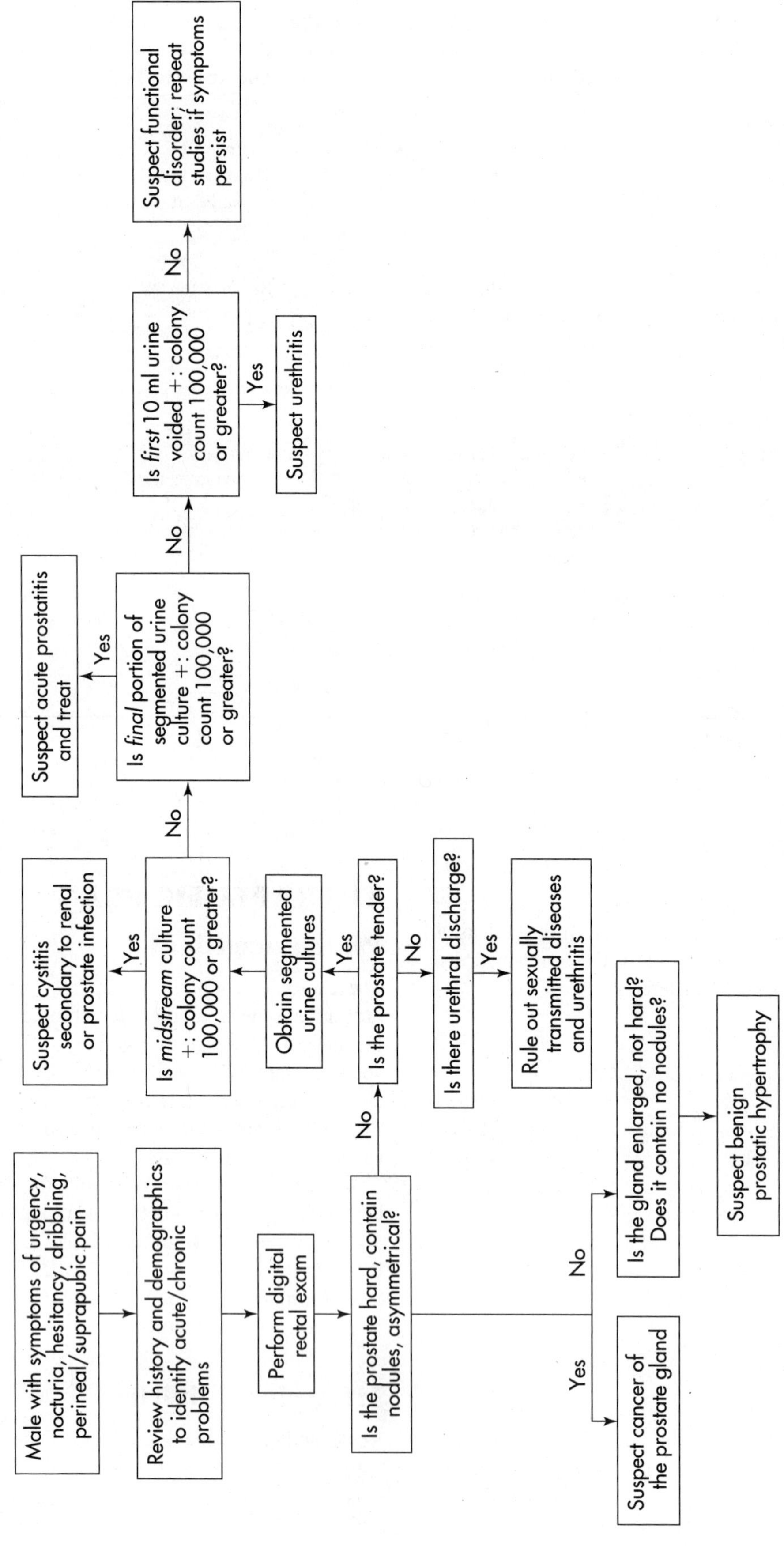

Figure 151-1 Differentiation of prostate symptoms in an adult male.

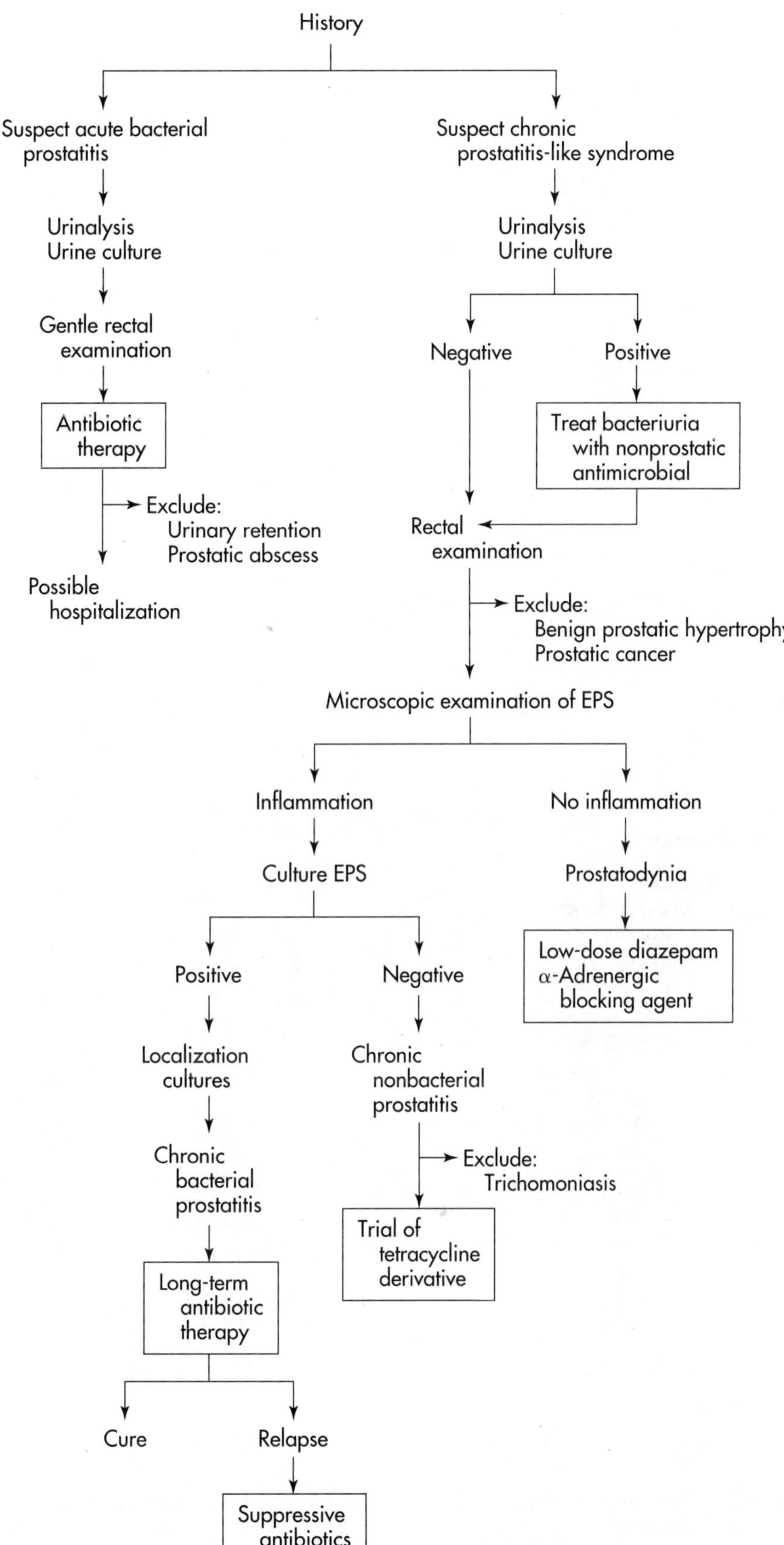

Figure 151-2 Algorithm for suspected prostatitis. *EPS,* Expressed prostatic secretion. (Adapted from Greene HL, Johnson WP, Lemcke D: *Decision making in medicine,* ed 2, St Louis, 1998, Mosby.)

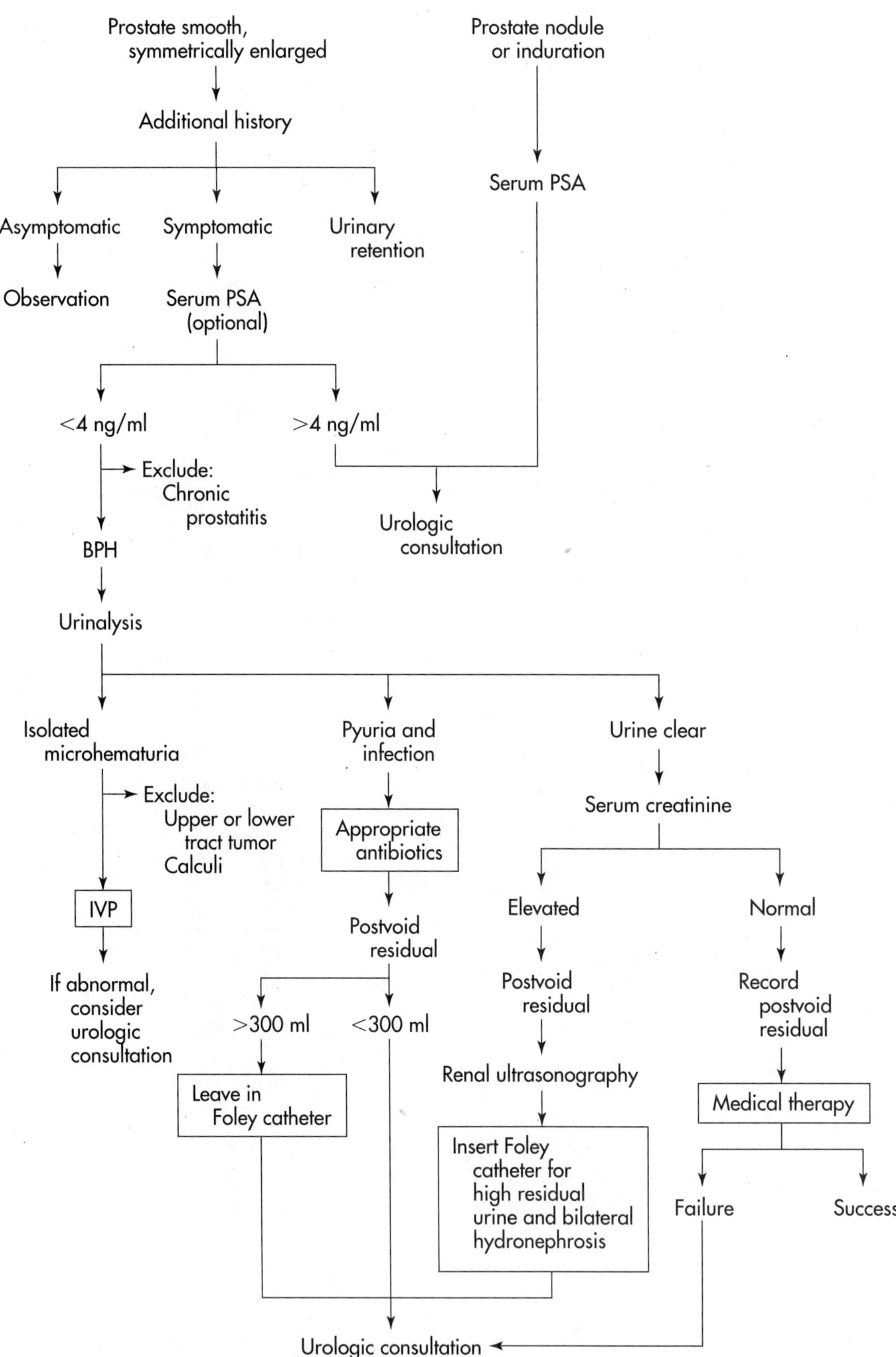

Figure 151-3 Algorithm for abnormal digital rectal examination. *BPH,* Benign prostatic hypertrophy; *IVP,* intravenous pyelography; *PSA,* prostate-specific antigen. (Adapted from Greene HL, Johnson WP, Lemcke D: *Decision making in medicine,* ed 2, St Louis, 1998, Mosby.)

TABLE 151-2 Differential Diagnosis: Prostate Problems

Diagnoses	Supporting Data
Nonbacterial prostatitis	Negative segmented urine cultures; EPS reveals increased leukocytes; most common prostatitis syndrome and is diagnosis of exclusion
Prostatodynia	Negative segmented urine cultures; EPS normal; if urodynamic tests done, may show spasms of urinary sphincter, high urethral pressure, and detrusor contraction without urethral relaxation
STDs	Sexually active, dysuria, penile discharge; by DNA probe
Urethral stricture	Initially minor slowness of stream; then frequent voiding of small amounts followed by chronic distention and overflow incontinence
Chronic urethritis	Sexually active; negative GC and chlamydia DNA probes; negative segmented urine cultures revealing tetracycline-resistant strains of *Ureaplasma urealyticum*
Pyelonephritis	Flank pain, fever with shaking chills, tachycardia, CVA tenderness UA: Pyuria, white cell casts, hematuria CBC: Leukocytosis with left shift
Acute diverticulitis	Acute abdominal pain, LLQ pain, fever, LLQ mass, N/V frequent, low-grade fever, positive stool occult blood

CBC, Complete blood count; *CVA,* costovertebral angle; *DNA,* deoxyribonucleic acid; *EPS,* expressed prostatic secretions; *GC,* gonorrhea culture; *LLQ,* left lower quadrant; *N/V,* nausea and vomiting; *STD,* sexually transmitted disease; *UA,* urinalysis.

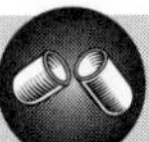

TABLE 151-3 Pharmaceutical Treatment: Prostate Problems

Drug	Adult Dose	Cost ($)	Prophylaxis
For Acute and Chronic Prostatitis			
Trimethoprim-sulfamethoxazole (TMP-SMZ)	160/800 mg (1 double strength tablet) BID ×14-30 days (chronic: for at least 12 weeks)	9-121	80/400 mg HS indefinitely
Norfloxacin (Noroxin)	400 mg BID ×14-30 days (chronic: for at least 12 weeks)	57	400 mg HS indefinitely
Ciprofloxacin (Cipro)	750 mg BID 14-30 days (chronic: 250-500 mg for at least 12 weeks)	572	Ciprofloxacin 250-500 mg HS indefinitely
Ofloxacin (Floxacin)	300-400 mg BID 14-30 days (chronic: for at least 12 weeks)	366-384	300-400 mg hs indefinitely
Cephalexin (does not concentrate as well in the prostate as other medications)	500 mg BID 14-30 days	31-253	
Amoxicillin	500 mg BID 14-30 days	17-49	
Doxycycline	100 mg BID 14-30 days	6-177	
Erythromycin	25-500 mg 14-30 days	22-41	250-500 mg hs indefinitely
For Prostate Cancer			
Leuprolide (Lupron)	1 mg SQ QD or IM depot 7.5-mg dose q mo	278-496	
Flutamide (Euflex)	250 mg q8h	269	
For BPH*			
Finasteride (Proscar)	5 mg QD	195	5 mg QD
Prazosin (minipress)†	Initially 1 mg HS; if dosage >2 mg, give in divided doses	6-48	1-20 mg QD
Doxazocin (Cardura)†	Initially, 1 mg HS; may increase to 8 mg QD	89	1-8 mg QD
Tamulosin (Flomax) (may take few months before clinical benefits are experienced)	Initially 0.4 mg QD 30 minutes after the same meal daily	Not available	Can increase to 0.8 mg after 2-4 weeks if needed
Terazosin (Hytrin)†	Initially 1 mg HS; may increased to 10 mg QD	136	1-10 mg QD, 10 mg is usually required for adequate response

*All drugs used to treat BPH cause postural hypotension. Geriatric patients are more sensitive to this side effect.

†Peripheral alpha blockers. Slowly titrate to avoid side effects. Usually immediate clinical effects.

TABLE 151-4 American Urological Association Symptom Index

	AUA Symptom Score (Circle 1 Number on Each Line)					
Questions To Be Answered	**Not At All**	**Less Than 1 Time in 5**	**Less Than Half the Time**	**About Half the Time**	**More Than Half the Time**	**Almost Always**
1. Over the past month, how often have you had a sensation of not emptying your bladder completely after you finished urinating?	0	1	2	3	4	5
2. Over the past month, how often have you had to urinate again less than 2 hours after you finished urinating?	0	1	2	3	4	5
3. Over the past month, how often have you found you stopped and started again several times when you urinated?	0	1	2	3	4	5
4. Over the past month, how often have you found it difficult to postpone urination?	0	1	2	3	4	5
5. Over the past month, how often have you had a weak urinary stream?	0	1	2	3	4	5
6. Over the past month, how often have you had to push or strain to begin urination?	0	1	2	3	4	5
7. Over the past month, how many times did you most typically get up to urinate from the time you went to bed at night until the time you got up in the morning?	0 (None)	1 (1 time)	2 (2 times)	3 (3 times)	4 (4 times)	5 (5 times or more)
Sum of 7 circled numbers (AUA Symptom Score): ________						

From Barry MJ et al: The American Urological Association symptom index for benign prostatic hyperplasia, *J Urol* 148(5):1549-1557, 1992. Used with permission.

leave the home for long periods of time because of irritative voiding symptoms.

Encourage men not to become isolated. Alpha adrenergic antagonists should be given HS because of initial hypotension.

Diet

Low fat

Avoid caffeinated/alcoholic beverages/highly spiced foods

Add lycopenes (tomatoes, sauces containing tomatoes) to diet

Patient Education

A seated position may enhance voiding with obstruction

Increase water intake

Sitz baths

Compliance with medication regimen should be stressed

Advise regarding chronic/relapsing nature of prostatitis

Isolated prostatitis does not cause impotency or infertility

Avoid over-the-counter antihistamines/decongestants

Family Impact

It is important to stress early treatment for symptoms and compliance of therapeutic regimen. Men should be educated about symptoms that may indicate prostate cancer and informed that early intervention is necessary and results in a better prognosis. If prostatectomy is performed, counsel men about possible incontinence and impotence and aids for these possible side effects.

Referral

Men with BPH, suspected prostate cancer, or chronic/relapsing cases of prostatitis should be referred to a urologist. Men with high fever, leukocytosis, and severe perineal pain may need hospitalization.

Consultation

Consider consulting with collaborating physician on any case of failed initial treatment.

Follow-up

Segmented urine cultures and examination of prostatic secretions should be performed after therapy is completed to ensure that therapy has eradicated the infection. BPH therapy should be checked periodically for treatment response, (i.e., monitored every 1 to 6 months) (Table 154-4). Men on alpha-adrenergic antagonists should also have periodic blood pressure checks.

EVALUATION

Indications for urologic investigation include treatment failures with appropriate medications, chronic/relapsing cases of prostatitis, BPH, or suspected prostate cancer.

SUGGESTED REFERENCES

Ellsworth A et al: *Mosby's 1998 Medical drug reference,* St Louis, 1998, Mosby.

Fugh-Berman A: A better way to shrink an enlarged prostate, *Health Confidential,* January 1996, p 10.

Goolsby MJ: Screening, diagnosis, and management of prostate cancer: improving primary care outcomes, *Nurse Pract* 23(3):11-36, 1998.

Gorroll AH, May LA, Mulley AG: *Primary care medicine: office evaluation and management of the adult patient,* ed 3, Philadelphia, 1995, JB Lippincott.

Healthcare Consultants of America, Inc: *1998 Physicians fee and coding guide,* Augusta, Ga, 1998, Healthcare Consultants of America, Inc.

Hollander JB, Diokno AC: Prostatism, *Urol Clin North Am* 23(1):75-86, 1995.

Hostetler RM, Mandel IG, Marshburn J: Prostate cancer screening. *Med Clin North Am* 80(1):83-99, 1996.

Liebman B: Clues to prostate cancer, *Nutr Action Healthletter,* March 1996, pp 12-13.

US Department of Health and Human Services: Benign prostatic hypertrophy: Diagnosis and treatment, AHCPR Publication No. 94-0583, Rockville, Md, 1994, US Department of Health and Human Services

Peters S: For men only: an overview of three top health concerns, *Adv Nurse Pract* 5:53-57, 1997.

Tierney LM, McPhee SJ, Papadakis MA: *Current medical diagnosis and treatment,* ed 37, Stamford, Conn, 1998, Appleton & Lange.

Uphold C, Graham M: *Clinical guidelines in family practice,* Gainesville, Fla, 1994, Barmarrae Books.

Vetrosky DT, Gerdom L, White GL: Prostate cancer: etiology, diagnosis, and management, *Clinician Rev* 7:79-100, 1997.

Zippe CD: Benign prostatic hyperplasia: an approach for the internist. *Cleveland Clin J Med* 63(4):26-36, 1996.

152 Proteinuria

ICD-9-CM

Proteinuria 791.0
Gestational 646.2
Orthostatic 593.6
Bence Jones Protein 791.0
Postural 593.6

OVERVIEW

Definition

Proteinuria is loss of an excessive amount of protein in the urine, usually defined as >150 mg/day. Normal people may lose a small amount of protein in the urine (<150 mg/day), which is below the threshold of the test for proteinuria via dipstick. Therefore even a trace of protein on a dipstick is considered proteinuria.

Glomerular proteinuria is a manifestation of primary or secondary glomerular disease. It is usually composed of albumins with globulins and other proteins. When the amount of protein is >3.5 g in 24 hours, the patient has nephrotic range proteinuria.

Tubular (or nonnephrotic) proteinuria normally is <1.5 g in 24 hours. It is caused from tubular cell damage with inability to resorb proteins. This is usually seen with tubulointerstitial injury.

Overflow proteinuria is usually composed of light-chain proteins and is caused by a plasma cell dyscrasia, with the finding of a paraprotein in the urine. The usual causes are multiple myeloma, amyloidosis, and light-chain nephropathy. Because the urine dipstick will detect only albumin, a large quantity of protein in a 24-hour sample with a trace dipstick reading should suggest a nonglomerular protein, often a light-chain. (e.g., Bence Jones proteinuria, multiple myeloma, myoglobinuria).

Transient proteinuria and *orthostatic proteinuria* are usually self-limited. Febrile illness, elevation in blood pressure. or exercise may lead to a mild proteinuria that will usually remit in the near future. Other patients have persistent proteinuria, but the bulk of the protein is associated with ambulation (e.g., congestive heart failure [CHF], fever, seizures, exercise).

Proteinuria in Pregnancy

Protein is not normally found in the urine. However, small amounts (traces) may be found in a specimen contaminated by vaginal secretions or blood. A large amount of protein (1 to 4+) is a common characteristic of renal dysfunction. In the **pregnant patient,** proteinuria may indicate a kidney or bladder infection, a sign of preeclampsia, or chronic/acute renal disease. Pregnant patients should have their urine dipped for protein at each visit.

Pathophysiology

Plasma albumin is normally restricted in its passage through the glomerulus due to its charge (albumin) or size (immunoglobulins). In minimal-charge disease the negative charges are lost, permitting large quantities of albumin to appear in the urine. In most other diseases, the size selective property of the glomerular capillary is disrupted, permitting all plasma proteins to pass through the barrier.

SUBJECTIVE DATA

History of Present Illness

Proteinuria is often found in asymptomatic patients on random urine dipstick. When found, ask about:

- A recent complaint of pharyngitis, gross hematuria, arthritis, skin rash, indicating a systemic illness
- Risk factors for human immunodeficiency virus
- Nonspecific complaints of renal insufficiency: Fatigue, anorexia, or weakness
- Hematuria, dysuria, frequency, nocturia, incontinence, or inability to start stream

Box 152-1

Drugs with Nephrotoxic Potential

Aminoglycosides
Nonsteroidal antiinflammatory drugs
Radiocontrast media
Angiotensin-converting inhibitors
Amphotericin B
Pentamidine
Cephalosporins
Lithium

- Weight loss, diffuse symptoms, fevers, bleeding, and severe pain
- Symptoms of CHF
- Peripheral edema
- Ascites
- Frothy or foamy urine
- Pain in flank area, ureter, bladder, urethra, or prostate
- Pain or burning on urination, urgency, frequency, fever, and/or chills
- Flank or suprapubic pain
- Headache
- Visual disturbances
- Epigastric pain
- Decreased urinary output
- Generalized edema
- Vaginal discharge, accompanying signs and symptoms of vaginitis

Past Medical History

Ask about:

- Diabetes and past diagnosis or treatment for hypertension (HTN)
- Past deep visceral infections, endocarditis, or hepatitis
- History of urinary tract infections or kidney problems (get details of treatment if available)

Medications

Many tubulointerstitial diseases are a result of toxins, abuse of analgesics, or exposure to industrial products (Box 152-1). When asking about analgesic use, it is important to quantify doses because chronic injury is usually seen only with large doses.

Family History

Ask about:

- A positive history of kidney disease
- Family history of diabetes, HTN, collagen vascular disease, nephrolithiasis, or polycystic kidney disease

Psychosocial History

Ask about:

- Smoking history
- Street drugs used, especially intravenous drug use
- Alcohol ingestion
- Occupational history with potential exposure to:
  - Volatile hydrocarbons
  - Benzine
  - Aniline
  - Xylene
  - Heavy metals
  - Ionizing radiation

OBJECTIVE DATA

Physical Examination

Perform a physical examination, with particular attention to:

- Vital signs: Especially blood pressure, temperature, weight
- Funduscopic examination; noting arteriolar narrowing, arterial-venous nicking, hemorrhages, exudates, or papilledema
- Assess neck for bruits, enlarged thyroid, jugular vein distention, enlarged lymph nodes
- Lungs: Crackles
- Heart: Note tachycardia, enlarged heart (shift in point of maximal impulse), precordial heave, thrills, murmurs, rubs, extra heart sounds
- Abdominal examination: Note bruits, enlarged kidneys, masses, hepatomegaly, splenomegaly, flank pain
- Assess extremities for abnormal pulses, edema, anascara, clubbing, arthritic changes
- External genitalia: Developmental anomalies
- Neurological: Deep tendon reflexes, hyperreflexia (pregnancy-induced HTN)

Diagnostics Procedures

Diagnostic procedures are outlined in Table 152-1 and Figure 152-1.

ASSESSMENT

Based on findings regarding specific body systems
Table 152-2 outlines the differential diagnoses for proteinuria

THERAPEUTIC PLAN

Based on 24-hour urine protein
24-hour protein <150 mg: No follow-up necessary

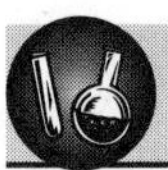

TABLE 152-1 Diagnostic Procedures: Proteinuria

Diagnostic Test	Finding/Rationale	Cost ($)
Urine dipstick (repeat if done previously) and do microscopic	Look for RBC casts, RBCs, WBCs, bacteria, and fat oval bodies (lipids present in nephrotic syndrome) Protein: Trace = 10-20 mg/dl; 3+ = 300 mg/dl 1+ = 30 mg/dl; 4+ = 500-1000 mg/dl 2+ = 100 mg/dl	15-20
24 hr urine	A 24-hour urine (may consider splitting collection into two groups: one done while patient is ambulating, and the other while patient is recumbent) to evaluate for recumbent proteinuria	21-26
Spot urine: protein/creatinine	Sensitive and specific for determining nephrotic range proteinuria (some think this test is better than 24-hr urine) <3.5 is considered nonnephrotic proteinuria	19-24/cr; 15-20/pro
Urine protein electrophoresis	Evaluates type of renal disease by identification of proteins	74-92
Renal sonogram	Determines size of kidneys (if acute, kidneys are usually normal, whereas small kidneys indicate chronic disease) and chronicity of disease; also rules out obstruction	346-416
Glucose, BUN, and creatinine; electrolytes	Baseline purposes and to determine the degree of renal impairment	28-39/metabolic panel
Microalbuminuria	For diabetics	25-33
HIV	Rule out HIV	41-52
Serum albumin, calcium, and phosphorus levels	For baseline purposes, and to determine any hypoalbuminemia	18-23/alb; 18-23/ca 16-20/ph
SSA test	Used to determine if Bence Jones proteins are present in the urine	N/A
ESR, ANA	If suspicious of vasculitis or glomerulonephritis, consider doing; both would be increased	16-20/ESR; 42-52/ANA

ANA, Antinuclear antibody; *BUN,* blood urea nitrogen; *ESR,* erythrocyte sedimentation rate; *GFR,* glomerular filtration rate; *HIV,* human immunodeficiency virus; *HTN,* hypertension; *N/A,* not available; *RBC,* red blood cell; *SSA,* sulfosalicylic acid; *WBC,* white blood cell.

24-hour protein 150 to 1000 mg:
- Rule out orthostatic proteinuria by splitting 24-hour urine
- <75 protein in recumbent specimen confirms orthostatic proteinuria
- Evaluate patient again in 6 to 12 months; watch for increasing proteinuria and hematuria

24-hour protein 1 to 3.5 g:
- Nonnephrotic, persistent proteinuria
- Evaluate patient for:
  - Tubular diseases:
    - Fanconi syndrome
    - Cystinosis
    - Hypokalemia
    - Galactosemia
    - Monocytic leukemia
    - Wilson's disease
    - Analgesic drugs
    - Myeloma
    - Bence-Jones protein myeloma
    - Glomerulonephropathy

24-hour protein >3.5 g: Nephrotic syndrome
- Check for systemic diseases: Diabetes mellitus, lupus, amyloidosis
- Primary glomerulonephritis: Most common in children and managed with steroids

Lifestyle/Activities

Dependent on extent of renal dysfunction

Diet

Dependent on the type of renal problems, extent of renal failure, degree of catabolism, and specific metabolic abnormalities

History and Physical Examination
Evaluate for chronic protein loss: peripheral edema, heart failure, ascites

↓

Urine dipstick test

↓

Repeat dipstick test
Obtain U/A microscopic, looking for:
RBC casts
WBCs
Bacteria
Fat oval bodies (nephrotic urinary sediment)

↓

Sulfosalicylic acid (SA) test
Used to determine if Bence Jones protein in urine

↓

Get urine protein (spot or 24-hr)
Get urine creatinine
Determine ratio of protein/creatinine; if >3.5, it is consistent with nephrotic range proteinuria
The spot test has supplanted 24-hr urine for protein

↓

Serum electrolytes, creatinine, BUN, glucose, CBC, albumin, calcium, phosphorus (baseline data)

↓

Categorize proteinuria into nephrotic/nonnephrotic range

Figure 152-1 Algorithm for patients with proteinuria.

Table 152-2 Differential Diagnosis: Proteinuria

Diagnosis	Supporting Data
Nephrotic Proteinuria	
Uncontrolled HTN	One of the most common causes of nephrotic range proteinuria
Diabetes mellitus (DM) (Ch. 55)	Nephrotic syndrome is almost always due to diabetes in patients with DM. First clue: Microalbuminuria predicts significant glomerular disease with 90% accuracy. History may reveal poor glycemic control or HTN.
Glomerulonephritis	Caused by immune complex deposition on the epithelial side of the basement membrane. May see HTN, proteinuria >10 g/day, or reduced GFR. May be seen with vasculitis, postinfectious (hematuria, HTN, pulmonary congestion, peripheral, and periorbital edema), or acute renal failure.
SLE (Ch. 110)	Usually present with hematuria, active urine sediment, proteinuria, some degree of urinary insufficiency, and HTN.
Exposure to heavy metals	Initially nonspecific findings: Fatigue, anorexia, or weakness. May note elevated creatinine, 2+ protein, history of relevant drug, or toxin exposure.
Nonnephrotic Proteinuria	
UTI (Ch. 187)	Dysuria, frequency, pyuria
Benign positional proteinuria	Mild proteinuria that occurs when the patient is in an upright position, but resolves when the patient is recumbent. Evident when 2- to 12-hr urine collections are done, one while recumbent, one upright. The recumbent sample will be normal.
Isolated	Normal urine sediment, no overt systemic disease that could damage glomeruli. Fever, CHF, and heavy exercise can cause proteinuria.
Pregnancy: PIH (Ch. 149)	Proteinuria, edema, HTN usually beginning in third trimester

CHF, Congestive heart failure; *GFR,* glomerular filtration rate; *HTN,* hypertension; *PIH,* pregnancy-induced hypertension; *SLE,* systemic lupus erythematosus; *UTI,* urinary tract infection.

Patient Education

Discuss the tests done, and why.
Describe how the kidneys work and what they do.
If more is known about cause of renal problem, explain findings.
Stress importance of proper perineal hygiene.

Referral

Refer to nephrologist for persistent proteinuria 1 to 3.5 mg or in cases of persistent or worsening proteinuria
Consult nephrologist or OB/GYN for pregnant woman with persistent proteinuria or other symptoms of PIH

EVALUATION/FOLLOW-UP

If no clear cause of proteinuria is determined (and <2 g/day) after consultation with nephrologist, do a urinalysis, electrolytes, blood urea nitrogen, and creatinine q4-6 mos.

SUGGESTED READINGS

Aiello J: Preventing diabetic nephropathy: the role of primary care, *Nurse Pract* 23(2):12-13, 1998.

Berg D: *Handbook of primary care medicine,* Philadelphia, 1993, JB Lippincott.

Driscoll C et al, editors: *The family practice desk reference,* ed 3, St. Louis, 1996, Mosby.

Lommel L: *Ambulatory obstetrics: protocols for nurse practitioners/nurse midwives,* ed 2, San Francisco, 1990, The Regents.

Poirier S: Reducing complications in type 2 DM, *Am Family Physician* 57(6):1238-1239, 1998.

153 Psoriasis

ICD-9-CM

Psoriasis, Any Type 696.1
Psoriasis, Guttate 696.1
Psoriasis, Vulgaris 696.1

OVERVIEW

Definition

Psoriasis vulgaris is the most common type of psoriasis. It is characterized by the presence of sharply demarcated dull-red scaly plaques, particularly on the extensor prominences and scalp. Psoriasis is enormously variable in duration and extent, with common morphological variants. Types of psoriasis are

- Guttate
- Plaque
- Palmar and pustular pustulosis
- Generalized pustular psoriasis
- Erythrodermic psoriasis

Incidence

Psoriasis is one of the most common skin disorders. It affects 1.5% to 2% of the population in western countries. It can begin at any age, but it commonly makes its first appearance in the late 20s and the seventh decade. However, approx. ⅓ of patients are affected before 20 years of age, especially females. Males and females are otherwise affected equally. There is a lower incidence in west Africans, Japanese, Eskimos, and North and South American Indians.

Pathophysiology

The principle abnormality is an alteration in cell kinetics of keratinocytes. The cell cycle is shortened from 311 hours to 36 hours, with an increase of 28 times the normal production of epidermal cells. The cause of this change in the production of cells is unknown. Results of this increased production are:

- Marked thickening and thinning of the epidermis
- Increased mitosis of keratinocytes, fibroblasts, and endothelial cells
- Inflammatory cells in the dermis and in the epidermis

Protective Factors Against

None

Factors That Increase Susceptibility

Positive family history: One parent with psoriasis: 8% of offspring will have psoriasis; both parents: 41%. Certain human leukocyte antigen groupings are also associated with an increased likelihood of having the disease.

Minor trauma (Koebner's phenomenon): rubbing and scratching stimulates the proliferative process.

Certain drugs: Systemic corticosteroids, lithium, alcohol, chloroquine, beta-adrenergic blockers.

Stress and obesity: Cause exacerbation of preexisting psoriasis in approximately 40% of people.

Infection (human immunodeficiency virus [HIV], streptococcal upper respiratory infection).

Endocrine factors.

SUBJECTIVE DATA

History of Present Illness

Ask about when symptoms noticed, where first noticed; if onset sudden (acute guttate), ask about previous treatment for psoriasis or other skin diseases.

Past Medical History

Ask about:

- Medication history
- Other skin disorders
- Trauma (surgeries, minor bumps)
- Infections

TABLE 153-1 Differential Diagnosis: Psoriasis

Diagnosis	Supporting Data
Seborrheic dermatitis	May be indistinguishable in sites involved and morphology
Lichen simplex chronicus	Specialized form of lichenification, usually occurring in circumscribed plaques; the main symptom is pruritus in spasms; the scratching becomes automatic and reflexive and an unconscious habit
Candidiasis	Superficial infection occurring on moist cutaneous site; common areas include axilla, inframammary, groin, diaper area
Psoriasiform drug eruptions	Most common drugs: Beta blockers, gold, and methyldopa
Secondary syphilis	Red macules and papules, round to oval, with generalized eruption on the trunk; may cause hair loss, scattered discrete lesions

Allergies
Sexually transmitted diseases
Associated risk factors
Sun overexposure
HIV (or at risk for HIV)

Medications

Ask about the use of corticosteroids, lithium, alcohol consumption, chloroquine, B-blockers, interferon-a.

Family History

Ask about family history of skin disorders.

Psychosocial History

Help patient identify stressors.

Diet History

Obtain diet history for calorie count, especially in the elderly (due to increased metabolic rate).

Description of Most Common Symptoms

Skin
- Pruritus, pustules, papules and "salmon pink" plaques
- Lesions: Single or localized to one area, regional involvement, or generalized
- Pattern: Bilateral, but rarely symmetrical, favors: elbows, knees, scalp, and intertriginous areas; facial region is usually uninvolved

Systemic
- Arthritis (resembles rheumatoid arthritis), fever, acute illness
- Nail involvement resembles fungal infection with stripping, pitting, fraying, or separation of the distal margin and thickening discoloration and debris under the nail plate
- Hair growth is usually unaltered

Associated Symptoms

Joint pain (psoriatic arthritis)
- Acute illness: Weakness, chills, fever (von Zumbusch syndrome)
- Elderly: Hypothermia
  - Hemodynamic changes (shunting of blood to the skin)

OBJECTIVE DATA

Physical Examination

A problem-oriented physical should be conducted, with particular attention to:

General appearance: Ranges from well to uncomfortable to toxic, based on type and involvement
Vital signs
Skin lesions: Type, shape, arrangement, and distribution of lesions
Hair and nails
Mucous membranes

Diagnostic Procedures

No consistent lab findings in uncomplicated psoriasis
Serum HIV to determine HIV sero status in at-risk individuals with sudden onset psoriasis ($52-$67)

ASSESSMENT

Differential Diagnoses

Differential diagnoses are outlined in Table 153-1.

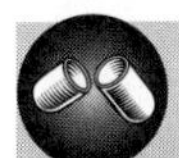

TABLE 153-2 Treatment Plan: Psoriasis

Location of Psoriasis	Drugs	Comments	Cost
Elbows, knees, and isolated plaques (treat only with topical agents)	Topical fluorinated corticosteroids in ointment base applied to affected area BID-TID Triamcinolone acetonide (Kenalog, Aristocort) Fluticasone Propionate (Cutivate) Hydrocortisone Valerate (Cortaid, Synacort, Westcort)	Apply after removing scales by soaking in water; ointment applied to wet skin, covered with plastic wrap, and left overnight Pregnancy: C	\$4-\$27/0.1% (60 g); \$4-\$37/0.5% (20 g)
	Hydrocolloid dressing	Leave on for 24-48 hours; helps prevent scratching; use class I and II fluorinated corticosteroid creams (see Appendix R); will develop tolerance over long periods; to avoid atrophy of skin, max. 50 g ointment/wk	
	Triamcinolone acetonide aqueous (e.g., Aristocort, Trilone) suspension into lesion	Intradermal injection; hypopigmentation can occur at the site	\$9/3 mg/ml (5 ml); \$7/10 mg/ml (5 ml)
	Anthralin preparations	Excellent when used properly Pregnancy: C	N/A
	Vitamin D analogs, calcipotriol (Dovonex)	Response is slower than corticosteroids, but long lasting; apply to <40% BSA and <100 g/wk Pregnancy: C	\$35/0.005% (30 g)
Scalp	Coal tar shampoos followed by betamethasone valerate (Betatrex, Valisone), 2× week	Mild scalp psoriasis: Superficial scaling, no thick plaques If refractory, clobetasol propionate 0.05% scalp application	\$2-\$16/0.1% (15 g)
	Vitamin D_3 analogs as lotion Fluocinolone cream or lotion applied, covered, and left on overnight	Severe: thick adherent plaques; plaques must be removed before active treatment: 2% to 10% salicylic acid in mineral oil covered with plastic cap	N/A
Trunk, palms, and soles	Treatment may include topical corticosteroids, anthralin, vitamin D_3 UVB phototherapy with emollients, PUVA, photochemotherapy, methotrexate given weekly, combination therapy with etretinate (Tegison) or methotrexate and PUVA	When generalized, refer to dermatologist; lesions on palms and soles are difficult to treat and are frequently refractory to treatment Etretinate: Pregnancy: X SE: Fatigue, headache, eye irritation, anorexia, alopecia	\$34-\$42/UVB; \$155-\$210/UVA \$60/Etretinate: 10 mg (30)
Facial and intertriginous areas	Beclomethasone Dipropionate Clobetasone butyrate Desonide Dexamethasone Fluocinolone acetonide	See Appendix R for more details	

BSA, Body surface area; *N/A*, not available; *SE*, side effects; *UVB*, ultraviolet B.

THERAPEUTIC PLAN

Pharmaceutical/Nonpharmaceutical

Treatment is based on location of the lesion. A treatment plan is outlined in Table 153-2.

Lifestyle/Activities

Consider stress-reducing techniques.
Limit sun exposure.

Diet

Elderly patients may need a high-calorie, high-protein diet due to increased metabolic rate.

Patient Education

Instruct the patient to avoid rubbing or scratching the lesions since trauma stimulates the psoriatic process.
Instruct about medication; effects/side effects.
Instruct about the disease process.
Reassure that disease is not contagious.

Referral

Refer to dermatologist:
- Patients with:
  - Erythrodermic psoriasis
  - Generalized pustular psoriasis
  - Subacute psoriasis
  - Extensive flexural psoriasis
  - Extensive psoriasis vulgaris
  - Psoriasis that interferes with function
- Elderly or incapacitated patient

EVALUATION/FOLLOW-UP

Initial follow-up in 2 weeks to assess effectiveness of treatment; follow up in 2-month intervals thereafter

SUGGESTED REFERENCES

Ellsworth A et al: *Mosby's 1998 medical drug reference,* St Louis, 1998, Mosby.

Fitzpatrick TB et al: *Color atlas and synopsis of clinical dermatology: common and serious diseases,* ed 3, New York, 1997, McGraw-Hill.

Habif T: *Clinical dermatology,* St Louis, 1996, Mosby.

Healthcare Consultants of America, Inc: *1998 Physicians fee and coding guide,* Augusta, Ga, 1998, Healthcare Consultants of America, Inc.

Marks R: *Skin disease in old age,* Philadelphia, 1987, JB Lippincott.

Parazzini LN et al: Dietary factors and the risk of psoriasis. Results of an Italian case-control study, *Br J Dermatol* 134:101-106, 1996.

Rectal Bleeding (Hematochezia) or Occult Gastrointestinal Bleeding

ICD-9-CM

Hemorrhoids 455.6
Anal Fissure 565.0
Colorectal Cancer 154.0

OVERVIEW

Definition

Rectal bleeding is bleeding that is visible on the toilet paper or in the toilet. Occult gastrointestinal (GI) bleeding may be detected by positive hemoccult or iron deficiency anemia. The most common cause is local anal disease, usually hemorrhoids or anal fissures. Less often the bleeding is from a more proximal source (10%).

Incidence

Greater than 10% of the general population report having blood on the toilet paper or in the toilet within the last 6 months

Pathophysiology

Bleeding usually occurs with a bowel movement, although oozing and spotting of the undergarments may occur. Local anal bleeding usually occurs after straining at stool. The patient notices streaking or coating of the stools with blood or blood on the toilet paper. Since blood can reflux proximal to the anus from hemorrhoids, blood mixed with stool is compatible with local anal disease. The passage of blood only or mixed with mucus is more suspicious for a more proximal source, usually the colon (Figure 154-1).

SUBJECTIVE DATA

History of Present Illness

Ask about duration of symptoms. Ask about weight loss and a change in bowel habits (e.g., constipation and straining). Make sure to ask about visible rectal bleeding.

Children and **adults:** Ask about the relationship of symptoms to bowel movements.

Past Medical History

Ask about:

- History of inflammatory bowel disease, colonic polyps, or hemorrhoids, constipation, liver disease, past anorectal surgery, diabetes, pregnancy
- Allergies
- Menstrual periods for women: Duration, amount of bleeding, frequency

Medications

Ask about:

- Recent use of antibiotics (possibility of pseudomembranous colitis)
- Any medications for constipation
- Use of acetylsalicylic acid (ASA) or nonsteroidal anti-inflammatory drugs (NSAIDs)

Family History

Ask about family history of colon cancer, colon polyps, rectal bleeding.

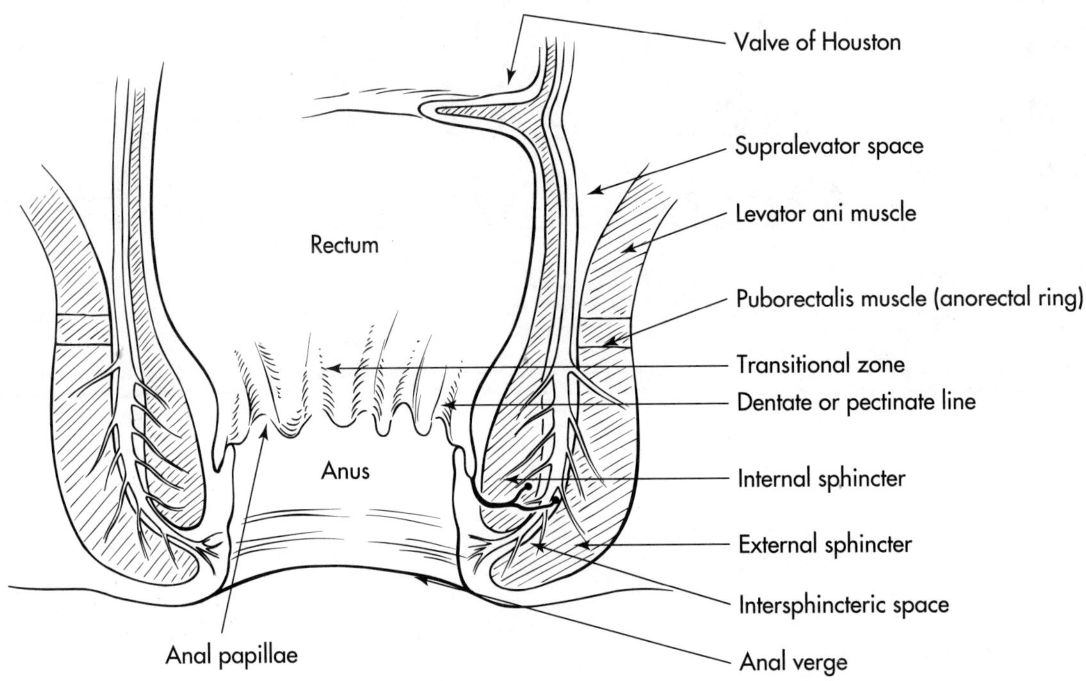

Figure 154-1 The anatomy of the anal canal. (From Pfenninger JL, Fowler GC: *Procedures for primary care physicians,* St Louis, 1994, Mosby.)

Psychosocial History

Diet: Ask about recent food ingestion: red meat, beets
Children: Consider possible child sexual abuse—may need to ask about this once relationship is established
Adult: Ask about employment (e.g., jobs that might increase the tendency for hemorrhoids or valsalva maneuvers such as lifting, driving a truck)

Description of Most Common Symptoms

Children: May cry during or after a bowel movement; may bring legs up to chest
Elderly: May be asymptomatic; fever is uncommon

Associated Symptoms

Anal pain, burning or itching, swelling, discharge, constipation, diarrhea, lack of bowel control, change in urination

OBJECTIVE DATA

Physical Examination

A problem oriented physical should be conducted, with particular attention to:

Vital signs and weight, general appearance, general hydration status, including orthostatic changes
Abdomen: Full abdominal examination
Rectal: Examine for fissures, hemorrhoids, or fistulae
Anoscopic examination: Assess for prostate tenderness or enlargement
Children: Assess for dehydration, activity level; physical examination may be essentially within normal limits in children

Diagnostic Procedures

Diagnostic procedures are outlined in Table 154-1.

ASSESSMENT

Differential diagnoses include:

Colorectal carcinoma, polyps, inflammatory bowel disease, colonic diverticulosis, and anal fissures; in 10% of cases with significant hematochezia, an upper GI source of bleeding (peptic ulcer) is found (Tables 154-2 and 154-3, Figure 154-2)
Children: Sexual abuse, constipation, appendicitis

THERAPEUTIC PLAN

The patient's volume should be assessed and fluids given as appropriate. Treatment is directed at the underlying cause.

Pharmaceutical Treatment

Once hemorrhoids are diagnosed, recommend over-the-counter products such as those outlined in Table 154-4.

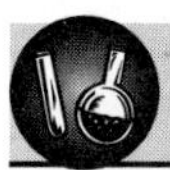

TABLE 154-1 Diagnostic Procedures: Rectal Bleeding

Diagnostic Tests	Findings/Rationale	Cost ($)
Fecal occult blood ×3-5	Should be done annually for patients >50	13-17
Anoscopy	Healthy patients <40 should have anoscopy done to look for evidence of anorectal disease	57-70; 248-297/ to control bleeding
Sigmoidoscopy	Healthy patients <40 should have sigmoidoscopy done to look for evidence of inflammatory bowel disease or infectious colitis; if no likely source of bleeding is found, no further evaluation is needed unless bleeding persists or is recurrent	254-302
Colonoscopy	Should be done on all patients with significant lower tract bleeding (fall in hematocrit); also should be test of choice in patient with ↓ hematocrit and iron deficiency anemia; considered test of choice because of accuracy and therapeutic capability	799-956
Barium enema	Should be done on all patients who have occult gastrointestinal bleeding or iron deficiency anemia in an adult	294-351
Nasogastric and lavage	Should be done on all patients with large bleed to look for site of upper gastrointestinal bleed; if blood is not seen and bile is aspirated, upper bleed is unlikely	Not available

TABLE 154-2 Differential Diagnosis: Rectal Bleeding

Diagnoses	Supporting Data
Hemorrhoids (Ch. 88)	Small amounts of bright red blood noted on toilet paper; bleeding is usually slight and seldom results in significant blood loss; painless bleeding is caused by internal hemorrhoids
Fissure	Intermittent pain associated with bowel movement; tenderness of rectal area; fissures are often noted near skin tags
Perirectal abscess	Extreme throbbing pain, perineal swelling; localized perirectal redness and tender swelling
Carcinoma	Third most frequent cause of lower gastrointestinal bleeding; usually asymptomatic change in bowel habits (diarrhea frequently seen in middle aged patients); blood streaked stool or blood may be mixed with stool itself; stool often positive for occult blood
Inflammatory bowel disease (Ch. 100) (Crohn's disease and ulcerative colitis)	Second most common cause of bleeding; frequent small stools or diarrhea with passage of blood, mucus, and pus; patient complains of tenesmus and urgency; with acute form, patients will appear toxic and have fever, dehydration, weight loss, anemia
Diverticulosis (Ch. 58)	The most common cause of lower tract bleeding; presents as an acute, painless, large-volume maroon or bright red hematochezia in patients >50

TABLE 154-3 Nature of Bleeding

Color of Bleeding	Diagnosis to Consider	Diagnostic Test
Dark red bleeding	Meckel's diverticulum	Meckel's scan
	Mild colitis	Stool culture, colonoscopy
	Inflammatory bowel disease	Erythrocyte sedimentation rate, culture, stool leukocytes, complete blood count, colonoscopy
Bright red bleeding	Anal fissure	Anoscopy
	Rectal lesion	Anoscopy
	Polyp	Colonoscopy

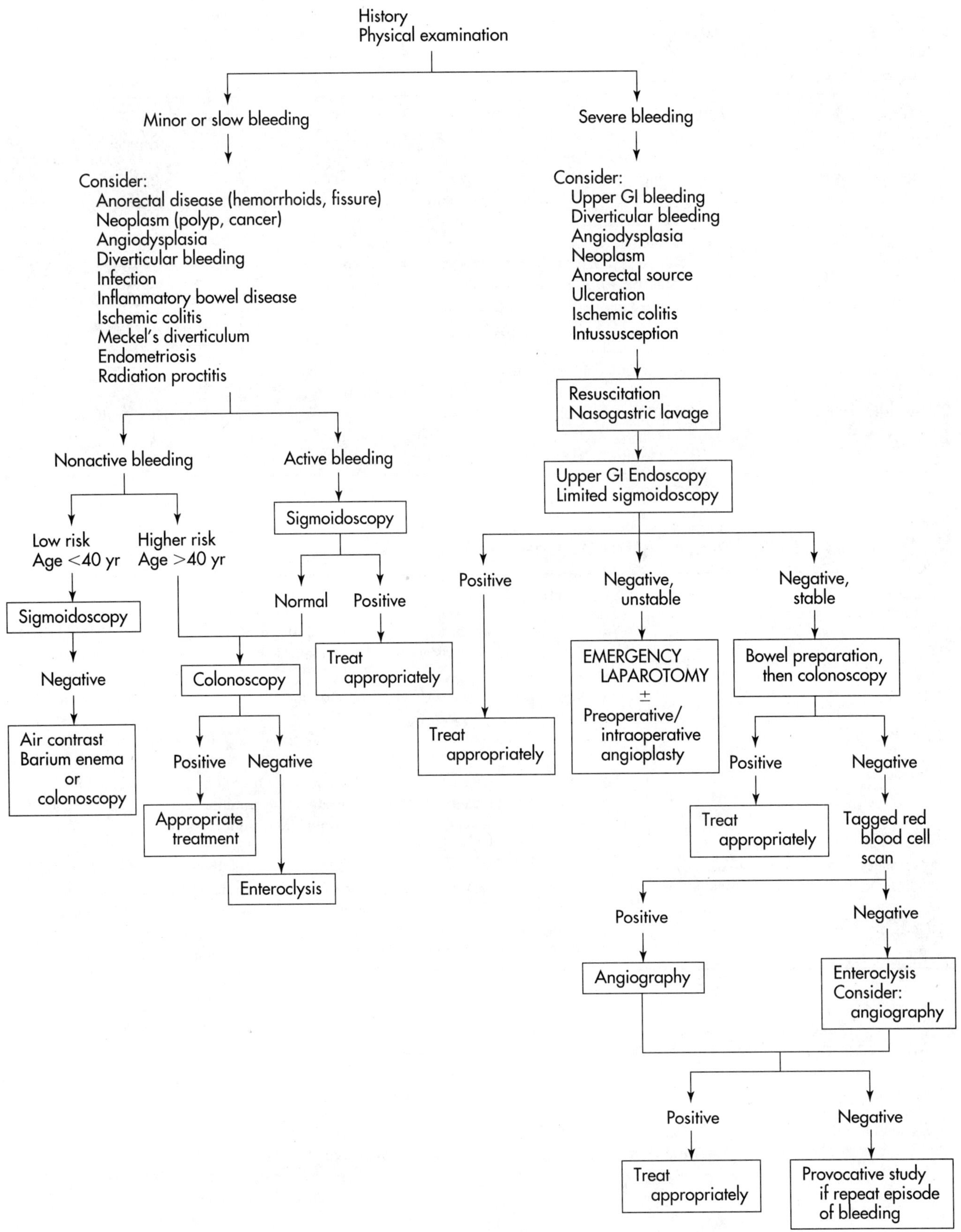

Figure 154-2 Algorithm for patient with rectal bleeding. (Adapted from Greene HL, Johnson WP, Lemcke D: *Decision making in medicine,* ed 2, St Louis, 1998, Mosby.)

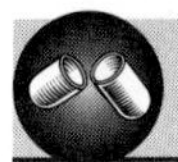

TABLE 154-4 Over-the-Counter Treatment of Hemorrhoids

Drug	Dose	Comments	Cost
Witch hazel 50%, glycerin 10%, gel (Tucks)	Apply pad or gel up to six times daily or as compress to affected area, replace q5-15 min	Not recommended for children	N/A
Phenylephrine 0.25%, petrolatum 71.9%, mineral oil 14%, shark liver oil 3% (Preparation H)	Apply up to QID daily Suppository: 1 rectally up to QID	Not recommended for children	N/A
Pramozine 1%, zinc oxide 12.5%, mineral oil (Anusol)	Apply up to five times daily	Once hemorrhoids are diagnosed Not recommended for children Precaution: Pregnancy SE: Burning sensation	N/A
Pramoxine with hydrocortisone 25 mg (Anusol HC)	1 rectally in AM and HS for 2 weeks; if severe, 1 rectally TID or 2 rectally BID	Not recommended for children Pregnancy: C SE: Dermal and epidermal atrophy, poor wound healing, local irritation	\$3/supp: 1%: (10); \$3/oint: 1% (30 g); \$14/foam: 1% (15 g)

N/A, Not available; *SE,* side effects.

Lifestyle/Activities

Discontinue ASA and other NSAIDs.
Sitz baths may be helpful for anorectal problems.
Exercise.

Diet

Increase fiber, fluids, exercise to prevent constipation.

Patient Education

Stress the importance of getting follow-up if blood is noted in toilet.
Stress the importance of fecal occult blood testing for patients >50.
Stress the importance of ANNUAL.

Family Impact

Approximately 15% of patients with GI bleeding have carcinoma; however, the threat of cancer must always be considered.

Referral

Referral to a GI specialist is appropriate if the bleeding continues and a site of bleeding is not identified. The most common cause of anemia in patients >50 is GI bleeding; invasive tests are needed in most cases to locate the source of bleeding (i.e., sigmoidoscopy). If the source of bleeding is found to be hemorrhoids or local anorectal problems, these problems can usually be handled by the primary provider.

Consultation

Discuss the need for further testing of any patient who presents with GI bleeding.

Follow-up

Do fecal occult blood testing annually on all patients >50.

EVALUATION

Monitor fecal occult blood periodically after diagnosis. Periodic hemoglobin or hematocrit may also be helpful.

SUGGESTED READINGS

Bassford T: Treatment of common anorectal disorders, *Am Family Physician* 45(4):1787-1794, 1992.

Ellsworth W et al: *Mosby's 1998 medical drug reference*, St. Louis, 1998, Mosby.

Healthcare Consultants of America, Inc: *1998 physicians fee and coding guide*. Augusta, Ga, 1998, Healthcare Consultants of America, Inc.

Hefand M et al: History of visible rectal bleeding in a primary care population: initial assessment and 10 year follow-up, *JAMA* 277 (1):44-48, 1997.

Janicke D, Pundt M: Anorectal disorders, *Emerg Med Clin North Am* 14(4):757-788, 1996.

Machicado G, Jensen D: Acute and chronic management of lower gastrointestinal bleeding: cost effective approaches, *Gastroenterologist* 5(3):189-201, 1997.

McQuaid K: Alimentary Tract. In Tierney L, McPhee S, Papadakis M, editors: *Current medical diagnosis & treatment,* ed 37, Stamford, Conn, 1998, Appleton & Lange.

Metcalf A: Anorectal disorders: five common causes of pain, itching, and bleeding. *Postgrade Med* 98(5):81-84, 1995.

Palley S: Rectal bleeding. In Greene H, Johnson W, Lemcke D, editors: *Decision making in medicine,* ed 2, St Louis, 1998, Mosby.

Pfenniger JL, Fowler GC: *Procedures for primary care physicians,* St Louis, 1994, Mosby.

Seller R: *Differential diagnosis of common complaints,* ed 3, Philadelphia, 1996, WB Saunders.

Sladden J, Thomson A: How do general practitioners handle rectal bleeding? *Aust Family Physician* 27(1-2):78-82, 1998.

Vernava A et al: Lower gastrointestinal bleeding, *Dis Colon Rectum* 40(7):846-858, 1997.

Wasson J: *The common symptom guide,* ed 4, New York, 1997, McGraw Hill.

155 Red Eye

ICD-9-CM

Conjunctivitis 372.30
Acute Atopic Conjunctivitis 372.5
Other Chronic Allergic Conjunctivitis 372.14
Herpes Simplex (HSV) with Ophthalmic Complications 054.40
Corneal Ulcer 370.0
Foreign Body, Eye (External) 930.9
Foreign Body, Eyelid 930.1

OVERVIEW

Definition

Red eye refers to conjunctival blood vessel injection with an unknown cause.

Incidence

Red eye is a frequent, common complaint seen in both the provider's office and Emergency Department. Approximately 5% of all patients requiring immediate care have eye complaints.

Approximately 1300 eye injuries occur each year from BB guns and air guns. In **young patients** the most common cause of visual blurring is refractive error.

Pathophysiology

Injection of the conjunctival blood vessels occurs in response to inflammation, trauma, allergies, increased pressure in the eye, as well as with eyelid abnormalities. The pathophysiology varies with each condition that presents with a red eye.

Protective Factors Against

Good aseptic technique/hand washing
Use of protective eye goggles

Factors That Increase Susceptibility

Environmental exposure to chemicals: cleaning agents, Super Glue
Unsupervised sports: increase risk of eye injury
Baseballs most common cause of ocular injury in sports
Not using protective eye goggles
Long-term use of topical steroids (>4 to 6 weeks): May produce glaucoma
Presence of systemic disease: Lyme, Kawasaki syndrome, juvenile rheumatoid arthritis

SUBJECTIVE DATA

History of Present Illness

Determine if:
- Onset is sudden or gradual
- Visual problem is present in one or both eyes
- Exposure to chemicals: *If chemical exposure to eye: begin flushing of eye immediately with copious amounts of water*
  - Cleaning chemicals, especially those containing lye or alkaline products
  - Recent use of Super Glue (cyanoacrylate glue)
  - Cosmetic use
- Any treatment done (e.g., flushing of eye)

Ask about:
- Trauma to eye via thrown objects (e.g., rocks, balls, darts, pencils)
- Foreign body (FB) in eye: Metal, sawdust, trees/bark, rust; ask if FB seen
- Tears overflowing onto the cheeks in newborn
- Mucoid material on eyelids
- Light sensitivity and excessive production of tears
- Itching of eyes, conjunctival edema and eye discharge; determine whether these symptoms are recurrent, bilateral or seasonal
- Skin rashes in other family members or exposure to skin rashes
- Symptoms of otitis media
- Vision: Blurry, photophobia, pain, inability to see, "floaters" in vision, double vision, halos around lights

Exposure to conjunctivitis in school/home settings
Last eye examination

Past Medical History

Ask about recent upper respiratory infection
Determine if patient has any systemic illnesses:
- Otitis media
- Kawasaki's syndrome
- Juvenile rheumatoid arthritis
- Ataxia-telangiectasia (Louis-Bar syndrome)
- Lyme disease
- Collagen disease (dry eyes)
- Diabetes mellitus: Ask about glucose level
- Hypertension
- Glaucoma
- Migraine headache

Ask about:
- Previous eye problems or refractory correction
- Contact lens use
- Previous eye surgery: Condition requiring, date performed, outcome
- Conditions that may cause patient to be immunocompromised:
  - Acquired immunodeficiency syndrome
  - Chemotherapy
  - **Children:** Ask if preterm, resuscitated, or oxygen used as newborn

Medications

Eye drops: Over-the-counter, prescription
- Vasoconstrictors or artificial tears

Oral medications:
- Use of diuretics, antihistamines, or antidepressant medications: Dry eyes
- Psychotropic agents
- Digitalis products: Yellow vision
- Drugs that dilate the pupil

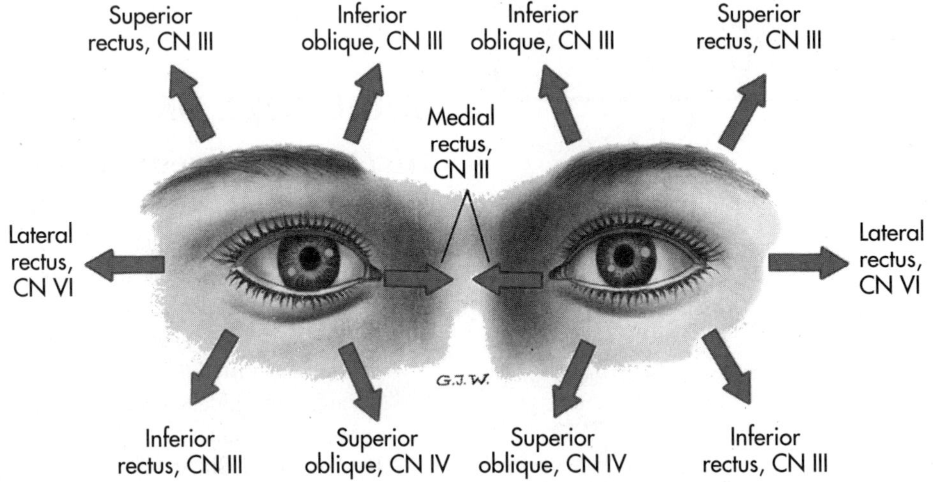

Figure 155-1 Cranial nerves and extraocular muscles associated with the six cardinal fields of gaze. (From Seidel HM: *Mosby's guide to physical examination,* ed 4, St Louis, 1999, Mosby.)

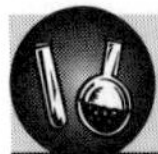

Table 155-1 Diagnostic Procedures: Red Eye

Diagnostic Test	Findings/Rationale	Cost ($)
Complete blood count	Rule out systemic disease	18-23
Thyroid studies	Rule out hyperthyroidism, which can cause certain oculomotor palsies	47-61
Blood glucose	Identify glucose level	16-20
Erythrocyte sedimentation rate	Rule out temporal arteritis	16-20
Fluorescein stain/blue filter light	To detect corneal abrasions/defects	Not available
Culture of eye discharge	Not routinely done, should be checked if gonorrhea is suspected. Swab done of conjunctival sac. Culture both eyes, even if only one affected.	31-39

TABLE 155-2 Conditions Causing Red Eye

Diagnoses	Supporting Data
Bacterial conjunctivitis (Ch. 43)	Discharge purulent, crusting along lid margins, matting of eye after sleeping. Onset in one eye, with second eye infected in 2-5 days. Eyelid may be swollen. Hyperemia of palpebral conjunctiva is seen often with preauricular lymph nodes.
Viral conjunctivitis	Approximately 20% of conjunctivitis is caused by virus. **Children** are primarily affected. Highly contagious, usually seen following upper respiratory infection or through direct contact with infection. Sometimes seen during summer through cross contamination via a swimming pool. Onset is abrupt and unilateral. Involvement of the other eye is within 2-3 days. Associated symptoms are excessive tearing, sneezing. Eye drainage is nonpurulent. Examination: Hypertrophy of lymphoid follicles on lower palpebral conjunctiva. Tender preauricular lymph nodes can be palpated.
Allergic conjunctivitis	History of past sensitivity to allergens. The patient complains of itchy, swollen, watery eyes with watery, nonpurulent discharge. Allergic conjunctivitis occurs more in the spring and fall. Large cobblestone papillae can be seen in both eyes. Allergic shiners may be noted. Nasal mucosa is pale and edematous.
Eye injury	Hyphema is blood in the anterior chamber, which occurs after trauma to the eye. Orbital fractures (if any suspicion, get computed tomography or Waters view of sinuses) usually are accompanied by an injury to the eye itself. Penetrating injuries appear as a small, protruding mass of iris accompanied by a distorted pupil and a flat anterior chamber. Always obtain an x-ray to rule out retained FB. Patient should be kept NPO until evaluated by ophthalmologist. Eyelid lacerations may also be seen with an eye injury.
Subconjunctival hemorrhage	Sudden onset of painless, bright red discoloration of all or part of bulbar conjunctiva. Vision is normal. Condition is benign and disappears in about 3 weeks.
Corneal disease (Ch. 46) or injury	History for FB reveals a sudden onset of discomfort, with intense pain. Symptoms include tearing, photophobia, and blurred vision. Signs of abrasion are pain, continued tearing, redness, and a sensation of FB in the eye. Herpetic keratitis: infection of the eye caused by herpes. Staining of cornea reveals a characteristic branching lesion. Any suspicion of herpes warrants referral to ophthalmologist. Ultraviolet and contact lens keratitis: keratitis can develop from anyone who does not protect the eyes from the glare of a welding torch or sunlamp; contact lens problems may also cause a keratitis. Fluorescein stain reveals a superficial punctate keratitis. Chemical burns: diagnosis is obvious from the history; photophobia and pain are present.
Acute narrow-angle glaucoma (Ch. 80)	Sudden increase in pressure in the eye. Patient complains of sudden intense pain, visual loss and often vomiting; intraocular pressure >20 mm Hg.
Uveitis	Less common than conjunctivitis but should suspect uveitis when a patient has a red eye with reduced vision, normal or slightly elevated intraocular pressure, and a cloudy anterior chamber.
Eyelid swelling (Ch. 22)/ problems	Acute dacryocystitis: inflammation inside the lacrimal sac. The sac appears as a red and tender mass that creates a lump under the skin on the side of the nose, below the inner canthus. Treat dacryocystis as you would any infection: warm compresses, antibiotics, and surgical drainage if necessary. Blepharitis: This condition is characterized by red-rimmed eyes, chronic mild irritation of the eyes, and granulated eyelids. Hordeolum (stye): Abscess at the root of an eyelash. Treat with warm compresses, local antibiotics and incision and drainage if necessary. Chalazion: Most chalazions feel like peas under the skin of the eyelid. This condition results from obstruction of one of the tarsal (meibomian) glands. Surgical removal may be necessary.

FB, Foreign body.

Family History

Family history of eye disease/problems
- Retinoblastoma or cancer of retina (autosomal-dominant disorder)
- Color blindness, cataracts, diabetes mellitus, glaucoma, retinitis, macular degeneration
- Refractory problems: Nearsighted, farsighted, strabismus

Psychosocial History

Ask about:

- Any changes in activities of daily living related to vision
- Activities or participation in sporting activities that may endanger eye

Associated Symptoms

Clear nasal discharge
Nausea and vomiting
Headache
Dizziness

OBJECTIVE DATA

It is critical to examine the patient in a well-lit room. It is important to follow the same routine for every patient with a red eye.

Physical Examination

Eye: Use ophthalmic anesthetic to facilitate examination
- Always assess visual acuity (V/A) when a patient presents with a red eye; it provides information about vision as well as a baseline against which to compare progress
- Visual fields
- Extra-ocular movements (Figure 155-1)
- Check pupil response
- **Children:** Cover/uncover test
- Eyelids: Examine for evidence of inflammation, edema, ptosis
- Inspect bulbar and palpebral conjunctiva for FB, discharge, color, lacrimal ducts, corneal arcus
- External eye: Examine for corneal clarity and FB, color of iris, size, shape, and reactivity
- Determine eye pressure: Use tonometer or via palpation
- Funduscopic examination: Check for red reflex, lens clarity; check disc margins, physiologic cup, blood vessels, retina, macula
- Use slit lamp to visualize anterior structures

Head/eyes/ears/nose/throat: Check for lymphadenopathy; examine face carefully for injuries, inflammation

Diagnostic Procedures

Diagnostic procedures are outlined in Table 155-1.

ASSESSMENT

Almost always, redness of the eye is caused by one of six conditions described in Table 155-2. Differential diagnoses for red eye are outlined in Table 155-3. See also Figures 155-2 and 155-3.

THERAPEUTIC PLAN

Pharmaceutical

Treatment depends on diagnosis. Pharmaceutical treatment for red eye is outlined in Table 155-4.

Lifestyle/Activities

Cool compresses may relieve some discomfort.
Eyelids should be washed daily with a gentle, neutral soap such as baby shampoo to remove crusting.

Diet

No specific diet needed

TABLE 155-3 Differential Diagnosis: Red Eye

Diagnosis	Disease	
	Infectious	**Noninfectious**
Conjunctivitis	Viral Herpes Bacterial	Allergic Dry eye Chemical Contact lens use Foreign body Idiopathic
Keratitis	Bacterial Viral Fungal Acanthamoeba	Recurrent epithelial erosion Foreign body
Eyelid abnormalities	Trichiasis Molluscum contagiosum	
Orbital disorders	Cellulitis Idiopathic orbital Inflammation	

Modified from Morrow et al: Conjunctivitis, *Am Family Physician* 57(4):735-746, 1998.

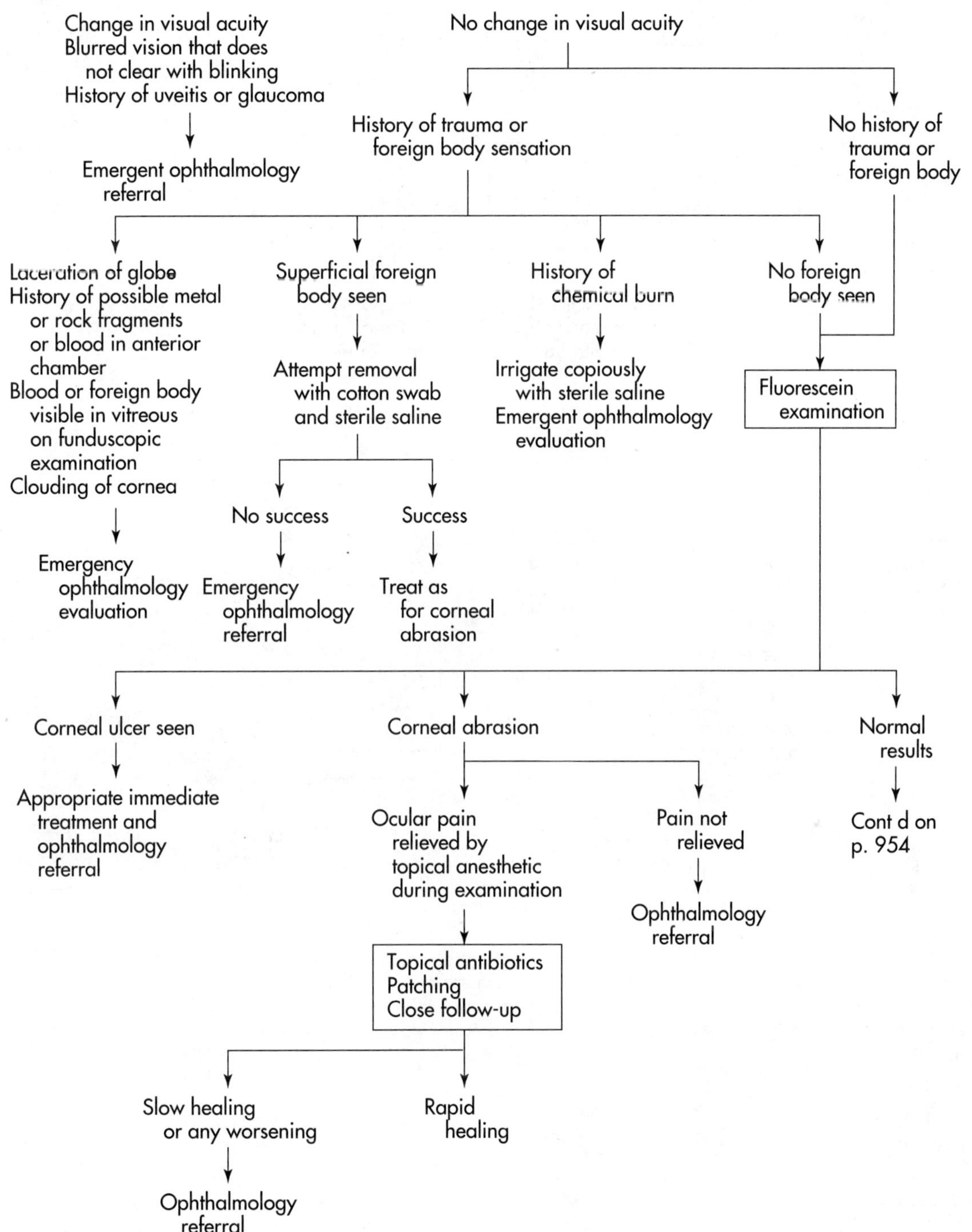

Figure 155-2 Algorithm for patient with acute red eye. (Adapted from Greene HL, Johnson WP, Maricic M: *Decision making in medicine,* St Louis, 1993, Mosby.)

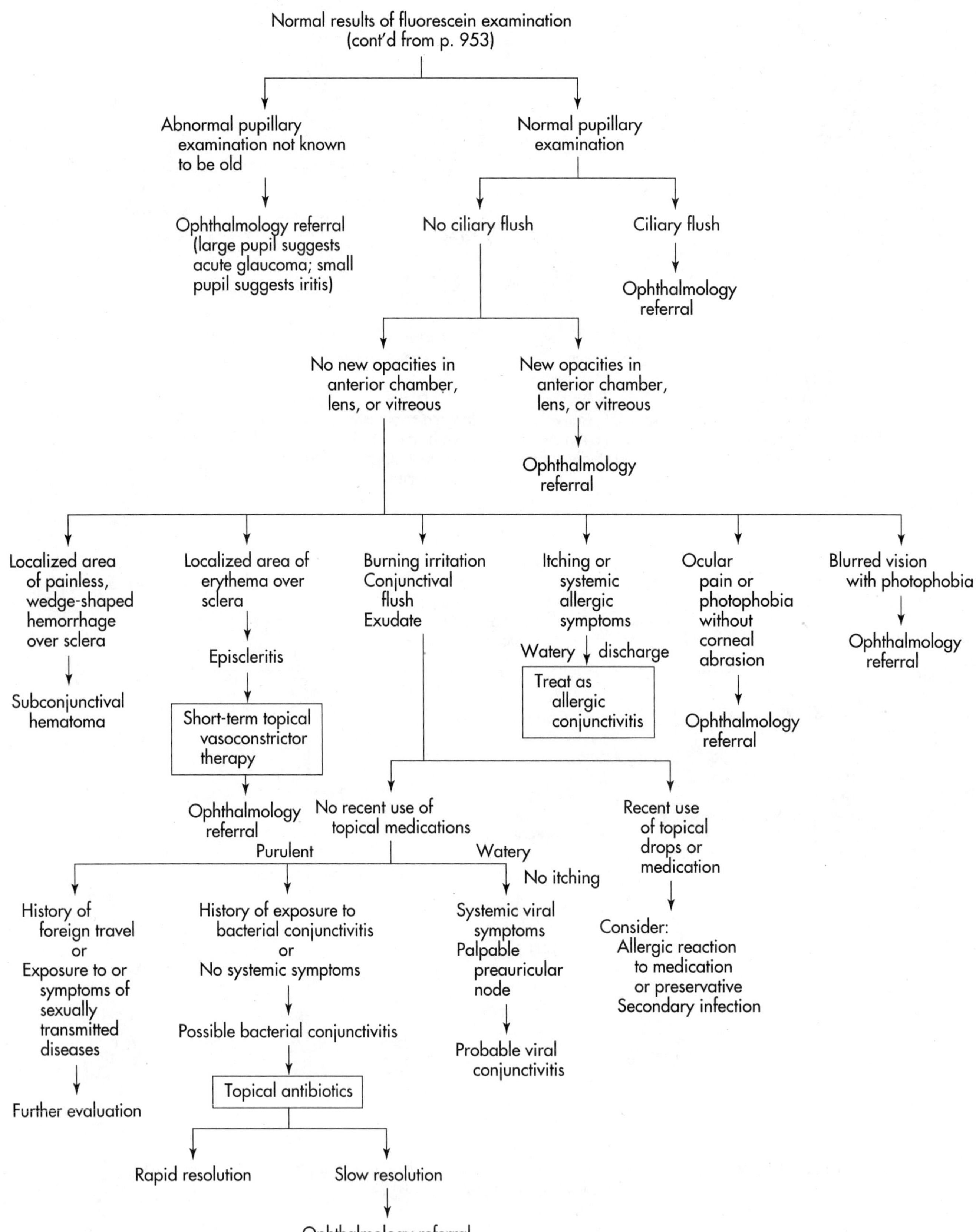

Figure 155-2, cont'd For legend see p. 953.

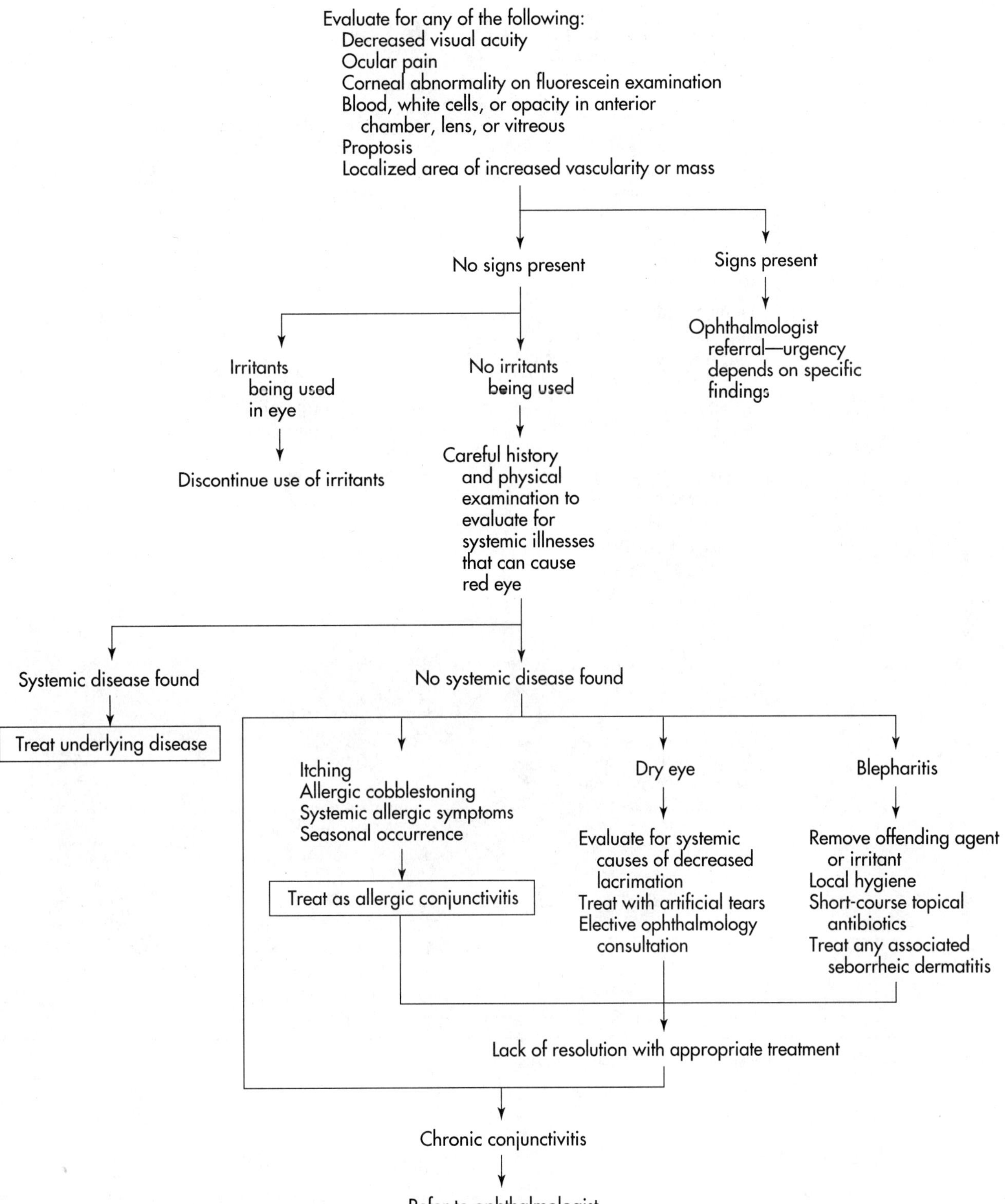

Figure 155-3 Algorithm for patient with chronic red eye. (Adapted from Greene HL, Johnson WP, Maricic M: *Decision making in medicine,* St Louis, 1993, Mosby.)

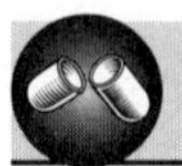

TABLE 155-4 Pharmaceutical Treatment: Red Eye

Drug	Examples	Comments	Cost
Ophthalmic antibiotic drops/ointments	Erythromycin, bacitracin-polymyxin (Polysporin); combination products: trimethoprim-polymyxin (Polytrim), Ofloxacin (Ocuflox)	Well tolerated, excellent coverage most conjunctival pathogens; for both children and adults Consider ointments for children who will complain less about blurring of vision Pregnancy: C SE: Burning, photophobia	
Viral topic agents	Trifluridine (Viroptic) 1 gtt 9× daily; idoxuridine (Herplex) 1 gtt q1h; vidarabine (Vira-A) 0.5 inch ointment 5× daily	Useful for ocular herpes infections Pregnancy: C SE: Visual haze, lacrimation, ocular discomfort, photophobia, edema, conjunctival injection	$48/10 mg/ml (7.5 ml)
Topical antihistamine/ decongestants	Levocabastine (Livostin) 1 gtt QID; iodoxamine (Alomide) 1 gtt QID; naphazoline (Naphcon) 1 gtt BID-QID; naphaxozine + pheniramine (Naphcon A) 1 gtt BID-QID; olopatadine (Patanol) 1-2 gtts BID	Useful for allergic conjunctivitis Pregnancy: C (Alomide B) SE: Burning, stinging, pruritus, blurred vision, dry eye, discharge, hyperemia	N/A
Mast cell stabilizer	Cromolyn sodium (Crolom) 1 gtt 4-6× daily	Useful for allergic conjunctivitis Pregnancy: B SE: Burning, stinging, or discomfort	$26-$28/0.5% (5 ml); $28/1% (5 ml)
Topical NSAIDs	Ketorolac (Acular) 1 gtt QID; diclofenac sodium (Voltaren) 1 gtt QID	Useful for allergic conjunctivitis Pregnancy: C SE: Stinging, burning, irritation, superficial keratitis or infections, allergic reactions	$6-$17/0.5% (15 ml)
Anesthetic agents	0.5% proparacaine (Alcaine); 0.4% benoxinate (Dorsicaine)	Local ocular anesthetic NEVER GIVE TO PATIENT TO TAKE HOME TO RELIEVE PAIN: Causes softening of corneal epithelium; prolonged use can lead to corneal damage and permanent loss of vision	

N/A, Not available; *NSAID,* nonsteroidal antiinflammatory drug; *SE,* side effects.

Patient Education

Meticulous hand washing after touching the eye

- Patient's towel and washcloth should be kept separate
- Discard any make-up to prevent reinfection/cross infection

Family Impact

Depending on cause, family may be affected by loss of ability to drive and participate in work activities. Some conditions are very painful. Diagnosis of glaucoma affects the family since glaucoma has a familial tendency.

Referral

Immediate referral to ophthalmologist:

- If intraocular FB or penetrating injury suspected
- Super Glue in eye
- Hyphema
- Closed-angle glaucoma

Herpes dendritic keratitis
Hyperacute bacterial conjunctivitis
Herpes zoster of ophthalmic branch of trigeminal nerve
Eyelid laceration if laceration crosses the eyelid margin or in the inner canthus involving the tear duct system; if fat is seen, the orbit has been entered
Vision loss caused by central retinal artery occlusion, retinal tears and detachments, traumatic injuries, and endophthalmitis; infection of eye usually caused by staphylococcus epidermis (occurs after ocular surgery; patient complains of pain and loss of vision)

Consultation

Consult with physician if unsure of diagnosis or if visual acuity reveals change in vision.

Follow-up

Corneal abrasions should be re-evaluated in 24 hours. Any change or non-improvement in visual acuity should be reevaluated.

EVALUATION

Reexamination of the eye should indicate that all tests have returned to normal baseline.

Use of visual acuity can provide protection both for patient and nurse practitioner.

Visual acuity should always be measured on any patient with eye problems.

SUGGESTED READINGS

Bertolini J, Pelucio M: The red eye, *Emerg Med Clin North Am* 13(3): 561-579, 1995.

Davey C (1996). The red eye, *Br J Hosp Med* 55(3):89-94, 1996.

Donnefield E, Kaufman H, Schwab I: Conjunctivitis: update on diagnosis and treatment, *Patient Care* 27(10):22-48, 1993.

Easterbrook M, Jonston R, Howcroft M: Assessment and management of ocular foreign bodies *Physician Sports Med* 25(2):77-87, 1997.

Ellsworth W et al: *Mosby's 1998 medical drug reference,* St Louis, 1998, Mosby.

Hara J: The red eye: diagnosis and treatment, *Am Family Physician* 54(8):2423-2430, 1996.

Healthcare Consultants of America, Inc: *1998 physicians fee and coding guide.* Augusta, Ga, 1998, Healthcare Consultants of America, Inc.

Michelson P: Red unresponsive to treatment, *West J Med* 166(2):145-147, 1997.

Morrow G, Abbott R: Conjunctivitis, *Am Family Physician* 57(4):735-746, 1998.

Ruppert S: Differential diagnosis of pediatric conjunctivitis (red eye), *Nurse Pract* 21(7):12-26, 1997.

Silverman H, Nunez L, Feller D: Treatment of common eye emergencies, *Am Family Physician* 45(5):2279-2287, 1992.

Small R: Five steps toward a differential diagnosis, *Consultant* 31:29-31, 1991.

Weber C, Eichenbaum J: Acute red eye, *Postgrad Med* 101(5):185-186, 1997.

Weinstock F, Weinstock M: Common eye disorders: six patients to refer, *Postgrad Med* 99(4):107-110, 1996.

156 Renal Failure

ICD-9-CM

Acute 584.9
Chronic 585

OVERVIEW

Definition

Acute renal failure is the sudden decrease, over days to weeks, in renal function, resulting in retention of urea nitrogen and creatinine in the blood. Many diseases that cause acute renal failure are reversible, and complete recovery is possible.

Chronic renal failure is the progressive inability, over months to years, of the kidneys to respond to changes in body fluid and electrolyte composition. The glomerular filtration rate (GFR) falls below 20 ml/min, producing serum creatinine levels greater than 5 mg/dl. Systemic symptoms related to biochemical abnormalities are present.

Incidence

Greater incidence is noted in **males** (30% to 40% higher) than in females. **Incidence peaks around the ages of 65 to 74 years.** Nonwhites are four times more likely to experience renal failure than whites.

Pathophysiology

Renal failure is divided into three categories: prerenal, renal, and postrenal.

Prerenal causes of renal failure result in hypoperfusion of the kidneys from conditions such as heart disease, shock, or hypertension. There is no structural damage to the kidneys; thus the urinalysis is normal. Prerenal is the most common form of renal failure.

Renal causes produce acute tubular necrosis from either renal ischemia or nephrotoxic injury. Common causes include antibiotics (most frequently aminoglycosides), radiographic contrast media, cyclosporine, and myoglobin from severe trauma or burns.

Postrenal failure results from obstruction of the urinary tract. Urine flow may be polyuric to anuric. Some postrenal causes of failure are bladder cancer, hydronephrosis, and prostatic disease.

Protective Factors Against

Control of diabetes mellitus and hypertension
Prevention of congestive heart failure through hypertension control
Absence of congenital kidney disorders (polycystic disease, hydronephrosis, and horeshoe-shaped kidneys)

Factor That Increases Susceptibility

Multiple traumatic injury

SUBJECTIVE DATA

History of Present Illness

Dysuria (polyuria or anuria)
Prerenal: Is the patient thirsty? Any avenue for fluid loss? Has the patient had recent weight changes?
Renal: Has the patient had an abnormal U/A in the past? Any new medications started?
Postrenal: Any symptoms of urinary hesitancy?

Past Medical History

Congestive heart failure
History of nephrolithiasis
Renal transplant recipient or donor
Cirrhosis
Nephrosis
Diabetes mellitus
Hypertension

Benign prostatic hypertrophy
Collagen vascular disorders

Medications

Diuretics
Unopposed estrogen use
Nonsteroidal antiinflammatory drugs
Antibiotics (aminoglycosides)
Cyclosporine
Angiotensin-converting enzyme inhibitors
Radiographic contrast media

Family History

Polycystic kidney disease
Medullary sponge kidney
Allport's syndrome
Hypertension
Diabetes mellitus
Renal failure
Renal carcinoma

Psychosocial History

Use of heroin

Associated Symptoms

The presence of associated symptoms depends on the degree of renal insufficiency and the GFR. Table 156-1 lists common symptoms and signs in renal failure.

OBJECTIVE DATA

Physical Examination

General appearance, including vital signs, weight; will appear chronically ill with sallow skin.
Refer to Table 156-1 for systems to assess and signs of renal failure.
Prerenal: Does the patient look dehydrated? Any ascites, edema or other indicators of cirrhosis or congestive heart failure?
Renal: Are there signs of diabetes? Is the patient hypertensive?
Postrenal: Does the patient have an enlarged bladder or prostate?

Diagnostic Procedures

Laboratory Tests

Urinalysis ($14-$18): Pay particular attention to the appearance of casts in the urine. Table 156-2 explains the

TABLE 156-1 Common Signs and Symptoms in Renal Failure

System	Symptom	Sign	Pathophysiology
Integument	Pruritus, easy to bruise	Pallor, yellow skin, edema, ecchymoses, uremic frost	Anemia, urochrome excretion, calcium and phosphate skin deposits, platelet dysfunction, urea skin crystals
Ear/nose/throat	Epistaxis, metallic taste	Urinous breath	Platelet dysfunction, nitrogen waste accumulation
Pulmonary	Shortness of breath	Crackles, pleural effusion, tachypnea	Left ventricle dysfunction, increased capillary permeability, fluid volume overload, metabolic acidosis
Cardiovascular	DOE, retrosternal pain on inspiration	Hypertension, S_3 or S_4, dysrhythmia	Hyperkalemia, hypocalcemia, fluid volume overload, increased sodium retention, activation of renin
Gastrointestinal	Anorexia, nausea and vomiting	Gastrointestinal bleeding	Breakdown of urea, release of ammonia, ammonia produces ulcerations, plus altered coagulation
Neurologic	Confusion, irritability, inability to concentrate	Change in level of consciousness, mini-mental state examination	Uremic toxin accumulation, metabolic acidosis
Neuromuscular	Restless legs, numbness, leg cramps	Tremors, hyperreflexia, hyperphosphatemia, hyperkalemia, hypocalcemia	Hyperkalemia, decreased calcium absorption from decreased conservation of vitamin D, decreased excretion of phosphate

TABLE 156-2 Significance of Specific Urinary Casts

Type	Significance
Hyaline casts	Concentrated urine, febrile disease, after strenuous exercise, in the course of diuretic therapy (not indicative of renal disease)
Red cell casts	Glomerulonephritis
White cell casts	Pyelonephritis, interstitial nephritis (indicative of infection or inflammation)
Renal tubular cell casts	Acute tubular necrosis, interstitial nephritis
Coarse, granular casts	Nonspecific; represent degeneration of cast with cellular element
Broad, waxy casts	Chronic renal failure (indicative of stasis in collecting tubule)

From Tierney LM, McPhee SJ, Papadakis MA: *Current medical diagnosis and treatment,* ed 37, Stamford, Conn., 1998, Appleton & Lange.

significance of casts. The persistent detection of protein may indicate the need for a 24-hour urine collection, since the concentration of the urine sample influences the detection of protein.

24-hour urine collection: Protein is a clinical marker. If elevated, check for other systemic causes. Levels greater than 3.5 g/24 hours is indicative of glomerulonephritis. The calculation of creatinine clearance also requires a 24-hour urine. A creatinine concentration of 15 to 25 mg/kg/24 hours is expected for males, and 10 to 20 mg/kg/24 hours is expected of females.

Calculating GFR: The GFR can be calculated using the creatinine clearance using the formula:

$$\frac{\text{U (urine creatinine in mg/dl)} \times \text{V (urine volume ml/24 hours)}}{\text{P (plasma creatinine concentration in mg/dl)}}$$

This number is further divided by 1440 (number of minutes in 24 hours) for ml/min GFR. Another formula can be used to calculate GFR when a 24-hour urine is not available but the serum creatinine level is available:

$$\frac{(140\text{-age}) \times \text{body weight in kg}}{72 \text{ (serum creatinine level)}}$$

Blood urea nitrogen (BUN) ($24-$30): It is an unreliable index of GFR. It will be elevated in renal failure, but it is nonspecific.

Complete blood count ($13-$16): Anemia will be present. Decreased neutrophils and platelets may be present.

Serum glucose ($16-$20) *and electrolytes* ($23-$30): Hypocalcemia, hyperkalemia, hyperphosphatemia, and hyperglycemia may be present in chronic renal failure.

Serum creatinine ($19-$24): This will be elevated. The BUN/creatinine ratio is important in diagnosing site of the problem (Table 156-3).

Special tests: Serum complement levels ($47-$59), antinuclear antibody ($40-$51), rheumatoid arthritis factor ($22-$28); tests such as systemic lupus erythematosus prep may be considered if an immunologic mediated disease is suspected.

Radiographic Tests

Common radiographic procedures are listed in Table 156-4.

ASSESSMENT

Because renal failure is caused by an underlying ailment, it is helpful to first isolate the type of renal failure and then diagnose the condition. Table 156-5 differentiates the types of renal failure. Box 156-1 lists conditions associated with types.

Renal carcinoma should be suspected when the patient has a history of unopposed estrogen use, cigarette smoking, and hypertension and a family history of renal cell carcinoma. Gross hematuria, palpable mass, and flank pain are classic symptoms.

Urinary tract infection is associated with painful urination (suprapubic or flank), hematuria, fever and chills (upper urinary tract).

THERAPEUTIC PLAN

Pharmaceutical

Adjust doses of medications to be consistent with level of renal function. Congestive heart failure patients may require inotropic or afterload reducing agents because diuretics may worsen prerenal renal failure. A pharmaceutical plan is outlined in Table 156-6.

Lifestyle/Activities

Chronic renal failure limits daily activities, particularly if the patient requires dialysis. Fatigue and shortness of breath are major factors in limiting activities.

Diet

Reduce intake of sodium (6 g NaCl—no added salt—diet), water, and potassium. Limit dietary protein to 1 g/kg/day. Foods rich in phosphorus should be avoided (eggs, dairy products, meat).

Patient Education

Teach patient:

To carefully track body weight, intake and output, and nutrition daily as necessary for condition

TABLE 156-3 Classification and Differential Diagnosis of Renal Failure

			Intrinsic Renal Disease			
	Prerenal Azotemia	**Postrenal Azotemia**	**Acute Tubular Necrosis (Oliguric)**	**Acute Tubular Necrosis (Polyuric)**	**Acute Glomerulonephritis**	**Acute Interstitial Nephritis**
Etiology	Hypovolemia, congestive heart failure	Obstruction of the urinary tract	Hypotension, nephrotoxins	Hypotension, nephrotoxins	Poststreptococcal; collagen vascular disease	Allergic reaction; drug reaction
Urinary indices						
Serum BUN: Cr	>20:1	>20:1	<20:1	<20:1	>20:1	<20:1
U_{Na} (meq/L)	<20	Variable	>20	>20	<20	Variable
FE_{Na} (%)	<1	>1	>1	>1	<1	<1; >1
Urine osmolality (mosm/kg)	>500	<400	250-300	250-300	>500	Variable
Urinary sediment	Hyaline casts	Normal or red cells, white cells, or crystals	Granular casts, renal tubular cells	Granular casts, renal tubular cells	Red cells, red cell casts	White cells, white cell casts ± eosinophiluria

From Tierney LM, McPhee SJ, Papadakis MA: *Current medical diagnosis and treatment,* ed 37, Stamford, Conn., 1998, Appleton & Lange.

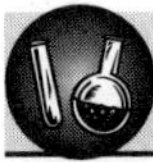

TABLE 156-4 Common Radiographic Tests

Radiographic Test	Significance	Costs ($)
Radionuclide scan	Measures renal function; can detect renovascular disease (renal artery stenosis) and obstruction	Not available
Renal ultrasound	Detects unilateral disease by estimating kidney size; detects masses and cysts	259-319
Computed tomography (CT) scan	Evaluation of solid or cystic lesions detected by ultrasound or intravenous pyelography; not first-line test	807-956
Magnetic resonance imaging	May be used instead of CT for staging of renal carcinoma or evaluation of a mass	1515-1790
Arteriography and venography	Useful in detecting stenosis, aneurysms, vasculitis	265-325
Renal biopsy	Used when no other test has revealed cause of renal failure, but a systemic illness is suspected (e.g., tuberculosis, systemic lupus erythematosus) or when transplant rejection is suspected	Not available
Intravenous pyelography	Best for detecting anatomical structural problem such as lithiasis, lacerations and tears due to trauma	280-333

TABLE 156-5 Types of Renal Failure

Prerenal	Renal	Postrenal
Patient may complain of thirst. Recent weight loss. No casts on U/A. Linked frequently to use of NSAIDs and ACE inhibitors.	Client may be hypertensive. History of trauma. Granular, and tubular casts are present in the U/A.	History of urinary colic, enlarged prostate. Urine flow may fluctuate from day to day. High BUN/creatinine ratio. Hematuria, pyuria, or crystals may be in the U/A.

ACE, Angiotensin-converting enzyme; *BUN*, blood urea nitrogen; *NSAID*, nonsteroidal antiinflammatory; *U/A*, urinalysis.

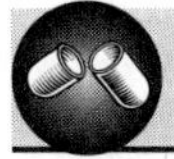

TABLE 156-6 Pharmaceutical Treatment: Renal Failure

Drug	Dose	Comments	Cost ($)
Sodium polystyrene sulfonate	15-30g QD in juice	Ion exchange resin for hyperkalemia	165/454 g
Sodium bicarbonate	650 mg TID	Prevents acidosis; do not use in conjunction with calcium carbonate	2-3
Erythropoietin	30-150 µg three times a week SQ	Used when hematocrit drops below 35%	24-30
Calcitriol	0.25 µg/day	Helps to normalize calcium	33/30 tablets
Calcium carbonate	650 mg TID	Acts as phosphate binding agent, use with hyperphosphatemia	3-8

Box 156-1

Classification of Kidney Diseases That May Result in Chronic Renal Failure

Prerenal Diseases

Renal artery stenosis S
Hepatorenal syndrome S

Renal Parenchymal Diseases

Glomerular diseases
- Membranous glomerulonephritis (GN) I
- Membranoproliferative GN I
- Focal glomerulosclerosis I
- HIV nephropathy S
- Rapidly progress GN I
- Goodpasture's syndrome I, S
- Lupus nephritis I, S
- IgA nephropathy I
- Alport's syndrome—hereditary nephritis H, S
- Diabetic glomerulosclerosis M, S

Tubulointerstitial diseases
- Drug-induced interstitial nephritis N
- Chronic pyelonephritis with reflux
- Analgesic nephropathy N
- Radiation nephritis N
- Polycystic kidney disease H, S
- Sickle cell nephropathy S
- Heavy metal nephropathy N
- Gouty nephropathy M, S
- Medullary cystic disease H
- Vascular diseases
- Thrombotic thrombocytopenic purpura S
- Hemolytic-uremic syndrome S
- Scleroderma kidney S
- Hypertensive nephropathy S
- Vasculitis I, S
- Wegener's granulomatosis I, S

Miscellaneous
- Myeloma kidney N, S
- Amyloidosis S

Postrenal Diseases

Nephrolithiases
Bilateral ureteral obstruction
Bladder outlet obstruction

From Barker L, Burton J, Zieve P: *Principles of ambulatory medicine,* ed 4, Baltimore, 1995, Williams & Wilkins.

H, Hereditary; *I,* immunologically mediated; *M,* metabolic; *N,* nephrotoxic; *S,* part of a systemic disorder.

To avoid magnesium-containing antacids.

Proper method of collecting 24-hour urine: begin collection on rising, void and discard first specimen, collect all other urine until the same time the following day when the patient voids and adds that last specimen to the total amount.

Introduce the ideas of dialysis or renal transplantation as indicated.

Family Impact

Family support is often needed for transportation to dialysis or in being screened as a potential donor.

Referral/Consultation

The nurse practitioner typically will order laboratory tests, except for the special tests identified in this chapter that are diagnostic for systemic disease. The practitioner may order a renal ultrasound test. Consultation is recommended for any patient with consistent proteinuria. A referral to a urologist should be made if acute or chronic renal failure is suspected. It is debatable whether a patient with asymptomatic hematuria should be referred to a urologist. Look for an association with proteinuria. If both are present, consider referral.

Follow-up

Patients with chronic renal failure who are being followed by the primary care provider for hypertension and diabetes will need 24- to 48-hour phone follow-up when new medications are introduced. Patients should be reevaluated in the office within 2 weeks.

EVALUATION

A urinalysis should be performed at each office visit. Serum creatinine should be monitored frequently. 24-hour urine collections should be made annually in stable patients.

SUGGESTED READINGS

Briefel G: Chronic renal insufficiency. In Barker L, Burton J, Zieve P, editors: *Principles of ambulatory medicine,* ed 4, Baltimore, Md, 1995, Williams & Wilkins.

Clive D: Azotemia. In Greene H et al, editors: *Clinical medicine,* ed 2, St Louis, 1996, Mosby.

Ellsworth W et al: *Mosby's 1998 medical drug reference*, St. Louis, 1998, Mosby.

Froom P, Froom J, Ribak J: Asymptomatic microscopic hematuria—is investigation necessary? *J Clin Epidemiol* 50:1197-1200, 1997.

Healthcare Consultants of America, Inc: *1998 physicians fee and coding guide.* Augusta, Ga, 1998, Healthcare Consultants of America, Inc.

Morrison G: Kidney. In Tierney L, McPhee S, Papadakis M, editors: *Current medical diagnosis and treatment,* ed 37, Stamford, Conn, 1998, Appleton & Lange.

Yamagata K et al: A long-term follow up study of asymptomatic hematuria and or proteinuria in adults, *Clin Nephrol* 45:281-288, 1996.

157 Rosacea

ICD-9-CM

Rosacea 695.3

OVERVIEW

Definition

Rosacea is a chronic facial disorder of middle-aged and older persons with three components: tendency to flush easily, pimples, and hyperplasia of the nose.

Incidence

Affects fair-skinned persons more often. Incidence is higher in **women (ages 30 to 50)** but the **men** tend to have more hyperplasia (rhinophyma) than the women with rosacea

Pathophysiology

The cause is unknown. There is a link between rosacea and how often and how strongly people blush. The greater the blush, the greater the likelihood of rosacea. Migraine headaches have also been associated with this condition. Repressing anger, fear, and other emotions is also linked to the condition.

Protective Factors Against

Youth
Dark or olive-toned skin

Factors that Increase Susceptibility

"Peaches and cream" complexion
Sensitivity to cosmetics

SUBJECTIVE DATA

History of Present Illness

Patient may ignore initial phase of rosacea in which the face appears flushed or sunburned.
May complain of easily flushing with burning or stinging.

Past Medical History

Migraine headaches

Medications

Use of topical corticosteroids on the face; may cause temporary change in cheek color

Family History

Noncontributory

Psychosocial History

NOT associated with alcoholism; alcohol may worsen flushing

Associated Symptom

Tearing of eyes

OBJECTIVE DATA

Physical Examination

Head/eyes/ears/nose/throat:
- Face: Dry facial skin
  - Small, red, possibly pus filled papules (Figure 157-1)
  - Telangiectasia

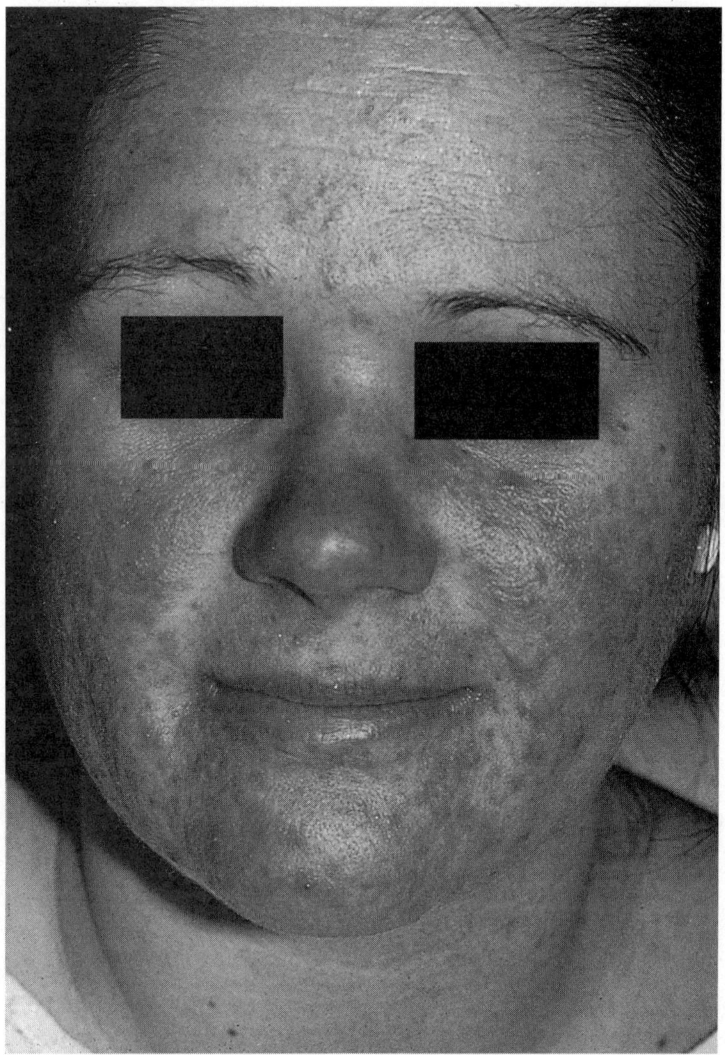

Figure 157-1 Rosacea. Generalized inflammation with multiple inflammatory papules and pustules, predominantly located on the central aspect of the face and nose. (From Hooper BJ, Goldman MP: *Primary dermatologic care,* St Louis, 1999, Mosby.)

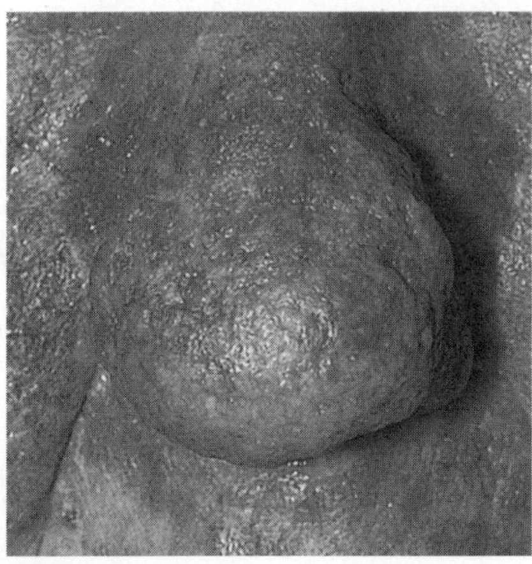

Figure 157-2 Pustular lesions and rhinophyma in rosacea. (From Cox NH, Lawrence CM: *Diagnostic problems in dermatology,* St Louis, 1998, Mosby.)

TABLE 157-1 Differential Diagnosis

Diagnosis	Supporting Data
Acne	Youth, comedones both black and white, no telangiectasia or rhinophyma

Nose: Enlarged, with bumps (Figure 157-2)
Eyes: Injected conjunctiva with tearing or discharge

Diagnostic Procedures

None

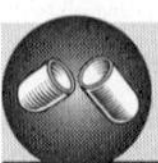

TABLE 157-2 Pharmaceutical Treatment: Rosacea

Drug	Dose	Comments	Cost ($)
Tetracycline	250-500 mg PO BID	Take on empty stomach	7-20
Erythromycin	250-500 mg BID	Take on empty stomach	14-20
Isoretinoin	0.5-1 mg/kg/day PO for 12-28 weeks	Use when other measures fail	333-395
Metronidazole	250 mg BID × 3 weeks	Disulfiram effect with alcohol	3-131
Metronidazole	0.75% gel applied BID	Start with this therapy first	32

Occasionally a mild topical corticosteroid (e.g., 1% hydrocortisone) may be used daily in the early weeks of treatment.

ASSESSMENT

Differential diagnois is listed in Table 157-1.

THERAPEUTIC PLAN

Pharmaceutical

Pharmaceutical treatment is outlined in Table 157-2.

Surgical

Surgery may be used to correct the rhinophyma.
Laser may be used to treat the telangiectasis.

Lifestyle/Activities

Facial flushing can be triggered by hard exercise.
Avoid stress, sunlight, extreme heat or cold.

Diet

Avoid hot drinks, alcohol, spicy foods.

Patient Education

Identify what triggers flushing and avoid the situtation.
Treatment does not cure the condition but keeps the condition from worsening. Rosacea usually returns within 1 week to 6 months following the cessation of drug therapy.
Avoid skin cleansing products that contain alcohol, acetone, oil, or perfumes.
Use moisturizer as needed.
Use a sunscreen with SPF15.
Avoid strong steroid creams.
Menopause may worsen the condition.

Family Impact

Relatively little impact.

Referral/Consultation

Consultation with a dermatologist and plastic surgeon may be warranted. Dermatologist may prescribe beta blockers to reduce redness and swelling.

Follow-up

Schedule for monthly visits until flushing is under control.

EVALUATION

Monitor for increasing swelling of nose and telangiectasis.

RESOURCES

National Rosacea Society
800 South Northwest Highway
Suite 200
Barrington, IL 60010
1-888-NO-BLUSH

SUGGESTED READINGS

Berger T, Goldstein S, Odom R: Skin and appendages. In Tierney L, McPhee S, Papadakis M, editors: *Current medical diagnosis and treatment,* ed 36, Stamford, Conn, 1998, Appleton & Lange.

Ellsworth W et al: *Mosby's 1998 medical drug reference,* St Louis, 1998, Mosby.

Roseola

Roseola infantum, Exanthem subitum

ICD 9-CM

Roseola 057.8
Roseola Infantum, Infantilis 057.8

OVERVIEW

Definition

Roseola is an acute viral illness of the herpes family (HHV-6).

Incidence

Infection occurs throughout the year. Mean incubation period is 9 to 10 days. Contagious before and during the febrile period. Rare before age 3 months and after 4 years. Peaks in second year of life. Most common in spring. Outbreaks are rarely recognized. Infection may occur without symptoms.

Pathophysiology

There are antibodies to HHV-6 in cord blood. Greater than 90% of children have antibodies to HHV-6 by age 3.

Mode of transmission is unknown, but the HHV-6 genome may be persistent in lymphocytes and salivary glands.

SUBJECTIVE DATA

History of Present Illness

There is an abrupt onset of fever as high as 41° C (106° F), lasts 3 to 5 days. The child may be mildly lethargic and irritable.

Past Medical History

Immunization history
Communicable disease history

Medications

Current/new medications

Family History

Illness among family members
Age of siblings

Psychosocial History

Environmental exposure (e.g., day care)

Description of Most Common Symptoms

An erythematous, maculopapular rash appears on the trunk following the fever, spreading to the extremities, neck and face. The rash fades within 24 hours.

Associated Symptoms

Occasionally the pharynx, tonsils, and tympanic membranes are injected. In immunocompromised hosts, HHV-6 infection has been associated with pneumonitis.

OBJECTIVE DATA

Physical Examination

Head/eyes/ears/nose/throat: Observe pharynx, tonsils, and tympanic membrane for injection.
Extremities: Observe trunk, arms, neck, face, and legs for erythematous, maculopapular, pin-point, nonpruritic rash.

TABLE 158-1 Differential Diagnosis: Roseola

Diagnoses	Supporting Data
Fifth disease	Warm, red, nontender, "slapped cheeks" rash. Spreads in 1 to 2 days to trunk, neck, and buttocks. Fades with central clearing, leaving a lacy, reticulated rash that lasts 2-40 days.
Impetigo	Honey-crusted lesions at the site of broken or irritated skin. Frequently around the mouth, nose, or hands. Not associated with fever.
Rubeola	Erythematous, maculopapular rash. Begins on face, becomes generalized. Sometimes ends in branny desquamation. Prodromal fever, conjunctivitis, coryza, cough, and Koplik spots on buccal mucosa.
Scabies	Burrows (raised lines or scratches), bumps, blisters, or scaly patches on hands, wrists, elbows, buttocks, genitals and between digits of children or adults. Infants are usually affected on the palms, soles, head, neck, and face.
Scarlet fever	A fine, erythematous rash that blanches on pressure; often felt easier than seen (sand papery). Most often on the neck, chest folds of the axilla, elbow, groin, and inner thighs. Cheeks may appear flushed and pale around the mouth. Follows a strep infection, usually streptococcal pharyngitis.
Meningitis	Headache, fever, stiff neck, rash: macular and erythematous at onset, then petechial or purpuric

Diagnostic Procedures

Not necessary

ASSESSMENT

Differential diagnoses include fifth disease, impetigo, rubeola, scabies, meningitis, and scarlet fever (Table 158-1).

THERAPEUTIC PLAN

Pharmaceutical

Treatment is directed at fever control for children at risk of febrile seizures (ages 6 months to 2 to 3 years, or previous history of febrile seizures). Pharmaceutical treatment is outlined in Table 158-2.

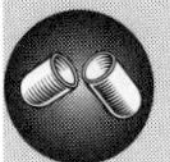

TABLE 158-2 Pharmaceutical Treatment: Roseola

Drug	Dose	Comments
Acetaminophen	See pediatric dosing chart in Appendix M	q4h, max. 5 doses/day

Lifestyle/Activities

Supportive care as needed
Keep child home
Adequate rest until fever ends

Diet

Regular. Encourage fluids

Patient Education

Self-limiting disease
High fever can cause seizures
Keep child well hydrated

Family Impact

None

Referral

Refer to MD:

Prolonged high fever
Febrile seizures
Signs of meningeal irritation

Consultation

Immunocompromised individuals

Follow-up

None

EVALUATION

None

SUGGESTED REFERENCES

American Academy of Pediatrics: Human herpesvirus 6 (including roseola). In Peter G, editor: *1997 Red Book: Report of the Committee on Infectious Disease,* ed 24, Elk Grove Village, Ill, 1997, American Academy of Pediatrics.

American Public Health Association: *Control of communicable diseases manual,* ed 16, Washington, DC, 1995, American Public Health Association.

Ellsworth W et al: *Mosby's 1998 medical drug reference,* St Louis, 1998, Mosby.

Rubella

German Measles, 3-day Measles

ICD-9-CM

Maternal Rubella Affecting Fetus or Newborn 760.2
Exposure to Rubella V01.4
Uncomplicated Postnatal Rubella 056.90
Postnatal Rubella with Specific Complications 56.79
Congenital Rubella 771.0
Vaccination, Prophylactic Against V04.3

OVERVIEW

Definition

German measles is a mild viral disease, important due to its teratogenicity. Congenital rubella syndrome (CRS) occurs in up to 90% of infants born to females who acquire rubella during the first trimester of pregnancy. The risk falls to 10% to 20% by the 16th week and is minimal after the 20th week.

Incidence

Late winter, early spring; 14- to 21-day incubation period
Contagious a few days before rash and 5 to 7 days after rash appears
Cases have decreased 99% from the prevaccine era

Pathophysiology

Spread by direct contact with infected people by their nasopharyngeal secretions and respiratory droplets
Replicates in nasopharynx and regional lymph nodes
Usually self-limiting and does not manifest complications
Infants with CRS can shed the virus in their urine and nasopharyngeal fluids for 1 year
Active immunity is acquired by natural infection (permanent) or immunization (thought to be lifelong); infants born to immune mothers are protected for 6 to 9 months
10% of young adults are susceptible primarily due to lack of vaccination

SUBJECTIVE DATA

History of Present Illness

Young children may experience mild coryza and diarrhea.
Older children and adults may have sore throat.
Prodromal symptoms last 1 to 5 days, followed by a rash that begins on the face and spreads downward to the trunk and extremities.
Lesions remain pink and discrete.

Past Medical History

Immunization history
Communicable disease history

Medications

Current/new medications

Family History

Rash or illness among household contacts
Family immunization history
Pregnancy of family members/close contacts

Psychosocial History

Known exposures

Description of Most Common Symptoms

Exanthem is a pink, maculopapular eruption. It begins on face and spreads down to trunk and extremities.
Facial rash clears as extremity rash erupts.
Rash usually clears by 3 to 5 days.
Lesions remain pink and discrete.

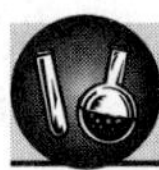

TABLE 159-1 Diagnostic Procedures: Rubella

Diagnostic Test	Findings/Rationale	Cost ($)
Complete blood count	Mild leukopenia with lymphocytosis	18-23
Rubella antibody titer	Draw antibody titers during the acute phase (7-10 days after onset) and convalescent sera (2-3 weeks later); 4× rise in titer; antibody titers are also a part of routine prenatal testing to identify at-risk status	36-44
Rubella virus culture from pharynx, nose, or blood	Positive for rubella virus	61-75

TABLE 159-2 Differential Diagnosis: Rubella

Diagnoses	Supporting Data
Kawasaki's syndrome	Similar to scarlet fever with additional signs of conjunctivitis, cracking lips, and diarrhea.
Roseola	An erythematous, maculopapular rash. Appears on the trunk following a fever as high as 106 degrees. Spreads to the extremities, neck and face. Rash fades within 24 hours.
Rubeola	An erythematous, maculopapular, discrete rash. Generalized lymphadenopathy. Slight fever.
Scarlet fever	A fine erythematous rash that blanches on pressure. Often felt rather than seen (sand papery). Most often on the neck, chest folds of the axilla, elbow, groin and inner thighs. Cheeks may appear flushed with circumoral pallor. Follows a streptococcal infection, usually streptococcal pharyngitis.

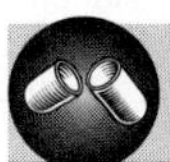

TABLE 159-3 Pharmaceutical Treatment: Rubella

Drug	Dose	Comments	Cost
Acetaminophen infant drops (80 mg/0.8 ml)	See pediatric dosing in Appendix M	q4h, max. 5 doses/day	See Appendix M
Ibuprofen suspension (100 mg/5 ml)	See pediatric dosing in Appendix M	q6-8h	

Associated Symptoms

Postauricular and suboccipital lymphadenopathy

OBJECTIVE DATA

Physical Examination

Skin: Inspect skin, noting characteristics of exanthem
To rule out other exanthems:
- Head/eyes/ears/nose/throat
  - Assess mouth for Koplik's spots
  - Check for nuchal rigidity
- Chest: Auscultate heart

Diagnostic Procedures

Clinical diagnosis is often inaccurate. Laboratory diagnosis is important. Diagnostic procedures are outlined in Table 159-1.

ASSESSMENT

Differential Diagnoses include Kawasaki's syndrome, roseola, rubeola, scarlet fever and are outlined in Table 159-2.

THERAPEUTIC PLAN

Pharmaceutical

Pharmaceutical treatment is outlined in Tables 159-3 and 159-4.

Lifestyle/Activities

Exclude from school/work/day care for at least 7 days after onset of rash.

Diet

Regular

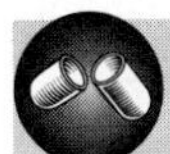

TABLE 159-4 Immunizations: Rubella

Drug	Dose	Comments	Cost ($)
Measles, mumps, and rubella (MMR)	Adults: 0.5 ml SQ Children: 0.5 ml SQ: first dose at 15-18 mos, second dose at 4-6 years or 11-12 years	All nonimmunized persons should receive MMR (live virus): ask about egg allergies or reaction to neomycin; do not give to pregnant women or patients with immunosuppression (e.g., acquired immunodeficiency syndrome, cancer patients) Pregnancy: C Recommend delaying pregnancy for 3 months after vaccination	43-52

Patient Education

Discuss need for preventive immunization (see Table 159-4).
Identify pregnant female acquaintances and avoid contact with them (explain why).

Family Impact

Need for ill child care may be difficult for working parents.

Referral

Pregnant females, especially in the first trimester.

Consultation

The Health Department is an important local resource in terms of identifying location of outbreeds and prophylactic measures for that community.

Follow-up

Return to have convalescent titer drawn.
Report to local health authority.
Phone contact in 72 hours.

EVALUATION

Possible complications: encephalitis, thrombocytopenic purpura, congenital rubella

SUGGESTED READINGS

American Academy of Pediatrics: Rubella. In Peter G, editor: *1997 Red Book: Report of the Committee on Infectious Disease,* ed 24, Elk Grove Village, Ill, 1997, American Academy of Pediatrics.

American Public Health Association: *Control of communicable diseases manual,* ed 16, Washington, DC, 1995, American Public Health Association.

Ellsworth W et al: *Mosby's 1998 medical drug reference*, St. Louis, 1998, Mosby.

Fenstermacher K, Hudson BT: *Practice guidelines for family nurse practitioners,* Philadelphia, 1997, WB Saunders.

Healthcare Consultants of America, Inc: *1998 physicians fee and coding guide,* Augusta, Ga, 1998, Healthcare Consultants of America, Inc.

Uphold C, Graham M: *Clinical guidelines in family practice,* ed 2, Gainesville, Fla, 1994, Barmarrae Books.

Rubeola

Measles, Hard Measles, Red Measles

ICD-9-CM

Rubeola (Measles) 055.9
Complicated 055.8

OVERVIEW

Definition

Measles is an acute, highly communicable viral disease caused by morbilli virus in the paramyxovirus family.

Incidence

Measles occurs in late winter and early spring. There is an 8- to 12-day incubation period. Those who contract the disease are contagious 1 to 2 days before any symptoms until 4 days after the rash appears. Since 1992 incidence in the United States has been low, less than 1000 reported cases per year. Cases occur in unimmunized populations; cases occurring in previously vaccinated adolescents and young adult in secondary schools and colleges are due to vaccine failure (failure to seroconvert after 1 dose). Male = female.

Pathophysiology

Spread by direct contact with nasal/throat secretions of infected person or contact with articles soiled with nose/throat secretions.

Immunization at 15 months of age produces immunity in 95% to 98% of recipients. A second dose may increase immunity levels to 99%. Acquired immunity after the illness is permanent.

SUBJECTIVE DATA

History of Present Illness

Fever (as high at 105° F) with conjunctivitis and photo phobia

Dry hacking or barking cough and cold symptoms followed by a deep red, blotchy rash beginning on the face; becomes generalized, confluent, and sometimes ends in branny desquamation

Past Medical History

Immunization history, including number of doses of vaccine and age at time of administration

Communicable disease history

Medications

Current/new medications

Family History

Illness or rashes among household members.

Immunization history of household members.

Psychosocial History

Environmental exposures

Description of Most Common Symptoms

Confluent red maculopapular rash beginning on face and moving down trunk

Associated Symptoms

Koplik spots (gray/white sand grain sized dots on red base on buccal mucosa opposite lower molars) appear about 2 days before rash appears

OBJECTIVE DATA

Physical Examination

Skin: Inspect skin, note characteristics of exanthem.
Head/eyes/ears/nose/throat: Note conjunctivitis, photophobia, Koplik spots and other findings.
Chest: Auscultate heart and lungs.
Neurological: Evaluate mental status and neurological system to rule out complications such as encephalitis.

Diagnostic Procedures

Usually none needed
Antibody titers at appearance of rash and 3 to 4 weeks later or measles specific immunoglobulin M antibodies 10 days after rash appears ($57-$70)

ASSESSMENT

Differential diagnoses include Kawasaki's syndrome, roseola, rubella, and scarlet fever and are outlined in Table 160-1.

THERAPEUTIC PLAN

Pharmaceutical

Pharmaceutical treatment is outlined in Table 160-2.

Lifestyle/Activities

Supportive care: Cool baths for fever control
Rest in semi-darkened room
Exclude from school/day care until 4 days after rash appears

TABLE 160-1 Differential Diagnosis: Rubeola

Diagnoses	Supporting Data
Kawasaki's syndrome	Similar to scarlet fever with additional signs of conjunctivitis, cracking lips, and diarrhea
Roseola	An erythematous, maculopapular rash; appears on the trunk following a fever as high as 106° F; spreads to the extremities, neck, and face; rash fades within 24 hours
Rubella	An erythematous, maculopapular, discrete rash; generalized lymphadenopathy; slight fever
Scarlet fever	A fine, erythematous rash that blanches on pressure; often felt rather than seen (sand papery); most often on the neck, chest folds of the axilla, elbow, groin, and inner thighs; cheeks may appear flushed with circumoral pallor; follows a streptococcal infection, usually streptococcal pharyngitis

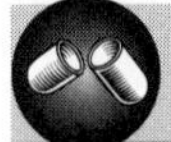

TABLE 160-2 Pharmaceutical Treatment: Rubeola

Drug	Dose	Comments	Cost
Acetaminophen	Adults: 325-650 mg Infants/children: See pediatric dosing in Appendix M		$1/325 mg (100)
Vitamin A	6 mos-1 yr: 100,000 IU PO >1 yr: 200,000 IU PO; repeat the next day and in 4 weeks.	Consider for patients 6 mos-2 yrs hospitalized with measles and complications *or* >6 mos with ophthalmologic or nutritional disorders or recent immigrants; given to increase vitamin A, which is reduced early in disease Pregnancy: X	$2/25,000 U (100); $3-$72/50,000 U (100)
Post exposure prophylaxis: Immune globulin	0.25 mg/kg IM, max. dose 15 ml; immunocompromised: 0.5 mg/kg, max. dose 15 ml	Prevents or modifies disease in person exposed to measles <6 days before administration; do not give in severe vitamin A deficiency or severe thrombocytopenia	$24-$30

TABLE 160-3 Immunization: Rubeola

Drug	Dose	Comments	Cost ($)
MMR	Adults: 0.5 ml SQ Children: 0.5 ml SQ; first dose at 12-15 mos, second dose at 4-6 years or 11-12 years	All nonimmunized persons should receive MMR (live virus); ask about egg allergies or reaction to neomycin; do not give to pregnant women; warn patients who are immunocompromised (acquired immunodeficiency syndrome) that, if a live virus is used in family members, the disease can be transmitted to them Pregnancy: C	43-52

Diet

As tolerated; encourage fluids to prevent dehydration

Patient Education

Encourage immunization. Table 160-3 contains an immunization schedule.

Postexposure globulin administered within 72 hours can offer protection.

Teach family to observe changes in level of consciousness and to monitor temperature and respirations daily.

Encourage thorough hand washing, disposal of tissues, covering mouth when coughing.

Family Impact

Need to care for ill child may be difficult for working parents

CAUTION: Alternate child care arrangements must be taken if family members are immunocompromised, since this is a live virus.

Referral

Exposed pregnant females

Consultation

Refer to MD before administering vitamin A or if complications develop.

Follow-up

Examine daily during acute phase and 3 to 4 days after onset of exanthem to monitor development of complications.

Report cases to local health authority.

EVALUATION

Complications include otitis media, bronchopneumonia, croup, diarrhea, encephalitis (1 in 1000 cases), and death (1 to 2 in 1000 cases).

SUGGESTED READINGS

American Academy of Pediatrics: Measles. In Peter G, editor: *1997 Red Book: Report of the Committee on Infectious Disease,* ed 24, Elk Grove Village, Ill, 1997, American Academy of Pediatrics.

American Public Health Association: *Control of communicable diseases manual*, ed 16, Washington, DC, 1995, American Public Health Association.

Ellsworth W et al: *Mosby's 1998 medical drug reference*, St. Louis, 1998, Mosby.

Fenstermacher K, Hudson BT: *Practice guidelines for family nurse practitioners,* Philadelphia, 1997, WB Saunders.

Healthcare Consultants of America, Inc: *1998 physicians fee and coding guide,* Augusta, Ga, 1998, Healthcare Consultants of America, Inc.

Uphold C, Graham M: *Clinical guidelines in family practice,* ed 2, Gainesville, Fla, 1994, Barmarrae Books.

161 Scabies

ICD-9-CM

Scabies (Any Site) 133.0

OVERVIEW

Definition

Scabies is an infestation of the skin with an obligate parasite, the human skin itch mite, *Sarcoptes scabiei var hominis*.

Incidence

Scabies is most commonly seen in children, young adults, institutionalized persons of all ages, and persons with acquired immunodeficiency syndrome (AIDS). A persistently high incidence is found in developing countries and in housing where overcrowding occurs.

Pathophysiology

The impregnated female mite burrows into the skin using chemical factors in the saliva to dissolve keratin on the skin surface. Once in the burrow, the female remains there her entire life, approximately 30 days, laying two to three eggs per day. The eggs hatch in 3 to 4 days; and the mites reach maturity in about 4 days, migrate to the skin surface, mate, and repeat the cycle.

Symptoms occur 4 to 6 weeks after the first infestation and are caused by a hypersensitivity reaction. This response is due to the mite saliva and feces (scybala), which is deposited in the skin. Those who are infested with scabies more than once will develop symptoms 24 to 48 hours after succeeding exposures.

Protective Factors Against

Hand washing and universal precautions are the best protection against scabies infestation for personnel involved in patient care. Scabies can be transmitted if, after direct skin-to-skin contact, there has been time for the mite to leave its burrow and walk from one body to another. Hand washing will remove scabies mites from the skin before they can burrow.

Factors That Increase Susceptibility

Sexual contact with an infested person
Close physical contact with an infested person
Overcrowding
Sharing linens and sleeping on a mattress after an infested person

Persons Most Susceptible

Children
Young adults
Elderly living in nursing homes
Institutionalized persons of all ages
Immunosuppressed persons

SUBJECTIVE DATA

Past Medical History

Ask about history of a previous similar episode.

Family History

Ask about family members or close contacts having the same symptoms.

Psychosocial History

Ask about:

Multiple sexual partners
Child enrolled in day care, school, or camp
Children or adults who are institutionalized
Elderly in nursing homes
Other members of the household with same symptoms

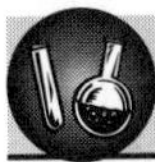

TABLE 161-1 Diagnostic Test: Scabies

Diagnostic Test	Findings/Rationale	Cost ($)
Microscopic examination of specimen	Procedure to obtain specimen: 1. Use a No. 15 scalpel and shave a paper thin 3- to 5-mm top off the burrow. 2. Place the shaving on a microscope slide, add a drop of mineral oil or immersion oil, then cover with a cover slip. 3. Examine each shaving under the microscope. Mites are an oval slightly spiny organism with several fine, short legs. Eggs are about ⅓ the size of the mite. Mite feces are seen as oval golden-brown objects and are ⅒ the size of the mite egg. Alternate procedure to obtain a specimen: Locate a tiny dark dot at one end of the burrow, gently remove with the point of a 16-22 gauge hypodermic needle and place on a microscope slide with a drop of oil; will need to magnify 10 times.	17-21

TABLE 161-2 Differential Diagnosis: Scabies

Diagnosis	Supporting Data
Atopic dermatitis	Erythematous papular lesions that are diffuse with scaling, usually in flexural areas associated with abnormally dry skin; may have episodes of itching
Allergic and contact dermatitis	Maculopapular to vesiculopapular lesions; may be grouped or linear lesions limited to area of contact
Pediculosis	Itching and skin excoriation from scratching, worse at night
Insect bites	Papule or vesicles on erythematous base with intense pruritus, scattered over body, usually in exposed areas
Secondary syphilis	Primary: Chancre, painless, indurated ulcer Secondary: Skin rash with enlarged lymph nodes, malaise

Description of Most Common Symptoms

Presents as a generalized pruritic rash, particularly on hands, flexor portion of wrists, elbows, axillary folds, buttocks, breasts, abdomen, and genitals

Intense intermittent itching, more intense with increased warmth of skin

Nocturnal itching is a classic symptom

Persons with a suppressed immune system may not have pruritus

Associated Symptoms

History of sleeplessness due to intense pruritus

OBJECTIVE DATA

Physical Examination

A problem-oriented physical should be conducted, using strong lighting and a hand-held magnifying lens to facilitate identification of the burrows. The examiner should always wear gloves when examining persons with skin diseases.

Assess all skin surfaces. Primary lesions are papules, vesicles, and burrows. Scabies appears as an erythematous, papular, symmetrical rash found on the trunk, often concentrated in skin folds, including axilla, nipples of women, waistline, buttocks, upper thighs, and external genitalia. The rash does not necessarily correspond to where the burrows and mites are found.

Assess interdigital areas of fingers and flexor aspects of wrists for burrows, using a magnifying lens. Burrows appear as gray-to-white linear ridges and contain the female mite. Eighty five percent of infested individuals have burrows on the fingers, interdigital areas, flexor aspects of wrists, lateral palms, nipples of females, and male genitalia. Burrows are indicative of the diagnosis.

Infants and **young children:** Assess for generalized skin eruptions on the scalp, face, palms, and soles. Vesicles, vesiculopustules, and papules are common. Burrow

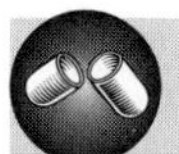

TABLE 161-3 Pharmaceutical Plan: Scabies

Drug	Dose	Comments	Cost
Permethrin 5% cream (Elimite)	30 g or 1 ounce	Considered the treatment of choice because of its low toxicity and high efficacy Pregnancy: B SE: Mild pruritus and transient burning; Permethrin safety for use in children under age 2 mos or pregnant or nursing women has not been established 1. Precede treatment with a warm shower or bath, scrubbing involved areas with soap and water. 2. Dry thoroughly and let the skin temperature cool down. 3. Apply cream to the entire body from the neck down. 4. Leave the cream on 8 to 12 hours and then remove by showering. 5. One ounce (30 g) of the cream is sufficient for one application, and a single application is usually effective. **Children** <2 years of age: Apply to the scalp and face, as well as the entire body. Avoid the eyes, nose, and mouth.	$17/5 % (60 g); $9/liq: 1% (60 ml)
Lindane 1% lotion (Kwell)		NOTE: This drug is considered an alternate treatment because of organism resistance and neurotoxic effects in **infants.** This medication should not be used on **infants, pregnant** or **nursing women,** or patients with neurological disorders or excoriated areas of skin. In geriatric patients and young children, neurotoxic effects such as seizures have occurred from overuse of the medication or ingestion of the drug. Ingestion of the drug can occur in children by thumb sucking. Pregnancy: B 1. Precede treatment with a shower or bath. 2. Dry thoroughly and allow the skin temperature to cool. 3. Apply lotion to the entire body from the neck down. 4. In **young children** apply lotion to the scalp and face as well as the entire body (avoid eyes, mouth, nose). 5. Leave the lotion on the skin for 8 hours, and then remove with a shower. 6. Repeat the treatment in 7 days.	$2-$6/lotion; $2-$5/shampoo: 1% (60 ml); $13/cream: (60 g)
Crotamiton 10% (Eurax)		Cream or lotion is considered safe for **infants** and **pregnant** or **nursing women.** It is less effective than permethrin. Pregnancy: C 1. Precede treatment with shower or bath. 2. Dry thoroughly and allow the skin temperature to cool. 3. Apply cream or lotion to the entire body from the neck down. 4. **Infants** and **young children:** Apply to the scalp, face, and entire body (avoid eyes, nose, mouth). 5. Reapply the treatment the second night without removing the first treatment. 6. Wash off the medication 24 hours after the second application. SE: Itching, rash, irritation, contact dermatitis	$11/lotion: 10% (60 g) $10/cream: 10% (60 g)
Sulfur preparation (Precipitated sulfur 5%-10%)		Treatment of choice for infants under age 2 months, pregnant or nursing women, and persons who cannot afford other treatments. 1. Apply every other night for three consecutive treatments. 2. Remove applications between treatments.	N/A
Ivermectin	200 µ/kg PO ×1	May be used as alternative treatment (Meinking et al, 1995); safety and efficacy has not been established in children <15 kg	N/A

N/A, Not available; *SE*, side effects.

lesions are most commonly found on the proximal half of the foot and heel. Nodules may be present in axilla and groin of young children.

Norwegian or crusted scabies: Thick, crusted plaques are present on the hands and feet, including palms and soles. This type of scabies is seen in neurologically or immunologically impaired hosts.

Associated Lesions

Excoriation from scratching

Impetigo

Reddish-brown firm nodules (nodular scabies) that persist up to 12 months after treatment are caused by a severe hypersensitive reaction to the scabies mites; nodules are most frequently found on the axilla, areolae and male genitalia

Diagnostic Procedures

To help identify burrows, place a drop of mineral oil on the skin surface in question. Oil sharpens the appearance of the lesion and makes the specimen adhere to the scalpel blade. An alternative method is to lightly go across the lesion with a black felt tip marker, then wipe dry. Burrows stand out as distinct black lines. Diagnostic procedures are outlined in Table 161-1.

Scrapings do not always yield mites, so the diagnosis of scabies may often be made on the basis of clinical presentation alone.

ASSESSMENT

Confirm the presence of the mite, eggs or mite feces under the microscope. If unable to identify the presence of any of these substances, confirm the presence of burrows. Differential diagnoses include those found in Table 161-2.

THERAPEUTIC PLAN

Pharmaceutical

Pharmaceutical treatment is outlined in Table 161-3.

Crusted Norwegian scabies—three treatments are required at 3 day intervals to ensure all the crusts have been penetrated. Permethrin 5% cream is the treatment of choice. Remove applications between treatments.

Oral antihistamines and mild topical corticosteroid agents may be needed after treatment to help control the pruritus.

Additional Treatment

All bed linens and clothing that have been worn in the past 3 days should be washed in hot water with detergent and dried in a hot dryer or dry cleaned. Bed linen should be washed in hot water daily until treatment course is finished. Items not washable may be sealed in a plastic bag for 7 days since the mite cannot survive off the host for more than 3 days. Mites can live 24 to 36 hours in room conditions and longer in humid environments.

Treat secondary bacterial infections.

Patient Education

Reassure that scabies is curable and is a common problem in all socioeconomic groups.

Onset of symptoms occurs 4 to 6 weeks after infestation and coincides with development of the immune response.

Because of the lag time between infestation and symptoms, unrecognized transmission may have occurred.

All infested family members should be treated simultaneously to avoid reinfestation.

Asymptomatic family members and close contacts should also be treated because of delay in symptoms.

In adults the scabicide should be applied from the neck down to the toes, with special attention to interdigital areas of the fingers and toes, umbilicus, and skin folds.

Treatment of infants and young children should include the scalp and face if lesions are present.

Relief from itching may not occur from 3 to 6 weeks after treatment. This is because of the hypersensitivity of the skin to the debris left in the burrow and itching will continue until the natural turnover of skin. Retreatment is not indicated for continued itching.

Family Impact

All family members need to be treated simultaneously.

Follow-up

Assess for new lesions 10 to 14 days after treatment. Assess for irritant dermatitis.

EVALUATION

Rash and intense itching should have disappeared in 4 weeks.

REFERENCE

Meinking T et al: The treatment of scabies with ivermectin, *N Engl J Med* 333(1):26-30, 1995.

SUGGESTED READINGS

Belkengren R, Sapala S: Pediatric management problems, *Pediatric Nursing* 21(2):164-165, 1995.

Cutter J: Scabies: Fighting the mite, *Nurse Prescriber* 2(8):44, 1996.

Elgart ML: Scabies: Diagnosis and treatment, *Dermatol Nurs* 5(6):464-468, 1993.

Ellsworth W et al: *Mosby's 1998 medical drug reference,* St Louis, 1998, Mosby.

Forsman KE: Pediculosis and scabies: What to look for in patients who are crawling with clues, *Postgrad Med* 98(6):94-100, 1995.

Goroll AH, May LA, AG Mulley Jr: *Primary care medicine*, Philadelphia, 1995, JB Lippincott.

Hicks LM, Lewis DJ: Management of chronic, resistive scabies: a case study, *Geriatric Nurs* 16(5):230-237, 1995.

Koda-Kimble M, Young L, editors: *Applied therapeutics: the clinical use of drugs,* ed 5, Washington, DC, 1993, Applied Therapeutics.

Mackey S, Wagner K: Dermatologic manifestation of parasitic diseases, *Infect Dis Clin North Am* 8(3):739-741, 1994.

Nurse practitioners drug handbook, Springhouse Pa, 1996, Springhouse Corp.

Pigott K: Lice and scabies, *Lippincott's Primary Care Practice* 1(1):93-111, 1997.

Reeves JRT, Maibach H.: *Clinical dermatology illustrated,* Philadelphia, 1991, FA Davis.

Uphold CR, Graham MV: *Clinical guidelines in family practice,* Gainesville, Fla, 1994, Barmarrae Books.

Scarlet Fever

Scarlatina

ICD-9-CM

Scarlet Fever 034.1
Scarlatina 034.1

OVERVIEW

Definition

Scarlet fever is a disease caused by group A (beta-hemolytic) streptococci (GAS), characterized by a skin rash. Other than the rash, the epidemiology, symptoms, sequelae, and treatment of scarlet fever are no different from those of streptococcal pharyngitis.

Incidence

There is a 2- to 5-day incubation period for scarlet fever. The patient is contagious 24 hours before symptoms until 24 hours after treatment with penicillin or 10 to 21 days in untreated, uncomplicated cases. Cases occur year round but peak in late winter and early spring. They are unusual under 2 to 3 years of age. Cases peak in **6- to 12-year-old children** and decline after that.

Pathophysiology

Spread by respiratory droplets or direct contact; rarely by indirect contact through objects

Rash occurs when the infecting strain of streptococcus produces a pyrogenic exotoxin and the patient is sensitized but not immune to the toxins. Complications include acute rheumatic fever and acute glomerulonephritis.

SUBJECTIVE DATA

History of Present Illness

Rash occurs 3 to 5 days after sudden onset of fever and sore throat

Exposure to group A streptococcus (GAS)

Past Medical History

Immunization history
Communicable disease history
Previous GAS infection
Allergies, especially antibiotics

Medications

Current medications, new medications
Over-the-counter medications used

Family History

Illness among family members, care takers.

Psychosocial History

Environmental exposure

Description of Most Common Symptoms

The rash is a fine, erythematous, papular rash that blanches on pressure, often felt rather than seen (like sandpaper). It appears most often on the neck, chest folds of the axilla, elbow, groin, and inner thighs. It usually does not involve the face, but cheeks may appear flushed with circumoral pallor. There is a distinctive odor to the breath.

Associated Symptoms

Nausea and vomiting often accompany severe infection
Chills
Anorexia
Headache

OBJECTIVE DATA

Physical Examination

General: Patient looks ill
Head/eyes/ears/nose/throat: Pharynx may be injected and edematous
Palatial petechia
Tonsils: Beefy red with exudate
Tongue: Coated or strawberry (protruding red papillae showing on coated surface)
Skin: Observe for rash. May see desquamation after 3-6 days of rash, especially on fingertips and creases

Diagnostic Procedures

Diagnostic procedures include those listed in Table 162-1.

ASSESSMENT

Differential diagnoses include fifth disease, Kawasaki's syndrome, and toxic shock syndrome and are outlined in Table 162-2.

THERAPEUTIC PLAN

Pharmaceutical

Pharmaceutical treatment is outlined in Table 162-3.

Lifestyle/Activities

Children should not return to school or day care until at least 24 hours after beginning antimicrobial treatment.
Avoid contact with other children during this time.

Diet

As tolerated. Push fluids to avoid dehydration.

Patient Education

Change toothbrush.
Wash hands frequently.
Properly dispose of items contaminated with throat and nasal secretions.
Stress the need to complete all antibiotics, even if all symptoms are gone.
Call immediately if symptoms of adverse reactions to penicillin.
Gargle with saline.
Instruct about symptomatic care (i.e., antipyretics).

Family Impact

Observe other family members for signs of disease.

TABLE 162-1 Diagnostic Tests: Scarlet Fever

Diagnostic Test	Findings/Rationale	Cost ($)
Rapid streptococcus	If positive, group A streptococcus; if negative, may follow with throat culture	20-25
Throat culture	Rapid streptococcus may be negative, but a culture may be positive for streptococcus	24-30
Mononucleosis spot	Streptococcus and mononucleosis coexist in about 25% of cases	20-25

TABLE 162-2 Differential Diagnosis: Scarlet Fever

Diagnoses	Supporting Data
Fifth disease	Warm, red, nontender, "slapped cheeks" rash; spreads in 1-2 days to trunk, neck and buttocks; fades with central clearing leaving a lacy, reticulated rash that lasts 2-40 days
Kawasaki's syndrome	Has additional signs of conjunctivitis, cracking lips, and diarrhea
Toxic shock syndrome	An erythematous, "sunburn-like" rash with sudden-onset high fever, vomiting, profuse, watery diarrhea, and myalgia
Rubeola	Koplik's spots, rash, cough, fever
Rubella	Postauricular adenopathy, mild illness
Roseola	Fever, child is not toxic, rash appears after fever

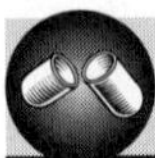

TABLE 162-3 Pharmaceutical Plan: Scarlet Fever

Drug	Dose	Comments	Cost
Penicillin (Pen Vee K)	Children: 15-56 mg/kg QID Adults: 125-500 mg QID	Pregnancy: B SE: Rash, anaphylaxis, superinfection	$11/125 (100); $4-$42/250 (100)
Penicillin G benzathine (Bicillin LA, Bicillin CR [includes Procaine])	<60 lbs: 600,000 U >60 lbs: 1,200,000 U	Intramuscularly Pregnancy: B SE: As for penicillin	$21/300,000 U/ml (10 ml); $7/600,000 U/ml
Erythromycin (Estolate)	30-50 mg/kg/day q6-8h ×10 days; take with food to decrease gastrointestinal upset	Pregnancy: B Used when patient is allergic to penicillin SE: Gastrointestinal upset, abdominal pain, hepatic dysfunction in adults, P450 interactions (see Appendix D)	$70/base: 333 (60)
Erythromycin ethyl succinate	40 mg/kg BID-QID ×10 days	Max. dose 1 g/day used when patient is allergic to penicillin Pregnancy: B SE: As for erythromycin	$13-$27/200 mg/ 5 ml (480 ml)

Referral

Refer to MD for complications, including acute rheumatic fever, glomerulonephritis, peritonsillar suppurative cervical adenitis, and retropharyngeal abscess.

Consultation

None needed unless complications or no improvement in 48 hours

Follow-up

If there is no significant improvement, recheck in 3 to 4 days.

EVALUATION

Post-treatment throat cultures for patients who have high risk for rheumatic fever or who are still symptomatic after treatment

A culture may be required for frequent episodes of GAS, including other family members (consider pets in multiple episodes)

SUGGESTED REFERENCES

American Academy of Pediatrics: Measles. In Peter G, editor: *1997 Red Book: Report of the Committee on Infectious Disease,* ed 24, Elk Grove Village, Ill, 1997, American Academy of Pediatrics.

American Public Health Association: *Control of communicable diseases manual,* ed 16, Washington, DC, 1995, American Public Health Association.

Ellsworth W et al: *Mosby's 1998 medical drug reference*, St Louis, 1998, Mosby.

Healthcare Consultants of America, Inc: *1998 physicians fee and coding guide,* Augusta, Ga, 1998, Healthcare Consultants of America, Inc.

Uphold C, Graham M: *Clinical Guidelines In Family Practice,* ed 2, Gainesville, Fla, 1994, Barmarrae Books, American Academy of Pediatrics.

Boyton R, Dunn E, Stephens G: *Manual of ambulatory pediatrics,* ed 4, Philadelphia, 1998, JB Lippincott.

163 Scoliosis

ICD-9-CM

Scoliosis (Acquired, Postural, Idiopathic) 737.30
Congenital 754.2

OVERVIEW

Definition

Scoliosis is a lateral S- or C-shaped curve of the thoracic and/or lumbar spine associated with a rotational deformity of the rib cage creating a rib hump or prominence.

Incidence

Scoliosis is most prevalent during prepubertal growth spurt **(10 years to adolescence).**

Scoliosis can progress during the growth spurt.

A greater number of **females** than males are affected; in cases with curves greater than 20%, girls outnumber boys 5 to 1.

Two percent of U.S. **children** have curves greater than 10%.

Types

Structural scoliosis, including congenital scoliosis, is secondary to a bony abnormality of the vertebrae.

Nonstructural scoliosis is seen in infants and is secondary to an intrauterine positional deformation.

Functional scoliosis is due to leg length discrepancy.

Neuromuscular scoliosis is secondary to the imbalance of paraspinal muscles caused by progressive neuropathic and myopathic disorders.

Idiopathic scoliosis is the most common type of scoliosis and is classified according to the patient's age at onset; **infantile** is under 3 years of age, **juvenile** is from 3 to 10 years of age, **adolescent** is from 10 years of age to skeletal maturity, and **adult** is after skeletal maturity.

Etiology

Eighty percent of cases of scoliosis are idiopathic and the cause is unknown. It is familial, with a **female**-to-male ratio of 4:1 for curves less than 20 degrees.

SUBJECTIVE DATA

History of Present Illness

Spinal column abnormalities, the age first detected, and how it was detected

Poor posture

Asymmetry of shoulder height and/or hip height

Back pain is usually not associated with idiopathic scoliosis and any complaints of pain warrants a complete neuromuscular evaluation

The most common types of idiopathic curves are the right thoracic curve, followed by the double right thoracic and left lumbar curve and the right thoracolumbar curve; a child with a left thoracic curve has an increased incidence of intraspinal disease (i. e., tumor)

Past Medical History

Neuromuscular disease, including family history (In such cases scoliosis is almost never the first or only clue, but rather a complication of a condition already known to exist.)

Family History

The incidence is greater in **children of women** with scoliosis and particularly in **daughters.**

OBJECTIVE DATA

Physical Examination

Assess gait.

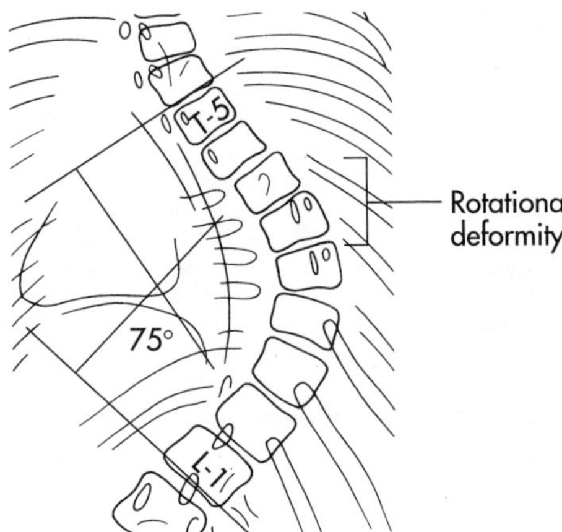

Figure 163-1 Use of the Cobb method to measure the scoliotic curve. First, lines are drawn along the end plates of the upper and lower vertebrae that are maximally tilted into the concavity of the curve. Next, a perpendicular line is drawn to each of the earlier drawn lines. The angle of intersection is the Cobb angle. (From Zitelli BJ, Davis HW: *Atlas of pediatric physical diagnosis,* ed 3, St Louis, 1997, Mosby.)

Have the patient stand up straight, feet slightly apart, looking straight ahead, with arms at the side. Stand behind the patient.
- Assess symmetry of shoulder height, scapula height, and hip height.
- Assess for scapula prominence.
- Assess for equal distance between the arms and sides.
- Assess for lateralization of the spine.

Have the patient bend forward with their head and hands down.
- Assess for rib hump or prominence.

Assess:
- Tanner stage of sexual development.
- Leg length symmetry.
- Skin for hairy patches, nevi, café au lait spots, lipomas, or dimples in the sacral area.

Neurological examination, including toe walk, heel walk, motor/sensory testing upper and lower extremities, reflexes.

Cardiac assessment for murmurs consistent with Marfan syndrome.

Screening Procedures

The forward bend test is the mainstay of most screening programs.

A scoliometer measures the angle of trunk rotation (ATR) while the patient is bending forward. An ATR <5 degrees is considered passing.

Diagnostic Procedures

A single anteroposterior x-ray of the spine will permit measurement of most minor curvatures. X-ray will also permit evaluation of bone age.

In more severe cases, x-rays of the entire length of the spine should be taken. This generally requires the use of an extra long cassette. Ideally the patient should be standing; if this is not possible, x-rays can be obtained sitting.

Curves are measured using the Cobb method (Figure 163-1).

Diagnostic procedures are listed in Table 163-1.

ASSESSMENT

Functional scoliosis corrects with forward bending (Adam's position).

Infantile, juvenile, adolescent, or adult scoliosis is determined according to age of onset.

Idiopathic scoliosis accounts for 80% of cases.

Scoliosis secondary to neuromuscular disease is not typically a primary finding, and systemic problems such as cerebral palsy or multiple sclerosis should be considered.

THERAPEUTIC PLAN

Nonpharmaceutical

Table 163-2 outlines a nonpharmaceutical treatment plan for scoliosis.

Curvatures greater than 30 degrees in **preadolescents** with a bone age less than 12 years generally progress, whereas curvature less than 20 degrees in skeletally mature **adolescents** rarely progress.

Those with curvatures greater than 50 to 60 degrees at maturity may progress during **adulthood.**

A curvature <10 degrees can be managed by observation only unless the patient has neuromuscular disease or a high rate of progression.

Progression is defined as a sustained increase of 5 degrees or more of the Cobb angle. The potential for error of measurement using the Cobb angle is 3 to 5 degrees; therefore it is considered significant if progression is greater than 5 degrees.

Curvatures 20 to 40 degrees in skeletally immature patients should be referred for orthotic therapy (Milwaukee brace).

The goal of brace therapy is to prevent further curve progression during the growth period. Braces do not afford long-term correction.

Contraindications to brace therapy include curves greater than 40 degrees because of the greater pressure that must be exerted to effect correction.

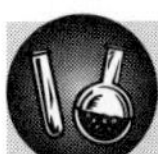

TABLE 163-1 Diagnostic Tests: Scoliosis

Symptoms	Findings	Diagnostic Tests	Costs ($)
Asymmetrical scapulas, hips	Lateralization of the spine	Spinal x-ray	104-135/C spine; 119-151/T spine 122-146/lumbosacral
Asymmetrical scapulas, hips with pain	Lateralization of the spine, neurological deficits	Magnetic resonance imaging	1805-1399/C spine; 1860-2204/T spine; 1815-2145/ lumbosacral spine

TABLE 163-2 Management of Scoliosis

<10 Degrees	>20 Degrees	>40 Degrees	Congenital Scoliosis
Observation only, unless patient has neuromuscular disease or high rate of progression	Skeletally immature, and/or rotational deformity, and/or positive family history; refer for orthotics	Refer for surgical evaluation	Atypical curve, rapid progression, or abnormal neurologic evaluation; refer for neurosurgical evaluation

Curvatures greater than 40 degrees should be referred for surgical evaluation. Historically the standard has been posterior fusion and Harrington rod instrumentation.

Curvatures greater than 60 degrees can cause cardiopulmonary compromise.

Patient Education

See pp. 986 to 988.

Children and adolescents will require psychosocial counseling and support because of self-image issues, the use of braces and casts, and possibly surgery.

Children and adolescents may have concerns about clothing and participation in sports.

Consultation/Referral

Referral to orthopedist or spine specialist indicated:

- With any degree of scoliosis accompanied by pain
- When curvature is progressive (change of 5%) or when a curve is greater than 20 degrees in a growing child (Tanner 2)

EVALUATION/FOLLOW-UP

Evaluate psychologic adjustment to treatment.

Evaluate degree of adherence to prescribed treatment.

Recheck a growing child with scoliosis within 6 months for progression.

Curves of 40 to 50 degrees should be checked for progression in adulthood every year.

Adults who have idiopathic scoliosis without signs of progression should be checked every 2 to 5 years.

SUGGESTED REFERENCES

Burns C et al: *Pediatric primary care: a handbook for nurse practitioners,* Philadelphia, 1996, WB Saunders.

Dershewitz R: *Ambulatory pediatric care*, ed 2, Philadelphia, 1993, JB Lippincott.

Healthcare Consultants of America, Inc: *1998 physicians fee and coding guide,* Augusta, Ga, 1998, Healthcare Consultants of America, Inc.

Nelson W: *Textbook of pediatrics,* Philadelphia, 1996, WB Saunders.

Skinner HB: *Current diagnosis & treatment in orthopedics,* Norwalk, 1995, Appleton & Lange.

RESOURCE

National Scoliosis Foundation
72 Mount Auburn St.
Watertown, MA 02172
(617) 926-0397

WHAT IS SCOLIOSIS?

Scoliosis is a sideways (lateral) curving of the spine.

One in 10 persons will have scoliosis. Two to three persons in every 1000 will need active treatment for a progressive condition. In one out of every 1000 cases, surgery may be necessary.

Frequent signs are a prominent shoulder blade, uneven hip and shoulder levels, unequal distance between arms and body, and clothes that do not "hang right."

Eighty percent of scoliosis cases are idiopathic (cause unknown). Scoliosis tends to run in families and affects more girls than boys.

Spinal curvature is best dealt with when a young person's body is still growing and can respond to one or a combination of treatments (e.g., body brace, electrostimulation).

You, your physician, and/or your school screening program (now required in many schools) can perform a 30-second annual screen during these growing years. Mild cases may not need treatment, but must be monitored.

Kyphosis (round back) may occur in developing adolescents. It should be screened for and may need to be treated.

An annual 30-second screening for scoliosis and kyphosis during the bone growing years can make the difference between a preventable condition and a disability in adult years.

SCREENING FOR SCOLIOSIS

1A: Normal

Head centered over buttocks
Shoulders level
Shoulder blades level, with equal prominence
Hips level and symmetrical
Equal distance between arms and body.

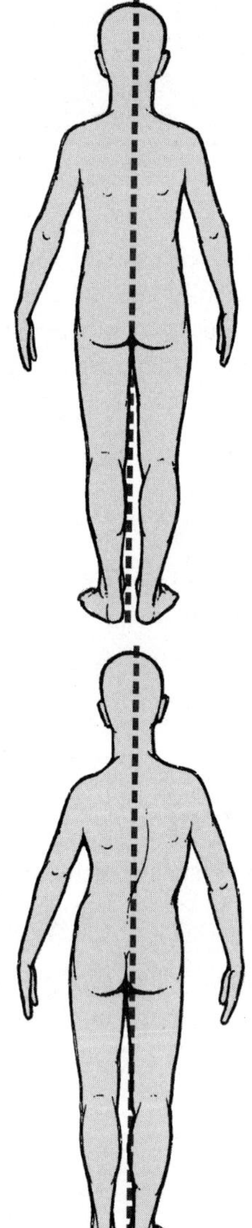

1B: Possible Scoliosis

Head alignment to one side of mid-buttocks
One shoulder higher
One shoulder blade higher, with possible prominence
One hip more prominent than the other
Unequal distance between arms and body

Text from National Scoliosis Foundation, Watertown, Massachusetts. Illustrations 1B, 1B, and 4B redrawn from Hilt NE, Schmitt EW: *Pediatric orthopedic nursing,* St. Louis, 1975, Mosby. In Wong DL et al: *Whaley & Wong's Nursing care of infants and children,* ed 6, St Louis, 1999, Mosby. Illustrations for 2A, 2B, 3A, and 3B from Fox JA: *Primary health care of children,* St Louis, 1997, Mosby.

2A: Normal

Both sides of upper and lower back symmetrical
Hips level and symmetrical

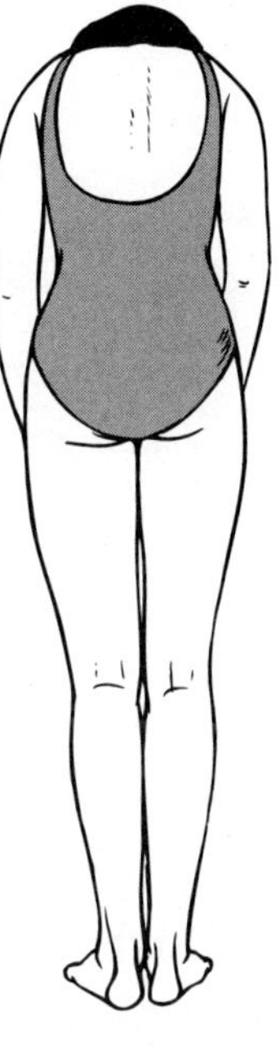

Normal

2B: Possible Scoliosis

One side of rib cage and/or the lower back showing uneven symmetry

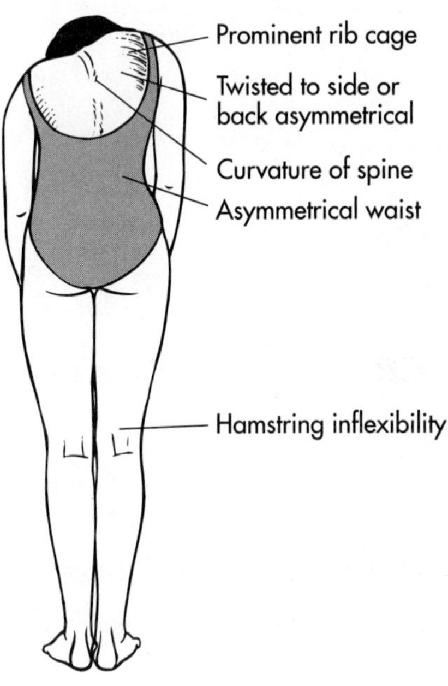

Abnormal

3A: Normal

Even and symmetrical on both sides of the upper and lower back

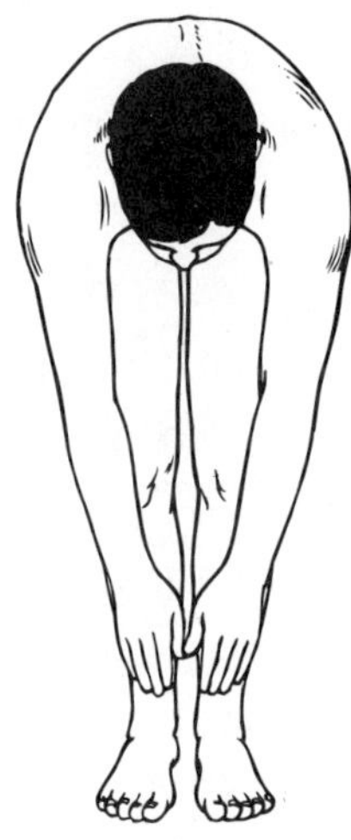

Normal

3B: Possible Scoliosis

Unequal symmetry of the upper back, lower back, or both

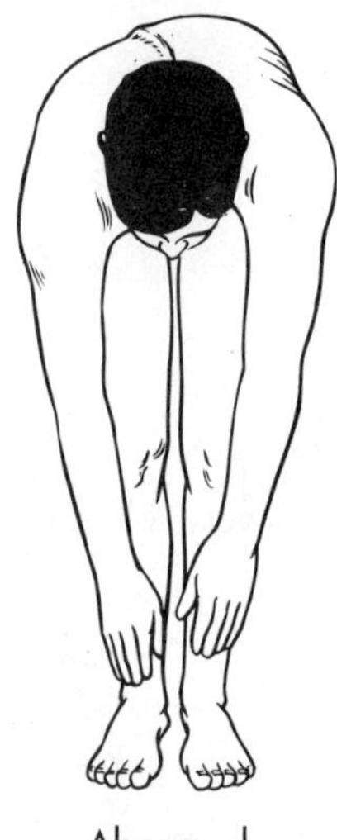

Abnormal

SCREENING FOR KYPHOSIS

4A: Normal

Smooth, symmetrical even arc of back

4B: Possible Kyphosis

Lack of smooth arc with prominence of shoulders and round back

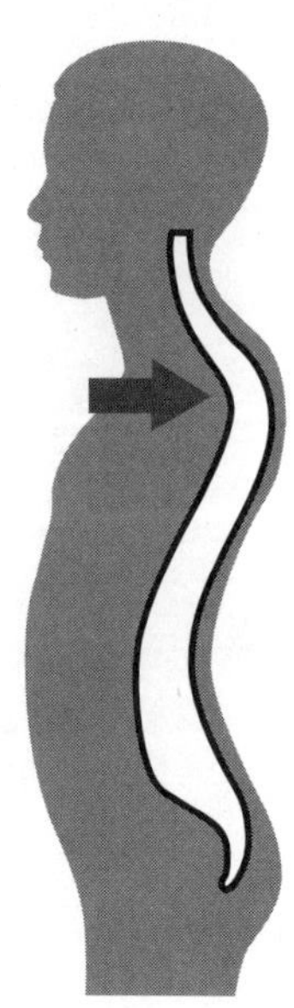

Screen out Scoliosis! If one or more physical features suggest scoliosis or kyphosis, professional diagnosis must be sought.

164 Seizure Disorders

ICD-9-CM

Seizure 780.39
Psychomotor 354.4
Febrile 780.31
Petit Mal 345.0
Jacksonian 345.5
Clonic Seizure 345.1
Generalized 345.9
Grand Mal 345.1
Partial 345.5

OVERVIEW

Definition

Seizure is a paroxysmal, abnormal discharge of neurons of the cerebral cortex that alters neurologic function.

Epilepsy is a heterogeneous condition characterized by recurrent, unprovoked seizures.

Incidence

About 2 million people in the United States may have epilepsy. An even larger number seek medical advice for a possible seizure disorder, generating about 5% of visits to physicians and 20% of visits to neurologists.

Seizures in **children** are not uncommon, and their incidence in children is much higher than in adults. Four to 6% of all children have seizures, including febrile seizures. The febrile seizure group alone may make up between 2.5% and 4% of that total.

Epilepsy is especially likely to affect the **elderly.** Common causes of epilepsy in the elderly are cerebrovascular disease and neoplasms, as well as metabolic derangements and head trauma.

Pathophysiology

The final common pathway of many epileptic seizures is a sudden electrical depolarization of cortical neurons that is usually seen on the surface electromyelogram (EEG) as a negative spike. This is frequently followed by a sustained inhibitory hyperpolarization usually seen as a slow wave on the surface EEG. No cause can be found in 40% to 70% of patients with seizures.

Factors Associated With Increased Risk

Space-occupying central nervous system (CNS) lesion
Lack of immunization
Premature birth
Birth trauma
Perinatal intracranial infection
Positive family history of epilepsy, neurocutaneous disease, sickle cell, febrile seizures, breath holding spells
Developmental delay
Chromosomal disorders
Illicit drug use
Chronic illness
Meningitis and encephalitis
Cardiac disease
History of severe head trauma

Etiology Based on Age

Neonatal seizures are often related to birth trauma or congenital malformation.

Seizures in **infancy to early childhood** (less than 6 years) are likely due to metabolic disorders, CNS infections, febrile seizures.

In **children** (ages 6 to 10 years) seizures are most often CNS infection, idiopathic epilepsy, CNS degeneration.

In **childhood to adolescence** (10 to 18 years) idiopathic epilepsy, trauma, and alcohol and drug abuse are likely causes.

Seizures in **older persons** are often related to trauma, neoplasm, or stroke.

Box 164-1

Epileptic Seizures: Classification and Characteristics (Proposed by the International Classification of Epileptic Seizures)

Partial Seizures (Focal Seizures)

Simple partial seizures
Complex partial seizures
 Simple partial onset followed by impairment of consciousness
 With impairment of consciousness at the onset
Partial seizures evolving to generalized seizures

Generalized Seizures (Convulsive or Nonconvulsive)

Absence seizures
 Typical absence seizures (petit mal)
Myoclonic seizures
Clonic seizures
Tonic seizures
Tonic-clonic seizures
Atonic seizures
Infantile spasms

Unclassified Epileptic Seizures

Includes all seizures that cannot be classified because of incomplete data or because they defy classification into the preceding categories (e.g., neonatal seizures with swimming movements).

Status Epilepticus

Modified from Leppik I: *Contemporary diagnosis and management of the patient with epilepsy,* ed 2, Newtown, Pa, 1996, Handbooks in Health Care.

Classification of Seizures

One of the major developments in epileptology of the last few decades has been the adoption of the International Classification of Epileptic Seizures (ICES). Much of the basis for this classification, as illustrated in Box 164-1 is the recognition that the brain is highly organized, with specific functions represented in discrete anatomical regions.

SUBJECTIVE DATA

Clinical Presentation

Partial Seizures

Simple Partial Seizures

Simple partial seizures (auras) usually last 20 to 180 seconds and are not associated with impairment of consciousness.

There are usually no postictal symptoms, but lethargy may occur.

Complex Partial Seizures

Associated with impairment, but no loss of consciousness.

Patients typically stare but do not respond to questions or commands.

Usual duration is 30 to 180 seconds.

Auras are common.

Postictal symptoms are common, but usually brief (<20 minutes); lethargy and confusion.

Partial Seizures Evolving to Secondarily Generalized Seizures

Patients may not recall aura, but witnesses may report patient described an aura or may observe focal movements or automatisms before the convulsion.

Generalized Seizures

Absence (Petit Mal)

Onset is usually 4 to 11 years
Paroxysmal onset and offset
Usually brief (<15 seconds) impairment of consciousness
Precipitated by hyperventilation
No aura, postictal confusion or lethargy
May be frequent (>100/day)

Myoclonic

Brief, shock like jerk of muscles or group of muscles
Two types
 Nonepileptic: Often unilateral
 Epileptic myoclonus: Usually bilateral, symmetrical movements

Tonic

Brief episode with sudden increase in tone in trunk or extremities
Usually <20 seconds

Tonic-clonic (Grand Mal)

May be partial (beginning focally) or primary generalized (bilateral symmetrical onset)
Initial brief tonic phase lasting 2 to 10 seconds with loss of consciousness, extensor rigidity, fall, often a cry; superior deviation of eyes and pupil dilation
Secondary clonic phase with bilateral jerking lasting 30 to 180 seconds; rate of jerking usually slows; often a large jerk followed by flaccidity and coma
There may be hypersalivation, tongue biting, and urinary incontinence
Postictal period lasting minutes to hours with lethargy, confusion, decreased attention, depression

Atonic

Brief episode with sudden decrease in tone in trunk or extremities
Onset usually in childhood
<15 Seconds
Sudden loss postural tone from head nod to fall with major trauma

May be accompanied by tonic seizures
Injury common and these patients often require helmets
Primarily seen in Lennox-Gastaut syndrome

Unclassified Seizures

Lennox-Gastaut Syndrome

Begins at ages 1 to 7 years
Often coexists with atonic seizures
Patient falls are common
Symmetrical jerking of proximal arms with twitching of facial muscles (mouth and eyes)

West Syndrome (Infantile Spasms)

Presents at 2 months of age to 1 year
Sudden flexion of extremities, head, and trunk for limited time
Untreated, infantile spasms subside within 1 to 4 years but often are replaced by other forms of seizures; prognosis is poor

Febrile Seizures

Usually occur between 6 months and 5 years and most commonly occur before 13 months of age
They are brief, generalized, short, and nonfocal
Patient is febrile before seizure and has no evidence of CNS infection
Prognosis is excellent since fewer than 3% of the children with simple febrile seizures will have nonfebrile seizures subsequently

Status Epilepticus

Characterized by a seizure that continues longer than 30 minutes or by repeated seizures associated with impaired awareness for more than 30 minutes
They are medical emergencies that can cause brain damage and death
Thus any tonic-clonic seizure lasting longer than 5 to 10 minutes should be treated.

History of Present Illness

Determine what type of seizure occurred by asking patient, family members, and witnesses.

Obtain a good description of the seizure.
Determine whether it was focal (involving only the face or one extremity or one side of the body); immediately generalized (involving all extremities); or started as a focal seizure and then generalized to involve the extremities; and how long it occurred.
Ask whether the patient lost consciousness.
When patient aroused, determine if there was any evidence of an aura.
Did the patient lose control of bowel or bladder?
Was there a period of postictal lethargy, and how long it occurred?
Describe how the patient acted after the seizure.
Is there any associated illness or fever or any sleep deprivation?
Determine the relationship of seizure to the time of day, meals, fatigue, emotional stress, excitement, menses, discontinuing medication, activity before attack, and frequency of occurrence.
Inquire about history of trauma, drug withdrawal, particularly alcohol, barbiturates, or benzodiazepines and any exposure to toxins.

Past Medical History

Birth history
Prenatal history for **children:** Infection, substance abuse, bleeding, preterm labor, diabetes, hypertension
Labor and delivery: Complications, oxygen needed
Neonatal: Gestation, infections, apnea, major complications, or congenital anomalies
Is there a history of cardiac arrhythmias, valve disease, stroke, and malignancies?
Is there any diabetes or renal disease?
Is there history of head trauma with loss of consciousness, febrile seizures?
If the patient has had seizures before, determine the following:
Precipitating factors
Whether the seizure is the same as past ones
Is there medication compliance?
Are the seizures occurring more frequently?

Medications

Determine what medications patient is taking.

Family History

Determine if there is a family history of seizures or neurological disorders.

Psychosocial History

Determine the following:

Any recent travel?
Occupation
Alcohol consumption with amount
Drug abuse with type and amount of drug or drugs
Type and age of dwelling: Lead screen
Description of attainment of development milestones/school performance

Diet History

Determine the type of foods patient has eaten in the recent past.

OBJECTIVE DATA

Physical Examination

Observe for an injury pattern.

Determine vital signs, head circumference in children, height, weight.

Do a complete neurological examination: Mental status, speech, cranial nerves, eye fundus, strength, tone, reflexes, cerebellar.

Do a complete cardiovascular examination: Bruits, murmurs, abnormalities of rhythm.

Observe the skin for any abnormalities (often associated with congenital disorders).

- Cafe-au-lait spots: Neurofibromatosis?
- Adenoma sebaceum (reddish nodules over the nose, cheeks, and occasionally the chin) or shagreen patch (like untanned leather) over the dorsum of the trunk: Tuberous sclerosis?
- Hemangioma involving one side of face or involving one side of body: Sturge Weber?

Abdomen: Liver size

Diagnostic Procedures

Diagnostic procedures are outlined in Table 164-1.

ASSESSMENT

Differential diagnoses are outlined in Table 164-2. See also Figure 164-1.

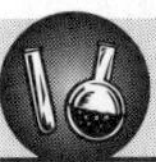

TABLE 164-1 Diagnostic Tests: Seizure Disorders

Diagnostic Test	Finding/Rationale	Cost ($)
Electrolytes, glucose, renal function, complete blood count (CBC) with differential, calcium, magnesium, phosphorus	Diagnostic tests should be tailored to individual patients. Basic laboratory tests focus on detecting systemic disturbances potentially associated with seizures. Rule out electrolyte imbalance, hypoglycemia, renal or metabolic dysfunction.	23-30; 32-43/comprehensive metabolic panel; 18-23/CBC; 20-25/mg; 19-23/ca; 16-20/ph
Lead level	If lead ingestion suspected	41-51
Drug screen	If drug use/abuse suspected	57-72
Electroencephalogram (EEG)	Used to detect epileptiform activity, strengthen the diagnosis, identify focal electrocerebral abnormalities suggesting a focal structural brain lesion, and document specific epileptic patterns associated with particular epilepsy syndromes. The EEG is also helpful in assessing the risk of recurrent seizures. It may be normal if patient is not presently having a seizure. An abnormal EEG does not necessarily confirm the diagnosis. Natural sleep is the best way to elicit an abnormal EEG, so have patient be sleepy if possible.	283-345
Computed tomography (CT) or magnetic resonance imaging (MRI)	May be warranted in the following cases: intractable seizures, focal neurological abnormalities, unprovoked seizure to detect underlying cerebral lesions (tumor, abscess, vascular malformation, stroke, or traumatic injury). In nonurgent cases MRI is the modality of choice since it is more sensitive than CT in identifying lesions. Emergent CT imaging is recommended for new focal deficits, persistent headache, and persistent altered mental state since it is more widely available and because of its superior ability to detect acute hemorrhage.	990-1175/CT; 1781-2004/MRI
Lumbar puncture	Essential if patient is suspected of having meningitis or encephalitis or in immunocompromised patients since occult meningitis is a common finding is this group.	172-208
Genetic studies	Based on congenital/family history.	315-695

THERAPEUTIC PLAN

Generally 80% of seizures can be controlled with anticonvulsants.

Immediate Management

Maintain clear airway by turning patient on his side with head down; remove vomitus or dentures.

Do not try to pry tight jaws open to place an object between the teeth.

Protect patient from injuries.

Administer oxygen if cyanotic.

Status epilepticus (seizure longer than 10-minute duration) necessitates Emergency Department transport and immediate consultation with physician.

Principles of Treatment

Consult physician for all first-time seizures.

The decision to treat a first-time seizure is difficult and should be based on the interpretation of the subtle clinical, historical, and /or laboratory findings. The final decision about treatment must be made individually for each patient and should take into account the potential psychological, vocational, and physical consequences of further seizures.

Box 164-2 outlines steps to follow when considering treatment of the first seizure. A *provoked seizure* is one in which factors that precipitated the episode can be identified and remedied, such as physical injury and drug overdose.

In *febrile seizures*, the initial treatment is lowering the temperature with acetaminophen, ibuprofen, or cool baths. (Generally, febrile seizures do not require anticonvulsant therapy; however, frequent recurrent febrile seizures may require prophylactic treatment with oral phenobarbital.)

Pharmaceutical

Antiepileptic drug (AED) selection is based on the preference of the health care provider. The nurse practi-

Table 164-2 Differential Diagnosis: Seizure Disorders

Diagnosis	Supporting Data
Syncope	
Vasovagal attack-hyperventilation-induced syncope	Cold hands, pallor, dimming vision, nausea, loss of balance, precipitated by fear or anxiety. Prodrome: Nausea, warmth, lightheadedness, diaphoresis, epigastric discomfort, and a sensation of impending faint.
Syncope: Cardiac	
Atrioventricular block	Generalized weakness, fatigue, pallor, worse when standing, improves when lying down, but can occur in any position.
Paroxysmal tachycardia	Increased heart rate, shortness of breath, anxiety, smothering feeling
Hypovolemia	Sudden loss of consciousness when patient stands up, weakness, increased heart rate.
Cerebrovascular ischemia	Longer duration, lack of spread than seizures. There is a loss of motor or sensory function (weakness or numbness).
Micturition syndrome	Fatigue, dizziness, syncope, low blood pressure while in process of urinating.
Other None Syncope Causes	
Nonepileptic seizures of psychogenic origin (pseudoseizures)	Term used to denote both hysterical conversion seizures and attacks due to malingering when they simulate seizures. Many patients with pseudoseizures also have a positive family history or may even have true seizures. Presents in many different ways: often with movement of limbs, closed eyes, then ending with lying limp. No incontinence, vital signs within normal range.
Breath-holding spells	Breath-holding spells occur in 5% of **children,** may start in infancy and tend to run in families. Children hold their breath in response to anger, frustration, or other external stimuli. The children hold their breath, become cyanotic, and may lose consciousness in association with clonic or tonic movements. 90% resolve by age 6.
Paroxysmal rapid eye movement sleep disorders	Sleep walking, night terrors, sleep apnea, head banging, myoclonic jerks (more common in men in 50s and older).
Panic attack	Hard to distinguish from simple or partial seizures unless evidence of psychopathologic disturbances between attacks; dyspnea, tachycardia, smothering feelings, nausea, choking are all common symptoms seen in panic attacks.

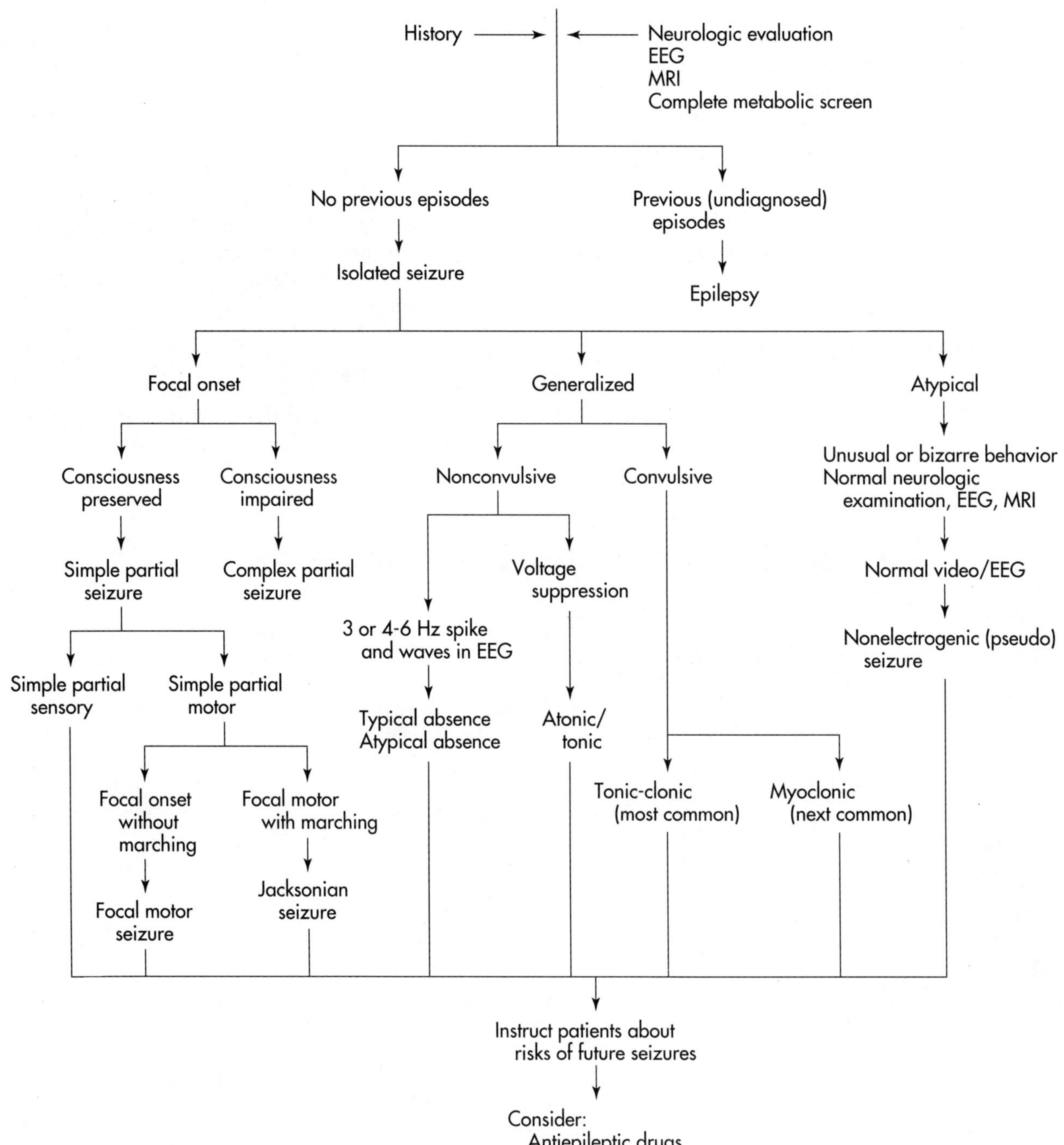

Figure 164-1 Algorithm for patient with seizures. *EEG,* Electroencephalogram; *MRI,* magnetic resonance imaging. (Adapted from Greene HL, Johnson WP, Lemcke D: *Decision making in medicine,* ed 2, St Louis, 1998, Mosby.)

tioner may actively participate in the process of selecting the AED, monitoring its administration, and assessing the patient's response, including side effects.

If AED treatment is chosen, consider the following:

The goal of AEDs is to prevent the recurrence or lessen seizures while avoiding side effects from the drugs (Tables 164-3 and 164-4).

Choose agent appropriate to the seizure type.

Initiate treatment with a single drug; consider cost and toxicity.

When dosing, consider the half-life of the drug in terms of how often the drug should be given and how long it takes to achieve a steady-state level.

Box 164-2

Antiepileptic Drug Treatment After First Seizure

Provoked

Adult and Children

Consider whether provoking factor can be corrected

If yes, antiepileptic drug (AED) treatment is unnecessary

If no, AED treatment should be considered

Unprovoked

Adult

Estimate recurrence risk and consequences (medical, social, occupational, psychologic)

Consider patient's preference

Evaluate risks vs benefits:

If yes, advise AED treatment

If no, withhold AED treatment

Child

No AED treatment unless consequence is grave

Modified from Uphold C, Graham M: *Clinical guidelines in adult health,* Gainesville, Fla, 1994, Barmarrae Books.

When you have to add additional drugs, add one at a time.

When you want to stop one or all drugs, taper them off; don't stop abruptly.

Hematologic/hepatic monitoring should be done at initiation of therapy, once during the first few months, whenever clinical symptoms occur, and annually.

Individualize treatment to seizure type, response to medication, and maintenance of appropriate blood levels.

Patients at high risk for recurrence should be treated for 2-year period.

Special Considerations

Reproductive Health and Pregnancy

Preconception counseling is imperative: if seizure free for 2 years, will consider an attempt at drug withdrawal before conception.

Fertility rates may be lower in women with localization-related epilepsy.

Family planning may be affected by the high failure rate of oral contraceptives and AEDs.

Changes in hormones over the menstrual cycle may influence the frequency of seizures.

Pregnancy causes a large increase in circulating serum proteins; since most drugs are protein bound, there may be a decrease in free or active blood levels, especially during the first trimester. Free drug levels rather than total serum drug level should be measured.

Pregnant women with epilepsy have more frequent seizures (30% to 50%), pregnancy complications (blunt abdominal trauma due to falls or motor vehicle accidents).

The probability of teratogenesis in fetuses of epileptic women treated with AEDs is higher than the probability of teratogenesis in fetuses of untreated epileptic women (rates of stillbirth, neonatal death and perinatal death is 3× greater) (200 to 300× risk of stillbirth, prematurity, developmental delay).

Table 164-3 Choice of Antiepileptic Drug Based on Type of Seizure

Type of Seizure	Antiepileptic Drugs to Consider
Simplex and complex, partial	Preferred: Carbamazepine, phenytoin, divalproex sodium, valproic acid; acceptable: gabapentin, lamotrigine, topiramate
Absence	Preferred: Ethosuximide, valproic acid, divalproex sodium; acceptable: methsuximide (Celontin Kapseals—no information available)
Tonic-clonic	Phenytoin, valproic acid, carbamazepine, divalproex sodium
Myoclonic and atonic	Clonazepam
Special considerations	Felbamate for treatment of Lennox-Gastaut syndrome; gabapentin for use as add-on therapy in refractory simple and complex partial seizures; lamotrigine for treatment of partial seizures and possibly also tonic-clonic, absence, and atonic seizures; vigabatrin for childhood forms of epilepsy

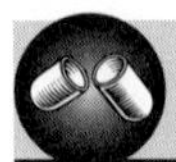

TABLE 164-4 Pharmaceutical Plan: Seizure Disorders

Drug	Dose	Comments	Cost
Phenytoin (Dilantin)	Adults: Begin 100 mg TID; may increase weekly to max 200 mg TID Children: 5 mg/kg/day in 2-3 divided doses; maintenance 4-8 mg/kg/day with max 300 mg daily; available in suspension: Dilantin-30 (30 mg/5 ml) and Dilantin-125 (125 mg/5 ml)	Monitor serum drug concentration 2-4 weeks after any dose increase; obtain annual CBC, LFTs, and platelets; periodic serum drug concentrations; need proper dental hygiene due to gingival hyperplasia Pregnancy: Not recommended *Potentiated* by ETOH, benzodiazepines, estrogen, fluoxetine, H_2 blockers, phenothiazines, INH, salicylates, sulfonamides, tolbutamide, trazodone; *antagonizes* tricyclic antidepressants, oral anticoagulants, OCPs, estrogens, corticosteroids, doxycycline, digitoxin, furosemide, theophylline, rifampin, quinidine SE: Nystagmus, drowsiness, ataxia, GI disturbances, blood dyscrasias, rash, hyperglycemia	\$20/chew: 50 mg (100); \$30/susp: 125/5 ml (240); \$6-\$22/100 mg (100)
Carbamazepine (Tegretol)	Adults: Begin 200 mg BID and increase dose 1× week if needed by increments of 200 mg/day in 3-4 divided doses; max 1.6 g Children over 6 years: Begin 100 mg chewable tablets BID and increase weekly 100 mg/day in 3-4 divided doses, maximum 1 g XR: Controlled release form for BID dosing	CBC and LFTs every 2-3 weeks for first 2 months, then every 3 months; Refer to an ophthalmologist for periodic slit-lamp examination Make sure patient knows to contact practitioner immediately for high fever or systemic symptoms of infection; periodic serum drug concentrations Pregnancy: C ↑ Plasma with CYP3A4 inhibitors: Cimetidine, INH, fluoxetine, terfenadine, ketoconazole; may ↑ lithium toxicity; may ↓ OCP effectiveness (see Appendix D) SE: N/V, aplastic anemia, bone marrow, depression, rash, Stevens-Johnson syndrome, drowsiness, liver and urinary disorders Toxicity: Nystagmus, ataxia, depression, drowsiness, N/V, megaloblastic anemia	\$16-21/100 mg (100); \$10-\$39/200 mg 100); \$23/susp: 100 mg/ 5 ml (450 ml)
Phenobarbital Control IV	Adults: Begin with 30 mg BID; maintenance 60-300 mg QD Children: Begin 15 mg BID; maintenance 3-5 mg/kg QD; HS dosing recommended	Annual CBC and LFTs; reserve for refractory patients; ETOH ↑ metabolism Pregnancy: D SE: Drowsiness, depression, fatigue, ↓ cognitive performance, paradoxical hyperactivity in children	\$3-\$8/15 mg (100); \$4-\$11/20 mg/ 5 ml (480)

CBC, Complete blood count; *CNS*, central nervous system; *ETOH*, ethanol; *GI*, gastrointestinal; *INH*, isoniazid; *LFT*, liver function test; *N/A*, not available; *N/V*, nausea and vomiting; *OCP*, oral contraceptive pill; *SE*, side effect; *TEN*, toxic epidermal necrolysis.

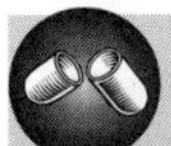

TABLE 164-4 Pharmaceutical Plan: Seizure Disorders—cont'd

Drug	Dose	Comments	Cost
Valproic acid (Depakene, Depakote)	Adults: Begin 15 mg/kg/day in divided doses and may increase weekly by 5-10 mg/kg/day to maximum of 60 mg/kg/day; BID dosing common Children: Same as adult dosage	Baseline LFT; then LFTs every 2-3 months for 2×; periodic serum drug concentrations Pregnancy: D SE: GI disturbances, weakness, blood dyscrasias, BM suppression, hepatotoxicity Toxicity: Tremor, weight gain, alopecia	$13-$116/250 mg (100); $34-$119/susp: 200 mg/5 ml (480 ml)
Clonazepam (Klonopin) Control IV	Adults: Begin 0.5 mg TID and increase every 3 days by 0.5-1 mg daily; max 20 mg daily Children under 10 years: Begin 0.01-0.03 mg/kg/day in 2-3 divided doses; increase if needed every 3 days by 0.25-0.5 mg daily; maintenance 0.1-0.2 mg/kg/day in 3 divided doses	Contraindicated in liver disease and narrow-angle glaucoma Pregnancy: C; not recommended during nursing Potentiation of CNS depression with ETOH SE: Abuse potential, CNS depression, ataxia, drowsiness, increased salivation, respiratory congestion, liver disorders, GI upset, blood dyscrasias	$57-$73/0.5 mg (100); $66-$83/1 mg (100)
Ethosuximide (Zarontin)	Adults: Begin with 500 mg daily; increase every 4-7 days by 250 mg daily; max 1.5 g daily in 2 divided doses Children over 3 years: 20-40 mg/kg/day in 2 divided doses; begin 250 mg QD, increasing by 125 mg every 4-7 days	Periodic CBC Pregnancy: D SE: Blood dyscrasias, drowsiness, ataxia, hepatic and renal problems, GI disorders, Stevens-Johnson syndrome, headache, rash, gingival hyperplasia	$63-$79/250 mg/5 ml (400 ml); $75/250 mg (100)
Gabapentin (Neurontin)	Adults: 300 mg QD to TID	Used for >12 years of age for localization related epilepsy (partial seizures) Pregnancy: C Antacids may interfere with absorption; separate dosing by 2 hrs SE: Somnolence, dizziness, ataxia, fatigue	$36/100 mg (100); $90/300 mg (100)
Lamotrigine (Lamictal)	Adults: 25 mg QOD to 25 mg BID; take with other epileptic medications	Used for localization related epilepsy in adults; do not use with valproic acid Pregnancy: C SE: *Black box warning: life-threatening rashes, including Stevens-Johnson syndrome and TEN; dizziness, ataxia, somnolence, headache, blurred vision, N/V*	$39/25 mg (25); $166/100 mg (100)
Tiagabine (Gabitril)	Adults: 4 mg QOD; adjunct to other epileptic agents; take with food	Used for >12 y/o with localization-related epilepsy Pregnancy: C SE: Dizziness, nervousness, asthenia, confusion, tremor	N/A

Continued

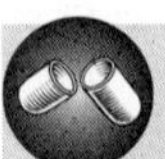

TABLE 164-4 Pharmaceutical Plan: Seizure Disorders—cont'd

Drug	Dose	Comments	Cost
Topiramate (Topamax)	Adults: 25 mg BID; adjunctive therapy for localization-related epilepsy and some generalized epileptics	Pregnancy: C Increases risk of nephrolithiasis SE: Somnolence, dizziness, ataxia, slurred speech, psychomotor slowing, cognitive problems	N/A
Fosphenytoin (Cerebyx)	IV phenytoin prodrug; used for staticus epilepticus	Easier to administer and better tolerated than phenytoin	$18/150 mg/2 ml
Felbamate (Felbatol)	Adults: 1200 mg q6-8h Children: 15-45 mg/kg/day q6-8h	Approved for partial seizures, Lennox-Gastaut syndrome Pregnancy: C SE: *Black box warning: Reserved for compassionate use due to serious toxicity: aplastic anemia, hepatic failure*	N/A

N/A, Not available.

Other problems associated with epilepsy in pregnancy:
- Increased risk of bleeding
- Decrease in fetal growth
- Decrease in childhood intelligence

Elderly Population

Common causes of epilepsy in elderly are cerebrovascular disease and neoplasms, as well as metabolic derangements and head trauma.

A slower metabolic rate often requires a decrease in dosage of AEDs.

The possibility of drug interactions is increased mainly due to the fact that many elderly take numerous medications.

The cost of AEDs may be of great concern to those on a fixed income.

Failing memory can make compliance difficult, especially when the drug requires multiple daily doses.

Lifestyle/Activities

The degree to which activities should be restricted is individualized for each person and depends on the type, frequency, and severity of the seizures; the response to therapy; and the length of time the seizures have been controlled.

The patient should be encouraged to follow a regular and moderate routine in lifestyle, diet, exercise, and rest. (Sleep deprivation may lower the patient's threshold to seizures.)

Normal healthy activities are encouraged for **children,** and participation in competitive sports is determined on an individual basis. Contact sports such as football, karate, or wresting are avoided, but basketball, baseball, and tennis are allowed.

Diet

There are a variety of special diets for the treatment of seizures. One of the recommendations is to eat a healthy, well-balanced diet. Also, the ketogenic diet that stimulates the ketosis and acidosis of starvation has been advocated as therapy for epilepsy, but no controlled studies have evaluated its effectiveness.

Excessive amounts of caffeine and alcohol should be avoided.

Patient Education

Make sure patient and or parent understands the goals and time frame of treatment and he or she has been provided with information and support about seizures.

Teach families what to do in the emergency management of seizures. To avoid unnecessary medical intervention and to ensure that observers respond appropriately to seizures, the patient may want to wear an identification bracelet that notes the condition and phone number of contact person.

Counseling in **children** is especially important, emphasizing the significance of seizures, that they can live a normal life within some limits, and that they must learn to cope with some of the attitudes of the public regarding seizures.

Areas of psychosocial difficulty should be identified early in the course of treatment so that disabilities related to epilepsy can be minimized by using the necessary social, educational, vocational, and psychological support services.

Review each state law concerning driving an automobile.

If patient has good control of seizures, minimum restrictions are needed such as swimming with a buddy or wearing a helmet with some sports.

Stress the importance of drug compliance and instruct patient about the actions and side effects of medications.
AEDs reduce effectiveness of oral contraceptives.
AEDs are teratogenic.
AEDs and other drugs may display numerous interactions.
Review with the patient that a number of factors tend to precipitate seizures insome patients and should be avoided:
Sleep deprivation
Fever
Strobe lights
Psychological stress
Excessive alcohol.
Patient who is not well-controlled should not have pertussis vaccine.

Family Impact

The complete cooperation of the patient and family is of the utmost importance. They must have a strong confidence in the value of the regimen that has been prescribed.
The burden on the family is great, and family problems run the gamut of outright rejection to overprotection.
It is important to encourage a healthy attitude toward the **child** and his or her disease and to help the parents feel competent in their ability to meet their responsibilities to the child. Many parents refrain from correcting or punishing the child, especially if in the past such an emotional stress precipitated an attack. The child should not be made to feel that he or she is different.
The **child** needs to learn about his disease and the role that the medication plays in contributing to his well-being. As soon as he or she is old enough, the child should assume responsibility for taking his or her own medication.
The family should know seizure first aid.

Referral

Consult specialist for treatment of patients with West syndrome and Lennox-Gastaut syndrome.
Consultation with a neurologist is recommended before **pregnancy** in those women contemplating pregnancy to ascertain that AED is indicated and to consider alteration of the current regimen to one that would have a lower risk to the fetus.
New options available for refractory seizures
Vagus nerve stimulator
Seizure surgery: Anterior lobe resection most common

Consultation

Consult physician on all first time seizures.
Consult physician about patients that have complicating factors such as persistent seizures, change in seizure pattern and serious infection.
Consult physician regarding patients that may require hospitalization such as children with a complex febrile seizure.

Follow-up

Follow-up is indicated according to the chosen AED.
In general, every 3 to 6 months to evaluate seizure control and side effects of drugs.
If seizures occur in patient on antiepileptic medications:
Draw blood level of drug
Consult with physician

EVALUATION

Follow-up is indicated according to the chosen AED for blood work related to liver function and serum drug concentrations.
Always ascertain any untoward side effects that the patient may be experiencing.
Reinforce education as described previously.
Patients who are seizure free for 2 years can be considered for medication withdrawal.
Focal motor seizures are more likely to recur than generalized seizures, and those with a prior history of neonatal seizures have a greater risk of seizure recurrence.

RESOURCES

Epilepsy Foundation of American (1-800-efa-1000) or on the internet: www.efa.org.

Epilepsy Foundation of America
800-efa-4050

Epilepsy information service
800 642-0500

National Institute of Neurological Disorders and Stroke
800-352-9424

Staying in Touch, quarterly publication published by Schuler, Sadowski, and Bloodgood. 227 Route 206, Building 2, 2nd floor, Flanders, NJ 07836

SUGGESTED READINGS

Celano R: Diagnosing pediatric epilepsy: an update for the primary care clinician, *Nurse Pract* 23(3):69-96, 1998.
Curry W, Kulling D: Newer antiepileptic drugs: gabapentin, lamotrigine, felbamate, topiramate and fosphenytoin, *Am Family Physician* 57(3): 513-520, 1998.
Ellsworth W et al: *Mosby's 1998 medical drug reference*, St. Louis, 1998, Mosby.
Healthcare Consultants of America, Inc: *1998 physicians fee and coding guide,* Augusta, Ga, 1998, Healthcare Consultants of America, Inc.

Henneman PL, DeRoos F, Lewis RJ: Determining the need for admission in patients with new-onset seizures, *Ann Emerg Med* 12(6):1108-1113, 1994.

Kaplan PW, Fisher RS: Seizure disorders. In Barker LR, Burton JR, Zieve PD, editors: *Principles of ambulatory medicine,* ed 4, Baltimore, 1995, Williams & Wilkins.

Kuhn BR, Allen KD, Shriver MD: Behavioral management of children's seizure activity. Intervention guidelines for primary care providers, *Clin Pediatr* 34(11):570-575, 1995.

Leppik IE: *Contemporary diagnosis and management of the patient with epilepsy,* ed 2, Newtown, Pa, 1996, Handbooks in Health Care.

Marks W, Garcia P: Management of seizures and epilepsy, *Am Family Physician* 57(7):1589-1604, 1998.

McLachlan RS: Managing the first seizure, *Can Family Physician* 39:885-888, 891-893, 1993.

Mikati M, Browne TR: Seizures and epilepsy. In Dershewitz RA, editor: *Ambulatory pediatric care,* ed 2, Philadelphia, 1993, JB Lippincott.

Moore-Sledge CM: Evaluation and management of first seizures in adults, *Am Family Physician* 56(4):1113-1120, 1997.

Morrell MJ: XII Epilepsy. In Dale DC, editor: *Scientific American medicine,* New York, 1994, Scientific American.

Oommen K: Seizures. In Greene H, Johnson W, Lemcke D, editors: *Decision making in medicine,* ed 2, St Louis, 1998, Mosby.

Percy AK, Percy PD: Acute management of seizures in children, *Nurse Pract* 11(2):15-28, 1986.

Rochester J: Epilepsy in pregnancy, *Am Family Physician* 56(6):1631-1638, 1997.

Scheuer ML, Pedley TA: The evaluation and treatment of seizures, *N Engl J Med* 323(21):1468-1473, 1990.

Sexual Dysfunction

ICD-9-CM

Psychosexual Dysfunction, Unspecified 302.70
Psychosexual Dysfunction with Inhibited Sexual Excitement (Frigidity, Impotence) 302.72
Psychosexual Dysfunction with Inhibited Female Orgasm 302.73
Psychosexual Dysfunction with Inhibited Male Orgasm 302.74
Psychosexual Dysfunction with Functional Dyspareunia 302.76
Vaginismus 306.51

OVERVIEW

Definition

Sexual dysfunction is a complaint involving a sexual issue or a specific sexual dysfunction.

Incidence

An estimated 40% of couples have a sexual problem at some time during their relationship. Many women report dissatisfaction with sexual relationships, citing the use of avoidance, infrequency, or noncommunication related to sexual issues. Most patients think that it is the role of the primary care provider to address sexual dysfunction.

Pathophysiology

Pathophysiology depends on the cause of the sexual dysfunction. The human sexual response is a complex response dependent on a variety of emotional and physiological factors. There are four phases of sexual response: excitement, plateau, orgasm, and resolution (Masters and Johnson, 1970).

The physiological components are mediated by two processes:

Changes in muscle tone, myotonic activity
Changes in blood flow, especially vasocongestion

SUBJECTIVE DATA

A complete sexual history is an important component to obtain when evaluating a sexual problem. Discuss these issues when patient is fully clothed, preferably in a consultation room. See sample sexual history and physical examination form, pp. 1005 and 1006.

History of Present Illness

See sexual history form, pp. 1005 and 1006.

Medications

Medications associated with sexual disorders: decreased libido, erectile dysfunction (Table 165-1)

OBJECTIVE DATA

Physical Examination

A detailed examination of the genitourinary system should be conducted (see sexual history and physical examination form, pp. 1005 and 1006)
Vital signs: General: Symptoms of androgen or estrogen excess or deficiency
Skin
Cardiovascular: Vascular disease
Abdominal: Bowel sounds, masses
Pelvic: Look for atrophic vaginitis, vaginal atresia, defective vaginal repair, pelvic inflammatory disease, endometriosis, signs of vaginitis, vulvitis

Diagnostic Procedures

Diagnostic procedures are outlined in Table 165-2.

TABLE 165-1 Medications Associated with Sexual Disorders

Decreased libido	Anorgasmia	Erectile dysfunction
Sympatholytics, both central and peripheral; alpha-blockers (Prazosin); angiotensin-converting enzyme inhibitors (minimal); tricyclics: carbonic anhydrase, inhibitors, tranquilizers, sleep medications	Monoamine oxidase (MAO) inhibitors; tricyclics; sympatholytics, both central and peripheral	Antihypertensives: Beta blockers (especially propranolol and other nonselective agents); calcium channel blocking agents; centrally acting sympatholytic agents (methyldopa); peripherally acting sympatholytic agents (reserpine); spironolactone; thiazide diuretics (most common) Central nervous system agents: MAO inhibitors, opioids (long-term use); phenothiazine antipsychotic agents; substances of abuse (alcohol, cocaine, marijuana); tricyclic antidepressants; elective serotonin reuptake inhibitors Miscellaneous agents: Disopyramide (Norpace); nicotine; sympathetic agents (epinephrine, phenylephrine, phenylpropanolamine, pseudo-ephedrine); cimetidine (Tagamet); estrogens; antiandrogens; metoclopramide (Reglan)

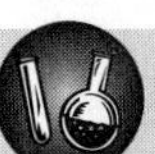

TABLE 165-2 Diagnostic Tests: Sexual Dysfunction

Diagnostic Test	Finding/Rationale	Cost ($)
Hemoglobin/hematocrit	Rule out anemia	11-14
Electrolytes, blood urea nitrogen, creatinine, glucose, liver function tests, thyroid function tests	Rule out endocrine, liver and renal disease	23-30/elec; 32-42/comprehensive metabolic panel; 86-109/thyroid
Serum estradial	<35 ng/ml is indicative of low sexual frequency	85-107
Follicle-stimulating hormone, prolactin, luteinizing hormone, and testosterone	To rule out hypothalamus dysfunction	61-76/LH; 62-78/FSH; 80-101/Tes
Sexual energy scale	Provides an objective means of measuring the change in a patient's subjective experience of vitality/sexual energy when androgens are used; the scale also provides a clinical indication of when androgens should be adjusted (Warnock, Bundren, Morris, 1997)	

TABLE 165-3 Differential Diagnoses: Sexual Dysfunction

Diagnosis	Supporting Data	
Organic factors	Gradual onset; rapid onset when associated with certain medications; no response to an adequate course of sex therapy	Conditions associated with sexual disorders: arthritis, joint disease; diabetes mellitus; liver or renal failure; mood disorders; peripheral neuropathy; respiratory disorders (chronic obstructive pulmonary disease); spinal cord injury; vascular disease
Situational factors	Rapid onset, sexual phobia, and aversion	
Medication related	See preceding list of medications related to sexual dysfunction	
Psychological factors	May play a part even when a medical cause is identified: performance anxiety, inadequate communication, fantasy intrapsychic causes (sexual trauma, guilt, fear, anxiety), relationship issues (lack of trust, anger at partner, infidelity), sociocultural factors (attitudes, values, religious beliefs), educational factors (myths, gender expectations, sexual ignorance)	
Low or absent sexual desire	May include discrepancy of partner's sexual desire; can be related to power struggles, childhood sexual, physical or emotional abuse; the disturbance causes distress or interpersonal difficulty; the most common chief complaint; factors associated with low sexual desire: drug side effects, diabetes mellitus, inflammatory bowel disease, heart disease, problems with intimacy, religious prohibitions	Treatment: Careful delineation of issues, listening exercises to improve communication, may be related to depressive disorder; low-dose methyltestosterone may be appropriate
Sexual arousal disorder	Persistent inability to attain or maintain an adequate response to sexual excitement, which causes marked distress or interpersonal difficulty; less of a problem than it used to be (lubrication-swelling response)	Treatment: Increase direct stimulation with partner, use of vaginal moisturizers (Astroglide, KY jelly, Replens), genital caressing, progressive relaxation, ways other than intercourse to pleasure partner; discuss a weekend away from children; set aside time to talk with partner
Orgasmic disorder	Persistent delay or absence of orgasm following normal sexual excitement; selective serotonin reuptake inhibitors (SSRIs) appear to have a dramatic effect on orgasm, particularly in the first 1 or 2 months; orgasmic quality also appears to be lower when SSRIs are taken. Other factors: performance anxiety, fear of loss of control, anger at partner, lack of attraction to a partner	Treatment: Listening exercises to improve communication, education, conflict resolution, treatment of depressive disorder, use of a vibrator may be helpful; oral vasodilator medications may be helpful in treating arousal and orgasmic disorders
Dyspareunia, vaginismus	Recurrent or persistent genital pain associated with sexual intercourse (dyspareunia); recurrent or persistent involuntary spasm of the outer ⅓ of the vagina that interferes with sexual intercourse (vaginismus)	Treatment: Listening exercises to improve communication, may be related to depressive disorder; emphasize the need to have adequate stimulation before penetration; give the woman control over when and how penetration occurs; Kegel exercises to increase awareness and control over pelvic muscles; vaginal self-dilation; artificial lubricants; estrogen creams to counteract postmenopausal thinning of vaginal walls (0.625 mg/g [45 g]: $29-$32)

ASSESSMENT

Differential diagnoses include those found in Table 165-3. See Chapter 98 for more specific diagnoses for men.

THERAPEUTIC PLAN

Pharmaceutical

Dependent on type of dysfunction

Nonpharmaceutical

Use of the PLISSIT model

P = Permission to deal with sexual issues, empathetic listening by nurse practitioner
  Reassurance to help normalize, inquiry into positive perceptions

LI = Limited information pertinent to situation (need to know information)

SS = Specific suggestions for action
  Temporary agreement not to have intercourse
  Focus on pleasurable touch, caressing
  Progressive muscle relaxation exercises
  Positive self talk
  Ways to improve general and sexual communication with partner

IT = Intensive therapy: referral to a specialist in sexual therapy (Bullard and Caplan, 1997)

Lifestyle/Activities

See Table 165-3.

Diet

Not applicable

Patient Education

Give information to patient on need-to-know basis. Do not overload with all information pertaining to disorder. Suggest the woman go to the library and get self-help books on sexual relationships (Barbach, 1976).

Offer communication suggestions with partner.
Teach progressive relaxation methods.

Referral/Consultation

A patient whose dysfunction is >1 year duration, consists of multiple disorders, or is in the context of an unstable relationship should be referred to a OB/GYN specialist or sex therapist. Those problems that are secondary (i.e., began after an interval of satisfactory sexuality) tend to be more likely to have a satisfactory outcome than those that are primary.

Follow-up

Follow-up after 1 month to see if progress has been made. If no progress has been made, consider referral.

EVALUATION

Satisfaction with self and partner's sexual relationship

REFERENCES

Barbach L: *For yourself, the fulfillment of female sexuality,* New York, 1976, Signet.

Bullard D, Caplan H: Sexual problems. In Feldman M, Christensen J, editors: *Behavioral medicine in primary care,* Stamford, Conn, 1997, Appleton & Lange.

Masters W, Johnson V: *Human sexual inadequacy,* Boston, 1970, Little Brown.

Warnock J, Bundren J, Morris D: Female hypoactive sexual desire disorder due to androgen deficiency: clinical and psychometric issues, *Psychopharmacol Bull* 33(4):761-766, 1997.

SUGGESTED READINGS

Ellsworth W et al: *Mosby's 1998 medical drug reference*, St. Louis, 1998, Mosby.

Healthcare Consultants of America, Inc: *1998 physicians fee and coding guide,* Augusta, Ga, 1998, Healthcare Consultants of America, Inc.

Gentili A, Mulligan T: Sexual dysfunction in older adults, *Clinical Geriatr Med* 14(2):383-393, 1998.

Labbate L et al: Sexual dysfunction induced by serotonin reuptake antidepressants, *J Sex Marital Ther* 24(1):3-12, 1998.

Read S, King M, Watson J: Sexual dysfunction in primary medical care: prevalence, characteristics, and detection by the general practitioner, *J Public Health Med* 19(4):387-391, 1997.

Segraves R: Antidepressant-induced sexual dysfunction, *J Clinical Psychiatry* 59(suppl 4):48-54, 1998.

SEXUAL HISTORY

Date: | Name: | DOB: | Allergies:

T: | P: | B/P: | Weight:

CC:

Medications:

Present illness:

Intro: One area that is often neglected is sexual health, yet it is an important part of women's lives. Do you have questions about sexual issues?

How are things sexually? Is there any way you would like your sex life to be different?

Are you sexually active now?

How many partners do you have now?

How old were you when you had sex the first time?

Are you sexually active with: (use partner instead of husband/wife)

Men ☐ Yes ☐ No

Women ☐ Yes ☐ No

Both ☐ Yes ☐ No

Past medical Hx:

☐ Surgeries

☐ Hospitalizations

☐ Treatment for
  depression
  anxiety
  eating disorders ____

______

______

☐ Illnesses: chronic

______

☐ History of STDs
  Trt ______

☐ Ever been tested for HIV?

Social:

☐ Smoke ____ PPD

☐ Alcohol ____ Day

☐ Drugs

☐ Employment Y N

☐ # years of school completed

☐ Living arrangements

☐ Significant other

☐ Children Y ____ N

Sexual experiences:

☐ How satisfied are you with your sexual experiences?

☐ Frequency

☐ Variety

☐ Who initiates

☐ Safe sex practices

☐ Have you ever had a difficult, disturbing, or abusive sexual experience?

Specific problem:

☐ Describe the problem you are having. Does it happen with masturbation or with a specific partner or any partner?

☐ How does your partner respond when the problem happens?

☐ Any situations when it is not a problem?

☐ Any specific worries right now?

☐ What have you tried so far to help the problem?

☐ Have you ever had sexual therapy or couple therapy?

☐ Have you discussed this openly with your partner?

ROS: Circle

Heent: head inj, seizures, H/A, glaucoma, cataracts, visual problems, hearing loss, infection, allergies/sinus, nosebleeds, chronic sore throats, difficulty swallowing

Lymph: swellings in neck, axilla, groin, anemia

Endocrine: thyroid problems, DM, wt loss

Pulmonary: asthma, pneumonia, hemoptysis

CV: murmur, rhythm disturb, HTN, C/P, angina

Breast: mass/lump/DC/pain

GI: GERD, hematemesis, PUD, abd. pain, chronic constipation or diarrhea, change in bowel movement, liver or GB problems, pancreatitis, melena or hemoatochesia, hemorrhoids, hepatitis

GU: dysuria, hematuria, UTI, STDs, warts, difficulty with urination or incontinence

MS: arthritis, gout, swelling, claudication, back pain

Neuro: numbness, weakness, chronic tingling, B/B incontinence, gait disturb, falling

Skin: changes in moles/warts, chronic rashes, acne

GYN: hot flashes, numbness, H/A, palpitations, drenching sweats, mood swings, vaginal dryness, itching

Frequent vaginal infections

Unusual vaginal discharge

Vaginal odor

Genital warts

STD (chlamydia, gonorrhea, syphilis, herpes)

Infection in uterus, tubes, ovaries (PID)

Pain or bleeding after intercourse

Missed periods

Bleeding b/w periods

Uterine abnormalities

Abnormal Pap smears

Cervical lesions/biopsy

Cysts/tumors on ovary

Premenstrual symptoms

FH:

☐ HTN ☐ MI

☐ CAD ☐ CVA

☐ DM ☐ CA

☐ Resp. ☐ Depression

☐ ETOH ☐ Seizures

Menstrual HX:

Age periods started ____

Periods last ____ days

Periods come q ____ days

Are periods:

☐ Regular

☐ Irregular

☐ Painful

☐ Light

☐ Moderate

☐ Heavy

LMP ______

Last Pap ______

Where: ______

Results: ______

Objective:

System	Norm	Abnormal	Comments
Skin	☐	☐	______
Head	☐	☐	______
Oral cavity	☐	☐	______
Neck	☐	☐	______
Thyroid	☐	☐	______
Chest	☐	☐	______
Heart	☐	☐	______
Breast	☐	☐	______
Abdomen	☐	☐	______
Neuro	☐	☐	______
Extremities	☐	☐	______
Pelvic	☐	☐	______
External	☐	☐	______
B.U.S.	☐	☐	______
Vagina	☐	☐	______
Cervix	☐	☐	______
Fundus	☐	☐	______
Adnexae	☐	☐	______
Rectal	☐	☐	______

Assessment:
- ☐ Normal exam
- ☐ Low sexual desire
- ☐ Sexual arousal disorder
- ☐ Orgasmic disorder
- ☐ Dyspareunia
- ☐ Vaginismus

Referral:
- ☐ OBG
- ☐ Sex therapy
- ☐ Counseling

Obstetric HX:

Number of preg: ______
Number of live birth ______
Stillbirth: ______
Miscarriage: ______
Abortion: ______
Any pregnancy complications?

DM	Y	N
HTN	Y	N
Toxemia	Y	N

Contraceptive HX:

Current birth control?
- ☐ None
- ☐ Pills
- ☐ IUD
- ☐ condoms (rubbers)
- ☐ BTL
- ☐ Depo
- ☐ Diaphragm/cervical cap

Plan:

Labs:
- ☐ H/H
- ☐ HIV
- ☐ RPR
- ☐ Electrolytes
- ☐ LFT
- ☐ BUN
- ☐ Creatinine
- ☐ GC/chlamydia
- ☐ Pap
- ☐ U/A
- ☐ Wet mount
  - ☐ KOH
  - ☐ NaCl
- ☐ HCG
- ☐ FSH
- ☐ LH
- ☐ Prolactin
- ☐ Estradial
- ☐ Androgen

Medications:

______
______
______
______
______

Instructions:

Counseled:
- ☐ Exercise 3-5x week
- ☐ Low fat, high carb, high fiber diet
- ☐ Smoking cessation
- ☐ Alcohol moderation

RTO: ______

Signature: ______

166 Sinusitis

ICD-9-CM

Acute Sinusitis, Unspecified 461.9
Chronic Sinusitis, Unspecified 473.9

OVERVIEW

Definition

Sinusitis is inflammation of the mucous lining of the paranasal sinuses. Sinusitis occurs when an undrained collection of pus accumulates in a sinus. The underlying causes are diseases that swell the nasal mucosal membranes such as a viral upper respiratory tract infection or allergic rhinitis. In addition, sinusitis is often associated with swimming or diving. *Acute sinusitis* is a symptomatic sinus infection lasting up to 3 weeks. *Chronic sinusitis* is a symptomatic sinus infection that persists for longer than 3 weeks, despite adequate treatment.

Incidence

A common health problem prevalent in all ages and equally prevalent in both sexes.

Pathophysiology

Protective Factors Against

A protective mucous blanket that traps bacteria and other irritants, covers the respiratory cilia, and is moved constantly along predetermined pathways to the sinus ostia.

Factors that Increase Susceptibility

Nasal polyps
Deviation of the nasal septum

Conditions Associated with Increased Risk for Development of Sinusitis

Diseases that swell the nasal mucous membrane or interfere with the normal cleansing of the mucosal cilia. Causes include:
- Response to a virus, bacterium or allergen
- Fungal infestation
- Mechanical obstruction
- Trauma
- Air pollution, tobacco smoke, or low humidity
- Rapid changes in altitude
- Dental infection

Common Pathogens

Similar pathogens occur in adults and children and are the same as those that cause acute otitis media.

Acute Sinusitis

Streptococcus pneumoniae (35%) and *Haemophilus influenzae* (35%)
Moraxella catarrhalis (5%) is a common cause in **children**
Streptococcus pyogenes and alpha-hemolytic streptococcus (10%)
Viruses (9%)
Staphylococcus aureus (6%)

Chronic Sinusitis

Anaerobic bacteria (>50%)
Staphylococcus aureus
Opportunistic pathogens

Common Sites

Maxillary and frontal sinusitis are common in **adults;** ethmoiditis is more common in **children.** The sinuses may be involved singly or, more frequently, in combination (Figure 166-1).

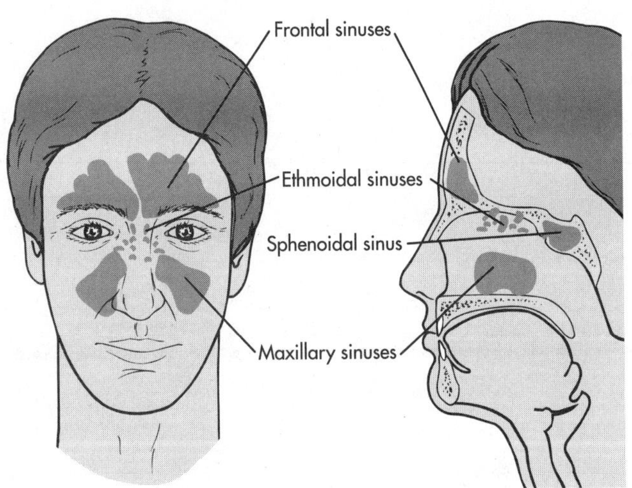

Figure 166-1 Location of sinuses. (From Lewis SM, Collier IC, Heitkemper MM: *Medical-surgical nursing: assessment and management of clinical problems,* ed 4, St Louis, 1996, Mosby.)

SUBJECTIVE DATA

History of Present Illness

Question about duration of symptoms, response to use of decongestants, and color of nasal drainage. Ask about halitosis with a metallic taste, pain with mastication, headache, toothache or facial pain, and frequent clearing of the throat. Inquire about self-treatment, especially duration and use of nasal sprays.

Children: Cough and nasal discharge are the most common symptoms of acute sinusitis and occur in 80% of the children. Headache and facial pain are unusual, especially in those younger than 10 years.

Elderly: May present with none or few of the characteristics listed in previous paragraphs. A fever with associated delirium and cognitive dysfunction may be the presenting symptoms.

Past Medical History

Ask about history of diabetes, asthma or immunosuppression, a seasonal relationship with symptoms, allergies, recent nose trauma, dental work or upper respiratory infection (URI), past sinusitis episodes, and treatments.

Medications

Recent use of antibiotics, steroids, decongestants, nasal sprays or antihistamines

Family History

Ask about a family history of asthma, allergies, and chronic sinusitis.

Psychosocial History

Children: Whether a smoker resides in the household, household pets

Adults: Smoker or whether a smoker resides in the household, household pets

Description of Most Common Symptoms

Persistent symptoms of URI for more than 10 days that have not begun to abate.

Acute

Adult: Nasal discharge (serous, mucoid, mucopurulent) cough, tooth and/or facial pain, jaw claudication, sore throat, decreased or loss of sense of smell, halitosis or a metallic taste in the mouth, and headaches that are often worse at night and early in the morning

Children: Often have more nonspecific complaints than adults. Suspect sinusitis if URI symptoms persist beyond 10 days without improvement, unusually severe, with persistent cough and nasal discharge; the allergic child may have an acute exacerbation of respiratory symptoms

Elderly: Fever with associated delirium and cognitive dysfunction may be the only presenting symptoms.

Chronic

Indolent symptoms of chronic nasal congestion, postnasal drip, cough, facial fullness, headache are present. Nasal drainage may vary in consistency and appearance. Taste and smell may be reduced, and bad breath is frequent.

Associated Symptoms

Early morning periorbital edema, fever, malaise, and increased pain with coughing, bending forward, and sudden head movement; high temperature and signs of acute toxicity are unusual, except in the most severe cases.

OBJECTIVE DATA

Physical Examination

A problem-oriented physical examination should be conducted, with particular attention to:

- Vital signs including temperature
- General appearance
- Eyes: Allergic shiners or periorbital edema
- Nasal mucosa for edema, erythema, mucopurulent discharge, and boggy turbinates; polyps; patency of both nasal nares and structures of the nasal septum
- Ears, throat, and mouth for signs of inflammation
- Frontal and maxillary sinuses: Pain on percussion, erythema, edema and inability to transilluminate

TABLE 166-1 Physical Findings in Sinusitis

Symptoms	Findings
Acute	
Nasal discharge, headache, cough, maxillary toothache, poor response to nasal decongestants, facial pain	Nasal mucosa erythematous, edematous with mucopurulent discharge; frontal or maxillary sinus pain on percussion, erythema
Chronic	
Indolent symptoms of chronic nasal congestion, postnasal drip, cough, facial fullness, headache, reduced taste/smell, malodorous breath	Physical findings are similar to those seen in acute sinusitis; anatomic abnormalities such as nasal polyps, septal deviation may be present

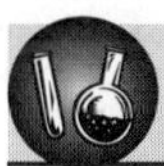

TABLE 166-2 Diagnostic Tests: Sinusitis

Diagnostic Test	Findings/Rationale	Cost ($)
Computed tomography (CT) scan or sinus films	If signs and symptoms have not resolved in 10 to 14 days of treatment, CT scan or sinus films should be obtained to confirm the diagnosis. CT scans have increasingly replaced sinus films for screening purposes. They are more sensitive to inflammatory changes and bone destruction and no more expensive than conventional films. Standard set of conventional sinus films: Caldwell (frontal), Waters (maxillary), lateral (sphenoid), and submentovertical (ethmoid).	146-173/sinus films; 704-834/CT without contrast; 1021-1271/with/without contrast
Allergy testing	Usually done as third-line test if recurrent acute sinusitis or chronic sinusitis.	4-15/test

sinuses (variations in soft tissue thickness and technique often make interpretation difficult)

Maxillary teeth: Percuss to check for a dental source of maxillary sinusitis

Neck and jaw for lymphadenopathy

Heart and lungs: Auscultate

Table 166-1 lists physical findings in sinusitis.

Diagnostic Procedures

It is often possible to make the diagnoses of sinusitis on clinical grounds. Table 166-2 outlines diagnostic tests for sinusitis.

ASSESSMENT

Differential diagnoses include those listed in Table 166-3:

Inflammatory rhinitis: Allergic (seasonal, perennial), viral rhinitis

Noninflammatory rhinitis: Vasomotor rhinitis, rhinitis medicamentosa, hormonal/endocrine

Anatomic obstruction: Deviated septum, adenoidal hypertrophy, sinus neoplasms, foreign body

Other: Dental pain, migraine headache, temporal arteritis

THERAPEUTIC PLAN

See Figure 166-2.

Pharmaceutical

Antibiotics

Antibiotic treatment for sinusitis is based on the acuteness or chronicity of the disease (Tables 166-4 and 166-5). Goals are management of infection, reduction of tissue edema, facilitation of drainage, relief of pain, and maintenance of the patency of the sinus ostia.

See the pediatric dosing chart in Appendix M.

Decongestants

Topical decongestants (Afrin or Neo-Synephrine spray) should not be used for more than 3 or 4 days.

Topical steroid nasal sprays (beclomethasone, flunisolide,

TABLE 166-3 Differential Diagnosis: Sinusitis

Diagnoses	Supporting Data
Noninflammarory Rhinitis	
Vasomotor rhinitis	Rapid onset of nasal congestion occurs, with abrupt changes in barometric pressure, odors, emotional stress
Rhinitis medicamentosa	With use of topical nasal decongestants for >3 days, a secondary vasodilation can occur, resulting in increased nasal congestion
Hormonal/endocrine	Hypothyroidism, pregnancy or oral contraceptive use
Inflammatory Rhinitis	
Allergic	Usually involves the triad of nasal congestion, sneezing and clear rhinorrhea; itchy, puffy eyes often accompany; nasal mucosa is pale and boggy, throat cobblestone appearance, allergic shiners may be present
Viral	Malaise, coryza, headache, temperature <100° F, mild cough worse at bedtime, pharynx erythematous without exudate or lymphadenopathy
Anatomic obstruction	Unilateral nasal discharge
Neuralgias	
Dental pain, migraine headache, temporal arteritis	Neuralgias usually accompanied by a burning or searing pain, jaw claudication

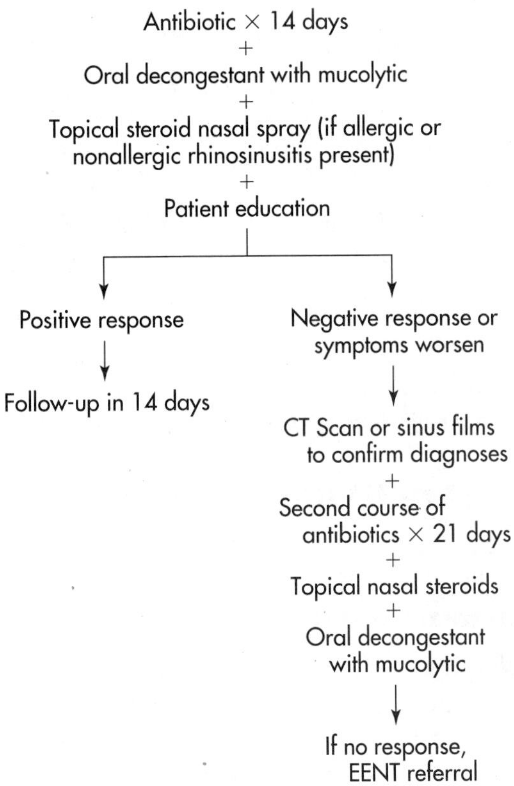

Figure 166-2 Algorithm for treatment of sinusitis. *CT,* Computed tomography; *EENT,* eyes, ears, nose, throat.

triamcinolone) can relieve symptoms of allergic and nonallergic rhinosinusitis without inducing adrenal suppression. Evidence suggests that this class of nasal sprays reaches affected areas by ciliary transport and can suppress inflammation of the nasal mucosa at the sinus ostia. In addition, these agents act to reduce inflammation and edema, decrease vascular permeability, inhibit leukotriene release, and suppress acute and late-phase reactions.

Oral decongestants in combination with mucolytics (Humibid, Zephrex, Entex) can thin sinus secretions and increase sinus drainage (Tables 166-6 to 166-8).

Antihistamines

The role of antihistamines is controversial. Classic antihistamines dry and thicken purulent sinus secretions but may be useful in patients with underlying allergy.

Analgesics and Antipyretics

As indicated for comfort measures

Lifestyle/Activities

Avoid allergens and excessively dry heat.
Avoid use of antihistamines unless there is an allergic basis to disease.
Cessation of smoking.

Diet

None

Patient Education

Overview of the disease process, causes and risk factors, and the potential side effects of the prescribed medications.
Orbital or facial swelling is a medical emergency that warrants immediate evaluation and treatment.
Humidify the air. Increase fluid intake.

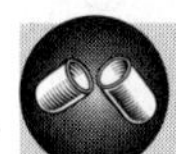

TABLE 166-4 Pharmaceutical Plan: Acute Sinusitis—14 Days' Duration

Drug	Dose	Comments	Cost
Amoxicillin (Amoxil, Trimox, Wymox)	500 mg TID for 14 days; may need to extend to 21 days Child: 40 mg/kg/day in 3 divided doses; can consider using an increased Amoxil dose of 60-80 mg/kg/day	Pregnancy: B Caution in penicillin or cephalosporin allergy	$8-$27/200 mg (100); $17-$49/500 (100); $3-$5/125 mg/5 ml (150 ml); $4-$8/250 mg/5 ml (150 ml)
Amoxicillin/potassium clavulanate (Augmentin)	500 mg q8 h for 14 days; 875 mg q12h Child: 13.3/3.3 mg/kg/day q8h	Pregnancy: B Caution in penicillin or cephalosporin allergy	$82/500 mg (30); $86/875 mg (30); $58/250 mg (30)
Cefaclor (Ceclor)	500 mg QID Child: 40 mg/kg/day in 3 divided doses; max 1 g/day	Pregnancy: B Caution in penicillin or other allergy SE: N/V/D, vaginitis, rash, urticaria	$365-$426/500 mg (100); $27-$31/125 mg/5 ml (150 ml); $48-$56/250 mg/5 ml (150 ml)
Cefixime (Suprax)	400 mg QD or 200 mg BID Child: Under 6 months not recommended; <50 kg and 6-12 years: 8 mg/kg/day in daily or twice daily doses	Pregnancy: B Caution in penicillin or other allergy SE: N/V/D, vaginitis, rash, urticaria	$322/200 mg (100); $663/400 mg (100); $31/100 mg/5 ml (50)
Clarithromycin (Biaxin)	500 mg BID Child: Under 6 months not recommended; 6-20 months see literature; 7.5 mg/kg twice daily	Pregnancy: C SE: N/V/D, vaginitis, rash, urticaria	$185/500 mg (60); $26-$49/125 mg/5 ml (100 ml)
Trimethoprim-sulfamethoxazole (TMP/SMZ, Bactrim)	160/800 mg (1 double strength tablet) BID Child: Under 2 months not recommended; 4 mg/kg T +20 mg/kg S BID	Pregnancy: C Caution in sulfa allergies SE: N/V/D, abdominal pain, rash, photosensitivity	$7-$74/reg. strength tab: (100); $9-$121/DS: (100); $27-$43/200 SMX/40 mg TMP/5 ml (450 ml)

N/V/D/, Nausea, vomiting, diarrhea; *SE,* side effects.

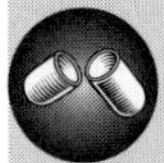

TABLE 166-5 Pharmaceutical Plan: Chronic Sinusitis—14 to 21 Days' Duration

Drug	Adult Dose	Child Dose	Cost
Amoxicillin/potassium clavulanate (Augmentin)	500 mg Amox/125 mg clavulanate q8h for 14 days	13.3 mg/3.3 mg/kg/day q8h	See Table 166-4
Cefixime (Suprax)	400 mg QD or 200 mg BID	Under 6 months not recommended; <50 kg and 6-12 years: 8 mg/kg/day in daily or twice daily doses	See Table 166-4
Clarithromycin (Biaxin)	500 mg BID	Under 6 months not recommended; 6-20 months, see literature; 7.5 mg/kg twice daily	See Table 166-4
Clindamycin HCL (Cleocin) CAUTION: Can promote severe antibiotic-associated colitis; limit to anaerobic infections only (Pregnancy C)	150-300 mg q6h	8-16 mg/kg/day in 4 divided doses	Adult: $75-$115/150 mg (100); $231/300 mg (100) Child: $13/75 mg/5 ml (100 ml)

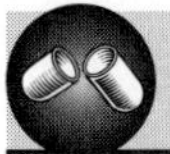

TABLE 166-6 Decongestants

Drug	Dose	Comments	Cost
Pseudoephedrine (Sudafed) tabs: 30, 60 mg; liq: 7.5 mg/0.81 15 mg/5 ml	adult: 60 mg q 4-6 h, max 240 QD 2-6: 15 mg (1.6 ml) q 4-6 h, max 4 doses/day 6-12: 30 mg q 4-6h	Not recommended <2 years of age Pregnancy: B Helpful for nasal congestion only SE: Central nervous system overstimulation, headache, palpitations, hypertension, nervousness, insomnia, tremor	$5-$7/syrup: 30 mg/5 ml (480 ml); $1-$11/30 mg (100); $3-$25/60 mg (100)

SE, Side effects.

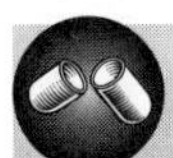

TABLE 166-7 Topical Nasal Corticosteroids

Drug	Dose	Comments	Cost
Beclomethasone dipropionate (Beconase AQ) 42 μg/spray (200 sprays)	>6 y/o: 1-2 sprays in each nostril BID	Needs to maintain regular regimen; may use decongestants if needed Pregnancy: C SE: Nasal discomfort, sneezing, headache, nausea, epistaxis, rhinorrhea	\$34/42 μg /spray (25 g); \$17-\$36/MDI nasal inh (6.7-7 g)
Fluticasone propionate (Flonase) 50 μg/spray (120 sprays)	Initially 2 sprays in each nostril 1× daily or 1 spray BID; maintenance: 1 spray in each nostril QD >4 y/o: 1 spray in each nostril	Needs to maintain regular regimen; may use decongestants if needed Pregnancy: C Caution: CYP3A4 inhibitors (ketoconazole) SE: Nasal discomfort, sneezing, headache, nausea, epistaxis, rhinorrhea	\$41/0.05 mg/inh (16 g)
Triamcinolone acetonide (Nasacort AQ) 55 μg/spray (120 sprays)	2 sprays in each nostril QD 6-12 y/o: 1 spray in each nostril QD	Needs to maintain regular regimen; may use decongestants if needed Pregnancy: C SE: Nasal discomfort, sneezing, headache, nausea, epistaxis, rhinorrhea	\$39/55 μg (10 g)
Flunisolide (Nasalide) 25 μg/spray (200 sprays) (Nasarel)	Blow nose Adults: 2 sprays in each nostril BID, max 8 sprays/nostril/day 6-14 y/o: 1 spray in each nostril TIC or 2 sprays BID, max 4/nostril/day	Needs to maintain regular regimen; may use decongestants if needed Pregnancy: C SE: Nasal discomfort, sneezing, headache, nausea, epistaxis, rhinorrhea, septal perforation	\$28/0.25 mg/ml (25 ml)
Mometasone furoate (Nasonex) 50 μg/spray (120 sprays)	2 sprays in each nostril QD; begin 2-4 weeks before anticipated start of pollen season	Needs to maintain regular regimen; may use decongestants if needed Pregnancy: C SE: Nasal discomfort, sneezing, headache, nausea, epistaxis, rhinorrhea	N/A
Budesonide (Rhinocort) 32 μg/spray (200 sprays)	Blow nose; initially 2 sprays in each nostril BID or 4 sprays QD; gradually reduce to lowest effective dose	Needs to maintain regular regimen; may use decongestants if needed Pregnancy: C SE: Nasal discomfort, sneezing, headache, nausea, epistaxis, rhinorrhea	\$28/32 μg/spray (200 sprays)
Beclomethasone dipropionate (Vancenase AQ Double Strength) 84 μg/spray (120-200 sprays)	>6 y/o: 1-2 sprays in each nostril QD	Needs to maintain regular regimen; may use decongestants if needed Pregnancy: C SE: Nasal discomfort, sneezing, headache, nausea, epistaxis, rhinorrhea, fungal overgrowth	\$42/84 μg/inh (19 g)

N/A, Not available; *SE,* side effects.

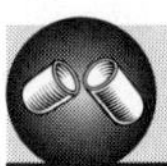

TABLE 166-8 Intranasal Decongestants

Drug	Dose	Comments	Cost
Naphazoline (Privine)	1-2 sprays of 0.05% solution in each nostril q6h PRN	Do not exceed 3-5 days Not recommended <12 y/o Caution: Pregnancy	$4/0.05% (20 ml)
Oxymetazoline (Afrin)	2-3 sprays of 0.05% solution in each nostril in AM and PM PRN	Do not exceed 3-5 days Not recommend <6 y/o Caution: Pregnancy SE: Central nervous system stimulation, palpitations, hypertension, headache	$3/0.025% (20 ml)
Phenylephrine (Neo-Synephrine)	2-3 sprays of 1% or 0.5% in each nostril q4h PRN	Do not exceed 3-5 days Not recommended <2 y/o Caution: Pregnancy SE: Rebound congestion, hypertension, nasal discomfort, insomnia, palpitations	$4/1% spray (15 ml)
Xylometazoline (Otrivin)	2-3 drops or sprays of 0.1% in each nostril q8-10h PRN, max 3 doses/24h or 3 days of use	Not recommended <2 y/o Caution: Pregnancy SE: As for phenylephrine	$3-$5/0.01% (20 ml)

SE, Side effects.

Steam inhalation and warm compresses to the face.
Blow nose gently with both nostrils at the same time.
Avoid swimming/diving during the acute phase.
Encourage smoking cessation.
Avoid allergens.

Family Impact

It may be necessary to remove pets from the household to avoid an allergen. Parents who smoke should be urged to quit.

Referral

Refer to ear/nose/throat specialist for recurrent sinusitis or complications of acute sinusitis.

Consultation

Extreme pain with palpation or percussion of face
Periorbital swelling, facial swelling, or possible cellulitis

Follow-up

Instruct to return if no improvement within 48 hours or swelling develops in the periorbital area.
Schedule return visit in 10 to 14 days

EVALUATION

As indicated by the initial precipitating factor and course of disease

SUGGESTED READINGS

Baker R: *Handbook of pediatric primary care,* Boston, 1996, Little, Brown.

Corren J: Making the clinical diagnosis of sinusitis, *Clin Focus,* December 1993, pp 11-17.

Douville L: Pharmacologic highlights. Management of acute sinusitis, *J Am Acad Nurse Pract* 7(8):407-411, 1995.

Ellsworth W et al: *Mosby's 1998 medical drug reference,* St. Louis, 1998, Mosby.

Evans K: Diagnosis and management of sinusitis, *Br Med J* 309:1415-1422, 1994.

Healthcare Consultants of America, Inc: *1998 physicians fee and coding guide,* Augusta, Ga, 1998, Healthcare Consultants of America, Inc.

Jackler R, Kaplan M: In Tierney L, McPhee S, Papadakis M, editors: *Current medical diagnosis & treatment,* ed 37, Stamford, Conn, 1997, Appleton & Lange.

Schwartz R: The diagnosis and management of sinusitis, *Nurse Pract* 19(12):58-63, 1994.

Uphold C, Graham M: *Clinical guidelines in family practice,* Gainesville, Fla, 1994, Barmarrae Books.

Wilder B: Management of sinusitis, *J Am Acad Nurse Pract* 8(11):525-529, 1996.

Skin Cancer and Other Sun-related Conditions

ICD-9-CM

Skin Abnormalities 757.9
Solar Radiation 990
Melanoma 172.8
Squamous Cell Carcinoma M8070/3
Seborrheic Keratosis 70219
Actinic Keratosis 370.24
Basal Cell Carcinoma M8090/3

OVERVIEW

Definition and Incidence

Benign or Premalignant Lesions

Seborrheic keratosis is a proliferation of immature keratinocytes and melanocytes. It affects mainly males 30 years and older. They are beige, brown or black plaques with a velvety or warty surface.

Actinic keratosis is damage to keratinocytes by sunlight, ultraviolet energy. It is common in fair-skinned persons during middle to old age. It affects the dorsum of the hands, forehead, scalp, nose, and ears. Rough, adherent crusts form on an erythematous base. 1:1000 lesions progress to become squamous cell carcinoma.

Nevi are hyperplasia and proliferation of melanocytes located in the epidermis, dermis, and occasionally subcutaneous tissue. They are more common in whites with a family history of nevi. They may be present from birth.

Cancerous Lesions

Half of all new cancers are skin cancers. Both basal cell and squamous cell carcinoma have a better than 95% cure rate if detected and treated early. Melanoma is more common than any nonskin cancer among people between 25 and 29 years old.

The three most common cancerous lesions are reviewed in Table 167-1.

Protective Factors Against

Dark skin
Youth

Factors That Increase Susceptibility to All Sun-related Lesions

Working outdoors
Frequent sun exposure without sunscreen
History of sunburn

Factors That Increase Susceptibility to Skin Cancer

Smoking
Immunosuppression
Industrial carcinogen exposure
Intense, intermittent sun exposure
Light hair and blue eyes
Inability to tan

SUBJECTIVE DATA

History of Present Illness

Ask about duration of lesions. Lesions present since birth are usually nonmalignant.

Noncancerous Lesions

Seborrheic keratosis: Complains of "stuck on" brown spots over trunk, may bleed when irritated by clothing or picking

Actinic keratosis: May seek treatment because there are multiple lesions and they are cosmetically unpleasing

Nevi: Usually seeks treatment because of increasing number of nevi or change in appearance of a nevus

Cancerous Lesions

Basal cell carcinoma: Reports that lesion got red, peels, or bleeds, then improves, only to repeat the cycle again.

Squamous cell carcinoma: May complain of firm, hard nodule

Melanoma: Usually reports change in color, size, or border of a preexisting lesion

Table 167-1 Comparison of Cancerous Skin Lesions

Type	Objective Data
Basal Cell Carcinoma	
Nodule-ulcerative	Small, firm, waxy papule often with telangiectasis, may ulcereate
Superficial	Erythematous, sharply circumscribed, scaly macule or thin plaque
Morpheaform	Scarlike lesion, whitish/yellow, smooth and shiny
Pigmented	Blue, brown, or black, waxy papule
Squamous Cell Carcinoma	
Common	Firm to hard, erthematous, scaly, or ulcerated nodule
Bowen's disease/in situ	Erythematous, sharply circumscribed, scaly macule or thin plaque
Melanoma	
Superficial, spreading	Usually brown but can be brown, black, blue, red, or white or any combination of these colors; flat papule, plaque, or macule, usually greater than 6 mm in diameter
Nodular	Symmetric, uniform papule or nodule in the colors noted immediately above
Lentigo maligna	Tan or brown with focal surface elevation usually on sun-exposed surface
Acral lentiginous	May be pigmented band in the nail fold (Hutchinson's sign) tan or brown macule similar to lentigo maligna

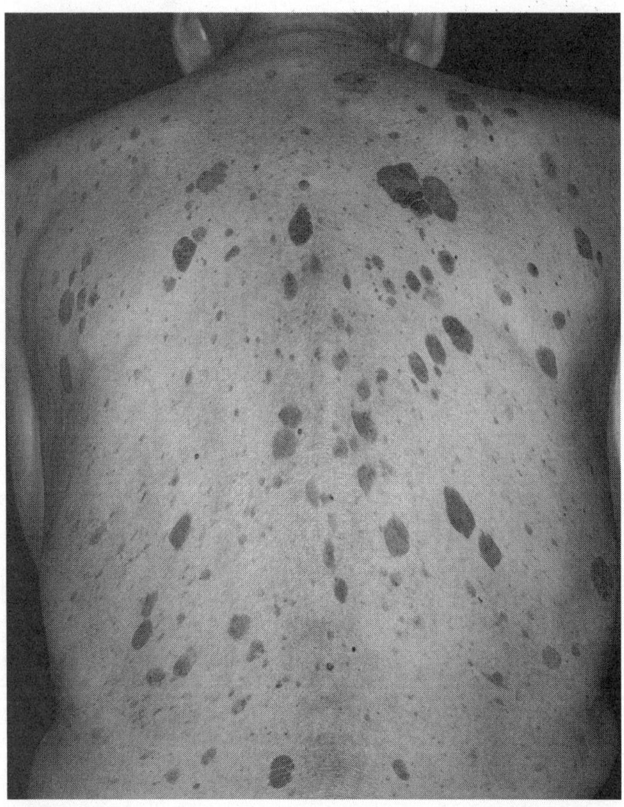

Figure 167-1 Seborrheic keratosis. Lesions are very common on the back; an individual may have numerous lesions on the sun-exposed back and none on the buttocks. (From Habif TP: *Clinical dermatology: a color guide to diagnosis and therapy,* ed 3, St Louis, 1996, Mosby.)

Past Medical History

Chronic illness or immunosuppression

Medications

Use of corticosteroids
Use of sunscreen

Family History

History of melanoma
FAMM: Familial atypical mole and melanoma syndrome (family history of melanoma in a first- or second-degree relative), multiple nevi (greater than 50), and atypical moles. These persons have a lifetime risk nearing 100% for the development of melanoma.

Psychosocial History

Recreational hobbies that involve the outdoors
Occupation with sun exposure

Associated Symptoms

Fatigue
Weight Loss

OBJECTIVE DATA

Physical Examination

Have patient undress and inspect entire body for lesions.

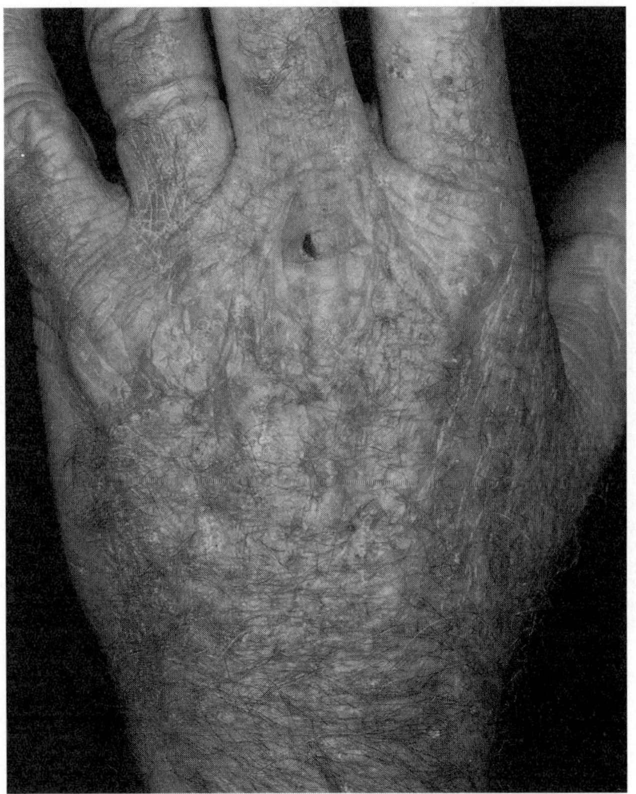

Figure 167-2 Actinic keratosis. Several oval-to-round, red, indurated lesions with adherent scale. (From Habif TP: *Clinical dermatology: a color guide to diagnosis and therapy,* ed 3, St Louis, 1996, Mosby.)

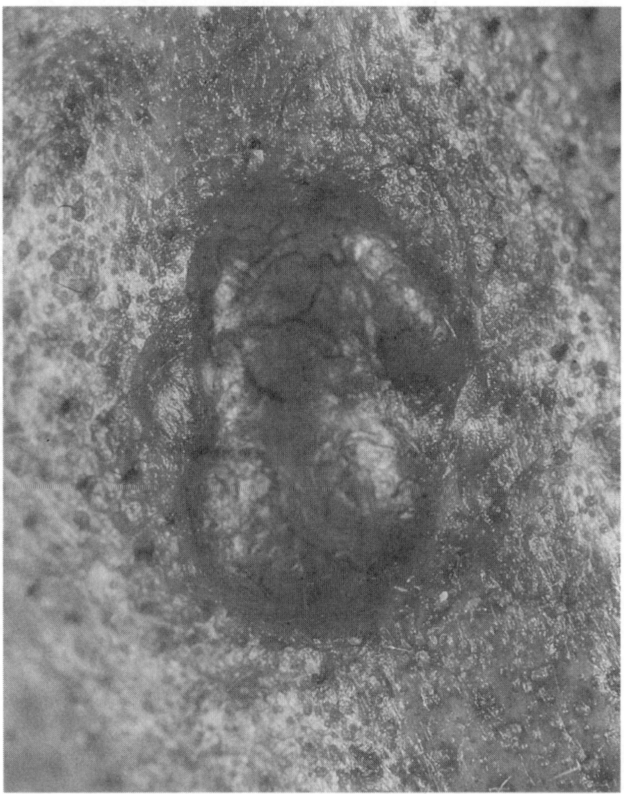

Figure 167-3 Basal cell carcinoma. Classic presentation. A pink pearly white papule with prominent telangiectatic vessels. (From Habif TP: *Clinical dermatology: a color guide to diagnosis and therapy,* ed 3, St Louis, 1996, Mosby.)

Noncancerous Lesions

Seborrheic keratosis: Size varies from 1 to 3 cm; may be skin colored, tan, brown, or black; usually oval shaped with a warty, greasy feel; distributed on face, neck, scalp, back, and upper chest (Figure 167-1).

Actinic keratosis: Multiple, flat or slightly elevated brownish or tan scaly lesions with "stuck-on" appearance; may be up to 1.5 cm; feel like sandpaper (Figure 167-2).

Nevi: Usually flat and symmetrical; brown or black in color.

Cancerous Lesions

Basal cell carcinoma: Can be nodular, ulcerative, pigmented, or superficial; usually whitish, brown, or black with will ill-defined borders; seen on face and other exposed areas; very slow growing (Figure 167-3).

Squamous cell carcinoma: Isolated, keratotic, eroded, ulcerated lesion (papule, plaque, or nodule); rapidly growing with a central ulcer and an indurated, raised border on a red base (Figure 167-4).

Melanoma: A pigmented lesion (usually brown, tan, blue, red, black, or white), that is asymmetrical with irregular borders; frequently greater than 6 mm (Figure 167-5). There are many forms of melanoma. One form in persons of African-descent results in Hutchinson's sign, which is

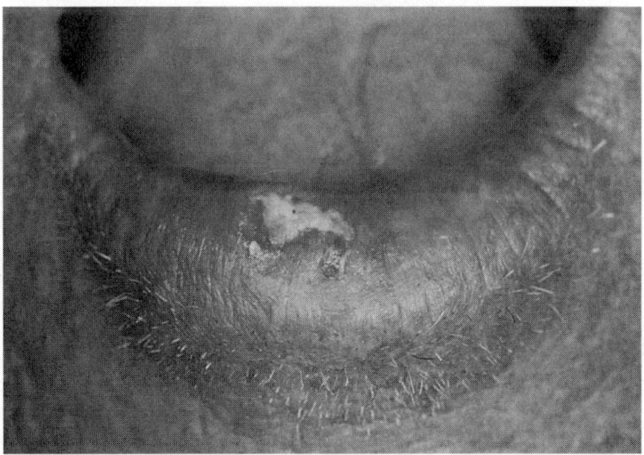

Figure 167-4 Squamous cell carcinoma. The sun-exposed lower lip is a common site. Palpation reveals a deep nodular mass. (From Habif TP: *Clinical dermatology: a color guide to diagnosis and therapy,* ed 3, St Louis, 1996, Mosby.)

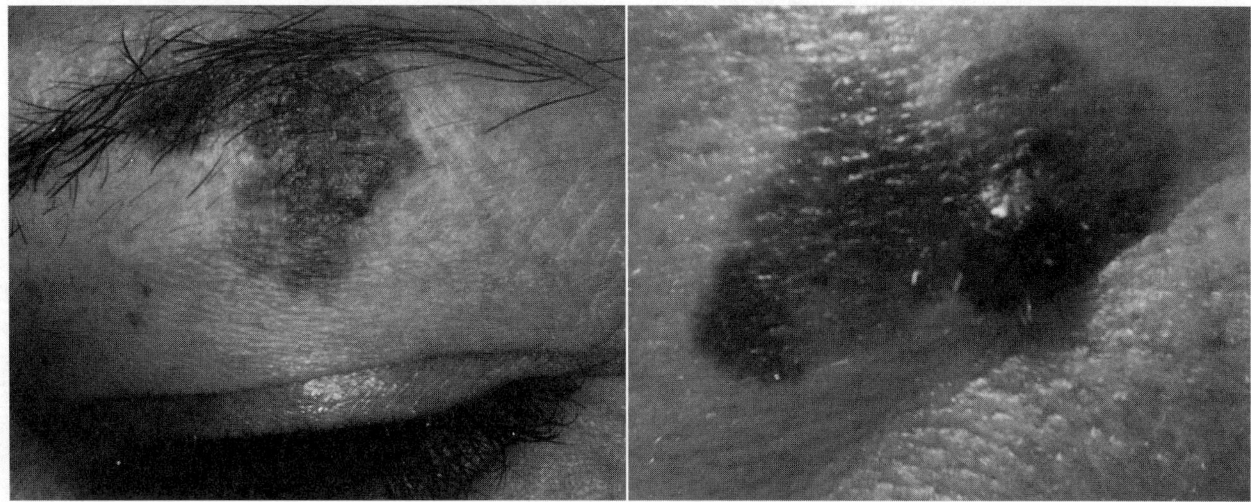

Figure 167-5 Lentigo maligna-melanoma. The lesions grow slowly and regress for several years, forming highly irregular borders. The color remains brown or black until the tumor stage is reached. (From Habif TP: *Clinical dermatology: a color guide to diagnosis and therapy,* ed 3, St Louis, 1996, Mosby.)

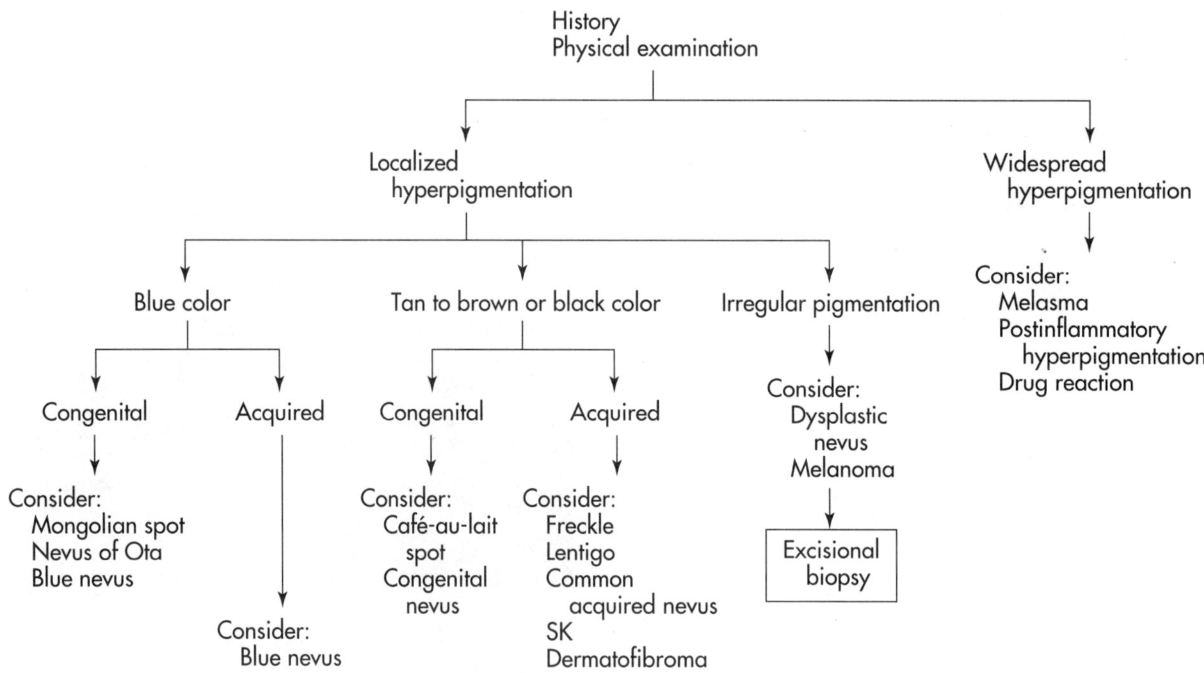

Figure 167-6 Algorithm for patient with pigmented lesions. *SK,* Seborrheic keratosis. (Adapted from Greene HL, Johnson WP, Lemcke D: *Decision making in medicine,* ed 2, St. Louis, 1998, Mosby.)

pigment extending onto nail fold with subungal pigmented lesion. It highly predictive of melanoma.

Use the ABCD approach to inspection:

A = Asymmetry
B = Border irregular
C = Color varies (usually brown, tan, blue, red, black, or white)
D = Diameter larger than 6 mm (pencil eraser)

TABLE 167-2 Differential Diagnosis: Warts

Diagnosis	Supporting Data
Wart	Most common in **children** and **young adults;** lesions disrupt normal skin lines and have a pinpoint black dot; they appear most commonly at sites of irritation; usually skin colored or pink and 1 mm in size

Diagnostic Procedure

Skin biopsy (usually performed by dermatologist)

ASSESSMENT

Differential diagnoses are all presented in this chapter except for warts (Table 167-2). See preceding paragraphs for discriminating information.

Figure 167-6 presents a decision tree for diagnosing pigmented lesions.

THERAPEUTIC PLAN

Pharmaceutical

None

Surgical

Removal of noncancerous lesions with electrocautery or liquid nitrogen; refer all patients with cancerous lesions for removal

TABLE 167-3 Sun-blocking Agents

Brand Name	Active Ingredient	SPF
Bain de Soleil	7% octyldimethyl PABA, 2.5% oxybenzone, 0.5% dioxybenzone	15
Cancer Garde-33	8% octyl-*p*-dimethylaminobenzoate, 7.5% octyl-*p*-methoxycinnamate, 5% titanium dioxide, 3% oxybenzone	33
Durascreen 15	Methoxycinnamate, salicylate, oxybenzone	15
Durascreen 30	Methoxycinnamate, salicylate, oxybenzone, titanium dioxide	30
PreSun-15	Octylmethoxycinnamate, oxybenzone, octylsalicylate	15
PreSun-29	Octylmethoxycinnamate, oxybenzone, octylsalicylate	29
Shade UVAGUARD	3% parsol 1789 (avobenzone), 7.5% octylmethoxycinnamate, 3% oxybenzone	15
Solbar PF 15 cream	Oxybenzone USP, octylmethoxycinnamate	15
Solbar PF 15 liquid	Oxybenzone USP, octylmethoxycinnamate, alcohol 40	15
Solbar PF 50	Oxybenzone USP, octylmethoxycinnamate, octrocrylene	50
Sundown-15	7% octyldimethyl PABA, 5% octylsalicylate, 4% oxybenzone	15
Sundown-24	Octyldimethyl PABA, oxybenzone	24
Sundown-30	Octylmethoxycinnamate, octylsalicylate, oxybenzone, titanium dioxide	30
Tis screen-15	3% 2-hydroxy-4-methoxybenzophenone	15
Total Eclipse-15	2.5% glyceryl PABA, 2.5% octyldimethyl PABA, 2.5% oxybenzone	15
Physical Sunscreens		
(Absorb all wavelengths of light)		
A-Fil	Titanium dioxide, zinc oxide, talcum, kaolin, iron oxide, or red veterinary petrolatum	6
Clinique		6
Covermark		6
Reflecta		6
RV Paque		6

From Habif TP: *Clinical dermatology: a color guide to diagnosis and therapy,* ed 3, St Louis, Mosby, 1996.
SPF, Sun protection factor.
NOTE: PABA and its esters and preservatives in sunscreens may occasionally cause allergic contact photodermatitis and allergic contact dermatitis. Allergic patients should be given a product containing a different active ingredient.

Lifestyle/Activities

Decrease sun exposure.
Change wearing apparel. Cover body with cotton clothing.
No tanning.

Diet

Noncontributory

Patient Education

After removal of lesions, area may be hypopigmented.
Perform skin self examination every month and report changes to health care provider.
Use sun blocking agents with PABA (P-aminobenzoic acid). Table 167-3 lists available agents and their respective sun protection factors.
Wear hats.
Teach what to look for in skin lesions that indicates need to see health care provider.

- Change in color
- Change in size
- Change in shape
- Change in elevation
- Change in surface
- Change in surrounding skin
- Change in sensation (itching, tenderness, pain)
- Change in consistency (softening, friability)

Family Impact

None

Referral/Consultation

Consider referral to dermatologist for removal of lesions and for biopsy.

Follow-up

Actinic keratosis: Skin check by provider every 6 months since new lesions frequently occur.

EVALUATION

Fewer sunburns
Fewer occurring lesions

SUGGESTED READINGS

Berger T, Goldstein S, Odom R: Skin and appendages. In Tierney L, McPhee S, Papadakis M, editors: *Current medical diagnosis and treatment,* ed 36, Stamford, Conn, 1998, Appleton & Lange.

Boynton R, Dunn E, Stephens G: *Manual of ambulatory pediatrics,* ed 4, Philadelphia, 1998, JB Lippincott.

Fernstermacher K, Hudson B: *Practice guidelines for family nurse practitioners,* Philadelphia, 1997, WB Saunders.

Whitmore E: Common problems of the skin. In Barker L, Burton J, Zieve P, editors: *Principles of ambulatory medicine,* ed 4, Baltimore, 1995, Williams & Wilkins.

168 Sleep Disorders

ICD-9-CM

Sleep Disturbances, Unspecified 780.50
Insomnia with Sleep Apnea 780.51
Other Insomnia 780.52
Psychogenic Apnea 306.1
Cataplexy and Narcolepsy 347.0

OVERVIEW

Definition

Sleep disorders include a variety of disorders that interfere with the quality and quantity of sleep. Common sleep problems include insomnia (restless legs syndrome, periodic leg movements, chronobiologic disorders); hypersomnias (narcolepsy, sleep apnea); and parasomnias (sleepwalking, nightmares). The average **adult** needs from 6 to 9 hours of sleep a night.

Insomnia is defined as involuntary sleeplessness severe enough to interfere with daytime alertness and energy level. Insomnia is classified as primary (no apparent cause) or secondary (identifiable cause). It may also be classified as transient (only a few nights), short term (lasting up to 3 weeks) and long term (lasting >3 weeks).

Incidence

One of three Americans has difficulty sleeping over the course of a year, and more than 50 million people have some type of sleeping disorder. Approximately ½ of all **elderly** >65 experience insomnia. Insomnia is the most frequent sleep complaint. **Women** >40 are more likely to complain of difficulty sleeping.

Pathophysiology

The average **newborn** sleeps 18 hours a day, with a high proportion of rapid eye movement (REM) sleep. Circadian patterns do not develop for at least several weeks or months. Sleep continues to be polyphasic, with daytime naps, until the child is 5 or 6. Amount of sleep decreases with age; the quality and quantity of sleep drops sharply with puberty. The **elderly** tend to sleep less, usually an average of 6.5 hours. The sleep tends to be lighter, with more arousals and near disappearance of slow wave sleep. Sleep onset and final awakening come earlier. Severe insomnia also increases with age, and excessive daytime sleepiness is also increased. Sleep apnea and periodic leg movements occur frequently in the **elderly,** disturbing nighttime sleep.

The sleep-wake cycle is controlled by the circadian rhythm located in the hypothalamus. Two of the neurotransmitters associated with sleep are serotonin and gamma-aminobuturic acid (GABA).

A normal sleep cycle is a complex electrophysiologic process consisting of alternating periods of wakefulness, REMs, and non-REM sleep (Table 168-1). A sleep cycle consists of two different types of sleep: REM and non-REM (NREM) sleep. Growth hormone is secreted, and the immune system is more active during NREM sleep.

A healthy adult progresses through non-REM stages 45 to 60 minutes before beginning the first REM sleep stage, which is brief. As the night progresses, less time is spent in slow-wave sleep, and the REM cycles are longer in duration. Overall, REM sleep makes up 20% to 25% of sleep time. The non-REM/REM cycle usually lasts 90 to 110 minutes, so there are usually four complete cycles per night.

Factors That Increase Risk

Previous history of sleep disorders
Diagnosis of psychiatric disorder
- Anxiety
- Depression

Alcohol and drug use
Tobacco use
Pain and discomfort
Orthopnea
Nocturia
Gastroesophageal reflux disease (GERD)
Asthma
Fibromyalgia

Table 168-1 Characteristics of Stages of Sleep

Sleep Stage	Characteristics
Awake	Low-voltage, high-frequency wave forms
Stage I	Brief transition from wakefulness to sleep; slow roving eye movements, low-voltage mixed EEG activity, and moderately high EMG (stage I tends to increase in **elderly**); disappearance of alpha waves, establishment of theta waves
Stage II	Considered the onset of true sleep; low-voltage EEG interspersed with brief, high voltage discharges (K waves) and vertex waves that are interspersed with low to moderate amplitude discharges on background of theta waves
Stage III	Considered deep sleep; high amplitude background activity of delta and theta waves, K complexes, and sleep spindles; eye movements infrequent or totally absent; this stage tends to decrease in the **elderly**
Stage IV	Considered a deep sleep phase; high voltage delta waves; eye movements infrequent or totally absent; this stage tends to decrease in the **elderly**
Stage V	Considered REM sleep; dreams occur that patients might remember; heart rate, BP, and respirations are similar to a waking state; EEG appears as a low-voltage, fast frequency activity observed during wakefulness or in stage I sleep; resembles a sawtooth wave pattern of moderately high amplitude or a triangular-shaped waveform; absence of DTRs; EMG activity is markedly suppressed or absent

BP, Blood pressure; *DTR,* deep tendon reflex; *EEG,* electroencephalogram; *EMG,* electromyelogram; *REM,* rapid eye movement.

SUBJECTIVE DATA

History of Present Illness

Complaints of
- Difficulty falling asleep
- Awakening in the middle of the night
- Awakening early in the morning

Fatigue
Irritability
Decreased concentration
Ask about length of time the insomnia has occurred
How long does it take you to fall asleep once you go to bed?
Do you remain asleep all night?
How much sleep do you get?
How sleepy are you during the day?
Do you feel well rested in the morning?
What type of bedtime routine do you have?
Do you exercise before bedtime?

Past Medical History

Ask about:
- History of psychiatric disorders: Anxiety, depression
- Thyroid disorders
- Renal disorders
- GERD
- Orthopnea
- Nocturia
- Fibromyalgia
- Chronic obstructive pulmonary disease
- Arthritic disorders
- Neurological disorders: Parkinson's disease, past head trauma, cerebrovascular accident

Medications

Ask about the use of:

- Melatonin
- Caffeine
- Sleep aids
- Cold/allergy medications
- Prescription drugs that may cause insomnia:
  - AntiParkinson's: Amantadine, dephendydramine, pergolide
  - Cardiovascular: Beta blockers, calcium channel blocking agents
  - Conjugated estrogens
  - Nonsteroidal antiinflammatory drugs
  - Psychotropics: Alprazolam (Xanax), clozapine (Klonapin), fluoxetine (Prozac)
  - Muscle relaxants: Cyclobenzaprine (Flexeril)
  - Beta adrenergics: Aminophylline, theophylline, alupent
  - Diuretics: If they cause nocturia

Family History

Ask about family history:

- Sleep disorders
- Restless legs syndrome or periodic leg movements

Psychosocial History

Alcohol ingestion
Tobacco use
Substance abuse/dependence

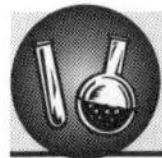

Table 168-2 Diagnostic Tests: Sleep Disorders

Diagnostic Test	Finding/Rationale	Cost ($)
Sleep diary	Keep a sleep diary for 2 weeks: document sleep onset and wake up times, rating sleep quality and daytime fatigue and sleepiness.	N/A
EEG	Identify the changes specific to psychiatric problems, as well as identification of the stages of sleep	283-345
EMG	Test that records the state of the muscle contraction when the muscle is stimulated	312-375
EOG	Helps correlate brain waves with eye movements	111-133
Polysomnographic recording (PSG)	All night sleep study: test that includes EEG, EOG, EMG of submental and anterior tibialis muscles, respiratory muscles, nasal airflow, ear oximetry and ECG; not helpful in most cases, save for refractory insomnia	879-1050
Sleep study	Record respiratory effort, HR, ECG, O_2 saturation	720-1080

ECG, Electrocardiogram; *EEG,* electroencephalogram; *EMG,* electromyelogram; *EOG,* electro-oculogram; *HR,* heart rate; *N/A,* not available; *PSG,* polysomnographic recording.

Recent stressors that may interfere with sleep
  Cold, noise, new baby, pain
Travel across time zones
Occupation: Shift work

OBJECTIVE DATA

Physical Examination

Rule out physical or organic causes of insomnia.

- Vital signs
- General appearance
- Head/eyes/ears/nose/throat: Nasal stuffiness, postnasal drip
- Lungs: Wheezing, shortness of breath
- Cardiovascular: Baseline assessment
- Abdominal: Assess for urinary tract infection: costovertebral angle tenderness, suprapubic tenderness

Diagnostic Procedures

Diagnostic procedures are outline in Table 168-2.

ASSESSMENT

Differential diagnosis include those found in Table 168-3. See also Figure 168-1.

THERAPEUTIC PLAN

The plan should identify specific short-term goals, such as:

- Shorter sleep latency
- Delayed morning wake-up
- Fewer nocturnal awakenings

In short-term insomnia:

- Short-term therapy
- Benzodiazepines should be used in conjunction with sleep-hygiene program

Pharmaceutical

Pharmaceutical treatment is outlined in Table 168-4.

Lifestyle/Activities

Sleep-hygiene measures:
- Maintain a regular wake/sleep schedule
- Regular bedtime routine: Bathing, story telling, rocking can facilitate a winding-down process
- Flexibility and compromise with teenagers: Adding naps, warning about driving while sleepy, avoid working late at night while in school
- Avoid caffeine, alcohol, and excessive time in bed while awake
- Use of a "white noise" machine may help to block out environmental noises.

For those with delayed sleep phase:
- Avoidance of late night activity
- Cognitive therapy

Chronobiologic treatment:
- Use of bright natural or artificial light carefully timed so the circadian rhythm is phase shifted to move sleep propensity to a later time. The patient needs to rise early to receive light therapy. Light fixtures and information is available from:
  The National Sleep Foundation
  122 South Robertson Blvd, third floor
  Los Angeles, CA 90048
  1-800-NSF-SLEEP

TABLE 168-3 Differential Diagnosis: Sleep Disorders

Diagnosis	Supporting Data
Anxiety (Ch. 13)	25% of people with chronic insomnia have an anxiety disorder. The patient complains of difficulty falling asleep and maintenance of sleep.
Depression (Ch. 52)	90% of all patients who have depression complain of insomnia. Electroencephalogram reflects a sleep disturbance.
Chronic insomnia	Diagnosis of exclusion; it may develop after a period of sleep disruption; sometimes it continues after the cause disappears. Long-term sedatives may cause chronic insomnia.
Restless legs syndrome (RLS)	An irresistible need to move, stretch, or rub the lower extremities. Creepy-crawly sensations are sometimes described. Periodic limb movements are also present, which can lead to further sleep disturbances. This syndrome affects approximately 5% of the population. It sometimes appears in females during pregnancy, but it can run in families and tends to worsen with age.
Periodic leg movements during sleep (PLMS)	These are repetitive myoclonic movements of the lower extremities that come in bursts lasting from a few seconds to minutes; they usually occur in the first ½ of the night. These movements are associated with brief arousals, leading to nonrestorative sleep and daytime sleepiness. The prevalence increases with age: 5% in those ages 30 to 50 and up to 44% in those over age 65. These are not the same as nocturnal leg cramps. They are best documented by polysomnography (PSG). A PLMS index of >5 muscle jerks an hour is considered positive.
Alcohol and drugs (Ch. 171)	Alcohol causes decreased alertness, but it also suppresses slow-wave sleep, making sleep lighter. Alcohol also tends to produce a rebound arousal effect in the second ½ of the night, thus producing less sleep overall. Amphetamines and cocaine also cause a decrease in sleep.
Medical disorders	Pain, rheumatic disorders, neuromuscular disease, cardiac disease, pulmonary disease, dyspepsia, inflammatory bowel disease, and nocturia are all causes of insomnia. Fibromyalgia is another disorder that inteferes with normal sleep patterns.
Neurodegenerative diseases	Alzheimer's and Parkinson's disease (PD) cause an interference with day-night differences. Akinesia in PD may cause physical discomfort, and the medication can cause arousal.
Snoring	Snoring may signify obstruction of the airway. Males > females, although more snoring is seen in postmenopausal females. Obesity, supine positions, alcohol, smoking, and possibly genetic factors may increase snoring.
Sleep apnea	Obstructive sleep apnea (OSA) is a major cause of cardiovascular morbidity and daytime sleepiness. OSA includes a wide range of upper airway narrowing. Two percent of women and 4% of men have OSA in midlife. Symptoms include loud snoring, getting worse with age and increased weight, snorting and gagging sounds, night sweats, abrupt awakenings with a feeling of choking, and profound sleep disruption (Singer and Sack, 1997). PSG confirms the diagnosis. Surgical uvuloplasty, tracheostomy, continuous positive airway pressure, and dental appliances are options for treatment.
Sleep terrors	These occur in **children,** usually ages 3 to 6, when they awaken with a scream, appear terrified, heart racing, sweating. They may last from a few minutes to 30 minutes. Attempts to comfort the child usually do not work, and finally the child goes back to a quiet sleep. In the morning the child does not remember the episode. Sleep terrors involve a partial arousal from stage IV (deep sleep).
Nightmares	True nightmares occur in rapid eye movement sleep. They are usually transient problems, usually triggered by personal events. Persistent nightmares may indicate a mental health problem and warrant referral to a mental health specialist.
Sleepwalking	Occurs during stage IV (deep sleep). Occasional sleep walking is common in **children** and may follow a personal stressor.

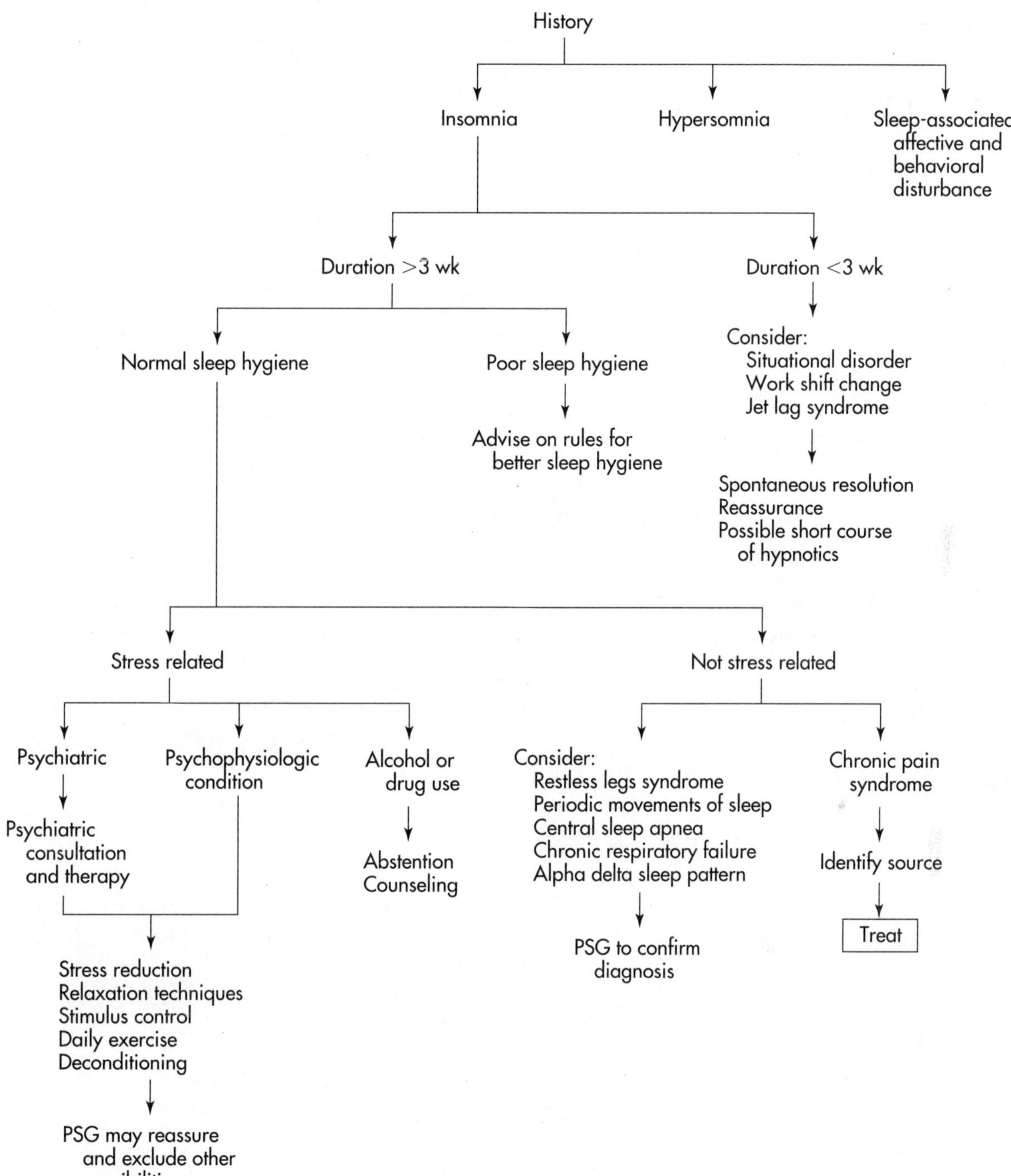

Figure 168-1 Algorithm for patient with sleep disturbance. *PSG,* Polysomnographic recording. (Adapted from Greene, HL, Johnson WP, Lemcke D: *Decision making in medicine,* ed 2, St Louis, 1998, Mosby.)

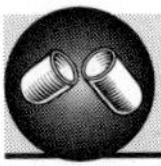

TABLE 168-4 Pharmaceutical Plan: Sleep Disorders

Drug	Dose	Comments	Cost
Benzodiazepines			
Temazepam (Restoril) Estazolam (Prosom)	7.5 mg-30 mg at HS; elderly 7.5 mg, max. treatment of 1 mo Initially 1 mg at HS; may increase to 2 mg at HS	Alter sleep structure: Reducing rapid eye movement and slow-wave sleep; generally safe for younger adults; use for short-term treatment of insomnia; patients with sleep apnea, severe respiratory problems, alcohol abuse should not be given these drugs Pregnancy: X SE: Abuse potential, central nervous system depression, somnolence, dizziness, confusion, anxiety, paradoxical excitement	\$47-\$462/7.5 mg (100); \$3-\$69/15 mg (100); \$4-\$77/30 mg (100)
Zolpidem (Ambien)	5-10 mg at HS	Short ½ life (1.4-3.8 hr); it preserves the normal sleep architecture; recommend getting into bed quickly due to swift onset Pregnancy: B SE: Dizziness, daytime fatigue, diarrhea, drugged feelings, amnesia	\$131/5 mg (100); \$160/10 mg (100)
Sedating Antidepressants			
Trazodone (Desyrel) Nefazodone (Serzone) Doxepin (Sinequan) Amitriptyline (Elavil)	50-150 mg q HS 200 mg in divided doses 75 mg at HS 50-100 mg at HS	Some think that these drugs are better choices for long-term treatment, although this has not been studied; less impairment of nighttime breathing and slow-wave sleep; special care in **elderly** Pregnancy: C SE: Nausea, insomnia, dizziness, constipation, blurred vision confusion	\$5-\$140/traz: 50 mg (100); \$12-\$242/100 mg (100); \$50/nefaz: 100-250 mg (100); \$10-\$96/dox: 75 mg (100); \$3-\$69/ami: 50 mg (100); \$4-\$91/100 mg (100)
Diphendydramine (Benadryl)	25-50mg q HS	Generally safe and effective for short-term use; tolerance develops quickly; CAUTION: anticholinergic effects Pregnancy: C	\$1-\$22/25 mg (100); \$2-\$29/50 mg (100)
Valerian root		Efficacy and safety not established	N/A
Melatonin	0.5 mg is a reasonable starting dose	Has sleep-promoting effects in many people; considered an experimental drug; greater than 0.5 mg produces plasma levels greater than would occur naturally; avoid "pineal extracts"; use synthetic melatonin; this may be helpful in cases of chronobiological disorders: jet lag; a person with delayed sleep phase may take melatonin early in the evening (8-9 PM), hours before endogenous melatonin is secreted, to reset the body clock to an earlier time	N/A

N/A, Not available; *SE,* side effects.

The Society for Bright Light and Biological Rhythms
10200 West 44th, Suite 304
Wheat Ridge, CO 80033
303-424-3697
Fax: 303-422-8894

Restless leg syndrome: As above plus: stretching before bedtime, opiods, L-dopa, and sedative-hypnotics may be helpful; there is a national support group for this disorder

Periodic leg movements during sleep: Benzodiazepines may be helpful in increasing the sleep continuity, but do not reduce the number of leg movements; opioids work well, but should be reserved for those with severe symptoms

Snoring: Losing weight, avoiding sedating medications or alcohol, using appliances to avoid sleeping on back (sew tennis ball to the back of the nightshirt); surgery may be considered an option; polysomnographic recording evaluation should be done before surgery

Sleep terrors: Reassurance of the parents; in persistent sleep terrors, medication may be justified

Sleepwalking: The concern here is accidental injury; protective measures should be taken (e.g., gates in front of stairwells, keep windows shut and locked)

Diet

Any foods/drink that seem to intensify insomnia or interfere with sleep should be avoided.

Sugary snacks and heavy meals late in the evening may stimulate metabolism, making it difficult to fall asleep or sleep restfully.

Patient Education

Caution patient about drinking alcohol with benzodiazepines: mixing them can cause death.

Cognitive therapy involves techniques to reduce anxiety and initiate behavioral changes to improve sleep hygiene. Examples include:

- Talking about the frustration of not falling asleep: Bed restriction (out of bed if awake for more than 30 minutes); no reading, eating, TV in bed
- Education about sleep and daytime napping (ok if midday and <1 hr): no caffeine, alcohol, or nicotine late in the day
- Reframe concept of poor sleep in a positive manner: Bright light exposure (especially in morning) and exercise in the afternoon (Singer and Sack, 1997)
- Biofeedback, muscle relaxation techniques, breathing exercises may be helpful as an adjunct to treatment

Referral

Any patient with refractory insomnia should be referred to a sleep disorder center. The American Sleep Disorders Association can supply the name of sleep disorder centers: 507-287-6008; the National Sleep Foundation can supply the name of sleep disorder centers: 1-800-NSF-SLEEP.

Consultation

Consultation may be appropriate before ordering expensive sleep tests or to order controlled substances.

Follow-up

Reevaluate patients who have been taking benzodiazepines for 2 to 3 weeks.

Reevaluate patient if insomnia continues for more than 3 weeks.

EVALUATION

Identify the relapse of insomnia.

Encourage lifestyle changes (e.g., exercise) as an adjunct to treatment

Identification of underlying depression or anxiety

RESOURCES

American Sleep Apnea Association
2025 Pennsylvania Ave. NW, Suite 905
Washington, DC. 20006
202-293-3650

Better Sleep Council
333 Commerce St.
Alexandria, VA, 22314
703-683-8371

Narcolepsy Network
PO Box 42460
Cincinnati, OH 45242
513-891-9936

National Foundation for Sleep and Related Disorders in Children
4200 W. Peterson Suite 109
Chicago, IL, 60646
708-353-4572

The Restless Legs Foundation (RLS) Foundation
1904 Banbury Rd.
Raleigh, NC 27609

Sleep Disorders Dental Society
11676 Perry Highway Building #1, Suite 1204
Wexford, PA 15090
412-935-0836

Sleep/Wake Disorders Canada
3089 Bathhurst Street, Suite 304
Toronto, Ontario, M6A 2A4 Canada
416-787-5374

National Sleep Foundation
1-800-NSF-SLEEP

REFERENCE

Singer C, Sack R: Sleep disorders. In Feldman M, Christensen J, editors: *Behavioral medicine in primary care,* Stamford, Conn, 1997, Appleton-Lange.

SUGGESTED READINGS

Bamford C: Sleep disturbance. In Greene H, Johnson W, Maricic M, editors: *Decision making in medicine*, St. Louis, 1993, Mosby.

Becker P, Jamimon A: Common sleep disorders in the elderly; diagnosis and treatment, *Geriatrics* 47(3):41-52, 1992.

Cupp M: Melatonin, *Am Family Physician* 56(5):1421-1425, 1997.

Ellsworth A et al: *Mosby's 1998 medical drug reference*, St. Louis, 1998, Mosby.

Healthcare Consultants of America, Inc: *1998 physicians fee and coding guide*. Augusta, Ga, 1998, Healthcare Consultants of America, Inc.

Insomnia: what to do when you can't get a good nights sleep, *Mayo Clin Health Let* 16(4):1-3, 1998.

Mosier W, Nelson S, Walgren K: Wanted: a good night's sleep, *Adv Nurse Pract* 6(5):30-35, 1998.

Phillips B, Amstead M, Gottlieb D: Monitoring sleep and breathing: Part I, monitoring breathing, *Clin Chest Med* 19(1):203-212, 1998.

Riedel B, Lichstein K: Objective sleep measures and subjective sleep satisfaction: how do older adults with insomnia define a good night's sleep? *Psychol Aging* 13(1):159-163, 1998.

Sack R, Lewy A, Hughes R: Use of melatonin for sleep and circadian rhythm disorders, *Ann Med* 30(1):115-121, 1998.

Sahelian R: Use of melatonin for insomnia, *Am Family Physician* 57(8):1783, 1998.

Wilson K, Watson S, Currie S: Daily diary and ambulatory activity monitoring of sleep in patients with insomnia associated with chronic musculoskeletal pain, *Pain* 75(1):75-84, 1998.

Stomatitis

ICD-9-CM

Stomatitis 528.0
Aphthous 528.2
Herpetic 054.2

OVERVIEW

Definition

Stomatitis is a general term for an ulcerative, inflammatory lesion or lesions of the oral mucosa. Gingivitis is an inflammatory infection of the gingiva or gum. *Gingivostomatitis* is an inflammatory infection of both the gingiva and any other part of the oral mucosa.

Incidence

Aphthous stomatitis is very common and is familial, affecting **women** slightly more than men, with a peak onset of 10 to 19 years.

Acute herpetic gingivostomatitis is extremely prevalent, commonly occurring in **children** 1 to 5 years of age.

Herpangina mainly affects **children** under 6 years of age.

Hand-foot-mouth disease is seen more commonly in **children** under 6 years of age.

Pathophysiology

The cause of aphthous stomatitis is unknown.

Suggested etiologies of the many forms of gingivostomatitis include hereditary factors, immunopathologic factors, food and drug allergies, stress and other psychologic factors, viral and bacterial causes, trauma, nutritional deficiencies, hormonal influences, side effects of medications, cancer, and systemic illness.

SUBJECTIVE DATA

History of Present Illness

Inquire about onset and duration of oral lesions and degree of pain.

Inquire about prodromal symptoms of burning or prickling.

Inquire about systemic symptoms of fever, malaise, headache.

Inquire about nutritional status and recent spicy or citrus foods.

Inquire about difficulty chewing or swallowing.

Inquire about smoking, pipes, chewing tobacco, trauma, dentures, braces.

Inquire about recent or current medication.

Inquire about last menstrual period if appropriate.

Past Medical History

Inquire about history of mouth sores and outcome.

Inquire about past or concurrent medical problems.

Inquire about last dental care.

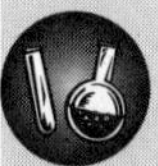

TABLE 169-1 Diagnostic Tests: Stomatitis

Diagnostic Test	Findings/ Rationale	Cost ($)
Complete blood count	Rule out anemias, neutropenias	13-16
Vitamin B_{12} Folate or iron levels	Suspected nutritional deficiencies	53-67/B_{12}; 49-62/folate; 23-28/iron
Culture (viral, fungal)	Confirm viral vs. fungal vs. idiopathic cause	27-34
Biopsy	Evaluate lesions with unusual clinical presentations; lesions unresponsive to treatment	Not available

TABLE 169-2 Differential Diagnosis: Stomatitis

Diagnosis	Etiology	Presentation	Treatment
Gingivitis (Ch. 51)	Bacterial plaque formation at the gingival margin	Swelling of the gingiva, possible bleeding; edges may become eroded; mouth odor	Dental gingival curettage, flossing, half-strength peroxide mouth rinse
Acute necrotizing ulcerative gingivitis (Vincent's infection, trench mouth)	Caused by spirochetes and fusiform bacilli	Painful, acute gingival swelling, necrosis, bleeding, halitosis, fever, cervical adenopathy	Dental gingival curettage, half-strength peroxide mouth rinse, oral penicillin
Acute herpetic gingivostomatitis	Caused by herpes simplex type 1; transmitted by close contact or oral secretions; incubation period is 3-4 days; occurs most commonly in children 1-5 years of age	Primary outbreak can present with high fever, malaise, refusal to eat or drink, drooling; vesicles are seen on the pharynx, tonsils, and soft palate, progressing to ulcers with yellow-gray membranes surrounded by a red halo; ulcers heal within 7-14 days; cervical adenopathy is common; recurrence is common and can present as a cold sore or fever blister at the lip margin	Acyclovir ($84-$98) may shorten the course of illness (not recommended in children under 2); only FDA-approved for immunocompromised patients; symptomatic treatment for the pain and fever
Angular stomatitis	Possible nutritional deficiency	Lesions appear at corner of mouth and range from erythema to crusted fissures; typically do not progress to ulcers	Treatment aimed at identifying and correcting nutritional deficiencies
Herpangina	Caused by coxsackie A virus	Mainly affects children; presents with small vesicular lesions on the pharynx, tonsils, and soft palate that ulcerate in 2-3 days; high fever, malaise, and sore throat are common; heals within 1 week	Symptomatic treatment
Hand-foot-mouth disease (Ch. 83)	Caused by coxsackie A virus	Presents with vesicular lesions on the buccal mucosa and palate but not the gingiva; concurrent maculopapular and vesicular rash of the hands and feet; fever, malaise, and adenopathy are common	Symptomatic treatment
Oral candidiasis (Ch. 51)	Caused by *Candida albicans*	Common in infancy; lesions are white, curdlike plaques on the buccal mucosa, tongue, gingiva, hard and soft palate	Nystatin ($3-$22) oral suspension PO QID × 14 days
Erythema multiforme	Caused by *Herpes simplex* and *Mycoplasma pneumoniae* infections and drug reactions	Common in children and adolescents; presents as erythematous macules with circumferential pallor; central portion develops epidermal necrosis, resulting in target lesions, which are symmetrically distributed, affecting the extensor surfaces of the extremities, palms, soles, and later the flexural surfaces, trunk, and ears	Treatment consists of removing offending agent if identifiable; symptomatic treatment of cool compresses, oral antihistamines, and antibiotics if secondary infection develops
Squamous cell carcinoma (Ch. 167) (accounts for 90% of oral cancers)	Alcohol and tobacco are contributing factors	Leukoplakia is any white lesions that cannot be removed from the mucosal surface by rubbing; erythroplakia is similar but has an erythematous component and accounts for 90% of dysplasias and carcinomas	Specialty referral is indicated for both diagnosis and treatment

OBJECTIVE DATA

Physical Examination

Assess vital signs including temperature.
Assess for lymphadenopathy of the head, neck, and clavicles.
Assess the mouth, noting number and description of lesions (papular, vesicular, or ulcerative), location (buccal mucosa, hard or soft palate, gingiva, and/or lip), and the presence of erythema and/or exudate.
Assess for inflammation of the gingiva.
Assess for mouth odor.
Assess ability to swallow and presence of drooling.

Diagnostic Procedures

Diagnosis is usually based on clinical presentation and are outlined in Table 169-1.

ASSESSMENT

Aphthous stomatitis (cold sore, canker sore) typically presents as a single, painful, 1- to 2-mm ulcerated lesion with yellow-gray exudate, surrounded by a red halo. It can present as multiple lesions. It is found on the labial and buccal mucosa. It rarely occurs on the hard palate or gingiva. The cause is unknown. Onset is most common between **ages 10-19 years.** It heals in 7-14 days. (See also Table 169-2.)

THERAPEUTIC PLAN

Pharmaceutical

Half-strength peroxide as a gargle
Liquid antacids as a gargle
Diphenhydramine Elixir ($2-$15) may also be used as a mouth rinse QID PRN pain
2% viscous lidocaine ($2-$16) 15-ml, swish and swallow or spit q3h PRN pain. **Children <3 years:** ¼ tsp applied directly to area q3h.
For severe cases consider topical triamcinolone 0.1% in orabase, applying a thin film to area TID after meals and at bedtime; **not recommended for children**
For recurrent cases of aphthous stomatitis use tetracycline 250 mg/10 ml ($9-$11) as a rinse for 2 minutes QID, then swallow, ×14 days; dexamethasone elixir ($8-$17) is prescribed concomitantly as a mouthwash for 2 minutes QID, then expectorated
Systemic prednisone can be used with extremely severe and recurring cases of aphthous stomatitis
Over-the-counter preparations can be used for relief of symptoms (e.g., viractin, oro-gel)
Vitamin, iron, and/or folic acid deficiencies should be treated with supplementation.

Patient Education

Educate patients about causes of stomatitis and treatment options
Usually resolves spontaneously

Diet

Includes smoking cessation, no chewing tobacco, and no spicy or salty foods
Cool, bland beverages such as milk or milk shakes are usually tolerated

Consultation/Referral

Usually not necessary.

EVALUATION/FOLLOW-UP

Severe cases should be reassessed in 48-72 hours, otherwise in 2-3 weeks.

SUGGESTED READINGS

Dershewitz RA: *Ambulatory pediatric care,* Philadelphia, 1988, JB Lippincott.
Doughty DB, Jackson DB: *Gastrointestinal disorders,* St Louis, 1993, Mosby.
Dunn SA: *Primary care consultant.* St Louis, 1998, Mosby.
Peterson MJ, Baughman RA: Recurrent aphthous stomatitis: primary care management, *Nurs Pract* 21(5):36-42, 1996.
Tierney LM, McPhee SJ, Papadakis MA: *Current medical diagnosis & treatment,* ed 35, Stamford, Conn, 1996, Appleton & Lange.
Uphold CR, Graham MV: *Clinical guidelines in family practice,* Gainesville, Fla, 1994, Barmarrae Books.
Ellsworth AJ et al: *Mosby's medical drug reference,* St Louis, 1998, Mosby.
Healthcare Consultants of America, Inc: 1998 physicians fee and coding guide, Augusta, Ga, 1998, Healthcare Consultants of America, Inc.

170 Strabismus

ICD-9-CM

Strabismus 378.9

OVERVIEW

Definition

Strabismus is the anatomic misalignment of the eyes that frequently is described as a "lazy eye" or a "squint." The eye may turn inward (esotropia), outward (exotropia), upward (hypertropia), or downward (hypotropia). Deviation of the eyes may be unilateral or bilateral, present all the time (tropia) or only when binocular vision is blocked as when one eye is covered (phoria), paralytic or nonparalytic. *Amblyopia* is defined as diminished vision in a structurally normal eye and can develop as a result of strabismus.

Incidence

Strabismus occurs in approximately 5% of **children.**

A family history of strabismus is common.

Strabismus is more common in **premature children** and **children** with developmental disabilities such as cerebral palsy.

Amblyopia develops in 30% to 50% of children with strabismus.

Pathophysiology

Binocular vision is the result of coordinated and simultaneous use of both eyes so that the images perceived by the brain are combined to appear as one single image.

Strabismus may interfere with the ability of the eyes to work together in unison as they focus on an object. As a result, the brain receives different messages. Deviation of an eye causes the focus of the image to occur outside of the macula of the retina, resulting in a blurred image. The brain attempts to correct this by focusing on the clearer image. The brain will then suppress the blurred image of the deviated eye and will rely more on the vision of the unaffected eye.

Amblyopia is a permanent loss of visual acuity. The concurrent loss of binocular vision also results in the loss of depth perception.

SUBJECTIVE DATA

History of Present Illness

Infants do not obtain coordinated eye muscle movement until about 3 to 5 months of age. **Infants** may have temporary deviation of the eyes, followed by subsequent realignment.

Any **infant** who has constant deviation of the eyes that persists for several weeks or who develops a constant deviation after 6 months of age should be evaluated for strabismus.

Inquire about a *family history* of eye problems, including strabismus, amblyopia, patching therapy, glasses, and eye muscle surgery.

Ask the parents if their child's eyes work together. Do the eyes appear crossed when focusing on an object up close or when the child is tired?

Ask the parent about a constant assumed head position such as tilting of the head.

Past Medical History

Strabismus may be associated with cerebral palsy, hydrocephalus, congenital cataracts, colobomas, retinoblastomas, and prematurity associated with intraventricular hemorrhage or regressed retinopathy.

OBJECTIVE DATA

Physical Examination (Table 170-1)

Ideally the infant or child should be awake and alert.

Observe for assumed head tilt.

TABLE 170-1 Screening Tests: Strabismus

Test	Findings
Red reflex	Absence of a red reflex may indicate a cataract, detached retina, or retinoblastoma
Pupillary reflex	Evaluates pupils for equality, roundness, accommodation, reaction to light
Hirschberg/corneal light reflex	The reflection of light in the eye should be symmetrical; asymmetry indicates a muscle imbalance
Cover/uncover test	Evaluate for abnormal deviation of the eye while one eye is covered, then uncovered
Snellen	Evaluate visual acuity for each eye and both eyes

Observe the eyes, including the eyelids, for size, symmetry, and general appearance.

Observe as to whether the infant or child will follow an object or the examiner's face.

Assess the red reflex for color, brightness, and symmetry. The room should be slightly darkened, and the ophthalmoscope should be set on +1 diopter.

Assess for pupillary reflex (infants >2 months). The pupils should constrict and remain constricted as a light is moved from one pupil to the other.

Assess the Hirschberg or corneal light reflex. The reflection of light from each cornea should be symmetrical and in the center of each pupil. In the presence of strabismus, the reflected light appears off center for the affected eye.

Assess for extraocular movements.

Assess an older infant or child by the cover/uncover test at a distance and at close range. One eye is covered by the examiner, who looks for movement in the contralateral eye. The covered eye is then uncovered, assessing for movement in that eye. Repeat the sequence on the other eye. The cover/uncover test differentiates phorias from tropias.

Assess for visual acuity of each eye and both eyes together.

ASSESSMENT

The diagnosis of *strabismus* is made by clinical inspection.

Nonparalytic strabismus is secondary to an imbalance in ocular tone. The deviation is constant in all directions of the gaze and is classified by the direction of the deviation.

Paralytic strabismus is secondary to weakness or paralysis of one or more of the ocular muscles. The deviation varies on the direction of the gaze.

Pseudostrabismus is defined as having the appearance of strabismus secondary to the presence of epicanthal folds and a wide, flat nasal bridge with more of the white of the eye being exposed temporally than nasally. Cover/uncover tests and corneal light reflexes are symmetrical.

THERAPEUTIC PLAN

Screening for strabismus and visual acuity should be a part of all routine examinations since strabismus may result in loss of visual acuity and depth perception, as well as psychological distress for the child.

Strabismus should be suspected on the basis of marked reduced visual in one eye.

Children with persistent head tilt may have strabismus with little apparent deviation of the eyes.

Treatment goals include the alignment of the eyes, the development of good visual acuity in each eye, and the preservation of binocular vision.

Surgery

Surgery may be considered to align the eyes. Children who attain proper alignment of the eyes by age 2 have the best chance of developing binocular vision.

Pharmaceutical

Ocutinune is a *medical alternative to surgery.* It works by preventing the release of acetylcholine from nerve terminals, which functionally paralyzes the muscle. This drug is meant to temporarily overcorrect the deviated eye. The hope is that, when the drug wears off in about 2 months, the eye will not revert to its original position. The success rate is approximately 50%. The most common side effect is drooping of the eyelid.

Patient Education

Infants <6 months of age may have temporary deviation, followed by realignment of the eyes, but it is important for parents to know that children older than 6 months will not outgrow strabismus.

Referral/Consultation

Refer to a *pediatric ophthalmologist* whenever a screening test indicates an abnormality or if the screening test is inconclusive.

Patch therapy consists of placing an occlusive patch over the unaffected eye to allow vision to develop in the affected eye.

Glasses may be prescribed to correct refractive errors.

EVALUATION/FOLLOW-UP

The child with pseudostrabismus <6 months of age should be reevaluated in 1 month. For an older child with pseudostrabismus, reevaluate for strabismus in 3 months.

SUGGESTED READINGS

Bates B: *A guide to physical examination.* (ed 5), Philadelphia, 1991, JB Lippincott.

Berman S: *Pediatric decision making,* St Louis, 1996, Mosby.

Castigilia PT: Strabismus, *J Pediatr Health Care,* St Louis, 1994, Mosby.

Graham MV, Uphold CR: *Clinical guidelines in child health.* Gainesville, Fla, 1994, Barmarrae Books.

Hay WW et al: *Current pediatric diagnosis treatment,* Norwalk, 1995, Appleton & Lange.

Substance Abuse

ICD-9-CM

Alcohol Addiction 648.6
Alcohol Dependence 291.8
Drug Dependence 292.0

OVERVIEW

Definition

Substance: Drug of abuse, a medication or toxin
Substance abuse: Recurrent use results in
  Failure to fulfill obligations
  Use in hazardous situations
  Legal problems
Substance dependence: Recurrent use over 12 months leads to three or more of the following:
  Tolerance: Need more of substance for same effect, or less effect with same amount
  Withdrawal: Symptoms typical for the substance when the substance is stopped
  Unsuccessful efforts to cut back in use
  Much time spent obtaining or recovering from effects of substance
  Continued use despite adverse physical or psychological effects
Meeting the definition of substance dependence supersedes the definition of substance abuse (American Psychiatric Association, 1994)

Incidence

8% to 20% of primary care patients (**adults** and **adolescents**) have problem drinking (abuse or dependence)
5:1 male/female ratio
Highest incidence ages **18 to 24 years** (17% to 24% of males, 4% to 10% of females) with decreased incidence for **older patients**
3% to 40% of **pregnant women** who are alcohol dependent give birth to infants with fetal alcohol syndrome (FAS)
In **adolescents** ages 12 to 17, 18% used alcohol in the past month, 35% in the past year
In the **elderly** with problem drinking, 70% have a chronic, long-standing problem, 30% with a late-onset problem
Alcohol abuse costs taxpayers $85.8 billion per year
Other drugs of abuse (besides alcohol) are more commonly used by teens and young adults, men, the unemployed, those living in urban areas, and those who have not completed high school; cost: $47 billion per year
Pregnant women: 5.5% used illicit drugs at least once during pregnancy, 1.1% used cocaine.

Pathophysiology

Addictive substances stimulate the neural reward pathway in the limbocortical region of the brain, which regulates basic emotions and behaviors. The substances stimulate the reward pathway and entice humans to sacrifice other pleasures or to endure pain to get substance. See Table 171-1 for effects and health consequences of drug abuse.

Factors Contributing to Substance Abuse

Positive family history
Genetics
Cultural attitudes
Availability of substances
Personal experience with the substance
Stress (APA, 1994)

Pregnant Women

Alcohol use
Cigarettes
Poverty
Poor nutrition
Inadequate prenatal care

TABLE 171-1 Effects and Health Consequences of Substance Abuse

Drug	Intoxicating effects	Health consequences
Alcohol	CNS depression, sedation Lack of coordination Altered mood Blood alcohol 150-200 mg/dl Legal driving level <100 mg/dl most states (some have changed limit to <80 mg/dl) 12-24 hours after use stops: weakness, sweating, hyperreflexia, GI symptoms, seizures, hallucinations, delirium tremens	Cirrhosis, peripheral neuropathy, dementia, cardiomyopathy, CHF, arrhythmia, pancreatitis, gastritis, thiamine deficiency **Women:** Adverse health effects develop sooner with less consumption than men **Pregnant women:** FAS with 7-14 drinks/wk; more risk early in pregnancy or with binge drinking; FAS: Fetal growth retardation, facial deformities, CNS dysfunction (microcephaly, mental retardation, behavior problems); any alcohol may cause risk **Adolescents and young adults:** Contributes to leading cause of death (MVA) and other problems (injuries, homicides, suicides, unsafe sex, legal problems) **Elderly:** Slowed metabolism: Elevated alcohol with less drinking; isolation, falls, malnutrition, dementia, self-neglect, suicide
Marijuana	Euphoria, increased taste perceptions, relaxation, drowsiness	Asthma, bronchitis, memory impairment, pharyngitis
Cocaine, amphetamine	Stimulates CNS: Euphoria, hyperactivity, alertness, grandiosity, anger, impaired judgment, altered pulse, blood pressure Other symptoms: Perspiration, chills, paranoia, seizures, chest pain, myocardial infarction, arrhythmia Acute withdrawal: Depression, suicidal ideation Withdrawal: Fatigue, unpleasant dreams, psychomotor retardation or agitation, increased appetite	Chronic use: Fatigue, social withdrawal, weight loss Snorting: Nasal mucosal irritation, perforated nasal septum Short-acting: Rapid dependence Dependence: Large amounts of money for repetitive use, prostitution; increased incidence of sexually transmitted diseases Amphetamine: Diaphoresis, flushing, hyperreflexia, insomnia, irritability, restlessness, tachycardia Chronic use: Confusion, depression, headache, paranoia
Opioids	CNS depressant: Drowsiness, decreased vital signs, dry mouth, constipation, euphoria, flushing, itchy skin	Tolerance within 2-3 days after prescribed use Withdrawal within 4-6 hours: CNS hyperactivity, anxiety, increased respirations, yawning, perspiration, lacrimation, rhinorrhea Dependence associated with high death rate from overdose, injuries, violence **Men:** Erectile dysfunction **Women:** Irregular menses **Pregnant women:** Withdrawal in newborn
Phencyclidine hydrochloride (PCP)	Ataxia, disinhibition, euphoria	Panic attacks, sweating, sensitivity to sensation
Hallucinogens	Altered visual perception	Hallucinations, flashbacks, panic attacks, psychosis IDU: Shared needles, hepatitis B, hepatitis C, hepatitis D, HIV, septicemia, bacterial endocarditis, localized cellulitis

Adapted from Schonberg S: *Substance abuse: a guide for health professionals*, Elk Grove Village, Ill, 1988, American Academy of Pediatrics/Pacific Institute for Research and Evaluation.; and Ash K, Schik M, Schwartz M: Helping the teenage drug user, *Patient Care* 23(20):614-627, 1989.
CHF, Congestive heart failure; *CNS,* central nervous system; *FAS,* fetal alcohol syndrome; *GI,* gastrointestinal; *HIV,* human immunodeficiency virus; *IDU,* injection drug use; *MVA,* motor vehicle accident.

SUBJECTIVE DATA

History of Present Illness

May need to confirm or get additional perspective for another family member if possible
Ask about quantity, frequency of use
Consider that patient might underreport (common)
May present with vague complaints
Frequently seen for gastrointestinal complaints
If patient admits to substance abuse/dependence, find out the following:
- Age substance use began
- Amount and pattern of use, including binges
- Method used to support habit (stealing, prostitution, employment, etc.)
- History of intravenous drug use or needle sharing
- Any treatment
- Length of substance-free periods and remissions
- Circumstance of remission (incarceration, inpatient unit)
- Legal history (DUI)
- Work history

Withdrawal symptoms:
- Alcohol: Morning shakes, seizures, hallucinations
- Opioids: Nausea, vomiting, diarrhea, abdominal pain/cramps, chills, runny nose and eyes, sweating, bone or muscle pain
- Cocaine: Depression, suicidal thoughts

Most Frequent Presenting Symptoms

Anxiety
Depression
Fatigue
Headache
Weight loss
Rhinorrhea
Dysphagia
Cough
Shortness of breath
Dysuria
Chest pain
Edema
Genital discharge
Rectal bleeding
Constipation
Rash
Paresthesia

Past Medical History

Ask about substance-related illnesses and hospitalizations related to:
- History of head injury
- Motor vehicle accident
- Other injuries/fractures
- Seizures
- Learning disorders
- Hypertension
- Cardiovascular disease
- Pneumonia
- Emphysema
- Pancreatitis
- Hepatitis (alcoholic or viral)
- Human immunodeficiency virus status
- Cirrhosis
- Cancer
- Sexual dysfunction
- Frequent sexually transmitted diseases
- Abuse: Physical, emotional, sexual

Psychiatric disorders: Depression, suicide, anxiety (alcohol, sedative/hypnotics, cocaine, opioids), bipolar disorder (alcohol, sedative/hypnotics, cocaine, opioids), paranoia (alcohol, cocaine, stimulants), hyperactivity/attention-deficit, hyperactivity disorder (alcohol, cocaine, stimulants), sleep disorders (alcohol, sedative/hypnotic, cocaine, stimulants, opioids), dementia (alcohol, sedative/hypnotics), amnesiac disorders (alcohol)
Gynecological history: Last menstrual period, birth control method, gravity, parity, abortions, ectopics, complications during pregnancy, source of prenatal care, history of drug use during pregnancy, health of newborns

Medications

Current medications
Psychotropics
Prescription drugs of abuse (opioids, benzodiazepines, barbiturates, stimulants)

Family History

Go back at least two generations and include current close relatives
Substance abuse/dependence
Effect of substance problem on family

Psychosocial History

Ask about (concentrate on losses related to substance abuse):

Losses: Jobs, property, relationships, children, self-respect, health
Marital history
Number and ages of children
Occupation (frequent absences from work)
Financial status
Legal problems
Adequacy of housing (consider homelessness)

TABLE 171-2 Substance Abuse Screening

Screening Test	Screening Questions	Findings
CAGE questionnaire (Ewing, 1984)	Ask first if the patient uses alcohol. If yes, ask: 1. Have you ever felt you ought to CUT down on drinking? 2. Have people ever ANNOYED you by criticizing your drinking? 3. Have you ever felt bad or GUILTY about your drinking? 4. Have you ever had a drink first thing in the morning to steady your nerves or get rid of a hangover (EYE OPENER)? Address other drug use after giving CAGE.	One "yes" response should raise suspicions of alcohol abuse. More than one "yes" response should be considered a strong indication that alcohol abuse exists. 100% specificity for those without alcohol abuse/dependence, 37% sensitivity of true cases (1 yes), 66% with 3 yes answers, 82% with 2 yes answers, and 90% with 1 yes answer.
Trauma scale	Since your 18th birthday: Have you had any fractures or dislocations? Have you ever been injured in a traffic accident? Have you injured your head? Have you been injured in an assault or fight? Have you been injured after drinking?	Two or more positive responses are the criteria for a positive test. 81% specificity for those who do not have a dependence/abuse problem; 68% sensitivity of true cases.
AUDIT (Alcohol Use Disorders Identification Test) (Saunders et al, 1993)	1. How often do you have a drink containing alcohol? Never (0) Monthly (1) 2-4 ×/mo (2) 2-3 ×/wk (3) >4 ×/wk (4) 2. How many drinks containing alcohol do you have on a typical day when you are drinking? 1 or 2 (0) 3 or 4 (1) 5 or 6 (2) 7 or 9 (3) >10 (4) 3. How often do you have 6 or more drinks at 1 time? Never (0) <1 mo (1) Monthly (2) Weekly (3) QD or almost QD (4) 4. How often during the last year have you found that you were not able to stop drinking once you had started? Never (0) <1 mo (1) Monthly (2) Weekly (3) QD or almost QD (4) 5. How often during the last year have you failed to do what was normally expected from you because of drinking? Never (0) <1 mo (1) Monthly (2) Weekly (3) QD or almost QD (4) 6. How often during the last year have you needed a first drink in the AM to get yourself going after a heavy drinking session? Never (0) <1 mo (1) Monthly (2) Weekly (3) QD or almost QD (4) 7. How often during the past year have you had a feeling of guilt or remorse after drinking? Never (0) <1 mo (1) Monthly (2) Weekly (3) QD or almost QD (4) 8. How often during the last year have you been unable to remember what happened the night before because you had been drinking? Never (0) <1 mo (1) Monthly (2) Weekly (3) QD or almost QD (4) 9. Have you or has someone else been injured as a result of your drinking? No (0) Yes, but not in last year (2) Yes, during last year (4) 10. Has a relative or friend, or health care professional been concerned about your drinking or suggested you cut down? No (0) Yes, but not in last year (2) Yes, during last year (4)	Questions are scored as indicated; total score 0-40. A score of ≥11 indicates a strong likelihood of hazardous or harmful alcohol consumption; most helpful for current alcohol problems, less so for past drinking problems.

Modified from Ewing J: Detecting alcoholism: the CAGE questionnaire, *JAMA* 252(14):1905-1907, 1984; National Institute on Alcohol Abuse and Alcoholism: Seventh Special Report to the US Congress on Alcohol and Health, Rockville, Md, 1990, US Department of Health and Human Services, USDHHS publication 90-1656; Saunders J et al: Development of the AUDIT, *Addiction* 88(6):791-804, 1993; Skinner H: The DAST, *Addict Behav* 7(4):363-371, 1982; and Clark W: The medical interview: focus on alcohol problems, *Hosp Pract* 20(11):59-65, 1985.

TABLE 171-2 Substance Abuse Screening—cont'd

Screening Test	Screening Questions	Findings
Drug Abuse Screening Test (DAST) (Skinner, 1982)	Have you ever used drugs other than those required for medical reasons? Have you abused prescription drugs? Do you abuse more than one drug at a time? Can you get through the week without using drugs? Are you always able to stop using drugs when you want to? Do you abuse drugs on a continuous basis? Do you try to limit your drug use to certain situations? Have you had "black outs" or "flashbacks" as a result of drug use? Do you ever feel bad about your drug use? Does your spouse (or parents) ever complain about your involvement with drugs? Do your friends or relatives know or suspect you abuse drugs? Has your drug use ever created problems between you and your partner? Has any family member ever sought help for problems related to your drug use? Have you ever lost friends because of your use of drugs? Have you ever neglected your family or missed work/school because of your use of drugs? Have you ever been in trouble at work/school because of drug use? Have you ever lost a job because of drug abuse? Have you ever gotten into fights when under the influence of drugs? Have you ever been arrested because of unusual behavior while under the influence of drugs? Have you ever been arrested for driving while under the influence of drugs? Have you engaged in illegal actions to obtain drugs? Have you ever been arrested for possession of illegal drugs? Have you ever experienced withdrawal symptoms as a result of heavy drug intake? Have you had any medical problems as a result of your drug use (memory loss, hepatitis, convulsions, bleeding?) Have you ever gone to anyone for help for a drug problem? Have you ever been in a hospital for medical problems related to your drug use? Have you ever been involved in a treatment program for drug use? Have you ever been treated as an outpatient for problems related to drug use?	Yes = 1; no = 0. A score of >5 requires further evaluation for substance abuse problems. 96% specificity for those without a substance abuse problem, 79% sensitivity.

Continued

Sexual preferences/practices
Cigarette smoking
Alcohol use: If a nondrinker, ask why, whether he or she ever drank in past, and when drinking stopped

Substance Abuse Screening

Screening tests for drugs and alcohol are found in Table 171-2. Special populations to screen are found in Table 171-3.

OBJECTIVE DATA

Physical Examination

Conduct a problem-oriented physical examination, guided by substance of abuse, symptoms, risk behaviors (Table 171-4).

Diagnostic Procedures

Diagnostic procedures are outlined in Table 171-5.

TABLE 171-2 Substance Abuse Screening—cont'd

Screening Test	Screening Questions	Findings
Follow-up questions to screening	Mnemonics: HALT BUMP Do you usually use drugs/drink to get HIGH? Do you sometimes drink or use drugs ALONE? Have you found yourself LOOKING forward to using substance? Have you noticed an increased TOLERANCE? Do you have memory lapses or BLACKOUTS that occur while drinking? Do you find yourself using/drinking in UNPLANNED ways? You use/drink when you feel anxious, stressed, or depressed for MEDICINAL REASONS? Do you work at PROTECTING your supply, having drugs or alcohol at all times?	Help determine preoccupation with substance abuse.
As above	Mnemonic FATAL DT Family history of alcohol or substance use problems? Alcoholics anonymous/other 12-step program attendance? Thoughts of having alcoholism or being drug dependent? Attempts or thoughts of suicide? Legal problems? Driving while intoxicated or using drugs? Tranquilizer or disulfiram (Antabuse) use?	Used to identify important information, including negative consequences that have resulted from substance abuse.

ASSESSMENT

Differential diagnoses are outlined in Table 171-6.

Categories of Use

Nonuser: Less than three drinks/month and use no illicit drugs
Light to moderate use: One to twelve drinks/week, fewer than four drinks/episode, and/or use other drugs once or twice a week in small quantities
Heavy users: Drink >12 drinks/week, four or more drinks three or more times a week, exhibit binge patterns of use, and or use illicit drugs more than two times/week
Problematic user: Problematic users have developed one or more alcohol- or drug-related problems, such as DUI, medical complications, family problems
Consider substance abuse/dependence when:
- Frequently missed appointments
- Frequent requests work excuses for missed work
- Report of lost prescriptions, or request for frequent refills
- Frequent Emergency Department visits for headache, stomach pain, tooth problems, fights, motor vehicle accidents
- Family history of substance use
- Social history of financial or marital problems, or loss of custody of children

THERAPEUTIC PLAN

The primary treatment approach is the use of brief intervention techniques that last approximately 5 to 10 minutes.

Discuss diagnosis with patient; discuss findings in a nonjudgmental, caring manner. State negative consequences of the patient's substance use; express concern that the patient may be developing a problem with drug/alcohol. Elicit the patient's reaction. When patient is ready to change his or her substance use behavior, a quit date can be negotiated, and a behavior contract developed. Follow-up calls to provide support have been found to be helpful. Referral to a person or program specific for substance abuse/dependence may be another option. Figure 171-1 identifies the initial management of a patient thought to have a substance problem.

Pharmaceutical

Pharmaceutical treatment for acute intoxication and withdrawal is found in Tables 171-7 and 171-8.
Consider inpatient detoxification if patient:
- Has a history of alcohol withdrawal seizures
- Does not have a stable home environment
- High potential for withdrawal problems:
  - Age >40 years
  - Male gender

Text continued on p. 1047

TABLE 171-3 Specific Populations to Screen

Population to Screen	Screening Questions	Findings
Pregnant women: All pregnant women should be screened for drugs and alcohol	Include questions of tolerance: How many drinks can you hold? Also ask about other substances/drugs	Tolerance: Three or more drinks to feel high or ability to drink 5 drinks at a time. Two or more drinks/day or binge drinking may result in fetal alcohol syndrome.
Adolescents: All adolescents should be screened for tobacco, alcohol, drug use	Ask about school, extracurricular activities, friends and nighttime activities, neighborhood, family life. Then screen for alcohol/drug use. Do you know anyone who smokes, drinks alcohol, or uses drugs? Does anyone in family smoke, drink, or use drugs? Do any of your friends smoke, drink, or use drugs? Have you ever used tobacco, alcohol, or drugs in past? Now? Ask directly about drug and alcohol use, specific substances, frequency, and duration of use. Ask if there is a problem and if he or she is interested in getting help.	If admits to substance abuse. determine the following: Tobacco dependence <17 y/o Poor grades (more than 2 Ds or Fs on two consecutive report cards) An experience of rape, incest, or physical abuse Frequent drunkenness in early adolescence Chronic deceptiveness, aggression, hostility, or resentment Staying away from home for ≥48 hours without parental permission Sexual promiscuity
Elderly	Alcohol is the most likely abused substance for elderly. 2%-10% of population. Screen patient with recent stresses in life and his or her ability to cope with stress. Then ask: Have you drunk any alcohol in past year? Have you used any drugs in past year? If yes: Use CHARM screen: Have you ever thought about CUTTING down? HOW: Do you have rules about drinking or drug use? Has your pattern of drinking/drugs changed recently? Has ANYONE expressed concern about your alcohol/drug use? What ROLE does alcohol/drugs play in your life? Have you ever used alcohol/drugs MORE than you intended? Have you ever had problems with your MEDICATIONS or taken more than prescribed?	

Adapted from Sumnicht G: *Sailing with horses: adventures with older substance abusers*, Madison, Wis, 1991, Prevention and Intervention Center for Alcohol and Other Drug Abuse.

TABLE 171-4 Physical Examination for Substance Abuse

System	Focus Area/Findings
General	Vital signs, temperature if infection suspected Hygiene, weight loss (stimulants, cocaine, opioids)
Mental status	Affect (full, flat, blunted, inappropriate, labile, restricted) alertness, orientation, mood (dysphoric, elevated, euthymic, restricted)
Skin	Lesions, scars, tracks, jaundice (alcohol, IV opioids), contusions and bruises (alcohol, sedative/hypnotic), petechiae, diaphoresis (sedative hypnotics), spider angiomas (alcohol, stimulants), burns, esp. on fingers (alcohol), needle marks (opioids), homemade tattoos (cocaine, IV opioids, increased vascularity of face (alcohol), piloerection (opioid withdrawal)
Head/eyes/ears/nose/throat	Eyes: Pupillary response (pinpoint: opioid intoxication, dilated: opioid withdrawal), accommodation EOM, nystagmus (vertical: PCP, lateral: alcohol, sedative/hypnotics), sclera (jaundice), funduscopy if blood pressure high Nose: Condition of mucosa and septum (perforated: cocaine), rhinorrhea (cocaine, opioids) Mouth and pharynx: Dentition (periodontal disease: alcohol), lesions, increased gag reflex (alcohol), excessive yawning (alcohol, opioid withdrawal) Neck: Thyroid size, asymmetry, mass, check carotid bruit (increased head/neck cancer with alcohol use)
Chest	Chest diameter, breath sounds, hoarseness (cocaine, opioids, nicotine), chest trauma (esp. rib fracture: alcohol, sedative/hypnotics), adventitious sounds: wheezing (nicotine, cocaine), gynecomastia (alcohol)
CV	Rate, rhythm, murmurs, rubs, gallops, arrhythmias (alcohol, cocaine, stimulants), hypertension (alcohol), cardiomyopathy (alcohol), subacute endocarditis (IV opioids, cocaine), thrombophlebitis (cocaine, opioids)
Abdomen	Bowel sounds, bruit, hepatosplenomegaly (alcohol), tenderness, esophagitis, gastritis, epigastric and right upper quadrant tenderness (alcohol)
Neuro	Tremors (alcohol, sedative hypnotics), sensation/symptoms of neuropathy (alcohol, sedatives/hypnotics), reflex sympathetic dystrophy (alcohol, sedative/hypnotics, opioids) coordination, gait, reflexes (hyperactive: alcohol, cocaine, opioids intoxication)
Genital/rectal	Examine if symptomatic, or if high-risk behavior Vaginitis (opioids, alcohol, cocaine)
GU	Penile scars or tracks (IV opioid), atrophic testes (alcohol)
Extremities	Check peripheral pulses, look for palmar erythema, compression syndromes ("Saturday night palsy"), peripheral edema, myopathies (alcohol)

Caulkner-Burnett I: Primary care screening for substance abuse, *Nurse Pract* 19(6):42-48, 1994.

CV, Cardiovascular; *EOM,* extraocular movements; *GU,* genitourinary; *IV,* intravenous; *PCP,* phencyclidine hydrochloride.

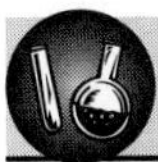

TABLE 171-5 Diagnostic Tests: Substance Abuse

Diagnostic Test	Finding/Rationale	Cost ($)
Gamma glutamyltransferase (GGT),* aspartate aminotransferase (AST),* alanine aminotransferase (ALT),* lactate dehydrogenase (LDH), alkaline phosphatase, total bilirubin, cholesterol, triglycerides, uric acid, mean corpuscular volume	Increased in chronic excessive alcohol intake Also sensitive: AST/ALT ratio >1 Other causes of elevated GGT: Drugs (anticonvulsants, tranquilizers) or metabolic diseases (diabetes mellitus, hyperlipidemia).	20-25/GGT; 17-23/ALT; 18-23/AST; 20-25/LDH; 19-24/alk phos; 23-30/total bili; 17-21/chol; 18-24/trigly; 18-24/uric; 18-24/MCV (as part of CBC)
Blood alcohol level	Provides level of intoxication. The following are indicators of abuse: 300 mg/100 ml at any time, 100 mg/100 ml during routine physical examination, 150 mg/100 ml without evidence of intoxication.	41-53
Complete blood count (CBC)	Screen for low hemoglobin/hematocrit from alcoholic gastritis and elevated MCV. Consider advanced disease with low white blood count and low platelets (bone marrow depression).	18-23
Human immunodeficiency virus screen (HIV) Hepatitis panel Rapid plasma reagin (RPR)	If high-risk behaviors.	108-151/hepatitis panel; 41-52/HIV; RPR 18-22
Thyroid-stimulating hormone (TSH), T4	Screening.	86-109/thyroid panel (with TSH); 56-70/TSH
Chest x-ray	Screen for adult smokers.	77-91
Toxicology tests	Excretion rates vary. Positive results occur for 1-4 days after use (several weeks for long-term marijuana use). Prevent false-positive with confirmatory tests on same sample (per routine lab procedure). Record list of current medications in case of cross reactivity. Consider direct observation of urine collection (prevent sample tampering). Newborn meconium toxicology confirms recent maternal use. Consider screening for those involved in serious motor vehicle accidents, a suicide attempt, unexplained seizure, violent outbursts of temper, antisocial acts, promiscuity, syncope, unexplained cardiac arrhythmia.	57-72

Adapted from American Medical Association: Scientific issues in testing, *JAMA* 257:3110-3114, 1987; and Ash K, Schiks M, Schwartz M: Helping the teenage drug user, *Patient Care* 23(20):614-627, 1989.
*Most sensitive.
MCV, Mean corpuscular volume.

Continued

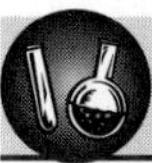

TABLE 171-5 Diagnostic Tests: Substance Abuse—cont'd

Diagnostic Test	Finding/Rationale	Cost ($)
Screening for Drugs of Abuse		
Color or spot tests	Easy to use, low cost, immediate results, but specific compounds difficult to identify. High concentration of drug required to achieve a color reaction.	Not available
Thin-layer chromatography (TLC)	High sensitivity rate, easy to use. Low specificity rate.	600-750
Enzyme-multiplied immunoassay (EMIT)	Can detect a number of drugs, rapid results, semi-quantitative. Cross reactivity with other drugs. Reagents expensive.	Not available
Fluorescent polarization immunoassay technique	Easy to use, high sensitivity rate, rapid results, quantitative.	Expensive
Radioimmunoassay (RIA)	Semiquantitative, but cross reactivity with other drugs, discrete testing only, special training and equipment required.	Not available
Confirmation Tests for Drugs of Abuse		
Gas chromatography (GC); GC/MS (mass spectrometry); high performance liquid chromatography (HPLC)	High sensitivity and specificity: GC, GC/MS Good sensitivity and high specificity: HPLC Special training and equipment required.	Not available

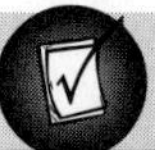

TABLE 171-6 Differential Diagnosis: Substance Abuse

Diagnosis	Supporting Data
Substance intoxication (specify substance)	Excessive use of substance, with expected symptoms of behavior/physical manifestations based on the substance used
Substance withdrawal (specify)	The development of a substance specific syndrome due to discontinuation or reduction in substance use that has been heavy and prolonged
Substance abuse	Maladaptive pattern of substance use leading to clinically significant impairment (during 12-month period); failure to fulfill major role obligations at work, school, home, recurrent use in situations in which it is physically hazardous (driving car); arrests for substance-related activities, continued use despite above problems; does not meet criteria for substance dependence
Substance dependence	Tolerance, withdrawal, inability to cut down on use of substance; great amount of time spent in procuring substance; decreased social, occupational, or recreational activities given up or reduced because of substance use; and substance use continued despite physical or psychological problems likely caused by the substance (during past 12 months)
With early remission:	Substance free >1 month <1 year
With full remission	Substance free >12 months; specify if in controlled environment

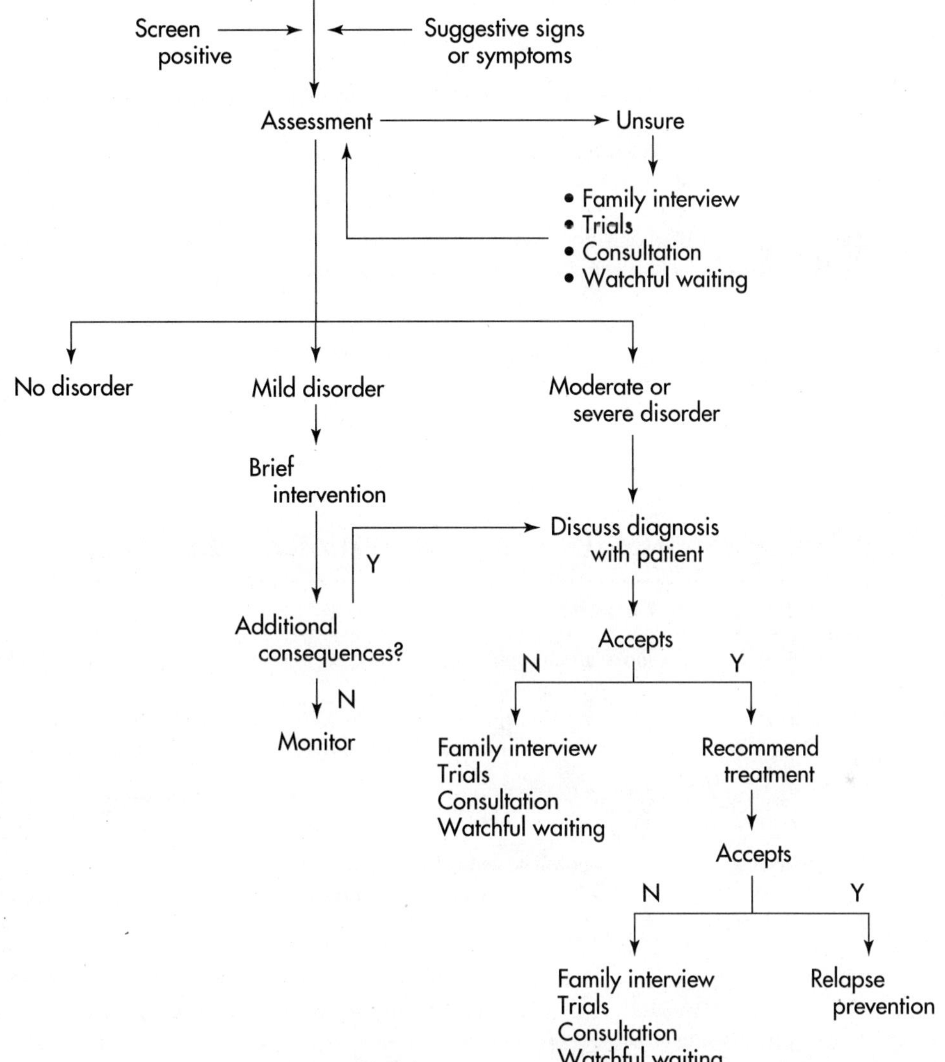

Figure 171-1 Specific approach to the initial management in patients thought to have an alcohol or drug problem based on classification of problematic use as mild moderate, or severe. Family interviews, cessation trials, consultation with other specialists, or watchful waiting can help clarify the diagnosis and ameliorate patient resistance. (From Fleming M, Barry K: *Addictive disorders*, St Louis, 1992, Mosby.)

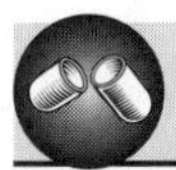

TABLE 171-7 Pharmaceutical Treatment: Acute Intoxication

Substance	Treatment
Alcohol and barbiturate intoxication	Supportive care is the rule
Benzodiazepine intoxication	The antagonist flumazenil (Mazicon, 0.1-0.2 mg/min IV up to 1 mg) can be used to reverse toxic effects
Opiate intoxication	If the patient is unconscious and respiration is depressed, the opiate antagonist naloxone (Narcan, 0.4-2 mg IV q 3 min) can be used to revive the patient. Narcan will cause physical withdrawal in dependent patients. If a total dose of 10 mg is given with a no response, a drug other than an opiate is involved.
Stimulant intoxication	Treated only if patient is overtly psychotic and agitated. Lorazepam (Ativan) 2-4 mg IM q30 min to 6h PRN agitation. Monitor cardiac function.
Hallucinogens, marijuana, inhalants	Reassurance or talk down therapy may be helpful. If not, use Lorazepam as described above.
Phencyclidine hydrochloride	Minimize sensory input; talk down therapy not recommended. More unpredictable; leave patient alone in dimly lit room. Lorazepam may be needed.

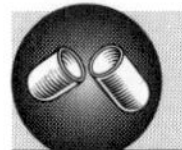

TABLE 171-8 Pharmaceutical Treatment: Withdrawal Protocols

Substance	Withdrawal Therapy
Alcohol	Detox: Chlordiazepoxide (Librium) 50 mg TID/QID or lorazepam 2 mg TID/QID; taper over 5-7 days Withdrawal: Hallucinations: Lorazepam 2 mg IM Seizures: Lorazepam 2 mg IM after seizure ends, use higher detox dosage and slower taper Supportive drugs: Thiamine 100 mg IM, then 100 mg PO QD, MVI QD, magnesium sulfate 1 g IM × 1-3 day Dependence: Disulfiram (Antabuse) used for sobriety; 250-500 mg PO QD; must abstain from alcohol for 12 hrs before using Naltrexone (ReVia) alcohol dependence; 25-50 mg PO QD
Benzodiazepines	Short to intermediate: Chlordiazepoxide 50 mg TID/QID or lorazepam 2 mg TID/QID, taper over 5-7 days Long acting: Chlordiazepoxide 50 mg TID/QID or lorazepam 2 mg TID/QID, taper over 10-14 days
Barbiturates	Pentobarbital tolerance test (administer 200 mg PO; after 1 hour, assess loss of consciousness and toxicity), initial detoxification at upper limit of tolerance; decrease dosage by 100 mg QD; (all patients who take 1 mg or more/day for more than 3 months develop varying degrees of physical dependence and are at risk for sedative withdrawal)
Opioids	Methadone 20-80 mg PO QD, taper by 5-10 mg QD or clonidine (Catapres) 2 μg/kg TID × 7 days, taper over additional 3 days Dependence: Naltrexone (ReVia) narcotic dependence; 25-50 mg QD; avoid if recent ingestion of opioids (past 7-10 days) (Pregnancy: C) SE: Weight loss, will precipitate withdrawal symptoms; cost: Not available Levomethadyl (LAAM, Orlaam) narcotic dependence; start 20-40 mg 3 ×/wk or QOD; do not give QD; Dispensed only in DEA, FDA or state-approved treatment programs (10 mg/ml)
Central nervous system stimulants	Supportive treatment only; bromocriptine 2.5 mg TID or higher may be helpful for severe craving associated with cocaine withdrawal

Box 171-1

Clinical Management Strategies for Prevention, Risk Reduction, and Early Interventions in Alcohol and Substance Abuse

Prevention Activities

Provide alcohol and substance use information routinely while providing medical care. Discuss alcohol and drug use and how it may relate to the condition being treated. Use opportunities such as school health physicals, sports physicals, or gynecological appointments to broach the subject of substance use.

Provide anticipatory guidance (e.g., counseling and discussion) before the occasions arise in which the patient must make decisions about alcohol and substance use. Especially applicable to young adolescents.

Develop office protocols concerning substance abuse.

Risk Reduction Activities

Identify patients at risk.

Initiate a risk reduction regimen and provide patient education.

Monitor patient's success in modifying high-risk practices.

Make a note in the agency or medical record about risk factors and efforts to reduce risk.

Early Intervention

Routine screening of all patients.

If positive screening results, arrange for evaluation and further work-up.

If patients report alcohol or substance use that is different from previously noted use, assess the implications.

If a problem exists, arrange for treatment.

Develop office policies on details such as prescription refills, lost prescriptions.

Follow-up Care to Prevent Recurrence

Be informed about and monitor compliance with aftercare plans.

Include the follow-up plan in medical record or agency chart.

Adopt a plan to respond to a relapse so that if one were to occur, important decisions do not need to be made during a crisis.

Modified from Kinney J: *Clinical manual of substance abuse*, ed 2, St Louis, 1996, Mosby.

Daily consumption of more than a fifth of liquor

Drinking around the clock to maintain a steady blood level

Excessive drinking >10 years

Development of tremulousness and anxiety within 6 to 8 hours of cessation

History of seizures, hallucinations, delusions with alcohol withdrawal

Box 171-2

Indicators for Inpatient vs. Outpatient Treatment

Indications for Inpatient Treatment Program

Prior unsuccessful outpatient treatment

Minimal social supports

Concomitant medical problems

Concomitant psychiatric illness

Ambivalence about need for treatment

Indications for Outpatient Treatment Program

Intact and supportive family

No previous formal treatment

No history of withdrawal difficulty

Insights into need for treatment

Absence of major medical problems

Presence of an acute medical problem such as pneumonia

Alcohol level >250 mg/dl

Lifestyle/Activities

Participation and commitment to treatment plan

Diet

Well-balanced diet is important to anyone who has nutritional deficits due to substance abuse/dependence.

Patient Education

Discuss with all patients the risks of driving while intoxicated with drugs or alcohol

All pregnant women should be encouraged to abstain from alcohol and drugs during pregnancy

Awareness of the need for repeated attempts to achieve goals

Have patient identify anxiety-provoking situations

Develop strategies for resisting temptations

Explain disease process

Discuss prevention strategies (Box 171-1)

Family Impact

Role of family members can be very important during substance abuse/dependence treatment. A sober and responsible family member or friend is an integral part of outpatient medical detoxification. Family and friends can encourage the patient to:

Table 171-9 Treatment by Specific Population

Population	Treatment
Pregnant women	Prenatal care, improved nutrition, child care, financial support, vocational services, educational services, and drug-free transitional housing for women and child are important features to consider
Adolescents	Parents need to be involved; consider outpatient, partial hospitalization, or residential treatment
Co-existing mental disorders	Patients may need crisis intervention, community case psychiatric stabilization, detoxification, assistance with housing, education, vocational rehabilitation, long-term residential treatment or relapse prevention

Treatment Resource Worksheet

1. AA information number: ______
2. Al-Anon information number: ______
3. Narcotics Anonymous information number: ______
4. Community mental health substance abuse services:
   Name ______ Phone ______
   Address ______ Hours ______
   Contact person ______
   Services available (circle) Counseling: Alcohol/other drugs
   Detoxification: Alcohol/other drugs
   Half-way house: Men/women
   Methadone program
   Adolescent program/family program
   Other ______
5. Fee-for-service treatment programs:
   Name ______ Phone ______
   Hours ______ Contact person ______
   Type of facility (circle) Residential/outpatient/evening
   Adolescent/adult
   Payment accepted: Insurance/sliding scale/indigent care
6. Individual therapist knowledgeable regarding substance abuse:
   Name ______ Phone ______
   Services (circle): Individual/families/interventions
   Name ______ Phone ______
   Services (circle): Individual/families/interventions
7. AA member contracts
   Name ______ Phone ______
   Name ______ Phone ______
   Name ______ Phone ______

Figure 171-2 The Treatment Resource Worksheet is a useful office guide when referring a patient to treatment. Completion of the worksheet may be facilitated by calling the local AA chapter and the community mental health center. (From Fleming M, Barry K: *Addictive disorders*, St Louis, 1992, Mosby.)

Attend Alcoholics Anonymous or Narcotics Anonymous meetings
Provide a safe, loving environment
Watch for serious withdrawal symptoms
Assist with medications
Drive the patient to appointments
Provide for massages and hot baths for muscle cramps and anxiety
Minimize the risk of relapse by keeping the patient away from situations that may lead to relapse
Dispose of drugs/alcohol in the home environment
Participate in a treatment program

Referral/Consultation

Federal law protects the confidentiality of persons receiving alcohol and drug abuse prevention and treatment services; a signed consent must be completed for release of information
Minors: Check state law regarding ability to treat without parental consent; exception: in medical emergencies, court orders, patient crime against staff or program, approved research, initial child abuse reports
Level of treatment: Match personality, background, mental condition, duration and extent of substance use and type of substance with level of treatment (Table 171-9)
Type of treatment: Inpatient vs. outpatient based on diagnosis (Box 171-2):
 Substance dependence: Formal inpatient or outpatient treatment is needed
 Substance abuse: Outpatient treatment may be appropriate
Those not meeting criteria for abuse or dependence: Intervention by primary care or community health staff. Formal treatment to achieve abstinence is not necessary.
Psychiatrist or addiction specialist for inpatient treatment care. For outpatient care, use of support groups, employee assistance programs, and individual or family counseling may be appropriate.

EVALUATION/FOLLOW-UP

Monitor the patient closely
If referred to an addiction specialist, be aware of progress and need to be consistent with interventions used
Do not refill prescriptions if lost or stolen
Convey a clear message regarding your feelings/policies concerning substance use. Development of an office policy regarding control substances is recommended. (See Sample Drug Control Policy, pp. 1051 to 1062.)

RESOURCES

The use of a treatment resource worksheet may be helpful with regard to options available to patients (Figure 171-2).
Alcoholics Anonymous (AA)
Cocaine Anonymous (CA)
Narcotics Anonymous (NA)
Al-Anon family groups
Alateen
Adult Children of Alcoholics
National Clearinghouse for Alcohol and Drug Information: 1-800-729-6686; www.health.org
Substance Abuse and Mental Health Services Administration (SAMHSA); www.samhsa.gov
Center for Substance abuse prevention (CSAP): 1-800-729-6686; www.samhsa.gov/csap/index.htm
Center for Substance abuse treatment: www.samhsa.gov/csat/index.htm
National Directory of Drug Abuse and Alcoholism Treatment and Prevention Programs: www.health.org/search/treatdir96.htm
Workplace Helpline (provides assistance for employers, unions, etc. in implementing substance abuse prevention programs): 1-800-967-5752

REFERENCES

American Psychiatric Association: Diagnostic and statistical manual of mental disorders, ed 4, Washington, DC, 1994, APA.

SUGGESTED READINGS

American Medical Association: Scientific issues in testing, *JAMA* 257:3110-3114, 1987.
Ash K, Schiks M, Schwartz M: Helping the teenage drug user, *Patient Care* 23(20):614-627, 1989.
Caulkner-Burnett I: Primary care screening for substance abuse, *Nurse Pract* 19(6):42-48, 1994.
Clark W: The medical interview: focus on alcohol problems, *Hosp Pract* 20(11):59-65, 1985.
Brown R: Identification and office management of alcohol and drug disorders. In Fleming M, Barry K, editors: *Addictive disorders*, St Louis, 1992, Mosby.
Chenitz W, Stone J, Salisbury S: *Clinical gerontological nursing: a guide to advanced practice*, Philadelphia, 1991, WB Saunders.
Ewing J: Detecting alcoholism: the CAGE questionnaire, *JAMA* 252(14): 1905-1907, 1984.
Fleming M, Barry K: *Addictive disorders*, St Louis, 1992, Mosby.
Grinspoon L: Treatment of drug abuse and addiction, part I, *Harv Med Let* 12(2), 1995.
Healthcare Consultants of America, Inc: *1998 physicians fee and coding guide*, Augusta, Ga, 1998, Healthcare Consultants of America, Inc.
Hoksema H, deBock M: The value of laboratory tests for the screening and recognition of alcohol abuse in primary care patients, *J Family Pract* 37(3):268-275, 1993.
National Institute on Alcohol Abuse and Alcoholism: *Seventh special report to the U.S. Congress on alcohol and health* (U.S. Department of Health and Human Services Publication No. ADM 90-1656), Rockville, Md, 1990, USDHHS.
Saunders J et al: Development of the AUDIT, *Addiction* 88(6):791-804, 1993.
Schonberg S: *Substance abuse: a guide for health professionals*, Elk Grove Village, Ill, 1988, American Academy of Pediatrics/Pacific Institute for Research and Evaluation.
Schulz J, Barry K: Alcohol and drug treatment and role of 12 step programs. In Fleming M, Barry K, editors: *Addictive disorders*, St Louis, 1992, Mosby.
Skinner H: The DAST, *Addict Behav* 7(4):363-371, 1982.
Stafford W: *Control drug policy*, Covington, Ky, 1997, Northern Kentucky Family Health Center.
Substance Abuse and Mental Health Services Administration: *Treatment for alcohol and other drug abuse: opportunities for coordination* (Technical Assistance Publication Series: 11 [DHHS Publication No SMA 94-2075]), Rockville, Md, 1994, U.S. Government Printing Office.
Sumnicht G: *Sailing with horses: adventures with older substance abusers*, Madison, Wis, 1991, Prevention and Intervention Center for Alcohol and Other Drug Abuse.

U.S. Department of Health and Human Services Public Health Service: *Clinician's handbook of preventive services: put prevention into practice*, Washington, DC, 1994, U.S. Government Printing Office.

U.S. Preventive Services Task Force: *Guide to clinical preventive services*, ed 2, Baltimore, 1996, Williams & Wilkins.

Warner A: *Drug testing-practices and pitfalls* (unpublished handout), Cincinnati, Ohio, 1996, University of Cincinnati Medical Center Division of Toxicology.

West D, Kinney J: An overview of substance use and abuse. In Kinney J, editor: *Clinical manual of substance abuse*, ed 2, St Louis, 1996, Mosby.

CONTROL DRUG POLICY SUMMARY FOR HEALTH PROVIDERS

Policy is voluntary with no sanctions for noncompliance.

We do not prescribe Xanax, Soma, Fiorinal with codeine, and Stadol Nasal Spray. See the full list on page 2 for others.

Treat acute pain for 1 to 5 days, but no refills for 60 days.

Benzodiazepine prescriptions for acute anxiety are OK for a maximum of two weeks with no refill before six months.

Patients already established on chronic benzodiazepine therapy must be tapered and prescription stopped.

If patients do not tolerate withdrawal or wish to stay on benzodiazepines, mental health consultation is required. There is a form letter you can use for this if you wish.

The taper and discontinue policy is stated in a contract for the patient to sign. It gives the patient three months to see the consultant and get a written report for their record.

If you want to continue to prescribe medications chronically for patients, have the chart sent to Adult Provider Committee for a group discussion and record of the outcome of that discussion.

There is a contract for chronic opioid therapy. It says: no phone refills, no replacement of lost rxs, bring in bottles of pills for review, and allows urine drug testing.

The opioid contract is very strict. Legitimate patients should be able to comply with no difficulty. If patients break the contract, no more prescriptions or dismiss from practice.

Document the outcome in the chart with an Alert Sheet.

Courtesy Northern Kentucky Family Health Centers, Inc., and William Stafford, MD.

NORTHERN KENTUCKY FAMILY HEALTH, INC.

Adult Provider's Policy on Use of Controlled Drugs
Effective Date 1/1/97

Employees/Staff Covered by This Policy:

Physicians and Nurse Practitioners who see adult patients

Supervisor(s):

Medical Director, physicians providing backup for Nurse Practitioners

Other Staff Affected by This Policy:

Executive Management Team, Executive Director, Nurses
Medical Records staff (for chart transport and return after review)

Purpose

To provide voluntary guidelines for NKFH health providers in the evaluation and treatment of patients that subjectively benefit from medications that have high potential for abuse or misuse.

To improve the efficiency of operations at the centers by clarifying telephone and appointment policy for patients using these medications.

To improve MD and NP job satisfaction by reducing the numbers of patients that utilize NKFH services and provider/patient relationships inappropriately.

To improve community health by increasing the identification of patients with drug or alcohol misuse/abuse/addiction, thus allowing appropriate treatment or referral.

Exclusions

This policy does not apply to the evaluation, care, and treatment of patients with pain due to cancer or terminal illness (i.e., end-stage COPD or AIDS), or to the use of controlled drugs in other pharmacotherapeutic classes, except those specifically named.

Background

It is the nature of Community Health Centers to often care for patients that circumstances and socioeconomic conditions place at risk for substance abuse. Additionally, patients often lack the family or social support, the personal skills, education, or resources to cope successfully with life stresses. However, those conditions are often denied by the patient and frequently unrecognized by their health care provider.

These preexisting conditions, along with health care provider's natural inclination to "want to help" creates an environment where patients may misuse certain medications and providers may prescribe them for inappropriate reasons. This may lead to stress in staff who feel manipulated, or overwhelmed by patient needs or even demands. Often the expedient solution is to treat with a prescription which the patient wants. Other providers may fear reprisal for overprescribing by regulatory agencies, thus undertreating patients.

Since the formation of the Adult Provider's Committee in 1995, this has been a primary topic of discussion and activity. This policy is the result of the committee's work to develop guidelines for the use of controlled drugs without compromising patient care.

Formal Statement of Policy (provider consensus position)

NKFH physicians agree not to prescribe or refill prescriptions of the following for any reason:

Equanil (meprobamate)
Stadol Nasal Spray (butorphanol)
Talwin (Pentazocine)
Artane (trihexphenidyl)

Dilaludid (hydromorphone)
Soma (Carisprodol)
Halcion (triazolam)
Fiorinal with Codeine (butalbital)
Xanax (alprazolam)

NKFH physicians agree that the narcotic or opioid pain medications listed are primarily prescribed for acute (new and recent) conditions. Refills for recurrent conditions (back pain, kidney stones, headaches) are not to be made more often than every 60 days for any reason.

Codeine (i.e., Tylenol #3)
Hydrocodone (i.e., Lorcet, Vicodin)
Methadone
Oxycodone (i.e., Percocet)
Propoxyphene (i.e., Darvon)
Morphine

While the following drugs are not technically narcotics, they are included in this policy.

Butalbital (i.e., Fioricet, Fiorinal)
Tramadol (i.e., Ultram)

NKFH physicians agree to treat chronic nonmalignant pain with narcotics only if a separate doctor's opinion is obtained and a specific medication contract is signed by the patient and provider. This opinion may be obtained via formal referral *or* by discussion of the case at a designated peer review session, so long as the review is documented in the patient's record.

NKFH physicians agree to prescribe the following medications for a maximum of two weeks in any six-month period. If more seems needed, a mental health referral is required, and the decision to continue medications will be determined by the consultant. For patients already established on these medications, the drug is to be slowly tapered and discontinued, which may require changing to one of the other drugs in this class to help reduce withdrawal symptoms. Patients who are unable to tolerate the withdrawal should be referred to a mental health consultant.

Valium (diazepam)
Dalmane (flurazepam)
Restoril (temazepam)
Halcion (triazolam)
Ativan (lorazepam)
Tranxene (clorazepate)
Librium (chlordiazepoxide)
Serax (oxazepam)
Klonopin (clonazepam)
Xanax (alprazolam)

NKFH providers recognize that certain situations exist with individual patients which may seem to require deviation with this voluntary policy. Providers agree to obtain second opinions on these cases by means of a designated peer review process *or* by referral to an outside consultant *and* to document this in the patient's medical record. Some nonexclusive examples are the use of chlordiazepoxide for familial tremor or clonazepam for restless leg syndrome.

NKFH providers agree that chart audits to determine compliance with this policy may be done on selected charts with the result of the audit to be reviewed at the Adult Provider's Committee or other designated peer review activities.

Specific Procedure for Benzodiazepine Prescriptions

New prescriptions only for 1 to 2 weeks, with refills allowed every 6 months.

If continued daily dosing seems appropriate, mental health consultation is required. Use of a formal letter of referral is recommended to insure clear communication and delineation of responsibility between NKFH and the consultant. A preprinted form letter is part of this document.

At the time the patient is notified of NKFH policy, they and provider should sign benzodiazepine medication contract which documents these dates and deadlines. It includes informed consent about withdrawal symptoms.

Established patients or new patients already on these medications who wish to continue on them may be given continued prescriptions for 3 months from the time they are notified of this policy to get a mental health consultation (in writing) regarding their medications.

Established or new patients who do not wish to obtain mental health consultation should begin tapering medications over 4 to 8 weeks starting with their next refill.

Patients who do not obtain the required consultation for any reason are to have their medication tapered and discontinued over four to eight weeks starting 3 months after their notification of our new policy, or sooner if they and their provider agree.

Continued

Patients on alprazolam or triazolam are to be changed to clonazepam on a mg for mg daily dose and have dose reduced by 1/8th every week. An initial dose of 2 to 3 times the initial mg dose may be appropriate for selected patients. Patients on other benzodiazepines are to have their dose reduced by 20-25% per week.

Patients who fail their withdrawal schedules should be referred to a mental health or chemical dependency specialist. Patients who are taking higher than usual doses of benzodiazepines may be tapered, but referral to a consultant is recommended.

If not following this policy seem medically indicated, schedule a discussion and chart review at Adult Provider's Committee. Then document the results of the discussion in the patient's chart. A form letter to send to the patient representative manager is included in this policy which asks that the chart be transported to the meeting location and returned to the proper center promptly. Providers are not to carry charts from center to center for any reason.

Prior to review and committee discussion, complete the Provider Checklist on Controlled Medications. A copy is part of this policy.

The preferred method of documenting the final decision about prescribing is to complete an Alert Sheet. This is a special progress note on a brightly colored paper to stand out in the progress notes. Less preferred alternatives are to highlight the appropriate progress note with a colored marker or flag the chart page with a colored tab. A copy of the Alert Sheet if included with this policy, but should be photocopied onto bright colored paper before use.

Specific Procedure for Narcotic (including butalbital and tramadol) Prescriptions

New prescriptions only for short term treatment of acute pain conditions.

Prescribe an adequate amount of medication for one to five days with no refills.

Advise the patient and document no refills in the medical record.

For recurrent painful conditions (i.e., kidney stones, headache, back pain), advise the patient of our policy of only issuing prescriptions every 60 days. Document this discussion. An Alert Sheet is recommended for the chart.

In patients for whom chronic prescriptions of narcotic pain medication for non-malignant pain seems appropriate, refer chart for peer review at Adult Provider's Committee. A form letter to the Medical Records Supervisor is part of this policy that can be used to request that charts be brought to the committee location.

Prior to review complete the Provider's Checklist for Controlled Medications.

If the decision is jointly made to prescribe narcotic medications for chronic non-malignant pain, a medication contract with the patient is mandatory. This needs to be completed as soon as practical with every patient receiving these prescriptions.

The preferred method of documenting the final decision about prescribing is to complete an Alert Sheet. This is a special progress note on a brightly colored paper to stand out in the progress notes. Less preferred alternatives are to highlight the appropriate progress note with a colored marker or flag the chart page with a colored tab. A copy of the Alert Sheet is included with this policy, but should be photocopied onto bright colored paper before use.

Specific Procedure for Peer Review

After selecting a patient to be reviewed, complete a Request for Chart Transport form giving the provider name, center, patient name, DOB, and date, time, and location of the scheduled review session. The copy of the form is included with this policy. Send the form to the Patient Business Supervisor at the Administrative Offices.

It is the responsibility of the Business Supervisor to arrange chart transport to and from the meeting.

Check off the boxes in a Provider Checklist for Controlled Drugs. It may be left with the patient's chart or carried to the review session by the provider. A copy of this form is included with this policy. It is not part of the patient's medical record.

Chart reviews are a scheduled part of Adult Provider's Committee. No chart will be reviewed unless the provider who requested the review is present. A maximum of four charts per provider will be discussed at any single meeting.

Separate peer review sessions may be scheduled at other times. These may be included in Quality Assurance activity or as required by the Medical Director.

NOTICE TO OUR PATIENTS
OUR POLICY ON PRESCRIBING NERVE AND PAIN PILLS

Physicians do not prescribe the following medications for any reason:

Equanil (meprobamate)	Soma (Carisprodol)
Talwin (Pentazocine)	Stadol Nasal Spray (butorphanol)
Xanax (alprazolam)	Artane (trihexphenidyl)
Dilaludid (hydromorphone)	Fiorinal with Codeine (butalbital)

Narcotic pain medications are only prescribed for acute (new and recent) conditions. Refills for recurrent conditions (such as back pain, kidney stones, headaches) are not given more often than every 60 days for any reason.

Codeine (i.e., Tylenol #3)	Oxycodone (i.e., Percocet)
Tramadol (i.e., Ultram)	Hydrocodone (i.e., Lorcet, Vicodin)
Propoxyphene (i.e., Darvon)	Butalbital (i.e., Fioricet)
Methadone	Meperidine (i.e., Demerol

A separate doctor's opinion and a signed agreement from you is required for chronic pain treatment with these drugs or medications that contain these drugs.

The following nerve or sleeping medications are only prescribed for a maximum of two weeks and no refills will be given before six months. If more seems to be required, a mental health referral is required, and the decision to continue medications will be made by the consultant.

Ativan (lorazepam)	Serax (oxazepam)
Librium (chlordiazepoxide)	Tranxene (clorazepate)
Klonopin (clonazepam)	Halcion (halazepam)
Restoril (temazepam)	Dalmane (flurazepam)
Valium (diazepam)	

If you have been on these medications for a long time and wish to continue them, we will assist you in obtaining the opinion of a mental health consultant. Otherwise, we will slowly taper and discontinue these medications, usually over four weeks. This tapering may require changing to one of the other drugs in this class to help reduce your withdrawal symptoms *which will occur*.

Courtesy Physicians and Nurse Practitioners at Northern Kentucky Health Centers

NORTHERN KENTUCKY FAMILY HEALTH, INC.
PATIENT AGREEMENT FOR BENZODIAZEPINE NERVE MEDICINES

I understand and agree to the following. I have asked any questions that I have about this contract and my medications.

NAME OF MEDICATION ____________________

DOSE: ____________ TIME(S) TO TAKE: ____________

NUMBER OF PILLS PRESCRIBED PER WEEK ______

1. **I agree to see a psychiatrist, psychologist, or mental health specialist and get their opinion in writing about my medication. I understand that NKFH must have a report from this specialist within THREE months from today's date or the medication above will automatically be tapered and stopped. Tapering may require substitution of a similar, but longer acting medication.**
2. I understand that it is my responsibility to keep or reschedule my appointment with the specialist so that a written report will be available to my provider here at Northern Kentucky Family Health within three months from today's date.
3. I agree that a psychiatrist or mental health specialist may assume the responsibility of prescribing my medication and I understand this is satisfactory to my provider at Northern Kentucky Family Health. The doctor here will only continue to prescribe this drug *if specifically recommended by that specialist.*
4. I agree that no later than 3 months from today, my doctor may taper and stop my medication. **I know that withdrawal symptoms such as increased nervousness and sleep problems *are normal and to be expected.* Other symptoms of withdrawal are: nausea, vomiting, loss of appetite, tremors, blurred vision and sweating. Suddenly stopping some of these drugs increases the risk of convulsions.**
5. I will bring all my medication bottles with me to my doctor's appointments. No refills will be given to me unless I bring the bottles.
6. If my prescription is lost or stolen, it *will not be replaced or refilled early.* It does not matter if you lose the written prescription or the pills themselves.
7. I will not request refills by phone and must keep my regular appointments. I will call and reschedule appointments if I cannot keep them.
8. If I get prescriptions of this or similar drugs from other doctors that I have not been referred to by my doctor, no more refills may be given and I may be discharged from this practice. This includes prescriptions from Emergency Rooms for any reason.
9. If the office or my doctor has to reschedule, postpone, or cancel my appointment, my doctor will determine if I must be seen or if my prescription can be refilled by phone.
10. My doctor will no longer prescribe this medication when they feel it is no longer medically necessary.
11. If I break this agreement, no refills of this or similar medications will be given by any physician at any of Northern KY Family Health Centers, and I may be discharged from the practice with 30 days notice.

____________________	____________________
patient	date
____________________	____________________
witness	doctor

Deadline for NKFH to receive written report from mental health consultant: ____________

Date when written report was received: ____________ ☐ Never obtained

Outcome: ☐ Taper and discontinue beginning ____________

☐ Specialist to prescribe for patient

☐ Specialist recommends that we continue prescribing ____________

☐ Other ____________

Date: ______________ Re: ______________________________ DOB: ______________

Dear ______________________________

I am referring my patient to you to request your evaluation and help in deciding if long term treatment with benzodiazepines is appropriate in this patient.

☐ This patient has been treated with a short course. ☐ This patient has never been treated with benzodiazepines.

☐ This patient has been on ______________________ for ______ years.
(drug, dose, and frequency)

☐ Please evaluate and manage therapy/prescriptions as you feel appropriate. I will prescribe psychotropic medications *only if you specifically approve and request in writing that I do so.*

☐ Please provide me with your opinion about this patient. I will continue to see and prescribe based on your recommendations.

This patient has these other conditions:

☐ h/o ethanol problems	☐ h/o depression	☐ h/o drug problems	☐ family stress	☐ heart disease
☐ chronic pain	☐ diabetes	☐ liver disease	☐ hypertension	☐ headaches
☐ arthritis	☐ seizures	☐ smoking	☐ social isolation	☐ lung disease
☐ Other ______________				

Thank you for your evaluation. Please send me a written response to be placed in this patient's chart. For your convenience, you may just check or fill in below as needed, sign below, then fax this form back to me. Thank you for your help with this patient.

Sincerely,

NOTE: It is the policy of NKFH that we do not prescribe alprazolam (Xanax) for any patient.

sign ______________________ print name ______________________

REPLY (check/fill in all that apply) *FAX back to* ______________________

☐ I will/did assume management of this patient's psychotropic medications on this date: ______________

☐ I will continue to follow and treat this patient for the following diagnosis(es):

____

☐ I recommend that NKFH taper and discontinue benzodiazepines.

☐ I recommend that NKFH prescribe and maintain the following prescription:

____

☐ I will NOT continue to follow this patient.

☐ I recommend evaluation by a specialist for the following diagnosis(es):

____

☐ I cannot make a recommendation on this patient for the follow reasons:

____

sign ______________________ print name ______________________

date ______________

NORTHERN KENTUCKY FAMILY HEALTH, INC.
PATIENT AGREEMENT FOR OPIOID PAIN MEDICINES

Patient Name: ______________________________ DOB: ______________

NAME OF DRUG: ______________ DOSE: __________ TIMES(S) TO TAKE: __________

NUMBER PRESCRIBED PER WEEK __________ OR PER MONTH __________

I have read, understand and agree to the following. I have asked any questions that I have about this contract and my medications.

I have the following problems now: ☐ Constipation ☐ Dizziness ☐ Itching ☐ Nausea ☐ Difficulty urinating

I am allergic or have had a bad reaction to the following medications: ______________________
(Write "none" if that is the case)

1. I understand that I am getting a prescription of a narcotic medication for a chronic pain condition. These drugs can be helpful to some patients with chronic pain. Some, but not all, patients say they can do more when taking these medications. Most patients report good, but not total, pain relief.
2. I understand that taking this drug may decrease my concentration and ability to think clearly. This side effect usually decreases with time. Other side effects from the drug that I may have are: dizziness, constipation, itching, nausea, and trouble passing urine.
3. **I understand that taking these drugs regularly usually causes physical dependence which means that I will have withdrawal symptoms if I suddenly stop the medication. Withdrawal symptoms include problems such as agitation, trouble sleeping, teary eyes, runny nose, nausea, vomiting, loss of appetite, diarrhea, cramps, sweating, or severe discomfort.** These symptoms may be uncomfortable, but are not life threatening.
4. I understand that taking this drug puts me at risk for developing an addiction to it. This means that I could become preoccupied with taking narcotics or other drugs to the point that other important aspects of my life, such as family, friends, work, and health could suffer or be harmed. I understand that people with addictions often do not realize they are addicted. Because of this, it will be important for my providers at NKFH to assess whether I am having a problem with addiction.
5. I give NKFH permission to determine whether I am developing an addiction. This includes checking my urine for narcotics and other drugs as well as contacting my family members, friends, or workplace. This is because others may see the signs of addiction before I recognize them myself. I know that I may be asked that a center staff member observe me when I urinate for the specimen.
6. I understand that if my prescription is lost or stolen, *it will not be replaced or refilled early*. I agree to bring all my medication bottles with me to my doctor's appointments, not just this drug. *No refills will be given to me unless I bring the bottles and all my unused pain medicine*.
7. I understand that my prescription will not be refilled outside of office hours. NKFH doctors and nurse practitioners on call for my regular provider will not refill my prescription without access to my medical record. My records are only available at one NKFH center during office hours.
8. It is my responsibility to keep my scheduled appointments and to call and reschedule appointments if I cannot keep them. If the office or my provider has to reschedule, postpone, or cancel my appointment, my provider will determine if I must be seen or if my prescription can be refilled by phone, or by a written prescription.
9. I agree to get prescriptions for addictive medications (narcotics, sleeping pills, nerve pills) from no one besides my regular provider or other NKFH providers. If I have an emergency that may require additional pain medicine, I will call my NKFH office first if at all possible. The only exception would be if an emergency requires that I go straight to an emergency room. If that happens, I will alert the doctor at the ER or hospital to my special arrangements for pain medicine and I will notify NKFH that I received pain medicine from another doctor.
10. I give permission for NKFH to receive information from *any health care provider or pharmacist* about use or possible misuse of alcohol and other drugs. This permission shall expire only with my written cancellation of this agreement.

11. I will have all of my prescriptions filled at one pharmacy: ______________________
    I give NKFH permission to contact all other pharmacies and physicians and ask them not to provide me with any addictive medications. This permission shall expire only with my written cancellation of this agreement.
12. My provider will no longer prescribe this medication when they feel it is no longer medically necessary or if I do not follow this plan of care. If I break this agreement, no refills of this or similar medications will be given by any physician at any of Northern KY Family Health Centers, and I may be discharged from the practice with 30 days notice.
13. I will not drink alcohol while I am taking narcotics. If I feel tired or mentally foggy, I agree not to drive, operate heavy machinery, or serve in any capacity related to public safety.
14. WOMEN ONLY: I understand that taking regular doses of narcotics during pregnancy can be harmful to developing babies. I am definitely not pregnant now and I make sure as best I can that I will not become pregnant while taking these drugs.

______________________	______________________
patient	date
______________________	______________________
witness	doctor

cd961121

Brown R, Fleming M, Patterson J: Chronic opioid analgesic therapy for chronic low back pain, *JABFP* 9(3):191-204, 1996.

PROVIDER CHECKLIST FOR PEER REVIEW: CONTROLLED MEDICATIONS

Patient Name ______________________________ DOB ____________________

Preexisting Conditions

Does the patient have any history of these conditions (either past or current)?

- ☐ Drug abuse (10)
- ☐ Alcohol abuse (10)
- ☐ Depression (9)
- ☐ Dysthymia (7)
- ☐ Anxiety (5)
- ☐ Schizophrenia (9)
- ☐ Personality Dis. (10)
- ☐ Family discord/distress (4)
- ☐ Suicide attempts (9)
- ☐ Bipolar disorder (7)
- ☐ Dementia (5)

If there were any positives in last question, how are they documented?

- ☐ Our chart notes
- ☐ Other outpatient records
- ☐ Hospital records
- ☐ Patient history form
- ☐ Letter(s) from consultant(s)
- ☐ Not documented

Warning Signs

How often has patient had a lost prescription?

☐ Never-0 ☐ Once-1 ☐ Rarely-2 ☐ Occasionally-4 ☐ Frequently-8

How often does patient request refills on the phone?

☐ Never-0 ☐ Once-1 ☐ Rarely-2 ☐ Occasionally-3 ☐ Frequently-7

Has the patient ever made a public display or outburst regarding their condition?

☐ Never-0 ☐ Once-1 ☐ Rarely-2 ☐ Occasionally-3 ☐ Frequently-4

Has the patient required an increase in the dose of their medication?

☐ Never-0 ☐ Once-1 ☐ Rarely-2 ☐ Occasionally-3 ☐ Frequently-5

Are we providing treatment/care for other problems besides this one?

- ☐ No, and does not see NKFH for any other care (8)
- ☐ Yes, but only episodic or acute problems (4)
- ☐ No, but does get routine health prevention visits (PAP, flu vax, etc.) (2)
- ☐ Yes, chronic medical problem(s) (i.e., DM, CAD, CHF, COPD) (1)
- ☐ Yes and at least one problem has a poor or terminal prognosis (0)

Comfort Level

What is the provider level of discomfort with *short term* treatment (<30 days)?

- ☐ None (0)
- ☐ Mild reservations, but no real discomfort (2)
- ☐ Moderate discomfort, but appropriate due to individual situation (4)
- ☐ Significant reservations, uncomfortable with current treatment (10)
- ☐ Strong reservations and discomfort with current treatment (12)

What is the provider level of discomfort with long term prescribing for this patient?

- ☐ None (0)
- ☐ Mild reservations, but no real discomfort (2)
- ☐ Moderate discomfort, but OK due to individual situation (4)
- ☐ Marked reservations, uncomfortable with chronic treatment (8)
- ☐ Strong reservations and discomfort with long term treatment (12)

Compliance with Therapy

How often does the patient miss or cancel appointments?

☐ Never-0 ☐ Once-0 ☐ Rarely-1 ☐ Occasionally-2 ☐ Frequently-4

How often does the patient request or receive early refills?

☐ Never-0 ☐ Once-1 ☐ Rarely-2 ☐ Occasionally-4 ☐ Frequently-6

How often does the patient fail to see consultants when referred by us?

☐ Never-0 ☐ Once-1 ☐ Rarely-2 ☐ Occasionally-4 ☐ Frequently-6

How often does the patient fail to get scheduled outpatient tests or therapy?

☐ Never-0 ☐ Once-0 ☐ Rarely-1 ☐ Occasionally-2 ☐ Frequently-4

Total score ______________________________ Date ____________________

____

Peer Review Recommendations

Date of Review ____________________

Benzodiazepines

☐ Discontinue benzodiazepines per policy
☐ Refer patient to Mental Health Consultant per policy
☐ Follow Mental Health Consultant recommendations
☐ Chronic prescription of ____________________ appears appropriate
☐ Discharge patient from practice
☐ Other (specify) ______________________________

Narcotics

☐ Discontinue prescription
☐ Chronic prescription of ____________________ appears appropriate
☐ Discharge patient from practice
☐ Other (specify) ______________________________

Committee Chairman ______________________________

NORTHERN KENTUCKY FAMILY HEALTH
REQUEST TO DISCHARGE PATIENT FROM PRACTICE

Patient Name: ______________________ DOB: ______________

Address: ______________________ Medicaid # ______________

Center: ☐ Cov. Med. ☐ Newport ☐ Dayton ☐ Ida Spence ☐ Dental ☐ WH ☐ OB/Gyn

I request that the patient listed above be discharged from our practice for the reasons indicated below.

Is this documented in a chart note? ☐ yes ☐ no If yes, date of note?

Are there other members of the patient's family that this may also affect? ☐ yes ☐ no

Has this been discussed in person with the patient? ☐ yes ☐ no

Has this been discussed by phone with the patient? ☐ yes ☐ no

Could the patient be referred to another provider within our system? ☐ yes ☐ no

Is the patient insured by Kentucky Medicaid? ☐ yes ☐ no (If yes, fill in the number above.)

Reason(s) for Discharge from Practice

☐ Non-compliance with appointments and follow-up ☐ NKFH ☐ Outside referrals

☐ Non-compliance with treatment plan ☐ Medication ☐ Substance abuse

☐ Patient states they require medications that are against our policies to prescribe

☐ Difficulty with the provider/patient relationship

☐ Patient has been ☐ verbally ☐ physically abusive to staff

☐ Other ______________________

______________________ signature ______________ date

172 Syncope

ICD-9-CM

Syncope 780.2

OVERVIEW

Definition

Syncope is a transient loss of consciousness accompanied by unresponsiveness and loss of postural tone with spontaneous recovery.

Incidence

Syncope is most likely to occur in the **elderly,** increasing with age from 2% in **ages 65 to 69** to 12% in those **greater than 85 years of age.**

The **pregnant woman** is more susceptible to syncopal episodes due to a hemodilution and vasodilation, particularly when changing position.

SUBJECTIVE DATA

History of Present Illness

Ask about the circumstances around the syncopal episode, what the patient was doing, where they were, and their description of the event.

Women of childbearing age, ask date of last menstrual period and of contraceptive use.

Timing of the syncopal episode is critical (i.e., does it occur after micturition, defecation, coughing, or swallowing). These events may lead to a transient hypotension that results in syncope.

Another cause of syncope is carotid sinus hypersensitivity. Syncope usually occurs with tight collars or neck turning as with shaving.

Medications can also cause carotid sinus hypersensitivity (e.g., digitalis, beta-blockers, alpha-methyldopa, and calcium channel blockers).

See sample detailed history form on p. 1066.

Past Medical History

Ask about hypotension, cardiovascular or peripheral vascular disease, atrial fibrillation, ventricular aneurysms, aortic stenosis, hypoglycemia, seizures, pulmonary disease, carotid artery disease.

Family History

History of cardiovascular disease, history of cerebral vascular accidents

Psychosocial History

Smoking, increased stress

Medication History

In the **elderly,** the medications most likely to cause syncope are phenothiazines, tricyclic antidepressants, and antihypertensive medications.

Diet History

Syncope can be precipitated by swallowing, so the timing in relationship to meals is important. Also, if the patient is taking antihypertensive medications with a meal or just before, hypotension can develop, causing a syncopal episode.

Poor nutrition can also cause dehydration and hypotension leading to syncope.

Associated Symptoms

Chest pain, shortness of breath, pleuritic chest pain, focal neurological deficits

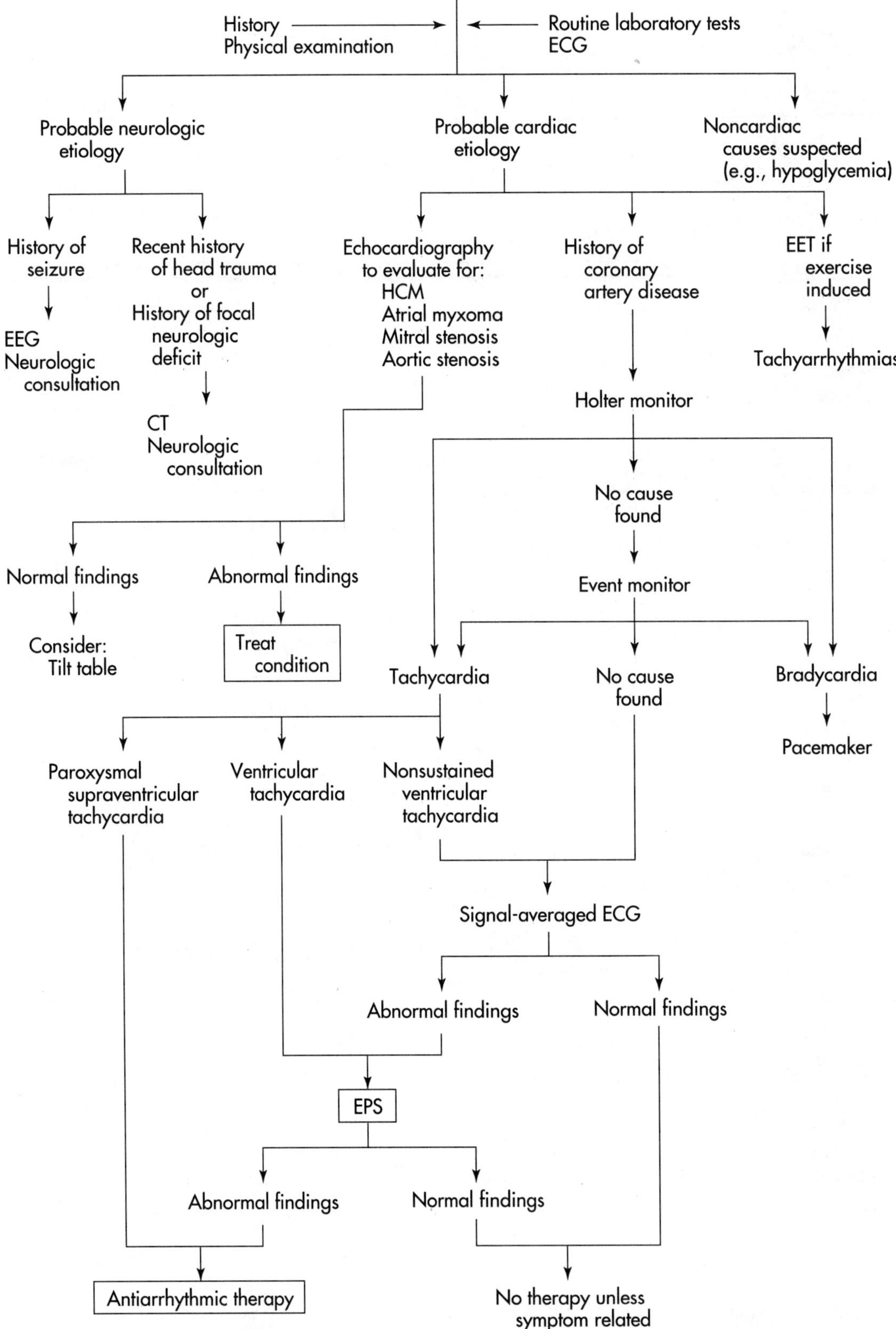

Figure 172-1 Algorithm for patient with syncope. *CT,* Computed tomography; *ECG,* electrocardiogram; *EEG,* electroencephalogram; *EPS,* electrophysological study; *ETT,* exercise treadmill test; *HCM,* hypertrophic cardiomyopathy. (Adapted from Greene HL, Johnson WP, Lemcke D: *Decision making in medicine*, ed 2, St Louis, 1998, Mosby.)

OBJECTIVE DATA

Physical Examination

A complete physical examination is indicated with a chief complaint of syncope.

Vital signs: Orthostatic vital signs should be taken, hydration status should be assessed.

Cardiovascular examination: Listen for arrhythmias (atrial fibrillation may cause syncope if new and uncontrolled ventricular response), murmurs (particularly those of aortic stenosis, may be cause of syncopal event), gallop rhythms.

Pulmonary examination: Listen for breath sounds.

Abdominal examination: Listen for bruit, palpate for pulsating mass.

Neurological examination: Usually there will not be any neurological deficits; if there are, watch for transient ischemic attack or stroke.

Extremities: Excess pretibial edema (may indicate a volume problem).

Diagnostic Procedures

Laboratory tests:

- Complete blood count ($13 to $16)
- Electrolytes ($23 to $30)
- Glucose ($16 to $20)
- Creatinine kinase ($23 to $29)
- May want to consider troponin I ($34 to $46) if possible myocardial infarction
- Thyroid-stimulating hormone (Cost not available)
- Radiologic tests
- Echocardiogram ($675) if history of heart disease
- May want to consider computed tomography of head if trauma to head during syncopal episode
- Consider carotid artery Doppler study if any indication of central nervous system problem
- Other tests:
  - Electrocardiogram ($56 to $65)
  - Consider doing 24-hour Holter monitor ($295 to $388)
  - Consider tilt table
  - Consider other electrophysiologic testing if all other tests are negative

ASSESSMENT

An algorithm for a patient with syncope is found in Figure 172-1. Differential diagnoses include:

Pulmonary embolus
Myocardial infarction
Vasovagal syncope
Situational syncope
Drug-induced syncope
Orthostatic hypotension
Postprandial hypotension
Aortic stenosis
Pulmonary hypertension
Idiopathic hypertrophic subaortic stenosis
Carotid sinus syncope
Subclavian steal
Coronary artery disease
Transient ischemic attack
Seizure
Psychogenic syncope
Left atrial myxoma
Tetralogy of Fallot
Arrhythmias
Hypoglycemia
Pregnancy

THERAPEUTIC PLAN

The therapeutic plan depends on the diagnosis. While performing a patient workup, the practitioner may consider using ASA 81 mg QD ($1 to $3) for platelet inhibition.

EVALUATION/FOLLOW-UP

Patients should be followed weekly until a cause is known for the syncopal episode. Patients should be educated to change positions slowly, waiting before actually moving after a position change has been made. Avoid dosing antihypertensive medications with meals. Beware of positive changes postprandial.

SUGGESTED READINGS

Ellsworth AJ et al: *Mosby's 1998 medical drug reference*, St Louis, 1998, Mosby.

Hart G: Evaluation of syncope, *Am Family Physician* 51:1941-1948, 1995.

Healthcare Consultants of America, Inc: *1998 physicians fee and coding guide*, Augusta, Ga, 1998, Healthcare Consultants of America, Inc.

Kapoor W: Evaluation and management of syncope, *Cont Int Med* 6:29-39, 1994.

McCance K, Huether S: *Pathophysiology: the biologic basis for disease in adults and children*, ed 2, St Louis, 1994, Mosby.

Reuben D, Yoshikawa T, Besdine R, editors: *Geriatrics review syllabus*, New York, 1995, American Geriatrics Society.

Uphold CR, Graham MV: *Clinical guidelines in family practice*, ed 2, Gainesville, Fla, 1994, Barmarrae Books.

Wilson J et al, editors: *Harrison's principles of internal medicine*, ed 2, New York, 1991, McGraw-Hill.

Woodley M, Whelan A, editors: *Manual of medical therapeutics*, ed 27, Boston, 1992, Little, Brown.

DETAILED HISTORY FOR SYNCOPE

Medications: ________ Diuretics ________ Antiarrhythmic ________

Antihypertensive ________ Anticonvulsant ________ Other ________

Previous episode: When ________

Duration of this episode ________

Position at onset ________

Sensation of impending attack (warning): darkening of vision ________ numbness ________ palpitations ________

pain ________ other ________

No warning ________

Change of skin color: flushed ________ pale ________ return of skin color: rapid ________ slow ________

Prodromal symptoms or activity ________

Trauma: ________ cause ________ or result ________

Associated symptoms: fever ________ ear pain/deafness ________ hyperventilation ________

other ________

Recent: illness ________ infection ________ surgery ________ trauma ________ emotional upset and/or stress ________ other ________

Potentiators of attack: ETOH ________ prolonged standing ________ excessive heat ________ micturation ________ eating ________

medication with meal ________ other ________

Pregnant: last menstrual period ________ normal period ________ abnormal ________

Post syncopal symptoms ________

Time span for recovery ________

173 Syphilis

ICD-9-CM

Syphilis 087.9
Congenital Syphilis 090.9
Early Syphilis 091.0
Latent Syphilis 097.1
Secondary Syphilis 091.9
Tertiary Syphilis 097.0
(Many more codes available depending on site involved)

OVERVIEW

Definition

Syphilis is a sexually transmitted disease (STD) that may effect multiple systems. It is characterized by periods of exacerbations followed by episodes of latency. It is caused by a motile spirochete, *Treponema Pallidum*. Incubation is 10 to 90 days, with an average of 21 days.

Syphilis is divided into six stages: primary syphilis, secondary syphilis, tertiary syphilis, early latent syphilis (syphilis acquired in the previous year), late latent syphilis, and syphilis of unknown duration.

Incidence

Syphilis is the third most commonly reported disease in the United States, with a higher prevalence in large, urban areas. **Young adults** are most commonly affected with primary syphilis.

Pathophysiology

The spirochete *T. pallidum* is transmitted during sexual contact through abraded areas in the skin (often microabrasions) or mucosal surfaces. Risk of infection appears to be about 30%, with women appearing to be at a higher risk for contracting syphilis than men engaged in the same high-risk behaviors. Individuals harboring the spirochete are capable of transmitting the infection for about 1 year. Syphilis is transmitted across the placenta to produce chronic infection in the fetus.

SUBJECTIVE DATA

Presenting Symptoms

Primary Syphilis

Patients will generally present with a painless lesion (chancre) with a granular base and well-formed edges. This lesion develops at the site of inoculation (penis, fourchette, cervix, anus, labia). There may be a serous discharge from the lesion. The untreated lesion may heal spontaneously in 1 to 5 weeks. Patients may complain of swollen lymph nodes in the groin.

Secondary Syphilis

Patients may complain of a low-grade fever, headache, sore throat, general malaise. Often there are bilateral, symmetrical macular, papular, or papulosquamous skin lesions on the palms, soles of the feet, and face, in addition to the trunk and the extremities. Patients complain of loss of hair (alopecia) and often a loss of the lateral third of the eyebrow. They may complain of white patches in the mouth and nose. Secondary syphilis is highly infectious.

Tertiary Syphilis

There is multisystem involvement with emphasis on cardiac, neurological, ophthalmic, auditory systems. Syphilis is often found during extensive work-up in the hospital setting.

Early Latent Syphilis

Patients usually have no presenting signs, and the diagnosis is made by serologic testing.

Late Latent Syphilis

Patients may develop cutaneous lesions called gummas, although rarely seen today. These lesions may develop in patients from 2 to 40 years after the initial infection.

History of Present Illness

Symptoms

When did the symptoms appear (acute or gradual onset)?
How many days, weeks months (be specific)?

Associated Symptoms

Discharge, odor, dysuria, lesion, genital itch, rash, abdominal or scrotal pain

Precipitating Factors

Lack of barrier protection?

Relieving Factors

Did anything make you feel better?

Treatment

What have you used so far?

Past Medical History

Prior STDs and when? Treatment? Did you complete treatment? Was your partner treated?

Sexual History

Last exposure (sexual act)
Number of partners in the past month? Past year?
Number of lifetime partners <5, 5 to 10, >10
Sexual preference: Male, female, both?
Sexual interaction with a bisexual partner
Type of intercourse: Oral, vaginal, anal?
Ever used sex to obtain money or drugs?

Gynecological History

Last Menstrual Period
Gravida_______ Para _______
Ectopic pregnancy?
Infertility?
Hysterectomy?
Last Pap smear? Results?
Pregnant? If yes, what trimester?

Contraceptive History

None, condom, intrauterine device, oral contraceptive pill, sterilization
How long? How often?

Medications

Prescribed, especially antibiotics in the past 2 weeks
Recreational drugs
Over-the-counter drugs

Psychosocial History

Socioeconomic status
Spouse or partner relationship
Substance abuse history
Intravenous or intramuscular drug use
Travel to Third World countries?

OBJECTIVE DATA

Physical Examination

A problem-focused physical examination should be performed, with particular attention to:

Hair: Patchy alopecia, pattern opposite of male pattern baldness (progresses from occiput to temples), loss of lateral third of eyebrows

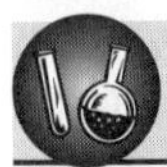

TABLE 173-1 Diagnostic Tests: Syphilis

Diagnostic Test	Findings/Rationale	Cost ($)
Nontreponemal Tests Complement fixation tests (VDRL or RPR)	Used for screening; they become positive 4-6 weeks after infection; they start in low titer and, over several weeks, may reach 1:32 or higher; after adequate treatment of primary syphilis, the titer falls fourfold and in most cases is nonreactive within 9-18 months; false-positives occur in hepatitis, mononucleosis, pregnancy, viral pneumonia, malaria, varicella, autoimmune diseases, diseases associated with increased globulins, narcotic addicts, leprosy, and old age	19-23
Treponemal Tests Includes the FTA-ABS test, TPI test, and microhemagglutination assay for *T. pallidum* (MHA-TP)	A treponemal test should be used to confirm a positive VDRL or RPR; treponemal tests are specific to treponema antibodies and will remain positive after treatment	42-54/FTA
HIV screen	All patients suspected of syphilis or who have syphilis should be tested for HIV	53-67
Dark-field examination	Can diagnose immediately if treponema seen	

HIV, human immunodeficiency virus; *RPR,* rapid plasma reagin; *TPI,* treponemal immobilization test; *VDRL,* Venereal Disease Research Laboratories.

Oropharynx: Ulcers, exudate, patches, pharyngitis
Mucous membranes: Pink to gray mucous patches, painless, dull erythematous patches of grayish-white erosion
Neck: Lymphadenopathy
Skin: Folliculitis, rash (especially of soles and palms), chancre, painless, nonpruritic lesions; symmetrical distribution of secondary syphilis
Lymph nodes: Check inguinal and cervical nodes looking for firm, movable, discrete, rubbery, nonfluctuant, painless, unilateral or bilateral nodes
Pubic hair: Patchy hair loss
Penis: Ulcer, chancre
Scrotum: Palpate the scrotum; note any lesions or tenderness
External female genitalia: Ulcer, chancre
Cervix: Lesion, leukoplakia
Bimanual: Check for discharge, erythema, cervical motion tenderness (signs of other STDs)
Perianal: Ulcer, chancre

Diagnostic Procedures

STDs are often superimposed on one another. Other physical findings may indicate multiple infections. Other tests needed will be based on history and physical examination. This section will concentrate only on the diagnostic testing for syphilis (Table 173-1).

TABLE 173-2 Differential Diagnosis: Syphilis

Diagnosis	Supporting Data
Syphilis	Clean, painless ulcer with a hard base
Chancroid	The combination of a painful ulcer and tender inguinal lymphadenopathy suggests a diagnosis of chancroid.
Lymphogranuloma venereum	Begins with an initial ulcerative or vesicular lesion, often unnoticed; lymph node enlargement, softening and suppuration with draining sinuses, positive groove sign
Granuloma inguinale	Uncommon in United States, painless, progressive, ulcerative lesions without regional lymphadenopathy; the lesions are vascular and bleed easily on contact
Impetigo	Vesicles that rupture, with release of honey-colored discharge/crust formation, painful

Pregnancy Screening

Congenital syphilis is preventable if maternal syphilis is treated in early pregnancy. Nontreponemal tests should be used for screening and positive results confirmed by treponemal testing.

ASSESSMENT

Differential diagnoses include primary syphilis, secondary syphilis, tertiary or latent syphilis, as well as differential diagnoses in Table 173-2.

THERAPEUTIC PLAN

Pharmaceutical

See Table 173-3 for treatment of primary and secondary syphilis. Treatment for early latent syphilis is found in Table 173-4, and treatment for late latent syphilis is found in Table 173-5.

Pregnant Patients

All pregnant patients should be treated with the penicillin (PCN) regimen appropriate for the stage of syphilis. Some experts recommend a second dose of benzathine penicillin 2.4 million U IM 1 week after the initial dose for women who have primary, secondary, or early latent syphilis.

All pregnant patients with PCN allergies should be desensitized (see CDC recommendations, 1998).

Neurosyphilis

Aqueous crystalline PCN G 18 to 24 million U/day per intravenous piggyback for 10 to 14 days.

Treatment of Sex Partners

Sexual transmission of *T. pallidum* occurs only when mucocutaneous syphilitic lesions are present; such manifestations are uncommon after the first year of infection. However, persons exposed sexually to a patient who has syphilis in any stage should be evaluated clinically and serologically according to the following recommendations.

Persons who were exposed within the 90 days preceding the diagnosis of primary, secondary, or early latent syphilis in a sex partner might be infected even if seronegative; therefore such persons should be treated presumptively.

Persons who were exposed >90 days before the diagnosis of primary, secondary or early latent syphilis in a sex partner should be treated presumptively if serologic tests results are not available immediately and the opportunity for follow-up is uncertain.

For purposes of partner notification and presumptive treatment of exposed sex partners, patients with syphilis of unknown duration who have high nontreponemal serologic test titers (i.e., >1:32) may be considered as having early syphilis. However, serologic titers should not be used to

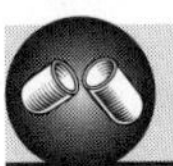

TABLE 173-3 Pharmaceutical Plan: Primary and Secondary Syphilis

Drug	Dose	Comments	Cost
Benzathine penicillin G (Wycillin)	Adults: 2.4 million U IM × 1 dose Children: 50,000 U/kg IM up to the adult dose of 2.4 million U	Observe for 20-30 minutes after injection Pregnancy: B SE: Rash, drug fever, anaphylaxis	$21/300,000 U/ml (10 ml) $7/600,000 U/ml (10 ml)
For patients with PCN allergy:		Doxycycline: Pregnancy: D SE: Photosensitivity, rash, GI upset, enterocolitis	$6-$177/100 mg (50)
Adults (Nonpregnant): Doxycycline (Doryx) *or* Tetracycline (Achromycin)	100 mg PO BID × 14 days *or* 500 mg PO QID × 14 days	Tetracycline: Pregnancy: D SE: Photosensitivity, GI upset, rash, hepatotoxicity	$11/500 mg (100)
Alternate regimen: Ceftriaxone	1 g QD ×5-10 days	Pregnancy: B SE: Diarrhea, pain at injection site, local reaction	$12/250 mg/vial; $21/500 mg/vial; $35/1 g/vial
Erythromycin	500 mg PO QID ×14 days	Pregnancy: B SE: GI upset, abdominal pain, rash, anorexia	$26-$154/500 mg (100)

GI, Gastrointestinal; *PCN*, penicillin; *SE*, side effects.

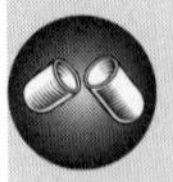

TABLE 173-4 Pharmaceutical Plan: Early Latent Syphilis

Age	Drug	Dose
Adults	Benzathine penicillin G	2.4 million U IM ×1 dose
Children	Benzathine penicillin G	50,000 U/kg IM up to the adult dose of 2.4 million Units

differentiate early from late syphilis for the purpose of determining treatment.

Long-term sex partners of patients who have late syphilis should be evaluated clinically and serologically for syphilis and treated on the basis of the findings of the evaluation.

The time periods before treatment used for identifying at-risk sex partners are

3 months plus duration of symptoms for primary syphilis
6 months plus duration of symptoms for secondary syphilis
1 year for early latent syphilis

Lifestyle/Activities

Safer sex/barrier protection

Diet

Not applicable

Patient Education

Jarisch-Herxheimer reaction: Thought to be a reaction to lysis of treponemes, occurs in approximately 30% of patients treated for primary syphilis and 70% of those treated for secondary syphilis. Usually presents with fever, chills, myalgia, headache, palpitations, and flushing, but may be severe enough to cause hypotension. Mild forms may be treated with aspirin. More severe forms require emergency care to prevent end organ damage.
Importance of compliance with medication if any of the multi-dose, multi-day therapies are initiated.
Barrier protection
Partner(s) notification
Abstinence during treatment and until symptoms subside
Identification of chancre and other signs of STDs in partner(s)
Limit number of partners
Information about STD transmission

Referral

Patients with PCN allergies
Children

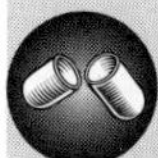

TABLE 173-5 Pharmaceutical Plan: Late Latent Syphilis, Latent Syphilis of Unknown Duration, or Tertiary without Neurosyphilis

Age	Drug	Dose
Adults	Benzathine penicillin G	7.2 million U total, administered as three doses of 2.4 million U IM, each at 1-week intervals
Children	Benzathine penicillin G	50,000 U/kg IM, up to the adult dose of 2.4 million U, administered as three doses at 1-week intervals (total 150,000 U/kg up to the adult dose of 7.2 million U)
Penicillin-allergic adults (Nonpregnant)	Doxycycline Tetracycline	100 mg PO BID ×14 days 500 mg PO QID ×14 days Both drugs should be administered for 2 weeks if the duration of the infection is known to have been <1 year; otherwise, they should be administered for 4 weeks

Human immunodeficiency virus (HIV)–positive patients
Persistent elevation of titers
Late latency syphilis
Tertiary syphilis (need cerebrospinal fluid evaluation)
Neurosyphilis
Congenital syphilis
Reportable to local/state health departments
- Can be helpful in identifying patients who have been treated and "forgot" or who were too embarrassed to disclose
- Can also stage syphilis, which determines treatment

Follow-up

Nontreponemal test at 1 month after treatment and every 3 months for at least 1 year is required for evaluation. Adequate treatment of primary or secondary syphilis is indicated by a fourfold decrease in titer by 3 months and by 6 months in latent syphilis. Some patients will have a Veneral Disease Research Laboratories (VDRL) that will remain unchanged on subsequent testing after treatment. These people are considered sero-fast or sero-resistant. For most patients the titer continues to decrease until nonreactive. A fourfold increase in the titer indicates a reinfection and requires further treatment.

A VDRL obtained on cord blood of a newborn may be reactive from the passive transfer of antibodies from the mother. A VDRL should be performed every month for 3 or 4 months to determine whether the titer is rising or falling. If the titer falls or becomes non-reactive, the infant had maternal transfer and not congenital syphilis.

HIV-positive patients should be evaluated via serology for treatment failures at 3, 6, 9, 12, and 24 months.

EVALUATION

Fourfold drop in VDRL titer signifies adequate treatment

RESOURCES

CDC/ STD Web site (includes copy of 1998 STD treatment guidelines): http://www.cdc.gov/nchstp/dstd/breaking_news.htm
American Social Health Association: http://sunsite.unc.edu/ASHA/
Ask Noah about STDs (Web site with multiple resources): http://www.noah.cuny.edu/illness/stds/stds.html

Journal of American Medical Association Women's Health STD Web site: http://www.ama-assn.org/special/std/support/support.htm

REFERENCES

Centers for Disease Control and Prevention: Guidelines for treatment of sexually transmitted diseases, *MMWR* 47(No RR-1):28-49, 1998.

SUGGESTED READINGS

Cherniak D: *STD handbook*, Montreal, 1995, Montreal Health Press.
Dunnihoo DR: *Fundamentals of gynecology and obstetrics*, ed 2, Philadelphia, 1992, JB Lippincott.
Ellsworth A et al: *Mosby's 1998 medical drug reference*, St Louis, 1998, Mosby.
Gunn R, Harper S: Emphasizing infectious syphilis partner notification, *Nurs Times* 25(4):218-219, 1998.
Hawkins JW, Roberto-Nichols DM, Stanley-Haney JL: *Syphilis protocols for nurse practitioners in gynecologic settings*, ed 5, New York, 1995, Tiresias Press.
Healthcare Consultants of America, Inc: *1998 physicians fee and coding guide*, Augusta, Ga, 1998, Healthcare Consultants of America, Inc.
Hook EW, Marra CM: Acquired syphilis in adults, *N Engl J Med* 326:1060-1067, 1992.
Johnson CA: Syphilis. In Johnson CA, Murray J, Johnson B, editors: *Women's health care handbook*, St Louis, 1996, Mosby.
Landers D, Sweet R: Sexually transmitted infection. In Glass RH, editor: *Office gynecology*, ed 4, Baltimore, 1993, Williams & Wilkins.
McMillan A: Sexually transmittable diseases. In Loudon N, Glesier A, Gebbie A: *Handbook of family planning and reproductive health*, ed 3, New York, 1995, Churchill Livingstone.
Rolfs RT: Treatment of syphilis, 1993, *Clin Infect Dis* 20(Suppl 1): S23-S38, 1995.
Sexually Transmitted Diseases: *Syphilis: Epidemiology and Laboratory Examinations,* STD Training Center, Cincinnati Ohio.
Weston A: Striking back at syphilis, *Nurs Times* 94(3):30-32, 1998.

174 Temporomandibular Joint Disorders

ICD-9-CM

Temporomandibular Joint Pain Dysfunction Syndrome 524.6
Bruxism 306.8

OVERVIEW

Definition

Temporomandibular joint (TMJ) disorder is a term that includes a number of clinical complaints involving the temporomandibular joint and associated orofacial structures. TMJ is a major cause of nondental pain and is considered a subclassification of musculoskeletal disorders.

Incidence

Approximately 3% to 7% of the population seeks care for TMJ disorders. There is a slightly greater incidence in women at a ratio from 3:1 to 9:1.

Pathophysiology

In most patients the TMJ complaint is not about the joint itself, but about the muscles of mastication associated with the joint. The primary signs and symptoms of TMJ originate from the masticatory structures and are associated with jaw function. The TMJ is a hinge joint and at the same time allows gliding movements in another plane. It is considered a ginglymoarthrodial joint. The joint is formed by the intersection of the mandibular condyle, which fits into the mandibular fossa of the temporal bone. Separating these two bones is the articular disk. During normal opening and closing, the disk is maintained between the condyle and fossa.

Four pairs of muscles move the mandible and permit function of the masticatory system (Table 174-1).

Pathophysiology in TMJ pain disorders occurs when the disk is altered and becomes elongated. The disk can then become dislocated from its normal position between the condyle and fossa. Muscle pain in TMJ seems to result from a CNS effect on the muscle that results from an increase in peripheral nociceptive activity. These conditions are further complicated when the patient has bruxism. Bruxism is the subconscious grinding and gnashing of the teeth.

SUBJECTIVE DATA

History of Present Illness (Box 174-1)

Complaints of:
- Facial muscle pain
- Preauricular pain
- TMJ sounds: Jaw clicking, popping, catching, locking
- Limited mouth opening
- Increased pain while chewing
- Some people may have difficulty talking or singing
- History of recent trauma or injury to neck, jaw, or mouth
- Previously been treated for unexplained facial pain or jaw pain problem?
- Have you ever been told by your dentist that you grind your teeth?
- Have you ever been treated for grinding your teeth?
- When was your last dental visit?

Associated Symptoms

Earache
Headache
Neck ache

Past Medical History

Use of dentures
Underlying conditions

TABLE 174-1 Muscles of Mastication and Their Function

Muscle	Function
Masseter; temporalis; medial pterygoid	Elevate the mandible: Major force in chewing (they can provide up to 975 lbs of biting force)
Lateral pterygoid	Provides protrusive movement of the mandible
Other muscles that are not considered to be muscles of mastication, but play an important role in mandibular function include the digastric muscles	Depress the mandible: Open the mouth

Medications

Current medications

Family History

Noncontributory

Psychosocial History

Stress levels
Coping patterns used
Use of alcohol to relieve stress
Chew gum frequently
Smokes cigarettes or uses smokeless tobacco

OBJECTIVE DATA

Physical Examination

A thorough evaluation of the head/neck and musculoskeletal system is warranted.

Vital signs
General
Head/eyes/ears/nose/throat: Assess for sinus pain with palpation
Ear: Evaluate for potential ear problems with otoscope
Throat: Assess for erythema
Neck: Assess for lymphadenopathy
Face: Assess for masseter, temporal muscles and preauricular area for pain or tenderness.
Inspect the face, jaw and dental arches for symmetry
Ask the patient to open and close the mouth keeping your fingers over the preauricular areas: Be alert for joint sounds
Mouth: Measure mouth opening: use millimeter rule on teeth and have patient open as wide as possible. Measure the distance between the maxillary and mandibular teeth (and other teeth in mouth). <40 mm is considered a restricted mouth opening. Inspect teeth for significant wear, mobility, or decay. Look at the buccal mucosa for riding and the lateral edges of the tongue for scalloping. These are signs of clenching and bruxism.

Box 174-1

Screening Questions for Patients with Temporomandibular Joint Disorders

Do you have difficulty, pain, or both when opening your mouth (e.g., when yawning)?
Does your jaw get stuck, locked, or go out?
Do you have difficulty or pain or both when chewing, talking, or using your jaws?
Are you aware of noises in the jaw joints?
Do your jaws regularly feel stiff, tight, or tired?
Do you have pain in or about the ears, temples, or cheeks?
Do you have frequent headaches, neck aches, or toothaches?

Diagnostic Procedures

No procedures are indicated. A panoramic dental x-ray might be appropriate, but can be done when seen by the dentist. Magnetic resonance imaging of the TMJ may be indicated for more information ($1101 to $1321)

ASSESSMENT

Differential diagnoses include those found in Table 174-2.

THERAPEUTIC PLAN

Pharmaceutical

Pharmaceutical treatment is outlined in Table 174-3.

Lifestyle/Activities

Night guard when sleeping
Stress reduction/relaxation techniques
Regular dental checkups
Rule of thumb: "If it hurts, don't do it"
Physical therapy: Use of moist heat or cold can be helpful
Exercise: Gently open the mouth to resistance and close; then move jaw laterally; if these exercises produce pain, they should be stopped

TABLE 174-2 Differential Diagnosis: Temporomandibular Joint Disorders

Diagnosis	Supporting Data
Dental pain	Facial pain, may radiate up into ear or mandible; may have visible swelling of jaw; pain increases with chewing/drinking
Trigeminal neuralgia	Unilateral, with severe pain in area of nerve affected: Eyes, upper lip, nose, cheek, or tongue/lower lip
Sinusitis	Pain over maxillary or frontal sinuses, usually rhinorrhea of yellow/green, fever
Condylar fracture or dislocation of mandible	History of trauma to jaw from falls and motor vehicle accidents; main complaint is that the teeth don't feel right; complaints of tenderness to palpation and pain with movement of jaw
Temporal arteritis	Headache, polymyalgia rheumatica, impaired vision, jaw claudication

Diet

Soft diet
Eat more slowly
Eat smaller bites

Patient Education

Reassurance that it is not a malignancy
Usually a self-limiting illness
Understand the role of emotional stress
Relaxation of the jaw: Let jaw muscles relax, keeping the teeth apart
Avoid activities that cause pain or disorder
Select activities that are less bothersome to the joint structures (e.g., chew on other side)

Referral/Consultation

If the patient has any of the following, consider a referral to a dental office:

- History of trauma to the face which coincides with the beginning of the pain
- Significant popping/crepitus sounds during jaw function
- Locking or catching of jaw when opening
- Change in the way the teeth fit together
- Significant tooth problems: Mobility, sensitivity, decay or wear
- Pain that has been present for >2 months

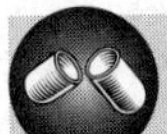

TABLE 174-3 Pharmaceutical Plan: Temporomandibular Joint Disorders

Drug	Dose	Comments	Cost
Ibuprofen	200-800 mg TID	See Appendix J for more detailed information; reduces pain, helps stop the cyclic effects of deep pain input Pregnancy: B SE: Gastrointestinal upset, bleeding or ulceration, edema, heartburn; take with foods	\$3-\$9/200 mg (100); \$4-\$80/600 mg (100)
Methocarbamol (Robaxin) or other muscle relaxants	500-750 mg at hs	To significantly relax the muscles, the amount needed will debilitate the person; it can be used on a short-term basis at night to help with sleep Pregnancy: C SE: Drowsiness, syncope, headache, dry mouth, nervousness	\$6-\$49/500 mg (100); \$8-\$72/750 mg (100)
Zolpidem (Ambien) or low-dose Trazodone (Desyrel)	5-10 mg hs 50 mg hs	Fewer side effects than cyclobenzaprine, especially in the elderly Zolpidem: Pregnancy: B SE: Dizziness, daytime drowsiness, diarrhea, drugged feelings Trazodone: Pregnancy: C SE: Drowsiness, anticholinergic effects (rare), fatigue, headache, impotence, seizures, altered liver tests	Zolpidem: \$130/5 mg (100); \$160/10 mg (100) Traz: \$5-\$139/5 mg (100); \$12-\$243/100 mg (100)

SE, Side effects.

Orthopedic appliances: Splints, bite guards, occlusal appliances may be helpful; the dentist should be consulted for this therapy

Follow-up

Follow-up in 2 weeks to determine the effectiveness of pain medications, and stress reduction techniques

EVALUATION

Most cases resolve without sequelae, although chronic pain is a potential complication

SUGGESTED READINGS

Ellsworth A et al: *Mosby's 1998 medical drug reference*, St Louis, 1998, Mosby.

Garofalo J et al: Predicting chronicity in acute temporomandibular disorders using research diagnostic criteria, *J Am Dent Assoc* 129(4): 438-447, 1998.

Halpern L et al: Temporomandibular disorders: clinical and laboratory analyses for risk assessment of criteria for surgical therapy, a pilot study, *Cranio* 16(1):35-43, 1998.

Healthcare Consultants of America, Inc: *1998 physicians fee and coding guide*, Augusta, Ga, 1998, Healthcare Consultants of America, Inc.

Israel H: Temporomandibular disorders: what the neurologist needs to know, *Semin Neurol* 17(4):355-366, 1997.

Moses A: Controversy in TMD: putting the issues in perspective, *Dental Today* 16(3):92, 1997.

Okeson J, deKanter R: Temporomandibular disorders in the medical practice, *J Family Practice* 43(4):347-356, 1996.

Orhback R, Dworkin S: 5-year outcomes in TMD: relationship of changes in pain to changes in physical and psychological variables, *Pain* 74(2-3):315-326, 1998.

Pettengill C et al: A pilot study comparing the efficacy of hard and soft appliances in the treatment of the patient with temporomandibular disorders, *J Prosthet Dent* 79(2):165-168, 1998.

Shankland W: Common causes of nondental facial pain, *Gen Dent* 45(3):246-253, 1997.

Talley R: Assessment of temporomandibular injury and orofacial pain, *J Okla Dent Assoc* 86(2):38-41, 1995.

Tendinitis/Bursitis

Impingement Syndromes

ICD-9-CM

Bursitis, Shoulder 726.0
Bursitis, Hip 726.5
Bursitis, Subacromial 726.19
Tenosynovitis, Elbow 727.09
Tenosynovitis, Supraspinatus 726.10

OVERVIEW

Definition

Tendinitis/bursitis is inflammation of tendons and bursae of involved joints.

Incidence

Joint pain is a common presentation with tendinitis/bursitis. The incidence depends on the location of the inflammation

Stages of impingement syndrome in the shoulder (Table 175-1)
- Bursitis (subacromial, subdeltoid)
- Tendinitis (rotator cuff, biceps tendon, calcific tendinitis)
- Rotator cuff tears

Pathophysiology

A bursa is a thin-walled sac lined with synovial tissue located where tendons rub against tendons. Its purpose is to act as a shock absorber and reduce friction. Bursitis is an inflammation of the synovium. Common locations include:

- Subacromial bursa: Located superior to the glenohumeral joint, above the supraspinatus muscle and below the acromion
- Olecranon bursa: Facilitates smooth movement of the skin over the olecranon during elbow flexion and extension
- Ischial bursa
- Trochanteric
- Prepatellar bursa

A tendon is a cord that attaches a muscle to a bone. Repetitive overuse causes micro tears of the tendons that become inflamed and painful. Common locations include:

- Epicondyle (tennis elbow or golf elbow)
- Rotator cuff: Consists of four muscles: subscapularis, supraspinatus, infraspinatus, and teres minor. The subacromial bursa provides lubrication for the rotator cuff. The rotator cuff is a stabilizer of the glenohumeral joint.

Factors That Increase Susceptibility

Age
Overuse
Instability of glenohumeral joint
Poorly vascularized tendons
Rotary motions of forearm
Diabetes mellitus

SUBJECTIVE DATA

History of Present Illness

Ask about:
- Dominant hand
- Frequent lifting overhead: Painting
- Frequent elbow flexing; swimming, gymnastics, weight lifting
- Direct trauma to the elbow
- Repeated rotary movements of the elbow
- Pain: Onset, location, radiation, interference with sleep
- Cause of pain: Lifting, fall, motor vehicle accident, injured at work, pulling, sports injury
- No apparent cause
- Pain with following movements: Putting on coat, combing hair, washing back, sleeping on side

TABLE 175-1 Stages of Impingement Syndrome in the Shoulder

Stage	Patients Most Likely Affected	Symptoms
Bursitis	Athletes <25 (swimmers, throwers)	Pain after exercise or activity; mild, dull achy pain
Tendinitis	Occurs most frequently in laborers ages 25-40 who reach overhead; golf and tennis elbow occur in patients who do not play on a regular basis; rare in professional athletes	Pain occurs during activity as well as after; pain vague, but increases in intensity, usually during sleep
Rotator cuff tear	Laborers >40 with long history of shoulder problems	Sudden severe episode of pain Pain occurs during, after activity, and during sleep; also complains of stiffness and weakness

Adapted from Brunet M, Norwood L, Sykes T: What to do for the painful shoulder, *Patient Care* 31(18):56-83, 1997.

Swelling
Fever
Is joint weak, stiff, or loose?
Limitations in range of motion (ROM) of affected joint
Are you able to currently work?
Relieving/aggravating factors
Treatments tried and results
Previous history of bursitis/tendinitis; any tests or injections done?

Past Medical History

Previous joint surgery of affected part
Arthritis

Medications

Use of nonsteroidal antiinflammatory drugs (NSAIDs) or other analgesics for pain
Other medications

Family History

Arthritis

Psychosocial History

History of alcohol use
History of smoking
Occupation: Mining, painting, or other occupations that require lifting or repetitive movements.

Description of Most Common Symptoms

Erythema
Pain with ROM
Swelling
Pain on palpation

OBJECTIVE DATA

Physical Examination

A focused physical examination is conducted, with particular attention to:

General: Overall appearance, response to pain
Extremities: Observe for swelling, erythema, atrophy or asymmetry
- Palpate joint area for tenderness or swelling
- Head compression test
  - Screen for cervical spine pathology; have patient sit; apply pressure gently but firmly on patient's head; pain localized to neck implies disk degeneration; burning pain or pain down shoulder or arm implies nerve root involvement: detailed neurological examination
- ROM
- Apley's scratch test
  - Have patient place arm and hand behind back to try to touch opposite scapula
- Impingement sign
  - Point of tenderness at greater tuberosity of humerus
  - Painful arc of abduction
  - Neer impingement: Bring arm into full flexion, positive with pain
  - Hawkins impingement: Positive with pain when flexing arm to 90 degrees; then bend elbow internally to rotate shoulder

Diagnostic Procedures

Diagnostic procedures are included in Tables 175-2 and 175-3.

ASSESSMENT

Differential diagnoses include those found in Table 175-4. The most likely diagnoses of shoulder pain are:

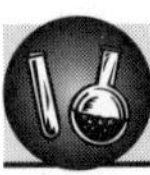

TABLE 175-2 Diagnostic Tests: Tendinitis/Bursitis

Diagnostic Test	Finding/Rationale	Cost ($)
X-ray	Not usually needed; diagnosis made on basis of physical examination; helpful in shoulder pain; rule out rotator cuff tear	106-134
MRI	May be helpful if problem is chronic or to identify rotator cuff tears or septic bursitis	Dependent on area: 1415-1670/LE; 1485-1755/UE
Arthrogram	May be helpful to diagnose rotator cuff tears	426-575
Complete blood count with differential	Helpful if septic bursitis or arthritis is a consideration	18-23
Joint aspiration	Analyze for uric acid crystals, cell count with differential, Gram stain, and cultures; white blood cell count ↑ with septic condition (70,000/mm^2 with ↑ polymorphonuclear neutrophils); culture commonly reveals *Staphylococcus aureus* (70%-100%)	31-39/culture; 26/sensitivity

LE, Lower extremity; *UE*, upper extremity.

TABLE 175-3 Physical Examination Findings Based on Etiology

Etiology	Characteristics	Key Physical Examination Tests
Subacromial/subdeltoid bursitis	Shoulder pain with insidious onset worse at night, no specific injury is recalled; overhead lifting is uncomfortable	↓ Range of motion (ROM) with ↓ elevation, internal rotation, and abduction; most painful motion is between 70 and 120 degrees of abduction; impingement sign: Forcibly forward flexing the internally rotated arm above 90 degrees; positive if pain produced
Rotator cuff injury	Pain, weakness and loss of motion; pain is ↑ with overhead or above the shoulder activities; pain worse at night (wakes from sleep) and ↑ when lying on shoulder	Anterior/lateral tenderness, assess for signs of impingement: Moving shoulder through passive ROM (forward flexion, internal and external rotation with arm abducted 90 degrees with 5-10 lb of force directed inferiorly on the acromion—narrowing the subacromial space)
Adhesive capsulitis (frozen shoulder)	Pain when putting on coat or washing back; decreased ability to go to sleep	Putting on a coat or washing the back is external rotation of the shoulder; + pain implies adhesive capsulitis
Little League shoulder	Pain with throwing motion	Injury to proximal humeral physis of an adolescent resulting from repetitive stress of throwing; later presents as tendinitis in adult
Olecranon bursitis	Tender, swollen area of redness on the back of the elbow; 40% give history of trauma to the bursa	Goose egg swelling at the tip of the elbow
Epicondylitis: medial (golf) or lateral (tennis)	Pain on medial or lateral aspect of elbow, worse by grasping; pain may radiate into arm or distally into forearm	Pain is most noticed at 1-2 cm distal to epicondyle; resisted dorsiflexion or volar flexion may ↑ pain; normal ROM, no swelling, normal x-ray
Trochanteric bursitis	Women > men, pain in lateral hip and proximal thigh; worsened when sitting in chair or car	Tenderness over the greater trochanter, pain on hip flexion and external rotation; leg length discrepancies may exist; ROM usually normal and painless
Prepatellar bursitis	Pain, swelling, and redness over knee; trigger is usually minor trauma (kneeling on floors)	Swelling over the patella, no distention of knee joint
Baker's cyst	Swelling behind knee, may have sense of fullness behind knee	Cystic swelling in popliteal space; if bursa ruptures: Acute swelling of lower leg, mimicking deep venous thrombosis

TABLE 175-4 Differential Diagnosis: Tendinitis/Bursitis

Diagnosis	Supporting Data
Arthritis/autoimmune disorders	More insidious onset, active and passive range of motion more limited in arthritis; small joints involved, progression centripetal and symmetric, deformities common; ↑ erythrocyte sedimentation rate, + antinuclear antibodies, + rheumatoid factor
Septic bursitis/ Arthritis	Most common sites olecranon and prepatellar bursae; fever, erythema, tenderness; usually present within week of developing symptoms; an overlying skin lesion may be present, as well as peribursal cellulitis; aspirate of fluid reveals *Staphylococcus aureus,* beta-hemolytic streptococcal and fungal agents; may appear ill, white blood cells ↑
Crystal deposition	Anterolateral tenderness, + impingement signs, + aspirate (crystals)
Reflex sympathetic dystrophy	Initially diffuse swelling, increased vascularity, temperature changes in involved extremity compared to uninvolved; if untreated for >3-6 months, atrophy may begin to develop; the third phase includes trophic changes, pale, cold painful extremity
Osteoarthritis	Pain relieved by rest, morning stiffness brief, articular inflammation minimal, narrowed joint space and osteophytes on x-ray, weight-bearing joints most affected
Fibromyalgia	Pain disorder, primarily affecting women 40-60 y/o; accompanied by fatigue and trigger points located near ligamentous and muscular attachments to bone; common sites include medial epicondyles and the medial aspect of the knees
Tumor	Patient presents with shoulder pain; presence of mass, history of smoking, chest x-ray may show Pancoast's tumor

- Impingement syndrome
- Bursitis: Subacromial, subdeltoid
- Tendinitis: rotator cuff, biceps tendon, calcific tendinitis
- Rotator cuff tear

Shoulder instability
Adhesive capsulitis (frozen shoulder)
Inflammation of the acromial clavicular joint

THERAPEUTIC PLAN

The treatment plan should address both pain management and facilitation of healing through rehabilitation. Use of the PRICEMM eponym may be helpful (Salzman, Lillegard, and Butcher, 1997):

- **P**rotection: Padding, braces, changes in technique to avoid future injury
- **R**est: Avoid activities that exacerbate pain
- **I**ce: Apply to affected site 20 minutes 3x/day
- **C**ompression: Ace dressings over swollen bursae (olecranon)
- **E**levation: Elevate affected limb above heart
- **M**odalities: Physical modalities: ultrasound, electric stimulation, and heat
- **M**edications: NSAIDs, acetaminophen, or injectable corticosteroids

Pharmaceutical

Pharmaceutical treatment is outlined in Table 175-5. See also detailed prescribing information on NSAIDs in Appendix J.

Myorelaxants may be helpful for pain related to muscle spasm and prescribed for short periods of time (3 to 5 days).

Lifestyle/Activity

Activity should be modified to prevent further injury
Pain should be guide as to extent of activity
ROM should be continued to prevent loss of function, especially in shoulder
Physical therapy:
- Specific exercises to strengthen the rotator cuff
- Flexibility exercises
- Ultrasound reduces inflammation by molecular vibration

Use of elbow cushion for olecranon bursitis
Hip stretching
Splinting of elbow in 90-degree flexion for epicondylitis for 3 to 5 days may be helpful
A compression band may be helpful for chronic epicondylitis
Leg length discrepancies may be part of etiology of trochanteric bursitis: shoe lifts may be helpful to reduce pain

Diet

Not applicable

Patient Education

Emphasize the importance of active rest (keep doing ROM of joint)

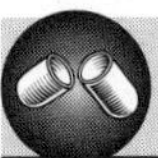

TABLE 175-5 Pharmaceutical Plan: Tendinitis/Bursitis

Drug	Dosage	Comments	Cost
Naproxen (Naprosyn)	250-500 BID	NSAIDs are indicated for musculoskeletal injury; NSAIDs inhibit prostaglandin synthesis, which decreases pain; DO NOT prescribe to those with peptic ulcer disease, allergy to NSAIDs/aspirin, renal dysfunction, or pregnant women Pregnancy: B (D if used near term)	$12-$80 /250 mg (100); $18-$126/500 mg (100); $100/SR 500 mg (75)
Ibuprofen (Motrin)	200-800 mg QID; max 3.2 g/day	See naproxen	$3-$9/200 mg (100); $4-$80/600 mg (100)
Etodolac (Lodine)	200-400 mg q6-8h	Pregnancy: C	$114/200 mg (100); $132/400 mg (100)
Diclofenac (Voltaren)	50 mg BID or TID	See naproxen	$84-$108/50 mg (100)
Acetaminophen (Tylenol)	325-650 mg q4-6h; max 5 doses/day	May be helpful in those conditions not associated with excessive inflammation Pregnancy: B SE: Rash, hepatotoxicity	$3/cap: 325 mg (24); $1/tab: 325 mg (100)

NSAID, Nonsteroidal antiinflammatory drug; *SE,* side effects.

A sling may be helpful initially (emphasize need to still do ROM of shoulder to prevent frozen shoulder)

NSAIDs

Exercises to restore normal function

- Begin with ROM exercises
- Work up to resistance exercises using rubber bands or light weights
- Resistance training with weight machines or free weights

Aerobic exercises help by increasing blood flow to site

Stop smoking

Surgery may be needed for tears to tendons when pain continues or if there is weakness

Referral

Corticosteroid injection

If conservative measures do not work in 3 to 4 weeks, consider referring to an orthopedist or collaborating MD (depending on joint involvement) for injection:

- Give no more than three injections in 12-week period
- Do not repeat series in less than 12 months from last injection

Surgery

- Consider referral to an orthopedist for surgery if no improvement in 3 months of therapy
- Arthroscopy to debride subacromial space

Rehabilitation exercises

Consultation

Discuss options of steroid injection

EVALUATION

Return as close as possible to normal ROM and pain free status

REFERENCE

Salzman K, Lillegard W, Butcher J: Upper extremity bursitis, *Am Family Physician* 56(7):1797-1808, 1997.

SUGGESTED READINGS

Benjamin J: Hip pain. In Greene H, Johnson W, Maricic M, editors: *Decision making in medicine*, St Louis, 1993, Mosby.

Brunet M, Norwood L, Sykes T: What to do for the painful shoulder, *Patient Care* 31:56-83, 1997.

Burckhardt C, Jones K, Clark S: Soft tissue problems associated with rheumatic disease, *Lippincott's Primary Care Pract* 2(1):20-29, 1998.

Ellsworth A et al: *Mosby's 1998 medical drug reference*, St Louis, 1998, Mosby.

Healthcare Consultants of America, Inc: *1998 physicians fee and coding guide*, Augusta, Ga, 1998, Healthcare Consultants of America, Inc.

Fongemie A, Buss D, Rolnick S: Management of shoulder impingement syndrome and rotator cuff tears, *Am Family Physician* 57(4):667-678, 1998.

Genovese M: Joint and soft tissue injections: a useful adjuvant to systemic and local treatment, *Postgrad Med* 103(2)125-128, 130-134, 225-228, 1998.

Rotator cuff injury: when your shoulder throws you a curve, *Mayo Clin Health Lett* 16(2):1-3, 1998.

Reveille J: Soft tissue rheumatism: diagnosis and treatment, *Am J Med* 102(1A):23S-29S, 1997.

Salzman K, Lillegard W, Butcher J: Lower extremity bursitis, *Am Family Physician* 55:2317-2324, 1996.

176 Testicular/Scrotal Mass

ICD-9-CM

Hydrocele 603.9
Varicocele 456.4
Testicular Cancer 186.9

OVERVIEW

Definition

A hydrocele is a result of the collection of fluid between the two layers of the tunica vaginalis in the scrotum. A varicocele is the result of dilation of the veins in the spermatic cord. Testicular cancer is a tumor of the testicles.

Incidence

Hydroceles are most common in **infants** but can form as a result of testicular pathology in adult men

Varicoceles are most common in **older boys** and **adolescents** and are rare before puberty they are present in up to 20% of all males

Testicular cancer is most common in **young men** with an average age of 32; it represents 1% of all cancers in males

Pathophysiology

Hydroceles are described as communicating and noncommunicating. In a communicating hydrocele the processus vaginalis is patent between the peritoneal cavity and the tunica vaginalis, allowing the peritoneal fluid to shift back and forth through this opening. In a noncommunicating hydrocele the processus vaginalis has closed, but there is residual fluid in the tunica vaginalis.

Communicating hydroceles can be associated with inguinal hernias and usually occur at birth or in the **neonatal** period.

Hydroceles in adulthood are usually associated with testicular pathology.

Varicoceles are caused by incompetent valves of the internal spermatic venous system. Left-sided varicoceles are most common, with an unknown etiology. Right-sided varicoceles may represent acute venous obstruction from a tumor or intraabdominal pathology.

Varicoceles are associated with male infertility. The exact cause is unknown but is speculated to be a result of alteration of scrotal temperature secondary to increased blood flow, which affects spermatogenesis and sperm motility.

Approximately 97% of testicular tumors are germinal in origin. Seminoma is the most common, followed by embryonal cell carcinoma, teratoma, and choriocarcinoma. Testicular tumors spread along the lymphatic system in predictable and preferential pathways.

There is a significant increase in the incidence of testicular cancer in patients with cryptorchidism (undescended testicles). Cancer can develop in both the undescended and the contralateral descended testis.

SUBJECTIVE DATA

History of Present Illness

Hydrocele

Inquire about onset and duration, constant or intermittent pattern of scrotal swelling, pain, color change.

Inquire about associated swelling or mass in the inguinal area.

A communicating hydrocele in an **infant** will often present with progressive swelling throughout the day only to resolve overnight.

A new onset of a hydrocele in an adult or scrotal hemorrhage after minor trauma may be a sign of testicular cancer.

Varicocele

Inquire about onset and duration; pattern of swelling, including intermittent or constant, left-sided or right-sided swelling; pain, including heaviness

Often described as feeling like a bag of worms

Most varicoceles are asymptomatic

Inquire about associated infertility if appropriate

Testicular Cancer

Inquire about:

- Onset and duration, increasing size of mass, presence of pain
- Associated symptoms of a hydrocele or hemorrhage from trauma
- The practice of testicular self-examination

Past Medical History

Inquire about past genitourinary surgeries or history of an undescended testis

OBJECTIVE DATA

Physical Examination

Assess for gynecomastia.

Perform an abdominal examination.

Palpate the inguinal area for swelling, masses, or pain. Assess for lymphadenopathy.

Inspect scrotum and testes for size, shape, symmetry, swelling, masses, lesions, and color both in a supine and standing position.

Palpate each testes specifically for the epididymis and vas deferens.

Assess swelling or masses by transillumination.

Diagnostic Procedures

Diagnostic procedures are outlined in Table 176-1.

ASSESSMENT

Figure 176-1 summarizes the relationship between diagnostic procedures and findings.

A hydrocele is most common in the **pediatric** age group and is a fluid collection between the two layers of the tunica vaginalis in the scrotum. A new onset of a hydrocele in an adult is often associated with testicular pathology.

A varicocele is most common in **adolescents** and is a result of dilated veins in the spermatic cord. It can be associated with infertility in adulthood.

Testicular cancer is a tumor of the testis and is most common in **young men.**

Differential diagnoses are outlined in Table 176-2.

THERAPEUTIC PLAN

Nonpharmaceutical

In **infancy,** a hydrocele usually resolves spontaneously during the first year of life and requires no specific therapy. Hydroceles produce brilliant transillumination.

If the hydrocele is associated with an inguinal hernia, referral to a surgeon is indicated at any age.

An adult with a hydrocele will need further evaluation to rule out testicular pathology. An ultrasound ($265 to $316) may be indicated.

Varicocele

Most varicoceles are asymptomatic and do not require treatment.

If pain is present, causing a dull ache or heavy sensation, refer for surgical evaluation.

A right-sided varicocele warrants evaluation of an intraabdominal obstruction at **any age.**

A left-sided varicocele with a sudden onset in an **older man** warrants evaluation for a possible renal tumor, with resultant occlusion of the spermatic vein.

If infertility is a concern and the patient has an abnormal semen evaluation, refer for surgical correction.

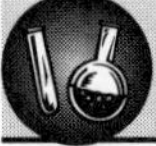

TABLE 176-1 Diagnotic Tests: Testicular/Scrotal Mass

Test	Findings	Cost ($)
Ultrasonography	Differentiates fluid from solid masses, intratesticular from extratesticular masses	259-319
Tumor marker screenings Serum alpha fetoprotein Human chorionic gonadotropin (HCG) Lactic dehydrogenase	Differentiates origin of testicular tumors	52-65/AFP; 20-25/LDH; 18-24/HCG
Semen analysis	Indicated when a patient has a varicocele and infertility is questioned	63-77

Testicular Cancer

Patient with a suspicious testicular mass may or may not have associated gynecomastia.

Testicular cancer does not transilluminate and is free of fixation from the scrotum.

The tumor often replaces the testicle making it difficult to discern on examination.

Ultrasound is indicated to help define suspicious masses.

Abdominal computerized tomographic (CT) scan may be indicated for staging of disease.

Chest films and a CT scan of the lungs may also be indicated to assess for metastatic disease.

Surgical management of testicular cancer consists of radical orchiectomy with high ligation of the spermatic cord via an inguinal approach.

Serum alpha-fetoprotein and human chorionic gonadotropin

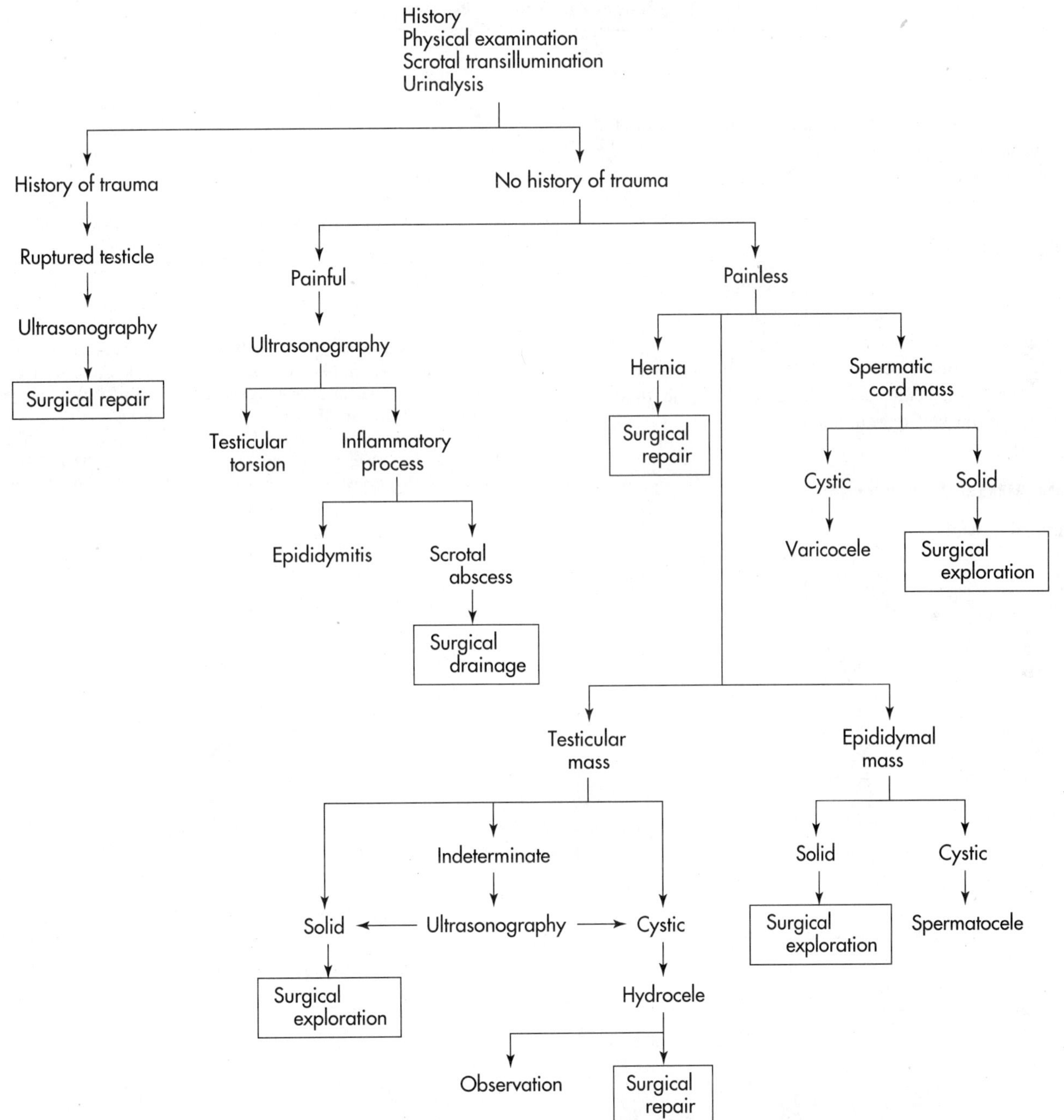

Figure 176-1 Algorithm for adult patient with scrotal mass. (Adapted from Greene HL, Johnson WP, Lemcke D: *Decision making in medicine*, ed 2, St. Louis, 1998, Mosby.)

TABLE 176-2 Differential Diagnosis: Testicular/Scrotal Mass

Differential Diagnosis	Supporting Data
Inguinal hernia	Commonly associated with a scrotal mass
Testicular torsion	Sudden onset of severe scrotal pain caused by twisting of the testicular appendages
Epididymitis	Most common cause of painful scrotal swelling in postpubertal males; associated with fever, urethral discharge, and urinary symptoms, including pyuria
Acute orchitis	Red, warm, painful, sudden swelling of the testes associated with viral parotitis (mumps)
Spermatocele	Cyst that contains sperm that is well-circumscribed, does not transilluminate, and persists when the patient is supine
Cryptorchidism	Failure of the testes to descend into the scrotum

levels, if previously elevated, can be followed to determine recurrence of disease.

Five-year survival rate exceeds 90% in most cases.

Patient Education

Educate parents about the benign nature of hydroceles

Educate parents and adolescents about varicoceles and the possible association of infertility. Caution adolescents about the importance of appropriate birth control.

Educate all adolescent and adult males about the importance of testicular self-examination.

Consultation/Referral

Surgical consult.

EVALUATION/FOLLOW-UP

Depends on diagnosis, age of onset, and associated symptoms

SUGGESTED READINGS

Junnila J, Lassen P: Testicular masses, *Am Family Physician* 57(4):685-692, 1998.

Ellsworth A et al: *Mosby's 1998 medical drug reference*, St Louis, 1998, Mosby.

Healthcare Consultants of America Inc: *1998 physicians fee and coding guide*, Augusta, Ga, 1998, Healthcare Consultants of America Inc.

Graham MV, Uphold CR: *Clinical guidelines in child health,* Gainesville, Fla, 1994, Barmarrae Books.

Gray M: *Genitourinary disorders*, St Louis, 1992, Mosby.

Hoekelman RA: *Primary pediatric care*, ed 2, St Louis, 1992, Mosby.

Hoekelman RA: *Primary pediatric care*, ed 3, St Louis, 1997, Mosby.

Thrombophlebitis

Superficial and Deep Venous Thrombophlebitis

ICD-9-CM

Phlebitis and Thrombosis 451.9
Phlebitis and Thrombosis of Superficial Vessels of Lower Extremities 451.0
Phlebitis and Thrombosis of Deep Vessels of Lower Extremities 451.19

OVERVIEW

Definition

Superficial

Partial or complete occlusion of a superficial vein by a thrombus, accompanied by inflammatory changes in the wall of the vein

Deep Vein

The partial or complete occlusion in the deep venous system by a thrombus with inflammatory changes in the wall of the vein

Incidence

A common vascular disorder that is diagnosed in up to 800,000 new patients per year. More common in women; all races affected equally; increases with advancing age. Although thrombophlebitis does occur in **children,** the incidence is low.

Pathophysiology

Protective Factors Against

Body's natural fibrinolytic system to prevent thrombus formation

Factors that Increase Susceptibility

Stasis of blood flow; endothelial injury; hypercoagulability

Conditions Associated with Increased Risk

Trauma
Old age
Varicosities
Prior thrombophlebitis
Immobility or paralysis
Cancer
Congestive heart failure
Myocardial infarction (MI)
Abdominal, pelvic, and lower extremity surgery
Obesity
Pregnancy
Oral contraceptives and hormone replacement therapy
Inherited disorders such as antithrombin III deficiency, protein C deficiency, sickle cell anemia, and polycythemia

Common Sites

Superficial: The greater or lesser saphenous veins or their tributaries are most often involved.

Deep Vein: The calf veins are most frequently affected but the popliteal, femoral, and iliofemorals are also common (Figure 177-1).

SUBJECTIVE DATA

History of Present Illness

Superficial thrombophlebitis: Question about current or recent pregnancy, varicose veins, or recent trauma such as a blow to the region or recent intravenous therapy

Ask about a dull pain in the region of the involved vein

Past Medical History

Question about conditions that predispose to immobility such as surgery, sedentary lifestyle, MI, or stroke. Inquire concerning previous superficial or deep vein thrombophlebitis (DVT), pregnancy, recent childbirth, or coagulopathies.

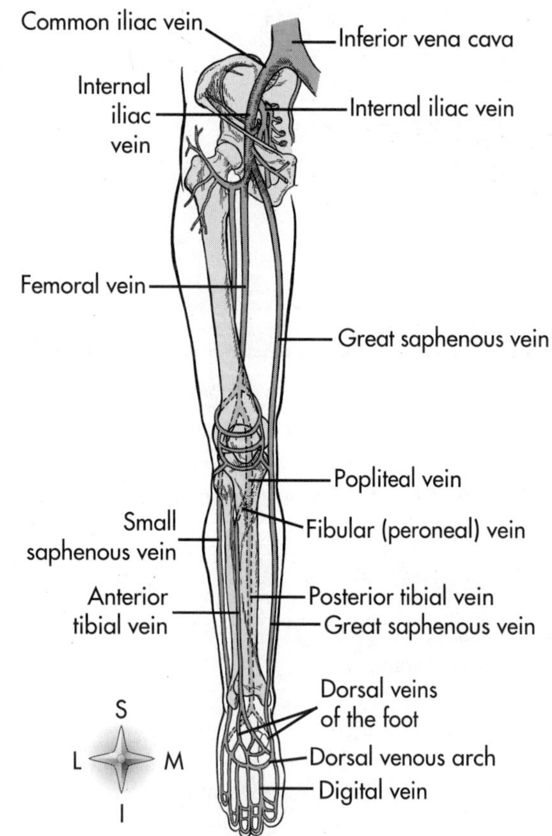

Figure 177-1 Major veins of the lower extremity. (From Thibodeau GA, Patton KT: *Anatomy and physiology*, ed 4, St. Louis, 1999, Mosby.)

Medications

Recent use of oral contraceptives or hormone replacement therapy

Family History

Ask about a family history of blood clotting disorders, varicose veins or DVTs

Psychosocial History

Tobacco use

Description of Most Common Symptoms

Superficial Thrombophlebitis

Induration, redness, and tenderness along a superficial vein. A tender palpable cord and/or low-grade fever may be present.

Deep Vein Thrombophlebitis

The physical signs for diagnosing DVTs are unreliable. Calf pain, tenderness, unilateral swelling, low-grade fever, warmth, erythema, engorged, prominent superficial veins, and pain during dorsiflexion (Homans' sign) may occur but are nonspecific. In the early stages approximately 50% of patients with DVT have no symptoms or signs in the extremity. Pulmonary embolism may be the first clinical indication of thrombosis.

Associated Symptoms

Slight fever and tachycardia; skin may be cyanotic if venous obstruction is severe or pale and cool if a reflex arterial spasm is superimposed

OBJECTIVE DATA

Physical Examination

A problem-oriented physical examination should be conducted, with particular attention to:

Vital signs, including temperature
Skin: Check for cyanosis, diaphoresis, paleness, or coolness
Lungs: Listen for crackles
Heart: Auscultate for accentuation of the pulmonary component of the second heart sound
Lower extremities: Examine for thigh or calf tenderness on palpation, warmth, erythema, swelling and palpable cord; palpate femoral, popliteal, post-tibial and pedal pulses
Feel for enlarged, tender inguinal lymph nodes; test for Homans' sign (considered unreliable by some sources)

Diagnostic Procedures

Deep Vein Thrombophlebitis

First line: Refer for venous Doppler studies: Measure blood flow and detect venous obstruction; good sensitivity and specificity ($257 to $300)

Second line: Venography is considered one of the most accurate means for diagnosis of deep vein thrombosis ($613 to $738)

Superficial Thrombophlebitis

Readily diagnosed on physical examination; if there is suspicion of progression toward the saphenofemoral junction or the process is not well localized, venous Doppler studies are indicated (Table 177-1)

ASSESSMENT

Differential diagnoses include:

Superficial: Calf muscle strain, cellulitis, severe muscle cramp, or trauma

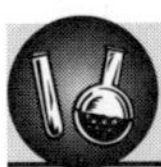

TABLE 177-1 **Diagnostic Tests: Superficial Thrombophlebitis**

Symptoms	Findings	Diagnostic Tests	Cost ($)
Dull pain in the area of the involved vein	Induration, redness, and tenderness along a superficial vein; a tender, palpable cord and/or low-grade fever may be present	Venous Doppler studies if indicated	257-300, but operator-dependent
Dull ache, a tight feeling, or frank pain in the calf or whole leg, especially when walking	Calf tenderness, unilateral swelling, low-grade fever, warmth, erythema, engorged, prominent superficial veins Positive Homans' sign may be present	Venous Doppler studies Venography is useful when the clinical picture strongly suggests calf vein thrombosis, but venous Doppler studies are inconclusive	As above 613-738, risky and uncomfortable
Abrupt onset of dyspnea, chest pain, apprehension, hemoptysis, or syncope; may or may not be accompanied by symptoms of DVT	Tachycardia, tachypnea, crackles, and accentuation of the pulmonary component of the second heart sound	Chest x-ray Ventilation/perfusion scan Venous Doppler studies	77-91 890-1100, cost-effective As above

Deep vein: Ruptured calf muscle, Baker's cyst, trauma, cellulitis, lymphedema, or acute arterial occlusion (Table 177-2)

THERAPEUTIC PLAN

Pharmaceutical

Treatment for thrombophlebitis is based on whether there is a superficial or deep vein thrombosis.

Superficial, well-localized and not near the saphenofemoral junction (Table 177-3).

Deep vein thrombosis or superficial thrombosis that is not well localized or near the saphenofemoral junction require a physician referral/ hospitalization for initiation of antithrombotic therapy (Table 177-4).

Oral anticoagulant therapy for DVT (initial episode without complications) is 3 months' duration. If this is the second episode, oral anticoagulant therapy is ongoing. See Chapter 12 for more complete details on anticoagulant therapy.

Lifestyle/Activities

Leg exercises, compression stockings, and walking for brief but regular periods and during long airplane and automobile trips

Discontinue oral contraceptives or hormone replacement therapy

Smoking cessation

Diet

Weight loss if indicated

Patient Education

Overview of the disease process, causes, and risk factors and the potential side effects of the prescribed medications

Proper use of compression stockings, avoid leg crossing at knees and prolonged inactivity, including sitting and standing; need for a balance of exercise/rest; effects of oral contraceptives and hormone replacement therapy on blood clotting; hazards of smoking

If on oral anticoagulants, see Chapter 12

Family Impact

See Chapter 12. Families with numerous members who have had DVT should be evaluated via genetic studies. Family members with this history should be aware that they are more at risk for initial and recurrent DVTs.

Referral

Superficial: Phlebitis of a varicose vein is generally an indication for surgical removal

Deep vein: Requires a physician referral and hospitalization

Pregnant women: Should be followed by OB/GYN as well

Children: Should be followed by a pediatrician

TABLE 177-2 Differential Diagnosis: Thrombophlebitis

Diagnoses	Supporting Data
Superficial thrombophlebitis	Linear lesion distributed along a superficial vein; a firm cord may be felt; edema and deep calf tenderness usually absent; positive venous Doppler studies
Deep vein thrombophlebitis	*Physical signs are unreliable;* calf pain, tenderness, unilateral swelling, engorged, prominent superficial veins; pulmonary embolism may be the first clinical indication of thrombosis; positive venous Doppler studies; positive venography if venous Doppler studies inconclusive; positive lung perfusion scan if pulmonary emboli suspected
Calf muscle strain, severe muscle cramp	Difficult to differentiate from thrombophlebitis; negative venous Doppler studies
Cellulitis, trauma	Usually an associated wound; inflammation of the skin is more marked and in a circular pattern; negative venous Doppler studies
Baker's Cyst	History of arthritis in the knee of the same leg On examination may find a palpable, cystic mass in the medial aspect of the popliteal fossa; impaired knee flexion; negative venous Doppler studies
Lymphedema	Unilateral swelling more chronic and painless; venous Doppler studies
Acute arterial occlusion	More painful; distal pulses are absent; usually no swelling; superficial veins in the foot fill slowly when emptied; negative venous Doppler studies

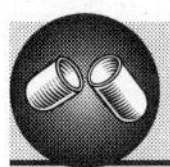

TABLE 177-3 Pharmaceutical Plan: Superficial Thrombosis

Drug	Adult Dose	Child Dose	Prophylaxis
Aspirin or other nonsteroidal anti-inflammatory drugs (NSAIDs); see Appendix J for more complete NSAID therapy information	Doses used to suppress inflammation are considerably larger than the doses used for analgesia or reduction of fever	Drug dependent; several are contraindicated in children; should be avoided entirely by children with flu or varicella symptoms	None

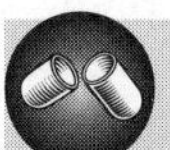

TABLE 177-4 Pharmaceutical Plan: Deep Vein Thrombosis

Drug	Adult Dose	Child Dose	Prophylaxis
Heparin*: Initial therapy with continuous or intermittent intravenous therapy (Pregnancy: C)	Titrate to keep activated partial thromboplastin time (APTT) between 1.5 and 2.5 times control	Titrate to keep APTT between 1.5 and 2.5 times control	Low-dose heparin is used to prevent postoperative venous thrombosis
Warfarin* (Pregnancy: X)	Titrate to maintain international normalized ratio (INR) between 2 and 3, the current recommended therapeutic range for deep vein thrombophlebitis (DVT) treatment and prophylaxis	Titrate to maintain INR between 2 and 3, the current recommended therapeutic range for DVT treatment and prophylaxis	Titrate to maintain INR between 2 and 3, the current recommended therapeutic range for DVT prophylaxis

*The current accepted therapeutic approach is to begin heparin and oral anticoagulants together at the time of diagnosis. Heparin is discontinued once patient is fully anticoagulated with warfarin.

Consultation

Consult with MD on any patient in whom you suspect DVT or nonlocal superficial thrombophlebitis, all **pregnant women,** and all **children.**

Follow-up

Superficial: Follow-up for symptom assessment
Deep vein: Patient should be managed in consultation with a physician

EVALUATION

All adults: Directed physical examination; migrating superficial thrombophlebitis may be a marker for a carcinoma and requires investigation

All patients on oral anticoagulant: See Chapter 12

Children: Hypercoagulability studies

Pregnant women: Should be followed by an OB/GYN

SUGGESTED READINGS

Creager MA, Dzau VJ: Vascular diseases of the extremities. In Isselbacher KJ et al, editors: *Harrison's principles of internal medicine*, ed 13, New York, 1994, McGraw-Hill.

Eftychiou V: Clinical diagnosis and management of the patient with deep venous thromboembolism and acute pulmonary embolism, *Nurse Pract* 21(3):50-62, 1996.

Ellsworth A et al: *Mosby's 1998 medical drug reference*, St Louis, 1998, Mosby.

Healthcare Consultants of America, Inc: *1998 physicians fee and coding guide*, Augusta, Ga, 1998, Healthcare Consultants of America, Inc.

Feied C, Stephen J: Venous thrombosis: lifting the clouds of misunderstanding, *Postgrad Med* 97(1):36-47, 1995.

Spittell JA, Spittell PC: Diseases of peripheral arteries and veins. In Alpert JS, editor: *Cardiology for the primary care physician*, ed 1, Philadelphia, 1996, Current Medicine.

Tierney L, Messina L: Blood vessels and lymphatics. In Tierney L, McPhee S, Papadakis M, editors: *Current medical diagnosis and treatment*, ed 37, Stamford, Conn, 1997, Appleton & Lange.

Uphold C, Graham M: *Clinical guidelines in family practice*, Gainesville, Fla, 1994, Barmarrae Books.

178 Thyroid Disorders

ICD-9-CM

Acquired Hypothyroid 244.9
Iatrogenic Hypothyroidism 244.3
Postsurgical Hypothyroid 244.0
Follicular Carcinoma of the Thyroid 193.0
Acute Thyroiditis 245.0
Toxic Diffuse Goiter 242.0
Hyperthyroidism 242.9
Hashimoto's Thyroiditis 245.2
Postpartum Thyroiditis 648.1

OVERVIEW

Definition

Hypothyroidism is defined as the undersecretion of thyroid hormone T3 and T4. It is termed cretinism when it causes brain damage as a congenital condition, and myxedema when it is a life-threatening complication of hypothyroidism in adults.

Hyperthyroidism is defined as the oversecretion of thyroid hormone.

Thyroid nodules refer to a tumor that occurs in a normal thyroid.

Incidence

Hyperthyroidism and hypothyroidism have a prevalence of 0.5% in the general population, but have a higher prevalence in selected groups. **Adults** have an incidence of approximately 11% to 15% of hypothyroidism. 85% of all cases of thyroid disease occur in women.

Postmenopausal women are more at risk for developing hypothyroidism. About 2% of the adult population has hyperthyroidism, most often in young women, although it can occur in men and at any age. **Children:** Approximately 1 in 500 children is treated for hypothyroidism in the United States.

Thyroid nodules occur in 2% to 3% of **adults,** usually three to four times more often in women than in men. There is a 5% to 10% lifetime risk for developing a palpable thyroid nodule. Only 5% of palpable thyroid nodules are malignant.

Pathophysiology

Two thyroid hormones are produced by the body, T3 and T4. Production and release of T4 by the thyroid is regulated by the anterior pituitary gland by the means of thyroid-stimulating hormone (TSH). Increases in T4 or T3 result in decreased production of TSH, whereas decreases in T4 or T3 result in increased TSH production. TSH production is primarily regulated by thyrotropin-releasing hormone (TRH), which is produced by the hypothalamus. These mechanisms produce a negative feedback loop maintaining T4 and T3 within therapeutic ranges.

Primary Hypothyroidism

Insufficient quantity of thyroid tissue or loss of functional thyroid tissue due to iatrogenic causes such as thyroidectomy or autoimmune responses (Hashimoto's disease)

Secondary Hypothyroidism

Less common, usually occurring along with other anterior pituitary deficiencies, and is most often caused by a pituitary tumor

Hyperthyroidism

Increased level of thyroid secretion, usually due to an autoimmune disorder in which the body produces thyroid-stimulating antibodies against TSH receptors on the thyroid cells, pathologically stimulating the thyroid cells (Graves disease). Graves disease is the cause of hyperthyroidism in approximately 90% of cases. Various types of thyroiditis cause the other 10% of hyperthyroidism cases.

Box 178-1

Common Symptoms of Hypothyroidism

Congenital

Infrequent crying
Hypoactivity
Poor feeding
Inconsistent bowel habits
Lethargy
Temperature instability

Adult

Early

Fatigue
Dry skin
Weight gain
Cold intolerance
Constipation
Heavy menstrual flow
Headache

Later

Excessively dry skin
Coarse hair texture
Alopecia
Increased weight gain
Decrease in mental awareness
Depression
Pain/swelling in neck
Hoarseness

Myxedema

Thick, dry, scaly skin
Enlarged tongue
Muscle weakness
Joint pain

Thyroid Nodules

Nodules on the thyroid are usually a thyroid adenoma, thyroid cyst, or thyroid carcinoma. Of these, only thyroid cancer poses a risk to the patient.

Factors That May Contribute to Thyroid Disorders

Newborns
Strong familial history of thyroid disease
Postpartum period
History of autoimmune disorders
Iatrogenic, surgery, x-ray treatments
Medications
Thyroid carcinoma: Men, young age, history of neck irradiation, positive family history
Obesity

Box 178-2

Signs and Symptoms of Hypothyroidism and Hyperthyroidism

Hypothyroid (in Order of Occurrence)	Hyperthyroid (in Order of Occurrence)
Weakness	Goiter
Dry skin	Dyspnea on exertion
Coarse skin	Tiredness
Lethargy	Hot hands
Slow speech	Palpitations
Edema of eyelids	Preference for cold
Sensation of cold	Hands sweating
Decreased sweating	Excessive sweating
Cold skin	Regular pulse rate over 90 beats/min
Thick tongue	Finger tremor
Edema of face	Lid lag
Coarseness of hair	"Nervousness"
Cardiac enlargement (x-ray)	Weight loss
Pallor of skin	Goiter, diffuse enlargement of thyroid gland
Memory impairment	Hyperkinesis
Constipation	Exophthalmos
Gain in weight	Goiter, nodular
Loss of hair	Increased appetite
Pallor of lips	Atrial fibrillation
Dyspnea	Scanty menses
Peripheral edema	Constipation
Hoarseness of aphonia	Diminished appetite
Anorexia	Diarrhea
Nervousness	Weight gain
Menorrhagia	Goiter, single adenoma
Palpitation	Excessive menses
Deafness	
Poor heart sounds	
Precordial pain	
Poor vision	
Fundus oculi changes	
Dysmenorrhea	
Loss of weight	
Atrophic tongue	
Emotional instability	

SUBJECTIVE DATA

Past Medical History

Allergies
Last menstrual period and characteristics
Past neck irradiation
Past thyroid problems

Medications

Taking any iodine containing medication or antithyroid medication during pregnancy
Kelp products

Family History

Ask about other family members with endocrine disorders

Psychosocial History

Ask about smoking, alcohol, substance use
Ask about ability to function in school, workplace

Diet History

Ask about the type of diet the patient usually eats: 24-hour recall

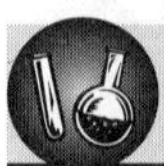

TABLE 178-1 Diagnostic Tests: Thyroid Disorders

Test	Findings	Cost ($)
Screening: TSH (sensitive assay) Do not use TSH if lower limit is 0; need sensitive test that can detect small amounts above 0	Hypothyroid: High in primary, low in secondary Hyperthyroid: Suppressed Nodules: Indicates thyroid dysfunction	56-70
T_3, T_4	Hyperthyroid: Elevated Hypothyroid: Decreased Screen done of all newborns in United States	47-61/thyroid panel
Thyroid antibody titers (antithyroglobulin and antimicrosomal)	Usually high in Hashimoto's thyroiditis	Not available
Iodine uptake and scan	Hyperthyroid: Increased diffuse areas vs "hot" areas, less valuable since FNA	356-428
Specific genetic testing/calcitonin	In patients with family history of medullary carcinoma, genetic testing and a calcitonin should be done	315-695/genetic; 84-105/calcitonin
Fine-needle aspiration (FNA)	Best diagnostic method for thyroid cancer	440-521
Ultrasound	Identifies solid vs. cystic nodules; pure cysts are not usually malignant; preferred over computed tomography or magnetic resonance imaging due to lower cost and ease of test; however, does not determine if nodule is malignant; not usually recommended unless used to guide FNA	309-365
Electrolytes, blood urea nitrogen, creatinine, glucose, calcium	Baseline tests	32-42/comprehensive metabolic panel
Lipids	May see increase in cholesterol in hypothyroid	49-62
Complete blood count	Anemia may be seen in hypothyroid	18-23
Other tests as appropriate for autoimmune diseases	Antinuclear antibodies, fasting blood glucose	42-52/ANA; 16-20/FBG

FNA, Fine-needle aspiration.

Description of Most Common Symptoms

Hypothyroidism

Common symptoms of hypothyroidism are described in Box 178-1.

Hyperthyroidism

Nervousness: Irritability, decreased concentration, restless, tremor
Weight loss, despite increased appetite, **elderly:** Anorexia
Heat intolerance: Sweating
Skin changes: Silky, hyperpigmentation over joints
Menstrual: Oligomenorrhea or amenorrhea
Hair loss: **Women:** Thinning of scalp
Neck mass
Eyes: Bulging
Shortness of breath
Symptoms of heart failure: Palpitations, angina
Gastrointestinal: Loose stools

Thyroid Nodules

Neck mass: A pattern of growth over weeks or months
Neck discomfort
Hoarseness
Dysphagia

OBJECTIVE DATA

Physical Examination

A problem-oriented physical should be conducted, with particular attention to vital signs and weight

Hypothyroidism

General appearance
  Slow movements, lethargy, and irritability
Head/eyes/ears/nose/throat
  Hair texture: Coarse
  Inspect neck/thyroid
  Dull facies
  Puffiness of face and eyelids
  Thickening of tongue
Cardiovascular: Cardiomegaly, slow heart rate
Abdominal: Decreased bowel sounds
Neurological: Delayed deep tendon reflexes, persistently opened posterior fontanelle, large anterior fontanel

TABLE 178-2 Interpreting Thyroid Function Test Results

TSH	T_4	T_3	Cause
High	Low	Low or normal	Primary hypothyroidism
Mildly high	Normal	Normal	Subclinical hypothyroidism
Normal	Low	Low or normal	Secondary hypothyroidism
Normal	High	High	Estrogen use or pregnancy
Low	High	High	Primary hyperthyroidism
Low	Normal	Normal	Subclinical hyperthyroidism

Skin: Plaques with sharp raised margin, complains of pruritus, "doughy-feeling" skin

Infant: Symptoms may appear as early as 2 weeks, but some newborns may be asymptomatic for up to 1 month; irreversible mental changes may occur before symptoms become evident

Evaluate for other autoimmune diseases since they frequently cluster together:
- Arthritis
- Systemic lupus erythematosus
- Diabetes mellitus
- Hypoparathyroid

Hyperthyroidism

Eyes
- Forward protrusion of globe
- Lid lag
- Stare
- Limitation in ability to converge

Thyroid
- Enlargement or asymmetric, goiter (often with bruit)
- **Young:** Enlargement
- **Elderly:** May not find enlargement
- Bruit

Cardiovascular
- Sinus tachycardia
- Atrial fibrillation
- Systolic flow murmurs
- Cardiac failure

Thyroid Nodule

Neck
- Enlargement: Give patient a drink of water; observe anterior neck during swallowing; the thyroid moves up with swallowing and may be visible in a thin neck; enlargement or asymmetry may be noted
- Best palpation: From behind neck; note any nodules, location, size, firmness, and tenderness, consistency, movement
- Check for lymphadenopathy and bruits

See Box 178-2 for symptoms and signs of hypothyroidism and hyperthyroidism.

TABLE 178-3 Differential Diagnosis: Hypothyroidism

Diagnoses	Supporting Data
Heart failure	Shortness of breath, peripheral edema, paroxysmal nocturnal dyspnea, hepatosplenomegaly
Depression	Feelings of sadness, guilt, low self-esteem, worthlessness, apathy, pessimistic thoughts, fearfulness, anxiety, and irritability, poor hygiene, psychomotor retardation, decreased libido, fatigue, constipation, sleep disturbances (insomnia or hypersomnia), changes in appetite with either weight gain or loss, impaired concentration, indecisiveness, and impaired cognitive reasoning
Nephrotic syndrome	Fatigue, weakness, malaise, anorexia, nausea and vomiting, decreased ability to concentrate, insomnia, irritability, restless legs, twitching. In later stages may see decreased libido, menstrual irregularities, pruritus, easy bruising
Liver disease	Fatigue, easy bruising, abdominal pain, jaundice, nausea and vomiting, flulike syndrome

Diagnostic Procedures

Diagnostic procedures are outlined in Tables 178-1 and 178-2.

ASSESSMENT

Differential diagnoses for hypothyroidism and hyperthyroidism are outlined in Tables 178-3 and 178-4.

Thyroid nodules
- Diagnosis primarily concerned with malignancy vs. benign nodule
- Types of malignancy include papillary, follicular, anaplastic and medullary (Table 178-5)

THERAPEUTIC PLAN

Pharmaceutical

Pharmaceutical treatment for hypothyroidism is outlined in Table 178-6. Treatment for Graves' disease involves a choice of the methods found in Box 178-3. Must treat with levothyroxine after patient becomes euthyroid

Nonpharmaceutical

Nodules
- Referral to surgeon for fine-needle aspiration (FNA)
- Most nodules are benign
- In **pregnancy,** nodules should be managed the same as in nonpregnant women
- **Children:** Nodules are less common in children and probably more often malignant than those in adults

Lifestyle/Activities

No restrictions

TABLE 178-4 Differential Diagnosis: Hyperthyroidism

Diagnoses	Supporting Data
Cancer	Hypermetabolism caused by various kinds of cancer: confusion is rarely noted
Cardiac	Atrial fibrillation refractory to treatment might be caused by underlying hyperthyroidism
Psychological problems	Anxiety or mania but thyroid not enlarged and thyroid function tests normal
Tremors: neurological problem	Rule out essential, physiological, cerebellar, or senile tremor

Diet

No special diet
Avoid constipation by eating a high-fiber diet
Weight loss diet if overweight
Decreased fat/cholesterol diet if hyperlipidemic

Patient Education

Congenital hypothyroidism
- Educate the family concerning the disease process and importance of early treatment to prevent brain damage and ensure normal physical growth
- Emphasize the importance of follow-up to obtain a euthyroid level

Adult hypothyroidism
- Educate the family concerning the side effects of medication and the signs and symptoms of hyperthyroidism
- Alert families to genetic component of thyroid disorders
- Alert families to increased oxygen needs of elderly patients: seek help right away if they experience chest pain

Hyperthyroidism
- Symptoms of thyroid storm (complication of increased thyroid level: symptoms include tachycardia, fever, nervousness, cardiovascular collapse, angina) and need for medical emergency care, fluids, beta blockers

Family Impact

The family may feel reassured knowing that the symptoms seen in their loved one were due to thyroid dysfunction.

If radioactive iodine is chosen as treatment, there will be no exposure to family members if preventive steps are taken.

Consultation/Referral

Congenital hypothyroidism: Refer to physician, pediatric endocrinologist

TABLE 178-5 Differential Diagnosis: Thyroid Nodules

Data	Low Index of Suspicion for Cancer	High Index of Suspicion for Cancer
History	Positive family history of goiter, lives in area with endemic goiters	Previous radiation to head/neck or chest, complains of hoarseness
Physical examination	Older women, soft nodule, multinodular goiter	Young adults, men, solitary, firm nodule, vocal cord paralysis, enlarged lymph nodes
Fine-needle aspiration	Colloid nodule or adenoma	One of four types of cancer: papillary, follicular, medullary, or anaplastic
Scan	"Hot" lesion, cystic lesion	"Cold" nodule, solid lesion
Thyroxine therapy	Regression after treatment for >6 mos	Increase in size

Modified from Fitzgerald P: Endocrinology. In Tierney L, McPhee S, Papadakis M, editors: *Current medical diagnosis, treatment*, ed 37, Stamford, Conn, 1998, Appleton & Lange.

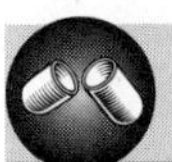

TABLE 178-6 Pharmaceutical Plan: Hypothyroid

Medications	Dose	Comments	Cost
Levothyroxine (drug of choice) (Synthroid) (Levoxyl) (Levothyroid) Half-life 7 days; do not substitute generic brands	50-100 μg daily, increasing by 25 μg every 1-3 weeks until stabilization (female: 0.05-0.075 mg; male: 0.075-0.1)	Elderly: Start with 25-50 μg Pregnancy: A Take before breakfast; sucralfate, aluminum hydroxide antacids, iron preparations, and phenytoin may interfere with absorption of thyroxine SE: Hyperthyroidism, tremors, palpitations, tachycardia, cardiopulmonary	\$4-\$24/0.25 mg (100); \$4-\$20/0.05 mg (100); \$6-\$25/0.1 mg (100); \$6-\$29/0.125 mg (100)

SE, Side effects.

Box 178-3

Pharmaceutical Plan: Graves' Disease

Propranolol

Propranolol: Symptomatic relief until hyperthyroidism is resolved. It effectively treats the tachycardia, tremor, and anxiety that occur. It is the initial treatment of choice for thyroid storm.
10 mg (100) $1-$33,
20 mg (100) $2-$35
Start dosage at 10 mg and increase until an adequate response is achieved, usually 20 mg QID. Keep resting heart rate (HR) between 60 and 70 and walking HR <100
Pregnancy: C
SE: Fatigue, dizziness, lethargy, bronchospasm

Thiourea Drugs

Thiourea drugs: Used for young adults, small goiters, or fear of radioisotopes. These drugs are used for preparation for surgery. These drugs do not permanently damage the thyroid.
50 mg (100) $5-$10

Propylthiouracil (PTU): preferred for **pregnant** women. 300 mg/d (100 mg TID). In severe hyperthyroidism or very large goiters, initial dose is 400 mg/day. Maintenance 100-150 mg/day. **Children:** (6-10 yrs) initial dose is 50-150 mg/day. Pregnancy: D
Methimazole (Tapazole): 15 mg daily (5 mg TID) for mild hyperthyroidism, 20-40 mg/day for moderate or severe hypothyroidism and 60 mg/day for severe hypothyroidism. Maintenance 5-15 mg/day
Children: 0.4 mg/kg/day
Agranulocytosis: monitor complete blood count monthly for first 3-4 mos
Pregnancy: D

Radioactive Iodine

Can receive radioactive iodine while taking propranolol. Patients may have hypothyroidism after being treated. Follow-up with TSH levels is necessary.

Pregnant women should not take radioactive iodine and should not become pregnant for 4 mos after treatment. Emphasize need to inform OB/GYN of past Graves' disease

Surgery

Less frequent treatment since radioactive iodine. Reserved for pregnant women whose thyrotoxicosis is not controlled or those with large goiters or with a potential for malignancy.

Complications include recurrent laryngeal nerve damage and damage to parathyroid. Thyroid replacement is necessary.

SE, Side effects.

Adult hypothyroidism: Refer to endocrinologist if myxedema present, cardiac disease, hypothyroidism due to pituitary or hypothalamus dysfunction

Hyperthyroidism: Pediatric endocrinologist for children and endocrinologist for adults

Follow-up

Congenital hypothyroidism

Monitor T4 and TSH every 2 to 4 weeks after therapy is begun, then monthly until 1 year, then bimonthly until 3 years.

Adult hypothyroidism

Reassess thyroid levels after 4 to 6 weeks after treatment.

There is a wide variation in the patient's set point (i.e., the TSH level at which the patient feels best), so the TSH can be fine-tuned within the normal range.

There is no need to raise the TSH above normal.

There is a circadian rhythm in TSH levels: they tend to be lowest around 11 AM and highest just before midnight.

Since oral contraceptive pills (OCPs) can cause need for ↑ thyroid, check 4 to 6 weeks after beginning OCPs.

Monitor thyroid every 6 to 12 months after stable dosage.

Pregnancy: Need to monitor thyroid level in first trimester. May need to increase by ¼ to ⅓ of normal dose. Thyroid hormones are influenced by the rising human chorionic gonadotropins (HCG) in early pregnancy. TSH levels should be monitored monthly. The pregnant thyroid patient should be followed by the OB/GYN.

Hyperthyroidism: Monitor TSH levels every 6 to 12 months.

Thyroid nodules

If FNA reveals benign nodule, the patient should still be followed closely. Many endocrinologists will repeat the biopsy after 6 to 24 months in nodules that remain unchanged and will rebiopsy any time the nodule enlarges or becomes suspicious.

EVALUATION

Patient should be euthyroid with treatment.

RESOURCES

National Graves' Disease Foundation: (904) 724-0770

Thyroid Foundation of America: (800) 832-8321

SUGGESTED READINGS

Adlin V: Subclinical hypothyroidism: deciding when to treat, *Am Family Physician* 57(4):776-780, 1998.

American Association of Clinical Endocrinologists: *AACE clinical practice guidelines for the diagnosis and management of thyroid nodules*, Mt Olive, NJ, 1997, Knoll Pharmaceuticals.

Bishnoi A, Sachmechi I: Thyroid disease during pregnancy, *Am Family Physician* 53(1):215-220, 1996.

Brody M, Reichard R: Thyroid screening: how to interpret and apply the results, *Postgrad Med* 98(2):54-66, 1995.

Costa A: Interpreting thyroid tests, *Am Family Physician* 52(8):2325-2330, 1995.

Ellsworth A et al: *Mosby's 1998 medical drug reference*, St Louis, 1998, Mosby.

Healthcare Consultants of America, Inc: *1998 physicians fee and coding guide*, Augusta, Ga, 1998, Healthcare Consultants of America, Inc.

Fitzgerald, P: Endocrinology. In Tierney L, McPhee S, Papadakis M, editors: *Current medical diagnosis, treatment*, ed 37, Stamford, Conn, 1998, Appleton & Lange.

Gregerman R: Thyroid disorders. In Barker R, Burton J, Zieve P, editors: *Principles of ambulatory medicine*, Baltimore, 1995, Williams & Wilkins.

Madison L: Pinpointing the cause of hypothyroidism, *Women's Health in Primary Care* 1(1):12-26, 1998.

Schubert M, Kountz D: Thyroiditis, *Postgrad Med* 98(2):101-112, 1995.

179 Tinea Infection

ICD-9-CM

Dermatophytosis of Scalp and Beard 110.0
Dermatophytosis of Body (Corporis) 110.5
Dermatophytosis, Cruris 110.3
Dermatophytosis, Pedis 110.4
Tinea Versicolor 111.0

OVERVIEW

Definition

Tinea is a fungal infection caused by an organism known as a dermatophyte, capable of colonizing keratinized tissues such as the epidermis, nails, hair, tissues of various animals, and the feathers of birds. The dermatophytes rarely affect deep layers of tissue or cause systemic infections.

Tinea capitis/ringworm of the scalp is a fungal infection of the hair follicles and surrounding skin.

Tinea barbae/ringworm of the beard is similar to tinea capitis but affects the beard and mustache.

Tinea corporis/ringworm of the glabrous skin of the trunk and extremities with the exclusion of the palms of the hands, soles of the feet, and the groin.

Tinea versicolor typically appears on the trunk, neck, and proximal extremities.

Tinea pedis/athletes foot is a fungal infection of the feet. It is the most common infection.

Tinea manuum is a fungal infection of the palmar and interdigital areas of the hand.

Tinea cruris ("jock itch") is a fungal infection of the groin areas, including genitalia, pubic area, and perineal and perianal skin.

Tinea unguium/onychomycosis is ringworm of the nails; it more commonly affects the toenails than the fingernails.

Incidence

Tinea infections are fairly common in the United States. They affect **all ages,** males and females equally. The estimated cost of treatment of fungal infections in 1994 was 400 million dollars.

Pathophysiology

Infection begins when a fungal spore adheres to the skin under suitable conditions (trauma to tissue and moist, occlusive environment). Within 4 to 6 hours the spore germinates. The germinating spores develop hyphae and complete the life cycle by producing more spores. As the dermatophyte grows on the skin, there may be no clinical signs of infection. Some individuals may be asymptomatic carriers. Dermatophyte colonizations are not highly infectious. Inflammation associated with the fungal growth is usually an allergic response to fungal antigens that have affected the epidermal layer composed of living cells.

Common Pathogens

Epidermophyton
Microsporum
Trichophyton rubrum

Protective Factors Against

Dryness
Loose-fitting clothes and nonocclusive footwear
Cotton undergarments and socks
Good hygiene
Wearing footwear in communal areas
Not sharing personal care items such as combs, brushes, mats, towels

SUBJECTIVE DATA

History of Present Illness

Duration of occurrence
Location of occurrence
Associated symptoms such as itching, burning, pain

Current treatments
Contact with infected animals or persons
History of shared combs, towels, and clothing
Recent travel
Use of communal showers or swimming areas
Environmental exposures such as contact sports, use of sports facilities, excessive sweating
Swimming
Gardening

Past Medical History

General medical condition, especially hepatic, renal, endocrine systems and immunosuppressive disorders
History of previous occurrence and past treatments
History of other skin disorders
Allergies

Medications

Current medications

Family History

History of tinea infections
History of other skin disorders
Other family members with skin disorder

Psychosocial History

Assess living conditions

Description of Most Common Symptoms

Hair loss
Mild itching, occasionally intense itching
Inability to tan in patchy areas

OBJECTIVE DATA

General Physical Examination of Involved Area

Careful skin evaluation: Use good lighting source, examine all body surfaces with clothes removed (Table 179-1)
Check for lymph node enlargement

Diagnostic Procedures

Diagnostic procedures are outlined in Table 179-2.

ASSESSMENT

Differential diagnoses are included in Table 179-3.

THERAPEUTIC PLAN

Pharmaceutical

Topical creams are the treatment of choice for all forms of tinea except tinea capitis, tinea barbae, and onychomycosis, which require topical and oral medications: oral agents penetrate the hair shaft, and topical agents limit the spread of spores.

Oral antifungal medications are used for tinea capitis and resistant infections. Common side effects are gastrointestinal complaints and headache (Table 179-4).

Lifestyle/Activities

Children in day care do not need to be isolated once treatment has begun.

Children may return to school after beginning oral therapy.

Diet

Not applicable

Patient Education

Side effects and drug interactions of oral antifungal medications
Clean environment and fomites to remove fungal scales
Avoid sharing brushes, combs, hat, towels, or other items that can transmit fungal scales
Search out infected animals/pets and treat appropriately
No oils to hair or scalp
Avoid braiding hair
Apply creams after bathing and reapply after swimming or exercising
Instruct patients with tinea versicolor that recurrence is high and treatment may be needed each spring before tanning season
Instruct patients to wear leather shoes or shoes that allow their feet to breathe
Remove wet swimsuits as soon as possible
Use drying powders on feet
Wear sandals or rubber shoes in communal areas
Keep skin dry

Family Impact

It may be necessary to culture and treat other family members. All family members can use selenium sulfide shampoo to prevent recurrence by asymptomatic carriers.

Referral/Consultation

Collaborate with MD:
Patient requiring long-term (>2 months) oral antifungal

Text continued on p. 1103

TABLE 179-1 Common Types of Tinea Infections

Type	Risk Factors	Classic Lesions	Differential Diagnosis
Tinea capitis/ tinea barbae	**Children** 2-10 y/o, males, blacks, contact with infected persons and animals, confined/crowded living quarters, sharing of combs, brushes, hats, day care, poor hygiene, immunosuppression, occlusive pomades, tight braiding, family history	Scalp/beard, mustache. Noninflammatory: areas of alopecia with characteristic black dots caused by the breaking of the hair shaft at the level of the follicle. Areas of hair loss are patchy and round. May have single or multiple erythematous plaques with follicular papules, nodules, crusting. Inflammatory: A swollen hairless purulent area develops, accompanied by suppurative folliculitis. Pus may be present at the site. Scarring and permanent hair loss can occur. Often associated with cervical adenopathy, an important finding to differentiate from other alopecias.	Seborrhea dermatitis Atopic dermatitis Psoriasis Alopecia areata Impetigo Bacterial folliculitis
Tinea corporis	**Children,** occlusive clothing, day care centers, pets, immunosuppression	Trunk and extremities, excluding palms of hands and soles of feet. Annular plaque with scaling, vesicle formations, and papules seen in an advancing border with hypopigmented or light brown center. May occur singly or in groups of three or four.	Nummular eczema Granuloma annular Psoriasis Lichen planus Seborrhea dermatitis Pityriasis rosea
Tinea versicolor	Humidity, warm temperatures, occlusive clothing, excessive sweating, sharing of footwear, tropical climates	Trunk, neck, proximal extremities. Presents as small oval or round hyperpigmented or hypopigmented macule, sharply marginated. Fine scales appear with scratching of the skin surface. Colors range from white to red/brown. Opportunistic infection caused by normal flora on the skin. May be periodic recurrence.	Pityriasis alba Seborrhea dermatitis Secondary syphilis Pityriasis rosea Vitiligo
Tinea pedis and tinea manuum	Communal showers and pools, occlusive footwear, excessive sweating, sharing of footwear, tropical climates	Surface of feet. Mild to moderate erythema between toes, macerated and scaly skin between toes, and plantar/ lateral surfaces of the feet. Vesicles/pustules in severe cases. Foot odor. Tinea manuum is associated with tinea pedis and is unilateral in nature.	Contact dermatitis Interdigital psoriasis Eczema

Continued

TABLE 179-1 Common Types of Tinea Infections—cont'd

Type	Risk Factors	Classic Lesions	Differential Diagnosis
Tinea cruris	Occlusive and tight clothing, athletic supporters, obesity, wet swimsuits, diagnosis of tinea pedis or tinea unguium, immunosuppression, males	Genitalia, pubic area, perineal and perianal skin. Annular formation of erythematous, raised, well-marginated border; area within the border is often pigmented red-brown. Lesions rarely extend beyond the genitocrural crease and medial upper thigh. Lateral or bilateral. First site involved is usually the left medial thigh adjacent to the scrotum.	Candidiasis Erythrasma Psoriasis Seborrhea Dermatitis Lichen simplex chronicus Benign familial chronic pemphigus Intertrigo
Tinea unguium/ onychomycosis	Tinea pedis, immunosuppression, diabetes, **elderly** with venous insufficiency, trauma to nails	Nails lose their luster and become opaque yellow in color, thicken, lifting up the nail bed; distal edge becomes brittle and crumbles.	Candidiasis Psoriasis

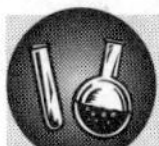

TABLE 179-2 Diagnostic Tests: Tinea Infection

Diagnostic Test	Findings/Rationale	Cost ($)
Potassium hydroxide preparation (KOH)	Obtain several hair roots. The proximal 5- to 6-cm is the most important area. Scalp scrapings from the active margin of the suspected infection may be used. Place the scrapings on a slide and add 10% aqueous KOH. Let the specimen sit for 5-10 minutes to clear the keratinous material. A drop of ink may be added to highlight the hyphae. Hyphae appear as long, translucent, branching filaments of uniform width. Septa may be visible as lines of separation at irregular intervals. Visualization of hyphae and spores under the standard light microscope should be suitable for diagnostic purposes.	19-23
Woods lamp	Fluoresce a yellowish color. Not all strains causing tinea will fluoresce.	Not available
Fungal culture	Several hairs or scrapings from an infected area may be obtained and placed on the appropriate test medium. Dermatophyte test media have a color indicator that changes the medium from yellow to pink/red in the presence of a dermatophyte. Although this yields a more precise diagnosis, the results take longer. Such precision is not usually necessary. For most clinical purposes, classification of fungal infection by anatomic site is preferred.	38-47

TABLE 179-3 Differential Diagnosis: Tinea Infection

Diagnosis	Data Supporting
Atopic dermatitis	Chronic pruritic inflammation of the epidermis and dermis, usually a positive family history of asthma, allergies, or atopic dermatitis. Physical examination reveals poorly defined erythematous patches with excoriations that come from scratching.
Psoriasis	Hereditary disorder, chronic scaling and plaques of scalp, elbows, forearms, knees, hands, and feet.
Alopecia areata	Localized loss of hair in round or oval areas without any visible inflammation, usually in scalp.
Folliculitis	Inflammation of hair follicles, with papule, pustule at hair follicle. Usually of beard, axilla, legs.
Lichen planus	Flat topped, shiny, pruritic papules on the skin.
Pityriasis rosea	Primary plaque (herald lesion), with 1-2 weeks later: A generalized eruption of fine scaling papules in a "Christmas tree" distribution.
Vitiligo	Totally white macules where there is an absence of melanocytes.

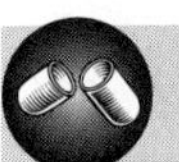

TABLE 179-4 Pharmaceutical Plan: Tinea Infection

Type of Tinea	Treatment	Comments	Cost
Tinea capitis/ tinea barbae	**Children:** CAUTION: need to specify Microsize or Ultramicrosize since formulations and dosing are different Griseofulvin: Ultramicrosize 14-23 kg: 31.25-82.5 mg q12h or 62.5-165 mg QD >23 kg: 125-330 mg QD Terbinafine (Lamisil): 3-6 mg/kg/day ×1-4 wks Ketoconazole is not recommended for children **Adults:** Griseofulvin 250-373 mg QD Ketoconazole (Nizoral): 3.3-6.6 mg/kg/day, up to 200 mg QD × 6-8 wks Lamisil: 250 mg QD ×2 wks Topical therapy/adjunctive therapy: 2.5% selenium sulfide shampoo to prevent spread of infection. Available by prescription only. 1% Selsun blue shampoo can be purchased over the counter Prednisone: 1-2 mg/kg day for 5-10 days in adults with inflammatory tinea capitis	Griseofulvin*: Ultramicrosize is better absorbed than microsize; photosensitivity reactions can occur, avoid ultraviolet light; rare occurrences of hepatotoxicity, granulocytopenia; absorption is enhanced with or after a fatty meal; not recommended for children under 2 years old; drug interactions include alcohol, oral contraceptives, warfarin and barbiturates; do not use if pregnant or lactating Ketoconazole (Nizoral): Hepatotoxicity is most important adverse effect; absorption is enhanced if taken on an empty stomach; absorption is decreased by antacids or H_2 blockers; **warning: itraconazole or ketoconazole are contraindicated in patients taking astemizole or terfenadine, as life-threatening arrhythmias may result; may also occur with cisapride, triazolam, and midazolam** Pregnancy: C Not recommended for use in children Terbinafine (Lamisil): Associated with hepatobiliary dysfunction, taste disturbances, rash, lymphocytopenia and neutropenia; clearance affected by cimetidine (potentiates) and rifampin (antagonizes) Pregnancy: B, not recommended for nursing mothers	Griseo ultramicrosize: \$33-\$44/ 125 mg (100); \$65-\$84/250 mg (100); \$35-\$60/165 mg (100); \$60-\$114/330 mg (100) Suspension: \$22/125/5 ml, 120 ml Keto: \$271-\$298/200 mg (100) Terbinafine: \$187/250 mg (100)
Tinea corporis	Topicals are usually effective. Miconazole nitrate 1% (Monistat) Clotrimazole 2% (Lotrimin) Econazole 1% (Spectazole) Ketoconazole 2% QD as above. (Nizoral) Terbinafine 1% QD ×7 days (Lamisil) Butenifine 1% QD ×2 weeks (Mentax) Oral agents are for widespread, inflammatory, or resistant infections Griseofulvin 500-1000 mg QD	Butenifine not recommended for children Apply BID ×2 wks after clinical signs and symptoms have disappeared	\$2-\$13/Monistat Cr: 2% (15 g); \$15-\$19/Lotrimin 1% Cr (30g); \$11/Econ: 1% (15 g); \$13/Keto: 20 mg/g (15 g); \$45/Terf: 1% (30 g)

*Griseofulvin not used as frequently since newer and safer antifungals are available.
SE, Side effects.

Continued

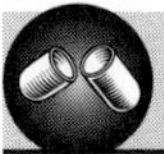

TABLE 179-4 Pharmaceutical Plan: Tinea Infection—cont'd

Type of Tinea	Treatment	Comments	Cost
Tinea versicolor	Topical: 2.5% Selenium sulfide lotion (Selsun) 2% Miconazole cream 1% Clotrimazole 25% Thiosulfate Ketoconazole 200-400 mg once or twice a month	Apply beyond borders of affected areas for 5-10 min daily for 2 wks; oral medication not usually needed for the usual case of tinea versicolor; may be used in resistant cases or for prophylaxis Pregnancy: C	\$3-\$13/2.5% (4 oz)
Tinea pedis and tinea manuum	Clotrimazole, miconazole, tolnaftate, terbinafine HCL; apply creams twice a day to feet. Apply for 2 wks after feet have cleared Butenifine 1% QD after bathing for 4 wks Talcum powder or antifungal powders (over-the-counter) Severe cases: Burrows solution for lesions that are oozing Oral: Griseofulvin 1 g in divided doses for 4-8 wks Fluconazole 150 mg q wk for 6 wks	Butenifine not recommended for children	\$2-\$4/powder (45 g); \$27/cream: 1% (15 g)
Tinea cruris	Clotrimazole, Miconazole topical creams applied twice a day for 3-4 wks Terbinafine 1% QD ×7 days in children Butenifine 1% QD after bathing ×2 wks Oral: For resistant cases Griseofulvin (Microsized) 500 mg QD in single or divided doses Ketoconazole 200 mg QD ×4 wks Fluconazole 150 mg wkly ×4-6 wks	Butenifine not recommended in children	See tinea capitis for oral drug costs
Onychomycosis	Topical medications are usually not effective Oral: Itraconazole (Sporanox) 200 mg daily for 90 days or pulse therapy: take 1 wk, off 3 wks for 3-6 rounds of therapy: 3-6 months Griseofulvin 1000 mg/day in divided doses for 4-6 mo for fingernails and 12-18 mo for toenails (not usually recommended since itraconazole and terbinafine are available and much less expensive) Terbinafine HCL 250 mg QD for 6 wks for fingernails, 12 wks toenails; pulse therapy also used	Pregnancy: C SE: Nausea, monitor liver function, avoid antacids within 2 hours; inhibits P450 cytochrome (see Appendix D)	Iatr: \$539/100 mg (100); griseo: see tinea capitis for oral drug costs

medications secondary to concerns for liver toxicity; monitor appropriately

Patient not showing improvement in 2 weeks

Follow-up

Reevaluate all tinea infections in 2 weeks for response to therapy.

Resistant infections and tinea capitis may require follow up visits every 2 to 4 weeks until clear.

Monitor hepatic, renal, and hematopoietic functions monthly while on oral antifungals.

Monitor for superimposed bacterial infections at follow-up visit. May need cultures and Gram stains to provide appropriate antibiotic therapy. Monitor patient for side effects and drug interactions associated with oral antifungals.

EVALUATION

Resolution of lesions

SUGGESTED READINGS

Abdel-Ranman SM, Nahata MC: Oral terbinafine: a new antifungal agent, *Ann Pharmacother* 31(4):445-456, 1997.

Bakos L et al: Open clinical study of the efficacy and safety of terbinafine cream: 1% in children with tinea corporis and tinea cruris, *Pediatr Infect Dis J* 16(6):545-548, 1997.

Bergus GR, Johnson JS: Superficial tinea infections, *Am Family Physician* 48(2):259-267, 1993.

Degreef HJ, DeDoncker PRG: Current therapy of dermatophytosis, *J Am Acad Dermatol* 31(3):S25-S29, 1994.

Drake LA et al: Guidelines of care for superficial mycotic infections of the skin: tinea capitis and tinea barbae, *J Am Acad Dermatol* 34(2):290-294, 1996.

Ellsworth A et al: *Mosby's 1998 medical drug reference*, St Louis, 1998, Mosby.

Faergemann J et al: A multicentre (double blind) comparative study to assess the safety and efficacy of fluconazole and griseofulvin in the treatment of tinea corporis and tinea cruris, *Br J Dermatol* 136(4):575-577, 1997.

Frieden IJ, Howard R: Tinea capitis: epidemiology diagnosis treatment and control, *J Am Acad Dermatol* 31(3):S42-S46, 1994.

Greer DL et al: A randomized trial to assess once-daily topical treatment of tinea corporis with Butanefrine, a new antifungal agent, *J Am Acad Dermatol* 37(2):231-235, 1997.

Healthcare Consultants of America Inc: *1998 physicians fee and coding guide*, Augusta, Ga, 1998, Healthcare Consultants of America Inc.

Hoffmann TJ, Schelkum PH: How I manage athlete's foot, *Physician Sportsmed* 23(4):29-32, 1995.

Lesher JL et al: Butanefrine 1% cream in the treatment of tinea cruris: a multicenter vehicle-controlled double blind trial, *J Am Acad Dermatol* 36(2):S20-S24, 1997.

Lesher J, Levine N, Treadwell P: Fungal skin infections; common but stubborn, *Patient Care* 28(2):16-30, 1994.

Martin AG, Kobayashi GS: Superficial fungal infection; dermatophytosis tinea nigra piedra. In Fitzpatrick TB et al, editors: *Dermatology in general medicine,* New York, 1993, McGraw Hill.

Martin AG, Kobayashi GS: Yeast infections: candidiasis pityriasis (tinea) versicolor. In Fitzpatrick TB et al, editors: *Dermatology in general medicine,* New York, 1993, McGraw Hill.

Pierard GE, Arrese JE, Pierard-Franchimont C: Treatment and prophylaxis of tinea infections, *Dis Management* 52(2):209-224, 1996.

Reilly K: Tinea versicolor. In Dambro M: *Griffith's 5-minute consult,* Baltimore, 1996, Williams & Wilkins.

Stevenson L, Brooke DS: Tinea capitis *J Pediatr Care* 8(4):189-190, 1994.

Tschen E et al: Treatment of interdigital tinea pedis with a 4-week once-daily regimen of Butanefrine hydrochloride 1% cream, *J Am Acad Dermatol* 36(2):S9-S14, 1997.

Uphold CR, Graham MV: *Clinical guidelines in family practice,* Gainesville, Fla, 1994, Barmarrae Books.

180 Tinnitus

ICD-9-CM

Tinnitus 388.3

OVERVIEW

Definition

Tinnitus is perception of abnormal ear or head noises.

Incidence

Most people suffer from an occasional intermittent tinnitus that lasts for several minutes; this occurs even in normal hearing persons. Continuing tinnitus usually means the person has suffered sensory hearing loss. Approximately 1% of the U.S. population suffers from chronic tinnitus that causes severe distress and requires some kind of management intervention. The overall prevalence of unexplained tinnitus is 11%. Tinnitus appears to be clearly associated with somatization disorders (42%) or hypochondriacal disorder (27%).

Pathophysiology

Some forms of tinnitus may be due to loss of the normal masking effect of ambient noise, with the emergence of otherwise subaudible tympanic, vascular, or muscular noises.

SUBJECTIVE DATA

History of Present Illness

Complains of ringing or buzzing in ears
Ask about:
- Involvement of one ear or both ears
- Ringing or buzzing associated with movement or rotation

Complaints of decreased hearing (90% of patients with decreased hearing also experience tinnitus)
Ask if hearing loss was gradual or sudden
Has hearing acuity fluctuated?
Associated symptoms such as vertigo, otalgia, or otorrhea
Ear pain
Ear discharge
Complaints of being nervous or depressed
Inability to sleep or concentrate due to noises
Ask about temporomandibular symptoms
- Facial muscle pain
- Preauricular pain
- Temporomandibular joint (TMJ) sounds: Jaw clicking, popping, catching, locking
- Limited mouth opening
- Increased pain while chewing
- Some people may have difficulty talking or singing
- History of recent trauma or injury to neck, jaw, or mouth
- Previously been treated for unexplained facial pain or jaw pain problem?
- Have you ever been told by your dentist that you grind your teeth?
- Have you ever been treated for grinding your teeth?
- When was your last dental visit?

Screening questions for patients with TMJ disorders:
- Do you have difficulty, pain, or both when opening your mouth (e.g., when yawning)?
- Does your jaw get stuck, locked, or go out?
- Do you have difficulty or pain or both when chewing, talking, or using your jaws?
- Are you aware of noises in the jaw joints?
- Do your jaws regularly feel stiff, tight, or tired?
- Do you have pain in or about the ears, temples, or cheeks?
- Do you have frequent headache, neck aches, or toothaches?

Past Medical History

Ask about:
- History of ear problems or disease

History of anxiety or depression
History of migraines
History of syphilis, diabetes, hypothyroidism, or head trauma as cause of hearing loss

Medications

Ask about use of aspirin or other ototoxic drugs
Aminoglycosides, diuretics, quinine, furosemide

Family History

Ask about:
Family history of hearing loss
Family history of migraines

Psychosocial History

Ask about exposure to excessive noise, use of ear plugs
Ask about coping strategies used so far to adjust to tinnitus

OBJECTIVE DATA

Physical Examination

The examination should concentrate on the head and neck.
Head/eyes/ears/nose/throat: Evaluate for an upper respiratory infection
Ear: Evaluate tympanic membrane (TM), external canal
Complete pneumatic otoscopy: Check for TM movement
Tympanogram
Face: Assess for masseter, temporal muscles, and preauricular area for pain or tenderness. Inspect the face, jaw, and dental arches for symmetry. Ask the patient to open and close the mouth, keeping your fingers over the preauricular areas: Be alert for joint sounds.
Mouth: Measure mouth opening: Use millimeter rule on teeth and have patient open as wide as possible; measure the distance between the maxillary and mandibular teeth; <40 mm is considered a restricted mouth opening; inspect teeth for significant wear, mobility, or decay; look at the buccal mucosa for riding and the lateral edges of the tongue for scalloping; these are signs of clenching and bruxism.
Neurological: Check sensation of face; note if facial movement is symmetrical, random alternating movements.
Hearing: Have patient repeat aloud words presented in a soft whisper, normal speaking voice, or a shout. Have the opposite ear occluded, then repeat on other side (Box 180-1).
Weber: Place the tuning fork on the forehead or front teeth; have the patient indicate where it is heard the best.

Box 180-1

Evaluation of Children's Hearing According to Age

0-3 mos: Response to noise
3-5 mos: Child turns to sound
6-10 mos: Child responds to name
10-15 mos: Child imitates simple words

Rinne: The tuning fork is placed alternately on the mastoid bone and in front of the ear canal

Diagnostic Procedures

Diagnostic procedures are outlined in Table 180-1.

ASSESSMENT

Differential diagnoses include those found in Table 180-2.

THERAPEUTIC PLAN

Pharmaceutical

Pharmaceutical treatment is outlined in Table 180-3.

Ongoing Research

The use of caroverine in patients with tinnitus has been evaluated in Austria. A single infusion of caroverine showed a reduction in subjective rating and psychoacoustic measurement immediately after the infusion. None of the control group showed a significant response to the placebo. Ongoing research will continue to evaluate the effectiveness of this treatment.

Lifestyle/Activities

The sound of a radio may help the patient go to sleep (FM radio delivers a broader spectrum of frequencies and is preferred)
Use of "white noise" may be helpful to mask sounds
Bedtime sedation to ensure adequate sleep
Some people with tinnitus recommend the following as being helpful:
Avoiding stress
Adequate rest
No alcohol
Ginkgo biloba at meals
Splint for TMJ disorders

Diet

Avoid caffeine

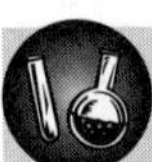

TABLE 180-1 Diagnostic Tests: Tinnitus

Diagnostic Test	Finding/Rationale	Cost ($)
Audiometric studies	Hearing test conducted in soundproof room. Pure-tone thresholds in decibels (dB) are obtained over the ranges of 250-8000Hz for both air and bone conduction; 25 dB or below is considered within normal limits. All patients with hearing loss should be referred for audiometric testing unless the cause is easily remediable (impacted cerumen). Patients can be referred directly to an audiologist. The location of an accredited audiologist can be obtained by calling the American Speech-Language Association at 1-800-638-8255.	119-159/comprehensive studies
Speech discrimination testing	Evaluates the clarity of hearing. Results are reported as percentage correct.	88-104
Tympanogram	Used to detect fluid in the middle ear and to determine the mobility of the tympanic membrane (TM). An electro-acoustic device is used to measure the compliance of the TM. Results are displayed in a graphic form. It is most reliable in children >6 mos.	31-37
Audiogram	Small hand-held audioscopes can provide a rough indication of hearing impairment. Usually four pure tones are emitted in sequence. This test can be affected by background noise, so the examination room must be quiet.	24-29
Tinnitus handicap inventory (THI)	A self-perceived rating scale to determine the effect of tinnitus on activities of daily living and the severity of the tinnitus handicap (Newman, Sandridge, Jacobsen, 1997)	Not available

TABLE 180-2 Differential Diagnosis: Tinnitus

Diagnosis	Supporting Data
Pulsatile tinnitus	Caused by conductive hearing loss; carotid pulsations are more apparent. May indicate a vascular abnormality such as gliomas tumor, carotid vaso-occlusive disease, arteriovenous malformation, or aneurysm
Sensory hearing loss (Ch. 85)	Conditions affecting the eighth cranial nerve leading to sensorineural hearing loss; the tinnitus can be caused by hyperirritability of the acoustic nerve
Acoustic neuroma	Unilateral tinnitus or hearing loss, mild positional vertigo, or sense of imbalance; audiometry demonstrates significant sensorineural hearing loss with poor discrimination

Patient Education

Reassurance that the sounds are not due to a serious intracranial condition

Tinnitus clinics and support groups are available

Tinnitus management training: Includes using "white noise" (i.e., a machine that makes a consistent steady noise—buzz, hum, ocean waves, birds—to help block out the tinnitus noise), biofeedback, and relaxation therapies; tinnitus was found to be less annoying, but the loudness of the tinnitus did not change, nor did the tinnitus awareness after the management therapy

Referral/Consultation

Noises that originate from the region of the patient's ear and are audible to the examiner should be referred to an otolaryngologist.

Patients that have tinnitus that lateralizes to one ear should also be referred to an otolaryngologist.

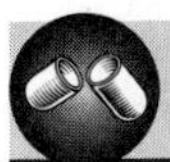

TABLE 180-3 Pharmaceutical Treatment: Tinnitus

Drug	Dose	Comments	Cost
Oral antidepressants: nortriptyline (Pamelor)	50 mg at HS	Treatment seems to be effective in reducing tinnitus; it may be due to treatment of underlying depression Pregnancy: C SE: Drowsiness, anticholinergic effects	\$21-\$178/50 mg (100)
Fluoxetine (Prozac)	20 mg at HS	Pregnancy: B SE: Central nervous system, stimulation, fatigue, headache, somnolence, sexual dysfunction	\$220/20 mg (100)
Misoprostol (Cytotec)	Dose not known	Pregnancy: X SE: Diarrhea, abdominal pain, flatulence, headache	\$51/100 μg (100); \$71/200 μg (100)
Melatonin	3 mg QHS	Melatonin appears to improve tinnitus according to tinnitus handicap inventory (THI), although not statistically significant; sleeping also appeared to improve; patients with high THI scores were most likely to benefit; side effects and safety profile has not been established; not FDA approved for use with tinnitus	Not available

FDA, Food and Drug Administration; *SE,* side effects.

Patients with temporomandibular disorders with co-existing tinnitus should be referred to a dentist; improvement in TMJ disorders also improves tinnitus.

Patients with severe tinnitus may benefit from surgery; cochlear resection and microvascular decompression are available, but clear-cut efficacy has not been shown.

Follow-up

Follow-up in 2 weeks to evaluate the effectiveness of antidepressant.

EVALUATION

Evaluation should determine how well the patient is sleeping.

Determine the effectiveness of masking tinnitus using biofeedback, relaxation, or "white noise."

RESOURCES

Tinnitus data registry
www.ohsu.edu/ohrc-otda/95-01

American Tinnitus Association
PO Box 5
Portland, OR 97207-0005
503-248-9985
www.teleport.com//~ata/

Tinnitus and Hyperacusis Centre
London, UK

J. Hazell homepage
www.tinnitus.org

REFERENCE

Newman C, Sandridge S, Jacobsen G: Psychometric adequacy of the tinnitus handicap inventory (THI) for evaluating treatment outcomes, *J Am Acad Audiol* 9(2):153-160, 1997.

SUGGESTED READINGS

Denk D et al: Caroverine in tinnitus treatment: a placebo-controlled blind study, *Acta Otolaryngol* 117(6):825-830, 1997.

Dineen R, Doyle J, Bench J: Managing tinnitus: a comparison of different approaches to tinnitus management training, *Br J Audiol* 31(5):331-344, 1997.

Ellsworth A et al: *Mosby's 1998 medical drug reference*, St Louis, 1998, Mosby.

Healthcare Consultants of America Inc: *1998 physicians fee and coding guide*, Augusta, Ga, 1998, Healthcare Consultants of America Inc.

Gelb H, Gelb M, Wagner M: The relationship of tinnitus and craniocervical mandibular disorders, *Cranio* 15(2):136-143, 1997.

Hiller W, Janca A, Burke K: Association between tinnitus and somatoform disorders, *J Psychosomatic Res* 43(6):613-624, 1997.

Meikle M: Electronic access to tinnitus data: the Oregon tinnitus data archive, *Otolaryngol Head Neck Surgery* 117(6):698-700, 1997.

Parnes S: Current concepts in the clinical management of patients with tinnitus, *Eur Arch Otorhinolaryngol* 254(9-10):406-409, 1997.

Rizzardo R et al: Psychological distress in patients with tinnitus, *J Otolaryngol* 27(1):21-25, 1998.

Rosenberg S et al: Effect of melatonin on tinnitus, *Laryngoscope* 108(3):305-310, 1998.

Shemin L: Fluoxetine for treatment of tinnitus, *Otolaryngol Head Neck Surgery* 118(3 Pt 1):421, 1998.

Tyler R: Perspective on tinnitus, *Br J Audiol* 31(6):381-386, 1997.

Wright E, Bifano S: Tinnitus improvement through TMD therapy, *J Am Dental Assoc* 128(10):1424-1432, 1997.

181 Toxic Shock Syndrome

ICD-9-CM

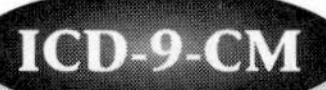

Toxic Shock Syndrome 040.89

OVERVIEW

Definition

Toxic shock syndrome (TSS) is an acute and potentially fatal multisystem illness that primarily affects menstruating women.

Incidence

Affects 3 to 14 **women** per 100,000 annually.
Primarily a disease of women but can affect **children** and adult men.

Pathophysiology

Caused by a toxin produced by *Staphylococcus aureus.*
The exact mechanism by which the toxin enters the body is unknown.
Enhances susceptibility to endotoxins that cause shock, as well as liver, kidney, and myocardial damage.

Factors That Increase Susceptibility

Superabsorbent tampon use, especially if the tampon is left in the vagina >24 hours
Postpartum infection
A diaphragm or contraceptive sponge that is left in the vagina >24 hours
Postsurgical infection
Soft tissue abscess
Osteomyelitis

SUBJECTIVE DATA

History of Present Illness

Inquire about symptoms consistent with a typical presentation, including acute onset of high fever (>39° C/ 102.2° F), vomiting, watery diarrhea, myalgia, headache, abdominal pain, conjunctivitis, and sometimes pharyngitis.
Recognize the importance of screening for hypotension (below 90 mm Hg systolic blood pressure); may progress to hypotensive shock within 48 hours.
Inquire about last menstrual period and current use of tampons. Presenting symptoms usually occur between days 2 and 4 of the menstrual cycle. Ask about possible burning sensation with a watery discharge at the onset of menstruation.
Inquire about a diffuse maculopapular erythroderma that will appear on the face, proximal extremities, and trunk. Typically the rash will progress over the next 5 days to 2 weeks. Desquamation of the skin, especially the palms and feet, is common.
Multisystem involvement is typical and a timely diagnosis is critical.

OBJECTIVE DATA

Physical Examination

Vital signs to assess for temperature elevation, hypotension, tachycardia.
Assess general observation and patient orientation.
A complete examination is indicated secondary to multisystem involvement.
Genitourinary examination; remove tampon, sponge, or diaphragm if present and culture.
Assess specifically for possible source, including soft tissue abscesses, osteomyelitis, or postsurgical infection if indicated.

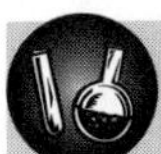

TABLE 181-1 Diagnostic Tests: Toxic Shock Syndrome

Diagnostic Test	Findings/Rationale	Cost ($)
Complete blood count (CBC), including platelets, peripheral smear	Evaluate for infection, anemia, and thrombocytopenia	13-16/CBC; 11-14/platelets
Comprehensive metabolic panel	Evaluate for multisystem involvement	32-42
Urinalysis	Evaluate for renal involvement, dehydration	14-18
Liver function	Evaluate liver function	29-41
Vaginal/cervical culture (culture of tampon)	Culture and sensitivity	31-39
Blood culture	Evaluate for bacteremia	31-39
Throat culture	May have concurrent pharyngitis; rule out scarlet fever	24-30
Lumbar puncture	Rule out meningitis	172-208
Wound culture	Rule out infection	31-39

Diagnostic Procedures

Diagnostic procedures are outlined in Table 181-1.

ASSESSMENT

Fever greater than or equal to 39° C (102° F)
Onset during menses with reported tampon use
Hypotension
Diffuse macular rash with desquamation of the palms and soles 1 to 2 weeks after onset
Multisystem involvement of three or more of the following: gastrointestinal, muscular, mucous membrane, renal, hepatic, hematologic, and/or central nervous system.
Differential diagnoses include:
- Meningococcal meningitis
- Mumps
- Rocky Mountain Spotted Fever
- Leptospirosis
- Postsurgical infection
- Soft tissue abscess
- Osteomyelitis
- Kawasaki's disease
- Gram negative sepsis

THERAPEUTIC PLAN

Pharmaceutical/Nonpharmaceutical

Hemodynamic stability is a priority.
Treatment must be instituted quickly and aggressively.
Consult with an emergency medical facility immediately. Transport via Emergency Medical Services.
Colloidal solutions are given intravenously.
Central and pulmonary edge pressures and urine output are monitored.
Vasopressor agents may be given to correct hypotension.
Mechanical ventilation may be necessary.
Arterial blood gases should be monitored if intubation is required.
Cephalosporins or beta-lactamase resistant penicillin should be administered.
Vancomycin or rifampicin is an alternative if the patient is allergic to penicillin.
Vaginal douching with an antibacterial iodine solution may be recommended.
Electrolyte imbalances should be corrected.
Hypocalcemia occurs in approximately half of patients. Intravenous calcium chloride is given to prevent seizures.
Myocarditis may develop in advanced stages.
Hemorrhage is a risk secondary to thrombocytopenia and coagulation disorders.
The mortality rate is 3% to 6%, with the three major causes of death being adult respiratory syndrome, intractable hypotension, and hemorrhage secondary to disseminated intravascular coagulopathy.

Patient Education

Desquamation of the skin can be quite dramatic.
Avoid tampon or contraceptive sponge use for 6 months after TSS.
Recurrence of TSS is common (approximately 30%).
Do not use tampons postpartum or postabortion.
Do not use superabsorbent tampons under the age of 24.
Frequently change the tampon or use pads at night.
Do not leave contraceptive sponges or diaphragms in place for more than 24 hours.
Always wash your hands before putting in a diaphragm.
Do not use a diaphragm during menses.
Do not use a diaphragm for 12 weeks' postpartum.
Wash the diaphragm after each use.

Consultation/Referral

Infectious disease specialists

EVALUATION/FOLLOW-UP

Obtain vaginal cultures monthly for 6 months.
May need long term follow-up.

SUGGESTED READINGS

Damien M: *Toxic shock syndrome.* In Friedman EA, Borten M, Chapin DS, editors: *Gynecological decision making,* ed 2, Philadelphia, 1998, BC Decker.

DeCherney AH, Pernoll ML: *Current diagnosis & treatment,* ed 8, Norwalk, Conn, 1994, Appleton & Lange.

Fogel CI, Woods NF: *Women's health care,* Thousands Oaks, Calif, 1995, Sage Publications.

Stenchever MA: *Office gynecology,* ed 2, St Louis, 1996, Mosby.

Ellsworth AJ et al: *Mosby's 1998 medical drug reference,* St Louis, 1998, Mosby.

Healthcare Consultants of America Inc: 1998 physicians fee and coding guide, Augusta, 1998, Healthcare Consultants of America, Inc.

182 Transient Ischemic Attacks

ICD-9-CM

Transient Ischemic Attacks 435.9

OVERVIEW

Definition

Transient ischemic attacks (TIAs) are defined as cerebral ischemia that is transient or reversible in nature. They present with acute focal neurologic deficit and usually last less than 20 minutes, but they may last up to 24 hours. Cerebral ischemia with signs that last more than 24 hours and fewer than 7 days is defined as reversible ischemic neurologic deficit (RIND).

Incidence

The incidence of cerebral ischemia has declined for patients under 70, probably as a result of aggressive hypertension and cardiovascular management. TIAs precede 50% to 75% of strokes caused by carotid artery thrombosis. However, among all stroke types, TIAs precede only about 10%. Approximately one third of patients who experience a TIA will experience a cerebral infarction within 5 years.

Pathophysiology

Atherosclerosis and inflammatory disease processes damage arterial walls, leading to the development of cerebral thrombosis. TIAs represent thrombotic particles causing an intermittent blockage of circulation. There is increased risk of vascular damage with prolonged hypertension, degeneration of the endothelial wall of vessels, and the adherence of platelets and fibrin.

SUBJECTIVE DATA

Past Medical History

Hypertension, diabetes, hyperlipidemia, cardiovascular or peripheral vascular disease, gout, atrial fibrillation, ventricular aneurysms, heart valve replacement

Family History

History of cardiovascular disease, history of cerebral vascular accidents

Medication History

Use of oral contraceptives

Psychosocial History

Smoking, increased stress levels

Diet History

Excessive intake of salt, carbohydrates, and fats

Description of Most Common Symptoms

Sudden onset of:

- Paralysis or paresis of one extremity or extremities on one side of the body
- Numbness
- Tingling
- Clumsiness of an extremity or both extremities on one side of the body
- Aphasia
- Visual disturbances
- Facial paralysis or drooping

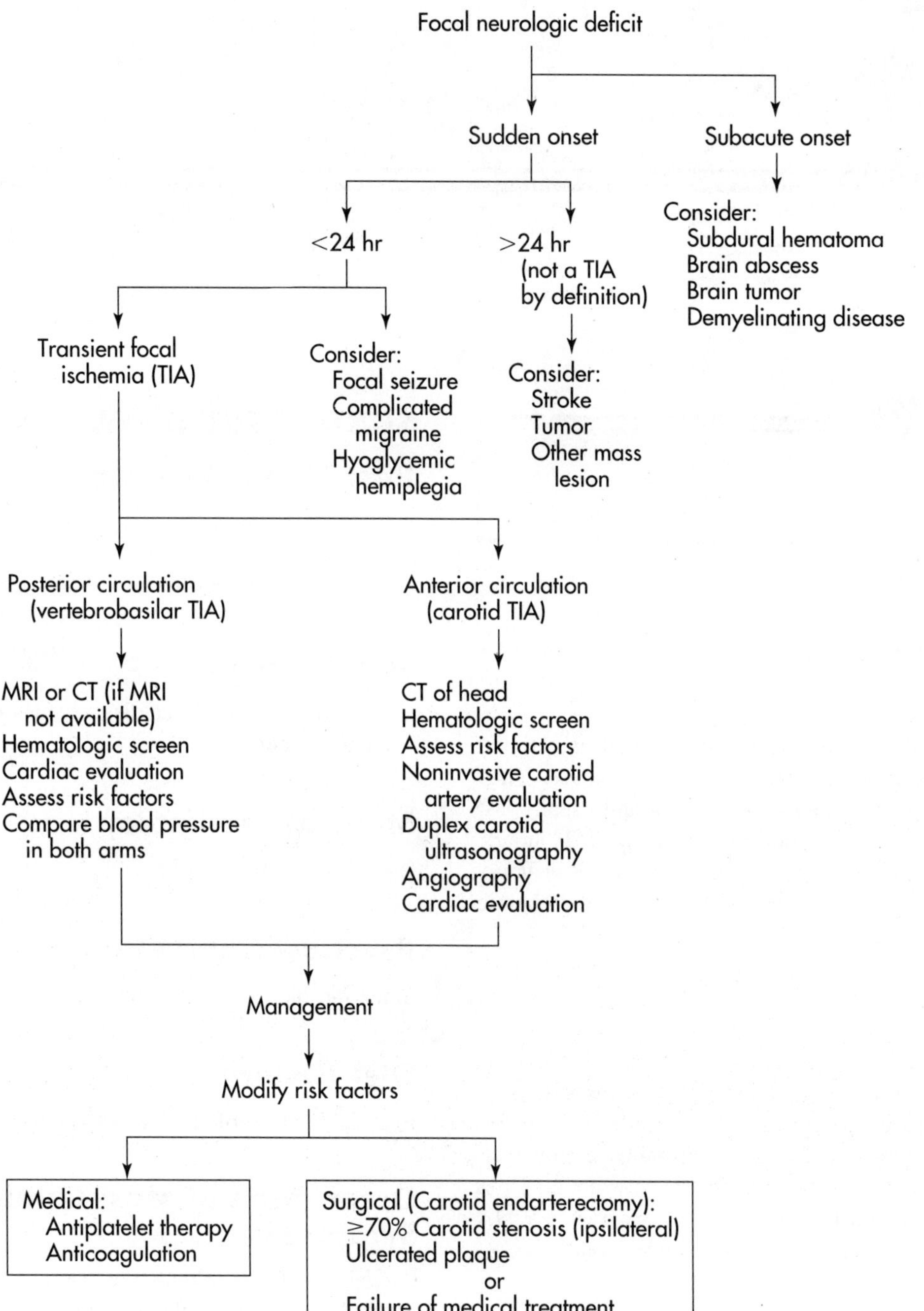

Figure 182-1 Algorithm for patient with suspected transient ischemic attack. *CT,* Computed tomography; *MRI,* magnetic resonance imaging; *TIA,* transient ischemic attack. (Adapted from Greene HL, Johnson WP, Lemcke D: *Decision making in medicine*, ed 2, St Louis, 1998, Mosby.)

Associated Symptoms

Headache, drooling, slurred speech

OBJECTIVE DATA

Physical Examination

General appearance: Confusion, facial drooping
Vital signs: Hydration status (dehydration can lead to hypovolemia and orthostatic hypotension), orthostatic changes (systolic blood pressure [BP] of 110 in normally hypertensive patient may in fact be hypotensive), hypertension (should not be based on BP but rather trending of the BP unless greater than 210 systolic and/or 120 diastolic)
Head/eyes/ears/nose/throat
- Eyes: Reactivity of pupils (remember in the **elderly** they may not have a brisk response) check for visual field deficit
- Throat: Check their ability to swallow

Neck: Supple, listen to carotid arteries for bruits, check for diminished or absent carotid pulsations
Cardiovascular
- Listen for irregular rhythms, murmurs, artificial heart valves (clicks)
- Check extremities for possible signs of deep venous thrombosis

Neurological
- Cranial nerve deficits, especially facial paresis or paralysis, possible abnormalities of the gag reflex, tongue, extraocular movements
- Deep tendon reflexes may be normal or hyperactive in upper extremities
- Level of consciousness, memory, speech, walking, balance (Romberg), sensory perception, and motor ability (e.g., hand grips, lifting leg off the table and holding against pressure)

Diagnostic Procedures

These patients need to either be referred to a physician, or at least consultation with a physician should occur. Other diagnostic tests should include electrocardiogram, computed tomography of the head (which should be normal) ($990-$1175), and lumbar puncture ($172-$208) if there is suspicion of septic embolism from bacterial endocarditis.

Laboratory Tests

Complete blood count ($13-$16), electrolytes ($23-$30), glucose ($16-$20), liver function ($29-$41), lipids ($49-$62)

Radiologic Tests

Another radiologic test that may be considered is a carotid artery duplex Doppler study ($257-$300) to determine the patency of the carotid arteries. If there is significant stenosis of the carotid arteries (>70%), arteriography should be performed.

Figure 182-1 is a decision tree for diagnostic procedures in a patient with a suspected TIA.

ASSESSMENT

Differential diagnoses (Table 182-1) include:
- TIA
- Reversible ischemic neurologic defect (RIND)
- Stroke (brain attack)

Underlying causes
- Atrial fibrillation
- Infective endocarditis

TABLE 182-1 Differential Diagnosis: Transient Ischemic Attack

Diagnosis	Findings	Evaluation
Stroke (rain attack)	Neurological deficit	None other than physical examination; need to be admitted for further evaluation; consult physician
Reversible ischemic neurologic deficit (RIND)	Neurological deficit	None other than physical examination; need admission to hospital to determine if RIND or brain attack
Transient ischemic attack (TIA)	History of unilateral weakness, confusion, clumsiness of arm or leg, visual disturbance, facial paralysis, aphasia, headache, slurred speech; physical examination normal; no neurological deficits; may have carotid bruit	12-Lead electrocardiogram; consider a computed tomography scan or magnetic resonance imaging scan of head, complete blood count, biochemical survey; may want to consider a carotid artery duplex to evaluate carotids for stenosis; arteriography is reserved for stenosis >70% on Doppler study

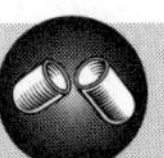

TABLE 182-2 Pharmacologic Treatment: Transient Ischemic Attack

Pharmacologic Agent	Dosage/Contraindications	Monitoring Parameters	Cost
Aspirin	81 mg QD (enteric-coated in the elderly)	Guaiac stool testing	$3/1-month supply
Dipyridamole (Persantine)	50 mg PO TID	Guaiac stool testing	$54/1-month supply
Clopidogrel (Plavix)	75 mg PO QD with or without food; use with caution in patients with gastrointestinal ulcers or hepatic disease; produces less neutropenia than ticlopidine	Complete blood count (CBC)	$87/1-month supply
Ticlopidine	250 mg BID; reserve for patients with aspirin intolerance	CBC, check for neutropenia	$114/1-month supply

Meningitis
Recent anteroseptal myocardial infarction
Valvular heart disease or heart valve replacement
Carotid stenosis, polycythemia
Blood dyscrasias, especially those resulting in hypercoagulable states
Connective tissue diseases
Hypertension
Chemical imbalances, particularly glucose and sodium

THERAPEUTIC PLAN

The therapeutic plan depends on whether an underlying condition such as carotid artery stenosis or uncontrolled hypertension is determined. Treatment of the underlying condition is imperative.

Pharmaceutical

Pharmaceutical treatment is outlined in Table 182-2.

Surgical

If carotid artery stenosis is significant, carotid endarterectomy may be indicated.

EVALUATION/FOLLOW-UP

Patients with TIAs should be followed at least weekly and told to call if any neurologic symptoms occur depending upon the symptoms of the underlying risk conditions. If unidentified, frequency of check-ups will vary from clinic to clinic. However, patients should be evaluated every 4 to 6 months and immediately should symptoms recur.

SUGGESTED READINGS

American Pharmaceutical Association: New Product Bulletin: Plavix (clopidogrel), 1998.

McCance K, Huether S: *Pathophysiology: the biologic basis for disease in adults and children,* ed 2, St Louis, 1994, Mosby.

Reuben D, Yoshikawa T, Besdine R: editors: *Geriatrics review syllabus,* New York, 1995, American Geriatrics Society.

Uphold CR, Graham MV: *Clinical guidelines in family practice,* ed 2, Gainesville, Fla, 1994, Barmarrae Books.

Wilson J et al, editors: *Harrison's principles of internal medicine,* ed 12, New York, 1991, McGraw-Hill.

Woodley M, Whelan A, editors: *Manual of medical therapeutics,* ed 27, Boston, 1992, Little, Brown.

183 Trigeminal Neuralgia

ICD-9-CM

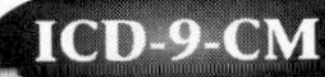

Trigeminal Neuralgia 350.1

OVERVIEW

Definition

Trigeminal neuralgia (Tic douloureux) is a recurrent unilateral facial pain syndrome. It most often affects the maxillary division of the trigeminal nerve. The attacks of pain may last several seconds and be repeated one after the other. They may come and go throughout the day and last for days, weeks, or months at a time and then disappear for the same length of time. It has no known cause.

Incidence

15,000 to 25,000 new cases in the United States each year; may be a low estimate because of difficulty of diagnosis in early stage and misdiagnosis as dental disease

More common in women than men

Occurs most often in **late middle age**

Associated with multiple sclerosis if younger in age and bilateral

Pathophysiology

Although there is no known cause, there is a compression hypothesis that attempts to explain the clinical findings. The pain may be due to electrical activity generated by compression of the trigeminal nerve. Demyelinated nerve fibers, hyperexcitability, and damaged axons combined with the discharge of nearby pain fibers may cause intense pain.

SUBJECTIVE DATA

History of Present Illness

Assess for duration, frequency, intensity of pain.

Identify what triggers the episode of pain.

Ask about associated headaches.

Past Medical History

Ask about:

- Last dental visit or dental problems
- Headaches and their treatment in past

Medications

Current medications

Ask about medications tried to decrease pain

Family History

Family history of headache, facial pain, neurological problems

Psychosocial History

Determine effects of stress, depression, and anxiety on pain.

Is patient able to sleep?

Description of Most Common Symptoms

Patients experience stabbing or clusters of stabbing pains that are restricted to one or more divisions of the trigeminal nerve. They will describe them as "electric-like shocks" of pain on one side of the face. These pains may last 20 to 30 seconds. Pain varies from mild to intense. Episodes may be brief and followed by long periods of remission. Trigger zones on the face or in the mouth are characteristic of this disorder. Activities involving the face, shaving, combing the hair, eating, drinking, and brushing the teeth may trigger the pain. The affected areas may be very sensitive to hot and cold. Patients are usually anxious when examined and may have a small degree of numbness in the affected area. Some patients experience atypical forms of trigeminal neuralgia, which has a less well-defined syndrome of pain. They may experience burning or aching over longer periods of time on one side of the face or forehead. There are usually no other neurological abnormalities.

OBJECTIVE DATA

Physical Examination

Perform a complete physical and neurological examination. Usually no abnormal physical findings are found. No evidence of sensory loss in the nerve distribution is usually found.

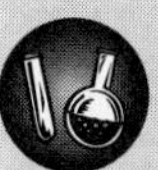

TABLE 183-1 Diagnostic Test: Trigeminal Neuralgia

Diagnostic Test	Finding/ Rationale	Cost ($)
Magnetic resonance imaging of head	To rule out multiple sclerosis or compression tumor (rare to find)	1781-2004

Diagnostic Procedures

There are no specific diagnostic tests; however, some tests may be needed to rule out other conditions (Table 183-1).

ASSESSMENT

Differential diagnosis include those found in Table 183-2.

THERAPEUTIC PLAN

Pharmaceutical

Medications take effect from 4 to 24 hours after initiation of therapy (Table 183-3).

Lifestyle/Activities

Avoidance of activities that trigger painful episodes

Diet

None specific unless certain foods trigger episode

Patient Education

Reassurance that trigeminal neuralgia is not fatal.
Connect patient with support group or national foundation.
Patient may require treatment from 3 months to over 1 year.
It may remit spontaneously.

TABLE 183-2 Differential Diagnosis: Trigeminal Neuralgia

Diagnosis	Supporting Data
Trigeminal neuralgia	Characteristic facial pain beginning near one side of mouth, and then shoots toward ear, eye or nose; physical examination, computed tomography, or magnetic resonance imaging usually normal
Herpes zoster/postherpetic neuralgia	Vesicular, painful lesions involving the trigeminal nerve; approximately 10% of patients suffer from postherpetic neuralgia
Dental disease	Temporomandibular joint (TMJ) disorder may cause facial pain as does a dental abscess
Trigeminal neuroma/acoustic neuroma/aneurism/multiple sclerosis/meningioma (these are secondary trigeminal neuralgias)	Pain radiates from the lesion to the periphery of the affected nerve and is usually intermittent but may become continuous and severe; these diagnoses should be considered, particularly if the patient is <40 y/o and has pain predominately in the upper division (forehead and eye) or has bilateral pain or evidence of bilateral sensory loss or associated motor weakness
Multiple sclerosis (MS)	MS should be considered as a contributing disease when a young person presents with trigeminal neuralgia
Cluster headache	Ipsilateral nasal congestion, rhinorrhea, lacrimation, redness of the eyes, Horner's syndrome; episodes usually occur at night, most often in men
Facial migraine	Pain about the eye, nausea and vomiting, diplopia
Sinus problems	History of upper respiratory infection, fever, tenderness to sinus palpation

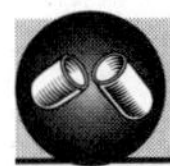

TABLE 183-3 Pharmaceutical Plan: Trigeminal Neuralgia

Drug	Dosage	Comments	Cost
Carbamazepine (Tegretol)	50 mg QID, then ↑ up to 200 mg/day until pain relieved Maintenance: 800-1.2 g/day ER: 100-200 mg QD or BID with meals, ↑ to 800-1200 mg/day	Pregnancy: C SE: aplastic anemia, bone marrow depression, photosensitivity, drowsiness Interactions with CYP3A4 inhibitors and CYP3A4 inducers (see Appendix D) Monitor: Complete blood count, iron, blood urea nitrogen, urinalysis, çarbamazepine levels, electrocardiogram, electrolytes, calcium, liver function tests; once pain controlled, dosage may be reduced to the minimum effective dose	\$10-\$39/200 mg (100); \$23/susp: 100 mg/5 ml (450 ml)
Phenytoin (Dilantin)	250 mg TID adjusting dose q7-10 days **Children:** 5 mg/kg/day in 2-3 doses; max 300 mg/day	Pregnancy: Not recommended SE: Nystagmus, drowsiness, gastrointestinal disturbances, gingival hyperplasia, hepatic disease; chewable and suspension not intended for once a day dosing; numerous drug interactions due to CYP-450 enzyme: see Appendix D Monitor: Phenytoin and thyroid levels	\$7-\$22/100 mg (100); \$20/chew: 50 mg (100); \$30/susp: 125 mg/5 ml (240 ml)
Baclofen (Lioresal)	5 mg TID initially, then ↑ by 5 mg/dose q3 days until desired response achieved; max 80 mg/day	Pregnancy: C SE: Drowsiness, dizziness, weakness, fatigue, increased urinary frequency	\$21-\$93/20 mg (100)
Neurontin (Gabapentin)	300 mg TID	Pregnancy: C Do not give within 2 hours of antacids SE: Somnolence, dizziness, ataxia, fatigue, nystagmus	Not available

ER, Extended release; *SE,* side effects.

Referral

Any patient experiencing atypical facial pain should be referred to a neurologist.

When the medical therapy is ineffective, subcutaneous injection of the ganglion with glycerol can provide relief and may be repeated if necessary.

Follow-up

A patient with typical/classic presentation may be treated and followed by the primary care physician unless response to medical management is ineffective.

Monitor appropriate laboratory values based on medication used.

Follow every 2 to 3 weeks for response to treatment.

EVALUATION

Complete resolution of pain is goal. Surgery is a last resort.

RESOURCES

Trigeminal Neuralgia Association
PO Box 340
Barnegat Light, NJ 08006
609-361-1014
www.neurosurgery.mgh.harvard.edu/tn-hfshp.htm

SUGGESTED REFERENCES

Bowsher D: Trigeminal neuralgia: an anatomically oriented review, *Clinical Anatomy* 10(6):409-415, 1997.

Ellsworth A et al: *Mosby's 1998 medical drug reference,* St Louis, 1998, Mosby.

Fields HL: Treatment of trigeminal neuralgia, *N Engl J Med* 334(17):1125-1126, 1996.

Healthcare Consultants of America, Inc: *1998 Physicians fee and coding guide,* Augusta, Ga, 1998, Healthcare Consultants of America, Inc.

Howard J: Tic douloureux, Parkinson's disease and the herpes connection, *Integr Phys Behav Sci* 32(3):257-264, 1997.

Johnson CJ: Headaches and facial pain. In Barker LR, Burton JR, Zieve PD, editors: *Principles of ambulatory medicine*, Baltimore, 1995, Williams & Wilkins.

Lawhern RA: Unexplained facial pain, 1998, Http://www.erols.com/lawhern/tn.html

Lincoff N, Rath P, Herano M: The treatment of periocular and facial pain with topical capsaicin, *J Neuroophthamol* 18(1):17-20, 1998.

Mabara G: Trigeminal neuralgia: a review of current therapeutic strategies, *J Phil Dental Assoc* 47(4):33, 1996.

Sist T et al: Gabapentin for idiopathic trigeminal neuralgia: report of two cases, *Neurology* 48:1467-1471, 1997.

Zakrzewska J et al: Lamotrigine (lamictal) in refractory trigeminal neuralgia: results from a double blind placebo-controlled crossover trial, *Pain* 73(2):223-230, 1997.

184 Tuberculosis

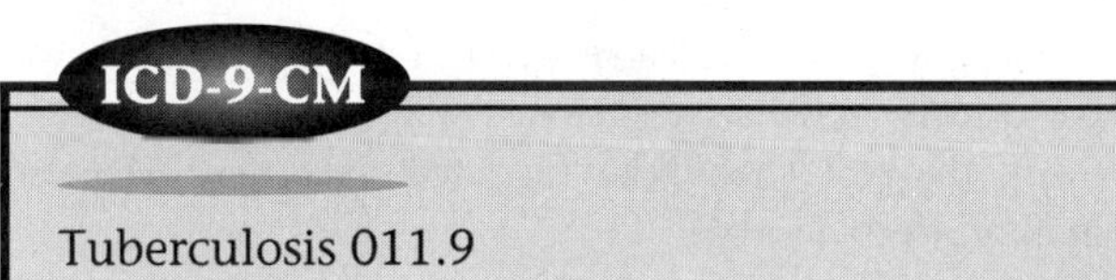

ICD-9-CM

Tuberculosis 011.9

OVERVIEW

Definition

Tuberculosis (TB) is a chronic, infectious, inflammatory, reportable disease. Patients infected with the bacillus are distinguished from those who have the disease. Tuberculosis usually infects the lungs but may occur in other tissues and organs in the body (extrapulmonary).

Incidence

The World Health Organization estimates that one third of the world population is infected with *Mycobacterium tuberculosis*. Tuberculosis cases in the United States in 1996 were 8 per 100,000. Those over age 65 have the highest case rate (16 per 100,000). The number of pediatric cases have increased 51% compared with an increase of 19% in all ages combined. Reasons for the increased incidence are:

- Human immunodeficiency virus (HIV) epidemic
- Immigration into the United States from countries where tuberculosis is common
- Inadequate public health efforts due to decreased funding
- Resistance to antibiotics due to misuse and noncompliance with therapy

Pathophysiology

Tuberculosis is caused by the bacteria *M. tuberculosis,* and it is transmitted by airborne droplets. The infected individual does not develop the disease unless the immune system is compromised. The disease can be pulmonary or extrapulmonary. Extrapulmonary disease includes meningitis, lymphadenitis, and renal, bone, and joint involvement.

Protective Factors Against

Living in uncrowded conditions with good ventilation
Avoid exposure to infected persons and at-risk populations
Intact immune system

Factors that Increase Susceptibility

Contact with infected persons, HIV-positive persons, people from Latin America, the Caribbean, Africa, and Asia (except Japan)
Living in homeless shelters, migrant farm camps, prisons, nursing homes, with health care workers
Alcoholism and drug abuse
Impaired immunity from chronic illness

SUBJECTIVE DATA

History of Present Illness

Chronic cough (usually with hemoptysis), lasts longer than 2 weeks
Night sweats
Unexplained weight loss
Children: Are less likely to have obvious symptoms

Past Medical History

Substance abuse
Diabetes
Silicosis
Cancer
Renal failure
Corticosteroid treatment or immunotherapy (e.g., transplant recipient)

Family History

Children do not transmit the disease to other children. However, more than one child can be exposed to the same source. Therefore all children in the home should be screened if one family member tests positive. They are generally infected by adults. A detailed family history is in order.

Ask about any chronic illness in family members since immunosuppression may allow the family member to have active tuberculosis disease.

Psychosocial History

Lifestyle/recreational drug use
Assess for alcoholism
Assess living conditions
Foreign travel

Associated Symptoms

Chest pain
Fatigue
Fever and chills
Anorexia

OBJECTIVE DATA

Physical Examination

General appearance, including vital signs (fever) (the examination may be negative, including the chest x-ray)
Chest
 Crackles upper posterior chest
 Bronchovesicular breathing
 Whispered pectoriloquy
 Supraclavicular and infraclavicular retraction
Lymph: Lymphadenopathy

Diagnostic Procedures

Laboratory

Complete blood count ($13-$16): Low hematocrit, normocytic and normochromic anemia
Urinalysis ($14-$18): Sterile pyuria suggests renal TB
Liver enzymes ($29-$41): If disseminated disease is present, these will be elevated
Sputum for culture and smear (acid-fast bacteria) ($23-$28) ×3: A positive smear is highly suggestive of TB, but only the culture is diagnostic. Cultures allow for testing for drug sensitivity to standard TB drugs.
TB Skin Test: 5 Tuberculin Unit dose of PPD-S (Mantoux test)

Who Should Be Tested

Any person who has spent time with a person who has infectious TB.
The patient who has a chronic illness that puts him or her at high risk for TB (e.g., HIV).
The patient who is from a country with a high rate of TB.

When Should the Test Be Done

If a person has been in contact with another person with active TB disease, it may take 10 to 12 weeks after exposure for the test to be positive. If you test earlier than 10 weeks, retest later.
Children should be tested based on the incidence of TB in their community. Guidelines recommend between 4 to 6 years and 11 to 16 years (Box 184-1).

Reading Results

If a person has received a BCG vaccination for TB, the person may have a positive TB test. The size of the reaction indicates the likelihood of active disease. Reactions from BCG get smaller over time. Results should be read between 48 and 72 hours after injection.
The basis of the reading is the presence or absence of induration determined from inspection and palpation. Record in millimeters.
If a multiple puncture test instead of a Mantoux test was performed, a positive test is vesicular in nature. If papules form, the test should be repeated using the Mantoux method (intradermal).

Positive Findings

Equal to or greater than 5 mm is positive for HIV-infected persons, persons who have had close contact with a person who has active TB disease, and persons who had healed TB as evidenced by chest x-ray.
Equal to or greater than 10 mm is positive in persons who are from countries with high incidence, and high-risk populations, including health care workers.
A reaction greater than or equal to 15 mm is positive in all persons.

Radiographic

Chest x-ray ($77-$91): Posteroanterior and lateral views
Apical scarring, hilar adenopathy with peripheral infiltrate, upper lobe cavitation may be present; a negative chest film rules out pulmonary tuberculosis

ASSESSMENT

Differential diagnoses are indicated in Table 184-1.

THERAPEUTIC PLAN

Pharmaceutical

Drug therapy is outlined in Tables 184-2 and 184-3.

Lifestyle/Activities

TB of the lungs and throat is infectious. The patient should stay home from work and school for at least 2 weeks after starting treatment.
If it is difficult for patient to remember to take the drugs, consider enrolling the patient in the directly observed therapy program at the health department.

Diet

If weight loss is present, high-calorie diet

Box 184-1

Tuberculin Skin Test Recommendations*

Children for Whom Immediate Skin Testing Is Indicated

Contacts of persons with confirmed or suspected infectious tuberculosis (contact investigation); this includes children identified as contacts of family members or associates in jail or prison in the last five years

Children with radiographic or clinical findings suggesting tuberculosis

Children immigrating from endemic countries (e.g., Asia, Middle East, Africa, Latin America)

Children with travel histories to endemic countries and/or significant contact with indigenous person from such countries

Children Who Should Be Tested Annually for Tuberculosis†

Children infected with human immunodeficiency virus (HIV) or living in household with HIV-infected persons

Incarcerated adolescents

Children Who Should Be Tested Every 2 to 3 Years†

Children exposed to the following individuals: HIV-infected, homeless, residents of nursing homes, institutionalized adolescents or adults, users of illicit drugs, incarcerated adolescents or adults, and migrant farm workers; foster children with exposure to adults in the preceding high-risk groups are included

Children Who Should Be Considered for Tuberculin Skin Testing at Ages 4 to 6 and 11 to 16 Years

Children whose parents immigrated (with unknown tuberculin skin test status) from regions of the world with high prevalence of tuberculosis; continued potential exposure by travel to the endemic areas and/or household contact with persons from the endemic areas (with unknown tuberculin skin test status) should be an indication for repeat tuberculin skin testing

Children without specific risk factors who reside in high-prevalence areas; in general, a high-risk neighborhood or community does not mean an entire city is at high risk; rates in any area of the city may vary by neighborhood or even from block to block; physicians should be aware of these patterns in determining the likelihood of exposure; public health officials or local tuberculosis experts should help clinicians identify areas that have appreciable tuberculosis rates

Children at increased risk of progression of infection to disease: Those with other medical risk factors, including diabetes mellitus, chronic renal failure, malnutrition, and congenital or acquired immunodeficiencies deserve special consideration; without recent exposure, these persons are not at increased risk of acquiring tuberculosis infection; underlying immune deficiencies associated with these conditions theoretically would enhance the possibility for progression to severe disease; initial histories of potential exposure to tuberculosis should be included on all of these patients; if these histories or local epidemiological factors suggest a possibility of exposure, immediate and periodic tuberculin skin testing should be considered; an initial Mantoux tuberculin skin test should be performed before initiation of immunosuppressive therapy in any child with an underlying condition that necessitates immunosuppressive therapy

From American Academy of Pediatrics: 1997 Red Book: Report of the committee on infectious diseases, ed 24, Elk Grove Village, Ill, 1997 American Academy of Pediatrics.

*BCG immunization is not a contraindication to tuberculin skin testing.

†Initial tuberculin skin testing is at the time of diagnosis or circumstance, beginning as early as age 3 months.

Table 184-1 Differential Diagnosis: Tuberculosis

Diagnoses	Supporting Data
Community-acquired pneumonia (fungal)	Fever, headache, sore throat, myalgia, nonproductive hacking cough, substernal chest pain
Chronic bronchitis	Productive cough >3 months in at least 2 consecutive years, smoker, shortness of breath with activity, digital clubbing, hyperinflation on chest film if emphysema is present

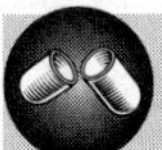

TABLE 184-2 Pharmaceutical Treatment for Active Tuberculosis

Drug	Dose	Comments	Cost ($)
Isoniazid (INH)	5-10 mg/kg PO QD up to 300 mg	Side effects include peripheral neuritis and hepatitis; warn patient NOT to drink alcoholic beverages; must be taken on an empty stomach Q AM	1-14
Rifampin (RIF)	10 mg/kg PO QD up to 600 mg	Side effects include hepatitis, purpura, reduces the effect of oral contraceptive pills and implants; use alternative contraceptive method; can turn saliva, tears, and urine orange; do not use soft contact lenses; can be taken on an empty stomach Q am	149-211
Streptomycin (strep)	15-20 mg/kg PO QD up to 1 g	Nephrotoxic, may damage hearing	Not available
Pyrazinamide (PZA)	15-30 mg/kg PO QD up to 2 g	Causes hyperuricemia	87-117
Rifater	Do not give if under 15 years of age; <44 kg/4 tabs, 44-54 kg/5 tabs, >55 kg 6 tabs PO QD	Used in initial phase of the 2-month treatment of pulmonary tuberculosis; continue to treat for 4 additional months with rifampin and INH	Not available
Ethambutol (ETB)	15-25 mg/kg PO QD	Can cause optic neuritis; check visual acuity often	47-159

NOTE: All of these drugs can be dosed on a twice or three times weekly schedule to promote adherence. Check additional drug reference for proper dosage. Drug treatment is for a 6-month period for adults. Children and people with HIV infection need longer treatment. Rifater is a newly approved drug that combines isoniazid, rifampin, and pyrazinamide.

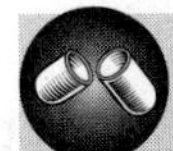

TABLE 184-3 Drug Therapy in Complicated Tuberculosis Cases

Situation*	Comment	Regimen
Multi-drug resistant tuberculosis (TB) (MDR) defined as resistant to at least two drugs	United States born, not living in area of high resistance	Months 1-2 INH 5 mg/kg/day PO or IM plus RIF 10 mg/kg/day PO plus PZA 25 mg/kg/day PO months 3-6 (16 wks); INH plus RIF at above dosage daily
TB during pregnancy		INH plus RIF plus ETB ×9 months; PZA not recommended; strep not used secondary to ototoxicity to the fetus
TB plus HIV/AIDS	Stop HIV protease inhibitor; RIF accelerates the metabolism of protease inhibitors while protease inhibitors increase the serum level of RIF increasing the likelihood of toxicity	INH plus RIF plus PZA plus ETB ×2 months followed by 4 months of INH plus RIF; if protease inhibitor is used, RIF is not used; indinavir ($338-$360) 800 mg q8h is the antiretroviral agent of choice; rifabutin ($371) is substituted for RIF

*These guidelines change rapidly but were current at time of publication. Check current source before prescribing.
ETB, Ethambutol; *INH,* isoniazid; *PZA,* pyrazinamide; *RIF,* rifampin; *strep,* streptomycin.

Patient Education

Explain the difference between TB infection and TB disease. Explain that in TB infection the person has no symptoms and cannot spread the disease to another person but he or she can develop active disease if not treated.

Warn patient about side effects of medications.

- No appetite
- Nausea and vomiting
- Yellowish skin or eyes
- Fever for more than 3 days
- Abdominal pain
- Tingling in fingers and toes
- Change in vision
- Rash

Stress need to complete drug therapy. Suggest reminder system: take same time each day around a routine activity (e.g., brushing teeth). Use a pill dispenser.

Family Impact

During infectious period, should sleep separately. Place a fan in the bedroom and air the room out.

Referral/Consultation

In cases of systemic disease, the patient should be referred to an infectious disease physician or an internal medicine specialist. A pulmonologist may also be consulted.

Follow-up

Monthly

EVALUATION

Monitor:

- Liver enzymes due to side effects of drug therapy
- Visual acuity
- Renal function

RESOURCES

Aepo-xdv-www.epo.cdc.gov/wonder/preguid
Update on Tuberculin skin testing, 1997

Http://hivinsite.UCSF.edu
AIDS knowledge base, 1998

SUGGESTED READINGS

Cornell S: Back from the dead: emerging and reemerging infectious diseases, *Adv Nurse Pract* 6(5):67-68, 1998.

Cornell S: Pediatric infectious disease: updates on three top offenders, *Adv Nurse Pract* 6(5):70-72, 1998.

Ellsworth AJ et al: *Mosby's 1998 medical drug reference*, St Louis, 1998, Mosby.

Healthcare Consultants of America, Inc: *1998 physicians fee and coding guide*, Augusta, Ga, 1998, Healthcare Consultants of America, Inc.

Murphy P: Tuberculosis in the ambulatory patient. In Barker L, Burton J, Zieve P, editors: *Principles of ambulatory medicine,* ed 4, Baltimore, 1995, Williams & Wilkins.

Upper Respiratory Tract Infections

ICD-9-CM

Common Cold 465.9
Allergic Rhinitis 477.9
Common Cold Pharyngitis 462
Croup 464.4
Epiglottitis 464.30
Upper Respiratory Infection 465.9

Definition

Upper respiratory tract infections (URI) are infections involving the nasopharynx and/or oropharynx.

COMMON COLD

OVERVIEW

Definition

The common cold is defined as a mild, self-limited viral syndrome involving the upper respiratory tract mucosa.

Incidence

It is the most common acute illness in the industrialized world and highly contagious. It is a common cause for seeking medical attention and absences from work and school. The number of colds per year tend to decrease with age:

- **Infants** and **preschool children:** 4 to 8 per year
- **School-age children:** 2 to 6 per year
- **Adults:** 2 to 4 per year
  - Households with children, adults tend to have higher rates, with mother having more than father

Pathophysiology

Viral

Transmission

Direct physical contact: Nasal mucosa to hand to another person's hand to eyes or nasal membranes
Large and small droplets produced by cough or sneeze

Common Pathogens

Most common:
- Rhinoviruses: Fall, mid-spring to summer
- Coronaviruses: Winter

Common:
- Parainfluenza: Fall, spring
- Respiratory syncytial virus: Winter to early spring
- Influenza: Winter

Infants: Respiratory syncytial virus (RSV) and rhinovirus

SUBJECTIVE DATA

Past Medical History

Usually noncontributory

Psychosocial History

Day care or school attendance
Children in the home
Smoker or exposure to second-hand smoke
Recent exposure to others with cold symptoms

Description of Most Common Symptoms

24-78 Hours:
- Dry scratchy throat
- Clear nasal discharge

Malaise
Sneezing
Loss of taste and smell
Low-grade fever
Redness and inflammation of nasal and pharyngeal membranes

4-7 Days:
Cough
Hoarseness
Thickening of nasal drainage

Neonates:
Minimal respiratory signs and symptoms
Nonspecific signs: Poor feeding and lethargy
Severe: Unexpected apnea episodes

Infants: Anorexia, vomiting, and diarrhea

Children: Filling of eustachian tubes causing obstruction and ear pain
Smokers: Symptoms usually worse with same outcome

OBJECTIVE DATA

Physical Examination

A problem-oriented examination should be performed, with special emphasis on tympanic membranes (TMs), mucous membranes, lymph nodes, and breath sounds.

Infants and **children:** Signs and symptoms of dehydration

Diagnostic Procedures

Sputum culture ($30-$37) if copious amount of sputum; consider acid-fast bacillus ($17-$21) if tuberculosis is in the differential diagnosis

CBC ($13-$16) if elevated temperature

Sinus x-rays if increased nasal congestion with sinus tenderness; it is difficult and unnecessary to identify the causative virus for management of the common cold

ASSESSMENT

Differential diagnosis include:

Pharyngitis
Influenza
Allergic rhinitis

Complications

Infants to 3 years
Otitis media associated 29% of the time

Infants
Sudden infant death syndrome (SIDS): 90% of the SIDS deaths have reported cold symptoms before death

Adults and **children**
Exacerbation of obstructive sleep apnea, disturbed sleep patterns, and bronchospasms

THERAPEUTIC PLAN

Pharmaceutical

Aspirin (EC-ASA $9-$37), ibuprofen ($3-$50), or acetaminophen ($2-$4): Relieves body aches and fever; aspirin and acetaminophen have been shown to excrete the virus more quickly from the mucous membranes

Aspirin products are not recommended in children under age 16 years.

Tylenol is the only recommended medication in pregnancy.

Antihistamines
Chlorpheniramine ($14-$18):
Action: Reduces sneezing, nasal mucus production
Side effect: Drowsiness
Diphenhydramine (Benadryl) ($20):
Action: No difference from placebo effect
Side effect: Drowsiness
Triprolidine (Actifed) (cost not available):
Action: No difference from placebo effect
Side effect: None
Astemizole (Hismanal) ($185)
Action: Reduces nasal mucus production
Side effect: Weight gain

Decongestants
Pseudoephedrine/phenylephrine ($5-$8) spray or oral preparations
Action: Reduces congestion, sneezing
Side effect: Tachycardia, palpitations, elevated diastolic blood pressure, fatigue, dizziness, bladder outlet obstruction
Oxymetazoline spray (Dristan, Afrin) ($4-$8)
Action: Improved nasal symptoms
Side effects: Rebound nasal congestion

Expectorants
Guaifenesin ($20-$80):
Action: Thinning of sputum, no reduction in cough
Side effects: None

Anticholinergics
Ipratropium spray: (Atrovent aerosol) ($30)
Action: Reduces sneezing and nasal discharge
Side effect: Dry throat

Combinations
Decongestant/antihistamine
Action: Decreases congestion, post nasal drip, rhinorrhea
Side effect: Dry mouth, nervousness, insomnia

Corticosteroids
Corticosteroids (Medrol Dose Pack)
Action: Reduction of inflammation (i.e., vocal cords)
Side effect: Weight gain, mood alteration

Nonpharmaceutical

Bed rest: Not necessary for a more rapid recovery
Steam or cool mist: Liquefies nasal secretions
Chicken noodle soup: Studies have shown chicken soup helps to clear nasal secretions.
Voice rest: Helps to decrease inflammation of vocal cords, which decreases hoarseness

Patient Education

Avoid touching nasal or eyes membranes
Wash hands after sneezing, coughing, or blowing nose
Throw away tissues
Cover nose and mouth during sneeze or cough
Avoid crowds
Do not use nasal preparations for over 5 days; avoids rebound congestion

Referrals

Infants: Infants with apnea episodes should be admitted for observation and evaluation and treatment of RSV
Children and **elderly:** Hospitalization may be required if pneumonia develops

EVALUATION/FOLLOW-UP

Worsening of symptoms
Increase in fever
Difficulty breathing, wheezing
Color change of nasal drainage or sputum

PHARYNGITIS

OVERVIEW

Definition

Pharyngitis is inflammation and pain within the oropharynx area.

Incidence

Pharyngitis tends to be one of the most common diseases treated by primary care providers in the United States. It is the fourth most common symptom seen and accounts for nearly 40 million primary care visits each year.

Pathophysiology

Bacterial and viral pathogens
Spread by person-to-person contact via droplets of oral, respiratory, and nasal secretions

Common Pathogens

Adults

Most common:
- Beta-hemolytic streptococci groups A (10% to 15%)
- *Mycoplasma pneumoniae*
- *Chlamydia pneumoniae*
- Influenza type A and B
- Parainfluenza
- Epstein-Barr virus
- Adenovirus
- Herpes simplex virus
- Enteroviruses

Less common:
- Beta-hemolytic streptococci groups (groups C, G)
- *Corynebacterium diphtheriae*
- *Neisseria gonorrhoeae*
- *Neisseria meningitidis*
- *Hemophilus influenzae*
- RSV

Children

Most common:
- Beta-hemolytic streptococci, group A
  - Age less than 2 years 3%
  - Ages 5 to 10 years most common cause
- Influenza A and B
- Parainfluenza
- Adenoviruses
- Herpes simplex virus
- Epstein-Barr virus

Less common:
- RSV
- Rhinovirus
- Coronaviruses
- Cytomegalovirus
- Rubeola
- Rubella
- *Candida* sp.
- *Toxoplasma gondii*

SUBJECTIVE DATA

Past Medical History

Previous streptococcal infections
Autoimmune disease
Sexually transmitted diseases
Rheumatic fever
Diabetes

Medications

Recent use of antibiotics and other medications
Drug allergies

Family History

Recent pharyngeal infections
History of rheumatic fever

Psychosocial History

Attendance in school/day care
Living conditions (crowded)
Smoking history
Sexual exposures
Drug use

Diet History

Recent decrease in oral intake, especially in young children due to pain

Description of Most Common Symptoms

Generally patients present with complaints of fever, sore throat, tender cervical nodes, cough, and general malaise.
Children may have abdominal pain, nausea and vomiting.
Infants may have excoriated nares.
See Table 185-1 for associated symptoms and treatment plan.

Associated Symptoms

Neisseria Gonorrhoeae

See also Chapter 81
Urethritis, vaginal itching and/or discharge

OBJECTIVE DATA

Figure 185-1 illustrates a typical workup for the complaint of sore throat.

Physical Examination

A problem-oriented physical examination should be conducted, with special attention paid to:

Vital signs, respiratory effort, general appearance, and hydration
Throat: Erythema, color of exudate, breath odor
Neck: Cervical and submandibular nodes
Ears: External otitis, otitis media
Nose: Drainage, excoriated nares (infants)
Skin: Rashes, lesions

See Figure 185-2 for decision tree regarding use of rapid streptococcal test vs. throat culture.

ASSESSMENT

Differential diagnoses include:

- Streptococcal (strep) infection
- Strep Score:
  - 1+ Tonsillar exudate
  - 1+ Anterior cervical adenopathy
  - 1+ Absence of cough
  - 1+ Fever
- The higher the score, the greater probability of strep infection
- Common cold
  - Influenza
  - Infectious mononucleosis
  - Herpangina
  - Herpetic pharyngitis
  - Mycoplasma
  - Acute human immunodeficiency virus
  - Diphtheria
  - Yersinia
  - Candida
  - Synthetic lupus erythematosus
  - Vincent's angina

THERAPEUTIC PLAN

Pharmaceutical

General: Tylenol ($2-$4) or ibuprofen ($3-$50) for fever and pain
Viral: Symptomatic and warm salt water gargle (see Table 185-1)

Patient Education

Rest
Drink fluids to stay hydrated
Cover mouth and nose during cough or sneeze
Wash hands after cough or sneeze
Avoid crowds
Dispose of tissues properly

Referral

Otolaryngology

Multiple recurrent episodes for possible tonsillectomy

TABLE 185-1 Associated Symptoms and Treatment Plan: Upper Respiratory Tract Infections

Pathogen	Fever	Exudate	Adenopathy	Oral Membranes	Other Symptoms	Diagnostic Studies	Treatment
Group A streptococcus	Yes ≥100° F	Yellow or creamy white	Anterior cervical		No cough; may have scarlatiniform rash	Rapid strep throat culture (throat culture for strep $39-$51)	**Adult:** Benzathine penicillin G: 1.2 million U IM ($10-$15) (if at high risk for rheumatic fever, repeat once a week for 4 weeks); pregnancy: B, *or* Penicillin V ($5-$42): 125 to 250 mg PO BID for 10 days; pregnancy: B, *or* Erythromycin ($14-$20): 250-500 mg PO QID for 10 days (if penicillin allergic); pregnancy: B **Children:** Penicillin VK: 25-50 mg/kg/day PO in divided doses q6h for 10 days (250 mg PO BID has also been shown effective), *or* Benzathine penicillin G: IM one time only: <30 kg: 300,000 U 31-60 kg: 600,000 U 61-90 kg: 900,000 U >91 kg: 1,200,000 U, *or* Erythromycin: 30 to 50 mg/kg/day PO in divided doses q8h for 10 days (10 mg/kg PO q12h has also been shown to be

							or Erythromycin estolate: Has less gastric upset and covers *Chlamydia;* 30 to 50 mg/kg/day PO in divided doses q6-8h for 10 days *or* Cefadroxil (Duricef): 30 mg/kg PO q day for 10 days; pregnancy: B
Epstein-Barr Virus	Yes ≥102° F	White, gray-green	Posterior cervical	Palatal petechiae	Fatigue, malaise (i.e., hepatosplenomegaly), headache	Atypical lymphocytes on peripheral smear ($54-$68); positive mono-spot ($57-$72)	Symptomatic; bed rest during acute phase (10-14 days)
Diphtheria	Yes; low-grade	Blue-white or gray-white	Cervical	Focal hemorrhagic raw surface under pseudomembranes	Weakness, malaise, elevated pulse disproportionate to fever	Fluorescent antibody stains ($51-$64)	Erythromycin 500 mg PO QID ×10 days; pregnancy: B *or* Penicillin G 1 g PO QID ×10 days; pregnancy: B
Chlamydia	Yes	None	None		Bronchitis, pneumonia	Negative strep culture; often associated with sexually transmitted diseases	Azithromycin ($16-$25) 1 g PO single dose; pregnancy: B *or* Doxycycline ($6-$125) 100 mg PO BID x 7 days; pregnancy: D *or* Tetracycline ($7-$20) 500 mg PO QID ×7 days; pregnancy: D *or* Erythromycin 500 mg PO QID ×7 days; pregnancy: B

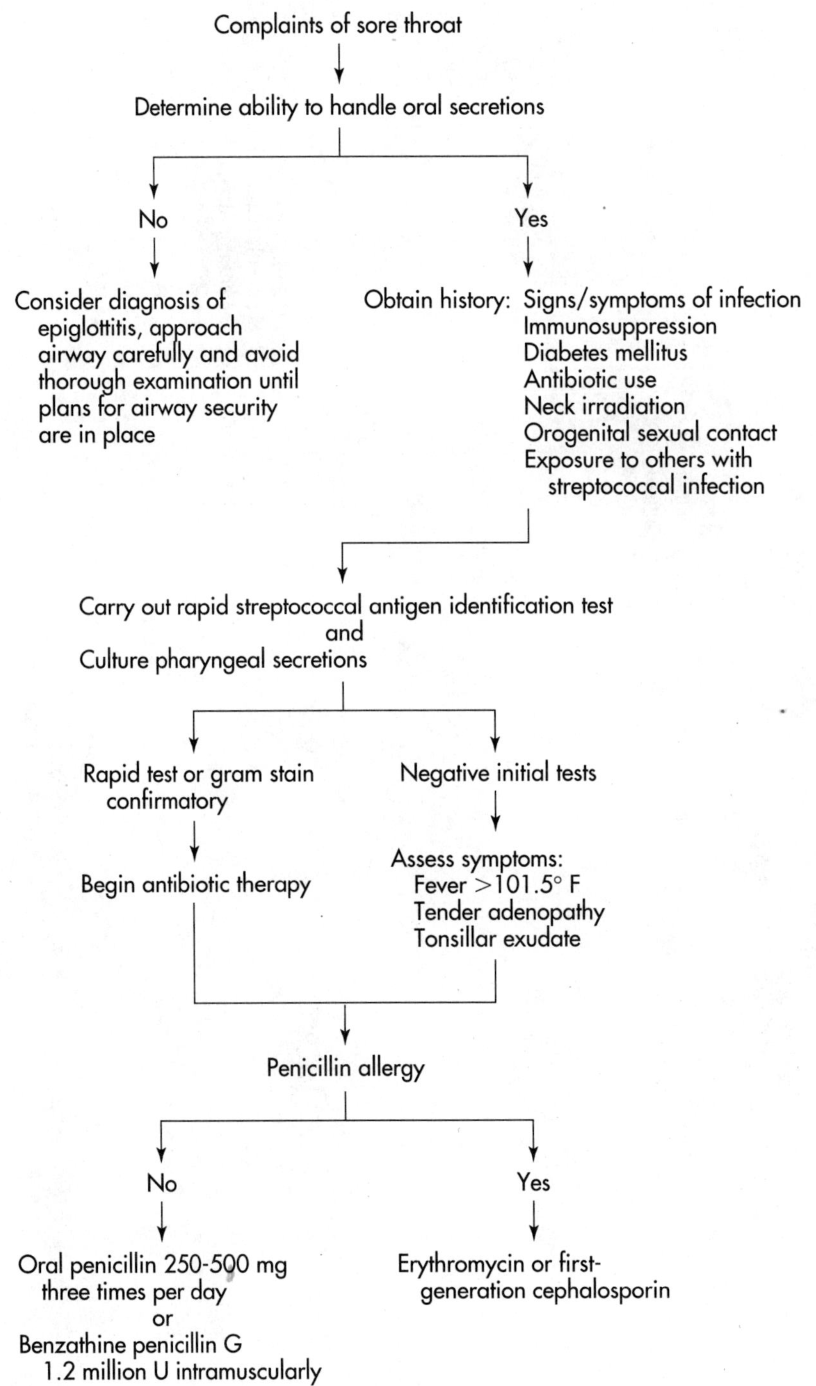

Figure 185-1 Diagnostic algorithm for sore throat pain in adults. (Adapted from Grodzin CJ, Schwartz SC, Bone RC: *Diagnostic strategies for internal medicine,* St Louis, 1996, Mosby.)

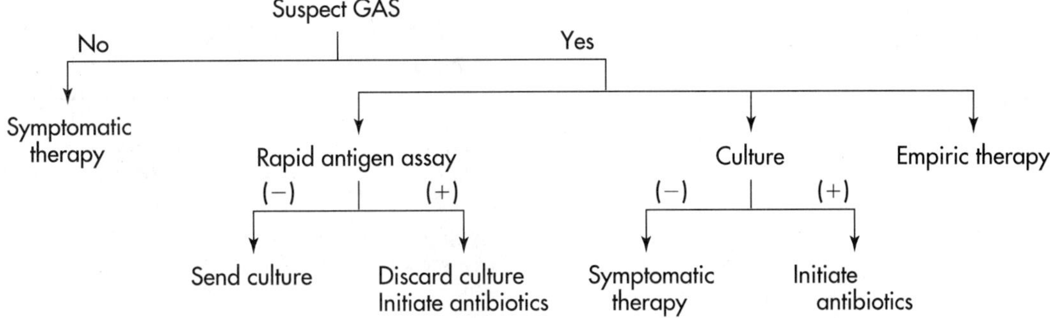

Figure 185-2 Management strategies in pharyngitis. *GAS,* Group A streptococcus. (From Rudolph A, Kamei R: *Rudolph's fundamentals of pediatrics*, ed 2, Stamford, Conn, 1998, Appleton & Lange.)

Severe episode of pharyngitis
Suspected abscess formation

Hospitalization

Unable to maintain hydration
Risk of sudden airway obstruction
IV antibiotic therapy if unable to take oral antibiotics due to airway obstruction, difficulty swallowing, or persistent nausea and vomiting
Surgical intervention (drainage of abscess)

EVALUATION/FOLLOW-UP

Continued fever
Inability to swallow medications
Development of new symptoms
Recurrent pharyngitis (more than 4 times in 12 months)

EPIGLOTTITIS AND CROUP

OVERVIEW

Definition

Epiglottitis is a rapid developing, life-threatening bacterial infection of the supraglottic area. This is a true medical emergency. It may or may not be proceeded by an upper respiratory infection (URI) syndrome.

Croup is an acute viral inflammatory disease of the subglottic mucosa. It is usually proceeded by a viral URI.

Incidence

Croup is at least ten times more common than epiglottitis.

Croup is most common in the fall and winter months, peaking between October and December.

Croup is the most common cause of stridor in **young children.**

Croup rarely occurs in **infants less than 1 month old** and **school-age children.** The most common age group is 6 months to 3 years and declines with age.

Boys are at higher risk than **girls.**

Croup is generally self-limited, epiglottitis is not.

Epiglottitis is rare and generally occurs in **children 2 to 6 years.** Adult cases do occur, and are most often seen between the second and fourth decade of life.

Epiglottitis can occur at any time of the year, and is most often seen in temperate climates.

Pathophysiology

Common Pathogens

Croup
- Parainfluenza virus, type 1 (most common)
- Parainfluenza virus, type 3
- RSV
- Adenoviruses
- Rubeola
- Influenza

Epiglottitis
- *Haemophilus influenzae:* The incidence is decreasing in **children** with the use of the *H. influenzae* vaccine, whereas the incidence is increasing in **adults.**

SUBJECTIVE DATA

Past Medical History

Recent viral infections
Exposures
Allergies
Medications
Immunization status

Family History

Recent illness

Psychosocial History

School/day care exposure
Smoking
Profession (possible exposure to inhaled irritants: paints, chemicals, dust particles, smoke, etc.)

Diet History

Decrease oral intake

Description of Most Common Symptoms

Croup
- Low-grade fever, rhinorrhea, barking cough especially during the night time hours

Epiglottitis
- High fever, drooling, difficulty swallowing
- **Children** may present with URI symptoms, sore throat, and voice change
- **Infants** may have a nonclassic presentation with URI symptoms, croupy cough, and low-grade fever

Associated Symptoms

Croup
- URI symptoms
- Hoarse voice
- Inspiratory and/or expiratory stridor

Epiglottitis
- Toxic looking
- Muffled voice
- Dysphagia
- Inspiratory stridor
- Prefers sitting position

OBJECTIVE DATA

Physical Examination

CAUTION: ENSURE THE AIRWAY IS NOT COMPROMISED BEFORE PROCEEDING WITH ANY PHYSICAL EXAMINATION! Have emergency life support equipment available!

A problem-oriented physical examination should be conducted, with particular attention to airway compromise, vital signs, general appearance, respiratory status, ears, nose, and lymph nodes (Table 185-2).

TABLE 185-2 Comparison of Signs: Croup and Epiglottitis

	Croup	Epiglottitis
Throat	Normal-appearing epiglottis	"Cherry Red" epiglottis
Appearance	Nontoxic	Toxic
Temperature	<103° F (39.5° C)	>103° F (39.5° C)
Breath sounds	Good air movement	Decreased air movement
Positioning	Variable	"Tripod" sitting

Diagnostic Procedures

CAUTION: DIAGNOSTIC PROCEDURES SHOULD NOT BE ATTEMPTED UNTIL THE AIRWAY IS SECURED!

Lateral neck x-ray:
- Croup: Normal epiglottis, with narrowing of the subepiglottis area
- Epiglottitis: "Thumb print" sign consistent with inflammation of the epiglottis (children near C_2—C_3, Adults near C_5—C_6)

Complete blood count with differential ($13-$16)
- Croup: Within normal limits
- Epiglottitis: White blood count 10,000 to 25,000 with elevated bands

Arterial blood gases and pulse oximetry
- Croup and epiglottitis: Results are variable, dependent on the degree of respiratory distress

Blood cultures ($39-$48)
- Croup and epiglottitis: results may vary, depending if an occult bacteremia coexists with the disease.

ASSESSMENT

Differential diagnoses include:

Foreign Body
Traumatic obstruction
Neoplasm
Angioneurotic edema
Laryngitis
RSV
Bacterial tracheitis
Inhalation injury

THERAPEUTIC PLAN

Pharmaceutical

Croup without stridor at rest:
- Acetaminophen or ibuprofen to control fever.

Croup with stridor at rest:
- Racemic epinephrine 2.25% solution ($10) via nebulizer

q2h while stridor continues at rest. (lasts approximately 4 hours, watch for rebound effect)
<20 kg: 0.25 ml in 2.25 ml saline
20 to 40 kg: 0.50 ml in 2.25 ml saline
>40 kg: 0.75 ml in 2.25 ml saline
Dexamethasone (Decadron): ($4-$25)
0.6 mg/kg/dose IV, IM, or PO for 1 to 4 doses q6 to 12h (it has also been used via hand-held nebulized (HHN) treatments with the same results)
Oxygen
Nasal cannula: 2 to 6 L/min (25% to 45% O_2)
Simple face mask: 5 to 10 L/min (35% to 50% O_2)
Nonrebreather mask: 8 to 15 L/min (60% to 90% O_2)
Epiglottitis: (requires ICU admission)
Oxygen at 100% followed by intubation
Antibiotics: IV for at least 5 days, then may switch to oral
Cefotaxime ($12-$22) 50 to 150 mg/kg/day divided q6-8h; pregnancy: B *or*
Ceftriaxone ($12): 50 to 75 mg/kg/day divided q12h; pregnancy: B *or*
Cefuroxime ($35-$124): 100 mg/kg/day divided q6-8h; pregnancy: B

Nonpharmaceutical

Oral fluids to maintain hydration
Cool mist humidifier

Patient Education

Croup
Keep room humidified with cool mist
Keep fever under control
Push oral fluids
If stridor begins, take child outside into the cool air for 5 min; if it does not resolve, take to clinic or Emergency Department
Epiglottitis
Explain need for intubation and procedures to family

Referral

Epiglottitis
Croup with stridor at rest
Dehydration or unable to drink fluids
If unable to control fever
If unable to maintain airway

EVALUATION/FOLLOW-UP

Recurrent croup episodes
If no improvement in 4 to 5 days
Increase in stridor
Stops drinking
Unable to control fever
New symptoms develop

SUGGESTED READINGS

Bamberger BM, Jackson MA: Upper respiratory tract infections: pharyngitis, sinusitis, otitis media and epiglottitis. In Niederman MS, Sarosi GA, Glassroth J: *Respiratory infections: a scientific basis for management,* Philadelphia, 1994, WB Saunders.

Barkin RM, Rosen R: Pulmonary disorders, In Barkin RM, Rosen R: *Emergency pediatrics: a guide to ambulatory care,* ed 4, St Louis, 1994, Mosby.

Berman S, Schmitt BD: Ear, nose and, throat. In Hay WW et al: *Current pediatric diagnosis and treatment,* ed 12, Norwalk, Conn, 1995, Appleton & Lange.

Casmmassima PS, Belanger GK:. Ear, nose, and throat disorders. In Barkin RM, Rosen R: *Emergency pediatrics: a guide to ambulatory care,* ed 4, Mosby, St Louis, 1994.

Ellsworth AJ et al: *Mosby's 1998 medical drug reference,* St Louis, 1998, Mosby.

Hall CB, McBride JT: Upper respiratory tract infections: the common cold, pharyngitis, croup, bacterial tracheitis and epiglottitis. In Pennington JE: *Respiratory infections: diagnosis and management,* ed 3, New York, 1994, Raven Press.

Healthcare Consultants of America, Inc: *1998 physicians fee and coding guide,* Augusta, Ga, 1998, Healthcare Consultants of America, Inc.

Jacoby DB: Adult epiglottitis, *J Am Acad Nurse Pract* 7(10):511-512, 1995.

Komaroff AL: Disease of the respiratory tract: pharyngitis, coryza, and related infections in adults. In Branch WT: *Office practice of medicine,* ed 3, Philadelphia, 1994, WB Saunders.

Koster FT, Barker LR: 1995 Respiratory tract infections. In Barker LR, Burton JR, Zieve PD: *Principles of ambulatory medicine,* ed 4, Baltimore, 1995, Williams & Wilkins.

Larsen GL et al: Respiratory tract and mediastinum. In Hay WW et al: *Current pediatric diagnosis and treatment,* ed 12, Norwalk, Conn, 1994, Appleton & Lange.

Paluzzi RG: Respiratory tract infections: pharyngitis. In Epstein KR: *Manual of office medicine,* Boston, 1995, Blackwell Scientific.

Urinary Incontinence

ICD-9-CM

Incontinence of Urine 788.3
Women
Stress Incontinence 625.6
Urge Incontinence 788.33
Urinary Retention or Stasis 788.20
Men
Stress Incontinence 788.32
Urge 788.33
Intermittent Stream 788.61

OVERVIEW

Definition

Urinary incontinence (UI) is the involuntary loss of urine, severe enough to have social and hygienic consequences.

Incidence

More than 13 million Americans suffer from UI. Women have UI twice a much as men. Ten percent to 30% of women ages 16 to 64 have some degree of UI. Approximately 50% of nursing home residents (>65 y/o) and homebound **elderly** have UI. Approximately 25% to 30% of hospitalized elderly have UI; incidence of UI in community dwelling **women >60** y/o is 25% to 35%. Ten percent to 15% of community dwelling **men >60** y/o have UI.

In women UI is predominantly of the mixed and stress types. In men UI is primarily a bladder irritation from benign prostatic hyperplasia, so urge incontinence predominates.

Pathophysiology

Anatomy of the Bladder and Urethra

The bladder is composed of a three-layer bundle of smooth muscle called the detrusor muscle. This muscle contracts in response to parasympathetic stimulation and relaxes under sympathetic and beta-andrenergic stimulation. Detrusor muscle activity is initiated by brain stem reflex unless inhibited by cortical control.

The bladder neck and proximal urethra contract in response to alpha-andrenergic stimulation. Two thirds of the proximal urethra lies intraabdominally and is supported by the pelvic floor. The pudendal nerve innervates and causes contraction of the pelvic floor. The urethra sphincter is made up of elastic tissue, blood vessels, and smooth muscles. Contraction of the sphincter is aided by increased intraabdominal pressure, which forces the proximal urethra forward against the pubic symphysis.

Types of Reversible Urinary Incontinence

Stress Incontinence

Most common type of incontinence, accounting for 80% of incontinence in women under the age of 60. Results from loss of anatomic support to the vesical neck and proximal urethra. Increases in intraabdominal pressure (e.g., coughing, sneezing, straining, laughing) causes the proximal urethra to no longer be pressed up against the pubic bone. Increased vesicular pressure overcomes the ability of the relatively weak proximal urethral sphincter mechanism to retain urine.

Urge Incontinence (a.k.a. Detrusor Instability)

Less common than stress incontinence; however, it is responsible for 70% of incontinence in the elderly, predominantly in men. Urge incontinence occurs when the urge to void is perceived by the individual, but the individual is unable to override the detrusor contraction effectively. This causes the individual to have a strong, sudden urge to void with a swift leakage of moderate to large amounts of urine. Detrusor instability may be caused by lesions of the central nervous system (e.g., strokes), demyelinating disorders, chronic cystitis, or tumors; or it may be idiopathic.

Overflow Incontinence

The least common type of incontinence. It occurs when the bladder, unable to void normally, becomes overdistended. This leads to frequent or constant urinary leakage. Causes include neurological problems that inhibit detrusor activity such as diabetes mellitus, vitamin B_{12} deficiency, or herniated disks; or obstruction of the outflow of urine such as urethral stricture, urethral sphincter contractions, tumors, or medications.

Functional Incontinence

Seen in elderly patients with a severe restriction in mobility or with severe cognitive impairment. These individuals either do not understand the urge to void or are unable to reach facilities.

Mnemonics for Remembering Causes of Incontinence

D: Delirium/dementia/depression *or*
R: Restricted mobility/retention/rectal impaction
I: Infection/Inflammation/irritation
P: Pharmaceuticals/polyuria

D: Delirium/dementia/depression
I: Infection
A: Atrophic urethritis/vaginitis
P: Pharmaceuticals/psychological
E: Endocrine (hypercalcemia/hyperglycemia)
R: Restricted mobility/retention
S: Stool impaction

SUBJECTIVE DATA

History of the Present Illness

Ask about:

Pattern of voiding: Frequency, timing, amount, precipitants, character of stream
Additional new symptoms: Polydipsia, fever, weight gain/loss, change in bowel habits or sexual function, sensomotor symptoms
Record of fluid intake, including time, type, amounts
Timing of incontinence (e.g., with exercise, cough, sexual intercourse)
Need to use an absorbent pad to protect clothing against loss of urine
Need to void so urgently with the inability to make it to the bathroom
Need to alter activities based on UI
Dysuria, hematuria, frequency (>7×/day) with urination
Symptoms of menopause (e.g., hot flashes, irritability)
Vaginal discharge or problems
Nocturia (in younger women >1× or in elderly >2 to 3× a night)

Past Medical History

Gynecologic/obstetric history: Parity, route of deliveries, operative vaginal deliveries (forceps, vacuum extraction, lacerations, episiotomy), contraceptives use, use of hormone replacement therapy, history of genital prolapse/repair, menstrual cycle history if not menopausal or date of menopause, previous anti-incontinence surgery, previous radical pelvic surgery
History of renal or urinary tract disease or recurrent UTIs
History of respiratory diseases: Chronic obstructive pulmonary disease, acute respiratory infection, chronic cigarette cough
Neurological disease: Stroke, multiple sclerosis, lumbar disk disease, neuropathies
History of sexual assault, abuse, incest
History of sexually transmitted diseases, especially those resulting in tissue destruction/scarring
History of circumcision

Medications

Medications, including over-the-counter: Sedative-hypnotics, diuretics, anticholinergics, alpha-adrenergics, calcium channel blockers, alpha antagonists (doxazosin, mesylate, terazosin hydrochloride, and prazosin hydrochloride—these drugs lower urethral pressures)
Estrogens
Drugs that can cause decreased bladder contractions with retention
- Anticholinergics: Antidepressants, anti-psychotics, sedative-hypnotics, antihistamines
- Nervous system depressants: Narcotics, alcohol, calcium channel blockers, alpha-adrenergic agonists, beta-adrenergic blockers

Drugs that cause stress incontinence by sphincter relaxation with urinary leakage
- Alpha-adrenergic incontinence

Drugs causing urge incontinence
- Diuretics (contractions stimulated by high urine flow)
- Caffeine (diuretic effect)

Sedative-hypnotics (depressed central inhibition of micturition)
Alcohol (diuretic effect and depressed central inhibition) (Seiss, 1998)

Family History

Family history of UI
Positive family history of death from coronary artery disease
Positive family history of osteoporosis or fractures

Psychosocial History

Use of tobacco, alcohol, or other drugs

Description of Most Common Symptoms

Complains of leaking urine
Pressure in pelvic area
Pain with defecation
Inability to empty bladder completely
Fecal incontinence
Dyspareunia

OBJECTIVE DATA

Physical Examination

A general examination is indicated to assess for systemic disease.

Vital signs: Blood pressure, temperature.

Mental status: Signs of dementia, delirium.

Respiratory: Assess for signs of chronic or acute disease, including chronic cough.

Cardiac: Assess for signs of cardiac disease, including congestive heart failure, edema.

Abdominal: Look for masses, suprapubic tenderness, fullness.

Pelvic examination: Look for signs of estrogen deprivation, pelvic relaxation, pelvic masses, observe for urine loss with Valsalva or uterine prolapse.

Hint: Break apart a plastic speculum. Then, using only the bottom portion, insert into the vagina. Place a small amount of pressure on the speculum and have the patient bear down. This will allow for complete viewing to evaluate for cystocele as well as for stress incontinence.

Rectal examination: Palpate for rectocele, obstruction, enlarged prostate, fecal impaction. Do a rectal-vaginal examination to assess the resting tone of the levator ani muscles, as well as the ability to contract these muscles.

Standing evaluation: With full bladder have patient stand and cough three times to confirm urine loss from urethra.

Neurological examination: Strength and sensation in lower extremities to assess the pudendal nerve (S3-S4) reflexes, including Babinski, light touch, deep tendon reflexes. Assess bulbocavernosus and clitoral reflex: stroke the labia majora or tap the clitoris; this should cause a visible contraction of the levator ani muscles and anal sphincter (may be absent in 20% of women who are neurologically intact).

Diagnostic Procedures

Diagnostic procedures are outlined in Table 186-1.

ASSESSMENT

Differential diagnoses include those found in Table 186-2.

THERAPEUTIC PLAN

Pharmaceutical

Pharmaceutical treatment is outlined in Table 186-3.

Lifestyle/Activities

See specific suggestions for each disorder and Table 186-4 for medication recommendation.

Stress Urinary Incontinence (SUI)

Pelvic floor exercises: Kegel exercises: hold muscle contraction for 10 seconds, do 10 to 20 contractions three to four times a day. A series of quick contractions combined with the sustained contractions gives even faster results. Kegels (when done correctly) help SUI in approximately 47% to 67% of women. Most women do not contract their muscles correctly, so initial instructions and close follow-up are essential to achieve good results.

Medications

Alpha agonists increase smooth muscle tone at the bladder outlet.

Tricyclics decrease detrusor contractility and increase outlet resistance.

Topical estrogen creams may be helpful in postmenopausal women.

Oral estrogen combined with alpha-agonists combined produce a greater decrease in the number of incontinent episodes and in the volume of leakage than dose of either agent individually.

Women who suffer incontinence only while doing vigorous exercise may benefit from taking an alpha agonist ½ hour before exercise and using a large or super size tampon for pelvic support.

Biofeedback (including vaginal cones, perineometry, or electromyelogram) has been shown to be effective in women in whom Kegel exercises help somewhat, but not enough. One study reported a 76% improvement rate in SUI in women using biofeedback. The most common and economical method is using vaginal cones.

Vaginal cones: Weighted cones are held in the vagina for 15 minutes twice a day. The cones range in weight between

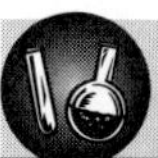

TABLE 186-1 Diagnostic Tests: Urinary Incontinence

Diagnostic Test	Finding/Rationale	Cost ($)
Urinalysis (U/A), culture and sensitivity (C&S)	Acute infection or asymptomatic bacteremia: treat and reevaluate in 2 weeks; hematuria, proteinuria, and glycosuria require further workup (urine cytology)	15-20/U/A; 31-39/C&S
Blood urea nitrogen (BUN), creatinine, calcium, glucose	Rule out underlying renal or metabolic problems	17-21/bun; 18-24/cr; 18-23/ca; 16-20/glu
Voiding diary:	Kept by the patient for 7 days. Should include frequency and amount of fluids, number and severity of incontinence episodes and associated events. Also include strength of stream. See voiding diary, Figure 186-1, and bladder diary on p. 1142.	Not available
Cotton swab test	Used to determine urethral hypermobility: patient is in the supine position; cleanse urethral meatus with povidone iodine and insert a sterile Q tip lubricated with anesthetic jelly into the urethra. Insert until the bladder is reached. A goniometer is used to determine the angle between the Q tip and the horizontal plane while resting and during a Valsalva maneuver. If the angle changes by more than 30 degrees from resting to straining, urethral hypermobility is present. This test is 90% sensitive in a woman with stress incontinence.	Not available
Postvoid residual (PVR)	Done to determine urine volume, either by catheterization or ultrasound. The most common method is in and out urethral catheterization done within a few minutes after the patient has urinated. The quantity of urine obtained is noted. PVR is normally <50 ml after voiding. Intermediate volumes (50-200 ml) are considered equivocal, and the test should be repeated.	36-43
Stress testing	These maneuvers can be performed after the bladder is filled during cystometry after the catheter is removed. The patient lies supine on the examination table and coughs forcefully. If leakage occurs onto a gauze pad during cough, a presumptive diagnosis of stress UI is made. Next, fingers should be placed on either side of the urethra to elevate the structure. The patient is again asked to cough. In patients with stress UI the urethral elevation prevents further urine leakage. These same maneuvers can be repeated with the patient in a standing position. If no urine leakage occurs, the patient probably does not have stress UI.	Not available
Cystometric testing	This is a simple office test that can help determine if the patient has detrusor instability. While the catheter is in place, a 50-ml syringe is attached. The syringe is filled with 50 ml of room temperature sterile water until the patient indicates an urge to void. Then 25-ml amounts are inserted until the patient is full. The first sensation to void is recorded. This usually occurs after 150 ml of water is instilled. Fullness is noted when the patient would like to void (usually 200-300 ml), and maximum capacity is when the patient cannot tolerate any more filling (400-700 ml). This test has a specificity of 75% and a sensitivity of 85%. The patient can also be asked to stand and cough with the bladder at maximum capacity to diagnose genuine stress incontinence.	57-79
Uroflowmeter testing	Done when diagnosis is not clear from the above evaluation. This test measures the voiding duration, amount, and rate of urine voided into a funnel with a urine flowmeter that records the information in a graphic format. Usually performed in combination with other tests.	80-108
Pad test	To help rule out other causes of soiling of underwear. The woman takes a Pyridium, which colors the urine orange. She uses a sanitary napkin, which is then checked for orange stains	Not available

Voiding Diary

This chart is a record of your voiding (urinating) and leakage (incontinence) of urine. It should also record all the liquids you drank while you were keeping this diary. Please complete this diary according to the accompanying instructions before your visit to our office.

Example

Time	Amount voided	Activity	Leak volume (circle)	Urge present? (circle)	Amount/type of intake
6:45 AM	10 oz	Awakening	0 1 2 3	Yes No	
7:00 AM		Turned on water	0 1 (2) 3	(Yes) No	2 cups coffee 6 oz orange juice

Your Diary

Time	Amount voided	Activity	Leak volume (circle)	Urge present? (circle)	Amount/type of intake
			0 1 2 3	Yes No	
			0 1 2 3	Yes No	
			0 1 2 3	Yes No	
			0 1 2 3	Yes No	
			0 1 2 3	Yes No	
			0 1 2 3	Yes No	
			0 1 2 3	Yes No	
			0 1 2 3	Yes No	
			0 1 2 3	Yes No	
			0 1 2 3	Yes No	
			0 1 2 3	Yes No	
			0 1 2 3	Yes No	
			0 1 2 3	Yes No	
			0 1 2 3	Yes No	
			0 1 2 3	Yes No	

Figure 186-1 Voiding diary. Instructions for patients: If possible, this voiding diary should be kept for 24 to 48 consecutive hours. Choose a time when it will be convenient for you to record your voiding, leakage, and liquid intake. If you are unable to keep the diary for at least 24 hours, try to keep it for as many hours as you can. For example, you may be able to record all of your voiding and leakage from early evening (after you get home from work) until you get up the next morning. Include all episodes of voiding or leakage, even if they occur in the middle of the night.

1. Record the time of all voiding, leakage, and intake of liquids.
2. Measure all intake and output in ounces or milliliters (30 ml = 1 oz.).
3. Describe what activity you were performing at the time of leakage. If you were not actively doing anything, record whether you were sitting, standing, or lying down.
4. Estimate the amount of leakage according to the following scale: 0 = no leakage; 1 = damp, few drops only; 2 = wet underwear or pad; 3 = soaked or emptied bladder.
5. If an urge to urinate accompanied (or preceded) the leakage, write "Yes." If you felt no urge to urinate when the leakage occurred, write "No."

(From Winkler H, Sand P: Stress incontinence: options for conservative treatment, *Women's Health Primary Care* 1(3):279-294, 1998.)

TABLE 186-2 Differential Diagnosis: Urinary Incontinence

Diagnosis	Supporting Data
Stress incontinence	Normal postvoid residual
Detrusor instability	Frequency, bedwetting, large bladder volume, normal postvoid residual, may have abnormal findings with neurological examination
Overflow incontinence	Poor stream, abnormal postvoid residual, large bladder capacity requires urodynamic testing
Functional	Evidence of impaired cognition, mobility without urinary complaints, normal bladder tone

20 and 100 g; these are used progressively. The cones are shaped in such a way that they are retained when a woman contracts her pelvis effectively, but fall out if intraabdominal pressure increases and the pelvic contraction is insufficient. About 70% of patients report that their incontinence is alleviated or cured after 1 month of use (Winkler & Sand, 1998).

Pelvic floor electrical stimulation: A probe is placed in the vagina or rectum, and electrical stimulation is applied BID. This method improved SUI at least 50% in most patients.

Pessaries may be used to control stress incontinence. Pessaries rest underneath the urethra, supporting and slightly obstructing it. The two most popular devices are the Continence Ring and the Introl device. Patients must be individually fitted with these devices and be taught how to insert and remove them properly. They are taught to remove the device each night and reinsert it each morning. It should be washed with soap and water before reinsertion.

Occlusive devices are used to occlude the urethra. These include the Reliance Catheter, the Fem-Assist, and the Impress Soft Patch. These devices are used to control stress incontinence but are contraindicated in women with high-pressure (>20 cm H_2O) detrusor overactivity. They obstruct the urethral meatus.

Surgery may be indicated in women who exhibit poor response to nonsurgical methods. Procedures include bladder neck suspension and urethral sling procedures (retropubic urethropexies such as Burch or Marshal-Marchetti have a cure rate of approximately 84%).

Urge Incontinence

Bladder retraining with gradual lengthening of time between voiding

Prompted voidings are used for patients with mobility problems or cognitively impaired individuals. The individual is asked at regular intervals about the need to void.

Medications

- Anticholinergics inhibit involuntary detrusor contractions.
- Smooth muscle agonists are direct acting smooth muscle depressants.
- Calcium channel antagonists inhibit bladder contractions. Efficacy has not been determined but may be an option for patients being treated simultaneously for hypertension or cardiac disease (not approved for this indication in United States).
- Hormone replacement therapy alleviates the sensory problems of urgency, frequency, dysuria, and nocturia in postmenopausal women. Women with an intact uterus should be cycled with progesterone.

Surgery has little role in urge incontinence. Denervation procedures and augmentation cystoplasty are done at tertiary care centers and are reserved for the most difficult cases.

Overflow Incontinence

A Crede or Valsalva maneuver may facilitate bladder emptying. Or have the patient place the flat of the hand over the bladder, apply pressure, and lean forward as he or she completes voiding.

Medications

- Alpha-antagonists reduce sphincter resistance.
- Cholinergics agents improve detrusor contractility.
- Hormonal therapy causes regression of hyperplastic prostate tissue through androgen suppression. Two to 6 months of therapy are required before improvement may be evident. (Pharmacologic therapy is not usually helpful in the long term and is not recommended.)

Intermittent or indwelling or suprapubic catheterization

Surgery: Transurethral resection of the prostate (TURP) is the procedure of choice in men with overflow due to benign prostatic hyperplasia. Newer approaches include transurethral incision of the prostate (TUIP) and transurethral ultrasound guided laser-induced prostatectomy (TULIP).

Referral/Consultation

Refer to urologist or gynecologist who specializes in urinary incontinence:

- Patients requiring urodynamic testing
  - Prostate nodules or asymmetry
  - Gross pelvic relaxation (beyond the hymen)
  - Systemic neurological disorders or spinal cord lesion
- Patients who do not improve with modalities tried
- For fitting with a female occlusive device
- For surgical intervention

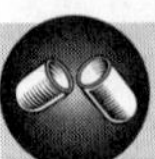

Table 186-3 Pharmaceutical Plan: Urinary Incontinence

Drug	Dose	Comments	Cost
Tricyclic Antidepressants			
Imipramine (Tofranil) (also has anticholinergic properties)	25-50 mg TID	Care with **elderly** due to long ½ life Pregnancy: C SE: Drowsiness, orthostatic hypotension, anticholinergic effects, restlessness, insomnia	\$2-\$44/imi: 25 mg (100); \$3-\$74/50 mg (100) \$5-\$44/dox: 25 mg (100); \$7-\$61/50 mg (100); \$10-\$96/100 mg (100)
Doxepin (Sinequan)	25-100 mg QHS		
Hormonal Therapy			
Estrogen vaginal cream (Premarin)	2-4 g QD for 1-2 weeks, then 1 g 1-3× week	Increases alpha receptors in the urethra; works well when combined with alpha agonists Pregnancy: X SE: N/V, breakthrough bleeding, edema, weight gain, swollen, tender breasts	\$29-\$32/crm: 0.625 mg/g (45 g); \$50/combo
Oral estrogen (cycled with progesterone)	0.3-1.25 QD		
Alpha-adrenergic Agonists			
Phenylpropanolamine (Dimetapp, Dexatrim)	25-50 mg q6-8h	Pregnancy: Caution SE: Anticholinergic effects, GI upset, insomnia, palpitations, anxiety	\$2-\$10/25 mg (100); \$2-\$10/50 mg (100)
Pseudoephedrine (Sudafed)	15-30 mg q6-8h		
Anticholinergics			
Propantheline (Pro-Banthine)	15 mg QID	Pregnancy: C SE: Headache, GI upset, rhinitis, abnormal vision, arrhythmias	\$23-\$71/15 mg (100)
Smooth Muscle Relaxants			
Oxybutynin (Ditropan)	2.5-5 mg BID-TID	Pregnancy: B SE: Anticholinergic effects	\$18-\$50/oxy: 5 mg (100); \$75/fla: 100 mg (100); \$3-\$35/dic: 20 mg (100)
Flavoxate (Urispas)	100-200 mg TID-QID		
Dicyclomine (Bentyl)	20 mg QID	SE: N/V, vertigo, headache, tachycardia	
Alpha-Antagonists			
Prazosin (Minipress)	1-5 mg TID	Pregnancy: C SE: Syncope (especially with first dose), headache, drowsiness, weakness, palpitations, blurred vision, nasal congestion, priapism; take first dose at HS to avoid hypotension	\$6-\$48/1 mg (100); \$7-\$61/2 mg (100); \$136/ter: all (100); \$89/dox: 1 mg (100); \$93/2 mg (100)
Terazosin (Hytrin)	1-10 mg QHS, usual dose is 10 mg, max. 20 mg/day		
Doxazosin (Cardura)	1 mg QD, increase to 16 mg QD if required, usual dose is 4-6 mg/day		
Cholinergics			
Bethanechol (Urecholine)	10-30 mg TID	Pregnancy: C SE: Hypotension, vomiting, cramps, headache, dyspnea, facial flushing, urinary urgency	\$2-\$68/10 mg (100); \$3-\$103/25 mg (100); \$7-\$79/50 mg (100)
Muscarinic Antagonist			
Tolterodine tartrate (Detrol) (also has anticholinergic properties)	2 mg BID, may decrease to 1 mg BID	Used for urge incontinence; increased residual urine, decreased detrusor pressure Pregnancy: C Interaction: CYP 3A4 (see Appendix D); contraindicated in patients with urinary retention	N/A

GI, Gastrointestinal; *N/A*, not available; *N/V*, nausea and vomiting.

TABLE 186-4 Medication Summary: Urinary Incontinence

Type of Incontinence	Summary of Medications Recommended
Urge	Oxybutynin (Ditropan) Imipramine (Tofranil) Flavoxate HCL (Urispas) Propantheline bromide (Pro-Banthine) Dicyclomine (Bentyl)
Stress	Estrogen Pseudoephedrine (Sudafed) Phenylpropanolamine (Dexatrim) Imipramine (Tofranil)
Overflow	Prazosin (Minipress) Bethanechol chloride (Urecholine)
Detrusor hyper-activity with impaired contractility	Oxybutynin (Ditropan)

EVALUATION/FOLLOW-UP

Monthly to evaluate therapies, then as needed

RESOURCES

American Foundation for Urologic Disease
The Bladder Health Council
1128 North Charles Street
Baltimore, MD 21201
(800) 242-2383 or (410) 468-1800

American Uro-Gynecologic Society
401 North Michigan Avenue
Chicago, IL 60611-4267
(312) 644-6610

Continence Restored, Inc.
407 Strawberry Hill Avenue
Stamford, CT 06902
(203) 348-0601 or (914) 285-1470

National Association for Continence
(formerly Help for Incontinent People, Inc.)
P.O. Box 8310
Spartanburg, SC 29305
(800) BLADDER or (803) 579-7900
http://www.nafc.org/

The Simon Foundation for Continence
P.O. Box 835
Wilmette, IL 60091
(800) 23-SIMON

National Institute of Diabetes, Digestive and Kidney Disease
http://www.NIDDK.nih.gov/health/health.htm

National Kidney and Urologic Diseases Information Clearinghouse
3 Information Way
Bethesda, MD 20892-3580
E-mail: nkudic@info.niddk.nih.gov

American Foundation of Urologic Disease
http://www.afud.org/

Agency for Health Care Policy and Research (AHCPR)
AHCPR Publications Clearinghouse, PO Box 8547, Silver Spring, MD 20907, 800-358-9295
http://www.ahcpr.gov

REFERENCES

Seiss B: Diagnostic evaluation of urinary incontinence in geriatric patients, *Am Family Physician* 57(11):2675-2684, 1998.

Winkler H, Sand P: Stress incontinence: options for conservative treatment, *Women's Health Primary Care* 1(3):279-294, 1998.

SUGGESTED READINGS

ACOG Technical Bulletin. Urinary Incontinence. No. 100, 1987.

Carlson K, Eisenstat S, Ziporyn T: *Incontinence, The Harvard guide to women's health,* Cambridge, Mass, 1996, Harvard Press.

Czarapata R: Urinary incontinence: proactive management, *Contemp Nurse Pract* 2(4):16-26, 1997.

Driscoll C et al: *The family practice desk reference,* ed 5, St Louis, 1996, Mosby.

Ellsworth AJ et al: *Mosby's 1998 medical drug reference*, St Louis, 1998, Mosby.

Fantl J, Newman D, Colling J: (1996). Urinary incontinence in adults: acute and chronic management. Clinical Practice Guideline No. 2. Rockville, Md, 1996, US Department of Health and Human Services, Public Health Service, Agency for Health Care Policy and Research, Publication No. 96-0682.

Hawkins J, Roberto-Nichols D, Stanley-Haney JL: *Loss of integrity of pelvic floor structures: protocols for nurse practitioners in gynecologic settings,* ed 5, New York, 1995, The Tiresias Press.

Healthcare Consultants of America, Inc: *1998 physicians fee and coding guide*, Augusta, Ga, 1998, Healthcare Consultants of America, Inc.

Jay J, Stashir D: Urinary incontinence, *Adv Nurs Pract* 6(10)32-37, 1998.

Peters S:. Don't ask, don't tell: breaking the silence surrounding female urinary incontinence, *Adv Nurse Pract* 5(5):41-44, 1997.

Rakel R: *Saunders manual of medical practice,* Philadelphia, 1996, WB Saunders.

Sulpik R, editor: Urinary incontinence. In Allison K: *American Medical Association complete guide to women's health,* New York, 1996 Random House.

Vail B: Urinary incontinence. In Johnson C, Murray J, Johnson B: *Women's health care handbook,* St Louis, 1996, Mosby.

Your Daily Bladder Diary

This diary will help you and your health care team. Bladder diaries help show the causes of bladder control trouble. The "sample" line (below) will show you how to use the diary.

Your name: ______________
Date: ______________

Time	Drinks		Urine		ACCIDENTS: Accidental leaks	Did you feel a strong urge to go?	What were you doing at the time?
	What kind?	How much?	How many times?	How much? (circle one)	How much? (circle one)	Circle one	Sneezing, exercising, having sex, lifting, etc.
Sample	*Coffee*	*2 cups*	✓✓	(sm) med lg	sm (med) lg	Yes (No)	*running*
6-7 a.m.				sm med lg	sm med lg	Yes No	
7-8 a.m.				sm med lg	sm med lg	Yes No	
8-9 a.m.				sm med lg	sm med lg	Yes No	
9-10 a.m.				sm med lg	sm med lg	Yes No	
10-11 a.m.				sm med lg	sm med lg	Yes No	
11-12 noon				sm med lg	sm med lg	Yes No	
12-1 p.m.				sm med lg	sm med lg	Yes No	
1-2 p.m.				sm med lg	sm med lg	Yes No	
2-3 p.m.				sm med lg	sm med lg	Yes No	
3-4 p.m.				sm med lg	sm med lg	Yes No	
4-5 p.m.				sm med lg	sm med lg	Yes No	
5-6 p.m.				sm med lg	sm med lg	Yes No	
6-7 p.m.				sm med lg	sm med lg	Yes No	

Time	Drinks		Urine		Accidental leaks	Did you feel a strong urge to go?	What were you doing at the time?
	What kind?	How much?	How many times?	How much? (circle one)	How much? (circle one)	Circle one	Sneezing, exercising, having sex, lifting, etc.
Sample	*Soda*	*2 cans*	✓✓	(sm) med lg	(sm) med lg	Yes (No)	*laughing*
7-8 p.m.				sm med lg	sm med lg	Yes No	
8-9 p.m.				sm med lg	sm med lg	Yes No	
9-10 p.m.				sm med lg	sm med lg	Yes No	
10-11 p.m.				sm med lg	sm med lg	Yes No	
11-12 midnight				sm med lg	sm med lg	Yes No	
12-1 a.m.				sm med lg	sm med lg	Yes No	
1-2 a.m.				sm med lg	sm med lg	Yes No	
2-3 a.m.				sm med lg	sm med lg	Yes No	
3-4 a.m.				sm med lg	sm med lg	Yes No	
4-5 a.m.				sm med lg	sm med lg	Yes No	
5-6 a.m.				sm med lg	sm med lg	Yes No	

I used ______ pads. I used ______ diapers today (write number).

Questions to ask my health care team: ______________________________

Let's Talk About Bladder Control for Women is a public health awareness campaign conducted by the National Kidney and Urologic Diseases Information Clearinghouse (NKUDIC), an information dissemination service of the National Institute of Diabetes and Digestive and Kidney Diseases (NIDDK), National Institutes of Health.

Urinary Tract Infection

ICD-9-CM

Cystitis 595.9
Chronic Cystitis 595.2
Pyelonephritis 590.80
Acute Pyelonephritis 590.10
Chronic Pyelonephritis 590.00

OVERVIEW

Definition

Cystitis is the presence of bacteria in urine causing a change in urinary patterns, considered a lower urinary tract infection (UTI). *Pyelonephritis* is an infection of the renal pelvis or parenchyma; it is an upper UTI.

Incidence

Second most common infection

20% of women complain of UTI symptoms/year; they become more common with increasing age.

Newborn males have UTIs more frequently than girls, but after the newborn period most UTIs occur in **girls.**

The highest prevalence of UTI or bacteriuria occurs in **women >65.**

20% of UTIs are recurrent; UTIs cost $1 billion per year

Pathophysiology

Protective Factors Against

Urinary acidity and osmolality
Antimicrobial properties of the mucosa
The "flushing" effect of urination
Cervical immunoglobulins

Factors That Increase Susceptibility

Bacterial virulence
Behavioral factors (poor hygiene, wiping back to front)
Abnormal urinary flow: Stones, benign prostatic hyperplasia, vesicoureteral reflux (structural abnormalities)
Long-term catheterization
Other host factors
- Decreased immunity, pregnancy, alcoholism, indwelling catheter, increased sexual activity, urinary instrumentation, bubble baths in girls have been found to be irritating and could lead to a UTI
- Decreased estrogen

Common Pathogens

70% to 85% of cystitisis caused by *Escherichia coli, Staphylococcus saprophyticus* (10% to 20%), or *Enterococcus* sp; 90% of pyelonephritis is caused by *E. coli.*

SUBJECTIVE DATA

History of Present Illness

Ask about duration of symptoms. If the patient has had UTI symptoms for more than 2 to 3 days, the likelihood of a more serious infection is present.

Adults: Ask about the relationship of symptoms to sexual activity.

Children: Symptoms will likely be more vague for children. Ask about more systemic symptoms.

Elderly: UTIs may precipitate delirium and somnolence in susceptible patients.

Past Medical History

Ask about:

- History of kidney stones, UTIs, kidney, bladder, or prostate disease
- Diabetes, hypertension, multiple sclerosis
- Last menstrual period, use of barrier birth control methods, birth control methods
- Allergies, date of last sexual contact, new sexual partner within last 6 months
- Pregnant female: Recent group A beta hemolytic streptococcal infection

Medications

Recent use of antibiotics, any other medications

Family History

Ask about family history of kidney problems

Psychosocial History

Diet: Ask about increased ingestion of caffeine or carbonated drinks, water intake

Decreased appetite may be seen in elderly

Children: Consider possible child sexual abuse; may need to ask about this once relationship is established

Description of Most Common Symptoms

Cystitis

Adults: Dysuria, frequency, urgency, hematuria, urine odor, suprapubic discomfort, pressure, acute onset.

Infants: Irritability, failure to thrive, systemic illness (fever), vomiting/diarrhea, abdominal pain and distention, decreased urination, change in urination pattern (enuresis), foul odor; UTI is the most common cause of fever of undetermined origin in infants; the younger the infant, the more likely that sepsis and structural abnormalities will be found

Toddlers: Abdominal discomfort, fever, altered voiding patterns, malodorous urine

Preschool: Voiding discomfort, enuresis

School age/teens: typical signs and symptoms

Elderly: may be asymptomatic; fever is uncommon

Pyelonephritis

Adults/school-age children, and **older:** Fever, malaise, prostration, and nausea, more gradual onset, toxic appearance

Children: Nonspecific symptoms similar to cystitis

Elderly: Generalized symptoms are common; 50% of women over age 65 may not have a fever until later in the course

Associated Symptoms

Back or flank pain, nausea/vomiting, incontinence in children (previously toilet trained) or older adults, fever, decreased force of urine stream, nocturia, diarrhea, constipation, vaginal discharge, urethral discharge, perianal itching

OBJECTIVE DATA

Physical Examination

A problem-oriented physical examination should be conducted, with particular attention to:

Vital signs and weight, general appearance, general hydration status, including orthostatic changes

Abdomen: Full abdominal examination; must check for costovertebral angle tenderness (common in pyelonephritis)

Genital/rectal

Female—Do complete pelvic examination if laboratory tests/examination don't clearly identify UTI

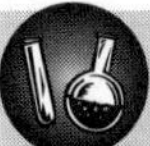

TABLE 187-1 Diagnostic Tests: Urinary Tract Infection

Symptoms	Findings	Diagnostic Tests	Cost ($)
Burning on urination, frequency, urgency, hematuria	Positive BS, abdomen soft, mild suprapubic tenderness, no CVA tenderness	Midstream urine for U/A C&S	 15-20 31-39
Flank pain, nausea and vomiting, fever, malaise	Toxic appearance, positive CVA tenderness, positive BS, ~ suprapubic tenderness	C&S More severely ill: CBC with differential Chemistry	31-39 18-23 32-42
Symptoms without pyuria or bacteriuria, complicated UTIs, failed prior treatment	As for Burning on urination	C & S	31-39
Males, children <8, renal colic, gross hematuria, persistent UTI, renal scarring	As for Burning on urination	IVP US with KUB, voiding cystourethrogram, cystoscopy	280-333 259-319 480-570 447-540

BS, Bowel sounds; *C&S,* culture and sensitivity; *CBC,* complete blood count; *CVA,* costovertebral angle; *IVP,* intravenous pyelography; *KUB,* kidneys, ureter, bladder; *U/A,* urinalysis; *US,* ultrasound; *UTI,* urinary tract infection.

Male—Do complete examination of external genitalia; assess for prostate tenderness or enlargement

Children: Assess for dehydration, activity level; physical examination may be essentially within normal limits in children.

Diagnostic Procedures

Diagnostic procedures are based on documented presence of pyuria/bacteriuria in clean-catch urine and are outlined in Table 187-1.

Children: May require catheterization or suprapubic tap (newborn) to obtain specimen

First line: Urine dipstick, microscopic urinalysis, urine culture

Second line: Complete blood count with differential, chemistry for toxic patient

Third line: Intravenous pyelogram; kidneys, ureter, and bladder with ultrasound, voiding cystourethrogram, cystoscopy

ASSESSMENT

Differential diagnoses include nephrolithiasis, pyelonephritis, trauma, prostatitis, diabetes, sexually transmitted diseases, acute urethral syndrome, tumor, pelvic inflammatory disease, vulvovaginitis, cervicitis, epididymitis, benign prostatic hypertrophy, renal tuberculosis, post streptococcal glomerular nephritis (Table 187-2, Figures 187-1 and 187-2). **Children:** Sexual abuse, constipation, appendicitis. **Elderly:** Menopause.

THERAPEUTIC PLAN

Pharmaceutical

Antibiotic treatment for UTI is based on how involved or complicated the infection is.

Simple, Uncomplicated UTI

3 days' duration

TABLE 187-2 Differential Diagnosis: Urinary Tract Infection

Diagnoses	Supporting Data
Cystitis, pyelonephritis	Urinalysis (U/A): Leukocyte + Nitrite + Blood + Microscopic urinalysis: >2-5 leukocytes/field >2-5 red blood cells/field >1+ bacteria White blood cell (WBC) casts in pyelonephritis (>0-5 epithelial cells contaminated: repeat) Culture and sensitivity: Colony-forming units 10^5 + Colony-forming units 10^2 + if female, symptomatic, + pyuria 15%-20% symptomatic women have negative culture
Sexually transmitted diseases/ vulvovaginitis	Vaginal discharge, odor, itching Wet-mount vaginal secretions + Trichomoniasis + Clue cells + Budding hyphae DNA probe + Gonorrhea + Chlamydia
Prostatitis	Sexually active men, swollen prostate, dysuria, frequency, low back, perineal pain Prostate secretions >10-20 WBCs/HPF Culture: *E. coli*
Epididymitis	Rare under 35 y/o, occurs in sexually active men, swollen, tender epididymitis, scrotum red and swollen; U/A, WBCs
Benign prostatic hyperplasia	Hesitancy, nocturia, males >40 y/o; may cause a UTI-related to obstruction

+, Positive; *HPF,* high-power field.

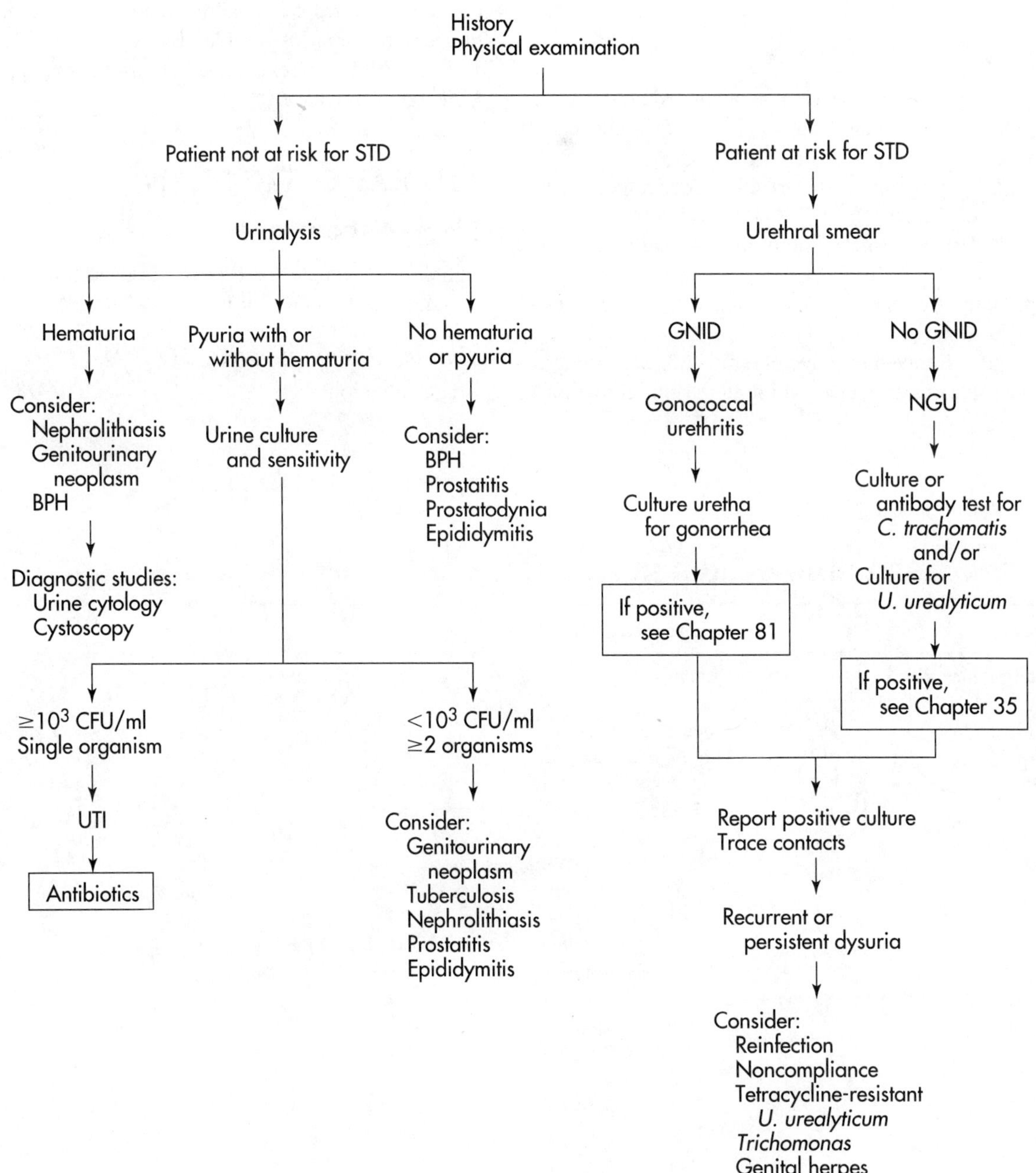

Figure 187-1 Algorithm for male patient with acute dysuria or pyuria. *BPH,* Benign prostatic hyperplasia; *CFU,* colony-forming units; *GNID,* gram-negative intracellular diplococci; *NGU,* nongonococcal urethritis; *STD,* sexually transmitted disease; *UTI,* urinary tract infection. (Adapted from Greene HL, Johnson WP, Lemcke D: *Decision making in medicine,* ed 2, St Louis, 1998, Mosby.)

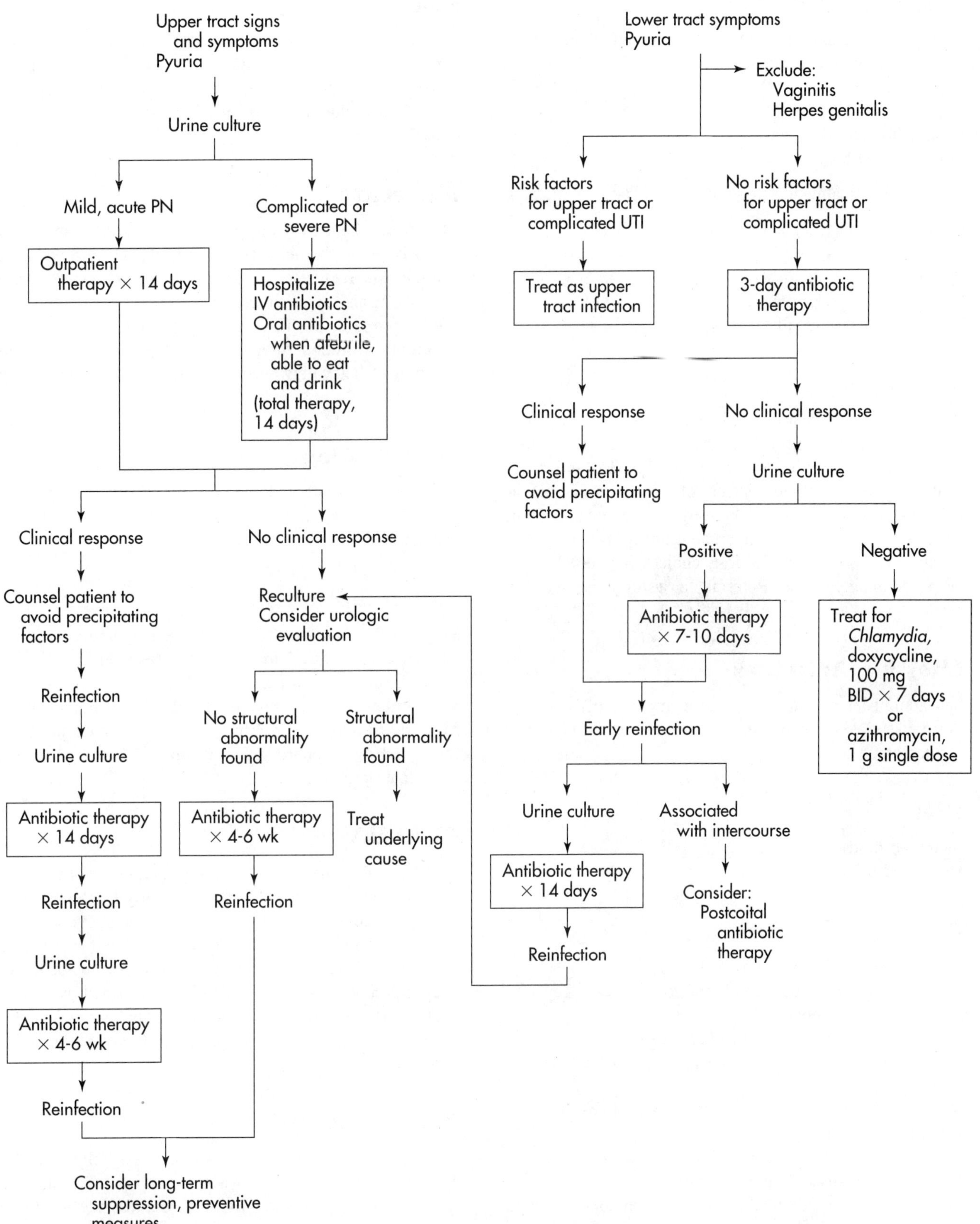

Figure 187-2 Algorithm for female patient with dysuria and frequent urination. *PN*, pyelonephritis; *UTI*, urinary tract infection. (Adapted from Greene HL, Johnson WP, Lemcke D: *Decision making in medicine*, ed 2, St Louis, 1998, Mosby.)

Complicated UTI

Male patients, children, and pregnant women
Nosocomial infections
After instrumentation
Abnormal urinary flow
Symptom duration >6 days
Compromised host

Antibiotic treatment for complicated UTIs: 7 to 14 Days

Diabetic patients, pregnant women: 7 to 10 days
Children: 10 days
Pyelonephritis: 10 to 14 days
Frequent relapses, prostatitis: 4 to 6 weeks
Large postvoid residual: Treat symptoms only
Permanent Foley: Treat symptoms only

Pyelonephritis

Patients who are healthy, at low risk for complications, with no nausea/vomiting can be treated on an outpatient basis. Those who are more ill, children, and pregnant women (increased chance of premature labor) at risk for complications will need to be treated with intravenous antibiotics with broad activity against gram-negative bacteria. Possible drug choices include Bactrim or an aminoglycoside. Referral to a urologist will be needed.

Lifestyle/Activities

Self-administered treatment at first symptoms of UTI
Postcoital doses for women with repeated UTIs after intercourse

Diet

Increased fluids
Decreased intake of caffeine

Patient Education

Incorrect post-voiding wiping technique
Use of barrier methods of birth control
Use of tampons, deodorants, douches
Need to void before and after intercourse
Local trauma (e.g., certain sexual positions, horseback riding)
Adequate fluid intake, increased when symptoms noted
Need for perineal hygiene
Effect of estrogen depletion on vaginal tissues
Pyridium: Red discoloration of urine
Children: Avoid full bladder; children in toilet training need regular schedule
Teach children not to delay urination: No bubble baths for children or sitting in soapy bath water

Family Impact

In children it is important to stress the implications of a UTI. Parents must understand that most infection-caused renal scarring occurs in infancy and childhood. The consequences of UTI in children is not the same as the "annoyance" experienced by adults.

Referral

Children: Children with symptomatic pyelonephritis or sepsis should be hospitalized and referred to a pediatric urologist. Also, refer children with severe vesicoureteral reflux or any other structural abnormalities.
Men: Men with a UTI should be referred to an urologist.
Pregnant women: Should be followed by OB/GYN/ urologist. They may need maintenance antibiotics during pregnancy.

Consultation

Consider consulting with MD on any patient in whom you suspect pyelonephritis or any patient who will require hospitalization.

Follow-up

Simple UTIs need no follow-up unless symptoms persist.
Children: Reculture 2 to 3 days after treatment is begun to check for sterile urine.
Pregnant women: Follow-up after course of treatment.
Men >50: Follow-up in 4 to 6 weeks is recommended.
Suspected pyelonephritis: Follow-up in 24 to 48 hours to evaluate progress.

EVALUATION

Children: Routine follow-up cultures should be done in 1 month, every 3 mos × 1 year, then yearly for 2 to 3 years.
Pregnant women: Should have cultures done every month after initial UTI. Women with sickle cell trait should also be screened every month due to a higher incidence of asymptomatic bacteruria. All UTIs confirmed by culture and treated should be reassessed by urinalysis in 2 weeks. Complicated UTIs need follow-up urine culture after treatment.

Pyelonephritis

Urinary output needs to be monitored. Follow-up for evaluation of symptom assessment and directed physical examination. Patient should also have a test of cure 2 to 4 weeks after antibiotic completion. Special diagnostic studies should be undertaken in men and children after an episode of pyelonephritis.

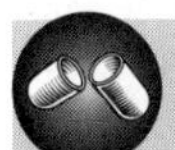

TABLE 187-3 Pharmaceutical Plan: Urinary Tract Infection

Drug	Dose	Prophylaxis	Comments	Cost
Trimethoprim-sulfamethoxazole (TMP-SMZ, Bactrim)	160 mg/800 mg (1 double strength tablet) BID **Child:** 4 mg/kg T +20 mg/kg S BID (>2 mo)	**Children*:** 1 mg/kg T + 5 mg/kg S BID; No bedwetting **Adult:** 40 mgT/200 mg S at HS (½ regular tablet)	Pregnancy: C CAUTION: Sulfa allergies SE: Nausea and vomiting, abdominal pain, photosensitivity; pay attention to skin rashes: could signify early Stevens-Johnson syndrome	$7-$74/reg strength: (100); $9-$121/DS: (100); $27-$43/susp: 200 mg, SMX/40 mg, TMP/5 ml (480 ml)
Trimethoprim (TMP, Proloprim)	100 mg BID	**Adult:** 100 mg QOD @ HS	Pregnancy: C	$16-$75/100 mg (100)
Nitrofurantoin macrocrystals (Macrodantin) Nitrofurantoin (Macrobid)	100 mg QID 100 mg BID **Child*:** 5-7 mg/kg q6h	**Children*:** 1-2 mg kg BID (>2 mos) **Adult:** 50 mg at HS	Pregnancy: B SE: Anorexia, nausea and vomiting, abdominal pain; food or milk may help with gastrointestinal upset; may cause brown discoloration of urine	$20/25 mg/5 ml (60 ml); $42-$56/25 mg (100); $58-$74/50 mg (100); $24/Macrobid 100 mg (100)
Cephalexin (Keflex)	500 mg BID		Pregnancy: B SE: Diarrhea	$15-$129/250 mg (100); $31-$253/500 mg (100); $5/100 mg/ml (10 ml); $10-$25/125 mg/5 ml (200 ml); $9-$48/250 mg/5 ml (200 ml)
Amoxicillin	500 mg BID **Child*:** 15 mg/kg TID		Pregnancy: B; not a good choice due to reduced bacterial sensitivity, but may be a choice with pregnancy and allergies	$17-$49/500 mg (100); $3-$5/125 mg/5 ml (150 ml); $4-$8/250 mg/5 ml (150 ml)
Ciprofloxacin (save for resistant pathogens)	250 mg BID		Pregnancy: C; do not take with antacids	$290/250 mg (100)
Phenazopyridine (Pyridium) consider use as urinary analgesic	100 mg TID for 2-3 days **Child >12 y/o:** 12 mg/kg/day TID		Pregnancy: B SE: Colors all body fluids: may stain contacts	$5-$53/100 mg (100)

*See Appendix M.
SE, Side effects.

Successful outcome is negative culture. Reinfection is considered a new infection, whereas relapse occurs when the focus of the infection was not completely eliminated, usually within weeks of the first infection.

SUGGESTED READINGS

Ahmed S, Swedlund S: Evaluation and treatment of urinary tract infections in children, *Am Family Physician* 57(7):1573-1582, 1998.

Barry H, Ebell M., Hickner J: Evaluation of suspected urinary tract infection in ambulatory women: a cost-utility analysis of office based strategies, *J Family Practice* 44(1):49-60, 1997.

Ellsworth AJ et al: *Mosby's medical drug reference*, St Louis, 1998, Mosby.

French M: UTI in elderly, *Adv Nurse Pract,* pp 25, 26, 28, 52.

Forland M: UTI- How its management has changed, *Postgrad Med* 93(5):71-86, 1993.

Healthcare Consultants of America, Inc: *1998 physicians fee and coding guide*, Augusta, Ga, 1998, Healthcare Consultants of America, Inc.

Hoffman R: Acute dysuria or pyuria in men. In Greene H, Johnson W, Lemcke D, editors: *Decision making in medicine,* ed 2, St Louis, 1998, Mosby.

Hooten T et al: Randomized comparative trial and cost analysis of 3-day antimicrobial regimens for treatment of acute cystitis in women, *JAMA* 273:41-45, 1995.

Johnson J: Recognizing and treating acute pyelonephritis, *Emerg Med* 24(3):25-33, 1992.

Katz M: Urinary tract infection in women. In Greene H, Johnson W, Maricic M, editors: *Decision making in medicine,* St Louis, 1993, Mosby.

Levin, M: Urinary tract infection: how best to diagnose and treat in elderly patients. *Consultant* 37(12):3061-3064, 1997.

Mulholland S: UTI in women, *Consultant* 35(4):534-540, 1995.

Nygaard I, Johnson M: UTI in elderly women, *Am Family Practice* 53(1):175-182, 1996.

Pollen J: Short-term course for uncomplicated UTI, *Contemp Nurse Pract* 1(2):21-30, 1995.

Valaitis S: Cystitis and pyelonephritis. In Zuspan F, Quilligan E, editors: *Handbook of obstetrics, gynecology, and primary care,* St Louis, 1998, Mosby.

Uterine Fibroids

aka Uterine Myomas, Leiomyomata, Fibromas

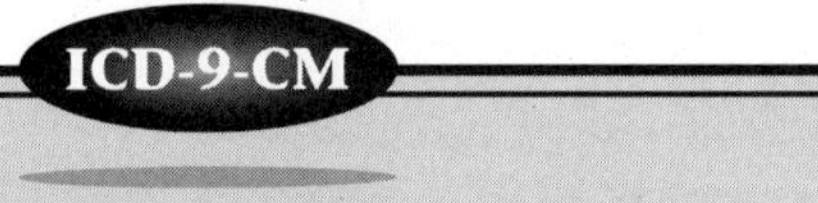

ICD-9-CM

Submucosa Leiomyoma of Uterus 218.9

OVERVIEW

Definition

Uterine fibroids are benign tumors that develop from the smooth muscle of the uterus. They may be inside, outside, or within the wall of the uterus, sometimes changing the shape of the uterus.

Incidence

Fibroids are the most common pelvic tumor in women, and as many as one in four are diagnosed during a woman's reproductive years. They are frequently found in women between the **ages of 30 and 50** and rarely occur before the age of 20 or after menopause. Approximately 30% to 50% of American women over age 30 have fibroids. For reasons unknown, **black women** have a higher incidence of fibroids.

Pathophysiology

Fibroids develop from the smooth muscle of the myometrium. The cause is unclear, although research points to a connection to estrogen. They may increase in size during pregnancy or while on oral contraceptives and may regress in menopause. There is also research pointing to a genetic predisposition.

Location of Fibroids

Submucous: Impinges on the endometrial lining
Pedunculated: On a stalk (inner or outer uterine surface)
Intramural: Within the uterine wall
Subserosal: Sticks through outer (serosal) surface
Parasitic: Lost connection to the uterus, blood from elsewhere

SUBJECTIVE DATA

History of the Present Illness

Many women are unaware they have fibroids and have no symptoms or complications. Fibroids inside the uterus itself or within the uterine wall may cause urinary frequency, dysmenorrhea, pelvic pain or pressure, or unusual menstrual bleeding. Patient may present with:

Acute or chronic pelvic pain; due to:
- Fibroid degenerates, causing a central infarction
- Uterine contractions, squeeze the myoma
- Pressure on nerves, ureters

Abnormal vaginal bleeding, cause is unknown, but theories are:
- Submucous fibroid increases surface area of uterine lining
- Uterine cavity distortion, which deforms normal uterine anatomy, which then leads to abnormal pressure on uterine blood vessels, or the uterus is unable to contract properly

Dyspareunia (painful coitus)

Pelvic pressure, which causes a mass effect, pressing on pelvic structures, leading to:
- Pelvic fullness and pressure sensation
- Urinary frequency/distention, secondary to decreased bladder filling
- Difficulty passing stools, leading to constipation

Past Medical History

Menstrual history
History of miscarriage
Menopausal symptoms
Last menstrual period
Use of hormone replacement therapy, infertility drugs
History of infertility

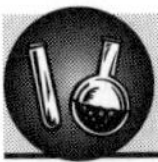

Table 188-1 Diagnostic Tests: Uterine Fibroids

Diagnostic Test	Finding/Rationale	Cost ($)
Hematocrit	To rule out anemia from heavy menstrual bleeding	11-14
Urine human chorionic gonadotropin	Rule out pregnancy	17-23
Transvaginal ultrasound	Can identify the presence of fibroids, helps to exclude ovarian masses	369-439
Endometrial biopsy	Removal of one or more areas of endometrium without cervical dilation to identify malignant changes	142-170
Abdominal x-ray	Flat plate shows "popcorn" calcifications, extrinsic compression of the bowel	121-151

History of premature births
History of pelvic surgery
Method and history of birth control

Family History

Ask about history of fibroids in family or menstrual irregularities.

OBJECTIVE DATA

Physical Examination

Perform a focused examination, looking at:

- Vital signs, including blood pressure, pulse, temperature
- Abdominal examination
  - Assess for guarding or tenderness, location of pain
  - Palpable bladder or distention
- Pelvic examination
  - Assess the cervix for any unusual tissue from the os, distortion of shape
  - Palpate the vagina for any masses
- Bimanual examination
  - Assess the uterus for tenderness, masses, enlargement, irregular contours, mobility; fibroids are usually smooth, and irregularly enlarge the shape of the uterus; the uterus is usually midline; the mass has a solid quality to it; the degree of enlargement is usually stated in terms of number of weeks' gestation
  - Assess for adnexal pain or tenderness
- Rectal examination
  - Palpate for any masses, tenderness

Diagnostic Procedures

Diagnostic procedures include those found in Table 188-1.

ASSESSMENT

Differential diagnosis includes those found in Table 188-2.

THERAPEUTIC PLAN

Nonpharmaceutical

If mass is small and causing little or no complaint; may monitor with bi-annual ultrasounds

If subsequent ultrasounds or examinations show rapid growth or if fibroids develop in postmenopausal women, they should be referred for a diagnostic laparotomy/laparoscopy

If masses are symptomatic, a referral for a laparoscopy/laparotomy is also indicated

Hysterectomy: Often indicated in symptomatic women whose uterus reaches the size of a 12-week pregnancy; it is considered the only definitive treatment; criteria include palpable fibroid, excessive uterine bleeding, anemia, and pelvic discomfort that is acute, severe, or chronic or causing bladder pressure/urinary frequency

Uterine myomectomy: Excision of the fibroids only Indicated for:
- Patient wants current or future fertility
- Patient wants to keep uterus
- Single, pediculated myoma
- Infertile, other diagnosis are excluded
- Habitual spontaneous abortions, other diagnosis excluded
- Patient is pregnant: Mass effect of pediculated fibroid

Hysteroscopy: If the fibroid is small, a procedure called a hysteroscopy may be used; a small telescoping instrument is inserted into the uterus via the cervix, and the fibroids are removed

Pharmaceutical

If surgical interventions are contraindicated or if the patient prefers medical management, GnRH agonists (Lupron, Synarel) may be an option. These produce a temporary "artificial menopause," thus causing the fibroids to shrink. This may also be an option before surgery if a patient has a particularly large fibroid, extreme pelvic pain, or extremely heavy blood loss. Side effects include hot flushing, insomnia, vaginal atrophy, and decreased bone mass and should be discontinued after 6 months.

TABLE 188-2 Differential Diagnosis: Uterine Fibroids

Diagnosis	Supporting Data
Pregnancy	Positive pregnancy test, tender swollen breasts, symmetrical enlargement of the uterus
Bladder tumor	Irritative voiding symptoms, hematuria, mass detected on bimanual examination
Uterine malignancy/leiomyosarcoma	Progressive irregular enlargement of the uterus in postmenopausal women, change in menstrual pattern and pelvic pain, positive endometrial biopsy; occurs in 3% of cancers involving uterus
Pelvic abscess	Fever, abdominal pain, cervical motion tenderness
Ovarian cyst or tumor	Vague gastrointestinal discomfort, pelvic pressure and pain, positive ultrasound
Ectopic pregnancy	Severe abdominal pain, hypotension, positive pregnancy test

Fibroids usually recur after completing this regimen, unless the patient is approaching menopause. Give Lupron 3.75 mg IM 1 q mo × 3-6 mos (3.75 mg/vial, $397). Pregnancy: X, SE: Edema, androgen-like effects, decreased libido.

Another consideration with Lupron is to give the medication until the fibroid shrinks; then add Premarin and Provera. This maintains the small uterine size indefinitely without the side effects. Probably the future treatment of choice.

Other drugs used to treat fibroids include Depo Provera, progestins, and danazol, although there is little research on their effectiveness. Give Depo (DMPA) 150 mg every month until bleeding is suppressed; then it is given 150 mg q 3 months. If a patient is 35 years or older, may consider an endometrial biopsy before initiating DMPA to rule out malignancy. See Chapter 198 for more details about DMPA. NSAIDs may also be used to help with the pelvic pain, but will have little effect on the bleeding.

Lifestyle/Activity

No changes needed

Diet

Increased iron in diet if anemia is present

Patient Education

Discussion about fibroids and their treatment

Need to follow every 6 months to monitor size, growth, symptoms

May need iron supplementation if anemic

Referral/Consultation

To a Gynecologist for surgical interventions or in consultation before initiating GnRH agonists

If there is a rapid change in size or symptoms

If there is compromise of adjacent organs

COMPLICATIONS

Infertility

Perhaps 40% of women with large fibroids are infertile.

Failure to conceive
- Blocked fallopian tubes from extrinsic pressure
- IUD-like effect within fundus, or by blocking the cervical canal
- Distorted endometrial surface

Spontaneous abortion
- Faulty implantation, abnormal contractions
- 18% of women who habitually abort have uterine fibroids
- Especially common in women with lower uterine segment fibroids

Pregnancy

2% of pregnant women have fibroids

Size change in pregnancy
- 59% changed by less than 10%
- 22% grew by >10% original size, but none were greater 25%
- 19% shrink by up to 20%

Serious complications develop in 10% to 30% of pregnant women
- Pain equals degeneration or hemorrhagic infarction of the myoma or placenta
  - 70% have general, mild abdominal pain
  - Also may see vaginal bleeding, nausea, vomiting, fever, increased white blood cells
  - Usually occurs in the second or third trimester
  - Symptoms are not linked to change in fibroid size
- Spontaneous abortion
- Premature labor and delivery
- Dystocia (obstructs labor)
- Postpartum hemorrhage and infection

EVALUATION/FOLLOW-UP

Every 6 months

As indicated by medical interventions used

BIBLIOGRAPHY

Carlson K, Eisenstat S, Ziporyn T: Uterine fibroids. *The Harvard Guide to women's health,* Cambridge, Mass, 1996, Harvard University Press.

Christiansen J: The facts about fibroids, *Postgrad Med* 94:129, 1993.

Ellsworth A et al: *Mosby's 1998 medical drug reference,* St Louis, 1998, Mosby.

Hawkins J, Roberto-Nichols D, Stanley-Haney JL: Uterine leiomyomatas, *Protocols for nurse practitioners in gynecological settings,* ed 5, New York, 1995, The Tiresias Press.

Healthcare Consultants of America, *1998 physicians fee and coding guide,* Augusta, Ga, 1998, Healthcare Consultants of America, Inc.

Muse K: Associate Professor, Division of Reproductive Endocrinology, UKMC, Lecture, April 23, 1998.

Strickland K: The primary care management of leiomyoma induced abnormal uterine bleeding, *Am Acad Nurse Pract* 8(11):541-545, 1996.

Sulpik R: Uterine fibroids. In Allison K, editor: *American Medical Association's Complete guide to women's health,* New York, 1996, Random House.

Treating fibroids, *Harvard Women's Health Watch* 5(8):2-3, 1998.

Uterine Prolapse/ Pelvic Relaxation

ICD-9-CM

Uterine Prolapse without Vaginal Wall Prolapse 618.1
Uterine Prolapse with Vaginal Wall Prolapse 618.4

OVERVIEW

Definition

Uterine prolapse is relaxation of the cardinal and uterosacral ligaments, which allows descent of the cervix and uterus into the vagina and beyond. Procidentia is prolapse of the uterus to the second degree or greater (i.e., the cervix is at the introitus or beyond).

Prolapse of the uterus is any descent of the uterus below its normal position in the pelvis. In first-degree prolapse, the uterus has descended to the point where the cervix is at the vaginal opening. When the cervix protrudes through the vaginal opening, a second-degree prolapse is present. In complete or third-degree prolapse, the entire uterus descends outside of the vagina (rare).

Incidence

Pelvic relaxation to some degree is found in 50% of parous women, with significant relaxation in about 25%.

Pathophysiology

The two large muscle groups (pubococcygeus and, most important, levator ani) are the muscles responsible for pelvic support. The levator ani muscles close off the pelvic floor so structures above them rest on their upper surface.

Pelvic relaxation is the weakening of the supporting structures of the female pelvis, which can cause varying degrees and combinations of prolapse, including the urethra (urethrocele), bladder (cystocele), rectum (rectocele), uterus (uterine prolapse), and posterior vaginal wall hernia (enterocele). Pelvic relaxation is generally caused from childbirth, although a genetic factor is frequently involved. Chronic and repetitive increases in intraabdominal pressure increase the risk of developing pelvic organ relaxation. Although it can occur at any time, it is most commonly seen during and after menopause because of the loss of hormonal support and generalized weakening of supporting tissues that occurs with aging.

Factors That Increase Susceptibility

Obstetrical trauma, chronic obstructive pulmonary disease, cigarette smoking, chronic cough, obesity, multiple pregnancies, multiple gestations, loss of elasticity through aging, and lack of estrogen

SUBJECTIVE DATA

History of Present Illness

The patient may complain of a bulge or lump in the vagina, which may be painful. Sometimes she may complain of pelvic pressure, which decreases when she lies down. On occasion, uterine prolapse interferes with sexual intercourse. She may complain of feeling like she's always "sitting on something."

Associated Symptoms

Usually a uterine prolapse is accompanied by either a cystocele or rectocele or both. Stress incontinence may also be present, so that coughing, sneezing, lifting, and pushing cause incontinence.

OBJECTIVE DATA

Physical Examination

Physical examination will focus on the pelvic examination, with attention also paid to the heart and lungs:

Vital signs, including weight
Heart: Assess for murmurs, rubs, extra heart sounds
Lungs: Assess lung excursion, A:P diameter, breath sounds
Pelvic examination: If possible, have the patient stand and Valsalva to assess degree of descent while standing
External genitalia: Assess introitus for presence of cervix at the vaginal opening
Speculum examination: Assess degree of prolapse, have the patient bear down to evaluate existing cystocele, rectocele; note length of cervix and any ulcerations on the uterus
Bimanual: Attempt to determine size of the uterus
Rectal examination: Note condition of the vaginal rectal septum; evaluate sphincter tone and condition of the levator ani muscles

Diagnostic Procedures

None

THERAPEUTIC PLAN

Nonpharmaceutical

Only symptomatic prolapse warrants treatment (see Chapter 186 for additional information on urinary incontinence)
Mild relaxation: Kegel exercises (purposeful squeezing of pubococcygeus muscle)
Pessaries are often useful for extreme relaxation when patient is unwilling or unable to have surgical correction

Indications for a Pessary

Symptomatic prolapse relieved by pessary
Symptomatic prolapse during and after pregnancy
When a patient wishes to delay surgical repair
After unsuccessful prolapse surgery
Useful as a preoperative diagnostic aid before reconstructive surgery

Fitting the Pessary

Adequate estrogenization should be achieved first (oral or topical) to prevent vaginal erosions with bleeding.
Start with either Ring pessary or Ring with Support. Sizes, like diaphragms, range from 0 to 13 (5, 6, and 7 are most common).
Determine the distance between the pubic symphysis and vaginal apex with bimanual examination as in fitting a diaphragm.
Try ring that most closely approximates this distance. If Valsalva causes pessary ring to pop out, choose the next larger size.
If the patient senses discomfort with pessary in place, remove it immediately. Walking, sitting, or lying should be tried to ensure that patient remains asymptomatic.
Caution patient that she may need to remove pessary to defecate and that urinary incontinence may occur when the pessary replaces the prolapse.
Recheck the patient in 72 hours.
Pessary may be removed for intercourse. Remove and wash pessary at least every 1 to 2 weeks.
Recheck the patient in 6 to 8 weeks for vaginal erosions or granulation tissue.

Discontinue Pessary

Recurrent vaginal erosions
Unacceptable urinary incontinence
Desire for surgery
Progression of symptoms and prolapse despite pessary use

Pharmaceutical

Antispasmodic drugs may help by relaxing the involuntary contractile nature of the bladder muscles (Table 189-1).

Lifestyle/Activities

Kegel exercises: Hold muscle contraction for 10 seconds, do 10 to 20 contractions three to four times/day. A series of

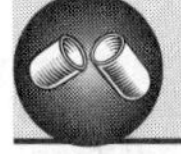

TABLE 189-1 Pharmaceutical Plan: Uterine Prolapse/Pelvic Relaxation

Drug	Dose	Comments	Cost
Oxybutyrin chloride (Ditropan)	Adults: 5 mg BID or TID, max 20 mg	Pregnancy: B SE: Anticholinergic effects CAUTION in **elderly:** May cause urinary retention, exacerbate glaucoma or ulcerative colitis; may cause drowsiness, blurred vision	\$18-\$50/5 mg (100)
Tolterodine (Detrol)	2 mg BID; use 1 mg/day with impaired liver function (affects P450 system)	For urinary frequency, urgency or urge incontinence; less likely to cause a dry mouth than oxybutynin	Not available

quick contractions combined with sustained contractions gives even faster results. If the woman experiences urinary incontinence during exercise, using a large or super size tampon may be helpful for pelvic support before exercise.

Diet

Not applicable

Patient Education

See Lifestyle/Activities

Referral

To MD for surgery
The usual treatment is hysterectomy.

EVALUATION/FOLLOW-UP

Since many women do not contract their muscles correctly, initial instructions and close follow-up are essential to achieve good results.

SUGGESTED REFERENCES

Ellsworth AJ et al: *Mosby's 1998 medical drug reference*, St Louis, 1998, Mosby.

Fritzinger K, Newman D, Dinkin E: Use of a pessary for the management of pelvic organ prolapse, *Lippincott's Primary Care Pract* 1(4):431-436, 1997.

Healthcare Consultants of America, Inc: *1998 physicians fee and coding guide*, Augusta, Ga, 1998, Healthcare Consultants of America, Inc.

Strohben K, Jakary J, Delancey J: Pelvic organ prolapse in young women, *Obstet Gynecol* 90(1):33-36, 1997.

Toozs-Hobson P, Boos K, Cardozo L: Management of vaginal vault prolapse, *Br J of Obstet Gynaecol* 105(1):13-17, 1998.

Varicose Veins

ICD-9-CM

Varicose Veins (Lower Extremity) 454.9

OVERVIEW

Definition

Varicose veins are dilated, tortuous, superficial veins in the lower extremities.

Incidence

Affects 1 out of 10 people, mostly **women** between the ages of 30 and 60

Pathophysiology

Failure of the valves within the saphenous veins and their tributaries to adequately close, allowing blood to flow back into the leg, producing distention; may also be due to a fundamental weakness in the walls of the vein

Primary: Caused by congenitally defective valves

Secondary: Occurs because another condition puts pressure on the veins that drain the legs (e.g., pregnancy, obesity, thrombophlebitis)

Protective Factors Against

Regular exercise to increase circulation
Proper weight for statue
Nulliparity

Factors that Increase Susceptibility

Family history of varicose veins
Prolonged standing or sitting
Heavy lifting
Excessive crossing of legs

SUBJECTIVE DATA

History of Present Illness

Fatigue, discomfort, or pain, heaviness in legs after standing
Muscle cramps of legs
Visible, enlarged veins
Swelling of the lower leg, with or without ulceration
Discoloration of skin in the lower extremities

Past Medical History

Obstetrical history
History of thrombophlebitis
Previous repair/treatment of varicose veins (increased risk of return of varicosities if not all veins with incompetent valves were resected)

Medications

Use of contraceptives (increases risk of postoperative thrombosis if veins are surgically repaired)
Use of anticoagulants (may increase bleeding during the surgical repair of varicose veins although reduced blood coagulation may also be beneficial in prevention of thrombosis)

Family History

Positive for varicose veins

Psychosocial History

Occupation that requires heavy lifting, prolonged sitting or standing.

Associated Symptoms

Usually none.

TABLE 190-1 Differential Diagnosis: Varicose Veins

Diagnoses	Supporting Data
Deep vein thrombophlebitis	Swelling of the leg will be unilateral. Fever and slight tachycardia may be present. Pain may be more severe than with varicosities. Skin may be cyanotic if venous obstruction is severe. Homans' sign may be positive.
Peripheral arteriosclerotic disease	Intermittent claudication. Coldness of feet. Diminished pedal pulses. Decrease hair on extremities. May have rubor of legs when dependent and blanching when elevated.
Chronic venous insufficiency	Progressive edema of the leg. Itching of the skin. Skin on lower extremities is thin, shiny, atrophic, with occasional superficial weeping.

OBJECTIVE DATA

Physical Examination

A physical examination should be performed, with attention to:

General appearance, including vital signs
Extremities
- Visible dilated, tortuous veins upon standing or palpation in the obese client
- Brownish pigmentation and thinning of the skin above the ankles
- Swelling, and ulceration of the legs may be present

Diagnostic Procedures

Duplex, ultrasound scan ($257-$300) of the lower extremities may be ordered for visual images of the veins and the direction of blood flow within the veins.
Transillumination with halogen light may also be used.

ASSESSMENT

Differential diagnoses include those found in Table 190-1.

THERAPEUTIC PLAN

Pharmaceutical

Usually none.

Lifestyle/Activities

Consistent aerobic exercise.

No heavy lifting (e.g. weight training)
Use of elastic stockings from the foot to below the knee during standing
Elevation of legs when possible

Diet

Low-calorie diet if patient is obese to relieve pressure

Patient Education

Instruct patient in proper posture and to avoid crossing legs.
Instruct in proper use of elastic stockings.
Teach signs and symptoms of thrombophlebitis.
Explain that varicose veins can recur even if surgically removed, although likelihood is less when they are treated with ambulatory phlebectomy or with ligation and stripping as compared with compression sclerotherapy.
Teach use of Valsalva maneuver during lifting to relieve pressure.

Family Impact

None

Referral/Consultation

Referral is not necessary unless the condition is painful or is causing skin ulcers. Referral to a dermatologist may be made for cosmetic repair using sclerotherapy. Referral to a surgeon may be made for surgical repair of the veins or if grafting for an ulcer is indicated. An enterostomal and wound care therapist may be consulted for ulcer healing.

Follow-up

Reevaluate in 24 to 48 hours if thrombophlebitis is suspected.

Reevaluate in 1 week if skin ulcer is present. For more information, refer to Chapter 109.

EVALUATION

Determine adherence to exercise routine and use of elastic stockings.

SUGGESTED READINGS

Tierney L, Messina L: Blood vessels and lymphatics. In Tierney L, McPhee S, Papadakis M, editors: *Current medical diagnosis and treatment,* ed 37, Stamford, Conn, 1998, Appleton & Lange.

Weiss R: State of the Art treatment for varicose and telangiectatic veins. Paper presented at the 56th Annual Meeting of the American Academy of Dermatology, March 25, 1998, Orlando, Fla.

191 Vertigo

ICD-9-CM

Vertigo 780.4
Benign Paroxysmal Positional 386.11
Meniere's Disease 386

OVERVIEW

Definition

Vertigo is a symptom commonly seen in vestibular disease. Vertigo is considered "either a sensation of motion when there is no motion, or an exaggerated sense of motion in response to a given bodily movement" (Jackler and Kaplan, 1998). It is different than dizziness or syncope which are usually non-vestibular in origin.

Incidence

Dependent on cause of vertigo

Pathophysiology

Dependent on cause of vertigo

SUBJECTIVE DATA

History of Present Illness

The initial symptom is vertigo. It may be associated with nausea and vomiting. The episode is often preceded by an aura of fullness or pressure in the ears lasting from 20 minutes to several hours. The symptom may present as a sense of tumbling, falling forward or backward, or the ground rolling under one's feet (earthquake-like).

Patients may present with complaints of difficulty hearing or family members may identify an inability of the patient to hear.

Ask about:
- Nausea and vomiting, tinnitus
- Loss of ability to "pop" ears
- Sense of fullness in ears
- Pulling at ears
- Diplopia
- Loss of equilibrium or loss of strength or sensation

May complain of foreign body in the ear

Ask about:
- Involvement of one ear or both

Was the onset gradual or sudden?

Has the hearing fluctuated since the hearing loss began?

Are there associated symptoms of: tinnitus, vertigo, otalgia, otorrhea, or facial weakness?

Past Medical History

Ask about:

- Hypertension
- Mumps
- Neurological problems
- Head trauma
- Diabetes
- Hypothyroidism
- Syphilis
- Migraine
- Heart problems or arrhythmias

Medications

Ask about use of:

- Aspirin (ASA) (high dose)
- Antibiotics: Aminoglycosides (gentamicin, streptomycin)
- Diuretics (loop-furosemide)
- Quinine

Family History

Ask about:

A family history of hearing loss
Ask about a familial disposition to Meniere's disease

Psychosocial Environment

Ask about:

Occupation: Exposure to loud noises, use of protective measures: ear plugs
Exposure to other sources of noise (e.g., music)

OBJECTIVE DATA

Physical Examination

The examination should be a complete screening examination to make sure it is related to vestibular function and not cardiovascular or cerebrovascular. In particular, the following areas should be emphasized:

Vital signs: Blood pressure, standing/lying
Head/eyes/ears/nose/throat: Evaluate for an upper respiratory infection
- Ear
  - Evaluate tympanic membrane (TM), external canal
  - Complete pneumatic otoscopy: check for TM movement
  - Tympanogram

Neck: Check for carotid bruit, auscultate over temporal and mastoid bones for bruits
Neurological: Check sensation of face, note if facial movement is symmetrical
- Random alternating movements, deep tendon reflexes
- Do Romberg test
- Evaluate gait
- Check for nystagmus: Nylen-Barany maneuver (limited use when the patient is able to visually fixate)
- Fukuda test (patient walks in place with eyes closed) can detect subtle defects. A positive response is when the patient rotates toward the diseased labyrinth.
- Fistula test: Place a pneumatic otoscope into the external canal; inflation causes TM fluctuation; if vestibulopathy is present, the result will be vertigo, nystagmus, and eye deviation

Hearing: Have patient repeat aloud words presented in a soft whisper, normal speaking voice, or shout; have the opposite ear occluded, then repeat on other side
- **Children**
  - 0-3 mos: Response to noise
  - 3-5 mos: Child turns to sound
  - 6-10 mos: Child responds to name
  - 10-15 mos: Child imitates simple words
- Weber: Place the tuning fork on the forehead or front teeth. Have the patient indicate where it is heard the best.
- Rinne: The tuning fork is placed alternately on the mastoid bone and in front of the ear canal.

Diagnostic Procedures

Diagnostic procedures are outlined in Table 191-1.

ASSESSMENT

Differential diagnoses include those found in Table 191-2.

Classification of hearing test and type of hearing loss is found in Tables 191-3 and 191-4.

THERAPEUTIC PLAN

Treatment is based on the cause of the vertigo

Pharmaceutical

For an acute attack, the aim is to sedate the vestibulo-brain stem; use only for 2 weeks and gradually wean (Table 191-5).

Lifestyle/Activities

Bed rest may reduce the severity of vertigo in an acute attack. In chronic vertigo, exercise is one of the most important therapies. It enhances the ability of the central nervous system to compensate for labyrinth dysfunction. The patient should begin exercise after the nausea and vomiting has resolved. Exercise should be performed until vertigo occurs.

Head maneuvers: A series of head maneuvers has been identified as a possible way to control positional vertigo; the maneuvers are intended to reposition free-floating otolithic particles to decrease the incidence of vertigo.

Diet

Low salt diet (< 2 g sodium daily); only effective if the cause of vertigo is Meniere's disease

Patient Education

Completely explain the disorder, indicating the expected course of the disease and medications.
Discuss the need to live with unpredictable illness.

Referral/Consultation

A variety of options for medical and surgical treatment are available if the patient is referred to an otolaryngologist.

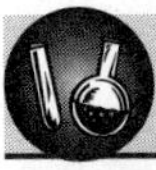

Table 191-1 Diagnostic Tests: Vertigo

Diagnostic Test	Finding/Rationale	Cost ($)
Rapid plasma reagin	Should be done to rule out syphilis, a known cause of Meniere's disease.	18-22
Magnetic resonance imaging (MRI) or computed tomography (CT)	MRI should be done if any focal signs are found on the examination. CT with contrast is the next best study	1781-2004/MRI; 990-1175/CT
Audiometric studies	Hearing test conducted in sound proof room. Pure-tone thresholds in decibels (dB) are obtained over the ranges of 250-8000 Hz for both air and bone conduction. All patients with hearing loss should be referred for audiometric testing unless the cause is easily remediable (impacted cerumen). Patients can be referred directly to an audiologist. The location of an accredited audiologist can be obtained by calling the American Speech-Language Association at 1-800-638-8255. An abnormal audiogram means there is a problem in either the trochlear nerve or the retrotrochlear apparatus.	119-154
Speech discrimination testing	Evaluates the clarity of hearing. Results are reported as percentage correct.	88-104
Brain stem auditory responses (BARE)	If sensorineural hearing loss is detected, further investigation should involve BARE. This examination tests the retrotrochlear apparatus. An abnormality suggests the presence of acoustic neuroma or other tumor. If the BARE is normal, possible diseases to consider include: Meniere's disease, labyrinthitis.	341-415
Tympanogram	Used to detect fluid in the middle ear and to determine the mobility of the tympanic membrane (TM). An electroacoustic device is used to measure the compliance of the TM. Results are displayed in a graphic form. It is most reliable in children >6 mos.	31-37
Audiogram	Small hand-held audioscopes can provide a rough indication of hearing impairment. Usually four pure tones are emitted in sequence. This test can be affected by background noise, so the examination room must be quiet.	24-29
Glycerol dehydration test	Measures the audiometric response to an oral dose of glycerol. Improvement in scores for hearing low frequency and discriminating speech is diagnostic as there is no other condition in which this change is observed.	Not available
Caloric testing	Reveals loss or impairment of nystagmus induced with cold substance in involved ear.	38-45
Electrocochleography	Presents with a highly characteristic waveform of Meniere's disease, although the results may be negative in the early and late stages of the disease.	141-169
Electronystagmography (ENG)	Objective recording of the nystagmus induced by head and body movements. It helps to quantify the degree of vestibular dysfunction. It should be done if the audiogram is normal. Benign positional vertigo and ototoxicity are supported by an abnormal ENG.	160-191

TABLE 191-2 Differential Diagnosis: Vertigo

Diagnosis	Supporting Data
Cerumen impaction (Ch. 62)	Occlusion of the external ear canal by cerumen. Usually self-induced via attempts at cleaning.
Serous otitis media (Ch. 134)	Dull tympanic membrane (TM), hypomobile TM. Air bubbles may be seen in the middle ear, with a conductive hearing loss present.
Acoustic neuroma	Hearing loss, vertigo, nausea and vomiting, deterioration of speech discrimination. Nystagmus is usually vertical, without latency, and unsuppressed by visual fixation. Look for cranial nerve 5, 7, 10 dysfunction.
Labyrinthitis	Acute episode of vertigo lasting several days to a week; it may follow an upper respiratory infection. There is usually accompanied hearing loss and tinnitus. Rapid head movement may bring on nausea and vomiting. The cause of labyrinthitis is unknown. The recovery period may last several weeks. Hearing loss may or may not resolve.
Meniere's disease (Ch. 114)	A triad of hearing loss, tinnitus, and vertigo.
Presbycusis	Progressive, mainly high frequency hearing loss of aging. Frequently with genetic predisposition. Patients complain of an inability to hear well (speech discrimination) in a noisy environment.
Noise trauma	Second most common cause of hearing loss. Sounds >85 dB are potentially damaging to the cochlea, especially with prolonged exposure. The loss typically occurs in the high frequencies (4000 Hz) and progresses to involve sounds in the normal speech frequencies. Sounds that have the potential for damage are industrial machinery, loud music, and weapons.
Ototoxicity	Hearing loss can be caused by substances that affect both the auditory and vestibular systems. Common causes: salicylates, aminoglycosides, loop diuretics and antineoplastic agents, especially cisplatin.
Traumatic vertigo	The most common cause of vertigo following a head injury is labyrinthine concussion. Basal skull fractures that involve the inner ear may result in severe vertigo that does not improve.
Benign positional vertigo (BPV)	Also known as benign paroxysmal positional vertigo. This vertigo is peripheral in origin. Transient vertigo occurs with head positioning and is the most common cause of vertigo. Symptoms include vertigo that lasts for several days, with the vertigo lasting 10 to 60 seconds after head positioning.
Central lesion of the central nervous system	Vertigo caused by these conditions is unrelenting and disabling. There are usually signs of other brain stem dysfunction such as cranial nerve palsies, motor, sensory or cerebellar deficits, or increased intraocular pressure. Auditory function is usually spared. Conditions include brain stem vascular disease, arteriovenous malformation, tumor of the brain stem, and multiple sclerosis.

TABLE 191-3 Classification of Hearing Test and Type of Hearing Loss

Classification	Rinne	Weber
Normal: both ears	AC> BC	Midline
Conductive loss Right ear	Rt ear: BC>AC Lt. Ear AC>BC	Lateralized to right ear
Left ear	Rt. Ear: AC>BC Lt. Ear: BC>AC	Lateralized to left ear
Both ears	Rt. Ear: BC>AC Lt. Ear: BC>AC	Lateralized to poorer ear of the two
Sensorineural loss Right ear	AC>BC both ears	Lateralized to left ear
Left ear	AC>BC both ears	Lateralized to right ear
Both ears	AC>BC both ears	Lateralized to better ear

AC, Air conduction; *BC*, bone conduction.

TABLE 191-4 Type of Hearing Loss

Category of Hearing Loss	dB level
Mild hearing loss	26-40 dB
Moderate hearing loss	41-55 dB
Moderately severe hearing loss	56-70 dB
Severe hearing loss	71-90 dB
Profound hearing loss	>91 dB

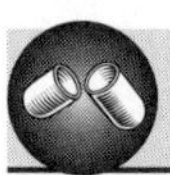

TABLE 191-5 Pharmaceutical Plan: Vertigo

Drug	Dose	Comments	Cost
Prochlorperazine (Compazine)	5-10 mg 3-4 ×/day or 10-30 mg spansule q AM or 10 mg spansule q12h (sustained release)	Pregnancy: C SE: Drowsiness, lowered seizure threshold, amenorrhea, photosensitivity,	\$34-\$60/5 mg (100); \$52-\$89/10 mg (100); \$79/SR: 15 mg (100)
Promethazine (Phenergan)	25-50 mg PO q6h **Children:** 12.5-25 mg Supp: 12.5, 25, 50 mg	Pregnancy: C SE: Sedation, sleepiness, dry mouth, lowered seizure threshold	\$3-\$33/25 mg (100); \$27/supp: 12.5 mg (12)
Diazepam	2-5 mg PO TID-QID available in solution 5 mg/5 ml	Many people with vertigo, particularly the **elderly,** respond well to the lower dosage and frequency Pregnancy: D Se: Dizziness, drowsiness, dry mouth, orthostatic hypotension	\$2-\$66/5 mg (100)
Meclizine (Antivert)	25 mg PO TID QID	Used for vertigo Pregnancy: B SE: Drowsiness, fatigue, dry mouth, blurred vision	\$3-\$49/25 mg (100)

SE, Side effects.

Medical options include intratympanic aminoglycosides to control vertigo. Surgical options include procedures that are not destructive to hearing: endolymphatic sac surgery (effective in approximately 80% to control vertigo), vestibular nerve section (effective in 90% to 95% to control vertigo; however, the surgery is major in that the posterior cranial fossa is opened), sacculotomy, cryosurgical treatment, and insertion of tympanostomy tubes. Other surgeries destroy any remaining hearing: labyrinthectomy, cochleosacculotomy, and vestibulocochlear neurectomy.

Follow-up

Usually done by otolaryngologist

EVALUATION

Improvement in vertigo with preserved hearing ability is the goal.

RESOURCES

The Meniere's Network: www.meniere2.htm

The Ear foundation: www.theearfound.com

REFERENCES

Jackler R, Kaplan M: Ear, nose and throat. In Tierney L, McPhee S, Papadakis M, editors: *Current medical diagnosis and treatment,* Stamford, Conn, 1998, Appleton & Lange.

SUGGESTED READINGS

Arts H, Kileny P, Telian S: Diagnostic testing for endolymphatic hydrops, *Otolaryngol Clin North Am* 30(6):987-1005, 1997.

Ellsworth AJ et al: *Mosby's 1998 medical drug reference*, St Louis, 1998, Mosby.

Healthcare Consultants of America, Inc: *1998 physicians fee and coding guide*, Augusta, Ga, 1998, Healthcare Consultants of America, Inc.

Epley J: Particle positioning maneuver for benign paroxysmal positional vertigo, *Otolaryngology Clin North Am* 29:323, 1996.

Fife T: Recognition and management of horizontal canal benign positional vertigo, *Am J Otolarynol* 19(3):345-351, 1998.

Gibson W, Arenberg I: Pathophysiologic theories in the etiology of Meniere's disease, *Otolaryngol Clin North Am* 30(6):961-967, 1997.

Grodzin C, Abrams, R: Case 1. In Grodzin C, Schwartz S, Bone R, editors: *Diagnostic strategies for internal medicine,* St Louis, 1996, Mosby.

Kartush J, Brackmann D: Acoustic neuroma update, *Otolaryngol Clin North Am* 29:377-380, 1996.

Lambert R: Evaluation of the dizzy patient, *Comp Ther* 23(11):719-723, 1997.

Mendel B et al: Living with dizziness: an explorative study, *J Adv Nurs* 26(6):1134-1141, 1997.

Pillsbury H: Benign paroxysmal positional vertigo and otolith repositioning: a cost-effective addition to the armamentarium. *Arch Otolaryngol Head Neck Surg* 124(2):226, 1998.

Vulvovaginitis

ICD-9-CM

Trichomoniasis 131.01
Vaginal Candidiasis or Monilial Vaginitis 112.1
Vulvovaginitis, Unspecified 616.10
Complicating Pregnancy or Puerperium 646.6

OVERVIEW

Definition

Vulvovaginitis is infection of the vagina, either inflammatory or noninflammatory.

Incidence

It is estimated that there are 20% to 25% of 10 million health care visits annually for vaginitis. Approximately 50% of vaginal infections are caused by bacterial vaginosis. It is not considered a sexually transmitted infection, yet it is uncommon in virginal women. Trichomoniasis causes approximately 25% of vulvovaginal infections. It is predominantly sexually transmitted; however, transmission by fomites does occur. Candidiasis accounts for approximately 35% of cases of vaginitis.

Pathophysiology

Vaginal secretions arise from several sources: mucus from the cervix (majority of liquid), exudates from Skene's and Bartholin's glands, and from vaginal transudate. Exfoliated squamous cells from the vagina wall give a white to off-white color. Approximately 1.5 g of vaginal fluid is produced on average per day in the asymptomatic woman. Normal vaginal secretions have no odor.

Bacterial vaginosis *(Gardnerella)* is caused from a change in the natural ecology of the vagina, resulting in an overgrowth of anaerobic bacteria *(Bacteroides* sp., *Peptococcus* sp., and *Mobiuncus* sp.) and a decrease in normal lactobacilli; whereas *Candida* infections occur when the natural flora of the vagina proliferates (*Candida albicans* and nonalbicans *Candida)*. Both are considered sexually associated *but not* sexually transmitted. Trichomoniasis is caused from the protozoan *Trichomonas vaginalis*. It is sexually transmitted.

Protective Factors Against

The normal vaginal ecosystem: Complex relationship between:
- Endogenous microflora (yeast, gram-positive and gram-aerobic, and obligate anaerobic bacteria)
- Metabolic products of the microflora and host
- Estrogen
- pH level (normal 3.5 to 4.5)

Factors That Increase Susceptibility

Antibiotics
Contraceptive preparation (oral and topical)
Vaginal medication
Sexually transmitted infections
Change in partners
Foreign body
Tight fitting clothes
Hormones (including steroids)
Douches or feminine hygiene sprays
Sexual intercourse
Stress
Latex allergy
Allergy to soap
Diet high in refined sugars (candidiasis)

SUBJECTIVE DATA

History of Present Illness

Relationship of symptoms to menses
Relationship of symptoms to intercourse

Partner symptoms
Complaints of discharge, itching, odor, vaginal irritation
Date of last sexual contact, number of sexual partners in last 6 months
Sexual activity (vaginal, oral, anal), use of vibrators or other paraphernalia

Past Medical History

Ask about previous vaginal infections and treatments. Ask if partner was treated
Ask about any chronic illness (especially diabetes, seizure disorders, human immunodeficiency virus)
Last menstrual period, use of barrier methods, type of birth control
Allergies

Medications

Ask about recent use of antibiotics and/or steroids. Ask about any over-the-counter treatment used.

Psychosocial History

Ask about:

Recent changes in lifestyle (stress, personal crisis)
Use of vaginal sprays, deodorant tampons, panty liners or pads, douches, perfumed toilet paper
Changes in laundry soaps, fabric softeners, body soap
Clothing: Consistent wearing of tight-crotch pants, nylon underwear, underwear to bed
Diet high in refined sugar

Family History

Not available

Description of Most Common Symptoms

Women with bacterial vaginosis may present with increased vaginal discharge, vaginal burning after intercourse and a strong, usually "fishy" odor. There are generally no associated symptoms of inflammation (hence the term *vaginosis* rather than *vaginitis* which indicates inflammation).
Women with candidiasis frequently complain of itching (often severe), burning with urination, and dyspareunia or burning during and/or after intercourse. Discharge is thick, white, and curdlike. Trichomoniasis often presents with a foul-smelling discharge, external itching and burning, dyspareunia, and postcoital bleeding. Partners may have similar symptoms.

OBJECTIVE DATA

Physical Examination

Examination components for vulvovaginitis are outlined in Table 192-1.

Diagnostic Procedures

Diagnostic procedures are outlined in Table 192-2.

ASSESSMENT

NOTE: Frequently, two or more vaginitis will co-exist.

Differential diagnoses include conditions that may mimic the following conditions (Table 192-3):

Candidiasis: Herpes, chemical dermatitis, contact dermatitis, candidiasis secondary to diabetes, other less frequently seen candidiasis, trichomoniasis, bacterial vaginosis, *Chlamydia*, gonorrhea, atrophic vaginitis

TABLE 192-1 Physical Examination

Examination Components	Candidiasis	Bacterial Vaginosis	Trichomoniasis
External genitalia	Excoriated, erythema, edema, ulcerations, lesions	Normal	Excoriated, erythema, edema, ulcerations, lesions
Vaginal mucosa	Erythema, irritated, white patches along walls	Normal	May notice red papules
Cervix	Normal	Normal	Strawberry-like appearance
Discharge	Thick, odorless, white, curdlike	Adherent homogenous; grayish in color with a fishy, musty odor	Greenish-yellow, malodorous and frothy

Bacterial vaginosis: *Chlamydia,* trichomoniasis, presence of a foreign body

Trichomoniasis: Candidiasis, bacterial vaginosis, urinary tract infection, *Chlamydia,* gonorrhea

THERAPEUTIC PLAN

Pharmaceutical

Candidiasis

Topical formulations are effective treatments, with the topically applied azole drugs being more effective than nystatin. Treatment with the azoles results in relief of symptoms and negative cultures in 80% to 90% of patients. The nonalbicans species (*C. glabrata* and *C. tropicalis)* is increasing in frequency and may account for approximately 35% of all infections. These species are less susceptible to the frequently prescribed agents such as clotrimazole and miconazole.

Recommended regimens are outlined in Tables 192-4 and 192-5.

If treatment is unsuccessful, may refill medications once; if still unsuccessful, consider treating partner and/or checking fasting blood sugar. Those with underlying disease may require 1 to 2 weeks of therapy. Recurrent infections should have the diagnosis confirmed by culture. Maintenance regimens include 100 mg PO fluconazole ×1 week, ketoconazole 200 mg/day, and clotrimazole 500 mg vaginal suppository, or ketoconazole 400 mg/day × 2 weeks, followed by 400 mg/day for 5 days beginning with onset of menses for 3 menstrual cycles (Elliott, 1998).

If blood sugar is normal and symptoms do not abate, consider a vulvar biopsy.

Treatment of Partner

Candidiasis is not acquired through sexual intercourse; treatment of sex partners is not recommended but may be considered for women who have recurrent infection, although it is controversial. A minority of male partners may have balanitis, which is characterized by anerythematous area on the glans in conjunction with pruritus or irritation. These partners may benefit from treatment with topical antifungal agents to relieve symptoms.

Pregnancy

Only topical azole should be used. Of these treatments, the most effective are butoconazole, clotrimazole, miconazole, and terconazole.

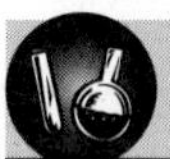

TABLE 192-2 Diagnostic Procedures: Vulvovaginitis

Diagnostic Test	Candidiasis	Bacterial Vaginosis	Trichomoniasis	Cost ($)
Microscopic examination (NS, KOH)	Hyphae, pseudo-hyphae, pH within 3.8-4.5	Clue cells >20%, positive whiff test, vaginal pH >4.5, absence of lactobacilli	Highly motile, oval cells	15-19
Gonorrhea and *Chlamydia* culture	Consider screening for gonorrhea and chlamydia when the woman complains of vaginal discharge/itching/or odor; increased rates of gonorrhea and *Chlamydia* have been reported with bacterial vaginosis			19-51/*chl:* 61-79/GC
Blood sugar	Consider blood sugar if candidiasis is recurrent or a severe case to rule out diabetes			16-20

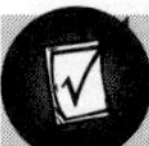

TABLE 192-3 Differential Diagnosis: Vulvovaginitis

Diagnosis	Supporting Data
Chlamydia	The disease is often asymptomatic, although if left untreated, patient may complain of vaginal pain, postcoital bleeding, abdominal pain, or the more serious pelvic inflammatory disease
Gonorrhea	Abnormal vaginal discharge, abnormal uterine bleeding, dysuria
Atrophic vaginitis	Vaginal epithelium becomes thin and cervical secretions diminish, complains of itching and burning
Foreign body	Foul odor, increased vaginal discharge (may be bloody), abdominal discomfort, uterine discomfort (usually "lost" tampon)
Urinary tract infection	Dysuria, frequency, urgency

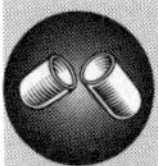

TABLE 192-4 Pharmaceutical Treatment of Vulvovaginitis With Intravaginal Agents

Drug	Dose	Comments	Cost
Butoconazole 2% cream (FemStat)	5 g (1 applicator) intravaginally for 3 days* at HS	Pregnancy: C SE: Vulvovaginal burning, vulvar itch, discharge, soreness, swelling	$13-$15/2%
Clotrimazole 1% cream (Gyne-Lotrimin, Mycelex F) 45 g	5 g intravaginally for 7-14 days* at HS	Not recommended in children Pregnancy: B SE: Vaginal burning, itching, rash, irritation, abdominal cramps, bloating, urinary frequency	$15/1% (45 g)
Clotrimazole (Mycelex G) 100 mg	Intravaginal tablet for 7 days* or 2 tablets for 3 days* at HS	Same as for clotrimazole 1%	$15/100 mg (7)
Clotrimazole 500 mg intravaginal tablet	1 tablet in a single dose* at HS	Same as for clotrimazole 1%	$13/500 mg (1)
Miconazole 2% cream (Monistat F) 45 g	5 g intravaginally for 7 days*	Not recommended in children Pregnancy: B SE: Vulvovaginal burning, itching, rash, urticaria	$13-$14/2% (45 g)
Miconazole (Monistat F) 100 mg vaginal suppository	1 suppository for 7 days*	Same as for miconazole 2%	$12/100 mg (7)
Tioconazole 6.5% ointment (Vagistat-1)	Intravaginally in a single application* q HS (4.6 g [1 applicator intravaginally])	Not recommended in children Pregnancy: C Complete relief of symptoms may take up to 7 days, may be less messy than other options SE: Vaginal burning, itching, dysuria, dyspareunia; better efficacy against non-albicans *Candida*	$24/6.5% (4.6-g single dose)
Terconazole 0.4% cream (Terazol 7)	5 g intravaginally for 7 days*	Not recommended in children Pregnancy: C SE: Vaginal burning, genital pain and fever, itching Better efficacy against non-albicans *Candida*	$23/0.4% (45 g)
Terconazole 0.8% cream (Terazol 3)	5 g intravaginally for 3 days*	Same as for terconazole 0.4%	$23/0.8% (20 g)
Terconazole 80-mg vaginal suppository	1 suppository for 3 days*	Same as for terconazole 0.4%	$23/80 mg (3)

*These creams and suppositories are oil-based and may weaken latex condoms and diaphragms.
SE, Side effects.

Patient Education

No intercourse until symptoms subside

No douching

Increase rest and reduce stress

Stress importance of completing therapy even if menses begin

Do not use tampons during treatment

Stress hygiene, cotton underwear, loose clothing, no underpants while sleeping, wipe from front to back

Do not use feminine hygiene sprays or deodorants

Alternative Strategies (Unsubstantiated)

Consider use of

Vitamin C 500 mg BID-QID to increase acidity of vaginal secretions or oral acidophilus tablets 40 million to 1 billion U QD (1 tablet)

Gentian violet 1% painted on the vagina 1/week for 4 or more weeks or monthly after menses for 4 months (may stain clothes)

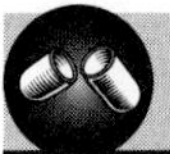

TABLE 192-5 Pharmaceutical Treatment of Vulvovaginitis With Oral Agent

Drug	Dose	Comments	Cost
Fluconazole (Diflucan)	150 mg PO in a single dose	Not recommended in children Pregnancy: C Lower potency against C. glabrata SE: Headache, nausea, abdominal pain, gastrointestinal upset, dizziness	$10-$15/150 mg (1 tablet)

SE, Side effects.

Vaginal application of yogurt 1 to 2 times QD ×7 days (use tampon for vaginal application)

Recurrent Vulvovaginitis from Persistent *Candida*

Recurrent vulvovaginitis from persistent *Candida* infections is defined as four or more episodes of symptomatic candidiasis annually. Risk factors include uncontrolled diabetes mellitus, immunosuppression, and corticosteroid use. Treatment guidelines suggest an initial intensive regimen continued for approximately 10 to 14 days, followed immediately by a maintenance regimen for at least 6 months. Maintenance ketoconazole 100 mg PO for 6 months is suggested. All cases of recurrent vulvovaginitis should be confirmed by culture before maintenance therapy is initiated. Follow-up is done by routine evaluations to monitor the effectiveness of therapy and the occurrence of side effects.

Bacterial Vaginosis

Recommended regimens are outlined in Table 192-6. Choose one regimen.

Treatment of Partners

Treatment of partners is not recommended. Consider treating if bacterial vaginosis is recurrent.

Pregnancy

Metronidazole 250 mg PO TID for 7 days
Metronidazole 2 g PO in a single dose
Metronidazole gel 0.075% 1 applicator QHS for 5 days
Clindamycin 300 mg PO BID for 7 days

A 1-month follow-up evaluation is recommended for pregnant patients. Complications include chorioamnionitis, premature rupture of membranes, premature labor, and postpartum endomyometritis.

Patient Education

No intercourse until symptoms subside
No douching
Stress importance of completing therapy even if menses begin
Do not use tampons during treatment
Stress hygiene, cotton underwear, loose clothing, no underwear while sleeping; wipe from front to back
Do not use feminine hygiene sprays or deodorants

Trichomoniasis

Recommended regimens are outlined in Table 192-7. Choose one regimen.

Treatment of Partner

Sex partners should be treated.
Recurrent trichomoniasis should be treated with a higher dose of metronidazole. If secondary treatment of trichomoniasis is unsuccessful, the patient should receive metronidazole 500 mg PO BID for 7 days. If treatment failure occurs repeatedly, the patient should be treated with the 2-g dose once a day for 3 to 5 days.

Pregnancy

Patients may be treated with 2 g of metronidazole in a single dose.

Lifestyle/Activities for All Types of Vulvovaginitis

Patients are advised to refrain from sexual activity until treatment is completed and symptoms are gone. Douching and use of "feminine hygiene" products are to be avoided. If the patient absolutely insists on douching, she is to be advised to douche no more than once a month, using only vinegar and water douche.

Diet

For patients prone to candidiasis infections, consider a diet low in refined sugars.
Consider the use of vitamin C 500 mg PO BID to QID or oral acidophilus tablets 40 million to 1 billion U QD (1 tablet).

Patient Education

Refrain from drinking alcohol for 24 hours before initiating treatment with metronidazole and for 48 hours after completing treatment.
Wear cotton underwear, loose clothing, no underwear while sleeping.

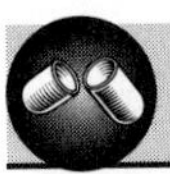

TABLE 192-6 Pharmaceutical Treatment of Bacterial Vaginosis

Drug	Dose	Comments	Cost
Metronidazole	500 mg PO BID for 7 days	Not recommended in children Pregnancy: B SE: Seizures, gastrointestinal upset, metallic taste, Candida overgrowth, anorexia, constipation, headache; patients who have a history of seizure disorders should not take metronidazole	$238/500 mg (100)
Metronidazole gel 0.75%	One applicator (5 g) intravaginally QD (QHS) or BID for 5 days	Same as for metronidazole	$25/0.75% (70 g)
Clindamycin (Cleocin)	300 mg BID ×7 days	Pregnancy: B SE: Diarrhea, colitis, rash, blood dyscrasias, gastrointestinal upset	$231/300 mg (100)
Clindamycin cream 2%	One applicator (5 g) intravaginally QHS for 7 days*	Not recommended in children Pregnancy: B; clindamycin vaginal cream is not recommended during pregnancy because studies have shown an increased risk of preterm births SE: Cervicitis, vaginitis, local irritation	$31/2% (40 g)
Alternative regimen: metronidazole 2 g PO in a single dose		See metronidazole; tend to have a higher recurrence rate	See metronidazole

*Clindamycin cream is oil-based and may weaken condoms.
SE, Side effects.

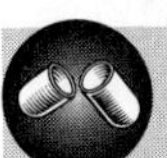

TABLE 192-7 Pharmaceutical Treatment of Trichomoniasis

Drug	Dose	Comments	Cost
Metronidazole (Flagyl)	2 g PO in a single dose	Not recommended in children Pregnancy: B SE: Seizures, gastrointestinal upset, metallic taste, Candida overgrowth, anorexia, constipation, headache	$7-$238/500 mg (100)
Metronidazole	500 mg PO BID for 7 days		

SE, Side effects.

Follow-up

Follow-up is only necessary if symptoms persist. A patient who continues to complain of vulvar itching after treatment for either candidiasis or trichomoniasis and who has no other signs should have a vulvar biopsy done.

REFERENCES

Elliott K: Managing patients with vulvovaginal candidiasis, *Nurse Pract* 23(3):44-52, 1998.

SUGGESTED REFERENCES

ACOG Technical Bulletin: Vaginitis, ACOG Technical Bulletin, No. 226, July 1996.

Caro-Paton T et al: Is metronidazole teratogenic? A meta-analysis, *Br J Clin Pharmacol* 44(2):79-182, 1997.

Centers for Disease Control and Prevention: Guidelines for treatment of sexually transmitted diseases, *MMWR* 47 (No. RR-1):59-69, 1998.

Colli E, Landoni M, Parazzini F: Treatment of male partners and recurrence of bacterial vaginosis: a randomized trial, *Genitourinary Med* 73(4): 267-270, 1997.

Davis J et al: Correlation between cervical cytologic results and Gram stain as diagnostic tests for bacterial vaginosis, *Am J Obstet Gynecol* 177(3):532-535, 1997.

Ellsworth AJ et al: *Mosby's medical drug reference*, St Louis, 1998, Mosby.

Hawkins JW, Roberto-Nichols DM, Stanley-Haney JL: *Protocols for nurse practitioners in gynecologic settings,* ed 5, New York, 1995, Tiresias Press.

Healthcare Consultants of America, Inc: *1998 physicians fee and coding guide*, Augusta, Ga, 1998, Healthcare Consultants of America, Inc.

Johnson CA: *Women's health care handbook,* St Louis, 1996, Mosby.

Majeroni B: Bacterial vaginosis: an update, *Am Family Physician* 57(6):1285-1290, 1998.

McMillan A: Sexually transmittable diseases. *Handbook of family planning and reproductive health,* ed 3, New York, 1995, Churchill Livingstone.

Wilkinson D et al: Tampon sampling for diagnosis of bacterial vaginitis: a potentially useful way to detect genital infections? *J Clin Microbiol* 35(9):2408-2409, 1997.

Warts (Nongenital)

ICD-9-CM

Common Warts 078.1
Plantar Warts 078.19

OVERVIEW

Definition

Warts are virus-induced epidermal tumors caused by human papillomavirus (HPV). More than 70 genotypes of HPV have been identified. There are three types of the HPV infections that occur in the general population: common wart, plantar wart, and flat wart. Warts can last for many months to several years.

Incidence

The common wart occurs in approximately 70% of all cutaneous warts; 20% occur in **school-age children.** Plantar warts are seen in older children and young adults, representing approx. 30% of cutaneous warts. Flat warts are also found in children and adults, representing 4% of cutaneous warts.

Pathophysiology

HPV is a double-stranded DNA virus of the papovavirus class. Minor trauma with breaks in the stratum corneum facilitates epidermal infection.

Factors That Increase Susceptibility

Being immunocompromised by human immunodeficiency virus or organ transplantation increases the risk of widespread cutaneous warts. There is an occupational risk associated with butchers and meat packers.

Transmission

Skin-to-skin contact

Minor trauma to skin facilitates infection; medical personnel may be exposed to the virus from the plume of warts treated by laser or electrosurgery, resulting in a nosocomial infection; Heredity is a factor in epidermodysplasia verruciformis (EDV)—most often an autosomal-recessive gene

SUBJECTIVE DATA

History of Present Illness

Ask about location, onset, duration, and symptoms

Description of Most Common Symptoms

Complaints of bleeding after shaving
Complaints of cosmetic disfigurement
May complain of pain on feet

Past Medical History

Ask about previous warts, treatments, and results.

Medication History

If previous HPV treatment, what was used, how often, was treatment completed?

Family History

History of EDV

Psychosocial

Not applicable

OBJECTIVE DATA

Physical Examination

Examine the lesion, looking for characteristic lesions
Use hand lens to assist in visualizing surface characteristics
Skin lesions: See Box 193-1 for description.

ASSESSMENT

Differential diagnoses include those outlined in Table 193-1; usually made on clinical findings

THERAPEUTIC PLAN

May resolve spontaneously in 12 to 24 months without treatment (approximately 50% do resolve spontaneously)

Pharmaceutical

Pharmaceutical treatment is outlined in Tables 193-2 and 193-3.

Lifestyle/Activities

Soaking warts in hot water for 10 to 30 minutes QD for 6 weeks may be effective in immunocompromised patients.

Diet

Not applicable

Patient Education

Reassure that in most cases warts will go away

Box 193-1

Characteristics of Types of Warts

Verruca Vulgaris (Common Warts)

Firm papules, 1-10 mm, skin color, round isolated or scattered discrete lesions; typically at site of trauma on hands, fingers, or knees

Verucca Plantaris (Plantar Warts)

Early stages are small, shiny papules; they later develop plaque with rough surface; skin colored, may have marked tenderness, confluence of many small warts, resulting in a mosaic wart; lesions may also occur on the two facing surfaces of toes; usually occurs on pressure points such as heads of metatarsal, heels, or toes

Verruca Plana (Flat Warts)

Flat papules, 1-5 mm on surface and 1-2 mm thick; skin colored, light brown; round, oval, polygonal or linear if caused by traumatic inoculation; may be discrete lesions, closely set; commonly on face, beard, dorsa of hand, shins

Epidermodysplasia Verruciformis

Flat wartlike lesions; lesions may be large, numerous, and confluent; skin colored, light brown, pink, or hypopigmented; occurs on face, trunk, extremities; premalignant and malignant occur most often on face

Table 193-1 Differential Diagnosis: Nongenital Warts

Diagnosis	Supporting Data
Molluscum contagiosum	Asymptomatic clusters of white papules caused by the molluscum virus; umbilicated waxy white/gray lesions
Condyloma lata	Flat wartlike lesions found in intertriginous areas and around the anal canal (associated with syphilis)
Lipomas, fibroma, adenomas	Round, soft fleshy nodules
Squamous cell carcinomas	History of sun exposure, enlarging and ulcerating red nodule
Nevi	Small (<1 cm), circumscribed, pigmented macules or papules located in the epidermis and dermis
Seborrheic keratoses	Flesh colored to pigmented papules or plaques; have an irregular, wartlike surface and "stuck on" appearance
Psoriatic plaques	Inflammatory skin disorder ranging from isolated plaques to involvement of the whole body; well-demarcated red plaques covered with thick silvery scales, distributed over the scalp, lower back, and extensor surfaces of the extremities

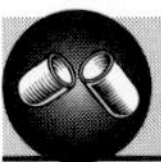

TABLE 193-2 Pharmaceutical Plan: Nongenital Warts

Drug	Dose	Comments	Cost
Salicylic acid 17% (Duofilm, Occlusal-HP, Compound W)	Apply thin coat to area, 1 or 2× daily; max 12 weeks Duofilm patch for **children:** Apply 1 patch, repeat q48h for up to 12 weeks	Soak wart in warm water 5 minutes, remove loose tissue, dry; contraindicated in patients with diabetes Pregnancy: Not indicated SE: Local irritation	\$16/gel: 6% (1 oz); \$24/plaster: 40% (25); \$3/sol: 13.6% (9.3 ml)
Liquid nitrogen	Applied to achieve thaw time of 20-45 seconds; two freeze-thaw times are given q2-4 weeks for several visits	Face, dorsal hands, and legs more sensitive than palms; useful on dry penile warts and filiform warts involving face and body	\$70-\$86
Resorcinol (RA lotion) (over-the-counter)	Per package directions Apply to affected areas; rub gently	Pregnancy: Can be systemically absorbed Wash hands immediately after applying; avoid contact with eyes; do not use other topical acne preparations or other products containing peeling agents; medication may darken light colored hair SE: Diarrhea, nausea, stomach pain, methemoglobinemia, redness or peeling of skin	Not available

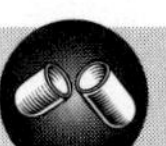

TABLE 193-3 Pharmaceutical Treatment Base on Type of Wart

Type Wart	Treatment	Cost ($)
Common	Topical salicylic preparations or cryotherapy	84-109/(14 lesions)
Filiform	Refer for removal by curette	Not available
Flat	Refer for removal; these warts are resistant to treatment and are usually located in cosmetically important areas	70-86/(14 lesions)
Plantar	Use 40% salicylic acid plasters (Mediplast); plaster is cut to size and applied to wart, removed in 48-72 hours, and repeated q 24-48h; any dead white keratin can be removed with pumice stone; this process can be continued up to 4-6 weeks until the wart is removed; pain relief results in first few days since a large part of the wart can be removed during that time; aggressive therapies may be painful and result in scarring Surgical removal, cryosurgery, electrosurgery, or laser may be considered	84-109

Family Impact

None significant

Referral

Dermatologist for excision

Follow-up

None may be indicated.

EVALUATION

Determined by clinical observations of resolving lesion

If lesion is on fingertips, return of fingerprint indicates resolution of wart

RESOURCES

Educational site about warts

http://www.nsc.gov.sg/commskin/viral.html

SUGGESTED REFERENCES

Ellsworth AJ et al: *Mosby's medical drug reference*, St Louis, 1998, Mosby.

Feldman S, Fleischer A, McConnell R: Most common dermatological problems identified by internists, *Arch Intern Med* 158(7):726-730, 1998.

Fitzpatrick T: *Color atlas and synopsis of clinical dermatology,* ed 3, New York, 1997, McGraw Hill.

Glass A, Solomon B: Cimetidine therapy for recalcitrant warts in adults, *Arch Dermatol* 32:680, 1996.

Healthcare Consultants of America, Inc: *1998 physicians fee and coding guide*, Augusta, Ga, 1998, Healthcare Consultants of America, Inc.

Landow, KV: Nongenital warts: when is treatment warranted? *Postgrad Med* 99:245, 1996.

Miller D, Brodell R: Human papillomavirus: treatment options for warts, *Am Family Physician* 53:135-148, 1996.

Sterling J: Treating the troublesome wart, *Practitioner* 239:44, 1995.

194 Weight Loss, Unintentional

ICD-9-CM

Weight Loss (Cause Unknown) 783.2

OVERVIEW

Definition

Involuntary weight loss is a nonspecific symptom that often suggests a serious physical or psychological illness. Unintentional weight loss greater than 5% within 6 months or greater or equal to 10% within a year is cause for concern and a starting point for evaluation. More than 95% of patients with an organic etiology will have lost at least that much weight. Involuntary weight loss should be distinguished from voluntary weight loss. Weight loss in **children** is determined by an altered weight maintenance or rate of weight gain compared to children of the same age. It is known as failure to thrive (see Chapter 71 for more detail).

Unintentional weight loss in the **elderly** of 10% or more over 10 years is strongly associated with increased mortality.

Pathophysiology

The three basic mechanisms of weight loss include decreased intake, increased rate of calorie use and excessive calorie loss. Whatever the underlying cause, decreased food intake is usually the most important mechanism, even when other mechanisms contribute.

SUBJECTIVE DATA

History of Present Illness

The first task is to document that weight loss has indeed taken place. Keep in mind that many patients who claim to have lost weight do not have their complaint corroborated by medical records or family members.

In the absence of recorded weights, historical data should include change in clothing size, especially belt size, ability to give exact weight change, and confirmation of history by a family member. To assist in determining amount of weight change when there is no documented weight for comparison: each notch on a belt represents approximately 5 lb.

Determine symptom pattern: Anorexia, difficulty eating, weight loss with normal intake, social problems.

Past Medical History

Information regarding potential social, psychological and physical factors should be identified.

History must always include alcohol/drug use and cigarette smoking. Smoking may increase the risk of cancer, ulcer disease, chronic pulmonary disease and tuberculosis.

Inquire about previous surgeries. Patients with prior abdominal surgery may have partial intestinal obstruction with pain, vomiting and weight loss. Those who have undergone a partial gastrectomy may have malabsorption and weight loss.

Ask about previous episodes of depression, anorexia or dementia.

Medication History

Many drugs have the potential for interfering with appetite by causing abdominal discomfort, diarrhea, nausea, loss of appetite and inhibition of gastric emptying.

Medications with central nervous system effects such as the selective serotonin reuptake inhibitors may suppress appetite. Digoxin, dilantin, theophylline, quinidine, and lithium may cause anorexia at toxic levels.

The risk of adverse effects is increased by polypharmacy, especially in the **elderly.**

Family History

A family history of chronic health problems, including psychiatric disorders and substance abuse should be elicited.

Diabetes and autoimmune diseases such as lupus have familial tendencies.

Psychosocial History

When decreased food intake is suspected, it is important to inquire about somatic symptoms of depression, excessive use of alcohol, and poor dentition.

If the patient is a **young woman,** it is necessary to ask about eating habits, self-image, and attitudes about weight, exaggerated fear of obesity, or inappropriate pursuit of thinness.

Question the **elderly** about social isolation, bereavement, physical impairment, and poverty. Ask about functional status.

Ask about risk factors for human immunodeficiency virus.

In determining how changes in physical activity have contributed to weight loss, it is advantageous to ask the patient to describe a typical day: time of awakening, time of going to bed, naps, total amount of sleep, and time spent engaged in physical activities.

Diet History

A food diary to include all meals and snacks is helpful.

Questioning about food availability, idiosyncratic food preferences, overzealous adherence to diets or real/presumed allergies to various foods may suggest a specific cause.

Unpleasant symptoms such as abdominal pain, dyspnea, dysphagia, or abnormal taste can curtail food intake and point to a possible solution to the dilemma.

Early satiety versus decreased appetite needs to be explored.

Associated Symptoms

Systemic causes will manifest symptoms other than weight loss; almost all physical causes are clinically evident during the initial evaluation

Review of systems
- Prostate disorders
- Cancers
- Depression and other mental illness
- Cognitive impairment
- Neurologic disorders

OBJECTIVE DATA

Physical Examination

Vital signs: Some patients may not realize that they have lost weight; thus it is important to document actual weights at each visit. Also include height, temperature, blood pressure, pulse (Table 194-1)

Mental status: Folstein Mini-Mental State Examination

Diagnostic Procedures

Because the number of potential causes is enormous, laboratory testing should be selective and directed toward areas of concern elicited from the history and physical examination. Keep in mind that cancer, depression, and

TABLE 194-1 Physical Examination: Weight Loss

System	Physical Examination Findings	Differentials
Skin	Pallor, ecchymoses, signs of Kaposi's sarcoma, rashes, jaundice	Anemia, HIV, connective tissue disease, liver disease
Head/eyes/ears/nose/throat	Glossitis or other mouth lesions, tooth enamel erosion, stomatitis, poor dentition, goiter, adenopathy, hair distribution	Endocrine and metabolic causes, gastrointestinal (GI) disease, oral disorders, connective tissue disease, cancer, eating disorders
Lungs	Crackles, wheezes, consolidation, effusion	Respiratory disorders, infection, cancer
Heart	Cardiomegaly, tachycardia, murmur, extra heart sounds	Cardiac disorders, infection, respiratory disorders
Abdomen	Surgical scars, organomegaly, hyperactive bowel sounds, focal tenderness, distention, ascites, masses	GI disease, liver disease, cardiac disorders, cancer, infection, respiratory disorders, renal disease, vitamin B_{12} deficiency
Rectum	Masses, tenderness, discharge, blood, color, character of stool	Cancer, GI disorders
Musculoskeletal	Soft tissue swelling, limited range of motion, functional disabilities	Rheumatoid arthritis, connective tissue disease, age-related factors
Neurologic	Signs of vitamin B_{12} deficiency, tremor, mania, depressive symptoms, signs of dementia, decreased taste and smell (CN I and VII)	Pernicious anemia, Parkinson's disease, dementia, delirium, depression, mania, behavioral causes

TABLE 194-2 Diagnostic Tests: Weight Loss

Diagnostic Test	Finding/Rationale	Cost ($)
Hemoccult	First-level test for basic screening: Cancer and gastrointestinal (GI) disorders	13-17
Complete blood count with differential	First-level test for basic screening: Anemia, alcohol abuse (↑ mean corpuscular volume), infection, neutropenia	18-23
Urinalysis	First-level test for basic screening: Glucose, infection, renal disease, liver disease	15-20
Chemistry	First-level test for basic screening: Glucose; diabetes, blood urea nitrogen/creatinine: renal disease, AST, ALT, GGT: liver, electrolyte imbalance, albumin: <3.4 mg/dl = malnutrition, serum prealbumin <18 mg/dl = malnutrition	32-42
Thyroid profile	First-level test for basic screening: Thyroid dysfunction; especially important to screeen **elderly** and early **postpartum**	47-61
Chest x-ray	First-level test for basic screening: Cancer, cardiac and lung disease	77-91
Colonoscopy, mammogram, Pap	First-level test for screening if suspicious of colon, uterine, breast cancer or if there is a history of these cancers in first-degree relatives	799-956/colo; 99-125/mam; 24-31/Pap
Drug screen	First-level test if patient is taking any of these drugs that can cause toxicity: Dilantin, digoxin, quinidine, theophylline or lithium levels	57-72
EGD or upper gastrointestinal (GI) series	Consider in the **elderly** or suspected human immunodeficiency virus (HIV); high yield of silent peptic ulcers in the **elderly,** upper GI mucosa is HIV infected	298-350/UGI
Screening tests for malabsorption	Consider when food intake is normal and there is no evidence of causes of increased metabolic rate from diabetes, thyroid, or tumor (Sudan stain, serum carotene, folic acid, 72-hour stool collection for fat)	Sudan: Not available; 37-45/caro; 49-62/folic; 66-83/stool

TABLE 194-3 Categories and Causes of Weight Loss

Categories of Weight Loss	Causes of Weight Loss
Anorexia (Ch. 63)	Depression, bereavement, alcoholism, dementia and delirium, medications, low-fat or sodium-restricted diets, gastrointestinal disorders such as peptic ulcer disease, gallbladder, gastroesophageal reflux disease, hyperparathyroidism, thyroid disorders, diabetes mellitus, congestive heart failure, and chronic obstructive pulmonary disease
Difficulty eating	Inability to consume enough calories because of oral problems, functional impairments, or swallowing disorders; drugs with anticholinergic effects cause xerostomia; inability to prepare meals
Weight loss, despite adequate caloric intake	Metabolic disorders (hyperthyroidism) and movement disorders (Parkinson's) increase caloric demands; Alzheimer's disease, diarrhea due to bacterial overgrowth, pancreatic abnormalities, celiac sprue
Social factors	Widowers are at risk for poor intake, eating alone

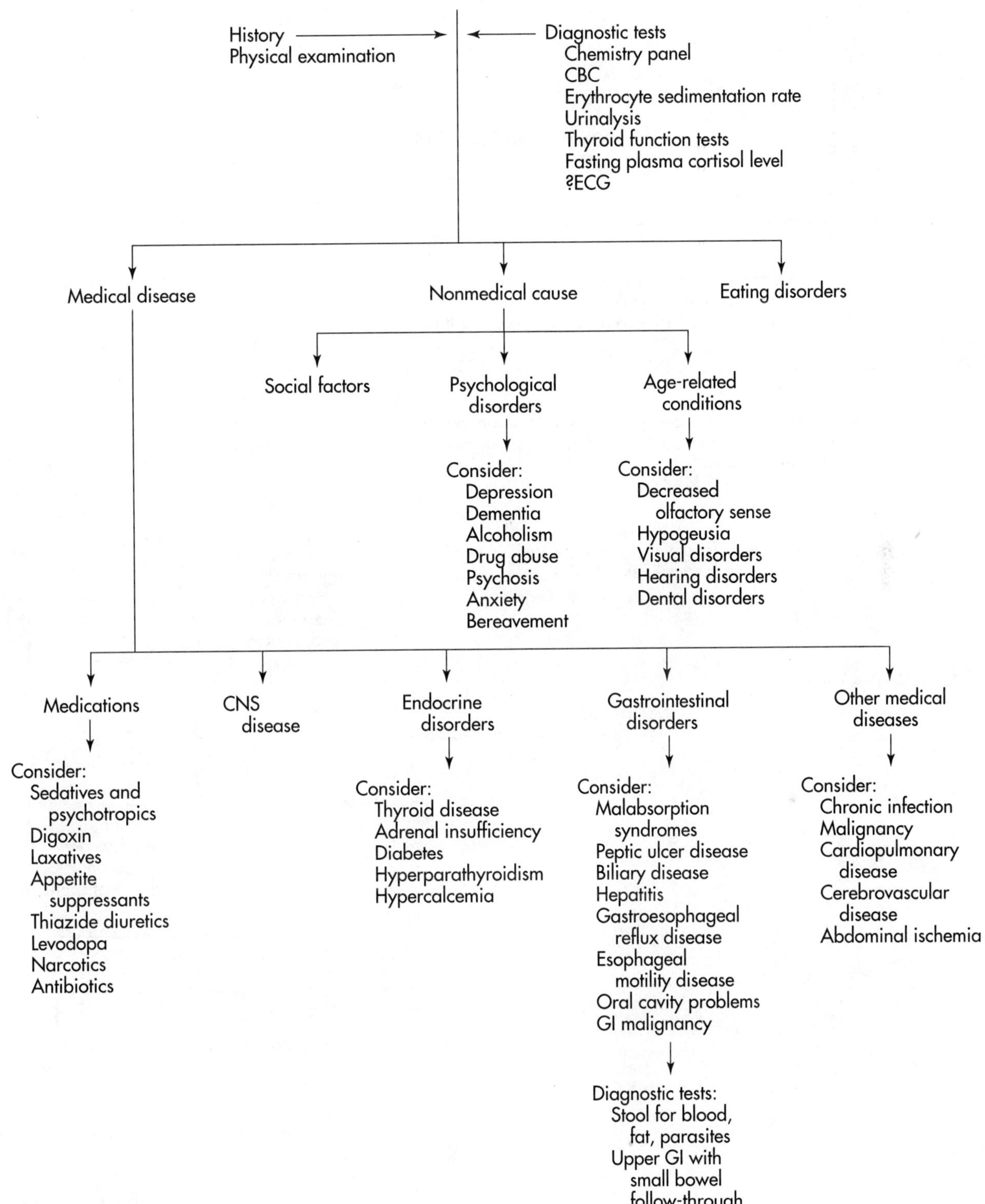

Figure 194-1 Algorithm for patient with anorexia. *CBC,* Complete blood count; *ECG,* electrocardiogram; *GI,* gastrointestinal. (Adapted from Greene HL, Johnson WP. Lemcke D: *Decision making in medicine,* ed 2, St Louis, 1998, Mosby.)

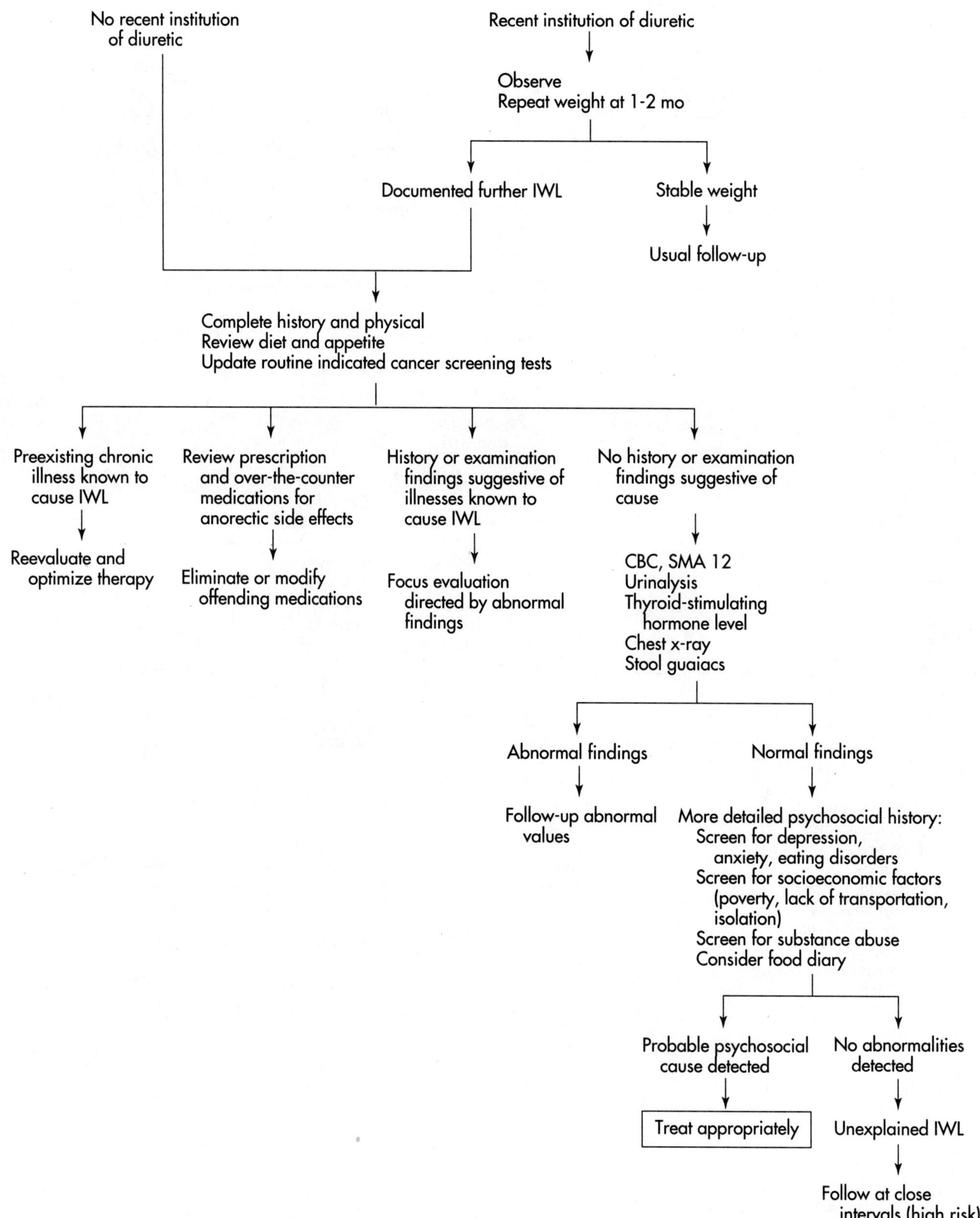

Figure 194-2 Algorithm for patient with documented involuntary weight loss. *CBC,* Complete blood count; *IWL,* involuntary weight loss; *SMA,* sequential multiple analyzer. (Adapted from Greene HL, Johnson WP. Lemcke D: *Decision making in medicine,* ed 2, St Louis, 1998, Mosby.)

gastrointestinal disorders are the most common causes in **adults.** Be alert to the possibility of a urinary tract infection in **infants** and **young children** presenting with unexplained weight loss (Table 194-2).

ASSESSMENT

The differential diagnosis of involuntary weight loss is extensive. Causes can be categorized into four categories (Table 194-3).

The most common causes in **adults** are cancer, depression, and gastrointestinal disorders. Growth failure (weight gain significantly below normal) in **children** includes a wide range of factors, including serious medical disease, dysfunctional child-caregiver interactions, poverty, parental misinformation, and child abuse. See Chapter 71 for complete information.

Indicators of malnutrition (Gazewood and Mehr, 1998) are:

Serum albumin: <3.4 mg/dl
Serum prealbumin: <18 mg/dl
Serum transferrin: <200 mg/dl
Total lymphocyte count: <1500/mm^3
Total cholesterol: <160 mg/dl
See Figures 194-1 and 194-2.

THERAPEUTIC PLAN

The first step to correcting weight loss is to treat the underlying medical, social, or psychiatric cause, if identified. In approximately 25% of involuntary weight loss cases, no cause of weight loss is ever found, despite extensive evaluation and prolonged follow-up. In the **elderly,** cancer is the most feared; however, social and psychiatric factors are also determinants. *Anyone with a weight loss in excess of 15 kg is likely to have a life-threatening condition and requires prompt work-up and hospitalization.*

Pharmaceutical

Poor intake associated with malignancy or use of antitumor agents can be overcome with amitriptyline (poorly suited for **patients** >**60** due to decrease in saliva production, dysphagia, adverse effects on cognition, and may lead to mental confusion), cyproheptadine (Periactin), corticosteroids or megestrol. Stomatitis is often helped with a mixture of Benadryl elixir and Kaopectate used as a mouth wash. Maldigestion due to pancreatic insufficiency can be counterbalanced with the use of oral pancreatic enzyme preparations. Poor appetite due to depression is eased with tricyclic therapy while bulimia has been helped with SSRIs. Weight loss associated with diabetes will improve as blood sugars normalize (Table 194-4).

Lifestyle/Activities

Lifestyle and activity are dictated by the cause of the weight loss. Functional disabilities may be improved with physical therapy. Depression can be amended by regular exercise, as can hyperglycemia (diabetes). Meals on wheels can help those who are unable to get out to buy groceries or who have functional impairments that prohibit meal preparation.

Referral

Appropriate referrals for the weight loss patient may include an endocrinologist, oncologist, gastroenterologist, cardiologist, rheumatologist, pulmonologist, social worker/agency, psychiatrist or dietitian.

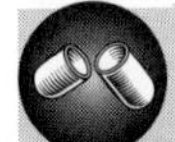

TABLE 194-4 Pharmaceutical Plan: Unintentional Weight Loss

Drug	Dose	Comments	Cost
Cyproheptadine (Periactin)	Adults: 4 mg TID with meals 2-6 y/o: 2 mg BID or TID with meals (max 8 mg/day) 2 mg/5 ml 6-14: 2 mg TID or QID with meals (max 16 mg)	Treatment should not exceed 6 mos Pregnancy: B SE: Drowsiness, dizziness, constipation, urinary retention, increased appetite Avoid alcoholic beverages	$2-$41/4 mg (100); $6-$31/syr: 2 mg/5 ml (480 ml)
Megestrol (Megace)	400-800 mg QD	Progesterone derivative Pregnancy: X Use contraception while taking SE: Seizures, paresthesia, confusion, palpitations, edema, alopecia	$85-$125/40 mg (100); $104/40 mg/ml (235 ml)

SE, Side effects.

Follow-up

Follow up is determined by the cause and severity of the weight loss. If no cause can be found, schedule the individual to return every 3 to 4 weeks.

EVALUATION

Monthly weights
Food diary to be brought to each visit
Medication list update at each visit to include OTC preparations

SUGGESTED READINGS

Boswell S: Evaluation of weight loss. In Goroll A, May L, Mulley A, editors: *Primary care medicine: office evaluation and management of the adult patient,* ed 3, Philadelphia, 1995, JB Lippincott.

Ellsworth AJ et al: *Mosby's 1998 medical drug reference*, St Louis, 1998, Mosby.

Fischer J, Johnson MA: Low body weight and weight loss in the aged, *Am Dietetic Assoc* 90:1697-1705, 1990.

Foster DW: Gain and loss in weight. In Isselbacher KJ et al, editors: *Harrison's principles of internal medicine,* ed 13, New York, 1994, McGraw-Hill.

Gazewood J, Mehr D: Diagnosis and management of weight loss in the elderly, *J Family Practice* 47(1):19-25, 1998.

Hassay K: Effective management of urinary discomfort, *Nurse Pract* 20(2):36-46, 1995.

Healthcare Consultants of America, Inc: *1998 physicians fee and coding guide*, Augusta, Ga, 1998, Healthcare Consultants of America, Inc.

Marton KL, Sox HC Jr, Krupp JR:. Involuntary weight loss: diagnostic and prognostic significance, *Ann Intern Med* 95:568, 1981 (classic article).

McPhee S, Schroeder S: Weight loss. In Tierney L, McPhee S, Papadakis M, editors: *1998 Current medical diagnosis & treatment,* ed 37, Stamford, Conn, 1997, Appleton & Lange.

Reife CM: Involuntary weight loss, *Med Clin North Am* 79:299, 1995.

Trujillo M: Anorexia. In Greene H, Johnson W, Lemcke D, editors: *Decision making in medicine,* St Louis, ed 2, 1998, Mosby.

195 Worms

ICD-9-CM

Uncinaria Americana 126.1
Pinworms (Enterobiasis) 127.4
Ascariasis (Roundworm) 133.9
Whipworm 127.3

OVERVIEW

Definition

Helminthiasis is the condition of being infected with parasitic worms.

Incidence

Helminthic infections endemic to the United States include hookworm (uncinariasis), pinworm (enterobiasis), roundworm (ascariasis), and whipworm (trichuriasis). Humans are the only vectors of these particular helminths. Pinworm infections are ubiquitous; however, the remaining types occur more commonly in the southeastern United States where the warm, moist climate is conducive to ova incubation or larva maturation in fecally contaminated soil. There is also a higher incidence in immigrants/travelers from warm, tropical regions.

Pathophysiology

Hookworms

Larvae in the soil penetrate the skin, migrate via the circulatory system to the cardiopulmonary bed, where they penetrate the alveoli, migrate up the bronchial tree, are coughed into the pharynx, and swallowed. In the gastrointestinal tract, larvae mature into adults and attach themselves to the intestinal mucosa; they can suck up to 0.5 ml of blood daily per worm. Hookworms also secrete an anticoagulant that contributes to additional blood loss.

Pinworms

Ingested eggs mature and live embedded in the wall of the cecum. Gravid females migrate to the anus to deposit eggs, which causes intense pruritus. Scratching often contaminates the fingers and enables reinfection of the host or other contacts. Chronic urinary tract infections in **girls** have infrequently been attributed to adult worms migrating up the urethra.

Roundworms

Larvae from ingested eggs penetrate the intestinal wall into the mesenteric venous system, migrate to the cardiopulmonary bed, where they penetrate the alveoli, migrate up the bronchial tree, are coughed into the pharynx and swallowed, and mature into adult worms. Adult roundworms live in the upper small intestine, and infections are often asymptomatic. Malnourishment and weight loss occur in more severe infections. Infrequently worms penetrate and block the common bile duct, or masses may cause intestinal obstruction.

Whipworms

Ingested eggs mature, then migrate to the cecum and colon, where they embed themselves in the intestinal mucosa. If infections are severe, the worms can consume enough blood to cause anemia and weight loss. In massive infestations, obstruction of the appendiceal lumen, bloody diarrhea, secondary infections of the colon may occur.

Factors that Increase Susceptibility

Children and institutionalized/disabled
Lower socioeconomic groups
Overcrowding
Poor hygiene practices and/or unsanitary conditions
Situations that contribute to soil contamination with human feces (e.g., flooding, open/untreated sewage)
Walking barefoot

SUBJECTIVE DATA

Many individuals with helminthiasis remain asymptomatic unless the infection becomes severe. Onset is usually insidious, and symptoms vague.

History of Present Illness

Ask about:

Pruitis of feet (hookworm) or anus/vagina (pinworm)
Transitory fever, cough, sore throat (hookworm, roundworm)
Abdominal discomfort, distention, nausea/vomiting, diarrhea (hookworm, roundworm, whipworm)

Past Medical History

Assess for pica, institutionalization, and/or disability.

Family Medical History

Signs/symptoms of helminthic infection in other family members will depend on age and degree of infestation.

Environmental

Inquire about:

Living situation relative to crowding
Sanitation and hygiene (washing of hands/food)
Exposure to raw sewage, human waste fertilizer
Not wearing shoes

Lifestyle/Activities

Assess for fatigue and unexplained weight loss; changes in elimination patterns; travel to susceptible regions.

Description of Most Common Symptoms

Table 195-1 outlines symptoms of helminthic infestation.

Associated Symptoms

Possible symptoms of urinary tract infection or vaginitis in extensive pinworm infections
Rectal prolapse can result from severe whipworm infections; adult worms may be visible in the prolapsed rectum

OBJECTIVE DATA

Physical Examination

General: Often do not appear symptomatic; may appear pale/anemic, underweight, malnourished; **children** may demonstrate retarded growth
Skin: Papulovesicular entry lesions (hookworm); pallor; clubbing if progressive anemia has occurred
Lungs: Wheeze, cough, and blood-tinged sputum may be present if larvae are in pulmonary migratory phase (roundworm, hookworm)
Heart: Increased force and lateral displacement of point of maximal impulse if anemia-induced hypertrophy has occurred

Diagnostic Tests

If a worm has been visualized, diagnostic tests are unnecessary. Table 195-2 outlines tests for worms.

ASSESSMENT

Visualization of worm in feces/emesis (roundworm); confirmation of ova in the feces (hookworm, roundworm, and whipworm); nocturnal anal pruritus and presence of ova on transparent tape (pinworm) (Table 195-3)

TABLE 195-1 Symptoms of Helminthic Symptoms

Type of Worm	Most Common Symptoms
Hookworms	Erythema and intense itching at site of entry—usually feet; papulovesicular lesion at entry site; fever, sore throat, cough, blood-tinged sputum associated with larvae in lungs; fatigue, weight loss, nausea/vomiting, uncontrolled diarrhea, melena
Pinworm	Intense anal pruritus, restlessness—especially at night; parents may report seeing adult worms on child's anal region
Roundworms	Fever, sore throat, cough, blood-tinged sputum associated with larvae in lungs; abdominal cramps and discomfort, weight loss, nausea, vomiting, diarrhea; presence of large white or reddish-round worm(s) in feces or vomitus
Whipworms	Heavy worm load (>30,000 ova/g feces) is associated with abdominal cramps and discomfort, flatulence, weight loss, bloody mucoid diarrhea

THERAPEUTIC PLAN

Unless symptomatic, patients with light hookworm (<1000 ova/g feces) or whipworm (<10,000 ova/g feces) infections do not require treatment. However, these infections are often accompanied by roundworm infections.

The potential complications from wandering roundworms require that they be treated, especially before elective surgery (anesthesia stimulates hypermotility) and after the third trimester of pregnancy.

Although annoying, pinworm infections are benign. Patients who are symptomatic for pinworms are treated; all members or household contacts are generally infected and also are treated to reduce the risk of reinfection.

Pharmaceutical

Pharmaceutical treatment is outlined in Tables 195-4 to 195-6.

Lifestyle/Activities

Careful hand washing after defecation and before meals is important
Keep fingernails short and clean
Avoid scratching perianal area
Wash bedding, towels, clothes of infected person
Snug fitting underwear may be helpful in children

Diet

Not applicable

Patient Education

Helminthic infections occur from the ingestion of ova, or penetration of larvae through the skin.

Explain the etiology and teach the importance of hand washing after defecation and before eating.

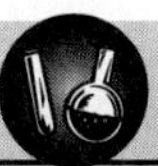

TABLE 195-2 Diagnostic Tests: Worms

Diagnostic Test	Findings/Rationale	Cost ($)
Stool sample for ova and parasites	Three stool samples for ova and parasites for diagnosis of hookworm, roundworm, and whipworm infections. Ova and parasites of pinworms may not be consistently present in feces; a piece of transparent tape on a tongue blade and applied to the perianal skin in the morning and examined microscopically will reveal the presence of pinworm ova	31-38
Blood tests	Are not requisite for diagnosis, although may confirm the associated presence of anemia and eosinophilia	18-23/complete blood count
Sputum specimen	Inconsistently larvae may be seen on microscopic sputum examination	31-38

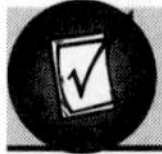

TABLE 195-3 Differential Diagnoses: Worms

Diagnosis	Helminth That Mimics	Supporting Data
Asthma, pneumonia	Hookworm, roundworm	Coughing, fever, hemoptysis, wheezing dyspnea
Duodenal ulcer, hiatal hernia, gallbladder, or pancreatic disease	Roundworm	Abdominal pain ranging from vague to sharp and spasmodic, vomiting, abdominal distention, intolerance for fats, pain that occurs when stomach empty
Allergic reaction; insect bites	Hookworm	Dermatitis, pruritus, erythema, papulovesicular eruption at site of bite
Nonspecific urinary/vaginal irritation or fungal infection, hemorrhoids, localized allergic response	Pinworm	Vaginal/perineal itching worse at night, rectal pain, restlessness, irritability
Appendicitis, enterogastritis	Hookworm, roundworm, whipworm	Abdominal pain, nausea, vomiting, flatulence, abdominal cramping, tenesmus, diarrhea, weight loss

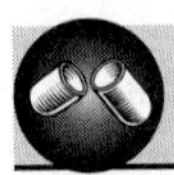

TABLE 195-4 Pharmaceutical Plan: Worms

Drug/Dose	Comments	Cost
Pyrantel pamoate (Antiminth) Available as suspension 50 mg/ml	May be taken without regard to food available as suspension 50 mg/ml; not recommended for **children <2 y/o** Pregnancy: C SE: Vomiting, diarrhea, headache, drowsiness; mild symptoms in up to 20%	$8-$38/50 mg/ml (60 ml)
Mebendazole (Vermox) Available as 100-mg chewable tablets	Administer before or after meals Hookworm: BID ×3 days Pregnancy: C Not recommended for **children <2 y/o;** chew tablet for best effect Pregnancy: Contraindicated For heavy whipworm infections, continue up to 6 days or repeat course if necessary	$52-$58/100 mg (12)
Levamisole (Ergamisol)	Available in United States, but not approved for this indication; highly effective Pregnancy: C **Children:** Caution SE: Occasional nausea, vomiting, abdominal pain, headache, dizziness	$194/50 mg (36)
Albendazole (Albenza) Available as 200-mg tablets	Available in United States, but not approved for this indication Pregnancy: Contraindicated SE: Migration of roundworm through nose or mouth is rare; may need to be repeated for 2-3 days in heavy infections	$98/200 mg (112)
Diethylcarbamazine (Hetrazan) Available as 50-mg tablets	Available for compassionate use (610-688-4400) Pregnancy: Unknown SE: Giddiness, nausea, and vomiting, malaise	Not available
Ivermectin (Stromectol) Tablets: 6 mg	Pregnancy: Unknown Safety not established in **children <15 kg** SE: Unknown	Not available
Thiabendazole (Mintezol) Tablets: 500 mg/suspension 500 mg/5 ml	Chewable tablets, take with food Pregnancy: C Safety not established in **children <13.6 kg;** monitor hepatic or renal dysfunction carefully SE: Dizziness, drowsiness, headache, anorexia, nausea, vomiting, diarrhea, pruritus, tinnitus	$21/susp: 500 mg/5 ml (120 ml); $36/500 mg (36)

SE, Side effects.

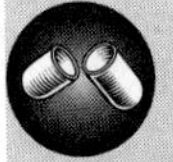

TABLE 195-5 Over-the-Counter Treatment: Worms

Over-the-Counter Pyrantel Formulations	Dose
Pin Rid Reese's Pinworm	180 mg pyrantel pamoate (equivalent to 62.5 mg pyrantel base)
Antiminth	Oral suspension (50 mg pyrantel/ml)
Pin Rid (cherry flavor) Pin-X (caramel flavor) Reese's Pinworm	Liquid 50 mg pyrantel/ml

Hygiene practices such as washing fruits and vegetables, changing underwear/linens daily (especially in pinworm infections), and regular housecleaning help prevent reinfection.

In hookworm infections, stress the importance of wearing shoes in endemic areas.

In pinworm infections children should bath daily (showers preferable to baths), nails should be kept short, and nail-biting discouraged.

Family Impact

A social stigma is often associated with helminthiasis. Infections may have occurred while traveling or children

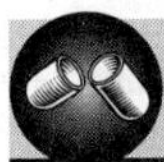

TABLE 195-6 Treatment Bases on Type of Helminth

Infecting Organism	Drug of Choice
Enterobius vermicularis (pinworm)	Albendazole 400 mg PO (1 dose) *or* Pyrantel pamoate 11 mg/kg PO single dose *or* Mebendazole 100 mg PO single dose, repeat after 2 weeks
Hookworm	Albendazole 400 mg PO (single dose) *or* Mebendazole 100 mg PO BID × 3 days *or* Pyrantel pamoate 11 mg/kg po qd × 3 days
Whipworm	Albendazole 400 mg PO (single dose) *or* Mebendazole 100 mg PO BID × 3 days
Roundworms	Albendazole 400 mg PO (single dose) *or* Mebendazole 100 mg PO BID × 3 days *or* Pyrantel pamoate 11 mg/kg single dose (max 1 g) *or* Thiabendazole <150 lbs: 10 mg/kg/dose BID × 2 days >150 lbs: 1.5 g/dose Diethylcarbamazine 13 mg/kg QD ×7 days (children: 6-10 mg/kg TID × 7-10 days)
Larva migrans	Diethylcarbamazine 2 mg/kg PO TID × 10 days (considered superior) *or* Albendazole 400 mg PO BID × 5 days *or* Mebendazole 100-200 mg po bid × 5 days

may have ingested eggs while playing outdoors or with contaminated objects. Families may need support.

Referral

Not needed unless refractory to treatment

Consultation

Pregnant woman (treat ascariasis after first trimester)

Follow-up

Roundworm: Recheck stool in 2 weeks; continue to retreat until worms are eradicated

EVALUATION

Eradication of helminths

SUGGESTED REFERENCES

Adreoli T et al: Infectious diseases of travelers; protozoal and helminthic infections. In *Cecil's essentials of medicine,* ed 4, Philadelphia, 1997, WB Saunders.

Ellsworth AJ et al: *Mosby's medical drug reference*, St Louis, 1998, Mosby.

Goldsmith R: Infectious diseases: Protozoal & helminthic. In Tierney L, McPhee S, Papadakis M: *Current medical diagnosis and treatment*, ed 3, Stamford, Conn, 1997, Appleton Lange.

Healthcare Consultants of America, Inc: *1998 physicians fee and coding guide*, Augusta, Ga, 1998, Healthcare Consultants of America, Inc.

Juckett G: Pets and parasites, *Am Family Physician* 56(7):1763-1774, 1997.

Roos M: The use of drugs in the control of parasitic nematode infections: must we do without? *Parasitology* 114(Supp):S137-144, 1997.

Sarinas P, Chitkara R: Ascariasis and hookworm, *Semin Respir Infect* 12(2):137, 1997.

Weinberg A, Levin M: Infections: parasitic & mycotic. In Hay W et al, editors: *Current pediatric diagnosis and treatment,* Stamford, Conn, 1997, Appleton & Lange.

Wound Management

ICD-9-CM

Injury, Superficial (Abrasion) 919.0
With Infection 919.1
Insect Bite 919.4; With Infection 919.5
Blister 919.2; With Infection 919.3
Scratch 919.0; With Infection 919.1
Superficial Foreign Body (Splinter) 919.6
Injury, Internal 869.0
Wound, Open 879.8

OVERVIEW

Definition

A wound is a structural alteration that results when energy is imparted during an interaction with a physical or chemical agent. It results in alteration in skin integrity.

Incidence

Nearly 10 million per year in the United States

Types of Wounds

Lacerations

Shearing

Eighty percent of soft tissue injuries are caused by shearing injuries. A sharp force is applied to the tissue by glass, metal, or blade. This results in a linear wound. A shearing injury may be superficial, extending through the dermis, or deep, extending through the subcutaneous tissue. This type of wound is the most resistant to infection.

Stellate

Caused by compression between tissues, which overlay bone, and an applied force to the tissue
Highly susceptible to infection
Most common type of scalp injury

Compression

Caused by collision of two bodies applying compression to soft tissue supported by bone
Often associated with a hematoma
Most common chin and eyebrow lacerations

Abrasion

The rubbing away of the dermal layer of skin against a firm surface; there may or may not be embedded material; similar to second-degree burn.

Avulsion

Full-thickness tearing away of the skin, exposing the underlying fat.
Most common tissue injury in **elderly.**

Puncture

Penetration of the skin by a sharp or pointed object; minimal bleeding; can cause serious injury to underlying tissues and structures

Bites

Includes puncture and possible tearing wounds of the skin; may be of human or animal origin

SUBJECTIVE DATA

History of Injury Event

Mechanism of injury: If related to a fall, what caused the fall? If caused by a syncopal episode, this patient must be further evaluated. Possibilities of syncope may include cardiac arrhythmias, dehydration, pregnancy, electrolyte imbalance, and anemia.
Puncture wounds:
- What was the instrument that caused the puncture wound?
- How long and wide was the instrument that caused the puncture wound? What position was the body in when

the puncture wound occurred? Knowing this information will aid in determining what underlying tissue, organs, bones, nerves, etc. may also be involved in this injury.

Time of injury: Wounds 6 to 24 hours old are more prone to infection and require special attention such as antibiotic treatment, excessive irrigation, or delayed closure.

First aid before arrival at health care provider.

Past Medical History

Tetanus status

Allergies especially to lidocaine, Betadine, tetanus, and antibiotics

Previous experiences with sutures

Immunity disorders

Diabetes

Last menstrual period (be sure patient is not pregnant before x-ray studies, antibiotic therapy, or tetanus injections)

Medication

Current medications, especially cardiovascular or asthma medications, may cause potential harmful side effects (elevation of heart rate or blood pressure) with the use of lidocaine with or without epinephrine.

Psychosocial History

Consider possibility of abuse (**child, elder,** or spousal) as cause of injury.

Associated Symptoms

Bleeding: Minimal to extensive

Pain, swelling

Decreased range of motion of function at site of injury, possibly due to tendon or ligament injury

Change in sensation at the site of injury or distal due to nerve injury

OBJECTIVE DATA

Physical Examination

A problem-oriented examination should be conducted, with particular attention to:

Vital signs

Heart rate: Increase may be due to infection; decrease may be due to a cardiac dysrhythmia

Blood pressure: An indication of potential shock

Temperature: An indication of infection

Diagnostic Procedures

Radiology

X-rays of the site of injury to rule out foreign bodies or bone involvement

Be aware that glass will only be visible on x-ray if it contains lead; wood will not be visible on x-rays

If an infection is involved, an x-ray may help to determine the depth and extent of the infection

Electrocardiogram

Especially in the **elderly** if the wound was caused by a fall or is unexplained; could possibly be due to cardiac arrhythmias

Wound Culture

If the wound appears infected, a wound culture should be obtained before any debridement or cleansing.

ASSESSMENT

Type of wound

Signs of infection

Sensory, motor (including range of motion of the joints above and below the wound) and vascular assessment distal to the injury

The presence of foreign bodies

Palpation of bony areas below and adjacent to injuries

THERAPEUTIC PLAN

Pharmaceutical

Tetanus Immunization

Tetanus immunization is outlined in Table 196-1.

Children

If less than 7 years, Diphtheria, Pertussis, Tetanus Toxoids Absorbed (DPT), or Diphtheria and Tetanus Toxoids absorbed (Td) if pertussis is contraindicated

Tetanus prone wounds include wounds that are:

Greater than 6 hours old

Stellate wound configuration

Injuries caused by missile, crush, burn, or frostbite

Greater than 1 cm in depth

Contaminated by debris (e.g., soil, feces, saliva)

Devitalized or ischemic tissue

Wound Cleansing

Irrigation under high pressure with normal saline is the most effective way to cleanse a wound. (An inexpensive and easy method is the use of a 35-ml syringe and a 19-gauge needle to create high flow irrigation.)

If Betadine solution is used to cleanse the wound, it must be irrigated completely in order not to cause tissue damage.

TABLE 196-1 Tetanus Immunization

History of Absorbed Tetanus Toxoid	Tetanus-Prone		Nontetanus Prone	
	Td	**TIG**	**Td**	**TIG**
Uncertain or less than three	Yes	Yes	Yes	No
Three or more (last dose within 5 years)	No	No	No	No
Three or more (last dose within 6-10 years)	Yes	No	No (Yes if greater than 10 years)	No

TIG, Human tetanus immune globulin; *Td,* tetanus and diphtheria absorbed.

Hair Removal

Hair should be clipped with scissors from around the wound. Hair in the wound acts like a foreign body and may delay the healing processes and potentiate the infectious process. Shaving the hair may cause injury to the hair follicle and increases the risk of infection.

Eyebrows should never be shaved. Shaving will alter the land marks, leading to possible misalignment of the wound edges. Eyebrows grow back very slowly, causing alteration in cosmetic looks.

Analgesia

Pharmacology

Local anesthetic agents prevent the influx of sodium across the nerve membrane. This in turn decreases the rate and amplitude of depolarization of the nerve membrane. When depolarization is decreased, an action potential cannot be formed. This results in the inability to transmit an impulse. A conduction blockade is achieved, resulting in local anesthesia.

Local anesthetics are classified as esters or amides. Esters are metabolized by plasma pseudocholinesterase. Amides are metabolized in the liver.

Esters: Procaine, chloroprocaine, cocaine, tetracaine
Amides: Lidocaine, mepivacaine prilocaine, bupivacaine, etidocaine

Topical

An excellent choice for use in small children and anxious adults; generally used on small superficial lacerations

TAC: A topical mixture of tetracaine 1%, topical adrenaline (epinephrine) 1:4000, and cocaine HCL 4%. A cotton ball is soaked with 10 cc of the solution and then applied to the wound. Anesthesia is achieved in approximately 10 to 15 minutes. It should never be used on mucous membranes or areas with poor perfusion. The person holding the TAC to the wound should wear an examination glove to avoid absorption of the mixture into his or her skin.

LET: A topical mixture of lidocaine 2% to 4%, topical epinephrine 1:4000, and tetracaine 1%. It is used in the same manner as TAC. Anesthesia is achieved within 20 to 25 minutes.

Infiltrative

The most common local anesthetics are outlined in Table 196-2. Other anesthetics include:

Diphenhydramine (Benadryl)
Concentration: 1 ml diphenhydramine 5% mixed with 4 ml normal saline to produce 1% solution
Onset: 5 to 10 minutes
Duration: 20 to 30 minutes
NOTE: Used only for patients who report an allergic reaction to caine-type drugs; it is a more painful solution then lidocaine; therefore it may be diluted into a 0.5% concentration if needed

Epinephrine
1:1000 can be added to lidocaine and bupivacaine; it aids in hemostatis of the wound and prolongs the effects of the anesthetic; it should never be used on fingers, toes, noses, tip of the ear, nipples, penis, or the tarsal plate of the eye

Sodium bicarbonate
May add to lidocaine in a 1:10 ratio to neutralize the pH of the lidocaine; this reduces the burning sensation that is felt during the infiltration of the lidocaine; the shelf-life of the mixture is 1 week
NOTE: 0.5% = 5 mg/ml
1% = 10 mg/ml
2% = 20 mg/ml

Anesthesia options are summarized in Table 196-3.

TABLE 196-2 Local Anesthesia

Agent	Concentration	Maximum Adult Dose	Maximum Pediatric Dose	Onset	Duration
Lidocaine	0.5% (5 mg/ml)	300 mg (60 ml)	4 mg/kg (0.8 ml/kg)	3-5 minutes	30-60 minutes
	1% (10 mg/ml)	300 mg (30 ml)	4 mg/kg (0.4 ml/kg)		
	2% (20 mg/ml)	300 mg (15 ml)	4 mg/kg (0.2 ml/kg)		
Lidocaine with epinephrine	0.5% (5 mg/ml)	500 mg (100 ml)	7 mg/kg (1.4 ml/kg)	2-5 minutes	60-120 minutes
	1% (10 mg/ml)	500 mg (50 ml)	7 mg/kg (0.7 ml/kg)		
	2% (20 mg/ml)	500 mg (25 ml)	7 mg/kg (0.35 ml/kg)		
Bupivacaine (Marcaine)	0.25% (2.5 mg/ml)	175 mg (70 ml)	Not recommended	5-10 minutes	90 120 minutes
Bupivacaine with epinephrine	0.25% (2.5 mg/ml)	225 mg (90 ml)	Not recommended	2-5 minutes	4-8 hours
Mepivacaine (Carbocaine)	0.5% (5 mg/ml)	400 mg (80 ml)	5 mg/kg (1 ml/kg)	5-10 minutes	75-150 minutes
Procaine	0.5% (5 mg/ml)	500 mg (100 ml)	7 mg/kg (1.4 ml/kg)	2-5 minutes	15-45 minutes
	1% (10 mg/ml)	500 mg (50 ml)	7 mg/kg (0.7 ml/kg)		
Procaine with epinephrine	0.5% (5 mg/ml)	600 mg (120 ml)	9 mg/kg (1.8 ml/kg)	2-5 minutes	15-45 minutes
	1% (10 mg/ml)	600 mg (60 ml)	9 mg/kg (0.9 ml/kg)		

TABLE 196-3 Anesthesia Options

Type of Anesthesia	Indications	Contraindications	Advantages	Disadvantages
Topical	**Young children;** lacerations <0.5 cm	Not to be used on fingers, toes, nose, ear, or penis	Painless; no distortion of wound edges; hemostasis	Must be held in place for at least 10-20 minutes; less effective on trunk and extremities
Infiltration	All age groups; laceration repair; excision of skin lesions; incision of an abscess	When large toxic amounts of anesthesia are required	Quick to do; generally considered safe; reliable	Distorts wound edges; requires a larger amount of medication; painful
Nerve block (Figures 196-1 to 196-11)	Large wounds; if distortion from infiltration compromises blood flow, or hampers wound closure	Patients who are taking monoamine oxidase inhibitors should not receive anesthesia with epinephrine; may lead to an exaggerated cardiac response	Provides anesthesia to a larger area with less medication and injections	May need to use local infiltrates if complete anesthesia is not obtained; potential to inject into a nerve bundle or blood vessel; painful

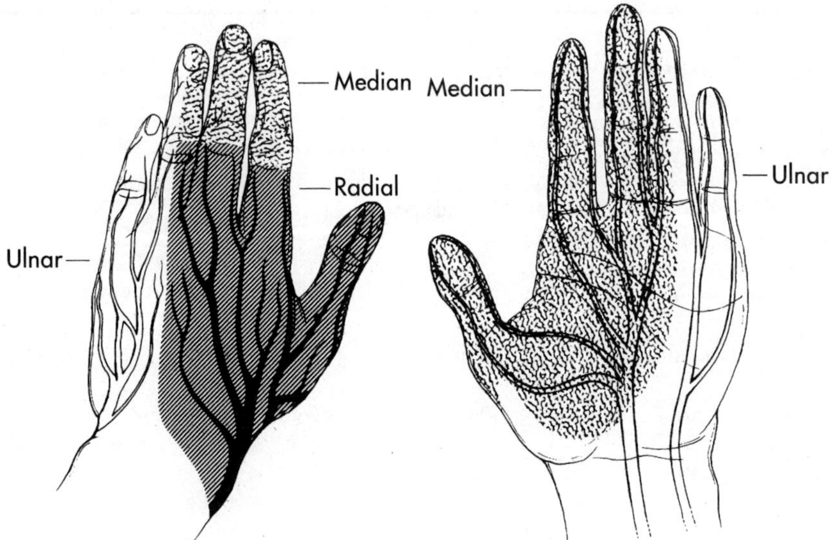

Figure 196-1 The sensory innervation of the hand. Note that there may be considerable overlap of the territories and considerable variation between individuals. (From Martin DS, Collins ED: *Manual of acute hand injuries,* St Louis, 1998, Mosby.)

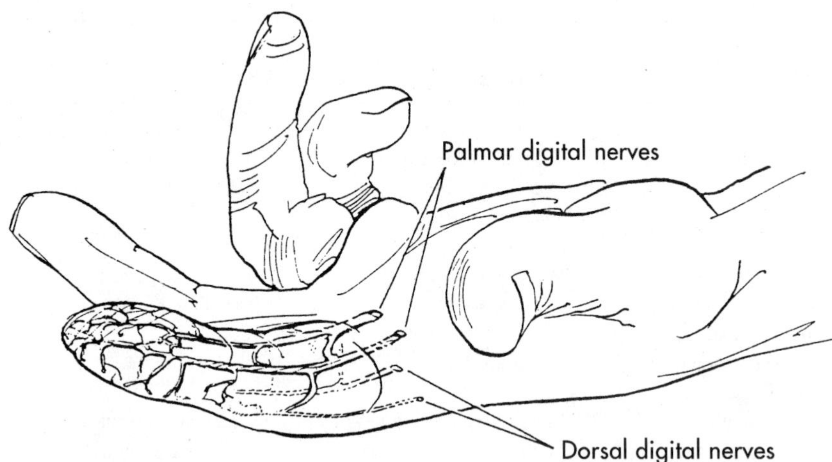

Figure 196-2 The four digital nerves of the digit. Note that the two palmar digital nerves are dominant and provide sensation to the volar surface of the finger, as well as the entirety of the volar pad and nail bed area. (From Trott AT: *Wounds and lacerations,* ed 2, St Louis, 1997, Mosby.)

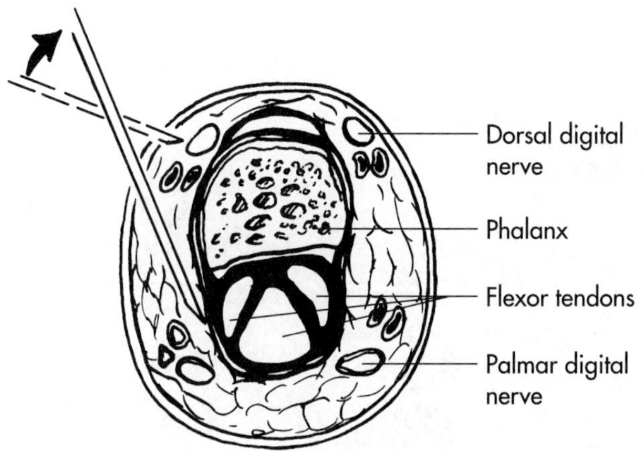

Figure 196 3 Digital nerve block. To effectively block a digit, all four nerves, dorsal and volar, are approached as illustrated. The needle is introduced dorsally to first anesthetize the dorsal nerve. Without reinserting the needle, it is redirected toward the volar nerve, and anesthetic is deposited. The same procedure is carried out on the opposite side of the same digit to complete the block. (From Trott AT: *Wounds and lacerations,* ed 2, St Louis, 1997, Mosby.)

Wound Closure

Absorable Suture

Biodegraded, last 2 to 6 weeks, used for internal sutures
- Gut: Made from sheep submucosa or beef serosa; rapidly degraded
  - Plain: May cause inflammatory reaction in the wound; lasts about 2 weeks
  - Chromic: Less tissue reactivity, but may potentiate wound infections; lasts about 4 weeks
- Synthetic: Dexon, Vicryl
  - Minimal tissue reaction; used for closures of dermal and subcutaneous layers and the ligation of blood vessels

Nonabsorbable Sutures

Will not degrade or may degrade very slowly; generally used for external closure
- Silk: Natural fiber; highly tissue reactive; slow absorbing suture
- Dacron: Synthetic, polyester; less reactive then silk; difficult to handle due to high friction
- Nylon: Synthetic; less reactive then Dacron; when used in contaminated wounds, there is a decreased risk of infection
  - Monofilament: Difficult to tie
  - Multifilament: Easy to tie
- Polypropylene and polyester: Synthetic; least tissue reactivity of all suture materials; the least chance of infection when used in contaminated wounds; hold knots better than nylon
- Staples: Made of stainless steel; cumbersome; not to be used over movable joints; excellent for scalp lacerations; increased infection rates when used in contaminated wounds

Wound Care

The wound should remain covered with a clean and dry dressing for 24 to 48 hours. It takes approximately 48 hours for a wound to become impermeable to bacteria.

The suture line should then be cleaned with soap and water two to three times a day to remove exudate and crusted blood from the site. This will aid in reducing the scarring.

An antibiotic ointment may be applied to the suture line. Note that neomycin may cause local reactions.

Wounds that are likely to become contaminated should remained covered for 1 week.

A joint should be immobilized in the position of function if movement of that joint will compromise the suture line integrity (Table 196-4).

Suture Removal

Face: 3 to 5 days
Scalp: 5 to 7 days
Neck: 4 to 6 days
Hand, foot: 7 to 14 days
Arm, leg: 7 to 14 days
Chest, abdomen, back: 6 to 12 days
Nail bed: Use absorbable suture and allow to absorb

Patient Education

Wound care instructions:
- Keep clean and dry
- Keep dressing in place for 24 to 48 hours
- Clean suture lines with soap and water; removing crusted material from suture line will ensure proper healing of wound

May apply antibiotic ointment, if desired

Keep sutured area elevated above heart to decrease swelling

Watch for signs of infection: Redness, red streaks, swelling, pus, fever

Prevention techniques:
- Home safety assessment
- Use of appropriate safety equipment

Referral

Depending on the extent and site of the wound (e.g., multi layer; large area) may need to refer to surgeon or plastic surgeon

If infection occurs, may need to refer to infectious disease physician

Text continued on p. 1202

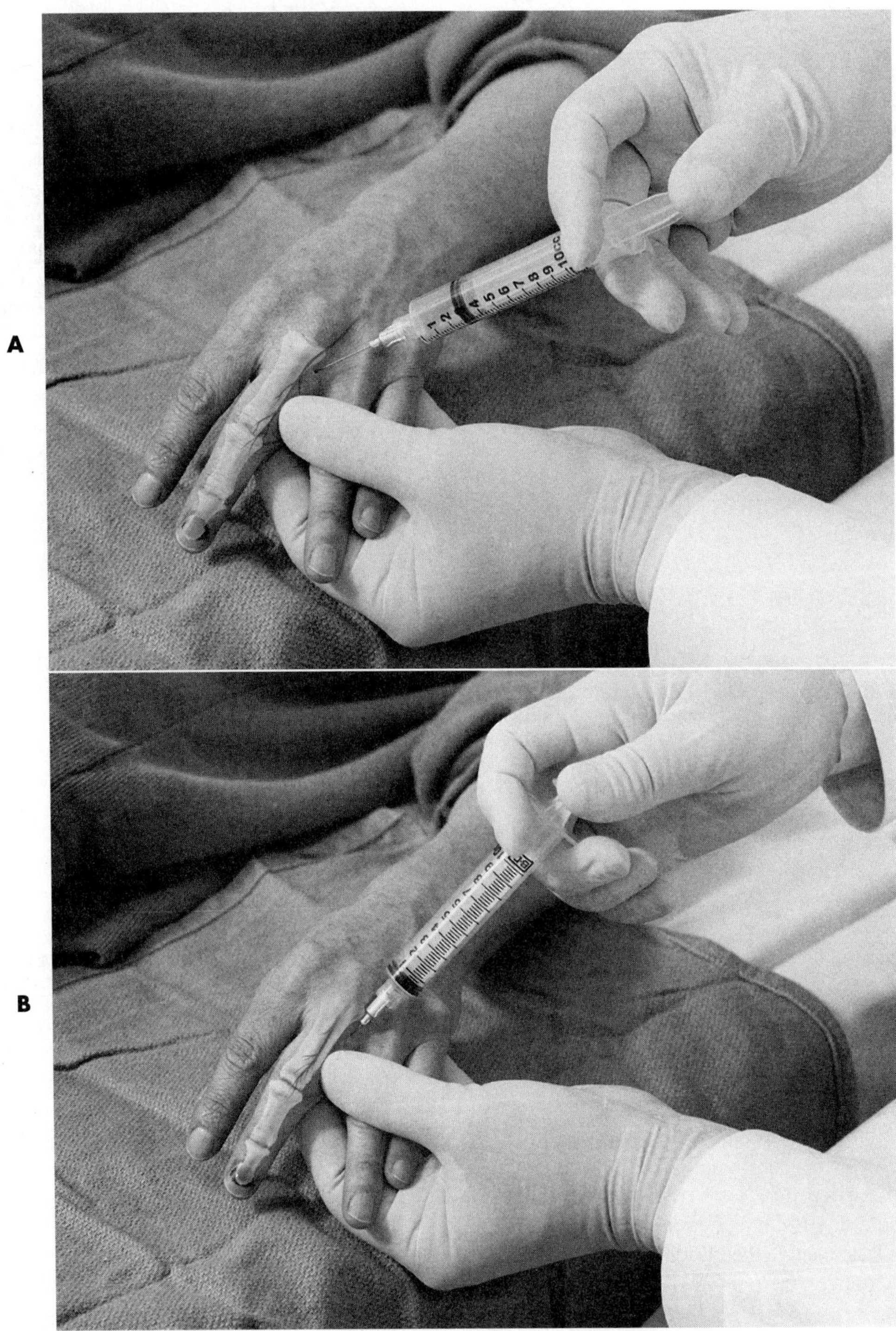

Figure 196-4 Digital nerve block. Note the course of the volar and digital nerves. **A,** Within the web space, the needle is introduce and advanced toward the dorsal digital nerve. **B,** After deposition of the anesthetic, the needle is redirected, without withdrawing it from the skin, toward the volar nerve, and anesthetic is deposited. (From Trott AT: *Wounds and lacerations,* ed 2, St Louis, 1997, Mosby.)

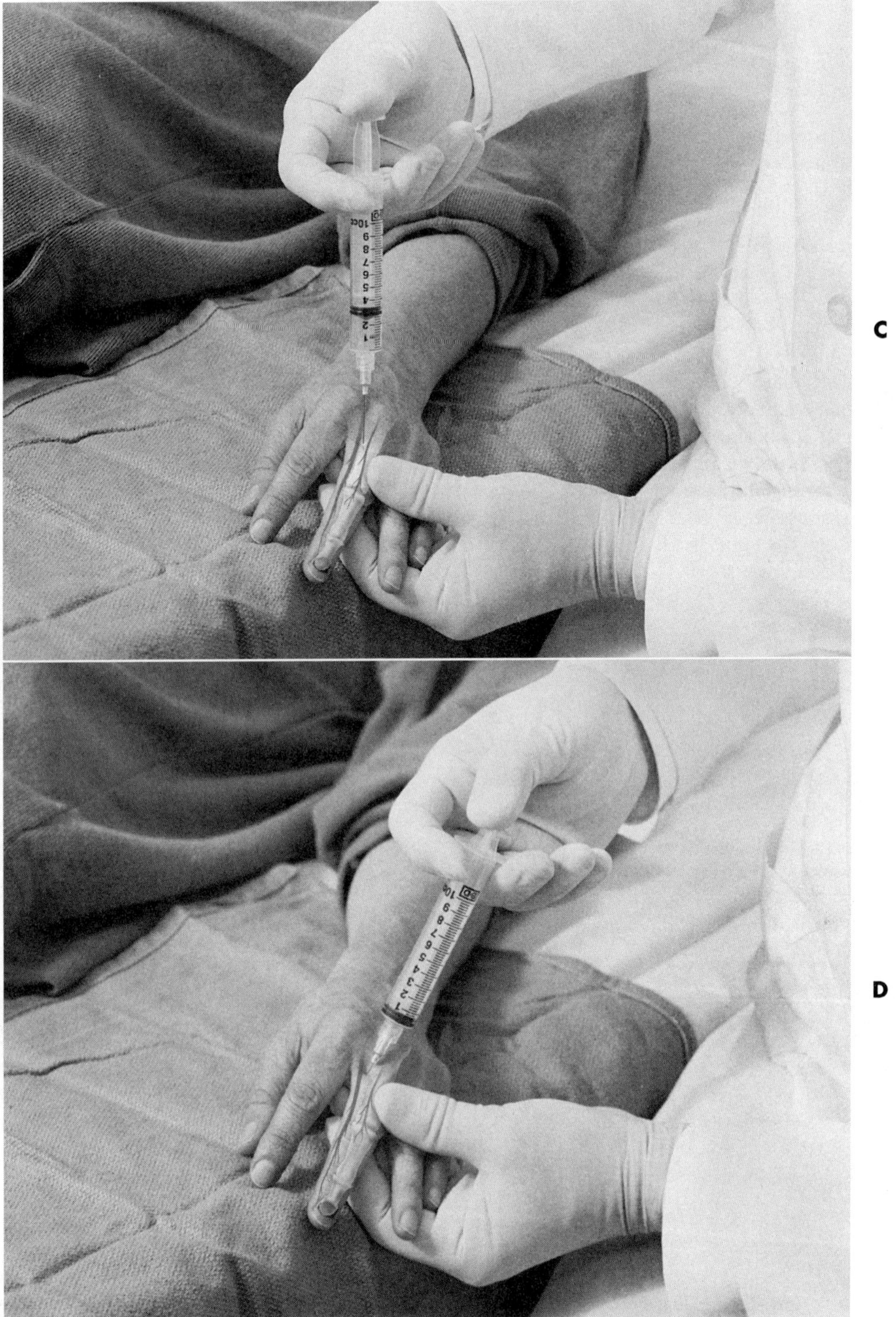

Figure 196-4, cont'd C and **D,** Repeat the same steps on the opposite side of the same digit. (From Trott AT: *Wounds and lacerations,* ed 2, St Louis, 1997, Mosby.)

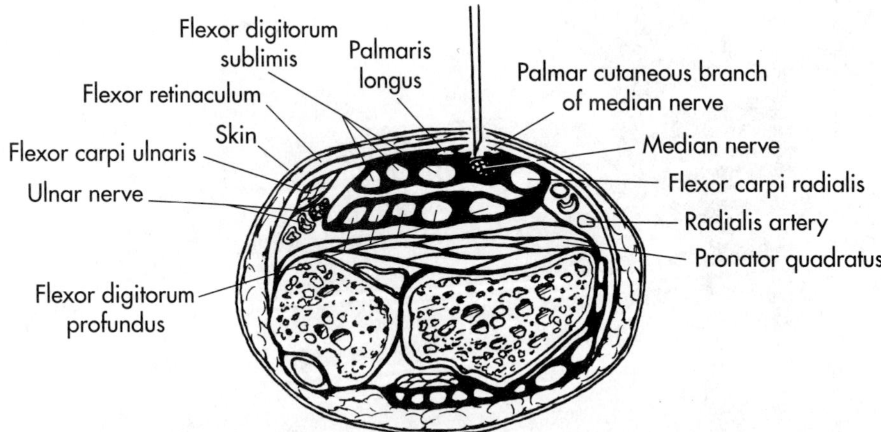

Figure 196-5 Cross-sectional anatomy of the wrist. Note the positions of the palmaris longus, flexor digitorum sublimis, and median nerve. (From Trott AT: *Wounds and lacerations,* ed 2, St Louis, 1997, Mosby.)

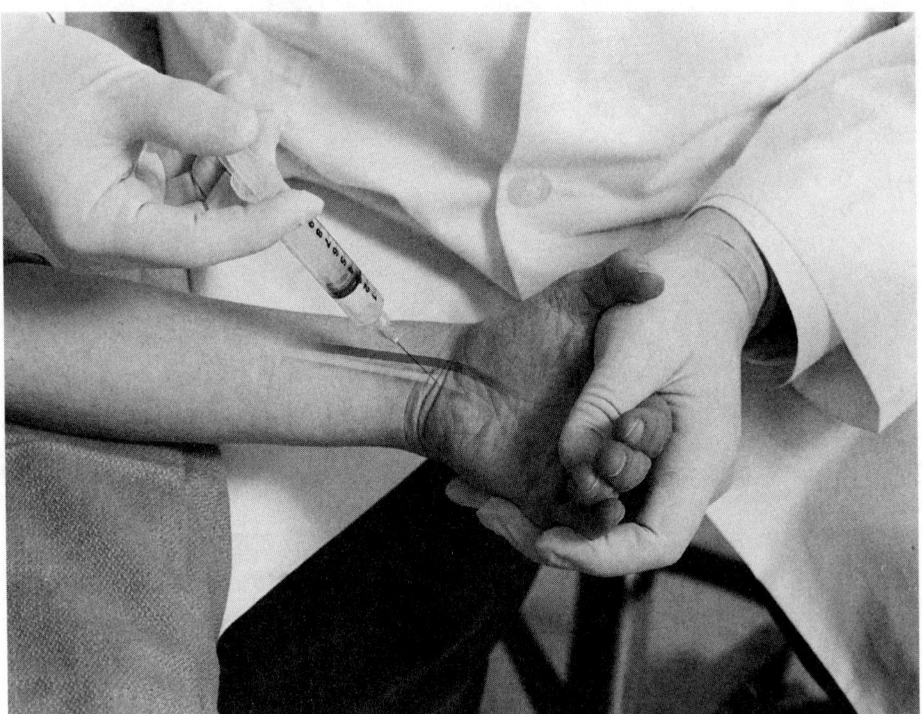

Figure 196-6 Median nerve block. Note the position and path of the palmaris longus and medial nerves. Immediately radial to the palmaris longus tendon, the needle is inserted throughout the flexor retinaculum toward the median nerve. (From Trott AT: *Wounds and lacerations,* ed 2, St Louis, 1997, Mosby.)

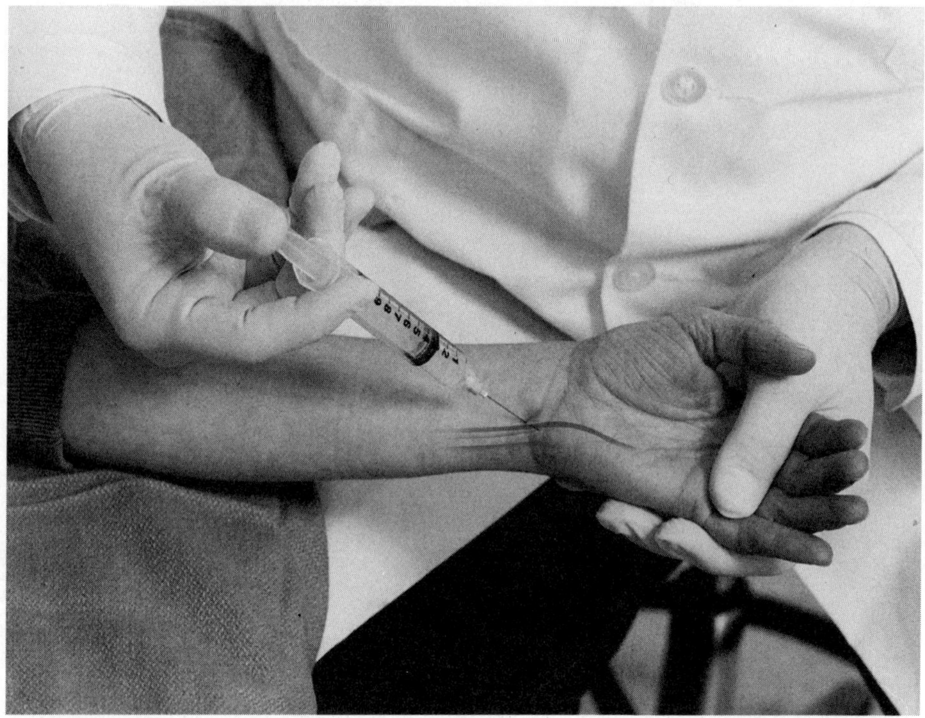

Figure 196-7 Ulnar nerve block. The ulnar nerve lies deep to the flexor carpi ulnaris tendon as shown. The needle is inserted at the radial border of the tendon and directed toward the nerve. Because the nerve lies adjacent to the ulnar artery, great care is taken to aspirate before injection. (From Trott AT: *Wounds and lacerations,* ed 2, St Louis, 1997, Mosby.)

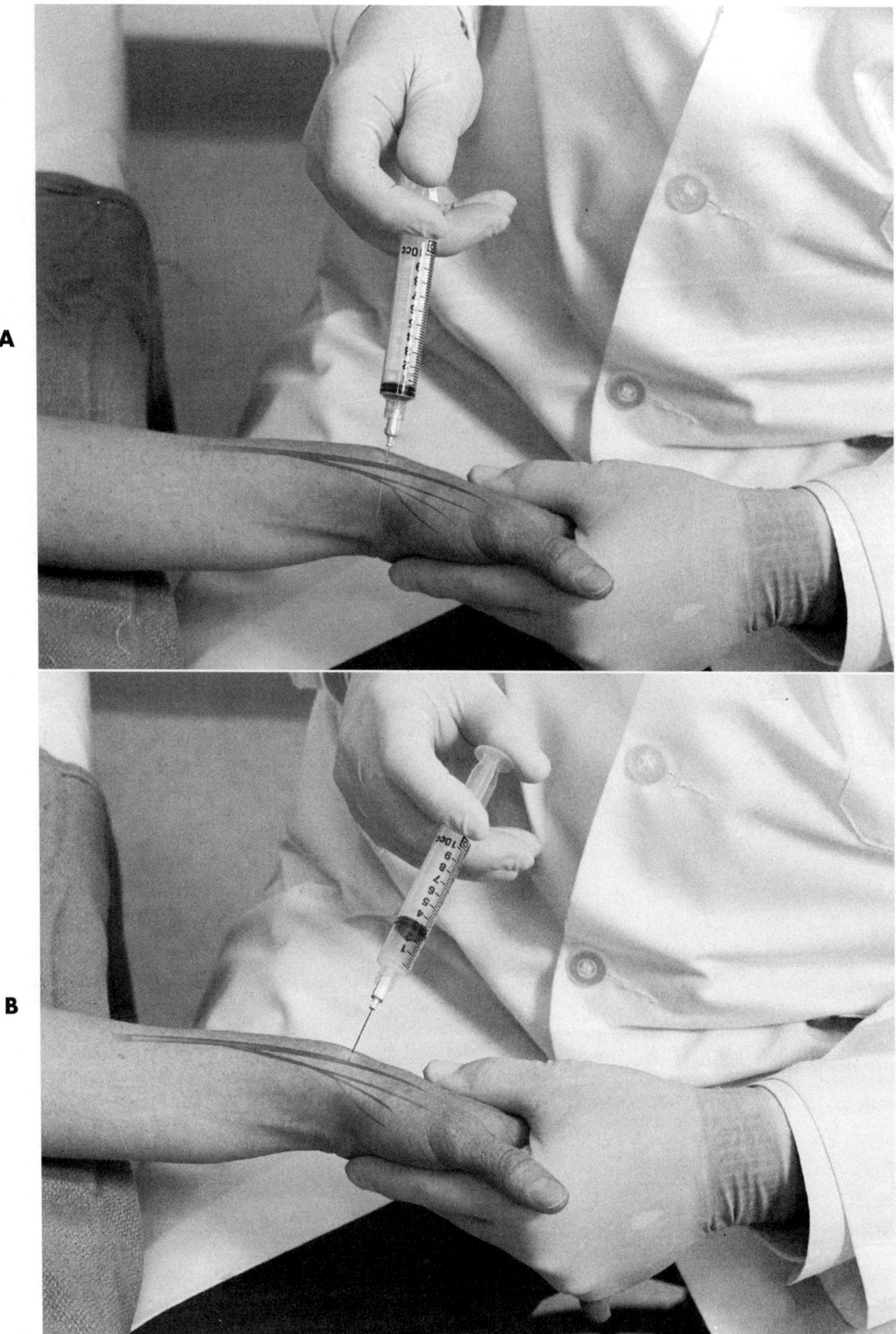

Figure 196-8 Radial nerve block. **A,** Note location and branching of the radial nerve. The needle is introduced to its hub. **B,** A continuous track of anesthetic is laid down as the needle is withdrawn across the branches of the radial nerve. (From Trott AT: *Wounds and lacerations,* ed 2, St Louis, 1997, Mosby.)

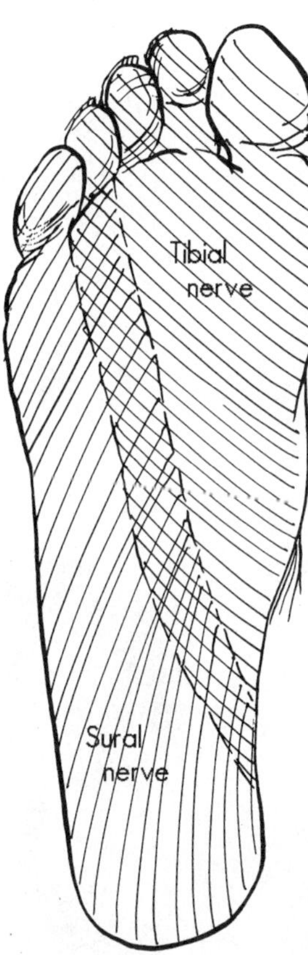

Figure 196-9 Plantar surface of the foot. Distribution of sural and tibial nerve sensory component. Note that there is overlap between the two distributions. (From Trott AT: *Wounds and lacerations,* ed 2, St Louis, 1997, Mosby.)

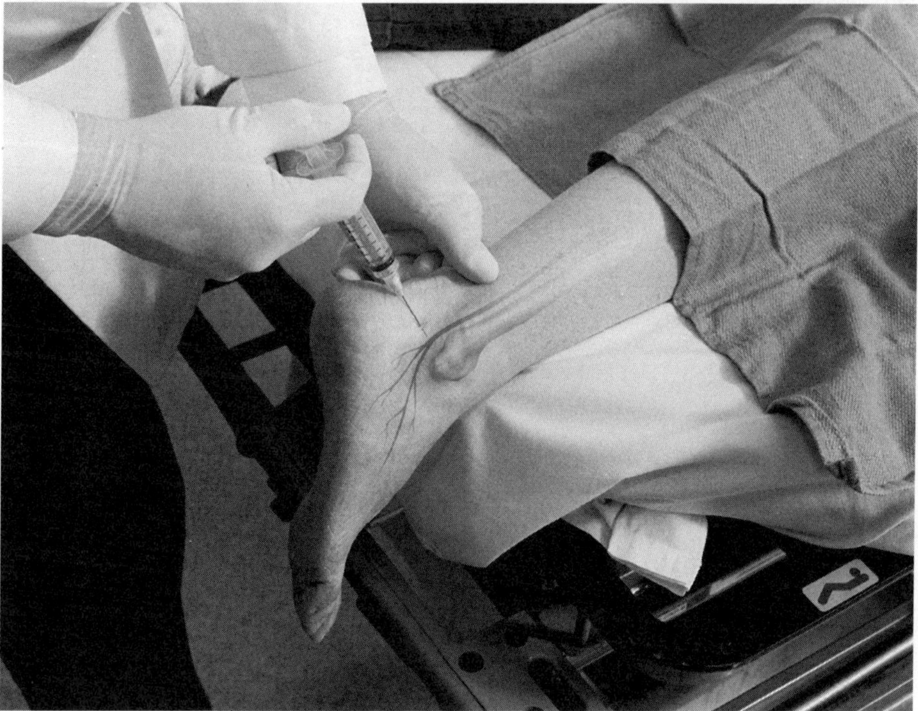

Figure 196-10 Sural nerve block. Note the path of the sural nerve and its relationship to the tip of the fibula. Because of the branching of the nerve, the injection is carried out in a fanlike manner to create an effective block. (From Trott AT: *Wounds and lacerations,* ed 2, St Louis, 1997, Mosby.)

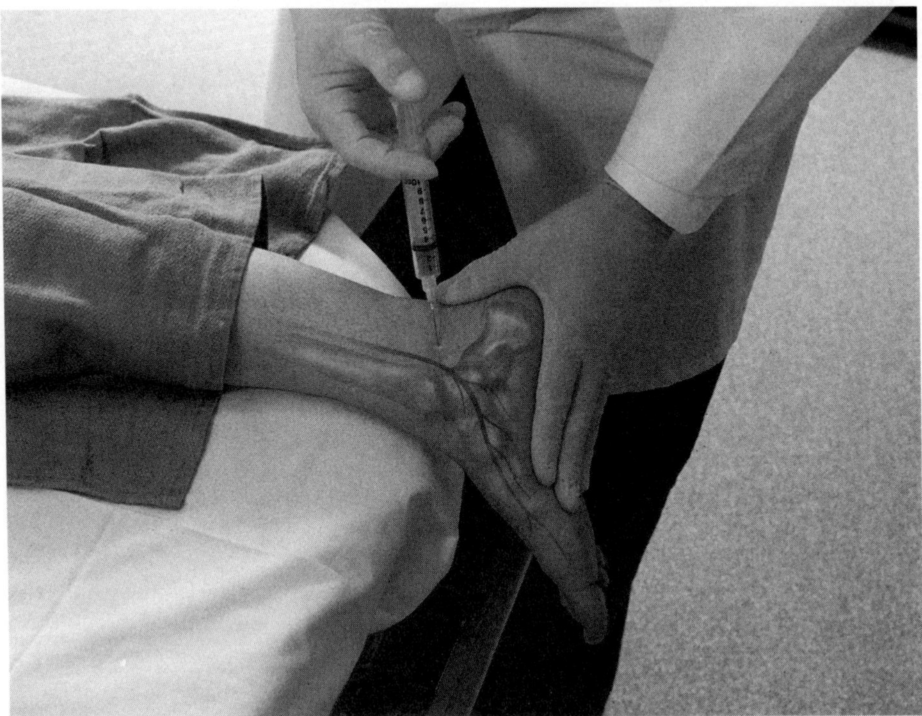

Figure 196-11 Posterior tibial nerve block. Note the path of the nerve and its relationship to the tibial medial malleolus. Because the nerve travels in conjunction with the posterior tibial artery, care is taken to aspirate before injection. (From Trott AT: *Wounds and lacerations,* ed 2, St Louis, 1997, Mosby.)

TABLE 196-4 Antibiotics Used in Wound Management

Type of Wound	Most Common Organism	Antibiotic	Adult Dose	Children's Dose*	Cost ($)
Laceration (grossly contaminated wounds)	*Staphylococcus aureus*	Amoxicillin/ clavulanate (Augmentin) Pregnancy: B	875/125 mg PO BID *or* 500/125 mg PO TID	45 mg/kg/day in two divided doses *or* 20-40 mg/kg/day in three divided doses*	35-86
		Cefuroxime (Ceftin) Pregnancy: B	250-500 mg PO BID	125 mg PO BID	29-124
		Cephalexin (Keflex) Pregnancy: B	250-500 mg PO TID	25-50 mg/kg/day in three divided doses	9-188
Puncture wounds	*S. aureus and Pseudomonas aeruginosa*	Cefuroxime (Ceftin) Pregnancy: B	250-500 mg PO BID	125 mg PO BID	29-124
		Amoxicillin/ clavulanate (Augmentin) Pregnancy: B	875/125 mg PO BID *or* 500/125 mg PO TID	45 mg/kg/day in two divided doses* *or* 20-40 mg/kg/day in three divided doses*	35-86
Human and animal bite	Multiple aerobic and anaerobic organisms (human, cat, dog, raccoon, bat, skunk)	Cefuroxime (Ceftin) Pregnancy: B	250-500 mg PO BID	125 mg PO BID	29-124
		Amoxicillin/ clavulanate (Augmentin) Pregnancy: B	875/125 mg PO BID *or* 500/125 mg PO TID	45 mg/kg/day in two divided doses* *or* 20-40 mg/kg/day in three divided doses*	35-86
		Ampicillin/ sulbactam (Unasyn) Pregnancy: B	1.5-3 g q6h IV	Doses of 200-400 mg/kg of ampicillin and 100-200 mg/kg of sulbactam QD in divided doses have been used*	Not available
		Cefuroxime (Zinacef) Pregnancy: B	750 mg-1.5 g q8h IV	50-100 mg/kg/day in three divided doses	6-14
		Penicillin G Pregnancy: B	2.5 million U q4h IV	400,000 U/kg/day in four divided doses	2-7

*Up to 12 years of age, dosage has not been established.

NOTE: Rabies prophylaxis: Should be administered if bitten by a wild animal or if by a domestic animal if the animal is unhealthy and unavailable to be observed for 10 days. The local public health department should have information on the incidence of rabies in your area.

Eye lid lacerations: Refer to ophthalmologist
Face injuries: Refer to plastic surgeon
Hand injuries: Refer to orthopedist, hand surgeon, or plastic surgeon (human bites to hand are usually admitted to the hospital for intravenous antibiotic therapy)

EVALUATION/FOLLOW-UP

All suture lines within 2 to 3 days to ensure proper healing without complication of infection
Any wound that becomes infected
All puncture wounds within 2 to 5 days
Any loss of function, change of sensation, or change in color at or distal to wound
Development of fever

SUGGESTED READINGS

Barkin RM, Rosen P: Bites. In Barkin, RM, Rosen P: *Emergency pediatrics: a guide to ambulatory care,* ed 4, St Louis, 1994, Mosby.

Dean E, Orlinsky M: Nerve blocks of the thorax and extremities. In Roberts JR, Hedges JR: *Clinical procedures in emergency medicine,* ed 3, Philadelphia, 1998, WB Saunders.

Hoole AJ et L: Emergencies. In Hoole AJ et al: *Patient care guidelines for nurse practitioners,* ed 4, Philadelphia, 1995, JB Lippincott.

Larsen JL, Wischman J: Tissue integrity: surface trauma. In Neff JA, Kidd PS: *Trauma nursing: the art and science,* St Louis, 1993 Mosby.

Markovchick VJ, Cantrill SV: Soft tissue injuries. In Barkin RM, Rosen P: *Emergency pediatrics: a guide to ambulatory care,* ed 4, St Louis, 1994, Mosby.

Martin DR: Soft-tissue injuries and lacerations. In Rund DA et al: *Essentials of emergency medicine,* ed 2, St Louis, 1996, Mosby.

Orlinsky M, Dean E: Anesthetic and analgesic techniques. In Roberts JR, Hedges JR: *Clinical procedures in emergency medicine,* ed 3, Philadelphia, 1998, WB Saunders.

Roberts JR: Pain control in the emergency department. In Roberts JR: *Robert's practical guide to common medical emergencies,* Philadelphia, 1996, Lippincott-Raven.

Uphold CR, Graham MV: *Clinical guidelines in family practice,* ed 2, Gainesville, Fla, 1994, Barmarrae Books.

II

Wellness Across the Lifespan

INTRODUCTION TO WELLNESS CARE

The intent of well care is to provide individualized care to patients who are healthy. At the same time, identification of risks for preventable illness, injuries, and deaths should be incorporated into well care. Evidence is abundant that the majority of deaths among Americans below the age of 65 are preventable, many through interventions introduced in the primary care office. Primary care providers have a key role in screening for many of these preventable problems. Equally important is the role of the provider in counseling patients to improve behaviors related to lifestyle issues such as diet, smoking, alcohol, exercise, injuries, and sexually transmitted diseases.

Although immunizations and screening tests are an important part of preventive services, the most promising arena for prevention lies in changing the personal health behaviors of patients long before a clinical disease develops. Smoking contributes to one of every five deaths in the United States, including coronary artery disease, chronic obstructive pulmonary disease, and cerebrovascular disease. Motor vehicle accidents and injuries are compounded by failure to use seat belts and the use of alcohol. Physical activity and dietary factors contribute to atherosclerosis, cancer, diabetes, and osteoporosis, leading to a continued cycle of inactivity. High-risk sexual behaviors result in unintended pregnancy and various sexually transmitted diseases, including acquired immunodeficiency syndrome. Approximately one half of all deaths in the United States can be attributed to these factors; there is a potential for risk reduction through changes in personal behaviors (McGinnis and Foege, 1993).

Clinical preventive medicine can be defined as "an integral part of preventive medicine concerned with the maintenance and promotion of health and the reduction of risk factors which result in injury and disease" (ACPM News, 1989). Components of clinical preventive care include:

- Assessment of individuals' risk for disease
- Implementation of interventions to modify or eliminate risk for disease/injury
- Integration and monitoring of personal prevention behaviors

From Kidd P, Robinson D: *Family nurse practitioner certification review,* St. Louis, 1999, Mosby.

Barriers to preventive care include:

- Failure of clinician to provide recommended clinical preventive services
- Inadequate reimbursement for preventive care
- Fragmentation of health care delivery
- Insufficient time allowed during appointment
- Recommendations from multiples sources, sometimes contradictory
- Uncertainty as to effectiveness of preventive services

The U.S. Preventive Services Task Force (USPSTF) was established in 1984 to address the issues of preventive care. This panel was charged with the task of developing preventive recommendations based on a systematic review of evidence of clinical effectiveness. The findings of USPSTF include the following:

- Interventions that address personal health practices are vitally important.
- Provider and patient should share decision-making.
- Clinician should be selective in ordering tests and providing preventive services.
- Every opportunity must be taken to deliver preventive services, especially in those with limited access to care.
- For some health problems, community level interventions may be more effective than clinical preventive services (U.S. Preventive Services Task Force, 1996).

Preventive care should be delivered by all nurse practitioners, regardless of specialty. One important component of preventive care is the periodic health examination. The periodic health examination describes a set of health prevention and promotion services that should be provided to an individual based on considerations of age, sex, risk factors, and other circumstances such as occupation and environment. This section reviews the recommendations for health prevention and health promotion for all age groups.

REFERENCES

ACPM News: *Newsletter Am Coll Prevent Med* 1:3, 1989.

McGinnis J, Foege W: Actual causes of death in the US, *JAMA* 270:2207-2212, 1993.

U.S. Preventive Services Task Force: *Guide to clinical preventive services,* ed 2, Baltimore 1996, Williams & Wilkins.

Coronary Artery Disease Management

ICD-9-CM

Counseling Without Complaints or Sickness V65.49
Dietary Counseling V65.3
Exercise Counseling V65.41

RISK FACTOR ANALYSIS FOR CARDIOVASCULAR DISEASE

Using risk factor interventions will improve the overall patient outcomes related to coronary artery disease (CAD). Compelling scientific evidence indicates that interventions can help extend overall survival, improve quality of life, decrease the need for interventional procedures, and help reduce the incidence of subsequent myocardial infarction.

All patients should be screened for CAD risk, with appropriate application of risk reduction in all eligible patients (Tables 197-1 and 197-2).

SUGGESTED READINGS

American Heart Association: Consensus Panel Statement Preventing Heart attach and death in patients with coronary disease, *J Am Col Cardiol* 26:292-294, 1995.

Castelli W, Ockene J, Roberts W: Cardiovascular risk reduction: what really works? *Patient Care* 31(10):47-60, 1997.

Manson J, Tosteson H, Ridker P: The primary prevention of myocardial infarction, *N Engl J Med* 326:1406-1416, 1992.

Roberts W: Preventing and arresting coronary atherosclerosis, *Am Heart J* 130:580-600, 1995.

TABLE 197-1 Risk Characteristics: Coronary Artery Disease

Risk Characteristics	Risk ID	Clinical Evidence of Atherosclerosis	Risk ID
Age	Age	Carotid disease	_Yes _No
		PVD	_Yes _No
Gender	_Male _Female		
Positive family history of premature CAD in first-degree relative (male <55, female <65)	_Yes _No	Other vascular disease	_Yes _No
Socioeconomic status	_Low _Not low	Coronary disease	_Yes _No
Weight	Weight___________	Myocardial infarction	_Yes _No
Height	Height___________	Stable angina	_Yes _No
Total cholesterol	_(mg/dl)	Unstable angina	_Yes _No
Triglycerides	_(mg/dl)	Coronary artery bypass graft	_Yes _No
Low-density lipoproteins	_(mg/dl)	Angioplasty	_Yes _No
High-density lipoproteins	_(mg/dl)	Angiography	_1 vessel
			_2 vessels
			_3 vessels
Smoker	_Yes _No	Stress test	_Ischemia
	_<20 cigarettes/day		_No ischemia
	_>20 cigarettes/day		
Exercise	_Yes _No	Left ventricular function	_Normal
	Type___________		_Mildly reduced
	Days/wk_________		_Severe reduced
Hypertension	_Yes _No	Arrhythmias	_Yes _No
controlled	_Yes _No	Atrial	_Yes _No
		Ventricular	_Yes _No
Diabetes	_Yes _No		
Insulin-dependent diabetes mellitus	_Yes _No		
Noninsulin-dependent diabetes mellitus	_Yes _No		
Comorbid conditions			

Adapted from Castelli W, Ockene J, Roberts, W: Cardiovascular risk reduction: what really works? *Patient Care* 31(10):47-60, 1997.

TABLE 197-2 Risk Reduction Recommendations

Risk	Goal	Recommendations
Smoking	Complete cessation	Strongly encourage cessation, use nicotine replacement via patch, nose spray or gum, Bupropion, commercial smoking cessation programs, and counseling as needed
Exercise	Minimum of 30 minutes three to four times/week	Assess risk to start exercise (stress test for those with CAD), develop exercise prescription; max 5-6 hours/week; for those high risk-monitored program
Weight management	Weight loss of 10%-15% may be helpful for those with hypertension or elevated lipids	Use a combination of exercise and diet for those >120% of ideal weight.
Lipid management	Low-density lipoproteins: <100 mg/dl if known CAD <130 mg/dl if two risk factors <160 if no risk factors	Advise smoking cessation, exercise, weight management; consider lipid lowering agents if above is not successful Secondary goal: High-density lipoproteins >35 mg/dl Triglycerides < 200 mg/dl
Antiplatelet agents/ anticoagulants	Prevention of thrombolic episodes	Begin ASA 80-325 mg/day if not contraindicated; consider warfarin use for those unable to take ASA or high-risk patients; titrate to international normalized ratio of 2-3.5
Estrogens	Consider in all post-menopausal women	Evaluate risk/benefit ratio dependent on other health risks
Blood pressure control	<140/90	Initiate lifestyle modification (weight loss, exercise, smoking cessation, alcohol moderation, moderate sodium restriction) in all patients with >140/90; medication should be started if above modifications do not lower blood pressure past goal; medications should be started in those if blood pressure is >160/100
Angiotensin-converting enzyme inhibitors	Start early in stable post myocardial infarction (MI) high-risk patients	High-risk patients (anterior MI, previous MI, rales, radiographic congestive heart failure, Killip Class II S3 gallop); continue indefinitely in all patients with left ventricular (LV) dysfunction (EJ <40) or symptoms of failure
Beta blockers	Start in high-risk post MI patients	High-risk patients (arrhythmia, LV dysfunction, inducible ischemia) at 5-28 days after MI; continue 6 mos minimum

Adapted from American Heart Association: Consensus Panel Statement on preventing heart attack and death in patients with coronary disease, *J Am Coll Cardiol* 26:292-294, 1995.

Family Planning

ICD-9-CM

Family Planning Advice V25.09
Gynecological Examination for Contraceptive Maintenance V25.40
Intrauterine Device V25.42
Oral Contraceptive Pills V25.41

When considering a method of contraception, it is important to offer patients information about risks, benefits, side effects, interactions, costs, failure rates, and ease of use. When choosing a method the patient should consider the questions in Box 198-1.

High effectiveness: Norplant, depot medroxyprogesterone acetate (Depo Provera), IUDs, combined oral contraceptive pills (OCPs)
Moderate effectiveness: Progestin-only OCPs, condoms (male and female), cervical cap, diaphragm, spermicides (combined use of two of these methods together increases their effectiveness to the highly effective group).
Low effectiveness: Periodic abstinence (rhythm method)
Discuss with patients their ability to be consistently compliant with daily pill use or consistent use of a barrier method. Discuss strategies to increase compliance.
Even if condoms are not to be used as the primary method of contraception, their use should be encouraged to decrease the risk of sexually transmitted infections.

PERMANENT METHODS OF CONTRACEPTION

Components of Presterilization Counseling

Alternative methods available
Reasons for choosing sterilization
Screening for risk indicators for regret
Details of the procedure, including anesthesia with attendant risks and benefits
The permanent nature of the procedure and information on reversal
The possibility of failure, including ectopic pregnancy

Male Sterilization (Vasectomy)

Vasectomies are performed in one of two ways; either through two incisions in the scrotum (one over each vas deferens) or by the "no scalpel vasectomy" in which the vas deferens is fixed externally, while a second specialized instrument is used to puncture the skin. This method has a higher acceptance rate and fewer complications. Both methods use the same method to occlude the vas. These include excising a segment of the vas and sealing the ends by ligation, electrocoagulation or thermocoagulation, or clips. Some surgeons further separate the severed ends by folding them back on one another or by burying one end in the scrotal fascia.

Advantages

Permanent, highly effective, no user action needed after azoospermia is verified

Disadvantages

Reversal is expensive and not consistently successful.
Short-term complications include a less than 2% incidence of infection, hematoma, sperm granuloma, and congestive epididymitis.
Long-term complications: Recent studies have suggested a possible increased risk of prostate cancer; however, no plausible explanation is available. The consensus is that screening for prostate cancer should not be any different for men who have had a vasectomy than for those who have not.

Bilateral Tubal Ligation

Bilateral tubal ligations (BTLs) are performed by one of several methods. These include excising a portion of each

Box 198-1

Considerations in Contraceptive Choice

How well will it fit into your lifestyle?
How compliant or exact do you have to be?
How effective will it be?
What degree of failure can I tolerate in my life?
How safe will it be?
How affordable will it be?
How reversible will it be?

fallopian tube and suturing the ends, excision of a portion, and then suturing the proximal end into the muscle of the uterus and the proximal end in the broad ligament, banding with silastic bands or clips, ligation of a loop of the tubes with nonabsorbable suture, and occlusion by electrocautery.

Advantages

Permanent, highly effective, no user action needed after the procedure

Disadvantages

When compared with vasectomy, the cost, invasiveness, and rates of complications and failure for BTLs are all higher. The procedure is performed under general anesthesia and the associated risks must be considered. Reversibility is expensive and not consistently successful.

Short-Term Complications

Occasionally bleeding or infection may occur.

Long-Term Complications

When failure occurs, the relative risk of ectopic pregnancy is increased.

NONPERMANENT METHODS

Intrauterine Device

An intrauterine device (IUD) is a small device made of flexible plastic that is inserted into the uterus. The IUD does not act as an abortifacient. Analysis of various white blood cells (WBCs), prostaglandins and enzymes in the uterine cavity will show a marked inflammatory response that likely interferes with sperm survival, motility, and/or capacitation. This inflammatory response also increases the ova's speed of transport in the fallopian tube and the inflammatory response in the endometrium itself.

Two types of IUDs are available in the United States. The Progestasert, which contains the hormone progestin, has a failure rate of 2%; the ParaGard Copper T380A, has a failure rate of 0.8%. Both IUDs trigger the inflammatory response, and each has additional attributes that affect the IUD's effectiveness. The Progestasert contains 38 mg of progestin in a delivery system that releases 65 μg per day. This slow release can reduce menstrual bleeding and cramping. The progestin in the Progestasert thickens cervical mucus, providing a barrier that prevents sperm from entering the uterus. It also affects the endometrial lining in ways that would prevent implantation in the unlikely event that an egg was fertilized. This device must be replaced annually. The copper in the ParaGard affects the behavior of enzymes in the lining of the uterus to prevent implantation. It also triggers an increase in the production of prostaglandins that affect the hormones that support pregnancy. The ParaGard has been approved for 10 years of continuous use.

Absolute Contraindications to IUD Placement

Confirmed or suspected pregnancy
Known or suspected pelvic malignancy
Undiagnosed vaginal bleeding
Known or suspected pelvic infections, acute or chronic, including sexually transmitted infections and genital actinomycosis
Reported behaviors placing an individual at risk for contracting sexually transmitted infections
Hyperbilirubinemia secondary to Wilson's disease, which is relevant only to use of the ParaGard IUD

Relative Contraindications to IUD Placement

Uterine size or shape incompatible with effective IUD use
Medical conditions requiring immunosuppression, which may increase the risk of infection (e.g., corticosteroid therapy, valvular heart disease)
Nulligravidity
Abnormal result to a Papanicolaou (Pap) smear (until managed)
History of ectopic pregnancy
Additional considerations: Cervical stenosis, endometrial polyps, impaired ability to check for presence of IUD strings

Initial Counseling Visit for IUD Placement

The patient should be scheduled for a complete physical examination, including either a complete history, if the patient is new to the practice, or an interim history if the patient is known. The pelvic examination is performed with attention to the size, consistency, and position of the uterus and any adnexal pain or fullness. A Pap smear, wet prep, and cultures for gonorrhea and chlamydial infection should be done during this visit. Additional testing based on history should also be considered (e.g., pregnancy test if menses are irregular, hemoglobin and platelet count if indicated).

An IUD consent form should be reviewed with the patient and signature obtained. A consent form should include definitions and mechanism of the IUD, risks, benefits, contraindications for use of IUDs, and alternative methods. Information regarding care of the IUD, including how to check strings and what to do if any adverse effects occur, should be included in both the consent form and printed handout the patient will be given to take home. Side effects that require immediate action must be noted, including late or absent menses, severe abdominal pain, especially with an elevated temperature; pain or bleeding after intercourse; and any unusual vaginal discharge and unusual vaginal bleeding, including passing of clots. The patient should be cautioned that she will probably experience heavier than normal menstrual flow and increased cramping (especially in the first month of IUD placement).

Scheduling the IUD Insertion

Patients may have an IUD inserted immediately at the time of a first trimester abortion, or with second normal menses afterward. If the IUD is to be inserted postpartum or after a second-trimester abortion, they should wait 8 weeks for the uterus to return to its nonpregnant size.

Many clinicians choose to insert the IUD during a patient's menses, because insertion of the IUD at another part of the cycle may cause a sudden resumption of menses with increased flow. The most comfortable time for IUD insertion is during menstruation, because the cervix is softest and the menstrual blood acts as additional lubricant. Also, the chances of interrupting or injuring a developing pregnancy is much less likely. However, there are some clinicians who prefer to insert an IUD midcycle, because the cervix is naturally dilated during ovulation.

Insertion

It is a good idea to instruct a woman to take an over-the-counter nonsteroidal antiinflammatory drug (NSAID) an hour or so before insertion to decrease cramping that may occur. Because infection with IUD use is most often associated with insertion, many clinicians recommend prophylactic administration of either doxycycline 200 mg PO 1 hour before insertion or erythromycin 500 mg PO 1 hour before and 6 hours after insertion. However, there is no evidence that prophylactic administration of antibiotics is necessary.

Box 198-2 outlines the procedure for inserting an intrauterine device.

Box 198-2

Procedure for Insertion of an IUD

Assess vital signs before and after procedure.
Don sterile gloves.
Determine uterine position by performing a bimanual examination.
Place a speculum for maximal exposure of the cervix.
Cleanse the cervix with a disinfectant such as povidone-iodine (Betadine), using well-soaked cotton balls and a ring forceps.
Administer a paracervical block as necessary to minimize insertional pain.
Place the tenaculum on the anterior lip of the cervix and apply gentle traction to stabilize the uterus and minimize flexion.
Sound the uterus, noting depth in centimeters (if less than 6 cm or greater than 9 cm, placement of an IUD is contraindicated).
Gently insert the IUD according to package directions. (NOTE: The manufacturer's physician information pamphlet should be read concerning the specifics of the IUD insertion.)
Remove the tenaculum.
Trim the strings of the IUD to about 2 cm. (Cutting the strings at a slight angle decreases sharp edges that may "stick" a partner.)
Charting should include the type of IUD used, depth of uterine sounding, length of strings, and description of how the patient tolerated the procedure.

Patient Education

The patient should be taught the following:

How to find the IUD strings and to promptly report the absence of the strings.
To abstain from sexual intercourse and not to insert anything (e.g., tampons, finger) into her vagina for 7 days. After 7 days she may resume sexual intercourse.
To use a second method of birth control for the first month.
To always check for strings after intercourse.
That there may be some spotting between periods during the first few months, and the first few periods may last longer and the flow may be heavier. Cramping or backache may occur for several days or weeks after insertion. Administration of NSAIDs usually resolves cramping and discomfort.
The need for a monogamous relationship and the use of barrier contraceptives to prevent STDs.

Postinsertion Follow-up

Patients should return for a checkup after their next menses to ensure that the IUD has not been expelled and to assess how the IUD is tolerated. Complications to be watchful for are outlined in Table 198-1.

Removing an IUD

If possible, remove the IUD during the patient's menses. Using a ring forceps, apply gentle, even traction and remove the IUD slowly.

Follow-up

Yearly Pap smears and pelvic examination
Whenever appropriate for replacement of IUD

TABLE 198-1 Potential Complications Associated with IUDs

Complication	Intervention
Pelvic infections	The risk of pelvic infection is increased during the first few months of IUD use, possibly because of introduction of organisms during insertion. Some researchers theorize that the pelvic tract is more susceptible to infections for the first few months because the acute inflammatory state of the uterus secondary to the presence of the IUD may increase susceptibility. This risk decreases within 3 months. If a patient is seen with suspected pelvic inflammatory disease (PID) or some other pelvic infection and her condition is otherwise stable, treat with antibiotics for 2 days before removing the IUD to prevent dissemination of the infection. After removing the IUD, continue the full course of antibiotics (see Chapter 140).
Expulsion	Objective findings when the cervix is visualized: IUD is seen protruding from the cervical os. IUD string is longer than at time of insertion (partial expulsion). IUD strings are missing (complete expulsion). If IUD is partially expelled, it should be removed. It may be reinserted immediately if there is no infection or chance of pregnancy. If it is completely expelled, a new IUD may be inserted during or after next menses.
Missing IUD strings	Perform a pregnancy test, since an intrauterine pregnancy can displace the IUD upward. If results are negative, gently insert a cytobrush as if obtaining an endocervical sample. Rotate the brush and slowly remove. This may locate strings that have migrated up toward the cervix. If strings still are not found, send for ultrasonography.
Actinomyces	This anaerobic, gram-positive bacterium is occasionally detected by cervical cytological evaluation in IUD users. If the patient is asymptomatic and wishes to continue IUD usage, treat with appropriate antibiotics. After treatment, a repeat Pap smear should be analyzed. If the results remain positive or if the patient is symptomatic, the IUD must be removed, and the patient should be referred to a physician.
Pregnancy	Consult with a physician.

Norplant

Norplant implants are flexible, silastic tubes filled with levonorgestrel, that are placed just under the skin on the inside of the upper arm. Each capsule contains 36 mg of levonorgestrel and releases a small amount of hormone over 5 years (declining over time from 85 μg/day to 30 μg/day).

Levonorgestrel causes genital tract changes typical of the luteal phase: Thickened cervical mucosa, decreased mobility of the uterine tube, and a disorganized endometrium. Ovulation is inconsistently suppressed.

Norplant is a highly effective, reversible form of birth control. Body weight of more than 70 kg (154 pounds) decreases its effectiveness slightly, although it still has the best user/effectiveness rate of any reversible birth control method.

Advantages

Highly effective, long duration
No user action required after insertion

Disadvantages

Clinician must be trained in implant technique
Frequent menstrual changes
High initial cost
Requires minor surgical procedure to insert and remove

Risks

The relative risk of ectopic pregnancy, in case of failure of the implant, may be increased. There are no known adverse effects on the fetus if pregnancy does occur. There is no permanent effect on fertility; serum levels of levonorgestrel are undetectable 48 hours after removal of the implant. There is minimal or no adverse effect on blood pressure, carbohydrate metabolism, liver function, coagulation, or blood lipid levels.

Side Effects

Bleeding: Many women complain of significant changes in menstrual patterns. Bleeding may occur daily for the first 6 to 9 months of use (the leading cause of patient dissatisfaction). After 9 months, irregular menses remain the rule, although the total amount of bleeding per year is comparable to that with no hormonal use.

Headaches: The mechanism is unknown. This is a common cause for Norplant removal.

Weight gain or loss: Neither is clearly directly related

to the hormone, although many women complain of weight gain.

Mastalgia, galactorrhea: More common when Norplant is inserted during lactation. Usually transitory and no treatment is needed.

Acne: Worst in the first year.

Other: Ovarian cysts, hirsutism, scalp hair loss, cervicitis, vaginitis, dizziness, abdominal pain, nausea, musculoskeletal pain, insertion-site pain, or pigmentation. All are usually self-limited, or, if severe, may be treated by removal of the Norplant.

Contraindications: Active thrombotic disease, undiagnosed vaginal bleeding, active liver disease, current breast or genital tract cancer; use caution in women who are depressed.

Drug interactions: Phenytoin, phenobarbital, carbamazepine, and rifampin significantly reduce the effectiveness of Norplant; their use should be considered a contraindication for implantation.

Consider a 6-month trial of norgestrel progestin-only pills (Ovrette) to predict tolerance of Norplant.

Management of Side Effects

Hypermenorrhea: May consider oral estrogen or transdermal patch; usually subsides in a year

Weight gain: Diet history, nutritional counseling, decrease snacking, increase exercise (average weight gain, 5 pounds [2.27 kg])

Mastalgia: Supportive bra, vitamin E 60 to 75 IU QD, not to exceed 300 IU/day

Galactorrhea: Decrease nipple stimulation (check bras for seams that cross over nipples)

Acne: Diet, skin cleansers, topical antibiotics, topical acne treatments

Follow-up

Check site after 2 weeks (usually done by clinician performing the insertion)

Evaluate tolerance to side effects in 3 months

Yearly annual examination, Pap smear

Depot Medroxyprogesterone Acetate (DMPA)

Depo Provera

Depo Provera works by inhibiting ovulation by suppression of pituitary secretion of luteinizing hormone (LH) and follicle-stimulating hormone (FSH). It also causes genital tract changes typical of the secretory phase (e.g., thickened cervical mucus, decreased uterine tube motility).

Effectiveness: Depo Provera has a failure rate of less than 1 pregnancy per 100 women per year.

Advantages

Highly effective, no user action required between injections

Use undetectable to partner

May be given immediately postpartum; does not interfere with lactation

Probably protective against ovarian and endometrial cancers

Increases hemoglobin concentration

Inhibits sickling in sickle cell anemia

Disadvantages

Return to fertility after last injection is variable: 50% at 6 months, 75% at 12 months, 85% at 18 months, 95% at 24 months.

Risks

No known tetrogenicity. No known carcinogenicity. Relative risk of ectopic pregnancy is increased in case of failure. Slight decrease in bone density with long-term use, reversible upon cessation of use. No known adverse effects on fetus in case of failure (although awareness of pregnancy may be delayed, leading to late prenatal care). No adverse effects on glucose, lipids, or blood pressure.

Side Effects

Menstrual irregularities are almost universal. Caution patients that daily spotting or bleeding may occur, especially between the first and second shots. If possible, have patients agree to a trial of 6 months, explaining that many side effects disappear after the second shot.

Bleeding usually decreases with time; 50% are amenorrheic after 6 months. Injection in the immediate postpartum period may cause prolonged, though not severe, postpartum bleeding.

Prolonged and heavy bleeding may be managed by:

- Ibuprofen 800 mg PO TID for 5 days
- Premarin 1.25 or 2.5 or Estrace 1 mg PO for 21 days/month for up to 3 months
- Estraderm 0.5 mg patch change every 3½ days for 3 months
- Climara 0.1 mg patch, change weekly for 3 weeks for up to 3 months

Weight gain of 3 to 6 lbs (1 to 3 kg) is common; however, some women lose weight.

Patients should be instructed that Depo Provera will increase their appetite, and if they give in to snacking, they will gain weight regardless of the method chosen.

Hair loss (or thinning) is fairly common, although easily managed with a multivitamin supplement.

PMS-like symptoms may occur with the first injection but will resolve spontaneously and are less severe with subsequent shots. These may be managed with supplements of vitamins E and B-complex, decreased caffeine and refined sugar intake, and increased complex carbohydrate intake.

Contraindications

Known or suspected pregnancy

Intention of becoming pregnant within the next year

Allergy to local anesthetics (same ingredient in carrier substance of local anesthetics and Depo Provera)

Known or suspected breast malignancy

Active liver dysfunction

Caution with patients taking antiseizure medications or who are depressed; these medications may decrease efficacy of DMPA

Before First Injection

History

Physical examination

Urine pregnancy test before first injection (even if on menses). Consider an HCG before second excretion if there is a history of irregular menses, if the first injection was given while not on menses, or if the woman is a poor historian or had symptoms of pregnancy.

Subsequent Visits

Measure blood pressure and weight at each visit.

Administration

The initial injection should be given during the menstrual cycle or within the first 5 days postpartum.

DMPA is safe to use while the patient is breastfeeding.

DMPA 150 mg is injected IM every 12 weeks into the gluteal or deltoid muscle.

Caution the patient not to massage the site.

Injections may be given anywhere from 9 to 13 weeks after the last injection.

If more than 13 weeks have passed since the last injection, perform two pregnancy tests 2 weeks apart, and caution the patient to have no sexual intercourse during the interim. Counsel the patient that pregnancy may occur and to use a back-up form of birth control. Repeat the pregnancy test before the next injection.

Diaphragm

A diaphragm is a shallow rubber cap with a flexible rim that is placed in the vagina so as to cover the cervix. It serves as both a mechanical barrier and a receptacle for spermicidal cream/jelly/film, which must be used to ensure effectiveness.

Advantages

This is a barrier method of birth control in which potential side effects associated with systemic medications are avoided. The diaphragm offers some protection against certain sexually transmitted infections, including gonorrhea, syphilis, herpes, and chlamydial infections when used with a spermicide.

Disadvantages

Moderately effective, depending on the woman's motivation to use the diaphragm each time she has intercourse

Proper use of spermicides is essential

Contraindications

Allergy to latex, rubber, or spermicidal agents

Uterine prolapse, severe cystocele, rectocele or substantial retroversion or anteversion of the uterus

Poor vaginal muscle tone

Recurrent urinary tract infections

Inability to insert or remove diaphragm

Before Use

Appropriate counseling is essential regarding diaphragm use and its advantages and disadvantages.

Strongly emphasize that this method's effectiveness depends on the individual's motivation and proper use of the diaphragm.

Obtain a complete history and perform a thorough physical examination.

A complete pelvic examination is necessary to rule out any pelvic anomalies that would contraindicate use of a diaphragm.

A set of fitting rings or complete diaphragms must be available for sizing.

Types of Diaphragms

Various types of diaphragms are compared in Table 198-2.

How to Fit a Diaphragm (Figure 198-1)

Hold the index and middle fingers together and insert into the vagina up to the posterior fornix. Raise the hand to bring the surface of the index finger in contact with the pubic arch.

Use the tip of the thumb to mark the point directly beneath the inferior margin of the pubic bone and withdraw the fingers in this position.

Place one end of the rim of the fitting diaphragm or ring on the tip of the middle finger. The opposite end should lie just in front of the thumb tip. This is the approximate diameter of the diaphragm needed.

Insert a fitting diaphragm or ring of the appropriate size into the vagina. Try both a larger and smaller size before making a decision.

The proper size diaphragm will fit snugly in the posterior fornix and behind the pubic arch without undue pressure.

Patient Education

Teach the patient the following:

- Examine the diaphragm carefully before each use and before putting it away by holding it up to a bright light. Make sure that it has no cracks or holes.
- Place 1 to 2 tablespoons of spermicidal jelly or cream into the dome of the diaphragm. Too much cream or jelly may make the diaphragm prone to slipping (patients may elect to use vaginal film instead of jelly; simply have them place a sheet of film into the dome of the diaphragm 5 to 10 minutes before intercourse).
- The diaphragm is to be left in place for 6 hours after the last intercourse.
- No douching for 6 hours after intercourse.
- Before repeated intercourse, additional jelly/cream should be applied with an applicator to outside of diaphragm or another vaginal film should be inserted.

TABLE 198-2 Types of Diaphragms

Type (in descending order of strength)	Ortho	Holland-Rantos	Schmid Products	Milex
Arching spring: Most used in the United States; thought to be easiest to insert, recommended for women with less than normal vaginal tone, mild to moderate cystocele or rectocele, prolapsed uterus, retroverted uterus; also good for nullipara women	Allflex Sizes 55-95	Koroflex Sizes 60-95	Rames Bendex Sizes 65-95	Wide Seal Sizes 60-95
Coil spring: Fits most women and is especially recommended for women with good vaginal support, no cystocele or rectocele, no pelvic floor relaxation, moderately protruding cervix in the anterior or midplane position	Ortho Diaphragm Sizes 50-95	Koromex Sizes 50-95	Rames Flexible Cushioned Sizes 50-95	Wide Seal Omniflex Sizes 60-95
Flat spring: Suitable for smaller women and is especially recommended for those with a very shallow notch or pocket behind the symphysis	Ortho White Sizes 55-95			

Do not remove the diaphragm to insert more spermicide! If the woman has difficulty removing, have her squat and try to remove.

Care of the Diaphragm

Wash with warm water and a mild soap after removal.

Allow to dry thoroughly before storing in its case.

Soak in rubbing alcohol for 30 minutes (no longer) after use following treatment for a vaginal infection.

Follow-up

The patient should be able to correctly insert and remove the diaphragm before leaving the office.

The patient should consider using a back-up method of birth control for the first month or so of use.

The patient should return to the office 1 week after initial fitting for a diaphragm check. During that week have the patient practice wearing the diaphragm for at least 8 hours. Have the patient wear the diaphragm to the office.

Instruct the patient to have her diaphragm refitted if she gains or loses more than 10 or 15 pounds, has a miscarriage, abortion, or baby, have any type of pelvic surgery, or if she experiences problems urinating or has trouble moving her bowels with the diaphragm in place.

At an annual examination, perform a pelvic examination and Pap smear.

Cervical Cap

The cervical cap is a thimble-shaped, deep-domed barrier device that fits over the cervix and is used in combination with a spermicidal jelly (Figure 198-2).

Effectiveness ranges from 92% to 96%, depending on proper usage.

Advantages

May be inserted up to 12 hours before intercourse and kept in place for up to 72 hours.

Additional spermicide is not necessary for repeated intercourse.

There is reduced risk of urinary tract infections and increased comfort compared with a diaphragm (Figures 198-3 and 198-4).

Disadvantages

Requires a clinician certified in fitting cervical caps.

Contraindications

An unusually long or short cervix
History of cervical lacerations or scarring
Current cervicitis
An unusually shaped or asymmetric cervix
Current pelvic, tubal, or ovarian infection
Current vaginal infection
Abnormal/unresolved abnormal Pap smear
History of toxic shock

RESOURCES

Additional information and caps may be ordered from:
Cervical Caps Ltd.
430 Montrey Avenue, Suite 1B
Los Gatos, CA 95030
(408) 358-6264

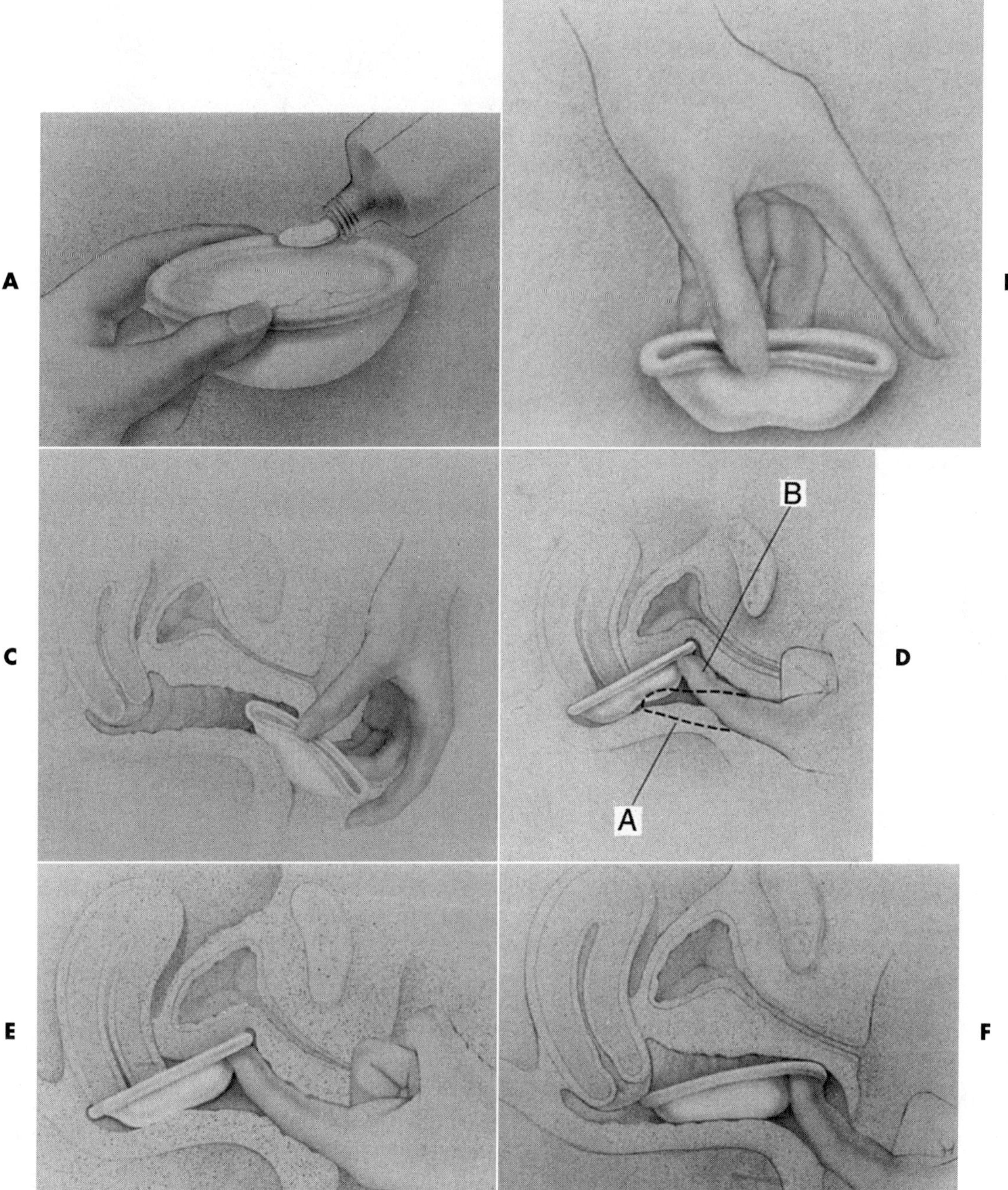

Figure 198-1 **A,** Proper application of spermicidal jelly to diaphragm and dome. **B,** Folding the diaphragm for insertion. **C,** Inserting the diaphragm. **D,** Proper positioning of the diaphragm: *A,* Cervix palpable behind the diaphragm; *B,* rim fits snuggly but without discomfort behind the symphysis pubis. Removal of the diaphragm: **E,** Hook finger under rim. **F,** Pull diaphragm out through the introitus. (Courtesy Ortho Pharmaceutical Co.)

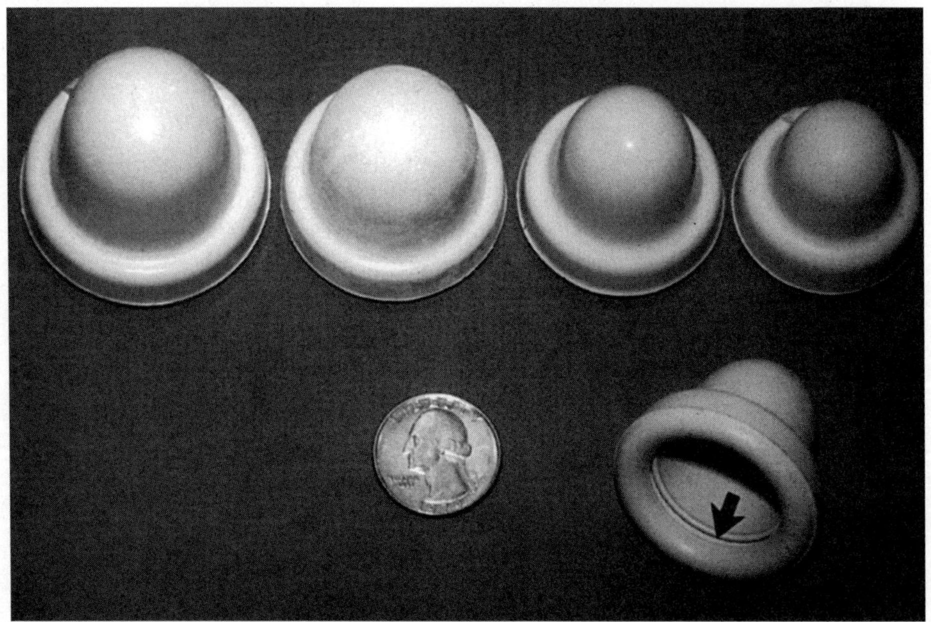

Figure 198-2 Four available sizes of Prentif Cavity-Rim Cervical Cap: 22, 25, 28, and 31 mm inside diameter. Arrow indicates hollow rim that creates suction to hold cap on cervix. (Quarter indicates relative size.) (From Stenchever MA: *Office gynecology,* ed 2, St Louis, 1996, Mosby.)

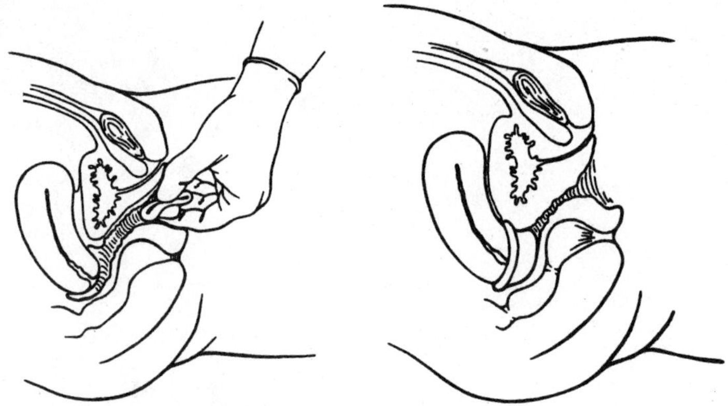

Figure 198-3 Properly fitted cervical cap. (From Pfenniger JL, Fowler GC: *Procedures for primary care physicians,* St Louis, 1994, Mosby.)

NATURAL FAMILY PLANNING

Fertility Awareness Methods

Overview

Definition

Fertility awareness methods (FAM) are techniques to help determine when a woman is most likely to be fertile. Couples who do not wish to have a child can then avoid sexual intercourse during the period of time when a woman is most likely to become pregnant. Couples who wish to conceive may engage in sexual intercourse during that time.

FAM usually involves abstinence during the fertile period, although some couples may elect to use barrier methods while having sexual intercourse during these times.

How It Works

Fertility awareness methods are based on the assumption that a woman is fertile only around the time of ovulation. The aim of FAM is to recognize when ovulation is approaching and when it has passed. FAM relies on the following facts:

An egg is usually released each cycle.

The egg is released about 14 days before menstruation.

The egg lives 12 to 24 hours.

Sperm may live for 5 days in a woman's body.

This means that a woman is fertile for as long as 5 days

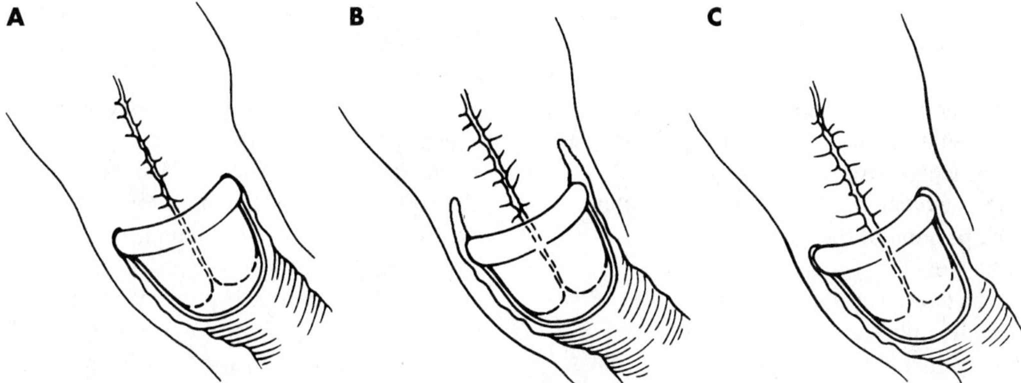

Figure 198-4 Properly and improperly fitted cervical caps. **A,** Properly fitted cap is closely applied to the cervix, and the rim of the cap fills the cervicovaginal fornix. **B,** The cap is too small. Although the dome of the cap is closely applied to the cervix, the rim does not reach into the fornix, leaving the base of the cervix exposed. **C,** The cap is too large. Although the dome covers the cervix and the rim extends into the fornix, the cap is not closely applied to the cervix and may easily be dislodged. (From Pfenniger JL, Fowler GC: *Procedures for primary care physicians,* St Louis, 1994, Mosby.)

before ovulation because of the length of sperm life. And after ovulation she is fertile for up to 3 days, because of the length of egg life. This amounts to 7 or 8 days of her cycle each month. The rest of the days are not considered fertile days, and intercourse during that part of the cycle should not result in pregnancy.

Each method can be used alone, but FAM is more reliable when the signs of one method is used to confirm the signs of another. When combining methods, it is important to have the woman keep a daily chart of body changes. The daily chart keeps a woman aware of what is going on in her current cycle, and helps her determine if ovulation is early and late.

The two most important things to check are cervical mucus and basal body temperature.

Cervical Mucus

A woman can learn to tell when ovulation is about to happen and when it has passed by checking her mucus discharge daily. She can check externally by touching the inner lips of the vagina and/or internally by putting her finger into her vagina. Several days after menstruation she will have no noticeable discharge and her vagina will feel relatively dry. Discharge will start to be noticeable as ovulation approaches. The mucus will be thick, white or yellow, and will feel tacky or pasty. The first sign of this tacky mucus will be the start of the fertile phase.

About the time of the start of ovulation, mucus increases to a peak, and there will be 1 or more days of clear, slippery, very wet mucus (similar to raw egg white) that can be stretched between two fingers. To prevent pregnancy a woman should avoid intercourse from the time she first notices the mucus to at least 4 days after the last day of the slippery mucus.

After ovulation, the mucus begins to dry up, and gets thick and pasty again. Often, it disappears completely until shortly before ovulation the next month. (NOTE: Vaginal infections or surgical procedures of the cervix may alter the production of mucus. Also, the use of spermicides may interfere with the pattern of mucus.)

Basal Body Temperature

Basal body temperature (BBT) is the temperature of the body after at least 3 hours of rest. Checking her temperature daily will teach the woman what is normal for her body and help determine her personal pattern of temperature shifts to maximize accurately pinpointing the fertile period.

Before ovulation, the BBT will be relatively lower. Within 12 hours following ovulation, the BBT usually rises several tenths of degrees and remains up until the menses begins. Keeping a BBT record helps indicate when an egg has been released When a woman sees her temperature rise and remain higher for at least 3 days, she knows it is likely that ovulation occurred shortly before her temperature rose, and she should no longer be fertile. When using the BBT method alone, a woman must abstain from intercourse from the end of menstruation until she is sure ovulation is past by at least 3 days.

Tips

Temperature may be disturbed by different things, including certain drugs, lack of sleep, travel, stress, and other factors. The patient should note these things in her daily chart; otherwise, it is possible to mistake an illness as a sign that ovulation has passed.

The temperature must be taken every morning immediately on awakening and before getting out of bed, smoking, eating, or drinking liquids.

A basal body thermometer is recommended, because it

registers small temperature changes more accurately than a fever thermometer.

Other Signs

Some women may notice physical signs of ovulation with changes of temperature and mucus. Recognizing these changes will benefit a woman in recognizing changes occurring around ovulation. These signs may include:

- Changes in the position of the cervix
- Softening of the cervix
- Slight aching in the lower abdomen in the area of the ovaries, usually unilateral
- Slight, temporary spotting
- Breast tenderness
- A feeling of heaviness in the lower abdomen

Calendar Method

The calendar method of FAM is relatively unreliable and involves guessing when ovulation will occur based on when it occurred in the past. While the method is unreliable alone, when combined with other methods it may be used to predict when ovulation may occur.

Effectiveness

FAM is most effective when used correctly, with no intercourse during the fertile days. About 24 of every 100 women who are average users of FAM become pregnant during the first year of this method's use.

Advantages

- There are no health risks or side effects.
- It can be used to prevent or plan a pregnancy.
- It can be fairly effective if used correctly by a woman with regular menses.
- It is acceptable to couples with religious concerns about birth control.
- It can lead to greater understanding and awareness of a woman's reproductive system.
- It is free, except for the cost of the basal body thermometer.

Disadvantages

- Learning FAM takes time and effort.
- Requires a commitment to keeping careful daily logs.
- Has a fairly high failure rate.
- Infections and use of spermicides may interfere with normal production of mucus.

COMBINED ORAL CONTRACEPTIVES

Overview

Oral contraceptive pills (OCPs) primarily suppress ovulation by inhibiting gonadotrophins. Secondarily, the progestin component produces changes in the cervical mucus and the endometrium that enhance the infertility effect of OCPs should ovulation occur. Because failure rates associated with OCP use relate to individual compliance, they range from less than 1 of 100 woman-years in women who are highly compliant, to greater than 15 of 100 woman-years among inner-city teenagers. Discontinuation rates in the United States during the first year range from 50% to 60%. Two thirds of patients discontinue use of their OCPs without consulting their health care provider.

Since 1992, all OCP preparations in the United States that contain 35 µg or less of estrogen use ethynyl estradiol (EE). Combined OCPs also include one of seven progestins: Norethindrone, levonorgestrel, norgestrel, norethindrone acetate, ethynodiol, and the two newest, norgestimate and desogestrel. Another new progestin, gestodene, may be available soon. A new OCP patch (EURA) is currently being tested.

Monophasic OCPs have a constant dose of estrogen and progestin in each of the 21 tablets of active hormones in each cycle pack. Phasic OCPs alter the dose of progestin (and in some combinations, estrogen) among the 21 active tablets in each pack. After the last pill in a 21-day pack is taken, a 7-day tablet-free period follows. In the 28-tablet packets, pills for the first 21 days contain active ingredients, and the remaining 7 pills contain inactive ingredients. In formulating phasic OCPs, manufacturers have lowered the monthly steroid dose with the aim of reducing metabolic effects while maintaining contraceptive efficacy and cycle control.

The forms of combined OCPs are outlined in Table 198-3.

Advantages

Combined OCPs are a highly effective method of birth control. Other noncontraceptive benefits are listed below

- Menstruation improvements
  - More regular and predictable menses
  - Reduced prevalence and severity of dysmenorrhea
  - Reduction in days and amount of menstrual flow
  - Increased iron stores in women with menorrhagia
  - Restoration of regular menses in anovulatory women
  - Reduction in symptoms of premenstrual syndrome (PMS)
- Prevention of benign conditions
  - Benign breast disease (fibroadenoma and cystic changes)
  - Pelvic inflammatory disease (PID)
  - Ectopic pregnancy
- Prevention of gynecological malignancies
  - Ovarian cancer
  - Endometrial adenocarcinoma
- Possible benefits
  - Prevention of functional ovarian cysts
  - Prevention of rheumatoid arthritis
  - Increased bone mineral density

TABLE 198-3 Combined Oral Contraceptive Pills

Type	Preparation	
Combination monophasic	Loestrin	Loestrin FE 1/20
	Loestrin 1.5/30	Loestrin FE 1.5/30
	BreviconNorethin 1/35E	Modicon
	Ortho Novum 1/35	Norinyl 1 + 35E
		Ovcon 35
	Ovcon 50	Alesse
	Levlen	Nordette
	Lo/Ovral	Ovral
	Demulen 1/35	Demulen 1/50
	Norethin 1/50M	Norinyl 1 + 50
	Desogen	Ortho-Cept
	Ortho-Cyclen	
Combination biphasic	Ortho-Novum 10/11	
	Jesest-28	
Combination triphasic	Ortho-Novum 7/7/7	
	Tri-Norinyl	
	Ortho Tri-Cyclen	
	Tri-Levlen	
	Triphasil	
Combination estrophasic	Estrostep 21	
	Estrostep FE	
Progestin-only pills (POP)	Micronor	Nor-QD
	Ovrette	

Disadvantages

Effectiveness depends on consistent daily use.

Risks

Small adverse effect on lipids, although probably not atherogenic.

Rare thrombotic events; usually limited to smokers and those with a preexisting (although often unknown) hypercoagulable state. In smokers over 35 years old, the risk of death from this cause exceeds the risk of death from accidental pregnancy, thus contraindicating the use of OCPs.

Between 1% and 5% of women develop hypertension, which is reversible with cessation of OCP use.

Previously controlled hypertension may worsen after use is initiated; however, a trial of OCPs is warranted.

The relative risk of an ectopic pregnancy is increased with failure of this birth control method.

The incidence of gallstones is increased.

There may be a slight increase in lifetime risk of cervical cancer.

Tricyclic preparations may increase the risk of functional ovarian cysts.

The relative risks of hepatic adenoma and hepatocellular carcinoma are increased, but absolute risk is negligible.

Concurrent use with antibiotics may decrease the effectiveness of OCPs. (See Appendix K.)

Side Effects (Boxes 198-3 and 198-4)

Systemic: Symptoms similar to those of early pregnancy (nausea, fluid retention, breast tenderness) may occur during the first two or three cycles. Some women report changes in libido and mood and frank depression. Increased appetite may lead to weight gain, though weight loss is equally common.

Reproductive tract: Breakthrough bleeding is common in the first three cycles. Menstrual bleeding is often scant. Amenorrhea may occur occasionally; if it persists for two or more consecutive cycles, test for pregnancy and then consider change of OCP formulation.

Neurological: New onset of migraine with pill use requires discontinuation. Preexisting common migraines are not necessarily a contraindication.

Dermatological: Oily skin and exacerbation of acne are fairly common, hair loss less so. Melasma occurs rarely.

Contraindications

Contraindications to the use of OCPs are listed in Table 198-4.

Counseling

Educate the patient about how OCPs work:

Describe advantages and disadvantages.

Ask her how she thinks the pills work. Correct any misconceptions.

Discuss use of backup contraception methods.

Show her the pill pack: Demonstrate how to start and how it works.

Help her to associate pill taking with everyday activities, such as brushing her teeth.

Review what she should do if she misses a pill.

Discuss side effects and how they might be dealt with.

Give written instructions (pill information has been written at a fifth-grade reading level since 1994).

Discuss the issue of emergency contraception.

For continuing users: Ask about pills at every visit: Are you taking a pill every day? What do you do if you miss a pill?

Interaction Between OCPs and Other Drugs

Possible drug interactions are outlined in Table 198-5.

Box 198-3

Relationship of Side Effects to Hormone Content

Estrogen Excess

General Symptoms

Chloasma
Chronic nasal pharyngitis
Gastric influenza and varicella
Hay fever and allergic rhinitis
UTIs

Premenstrual Syndrome

Bloating
Dizziness, syncope
Edema
Headaches (cyclic)
Irritability
Nausea and vomiting
Leg cramps
Visual changes (cyclic)
Weight gain (cyclic)

Reproductive System

Breast cystic changes
Cervical ecstrophy
Dysmenorrhea, menstrual cramps
Hypermenorrhea, menorrhagia, heavy flow and clots
Increase in breast size
Mucorrhea
Uterine enlargement
Uterine fibroid growth
Cervicitis
Flow length decreased
Moniliasis

Cardiovascular System

Capillary fragility
CVA
DVT, hemiparesis
Telangiectasis
Thromboembolic disease
Vascular headaches

Progestin Excess

Progestinal Symptoms

Appetite increased
Depression
Fatigability
Hyperglycemic symptoms
Libido decreased
Neurodermatitis
Tiredness
Weight gain (noncyclic)

Cardiovascular System

Hypertension
Leg veins dilated
Hyperlipidemia

Androgenic Symptoms

Acne
Cholestatic jaundice
Hirsutism
Libido increased
Oily skin and scalp
Rash and pruritus

Box 198-4

Progestin Androgenic Activity

Low

30-35 μEE

Cyclen, Tri-Cyclen, Ortho-Cept, Desogen, Modicon, Brevicon, Nelova 0.5/35, NEE 0.5/35, Ovcon 35

Medium

50 μg EE

Ovcon 50, Genora 1/50, Norethin 1/50, Norethin 1/50M, Norinyl 1+50, Demulen

30-35 μg EE

Triphasil, TriLevlen, ON 1/35, Norinyl 1+35, Genora 1/35, Norethin 1/35E, Norcept 1/35, Nelova 1/35, NEE 1/35, ON777, Tri-Norinyl, Estrastep, Demulen 1/35

20 μg EE

Alesse, Loestrin 1/20

High

50 μg EE

Norlestrin 2.5/50

30-35 μg EE

LoOvral, Loestrin 1.5/30, Nordette, Levlen

EE, Ethinyl estradiol.

Laboratory Tests Affected by OCPs

Values That Are Increased (Serum Values Unless Otherwise Stated)

α_1-Antitrypsin
Erythrocyte sedimentation rate (ESR), sometimes hematocrit, WBC, platelets
Alkaline phosphatase
Clotting factors I, II, VII, VIII, IX, X, and XII; also increased antiplasmins and antiactivators of fibrinolysis
Coproporphyrin (feces and urine) and porphobilinogen (urine)
C-reactive protein
Globulins (α_1 and α_2)
Increase in various binding proteins (transferrin, transcortin, thyroxine-binding globulin)
Insulin, growth hormone, and blood glucose
Positive ANA and LE preparation
Renin-angiotensin, angiotensinogen, and aldosterone
Serum copper and ceruloplasmin
Serum glutamic oxaloacetic transaminase, serum glutamic pyruvic transaminase, and serum γ-glutamyl transpeptidase
Serum iron and iron-binding capacity
Sulfobromophthalein and sometimes bilirubin
Total estrogens (urine)
Total T_4

TABLE 198-4 Contraindications to OCP Use

Type of Contraindication	Condition
Absolute	Current or past thrombolytic disease, cerebrovascular event, coronary artery disease; breast, liver, or reproductive tract carcinoma; smoker over 35 years old; current liver dysfunction; diabetes with clinical vascular disease (nephropathy, neuropathy, retinopathy, peripheral)
Relative	Undiagnosed vaginal bleeding; total cholesterol > 300 mg/dl or LDL cholesterol >140 mg/dl; acute phase of mononucleosis; elective surgery planned within the next 4 weeks or major surgery requiring immobilization planned; long leg casts or major injury to lower legs

LDL, Low-density lipoproteins.

TABLE 198-5 Interactions Between OCPs and Other Drugs

Contraceptive Unchanged, Drug Decreased	Contraceptive Unchanged, Drug Increased	Contraceptive Increased, Drug Unchanged	Contraceptive Decreased, Drug Unchanged
Acetaminophen*	Chlordiazepoxide	Ascorbic acid	Antibiotics‡ (see Appendix K)
Aspirin*	Corticosteroids†	Co-trimoxazole	Anticonvulsants‡
Clofibrate	Diazepam†		Griseofulvin§
Lorazepam	Imipramine HCl†		Purgatives
Morphine*	Meperidine†		Rifampin§
Oxazepam*	Metoprolol tartrate†		
Temazepam*	Theophylline†		
	Triazolam†		
	Vitamin A		

*Increase the dose of the drug.
†Decrease dose of drug needed, decrease by about one third.
‡With spotting, increase OCP dose; otherwise no management change needed.
§Increase OCP dose or change contraceptive method to avert contraception.

Triglycerides, phospholipids, and high-density lipoproteins (HDL); sometimes total cholesterol
Vitamin A
Xanthurenic acid (urine)

Values That Are Decreased

Antithrombin II
Ascorbic acid
Cholinesterase
Fibrinolytic activity
Folate and vitamin B_{12}
Glucose tolerance
Haptoglobin
LH and FSH
Pregnanediol and 17-ketosteroids
T_3 resin uptake
Zinc and magnesium

Choosing the Appropriate Combined OCP

Suggestions for which OCP to choose are outlined in Table 198-6.

Common complaints: Do not change pills until 3 months of pills have been taken.
Spotting: Remind the patient to take a pill at the same time each day. Allow three menstrual cycles for spotting to resolve; rule out missed doses, drug interactions, and pathological conditions.
Breakthrough bleeding in the first 2 weeks of the cycle: Change to a pill with higher estrogen.
Breakthrough bleeding in the last 2 weeks of the cycle: Change to a pill with higher progestin.

Patient Instructions

Sunday starters: Instruct the patient to begin the first package of pills the Sunday after her period begins. If her period starts on Sunday, she should begin the package of pills then.
First-day starters: Instruct the patient to begin the first package of pills on the first day of the period. Whichever day of the week the patient starts her first package of pills, instruct her to start each new pack on the same day.
Whenever the patient starts or restarts taking the pill, she is to use a back-up method of birth control for 1 week.

TABLE 198-6 Choosing a Combined Oral Contraceptive Pill

Patient Characteristics	First Choice	Second Choice
Average/teenager	Low androgenic (Ortho-Novum 1/35, Ortho-Novum 7/7/7, LoOvral)	Medium androgenic <35 μg EE
Obese with heavy periods/dysmenorrhea	High androgen (Nordette, Loestrin 1.5/30, Loestrin 1/20, Demulen 1/35)	
Perimenopausal	Low androgenic, may need to switch to a pill with a different type of progestin (Loestrin 1/20, Ortho-Novum 7/7/7)	Medium androgenic
Postpartum (lactating)	If no supplemental feedings and no menses, conception unlikely for 3 mo; POP for 6 weeks after delivery	May replace with OCP when feeding supplements are initiated
Postpartum (nonlactating)	Low androgenic; may need to switch to pill with a different type of progestin	Medium androgenic
Break-through bleeding (BTB)	Lowest incidence of BTB: 30-35 μg estrogen with either levonorgestrel, norgestimate, or desogestrel (Triphasil [levo], TriLevlen [levo], Levlen [levo], Nordette [levo], Cyclin [norg], TriCyclin [norg], Desogen [deso], Ortho-Cept [deso])	
Weight gain/obesity	Low androgenic (change to lower estrogen: Triphasil, Tri-Levlen, Brevicon, Ovcon 35)	Medium androgenic
Headache, common migraine	Low androgenic (may need to switch to different progestin pill); if headache occurs during pill-free interval, consider once-daily continuous combined OCPs to avoid cycling	Medium androgenic
Nausea	Low androgenic; nausea usually related to estrogenic activity; try 20-μg EE pill or Estrastep	
Breast tenderness	Low androgenic	
Mood changes	Low androgenic (may need to switch to different progestin pill)	Medium androgenic
Acne/hirsutism	Low androgenic. Tri-Cyclen is the only OCP with FDA approval for acne	Medium androgenic
Adverse lipid effects (except triglycerides)	Low androgenic	Medium androgenic
Hypertension (controlled)	Low androgenic	Medium androgenic
↑ Triglycerides	OCPS are contraindicated >350-600 mg/dl With mild elevations: Cyclen or Tri-Cyclen	
Smoker 30-35 years old	Low androgenic or medium androgenic <50 μg EE	
Heavy smoker <30 years old	Low androgenic or medium androgenic <50 μg EE	
+FH of CAD	Low androgenic	Medium androgenic
Classic migraine	Contraindicated	
Depression	Low androgenic, may need to switch to different progestin	Medium androgenic
+ FH breast cancer	Low androgenic	Medium androgenic
PMH of breast cancer	Contraindicated	
Benign breast disease	Low androgenic	Medium androgenic
Uterine fibroids	Low androgenic	Medium androgenic
DM	Low androgenic	Medium androgenic

Modified from Pfaff R: Untitled, Covington, Ky, 1997, Northern Kentucky Family Health Centers, Inc.

CAD, Coronary artery disease; *DM*, diabetes mellitus; *EE*, ethinylestradiol; *+FH*, positive family history; *OCP*, over-the-counter pill; *POP*, progestin-only pill; *PMH*, past medical history.

TABLE 198-6 Choosing a Combined Oral Contraceptive Pill—cont'd

Patient Characteristics	First Choice	Second Choice
Antiepileptic drugs	Formulations containing 50 μg may be preferable	
+FH of ovarian disease	Low androgenic	Medium androgenic
Sickle cell	Low androgenic	Medium androgenic
Prosthetic heart valves, anticoagulant user, mitral valve prolapse	Low androgenic	Medium androgenic
Menstrual cycle irregularities	Low androgenic	Medium androgenic
Persistent anovulation	Low androgenic	Medium androgenic
Premature ovarian failure	Low androgenic	Medium androgenic
Dysmenorrhea	Low androgenic	Medium androgenic
Functional ovarian cysts	Low androgenic (monophasic only)	Medium androgenic
Mittelschmerz	Low androgenic	Medium androgenic
Endometriosis	Medium androgenic (monophasic, continuous) (Ovral)	High androgenic (monophasic, continuous)
Bleeding with blood dyscrasias	Medium androgenic (continuous)	High androgenic (continuous)
Loss of libido	High androgenic activity	

After she has finished the packet of pills, she is to take the first tablet from the next packet the following day. *She is to take a pill every day of the week.*

Instruct her to take one pill every day around the same time.

What To Do if the Patient Misses a Pill

If she misses one pill: Take the pill immediately as soon as she remembers. A backup method is recommended

If she misses two pills in a row during the first 2 weeks: Take two pills on the day she remembers and two pills the next day. Take one pill a day until the pack is empty. Use a back-up contraceptive method for 7 days after the pills are missed.

If she misses two pills in a row in the third week or misses three or more pills in a row at any time:

Sunday starter: Instruct the patient to keep taking a pill every day until the next Sunday. On Sunday she is to throw away the unused portion of the packet and start a new pack and must use a back-up contraceptive method for 7 days after the pills are missed.

First-day starter: Instruct the patient to throw out the rest of the current packet of pills and to start a new packet on the usual start day. She must use a back-up contraceptive method for 7 days after the pills are missed.

Common Side Effects

Nausea: Take pills with a meal. Take at night before going to bed.

Bleeding or spotting between periods: Common during the first 3 months. If spotting continues after 3 months, consider changing pills. Use a back-up contraceptive method when spotting occurs.

Danger Signs While Taking the Pill

A Abdominal pain, new, severe
C Chest pain, new, severe
H Headaches, new or more frequent
E Eye problems, blurred or loss of vision
S Severe pain, swelling, numbness in an arm or leg
Also jaundice or extreme depression

Follow-up

Patients should return 3 months after starting a pill or after changing the pill to check blood pressure and tolerance of the pill. Thereafter she should be given a prescription for 13 months (a years' worth of pills) plus one additional packet (for emergencies). Yearly Pap and breast examinations should be done.

PROGESTIN-ONLY PILLS

Overview

Progestin-only pills (POPs) primarily work by inducting genital tract changes associated with the luteal phase. Ovulation is inconsistently suppressed.

Effectiveness

The first-year failure rate is 0.5% with perfect use, 3% with typical use. The 1-year continuation rate is 72%.

Advantages

POPs are highly effective with consistent use. They eliminate estrogenic and thrombotic side effects and the risks associated with combined OCPs. POPs may be used immediately postpartum with no adverse effects if breastfeeding.

Disadvantages

Effectiveness is dependent on consistent, daily use, which may be difficult. This is even more important with POPs than with OCPs, where an occasional missed pill is better tolerated.

Risks

There are no known carcinogenics or teratogenicity associated with POPs. The relative risk of ectopic pregnancy is increased in case of failure. There is an increased rate of functional ovarian cysts.

Side Effects

Menstrual irregularities indicate consistent or intermittent anovulation (and higher efficacy); many women continue having regular ovulatory cycles. Any of the side effects listed for combined OCPs may occur with POPs, although incidence is much lower.

Contraindications

Undiagnosed irregular vaginal bleeding, current genital tract cancer, active liver disease

Drug Interactions

None of clinical significance

Pill Selection

Only two formulations are available in the United States: Norethindrone and norgestrel (Micronor, Nor-QD, and Ovrette respectively). There is no compelling reason to choose one over the other.

Patient Education

Emphasize consistency of use.

Stress that unlike combined OCPs, there are no monthly pill-free intervals and no placebo pills that can be ignored. *A pill must be taken daily, without exception.*

Follow-up

Schedule a follow-up visit for 3 months after starting POPs to evaluate the patient's blood pressure and tolerance to the pill.

If the patient is taking POPs because she is breastfeeding, consider changing to a combined OCP when she begins supplemental feedings.

EMERGENCY CONTRACEPTION

Overview

Definition

Emergency Contraceptive Pills

The emergency contraceptive pill (ECP) is sometimes known as the "morning-after pill" or "postcoital" contraception. There are three primary methods of emergency contraception:

ECPs: The most commonly used emergency contraceptive method; safe for most women. Treatment must be initiated within 72 hours after unprotected intercourse and requires two elevated doses of regular combined OCPs taken 12 hours apart. This effective and well-researched method is known as the "Yuzpe regimen" (Table 198-7).

Progestin-only Pills

POPs can also be used for emergency contraception; treatment must be initiated within 48 hours after unprotected intercourse; requires two doses taken 12 hours apart. Limited data suggest POPs are equal in effectiveness to the Yuzpe regimen but cause fewer side effects. A much larger number of pills must be taken.

Copper T IUD

Insertion of a Copper T IUD within 5 days after unprotected intercourse also can prevent pregnancy. Advan-

TABLE 198-7 Types of Emergency Contraceptive Pills*

ECP	Number of Pills to Be Taken Immediately	Number of Pills to Be Taken 12 Hours Later
Ovral	2 White pills	2 White pills
LoOvral	4 White pills	4 White pills
Levlen	4 Light orange pills	4 Light orange pills
Nordette	4 Light orange pills	4 Light orange pills
Tri-Levlen	4 Yellow pills	4 Yellow pills
Triphasil	4 Yellow pills	4 Yellow pills
Ovrette	20 Pills	20 Pills

*Commercial products are now available that package the needed pills together (approximate cost, $20). "Preven" contains levonorgestrel, 25 mg plus ethinyl estradiol, 50 μg (4 tablets), plus one urine HCG pregnancy test.

tages of the IUD include the wider time interval for administration, the ongoing contraception benefit it offers to women who elect to leave the IUD in place, and a very low failure rate. The IUD is generally not recommended for women at risk for sexually transmitted infections.

Mechanism of Action

The mechanism of action of ECPs has not been clearly established. Several studies have shown that ECPs can inhibit or delay ovulation. It has also been suggested that ECPs may inhibit ovulation or delay ovulation. It has also been suggested that ECPs may prevent implantation by altering the endometrium. ECP may also prevent fertilization or transport of sperm or ova, but no data exist regarding these possible mechanisms. ECPs do not interrupt an existing pregnancy.

Information to Obtain

Date of last menstrual period (LMP)
Was this a normal period?
Are menstrual cycles regular?
Usual method of birth control
When did the patient have unprotected intercourse? (Date and time)
Were there other instances of unprotected intercourse since her last period?
Are there any contraindications to birth control pills?
Circumstance of unprotected intercourse (rape, consensual intercourse)
Any other medications?
Feelings about possibility of unintended pregnancy
Knowledge of contraception and experience in use of contraceptive methods

Laboratory Data

Urine pregnancy test ($18 to $24)
Other testing as deemed appropriate in case of rape

Drug Interactions

The effectiveness of combined OCPs is reduced for women who concurrently use anticonvulsants or the antibiotics rifampin or griseofulvin. Combined OCP use can also affect the potency of some medications such as anticoagulants and antidepressants. It is not known whether similar drug interactions are associated with one-time, short-term ECP use. In patients taking drugs that reduce combined OCP effectiveness, the ECP dose can be doubled.

Management of Side Effects

Nausea is a common side effect of ECP use. If vomiting occurs 1 hour after taking the pills, it is likely that sufficient quantities of the hormone have been absorbed. If vomiting occurs in less than 1 hour, or if the pills are visible in the emesis, a replacement dose may be warranted. Nonprescription antiemetic agents are listed in Table 198-8.

Special Circumstances

Presenting After 72 Hours

The effectiveness of ECP treatment later than 72 hours after unprotected intercourse has not been well documented. It is not likely that the efficacy drops to zero, so treatment after 72 hours may be reasonable. Unprotected intercourse that occurred more than 72 hours before ECP treatment may have resulted in pregnancy. If a woman is pregnant, ECP will not interrupt or harm the pregnancy. The Copper T IUD may be a more appropriate choice.

Multiple Acts of Unprotected Intercourse

There may be some situations in which the patient had unprotected intercourse more than once, with some acts of intercourse occurring more than 72 hours before seeking treatment and some occurring within the 72 hour window. If the interval since the first unprotected intercourse is more than 72 hours, the ECP treatment may not be effective in preventing pregnancy. In this case, however, using ECPs

TABLE 198-8 Nonprescription Antiemetics

Drug	Dose	Timing of Administration	Cost
Meclizine HCl (Dramamine II, Bonine)	1-2 25-mg tablets	1 hr before each ECP dose	$3-$31/12.5 mg (100); $3-$49/25 mg (100)
Diphenhydramine HCl (Benadryl)	1-2 25-mg tablets	1 hr before first ECP dose; repeat as necessary q4-6h	$2-$22/25 mg (100)
Dimenhydrinate (Dramamine)	1-2 50-mg tablets or 4-8 tsp Dramamine liquid	30 min to 1 hr before first ECP dose, repeat as needed every 4-6 hr	$2-$6/50 mg (100)
Cyclizine HCl (Marezine)	1 50-mg tablet	30 min before first ECP dose; repeat as needed q4-6h	Not available

will not disrupt or harm the pregnancy, and ECP treatment can reduce the risk of pregnancy resulting from later unprotected sex that occurred within the 72-hour window.

Initiating Regular Contraception After ECP Use

Condom: May be used immediately.
Diaphragm: May be used immediately.
Spermicide: May be used immediately.
OCPs: Consider starting regular OCPs immediately after ECP treatment. After taking both ECP dosages from a new pill pack, patients using LoOvral, Levlen, or Nordette can initiate regular use of these pills by taking one pill a day until the pack is finished. Patients should be advised to use a condom for added protection for the first week they are taking the pills. High-dose and triphasic formulations are not recommended for this follow-up regimen.
Depo Provera: Initiate during next menstrual cycle.
Implants: Initiate during next menstrual cycle.
IUD: Initiate during the next menstrual period if an IUD was not used as emergency contraception.
FAM: Initiate this method after onset of menstrual cycle if the next period is normal. If FAM is new to the patient, initiate after proper instruction and monitoring.
Sterilization: Perform any time after next menstrual cycle.

Follow-up

If no menses begins after 4 weeks, advise the patient to return for a pregnancy test. Have patient schedule an appointment for a pelvic examination, Pap smear, and cultures if she is going to initiate contraceptives.

SUGGESTED READINGS

ACOG Practice Patterns: *Emergency oral contraception,* No 2, 1996.

ACOG Technical Bulletin: *Hormonal contraception,* No 198, 1994.

ACOG Technical Bulletin: *The intrauterine device,* No 164, 1992.

ACOG Technical Bulletin: *Sterilization*, No 222, 1996.

Dickey R: *Managing contraceptive pill patients,* ed 9, Durant, Okla, 1994, Essential Medical Information Systems.

Emergency contraception: a resource manual for providers, Seattle, 1997, Path.

Hawkins J, Roberto-Nichols D, Stanley-Haney J: *Methods of family planning: protocols for nurse practitioners in gynecologic settings,* New York 1995, Tiresias Press.

Hatcher R et al: *Contraceptive technology,* ed 16, New York, 1994, Irvington Publishers.

Geruts T, Goorissen E, Sitsen J: *Summary of drug interactions with oral contraceptives*, New York, 1993, Parthenon Publishing Group.

Gold M, Coupey S: Young women's attitudes toward injectable and implantable contraceptives, *J Pediatr Adolesc Gynecol* 11:17-24, 1998.

Kauntiz A, Benrubi G: The good news about hormonal contraception and gynecologic cancer, *Female Patient* vol 23, 1998.

Kaunitz A, Ory H: Estrogen component of OC selection, *Dialog Contracept* vol 5, 1997.

Matheson C et al: Over-the-counter emergency contraception: a feasible option, *Family Practice* 15:38-43, 1998.

Mishell D et al: Practice guidelines for OC selection: update, *Dial Contracept* vol 5, 1997.

Long-term reversible contraception: twelve years of experience with the TCu380A and TCu220C, *Contraception* 56:341-352, 1997.

O'Dell C: Depot medroxyprogesterone acetate or oral contraception in postpartum adolescents, *Obstet Gynecol* 91:609-614, 1998.

Wysocki S: Improving patient success with oral contraceptives: the importance of counseling, *Nurse Pract* 23:51-62, 1998.

Lifestyle Changes

Smoking Cessation, Nutrition, Stress Management, and Exercise

ICD-9-CM

Tobacco Abuse 305.1
Dietary Counseling V65.3
Exercise Counseling V65.41
Health Advice Counseling V65.49
Counseling Injury Prevention V65.43

SMOKING CESSATION

The adverse effects of smoking tobacco are well known. Approximately 430,000 deaths are caused by cigarette smoking in the United States (Fiore, 1991). The prevalence of smoking in adolescents has stabilized since 1987; today approximately 21% of high school seniors smoke vs. 19% in 1987. However, the age of initiation of the habit is occurring at younger ages. Experimenting with smoking occurs most frequently in sixth grade, and the initiation of daily smoking occurs most often in grades 7 to 9 (Rasco, 1992).

Associated Risks of Smoking

Lung cancer
Other cancers
Emphysema
Respiratory infections
Coronary artery disease (CAD)
Cerebrovascular accident (CVA)
Pregnant women: Adverse effects on fetus, increasing risk of miscarriage, stillbirth, and low–birth-weight infant
Secondhand or passive smoke exposure
Bronchitis, pneumonia
Colds, ear infections
Asthma in infants and young children

Benefits of Smoking Cessation

Increases life expectancy
Reduces risk of:
- Dying within next 15 years by half if the individual quits before age 50
- Premature death in all ages
- Lung cancer, and cancer of larynx, oral cavity, esophagus, pancreas, bladder and uterine cervix
- Coronary artery disease (CAD)
- Peripheral vascular disease (PVD)
- Ischemic stroke and hemorrhage
- Respiratory symptoms

Why Smokers Smoke

Smoking cues/triggers
Peer pressure/socialization
Emotional dependence
Oral gratification
Relaxation and stress reduction
Need for reward
Physiological addiction to nicotine

The opportunity exists for nurse practitioners to reach millions of people with smoking-cessation advice, since 70% of all smokers are seen by a health care provider. Consider evaluation of smoking status to be a vital sign, along with blood pressure, pulse, respirations, and temperature (Robinson, et al, 1995).

ASSESSMENT OF SMOKING STATUS

Current smoker
- Determine whether the patient has ever tried to quit before
- Determine length of time off cigarettes, problems encountered, reasons for relapse

Former smoker
- Ask these questions about smoking:
  - Number of years smoked daily
  - Number of years as smoker
  - Depth of inhalation
- Review symptoms related to smoking:
  - Cough
  - SOB
  - Sputum production
  - Recurrent respiratory infections
- Family history of tobacco related diseases:
  - CAD
  - Chronic obstructive pulmonary disease
  - Cancer

Never smoked

Physical Examination

Make the physical examination an intervention

Highlight the relationship of the cardiovascular system and lungs

Relate relevant findings: Hoarse cough, diminished breath sounds, wheezes

Correlate peak expiratory flow rate findings to smoking

OPPORTUNITIES FOR INTERVENTION

Each time a smoker makes a visit: advise about smoking cessation

Ask if the patient has ever thought about quitting

The smoking cessation stages are outlined in Table 199-1.

Most smokers cycle through these stages three to four times before they quit for good. Relapse is a normal part of the smoking cessation process and should not be viewed as failure (Figure 199-1).

How to Intervene

Ask all patients if they smoke

Mark charts

Advise all smokers to stop

Strong, unequivocal message:
- "You must stop smoking now. Let's figure out how you can do it."
- "I am concerned about your smoking. I must highly recommend that you quit."

Personalize message: Relate to their disease, social role, etc.

Assist smokers who want to quit

Identify a quit date

Administer the Fagerstrom Test for Nicotine Dependence (Table 199-2)

Develop a stop-smoking contract

Provide self-help materials

Smoking cessation programs

Pharmacological therapy

Arrange follow-up visits

Phone the patient within 7 days of initial visit to remind the patient of quit date; reinforces decision to quit

Follow-up within first 2 weeks: Support and encouragement

Identify relapse risks

Help patient identify specific tempting situations and discuss ways to avoid these situations

Help patient to find something else to do instead of smoke in these situations

Set up a reward system

Nonpharmacological Strategies

Aversive conditioning

Hypnosis

Acupuncture

Behavior modification

TABLE 199-1 Stages of Smoking Cessation

Stage	Description
Precontemplation	Smoker is not considering quitting in the next 6 months. May rebuff efforts to advise him or her to quit. Nurse practitioner should back off and approach another visit. Pushing before the patient is ready is not a good idea. Patient may be set up for failure if he or she tries to quit before ready, which discourages desire to try again.
Contemplation	Smoker is seriously considering quitting within next 6 months. Amenable to advice, educational materials, and information about adverse effects of smoking. Often motivated by thoughts of cleaner teeth, better breath, no smoking odors on clothing, and improved self-esteem if he or she stops.
Preparation	Smoker is ready to change and intends to quit within next 30 days. Ready for information about behavioral counseling or pharmacological therapy
Action	Characterized by cessation and abstinence for 6 months.
Maintenance	Maintenance begins after 6 months and continues for up to 3 years. Important to understand the process from current smoker to former smoker is a long-term process.

Modified from Fiore M: Smoking status: the new vital sign, *JAMA* 266:3183-3184, 1991.

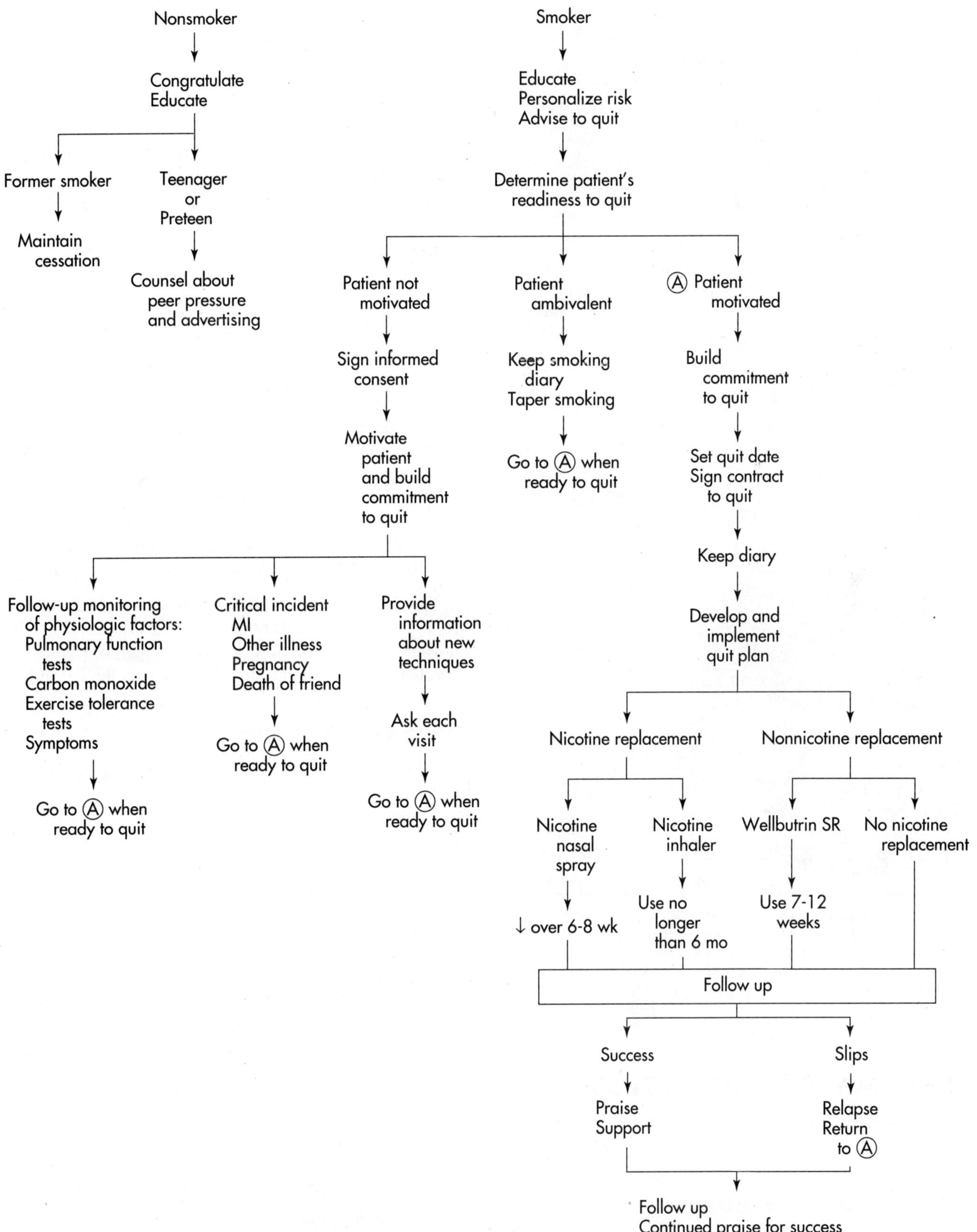

Figure 199-1 Algorithm for patient undergoing smoking prevention or cessation. (Modified from Greene HL, Johnson WP, Lemcke D: *Decision making in medicine,* ed 2, St Louis, 1998, Mosby.)

TABLE 199-2 The Fagerstrom Test for Nicotine Dependence

	Score
How soon after you wake up do you smoke your first cigarette?	
Within 5 minutes	3
6-30 minutes	2
31-60 minutes	1
After 60 minutes	0
Do you find it difficult to refrain from smoking in places where it is forbidden (e.g., in church, at the library, in the theater)?	
Yes	1
No	0
Which cigarette would you hate most to give up?	
The first one in the morning	1
All others	0
How many cigarettes do you smoke per day?	
<10	0
11-20	1
21-30	2
>31	3
Do you smoke more frequently during the first hours after waking than during the rest of the day?	
Yes	1
No	0
Do you smoke if you are so ill that you are in bed most of the day?	
Yes	1
No	0
Score:	
0-2 = very low	
3-4 = low	
5 = medium	
6-7 = high	
8-10 = very high	

Adapted from Heatherton TF, et al: The Fagerstrom test for nicotine dependence: a revision of the Fagerstrom Tolerance Questionnaire, *Br J Addict* 86:1119-1127, 1991; and Fagerstrom KO, Heatherton TF, Kozlowski LT: Nicotine addiction and its assessment, *Ear Nose Throat J* 69:763-768, 1990.

PHARMACOLOGICAL STRATEGIES

Pharmaceutical treatment approaches are outlined in Table 199-3.

Withdrawal Symptoms

Symptoms last days or weeks (Table 199-4):

- Craving for nicotine
- Irritability
- Restlessness
- Increased appetite
- Decreased concentration

NUTRITION

Increasing emphasis is being placed on the importance of nutrition. Eating healthy, along with exercise and weight control, is a big emphasis of the Healthy People 2000 goals. Lifestyle changes in dietary patterns can make substantial contributions to reductions in illness and preventable death. Some of the goals identified by Health People 2000 are:

- Reduce dietary fat intake.
- Increase complex carbohydrate and fiber-containing foods.
- Increase sound dietary practices combined with regular physical activity to attain appropriate body weight.
- Reduce overweight to a prevalence of no more than 20% among people aged 20 and older, and no more than 15% among adolescents aged 12 through 19.
- Increase the number of primary care providers who offer nutritional assessment and counseling and referral to qualified nutritionists or dietitians.

The largest group at risk for malnutrition is the **elderly** (Stark, 1994). Nutrition screening should be conducted for anyone who is 20% below desirable weight, or who has an involuntary loss of more than 10 pounds in the last month.

Nutrition Screening

Nutrition screening may include the following (Seidel et al, 1995):

- Anthropometric measurements
  - Body mass index
  - Desirable weight
  - Elbow breadth
  - Height/weight
  - Midarm circumference
  - Triceps skinfold
  - Waist/hip circumference
- Biochemical measurement
  - Cholesterol
  - Electrolytes
  - HDLs
  - Hematocrit
  - Hemoglobin
  - LDL/HDL ratio
  - LDLs
  - Nitrogen balance
  - Serum albumin
  - Serum transferrin
  - Triglycerides
  - Vitamin levels

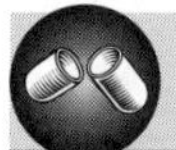

TABLE 199-3 Pharmaceutical Treatment: Smoking Cessation

Drug	Dosage	Comments	Cost
Nicotine gum	<25 cigarettes/day: 2 mg >25 cigarettes/day: 4 mg Chew one piece of gum slowly and intermittently over 30 min every 1-2 hr for 6 wk, then q2-4h for 3 wk, then q4-8h for 3 wk, then discontinue	Stop smoking. Do not eat or drink for 15 min and during use. Avoid acidic foods and beverages. Pregnancy: D Trauma to oral mucosa, teeth and dental work, jaw ache, GI discomfort, hiccups, tachycardia	$38/2 mg (96); $65/4 mg (96)
Nicotine transdermal patch (Habitrol)	Healthy patients: Begin with 21-mg patch QD for 4-8 wk, then 14 mg QD for 2-4 wk, then 7 mg QD for 2-4 wk, then discontinue Other patients: Begin with 14 mg/day	Stop smoking. Apply to clean, dry, nonhairy site on trunk or upper outer arm. Some patches should be removed after 16 hr. Dose may need to be adjusted by amount person smoked. Pregnancy: D SE: Local erythema, contact hypersensitivity, tobacco withdrawal symptoms, tachycardia, spontaneous abortion	$110/7 mg (30); $116/14 mg (30); $122/21 mg (30)
Nicoderm CQ	Healthy patients or if smoke >10 cigarettes/day: 21 mg/day for 6 wk, then 14 mg/day for 2 wk, then 7 mg/day for 2 wk Other patients or those who smoke <10 cigarettes/day: 14 mg/day for 6 wk, then 7 mg/day for 2-4 wk	As for Habitrol	$50/7 mg (14); $54/14 mg (14); $58/21 mg (14)
Nicotrol	15 mg/day for 4-12 wk, then 10 mg/day for 2-4 wk then 5 mg/day for 2-4 wk	As for Habitrol	$27/15 mg (7)
Prostep	100 lb: 22 mg/day for 4-8 wk, then 11 mg/day for 2-4 wk >100 lb: 11 mg/day for 4-8 wk	As for Habitrol	$30/11 mg (7); $32/22 mg (7)
Nicotine nasal spray (Nicotrol)	Usually 1-2 doses/hr Maximum: 5 sprays/hr or 40/day; set quit date Gradually decrease over 6-8 wk	Do not sniff, swallow, or inhale spray. Pregnancy: D SE: Local effects, nasopharyngeal irritation, tobacco withdrawal symptoms, tachycardia	$36/1% (10 ml)
Nicotine inhaler	Each puff delivers 4 mg of nicotine Self-titrate to level of nicotine required Initially 6-16 cartridges during the day Inhale using shallow, frequent puffs or deep inhalations Use should not continue past 6 mo	Each cartridge holds 300-400 puffs, but once opened it is good for only 1 day (thought to mimic hand-to-mouth ritual). Use with caution in patients with bronchospastic disease. Pregnancy: D SE: Dyspepsia, irritation, soreness in mouth and throat, oral burning, coughing after inhalation, rhinitis.	N/A
Bupropion (Zyban)	150 mg QD for 3 days, then increase to 150 mg BID Maximum: 300 mg/day Dispense behavioral modification kit in first treatment visit Stop if no progress toward abstinence within 7 wk	Avoid bedtime dosing Pregnancy: B SE: Dry mouth, insomnia, CNS effects, headache, constipation Interaction: CYP drugs (see Appendix D)	N/A

CNS, Central nervous system; *CYP,* cyproheptadine; *GI,* gastrointestinal; *N/A,* not available; *SE,* side effects.

TABLE 199-4 Ways to Cope with Withdrawal Symptoms

Withdrawal Symptom	Ways to Cope
Craving for cigarettes	Do something else, take slow deep breaths, take a walk, keep your hands busy, doodle, handle a worry stone, avoid alcohol and coffee, brush your teeth, use mouthwash
Anxiety	Slow deep breaths, decrease caffeine drinks, exercise, relaxation exercises
Irritability	Walk, do other things, use relaxation exercises
Constipation	Drink lots of water, exercise, eat high-fiber foods such as vegetables or fruits
Hunger	Eat a well-balanced meal, keep low-calorie foods available, such as carrots, rice cakes; drink water

Clinical Evaluation

Check for alopecia, cheilosis, glossitis, swollen, bleeding gums, dry and scaly skin, petechia/ecchymosis, bilateral dermatitis, edema, muscle wasting, arthralgia, disorientation, confabulation, neuropathy, and paresthesia.

Dietary Analysis

Amount of money spent on food
Ethnic/cultural background
Food allergies
Food intake history (24-hour)
Food preferences
Food restrictions
Meals skipped
Medications
Participation in food programs
Preparation of meals
Religion
Transportation to grocery store
Vitamin/mineral supplements

Measurements That Suggest Malnutrition

Triceps skinfold thickness <10th percentile
Midarm, muscle circumference <10th percentile
Serum albumin <3.5 g/dl
Evidence of osteoporosis or mineral deficiency
Evidence of vitamin deficiency

Obesity in Children

An alarming increase has been noted in childhood obesity in the U.S. population. Today nearly 5 million **children** 6 to 17 years old are overweight (Clinician Reviews, 1996). (See Chapter 136.)

Recommendations by the "Physical Activity, Genetic and Nutritional Considerations in Childhood Weight Management" include:

Children older than 5 years of age should limit fat to no more than 30% of daily caloric intake.

Children and adolescents should eat more fruit, vegetables, and grains in their regular diet.

Snacking should be less frequent. Snacks should be of more healthy, low-fat choices.

Recognition of the importance of serving sizes.

DIETARY GUIDELINES FOR AMERICANS*

Eat a variety of foods
Maintain healthy weight
Choose a diet low in fat, saturated fat, and cholesterol
Suggested total fat less than 30% of calories
Suggested saturated fat less than 10% of calories
Eating less fat from animal sources to reduce cholesterol levels
Eat more vegetables, fruits, and grain products
Use sugars only in moderation
Use salt and sodium only in moderation
Drink alcoholic beverages in moderation
One drink per day

USE OF THE FOOD GUIDE PYRAMID†

Replaces the four food groups (Figure 199-2)
Emphasizes food from five major food groups
All food groups are needed for a balanced diet

Bread, cereal, and rice	6-11 servings
Fruits	2-4 servings
Vegetables	3-5 servings
Meat/poultry, fish	2-3 servings
Milk/yogurt, cheese	2-3 servings
Fats/oils/sweets	Use sparingly

STRESS MANAGEMENT

Many visits made to health care providers are prompted by stress-related illnesses; some estimate that 60% to 90% of visits may be related to stress (Pelletier et al, 1988).

*USDA, 1990.
†USDA, 1992.

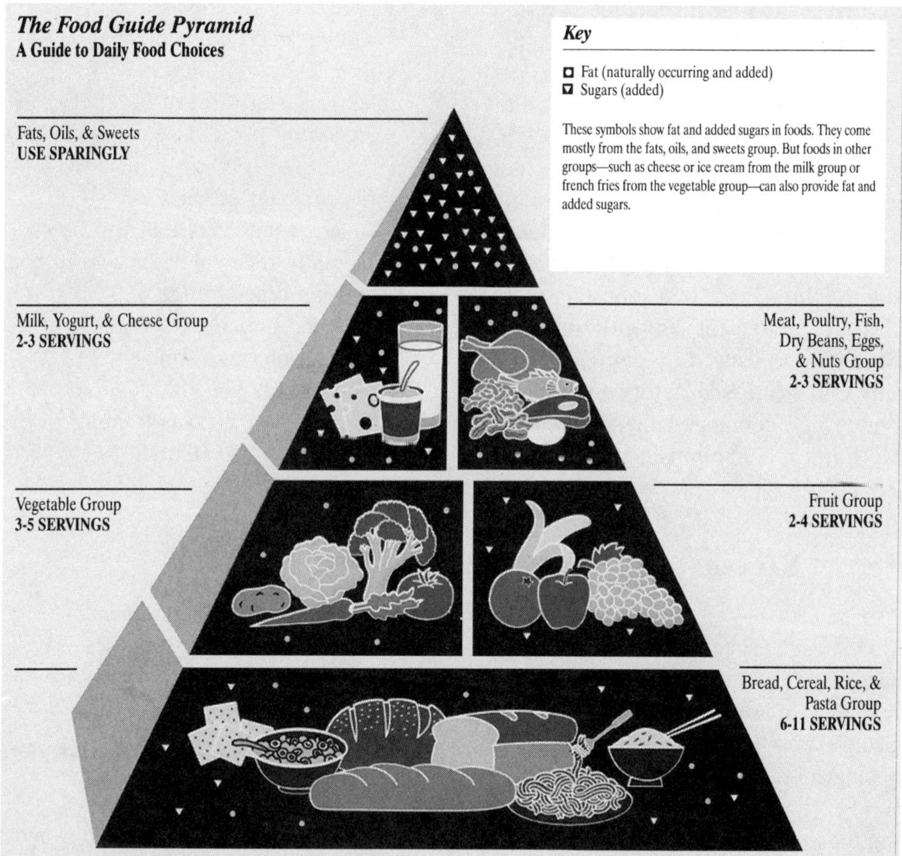

Figure 199-2 Food guide pyramid: a guide to daily food choices and number of servings. (From US Department of Agriculture and the US Department of Health and Human Services.)

Holmes and Rahe (1967) developed a method to identify the relationship between social readjustment, stress, and susceptibility to illness using their Social Readjustment Rating Scale. Strategies for health promotion and reduction of stress are important in the NP's armamentarium in primary care. Goals identified by Healthy People 2000 include:

Decrease to no more than 5% of the proportion of people aged 18 and older who report significant levels of stress who do not take steps to reduce or control stress.

Reduce to less than 35% the proportion of people age 18 and older who experienced adverse health effects from stress within the past year.

Increase to at least 40% the proportion of worksites employing 50 or more people that provide programs to reduce employee stress.

Stress has been defined as the "nonspecific response of the body to any demand made on it" (Selye, 1975). Physiological responses of the body to stress include:

Dilation of pupils
Increased respiratory rate
Increased heart rate
Peripheral vasoconstriction
Increased perspiration
Increased blood pressure
Increased muscle tension
Increased gastric motility
Release of adrenalin
Increased glucose levels

These reactions prepare the body for the "flight or fight" mechanism. Stress is associated with decreased life satisfaction, the development of mental disorders, increased incidence of stress-related illnesses, and decreased immunological functioning (Pender, 1996). Stressors are interpreted differently by each individual. Some stressors are considered positive and challenging, whereas others are viewed as negative and undesirable. Coping strategies assist the individual in dealing with the stressors. Coping strategies can be described as "learned and purposeful cognitive, emotional, and behavioral responses to stressors used to adapt to the environment or to change it" (Lazarus and Folkman, 1984).

Children experience stress and develop coping patterns early in life. Factors such as poverty, chronic illness, and parental dysfunction may influence the ability to develop effective coping strategies in children. Most stress research has been conducted with adults, and may or may not be applicable to children. Five of the most frequent stressors identified by **children** are feeling sick, having nothing to do, not having enough money to spend, being pressured to get good grades, and feeling left out of the group (Ryan, 1988).

Stressors in adulthood relate to initiating a career, establishing and maintaining a relationship, and child rearing. Work is often cited as a source of stress. Single parents are especially vulnerable to stress, trying to balance child rearing with the demands of the job. Loss is the primary stressor for **aging adults**. Loss of a spouse or close family member and even retirement are described as negative life events. Limitations caused by aging, such as decreased visual acuity and decreased ability to perform activities of daily living, may compound the individual's reaction to stressors, further compromising his or her immune system.

Primary Modes of Stress Management

The primary modes of stress management consist of the following goals, according to Pender (1996):
- Minimizing the frequency of stressors
- Increasing resistance to stress
- Avoiding the physiological arousal from stress

In general, minimizing the frequency of stressors is the first line of defense. If that is not possible, strengthening family and individual coping resources is the next step.

Minimizing Frequency of Stressors

- Changing the environment (most proactive approach)
- Flextime at work
- Job sharing
- Child care at worksite
- Changing job
- Avoiding excessive change
- Time blocking (Girdano and Everly, 1979)
- Taking time to focus on a specific change, developing strategies for adjustment by ensuring that necessary time is given to address critical tasks
- Managing time effectively
  - Identifying values/goals; prioritizing goals
  - Identifying time wasted, overcommitment, and unrealistic expectations
  - Learning to say "no" to demands that do not match goals
  - Reduction of tasks into smaller parts
  - Avoiding overload; delegating responsibilities
  - Reducing sense of time pressure and urgency

Increasing Resistance to Stress

- Physical conditioning
  - Promoting exercise; exercise seems to provide some stress resistance benefits (Norris et al, 1992)
  - Getting adequate sleep
  - Practicing good nutrition
- Psychological conditioning
  - Enhancing self-esteem
    - Practicing positive verbalization: Identify positive aspects of self
  - Enhancing self-efficacy
    - Undertaking tasks that can be successfully completed
    - Mentally rehearsing successful completion of task
  - Increasing assertiveness
    - Greeting patients by name
    - Maintaining eye contact
    - Commenting on the positive characteristics of others
    - Taking assertiveness training
  - Developing goal alternatives
  - Developing coping resources
    - Self-disclosure
    - Self-directedness
    - Acceptance
    - Finding social support
    - Assessing coping resources via Coping Resources Inventory (Matheny, 1993)

Avoiding the Physiological Arousal from Stress

- Goal is to replace muscle tension and heightened sympathetic nervous system activity with muscle relaxation and increased parasympathetic functioning (Pender, 1996)
- Deep-breathing exercises
- Relaxation training
- Biofeedback
- Imagery
- Meditation

EXERCISE

Physical activity is defined as "any bodily movement produced by skeletal muscles and resulting in calorie expenditure" (Bouchard, 1990). "Lifestyle exercise" has been characterized as the integration of short bouts of exercise into daily living (Gordon, 1993). Healthy People 2000 has set goals that 20% of adults and 75% of children engage in vigorous physical activity on 3 or more days per week for 20 or more minutes, and at least 30% of children 6 years of age and older to engage in light to moderate activity daily for at least 30 minutes. Physical activity appears to significantly decrease during adolescence in the United States (Stephens, 1985), with a decline of almost 50% from childhood through adulthood; females being more sedentary than males (Rowland, 1990). Because exercise or lack of exercise plays a major role in many disease states, it is imperative that all primary care providers assess and counsel their patients regarding the frequency, duration, and intensity of lifestyle exercise. A goal identified by Healthy People 2000 recommends that at least 50% of primary care providers should routinely assess and counsel patients regarding physical activity practices.

Benefits of Exercise*

Increase in lean muscle mass
Increase in bone mass or prevention of bone loss
Reduction in systolic and diastolic blood pressure
Higher HDLs
Reduction in excess body fat
Lowering of insulin levels and improved glucose tolerance
Lower incidence of breast cancer and cancer of reproductive tract
Improved pulmonary function
Decrease sympathetically mediated cardiovascular response to stress
Improvement of anxiety and depression
Reduction of resting heart rate
Increase circulating leukocytes
Enhance general mood and psychological well-being

Exercise Guidelines

At every visit, promote lifestyle exercise of at least 20 to 30 minutes of vigorous activity three times a week (vigorous activity describes an intensity sufficient enough to produce fatigue in 20 minutes).

Intensity: 60% or more of maximum heart rate, although recent research proposes that moderate exercise can be just as effective in terms of health benefits (Marcus, Selby, and Niaura, 1992). Moderate activity has higher compliance rates, meshes better with daily lifestyle, and is well maintained over time (Duncan, 1991).

Maximum heart rate: 220 – age, then multiply desired intensity by 60% to 85%. This does not work when the patient is taking beta blockers, since the medication lowers heart rate.

Maximal heart rate as determined from a maximal exercise test (Table 199-5). This method has a range of ± 15 beats and is more desirable than an estimated heart rate, especially if the patient is receiving beta blockers.

Risk of Exercise

Most adverse effects are related to injury during exercise. Potential adverse effects include: injury, osteoarthritis, myocardial infarction and rarely, sudden death.

Running/jogging has a high risk of injury of 35% to 65%, as does aerobic dancing, which increases with frequency of classes (U.S. Preventive Services Task Force, 1996). Injuries can be prevented by avoiding:

Excessive levels of exercise
Sudden dramatic increases in activity level (especially in those with poor fitness baseline)

*Bouchard, Shepard, and Stephens, 1990.

Table 199-5 Maximal Heart Rate

Age	Estimated Maximal Heart Rate	95% Confidence Intervals
20	200	170-220
30	190	160-220
40	180	150-210
50	170	140-200
60	160	130-190
70	150	120-180

From Kirkendall D: A program for fitness. In Matzen R, Lang R, editors: *Clinical preventive medicine,* St Louis, 1993, Mosby.

Improper exercise technique or equipment
Intense exercise can cause amenorrhea, bone loss, and increased risk of fracture
Long-term exercise does not seem to increase the prevalence of osteoarthritis in weight-bearing joints.

The risk of adverse cardiovascular events is greater in those who are sedentary who engage in vigorous activity. The risk of sudden death is lower for those who exercise regularly, when compared with sedentary counterparts.

Clinical Intervention*

Promote regular exercise in all children and adults.
Determine each patient's activity level.
Ascertain barriers to exercise.

Risk assessment: A male over 40 years old with two or more risk factors for CAD should have a resting ECG or stress test, others with known (previous MI, pulmonary disease) or possible risk (hypertension, cigarette smoking, high blood cholesterol, abuse of drugs, or diabetes) should have a thorough examination prior to the beginning of an exercise program (Woolf, 1996).

Provide information on the role of exercise in disease prevention.

Assist in selecting appropriate type of exercise (consider factors such as medical limitations and activity characteristics that improve health and enhance compliance).

Exercise: Regular, moderate intensity is reasonable for sedentary persons.

Short-term goal: Small increase over current activity level with progression to level to achieve cardiovascular fitness; 30 minutes of brisk walking most days of the week is ideal.

Sporadic exercise should be discouraged, especially for sedentary individual: regular is more important than the type of exercise.

*U.S. Preventive Services Task Force, 1996.

Interventions to Promote Exercise*

Contracts
Maintaining self-monitoring diaries and periodic discussion with provider
Providing personalized feedback and praise
Setting flexible goals
Providers who model active lifestyles are more likely to be effective with counseling
Encouragement of patient to "take control"
Periodic awards
Gradual change promotes permanent change[1]

REFERENCES

Bouchard C, Shepard R, Stephens T: *Exercise, fitness, and health*, Champaign, Ill, 1990, Human Kinetics Books.

Combatting childhood obesity, *Clin Rev* 6:109-110, 1996.

Duncan J, Gordon N, Scott C: Women walking for health and fitness: how much is enough? *JAMA* 266:3295-3299, 1991.

Fagerstrom K, Heatherton T, Kozlowski L: Nicotine addiction and its assessment, *ENTJ* 69:763-768, 1990.

Fiore M: The new vital sign: assessing and documenting smoking status, *JAMA* 266:3183-3184, 1991.

Girdano D, Everly G: *Controlling stress and tension*, Englewood Cliffs, NJ, 1979, Prentice-Hall.

Gordon N, Kohl H, Blair S: Lifestyle exercise: a new strategy to promote physical activity for adults, *J Cardiopulm Rehabil* 13:161-163, 1993.

Greene H., Garcia L: Smoking cessation. In Greene H, Johnson W, Lemcke D, editors: *Decision making in medicine*, St Louis, ed 2, 1998, Mosby.

Hobfoll S: *The etiology of stress*, Washington, DC, 1988, Hemisphere.

Holmes T, Rahe R: The social readjustment rating scale, *J Psychosom Res* 11:213-218, 1967.

Husten C, Manley M: How to help your patients stop smoking, *Am Family Physician* 42:1017-1026, 1990.

Lazarus S, Folkman S: *Stress, appraisal and coping*, New York, 1984, Springer.

Marcus B, Selby V, Niaura R: Self efficacy and the stages of exercise behavior change. *Res Q Exercise Sport* 63:60-66, 1992.

Matheny K et al: The coping resource inventory for stress: a measure of perceived resourcefulness, *J Clin Psychol* 49:815-829, 1993.

Norris R, Carroll D, Cochrane R: The effects of physical activity and exercise training on psychological stress and well-being in an adolescent population, *J Psychosom Res* 36:55-65, 1992.

*Marcus, Selby, and Niaura, 1992.

Pelletier K, Lutz R: Healthy people-health business: a critical review of stress management programs in the workplace. *Am J Health Promotion* 5:12-19, 1988.

Pender N: *Health promotion in nursing practice*, ed 3, Norwalk, Conn, 1996, Appleton & Lange.

Prochaska J, DiClemente C: Stages of change in the modification of problem behaviors, *Progressive Behavior Modification* 28:183-218, 1992.

Rasco C: Discouraging smoking: interventions for pediatric nurse practitioners, *J Pediatr Healthcare* 6:200-207, 1992.

Robinson M, Laurent S, Little J: Including smoking status as a new vital sign: it works, *J Family Practice* 40:556-563, 1995.

Rowland T: *Exercise and children's health*, Champaign, Ill, 1990, Human Kinetics.

Ryan N: The stress-coping process in school-aged children: gaps in the knowledge needed for health promotion, *Adv Nurs Sci* 11:1-12, 1988.

Selye H: *Stress without distress*, New York, 1975, NAL Dutton.

Sloane P, Hicks M: Preventive care: an overview. In Sloane P, Slatt L, Curtis P, editors: *Essentials of family medicine*, Baltimore, 1993, Williams & Wilkins.

Smith K, Johnson S, Mandle C: Stress management and crisis intervention. In Edelman C, Mandle C, editors: *Health promotion throughout the lifespan*, ed 3, St Louis, 1994, Mosby.

Smoking status: the new vital sign, New York, 1993, Medical Information Services.

Spark A: Nutrition counseling. In Edelman C, Mandle C, editors: *Health promotion throughout the lifespan* ed 3, St Louis, 1994, Mosby.

Stephens T, Jacobs D, White C: A descriptive epidemiology of leisure time physical activity, *Public Health Reports* 100:147-158, 1985.

Swanson J, Albrecht M: *Community health nursing: promoting the health of aggregates*, Philadelphia, 1993, WB Saunders.

US Department of Agriculture: *The food guide pyramid* (Home and Garden Bulletin 252), Washington, DC, 1992, US Government Printing Office.

US Department of Agriculture and US Department of Health and Human Services: *Nutrition and your health: dietary guidelines for Americans* (Home and Garden Bulletin 232), Washington, DC, 1990, US Government Printing Office.

US Department of Health and Human Services: *Nurses: Help your patients stop smoking* (NIH Publication No 92-2962), Washington, DC, 1993, US Government Printing Office.

US Department of Health and Human Services: *Healthy people 2000: National health promotion and disease prevention objectives for the year 2000*, Washington, DC, 1990, US Government Printing Office.

US Preventive Services Task Force: *Guide to clinical preventive services*, ed 2, Baltimore, 1996, Williams & Wilkins.

US Public Health Service: Smoking cessation in adults, *Am Family Physician* 51:1914-1918, 1995.

Woolf S, Jonas S, Lawrence R: *Health promotion and disease prevention in clinical practice*, Baltimore, 1996, Williams & Wilkins.

Department of Transportation Examination

ICD-9-CM

Occupational Examination V70.5
Preemployment Screening V70.5
Driving License Examination V70.3

OVERVIEW

Definition

The purpose of the Department of Transportation (DOT) examination is to certify that a commercial truck driver is healthy and capable of safe performance of his or her duties. The primary responsibility of the examiner performing DOT examinations is to protect the public to ensure public safety. The Federal Motor Carriers Safety Regulations (FMCSR) identify that the intent of the examination is to detect physical or mental defects of "such a character and extent as to affect the applicant's ability to operate a motor vehicle safely" (FMCSR, 1997). The FMCSR guidelines detail the conditions that may be disqualifying. Nurse practitioners, since 1992, have been able to perform DOT examinations if their state regulatory agency permits them to carry out examinations of this type.

Incidence

Approximately 6 million drivers operate commercial vehicles in interstate commerce.

SUBJECTIVE DATA

History

The history is the most important portion of the certification process because it directs the specific parts of the examination that should be completed.

Ask whether the person has any current medical problems or concerns.

Determine whether the person is under a health provider's care, and for what reason.

A comprehensive history and review of systems is recommended.

In particular, ask about the following potentially disqualifying medical conditions:
- History of seizures
- Diabetes controlled by insulin
- History of cardiovascular disease
- Respiratory problems that require treatment
- Hypertension
- Musculoskeletal, neurological, or vascular diseases (if severe enough, these can be disqualifiers)
- Mental disorders
- Vision problems, date of last eye examination
- Hearing problems, date of last examination
- Current diagnosis of alcoholism (i.e., not in remission)
- Loss of foot, arm, hand, or leg
- Ask about any hospitalizations or surgeries

Family History

Ask about family history of:
- Insulin-dependent diabetes mellitus
- Cardiovascular disease
- Mental illness
- Respiratory problems

Medications

Determine whether the person is taking any medications.

Determine use of street or prescribed drugs that may alter consciousness.

Psychosocial History

Ask about smoking patterns

Ask about alcohol

OBJECTIVE DATA

Physical Examination

See the Medical Examiner's Certificate, p. 1241 to 1243
Vital signs, height, weight
Visual acuity (with corrective lenses) and color vision
Hearing examination: Whispered voice test or audiometry
General appearance, gait, range of motion, coordination, posture
Concentrate the examination on:
- Head/eyes/ears/nose/throat
  - Ears: Note any discharge, symptoms of aural vertigo or Meniere's disease
  - Eyes: Note discharge, visual fields, exophthalmos, or strabismus; note use of contact lenses
  - Throat: Note any deformities that may interfere with eating or breathing
- Cardiovascular
  - Have the person jog in place for 2 minutes and record the pulse afterward.
- Assess for SOB or arrhythmias.
- Pulmonary: Assess breath sounds or adventitious sounds.
- Abdomen: Note any wounds, injuries, scars, or weakness of abdominal muscles. Note hernia if present.
- Neurological: Note tremor, pupils equal, round, reactive to light and accommodation (PERRLA), deep tendon reflexes (DTRs).
- Musculoskeletal:
  - Conduct 2-minute screening examination (see p. 1250)
  - Identify loss or impairment of extremity. Note any and all deformities, atrophy, semiparalysis or paralysis or varicose veins. If hand or finger deformity, determine if sufficient grasp is present to maintain grip on wheel.
- Spine: Note deformities, ROM, pain, injuries.
- Peripheral vascular: Check peripheral pulses, presence of edema, changes related to peripheral vascular disease.

Diagnostic Procedures

Additional testing should concentrate on conditions that have the potential to cause sudden loss of consciousness, risk factors for disqualifying conditions, or target organ damage. The purpose is not to diagnose a condition but to determine whether the person can operate a vehicle safely (Table 200-1).

ASSESSMENT

The conditions detailed in Table 200-2 may preclude a driver's being certified.
Approximately 5% to 10% of drivers may initially be denied certification pending the results of additional studies or verification of medical records.

THERAPEUTIC PLAN

Determine qualification of driver:
- Fully qualified for up to 2 years
- Temporary certification for 3 months
- No certification is allowed

Identify whether intrastate (within a state and not across state lines) or interstate (across state lines).
Each state has its own rules/regulations for licensing and certifying drivers who operate intrastate.
Be cautious not to certify a driver for interstate driving when the waiver/certification is intended only for intrastate driving. Do not write intrastate on the DOT card.
It is the driver's responsibility to provide test results, clearances from specialists, and any needed documentation.

Referral

To help clarify borderline or complex cases, refer the individual to a specialist when the problem is outside your area of expertise.

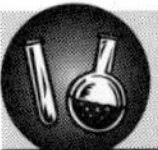

TABLE 200-1 Diagnostic Procedures: DOT Examination

Test	Finding/Rationale	Cost
Drug screening (using chain of custody)	To identify use of drugs	\$57-\$72
Urinalysis (required)	To identify renal disease or hyperglycemia	\$15-\$20
FPG or Hgb A1C	If urine dipstick reveals glucose, follow up with FPG or Hgb A1C	\$16-\$20/ FPG \$34-\$43/Hgb
Pulse oximetry, PFT, ABGs	Ordered if pulmonary status is in question	\$28-\$33/Pulse \$27-\$323/PFT \$78-\$98/ABGs
ECG	Ordered if any dysrhythmias, tachycardia, or bradycardia are found on examination or after exercise	\$56-\$65

ABGs, Arterial blood gases; *ECG,* electrocardiogram; *FPG,* fasting plasma glucose; *Hgb,* hemoglobin; *PFT,* pulmonary function test.

Table 200-2 Conditions That Preclude Certification

Condition	Recommendation
Loss of foot, leg, hand or arm	The driver is medically disqualified unless a waiver is obtained from the regional director of motor carriers. If the driver is otherwise medically qualified, check the statement "medically unqualified unless accompanied by a waiver" on the examination form and certification. See 391.49 of the FMSR for waiver information.
Impairments of hand or lower extremity	Any significant limb defect that interferes with the ability to perform tasks associated with operating a motor vehicle is disqualifying or requires a waiver (e.g., fused or immobile knee or hip, partial paralysis, a hand or finger that interferes with prehension or power grasping, etc.).
Insulin-controlled diabetes mellitus	A driver taking insulin cannot be certified for interstate driving. However, a driver who is well controlled by oral medications and diet may be qualified if the disease is well controlled and the driver is under medical supervision. Documentation from the driver's health care provider should be obtained. If diabetes is untreated or uncontrolled, certification should not be given. Carefully evaluate the potential for hypoglycemic reactions, even with individuals who have type 2 diabetes.
Current diagnosis of CV disease	Any condition accompanied by sudden and unexpected syncope, collapse, or congestive heart failure is disqualifying. Conditions such as myocardial infarction (MI), angina, or dysrhythmias should be evaluated completely by a cardiologist before certification is issued. Holter monitors and exercise stress tests may be needed when a driver has multiple risk factors and other questions need to be answered. Tachycardia or bradycardia should be investigated to rule out underlying cardiac disease. Asymptomatic dysrhythmia should not be disqualifying.
Established diagnosis of respiratory dysfunction	If a driver has clear symptoms of significant pulmonary disease, basic spirometry and lung volume tests are recommended. If the FEV_1 is <65% of predicted value, the FVC is <60% of predicted, or the ratio of FEV_1 to FVC is <65%, pulse oximetry should be done. If the pulse oximetry on room air is <92%, an ABG evaluation is recommended. If the Pao_2 is <65 mm Hg or $Paco_2$ is >45 mm Hg, disqualification is recommended.
Hypertension	If blood pressure is 160/90 or lower, a full 2-year certification is appropriate. If blood pressure is >160/90 but <181/105, a temporary certification for 3 months may be given to allow time for the driver to be evaluated and treated. If the initial blood pressure is >181/105, the driver should not be certified. Once treatment has brought the driver's blood pressure under control, certification should be issued for no more than 1 year at a time. Note that several readings should be taken over several days to rule out "white-coat hypertension." Significant target organ damage and additional risk factors increase the risk of sudden collapse and should be disqualifying
Musculoskeletal, neurological, or vascular diseases	Depending on severity, any condition can be disqualifying if it can significantly impair a driver's ability to control a motor vehicle or react in an emergency situation. Consider the driver's ability to control and operate a commercial motor vehicle safely if the following are present: rheumatic, arthritic, orthopedic, neuromuscular, or vascular conditions.
Epilepsy	A driver with a clinical diagnosis of epilepsy and recurrent seizures of any cause should never be certified. A driver who has an isolated seizure or episode of syncope may be certified, but only if the driver is not taking medications and has been free of seizures for 5 years following an isolated idiopathic seizure, and for 10 years following multiple seizures. Febrile seizures of childhood are not disqualifying. All questionable cases should be cleared by a neurologist.
Mental, nervous or psychiatric disorders	Mental conditions that can affect judgment, perception of reality, and reaction times may be disqualifying. When in doubt, the examiner should have the driver obtain a clearance from a psychiatrist or neurologist. Medications required for mental conditions may be disqualifying if they can alter consciousness or reaction times.
Vision <20/40 in each eye	Vision must be at least 20/40 in each eye with or without correction, field of vision of at least 70 degrees in the horizontal meridian in each eye, and the ability to recognize the colors of traffic signals and devices showing red, green, and amber. Certification can be given only once vision has been corrected. The driver should be advised to have his or her eyes evaluated, obtain corrective lenses, and then return for certification.
Hearing loss	The driver should pass a whispered voice test at 5 feet in at least one ear. A hearing aid may be worn for the test. If the test result is questionable, audiography is recommended. The better ear must not have an average hearing loss of >40 dB at 500, 1000, and 2000 Hz (assess ×3 and take average).

Adapted from Pommerenke F, Hegmann K, Hartenbaum N: DOT examinations: practical aspects and regulatory review, *Am Family Physician* 58:415-426, 1998; and Federal Motor Carrier Safety Regulations, regulation 391.41-49.

Continued

Table 200-2 Conditions That Preclude Certification—cont'd

Condition	Recommendation
Use of schedule 1 drugs and consciousness altering drugs	Use of a schedule 1 drug or any other consciousness-altering substance, an amphetamine, a narcotic, or any other habit-forming drug is cause for the driver to be found medically unqualified. Use of other prescription medications is not an automatic disqualifier; however, the condition being treated, the medications prescribed, and the dosage level must be consistent with the safe performance of the driver's duties.
Current diagnosis of alcoholism	The term "current diagnosis" is meant to encompass those instances in which the physical and mental condition of the driver with alcoholism has not fully stabilized, regardless of the time element. If the severity or extent of the problem is uncertain, the examiner may refer the driver to substance abuse counseling for evaluation and clearance.

Do not refer the individual when the condition is known to be disqualifying.

Following most significant cardiac events, the person should be cleared by a cardiologist.

A driver with significant musculoskeletal or neurological disorders should be cleared by a neurologist or psychiatrist.

RESOURCES

Federal Highway Administration
Office of Motor Carrier Research and Standards
400 7th Street, SW
Washington, DC 20590
(202) 366-1790
FAX: (202) 366-8842

National Technical Information Service
5285 Port Royal Rd.
Springfield, VA 22161
(703) 605-6000
FAX: (703) 321-8547

http://www/fhwa.dot.gov

http://www.acoem.com/dot/dotregs/html

http://mcregis.fhwa.dot.gov/39143.htm#391.43

SUGGESTED READINGS

Federal Motor Carrier Safety Regulations: 49 CFR, Part 391.41-49, *Subpart E—physical qualification and examination,* Washington DC, 1997, U.S. Department of Transportation.

Healthcare Consultants of America, Inc: *1998 Physicians fee and coding guide,* Augusta, Ga, 1998, Healthcare Consultants of America, Inc.

Pommerenke F, Hegmann K, Hartenbaum N: DOT examinations: practical aspects and regulatory review, *Am Family Physician* 58:415-426, 1998.

Wells J, Ferreira D: Guidelines for the Department of Transportation physical examination, *Nurse Pract* 24(5)78-98, 1999.

EXAMINATION TO DETERMINE PHYSICAL CONDITION OF DRIVERS		
Driver's name		
	[ ] New Certification	[ ] Recertification
Address		
Social Security No		
Date of birth	Age	
HEALTH HISTORY		
Yes No	Review of systems	Comments
[ ] [ ]	Head or spinal injuries	
[ ] [ ]	Seizures, fits, convulsions, or fainting	
[ ] [ ]	Extensive confinement by illness or injury	
[ ] [ ]	Cardiovascular disease	
[ ] [ ]	Tuberculosis	
[ ] [ ]	Syphillis	
[ ] [ ]	Gonorrhea	
[ ] [ ]	Diabetes	
[ ] [ ]	Gastronintestinal ulcer	
[ ] [ ]	Nervous stomach	
[ ] [ ]	Rheumatic fever	
[ ] [ ]	Asthma	
[ ] [ ]	Kidney disease	
[ ] [ ]	Muscular disease	
[ ] [ ]	Suffering from any other disease	
[ ] [ ]	Permanent defect from illness, disease or injury	
[ ] [ ]	Psychiatric disorder	
[ ] [ ]	Any other nervous disorder	
If answer to any of the above is yes, explain:		
PHYSICAL EXAMINATION		
General appearance and development:		
Good	Fair	Poor
Vision: For distance: Right 20/ Left 20/ [ ] Without corrective lenses	[ ] With corrective lenses if worn	
Evidence of disease or injury: Right	Left	
Color Test		
Horizontal field of vision: Right °	Left °	
Hearing: Right ear Left ear Disease or injury		

Continued

Audiometric Test (complete only if audiometer is used to test hearing) decibel loss at 500 Hz	at 1000 Hz	at 2000 Hz
Throat		

Thorax:

Heart ______

If organic disease is present, is it fully compensated: ______

______

______

Blood pressure:

Systolic ______ Diastolic ______

Pulse:

Before exercise ______ Immediately after exercise ______

Lungs		

Abdomen:

Scars ______ Abnormal masses ______

Tenderness

Hernia: Yes ______ No ______

If so, where? ______

Is truss worn?

Gastrointestinal:

Ulceration or other disease? Yes ______ No ______

Genito-Urinary:

Scars ______

Urethral discharge

Reflexes:

Romberg ______

Pupillary ______ Light R ______ L ______

Accommodation Right ______ Left ______

Knee Jerks:

Right: Normal ______ Increased ______ Absent ______

Left: Normal ______ Increased ______ Absent ______

Remarks ______

______

Extremities: Upper ______ Lower ______ Spine ______

Laboratory and other Special Findings:

Urine: Spec. Gr. Alb.

Sugar

Other laboratory date (e.g., serology) Radiological data Electrocardiograph		
General comments		
(Date of examination)	(Address of medical examiner)	
(Name of medical examiner [Print])	(Signature of medical examiner)	
(Title)	(License or Certification No)	(State)
Note: This section to be completed only when visual test is conducted by a licensed ophthalmologist or optometrist		
(Date of examination)	(Address of ophthalmologist or optometrist)	
(Name of ophthalmologist (or optometrist)	(Signature of ophthalmologist or optometrist [Print])	

(g) If the medical examiner finds that the person he/she examined is physically qualified to drive a commercial motor vehicle in accordance with 391.41(b), he/she shall complete a certificate in the form prescribed in paragraph (g) of this section and furnish one copy to the person who was examined and one copy to the motor carrier that employs him/her.

(h) The medical examiner's certificate shall be in accordance with the following form. Existing forms may be used until current printed supplies are depleted or until March 31, 1997, provided that the medical examiner writes down in pen and ink any applicable information contained in the following form:

Medical Examiner's Certificate I certify that I have examined

____

(Driver's Name—Print)

In accordance with the Federal Motor Carrier Safety Regulations (49 CFR 391.41 through 391.49) and with knowledge of his/her duties, I find him/her qualified under the regulations.

—Qualified only when wearing corrective lenses

—Qualified only when wearing a hearing aid

—Qualified by operation of 49 CFR 391.64

—Medically unqualified unless accompanied by a ______________ waiver

—Medically unqualified unless driving within an exempt intracity zone

A completed examination form for this person is on file in my office.

Area Code and Telephone Number ______________________________

(License or Certificate No) ______________________________

(State in Which Licensed) ______________________________

(Expiration Date)

____

(Name and Title of Medical Examiner—Print)

____

(Signature of Medical Examiner) ______________________________

(Signature of Driver)

____

(Address of Driver)

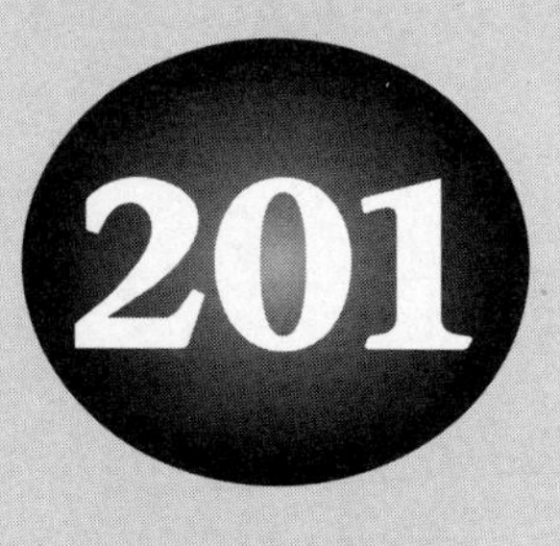

Preparticipation Sports Examination

ICD-9-CM

Sport Competition Examination V70.3

OVERVIEW

Definition

The purpose of the preparticipation sports examination (PSE) is to identify any individual who is at risk for worsening preexisting medical conditions, to identify general health and those at risk for future medical problems, and to provide information concerning safe, healthy athletic participation. Ideally the sports physical examination (PE) should take place at least 6 weeks before the individual's participation in sports to allow for follow-up if needed. In some states these examinations must be performed by a physician, or contain a physician's signature. Check with your state regulations for requirements concerning PSE.

Box 201-1 lists classifications of sports by level of contact, and Table 201-1 details the strenuousness of various sports.

Incidence

Approximately 30 million **children** participate in sports activities. The incidence of significant findings in PSE ranges from approximately 3.4% in junior high, 15% in high school, and 34% in college athletes. However, only 1.7% of all athletes were disqualified from participating in sports, regardless of age. The most common reasons for restriction with follow-up included musculoskeletal problems, asthma, vision difficulty, heart murmur, and elevated blood pressure (Rifat and Ruffin, 1995).

In many cases, the sports PE is the only contact that the person may have with the health care provider, so data that are important, but not relevant to athletic participation, should be included. This PSE may be the only opportunity to discuss health issues unrelated to sports participation. Access and cost may be an issue for others so the PSE is the only opportunity for some athletes to receive care.

Adolescents are more at risk for developing injuries because of an imbalance of strength and flexibility. In addition, significant changes are taking place in the biochemical properties leading to increased stiffness in bone and decreased resistance to impact.

SUBJECTIVE DATA

It is important to conduct a private interview with the **adolescent** to encourage truthful responses to sensitive subjects.

Information About Planned Sports Activities

Extent of participation
Level of competition
Planned training schedule
Protective equipment to be used

History of Present Illness

History of exercise induced syncope, near syncope, chest pain, or palpitations during exercise (any of these symptoms requires exclusion from sports until extensive work-up is done)
Allergies
History of concussion or loss of consciousness
Current level of conditioning
Normal health maintenance activities
Past injuries causing the athlete to miss a game
Previous exclusion from sports for any reason
Menstrual history in female athletes

Past Medical History

Chronic diseases
Any hospitalizations
Any surgeries
Immunization status: Tetanus
Use of glasses, contacts, hearing aids, braces
Recent history (within 3 months) of mononucleosis

Box 201-1

Classification of Sports by Contact

Contact/Collision

Basketball
Boxing*
Diving
Field hockey
Football (flag and tackle)
Ice hockey
Lacrosse
Martial arts
Rodeo
Rugby
Ski jumping
Soccer
Team handball
Water polo
Wrestling

Limited Contact

Baseball
Bicycling
Cheerleading
Canoeing/kayaking (white water)
Fencing
Field (high jump and pole vault)
Floor hockey
Gymnastics
Handball
Horseback riding
Racquetball
Skating (ice, incline, roller)
Skiing (cross-country, downhill, water)
Softball
Squash
Ultimate Frisbee
Volleyball
Windsurfing/surfing

Noncontact

Archery
Badminton
Bodybuilding
Bowling
Canoeing/kayaking (flat water)
Crew/rowing
Curling
Dancing
Field (discus, javelin, shot put)
Golf
Orienteering
Power lifting
Race walking
Riflery
Rope jumping
Running
Sailing
Scuba diving
Strength training
Swimming
Table tennis
Tennis
Track
Weight lifting

Reprinted with permission from Committee on Sports Medicine: Medical conditions affecting sports participation, *Pediatrics* 94:757-760, 1994.

*Participation not recommended.

Medications

Any regularly prescribed medications: Ask about anticholinergics, beta blockers, decongestants, and diuretics
Ask about over-the-counter medications or agents used to control weight: Laxatives, stimulants

Family History

Ask about myocardial infarction (MI) in family members younger than 50 years of age

Psychosocial History

Use of illegal substances: alcohol, street drugs, anabolic steroids

OBJECTIVE DATA

Physical Examination

The athlete should be in shorts and a shirt that allows inspection of the shoulders (see p. 1250).
An overall screening examination should be conducted with particular attention to:
- Vital signs
  - General appearance
  - Visual acuity
- Skin: Assess for infections such as impetigo
- HEENT: Not needed unless specific problems have been identified
- Lungs/heart: Be alert for a systolic murmur that increases with the patient standing and with a Valsalva maneuver and decreases with squatting (hypertrophic cardiomyopathy)
- Abdomen: Organomegaly or single kidney, assess for hernia
- Genitalia
  - Assess sexual maturity using Tanner's staging
  - Assess for descended testes
  - Genitalia in females do not require examination unless there is a specific complaint
- Neurological: Assess mental maturity
- Musculoskeletal: Conduct 2-minute screening examination (see p. 1250)

Diagnostic Testing

No routine testing is necessary. Tests performed will depend on the findings of the history and physical examination. Some diagnostic procedures are outlined in Table 201-2.

ASSESSMENT

Significant diagnoses to identify in PSE are those which may place the athlete at risk for sudden death. They are identified in Table 201-3. Table 201-4 details medical conditions that could affect the athlete's fitness to play.

THERAPEUTIC PLAN

The athlete should be given one of the following recommendations:
- Full clearance for participation
- Participation with limitations (identify restrictions)
- Clearance held pending further evaluation

Athletes in whom syncope or near syncope, chest pain, or palpitations are identified should be excluded from exercise until a complete workup is done. This evaluation should include an ECG, Holter monitor, echocardiogram, and a maximal stress test. Invasive electrophysiological testing should be considered in athletes in whom no cause is identified. Referral to a cardiologist would be appropriate.

TABLE 201-1 Classification of Sports by Strenuousness

High to Moderate Intensity			Low Intensity
High to Moderate Dynamic and Static Demands	**High to Moderate Dynamic and Low Static Demands**	**High to Moderate Static and Low Dynamic Demands**	**Low Dynamic and Low Static Demands**
Boxing*	Badminton	Archery	Bowling
Crew/rowing	Baseball	Auto racing	Cricket
Cross-country skiing	Basketball	Diving	Curling
Cycling	Field hockey	Equestrian	Golf
			Riflery
Downhill skiing	Lacrosse	Field events (jumping)	
Fencing	Orienteering	Field events (throwing)	
Football	Race walking	Gymnastics	
Ice hockey	Racquetball	Martial arts (karate, judo)	
Rugby	Soccer	Motorcycling	
Running (sprint)	Squash	Rodeoing	
Speed skating	Swimming	Sailing	
Water polo	Table tennis	Ski jumping	
Wrestling	Tennis	Water skiing	
	Volleyball	Weight lifting	

Reprinted with permission from Committee on Sports Medicine: Medical conditions affecting sports participation, *Pediatrics* 94:757-760, 1994.
*Participation not recommended.

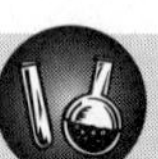

TABLE 201-2 Diagnostic Procedures: Preparticipation Sports Examination

Test	Findings/Rationale	Cost ($)
Hemoglobin and hematocrit	Consider only in teenagers who do not have ongoing health care. Also may consider in menstruating females if they run long-distance events.	11-14
Urine dipstick test for protein, glucose, and blood	Consider only if the athlete is symptomatic.	15-20

TABLE 201-3 Conditions Placing Athletes at Risk

Diagnosis	Supporting Data
Hypertrophic cardiomyopathy	A cause of sudden death in athletes. Associated with systolic murmur which increases with standing and during a Valsalva maneuver, and decreases with squatting. Patient may also have chest pain with exercise. A family history of sudden cardiac death before age 35 suggests disorders that may be transmitted in an autosomal-dominant fashion.
Marfan syndrome	Tall stature, myopia, arachnodactyly.

Table 201-4 Medical Conditions and Sports Participation*†

Condition	Explanation	May Participate?
Atlantoaxial instability (instability of the joint between cervical vertebrae 1 and 2)	Athlete needs evaluation to assess risk of spinal cord injury during sports participation; increased risk in those with Down's syndrome	Qualified yes
Bleeding disorder	Athlete needs evaluation	Qualified yes
Cardiovascular diseases		
Carditis (inflammation of the heart)	Carditis may result in sudden death with exertion	No
Hypertension (high blood pressure)	Those with significant essential (unexplained) hypertension should avoid weight and power lifting, body building, and strength training; those with secondary hypertension (hypertension caused by a previously identified disease), or severe essential hypertension, need evaluation	Qualified yes
Congenital heart disease (structural heart defects present at birth)	Those with mild forms may participate fully; those with moderate or severe forms or who have undergone surgery need evaluation	Qualified yes
Dysrhythmia (irregular heart rhythm)	Athlete needs evaluation because some types require therapy or make certain sports dangerous, or both	Qualified yes
Mitral valve prolapse (abnormal heart valve)	Those with symptoms (chest pain, symptoms of possible dysrhythmia) or evidence of mitral regurgitation (leaking) on physical examination need evaluation; all others may participate fully	Qualified yes
Heart murmur	If the heart murmur is innocent (does not indicate heart disease), full participation is permitted; otherwise, the athlete needs evaluation (see Congenital heart disease and Mitral valve prolapse)	Qualified yes
Cerebral palsy	Athlete needs evaluation	Qualified yes
Diabetes mellitus	All sports can be played with proper attention to diet, hydration, and insulin therapy; particular attention is needed for activities that last 30 minutes or more	Yes
Diarrhea	Unless disease is mild, no participation is permitted because diarrhea may increase the risk of dehydration and heat illness (see Fever)	Qualified no
Eating disorders (anorexia nervosa, bulimia nervosa)	These patients need both medical and psychiatric assessment before participation	Qualified yes
Eyes (functionally one-eyed athlete, loss of an eye, detached retina, previous eye surgery, or serious eye injury)	A functionally one-eyed athlete has a best corrected visual acuity of <20/40 in the worse eye; these athletes would suffer significant disability if the better eye was seriously injured as would those with loss of an eye; some athletes who have previously undergone eye surgery or had a serious injury may have an increased risk of injury because of weakened eye tissue; availability of eye guards approved by the American Society for Testing Materials and other protective equipment may allow participation in most sports, but this must be judged on an individual basis	Qualified yes
Fever	Fever can increase cardiopulmonary effort, reduce maximum exercise capacity, make heat illness more likely, and increase orthostatic hypotension during exercise; fever may rarely accompany myocarditis or other infections that may make exercise dangerous	No
Heat illness, history of	Because of the increased likelihood of recurrence, the athlete needs individual assessment to determine the presence of predisposing conditions and to arrange a prevention strategy	Qualified yes

*Adapted and reprinted with permission from Committee on Sports Medicine. Medical conditions affecting sports participation, *Pediatrics* 94:757-760, 1994. Copyright © 1994, American Academy of Pediatrics.

†This table is designed to be understood by medical and nonmedical personnel. In the "Explanation" section, "needs evaluation" means that a physician with appropriate knowledge and experience should assess the safety of a given sport for an athlete with the listed medical condition. Unless otherwise noted, this is because of the variability of the severity of the disease or the risk of injury in specific sports or both.

Continued

Table 201-4 Medical Conditions and Sports Participation*†—cont'd

Condition	Explanation	May Participate?
Human immunodeficiency virus infection	Because of the apparent minimal risk to others, all sports may be played that the state of health allows; in all athletes, skin lesions should be properly covered, and athletic personnel should use universal precautions when handling blood or body fluids with visible blood	Yes
Kidney, absence of one	Athlete needs individual assessment for contact/collision and limited contact sports	Qualified yes
Liver, enlarged	If the liver is acutely enlarged, participation should be avoided because of the risk of rupture; if the liver is chronically enlarged, individual assessment is needed before contact/collision or limited contact sports are played	Qualified yes
Malignancy	Athlete needs individual assessment	Qualified yes
Musculoskeletal disorders	Athlete needs individual assessment	Qualified yes
Neurologic		
History of serious head or spine trauma, severe or repeated concussions, or craniotomy	Athlete needs individual assessment for contact/collision or limited contact sports, and also for noncontact sports if there are deficits in judgment or cognition; recent research supports a conservative approach to management of concussions	Qualified yes
Convulsive disorder, well controlled	Risk of convulsion during participation is minimal	Yes
Convulsive disorder, poorly controlled	Athlete needs individual assessment for contact/collision or limited contact sports; avoid the following noncontact sports; archery, riflery, swimming, weight or power lifting, strength training, or sports involving heights—in these sports, occurrence of a convulsion may be a risk to self or others	Qualified yes
Obesity	Because of the risk of heat illness, obese persons need careful acclimatization and hydration	Qualified yes
Organ transplant recipient	Athlete needs individual assessment	Qualified yes
Ovary, absence of one	Risk of severe injury to the remaining ovary is limited	Yes
Respiratory		
Pulmonary compromise including cystic fibrosis	Athlete needs individual assessment but generally all sports may be played if oxygenation remains satisfactory during a graded exercise test; patients with cystic fibrosis need acclimatization and good hydration to reduce the risk of heat illness	Qualified yes
Asthma	With proper medication and education, only athletes with the most severe asthma will have to modify their participation	Yes
Acute upper respiratory infection	Upper respiratory obstruction may affect pulmonary function; athlete needs individual assessment for all but mild disease (see "fever" above)	Qualified yes
Sickle cell disease	Athlete needs individual assessment; in general, if status of the illness permits, all but high exertion, contact/collision sports may be played; overheating, dehydration, and chilling must be avoided	Qualified yes
Sickle cell trait	It is unlikely that individuals with sickle cell trait have an increased risk of sudden death or other medical problems during athletic participation except under the most extreme conditions of heat, humidity, and possibly increased altitude; these individuals, like all athletes, should be carefully conditioned, acclimatized, and hydrated to reduce any possible risk	Yes
Skin: boils, herpes simplex, impetigo, scabies, molluscum contagiosum	While the patient is contagious, participation in gymnastics with mats, martial arts, wrestling, and other contact/collision or limited contact sports is not allowed; herpes simplex virus probably is not transmitted by mats	Qualified yes
Spleen, enlarged	Patients with acutely enlarged spleens should avoid all sports because of risk of rupture; those with chronically enlarged spleens need individual assessment before playing contact/collision or limited contact sports	Qualified yes
Testicle: absent or undescended	Certain sports may require a protective cup	Yes

Lifestyle/Activities

Encourage the athlete to adequately warm up and cool down. Regular training is also important.

Diet

Recommend that the athlete follow the food pyramid for good food choices. More information is described below.

Patient Education

Safety

Emphasize the importance of safety and protection gear. Headgear and mouth guards have significantly reduced the incidence and severity of orofacial and head injuries.

Stress the importance of first aid and evaluation during sports activities.

The following injuries should be evaluated immediately:
- Loss of consciousness
- Loss of teeth
- Major head impact
- All potentially severe injuries

Emphasize the importance of adequate warm-up and cool-down.

Encourage the athlete and parents to be involved in evaluating and maintaining playing surfaces and athletic equipment.

Endurance training will enhance performance and increase endurance during a sporting event (20 to 30 minutes of physical activity every day).

Athletes who wear glasses should have glasses with shatter-proof lenses and flexible frames (sports glasses). They should also wear a strap to secure their glasses.

Nutrition

Encourage the athlete to eat breakfast before participating in sports.

Snacks should be nutritious: Raw vegetables, fruits, peanut butter, or cheese.

Fluid replacement: Encourage the athlete to drink 8 ounces of water every 25 to 30 minutes during exercise. The best choice for fluid replacement is water. Sports drinks are also acceptable.

Do not take salt tablets.

Review signs and symptoms of heat intolerance. **Children** are more at risk due to higher metabolic rate, poor sweating capacity, larger surface to mass ration, and immature cardiovascular system. Symptoms include: painful muscle cramps, moist skin, muscle twitching. Heat exhaustion symptoms include: increased temperature and heart rate, moist skin, thirst, weakness, headache, impaired judgment. Heat stroke symptoms include diarrhea, convulsions, blurred vision, hot skin, dizziness, and eventually collapse and unconsciousness.

Treatment includes shaded area, increased cool fluids, evaporative cooling, and lying down.

Health Maintenance

Preventive issues should also be discussed: Alcohol, smoking, drugs (steroids), safe sex.

High school athletes tend to engage in more risk taking than their nonathletic counterparts. (See Chapters 203 and 204 for more anticipatory guidance.)

Referral/Consultation

Refer any patients with syncope/near syncope, chest pain, or palpitations to a cardiologist.

Any patients with musculoskeletal problems or weakness should be seen by an orthopedist or physical therapist for strengthening exercises.

EVALUATION

The majority of athletes do not have conditions that will limit their participation in sports. Consider discussing other issues with the athletes, since this may be the only well visit they have.

SUGGESTED READINGS

Bratton R, Agerter D: Preparticipation sports examinations, *Postgrad Med* 98:123-132, 1995.

Briner W, Farr C: Athlete age and sports physical examination findings, *J Family Pract* 40:370-375, 1995.

Ellsworth A et al: *Mosby's 1998 medical drug reference,* St Louis, 1998, Mosby.

Healthcare Consultants of America, Inc: *1998 Physicians fee and coding guide,* Augusta, Ga, 1998, Healthcare Consultants of America, Inc.

Hergenroeder A: The preparticipation sports examination, *Pediatr Clin North Am* 44:1525-1540, 1997.

Krowshuk D: The preparticipation athletic examination: a closer look, *Pediatr Ann* 26:37-49, 1997.

Lowery-Ott J: Protecting young athletes, *Adv Nurse Pract* 6:46-54, 1998.

Nattive A, Puffer J, Green G: Lifestyles and health risks of collegiate athletes: a multi-center study, *Clin J Sports Med* 7:262-272, 1997.

Rifat S, Ruffin M, Gorenflo D: Disqualifying criteria in a preparticipation sports evaluation, *J Family Practice* 41:42-50, 1995.

SPORTS EXAMINATION FORM

Date:		Name: DOB:		Allergies:
T:	P:	B/P:	Weight:	
Interim History: Hospitalizations? Surgery?		Sport to be played? ____________ ____________	Medications:	

History:
Last dental exam ____
Last eye exam ____
Last hearing ex ____
☐ dT ________
☐ PPD ________
☐ Flu ________
☐ Pneumovax ____

____

FH:
Any one in your family ever died suddenly before 50? Y N
History of heart disease? Y N
Diabetes Y N
Asthma Y N

Past Medical
Diabetes Y N
Mono Y N
Bleeding prb Y N
Bruise easy Y N
Eye problem Y N
Both kidneys Y N
Both testicles Y N
Seizures Y N
Sting allergy Y N
Menstrual problems Y N

Social:
☐ Smoke ____ PPD
☐ Alcohol ____ Day
☐ Drugs (cocaine, steroids)
☐ Employment Y N
☐ Living arrangements
☐ School performance

Subjective:
Have you ever had any of these problems after exercising:
Fainting Y N
Dizziness Y N
Coughing Y N
Wheezing Y N
Short of breath Y N
Knocked out Y N
Neck pain/injury Y N
Back pain/injury Y N
Joint injury Y N
Broken bone Y N
Muscle strain Y N
Heat exhaustion Y N

Level of conditioning:
Are you able to run $1/2$ mile (2 x around a track) without stopping?
Y N
Describe your current conditioning/exercising
How often do you exercise?
____
For how long?
____
What do you do to get in shape?
____

Objective:

System	**Norm**	**Abnormal**	**Comments**
Skin	☐	☐	
Head	☐	☐	
Oral cavity	☐	☐	
Ear	☐	☐	
Nose	☐	☐	
Visual acuity		☐	
OD	____	☐	
OS	____	☐	
OU	____	☐	
Neck	☐	☐	
Chest	☐	☐	
Heart	☐	☐	
Abdomen	☐	☐	
Hernia	Y N	☐	
Neuro	☐		
Extremities	☐		
Tanner:	1 ☐		
	2 ☐		
	3 ☐		
	4 ☐		
	5 ☐		

Musculoskeletal exam:

Gait	WNL	Abn
Turn head (spine)	WNL	Abn
Shoulder	WNL	Abn
Abduct shoulders 90°	WNL	Abn
Rotate arms externally	WNL	Abn
Flex/extend elbows	WNL	Abn
Pronate/supinate wrist	WNL	Abn
Spread fingers/make	WNL	Abn
a fist	WNL	Abn
Tighten quadriceps	WNL	Abn
Duck walk	WNL	Abn
Touch toes	WNL	Abn
Raise up on toes/heels	WNL	Abn
Scoliosis check	WNL	Abn

Plan:
Labs:
☐ Lipid panel
☐ Hgb/Hct
☐ HIV
☐ Urine dip for protein/blood/glucose

Check-Up needed
☐ Vision
☐ Hearing
☐ Dental
☐ EKG
☐ Echocardiogram
☐ Holter monitor
☐ Stress test
Immunizations:
☐ dT
☐ Flu
☐ Pneumovax
☐ Varicella
☐ Hep A
☐ Hep B
☐ MMR

	Resting heart rate ______________ **Medications:** ______________ ______________ ______________ ______________ ______________ Heart rate after 2 minutes of aerobic exercise ______________ Adapted from American Academy of Pediatrics
Assessment: ☐ Full clearance ☐ Collision ☐ Contact ☐ Non-contact ☐ Participation with limitations ______________ ☐ Clearance held pending further evaluation ☐ Other: ______________	**Counseled:** ☐ Exercise 3-5x week ☐ Well balanced diet ☐ Smoking cessation ☐ Alcohol moderation or abstinence ☐ Sports safety: safety gear, warm-up/cool down ☐ Endurance training ☐ Reviewed symptoms of heat intoleranco ☐ Emphasized need for fluid replacement **Referral** ☐ Cardiologist ☐ Orthopedist ☐ ______________ RTO: ______________

Signature: ______________

202 Primary Care Related to Pregnancy

ICD-9-CM

Pregnancy (Unconfirmed) (Possible) V72.4
Prenatal Examination V22.1
First Pregnancy V22.1
High-risk Pregnancy V23.9
Postpartum Examination Immediately After Delivery V24.0
Postpartum Examination V24.2
Examination of Lactating Mother V24.1

PRECONCEPTION CARE

OVERVIEW

The purpose of preconception care is to assist women to make informed decisions for a healthy reproductive future. Three basic elements of preconception care are appropriate and ongoing risk assessment, health promotion, and medical and psychosocial interventions and follow-up (Summers and Price, 1993). Preconception counseling should be included as part of all ongoing primary care. Each visit should include questions about child-bearing plans and contraception (see the preconception health appraisal form, pp. 1259-1260).

SUBJECTIVE DATA

Historical Data

Past medical history
Family history
Medical-surgical history
Environmental exposure
Occupation
Psychosocial history
Obstetrical history: Gravidity and parity, date of each birth, outcome (gestational age at birth, type of delivery, length of labor, birth weight, gender, complications during pregnancy, delivery, postpartum)
Names and location of children
Feelings about loss, whether perinatal, adoption relinquishment, or infant or child death

Current Health Status

Medications: Prescription, over-the-counter (OTC), herbal products, vitamins
Dietary intake
Dietary supplementation
Physical activity
Contraception
Sexual practices—high risk for sexually transmitted diseases (STDs)

Safety

Abuse (physical, emotional, sexual)
Smoke and carbon monoxide detectors
Seat belt use and safety gear for hobbies

Psychosocial History/Habits

Smoking, alcohol, illicit drugs, or gambling

OBJECTIVE DATA

Physical Examination

A complete physical examination should be performed, with particular attention to:
- Height, weight, blood pressure, and pulse
- Skin
- Thyroid
- Lungs, heart
- Breast, abdomen, extremities
- Pelvic area, clinical pelvimetry

Laboratory/Diagnostic Testing

Laboratory and diagnostic tests should include:

- Complete blood count (CBC) ($18-$23)
- Genetic testing (indications include advanced maternal age, advanced paternal age, family history or previous child with genetic abnormality, ethnic background or as otherwise indicated by history)
- Gonococcal/chlamydial infection (gon: $23-$39; chlam: $63-$81)
- Hepatitis B surface antigen ($38-$48; hepatitis panel: $111-$156)
- Offer screening for illicit drugs and testing for human immunodeficiency virus (HIV) (HIV: $60-$77)
- Papanicolaou (Pap) smear ($28-$35)
- Purified protein derivative ($15-$20)
- Rh factor ($16-$22)
- Rubella and varicella titer (rubella: $37-$45; varicella: $49-$61)
- Syphilis ($19-$23)
- Urine dipstick test for protein, glucose ($15-$21)

Interventions

Follow up on abnormal findings on laboratory or physical examination.

Encourage the following:

- Keep menstrual calendar.
- Eat a well-balanced diet, and decrease caffeine intake.
- Start taking one prenatal multivitamin and 0.4 mg of folic acid daily. Women who have a child with neural tube defects should take 0.4 mg/day to decrease the likelihood of recurrence.
- Update immunizations: Advise the woman to delay pregnancy by 3 months if live-virus vaccines are used (measles/mumps/rubella [MMR], polio, and varicella [VZV]). If the woman has been immunized recently, no increased risk for congenital rubella has been documented if pregnancy occurs earlier than 3 months or even with vaccination during pregnancy. If the woman already had MMR >3 months, if exposed there is no risk due to lifelong immunity. Approximately 95% of all adults are immune to VZV resulting from prior infection. Even in those who don't recall a primary infection, up to 80% are immune. Therefore the occurrence of varicella in pregnancy is rare. If a woman is exposed to VZV, she should be offered VZIG within 96 hours to prevent maternal infection.
- Hepatitis immunization can be started before pregnancy and continued through the pregnancy without ill effects.
- Consider smoking cessation.
- Avoid environmental toxins (hyperthermia resulting from hot tub use or a febrile illness; handling of pesticides, anesthetic agents, heavy metals), illicit drug use, alcohol, OTC medications, prescription, and homeopathic medicines until their use is discussed with the health care provider.
- Exercise at least four times a week for 20 to 30 minutes.
- Limit risk of congenital toxoplasmosis by having someone else empty cat's litter box. For those who work in nurseries, day care centers, or schools, offer cytomegalovirus (CMV) status testing to precautions can be taken during pregnancy if needed.

Special Populations for Preconception Counseling

Diabetes

For patients with diabetes who are contemplating pregnancy, the goal is strict control or euglycemia. Oral hypoglycemic agents should be discontinued due to an increased risk of congenital malformations and since they do not provide adequate glucose control. Insulin needs may increase by two times during pregnancy—strict glycemic control is needed to decrease complications during pregnancy. Ideally this euglycemia occurs during organogenesis of the fetus.

Ophthalmic, renal, and cardiovascular evaluations may be needed to determine any target organ damage. Women who have a creatinine clearance of less than 30 ml/min, creatinine level of more than 2 mg/dl, or coronary artery disease should be counseled to avoid pregnancy because of the potential for increased morbidity and mortality.

Hypertension

For hypertensive women, blood pressure should be controlled with the use of drugs that have been studied in pregnancy: Methyldopa, beta blockers, calcium channel blockers, hydralazine, and clonidine are preferred. ACE inhibitors should be discontinued before pregnancy because of their teratogenic effect on the fetus. Diuretics should also be discontinued because they disrupt normal plasma volume expansion.

Asthma

Asthma medications are usually well tolerated and safe in pregnancy. Women may see an increase in the frequency of asthma symptoms. Approximately one third of women have an increase in the severity of their disease, while a third remain the same and a third improve.

Systemic Lupus Erythematosus

For women with systemic lupus erythematosus (SLE), the level of disease activity has an impact on pregnancy outcome. Renal function and antibody level should be assessed before pregnancy to help predict outcome. Women with SLE should be counseled to avoid pregnancy until they have been in remission 6 months.

Sickle Cell Disease

Women with sickle cell disease may develop vascular-occlusive crises, have increased risk of preeclampsia, urinary tract infections (UTIs), and placental disruption during their pregnancy. Genetic counseling should include the risk of transmission of sickle cell to the fetus, and the ability to diagnose this disease in utero should be discussed.

Epilepsy

Women who are taking antiepileptic medications should be counseled about the fetal effects. Ideally, if the women is seizure free for 2 or more years, withdrawal of the seizure medication may be attempted. If antiepileptic medication is necessary, using the least number of drugs possible is the goal. Folate supplementation is recommended before conception to decrease the possibility of neural tube defects. Seizures may increase in pregnancy.

Thyroid Dysfunction

For women with thyroid disorders, the goal is high-normal function. The preferred drug for hyperthyroidism is propylthiouriacil (PTU). Levothyroxine is the drug of choice for hypothyroidism during pregnancy.

PRENATAL CARE: THE INITIAL VISIT

OVERVIEW

The purpose of prenatal care is to promote the following: (1) A healthy pregnancy for mother and fetus, (2) health promotion, (3) parenting skills, (4) well child care, (5) family planning, and (6) decrease of family violence and neglect (Byrd, 1996). The initial visit should take place as early in the pregnancy as feasible.

SUBJECTIVE DATA

Historical Data

Update preconception history,- especially menstrual history, contraceptive history, psychosocial history, sexual practices, medications (prescription, OTC, herbal), dietary supplements, dietary intake, physical activity, hours of sleep, safety, and habits.

Determine the estimated date of delivery (EDD) via Nägele's rule: Add 9 months and 7 days to the first day of the last normal menstrual period, or subtract 3 months then add 7 days and 1 year. If the menstrual cycle varies by 7 or more days from the norm of 28 days, the EDD must be adjusted the same number of days.

OBJECTIVE DATA

Physical Examination

A physical examination should be performed, with particular attention to:

- Height, weight, blood pressure, pulse
- Skin
  - Chloasma: increased and pigmentation over face
  - Linea nigra: Brownish/brown streak down midline of abdomen
- Thyroid
- Lungs, heart
- Breast: Areola deepens in color, sebaceous glands hypertrophy; Montgomery's glands and vascularity visible, increased size of breast tubercles
- Abdomen, extremities
- Pelvic, clinical pelvimetry
  - Chadwick's sign: Vagina deeply congested/cyanotic
  - Hegar: Softening of the cervix
- Other elements as indicated

Laboratory/Diagnostic Procedures

Laboratory and diagnostic procedures should include:

- Antibody screen
- CBC ($18-$23)
- Genetic testing (see Table 202-1)
- Hepatitis B surface antigen (hepatitis panel: $111-$156)
- HIV($60-$77)
- Purified protein derivative ($15-$20)
- Random blood glucose level ($16-$21)
- Rh factor ($16-$22)
- Rubella titer ($37-$45)
- Syphilis ($19-$23)
- Titers for toxoplasmosis, rubella, cytomegalovirus, herpes, and hepatitis as indicated (TORCH antibody panel: $102-$132)
- Urine culture ($30-$38)
- Urine dipstick test for protein and glucose ($15-$21)
- Ultrasonography as indicated (dating, vaginal bleeding, maternal pelvic masses, uterine abnormalities, ectopic pregnancy, multiple gestation) (transvaginal: $376-$446; complete [uterus] $362-$430)

Interventions

Follow up on abnormal findings on laboratory tests or physical examination.

Encourage the following:

- Eat a well-balanced diet and decrease caffeine intake.
- Start/continue taking 1 prenatal multivitamin and 3 tablets containing 1 mg of folic acid daily.
- Update immunizations and consider smoking cessation.
- Exercise at least four times a week for 20 to 30 minutes.

Box 202-1

Frequency of Prenatal Visits

From 6 to 32 weeks: Every 4 weeks or sooner if indicated.
From 32 to 34 weeks: Every 2 weeks or sooner if indicated.
From 34 to 41 weeks: Every week or sooner if indicated
From 41 weeks to delivery: Twice a week

Provide health education on warning signs requiring notification of the health care provider:
- Vaginal bleeding
- Gush or leakage of fluid from the vagina
- Cramping or contractions
- Severe or persistent abdominal pain
- Fever greater than 38° C or 100.4° F
- Marked change in fetal activity
- Severe or persistent headaches
- Blurred vision
- Dizziness
- Edema of the face and or hands
- Dysuria, especially with low back or costovertebral back pain
- Nausea and vomiting lasting longer than 24 hours

Provide health education on what to avoid:
- Illicit and recreational drugs
- Smoking and second-hand smoking
- Alcohol beverages
- OTC, prescription, and homeopathic medicines until their use is discussed with the health care provider
- Undercooked meat
- Environmental toxins
- Changing cat litter boxes
- Gardening without gloves
- Dehydration and hyperthermia
- Dangerous sports
- Permitting air to be blown in the vagina
- Provide instructions on what to do in case of an emergency.
- Identify procedure to follow in case of emergency. This would include who to contact, depending on time of day, weekday, weekends, and holidays.
- Discuss frequency of prenatal visits (Box 202-1).
- Provide psychosocial support/referrals as needed.
- Provide information to relieve discomforts of pregnancy.

Physiological Changes During Pregnancy

First Trimester

Breast tenderness: Wear supportive bra. Discuss with partner need for gentleness in touching breasts during lovemaking. Acetaminophen may be used.

Constipation: Regular exercise. Increase consumption of water and other liquids. Add fiber to diet, such as fresh fruit and whole-grain breads. Drink prune juice. Laxatives (milk of magnesia), stool softeners, and bulk producers may be used.

Headaches: Rest, relaxation exercises, warm bath, warm or cold compresses to forehead, face, head, and shoulder massage, aroma therapy. Acetaminophen may be used.

Hemorrhoids: Avoid constipation and prolonged sitting. Take warm sitz baths, followed by an application of witch hazel.

Nausea/vomiting: Reassure the patient that this is self-limiting. Small, frequent meals and a protein snack at bedtime may help. Try hard candy, raspberry leaf tea, or 10 gtt of peppermint spirits in half of a glass of water. Avoid greasy and spicy foods. Keep dry crackers at bedside. Drink carbonated beverages. If dehydration, ketosis, or electrolyte abnormalities are present, antiemetics (meclizine, diphenhydramine, and metoclopramide) or pyridoxine may be used.

Urinary frequency: Decrease caffeine intake.

Varicosities: Wear supportive stockings or TEDS. Rest and elevate legs when possible. Perineal pads may help vulvar varicosities.

Second Trimester

Backache/musculoskeletal strain: Avoid excessive weight gain, be conscious of posture, use good body mechanics, wear flat or low-heeled shoes. Place a footstool under one foot while standing, a pillow in the lumbar area while sitting, and a pillow between the knees while lying on your side. Massage, apply ice or heat.

Backache/sacroiliac dysfunction: Place a wedge-shaped pillow underneath abdomen while lying on side. Perform back exercises.

Dizziness/faintness: Avoid lying flat on back, dehydration, and prolonged standing or sitting. Change position slowly. Lie in left lateral position.

Leukorrhea: Bathe daily and wear cotton underwear and change frequently.

Leg cramps: Exercise, calf stretch exercises, walks. Keep legs warm. Decrease phosphate intake by decreasing milk intake. Increase magnesium intake via magnesium tablets: 122 mg every morning and 244 mg every evening.

Round ligament pain: Avoid twisting and sudden movements. Bend over or raise knee to chest on affected side. Rest and apply warm compresses.

Third Trimester

Braxton-Hicks contractions: Teach patient to differentiate between true and false labor.

Empty bladder frequently. Increase fluid intake. Resting in a left lateral recumbent position or exercising lightly may help to relieve discomfort. Use relaxation techniques. Advise warm tub baths.

Edema: Avoid prolonged sitting or standing. Lie in left lateral recumbent position for 1 to 2 hours twice a day and sleep in that position. Elevate legs when possible. Refrain from wearing clothes that constrict the extremities. Increase fluid intake and decrease intake of sugar or fats. Advise moderate sodium intake.

Heartburn: Small, frequent meals. Try papaya or raw almonds after meals. Refrain from lying recumbent after eating. Avoid fried and gas-producing foods. Sleep with head raised using stacked pillows. Antacids with magnesium hydroxide or magnesium trilisate may be used. Avoid antacids with baking soda, aluminum, or high sodium contents.

Skin rashes: Apply ice. Diphenhydramine may be used. If relief not obtained, refer to dermatologist.

PRENATAL CARE: RETURN VISITS

SUBJECTIVE DATA

Historical Data

Fetal movement
Nausea and/or vomiting
Vaginal bleeding or discharge
Contractions, cramping, or pelvic pressure
Dysuria or frequency
Headaches
Scotoma or blurred vision
Edema
Preterm labor symptoms
Pain: Chest, abdomen, back, legs
Skin changes
Fever or exposure to infectious disease
Numbness or tingling of hands or wrists
Genital lesions, sores, or growths
Trauma
Medications taken

OBJECTIVE DATA

Physical Examination

A physical examination should be performed ,with particular attention to:

- Blood pressure, weight
- Fundal height
- Fetal heart tone, presentation
- Edema
- Other elements as indicated

Laboratory/DiagnosticTesting

Laboratory and diagnostic tests should include proteinuria, glucosuria, and ketonuria. Perform ultrasound as indicated. Specific tests are outlined in Table 202-1.

Interventions

The fundal height in centimeters should be equal to the number of weeks gestation plus or minus 2 cm. If the fundal height is 3 to 4 cm smaller or larger than the gestational age in weeks, review dating parameters and order ultrasonography.

Follow up on other abnormal results to laboratory tests or physical examination findings. Rhogam at 28 weeks as indicated.

Provide information to relieve discomforts of pregnancy.

Continue to encourage health promotion activities.

Provide education on the following topics:

- Planning for labor and birth
- Sibling preparation
- Warning signs
- Infant feeding and care

Provide psychosocial support/referrals as needed.

TABLE 202-1 Specific Laboratory/Diagnostic Tests

Weeks of Gestation	Laboratory/Diagnostic Test	Cost
9 to 11	Chorionic villi sampling as indicated	712-848
12 to 14	Early amniocentesis as indicated	456-543
15 to 16	Traditional amniocentesis as indicated	456-543
15 to 18	Maternal serum fetal alpha-protein or maternal serum multiple marker screening	54-67
24 to 28	Hemoglobin or hematocrit, diabetes and antibody screening	23-39;
32	Group B streptococcus culture, gonococcus, chlamydia, VDRL	18-23/Hgb-Hct; 69-87/insulin antibodies

POSTDATE OR POSTTERM PREGNANCY CARE

OVERVIEW

A prolonged pregnancy is one that continues past 295 days. Unreliable dates is cited as the most frequent cause for the diagnosis of postdate pregnancy. The purpose for increased monitoring of the woman experiencing a prolonged pregnancy is to prevent neonatal morbidity. The rate of neonatal morbidity has been shown to increase at 41 weeks of gestation.

SUBJECTIVE DATA

Historical Data

Fetal kick counts: Mother lying comfortably counts fetal kicks for 60 min; a minimum of 4 kicks /hour is normal
Nausea and/or vomiting
Vaginal bleeding or discharge
Contractions, cramping, or pelvic pressure
Dysuria or frequency
Headaches, scotoma, or blurred vision
Edema
Pain: Chest, abdomen, back, legs
Skin changes
Fever or exposure to infectious disease
Numbness or tingling of the hands or wrists
Genital lesions, sores, or growths
Trauma
Medications taken

OBJECTIVE DATA

Physical Examination

A physical examination should be performed with particular attention to:
- Blood pressure, weight
- Fundal height
- Fetal heart tone, presentation
- Edema
- Other elements as indicated

Laboratory/DiagnosticTesting

Laboratory and diagnostic tests should focus on:
- Proteinuria, glucosuria, ketonuria ($15-$21)
- Fetal well-being: Nonstress test ($223-$273), contraction stress test ($246-$314), amniotic fluid index, biophysical profile ($342-$410)

Interventions

Explain induction vs. expectant management.
Provide psychosocial support/referrals as needed.

POSTPARTAL CARE

OVERVIEW

The purpose of postpartal care is to promote (1) maternal physiological adaptation, (2) parenting skills, (3) well child care, (4) family planning, and (5) decrease of family violence and neglect.

SUBJECTIVE DATA

Historical Data

Physical problems: Fever, chills, breast engorgement, breast care, breastfeeding, nipple soreness, lochia/return of menses, incisional or perineal discomfort, dysuria, urinary frequency
Adaptation to motherhood: Rest and sleep habits, appetite and dietary habits, exercise, coping, sexual activity
Desired birth control method
Baby: Feeding, care, health, first examination, problems
Family adjustments

OBJECTIVE DATA

Physical Examination

A physical examination should be conducted with particular attention to:
- Thyroid
- Breasts
- Abdomen
- Extremities
- Pelvic region (uterus returns to normal size by 6 weeks)

Laboratory/Diagnostic Testing

Laboratory and diagnostic tests should include the following:
- Hemoglobin or hematocrit levels
- Fasting blood sugar for patients with diabetes or gestational diabetes
- Thyroid function tests for women whose thyroid dosage changed during the pregnancy (TSH: $58-$72; thyroid panel [does not include TSH]: $48-$62; thyroid panel with TSH: $89-$112)

Interventions

Follow up on abnormal laboratory or physical findings from pregnancy and this visit.

Provide method of contraception as requested.

Exercise can be started soon after birth. Start with simple activities and gradually advance to more strenuous ones.

Give weight reduction guidance.

Encourage health promotion activities.

Provide psychosocial support/referrals as needed. Distinguish postpartum blues from postpartum depression.

Provide information to relieve discomforts of postpartum period.

Breast engorgement: Encourage all mothers to wear a well-fitted supportive bra 24 hours a day.

Breastfeeding mothers: Frequent nursing and the use of warm compresses and a mild analgesic are recommended. Mother may need to manually express a small amount of milk before offering breast to baby.

Bottle-feeding mothers: May apply ice to breast and use a mild analgesic.

Nipple soreness: Avoid soap or other drying agents on the nipple. Allow nipples to be exposed to air after completing a feeding. Change nursing pads frequently. Determine whether (1) baby is properly positioned at the breast, (2) mother is properly breaking suction during feeding, or (3) baby has thrush or diaper candidiasis. Examine breasts for evidence of monilial, bacterial, or HSV infections. Treat condition based on data collected. See Chapter 25.

Perineal discomfort: Encourage proper perineal hygiene. Side-lying positioning or use of pillows may help to lessen discomfort. May use cool sitz baths or apply ice to perineum during the first 24 hours. Afterward, the use of heat may provide some relief. Heat sources may include a warm sitz bath, heat lamp, or shower. Mild analgesics may be used.

RESOURCES

The Reproductive Toxicology Center (REPROTOX) can be contacted to obtain summaries of the developmental effects of medications (202-687-5137).

REFERENCES

Byrd J: Content of prenatal care. In Ratcliffe SD, Byrd JE, Sakornut EL, editors: *Handbook of pregnancy and perinatal care in family practice: science and practice,* Philadelphia, 1996, Hanley & Belfus.

Summers L, Price RA: Preconception care: an opportunity to maximize health in pregnancy, *J Nurse-Midwifery* 38:188-198, 1993.

SUGGESTED READINGS

Akridge KM: Postpartum and lactation. In Youngkin EQ, Davis MS, editors: *Women's health: a primary care clinical guide,* Norwalk, Conn, 1994, Appleton & Lange.

Baxley E: Postpartum biomedical concerns. In Ratcliffe SD, Byrd JE, Sakornut EL, editors: *Handbook of pregnancy and perinatal care in family practice: science and practice,* Philadelphia, 1996, Hanley & Belfus.

Corder-Mabe J: Complications of pregnancy. In Youngkin EQ, Davis MS, editors: *Women's health: a primary care clinical guide,* Norwalk, Conn, 1994, Appleton & Lange.

Fontaine P, Sayres W: Obstetric risk assessment. In Ratcliffe SD, Byrd JE, Sakornut EL, editors: *Handbook of pregnancy and perinatal care in family practice: science and practice,* Philadelphia, 1996, Hanley & Belfus.

Fuqua MH: Assessing fetal well-being. In Youngkin EQ, Davis MS, editors: *Women's health: a primary care clinical guide,* Norwalk, Conn, 1994, Appleton & Lange.

Remich M: Promoting a healthy pregnancy. In Youngkin EQ, Davis MS, editors: *Women's health: a primary care clinical guide,* Norwalk, Conn, 1994, Appleton & Lange.

Walker MPR, Resnik R: Prolonged pregnancy, cervical ripening, and induction of labor. In Moore TR et al, editors: *Gynecology & obstetrics: a longitudinal approach,* New York, 1993, Churchill Livingstone.

Wheeler L: *Nurse-midwifery handbook: a practical guide to prenatal and postpartum care,* Philadelphia, 1997, JB Lippincott.

Youngkin EQ, Davis MS: Assessing women's health. In Youngkin EQ, Davis MS, editors: *Women's health: a primary care clinical guide,* Norwalk, Conn, 1994, Appleton & Lange.

Preconceptional Health Appraisal

Directions: Please mark an "X" next to any item that is true for you.

Nutrition:

_________ Are you underweight or overweight?
_________ Do you practice vegetarianism? (eat few or no meat)
_________ Do you crave unusual substances such as starch, dirt, or clay?
_________ Have you ever used extreme behaviors to control your weight such as fasting for longer than a day, make yourself vomit, or use diuretics or laxatives?
_________ Do you eat a special diet?
_________ Do you take vitamins?
_________ Do you take birth control pills?

Social History:

_________ Are you 34 years or older?
_________ Are you 18 years or younger?
_________ Have you finished high school?
_________ Do you smoke cigarettes or use tobacco products?
_________ Have you ever drunk beer, wine, or hard liquor?
_________ Have you drunk beer, wine, or hard liquor in the past month?
Type and amount ____________________
_________ Have you ever used marijuana, crack, cocaine, uppers, downers, IV drugs, or any recreational drugs?
Type and when last used ____________________
_________ Does anyone in your family have alcohol or drug problems?
_________ Have you ever been physically, sexually, or emotionally abused?
_________ Are you currently in an abusive or unhealthy relationship?
_________ Are you unemployed?
_________ Do you lack insurance?
_________ Do you use or work with lead or chemicals at your home or work?
_________ Do you work with radiation?

Medication History:

_________ Do you routinely or occasionally take prescribed medication?
If yes, list names and doses.

_________ Do you routinely or occasionally take over-the-counter medications?
If yes, list names and doses.

Medical History: Do you have or have you ever had:

_________ Diabetes
_________ Asthma
_________ Epilepsy
_________ Cancer
_________ Heart disease
_________ Thyroid disease
_________ Ulcerative colitis
_________ Crohn's disease
_________ Phenylketonuria (PKU)
_________ High blood pressure
_________ Deep vein thrombosis
_________ Kidney disease
_________ Systemic lupus erythematosus
_________ Sickle cell trait or disease
_________ Drug addiction
____

Other health problems that required medical or surgical care
If yes, please explain ____________________

Reproductive History: Have you ever had:

_______ Surgery on your ovaries, tubes, uterus, or cervix; or problems with your uterus or cervix including an abnormal Pap smear?
_______ History of your mother receiving DES (a drug to stop miscarriages) when she was pregnant with you?
_______ Two or more miscarriages/abortions in the first trimester?
_______ One or more pregnancies that ended between 14 and 28 weeks gestation?
_______ One or more fetal deaths (stillborn)?
_______ One or more neonatal deaths (infant died before one month of age)?
_______ Five or more confirmed pregnancies?
_______ One or more infants die of SIDS?
_______ Less than 12 months since last birth?
_______ One or more infants with a birth defect?
_______ One or more infants requiring a stay in NICU?
_______ An infant less than $5^1/_2$ pounds?
_______ An infant more than 9 pounds?

Infectious Disease History: Have you or your partner ever had:

_______ Gonorrhea
_______ Chlamydia
_______ Genital herpes
_______ Genital warts
_______ Syphilis
_______ Viral hepatitis
_______ Trichomonias
_______ HIV/AIDS
_______ High risk behavior including use of intravenous street drugs, intimate bisexual/homosexual contact, or multiple sexual partners (more than six partners in your lifetime)?
_______ Occupational exposure to blood or body secretions of others?
_______ Blood transfusion
_______ Are your immunizations deficient or not up-to-date?
_______ Do you own or work with cats?

Family History: Do you, your partner, or members of either family, including your children have:

_______ Hemophilia
_______ Fragile X
_______ Tay-Sachs disease
_______ Sickle cell disease or trait
_______ Birth defects
_______ Heart defects
_______ Blindness
_______ Deafness
_______ Mental retardation
_______ Phenylketonuria (PKU)
_______ Cystic fibrosis
_______ Kidney disease
_______ Multiple sclerosis
_______ Leukemia
_______ Neurofibromatosis
_______ Huntington's chorea
_______ Osteogenesis
_______ Alcoholism/drug addictions
_______ Are you and your partner related outside of marriage?

Identified Preconceptional Health Risks; Patient Education/Recommendations/Referrals:

1.
2.
3.
4.
5.

203 Well Child

ICD-9-CM

Infant Examination V20.2
Examination for Preschool Children V70.5
Examination for Admission to School V70-3
School Examination V70.5
Developmental Testing of Child or Infant V20.2
Annual Examination V70.0
Child Care (Routine) Examination V20-2

INFANT BIRTH TO 12 MONTHS

Growth and Development

The growth and developmental guidelines and milestones across the body systems are outlined in Table 203-1.

Well Child Care

SOAPE guidelines for development of infants from birth to 12 months of age are outlined in Table 203-2. Sample well infant examination forms are found on pp. 1272 to 1283.

CHILD 1 TO 10 YEARS

Growth and Development

The growth and developmental guidelines and milestones across the body systems are outlined in Table 203-3.

Well Child Care

SOAPE guidelines for development of the child age 1-10 years are outlined in Table 203-4.

Sample well child examination forms are found on pp. 1284 to 1297.

SUGGESTED READINGS

ACPM News, the newsletter of the American College of Preventive Medicine 1:3, 1989. American Academy of Pediatrics: Active and passive immunizations. In Peter G, editor: *1997 Redbook: report of the Committee on Infectious Disease,* ed 24, Elk Grove Village, Ill, 1997, The Academy.

Baker R: *Handbook of pediatric primary care,* Boston, 1996, Little Brown.

Barkauskas V et al: *Health and physical assessment,* St Louis, 1994, Mosby.

Behrman RE, Kleigman R: *Nelson's essentials of pediatrics,* ed 14, Philadelphia, 1992, WB Saunders.

Brady M: Patient management exchange: educating youths and their parents about the prevention of firearm injury, *J Pediatr Health Care* 8:127-129, 1994.

Hoekelman RA et al: *Primary pediatric care,* ed 2, St Louis, 1997, Mosby.

McGinnis J, Foege W: Actual causes of death in the US, *JAMA* 270:2207-2212, 1993.

Ramos AG, Tuchman DN: Persistent vomiting, *Pediatr Rev* 5:24-31, 1994.

Schmitt B: *Your child's health,* New York, 1987, Bantam.

US Preventive Services Task Force: *Guide to clinical preventive services,* ed 2, Baltimore, 1996, Williams & Wilkins.

TABLE 203-1 Growth and Development: 0 to 12 Months

System	0-3 Months	4-6 Months	7-12 Months
Neurological	Turns head side to side by 1 mo. Head lag when pulled from supine to sitting until 2-3 mo. Upright head control should be obtained. Landau (ventral suspension): Flexion position Reaching/grasping; palmar grasp at birth until about 2 mo By 3 mo, growing hand-eye coordination and infant attempts contact with objects and holds briefly.	Raises head and chest with arms extended. Raises head on vertical axis and turns head from side to side. Pulled from supine to sitting with no head lag. In a sitting position, head may tilt a little forward but no head bobbing. Head is erect by 5 mo. By 5-6 mo, infant is purposefully rolling over, first front to back and then back to front. By 4 mo, infant loses tonic neck reflex and head stays midline with extensors in more of a symmetric position. Infant regards hands, brings them to midline and mouth (symmetrotonic posture). Infant bears the weight of an erect head and enjoys being supported in upright position. At 4 mo, infant has increased attention for various objects. By 6 mo, infant reaches out for, retrieves, and transfers object from hand to hand. After discovering hands, discovers rest of body: face, head, trunk, lower extremities, and genitals. At 4 mo, enjoys standing erect. By 5-6 mo, can pull from sitting to a standing position and can bear weight by holding hands. By 6½ mo, can do this and then flex their knees momentarily. Infant sits alone with head erect.	By 7 mo, is able to pivot in pursuit of an object. By 8-9 mo, many infants stand for a few seconds independently, cruising by 9 mo. By 9-10 mo, takes a few steps with hands held. Between 6-9 mo, radial-palmar grasp moves to thumb and forefinger (pincher) grasp; by 12 mo, pincher grasp is used without the ulnar surface. At 9 mo, uses finger to poke at objects. By 9 mo, is able to release an object by request; looks for objects (object permanency) and finds hidden objects if in sight. By 12 mo, is able to release object into hand.
Vision	Neonates fixate and track an object to midline. By 2 mo, objects are followed past midline. By 3 mo, objects are tracked 180 degrees; peripheral vision is 180 degrees by 2 mo. By 6 wk, binocular vision begins, and it is well established by 4 mo. Acuity at birth is 200/200-200/400; by 3-4 mo, it is 20/200-20/300.	Visual accommodation equals that of adults; infant follows objects 180 degrees; perceives the color spectrum similar to adults; visual acuity 20/200 to 20/300. Infant prefers moving objects. By 5-6 mo, visual acuity is 20/40-20/60. EOMI, cover-uncover test WNL.	Equal tracking; EOMI, improving eye-hand coordination
Hearing	Responds to human voice; positive startle reflex with loud noises. By 2 mo, turns head to side when sound is made at ear level. By 3 mo, makes initiative to look toward sounds; can discriminate between pitch.	Turns to sound; responds to human voice, discriminates between pitch sounds.	Infants can locate sounds, recognize their name, understand commands, but usually do not obey. By 12 mo, will follow some simple commands

Dental	There is increase in salivation at 3 mo. May begin teething as early as 3-4 mo.	Infant may begin teething; teeth eruption.	Lower and upper incisors usually are present; lateral incisors should be erupting or present.
Nutrition	Intake of 110 kcal/kg/day is needed.	Intake of 110 kcal/kg/day is needed, with feeding 4-6 times per day, 4-6 oz q 4-6 hr (24-32 oz).	Eating time is a socialization process at 9-12 mo. Infants want to be a part of family meal times.
Breast-feeding	Neonate: Feeds q 1-2 hr 2 wk to 1 mo: Feeds q 2-4 hr 1-2 mo: Feeds q 4-6 hr	By 4 mo, tongue thrusting diminishes and infants turn their heads if full.	Infant shows interest in drinking from a cup, attempts to feed self. By 12 mo, drinks from a cup; feeds self. Needs approximately 12-16 oz milk/day.
Formula	Neonate: Feeds 2-3 oz q 2-3 hr 2 wk-1 mo: Feeds 3-4 oz q 3-4 hr 2-3 mo: Feeds 4-6 oz q 4-6 hr		By 12 mo, infant is self-feeder, there is decrease in growth demands, therefore decrease in appetite. May be picky eater.
Sleep	Neonates alert 1 hr/10 hr. Neonates are awake 3-4 hr/24 hr. By 2 mo, infants may be awake as long as 10 hr/day. Usually infant sleeps 4-6 hr at night. By 3 mo, infant should be sleeping 3-8 hr at night.	Infant sleeps in own bed, own room; sleeps 6-8 hr; by 5-6 mo, sleeps 8-10 hr, 1-2 naps, begins to resist separation; begins to experience night awakening (does not need night-time bottle) by 5-6 mo.	Infants may have decreased naps to 1 per day. They have more wakeful periods at night. A bedtime routine should be established.
Elimination	Stools begin as loose and watery; as infant matures, stools become more formed. Breast-fed infants: Stools with every feeding, UOP 6-8 wet diapers Formula-fed infant: Stools 1×/day, 1 every other day or 1 every 3rd day; UOP 6-8 wet diapers	Stools are formed; color changes are related to solids; bladder capacity is increasing, urination decreasing.	Stools are formed, 1-2 per day. UOP is same as at 4-6 mo.
Speech/Language	By 4 wk, makes throaty noises. Infant focuses on significant other and imitates. By 2 mo, makes vowel sounds and cooing. By 3 mo, infant attempts to make sounds in relation to socialization.	Infant continues to imitate; coos, babbles, squeals, laughs, vocalizes to mirror.	By 6½ mo, infant produces repetitive vowel sounds. By 9 mo, infant enjoys imitating sounds like-"mama" and "dada" with babbling. Infant recognizes words said by others (mom, dog, etc.). By 8-9 mo, infant responds to own name. By 1 yr, infant says 1-3 words related to object.
Psychosocial	Social smile is fully developed by 3-5 wk. (Infants who do not develop social smile by 3 mo may be an early identification of problems.) Neonate makes eye-to-eye contact and focuses on faces. By 3 mo, infant can recognize familiar faces.	Infants 4 mo old begin to laugh, squeal, or blow bubbles as part of social exchange; they are able to show displeasure by facial expressions. By 4-7 mo, infant responds to emotional tones of social contacts. By 6 mo, demonstrated social preference to caregivers; when mom is around, can display stranger anxiety. Development of separation anxieties may depend on infant's comfort with communication and emotional exchange.	Infant is developing into very social being; plays games and enjoys books and being read to for very short periods. Infant tries to figure out how things work, likes to manipulate objects. Infant imitates activities of caregiver; interacts with others; parallel play, separation anxiety, stranger anxiety are seen.

EOMI, Extraocular movements intact; *WNL,* within normal limits; *UOP,* Urinary output.

TABLE 203-2 Well Child Care: 0 to 12 Months

	0-3 Months	4-6 Months	7-12 Months
S	History: Determine any problems or changes since last seen. Ask about sleeping, elimination, immunizations, concerns of parents, birth history if has never been seen before. Nutrition: How often, how much formula or breast milk, feeding problems. Development: Infant cuddles, follows to midline, responds to sound, smiles with parent-child interaction. Family: Mom's health and rest, family adjustment to baby, child care issues, dad's involvement, support system, parents getting out and getting rest.	History: Determine any problems or changes since last seen. Ask about sleeping, elimination, immunization reactions and what immunizations have been completed, birth history if never seen before, parents' concerns. Nutrition: How often, how much formula or breast milk, feeding problems, solids Development: Infant follows 180 degrees, responds to voice, grasps rattle, rolls over one way, lifts head to 90 degrees, babbles, no head lag, coos, transfers, rolls over, sits up with minimal support. Family: Mom's health, dad's involvement, sibling adjustment.	History: Determine any problems or changes since last seen. Ask about sleeping, elimination, immunization reactions and what immunizations have been completed, birth history if never seen before, parents' concerns. Nutrition: How often, how much formula or breast milk, feeding problems, solids, feeding self with finger foods, fluoride Development: Infant plays peek-a-boo, looks for fallen object, pincher grasp, "mama, dada," crawls, sits without support, stands holding on, pat-a-cake, bangs 2 blocks together, imitates sounds, understands "no," cruises, stands alone 2-3 sec. Family: Family schedule, outside supports.
O	Physical examination (child is usually not fearful of strangers): 2 weeks: Infant gains 15-30 g, back to birth weight. Height, weight, HC. Skin, nodes, head, fontanelles, (flat, soft), eye (red reflex), ears, nose, oropharynx, neck, chest/breast, lungs, heart, abdomen, umbilicus: cord off, genitalia (testes descended), femoral pulse, musculoskeletal, hips (clicks/clunks), Moro's reflex, palmar reflex, plantar grasp, spine 2 months: Weight gain 15-30 g (1 oz/day), 1 inch/mo. Skin, nodes, head, fontanelles (posterior fused), eye (red reflex), ears, nose, oropharynx, neck, chest/breast, lungs, heart, abdomen, umbilicus (cord off), genitalia (testes descended), femoral, pulse, musculoskeletal, hips (clicks/clunks), Moro's reflex, plantar grasp (less intense).	Physical examination (child is not usually fearful of strangers): Height, weight, HC. Skin, nodes, head, fontanelles (flat soft), eye (red reflex), visual tracking (cover-uncover at 6 mo), ears, nose, oropharynx, teeth and gums, neck, chest/breast, lungs, heart, abdomen, genitalia (testes descended), femoral pulse, musculoskeletal, hips (clicks/clunks), Moro's and tonic neck reflexes (disappear by 6 mo), plantar grasp	Physical examination (child is usually fearful of strangers): Height, weight, HC. Skin, nodes, head, fontanelles (flat, soft), eye (cover-uncover), ears, nose, oropharynx, neck, chest/breast, lungs, heart, abdomen, genitalia (testes descended), femoral pulse, musculoskeletal, plantar grasp (disappears by 8 mo), positive pincher, positive parachute reflex

Dx	WCC Possible problems: Metabolic disorders, intestinal obstruction, cardiac anomalies, congenital defects, apnea, gastroesophageal reflux, FTT, STD (congenital syphilis, HIV, *Chlamydia*), abuse	WCC Possible problems: FTT, URI, OM, viral exanthem, diaper dermatitis, candidiasis diaper rash, atopic dermatitis, gastroenteritis, dacryostenosis, conjunctivitis, abuse	WCC Possible problems: OM, diaper dermatitis, URI, amblyopia, tibial torsion, genu varum; developmental delay, trained night feeders, undescended testicles, hypospadias, abuse
P	Immunizations DPT 1, HIB 1, IPV 1, HBV 2 Check neonatal screening results at 2 wk.	Immunizations 4 mo: DPT 2, HIB 2, IPV 2 6 mo: DPT 3, HIB 3, HBV 3 Sickle preparation if indicated	Immunizations 9 mo: Up to date 12 mo: DPT 4, HIB 4, oral polio vaccine 4, MMR 1; can offer varicella. Screen for lead level and CBC (or Hct) TB if indicated
E	Follow-up: 2 mo; next visit at 4 mo	Follow-up: 6 mo, 9 mo	Follow-up: 12 mo, 15-18 mo
Guidance	Assess parental ability to learn, previous experience as parent, educational level. Development: Review expected developmental changes, basic trust vs mistrust. Nutrition: Continue formula/breast, (25 oz formula/day 4-6 oz/time). Safety: Car, crib, falls, smoke alarm Parenting: Cuddling, talking to baby, music Potential problems: Possible diaper rash, spitting up, colic and crying	Assess parental ability to learn, previous experience as parent, educational level. Development: Review expected developmental changes, basic trust vs mistrust. Nutrition: Continue formula/breast (5 feedings, 6-8 oz/time), can offer water especially during hot weather. At 6 mo, add 1 new food at a time/week for allergies. Can begin cereal* with iron (1-2 tbsp 1 time/day) increasing up to ⅓-½ cup (2 times/day), then add fruits and vegetables (1 tsp at a time). Safety: Car, crib, falls, smoke alarm, babyproof house, all objects go into mouth, choking, bathing, Poison Control number Parenting: Call child by name, use soft music, touching games such as "little piggy." Potential problems: Possible diaper rash, teething, susceptible to infections, sleep patterns (night awakening), dental hygiene (no bottle in bed)	Assess parental ability to learn, prior experience as parent, educational level. Development: Review expected developmental changes, basic trust vs mistrust. Nutrition: Decrease in formula to 12-16 oz/day (8 mo), introduce cup, tolerance and acceptance of new foods. Introduce meat, breads, rice, macaroni, soft cheese, and egg yolks; decrease calorie intake, child will eat if hungry. Balanced diet, uses cup; use high chair to make child part of family mealtime. Safety: Check lead risks, gates on stairs, electrical outlets capped, car seat, playpen or crib for safe place, constant watching, falls and burns, poison (ipecac). Parenting: Reinforce positive behavior, stimulation (toy phone, name body parts, blowing games, noisy push/pulls, hugs/kisses), discipline, bedtime routine, separation and stranger anxiety, reading, dental care (no toothpaste). Prevention: Dental hygiene, weaning from bottle, pacifier

*Rice cereal is less allergenic.

CBC, Complete blood cell count; *DPT*, diphtheria-pertussis-tetanus vaccine; *FTT*, failure to thrive; *HC*, Head circumference; *Hct*, hematocrit; *HIB*, *Haemophilus influenzae* B vaccine; *MMR*, measles-mumps-rubella vaccine; *IPV*, inactivated poliomyelitis vaccine; *OM*, otitis media; *STD*, sexually transmitted disease; *TB*, tuberculosis; *URI*, upper respiratory tract infection; *WCC*, well-child check.

TABLE 203-3 Growth and Development: 1 to 10 Years

System	12-24 Months	24-35 Months	3-5 Years	5-10 Years
Neurological	By 12 mo, infant moves to an upright stance, takes a few independent steps or should be walking; walking should be accomplished by no later than 15-18 mo. By 15 mo, gait is ataxic but symmetric stoops and recovers. By 18 mo, infant walks up stairs holding on; runs; walks backward, By 20 mo, goes down stairs. At 24 mo, able to run about; kicks ball. By 12 mo, infant can release object into hand. By 15 mo, can place raisin into bottle. By 18 mo, infant can remove raisin by dumping it out. Infant can make a tower of blocks of 2 cubes at 15 mo; at 18 mo, can make a tower of 4 cubes; by 24 mo, makes a tower of 6 cubes.	At 2 yr, child is able to kick a ball without falling. Child progresses to being able to kick a ball 10 feet at 3 yr. Child runs and jumps with both feet, jumps from chair or step, rides a push toy to pedaling a tricycle at 3 yr. By 3 yr, fine and gross motor skills are becoming more refined, smoother, and more coordinated. Child enjoys physical play. Child is able to walk upstairs and downstairs holding onto railing with 2 feet on step. Child begins to scribble at 2 yr. Child draws a circle, matches colors; crosses midline; can use scissors by age 3 yr. By 3 yr, child can make a tower of 8 blocks; makes a bridge after demonstration.	Preschooler is slender but sturdy, graceful, and agile, with erect posture. Hops, skips and climbs. Child advances with fine motor skills; copies figures and draws recognizable pictures.	At 6-8 yr, gross and fine motor skills become more controlled, with improved eye-hand coordination; child prints, colors in lines, ties bow; rides bike, hops, jumps. By 10 yr, gross and fine motor skills are more precise; child does tricks with bicycle, cursive writing, makes crafts, organized sports.
Vision	Smooth ocular movements; depth perception, good eye-hand coordination; intense interest in bright colors and different shapes.	Visual acuity is 20/80, with depth perception. Child copies a vertical line; color recognition not until 3½ to 4 yr.	Visual capabilities continue to undergo refinement during preschool period. Color vision and depth perception are fully established. Visual acuity: 3 yr—20/50; 4 yr—20/40; 5 yr—20/30; hyperopic	At 6-8 yr, visual acuity 20/20; no color blindness
Hearing	Infant is reactive to whispering, localizes sounds well, understands most commands, recognizes name readily, and recognizes familiar words.	By 3 yr, acuity is at adult level; child is aware of pitch and tone.	Hearing develops to adult level; child is able to make fine discriminations among similar speech sounds, such as the differences between *f, th,* and *s.*	Normal

Dental	Infant may have as many as 6 teeth; during second year, 8 more teeth should erupt. First-year molars, cuspids, then second-year molars come in. Brush teeth bid with a washcloth until infant is able to spit. Infant no longer uses bottle by 15-18 mo.	Between 24-36 mo, dentition is completed.	Twenty deciduous teeth are present; primary teeth are important for chewing, speech, and to hold spaces for secondary teeth. Older preschoolers can be responsible for brushing with gentle reminding from parents.	Permanent teeth continue to erupt; continue brushing and flossing with regular dental visits.
Nutrition	By 1 yr, change to whole milk until 2 yr. Give soft table foods, with more textured foods by 15-18 mo. Infant usually eats one balanced meal, with decreased food intake related to decreased growth rate.	Average need at 2-3 yr is 100 kcal/kg/day. Fat should be approximately 30% or less. Calcium needs to be approximately 700 mg/day.	Average preschooler needs 95 kcal/kg/day. Child has definite food preferences; is likely to refuse new foods.	At 5-8 yr, child needs approximately 80 kcal/kg/day. Increased appetite, 3 meals/day plus 1-2 snacks. At 8-10 yr, nutrition is still under primary control of parent, but child is eating away from home more and more and influenced by peers and TV. Child likes a variety of foods, especially fast foods and snacks.
Sleep	Sleep is fitful at night; more REM periods. Increased tension; infant may have fits or energy bursts at night, rock crib, bang head. Infant naps, usually once per day. Infant sleeps 10-12 hr/day.	Child usually sleeps 10-12 hr; may still take afternoon naps; sleeps all night; enjoys sleeping with favorite toy or blanket; begins to be afraid of the dark. Bed should have side rails.	Average sleep is 8-12 hr/night. Bedtime rituals are still important; nightmares and night terrors can be common in this age group because of active imaginations.	Average sleep is 8-10 hr/night. Child usually resists bedtime, develops stall tactics.
Elimination	Stools are formed, urine more concentrated; infant may show interest in potty.	Maturation of cortex layers is seen; sensory development for bladder and bowel control; elimination, especially of stool, is expression of pleasure in what a child of 2-3 yr has to produce. Nighttime wetting is not expected to end until 3-6 yr.	Child should have established daytime bowel and bladder control. Nighttime bladder control is usually accomplished by 3-6 yr. Around 5 yr, child should be able to manage toileting independently.	Normal patterns are established.

Continued

TABLE 203-3 Growth and Development: 1 to 10 Years—cont'd

System	12-24 Months	24-35 Months	3-5 Years	5-10 Years
Speech and language	By 18 mo, vocabulary is about 10 words. Rapid learning of words and meanings usually develops by this time.	By 2 yr, >50 words is common vocabulary; child uses 2 word sentences, knows 5-6 body parts. Dysfluencies are common, child uses plurals, present verb tense; recognizes 3 colors. By 3 yr, child speaks in 3-4 word sentences; speech is clear. Child uses pronouns, negatives, past tense, understands some adjectives (e.g., big or little).	Language is sophisticated and complex; 3-4 yr, 3-4 word sentences; 4-5 yr, 4-5 word sentences with lots of why questions. Speech often has hesitations, repetitions, and revisions. Stuttering and stammering should be evaluated if lasting longer than 6 mo. Quality and quantity of language in home have the most important impact on the child's language development.	At 5 to 8 yr, child uses all parts of speech; learns to read; arranges story in sequence; composes stories; defines words according to related action. By 10 yr, uses metaphors, personifications; speech understandable. Quick to use slang; loves jokes and humor.
Psychosocial	Toddlers develop sense of control over their bodies and expressively demonstrate this (temper tantrums, breath-holding spells, and biting). Infant is developing sense of self separate from others, striving for independence by taking initiative in making choices about behaviors.	Child is egocentric, has better sense of time, anticipates consequences from parents to form more careful actions, pretends, with magical thinking, dramatic-imitation play. Child moves from sensory to intuitive learning, with development of memory, symbolic play, global organization.	Child separates with some apprehension at 3 yr. By 4-5 yr, child relates to unfamiliar people easily, tolerates periods of separation. Child enjoys playing and interacting with other children. Child progresses from associative play to cooperative play. Egocentric behaviors are still present; role play, make-believe, or fantasy play.	Child is very sociable, group play increases, becomes competitive, learns to share, cooperates in organized manner. By 8-10 yr, child enjoys team sports, parties, sleepovers. Child needs time for free play; do not overschedule.

Table 203-4 Well-Child Care: 1 to 10 Years

	12-24 Months	24-36 Months	3-5 Years	5-10 Years
S	History: Determine any problems since last seen, any parental concerns. Ask about sleeping, elimination, illnesses, injuries, immunizations, birth history if never seen before.	History: Determine any problems since last seen, any parental concerns. Ask about sleeping, elimination, illnesses, injuries, immunizations, birth history if never seen before.	History: Determine any problems since last seen, any parental concerns. Ask about sleeping, elimination, illnesses, injuries, immunizations, birth history if never seen before.	History: Determine any problems since last seen, any parental concerns. Ask about sleeping, elimination, illnesses, injuries, immunizations, birth history if never seen before. Ask about menses for girl, sexual activity.
	Nutrition: Number of meals/day, varied diet, balanced diet, fluoride, mealtime problems	Nutrition: Number of meals/day, varied diet, balanced diet, fluoride, mealtime problems.	Nutrition: Number of meals/day, varied diet, balanced diet, fluoride, mealtime problems; child enjoys helping prepare meals.	Nutrition: Number of meals/day, varied diet, balanced diet, fluoride, mealtime problems
	Development: Child drinks from cup, crawls up stairs, throws ball, walks well, removes clothes, stacks 2-3 blocks, walks up steps with help, knows body parts, uses 2-3 word sentences, handles spoon well.	Development: Child follows simple directions, knows full name, sex; knows 1 color, uses plurals, rides tricycle.	Development: Child puts toys away, knows prepositions, knows 3-4 colors, uses verbs and full sentences, hops on 1 foot, dresses alone, understands opposites, copies square and triangle, draws man (3-6 parts), uses heel-to-toe walk. Assess school readiness.	Developmental: Behavior includes chores, outside activities, reading for pleasure. Child knows days of week, skips rope, tells time, peer interaction, and organized sports.
	Family: Parents agree on discipline, child care, sibling rivalry.	Family: Discipline, child care, sibling rivalry, playmates, family activities, FH of early MI, high cholesterol Ask child questions and have him or her follow directions to test hearing.	Family: Mom and dad's work, family happy, discipline, any new family members, smokers or alcohol or drug use	Family: Family schedule, family activities, discipline, new family members, any smokers or alcohol or drug use, after-school care, firearms at home, sibling problems or rivalry
O	Physical examination (fear of strangers):	Physical examination (fear of strangers):	Physical examination (may be cooperative; parents close):	Physical examination (usually cooperative, older child may want privacy):
	Height, weight HC	Height, weight (3 inches of height, 5 lb of weight per yr), HC	Height (±3 inches per yr), weight, vital signs, vision screening, hearing	Height, weight, vital signs, vision and hearing screening
	Skin, nodes, head, fontanelles, eye (cover-uncover), ears, nose, oropharynx, teeth and gums, neck, chest/breast, lungs, heart, abdomen, genitalia, musculoskeletal, neurologic	Skin, nodes, head, eye (fundi, cover-uncover), ears (whisper test), nose, oropharynx, teeth and gums, neck, chest/breast, lungs, heart, abdomen, genitalia	Skin, nodes, head, eye (fundi, cover-uncover), ears, nose, oropharynx, teeth and gums, neck, chest/breast, lungs, heart, abdomen, genitalia	Skin, nodes, head, eye (fundi, cover-uncover), ears, nose, oropharynx, teeth and gums, neck, chest/breast, lungs, heart, abdomen, genitalia, Tanner staging, scoliosis screening

FH, Family history; *HC*, head circumference; *MI*, myocardial infarction; *HBV*, hepatitis B virus; *MMR*, measles-mumps-rubella vaccine; *OPV*, oral polio vaccine; *TB*, tuberculosis.

Continued

TABLE 203-4 Well-Child Care: 1 to 10 Years—cont'd

	12-24 Months	24-36 Months	3-5 Years	5-10 Years
Dx	WCC Possible problems: Dental caries, developmental delays, intoeing, chronic OM, conductive hearing loss, croup, pica, impetigo	WCC Possible problems: Speech delays, tibial torsion, nurse-maid elbow, sexual abuse, stomatitis, pinworms, septic arthritis	WCC Possible problems: Hypertension, primary enuresis, masturbation, night terrors, coxsackievirus, varicella, osteomyelitis, dental caries	WCC Possible problems: Enuresis, poor school performance, sibling rivalry, abuse, dental caries, vision or hearing problems, eating disorders
P	MMR 1; offer varicella vaccine if child has not had chickenpox. Start HBV series if child has not gotten. Screen for TB exposure. Do lead screen if not already done.	Screen for TB exposure. Offer varicella vaccine if child has not had chickenpox.	Offer varicella vaccine if child has not had chickenpox. Immunizations (5 yr): DTAP 5, OPV 4, MMR 2	Offer varicella vaccine if child has not had chickenpox. Assess for TB. Assess for HBV.
E Guidance	Follow-up: 15-18 mo, 2 yr Assess parental ability to learn, previous experience as parent, educational level. Development: Review expected developmental changes, autonomy vs shame.	Follow-up: 3 yr Assess parental ability to learn, previous experience as parent, educational level. Development: Review expected developmental changes, autonomy vs shame.	Follow-up: Yearly check Assess parental ability to learn, previous experience as parent, educational level. Development: Review expected developmental changes, initiative vs guilt.	Follow-up: Yearly check Assess parental ability to learn, previous experience as parent, educational level. Development: Review expected developmental changes, industry vs inferiority. Child goes from learning through intuition to learning through concrete experiences; discuss expected pubertal changes, body odor.
	Nutrition: Stress need for balanced diet, milk intake 12-16 oz; decreased growth so decreased intake. Avoid soda, give fruit juice, not fruit drinks, discontinue bottle; decrease junk food.	Nutrition: Stress need for balanced diet, milk intake 12-16 oz; decreased growth so decreased intake. Avoid soda, give fruit juice, not fruit drinks, discontinue bottle; decrease junk food; no potato chips, coconut, nuts, whole kernel corn, hot dogs, raw carrots (aspiration).	Nutrition: Stress need for balanced diet, milk intake 12-16 oz. Offer raw vegetables during day; avoid soda, give fruit juice, not fruit drinks, discontinue bottle; decrease junk food.	Nutrition: Stress need for balanced diet. Avoid soda, give fruit juice, not fruit drinks; decrease junk food.

	Safety: Aspiration, pets, plastic bags, outdoors, climbing out of crib, poison (ipecac), drowning	Safety: Aspiration, pets, plastic bags, outdoors, climbing out of crib, poison (ipecac), drowning	Safety: Pets, plastic bags, outdoors, poison (ipecac), strangers, tricycle/bike (helmets), drowning, matches, guns	Safety: Outdoors, bike (helmet), strangers, car, drowning, guns
	Parenting: Consistent discipline; reinforce positive behavior, set limits; let child problem solve, play; read to child. Issues may include thumb sucking; dental care; naps.	Parenting: Toilet training, dental care, play, reading books, TV limits, 1 long nap/day, need for large-muscle use activity, anticipating consequences, dramatic play, discipline (limit setting), positive role model	Parenting: Ignore stuttering, provide positive role model for speech, provide a listener to allow child to express ideas and feelings, set TV limits, use consistent schedule, positive reinforcement, develop and enforce family rules, give chores; at 5 yr, child should learn/know telephone number and address.	Parenting: Consistent schedule, positive reinforcement, family rules developed and enforced, chores, positive role model, participation in school activities, limit on TV, time to talk with child, new responsibilities given with appropriate supervision, allowance, respect, communication
			Nightmares: Need lots of reassurance, explain difference between real and pretend; monitor TV viewing.	
			Preventive: Dental appointment, brushing at least bid	Preventive: Dental appointment, brushing teeth at least bid, emergency plan developed, discussion of drugs, alcohol, and smoking

WELL-CHILD VISIT
1-4 WEEKS

Date of visit: Name: Age in weeks: Allergies:

Key: ☑ Addressed ☒ Abnormal/see comments ☐ Not discussed

SUBJECTIVE

Assessment of parental concerns ______

______

Chief complaint ______

Interval history (problems/illness/hospitalizations) ______

______

Prenatal history:

Prenatal care: ______

______

STI: ______

______

Substance abuse: ______

______

Problems: ______

______

Birth history:*

Intrapartum information

Delivery: ☐ Vaginal ☐ C/S

Complications: ______

Apgar scores: ______

Birth weight: ______

Gestational age: ______

Hospital name: ______

*Birth history should be included in every new visit

Environmental history:

Type of home: ______

PB exposure	☐ Yes	☐ No
TB exposure	☐ Yes	☐ No
Tobacco exposure	☐ Yes	☐ No
Fluoridated water	☐ Yes	☐ No
Bed: type of crib ______		
Crib slats ≤2" apart	☐ Yes	☐ No
No lead paint	☐ Yes	☐ No

Family assessment:

Number of household members: ______

Sibling ages: ______

Mom's health/rest: ______

Dad's health/rest: ______

Siblings' health/feelings/adjustment: ______

______

Child/day care: ______

Outside support systems: ______

______

Dad/Mom support each other: ______

______

Substance use: ETOH ☐ Drugs ☐ Tobacco ☐

Interaction with infant: ______

______

How do parents describe infant?: ______

______

______

______

Nutritional assessment:

Breastfeeding		
Feeding Q 1-2 hours	☐ Yes	☐ No
How long on each breast? ______		
BMs Q day	☐ Yes	☐ No
6 to 8 wet diapers	☐ Yes	☐ No
Breast care: ______		
Formula		
Type of formula: ______		
Feeding Q 1-3 hours	☐ Yes	☐ No
BMs Q day	☐ Yes	☐ No
6 to 8 wet diapers	☐ Yes	☐ No
Sterilizing water	☐ Yes	☐ No

Bottle cleaning/preparation: ______

______

Feeding problems: ______

Sleeping patterns:

Sleeping 2 to 4 hour intervals? ☐ Yes ☐ No

OBJECTIVE

Development:

	Present	Not present	Comments
Regards face	☐	☐	______
Equal movements	☐	☐	______
Follows to midline	☐	☐	______
Startle/Moro reflex	☐	☐	______
Responds to voices	☐	☐	______
Lifts head/turns side to side	☐	☐	______
Smiles responsively	☐	☐	______
Vocalizes	☐	☐	______

	Normal	Abnormal	Comments
Appearance	☐	☐	______
Skin	☐	☐	______
Head/fontanel	☐	☐	______
Eyes/red reflex	☐	☐	______
Ears	☐	☐	______
Nose/patency	☐	☐	______
Oropharynx soft/hard palate	☐	☐	______
Neck	☐	☐	______

Physical exam:

WT ______ % ______ T ______
HT ______ % ______ P ______
HC ______ % ______ R ______

PLAN

Immunizations:

Reaction: ______

HBV#1 ☐ (√ in hospital)
HBV#2 ☐
Reviewed risks/benefits/literature given ☐
Immunization schedule reviewed ☐

Labs/screening tests

______
______

Medications

______
______

ASSESSMENT

☐ WCC ☐ Colic ☐ FTT ☐ Constipation

Breasts/neonatal hypertrophy	☐	☐	______
Thorax/lungs	☐	☐	______
Heart	☐	☐	______
Femoral pulses	☐	☐	______
Musculoskeletal	☐	☐	______
Spine	☐	☐	______
Abdomen	☐	☐	______
Genitals:			______
Male phallus length; circ/uncirc; testes descended	☐	☐	______
Female clitoral size; virilization; introitus	☐	☐	______
Anus/rectum	☐	☐	______

Neuro-primitive reflexes: ☐ Moro ☐ Stepping ☐ Rooting ☐ Plantar grasp ☐ Palmar grasp ☐ Tonic neck (at approx. 1 month) ☐ Babinski

Hip clicks/clunks: ☐ Yes ☐ No

ANTICIPATORY GUIDANCE

Sleep:

No bottles in bed ☐
No bottle propping ☐
No pillows ☐
Infant sleeps in own bed/crib ☐
Placing infant in bed when awake ☐

Safety:

Babysitters/parents time out ☐
Not leaving infant unattended with young siblings/pets ☐
Sibling aggression ☐
Car seat: rear facing ☐
Hot water heater: 120° ☐
Carrying child safely ☐
Emergency phone #s ☐
Crib slats ≤2" apart ☐
No bean bag chairs ☐

Hygiene:

Skin care/baths/nail care ☐
Diaper hygiene:
  Wash diaper area Q change ☐
  Do not use wipes if irritated ☐
Umbilicus/cord care:
  Wash with soap/H_2O QD ☐
  Apply ABX oint. TID ☐
  Clean w/alcohol QD ☐
  Check for oozing, odor, bleeding, or inflammation ☐

Illness:

Taking infant out in public ☐
Fever measurement and control: acetaminophen ☐
How and when to call your doctor/nurse practitioner ☐

Bonding:

Nonnutritive sucking ☐
Cuddling/holding/talking ☐
Cry/temperament ☐

Nutrition:

Spitting/bubbling ☐
Delay solids ☐
Vitamins ☐
Amount: ______
Frequency: ______
Fluoride ☐
Amount: ______
Frequency: ______
Iron ☐
Amount: ______
Frequency: ______

RTO:
☐ 2 weeks for HBV #2
☐ 2 months for WCC
☐ ______

F/U NEXT VISIT:
______
______
______

Signature: ______

WELL-CHILD VISIT
2 Months

Date of visit:			Name:	DOB:	Allergies:
T:	P:	R :	Medications:	Weight:	
Interim history:				Length:	
Problems/hospitalizations:				Head circ:	
Illness?				Age in weeks:	

Key: ☑ Addressed ☒ Abnormal/see comments ☐ Not discussed

SUBJECTIVE

Assessment of parental concerns ____________________

____

Chief complaint ____________________

____

Environmental history:

Type of home: ____________________

PB exposure ☐ Yes ☐ No

TB exposure ☐ Yes ☐ No

Tobacco exposure ☐ Yes ☐ No

Fluoridated water ☐ Yes ☐ No

Bed: type of crib ____________________

Crib slats $\leq$2" apart ☐ Yes ☐ No

No lead paint ☐ Yes ☐ No

Family assessment:

Number of household members: ____________________

Sibling ages: ____________________

Mom's health/rest: ____________________

Dad's health/rest: ____________________

Siblings' health/feelings/adjustment: ____________________

____

Child/day care: ____________________

Outside support systems: ____________________

____

Dad/Mom support each other: ____________________

____

Substance use: ETOH ☐ Drugs ☐ Tobacco ☐

How do parents describe infant?: ____________________

____

____

____

____

Nutritional assessment:

Breastfeeding

Feeding Q 1-2 hours ☐ Yes ☐ No

How long on each breast? ____________________

BMs Q day ☐ Yes ☐ No

6 to 8 wet diapers ☐ Yes ☐ No

Breast care: ____________________

Formula

Type of formula: ____________________

Feeding Q 1-3 hours ☐ Yes ☐ No

BMs Q day ☐ Yes ☐ No

6 to 8 wet diapers ☐ Yes ☐ No

Sterilizing water ☐ Yes ☐ No

Vitamins ☐ Yes ☐ No

Bottle cleaning/preparation: ____________________

____

Feeding problems: ____________________

Sleeping patterns:

Goes to bed at: __________ Gets up at: __________

OBJECTIVE

Development:

	Present	Not present	Comments
Vocalizes/responds to voices	☐	☐	__________
Coo's/OOO/AAH	☐	☐	__________
Head up at 45°	☐	☐	__________
Follows past midline	☐	☐	__________
Turns head toward sound	☐	☐	__________

Physical exam:

	Normal	Abnormal	Comments
Skin	☐	☐	__________
Head/fontanel	☐	☐	__________
Eyes/red reflex	☐	☐	__________
Ears	☐	☐	__________
Nose/gums	☐	☐	__________
Oropharynx	☐	☐	__________
Breast hypertrophy	☐	☐	__________

ASSESSMENT
☐ WCC ☐ Diagnosis

PLAN
Immunizations:
NB screening results: ____________
Reaction: ____________
DTAP#1 site: ____________
IPV#1 site: ____________
HIB#1 site: ____________
HBV#2 site: ____________
Reviewed risks/benefits/literature given ☐
Immunization schedule reviewed ☐

Labs/screening tests
____
____

Medications
____
____

Thorax/lungs	☐	☐	____________
Heart	☐	☐	____________
Abdomen	☐	☐	____________
Genitals	☐	☐	____________
Femoral pulses	☐	☐	____________
Musculoskeletal	☐	☐	____________
Neuro:			
Startle less intense	☐	☐	____________
Tonic neck	☐	☐	____________
Toes downgoing	☐	☐	

ANTICIPATORY GUIDANCE

Sleep:
No bottles in bed ☐
No bottle propping ☐
No pillows ☐
Infant sleeps in own bed/crib ☐
Placing infant in bed when awake ☐

Illness:
Taking infant out in public ☐
Fever measurement and control: acetaminophen ☐
How and when to call your MD/NP ☐

Hygiene:
Skin care/baths/nail care ☐
Diaper hygiene:
Wash diaper area Q change ☐
Do not use wipes if irritated ☐

Safety:
Babysitters/parents time out ☐
Not leaving child unattended with younger children or pets ☐
Use play pen as safe place ☐
Sibling aggression ☐
Car seat: rear facing ☐
Hot water heater: 120° ☐
Carrying child safely ☐
Emergency phone #s ☐
Crib slats ≤2" apart ☐
No bean bag chairs ☐
Toys: no detachable parts/unbreakable ☐
Discourage walker ☐
Avoid holding infant and drinking hot liquids ☐
Smoke detector/evacuation plan ☐

Bonding:
Nonnutritive sucking ☐
Cuddling/holding/talking ☐
Cry/temperament ☐

Nutrition:
No solids in bottle ☐
Review feeding patterns ☐

Development:
Crib toys: music, mobile ☐
Hiccups/sneezing ☐
Immunization schedule ☐
Colic ☐
Neurodevelopment reviewed for the next 2 months ☐

RTO:
☐ 4 months for WCC
☐ ____________
☐ ____________

F/U NEXT VISIT:
____
____
____

Signature: ____________

WELL-CHILD VISIT
4 Months

Date of visit:	Name:	DOB:	Allergies:
T: P: R :	Medications:	Weight:	
Interim history:		Length:	
Problems/hospitalizations:		Head circ:	
Illness?		Age in weeks:	

Key: ☑ Addressed ☒ Abnormal/see comments ☐ Not discussed

SUBJECTIVE

Assessment of parental concerns ____________________

Chief complaint ____________________

Environmental history:

Home ☐ Apartment ☐

PB exposure	☐ Yes	☐ No
TB exposure	☐ Yes	☐ No
Tobacco exposure	☐ Yes	☐ No
Fluoridated water	☐ Yes	☐ No
Bed: type of crib ________		
Crib slats ≤2" apart	☐ Yes	☐ No
No lead paint	☐ Yes	☐ No

Family assessment:

Number of household members: ____________________

Sibling ages: ____________________

Mom's health/rest: ____________________

Dad's health/rest: ____________________

Siblings' health/feelings/adjustment: ____________________

Child/day care: ____________________

Outside support systems: ____________________

Dad/Mom support each other: ____________________

Substance use: ETOH ☐ Drugs ☐ Tobacco ☐

How do parents describe infant?: ____________________

Nutritional assessment:

Breastfeeding		
Feeding Q 1-2 hours	☐ Yes	☐ No
How long on each breast? ________		
BMs Q day	☐ Yes	☐ No
6 to 8 wet diapers	☐ Yes	☐ No
Breast care: ________		
Formula		
Type of formula: ________		
Feeding Q 1-3 hours	☐ Yes	☐ No
BMs Q day	☐ Yes	☐ No
6 to 8 wet diapers	☐ Yes	☐ No
Sterilizing water	☐ Yes	☐ No
Bottle cleaning/preparation: ________		
Feeding problems	☐ Yes	☐ No
Starting diluted juice	☐ Yes	☐ No
Introducing solids w/spoon	☐ Yes	☐ No
WIC	☐ Yes	☐ No
Vitamins	☐ Yes	☐ No

Sleeping patterns:

Goes to bed at: ________ Gets up at: ________

OBJECTIVE

Development:

	Present	Not present	Comments
Squeals/laughs/ vocalizes to mirror	☐	☐	________
Recognizes mom	☐	☐	________
Follows object 180°	☐	☐	________
Grasps object, brings to mouth	☐	☐	________
Hands midline	☐	☐	________

Physical exam:

	Normal	Abnormal	Comments
Skin	☐	☐	________
Head/fontanel	☐	☐	________
Eyes/red reflex	☐	☐	________
Ears	☐	☐	________
Nose/gums	☐	☐	________
Oropharynx	☐	☐	________
Breast hypertrophy	☐	☐	________

Head midline on sitting/no head lag	☐	☐	____
Pulls to sit/no head lag	☐	☐	____
Stands erect with support	☐	☐	____
Chest up-arm support 90°	☐	☐	____

Thorax/lungs	☐	☐	____
Heart	☐	☐	____
Abdomen	☐	☐	____
Genitals	☐	☐	____
Femoral pulses	☐	☐	____
Musculoskeletal	☐	☐	____
Hips/clicks/clunks	☐	☐	____
Neuro:			
Startle less intense	☐	☐	____
Tonic neck	☐	☐	____
Toes downgoing	☐	☐	____

ASSESSMENT

☐ WCC ☐ ____

PLAN

Immunizations:

Reaction: ____

DTAP#2 site: ____

IPV#2 site: ____

HIB#2 site: ____

Reviewed risks/benefits/literature given ☐

Immunization schedule reviewed ☐

Labs/screening tests

____

____

Medications

____

____

ANTICIPATORY GUIDANCE

Sleep:

- No bottles in bed ☐
- No bottle propping ☐
- No pillows ☐
- Infant sleeps in own bed/crib ☐
- Placing infant in bed when awake ☐
- Sleep patterns some predictable schedule ☐

Illness:

- Fever measurement and control ☐
- When to call your MD/NP ☐

Hygiene:

- Skin care/baths/nail care ☐
- Diaper hygiene:
  - Wash diaper area Q change ☐
  - Do not use wipes if irritated ☐

Safety:

- Review previous safety guidance ☐
- Car/houseproofing/bathing water temperature ☐
- Discourage walkers ☐
- Don't leave unattended w/younger siblings/pets ☐
- Play/toys/no removable parts or swallowable objects ☐
- Thumbsucking ☐
- Drooling/teething ☐
- Stranger anxiety ☐
- No physical punishment ☐
- Babysitters/parents time out ☐
- Avoid holding infant and drinking hot liquids ☐
- Smoke detector/evacuation plan ☐

Bonding:

- Nonnutritive sucking ☐
- Cuddling/holding/talking ☐
- Cry/temperament ☐

Nutrition:

- Introduce cereal, iron-fortified ☐
- First vegetables ☐
- First fruits ☐
- Introduce new food one at a time ☐

Development:

- Crib toys: music, mobile ☐
- Hiccups/sneezing ☐
- Talking to infant ☐
- Neurodevelopment reviewed for the next 2 months ☐

RTO:

☐ 6 months for WCC

☐ ____

☐ ____

F/U NEXT VISIT:

____

____

____

Signature: ____

WELL-CHILD VISIT
6 Months

Date of visit:			Name:	DOB:	Allergies:
T:	P:	R :	Medications:	Weight:	
Interim history:				Length:	
Problems/hospitalizations:				Head circ:	
Illness?				Age in weeks:	

Key: ☑ Addressed ☒ Abnormal/see comments ☐ Not discussed

SUBJECTIVE

Assessment of parental concerns ______________________________

Chief complaint ______________________________

Environmental history:

Home ☐ Apartment ☐

PB exposure	☐ Yes	☐ No
TB exposure	☐ Yes	☐ No
Tobacco exposure	☐ Yes	☐ No
Fluoridated water	☐ Yes	☐ No

Bed: type of crib ______________

Crib slats ≤2" apart	☐ Yes	☐ No
No lead paint	☐ Yes	☐ No

Family assessment:

Number of household members: ______________

Sibling ages: ______________

Mom's health/rest: ______________

Dad's health/rest: ______________

Siblings' health/feelings/adjustment: ______________

Child/day care: ______________

Outside support systems: ______________

Dad/Mom support each other: ______________

Substance use: ETOH ☐ Drugs ☐ Tobacco ☐

How do parents describe child?: ______________

Nutritional assessment:

Breastfeeding

Feeding Q 1-2 hours	☐ Yes	☐ No

How long on each breast? ______________

BMs Q day	☐ Yes	☐ No
6 to 8 wet diapers	☐ Yes	☐ No

Breast care: ______________

Formula

Type of formula: ______________

Feeding Q 1-3 hours	☐ Yes	☐ No
BMs Q day	☐ Yes	☐ No
6 to 8 wet diapers	☐ Yes	☐ No
Sterilizing water	☐ Yes	☐ No

Bottle cleaning/preparation: ______________

Feeding problems	☐ Yes	☐ No
Uses cup	☐ Yes	☐ No
Drinking juice	☐ Yes	☐ No
Taking solids w/spoon	☐ Yes	☐ No
Vitamins	☐ Yes	☐ No

Sleeping patterns:

Goes to bed at: ______________ Gets up at: ______________

OBJECTIVE

Development:

	Present	Not present	Comments
Babbles/imitates	☐	☐	______________
Vocalizes some defined syllables/ ba, da	☐	☐	______________
Turns to voice	☐	☐	______________
Reaches out and grasps	☐	☐	______________

Physical exam:

	Normal	Abnormal	Comments
Skin	☐	☐	______________
Head/fontanel	☐	☐	______________
Eyes/red reflex	☐	☐	______________
Ears	☐	☐	______________
Nose/gums	☐	☐	______________
Oropharynx	☐	☐	______________
Breast hypertrophy	☐	☐	______________

Transfers	☐	☐	______
Pulls from sitting to standing	☐	☐	______
Sits alone/head erect	☐	☐	______

Thorax/lungs	☐	☐	______
Heart	☐	☐	______
Abdomen	☐	☐	______
Genitals	☐	☐	______
Femoral pulses	☐	☐	______
Musculoskeletal	☐	☐	______
Spine	☐	☐	______
Neuro	☐	☐	______

ASSESSMENT

☐ WCC ☐ ______

PLAN

Immunizations:

Reaction: ______

DTAP#3 site: ______

HIB#3 site: ______

HBV#3 site: ______

Reviewed risks/benefits/literature given ☐

Immunization schedule reviewed ☐

Labs/screening tests

PB test (if positive risk assessment) ______

Sickle prep (if indicated) ______

______

Medications

______

______

ANTICIPATORY GUIDANCE

Sleep:

- Bedtime routine ☐
- Nighttime awakenings ☐
- Resistance to sleep/ using favorite toy ☐

Illness:

- Fever measurement and control ☐
- When to call your MD/NP ☐

Nutrition:

- Introduce to finger foods ☐
- Begins using cup ☐

Hygiene:

- Skin care/baths/nail care ☐
- Diaper hygiene:
  - Wash diaper area Q change ☐
  - Do not use wipes if irritated ☐

Safety:

- Review previous safety guidance ☐
- Mobility between 6-9 mo. means injury prevention is *crucial* ☐
- Child-proof home:
  - Gates on stairs ☐
  - Electrical outlets covered ☐
  - Poisons out of reach ☐
  - Sharp objects out of reach ☐
  - Window guards ☐
  - Syrup of Ipecac ☐
  - Discourage walker ☐
  - Bathtub safety ☐
  - Car restraint ☐

Behavior/discipline:

- Discourage hand slapping, use sharp "NO" ☐
- Correct behavior harmful to self ☐

Development:

- Pull to standing ☐
- Plays games, i.e., peek-a-boo, patty-cake ☐
- Toys/age appropriate ☐
- Shoes/soft, flexible ☐
- Separation/stranger anxiety ☐

RTO:

☐ 9 months for WCC

☐ ______

☐ ______

F/U NEXT VISIT:

______

______

______

Signature: ______

WELL-CHILD VISIT
9 Months

Date of visit:			Name:	DOB:	Allergies:
T:	P:	R :	Medications:	Weight:	
Interim history:				Length:	
Problems/hospitalizations:				Head circ:	
Illness?				Age in weeks:	

Key: ☑ Addressed ☒ Abnormal/see comments ☐ Not discussed

SUBJECTIVE

Assessment of parental concerns ______________________________

Chief complaint ______________________________

Environmental history:

Home ☐ Apartment ☐

PB exposure ☐ Yes ☐ No

TB exposure ☐ Yes ☐ No

Tobacco exposure ☐ Yes ☐ No

Fluoridated water ☐ Yes ☐ No

Bed: type of crib ______________

Crib slats ≤2" apart ☐ Yes ☐ No

No lead paint ☐ Yes ☐ No

Family assessment:

Parents describe child ______________________________

Family functioning ______________

Family routine/schedule ______________

Social changes ______________

Parent/child interaction ______________

Sleeping patterns:

Goes to bed at: ______________

Gets up at: ______________

Naps ______________

Nighttime awakenings ______________

Nutritional assessment:

Breastfeeding every ________ hours

Plans for weaning ______________

Formula/type ______________

Feeds every ________ hours

WIC ☐ Yes ☐ No

Vitamins ☐ Yes ☐ No

amount ________ frequency ________

Iron ☐ Yes ☐ No

amount ________ frequency ________

Eating finger foods ☐ Yes ☐ No

Using cup ☐ Yes ☐ No

Eating solids (fruit, cereal, vegetables) ☐ Yes ☐ No

OBJECTIVE

Development:

	Present	Not present	Comments
Plays peek-a-boo/ waves bye-bye	☐	☐	________
Jabbers	☐	☐	________
Combines syllables	☐	☐	________
Mama/dada nonspecific	☐	☐	________
Pulls to stand/stands for a few seconds	☐	☐	________

Physical exam:

	Normal	Abnormal	Comments
Skin	☐	☐	________
Head/fontanel	☐	☐	________
Eyes/cover/uncover	☐	☐	________
Ears	☐	☐	________
Nose/gums/teeth	☐	☐	________
Oropharynx	☐	☐	________
Breast hypertrophy	☐	☐	________
Thorax/lungs	☐	☐	________

Release object on command	☐	☐	________
Object permanency	☐	☐	________
Pincher grasp	☐	☐	________
Sits without support	☐	☐	________
Bangs two cubes together	☐	☐	________

Heart	☐	☐	________
Abdomen	☐	☐	________
Genitals	☐	☐	________
Femoral pulses	☐	☐	________
Musculoskeletal	☐	☐	________
Hips/clicks/clunks	☐	☐	________
Neuro:			
Toes downgoing	☐	☐	________
DTRs	☐	☐	________

ASSESSMENT

☐ WCC ☐ ________

PLAN

Immunizations:

None, if up to date

Labs/screening tests

PB level (if highrisk) ________

CBC/Hct ________

Subjective hearing/vision ________

____

____

Medications

____

____

____

ANTICIPATORY GUIDANCE

Sleep:

- Bedtime routine ☐
- No nighttime bottle ☐
- Resistance to sleep/ using favorite toy ☐

Nutrition:

- Finger foods/table foods ☐
- Meals with family at the table ☐
- Use of high chair ☐
- Weaning from bottle or breast/using cup ☐
- Decrease appetite ☐
- Introduce cow's milk at 12 months ☐
- No small foods: peanuts/grapes/hot dogs (choking) ☐

Hygiene:

- Dental: scrub teeth with washcloth ☐
- No bottles in bed ☐

Safety:

- Review previous safety guidance ☐
- Car restraint/change to toddler seat ☐
- Air bag safety ☐
- Avoid access to sharp objects/ingestion ☐
- Syrup of Ipecac ☐
- Anticipate mobility issues of toddlerhood ☐

Behavior/discipline:

- Discipline/setting limits/ no spanking ☐
- Consistency ☐

Development:

- Plays social games with parents/siblings ☐
- Separation anxiety/ stranger anxiety ☐
- Imitation ☐
- Review skills and anticipated neuro-development by 12 months ☐

RTO:

☐ 12 months WCC

☐ ________

☐ ________

F/U NEXT VISIT:

____

____

____

Signature: ________

WELL-CHILD VISIT
12 Months

Date of visit:			Name:	DOB:	Allergies:
T:	P:	R :	Medications:	Weight:	
Interim history:				Length:	
Problems/hospitalizations:				Head circ:	
Illness?				Age in weeks:	

Key: ☑ Addressed ☒ Abnormal/see comments ☐ Not discussed

SUBJECTIVE

Assessment of parental concerns ______________________________

Chief complaint ______________________________

Environmental history:

Home ☐ Apartment ☐ Moved? ☐

PB exposure	☐ Yes	☐ No
TB exposure	☐ Yes	☐ No
Tobacco exposure	☐ Yes	☐ No
Fluoridated water	☐ Yes	☐ No
Bed type ______		
Crib slats ≤2" apart	☐ Yes	☐ No
No lead paint	☐ Yes	☐ No

Sleeping patterns:

Goes to bed at: ______________________________

Gets up at: ______________________________

Naps ______________________________

Family assessment:

Parents describe child ______________________________

Family /work changes ______________________________

Parents time together ______________________________

Parental stresses ______________________________

Support systems ______________________________

Family interaction ______________________________

Assess for abuse: substance/physical/sexual

Nutritional assessment:

Breastfeeding every ________ hours

Plans for weaning ______________________________

Bottle/formula type ______________________________

Feeds ________ oz. every ________ hours

Feedings:

Meals per day ______________________________

Using spoon	☐ Yes	☐ No
Self feeding	☐ Yes	☐ No
Finger foods	☐ Yes	☐ No
Vitamins	☐ Yes	☐ No
amount ________ frequency ________		
Fluoride	☐ Yes	☐ No
amount ________ frequency ________		
Eating problems	☐ Yes	☐ No
WIC	☐ Yes	☐ No

Elimination:

Bowel movements ______________________________

Urination ______________________________

OBJECTIVE

Development:

	Present	Not present	Comments
Plays patty-cake/ waves bye-bye	☐	☐	________
Bangs 2 blocks	☐	☐	________
together	☐	☐	________
Puts block in cup			
Indicates wants	☐	☐	________
Says Mama/Dada (specific)	☐	☐	________

Physical exam:

	Normal	Abnormal	Comments
Skin	☐	☐	________
Head/fontanel	☐	☐	________
Eyes/red reflex	☐	☐	________
Ears	☐	☐	________
Nose/gums	☐	☐	________
Oropharynx	☐	☐	________
Breast hypertrophy	☐	☐	________
Thorax/lungs	☐	☐	________

Says 1-3 words related to object	☐	☐	______
Follows some simple tasks	☐	☐	______
Understands "no"	☐	☐	______
Cruises	☐	☐	______
Stands 2-3 seconds without support	☐	☐	______

Heart	☐	☐	______
Abdomen	☐	☐	______
Genitals	☐	☐	______
Femoral pulses	☐	☐	______
Musculoskeletal	☐	☐	______
Neuro:			
Toes downgoing	☐	☐	______
DTRs	☐	☐	______

ASSESSMENT

☐ WCC ☐ ______

PLAN

Immunizations:

Reactions ______

DTAP#4* site: ______

OPV#3* site: ______

HIB#4* site: ______

MMR#1 site: ______

Varicella site: ______

*Can be given now or at 15 mo or 18 mo visit

Reviewed risks/benefits/literature given ☐

Labs/screening tests

PB test (if at risk, repeat) ______

CBC/HCT ______

TB (PPD) (if at risk) ______ site: ______

______

______

Medications

______

______

______

ANTICIPATORY GUIDANCE

Sleep:

- Bedtime routine ☐
- Sleep patterns ☐
- No nighttime bottle ☐
- Resistance to sleep; using favorite toy ☐

Nutrition:

- 3 cups homogenized whole milk per day* ☐
- Decrease calorie requirements/decrease appetite ☐
- Finger foods/minimal sweets/no soft drinks ☐
- No reduced fat milk ☐
- Wean from bottle ☐

*can substitute yogurt or cheese for milk

Behavior/discipline:

- Discipline/consistent limits/discourage physical punishment ☐
- Physically remove from danger ☐
- Does not remember limits/needs reminding, not scolding ☐
- Don't use food as reward ☐

Safety:

- No small foods: peanuts, hot dogs, grapes ☐
- Never leave unattended ☐
- Water temperature ☐
- Air bag safety/car restraint ☐
- Stair safety ☐
- Poison-proof home ☐
- Syrup of Ipecac ☐
- Poison control # ☐

Hygiene:

- Dental: scrub teeth with washcloth ☐
- No toothpaste ☐

Development:

- Behaviors: likes to give/receive hugs ☐
- Understands praise ☐
- Plays alone/with others ☐
- Developing autonomy ☐
- Separation anxiety ☐
- Encourage speech development ☐
- Picture books ☐
- Review skills/anticipated neurodevelopment by 15 months ☐

RTO:

☐ 15 months WCC

☐ ______

☐ ______

F/U NEXT VISIT:

______

______

______

Signature: ______

WELL-CHILD VISIT
15 Months

Date of visit:			Name:	DOB:	Allergies:
T:	P:	R :	Medications:	Weight:	
Interim history:				Length:	
Problems/hospitalizations:				Head circ:	
Illness?					
Key: ☑ Addressed ☒ Abnormal/see comments ☐ Not discussed					

SUBJECTIVE

Assessment of parental concerns ______________________________

____

Chief complaint ______________________________

____

Environmental history:

Home ☐ Apartment ☐

Lead exposure	☐ Yes	☐ No
TB exposure	☐ Yes	☐ No
Fluoridated water	☐ Yes	☐ No
Bed type ______________		
Crib slats ≤2" apart	☐ Yes	☐ No
No lead paint	☐ Yes	☐ No

Family assessment:

Parents describe child ______________________________

____

Review ETOH/drug/tobacco use ______________

Assess for abuse/neglect ______________

Parental discipline/consistent with all care givers ______________

Child care/day care ______________

Family support systems ______________

Family functioning/stressors ______________

Nutritional assessment:

Meals per day ______________

Snacks per day ______________

Breastfeeding ________ times/day

Whole milk ________ oz/day

Self feeding/using a spoon with frequent spilling	☐ Yes	☐ No
Using a cup/weaned from bottle	☐ Yes	☐ No
Highchair/booster sit	☐ Yes	☐ No
Mealtime problems	☐ Yes	☐ No

**Vitamins/fluoride usually not needed

Sleeping patterns:

Goes to bed at: ______________

Gets up at: ______________

Naps ______________

Nighttime awakenings ______________

OBJECTIVE

Development:

	Present	Not present	Comments
Drinks from cup (little spilling)	☐	☐	________
Uses spoon	☐	☐	________
Indicates wants	☐	☐	________
Imitates activities	☐	☐	
Vocabulary			________
1-3 words	☐	☐	
Plays/throws ball	☐	☐	________

Physical exam:

	Normal	Abnormal	Comments
Skin	☐	☐	________
Head/fontanel	☐	☐	________
Eyes/red reflex	☐	☐	________
Ears	☐	☐	________
Nose/gums	☐	☐	________
Oropharynx	☐	☐	________
Breast hypertrophy	☐	☐	________
Thorax/lungs	☐	☐	________

Scribbles	☐	☐	________
Stoops and recovers	☐	☐	________
Walks	☐	☐	________

Heart	☐	☐	________
Abdomen	☐	☐	________
Genitals	☐	☐	________
Femoral pulses	☐	☐	________
Musculoskeletal	☐	☐	________
Hips/clicks/clunks	☐	☐	________
Neuro:			
Startle less intense	☐	☐	________
Tonic neck	☐	☐	________
Toes downgoing	☐	☐	________

ASSESSMENT

☐ WCC ☐ ________

PLAN

Immunizations:

Reactions ________

DTAP#4 site: ________

Can be given now or at the 18 mo visit

OPV#3 site: ________

Can be given now or at the 18 mo visit

HIB#4 site: ________

Varicella site: ________

Optional

Labs/screening tests

PB level ________

If at risk may need to repeat

TB (PPD) site ________

If at risk

CBC ________

If not done

____

Medications

____

____

ANTICIPATORY GUIDANCE

Sleep:

- No bottle in bed ☐
- Bed time routine ☐
- Use favorite toy ☐
- Routine naps ☐

Nutrition:

- Encourage self feeding/ using cup and spoon ☐
- Safe snacks ☐
- Discourage junk food ☐

Behavior/discipline:

- Discuss temper tantrums ☐
- Appropriate limit setting autonomy/ curiosity are nl ☐
- Give lots of praise/build self esteem ☐
- Ignore unwanted behavior ☐
- Consistency from all care givers ☐

Safety:

- Crib/lower mattress ☐
- Secure gates/doors of stairs ☐
- Toddler car restraints/air bag safety ☐
- Water temperature/drowning ☐
- Never leave unattended ☐
- Electrical dangers/plastic safety ☐
- Injury/burn care ☐

Hygiene:

- Dental care: Clean teeth with washcloth or soft toothbrush ☐
- Choose dentist ☐

Development:

- Tantrums ☐
- Self comforting behaviors thumb sucking/blanket/ stuff toy ☐
- Play/appropriate toys/ dolls/pots/pans/musical toys/riding toys/books ☐
- Supervise exploration ☐
- Reading/singing ☐
- Review skills/anticipated development 18 mos ☐

RTO:

☐ 18 months WCC

☐ ________

☐ ________

F/U NEXT VISIT:

____

____

____

Signature: ________

WELL-CHILD VISIT
18 Months

Date of visit:			Name:	DOB:	Allergies:
T:	P:	R :	Medications:	Weight:	
Interim history:				Length:	
Problems/hospitalizations:				Head circ:	
Illness?					

Key: ☑ Addressed ☒ Abnormal/see comments ☐ Not discussed

SUBJECTIVE

Assessment of parental concerns ______________________

Chief complaint ______________________

Environmental history:

Home ☐ Apartment ☐

Lead exposure	☐ Yes	☐ No
TB exposure	☐ Yes	☐ No
Fluoridated water	☐ Yes	☐ No
Bed type ______		
Crib slats ≤2" apart	☐ Yes	☐ No
No lead paint	☐ Yes	☐ No

Nutritional assessment:

Breastfeeding ______ times/day

Whole milk ______ oz/day

Meals/day ______

Snacks/day ______ type ______

Self-feeding/using cup/spoon/fork	☐ Yes	☐ No
Eating with family	☐ Yes	☐ No

PICA ______

Family assessment:

Parents describe child ______

Review ETOH/drug/tobacco use ______

Assess for abuse/neglect ______

Enjoyment of child by family ______

Parental relationship ______

Family changes (stresses) ______

Sleeping patterns:

Goes to bed at: ______

Gets up at: ______

Naps ______

Nighttime awakenings ______

Hygiene:

Dental hygiene/dental visit ______

Elimination:

Stool patterns/toilet training ______

OBJECTIVE

Development:

	Present	Not present	Comments
Mimic household tasks	☐	☐	
Removes clothes	☐	☐	______
Stacks 2-3 blocks	☐	☐	______
Runs (with little falling)	☐	☐	______
Walks up steps with help	☐	☐	______
Walks backward	☐	☐	______

Physical exam:

	Normal	Abnormal	Comments
Skin	☐	☐	______
Head/fontanel	☐	☐	______
Eyes/red reflex	☐	☐	______
Ears	☐	☐	______
Nose/gums	☐	☐	______
Oropharynx	☐	☐	______
Breast hypertrophy	☐	☐	______
Thorax/lungs	☐	☐	______

ASSESSMENT
☐ WCC ☐ Diagnosis

Heart	☐	☐	______
Abdomen	☐	☐	______
Genitals	☐	☐	______
Femoral pulses	☐	☐	______
Musculoskeletal	☐	☐	______
Hips/clicks/clunks	☐	☐	______
Neuro:			
Startle less intense	☐	☐	______
Tonic neck	☐	☐	______
Toes downgoing	☐	☐	______

PLAN
Immunizations:
Reactions ______
DTAP#4 site: ______
OPV#3 site: ______
Varicella site: ______

Labs/screening tests
PB level ______
Assess risk factors
TB ______
Assess risk factors
______
______

Medications
______
______

ANTICIPATORY GUIDANCE

Sleep:
Sleep patterns ☐
Bedtime rituals/ nightmares ☐
Nighttime awakening ☐
No bottle at bedtime ☐

Nutrition:
Nutritional patterns ☐
Eat meals as a family ☐
Discourage sweets, fast food, frequent snacks ☐
No force feeding ☐
Prevention of mealtime battles ☐
"Picky eater" normal behavior ☐

Behavior/discipline:
Discourage physical punishment ☐
Consistency between parents ☐
Praise accomplishments/ignore negative behaviors ☐
Temper tantrums ☐
Discourage food as rewards ☐

Safety:
Review previous precautions ☐
Poison control phone # ☐
Syrup of Ipecac ☐
Drawer safety locks ☐
Don't leave unattended ☐
Drowning/water safety ☐
Supervised play ☐

Hygiene:
Dental care ☐

Development:
Review skills and anticipated neurodevelopment by 2 yrs. ☐
Clinging behaviors normal ☐
Difficulty sharing ☐
Encourage parent to play games/pretend play ☐
Toys to take apart/no small parts ☐
Books/one word ☐
Encourage affection ☐
Toilet training readiness ☐
Masturbation normal behaviors ☐

RTO:
☐ 24 months WCC
☐ ______
☐ ______

F/U NEXT VISIT:
______
______
______

Signature: ______

WELL-CHILD VISIT
2 Years

Date of visit:			Name:	DOB:	Allergies:
T:	P:	R :	Medications:	Weight:	
Interim history:				Height:	
Problems/hospitalizations:					
Illness?					
Key: ☑ Addressed ☒ Abnormal/see comments ☐ Not discussed					

SUBJECTIVE

Assessment of parental concerns ______________________________

Chief complaint ______________________________

Environmental history:

Home ☐ Apartment ☐ Change ☐

Lead exposure	☐ Yes	☐ No
TB exposure	☐ Yes	☐ No
Fluoridated water	☐ Yes	☐ No
Bed type ______		
Crib slats ≤2" apart	☐ Yes	☐ No
No lead paint	☐ Yes	☐ No

Nutritional assessment:

Milk ______ oz/day

Meals ______ times/day

Snacks ______ /day types ______

**Calcium; vitamin D sources if does not drink milk

"Picky eater" ☐ Yes ☐ No

PICA ______

Family assessment:

Parents describe child ______

Assess substance/ETOH/physical/ sexual abuse ______

Parental relationships/personal time ______

Family changes ______

Enjoyment of child ______

Preschool enrollment/day care ______

Sleeping patterns:

Goes to bed at: ______

Gets up at: ______

Naps ______

Nighttime awakenings ______

Elimination:

Urine ______

BM ______

OBJECTIVE

Development:

	Present	Not present	Comments
Washes and drys hands	☐	☐	______
Brushes teeth with help	☐	☐	______
Tower of 4-6 cubes	☐	☐	
Handles spoon well	☐	☐	______
Knows 6 body parts	☐	☐	______
Combines words	☐	☐	______

Physical exam:

	Normal	Abnormal	Comments
Skin/nails	☐	☐	______
Head/fontanel	☐	☐	______
Eyes/red reflex/	☐	☐	______
EOMI	☐	☐	______
Ears	☐	☐	______
Nose/gums/teeth	☐	☐	______
Oropharynx	☐	☐	______
Breast hypertrophy	☐	☐	______

2 to 3 word sentences	☐	☐	______
Points to 2 pictures	☐	☐	______
Walks up steps	☐	☐	______
Throws ball	☐	☐	______
Kicks ball	☐	☐	______

Thorax/lungs	☐	☐	______
Heart	☐	☐	______
Abdomen	☐	☐	______
Genitals	☐	☐	______
Femoral pulses	☐	☐	______
Musculoskeletal	☐	☐	______
Hips/clicks/clunks	☐	☐	______
Neuro:			
DTRs	☐	☐	______
Toes downgoing	☐	☐	______
CNIII-XII	☐	☐	______

ASSESSMENT

☐ WCC ☐ ______

PLAN

Immunizations:

Reactions ______

Immunization schedule ______

Varicella ______

Labs/screening tests

Optional

PB level ______

Repeat if at risk

TB ______

If at risk/not tested

Cholesterol ______

If positive family history

______

______

Medications

______

______

ANTICIPATORY GUIDANCE

Sleep:

Sleep patterns/variable naps ☐

Discuss move to regular bed ☐

Behavior/discipline:

Encourage exploration ☐

Discipline with a firm no ☐

Needs frequent reminding ☐

Consistent limits-age appropriate ☐

Temper tantrum management ☐

Limit TV ☐

Nutrition:

Discuss family being together at meals ☐

Eating and sitting at table during mealtime ☐

Avoid battles over eating ☐

Encourage self-feeding with spoon, fork, cup ☐

Avoid control issues with feeding ☐

Avoid excessive snacks/juice/fast foods/sweets ☐

Safety:

Car/stairs/windows/ingestions ☐

Never leave unattended ☐

Development:

Encourage playing with peers ☐

Play groups ☐

Simple chores ☐

Read to child ☐

Intelligible speech to parents ☐

Review previous guidance issues ☐

Toilet training readiness - does child show interest ☐

RTO:

☐ 3 years WCC

☐ ______

☐ ______

F/U NEXT VISIT:

______

______

______

Signature: ______

WELL-CHILD VISIT
3 Years

Date of visit:			Name:	DOB:	Allergies:
T:	P:	R :	Medications:	Weight:	
Interim history:				Height:	
Problems/hospitalizations:					
Illness?					
Key: ☑ Addressed ☒ Abnormal/see comments ☐ Not discussed					

SUBJECTIVE

Assessment of parental concerns ____________________

____

Chief complaint ____________________

____

Environmental history:

Home ☐ Apartment ☐

Lead exposure	☐ Yes	☐ No
TB exposure	☐ Yes	☐ No
Fluoridated water	☐ Yes	☐ No
Bed type ____________________		
Crib slats ≤2" apart	☐ Yes	☐ No
No lead paint	☐ Yes	☐ No

Nutritional assessment:

Milk ________ oz/day

Meals ________ times/day

Snacks ________ /day types ____________

**Calcium sources if not drinking milk ____________

Mealtime problems ____________

Family assessment:

Parents describe child ____________________

____

Assess substance/ETOH/physical/____________
sexual abuse ____________________

Family changes/stresses ____________________

Family activities ____________________

Sleeping patterns:

Goes to bed at: ____________________

Gets up at: ____________________

Naps ____________________

Elimination:

Urine ____________________

BM ____________________

OBJECTIVE

Development:

	Present	Not present	Comments
Wash/dry hands	☐	☐	________
Brushes teeth	☐	☐	________
Puts on clothing	☐	☐	________
Names a friend/ knows full name	☐	☐	________
Knows age	☐	☐	________
Imaginary friend	☐	☐	________
Copies vertical line	☐	☐	________
Knows 1 color	☐	☐	________

Physical exam:

	Normal	Abnormal	Comments
Appearance	☐	☐	________
Skin/nodes	☐	☐	________
Head	☐	☐	________
Eyes/red reflex/	☐	☐	________
EOMI	☐	☐	________
Eyes/cover-uncover	☐	☐	________
Ears	☐	☐	________
Neck	☐	☐	________
Nose/OP	☐	☐	________

Speech is understandable	☐	☐	________
Knows 2 actions	☐	☐	________
Names 4 pictures	☐	☐	________
Balances on 1 foot (1 sec)	☐	☐	________
Broad jumps	☐	☐	________
Rides tricycle	☐	☐	________

ASSESSMENT

☐ WCC ☐ ________

Teeth/gums	☐	☐	________
Lungs	☐	☐	________
Heart	☐	☐	________
Abdomen	☐	☐	________
Genitals	☐	☐	________
Musculoskeletal	☐	☐	________
Spine/scoliosis	☐	☐	________
Neuro/CNII-CNXII symmetrical:			
DTRs	☐	☐	________
Toes downgoing	☐	☐	________

PLAN

Immunizations:

None

Labs/screening tests

Cholesterol screening

PB level ________

If >10 ug/dl

TB screening PPD ________

Repeat if at risk

Medications

____

____

ANTICIPATORY GUIDANCE

Sleep:

Regular bedtime rituals ☐

Napping optional ☐

Behavior/discipline:

Limit TV and watch TV with children ☐

Assigns chores appropriate for age ☐

Nutrition:

Nutritional patterns ☐

Avoiding junk foods/fast foods/poor nutrition ☐

Review healthy eating habits/self feeding/learning table manners/eating at table ☐

Safety:

Car/seat belt at 4 yr. and 40 lbs. ☐

Use booster seat ☐

Supervision for outside play ☐

Discuss strangers, dogs, and other animals ☐

Water/street safety ☐

Hygiene:

Dental hygiene/regular visits ☐

Development:

Review skills and anticipated neurodevelopment by 4 yrs. ☐

Toilet behaviors/hygiene (70% incontinent) ☐

Masturbation normal behavior/correct terms for genitals ☐

Curiosity about sexual differences ☐

Speech complete sentences and intelligible/some dysfluency normal ☐

Encourage independence/self play ☐

Encourage playmates/sharing ☐

Positive sibling relationships ☐

Preschool readiness ☐

RTO:

☐ 4 years WCC

☐ ________

☐ ________

F/U NEXT VISIT:

____

____

____

Signature: ________

WELL-CHILD VISIT
4 Years

Date of visit:			Name:	DOB:	Allergies:
T:	P:	R :	Medications:	Weight:	
Interim history:				Height:	
Problems/hospitalizations:					
Illness?					
Key: ☑ Addressed ☒ Abnormal/see comments ☐ Not discussed					

SUBJECTIVE

Assessment of parental concerns ____________________

____

Chief complaint ____________________

____

Environmental history:

Home ☐ Apartment ☐ Changes ☐

PB exposure	☐ Yes	☐ No
TB exposure	☐ Yes	☐ No
Tobacco exposure	☐ Yes	☐ No
Fluoridated water	☐ Yes	☐ No

Nutritional assessment:

Milk ________ oz/day

Meals ________ times/day

Snacks ________ /day

Elimination:

Urine ____________________

BM ____________________

Enuresis ____________________

Hygiene:

Brushing teeth

AM ____________________

PM ____________________

Dental examination ☐ Yes ☐ No

Sleeping patterns:

Goes to bed at: ____________________

Gets up at: ____________________

Naps ____________________

Family assessment:

Parents describe child's behavior ____________________

____

____

R/O abuse/neglect ____________________

Family changes ____________________

Parental relationship ____________________

Parental interaction with child ____________________

Family activities ____________________

Sibling relationship/friendships ____________________

OBJECTIVE

Development:

	Present	Not present	Comments
Dresses self with little or no help	☐	☐	________
Names friends	☐	☐	________
Enjoys playing cards/board games	☐	☐	________
Draws 3 part person	☐	☐	________
Copies letters T, O	☐	☐	________
Picks longer line	☐	☐	________
Names 4 colors	☐	☐	________

Physical exam:

	Normal	Abnormal	Comments
Skin	☐	☐	________
Head/fontanel	☐	☐	________
Eyes/red reflex	☐	☐	________
Ears	☐	☐	________
Nose/gums	☐	☐	________
Oropharynx	☐	☐	________
Breast hypertrophy	☐	☐	________
Lungs/thorax	☐	☐	________
Heart	☐	☐	________

Balances on each foot for 3 sec.	☐	☐	______
Hops	☐	☐	______
Complete sentences/ knows verbs and prepositions	☐	☐	______

Vision acuity OD ____ OS ____ OU ____

Hearing screening results ______

ASSESSMENT

☐ WCC ☐ ______

Abdomen	☐	☐	______
Genitals	☐	☐	______
Femoral pulses	☐	☐	______
Musculoskeletal	☐	☐	______
Hips/clicks/clunks	☐	☐	______
Neuro:			
DTRs	☐	☐	______
Toes downgoing	☐	☐	______
CNII-XII	☐	☐	______

PLAN

Immunizations:

Reactions ______

DTAP#5 site: ______

(Needs to be given before 7 yrs of age)

OPV#4 site: ______

(Need to give before 6th birthday)

MMR#2 site: ______

(Needs to be given before age 12)

Labs/screening tests

Urine ______

Optional

Cholesterol ______

If positive family history

TB (PPD) ______

If positive risk factors

Medications

______

______

ANTICIPATORY GUIDANCE

Sleep:

Bedtime ritual/routine ☐

Behavior/discipline:

Develop independence with structured limits ☐

Reprimand away from friends ☐

Nutrition:

Balanced diet ☐

Small portions ☐

Avoid conflict at mealtime ☐

Provide a family social hour during meals ☐

Safety:

Car seat /air bag ☐

Street safety/stranger safety ☐

Continue close supervision ☐

Inappropriate touching ☐

Bicycle helmet/safety ☐

Development:

Encourage board games/pretend play ☐

Encourage parents to go on child outings ☐

Limit TV/video games ☐

Daily exercise/fun ☐

Teach name/address ☐

Encourage peer activities ☐

Toilet hygiene (75% dry at night) ☐

Masturbation ☐

Encourage privacy for dressing/ bathing ☐

Sexuality education ☐

RTO:

☐ 5 years WCC

☐ ______

☐ ______

F/U NEXT VISIT:

______

______

______

Signature: ______

WELL-CHILD VISIT
5 Years

Date of visit:			Name:	DOB:	Allergies:
T:	P:	R :	Medications:	Weight:	
Interim history:				Height:	
Problems/hospitalizations:					
Illness?					
Key: ☑ Addressed ☒ Abnormal/see comments ☐ Not discussed					

SUBJECTIVE

Assessment of parental concerns ______________________________

Chief complaint ______________________________

Environmental history:

Home ☐ Apartment ☐

Lead exposure	☐ Yes	☐ No
TB exposure	☐ Yes	☐ No
Fluoridated water	☐ Yes	☐ No
Bed	☐ Yes	☐ No

Nutritional assessment:

Balanced meals	☐ Yes	☐ No
Family together at mealtimes	☐ Yes	☐ No
Pleasant mealtimes/social time for family	☐ Yes	☐ No
Behavior problems at mealtimes	☐ Yes	☐ No

Elimination:

Urine ______________________________

BM ______________________________

Enuresis ______________________________

Sleeping patterns:

Goes to bed at: ______________________________

Gets up at: ______________________________

Family assessment:

Parents describe child's behavior ______________________________

R/O abuse/neglect ______________________________

Family relationships ______________________________

Family changes/stresses ______________________________

Child care/preschool ______________________________

OBJECTIVE

Development:

	Present	Not present	Comments
School readiness	☐	☐	________
Dresses self	☐	☐	________
Prepares cereal	☐	☐	________
Brushes teeth	☐	☐	________
Plays board and card games	☐	☐	________
Copies a square	☐	☐	________
Draws 6 part person	☐	☐	________
Defines 1 word	☐	☐	________
Counts to 5	☐	☐	________

Physical exam:

	Normal	Abnormal	Comments
Skin	☐	☐	________
Head/fontanel	☐	☐	________
Eyes/red reflex	☐	☐	________
Ears	☐	☐	________
Nose/gums	☐	☐	________
Oropharynx	☐	☐	________
Breast hypertrophy	☐	☐	________
Lungs/thorax	☐	☐	________
Heart	☐	☐	________
Abdomen	☐	☐	________
Genitals	☐	☐	________

Balances on each foot for 4 seconds	☐	☐	______
Rides a bicycle (may use training wheels)	☐	☐	______
School readiness:			
Feels good about self	☐	☐	______
Separates from parent easily	☐	☐	______
Gets along with others	☐	☐	______
Listens	☐	☐	______
Follows commands/ directions	☐	☐	______
Verbally communicates	☐	☐	______
Dresses self	☐	☐	______
Dental visits	☐	☐	______
Nutritional concerns	☐	☐	______
Bowel/bladder habits	☐	☐	______

Femoral pulses	☐	☐	______
Musculoskeletal	☐	☐	______
Hips/clicks/clunks	☐	☐	______
Neuro:			
DTRs	☐	☐	______
Toes downgoing	☐	☐	______
CNII-XII	☐	☐	______

Vision acuity OD ____ OS ____ OU ____
Hearing screening results ______

ASSESSMENT
☐ WCC ☐ ______

PLAN
Screening tests/immunizations:
Reactions ______
DTAP#5 site: ______
OPV#4 site: ______
MMR#2 site: ______
(Needs to be given before age 12)
Varicella site: ______
(Optional)

ANTICIPATORY GUIDANCE

Sleep:
Bedtime routine ☐

Nutrition:
Balanced diet ☐

Behavior/discipline:
Review independence with limit setting ☐
Offer choices ☐
Play by rules ☐
Discipline in private ☐
Assign chores ☐

Hygiene:
Dental visits ☐
Tooth brushing ☐

Safety:
Car/seatbelts/airbag ☐
Supervision around water ☐
Bicycle safety-helmet ☐
Strangers/dogs/stray animals ☐
Street safety ☐
Firearms ☐

Development:
Praise accomplishments at school, home, with friends ☐
Encourage parent to communicate with teacher, participate in school ☐
Show affection ☐
Encourage parent-child-family interaction ☐
Plans for next visit ☐
Sexual curiosity ☐
Masturbation ☐
Promote interaction with peers ☐

RTO:
☐ 6 years WCC
☐ ______
☐ ______

F/U NEXT VISIT:
______
______
______

Signature: ______

WELL-CHILD VISIT
6-10 Years

Date of visit:			Name:	DOB:	Allergies:
T:	P:	R :	Medications:	Weight:	
Interim history:				Height:	
Problems/hospitalizations:					
Illness?					
Key: ☑ Addressed ☒ Abnormal/see comments ☐ Not discussed					

SUBJECTIVE

Assessment of parental concerns ______________________________

____

Chief complaint ______________________________

____

Environmental history:

Home/housing changes	☐ Yes	☐ No
PB/TB/Tobacco exposure	☐ Yes	☐ No
R/O substance abuse/ETOH	☐ Yes	☐ No

Nutritional assessment:

Describe eating habits ______________________________

Eating behaviors/problems ______________________________

Body image ______________________________

Elimination:

Urine ______________________________

BM ______________________________

Enuresis ______________________________

Family assessment:

Parents describe child's behavior ______________________________

____

____

Marital changes ______________________________

Family changes ______________________________

Family activities ______________________________

After school care ______________________________

Sibling problems ______________________________

OBJECTIVE

Development:

	Present	Not present	Comments
School activities (outside of classroom)	☐	☐	______
Peers/friendships	☐	☐	______
Tells time/knows days of week	☐	☐	______
Reads for pleasure	☐	☐	______
Learns to swim	☐	☐	______

Physical exam:

	Normal	Abnormal	Comments
Appearance	☐	☐	______
Skin/nodes	☐	☐	______
Head	☐	☐	______
Eyes/red reflex/	☐	☐	______
EOMI	☐	☐	______
Ears	☐	☐	______
Nose	☐	☐	______
Teeth/gums	☐	☐	______
Neck	☐	☐	______
Lungs	☐	☐	______
Heart	☐	☐	______
Abdomen	☐	☐	______
Genitalia	☐	☐	______
Musculoskeletal	☐	☐	______
Spine/scoliosis	☐	☐	______
Neuro:			
DTRs	☐	☐	______
Toes downgoing	☐	☐	______
CNII-XII symmetrical	☐	☐	______

PLAN

Immunizations:

Td site: ____________________

(5-10 years after DTAP#5)

Varicella site: ____________________

(If has not contracted varicella)

Tanner stage

Labs/screening tests

Cholesterol ____________________

If positive family history

U/A ____________________

Optional

TB (PPD) site: ____________________

Assess for at risk

Medications

____

____

ANTICIPATORY GUIDANCE

Sleep:

- Adequate sleep ☐

Behavior/discipline:

- Self-independence with age appropriate limits ☐
- Establish rules and consequences for house/school/outside activities ☐
- Chores/responsibilities ☐

Hygiene:

- Dental visit ☐
- Brush teeth 2x/day ☐
- Dental visit 2x/yr ☐

Nutrition:

- Review balance meals with snacks ☐
- Review family eating behaviors ☐
- Avoid junk food ☐
- Breakfast ☐

Safety:

- Car/seat belt/air bag ☐
- Street safety ☐
- Swimming ☐
- Fire arms ☐
- Bike safety/helmet ☐
- Sport safety ☐
- Drugs/alcohol/tobacco ☐

Development:

- Allowance ☐
- Show affection/praise child's accomplishments ☐
- Limit TV, videos/movies, video games, and music ☐
- Encourage reading, peer interaction, school activities, sports ☐
- Exercise regularly ☐
- Library card ☐
- Encourage sports/hobbies/outside activities ☐

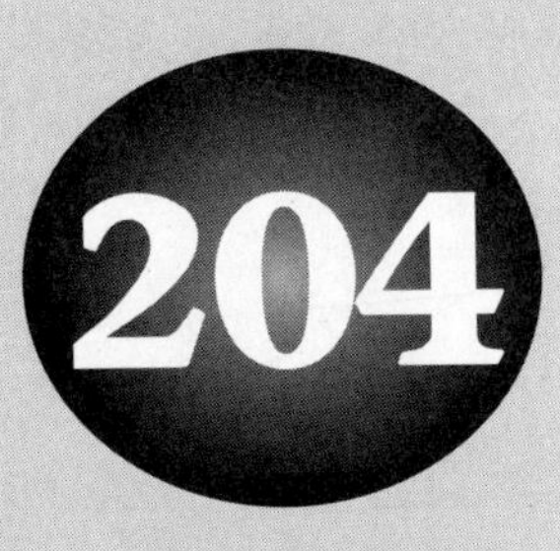

Well Adolescent

ICD-9-CM

Annual Examination V70.0
Routine Child Care Examination V20.2
School Examination V70.5
Routine Gynecological Examination V72.3
Family Planning Advice V25.09

OVERVIEW

Definition

Adolescence is a period of accelerated growth encompassing both physical and psychological development, resulting in the ability of a teenager to become an independent and responsible member of society.

Growth and Development

Pubertal changes occur in a predictable sequence for all adolescents. The age at which changes begin varies based on genetic, socioeconomic, and nutritional factors. The rate at which the changes occur is regarded as the tempo; there may be individual variances in tempo as well. Although the most evident changes are in the secondary sexual characteristics, changes occur in the endocrine glands, lymphatic system, brain, and body fat composition as well (Table 204-1).

Tanner Stages

Tanner stages are outlined in Tables 204-2 and 204-3 and in Figure 204-1.

Coping Mechanisms of Adolescents

Coping mechanisms of adolescents are outlined in Table 204-4.

GUIDELINES FOR ADOLESCENT PREVENTIVE SERVICES

Guidelines for Adolescent Preventive Services (GAPS) (AMA, 1995) offer the following:

- Purpose
  - To deter adolescents from participating in behaviors that jeopardize health
  - To detect physical, emotional, and behavioral problems early and to intervene immediately
  - To reinforce and encourage behaviors that promote healthy living
  - To provide immunizations against infectious disease
- Recommendations include yearly visits between 11 and 21 years to identify those who have begun high-risk behaviors and to provide information supporting healthy habits.
- Care should be age/developmentally appropriate and socioculturally sensitive.
- NP and adolescent should have a time alone without a parent to discuss issues that otherwise might never be addressed.

RECOMMENDATIONS FOR COMMUNICATION WITH ADOLESCENT

Recommendations for communication with an adolescent (Levenberg, 1998) include the following:

- Remind the adolescent that information discussed will be confidential unless they are engaged in at-risk behaviors.
- Use nonthreatening open-ended questions to establish rapport.
- Be matter of fact.
- Do not lecture; instead, involve the adolescent in health education and development of a plan of action.
- Acknowledge that it is uncomfortable talking about sensitive subjects, but learning to talk about difficult subjects is an important part of growing up.

TABLE 204-1 Pubertal Changes

Major Events of Puberty	Skeletal Growth	Secondary Sex Characteristics	Sequence of Events: Males	Sequence of Events: Females
Typical age for onset of puberty: Males 11-12 yr, normal range 9-14 yr Females 10-11 yr, range 8-13 yr	Body attains one fourth of total adult height with growth occurring in distal portions of limbs before proximal portions and trunk	Females enter puberty earlier than males and take longer to complete process; average length of pubertal events for males is 3-4 yr; for females 4-5 yr	Growth of testicles Pubic hair appears Growth of penis and scrotum Axillary hair First ejaculations (average, 13-14 yr) Growth spurt Facial hair Adult height	Ovaries increase in size Breast buds appear and/or pubic hair appears Growth spurt Pubic hair matures Breasts mature Axillary hair Menarche (range 10-16 yr) Adult height

From Kidd PS, Robinson DL: *Family nurse practitioner certification review,* St Louis, 1999, Mosby.

TABLE 204-2 Tanner Stages: Adolescent Female

Tanner 1	Tanner 2	Tanner 3	Tanner 4	Tanner 5
Tanner stage 1 is prepubertal; no observable change.	Small raised breast buds, sparse growth of fine downy pubic hair, usually along the sides of the labia	General enlargement of breasts with elevation of entire breast and areola from general chest contour; breast development is best assessed from side view; pubic hair is darker, coarser, and curlier and extends over the middle of the pubic bone; usually period of most rapid growth	Areola and papillae form contour that is separate from rest of breast; pubic hair has adult characteristics but does not extend to medial thigh; menarche generally occurs during this stage	Areola has same contour as rest of breast, with increase in overall size of breasts; pubic hair extends from thigh to thigh; some females may have additional growth at midline to form a triangle shape

Adapted from Kidd PS, Robinson DL: *Family nurse practitioner certification review,* St Louis, 1999, Mosby.

TABLE 204-3 Tanner Stages: Adolescent Male

Tanner 1	Tanner 2	Tanner 3	Tanner 4	Tanner 5
No pubic hair growth; prepubertal in appearance; testes 1 cm	Sparse growth of fine downy hair along base of penis; slight enlargement, increased texture of scrotum; testes 2-3.2 cm	Hair becomes darker, coarser, and curlier and spreads over middle of pubic bone; further growth and enlargement; testes 3.3-4 cm	Hair takes on adult characteristics but does not extend to thighs; penis significantly enlarged in length and circumference; increased size of testes (4-4.9 cm) and darkening of scrotal skin	Hair distributed from thigh to thigh and may extend up to navel; adult-size genitalia (testes 5 cm)

Adapted from Kidd, PS, and Robinson, DL: *Family nurse practitioner certification review,* St Louis, 1999, Mosby.

TABLE 204-4 Coping Mechanisms of Adolescents

Coping Mechanism	Strategy
Cognitive mastery	Teen attempts to learn as much as possible about situation or stressor
Conformity	Teen attempts to be image of peers: This includes language, dress, attitude, and actions
Controlling behaviors	The teen needs to be in control of some aspect of his or her life
Fantasy	Used more frequently by younger teens to deal with unpleasant situations
Motor activity	Serves as a safe tension-releasing strategy through release of energy

Ask sensitive questions using the third person: "Many teenagers go to parties where alcohol is served—do you?"

Mnemonics for History Taking and Assessment

Use mnemonics to help recall information to obtain from teens (Montalto, 1998):

HEADS
H Home, habits
E Education, employment, exercise
A Accidents, ambition, activities, abuse
D Drugs (tobacco, alcohol, others), diet, depression
S Sex, suicide

SAFE TEENS
S Sexuality
A Accident, abuse
F Firearms, suicide
E Emotions (suicide/depression)
T Toxins (tobacco, alcohol, others)
E Environment (school, home, friends)
E Exercise
N Nutrition
S Shots, school performance

HISTORY AND PHYSICAL EXAMINATION FORM

Using the history and physical examination form helps with consistency of approach and assists the nurse practitioner in making sure all components are included in each examination (see pp. 1307 to 1310).

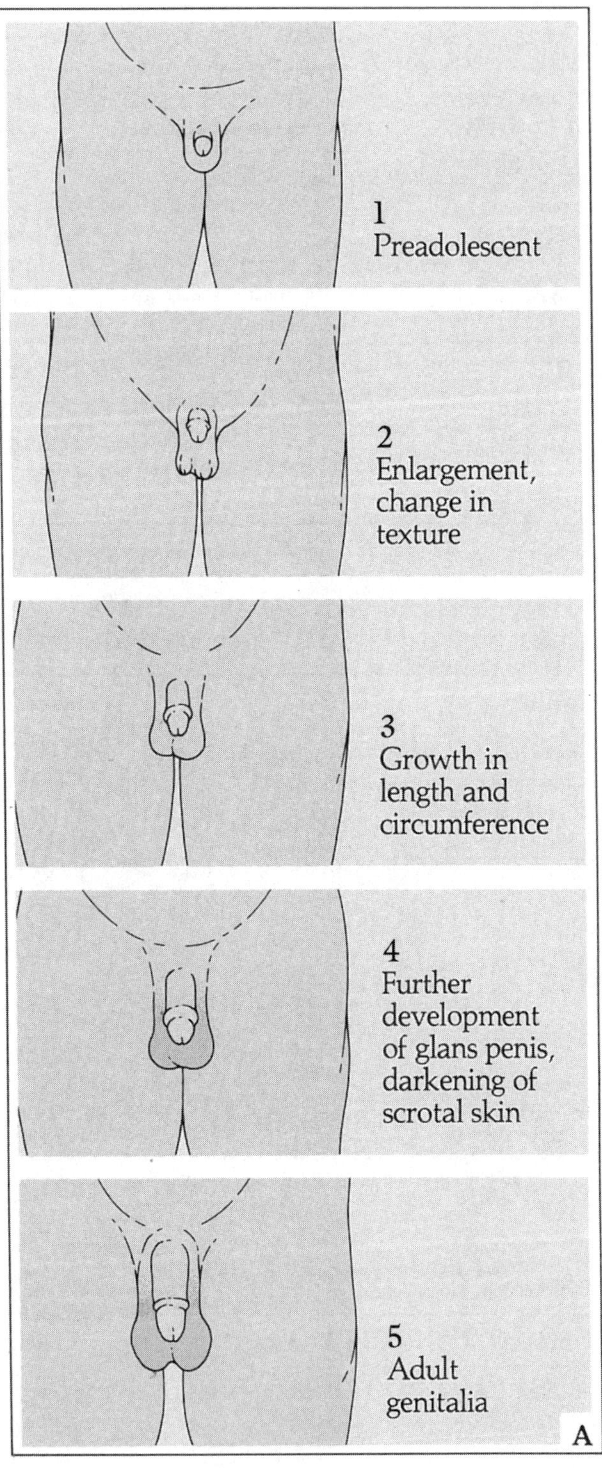

Figure 204-1 Male and female Tanner stages. **A,** Male genital development. (Adapted from Johnson TR, Moore WM, Jeffries JE: Children are different: development physiology, ed 2, Columbus, Ohio, 1978, Ross Laboratories.)

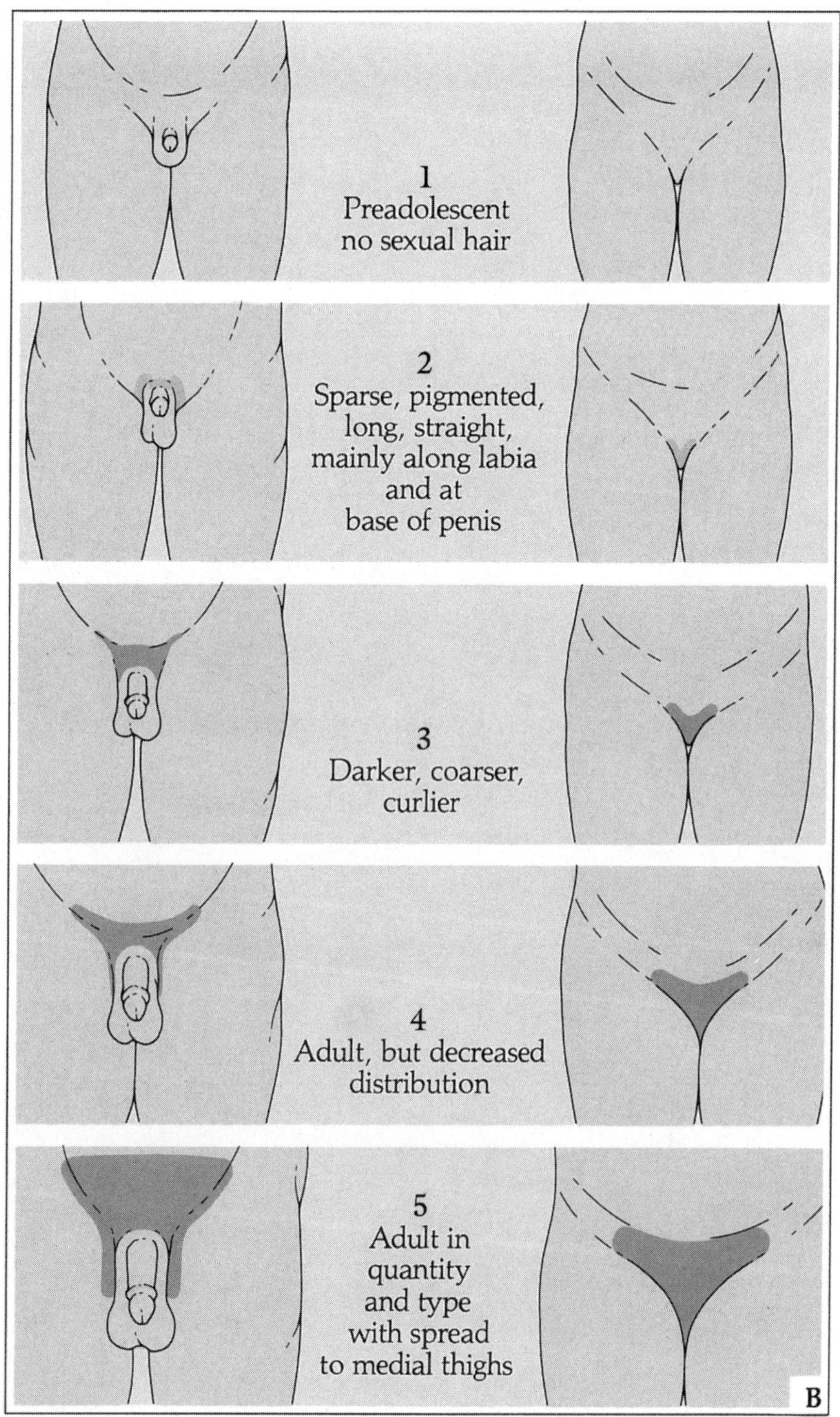

Figure 204-1, cont'd **B,** Pubic hair development.

Continued

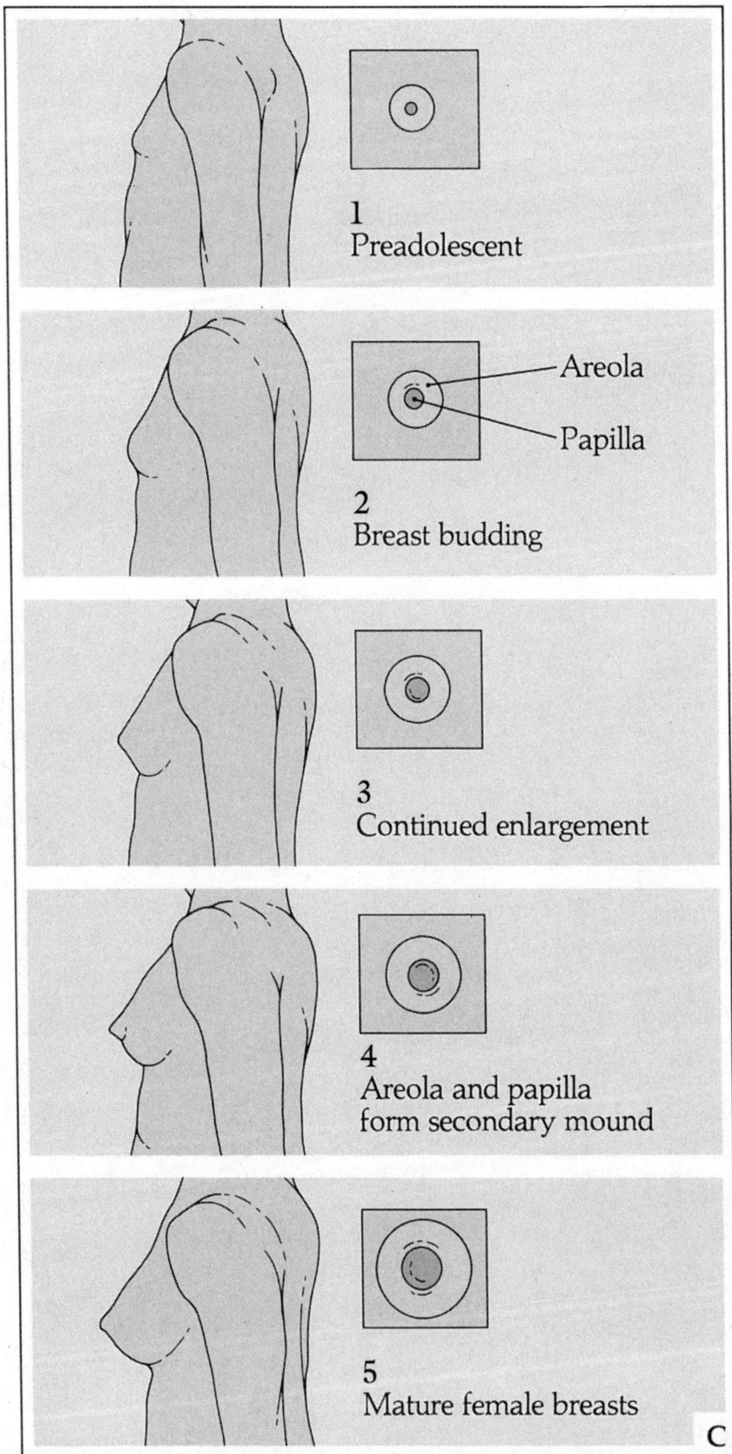

Figure 204-1, cont'd C, Breast development. (Adapted from Johnson TR, Moore WM, Jeffries JE: Children are different: development physiology, ed 2, Columbus, Ohio, 1978, Ross Laboratories.)

TABLE 204-5 Well Adolescent: 11-21 Years

	Early Adolescent (11-14)	Middle Adolescent (15-17)	Late Adolescent (18-21)
S	Lifestyle: Relationships: family, peer, school, peer group activities, tobacco, drug and alcohol usage, sexual involvement, legal history HEADS: Home setting: Who lives with patient, own room, relationships at home, what do parents do for a living, recent moves, running away, new people in home? Education/employment: School grade performance/changes, favorite/worst subjects, repeated classes, suspension, dropping out, future education plans, relations with teachers, employers, attendance Activities: Activities for fun—with whom, when, where, sports, church attendance, clubs, hobbies, TV, car seat belts, history of arrests, acting out Drugs: Use by peers, or patient, family members—amounts, frequency, patterns, car driving while using, source: How paid for Sexuality: Menarche, spermarche, orientation, degree and type of sexual experience, number of partners, masturbation (normalize), history of pregnancy, abortion, STD, contraception, comfort with sexual activity, history of sexual/physical abuse Nutrition: Body image, screen for eating disorders, typical daily intake Mental health: Suicide assessment, coping skills assessment	Lifestyle: Family relationships, employment, school, peer activities, substance use, sexual involvement, sexual orientation, weapon use, legal history HEADS: Home setting: Who lives with patient, own room, relationships at home, what do parents do for a living, recent moves, running away, new people in home? Education/employment: School grade performance/changes, favorite/worst subjects, repeated classes, suspension, dropping out, future education plans, relations with teachers, employers, attendance Activities: Activities for fun—with whom, when, where, sports, church attendance, clubs, hobbies, TV, car seat belts, history of arrests, acting out Drugs: Use by peers, or patient, family members, amounts, frequency, patterns, car driving while using, source: how paid for Sexuality: Orientation, degree and type of sexual experience, number of partners, masturbation (normalize), history of pregnancy, abortion, STD, contraception, comfort with sexual activity, history of sexual/physical abuse Nutrition: Body image, screen for eating disorders, typical daily intake Mental health: Depression, suicide assessment, coping skills assessment	Lifestyle: Family relationships, career plans, peer activities, substance use, sexual involvement, sexual orientation, weapon use, legal history HEADS: Home setting: who lives with patient, own room, relationships at home, what do parents do for a living, recent moves, running away, new people in home? Education/employment: School grade performance/changes, favorite/worst subjects, repeated classes, suspension, dropping out, future education plans, relations with teachers, employers, attendance Activities: Activities for fun—with whom, when, where, sports, church attendance, clubs, hobbies, TV, car seat belts, history of arrests, acting out Drugs: Use by peers, or patient, family members, amounts, frequency, patterns, car driving while using, source: how paid for Sexuality: Orientation, degree and type of sexual experience, number of partners, masturbation (normalize), history of pregnancy, abortion, STD, contraception, comfort with sexual activity, history of sexual/physical abuse, violence in dating relationships Nutrition: Screen for eating disorders especially bulimia, body image, typical daily intake Mental health: Depression, suicide assessment, coping skills assessment

Adapted from Kidd PS, Robinson DL: *Family nurse practitioner certification review,* St Louis, 1999, Mosby.

BP, Blood pressure; *BMI,* body mass index; *F,* female; *HBV,* hepatitis B virus; *M,* male; *MMR,* measles-mumps-rubella; *NSAIDs,* nonsteroidal antiinflammatory drugs; *STD,* sexually transmitted disease; *STI,* sexually transmitted infection, *TB,* tuberculosis; *Td,* tetanus-diphtheria toxoid (pediatric).

Continued

TABLE 204-5 Well Adolescent: 11-21 Years—cont'd

	Early Adolescent (11-14)	Middle Adolescent (15-17)	Late Adolescent (18-21)
O	One complete physical examination during early adolescence; BP, BMI; vision/hearing screen; dental screen; scoliosis screen; assess pubertal development; Tanner stage; screen for STI if sexually experienced, including Pap smear; TB screening if risk factors present; cholesterol screen if family history positive for early cardiovascular disease or hyperlipidemia	One complete physical examination during middle adolescence; BP, BMI; vision/hearing screen; dental screen; scoliosis screen; assess pubertal development; Tanner stage; screening for STIs if sexually experienced, including Pap smear, HIV screening if risk factors present; TB screening if risk factors present; cholesterol screen if family history positive for early cardiovascular disease of hyperlipidemia	One complete physical during late adolescence; Pap smear for all females, regardless of sexual experience; BP, BMI; vision/hearing screen; dental screen; hemoglobin screen; urinalysis screen; screening for STIs if sexually experienced, HIV screening if risk factors; TB screening if risk factors present; cholesterol screening if family history positive
A	Well adolescent Possible findings: gynecomastia, irregular menses, decreased school performance in junior high, myopia	Well adolescent Possible findings: Acne, dysmenorrhea, sports injuries, increased conflict at home	Well Adolescent Possible findings: Acne, chlamydia, obesity
Major morbidities	Consequence of sexual behavior (STIs, pregnancy), drug/alcohol/smoking, and effects of adolescent mental illness	Same	Same
Leading causes of death	Accidents (M > F), homicide (M > F), suicide (M > F), cancers (M > F), and heart disease (M > F)	Increase in homicide rates by 400% and 600%; increase in suicide rates compared with 10- to 14-yr olds Alcohol involved in 50% of above	Same
P	Immunizations: Td; hepatitis B series if not given in childhood; varicella if no reliable history of chickenpox or not given in routine childhood schedule; MMR if two vaccinations not documented earlier in childhood Gynecomastia: Reassurance Irregular menses: education about anovulatory cycles, reassurance, hormonal treatment if disruptive	Immunizations: None if updated at early adolescent visit Acne treatment: Begin with topical medications Dysmenorrhea: NSAIDs before onset of menses and every 6-8 hr for first 2 days of menses Eating disorder: Refer for dietary assessment if BMI <5th percentile Rehab all sports injuries before return to play	Immunizations: None if updated at early adolescent visit Acne treatment: Consider combination therapies Chlamydia: Single-dose therapy, partner notification Obesity: Low-fat diet, increased exercise. Refer for dietary counseling if BMI >95th percentile for age and gender

TABLE 204-5 Well Adolescent: 11-21 Years—cont'd

	Early Adolescent (11-14)	Middle Adolescent (15-17)	Late Adolescent (18-21)
Education	Education approach for a concrete thinker Development: Review normal physical changes, timing of menarche for females, peer pressure Injury prevention: Bike helmet use, protective equipment with sports, seat belt use Diet and physical activity: Calcium, iron sources in diet	Education approach for a early abstract thinking style; under stress this ability may be lost; adolescents feel invulnerable: things happen to others, but never to them Development: Skin care for acne, menstrual calendar, begin career planning Injury prevention: Stretching before physical activity, seatbelts, no driving while intoxicated or riding with intoxicated driver, violence prevention and conflict resolution	Education approach for abstract thinking; abstract thoughts and increased ability to set limits and understand consequences are established by late adolescence Development: Skin care, job/school/college search; leaving nest Injury prevention: Occupational safety, seatbelts, no driving while intoxicated or riding with intoxicated driver, conflict resolution Diet and physical health: Folic acid before planned pregnancy; calcium requirements; low-fat, high-fiber diet; exercise
	Healthy lifestyle: Contraception and condom usage, obtaining partner sexual activity to decrease risk, no alcohol, smoking cessation, substance use avoidance	Healthy lifestyle: Contraception and condom usage, obtaining partner sexual activity to decrease risk, no alcohol, smoking cessation, substance use avoidance	Healthy lifestyle: Contraception and condom usage, obtaining partner sexual activity to decrease risk, moderation with alcohol, smoking cessation, substance use avoidance; instruct in breast self-examination; instruct in testicular self examination, dental care
Follow-up	Return in 3 mo if menses remain irregular Return in 1 mo for second in HBV series	Return in 2 mo to evaluate dysmenorrhea resolution Consider oral contraceptive pills if dysmenorrhea continues Return in 2 mo for acne follow-up if pustules continue; begin combination treatment	Return in 3 mo to rescreen for STIs and reevaluate acne Return in 1 mo for further nutrition education; refer to dietitian if patient interested

WELL ADOLESCENT: 11 TO 21 YEARS

SOAPE guidelines for development of the adolescent 11 to 21 years old are outlined in Table 204-5.

REFERENCES

American Medical Association: *Guidelines for adolescent preventive services (GAPS) recommendations (monograph),* Chicago, Ill, 1995, The Association.

Levenberg P: GAPS: an opportunity for nurse practitioners to promote the health of adolescents through clinical preventive services, *J Pediatr Healthcare* 12:2-9, 1998.

Monalto N: Implementing the guidelines for adolescent preventive services, *Am Family Physician* 57:2181-2190, 1998.

SUGGESTED READINGS

American Psychiatric Association: *Diagnostic and statistical manual of mental disorders,* ed 4, (DSM4), Washington DC, 1994, The Association.

Bienfang DC et al: Ophthalmology, *N Engl J Med* 323:956-959, 1990.

Biro F et al: Adolescent girls' understanding of Papanicolaou smear results, *J Pediatr Adolesc Gynecol* 10:209-212, 1997.

Campbell M, McGrath P: Use of medication by adolescents for the management of menstrual discomfort, *Arch Pediatr Adolesc Med* 151:905-913, 1997.

Dawood MY: Dysmenorrhea, *Clin Obstet Gynecol* 33:168-178, 1990.

Draelos ZK: Patient compliance: enhancing clinician abilities and strategies, *J Am Acad Dermatol* 32:S42-48, 1995.

Dull P, Blythe M: Preventing teenage pregnancy, *Primary Care* 25:111-122, 1998.

Elster A, Kuznets N: *AMA guidelines for adolescent preventive services (GAPS): recommendations and rationale,* Baltimore, 1994, Williams & Wilkins.

Glass AP: Gynecomastia, *Endocrinol Metabol Clin North Am* 23:825-837, 1994.

Green M: *Bright futures: guidelines for health supervision of infants children and adolescents,* Arlington, Va, 1994, National Center for Education in Maternal and Child Health.

Hurwitz S: Acne treatment for the '90s, *Contemp Pediatr* 12:19-32, 1995.

Kidd PS, Robinson DL: *Family nurse practitioner certification review,* St Louis, 1999, Mosby.

Malat B: Reducing teen health risks, *Adv Nurse Pract* 6:47-50, 1998.

Moore P, Adler N, Kegeles S: Adolescents and the contraceptive pill: the impact of beliefs on intentions and use, *Obstet Gynecol* 88:48S-56S, 1996.

Neinstein LS: *Adolescent health care: a practical guide,* ed 3, Baltimore, 1996, Urban & Schwarzenberg.

Tanner JM: Issues and advances in adolescent growth and development, *J Adolesc Health Care* 8:470-478, 1987.

Wheeler MD: Physical changes of puberty, *Endocrinol Metabol Clin North Am* 20:1-14, 1991.

ADOLESCENT QUESTIONNAIRE

This form will be torn up and thrown away. The answers will not be told to anyone. The conversations that you have with the nurse practitioner or doctor will also not be discussed with anyone else except for matters that may be serious health problem for you or cause harm to others.

I have a problem with: Please circle yes or no

Breast	Yes	No	Heart	Yes	No	Sex organs	Yes	No
Chest	Yes	No	Joints/bones	Yes	No	Stomach	Yes	No
Ears	Yes	No	Lungs/breathing	Yes	No	Teeth	Yes	No
Eyes	Yes	No	Nose/throat	Yes	No	Urination	Yes	No
Head/neck	Yes	No	Periods	Yes	No	Other	Yes	No

Please circle answer:

1. I am having problems at home with parents, step parents, others	Yes	No	Some
2. I am having problems at school with friends, teachers or grades	Yes	No	Some
3. I drink alcoholic drinks such as beer, wine, liquor	Yes	No	Some
4. I smoke, dip or chew tobacco	Yes	No	Some
5. A friend or a family member has a problem with drugs or alcohol	Yes	No	Maybe
6. I have questions about sex, AIDS, or sexually transmitted diseases	Yes	No	Maybe
7. Have you had sex?	Yes	No	
8. Are you having sex now?	Yes	No	
9. I have questions about birth control or pregnancy	Yes	No	Maybe
10. I have been pregnant or have made someone pregnant	Yes	No	
11. I think I am underweight (skinny)	Yes	No	Maybe
12. I think I am overweight	Yes	No	Maybe
13. I am on a diet	Yes	No	
14. I use street drugs, huff or sniff chemicals, or take steroids	Yes	No	Some
15. I have experienced violence or abuse	Yes	No	Some
16. Do you have/own a gun?	Yes	No	
17. A family member has a gun in the house	Yes	No	
18. Have you been in trouble with the cops?	Yes	No	
19. There are times when I feel very sad, down or depressed	Yes	No	Some
20. I have trouble sleeping	Yes	No	Some
21. Have you missed more than 7 school days this year?	Yes	No	
22. I am involved in school groups or church groups	Yes	No	Some
23. I have a job	Yes	No	

24. I attend ____________ School in ________ Grade

25. After high school I want to: ______________________________

26. If you could have 3 wishes, what would you wish for? 1. ______________
2. ______________
3. ______________

27. Some teens have concerns about problems or issues they might have. I have a concern about: ______________

WELL ADOLESCENT VISIT

Date:		Name: DOB:		Allergies:
T:	P:	B/P:	Weight:	
Interim History:			Medications:	

History:
Last dental exam ________
Last eye exam ________
Last hearing ex ________
☐ dT ________
☐ PPD ________
☐ Surgeries
____
☐ Hospitalizations
____
☐ Illnesses: acute
____
☐ Illnesses: chronic
____
Home: Who lives with patient: ________
Have own room ☐ Y ☐ N
Recent moves ☐ Y ☐ N
Running away ☐ Y ☐ N
Education:
Level: ________
Grades: ________
Fav subject: ________
Worst subject: ________
Suspensions: ________
Relations with teachers:
____
Attendance: ________
Future education plans:
____
Activities:
Activities for fun: ________
____
Sports: ________
Church: ________
Arrests: ________
Have car: ☐ Y ☐ N
Employment ☐ Y ☐ N
Drugs:
Use by peers ________
Use by family ________
Use by patient ________
☐ Smoke ________ PPD
☐ Alcohol ________ Day
☐ Drug ________

Sexuality:
Menarche ________
Sexual orientation
☐ men
☐ women
☐ men and women
# of partners ________
Pregnancy ☐ Y ☐ N
Contraception ☐ Y ☐ N
Abortion ☐ Y ☐ N
Sexual/physical abuse ☐ Y ☐ N
☐ STDs Yes No
☐ Sex <18 Yes No
☐ >4 partners Yes No
☐ High risk sexual practices:
>1 partner past 6 mos ☐
☐ IVDA

Nutrition
Body image ________
Typical daily intake:
B ________
L ________
D ________
S ________

Lifestyle:
Family relationships:
____
____
Legal history: ________
____

Safety Assess/Counseling:
☐ Seat belts
☐ Firearms
☐ Smoke detectors
☐ Driving Hx
☐ Helmet use

Health habits:
Exercise: Yes No
Sleep problems Yes No

ROS: Circle
Heent: head inj, seizures, H/A, glaucoma, cataracts, visual problems, hearing loss, infection, allergies/sinus, nosebleeds, chronic sore throats, difficulty swallowing
Lymph: swellings in neck, axilla, groin, anemia
Endocrine: thyroid problems, DM, wt loss
Pulmonary: asthma, pneumonia, hemoptysis
Mental Health: depression, ADHD, thought of hurting self, ever been hospitalized for emotions

ROS: Circle
CV: murmur, rhythm disturb, HTN, C/P, angina
Breast: mass/lump/DC/pain
GI: GERD, hematemesis, PUD, abd. pain, chronic constipation or diarrhea, change in Bms, liver or GB problems, pancreatitis, melena or hematochezia, hemorrhoids, hepatitis
GU: dysuria, hematuria, UTI, STDs, warts, difficulty with urination or incontinence
MS: arthritis, gout, swelling, claudication, back pain
Neuro: numbness, weakness, chronic tingling, B/B incontinence, gait disturb, falling
Skin: changes in moles/warts, chronic rashes, acne
GYN: hot flashes, numbness, H/A, palpitations, drenching sweats, mood swings, vaginal dryness, itching
Frequent vaginal infections
Unusual vaginal discharge
Vaginal odor
Genital warts
STD (chlamydia, gonorrhea, syphilis, herpes)
Infection in uterus, tubes, ovaries (PID)
Pain or bleeding after intercourse
Missed periods
Bleeding b/w periods
Abnormal pap smears
Premenstrual symptoms
Satisfied with sexual relationship?
Questions/concerns about sexual issues?

FH:
- ☐ HTN ☐ MI
- ☐ CAD ☐ CVA
- ☐ DM ☐ CA
- ☐ Resp. ☐ Depression
- ☐ ETOH ☐ Seizures
- ☐ Substance abuse

OCP risks:
- ☐ Smoker ☐ Nonsmoker
- ☐ H/A ☐ HTN
- ☐ DVT ☐ Fibroids

Menstrual HX:

Age periods started ____

Periods last ________ days

Periods come q ____ days

Are periods:
- ☐ Regular
- ☐ Irregular
- ☐ Painful
- ☐ Light
- ☐ Moderate
- ☐ Heavy

LMP ____________

Last Pap ____________

Where: ____________

Results: ____________

Obstetric HX:

Number of preg: ________

Number of live birth ______

Stillbirth: ________

Miscarriage: ________

Abortion: ________

Any pregnancy complications?

DM	Yes	No
HTN	Yes	No
Toxemia	Yes	No

Contraceptive HX:

Current birth control?
- ☐ None
- ☐ Pills
- ☐ IUD
- ☐ Condoms (rubbers)
- ☐ BTL
- ☐ Depo
- ☐ Trying to become pregnant

Objective:

System	Norm	Abnormal	Comments
Skin	☐	☐	________
Head	☐	☐	________
Oral cavity	☐	☐	________
Ear	☐	☐	________
Nose	☐	☐	________
Eye	☐	☐	________
Neck	☐	☐	________
Thyroid	☐	☐	________
Chest	☐	☐	________
Heart	☐	☐	________
Breast	☐	☐	________
Abdomen	☐	☐	________
M/S	☐	☐	________
Scoliosis	☐	☐	________
Neuro	☐	☐	________
Extremities	☐		
Tanner	☐ 1	☐	________
	☐ 2	☐	________
	☐ 3	☐	________
	☐ 4	☐	________
	☐ 5	☐	________
Pelvic		☐	________
External	☐	☐	________
B.U.S.	☐	☐	________
Vagina	☐	☐	________
Cervix	☐	☐	________
Fundus	☐	☐	________
Adnexae	☐	☐	________
Rectal	☐		

BMI ____________

Plan:

Labs:
- ☐ Lipid panel
- ☐ HIV
- ☐ RPR
- ☐ Electrolytes
- ☐ LFT
- ☐ H/H
- ☐ GC/Chlamydia
- ☐ Pap
- ☐ U/A
- ☐ Wet mount
  - ☐ KOH
  - ☐ NaCl
- ☐ HCG

Screening:
- ☐ Vision
  - OD ________
  - OS ________
  - OU ________
- ☐ Hearing
- ☐ PPD

Immunizations:
- ☐ dT
- ☐ Flu
- ☐ Varicella
- ☐ Hep A
- ☐ Hep B
- ☐ MMR

Medications:

____

____

____

____

____

____

____

____

Instructions:

Assessment:		**Health promotion:**	F/U next visit:
☐ Normal exam	☐ Contraceptive counseling	☐ Exercise 3-5x week	__________
☐ Tobacco abuse	☐ Alcohol abuse	☐ Low fat, high carb high fiber diet	__________
☐ Acne	☐ Family planning	☐ Smoking cessation	__________
☐ Dysmenorrhea	☐ OCPs	☐ Alcohol moderation	__________
☐ Obesity	☐ Depo provera	☐ Use seat belts	
☐ Other: __________	☐ Vaginitis __________	☐ Sun protection	
__________	☐ UTI	☐ BSE	RTO: __________
__________	☐ Gynecomastia	☐ Dental care	
	☐ Myopia		

Signature: ____________________

Well Adult: Man

ICD-9-CM

Annual Examination V70.0
Preemployment Screening Examination V70.5

OVERVIEW

Definition

Comprehensive care can be provided across the lifespan for men based on knowledge of men's diverse lives. (See Table 205-1 and the well male examination sample form on pp. 1316 to 1317.)

PRACTICE GUIDELINES FOR PREVENTIVE CARE

Indications for Screening

Hearing: Presbycusis is the most frequent type of hearing loss for the elderly (Scheitel, 1996). Annual hearing tests should be conducted. Hearing loss can affect social, religious, and personal aspects of the individual.

Vision: Cataracts are common in the elderly. Counseling on what to look for will assist the individual in early detection. Periodic vision screening with a Snellen chart is appropriate. A dilated eye examination is recommended every 2 years.

Blood pressure: With individuals 75 years old and older, heart disease and cerebrovascular disease are among the top five causes of death. Although the United States Preventive Services Task Force recommends that blood pressure be measured every 2 years for individuals with normal readings, it is a quick, effective, measurement and is easily obtained during an office visit in screening for elevated pressure.

Skin: Skin examination for early detection of cancer, especially those **elders** who are exposed to the sun

Purified protein derivative (PPD): Close contacts of persons with known or suspected tuberculosis (TB), health care workers, persons with medical risk factors associated with TB, immigrants from countries with a high prevalence of TB, medically underserved low-income populations (including homeless persons), alcoholics, injection-drug users, and residents of long-term care facilities.

HIV: Men who have/had sex with men after 1975, past or present injection-drug users, persons who exchange sex for money or drugs, and their sex partners, bisexual or HIV-positive sex partners, currently or in the past, blood transfusion during 1978-1985, persons seeking treatment for sexually transmitted diseases (STDs).

Rapid plasma reagin (RPR): Persons who exchange sex for money or drugs and their sex partners, persons with other STDs (including HIV), and sexual contacts of persons with active syphilis.

Total cholesterol: Assess every 5 years, starting at age 25.

Digital rectal examination (DRE): Annually for prostate and colorectal cancer starting at age 50.

Prostate-specific antigen (PSA): Annually starting at age 40 for African-Americans and those with a family history of prostate cancer, and starting at age 50 for all others. After age 75, the screening has to be individualized based on level of activity, since it is theorized the disease is less virulent. More aggressive treatment of prostate cancer versus cautious observation has to be weighed with expected morbidity and/or mortality outcomes.

Fecal occult blood (FOB): Annually.

Sigmoidoscopy: Every 5 years.

Glaucoma: Annual screening by eye specialist for blacks >40 years old and whites >65 years old, those with a positive family history of glaucoma, and those with severe myopia.

Oral cavity: Individuals who smoke and/or drink alcohol regularly.

Chapter adapted with permission from Kidd P, Robinson D: *Family nurse practitioner certification review,* St Louis, 1999, Mosby.

Table 205-1 Well Male Care

SOAP	18-24 Years Old	25-65 Years Old	65 Years Old and Older
S	PMH, PSH, FH, medications, allergies Genogram to identify risk factors for CAD, DM, CA, asthma, psychiatric illnesses Lifestyle: Healthy diet and exercise, dental care, fluoridated water, risk for STDs, risk taking Habits: Alcohol/tobacco/illicit drugs, IV drug use Safety: Lap/shoulder belts, bike/motorcycle helmets; smoke detector, firearms: safe storage; alcohol while driving, swimming, boating Hot water and heater settings Use of space heaters Safety with hobbies Blood transfusion b/w 1978-1985 Ethnic background: Native American/Alaska Native, African-American Health maintenance: Last vision, hearing, and dental examination Pneumovax or influenza vaccine Social: Family relationships, employment, living arrangements, significant other Developmental tasks: Identity versus role confusion (adolescence)	PMH, PSH, FH, Medications, allergies Genogram to identify risk factors for CAD, DM, CA, asthma, psychiatric illnesses Lifestyle: Healthy diet and exercise, dental care, fluoridated water, risk for STDs Habits: Alcohol/tobacco/illicit drugs, IV drug use Safety: Lap/shoulder belts, bike/motorcycle helmets Smoke detector, firearms: safe storage Alcohol while driving, swimming, boating Hot water and heater settings Use of space heaters Safety with hobbies Blood transfusion b/w 1978-1985 Ethnic background: Native American/Alaska Native, African-American Health maintenance: Last vision, hearing. and dental examination Pneumovax or influenza vaccine Social: Family relationships, children, employment, living arrangements, health of parents Developmental tasks: Intimacy versus isolation (early adulthood) Generativity vs. stagnation (middle adulthood)	PMH, PSH, FH, Medications, allergies Genogram to identify risk factors for CAD, DM, CA, asthma, psychiatric illnesses Lifestyle: Healthy diet and exercise, dental care, fluoridated water, risk for STDs Habits: Alcohol/tobacco/illicit drugs, IV drug use Safety: Lap/shoulder belts, bike/motorcycle helmets Smoke detector, firearms: safe storage Alcohol while driving, swimming, boating Hot water and heater settings Use of space heaters Safety with hobbies Blood transfusion b/w 1978-1985 Ethnic background: Native American/Alaska Native, African-American Health maintenance: Last vision, hearing, and dental examination Pneumovax or influenza vaccine Social: Loss issues, family relationships, social activities Developmental task: Ego integrity versus despair
O	HT, WT, VS Skin Oral cavity Adenopathy Hearing Snellen test Heart/lung Testes Other systems dependent on risk factors and history	HT, WT, VS Skin Oral cavity Adenopathy Hearing Snellen test Heart/lung DRE Testes Other systems dependent on risk factors and history	HT, WT, VS Skin Oral cavity Adenopathy Hearing Snellen test Heart/lung DRE Testes Other systems dependent on risk factors and history

abd, Abdomen; *BM,* bowel movement; *BPH,* Benign prostatic hyperplasia; *CA,* cancer; *CAD,* coronary artery disease; *CBC,* complete blood cell count; *CP,* cardiopulmonary; *CV,* cardiovascular; *DM,* diabetes mellitus; *dT,* deoxythymidine; *ECG,* electrocardiogram; *FH,* family history; *FOB,* fecal occult blood; *GERD,* gastroesophageal reflux disease; *GI,* gastrointestinal; *GU,* genitourinary; *HEENT,* head/eyes/ears/nose/throat; *HIV,* human immunodeficiency virus; *HTN,* hypertension; *IVDA,* intravenous drug abuser; *LFT,* liver function test; *MI,* myocardial infarction; *MMR,* measles/mumps/rubella; *M/S,* musculoskeletal; *PMH,* past medical history; *PPD,* purified protein derivative; *PSA,* prostate-specific antigen; *PSH,* past surgical history; *PUD,* peptic ulcer disease; *ROS,* review of systems; *RPR,* rapid plasma reagin; *RTO,* return to office; *SE,* side effects, *STDs,* sexually transmitted diseases; *UTI,* urinary tract infection.

TABLE 205-1 Well Male Care—cont'd

SOAP	18-24 Years Old	25-65 Years Old	65 Years Old and Older
A	Well male Leading causes of death: Motor vehicle/other unintentional injuries, homicide, suicide, malignant neoplasms, heart disease, HIV, homicide	Well male Leading causes of death: Malignant neoplasms, heart disease, MVA, or other unintentional injuries, HIV, suicide and homicide	Well male Leading causes of death: Heart disease, malignant neoplasms (lung, colorectal, prostate), cerebrovascular disease, COPD, pneumonia, influenza
P	Screening: Lipid, HIV, PPD, RPR, GC, chlamydia Immunizations: dT, Hep B, Hep A, Flu, MMR, varicella Counseling: Problem drinking, illicit drug use, smoking cessation, alcohol/drug cessation, no drinking/drugs while driving, healthy diet and exercise, seat belts, bike helmets, firearm safety, STD prevention and protection, contraception, regular dental and vision care Skin cancer prevention	Screening: Lipid, HIV, PPD, RPR, GC, PSA, FOB, sigmoidoscopy, glaucoma Immunizations: dT, Hep B, Hep A, Flu, MMR, varicella Counseling: Problem drinking, illicit drug use, smoking cessation, alcohol/drug cessation, no drinking/drugs while driving, healthy diet and exercise, seat belts, bike helmets, firearm safety, STD prevention and protection, contraception, regular dental and vision care Skin cancer prevention	Screening: Lipid, FOB, HIV, PPD, RPR, PSA, sigmoidoscopy, glaucoma, hearing, mini-mental Immunizations: dT, Hep B, Hep A, Flu, MMR, varicella Counseling: Problem drinking, illicit drug use, polypharmacy, smoking cessation, healthy diet and exercise, seat belts, bike helmets, firearm safety, STD prevention, regular dental & vision care Skin cancer prevention Hot water heater <120° F, CPR for household members, emergency phone number available, fall prevention

TABLE 205-2 Immunization Guidelines: Adult Males

Immunizations	High-Risk Groups
Influenza	Annual vaccination of residents of long-term care facilities, persons with chronic cardiopulmonary disorders, metabolic diseases, hemoglobinopathies, renal dysfunction, or immunosuppression and health care providers for high-risk individuals
Pneumococcal	Immunocompromised institutionalized persons, immunocompromised persons with disorders such as chronic cardiac or pulmonary disease, diabetes mellitus, and anatomical asplenia. Immunocompromised persons who live in high-risk environments or social settings (e.g., certain Native American and Alaska Native populations); all persons >65 years old; no current recommendations for need of more than one vaccine
Tetanus	Every 10 years and in cases of severe or contaminated wounds
Hepatitis A	Persons living/working in or traveling to areas where the disease is endemic and where periodic outbreaks occur (certain Alaska Native, Pacific Island, Native American, and religious communities), men who have sex with men, injection/street drug users Consider for institutionalized persons and workers in these institutions, military personnel, and day care, hospital, and laboratory workers
Hepatitis B	Blood product recipients (including hemodialysis patients), persons with frequent occupational exposure to blood or blood products, men who have sex with men, injection drug users and their sex partners, persons with multiple recent sexual partners, persons with other STDs, travelers to countries with endemic hepatitis B
Varicella	Healthy adults without a history of chickenpox or previous immunization Consider serological testing for adults who are presumed susceptible

TABLE 205-3 Lifestyle Recommendations: Adult Males

Issue	Recommendation
Exercise/nutrition	Based on individual but periodic evaluation of weight gain/loss and counseling of dietary intake is appropriate. Examples of disease processes or related factors that can alter appetite or ability to eat and exercise are strokes, parkinsonism, dementia, depression, immobility, constipation, alcoholism, dental problems, medications, and impaired taste.
Medications	There should be a periodic review of all medications taken, including over the counter drugs, which can interact with prescription medications.
Smoking/tobacco	Recommend smoking/tobacco cessation to all individuals (see smoking cessation, Chapter 199)
Burns	Hot water heaters should be turned down to 48.9º C (120º F). Counsel to not smoke in bed. The main types of burns in the elderly are flame and scald injuries (Scheitel, 1996). Counsel the patient about fire extinguishers and fire alarms (see note under Home Safety Issues)
Motor vehicle accidents	Individuals over the age of 70 are at an increased risk for MVAs, especially if wearing bilateral hearing aids (Scheitel, 1996; McCloskey, 1994). Polydisease entities and subsequent polypharmocological management alone with normal aging processes, render the elderly at higher risk when operating a motor vehicle. Slowing of reflexes and a decrease in motor strength make the elderly more susceptible to accidents in situations which require rapid thinking and decision making such as at intersections. Decreased hepatic mass, blood flow, and enzyme activity as well as increased receptor site sensitivity make the elderly more susceptible to side effects of medications. Even if they are not at risk for causing the accident, all elderly tend to have more severe injuries and require hospitalizations more frequently. The heart and lungs become less pliant with age. Osteoporosis renders the elderly more vulnerable to fractures in what may seem to be a minor accident.
Driving assessment	A periodic review of driving history, including "near misses," is appropriate. Referral for formal, behind-the-wheel evaluation may be appropriate. There are some community resources that test driving skills without going through the State Department of Transportation. These programs bill based on "on-road" time and "class" time, with a general fee of $300 to $600. Some insurance companies offer reduced rates for individuals who go through formal programs and testing. Some automobile and other associations offer refresher course specifically designed for the elder driver; some at minimal or no cost. Get input from family members who have ridden in the vehicle with the elder. A Mini-Mental Examination will give an indication of the elder's cognitive function. Complete a hearing examination and range of motion/strength assessment as part of the physical. Review medications and alcohol use to assess for potential/actual side effects the elder may be experiencing.

Family Violence

A nurse practitioner must be alert to signs and symptoms of adult abuse. We need to find a comfort level in interview techniques that can assist in identifying family violence. Explore how things are going at home, work, and so on. Identify changes, good and bad. Is the patient anxious? How does he feel about life at work, at home, in general? Be empathetic. Support the feelings of the involved parties by identifying that other people are struggling with the same issues. Remain objective.

Use statements such as these:
"That sounds like it can be a very difficult situation."
"Is there anything you may want to change?"
"What kind of worries are most bothersome to you?"
"How do you manage this problem?"
"How have you managed similar problems in the past?"
"Who supports you?"

Immunizations

Immunizations for adult males are outlined in Table 205-2.

Lifstyle/Activities

Lifestyle recommendations are outlined in Table 205-3.

HOME SAFETY ISSUES

Areas to Assess

Security systems
Use of throw rugs, extension cords, or appliances with frayed cords
Use of space heaters or wood-burning stoves
Torn or frayed carpeting on stairways
Presence of pets that could get in the way of ambulation
Adequate lighting inside and outside
Whether the individual parks his car outside or in a garage and/or what time he gets home when he parks on the street

Recommendations

In general, there should be an ABC fire extinguisher and smoke detector for each level of the home. The fire extinguisher should be a 5-lb extinguisher to allow for some error in usage. If there is a high hazard area, there should be an additional fire extinguisher and smoke detector.

See Chapter 207 for wellness and health promotion guideline summaries.

REFERENCES

McCloskey L et al: Motor vehicle collision injuries and sensory impairments of older drivers, *Age Aging* 23:267-273, 1994.

Scheitel S et al: Geriatric health maintenance, *Mayo Clin Proc* 71:289-302, 1996.

SUGGESTED READINGS

Branch W, Jacobson T: Routine preventive studies: what to include and how often, *Consultant* 36:2401-2410, 1996.

Goldstein A: Health promotion. In Sloane P, Slatt L, Curtis P, editors: *Essentials of family medicine,* Baltimore, 1993, Williams & Wilkins.

Hicks M: Well adult care. In Sloane P, Slatt L, Curtis P, editors: *Essentials of family medicine,* Baltimore, 1993, Williams & Wilkins.

Kidd P, Robinson D: *Family nurse practitioner certification review,* St Louis, 1999, Mosby.

Leading causes of death, *Women's Health Primary Care* 1:38, 1998.

Murray SL: What's happening: driving and the elderly, *J Am Acad Nurse Pract* 9:133-136, 1997.

Nichol K et al: Effectiveness of influenza vaccine in the elderly, *Gerontology* 42:274-279, 1996.

Sloane P, Hicks M: Preventive care: an overview. In Sloane P, Slatt L, Curtis P, editors: *Essentials of family medicine,* Baltimore, 1993, Williams & Wilkins.

Uphold C, Graham M: *Periodic health evaluation for adults: clinical guidelines in family practice,* ed 2, Gainesville, Fla, 1994, Barmarrae Books.

US Preventive Services Task Force: *Guide to clinical preventive services,* ed 2, Baltimore, 1996, Williams & Wilkins.

Weingarten S et al: The adoption of preventive care practice guidelines by primary care physicians: do actions match intentions? *J Gen Intern Med* 10:138-144, 1995.

White P: Pearls for practice: polypharmacy and the older adult, *J Am Acad Nurse Pract* 7:545-548, 1995.

WELL MALE VISIT

Date:		Name:	DOB:	Allergies:
T:	P:	B/P:	Weight:	
Interim History:			Medications:	

History:
Last dental exam ____
Last eye exam ____
Last hearing ex ____
☐ dT ____
☐ PPD ____
☐ Flu ____
☐ Pneumovax ____
☐ X-ray trt to upper body
☐ Surgeries
____
____
☐ Hospitalizations
____
____
____
☐ Illnesses: acute
____
____
☐ Illnesses: chronic
____
____
____
____
____

Social:
☐ Smoke ____ PPD
☐ Alcohol ____ Day
☐ Drugs
☐ Employment Y N
☐ # years of school completed
☐ Living arrangements
☐ Significant other
☐ Children Y N

Safety: Assess/Counseling:
☐ Hot H_2O heater
☐ Seat belts
☐ Firearms
☐ Smoke detectors
☐ Driving Hx (.70)
☐ Fall assessment
☐ Helmet use

Subjective:
☐ **BPH symptoms:**
Dribbling, incontinence, diff. starting stream
☐ **CAGE**
☐ Have you ever felt you should cut down your drinking?
☐ Have people annoyed you by criticizing your drinking?
☐ Have you ever felt guilty about your drinking?
☐ Do you have an eye opener in the AM to steady your nerves?
HIV risk factors:
☐ High risk sexual practices:
> 1 partner past 6 mos Y N
Sexual relationships with:
☐ men
☐ women
☐ both men and women
☐ IVDA
☐ blood transfusion b/w 1978-1985

ROS: Circle
Heent: head inj, seizures, H/A, glaucoma, cataracts, visual problems, hearing loss, infection, allergies/sinus, nosebleeds, chronic sore throats, difficulty swallowing
Lymph: swellings in neck, axilla, groin, anemia
Endocrine: thyroid problems, DM, wt loss
Pulmonary: asthma, pneumonia, hemoptysis
CV: murmur, rhythm disturb, HTN, C/P, angina
GI: GERD, hematemesis, PUD, abd. pain, chronic constipation or diarrhea, change in Bms, liver or GB problems, pancreatitis, melena or hematochezia, hemorrhoids, hepatitis
GU: dysuria, hematuria, UTI, STDs, warts, diff. urination, incontinence
MS: arthritis, gout, swelling, claudication, back pain
Neuro: numbness, weakness, chronic tingling, B/B incontinence, gait disturb, falling
Skin: changes in moles/warts, chronic rashes, acne
Sexuality: Satisfied with sexual relationship? Question/concerns about sexual issues?

FH: Identify age current status

☐ HTN	☐ MI	____
☐ CAD	☐ CVA	____
☐ DM	☐ CA	____
☐ Resp.	☐ Depression	____
☐ ETOH	☐ Seizures	____

Objective:

System	Norm	Abnormal	Comments
Skin	☐	☐	____
Head	☐	☐	____
Oral cavity	☐	☐	____
Ear	☐	☐	____
Nose	☐	☐	____
Eye	☐	☐	____
Neck	☐	☐	____
Chest	☐	☐	____
Heart	☐	☐	____

Plan:
Labs:
☐ Lipid
☐ PSA
☐ HIV
☐ FOB
☐ RPR
☐ Electrolytes
☐ LFT
☐ Uric acid
☐ CBC
☐ Glucose

Immunizations:
☐ dT
☐ Flu
☐ Pneumovax
☐ Varicella
☐ Hep A
☐ Hep B
☐ MMR

Medications:
____
____

Abdomen ☐ ☐ ______ Prostate ☐ ☐ ______ M/S ☐ ☐ ______ Neuro ☐ ☐ ______ Extremities ☐ ☐ ______	**Screening:** ☐ Sigmoidoscopy ☐ Vision ☐ Hearing ☐ Dental ☐ EKG ______ ______ ______ Instructions:
Assessment: ☐ Normal exam ☐ BPH ☐ Tobacco abuse ☐ Alcohol abuse ☐ Hyperlipidemia ☐ HTN ☐ Other: ______ ______ ______	**Counseled:** ☐ Exercise 3-5x week ☐ Low fat, high carb high fiber diet ☐ Smoking cessation ☐ Alcohol moderation ☐ Use seat belts ☐ Sun protection ☐ Testicular SE F/U next visit: ______ ______ ______ ______ RTO: ______

Signature: ______

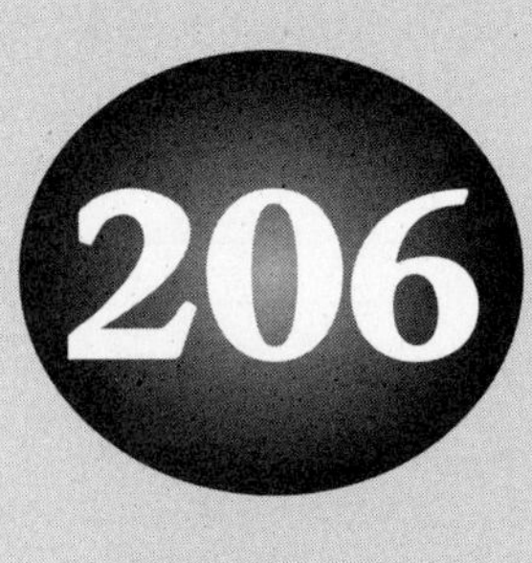

Well Adult: Woman

ICD-9-CM

Cervical Papanicolaou Smear V76.2
As Part of Routine Gynecological Examination V72.3
Gynecological Examination for Contraceptive Maintenance V25.42
IUD V25-42
Pill V25.41
Health Checkup V70.0
Occupational Examination V70.5
Preemployment Screening V70.5

OVERVIEW

Definition

Comprehensive care can be provided across the lifespan for women, based on knowledge of women's diverse everyday lives. See pp. 1325 to 1327 for sample well women examination forms.

SUBJECTIVE DATA

Past History

Family history
Medical history
Surgical history
Mental health history
Menstrual history
Gynecological and obstetrical history
Contraceptive history
Immunizations and infectious disease history
Allergies
Blood transfusion between 1978 and 1985
Occupational blood and body fluid exposure
Dental care

For women after age 65, ask about prior symptoms of transient ischemic attack and driving assessment, including near misses

Current Health Status

Ask the patient about:
- Medications and herbal uses
- Dietary intake
- Dietary supplementation
- Physical activity
- Contraception
- Sexual practices: High risk for sexually transmitted diseases

For women older than 65 years of age, ask about functional status at home

Safety

Ask about abuse (physical, emotional, sexual). Sample questions include:
- How are things going at home?
- Have you ever felt unsafe with your partner?
- Has your partner ever hurt you or controlled you or your finances?
- At any time has your partner ever hit or threatened you? (See Chapter 3 for more information.)

Ask about smoke and carbon monoxide detectors and fire extinguishers

Ask about seat belt use and safety gear for hobbies.

For women older than 65 years of age:
- Assess the potential for falls in the home:
  - Use of throw rugs, carpeting on stairways
  - Use of extension cords
  - Use of space heaters
  - Inadequate lighting
  - Low chairs
  - Incorrect footwear

Determine whether multifactorial risks are present:
- Psychoactive medications
- More than four prescription medications

Impaired cognition, strength, and balance or gait
Hot water heater temperature
Assess driving skills:
Driving history, including near misses
Get input from family members who have ridden in the vehicle
Complete a hearing assessment if assessment reveals near crashes
Review medications and alcohol use

Habits

Ask about alcohol, tobacco, illicit drugs, intravenous (IV) drug use, and gambling.

Psychosocial History

Ask about:

Religion
Ethnicity
Relations with family and friends
Occupation/employment status
Interests
Meaningful life changes

OBJECTIVE DATA

Physical Examination

A complete physical examination should be performed, with particular attention to:

Height, weight, blood pressure
Head/eyes/ears/nose/throat:
Adenopathy, thyroid
For women over age 65: visual acuity, hearing and hearing aids
Chest: Lungs, heart, breast
Abdomen
Pelvic examination
Digital rectal examination
Other elements are included based on history

Screenings: Indications and Frequency

Oral cavity examination: Suspicious symptoms or exposure to tobacco or increased amounts of alcohol
Skin: Suspicious lesions or personal or familial history of skin cancer or increased sunlight exposure
Dental examination: Every year
Eye examination with tonometry: Baseline during age 18 to 39, then every 3 to 5 years or more frequently if risk factors are present, annually after 65
Hearing: Regular exposure to excessive noise; baseline at age 40, repeat at 50; after age 60, every year
Carotid bruits: History of cerebrovascular disease or neurological symptoms or risk factors for cardiovascular or cerebrovascular disease
Pap smear/pelvic examination: Start when sexually active or at age 18; continue every year until age 60, then every 1 to 2 years; the specimen is collected from the transformation zone, which changes in various age groups; a sample at-risk form can be found on p. 1327
Proctoscopy/sigmoidoscopy: Family history of familial polyposis coli or cancer family syndrome or starting at age 50; obtain two consecutive annually negative examinations before intervals of every 3 to 5 years
Rectal examination: Every year (there is some controversy about this; some research has shown a low yield in patients under 40 years old; Campbell, Shaughnessy, 1998)

Laboratory/Diagnostic Procedures

Laboratory and diagnostic procedure screenings by age group are outlined in Table 206-1.

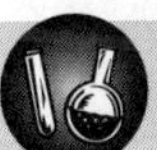

TABLE 206-1 Diagnostic Tests: Screenings by Age Group

18-39 Years	40-64 Years	65+ Years
Screening: Pap smear annually (see Pap follow-up table) History-dependent screening: PPD, fasting plasma glucose, rubella antibodies, U/A for bacteriuria, HIV, RPR, gonococcal /chlamydial infection, hearing, mammogram colonoscopy	Screening: Pap smear annually, mammogram every other year or annually History dependent screening: PPD, fasting plasma glucose, rubella antibodies, U/A for bacteriuria, HIV, RPR, hearing, gonococcal/ chlamydial infection, FOB/ sigmoidoscopy, fecal occult colonoscopy, bone mineral content.	Annual screening: dipstick urinalysis, Pap smear, mammogram, thyroid function tests History-dependent screening: Glaucoma testing

FOB, Fecal occult blood; *HIV,* human immunodeficiency virus; *PPD,* purified protein derivative; *RPR,* rapid plasma reagin; *U/A,* urinalysis.

Screenings: Indications and Frequency

Cholesterol: Baseline during age 18 to 39 and every 5 years; after age 40, every 3 to 5 years

Glucose: Every 3 years beginning at age 45 if asymptomatic; screening may need to begin earlier if the patient is obese, has a first-degree relative with diabetes mellitus (DM), is a member of a high-risk ethnic population (African-American, Hispanic, Native American, Asian), is hypertensive, has a high cholesterol or triglyceride level, or on previous testing had impaired glucose tolerance or impaired fasting glucose

Gonococcal/chlamydial infection: If the woman engages in or has partners who engage in high-risk sexual behavior or contact with person diagnosed with a chlamydial infection; highest risk in teens and twenties

Hematocrit/hemoglobin: Every 2 years from age 18 to 50, then every 5 years

Human immunodeficiency virus (HIV): If the woman engages in or has partners who engage in high-risk sexual behavior or contact with a person who is HIV positive; IV drug users; women who have male partners who have had sex with men or are injection-drug users; long-term residence or birthing in an area with high prevalence of HIV infection; or a history of transfusion between 1978 and 1985

Mammography: Baseline at age 35 to 40, then repeat every 1 to 2 years from age 40 to 49, every year after age 50; women with a family history of breast cancer should receive mammograms 5 years earlier than the age of breast cancer diagnosis in a first-degree relative

Papanicolaou smear: Every year until age 60, then every 1 to 2 years. Instruct the woman not to douche, use vaginal creams or have intercourse for at least 24 hours before a Pap smear (Table 206-2)

Purified protein derivative: household members of persons diagnosed with tuberculosis or other close contact with known or suspected TB; health care workers; risk factors associated with TB (HIV+); immigration from country with high TB prevalence; medically undeserved low-income population; alcoholism; IV drug use; residents of long-term care facility

Rapid plasma reagin: If the woman engages in or has partners who engage in high-risk sexual behavior or contact with a person diagnosed with active syphilis

Rubella antibodies: Lack of evidence of immunity

Stool hemoccult: Every year

Thyroid function: Starting at age 50, every 3 to 5 years

ASSESSMENT

Leading Health Problems by Age Group

Leading health problems by age group are outlined in Table 206-3.

THERAPEUTIC PLAN

Immunizations

Immunizations by age group are outlined in Table 206-4.

Indications for Immunizations

Influenza: Annual vaccination of: Residents of long-term care facilities, persons with chronic cardiopulmonary disorders, metabolic diseases, hemoglobinopathies, immunosuppression, renal dysfunction, and health care providers for high-risk patients

Hepatitis A: Women who reside in, travel to, or work in areas where the disease is endemic and where periodic outbreaks occur (e.g., countries with high or intermediate endemicity; certain Alaska Native, Pacific Island, Native American, and religious communities); women who have male partners who have had sex with men or are injection-drug users; consider for institutionalized persons and workers in these institutions, military personnel, and day care, hospital, and laboratory workers

Hepatitis B: Blood product recipients (including hemophiliacs and hemodialysis patients), persons with frequent occupational exposure to blood or blood products, travel to countries with endemic hepatitis B, household and sexual contacts of HBV carriers, multiple recent sex partners or multiple recent sex partners diagnosed with other recently acquired STDs, inmates of long-term correctional institutions, prostitutes, women who have male partners who have had sex with men or are IV drug users

MMR: Women who were born after 1956 and lack evidence of immunity to measles (e.g., documented administration of live vaccine on or after the first birthday, laboratory evidence of immunity, or a history of diagnosed measles)

Pneumococcal: Medical conditions that increase the risk of pneumococcal infections (e.g., diabetes mellitus, sickle cell disease, nephrotic syndrome, chronic cardiac or pulmonary disease, Hodgkin's disease, anatomical asplenia, alcoholism, cirrhosis, multiple myeloma, renal disease, conditions associated with immunosuppression); immunocompetent institutionalized persons over 50 years old; immunocompetent persons who live in high-risk environments or social settings (e.g., certain Native American and Alaska Native populations); all those over 65 years old

Tetanus-diphtheria: Every 10 years

Varicella: Healthy adults without a history of chickenpox or previous immunization; consider serological; testing for adults who are presumed susceptible

Counseling for All Women

Diet instruction related to fat, cholesterol, complex carbohydrate, fiber, sodium, iron, and calcium intake

TABLE 206-2 Classification and Management of Pap Smear Results

Bethesda System Result	Comment	Patient Management	Repeat
Adequacy of Specimen			
Within normal limits			1 year
Satisfactory, but limited by (reason specified)		If normal or benign result reported	At next normal interval: 1 year
Unsatisfactory for evaluation	Assumes no diagnosis included in Pap smear report	Repeat no sooner than 6 weeks after previous one; post-menopausal women: vaginal atrophy: apply topical vaginal estrogen for 4-6 wks	6-12 wks during midcycle; repeat Pap 1 week or more after finishing medication
Infection/Abnormal Descriptions			
Trichimoniasis	Highly specific	Offer*; if treated recently, no action	1 year
Fungus consistent with Candida		Offer therapy if symptomatic*; repeat only if inflammation is severe and a repeat smear is recommended	1 year
Coccobacilli with flora shift	Poor diagnostic accuracy for BV	Offer therapy if symptomatic*; management is controversial	1 year
Actinomyces	Significant if IUD in situ	Re-examine; if symptoms or physical examination suggests pelvic actinomycosis, removal of IUD is suggested, along with intensive antibiotic therapy	Dependent on symptoms; may warrant more frequent follow-up
Herpes simplex	Diagnostic of HSV shedding	HSV culture not necessary. Risk of vertical transmission to newborn†	1 year
Reactive Changes			
Inflammation	May be due to gonorrhea, chlamydia, other pathogens, or benign changes	Unless recently performed, contact patient and offer testing for gonorrhea and chlamydia; persistent inflammation may warrant colposcopic evaluation*	Repeat Pap q6mos × 2; refer for colposcopy if reactive changes found on any 2 Paps with 12 months after treatment of proven infection or if no infection documented
Atrophy with inflammation	Common in postmenopausal women	Offer estrogen vaginal cream QD × 6 weeks if symptomatic; then repeat Pap no sooner than 1 week after medication completed	Minimum of 7 wks after initial Pap
IUD	Normal finding in IUD wearers	No therapy	1 year

From Hatcher R, Trussell J, Stewart F: *Contraceptive technology,* New York, 1994, Irrington Publishers; Gries-Griffin J: Abnormal Pap test results, *Adv Nurse Pract* 3(7):16-21, 1995.

*The patient's medical record should be reviewed to determine whether evaluation or treatment of a specified condition was provided at the time of the Pap smear or during another visit. If not, a single contact by letter or telephone is deemed sufficient.

†The patient must be notified of the result and given additional information. A single contact by letter or telephone is deemed sufficient.

Continued

TABLE 206-2 Classification and Management of Pap Smear Results—cont'd

Bethesda System Result	Comment	Patient Management	Repeat
Epithelial Changes/Squamous Cell Abnormalities			
Atypical cell of undetermined significance (ASCUS)	Significant only if ASCUS/premalignant change; ASCUS/reactive considered benign	Reactive changes: no further evaluation needed; ASCUS premalignant should be considered equivalent to a reading of LSIL†	1 year
Low-grade squamous intraepithelial lesion (SIL)	Includes human papillomavirus/ condylomatous atypia cervical intraepithelial lesion (CIN I)	Only 15%-20% progress to higher grade lesion; if Pap shows ASCUS premalignant change or SIL on follow-up, refer for colposcopy†; determine what your organization prefers for follow-up: some want colposcopy right away	Repeat q 4-6 mos for 3 intervals; if poor compliance: colposcopy
High-grade SIL	Includes CIN II, III	Refer for colposcopy (even during pregnancy)†	Not applicable
Squamous cell carcinoma	High specificity for squamous cancer	Refer to MD experienced in the management of gynecological cancers†	Not applicable
Glandular Changes			
Endometrial cells in postmenopausal women	May be benign, hormonal replacement therapy, hyperplasia, or malignancy	Sample the endometrium†	Return in 1 year if endometrial sample is normal
Atypical glandular cells of undetermined significance (AGCUS)	Evaluate if AGCUS/ premalignant change	Refer for colposcopy†	Increased frequency of Pap smear screening × 15 mos
Adenocarcinoma	High specificity for adenocarcinoma of endocervix or endometrium	Refer to MD experienced in the management of gynecological cancers†	
Follow-up After Colposcopy	Figure 206-1		

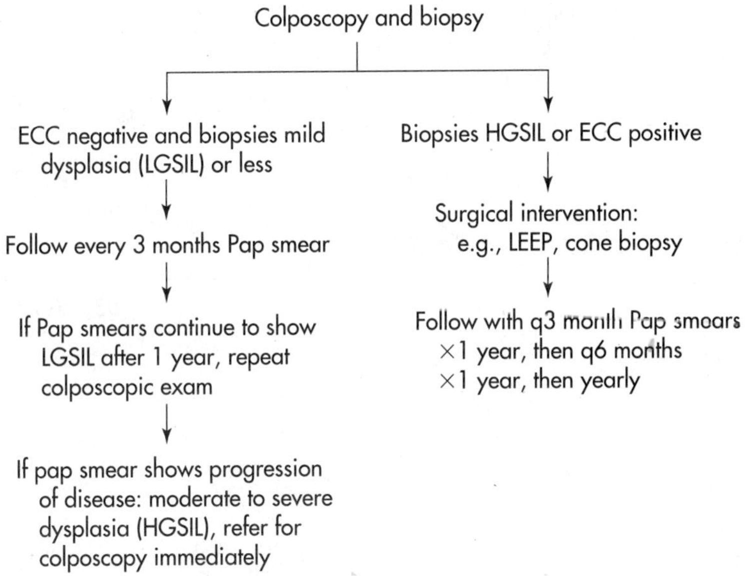

Figure 206-1 Follow-up after colposcopy and biopsy. *ECC,* Endocervical curettage; *HGSIL,* high-grade squamous intraepithelial lesion; *LEEP,* loop electrical excision procedures; *LGSIL,* low-grade squamous epithelial lesion.

TABLE 206-3 Leading Health Problems by Age Group

18-39 Years	40-64 Years	65+ Years
Injuries; viral, bacterial, and parasitic infections; acute UTIs; eating disorders; violence, rape; substance abuse	Osteoporosis and arthritis; orthopedic deformities and impairments of back, arms, and legs; cardiovascular diseases; hearing and vision impairments	Osteoporosis and arthritis; hypertension; urinary incontinence; cardiovascular diseases; injuries; hearing and vision impairment

TABLE 206-4 Immunizations by Age Group

18-39 Years	40-64 Years	65+ Years
Tetanus-diphtheria; HIGH-RISK: hepatitis B, influenza, MMR, pneumococcal vaccine	Tetanus-diphtheria; HIGH-RISK: hepatitis B, influenza, pneumococcal vaccine	Tetanus-diphtheria, influenza, pneumococcal vaccine, HIGH-RISK: hepatitis B

MMR, Measles/mumps/rubella.

TABLE 206-5 Specific Counseling by Age Group

18-39 Years	40-64 Years	65+ Years
Contraceptive options	Contraceptive options and hormone replacement therapy; use of products for lubricating thinning vaginal tissues; other counseling related to menopausal symptoms	Advance directives/living will/durable power of attorney Motor vehicle accidents: Refresher course for older drivers Specific counseling related to aging, osteoporosis, sexuality, depression of elderly

TABLE 206-6 Leading Causes of Death by Age Group

18-39 Years	40-64 Years	65+ Years
MVA; homicide; coronary artery diseases; AIDS; breast cancer, cervical and other uterine cancers	Coronary artery diseases; breast cancer; lung cancer; colorectal cancer; ovarian cancer; COPD; diabetes	Pneumonia and influenza; COPD; colorectal cancer; breast cancer; lung cancer; diabetes; accidents

AIDS, Acquired immunodeficiency syndrome; *COPD,* chronic obstructive pulmonary dysfunction; *MVA,* motor vehicle accidents.

Exercise program
Smoking cessation
Limiting alcohol consumption
Identification and treatment for abuse
Safer sex practices
Breast self-examination
Skin protection from ultraviolet light
Specific counseling for each age group is outlined in Table 206-5.
Leading causes of death for each age group are outlined in Table 206-6.

REFERENCES

Campbell K, Shaughnessy A: Diagnostic utility of the digital rectal examination as part of the routine pelvic examination, *J Family Practice* 46:165-167, 1998.

SUGGESTED READINGS

American Academy of Family Physicians (1997) American Academy of Family Physicians' age charts for periodic health examination. In Murray RB, Zentner JP, editors: *Health assessment & promotion strategies,* ed 6, Norwalk, Conn, 1997, Appleton & Lange.

Clinical Guidelines: Hepatitis B immunization/prophylaxis, *Nurse Pract* 21:64-70, 1997.

Gray-Miceli D: Falling among the aged, *Adv Nurse Pract* 5:41-42, 44, 1997.

Hahn MS: Matters of the heart, *Adv Nurse Pract* 3:13-19, 1995.

Murray RB et al: Assessment and health promotion for the person in later maturity. In Murray RB, Zentner JP, editors: *Health assessment & promotion strategies,* ed 6, Norwalk, Conn, 1997, Appleton & Lange.

Poirier L: The importance of screening for domestic violence in all women, *Nurse Pract* 22:105-122, 1997.

Prevention: Harvard Women's Health Watch, Newsletter, 5(12):2-4, 1997.

Shah MA: The nurse-midwife as primary care provider, *J Nurse-Midwife* 38:185-187, 1993.

Tetanus and diphtheria immunization/prophylaxis adults and older adults, *Nurse Pract* 22:116-120, 1997.

Treinen AD: Breast cancer screening: making sense of controversies, *Adv Nurse Pract* 5:17-23, 1997.

Writing Group of the 1996 AAN Expert Panel on Women's Health: Women's health and women's health care: recommendations of the 1996 AAN Expert Panel on Women's Health, *Nurs Outlook* 45:7-15, 1997.

Youngkin EQ, Davis MS: Assessing women's health. In Youngkin EQ, MS Davis MS, editors: *Women's health: a primary care clinical guide,* Norwalk, Conn, 1994, Appleton & Lange.

US Preventive Services Task Force: *Guide to clinical preventive services,* Baltimore, 1996, Williams & Wilkins.

WELL WOMAN VISIT

Date:		Name:	DOB:	Allergies:
T:	P:	B/P:	Weight:	
Interim History:			Medications:	

History:
Last dental exam ____
Last eye exam ____
Last hearing ex ____
☐ dT ____
☐ PPD ____
☐ Flu ____
☐ Pneumovax ____
☐ Irradiation to upper body
☐ Surgeries
____
____
☐ Hospitalizations
____
____
____
☐ Illnesses: acute
____
____
☐ Illnesses: chronic
____
____
____
____
____

Social:
☐ Smoke ____ PPD
☐ Alcohol ____ Day
☐ Drugs
☐ Employment Y N
☐ # years of school completed
☐ Living arrangements
☐ Significant other
☐ Children Y N

Safety: Assess/Counseling:
☐ Hot H_2O heater
☐ Seat belts
☐ Firearms
☐ Smoke detectors
☐ Driving Hx (.70)
☐ Fall assessment
☐ Helmet use

Health Habits:
Exercise: Y N
Sleep problems Y N
Calcium suppl Y N
BSE Y N
Have you ever been frightened of your partner? Y N
Have you ever been threatened by your partner? Y N

Subjective:
☐ **CAGE**
☐ Have you ever felt you should cut down your drinking?
☐ Have people annoyed you by criticizing your drinking?
☐ Have you ever felt guilty about your drinking?
☐ Do you have an eye opener in the AM to steady your nerves?
☐ High risk sexual practices:
> 1 partner past 6 mos Y N
Sexual relationships with:
☐ men
☐ women
☐ both men and women
☐ IVDA/partner who is IVDA
☐ blood transfusion b/w 1978-1985

ROS: Circle
Heent: head inj, seizures, H/A, glaucoma, cataracts, visual problems, hearing loss, infection, allergies/sinus, nosebleeds, chronic sore throats, difficulty swallowing
Lymph: swellings in neck, axilla, groin, anemia
Endocrine: thyroid problems, DM, wt loss
Pulmonary: asthma, pneumonia, hemoptysis

ROS: Circle
CV: murmur, rhythm disturb, HTN, C/P, angina
Breast: mass/lump/DC/pain
GI: GERD, hematemesis, PUD, abd. pain, chronic constipation or diarrhea, change in Bms, liver or GB problems, pancreatitis, melena or hematochezia, hemorrhoids, hepatitis
GU: dysuria, hematuria, UTI, STDs, warts, diff. urination, incontinence
MS: arthritis, gout, swelling, claudication, back pain
Neuro: numbness, weakness, chronic tingling, B/B incontinence, gait disturb, falling
Skin: changes in moles/warts, chronic rashes, acne
GYN: Hot flashes, numbness, H/A, palpitations, drenching sweats, mood swings, vaginal dryness, itching
Frequent vaginal infections
Unusual vaginal discharge
Vaginal odor
Genital warts
STD (chlamydia, gonorrhea, syphilis, herpes)
Infection in uterus, tubes, ovaries (PID)
Pain or bleeding after intercourse
Missed periods
Bleeding b/w periods
Uterine abnormalities
Abnormal Pap smears
Cervical lesions/biopsy
Cysts/tumors on ovary
Premenstrual symptoms
Satisfied with sexual relationship?
Questions/concerns about sexual issues?

FH:
☐ HTN ☐ MI
☐ CAD ☐ CVA
☐ DM ☐ CA
☐ Resp. ☐ Depression
☐ ETOH ☐ Seizures

OCP risks:
☐ Smoker ☐ Nonsmoker
☐ H/A ☐ HTN
☐ DVT ☐ fibroids

Menstrual HX:
Age periods started ____
Periods last ____ days
Periods come q ____ days
Are periods:
☐ Regular
☐ Irregular
☐ Painful
☐ Light
☐ Moderate
☐ Heavy

Obstetric HX:
Number of preg: ____
Number of live birth ____
Stillbirth: ____

Contraceptive HX:
Current birth control?
☐ None
☐ Pills

Cancer risks:
- ☐ M/GM/aunt/sib breast
- ☐ M/GM/aunt/sib uterine
- ☐ H/o uterine, breast, cervical cancer
- ☐ STDs Y N
- ☐ Sex <18 Y N
- ☐ >4 partners Y N

LMP ____
Last Pap ____
Where: ____
Results: ____

Miscarriage: ____
Abortion: ____
Any pregnancy complications?
DM Y N
HTN Y N
Toxemia Y N

- ☐ IUD
- ☐ condoms (rubbers)
- ☐ BTL
- ☐ Depo
- ☐ Trying to become pregnant
- ☐ Satisfied with current BC? Y N

Objective:

System	**Norm**	**Abnormal**	**Comments**
Skin	☐	☐	____
Head	☐	☐	____
Oral cavity	☐	☐	____
Ear	☐	☐	____
Nose	☐	☐	____
Eye	☐	☐	____
Neck	☐	☐	____
Thyroid	☐	☐	____
Chest	☐	☐	____
Heart	☐	☐	____
Breast	☐	☐	____
Abdomen	☐	☐	____
M/S	☐	☐	____
Neuro	☐	☐	____
Extremities	☐	☐	____
Pelvic	☐	☐	____
External	☐	☐	____
B.U.S.	☐	☐	____
Vagina	☐	☐	____
Cervix	☐	☐	____
Fundus	☐	☐	____
Adnexae	☐	☐	____
Rectal	☐	☐	____

Plan:
Labs:
- ☐ Lipid panel
- ☐ HIV
- ☐ FOB
- ☐ RPR
- ☐ Electrolytes
- ☐ Glucose
- ☐ LFT
- ☐ Uric acid
- ☐ CBC
- ☐ GC/chlamydia
- ☐ Pap
- ☐ U/A
- ☐ Wet mount
  - ☐ KOH
  - ☐ NaCl
- ☐ HCG

Screening:
- ☐ Sigmoidoscopy
- ☐ Vision
- ☐ Hearing
- ☐ Dental
- ☐ EKG

Immunizations:
- ☐ dT
- ☐ Flu
- ☐ Pneumovax
- ☐ Varicella
- ☐ Hep A
- ☐ Hep B
- ☐ MMR

Medications:
____
____
____
____
____

Instructions:

Assessment:
- ☐ Normal exam
- ☐ Tobacco abuse
- ☐ Hyperlipidemia
- ☐ Other: ____
____
____
- ☐ Contraceptive counseling
- ☐ Alcohol abuse
- ☐ HTN
- ☐ Family planning
- ☐ OCPs
- ☐ Depo Provera
- ☐ Vaginitis ____
- ☐ UTI

Health Promotion:
- ☐ Exercise 3-5x week
- ☐ Low fat, high carb high fiber diet
- ☐ Smoking cessation
- ☐ Alcohol moderation
- ☐ Use seat belts
- ☐ Sun protection
- ☐ BSE

F/U next visit:
____
____
____
____

RTO: ____

Signature: ____

CERVICAL CANCER: ARE YOU AT RISK?

☐ Extremely low risk for cervical cancer

- ☐ I have never had sex.
- ☐ I have had one sexual partner in my lifetime, and he has had one sexual partner.
- ☐ I have a yearly Pap smear.
- ☐ I have never had an abnormal Pap.
- ☐ I have had more than ten normal Pap smears.
- ☐ I am older than 65 years.
- ☐ I have never smoked.

☐ Low risk for cervical cancer

- ☐ I started having sex when I was 20 years old or older.
- ☐ I have had fewer than three sexual partners in my lifetime.
- ☐ I have never had a sexually transmitted infection, including genital warts.
- ☐ I use condoms.
- ☐ I am a nonsmoker.
- ☐ My last Pap smear was within 1 year and was normal.

☐ High risk for cervical cancer

- ☐ I started having sex before I was 20 years old.
- ☐ I have had more than three sexual partners in my lifetime.
- ☐ I have been treated for a sexually transmitted infection.
- ☐ I have the virus that causes genital warts.
- ☐ I have sex without using a condom.
- ☐ I have never asked my partner about his sexual history.
- ☐ My sexual partner has been treated for sexually transmitted infections including genital warts.
- ☐ I smoke cigarettes.
- ☐ I have had an abnormal Pap smear.
- ☐ I have been treated for an abnormal Pap smear.
- ☐ I have had an abnormal Pap smear and failed to keep my appointments for treatment and follow up.
- ☐ My mother took DES during her pregnancy with me.

Developed by KM Rogers, ARNP, with help from Dianne Forst, RN.

Wellness and Health Maintenance Guideline Summaries

ICD-9-CM

Counseling on Injury Prevention V65.43
Exercise Counseling V65.41
Routine General Medical Examination of Adult V70.0
Routine General Examination of Child V20.2

HEALTH MAINTENANCE GUIDELINES FOR CHILDREN

Principles of Preventive Care

Promote prevention (Table 207-1)
Share decision-making with patient and family
Be selective in ordering tests and services
Deliver preventive services at every available opportunity
Participate in community-level interventions

HEALTH MAINTENANCE GUIDELINES FOR ADULTS

Principles of Preventive Care

Promote prevention (Table 207-2)
Share decision-making with patient and family
Be selective in ordering tests and services
Deliver preventive services at every available opportunity
Participate in community-level interventions

GROWTH AND DEVELOPMENT OF ADULTS 65 YEARS AND OLDER

Physiological changes in adults 65 years of age and older are outlined in Table 207-3.

SUMMARY: CLINICIAN'S ALERT

A summary of conditions throughout the lifespan of which the clinician should be aware is outlined in Table 207-4.

RESOURCES

Agency for Health Care Policy and Research
www.ahcpr.gov/guide
American Academy of Family Physicians
www.aafp.org
American Academy of Pediatrics
www.aap.org/search
American Cancer Society
www.cancer.org
American College of Preventive Medicine
www.acpm.org
American Diabetes Association
www.diabetes.com
American Heart Association
www.amhrt.org
American Medical Association
www.ama-assn.org
Centers for Disease Control and Prevention
www.cdc.gov/prevguid.htm
Guide to Clinical Preventive Services
http://158.72.20.10/pubs/guidecps
Guidelines for Adolescent Preventive Services
www.ama-assn.org/ADOLhlth/ADOLhlth.htm
National Coalition for Adult Immunization
www.medscape.com/affiliates/ncai
Office of Disease Prevention and Health Promotion
http://odphp.osophs.dhhs.gov/pubs/guidecps
www.brightfutures.org

SUGGESTED READINGS

Branch W, Crouch M: Periodic health exams: what really matters? *Patient Care* 15:21-45, 1998.
US Preventive Services Task Force: *Guide to clinical preventive services*, ed 2, Baltimore, 1996, Williams & Wilkins.

TABLE 207-1 Recommendations for Screening for Asymptomatic Children

Health Item	Age	Recommendation
History and physical examination	0-18 yr	2 wk, 2 mo, 4 mo, 6 mo, 9 mo, 12 mo, 15 mo, 18 mo; 2-6, annually; 7-10, q1-2 yr; 11-18, q1 yr
Immunizations	0-18 yr	Per current immunization schedule (see schedule in Appendix H); influenza and pneumococcal vaccines for children at risk
Vision	4-18 yr	Annually
Hemoglobin/hematocrit levels	6-12 mo	One time
Lead screen	12 mo	Screen for children at high risk
Blood pressure	3-18 yr	Annually
Cholesterol		Only if there is a positive family history of hyperlipidemia or early sudden death
Hearing	3-5 yr	Annually
Scoliosis	10-18 yr	Screen during history and physical examination
Pap smear	10-18 yr	Annually for any female who is sexually active
Chlamydia	> 10 yr	Should be done for any female <20 yr who is sexually active
Tobacco, alcohol, and drugs	10-18 yr	Screen all adolescents for tobacco, alcohol, and drug use
Suicide/depression	10-18 yr	Screen all adolescents for symptoms of depression and suicide
Family violence	0-18 yr	Be alert to signs and symptoms of physical and sexual abuse; teens should be routinely assessed for emotional, physical, and sexual abuse; all suspected cases must be reported
Counseling		
Safety	0-18 yr	Seat belts, bike helmets, no drinking/driving, stranger safety, poisons, accidents, pools, guns
Nutrition	0-18 yr	Under 1 yr: Formula or breast milk >1 yr: Whole milk and healthy diet >2 yr: Limit dietary intake of fat and cholesterol, emphasize foods containing fiber (fruits, vegetables, grain products)
Physical activity	2-18 yr	Incorporate physical activity into daily routine
Dental care	1-18 yr	Recommend regular dental visits and brushing/flossing of teeth; do not give bottle at bedtime
Skin	0-18 yr	Avoid excess sun exposure, use sunscreen
STD	10-18 yr	Measures to avoid or decrease infection
Unintended pregnancy	10-18 yr	Counsel about contraceptive methods if sexually active

TABLE 207-2 Recommendations for Screening for Asymptomatic Adults

Health Item	Age	Recommendation
History and physical examination (to include height and weight)	19-64 65+	Every 1-3 yr Annually
Immunizations	≥19	Second MMR for adults born after 1956; Td every 10 yr; influenza: every year for those with chronic disease; consider for health care workers or others who come in contact with other people (e.g., school teachers, day care workers); reduces incidence of URI; pneumonia: one time for those at risk; hepatitis B: recommended for sexually active persons and anyone who might have exposure to blood-borne pathogens
Vision	≥19	Diabetic patients annually; all others: q 2 yr for complete ophthalmic examination; visual acuity test should be included in regular check-up
Hemoglobin/ hematocrit	Pregnancy	All pregnant women should be screened for anemia; for others: only patients with signs/symptoms of anemia should be tested
B/P	≥19	Annually/every visit
Cholesterol (to include HDL measurement)	≥19-79	Initial screening at 19, then q 5yr
Glucose	>45	American Diabetes Association recommends screening q3yr for asymptomatic persons Screen earlier and more often for those at high risk: Native Americans, blacks, Asians, Hispanics, those with a positive family history of diabetes, obesity, birth of a child >9 lb
Hearing	≥19	Only as part of physical examination More detailed testing should be done if decreased hearing ability is noted
Clinical breast examination	19-39 ≥40	Every 1-3 yr Annually
Mammogram	≥40-75	Annually
Pap smear	≥19	Annually
ECG	Variable	Some organizations recommend for anyone with >2 risk factors, or anyone >40 who begins an exercise program
Rectal examination	≥50	Annually, to include FOB testing, and sigmoidoscopy q3-5 yr
Prostate examination	≥50	Consensus unclear; PSA currently not recommended; discuss known benefits and risks (pros and cons) of screening; American Cancer Society recommends beginning screening at 40 yr for all men; PSA should be included >50 yr; black men or those with a positive family history of prostate cancer should begin PSA screening at 40 yr
Tobacco, alcohol, and drugs	≥19	Screen all adults and pregnant women for tobacco, alcohol, and drug use; perform thorough oral examination for any one who uses tobacco or alcohol
Suicide/depression	≥19	Be alert for symptoms of depression and suicide; if detected, administer specific mental health instrument
Family violence	≥19	Be alert for signs and symptoms of emotional, physical, and sexual abuse; all suspected cases of elder abuse must be reported
Counseling		
Safety	≥19	Seat belts, bike helmets, no drinking/driving, accidents, diving in shallow pools or ponds, guns, falls, smoke detectors, hot water temperature
Nutrition	≥19	Limit dietary intake of fat, and cholesterol, emphasize foods containing fiber (fruits, vegetables, grain products)

BSE, Breast self-examination; *FOB,* fecal occult blood; *HDL,* high-density lipoprotein; *HRT,* hormone replacement therapy; *PSA,* prostate-specific antigen; *Td,* tetanus toxoid; *TSE,* testicular self-examination.

TABLE 207-2 Recommendations for Screening for Asymptomatic Adults—cont'd

Health Item	Age (yr)	Recommendation
Physical activity	≥19	Incorporate physical activity into daily routine
Dental care	≥19	Recommend regular dental visits and brushing/flossing of teeth
Skin	≥19	Avoid excess sun exposure, use sun screen; incorporate skin examination in check-up; teach skin self-examination if at increased risk
STD prevention	≥19 yr	Measures to avoid or decrease infection
Unintended pregnancy	≥19 yr	Counsel about contraceptive methods if sexually active
Tobacco cessation	All smokers	Counsel all patients who use tobacco to stop
Alcohol use	≥19	Counsel moderation in anyone who drinks alcohol on a regular basis, or does binge drinking; caution about drinking/driving
Drug abuse	≥19	Pregnant women should be asked specific questions related to tolerance
Hormone replacement therapy	≥ Menopause	Discuss positives and negative consequences of HRT
Osteoporosis	≥ Menopause	Discuss HRT in relation to prevention of osteoporosis; recommend smoking cessation, physical exercise, and adequate calcium intake; check height annually as indicator of osteoporosis
Breast or testicle self exam	≥19	Recommend BSE for all women >19 yr Recommend TSE for men with a history of cryptorchidism
Advance directives	All patients	Discuss advance directives with all patients

TABLE 207-3 Growth and Development: 65 Years and Older

System	Overview of Developmental Changes
Heart and circulatory	Heart weight remains relatively constant after 25 yr. CO decreases 30%-40%. Cardiac power is decreased. Capacity to increase rate and strength is diminished. Women have a slightly higher resting HR than men. Maximal HR decreases. There is increased calcification and fibrosis of the aortic valve cusps.
Renal	Glomerular filtration rate decreases about 30%-47% from 20 to 90 yr. Renal mass decreases with age. Renal flow decreases 53% (perhaps to compensate for decreased CO). Urinary incontinence affects 15%-30% of ambulatory older adults, more women than men. Decreased muscle tone of ureters, bladder and urethra may contribute to incidence of incontinence. Bladder capacity decreases as much as 50%. Prostate increases in size.
Gastrointestinal	Salivary gland secretion decreases; saliva is more alkaline. Esophageal motility is decreased. Generalized atrophy of gastrointestinal tract is seen with advancing age. Acidity of gastric juices decreases with age, taste is also diminished. Hepatic blood flow is decreased. Abdomen is more protruberant. Abdominal wall is thinner and less taut. Sphincter control is decreased, with relaxation of perineal musculature.
Eyes	Approximately 95% of those older than 60 yr have some opacification of lens. Decreased visual acuity occurs in 50% of those older than 75 yr as a result of cataracts. There is decreased ability to accommodate (presbyopia). Cells responsible for lubricating conjunctiva decrease (dry eye syndrome). Arus senilus is common. Pupils decrease in size, react more slowly to light, and dilate more slowly in dark. Loss of fat pads from orbit of eye gives sunken appearance.
Ears	Skin of ear becomes dry and less resilient. Cerumen production is decreased. Hair growth increases, pinna increases in length. Presbycusis may result from degeneration of organ of Corti (loss of high frequency sounds).
Nose/mouth	Olfactory function decreases; with no loss or change in taste buds; there is decrease in salt/sweet taste perception.
Adipose tissue	There is increase of body fat, with corresponding decrease of lean muscle mass. Sharpness of contours increases, with increasingly bony landmarks. Adipose tissue is redistributed from extremities to hips and abdomen.

Kidd P, Robinson D: *Family nurse practitioner certification review,* St Louis, 1999, Mosby.
CO, Cardiac output; *HR,* heart rate.

Continued

TABLE 207-3 Growth and Development: 65 Years and Older—cont'd

System	Overview of Developmental Changes
Lymphoid tissue	Only very small changes occur.
Respiratory	Lung size and weight decrease. Basal metabolic rate decreases (ratio higher in men than women). Chest wall becomes less compliant.
Skeletal	Vertebral disks thin, spinal column shortens, kyphosis is seen with spinal column compression, osteoporosis increases. Loss of stature begins at approximately 50 yr. Women lose an average of 4.9 cm and men lose an average of 2.9 cm. Bones decrease in density and weight by 12% in men and 25% in women (Barkauskas, Stoltenberg-Allen, Baumann, & Darling-Fisher, 1994). There is loss of resilience and elasticity of ligaments, cartilage, and some tissues.
Muscular	Atrophy and loss of muscle tone by 30%-40% is seen between 30 and 80 yr. Exercise does help limit reduction of muscle mass.
Nervous	There is possible decrease in number of brain cells, decrease in myelin sheath. Impulses decrease, slowing down speed of action and reaction. Vibratory sense decreases, especially for feet and ankles; ankle jerk may be absent.
Reproductive	Estrogen and testosterone secretion are decreased. There is decreased pubic hair. Involution of uterus follows menopause frequently, with relaxation of the sacral ligaments so the uterus may be in a dropped position. Breasts atrophy with advancing age, becoming pendulous and with decreased fullness as a result of loss of fat. Penis decreases in size and has fewer sustained erections. Testes decrease in size and hang lower.
Integumentary	Regenerative powers are decreased. Dermis and epidermis thin, with loss of collagen and elastic fibers and less support for capillary walls so vessels dilate, diminished sebum production, and decreased subcutaneous fat.
Hair and nails	Scalp, axillary, and pubic hair thins and decreases. Eyebrow, nostril, and ear hair becomes coarser. Loss of hair pigment contributes to graying. Nail growth slows; nails become more yellow. Toenails commonly thicken.
Endocrine	All endocrine functions decline.

Kidd P, Robinson D: *Family nurse practitioner certification review,* St Louis, 1999, Mosby.

TABLE 207-4 Summary of Conditions for Which Clinicians Should Be Alert

Condition	Population
Symptoms of peripheral vascular disease	Older persons, smokers, persons with diabetes
Skin lesions with malignant features	General population, but especially with risk factors (light hair, eyes, and skin; severe sun burns as child; excessive sun exposure; malignant precursors; certain congenital nevi; freckles; FH, or personal history, immunosuppression)
Oral cancer and premalignancy	Those who use tobacco (cigarettes, pipes, cigars, chewing tobacco, snuff), older persons who use alcohol regularly
Thyroid impairment	Older persons, postpartum women, persons with Down syndrome
Hearing impairment	Older persons, infants, and young children (younger than 3 yr)
Ocular misalignment	Infants and children
Spinal curvatures	Adolescents
Changes in functional performance	Older adults
Depressive symptoms	Adolescents, young adults, persons at increased risk (personal history or positive FH of depression), those with chronic illnesses, those with recent loss, and those with sleep disorders, chronic pain, or multiple unexplained somatic complaints
Suicide risk	Those with established risks for suicide (depression, drug or alcohol abuse, other psychiatric disorders, previous attempted suicide, recent divorce, separation, unemployment, recent bereavement)
Family violence	General population
Drug abuse	General population
Dental problems	General population

Modified from U.S. Preventive Services Task Force: *Guide to clinical preventive services,* ed 2, Baltimore, 1996, Williams & Wilkins.

Appendix

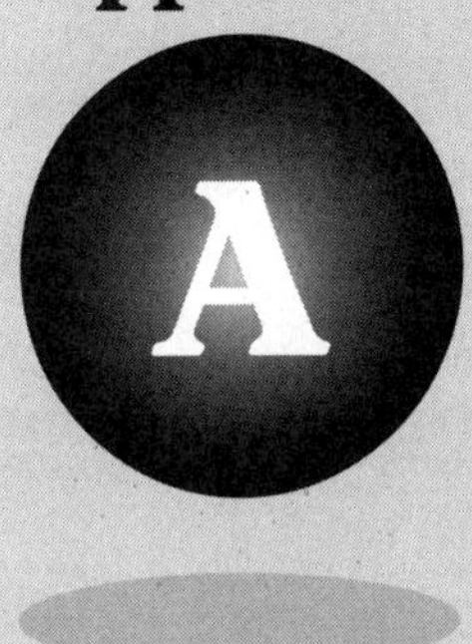

Body Mass Index

BODY MASS INDEX (BMI)

$$\text{BMI} = \frac{\text{Weight (kg)}}{\text{Height}^2 \text{ (m)}}$$

Normal range:

Male	21.9-22.4
Female	21.3-22.1

IDEAL BODY WEIGHT

Adults (>18 years):

Male IBW (kg) = 50 + 2.3 for each inch over 60 inches

Female IBW (kg) = 45.5 + 2.3 for each inch over 60 inches

Children:

Age 1 to 18 years, height <60 inches: IBW (kg) + [1.65 × height^2 (cm)]/1000

From Ellsworth AJ, Dugdale DC, Witt DM: *Mosby's medical drug reference,* 1998, St Louis, Mosby.

	Height (ft, in)																
Weight (lb)	**4′10″**	**4′11″**	**5′0″**	**5′1″**	**5′2″**	**5′3″**	**5′4″**	**5′5″**	**5′6″**	**5′7″**	**5′8″**	**5′9″**	**5′10″**	**5′11″**	**6′0″**	**6′1″**	**6′2″**
125	26	25	24	24	23	22	22	21	20	20	19	18	18	17	17	17	16
130	27	26	25	25	24	23	22	22	21	20	20	19	19	18	18	17	17
135	28	27	26	26	25	24	23	23	22	21	21	20	19	19	18	18	17
140	29	28	27	27	26	25	24	23	23	22	21	21	20	20	19	19	18
145	30	29	28	27	27	26	25	24	23	23	22	21	21	20	20	19	19
150	31	30	29	28	27	27	26	25	24	24	23	22	22	21	20	20	19
155	32	31	30	29	28	28	27	26	25	24	24	23	22	22	21	20	20
160	34	32	31	30	29	28	28	27	26	25	24	24	23	22	22	21	21
165	35	33	32	31	30	29	28	28	27	26	25	24	24	23	22	22	21
170	36	34	33	32	31	30	29	28	28	27	26	25	24	24	23	22	22
175	37	35	34	33	32	31	30	29	28	27	27	26	25	24	24	23	23
180	38	36	35	34	33	32	31	30	29	28	27	27	26	25	25	24	23
185	39	37	36	35	34	33	32	31	30	29	28	27	27	26	25	24	24
190	40	38	37	36	35	34	33	32	31	30	29	28	27	27	26	25	24
195	41	39	38	37	36	35	34	33	32	31	30	29	28	27	27	26	25
200	42	40	39	38	37	36	34	33	32	31	30	30	29	28	27	26	26
205	43	41	40	39	38	36	35	34	33	32	31	30	29	29	28	27	26
210	44	43	41	40	38	37	36	35	34	33	32	31	30	29	29	28	27
215	45	44	42	41	39	38	37	36	35	34	33	32	31	30	29	28	28
220	46	45	43	42	40	39	38	37	36	35	34	33	32	31	30	29	28
225	47	46	44	43	41	40	39	38	36	35	34	33	32	31	31	30	29
230	48	47	45	44	42	41	40	38	37	36	35	34	33	32	31	30	30

BMI:	What it means to your health (adults ages 20-65 years)
18.5-24.9	Good weight for most people
≥25	Risk for cardiovascular and other diseases increases
≥30	Risk of death increases

Appendix

Common Cardiovascular Drug Pearls

ADMINISTRATION OF ANGIOTENSIN-CONVERTING ENZYME INHIBITORS

Always ensure adequate renal function (serum creatinine) before starting.

Monitor throughout therapy.

Beware of hyperkalemia, particularly if patient is receiving potassium supplement or potassium-sparing diuretic.

Diuretics will potentiate angiotensin-converting enzyme inhibitors. Start low.

First- or second-line agent in congestive heart failure, third- or fourth-line agent in hypertension.

CHARACTERISTICS AND USES OF BETA-BLOCKING AGENTS

Cardioselective

Best for patients with asthma, for patients with diabetes, and for peripheral vascular disease

Atenolol
Metoprolol
Betaxolol
Acebutolol

Antiarrhythmic Quality (Membrane Stabilization)

Use for patients with hypertension and dysrhythmia

Acebutolol
Labetalol
Propranolol

Low Lipid Solubility

Produces fewer central nervous system side effects and sleep disturbances

Nadolol
Carteolol
Acebutolol
Betalol

Precautions

Beta-blockers are contraindicated in congestive heart failure.

Avoid abrupt cessation of beta-blockers.

ADMINISTRATION OF CALCIUM CHANNEL BLOCKING AGENTS

Avoid use in patients with cystic fibrosis.

These agents are used as third- or fourth-line agents in patients with hypertension.

Monitor liver function while patient is taking the drug.

From Kidd PS, Robinson DL: Family nurse practitioner certification review, St Louis, 1999, Mosby.

Appendix

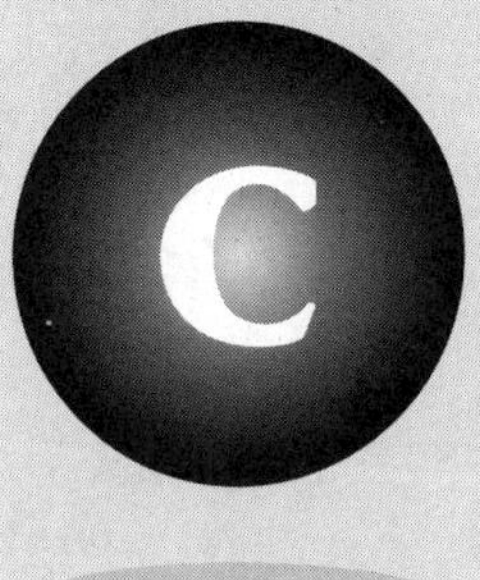

Conversion Tables

TEMPERATURE: FAHRENHEIT AND CELSIUS EQUIVALENTS

To convert centigrade or Celsius degrees to Fahrenheit degrees: multiply the number of centigrade degrees by 9/5 and add 32 to the result. *To convert Fahrenheit degrees to centigrade degrees:* Subtract 32 from the number of Fahrenheit degrees and multiply the difference by 5/9.

Fahrenheit and Celsius Equivalents: Body Temperature Range

F°	C°	F°	C°	F°	C°	F°	C°	F°	C°
94.0	34.44	97.0	36.11	100.0	37.78	103.0	39.44	106.0	41.11
94.2	34.56	97.2	36.22	100.2	37.89	103.2	39.56	106.2	41.22
94.4	34.67	97.4	36.33	100.4	38.00	103.4	39.67	106.4	41.33
94.6	34.78	97.6	36.44	100.6	38.11	103.6	39.78	106.6	41.44
94.8	34.89	97.8	36.56	100.8	38.22	103.8	39.89	106.8	41.56
95.0	35.00	98.0	36.67	101.0	38.33	104.0	40.00	107.0	41.67
95.2	35.11	98.2	36.78	101.2	38.44	104.2	40.11	107.2	41.78
95.4	35.22	98.4	36.89	101.4	38.56	104.4	40.22	107.4	41.89
95.6	35.33	98.6	37.00	101.6	38.67	104.6	40.33	107.6	42.00
95.8	35.44	98.8	37.11	101.8	38.78	104.8	40.44	107.8	42.11
96.0	35.56	99.0	37.22	102.0	38.89	105.0	40.56	108.0	42.22
96.2	35.67	99.2	37.33	102.2	39.00	105.2	40.67		
96.4	35.78	99.4	37.44	102.4	39.11	105.4	40.78		
96.6	35.89	99.6	37.56	102.6	39.22	105.6	40.89		
96.8	36.00	99.8	37.67	102.8	39.33	105.8	41.00		

From Anderson K, Anderson L, editors: *Mosby's medical, nursing, and allied health dictionary,* ed 5, St Louis, 1998, Mosby.

GRAMS TO POUNDS AND OUNCES CONVERSION FOR WEIGHT OF NEWBORNS

1 pound = 453.59 grams. 1 ounce = 28.35 grams. Grams can be converted to pounds and tenths of a pound by multiplying the number of grams by .0022.

	Ounces 0	1	2	3	4	5	6	7	8	9	10	11	12	13	14	15
Pounds																
0	—	28	57	85	113	142	170	198	227	255	283	312	430	369	397	425
1	454	482	510	539	567	595	624	652	680	709	737	765	794	822	850	879
2	907	936	964	992	1021	1049	1077	1106	1134	1162	1191	1219	1247	1276	1304	1332
3	1361	1389	1417	1446	1474	1503	1531	1559	1588	1616	1644	1673	1701	1729	1758	1786
4	1814	1843	1871	1899	1928	1956	1984	2013	2041	2070	2098	2126	2155	2183	2211	2240
5	2268	2296	2325	2353	2381	2410	2438	2466	2495	2523	2551	2580	2608	2637	2665	2693
6	2722	2750	2778	2807	2835	2863	2892	2920	2948	2977	3005	3033	3062	3090	3118	3147
7	3175	3203	3232	3260	3289	3317	3345	3374	3402	3430	3459	3487	3515	3544	3572	3600
8	3629	3657	3685	3714	3742	3770	3799	3827	3856	3884	3912	3941	3969	3997	4026	4054
9	4082	4111	4139	4167	4196	4224	4252	4281	4309	4337	4366	4394	4423	4451	4479	4508
10	4536	4564	4593	4621	4649	4678	4706	4734	4763	4791	4819	4848	4876	4904	4933	4961
11	4990	5018	5046	5075	5103	5131	5160	5188	5216	5245	5273	5301	5330	5358	5386	5415
12	5443	5471	5500	5528	5557	5585	5613	5642	5670	5698	5727	5755	5783	5812	5840	5868
13	5897	5925	5953	5982	6010	6038	6067	6095	6123	6152	6180	6290	6237	6265	6294	6322
14	6350	6379	6407	6435	6464	6492	6520	6549	6577	6605	6634	6662	6690	6719	6747	6776
15	6804	6832	6860	6889	6917	6945	6973	7002	7030	7059	7087	7115	7144	7172	7201	7228
16	7257	7286	7313	7342	7371	7399	7427	7456	7484	7512	7541	7569	7597	7626	7654	7682
17	7711	7739	7768	7796	7824	7853	7881	7909	7938	7966	7994	8023	8051	8079	8108	8136
18	8165	8192	8221	8249	8278	8306	8335	8363	8391	8420	8448	8476	8504	8533	8561	8590
19	8618	8646	8675	8703	8731	8760	8788	8816	8845	8873	8902	8930	8958	8987	9015	9043
20	9072	9100	9128	9157	9185	9213	9242	9270	9298	9327	9355	9383	9412	9440	9469	9497
21	9525	9554	9582	9610	9639	9667	9695	9724	9752	9780	9809	9837	9865	9894	9922	9950
22	9979	10007	10036	10064	10092	10120	10149	10177	10206	10234	10262	10291	10319	10347	10376	10404

From Wong DL: *Whaley & Wong's essentials of pediatric nursing*, ed 5, St Louis, 1997, Mosby.

POUNDS TO KILOGRAMS CONVERSION

Numbers in the farthest left column are 10-pound increments; numbers across the top row are 1-pound increments. The kilogram equivalent of weight in pounds is found at the intersection of the appropriate row and column. For example, to convert 34 pounds, read down the left column to 30 and then across that row to 4: 34 pounds = 15.42 kilograms.

Pounds	0	1	2	3	4	5	6	7	8	9
0	0.00	0.45	0.90	1.36	1.81	2.26	2.72	3.17	3.62	4.08
10	4.53	4.98	5.44	5.89	6.35	6.80	7.25	7.71	8.16	8.61
20	9.07	9.52	9.97	10.43	10.88	11.34	11.79	12.24	12.70	13.15
30	13.60	14.06	14.51	14.96	15.42	15.87	16.32	16.78	17.23	17.69
40	18.14	18.59	19.05	19.50	19.95	20.41	20.86	21.31	21.77	22.22
50	22.68	23.13	23.58	24.04	24.49	24.94	25.40	25.85	26.30	26.76
60	27.21	27.66	28.12	28.57	29.03	29.48	29.93	30.39	30.84	31.29
70	31.75	32.20	32.65	33.11	33.56	34.02	34.47	34.92	35.38	35.83
80	36.28	36.74	37.19	37.64	38.10	38.55	39.00	39.46	39.91	40.37
90	40.82	41.27	41.73	42.18	42.63	43.09	43.54	43.99	44.45	44.90
100	45.36	45.81	46.26	46.72	47.17	47.62	48.08	48.53	48.98	49.44
110	49.89	50.34	50.80	51.25	51.71	52.16	52.61	53.07	53.52	53.97
120	54.43	54.88	55.33	55.79	56.24	56.70	57.15	57.60	58.06	58.51
130	58.96	59.42	59.87	60.32	60.78	61.23	61.68	62.14	62.59	63.05
140	63.50	63.95	64.41	64.86	65.31	65.77	66.22	66.67	67.13	67.58
150	68.04	68.49	68.94	69.40	69.85	70.30	70.76	71.21	71.66	72.12
160	72.57	73.02	73.48	73.93	74.39	74.84	75.29	75.75	76.20	76.65
170	77.11	77.56	78.01	78.47	78.92	79.38	79.83	80.28	80.74	81.19
180	81.64	82.10	82.55	83.00	83.46	83.91	84.36	84.82	85.27	85.73
190	86.18	86.68	87.09	87.54	87.99	88.45	88.90	89.35	89.81	90.26
200	90.72	91.17	91.62	92.08	92.53	92.98	93.44	93.89	94.34	94.80

From Anderson F, Anderson L, editors: *Mosby's medical, nursing, and allied health dictionary*, ed 5, St Louis, 1998, Mosby.

Appendix

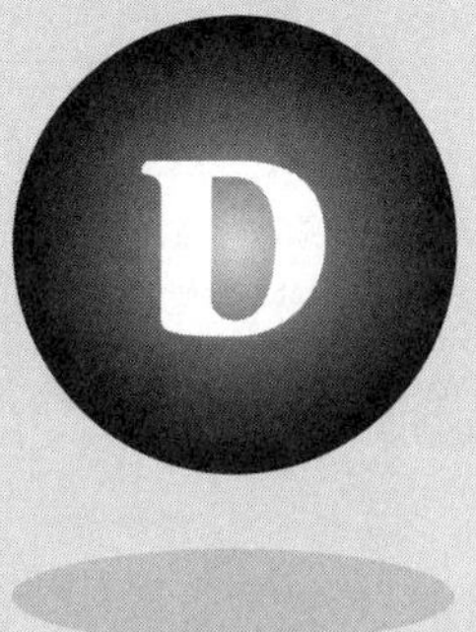

Drug Activity of Cytochrome P-450 Isoenzymes

The cytochrome P-450 (CYP) system is a system of 30 enzymes located in the reticulum of the hepatocytes. These enzymes are important, since they play a large role in many drug interactions. The reactions are not entirely predictable; factors such as genetics of the patient, dosage of the drugs, nutritional status, and the therapeutic index will influence the incidence and severity of the interaction. The CYP system has been classified into 11 isoenzyme families based on the chemical structure. Each family is referred to by the number of the family followed by a subfamily letter and a number for individual form. Each isoenzyme has a unique drug activity. CYP 1 and 3 are the ones most involved with drug metabolism. CYP2C19 and CYP2D6 exhibit polymorphism, so up to 10% of a population may totally lack a particular isoenzyme. This may account for drug responses seen in some racial or ethnic groups. Some drugs are both substrates and inhibitors, meaning that they both affect and are affected by other drugs. **If possible, avoid administration of drugs that interact as inhibitor and substrate in the same isoenzyme system.** If this cannot be avoided, be aware of potential interactions, and monitor the patient carefully.

Isozyme	Substrates (Drugs Affected by Inhibitors and Inducers)	Inhibitors (Slow the Elimination of Drugs; May Cause an Accumulation of the Drug)	Inducers (Speed the Elimination of Drugs, Which May Result in Therapeutic Failure)
CYPIA2	Caffeine	Fluvoxamine (Luvox)	Charcoal-broiled foods
	Clomipramine (Anafranil)	Cimetidine (Tagamet)	Cigarette smoke
	Clozapine (Clozaril)	Mexiletine (Mexitil)	Cruciferous vegetables (cabbage, brussel sprouts)
	Impramine (Tofranil)	Ciprofloxacin (Cipro)	Phenytoin (Dilantin)
	Olanzapine (Zypyrexa)	Erythromycin	Omeprazole (Prilosec)
	Tacrine (Cognex)	Tacrine (Cognex)	Rifampin
	Theophylline	Enoxacin (Penetrex)	
	Warfarin (Coumadin)	Ethinyl Estradiol	
	Zileuton (Zyflo)	Isoniazid (INH)	
	Oxycodone	Norethindrone	
	Methadone	Zileuton (Zyflo)	
	Acetominophen		
CYP2C9	Diclofenac (Voltaren)	Amiodarone (Cordarone)	Barbiturates
	Dronobinol (Mariol)	Cimetidine (Tagamet)	Carbamazepine (Tegretol)
	Flurbiprofen (Ansaid)	Cotrimoxazole (Bactrim)	Phenytoin (Dilantin)
	Fluvastatin (Lescol)	Disulfiram (Antabuse)	Primidone (Mysoline)
	Glimepriride	Fluconozole (Diflucan)	Rifampin (Rimactane)
	Glipizide (Glucotrol)	Fluoxetine (Prozac)	
	?Glibenclamide	Fluvoxamine (Luvox)	
	Ibuprofen (Motrin)	Isoniazid (INH)	
	Indomethacin (Indocin)	Itraconazole (Sporonax)	
	Losartan (Cozaar)	Ketoconazole (Nizoral)	
	Naproxen (Naprosyn)	Metronidazole (Flagyl)	
	Phenytoin (Dilantin)	Sulfinpyrazone (Anturane)	
	Piroxicam (Feldene)	Ticlopidine (Ticlid)	
	Tobutamide (Orinase)	Zafirlukast (Accolate)	
	Torsemide (Demadex)		
	Warfarin (Coumadin)		

Adapted from Hansten P et al: The Perils of P-450. *The clinical letter for nurse practitioners,* 1(1):7-8, 1997.
?, Questionable effect.

Continued

Isozyme	Substrates (Drugs Affected by Inhibitors and Inducers)	Inhibitors (Slow the Elimination of Drugs: May Cause an Accumulation of the Drug)	Inducers (Speed the Elimination of Drugs, Which May Result in Therapeutic Failure)
CYP2C19	Amitriptyline (Elavil)	Fluoxetine (Prozac)	
	Carisoprodol (Soma)	Omepraxole (Prilosec)	
	Clomipramine (Anafranil)	Flucanazole (Diflucan)	
	Diazepam (Valium)	Fluvoxamine (Luvox)	
	Imipramine (Tofranil)	Felbamate (Felbatol)	
	Lansoprazole (Prevacid)	Ticlopidine (Ticlid)	
	Mephenytoin		
	Naproxen (Naprosyn)		
	Omeprazole (Prilosec)		
	Pentamidine (Pentam)		
	Propranolol (Inderal)		
	Tolbutamide (Orinase)		
	Warfarin (Coumadin)		
CYP2D6	Amitriptyline (Elavil)	Amiodarone (Cordarone)	? Rifampin
	Bupropion (Wellbutrin, Zyban)	Chloroquine (Aralen)	? Dexamethasone
	Carvedilol (Coreg)	Cimetidine (Tagamet)	
	Clomipramine (Anafranil)	Fluoxetine (Prozac)	
	Codeine to Morphine	Haloperidol (Haldol)	
	Despramine (Norpramin)	Mibefradil (Posicor)	
	Dextromethorphan	Quinidine (Quinidex)	
	Encainide (Enkaid)	Paroxetine (Paxil)	
	Flecainide (Tambocor)	Perphenazine (Trilafon)	
	Fluoxetine (Prozac)	Propafenone (Rhythmol)	
	Fluvoxamine (Luvox)	Propoxyphene (Darvon)	
	Haloperidol (Haldol)	Ranitidine (Zantac)	
	Hydrocodone	Ritonavir (Norvir)	
	Imipramine (Tofranil)	Sertraline (Zoloft) weak	
	Maprotiline	Thioridazine (Mellaril)	
	Methamphetamine	Venlafaxine (Effexor)	
	Metoprolol (Lopressor)		
	Mexiletine (Mexitil)		
	Nortriptyline (Pamelor)		
	Oxycodone		
	Parxetine (Paxil)		
	Perphenazine (Trilafon)		
	Propafenone (Rhythmol)		
	Propranolol (Inderal)		
	Risperidone (Risperdal)		
	Thioridazine (Mellaril)		
	Timolol (Blocaden)		
	Tramadol (Ultram)		
	Trazodone (Desyrel)		
	Venlafaxine (Effexor)		
CYP3A4	Alfentanil (Alfenta)	Clarithromycin (Biaxin)	Aminoglutethimide (Cytandren)
	Alprazolam (Xanax)	Cimetidine (Tagamet)	Barbiturates
	Amlodipine (Norvasc)	Ciprofloxacin (Cipro)	Cabamazepine (Tegretol)
	Amiodarone (Cordarone)	Cylcosporine (Neoral)	Dexamethasone
	Astemizole (Hismanol)	Danazol (Danocrine)	Glucocorticoids
	Atorvastatin (Lipitor)	Delavirdine (Rescriptor)	Glutethimide
	Bepridil (Vascor)	Diltiazem (Cardizem)	Griseofulvin (Fulvicin)
	Bromocriptine (Parlodel)	Erythromycin	Nafcillin (Unipen)
	Carbamazepine (Tegretol)	Ethinyl estradiol	Phenytoin (Dilantin)
	Cisapride (Propulsid)	Fluconazole (Diflucan)	Primidone (Mysoline)
	Clarithromycin (Biaxin)	Fluvaxamine (Luvox)	Rifabutin (Mycobutin)
	Cyclophosphamide	Fluoxetine (Prozac)	Rifampin (Rimactane)
	Cyclosporine (Neoral)	Grapefruit juice	Troglitazone (Resulin)

Adapted from Hansten P et al: (1997) The Perils of P-450. *The clinical letter for nurse practitioners* 1(1):7-8, 1997.

Isozyme	Substrates (Drugs Affected by Inhibitors and Inducers)	Inhibitors (Slow the Elimination of Drugs: May Cause an Accumulation of the Drug)	Inducers (Speed the Elimination of Drugs, Which May Result in Therapeutic Failure)
CYP3A4—cont'd	Dapsone	Indinavir (Crixivan)	
	Delavirdine (Rescriptor)	Isoniazid (INH)	
	Dexamethasone	Itraconazole (Sporanox)	
	Diazepam (Valium)	Ketoconazole (Nizoral)	
	Diltiazem (Cardizem)	Metronidazole (Flagyl)	
	Dispyramide (Norpace)	Methylprednisone	
	Doxorubicin (Adriamycin)	Mibefradil (Posicor)	
	Ergotamine (Ergomar)	Miconazole (Monistat)	
	Erthromycin (E mycin)	Nefazodone (Serzone)	
	Ethinyl estradiol	Nelfinavir (Viracept)	
	Etoposide (Vepesid)	Nicardipine (Cardene)	
	Felodipine (Plendil)	Nifedipine (Adalat)	
	Fenofexadine (Allegra)	Norethindrone	
	Fentanyl (Sublimaze)	Norfloxacin (Norflox)	
	Finasteride (Proscar)	Oxiconazole	
	Flutamide (Eulexin)	Prednisone	
	Ifosfamide (Ifex)	Quinine	
	Indinavir (Crixivan)	Ritonavir (Norvir)	
	Isradipine (DynaCirc)	Saquinavir (Invirase)	
	Itraconazole (Sporanox)	Troleanodomycin	
	Keoconazole (Nizoral)	Verapamil (Calan)	
	Lidocaine	Zafirlukast (Accolate)	
	Loratadine (Claritin)		
	Losartan (Cozaar)		
	Lovastatin (Mevacor)		
	Methadone		
	Methylprednisolone		
	Mibefradil (Posicor)		
	Miconazole (Monistat)		
	Midazolam (Versed)		
	Nefazadone (Serzone)		
	Nicardipine (Cardene)		
	Nifedipine (Adalat)		
	Nimodipine (Nimotop)		
	Nisoldipine (Sular)		
	Nitrendipine		
	Paclitaxel (Taxol)		
	Pimozode (Orap)		
	Prenisolone		
	Quinidine (Quinidex)		
	Quinine		
	Rifabutin (Mycobutin)		
	Ritonavir (Norvir)		
	Squinavir (Invirase)		
	Sertraline (Zoloft)		
	Simvastatin (Zocor)		
	Tacrolimus (Prograf)		
	Tamoxifen (Nolvadex)		
	Terfenadine (Seldane)		
	Testosterone		
	Verpamil (Calan)		
	Triazolam (Halcion)		
	Verapamil (Calan)		
	Vinblastine (Oncovin)		
	Warfarin (Coumadin)		
	Zolpidem (Ambien)		

Appendix

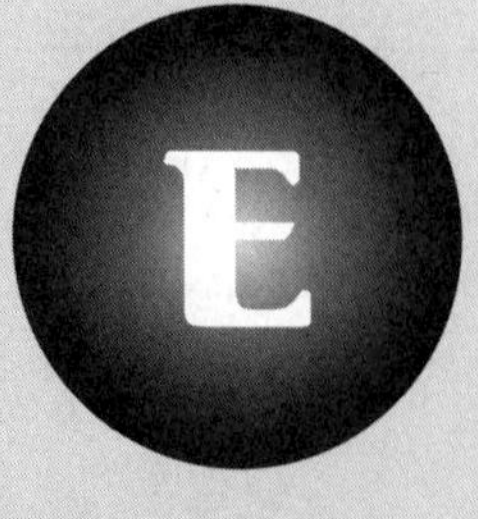

Medications and Drugs Commonly Used During Pregnancy

PREGNANCY CATEGORIES FOR DRUGS AND MEDICATIONS

Category A

Controlled studies in humans have demonstrated no fetal risks. There are few category A drugs. Examples include multivitamins or prenatal vitamins, but not megavitamins.

Category B

Animal studies indicate no fetal risks, but there are no human studies; or adverse effects have been demonstrated in animals, but not in well-controlled human studies. Several classes of commonly used drugs are in this category. An example is the penicillins.

Category C

There are either no adequate studies, either animal or human, or there are adverse fetal effects in animal studies but no available human data. Many drugs or medications commonly taken during pregnancy are in this category.

Category D

There is evidence of fetal risk, but benefits are thought to outweigh the risks. Examples include carbamazepine and phenytoin.

Category X

Proven fetal risks clearly outweigh any benefit. Accutane is an example. Multiple central nervous system, facial, and cardiovascular anomalies have been documented.

Drug	Category A	Category B	Category C	Category D	Category X
Antimicrobial					
Acyclovir			X		
Aminoglycosides			X	X	
Amantadine			X		
Amphotericin		X			
Azithromycin		X			
Cephalosporins		X			
Clindamycin		X			
Erythromycin		X			
Fluconazole			X		
Fluoroquinolones			X		

ACE, Angiotensin-converting enzyme; *MAO*, monoamine oxidase inhibitor; *NSAID*, nonsteroidal antiinflammatory drug; *OCP*, oral contraceptive pill; *SSRI*, selective serotonin reuptake inhibitor.

Drug	Category A	Category B	Category C	Category D	Category X
Antimicrobial					
Lindane		X			
Mebendazole			X		
Metronidazole		X			
Nitrofurantoin		X			
Nystatin		X			
Penicillins		X			
Ribavirin					X
Sulfonamides		X			
Tetracyclines				X	
Trimethoprim			X		
Vanconmycin			X		
Zidovudine			X		

Drug	Category A	Category B	Category C	Category D	Category X
Cardiovascular					
ACE inhibitors			X	X	
β-blockers			X		
Bretylium			X		
Ca channel antagonists			X		
Coumarins				X	
Digoxin			X		
Flurosemide			X		
Heparin			X		
Methyldopa			X		
Quindine			X		
Thiazides				X	

Drug	Category A	Category B	Category C	Category D	Category X
Asthma					
Albuterol			X		
Corticosteriods			X		
Cromolyn		X			
Epinephrine			X		
Terbutaline		X			
Theophylline			X		

Drug	Category A	Category B	Category C	Category D	Category X
Anticonvulsant					
Carbamazepine			X		
Phenobarbital				X	
Phenytoin				X	
Valproric acid				X	

Drug	Category A	Category B	Category C	Category D	Category X
Psychiatric					
Alprazolam				X	
Benzodiazepine				X	
Lithium				X	
MAOs			X		
SSRIs		X			

Drug	Category A	Category B	Category C	Category D	Category X
Analgesia					
Acetaminophen		X			
Aspirin			X		
Codeine			X		
Morphine		X			
NSAIDs		X			

Drug	Category A	Category B	Category C	Category D	Category X
Local Anesthetic					
Lidocaine			X		

Drug	Category A	Category B	Category C	Category D	Category X
Antiemetics					
Compazine			X		
Phenergan			X		

ACE, Angiotensin-converting enzyme; *MAO,* monoamine oxidase inhibitor; *NSAID,* nonsteroidal antiinflammatory drug; *OCP,* oral contraceptive pill; *SSRI,* selective serotonin reuptake inhibitor.

Drug	Category A	Category B	Category C	Category D	Category X
Hormones					
Danazol					X
OCPs					X

Drug	Category A	Category B	Category C	Category D	Category X
Social and Illicit Drugs					
Alcohol					X
Cocaine			X		
Marijuana			X		
Methamphetamines			X		
Nicotine			X		
Heroin		X			

Drug	Category A	Category B	Category C	Category D	Category X
Antihistamine Decongestants Expectorants					
Cetirizine		X			
Diphenhydramine			X		
Guaifenesin			X		
Loratadine		X			
Phenylpropanolamine			X		
Pseudoephedrine			X		

Drug	Category A	Category B	Category C	Category D	Category X
Thyroid					
Levothyroxine	X				

Appendix

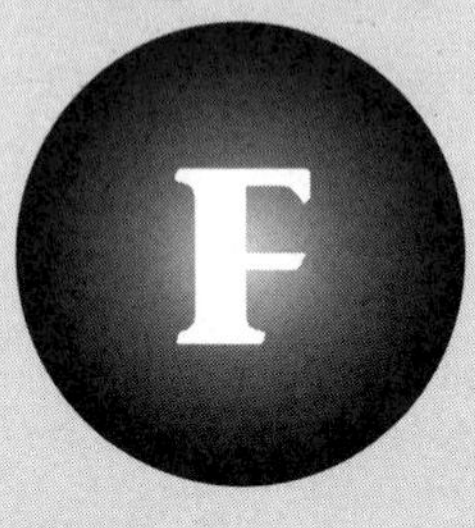

Effect of Food on Common Antiinfectives

Antiinfective	Effect of Food	Management
Amoxicillin (e.g., *Amoxil*)	Delayed absorption.	May take without regard to food.
Amoxicillin/Potassium Clavulanate (*Augmentin*)	No effect on absorption.	Take with food to decrease gastric irritation.
Ampicillin (e.g., *Omnipen*)	Decreased absorption.	Take on an empty stomach.
Azithromycin (*Zithromax*)	Decreased absorption.	Take on an empty stomach.*
Atovaquone (*Mepron*)	Increased absorption.	Take with food.
Bacampicillin (*Spectrobid*)		
Tablets	No effect.	May take without regard to food.
Suspension	Decreased absorption.	Take on an empty stomach.
Carbenicillin (e.g., *Geopen*)	Decreased absorption.	Take on an empty stomach.*
Cefaclor (*Ceclor*)	No significant effect.	May take without regard to food.
Cefadroxil (e.g., *Duricef*)	No effect.	May take without regard to food.
Cefuroxime (*Ceftin*)	Increased bioavailability.	Take with food.
Cefpodoxime (*Vantin*)	Increased absorption.	Take with food.
Cefradine (*Velosef*)	Delayed absorption.	May take without regard to food.
Cephalexin (*Keflex*)	Delayed absorption.	May take without regard to food.
Chloramphenicol (e.g., *Chloromycetin*)	Decreased absorption. May cause gastric irritation.	Take on an empty stomach.*
Chloroquine (*Aralen*)	Increased absorption.	Take with food to decrease gastric irritation.
Ciprofloxacin (*Cipro*)	Delayed absorption.	Take on an empty stomach.*
Clindamycin (*Cleocin*)	Delayed absorption.	May take without regard to food.
Clofazamine (*Lamprene*)	Increased absorption.	Take with food.
Cloxacillin (e.g., *Tegopen*)	Decreased absorption.	Take on an empty stomach.*
Clarithromycin (*Biaxin*)	Increased absorption.	May take without regard to food.
Colistin (*Coly-Mycin S*)	No effect.	May take without regard to food.
Cycloserine (*Seromycin*)	No effect.	May take without regard to food.
Dicloxacillin (*Dynapen*)	Decreased absorption.	Take on an empty stomach.*
Didanosine (*Videx*)	Decreased absorption.	Take on an empty stomach.
Doxycycline (e.g., *Vibramycin*)	Slightly decreased absorption.	May take with food or milk.
Enoxacin (*Penetrex*)	Decreased absorption.	Take on an empty stomach.*
Erythromycin base		
Enteric-coated (e.g., *E-Mycin*)	No effect.	May take with food if gastric upset occurs.
Uncoated	Decreased absorption due to degradation.	May take with food if gastric upset occurs.
Erythromycin estolate (e.g., *Ilosone*)	Increased or no effect on absorption.	May take with food if gastric upset occurs.
Erythromycin ethylsuccinate (*EES, EryPed*)	No effect.	May take with food if gastric upset occurs.

Reprinted with permission from Prescriber's Letter. Prescriber's Letter is a totally independent newsletter providing unbiased drug information to physicians and other prescribers who subscribe.

*1 hour before or 2 hours after food.

PRESCRIBER'S LETTER

2453 Grand Canal Blvd., Suite A, P.O. Box 8190 • Stockton CA 95208
TEL (209) 472-2240 • FAX (209) 472-2249

Antiinfective	Effect of Food	Management
Erythromycin stearate (e.g., *Erythrocin*)	Decreased absorption.	Take on an empty stomach.* If gastric upset occurs, take with food.
Ethambutol (*Myambutol*)	No effect.	May take with food if gastric upset occurs.
Ethionamide		May take with food to decrease gastric irritation.
Furazolidone (*Furoxone*)	Furazolidone is a potent MAO inhibitor.	Avoid tyramine containing foods while taking furazolidone and for several weeks after stopping.
Griseofulvin (e.g., *Gris-PEG*)	Fatty meals increase absorption.	Take with food.
Hydroxychloroquine (*Plaquenil*)		Take with food to decrease gastric irritation.
Isoniazid (*Nydrazid*)	Decreased absorption. Isoniazid may cause pyridoxine deficiency.	Take on an empty stomach.* If gastric irritation occurs, take with food.
Itraconazole (*Sporanox*)	Increased absorption.	Take with food.
Ketoconazole (*Nizoral*)	Decreased absorption.	Take with food to decrease gastric irritation.
Lincomycin (*Lincocin*)	Decreased absorption.	Take on an empty stomach.*
Lomefloxacin (*Maxaquin*)	No effect.	May take without regard to food.
Loracarbef (*Lorabid*)	Slowed absorption.	Take on an empty stomach.*
Mebendazole (*Vermox*)	Increased absorption.	Chew or crush tablet and take with food.
Mefloquine (*Lariam*)		Take with food and a full glass of water.
Methenamine (e.g., *Mandelamine*)		Take with food to decrease gastric irritation.
Metronidazole (*Flagyl*)	Delayed absorption.	Take with food to decrease gastric irritation.
Minocycline (*Minocin*)	No effect.	May take with food or milk.
Nafcillin (e.g., *Unipen*)	Decreased absorption.	Take on an empty stomach.*
Nalidixic acid (e.g., *NegGram*)		Take with food to decrease gastric irritation.
Neomycin (e.g., *Mycifradin*)	Chronic use may decrease fat soluble vitamin absorption.	Vitamins A, D, E and K supplements may be needed.
Niclosamide (e.g., *Niclocide*)		Take with a light meal to decrease gastric upset.
Nitrofurantoin (e.g., *Macrodantin*)	Increased absorption.	Take immediately after food. Food will also decrease gastric irritation.
Norfloxacin (*Noroxin*)	Decreased absorption.	Take on an empty stomach.*
Novobiocin (*Albamycin*)	Delayed absorption.	May take without regard to food.
Ofloxacin (*Floxin*)	Decreased absorption.	Take on an empty stomach.*
Oxacillin (e.g., *Prostaphlin*)	Decreased absorption.	Take on an empty stomach.*
Penicillin G	Decreased absorption.	Take on an empty stomach.*
Penicillin V	Delayed absorption.	May take without regard to food.
Piperazine (e.g., *Antipar*)	Contact between drug and parasite decreased by food.	Take on an empty stomach.*
Praziquantel (e.g., *Biltricide*)		Bitter taste may cause gagging or vomiting. Take with liquid during meals.
Primaquine		May take with food if gastric upset occurs.
Pyrimethamine (*Daraprim*)		Take with food to decrease gastric irritation.
Quinacrine (*Atabrine*)		Take after meals with a full glass of water to decrease gastric irritation.
Quinine		Take with food to minimize gastric irritation.
Rifabutin (*Mycobutin*)		Take with food to decrease gastrointestinal distress.
Rifampin (e.g., *Rimactane*)	Decreased absorption. Rifampin may decrease vitamin D absorption.	Take on an empty stomach.* Give vitamin D if needed.
Sulfonamides, e.g., Sulfisoxazole (*Gantrisin*) Sulfmethoxazole (*Gantanol*)	Delayed absorption.	Take on an empty stomach with a full glass of water.
Sulfasalazine (e.g., *Azulfidine*)	Sulfasalazine may decrease folate absorption.	Give folic acid if needed. Take with food if gastric irritation occurs.
Tetracycline	Decreased absorption of most tetracyclines.	Take on an empty stomach and 3 hours before or after dairy products.
Thiabendazole (*Mintezol*)		May take with food to decrease gastric irritation.
Trimethoprim (e.g., *Proloprim*)	No effect.	May take without regard to food.
Troleandomycin (*Tao*)	No effect.	May take without regard to food.
Vancomycin (e.g., *Vancocin*)	No effect.	May take without regard to food.
Zidovudine (*Retrovir,* AZT)	Fatty foods decrease absorption.	Avoid taking with fatty foods.
Zalcitabine (*Hivid,* ddc)	Decreased absorption.	Take on an empty stomach.

Appendix

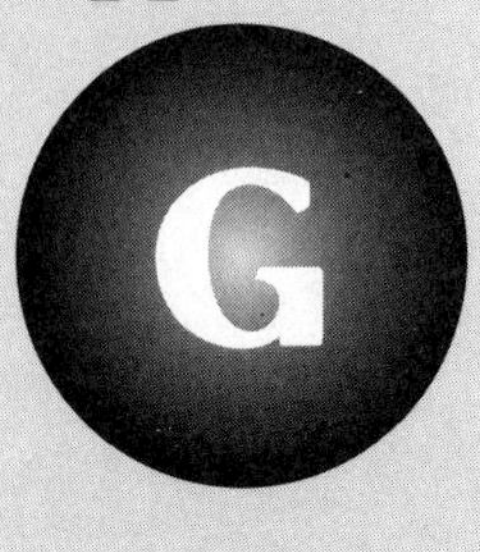

Heart Sounds: Abnormal

Summary of Abnormal Heart Sounds

Sound	Location	Significance
Split S_1	LLSB	Heard elsewhere or with S_2 split; may indicate right bundle-branch block and premature ventricular contractions
Split S_2	Second, third left ICS	Normal if accentuated by inspiration, absent with expiration or sitting up Widens with pulmonic valve closure delays Fixed with atrial septal defect and right ventricular failure Parodoxical with left bundle-branch block
Systolic click	LLSB, medial to apex Diaphragm, midsystole	Mitral valve prolapse
Opening snap	LLSB, medial to apex Diaphragm, early diastole	Mitral valve stenosis
S_3	Apex, left lateral position Louder on inspiration	Rapid ventricular filling, healthy children Ventricular gallop—overloaded left ventricle as in mitral or tricuspid regurgitation
S_4	Apex, left lateral position	Normal athletes and aged Atrial gallop—represents increased resistance to ventricular filling as in hyperparathyroidism, coronary artery disease, aortic stenosis
Innocent murmur	LLSB, systolic	No radiation, grade 1 to 2, medium-pitched May resolve on sitting, no other findings
Midsystolic Murmurs		
Physiologic murmur	LLSB, systolic	As with innocent murmur Common in anemia, pregnancy, fever, and hyperthyroidism
Aortic stenosis	Right second ICS; radiates to neck Medium, harsh; associated with thrill	Stiffening of aortic valve, dilated aorta, aortic regurgitation
Cardiomyopathy	Crescendo-decrescendo third, fourth ICS; radiates to apex or base, not to neck Harsh, medium	Left ventricular hypertrophy causes rapid systolic ejection of blood May also cause mitral regurgitation
Pulmonic stenosis	Second, third ICS, radiates to shoulder and neck Medium, soft Crescendo-decrescendo	Associated with split S_2 or right S_4

From Kidd PS, Robinson, DL: *Family nurse practitioner certification review,* St Louis, 1999, Mosby.
ICS, Intercostal space; *LLSB,* left lower sternal border.

Summary of Abnormal Heart Sounds—cont'd

Sound	Location	Significance
Holosystolic Murmurs		
Mitral regurgitation	Apex, axilla radiation	Volume overload on left ventricle
	Plateau (same intensity throughout cardiac cycle)	Decreased S_1, increased apical impulse
Tricuspid regurgitation	LLSB; radiates to xiphoid and right of sternum	Right ventricular failure and dilation
	Plateau	Associated with S_3 at LLSB, jugular venous distention
Ventricular septal defect	Third, fourth, fifth left ICS; wide radiation	Congenital hole between left and right ventricles
	Loud, thrill, high-pitched, harsh	
Diastolic Murmurs		
Aortic regurgitation	Second through fourth ICS, grade 1 to 3	Volume overload left ventricle
	High pitch, apex radiation	Associated with ejection sound, bounding pulses
	Blowing quality; heard best sitting forward with held exhalation decrescendo	
Mitral valve stenosis	Apex, no radiation grade 1 to 4	Thickened, stiffened mitral valve
	Low pitch	Associated with opening snap
	Listen at apical impulse in left lateral position, with exhalation	S_1 palpable at apex
	Crescendo-decrescendo	
Systolic/Diastolic Abnormalities		
Pericardial friction rub	Third ICS, left of sternum, no radiation	Pericardial inflammation as with pericarditis
	Scratchy, high pitch	
Patent ductus arteriosus	Loud in late systole	Persistent fetal structure
	Left second ICS, left clavicle radiation	Open channel between aorta and pulmonary artery
	Harsh, medium pitch	
Venous hum	Loudest in diastole	Turbulence of blood in jugular veins, common in children
	Above clavicles, especially on right, first and second ICS	
	Humming, roaring, low pitch	

Appendix

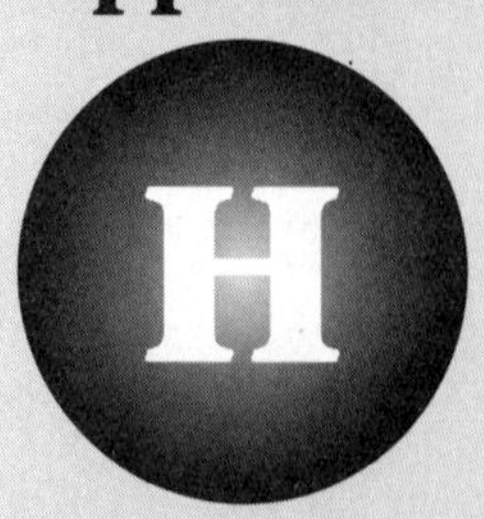

Immunization Guidelines

Table H-1 Summary of Rules for Childhood Immunization*

Vaccine	Ages Usually Given, Other Guidelines	If Child Falls Behind—Minimum Intervals	Contraindications (Remember, Mild Illness Is Not a Contraindication.)
DTaP contains acellular pertussis **DTP** contains whole cell pertussis Give IM	• DTaP is preferred over DTP for all doses in the series. • Give at 2m, 4m, 6m, 15-18m, 4-6yrs of age. • May give No. 1 as early as 6wks of age. • May give No. 4 as early as 12m of age if 6m has elapsed since No. 3 and the child is unlikely to return at age 15-18m. • If started with DTP, complete series with DTaP. • Do not give DTaP or DTP to children 7 yrs of age (give Td). • DTaP/DTP may be given with all other vaccines but at a separate site. • It is preferable but not mandatory to use the same DTaP product for all doses.	• No. 2 and No. 3 may be given 4wks after previous dose. • No. 4 may be given 6m after No. 3. • If No. 4 is given before 4th birthday, wait at least 6m for No. 5. • If No. 4 is given after 4th birthday, No. 5 is not needed. • Don't restart series, no matter how long since previous dose.	(DTaP and DTP have the same contraindications and precautions.) • Anaphylactic reaction to a prior dose or to any vaccine component. • Moderate or severe acute illness. Don't postpone for minor illness. • Previous encephalopathy within 7 days after DTP/DTaP. • Unstable progressive neurologic problem. **Precautions:** The following are precautions not contraindications. Generally when these conditions are present, the vaccine shouldn't be given. But, there are situations when the benefit outweighs risk so vaccination should be considered (e.g., pertussis outbreak). • Previous T≥105° F (40.5° C) within 48 hrs after dose. • Previous continuous crying lasting 3 or more hours within 48 hrs after dose. • Previous convulsion within 3 days after immunization. • Previous pale or limp episode, or collapse within 48 hrs after dose.
DT Give IM	• Give to children <7 yrs of age if the child has had a serious reaction to the "P" in DTaP/DTP, or if the parents refuse the pertussis component. • DT can be given with all other vaccines but at a separate site.	• For children who have fallen behind, use information directly above.	• Anaphylactic reaction to a prior dose or to any vaccine component. • Moderate or severe acute illness. Don't postpone for minor illness.

Adapted from ACIP, AAP, and AAFP by the Immunization Action Coalition, March 1999. Used with permission from the Immunization Action Coalition, St. Paul, Minnesota.

*Hepatitis A, influenza, pneumococcal, and Lyme disease vaccines are indicated for many children and teens, so make sure you provide these vaccines to at-risk children. The newer combination vaccines are not listed on this table but may be used whenever administration of any component is indicated and none are contraindicated. Read the package inserts. For full immunization information, see recent ACIP statements published in the *MMWR;* for the latest AAP Committee on Infectious Diseases' recommendations, see the *AAP's 1997 Red Book* and the journal, *Pediatrics.*

This table was developed to combine the recommendations for childhood immunization and to assist health care workers in immunization clinics to determine the appropriate use and scheduling of vaccines. It can be posted in immunization clinics or clinicians' offices.

Thank you to the following individuals for their review: William Atkinson, MD, Jane Seward, MBBS, Robert Sharrer, MD, Thomas Vernon, MD, Richard Zimmerman, MD, Harold Margolis, MD, and Linda Moyer, RN. Final responsibility for errors lies with the editors.

Your comments are welcome. Please send them to Lynn Bahta, PHN, or Deborah Wexler, MD, Immunization Action Coalition, 1573 Selby Ave., St. Paul, MN 55104 or call 612-647-9009, fax 612-647-9131, or e-mail: mail@immunize.org.

This table is revised yearly. The most recent edition of this table is available on our *website at <www.immunize.org>*

Continued

TABLE H-1 Summary of Rules for Childhood Immunization—cont'd

Vaccine	Ages Usually Given, Other Guidelines	If Child Falls Behind—Minimum Intervals	Contraindications (Remember, Mild Illness Is Not a Contraindication.)
Td Give IM	• Use for persons ≥7 yrs of age. • A booster dose is recommended for children 11-12yrs of age if 5yrs have elapsed since previous dose. Then boost every 10 years. • Td may be given with all other vaccines but at a separate site.	• For those never vaccinated or behind, or if the vaccination history is unknown, give dose No. 1 now; dose No. 2 4wks later; dose No. 3 6m after No. 2; and then boost every 10 years.	• Anaphylactic reaction to a prior dose or to any vaccine component. • Moderate or severe acute illness. Don't postpone for minor illness.
Polio **IPV** and **OPV** Give IPV SQ or IM Give OPV PO	• Give at 2m, 4m, 6-18m and 4-6yrs of age. • Give IPV for doses #1 and #2 (except in special circumstances, e.g., parent's refusal, imminent travel to polio-endemic area). • ACIP says for dose #3, give OPV at 12-18m, and for dose #4, give OPV at 4-6yrs. An all-IPV schedule is also acceptable. If an all-IPV or all-OPV schedule is used, dose #3 may be given as early as 6m of age. • AAP/AAFP say give either IPV or OPV for doses #3 and #4. Dose #3 is given at 6-18m of age and dose #4 at 4-6yrs. • ACIP/AAP/AAFP say IPV is acceptable for all 4 doses • Not routinely given to anyone ≥18yrs of age (except certain travelers). • IPV may be given with all other vaccines but at a separate site. • OPV may be given with all other vaccines.	• #1, #2, & #3 (IPV or OPV) should be separated by at least 4wks. • All IPV: a 6m interval is preferred between dose #2 and #3 for best response. • #4 (IPV or OPV) is given between 4-6yrs of age. • If #3 of an all-IPV or all-OPV series is given at ≥4yrs of age, dose #4 is not needed. • Children who receive any combination of IPV and OPV doses must receive all 4 doses, regardless of the age when first initiated. • Don't restart series, no matter how long since previous dose.	• Anaphylactic reaction to a prior dose or to any vaccine component. • Moderate or severe acute illness. Don't postpone for minor illness. • Use IPV when an adult in the household or other close contact has never been vaccinated against polio. • In pregnancy, if immediate protection is needed, see the ACIP recommendations on the use of polio vaccine. **The following are contraindications for OPV so use IPV in these situations:** • Cancer, leukemia, lymphoma, immunodeficiency, including HIV/AIDS. • Taking a drug that lowers resistance to infection, e.g., anti-cancer, high-dose steroids. • Someone in the household has any of the above medical problems.

Varicella **Var** Give SQ.	• Routinely give at 12-18m. • Vaccinate all children ≥12m of age including adolescents who have not had prior infection with chickenpox. • If Var and MMR (and/or yellow fever vaccine) are not given on the same day, space them ≥28d apart. • Var may be given with all other vaccines but at a separate site.	• Do not give to children <12m of age. • Susceptible children <13 yrs of age receive 1 dose. • Susceptible persons ≥13 yrs of age receive 2 doses 4-8wks apart. • Don't restart series, no matter how long since previous dose.	• Anaphylactic reaction to a prior dose or to any vaccine component. • Moderate or severe acute illness. Don't postpone for minor illness. • Pregnancy, or possibility of pregnancy within 1 month. • If blood, plasma, or immunoglobulin (IG or VZIG) have been administered during the past 5 months, consult ACIP recommendations or *AAP's 1997 Red Book* (p. 353) regarding time to wait before vaccinating. • Immunocompromised persons due to high doses of systemic steroids, cancer, leukemia, lymphoma, immunodeficiency. NOTE: For patients on high doses of systemic steroids or for patients with leukemia, consult ACIP recommendations. NOTE: Manufacturer recommends "no salicylates" for 6wks following this vaccine.
MMR Give SQ	• Give No. 1 at 12-15m. Give No. 2 at 4-6yrs. • Make sure that all children (and teens) over 4-6 years of age have received both doses of MMR. • If a dose was given before 12m of age, give No. 1 at 12-15m of age with a minimum interval of 1m between these doses. • If MMR and Var (and/or yellow fever vaccine) are not given on the same day, space them ≥28d apart. • May give with all other vaccines but at a separate site.	• Two doses of MMR are recommended for all children ≤18 years of age. • Give whenever behind. Exception: If MMR and Var (and/or yellow fever vaccine except polio) are not given on the same day, space them ≥28d apart. • There should be a minimum interval of 28days between MMR No. 1 and MMR No. 2. • Dose No. 2 can be given at any time if at least 28days have elapsed since dose No. 1, and both doses are administered after 1 year of age. • Don't restart series, no matter how long since previous dose.	• Anaphylactic reaction to a prior dose or to any vaccine component. • Pregnancy or possible pregnancy within next 3m (use contraception). • Moderate or severe acute illness. Don't postpone for minor illness. • If blood, plasma, or immunoglobulin have been administered during the past 11 months, consult ACIP recommendations or *AAP's 1997 Red Book* (p. 353) regarding time to wait before vaccinating. • HIV positivity is NOT a contraindication unless severely immunocompromised. • Immunocompromised persons, e.g., cancer, leukemia, lymphoma NOTE: For patients on high-dose immunosuppressive therapy, consult ACIP recommendations regarding delay time. NOTE: MMR is NOT contraindicated if a PPD test was done recently, but PPD should be delayed if MMR was given 1-30 days before the PPD.

Continued

TABLE H-1 Summary of Rules for Childhood Immunization—cont'd

Vaccine	Ages Usually Given, Other Guidelines	If Child Falls Behind—Minimum Intervals	Contraindications (Remember, Mild Illness Is Not a Contraindication.)
Hib Give IM	• HibTITER (HbOC) & ActHib (PRP-T): give at 2m, 4m, 6m, 12-15m. • PedvaxHiB (PRP-OMP): give at 2m, 4m, 12-15m. • Dose No. 1 of Hib vaccine may be given as early as 6wks of age but not earlier. • May give with all other vaccines but at a separate site. • All Hib products licensed for the primary series are interchangeable. • Any Hib vaccine may be used for the booster dose. • Hib is not routinely given to children ≥5 years of age.	**Rules for all Hib vaccines:** • The last dose (booster dose) is given no earlier than 12 months of age and a minimum of 2 months since the previous dose. • For children ≥15m and less than 5yrs who have NEVER received Hib vaccine, only 1 dose is needed. • Don't restart series, no matter how long since previous dose. **Rules for HbOC (HibTITER) & PRP-T (ActHib) only:** • #2 and #3 may be given 4 wks after previous dose. • If #1 was given at 7-11m only 3 doses are needed: #2 is given 4-8wks after #1, then boost at 12-15m. • If #1 was given at 12-14m, give a booster dose in 2 m. **Rules for PRP-OMP (PedvaxHiB) only:** • #2 may be given 4 wks after dose #1. • If #1 was given at 12-14m, boost 8wks later.	• Anaphylactic reaction to a prior dose or to any vaccine component. • Moderate or severe acute illness. Don't postpone for minor illness.

Hep-B Give IM	• Vaccinate all infants at 0-2m, 1-4m, 6-18m. • Vaccinate all children 0-18 years of age. • For older children/teens, spacing options include: 0m, 1m, 6m; 0m, 2m, 4m; or 0m, 1m, 4m. • Children who were born or whose parents were born in countries of high HBV endemicity or who have other risk factors should be vaccinated as soon as possible. • **If mother is HBsAg positive:** give HBIG and hep-B No. 1 within 12 hrs of birth, No. 2 at 1-2m, and No. 3 at 6m of age. • **If mother's HBsAg status is unknown:** give hep B No. 1 within 12 hrs of birth, No. 2 at 1-2m, and No. 3 at 6m of age. If mother is later found to be HBsAg-positive, her infant should receive the additional protection of HBIG within the first 7 days of life. • May give with all other vaccines but at a separate site. • Hepatitis B vaccine brands are interchangeable.	• **Don't restart series, no matter how long since previous dose.** • 3-dose series can be started at any age. • Minimum spacing for children and teens: 4wks between No. 1 and No. 2, and 2m between No. 2 and No. 3. Overall there must be 4m between No. 1 and No. 3. • Dose No. 3 should not be given earlier than 6 months of age. **Dosing of Hepatitis B vaccine:** For Energix B, use 10 μg (0.5 ml) for 0-19 years of age. For Recombivax HB, use 5 μg (0.5 ml) for 0-19 years of age.	• Anaphylactic reaction to a prior dose or to any vaccine component. • Moderate or severe acute illness. Don't postpone for minor illness.
Rotavirus Rv Give PO	• Give at 2m, 4m, and 6m. • Dose #1 should not be given before 6wks or at ≥7m. • No dose should be given on or after the first birthday. • Do not readminister a regurgitated dose. • May give with all other vaccines.	• Minimum interval is 3wks between doses. • Use minimum intervals to achieve protection prior to rotavirus season or if behind schedule. • Don't restart the series no matter how long since previous dose.	• Moderate or severe acute illness, including persistent vomiting. Don't postpone for minor illness. • Anaphylactic reaction to a prior dose or to any vaccine component. • Known or suspected altered immunity, including infants born to HIV+ mothers unless it is known that the child is not HIV infected. • For infants with pre-existing chronic GI conditions, see ACIP statement.

*As of July 15, 1999, the Centers for Disease Control and Prevention recommends that healthcare providers and parents postpone use of the rotavirus vaccine for infants, at least until November 1999, based on early surveillance reports of intussusception among some infants who received rotavirus vaccine. For more information, visit the CDC's website at www.cdc.gov.

TABLE H-2 Recommended Childhood Immunization Schedule,* United States, January, 1999

Vaccine	Age: Birth	1 Mo.	2 Mos.	4 Mos.	6 Mos.	12 Mos.	15 Mos.	18 Mos.	4-6 Yrs.	11-12 Yrs.	14-16 Yrs.
Hepatitis B†§	Hep B									*Hep B*	
		Hep B			Hep B-3						
Diphtheria and tetanus toxoids and pertussis¶			DTaP	DTaP	DTaP		DTaP		DTaP	Td	
Haemophilus influenzae type b**			Hib	Hib	Hib	Hib					
Poliovirus††			IPV	IPV	Polio				Polio		
Measles-mumps-rubella§§						MMR			MMR	*MMR*	
Varicella virus¶¶						Var				*Var*	
*Rotavirus****			RV	RV	RV						

Example	Range of Acceptable Ages for Vaccination
Example	Vaccines to Be Assessed and Administered if Necessary

Source: Advisory Committee on Immunization Practices (ACIP), American Academy of Pediatrics (AAP), and American Academy of Family Physicians (AAFP).

*This schedule indicates the recommended age for routine administration of currently licensed childhood vaccines; vaccines are listed under the ages for which they are routinely recommended. Catch-up immunization should be done during any visit when feasible. Some combination vaccines are available and may be used whenever administration of all components of the vaccine is indicated. Providers should consult the manufacturers' package inserts for detailed recommendations.

†Infants born to hepatitis B surface antigen (HBsAg)-negative mothers should receive the second dose of hepatitis B vaccine at least 1 month after the first dose. The third dose should be administered at least 4 months after the first dose and at least 2 months after the second dose, but not before 6 months of age. Infants born to HBsAg-positive mothers should receive hepatitis B vaccine and 0.5 mL hepatitis B immunoglobulin (HBIG) within 12 hours of birth, at a separate site. The second dose is recommended at age 1 to 2 months, and the third dose at age 6 months. Infants born to mothers whose HBsAg status is unknown should receive hepatitis B vaccine within 12 hours of birth. Blood should be drawn at the time of delivery to determine the mother's HBsAg status; if it is positive, the infant should receive HBIG as soon as possible (no later than age 1 week). The dosage and time of subsequent vaccine doses should be based on the mother's HBsAg status.

§Children and adolescents (through 18 years of age) who have not been vaccinated against hepatitis B may begin the series during any visit. Special efforts should be made to immunize children who were born in areas of the world with moderate or high endemicity of HBV infection.

¶Diphtheria and tetanus toxoids and acellular pertussis vaccine (DTAP) is the preferred vaccine for all doses in the vaccination series, including completion of the series in children who have received one or more doses of whole-cell diphtheria and tetanus toxoids and pertussis vaccine (DTP). Whole-cell DTP is an acceptable alternative to DTaP. The fourth dose (DTP or DTaP) may be administered as early as age 12 months, provided 6 months have elapsed since the third dose and if the child is unlikely to return at age 15-18 months. Tetanus and diphtheria toxoids, absorbed, for adult use (Td), is recommended at age 11-12 years if at least 5 years have elapsed since the last dose of DTP, DTaP, or diphtheria and tetanus toxoids, absorbed, for pediatric use (DT). Subsequent routine Td boosters are recommended every 10 years.

**Three *H. Influenzae* type b (Hib) conjugate vaccines are licensed for infant use. If *Haemophilus* b conjugate vaccine (meningococcal protein conjugate) (PRP-OMP) (PedvaxHIB® [Merck]) is administered at ages 2 and 4 months, a dose at age 6 months is not required.

††Two poliovirus vaccines currently are licensed in the United States: inactivated poliovirus vaccine (IPV) and oral poliovirus vaccine (OPV).

The ACIP, AAP, and AAFP now recommend that the first two doses of poliovirus vaccine should be IPV. The ACIP continues to recommend a sequential schedule of two doses of IPV administered at ages 2 and 4 months, followed by two doses of OPV at 12-18 months and 4-6 years. Use of IPV for all doses also is acceptable and is recommended for immunocompromised persons and their household contacts.

OPV is no longer recommended for the first two doses of the schedule and is acceptable only for special circumstances such as: children of parents who do not accept the recommended number of injections, late initiation of immunization which would require an unacceptable number of injections, and imminent travel to polio-endemic areas. OPV remains the vaccine of choice for mass immunization campaigns to control outbreaks due to wild poliovirus.

§§The second dose of measles-mumps-rubella vaccine (MMR) is recommended routinely at ages 4 to 6 years, but may be administered during any visit, provided at least 1 month has elapsed since receipt of the first dose and that both doses are administered beginning at or after age 12 months. Those who have not previously received the second dose should complete the schedule no later than the routine visit to a health care provider at ages 11 to 12 years.

¶¶Susceptible children may receive varicella vaccine (Var) at any visit after the first birthday and those who lack a reliable history of chickenpox should be vaccinated during the routine visit to a health care provider at age 11 to 12 years. Susceptible children aged ≥13 years should receive two doses at least 1 month apart.

Use of trade names and commercial sources is for identification only and does not imply endorsement by CDC or the U.S. Department of Health and Human Services.

***Rotavirus (Rv) vaccine is shaded and italicized to indicate: 1) health care providers may require time and resources to incorporate this new vaccine into practice; and 2) the AAFP feels that the decision to use rotavirus vaccine should be made by the parent or guardian in consultation with their physician or other health care provider. The first dose of Rv vaccine should not be administered before 6 weeks of age, and the minimum interval between doses is 3 weeks. The Rv vaccine series should not be initiated at 7 months of age or older, and all doses should be completed by the first birthday. NOTE: As of July 15, 1999, the CDC recommends that healthcare providers and parents postpone use of the rotavirus vaccine for infants, at least until November 1999, based on early surveillance reports of intussusception among some infants who received rotavirus vaccine. For more information, visit the CDC's website at www.cdc.gov.

TABLE H-3 Recommended Accelerated Immunization Schedule for Infants and Children <7 Years of Age Who Start the Series Late* or Who Are >1 Month Behind in the Immunization Schedule† (i.e., Children from Whom Compliance with Scheduled Visits Cannot Be Assured)

Timing	Vaccine	Comment
First visit (≥4 months of age)	DTaP,§ OPV,¶ Hib,‡ hepatitis B, MMR, Varicella	Must be ≥12 months of age to receive MMR and varicella. If ≥5 years of age, Hib is not normally indicated.
Second visit (1 month†† after first visit	DTaP,§ OPV,¶ Hib,‡ hepatitis B	
Third visit (1 month after second visit)	DTaP,§ OPV,¶ Hib‡	
Fourth visit (≥6 months after third visit)	DTaP,§ Hib,‡ hepatitis B	
4-6 years of age	DTaP,§ OPV, MMR	Preferable at or before school entry. DTaP is not necessary if fourth dose given on or after fourth birthday. OPV not necessary if third dose given on or after fourth birthday.
11-12 years of age	Varicella, MMR, and/or hepatitis B (if not already received), Td if >5 years since last dose	Repeat Td every 10 years throughout life.

*If initiated in the first year of life, administer DTaP doses 1, 2, and 3 and OPV doses 1, 2, and 3 according to this schedule; administer MMR and varicella when the child reaches 12 to 15 months of age. All vaccines should be administered simultaneously at the appropriate visit.

†See individual ACIP recommendations for detailed information on specific vaccines.

§Diphtheria and tetanus toxoids and acellular pertussis vaccine (DTaP) is preferred for all doses of the series. A vaccine containing whole cell pertussis vaccine is an acceptable alternative.

¶If the polio vaccine series is begun before 6 months of age, ACIP recommends the first two doses be administered as inactivated polio vaccine (IPV) and the third dose (OPV) be administered at 12-18 months of age.

‡Recommended Hib schedule varies by vaccine manufacturer and age of the child when vaccination series is started. If series is begun at age <6 months of age, 4 doses are needed (only 3 doses are needed if all doses are PRP-OPM [PedvaxHIB, Merck]). The fourth dose must be >2 months after the third dose and on or after the first birthday. If series started at age 12 to 14 months, 2 doses are needed, >2 months apart. If series started at age >15 months, 1 dose of any licensed conjugate Hib vaccine is recommended.

††An interval of 28 or more days.

Based on General Recommendations on Immunization (1994), with modifications from subsequent ACIP statements.

TABLE H-4 Minimum Age for Initial Vaccination and Minimum Interval Between Vaccine Doses by Type of Vaccine

Vaccine	Minimum Age for First Dose*	Minimum Interval From Dose 1 to 2*	Minimum Interval From Dose 2 to 3*	Minimum Interval From Dose 3 to 4*
DTP/DTaP (DT)†	6 weeks	4 weeks	4 weeks	6 months
Combined DTP-Hib	6 weeks	1 month	1 month	6 months
Hib (primary series)				
HbOC	6 weeks	1 month	1 month	§
PRP-T	6 weeks	1 month	1 month	§
PRP-OMP	6 weeks	1 month	§	
Polio¶	6 weeks	4 weeks	4 weeks**	††
MMR	12 months§§	1 month		
Hepatitis B	birth	1 month	2 month¶¶	
Varicella	12 months	4 weeks		

*These minimum acceptable ages and intervals may not correspond with the optimal recommended ages and intervals for vaccination. See Tables 3 to 5 in ACIP's General Recommendations on Immunization and ACIP's "Recommended Childhood Immunization Schedule, United States, January to December 1998" for the current recommended routine and accelerated vaccination schedules.

†The total number of doses of diphtheria and tetanus toxoids should not exceed six each before the seventh birthday.

§The booster dose of Hib vaccine that is recommended following the primary vaccination series should be administered no earlier than 12 months of age and at least 2 months after the previous dose of Hib vaccine (Tables 3 and 4 of ACIP's General Recommendations on Immunization).

¶Sequential IPV/OPV, all-OPV, or all-IPV.

**For unvaccinated adults at increased risk of exposure to poliovirus with <3 months or >2 months available before protection is needed, three doses of IPV should be administered at least 1 month apart.

††If the third dose is given after the fourth birthday, the fourth (booster) dose is not needed.

§§Although the age for measles vaccination may be as young as 6 months in outbreak areas where cases are occurring in children <1 year of age, children initially vaccinated before the first birthday should be revaccinated at 12 to 15 months of age, and an additional dose of vaccine should be administered at the time of school entry or according to local policy. Doses of MMR or other measles-containing vaccines should be separated by at least 1 month.

¶¶This final dose is recommended at least 4 months after the first dose and no earlier than 6 months of age.

This table reflects changes that have not yet been published in the ACIP's General Recommendations on Immunization. It is taken from CDC's Epidemiology and Prevention of Vaccine-Preventable Diseases, ed 4.

TABLE H-5 Immunizations During Pregnancy

An immunization history is an important part of preconceptional and obstetric care. Immunizations during pregnancy are recommended when the risk for disease exposure is high, the infection would pose a significant risk to mother or fetus, and when the vaccine is unlikely to cause harm.

Immunization	Adult Dose	Recommendations	Comments
Toxoids			
Tetanus-diphtheria	0.5 ml IM *Primary series* consists of 3 doses 1-2 months apart with a fourth dose 6-12 months after the third; *boosters* every 10 years	Recommended during pregnancy if the patient lacks a primary series or no booster within past 10 years	The only immunobiologic agent that is recommended for routine administration during pregnancy
Inactivated Virus Vaccines			
Influenza Peak incidence October through March	0.5 ml IM annually Considered safe at any stage of pregnancy	Recommended during pregnancy in women with underlying health problems such as cardiopulmonary disease	Women in their second and third trimester or during puerperium during peak influenza season, even in the absence of underlying disease, are at risk for complications from influenza and should be considered for influenza vaccine
Hepatitis B	1 ml IM (dose depends on manufacturer) 2 doses 4 weeks apart with the third dose 5 months later	Recommended in pregnancy if high risk: history of parental drug use, multiple sex partners, concurrent STDs, or employed as a health care worker	Infection could result in severe disease for both the mother and infant; screening for hepatitis B surface antigen should be a part of routine prenatal testing
Inactivated Bacterial Vaccines			
Pneumococcus	0.5 ml IM or SQ q6 years for high-risk patients	Recommended for high-risk patients; DM, asthma, splenectomy, or SS anemia	
Live Virus Vaccines			
Measles, mumps, and rubella	0.5 ml SQ 1 dose	**Contraindicated** during pregnancy; based on theoretical risk; no case of embryopathy caused by rubella vaccine has been reported	Administer during preconceptional counseling or at postpartum; advise patient to delay pregnancy for 3 months

DM, Diabetes mellitus; *IPV*, inactivated poliovirus vaccine; *OPV*, oral poliovirus vaccine; *SS*, sickle cell; *STD*, sexually transmitted disease.

Continued

TABLE H-5 Immunizations During Pregnancy—cont'd

Immunization	Adult Dose	Recommendations	Comments
Live Virus Vaccines—cont'd			
Poliomyelitis	*Primary series* consists of 2 doses IPV at 4- to 8-week intervals with third dose 6-12 months after the second; 1 dose OPV is recommended when immediate protection is desired during an outbreak	Generally **contraindicated** during pregnancy; travel to foreign countries poses a risk of exposure; IPV should be given if series can be completed before travel; otherwise give OPV	Routine vaccination of adults with documentation of primary series is not indicated
Varicella	0.5 ml SQ 2 doses 1 month apart	**Contraindicated** during pregnancy; effects of varicella vaccine on fetus is unknown	Screen for history of varicella during preconceptional counseling and administer if indicated
Specific Immune Globulin	Depends on exposure	Postexposure prophylaxis for hepatitis B, rabies, tetanus, and varicella	Considered safe during pregnancy when compared to risk from disease
Standard Immune Globulin	Depends on exposure	Postexposure prophylaxis for hepatitis A and measles	Considered safe during pregnancy when compared to risk from disease

SUGGESTED READINGS

ACOG Technical Bulletin No. 160: *Immunizations during Pregnancy.* Washington DC, October 1991, American College of Obstetricians and Gynecologists.

American Academy of Pediatrics (active and passive immunizations). In Peter G editor: *1997 Red Book: Report of the Committee on Infectious Diseases,* ed 24, Elk Grove Village, Ill, 1997, American Academy of Pediatrics, pp 45-50.

Cunningham FG et al: *Williams obstetrics* ed 20, Stamford, Conn, 1997, Appleton & Lange, pp 242-243.

Gall S: *Immunization for obstetrical patients and health care workers,* Louisville, Ky, 1997, University of Louisville PCC News, 24(9).

Appendix

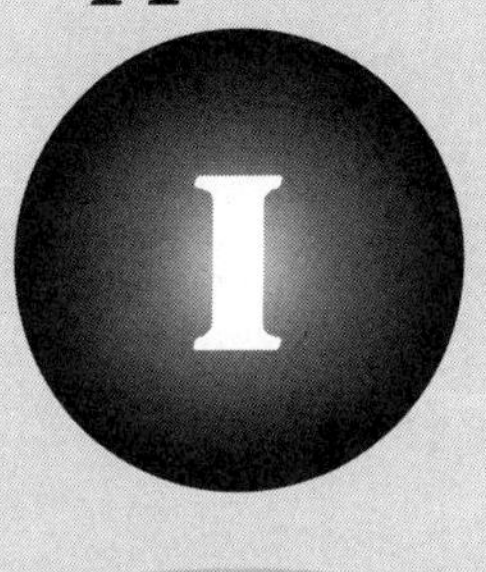

Laboratory Values: Normal Reference Values Across the Lifespan

Table I-1 Normal Reference Laboratory Values (Adult)
Blood, Plasma, or Serum Values

Test	Reference Range: Conventional Values	Reference Range: SI Units*
Acetoacetate plus acetone	0.30-2.0 mg/dl	3-20 mg/l
Acetone	Negative	Negative
Acid phosphatase	Adults: 0.10-0.63 U/ml (Bessey-Lowry)	28-175 nmol/s/L
	0.5-2.0 U/ml (Bodansky)	
	1.0-4.0 U/ml (King-Armstrong)	
	Children: 6.4-15.2 U/L	
Activated partial thromboplastin time (APTT)	30-40 sec	30-40 sec
Adrenocorticotropic hormone (ACTH)	6 AM 15-100 pg/ml	10-80 ng/L
	6 PM <50 pg/ml	<50 ng/L
Alanine aminotransferase (ALT)	5-35 IU/L	5-35 U/L
Albumin	3.2-4.5 g/dl	35-55 g/L
Alcohol	Negative	Negative
Aldolase	Adults: 3.0-8.2 Sibley-Lehninger units/dl	22-59 mU/L at 37°C
	Children: approximately 2 × adult values	
	Newborns: approximately 4 × adult values	
Aldosterone	Peripheral blood:	
	Supine: 7.4 ± 4.2 ng/dl	0.08-0.3 nmoL/L
	Upright: 1-21 ng/dl	0.14-0.8 nmol/L
	Adrenal vein: 200-800 ng/dl	
Alkaline phosphatase	Adults: 30-85 ImU/ml	
	Children and adolescents:	
	<2 years: 85-235 ImU/ml	
	2-8 years: 65-210 ImU/ml	
	9-15 years: 60-300 ImU/ml (active bone growth)	
	16-21 years: 30-200 ImU/ml	

From Pagana KD, Pagana TJ: Diagnostic testing and nursing implications: a case study approach, ed 5, St Louis, 1998, Mosby.

*The use of the System of International Units (SI) was recommended at the 30th World Health Assembly in 1977 to implement an international language of measurement. Because this system is being adopted by numerous laboratories, many of the common values are expressed in both conventional and SI units. SI units are calculated by multiplying the conventional unit by a number factor. The SI measurement system used moles as the basic unit for the amount of a substance, kilograms for its mass, and meter for its length.

Continued

TABLE I-1 Normal Reference Laboratory Values (Adult)—cont'd
Blood, Plasma, or Serum Values

	Reference Range	
Test	**Conventional Values**	**SI Units***
Alpha-aminonitrogen	3-6 mg/dl	2.1-3.9 mmol/L
Alpha-1-antitrypsin	>250 mg/dl	
Alpha-fetoprotein (AFP)	<25 ng/ml	
Ammonia	Adults: 15-110 μg/dl	47-65 μmol/L
	Children: 40-80 μg/dl	
	Newborns: 90-150 μg/dl	
Amylase	56-190 IU/L	25-125 U/L
	80-150 Somogyi units/ml	
Angiotensin-converting enzyme (ACE)	23-57 U/ml	
Antinuclear antibodies (ANA)	Negative	
Antistreptolysin O (ASO)	Adults: ≤160 Todd units/ml	
	Children:	
	Newborns: similar to mother's value	
	6 months-2 years: ≤50 Todd units/ml	
	2-4 years: ≤160 Todd units/ml	
	5-12 years: ≤200 Todd units/ml	
Antithyroid microsomal antibody	Titer <1:100	
Antithyroglobulin antibody	Titer <1:100	
Ascorbic acid (vitamin C)	0.6-1.6 mg/dl	23-57 μmol/L
Aspartate aminotransferase (AST, SGOT)	12-36 U/ml	0.10-0.30 μmol/s/L
	5-40 IU/L	5-40 U/L
Australian antigen (hepatitis-associated antigen, HAA)	Negative	Negative
Barbiturates	Negative	Negative
Base excess	Men: −3.3 to +1.2	0 ± 2 mmol/L
	Women: −2.4 to +2.3	0 ± 2 mmol/L
Bicarbonate (HCO_3^-)	22-26 mEq/L	22-26 mmol/L
Bilirubin		
Direct (conjugated)	0.1-0.3 mg/dl	1.7-5.1 μmol/L
Indirect (unconjugated)	0.2-0.8 mg/dl	3.4-12.0 μmol/L
Total	Adults and children: 0.1-1.0 mg/dl	5.1-17.0 μmol/L
	Newborns: 1-12 mg/dl	
Bleeding time (Ivy method)	1-9 min	
Blood count (see complete blood count)		
Blood gases (arterial)		
pH	7.35-7.45	
Pco_2	35-45 mm Hg	4.7-6.0 kPa
HCO_3^-	22-26 mEq/L	21-28 nmol/L
Po_2	80-100 mm Hg	11-13 kPa
O_2 saturation	95%-100%	
Blood urea nitrogen (BUN)	5-20 mg/dl	3.6-7.1 mmol/L
Bromide	Up to 5 mg/dl	0-63 mmol/L
Bromosulfophthalein (BSP)	<5% retention after 45 min	
CA 15-3	<22 U/ml	
CA-125	0-35 U/ml	
CA 19-9	<37 U/ml	
C-reactive protein (CRP)	<6 μg/ml	
Calcitonin	<50 pg/ml	<50 pmol/L
Calcium (Ca)	9.0-10.5 mg/dl (total)	2.25-2.75 mmol/L
	3.9-4.6 mg/dl (ionized)	1.05-1.30 mmol/L
Carbon dioxide (CO_2) content	23-30 mEq/L	21-30 mmol/L
Carboxyhemoglobin (COHb)	3% of total hemoglobin	

From Pagana KD, Pagana TJ: Diagnostic testing and nursing implications: a case study approach, ed 5, St Louis, 1998, Mosby.

Table I-1 Normal Reference Laboratory Values (Adult)—cont'd
Blood, Plasma, or Serum Values

Test	Reference Range	
	Conventional Values	**SI Units***
Carcinoembryonic antigen (CEA)	<2 ng/ml	0.2-5 μg/L
Carotene	50-200 μg/dl	0.74-3.72 μmol/L
Chloride (Cl)	90-110 mEq/L	98-106 mmol/L
Cholesterol	150-250 mg/dl	3.90-6.50 mmol/L
Clot retraction	50%-100% clot retraction in 1-2 hours, complete retraction within 24 hours	
Complement	C_3: 70-176 mg/dl	0.55-1.20 g/L
	C_4: 16-45 mg/dl	0.20-0.50 g/L
Complete blood count (CBC)		
Red blood cell (RBC) count	Men: 4.7-6.1 million/mm^3	
	Women: 4.2-5.4 million/mm^3	
	Infants and children: 3.8-5.5 million/mm^3	
	Newborns: 4.8-7.1 million/mm^3	
Hemoglobin (Hgb)	Men: 14-18 g/dl	8.7-11.2 mmol/L
	Women: 12-16 g/dl (pregnancy: >11 g/dl)	7.4-9.9 mmol/L
	Children: 11-16 g/dl	1.74-2.56 mmol/L
	Infants: 10-15 g/dl	
	Newborns: 14-24 g/dl	2.56-3.02 mmol/L
Hematocrit (Hct)	Men: 42%-52%	
	Women: 37%-47% (pregnancy: >33%)	
	Children: 31%-43%	
	Infants: 30%-40%	
	Newborns: 44%-64%	
Mean corpuscular volume (MCV)	Adults and children: 80-95 μ^3	80-95 fl
	Newborns: 96-108 μ^3	
Mean corpuscular hemoglobin (MCH)	Adults and children: 27-31 pg	0.42-0.48 fmol
	Newborns: 32-34 pg	
Mean corpuscular hemoglobin concentration (MCHC)	Adults and children: 32-36 g/dl	0.32-0.36
	Newborns: 32-33 g/dl	
White blood cell (WBC) count	Adults and children >2 years: 5,000-10,000/mm^3	
	Children ≤2 years: 6,200-17,000/mm^3	
	Newborns: 9000-30,000/mm^3	
Differential count		
Neutrophils	55%-70%	
Lymphocytes	20%-40%	
Monocytes	2%-8%	
Eosinophils	1%-4%	
Basophils	0.5%-1%	
Platelet count	150,000-400,000/mm^3	
Coombs' test		
Direct	Negative	Negative
Indirect	Negative	Negative
Copper (Cu)	70-140 μg/dl	11.0-24.3 μmol/L
Cortisol	6-28 μg/dl (A.M.)	170-635 nmol/L
	2-12 μg/dl (P.M.)	82-413 nmol/L
CPK isoenzyme (MB)	<5% total	
Creatinine	0.7-1.5 mg/dl	<133 μmol/L
Creatinine clearance	Men: 95-104 ml/min	<133 μmol/L
	Women: 95-125 ml/min	

Continued

TABLE I-1 Normal Reference Laboratory Values (Adult)—cont'd
Blood, Plasma, or Serum Values

Test	Reference Range	
	Conventional Values	**SI Units***
Creatinine phosphokinase (CPK)	5-75 mU/ml	12-80 units/L
Cryoglobulin	Negative	Negative
Differential (WBC) count (see CBC)		
Digoxin	Therapeutic level: 0.5-2.0 ng/ml	40-79 μmol/L
	Toxic level: >2.4 ng/ml	>119 μmol/L
Erythrocyte count (see complete blood count)		
Erythrocyte sedimentation rate (ESR)	Men: up to 15 mm/hour	
	Women: up to 20 mm/hour	
	Children: up to 10 mm/hour	
Ethanol	80-200 mg/dl (mild to moderate intoxication)	17-43 mmol/L
	250-400 mg/dl (marked intoxication)	54-87 mmol/L
	>400 mg/dl (severe intoxication)	>87 mmol/L
Euglobulin lysis test	90 min-6 hours	
Fats	Up to 200 mg/dl	
Ferritin	15-200 ng/ml	15-200 μg/L
Fibrin degradation products (FDP)	<10 μg/ml	
Fibrinogen (factor I)	200-400 mg/dl	5.9-11.7 μmol/L
Fibrinolysis/euglobulin lysis test	90 min-6 hours	
Fluorescent treponemal antibody (FTA)	Negative	Negative
Fluoride	<0.05 mg/dl	<0.027 mmol/L
Folic acid (Folate)	5-20 μg/ml	14-34 mmol/L
Follicle-stimulating hormone (FSH)	Men: 0.1-15.0 ImU/ml	
	Women: 6-30 ImU/ml	
	Children: 0.1-12.0 ImU/ml	
	Castrate and postmenopausal: 30-200 ImU/ml	
Free thyroxine index (FTI)	0.9-2.3 ng/dl	
Galactose-1-phosphate uridyl transferase	18.5-28.5 U/g hemoglobin	
Gammaglobulin	0.5-1.6 g/dl	
Gamma-glutamyl transpeptidase (GGTP)	Men: 8-38 U/L	5-40 U/L at 37°C
	Women: <45 years: 5-27 U/L	
Gastrin	40-150 pg/ml	40-150 ng/L
Glucagon	50-200 pg/ml	14-56 pmol/L
Glucose, fasting (FBS)	Adults: 70-115 mg/dl	3.89-6.38 mmol/L
	Children: 60-100 mg/dl	
	Newborns: 30-80 mg/dl	
Glucose, 2-hour postprandial (2-hour PPG)	<140 mg/dl	
Glucose-6-phosphate dehydrogenase (G-6-PD)	8.6-18.6 IU/g of hemoglobin	
Glucose tolerance test (GTT)	Fasting: 70-115 mg/dl	
	30 min: <200 mg/dl	
	1 hour: <200 mg/dl	
	2 hours: <140 mg/dl	
	3 hours: 70-115 mg/dl	
	4 hours: 70-115 mg/dl	
Glycosylated hemoglobin	Adults: 2.2%-4.8%	
	Children: 1.8%-4.0%	
	Good diabetic control: 2.5%-6%	
	Fair diabetic control: 6.1%-8%	
	Poor diabetic control: >8%	
Growth hormone	<10 ng/ml	<10 μg/L

From Pagana KD, Pagana TJ: Diagnostic testing and nursing implications: a case study approach, ed 5, St Louis, 1998, Mosby.

TABLE I-1 Normal Reference Laboratory Values (Adult)—cont'd
Blood, Plasma, or Serum Values

Test	Reference Range	
	Conventional Values	**SI Units***
Haptoglobin	100-150 mg/dl	16-31 μmol/L
Hematocrit (Hct)	Men: 42%-52%	
	Women: 37%-47% (pregnancy: >33%)	
	Children: 31%-43%	
	Infants: 30%-40%	
	Newborns: 44%-64%	
Hemoglobin (HgB)	Men: 14-18 g/dl	8.7-11.2 mmol/L
	Women: 12-16 g/dl (pregnancy: >11 g/dl)	7.4-9.9 mmol/L
	Children: 11-16 g/dl	
	Infants: 10-15 g/dl	
	Newborns: 14-24 g/dl	
Hemoglobin electrophoresis	Hgb A_1: 95%-98%	
	Hgb A_2: 2%-3%	
	Hgb F: 0.8%-2%	
	Hgb S: 0	
	Hgb C: 0	
Hepatitis B surface antigen (HBsAG)	Nonreactive	Nonreactive
Heterophil antibody	Negative	Negative
HLA-B27	None	None
Human chorionic gonadotropin (HCG)	Negative	Negative
Human placental lactogen (HPL)	Rise during pregnancy	
5-Hydroxyindoleacetic acid (5-HIAA)	2.8-8.0 mg/24 hours	
Immunoglobulin quantification	IgG: 550-1900 mg/dl	5.5-19.0 g/L
	IgA: 60-333 mg/dl	0.6-3.3 g/L
	IgM: 45-145 mg/dl	0.45-1.5 g/L
Insulin	4-20 μU/ml	36-179 pmol/L
Iron (Fe)	60-190 μg/dl	13-31 μmol/L
Iron-binding capacity, total (TIBC)	250-420 μg/dl	45-73 μmol/L
Iron (transferrin) saturation	30%-40%	
Ketone bodies	Negative	Negative
Lactic acid	0.6-1.8 mEq/L	
Lactic dehydrogenase (LDH) isoenzymes	90-200 ImU/ml	0.4-1.7 μmol/s/L
	LDH-1: 17%-27%	
	LDH-2: 28%-38%	
	LDH-3: 19%-27%	
	LDH-4: 5%-16%	
	LDH-5: 6%-16%	
Lead	120 μg/dl or less	<1.0 μmol/L
Leucine aminopeptidase (LAP)	Men: 80-200 U/ml	
	Women: 75-185 U/ml	
Leukocyte count (see Complete blood count)		
Lipase	Up to 1.5 units/ml	0-417 U/L
Lipids		
Total	400-1000 mg/dl	4-8 g/L
Cholesterol	150-250 mg/dl	3.9-6.5 mmol/L
Triglycerides	40-150 mg/dl	0.4-1.5 g/L
Phospholipids	150-380 mg/dl	1.9-3.9 mmol/L
Long-acting thyroid-stimulating hormone (LATS)	Negative	Negative
Magnesium (Mg)	1.6-3.0 mEq/L	0.8-1.3 mm/L
Methanol	Negative	Negative
Mononucleosis spot test	Negative	Negative

Continued

TABLE I-1 Normal Reference Laboratory Values (Adult)—cont'd
Blood, Plasma, or Serum Values

Test	Reference Range: Conventional Values	Reference Range: SI Units*
Nitrogen, nonprotein	15-35 mg/dl	10.7-25.0 mmol/L
Nuclear antibody (ANA)	Negative	Negative
5'-Nucleotidase	Up to 1.6 units	27-233 nmol/s/L
Osmolality	275-300 mOsm/kg	
Oxygen saturation (arterial)	95%-100%	0.95-1.00 of capacity
Parathormone (PTH)	<2000 pg/ml	
Partial thromboplastin time, activated (APTT)	30-40 sec	
Pco_2	35-45 mm Hg	
pH	7.35-7.45	7.35-7.45
Phenylalanine	Up to 2 mg/dl	<0.18 mmol/L
Phenylketonuria (PKU)	Negative	Negative
Phenytoin (Dilantin)	Therapeutic level: 10-20 µg/ml	
Phosphatase (acid)	0.10-0.63 U/ml (Bessey-Lowry) 0.5-2.0 U/ml (Bodansky) 1.0-4.0 U/ml (King-Armstrong)	0.11-0.60 U/L
Phosphatase (alkaline)	Adults: 30-85 ImU/ml Children and adolescents: <2 years: 85-235 ImU/ml 2-8 years: 65-210 ImU/ml 9-15 years: 60-300 ImU/ml (active bone growth) 16-21 years: 30-200 ImU/ml	20-90 units/L
Phospholipids (see Lipids)		
Phosphorus (P, PO_4)	Adults: 2.5-4.5 mg/dl Children: 3.5-5.8 mg/dl	0.78-1.52 mmol/L 1.29-2.26 mmol/L
Platelet count	150,000-400,000/mm^3	
Po_2	80-100 mm Hg	
Potassium (K)	3.5-5.0 mEq/L	3.5-5.0 mmol/L
Progesterone	Men, prepubertal girls, and postmenopausal women: <2 ng/ml Women, luteal: peak >5 ng/ml	6 nmol/L >16 nmol/L
Prolactin	2-15 ng/ml	2-15 µg/L
Prostate-specific antigen (PSA)	<4 ng/ml	
Protein (total)	6-8 g/dl	55-80 g/L
Albumin	3.2-4.5 g/dl	35-55 g/L
Globulin	2.3-3.4 g/dl	20-35 g/L
Prothrombin time (PT)	11.0-12.5 sec	11.0-12.5 sec
Pyruvate	0.3-0.9 mg/dl	34-103 µmol/L
Red blood cell count (see Complete blood count)		
Red blood cell indexes (see Complete blood count)		
Renin		
Reticulocyte count	Adults and children: 0.5%-2% of total erythrocytes Infants: 0.5%-3.1% of total erythrocytes Newborns: 2.5%-6.5% of total erythrocytes	
Rheumatoid factor	Negative	Negative
Salicylates	Negative Therapeutic: 20-25 mg/dl (to age 10: 25-30 mg/dl) Toxic: >30 mg/dl (after age 60: >20 mg/dl)	 1.4-1.8 mmol/L >2.2 mmol/L

From Pagana KD, Pagana TJ: Diagnostic testing and nursing implications: a case study approach, ed 5, St Louis, 1998, Mosby.

TABLE I-1 Normal Reference Laboratory Values (Adult)—cont'd
Blood, Plasma, or Serum Values

Test	Reference Range: Conventional Values	Reference Range: SI Units*
Schilling test (vitamin B_{12} absorption)	8%-40% excretion/24 hours	
Serologic test for syphilis (STS)	Negative (nonreactive)	
Serum glutamic oxaloacetic transaminase (SGOT, AST)	12-36 U/ml 5-40 IU/L	0.10-0.30 μmol/s/L
Serum glutamic-pyruvic transaminase (SGPT, ALT)	5-35 IU/L	0.05-0.43 μmol/s/L
Sickle cell	Negative	
Sodium (Na^+)	136-145 mEq/L	136-145 mmol/L
Sugar (see glucose)		
Syphilis (see Serologic test for syphilis, Fluorescent treponemal antibody, Venereal Disease Research Laboratory)		
Testosterone	Men: 300-1200 ng/dl Women: 30-95 ng/dl Prepubertal boys and girls: 5-20 ng/dl	10-42 nmol/L 1.1-3.3 nmol/L 0.165-0.70 nmol/L
Thymol flocculation	Up to 5 units	
Thyroglobulin antibody (see Antithyroglobulin antibody)		
Thyroid-stimulating hormone (TSH)	1-4 μU/ml Neonates: <25 μIU/ml by 3 days	5 m U/L
Thyroxine (T_4)	Murphy-Pattee: neonates: 10.1-20.1 μg/dl 1-6 years: 5.6-12.6 μg/dl 6-10 years: 4.9-11.7 μg/dl >10 years: 4-11 μg/dl Radioimmunoassay: 5-10 μg/dl	50-154 nmol/L
Thyroxine-binding globulin (TBG)	12-28 μg/ml	129-335 nmol/L
Transaminase (see Serum glutamic-oxaloacetic transaminase, Serum glutamic pyruvic transaminase)		
Triglycerides	40-150 mg/dl	0.4-1.5 g/L
Triiodothyronine (T_3)	110-230 ng/dl	1.2-1.5 nmol/L
Triiodothyronine (T_3) resin uptake	25%-35%	
Tubular phosphate reabsorption (TPR)	80%-90%	
Urea nitrogen (see Blood urea nitrogen)		
Uric acid	Men: 2.1-8.5 mg/dl Women: 2.0-6.6 mg/dl Children: 2.5-5.5 mg/dl	0.15-0.48 mmol/L 0.09-0.36 mmol/L
Venereal Disease Research Laboratory (VDRL)	Negative	Negative
Vitamin A	20-100 g/dl	0.7-3.5 μmol/L
Vitamin B_{12}	200-600 pg/ml	148-443 pmol/L
Vitamin C	0.6-1.6 mg/dl	23-57 μmol/L
Whole blood clot retraction (see Clot retraction)		
Zinc	50-150 μg/dl	

Continued

TABLE I-1 Normal Reference Laboratory Values (Adult)—cont'd
Urine Values

	Reference Range	
Test	**Conventional Values**	**SI Units***
Acetone plus acetoacetate (ketone bodies)	Negative	Negative
Addis count (12-hour)	Adults: WBCs and epithelial cells: 1.8 million/12 hours RBCs: 500,000/12 hours Hyaline casts: Up to 5000/12 hours Children: WBCs: <1 million/12 hours RBCs: <250,000/12 hours Casts: >5000/12 hours Protein: <20 mg/12 hours	Negative
Albumin	Random: ≤8 mg/dl 24-hour: 10-100 mg/24 hours	Negative 10-100 mg/24 hr
Aldosterone	2-16 μg/24 hours	5.5-72 nmol/24 hours
Alpha-aminonitrogen	0.4-1.0 g/24 hours	28-71 nmol/24 hours
Amino acid	50-200 mg/24 hours	
Ammonia (24-hour)	30-50 mEq/24 hours 500-1200 mg/24 hours	30-50 nmol/24 hours
Amylase	≤5000 Somogyi units/24 hours 3-35 IU/hour	6.5-48.1 U/hr
Arsenic (24-hour)	<50 μg/L	<0.65 mmol/L
Ascorbic acid (vitamin C)	Random: 1-7 ng/dl 24-hour: >50 mg/24 hours	0.06-0.40 mmol/L >0.29 mmol/24 hours
Bacteria	None	None
Bence Jones protein	Negative	Negative
Bilirubin	Negative	Negative
Blood or hemoglobin	Negative	Negative
Borate (24-hour)	<2 mg/L	<32 μmol/L
Calcium	Random: 1 + turbidity 24-hour: 1-300 mg (diet dependent)	1 + turbidity
Catecholamines (24-hour)	Epinephrine: 5-40 μg/24 hours Norepinephrine: 10-80 μg/24 hours Metanephrine: 24-96 μg/24 hours Normetanephrine: 75-375 μg/24 hours	<55 nmol/24 hours <590 nmol/24 hours 0.5-8.1 μmol/24 hours
Chloride (24-hour)	140-250 mEq/24 hours	140-250 mmol/24 hours
Color	Amber-yellow	Amber-yellow
Concentration test (Fishberg test)	Specific gravity: >1.025 Osmolality: 850 mOsm/L	>1.025 >850 mOsm/L
Copper (CU) (24-hour)	Up to 25 μg/24 hours	0-0.4 μmol/24 hours
Coproporphyrin (24-hour)	100-300 μg/24 hours	150-460 nmol/24 hours
Creatine	Adults: <100 mg/24 hours or 6% creatinine Pregnant women: ≤12% Infants <1 year: equal to creatinine Older children: ≤30% of creatinine	
Creatinine (24-hour)	15-25 mg/kg body wt/24 hours	0.13-0.22 nmol/kg^{-1} body wt/24 hours
Creatinine clearance (24-hour)	Men: 90-140 ml/min Women: 85-125 ml/min	90-140 ml/min 85-125 ml/min

From Pagana KD, Pagana TJ: Diagnostic testing and nursing implications: a case study approach, ed 5, St Louis, 1998, Mosby.

TABLE I-1 Normal Reference Laboratory Values (Adult)—cont'd
Urine Values

Test	Reference Range: Conventional Values	Reference Range: SI Units*
Crystals	Negative	Negative
Cystine or cysteine	Negative	Negative
Delta-aminolevulinic acid (ΔALA)	1-7 mg/24 hours	10-53 µmol/24 hours
Epinephrine (24-hour)	5-40 µg/24 hours	
Epithelial cells and casts	Occasional	Occasional
Estriol (24-hour)	>12 mg/24 hours	
Fat	Negative	Negative
Fluoride (24-hour)	<1 mg/24 hours	0.053 mmol/24 hours
Follicle-stimulating hormone (FSH) (24-hour)	Men: 2-12 IU/24 hours Women: During menses: 8-60 IU/24 hours During ovulation: 30-60 IU/24 hours During menopause: >50 IU/24 hours	
Glucose	Negative	Negative
Granular casts	Occasional	Occasional
Hemoglobin and myoglobin	Negative	Negative
Homogentisic acid	Negative	Negative
Human chorionic gonadotropin (HCG)	Negative	Negative
Hyaline casts	Occasional	Occasional
17-Hydroxycorticosteroids (17-OCHS) (24-hour)	Men: 5.5-15.0 mg/24 hours	8.3-25 µmol/24 hours
	Women: 5.0-13.5 mg/24 hours	5.5-22 µmol/24 hours
	Children: lower than adult values	
5-Hydroxyindoleacetic acid (5-HIAA, serotonin) (24-hour)	Men: 2-9 mg/24 hours	10-47 µmol/24 hours
	Women: lower than men	
Ketones (see acetone plus acetoacetate)		
17-Ketosteroids (17-KS) (24-hour)	Men: 8-15 mg/24 hours	21-62 µmol/24 hours
	Women: 6-12 mg/24 hours	14-45 µmol/24 hours
	Children: 12-15 yr: 5-12 mg/24 hours <12 yr: <5 mg/24 hours	
Lactose (24-hour)	14-40 mg/24 hours	41-116 µm
Lead	<0.08 g/ml or <120 g/24 hours	0.39 µmol/L
Leucine aminopeptidase (LAP)	2-18 U/24 hours	
Magnesium (24-hour)	6.8-8.5 mEq/24 hours	3.0-4.3 mmol/24 hours
Melanin	Negative	Negative
Odor	Aromatic	Aromatic
Osmolality	500-800 mOsm/L	38-1400 mmol/kg water
pH	4.6-8.0	4.6-8.0
Phenolsulfonphthalein (PSP)	15 min: at least 25%	At least 0.25
	30 min: at least 40%	At least 0.40
	120 min: at least 60%	At least 0.60
Phenylketonuria (PKU)	Negative	Negative
Phenylpyruvic acid	Negative	Negative
Phosphorus (24-hour)	0.9-1.3 g/24 hours	29-42 mmol/24 hours
Porphobilinogen	Random: negative 24-hour: up to 2 mg/24 hours	Negative

Continued

Table I-1 Normal Reference Laboratory Values (Adult)—cont'd
Urine Values

Test	Reference Range	
	Conventional Values	**SI Units***
Porphyrin (24-hour)	50-300 mg/24 hours	
Potassium (K^+) (24-hour)	25-100 mEq/24 hours	25-100 nmol/24 hours
Pregnancy test	Positive in normal pregnancy or with tumors producing HCG	Positive in normal pregnancy or with tumors producing HCG
Pregnanediol	After ovulation: >1 mg/24 hours	
Protein (albumin)	Random: ≤8 mg/dl	
	10-100 mg/24 hours	>0.05 g/24 hours
Sodium (Na^+) (24-hour)	100-260 mEq/24 hours	100-260 nmol/24 hours
Specific gravity	1.010-1.025	1.010-1.025
Steroids (see 17-Hydroxycorticosteroids, 17-Ketosteroids)		
Sugar (see Glucose)		
Titratable acidity (24-hour)	20-50 mEq/24 hours	20-50 mmol/24 hours
Turbidity	Clear	Clear
Urea nitrogen (24-hour)	6-17 g/24 hours	0.21-0.60 mol/24 hours
Uric acid (24-hour)	250-750 mg/24 hours	1.48-4.43 mmol/24 hours
Urobilinogen	0.1-1.0 Ehrlich U/dl	0.1-1.0 Ehrlich U/dl
Uroporphyrin	Negative	Negative
Vanillylmandelic acid (VMA) (24-hour)	1-9 mg/24 hours	<40 μmol/day
Zinc (24-hour)	0.20-0.75 mg/24 hours	

From Pagana KD, Pagana TJ: Diagnostic testing and nursing implications: a case study approach, ed 5, St Louis, 1998, Mosby.

TABLE I-2 Selected Neonatal and Pediatric Reference Values

Test/Specimen	Age/Sex/ Reference	Conventional Units		International Units (SI)	
		Normal Ranges			
Acetaminophen					
Serum or plasma	Therap. conc.	10-30 μg/ml		66-200 μmol/L	
	Toxic Conc.	>200 μg/ml		>1300 μmol/L	
Ammonia nitrogen					
Plasma or serum	Newborn	90-150 μg/dl		64-107 μmol/L	
	0-2 weeks	79-129 μg/dl		56-92 μmol/L	
	>1 month	29-70 μg/dl		21-50 μmol/L	
	Thereafter	15-45 μg/dl		11-32 μmol/L	
Urine, 24-hour		500-1200 mg/d		36-86 mmol/d	
Antistreptolysin O titer (ASO)					
Serum	2-4 years	<160 Todd units			
	School-age children	170-330 Todd units			
Base excess					
Whole blood	Newborn	(−10) - (−2) mEq/L		(−10) - (−2) mmol/L	
	Infant	(−7) - (−1) mEq/L		(−7) - (−1) mmol/L	
	Child	(−4) - (+2) mEq/L		(−4) - (+2) mmol/L	
	Thereafter	(−3) - (+3) mEq/L		(−3) - (+3) mmol/L	
Bicarbonate (HCO_3)					
Serum	Arterial	21-28 mEq/L		21-28 mmol/L	
	Venous	22-29 mEq/L		22-29 mmol/L	
		Premature (mg/dl)	**Full Term (mg/dl)**	**Premature (μmol/L)**	**Full Term (μmol/L)**
Bilirubin, total					
Serum	Cord	<2.0	<2.0	<34	<34
	0.1 day	8.0	<6.0	<137	<103
	1-2 day	12.0	<8.0	<205	<137
	2-5 day	16.0	<12.0	<274	<205
	Thereafter	2.0	0.2-1.0	<34	3.4-17.1
Bilirubin, direct (conjugated)					
Serum		0.0-0.2 mg/dl		0-3.4 μmol/L	
Bleeding time					
Blood from skin puncture					
Ivy	Normal	2-7 min		2-7 min	
	Borderline	7-11 min		7-11 min	
Simplate (G-D)		2.75-8 min		2.75-8 min	
Blood volume					
Whole blood	Male	52-83 ml/kg		0.052-0.083 L/kg	
	Female	50-75 ml/kg		0.050-0.075 L/kg	
C-reactive protein (CRP)					
Serum	Cord	52-1330 ng/ml		52-1330 μg/L	
	Adult	67-1800 ng/ml		67-1800 μg/L	

Modified from Behrman RE et al: *Nelson's textbook of pediatrics,* ed 14, Philadelphia, 1992, WB Saunders. In Wong DL: *Whaley & Wong's essentials of pediatric nursing,* ed 5, St Louis, 1997, Mosby.

Cholesterol, total serum or plasma reference National Cholesterol Education program: Report of the expert panel on blood cholesterol levels in children and adolescents, *Pediatrics* 89 (3 pt. 2): 527, 1992.

Potassium ranges are referenced from Johns Hopkins Hospital: The Harriet Lane handbook, ed 12, St Louis, 1992, Mosby.

Continued

TABLE I-2 Selected Neonatal and Pediatric Reference Values—cont'd

Test/Specimen	Age/Sex/ Reference	Conventional Units	International Units (SI)
		Normal Ranges	
Calcium, ionized			
Serum, plasma, or whole blood	Cord	50-60 mg/dl	1.25-1.50 mmol/L
	Newborn, 3-24 hours	4.3-5.1 mg/dl	1.07-1.27 mmol/L
	24-48 hr	4.0-4.7 mg/dl	1.00-1.17 mmol/L
	Thereafter	4.8-4.92 mg/dl or 2.24-2.46 mEq/L	1.12-1.23 mmol/L
Calcium, total			
Serum	Cord	9.0-11.5 mg/dl	2.25-2.88 mmol/L
	Newborn, 3-24 hours	9.0-10.6 mg/dl	2.3-2.65 mmol/L
	24-48 hours	7.0-12.0 mg/dl	1.75-3.0 mmol/L
	4-7 days	9.0-10.9 mg/dl	2.25-2.73 mmol/L
	Child	8.8-10.8 mg/dl	2.2-2.70 mmol/L
	Thereafter	8.4-10.2 mg/dl	2.1-2.55 mmol/L
Carbon dioxide, partial pressure (Pco_2)			
Whole blood, arterial	Newborn	27-40 mm Hg	3.6-5.3 kPa
	Infant	27-41 mm Hg	3.6-5.5 kPa
	Thereafter: Male	35-48 mm Hg	4.7-6.4 kPa
	Female	32-45 mm Hg	4.3-6.0 kPa
Carbon dioxide, total (tCO_2)			
Serum or plasma	Cord	14-22 mEq/L	14-22 mmol/L
	Premature (1 week)	14-27 mEq/L	14-27 mmol/L
	Newborn	13-22 mEq/L	13-22 mmol/L
	Infant, child	20-28 mEq/L	20-28 mmol/L
	Thereafter	23-30 mEq/L	23-30 mmol/L
Cerebrospinal fluid (CSF)			
Pressure		70-180 mm water	70-180 mm water
Volume	Child	60-100 ml	0.06-0.10 L
Chloride			
Serum or plasma	Cord	96-104 mEq/L	96-104 mmol/L
	Newborn	97-110 mEq/L	97-110 mmol/L
	Thereafter	98-106 mEq/L	98-106 mmol/L
Sweat	Normal (homozygote)	<40 mEq/L	<40 mmol/L
	Marginal (e.g., asthma, Addison disease, malnutrition)	45-60 mEq/L	45-60 mmol/L
	Cystic fibrosis	>60 mmol/L	>60 mmol/L
Cholesterol, total			
Serum or plasma*	Acceptable	<170 mg/dl	<4.4 mmol/L
	Borderline	170-199 mg/dl	4.4-5.1 mmol/L
	High	≥200 mg/dl	≥5.2 mmol/L

Modified from Behrman RE et al: *Nelson's textbook of pediatrics,* ed 14, Philadelphia, 1992, WB Saunders. In Wong DL: *Whaley & Wong's essentials of pediatric nursing,* ed 5, St Louis, 1997, Mosby.

Table I-2 Selected Neonatal and Pediatric Reference Values—cont'd

Test/Specimen	Age/Sex/ Reference	Conventional Units (Normal Ranges)	International Units (SI) (Normal Ranges)
Clotting time (Lee-White)			
Whole blood		5-8 min (glass tubes)	5-8 min
		5-15 min (room temp)	5-15 min
		30 min (silicone tube)	30 min
Creatine kinase (CK, CPK)			
Serum	Cord blood	70-380 U/L	70-380 U/L
	5-8 hours	214-1175 U/L	214-1175 U/L
	24-33 hours	130-1200 U/L	130-1200 U/L
	72-100 hours	87-725 U/L	87-725 U/L
Creatinine			
Serum	Cord	0.6-1.2 mg/dl	53-106 μmol/L
	Newborn	0.3-1.0 mg/dl	27-88 μmol/L
	Infant	0.2-0.4 mg/dl	18-35 μmol/L
	Child	0.3-0.7 mg/dl	27-62 μmol/L
	Adolescent	0.5-1.0 mg/dl	44-88 μmol/L
Urine, 24-hour	Premature	8.1-15.0 mg/kg/24 hr	72-133 μmol/kg/24 hr
	Full term	10.4-19.7 mg/kg/24 hr	92-174 μmol/kg/24 hr
	1.5-7 years	10-15 mg/kg/24 hr	88-133 μmol/kg/24 hr
	7-15 years	5.2-41 mg/kg/24 hr	46-362 μmol/kg/24 hr
Creatinine clearance (endogenous)			
Serum or plasma and urine	Newborn	40-65 ml/min/1.73 m^2	
	<40 years: Male	97-137 ml/min/1.73 m^2	
	Female	88-128 ml/min/1.73 m^2	
Digoxin			
Serum, plasma; collect at least 12 hr after dose	Therap. conc.		
	CHF	0.8-1.5 ng/ml	1.0-1.9 nmol/L
	Arrhythmias	1.5-2.0 ng/ml	1.9-2.6 nmol/L
	Toxic conc.		
	Child	>2.5 ng/ml	>3.2 nmol/L
Eosinophil count			
Whole blood, capillary blood		50-350 cells/mm^3 (μl)	50-350 × 10^6 cells/L
Erythrocyte (RBC) count			
Whole blood	Cord	3.9-5.5 million/mm^3	3.9-5.5 × 10^{12} cells/L
	1-3 days	4.0-6.6 million/mm^3	4.0-6.6 × 10^{12} cells/L
	1 week	3.9-6.3 million/mm^3	3.9-6.3 × 10^{12} cells/L
	2 weeks	3.6-6.2 million/mm^3	3.6-6.2 × 10^{12} cells/L
	1 month	3.0-5.4 million/mm^3	3.0-5.4 × 10^{12} cells/L
	2 months	2.7-4.9 million/mm^3	2.7-4.5 × 10^{12} cells/L
	3-6 months	3.1-4.5 million/mm^3	3.1-4.5 × 10^{12} cells/L
	0.5-2 years	3.7-5.3 million/mm^3	3.7-5.3 l× 10^{12} cells/L
	2-6 years	3.9-5.3 million/mm^3	3.9-5.3 × 10^{12} cells/L
	6-12 years	4.0-5.2 million/mm^3	4.0-5.2 × 10^{12} cells/L
	12-18 years: Male	4.5-5.3 million/mm^3	4.5-5.3 × 10^{12} cells/L
	Female	4.1-5.1 million/mm^3	4.1-5.1 × 10^{12} cells/L

Continued

Table I-2 Selected Neonatal and Pediatric Reference Values—cont'd

Test/Specimen	Age/Sex/Reference	Conventional Units		International Units (SI)	
		Normal Ranges			
Erythrocyte sedimentation rate (ESR)					
Whole blood					
Westergren (modified)	Child	0-10 mm/hr		0-10 mm/hr	
	<50 years: Male	0-15 mm/hr		0-15 mm/hr	
	Female	0-20 mm/hr		0-20 mm/hr	
Wintrobe	Child	0-13 mm/hr		0-13 mm/hr	
Fibrinogen					
Plasma	Newborn	125-300 mg/dl		1.25-3.00 g/L	
	Thereafter	200-400 mg/dl		2.00-4.00 g/L	
Galactose					
Serum	Newborn	0-20 mg/dl		0-1.11 mmol/L	
	Thereafter	<5 mg/dl		<0.03 mmol/L	
Urine	Newborn	≤60 mg/dl		≤3.33 mmol/L	
	Thereafter	<14 mg/dl		<0.08 mmol/d	
Glucose					
Serum	Cord	45-96 mg/dl		2.5-5.3 mmol/L	
	Newborn, 1 d	40-60 mg/dl		2.2-3.3 mmol/L	
	Newborn, >1 d	50-90 mg/dl		2.8-5.0 mmol/L	
	Child	60-100 mg/dl		3.3-5.5 mmol/L	
	Thereafter	70-105 mg/dl		3.9-5.8 mmol/L	
Urine (quantitative)		<0.5 g/d		<2.8 mmol/d	
(Qualitative)		Negative		Negative	
Glucose tolerance test (GTT), oral					
Serum					
Dosages		**Normal**	**Diabetic**	**Normal**	**Diabetic**
Child: 1.75 g/kg of ideal weight up to maximum of 75 g	60 min	120-170 mg/dl	≥200 mg/dl	6.7-9.4 mg/dl	≥11 mmol/L
	90 min	100-140 mg/dl	≥200 mg/dl	5.6-7.8 mg/dl	≥11 mmol/L
	120 min	70-120 mg/dl	≥140 mg/dl	3.9-6.7 mg/dl	≥7.8 mmol/L
Growth hormone (hGH, somatotropin)					
Plasma	Cord	10-50 ng/ml		10-50 μg/L	
Fasting, at rest	Newborn	10-40 ng/ml		10-40 μg/L	
	Child	<5 ng/ml		<5 μg/L	
Hematocrit (HCT, Hct)					
Whole blood	1 day (cap)	48%-69%		0.48-0.69 vol. fraction	
	2 day	48%-75%		0.48-0.75 vol. fraction	
	3 day	44%-72%		0.44-0.72 vol. fraction	
	2 month	28%-42%		0.28-0.42 vol. fraction	
	6-12 years	35%-45%		0.35-0.45 vol. fraction	
	12-18 years: Male	37%-49%		0.37-0.49 vol. fraction	
	Female	36%-46%		0.36-0.46 vol. fraction	

Modified from Behrman RE et al: *Nelson's textbook of pediatrics,* ed 14, Philadelphia, 1992, WB Saunders. In Wong DL: *Whaley & Wong's essentials of pediatric nursing,* ed 5, St Louis, 1997, Mosby.

TABLE I-2 Selected Neonatal and Pediatric Reference Values—cont'd

Test/Specimen	Age/Sex/ Reference	Conventional Units	International Units (SI)
		Normal Ranges	
Hemoglobin (Hb)			
Whole blood	1-3 day (cap)	14.5-22.5 g/dl	2.25-3.49 mmol/L
	2 months	9.0-14.0 g/dl	1.40-2.17 mmol/L
	6-12 years	11.5-15.5 g/dl	1.78-2.40 mmol/L
	12-18 years: Male	13.0-16.0 g/dl	2.02-2.48 mmol/L
	Female	12.0-16.0 g/dl	1.86-2.48 mmol/L
Hemoglobin A			
Whole blood		>95% of total	0.95 fraction of Hb
Hemoglobin F			
Whole blood	1 day	63%-92% HbF	0.62-0.92 mass fraction HbF
	5 days	65%-88% HbF	0.65-0.88 mass fraction HbF
	3 weeks	55%-85% HbF	0.55-0.85 mass fraction HbF
	6-9 weeks	31%-75% HbF	0.31-0.75 mass fraction HbF
	3-4 months	<2%-59% HbF	<0.02-0.59 mass fraction HbF
	6 months	<2%-9% HbF	<0.02-0.09 mass fraction Hbf
	Adult	<2.0% HbF	<0.02 mass fraction HbF
Immunoglobulin A (IgA)			
Serum	Cord blood	1.4-3.6 mg/dl	14-36 mg/L
	1-3 months	1.3-53 mg/dl	13-530 mg/L
	4-6 months	4.4-84 mg/dl	44-840 mg/L
	7 months-1 year	11-106 mg/dl	110-1060 mg/L
	2-5 years	14-159 mg/dl	140-1590 mg/L
	6-10 years	33-236 mg/dl	330-2360 mg/L
Immunoglobulin D (IgD)			
Serum	Newborn	None detected	None detected
	Thereafter	0-8 mg/dl	0-80 mg/L
Immunoglobulin E (IgE)			
Serum	M	0-230 IU/ml	0-230 kIU/L
	F	0-170 IU/ml	0-170 kIU/L
Immunoglobulin G (IgG)			
Serum	Cord blood	636-1606 mg/dl	6.36-16.06 g/L
	1 month	251-906 mg/dl	2.51-9.06 g/L
	2-4 months	176-601 mg/dl	1.76-60.1 g/L
	5-12 months	172-1069 mg/dl	1.72-10.69 g/L
	1-5 years	345-1236 mg/dl	3.45-12.36 g/L
	6-10 years	608-1572 mg/dl	6.08-15.72 g/L
Immunoglobulin M (IgM)			
Serum	Cord blood	6.3-25 mg/dl	63-250 mg/L
	1-4 months	17-105 mg/dl	170-1050 mg/L
	5-9 months	33-126 mg/dl	330-1260 mg/L
	10 months-1 year	41-173 mg/dl	410-1730 mg/L
	2-8 years	43-207 mg/dl	430-2070 mg/L
	9-10 years	52-242 mg/dl	520-2420 mg/L

Continued

TABLE I-2 Selected Neonatal and Pediatric Reference Values—cont'd

Test/Specimen	Age/Sex/Reference	Conventional Units		International Units (SI)
		Normal Ranges		
Iron				
Serum	Newborn	100-250 μg/dl		17.90-44.75 μmol/L
	Infant	40-100 μg/dl		7.16-1790 μmol/L
	Child	50-120 μg/dl		8.95-21.48 μmol/L
	Thereafter: Male	50-160 μg/dl		8.95-28.64 μmol/L
	Female	40-150 μg/dl		7.16-26.85 μmol/L
	Intoxicated child	280-2550 μ/dl		50.12-456.5 μmol/L
	Fatally poisoned child	>1800 μg/dl		>322.2 μmol/L
Iron-binding capacity, total (TIBC)				
Serum	Infant	100-400 μg/dl		17.90-71.60 μmol/L
	Thereafter	250-400 μg/dl		44.75-71.60 μmol/L
Lead				
Whole blood	Child	<10 μg/dl		<0.48 μmol/L
Urine, 24 hr		<80 μg/L		<0.39 μmol/L
Leukocyte count (WBC count)		**$\times$1000 cells/mm^3 (μl)**		**$\times 10^9$ cells/L**
Whole blood	Birth	9.0-30.0		9.0-30.0
	24 hours	9.4-34.0		9.4-34.0
	1 month	5.0-19.5		5.0-19.5
	1-3 years	6.0-17.5		6.0-17.5
	4-7 years	5.5-15.5		5.5-15.5
	8-13 years	4.5-13.5		4.5-13.5
		$\times$1000 cells/mm^3 (μl)		**$\times 10^6$ cells/L**
CSF	Premature	0-25 mononuclear		0-25
		0-100 polymorphonuclear		0-100
		0-1000 RBC		0-1000
	Newborn	0-20 mononuclear		0-20
		0-70 polymorphonuclear		0-70
		0-800 RBC		0-800
	Neonate	0-5 mononuclear		0-5
		0-25 polymorphonuclear		0-25
		0-50 RBC		0-50
	Thereafter	0-5 mononuclear		0-5
Leukocyte differential count				
Whole blood	Myelocytes	0%	0 cells/mm^3 (μl)	Number fraction 0
	Neutrophils—"bands"	3%-5%	150-400 cells/mm^3 (μl)	Number fraction 0.03-0.05
	Neutrophils—"segs"	54%-62%	3000-5800 cells/mm^3 μl)	Number fraction 0.54-0.62
	Lymphocytes	25%-33%	1500-3000 cells/mm^3 (μl)	Number fraction 0.25-0.33
	Monocytes	3%-7%	285-500 cells/mm^3 (μl)	Number fraction 0.03-0.07
	Eosinophils	1%-3%	50-250 cells/mm^3 (μl)	Number fraction 0.01-0.03
	Basophils	0%-0.75%	15-50 cells/mm^3 (μl)	Number fraction 0-0.0075

Modified from Behrman RE et al: *Nelson's textbook of pediatrics,* ed 14, Philadelphia, 1992, WB Saunders. In Wong DL: *Whaley & Wong's essentials of pediatric nursing,* ed 5, St Louis, 1997, Mosby.

TABLE I-2 Selected Neonatal and Pediatric Reference Values—cont'd

Test/Specimen	Age/Sex/Reference	Conventional Units	International Units (SI)
		Normal Ranges	
Mean corpuscular hemoglobin (MCH)			
Whole blood	Birth	31-37 pg/cell	0.48-0.57 fmol/L
	1-3 days (cap)	31-37 pg/cell	0.48-0.57 fmol/L
	1 week-1 month	28-40 pg/cell	0.43-0.62 fmol/L
	2 months	26-34 pg/cell	0.40-0.53 fmol/L
	3-6 months	25-35 pg/cell	0.39-0.54 fmol/L
	0.5-2 years	23-31 pg/cell	0.36-0.48 fmol/L
	2-6 years	24-30 pg/cell	0.37-0.47 fmol/L
	6-12 years	25-33 pg/cell	0.39-0.51 fmol/L
	12-18 years	25-35 pg/cell	0.39-0.54 fmol/L
Mean corpuscular hemoglobin concentration (MCHC)			
Whole blood	Birth	30%-36% Hb/cell or Hb/dl RBC	4.65-5.58 mmol or Hb/L RBC
	1-3 days (cap)	29%-37% Hb/cell or g Hb/dl RBC	4.50-5.74 mmol or Hb/L RBC
	1-2 weeks	28%-38% Hb/cell or g Hb/dl RBC	4.34-5.89 mmol or Hb/L RBC
	1-2 months	29%-37% Hb/cell or g Hb/dl RBC	4.50-5.74 mmol or Hb/L RBC
	3 months-2 years	30%-36% Hb/cell or g Hb/dl RBC	4.65-5.58 mmol or Hb/L RBC
	2-18 years	31%-37% Hb/cell or g Hb/dl RBC	4.81-5.74 mmol or Hb/L RBC
Mean corpuscular volume (MCV)			
Whole blood	1-3 days (cap)	95-121 μm^3	95-121 fl
	0.5-2 years	70-86 μm^3	70-86 fl
	6-12 years	77-95 μm^3	77-95 fl
	12-18 years: Male	78-98 μm^3	78-98 fl
	Female	78-102 μm^3	78-102 fl
Osmolality			
Serum	Child, adult:	275-295 mOsmol/kg H_2O	
Urine, random		50-1400 mOsmol/kg H_2O, depending on fluid intake; after 12 hr fluid restriction: >850 mOsmol/kg H_2O	
Urine, 24 hr		≈ 300-900 mOsmol/kg H_2O	
Oxygen, partial pressure (Po_2)			
Whole blood, arterial	Birth	8-24 mm Hg	1.1-3.2 kPa
	5-10 min	33-75 mm Hg	4.4-10.0 kPa
	30 min	31-85 mm Hg	4.1-11.3 kPa
	>1 hour	55-80 mm Hg	7.3-10.6 kPa
	1 day	54-95 mm Hg	7.2-12.6 kPa
	Thereafter (decreased with age)	83-108 mm Hg	11-14.4 kPa
Oxygen saturation (Sao_2)			
Whole blood, arterial	Newborn	85%-90%	Fraction saturated 0.85-0.90
	Thereafter	95%-99%	Fraction saturated 0.95-0.99

Continued

Table I-2 Selected Neonatal and Pediatric Reference Values—cont'd

Test/Specimen	Age/Sex/Reference	Conventional Units (Normal Ranges)	International Units (SI) (Normal Ranges)
Partial thromboplastin time (PTT)			
Whole blood (Na citrate)			
Nonactivated		60-85 s (Platelin)	60-85 s
Activated		25-35 s (differs with method)	25-35 s
pH			H^+ concentration:
Whole blood, arterial	Premature (48 hours)	7.35-7.50	31-44 nmol/L
	Birth, full term	7.11-7.36	43-77 nmol/L
	5-10 min	7.09-7.30	50-81 nmol/L
	30 min	7.21-7.38	41-61 nmol/L
	>1 hour	7.26-7.49	32-54 nmol/L
	1 day	7.29-7.45	35-51 nmol/L
	Thereafter	7.35-7.45	35-44 nmol/L
	Must be corrected for body temperature		
Urine, random	Newborn/neonate	5-7	0.1-10 µmol/L
	Thereafter	4.5-8	0.01-32 µmol/L
	(average ≃ 6)	7.0-7.5	(average ≃ 1.0 µmol/L)
Stool			31-100 nmol/L
Phenylalanine			
Serum	Premature	2.0-7.5 mg/dl	120-450 µmol/L
	Newborn	1.2-3.4 mg/dl	70-210 µmol/L
	Thereafter	0.8-1.8 mg/dl	50-110 µmol/L
Urine, 24-hour	10 days-2 weeks	1-2 mg/d	6-12 µmol/d
	3-12 years	4-18 mg/d	24-110 µmol/d
	Thereafter	trace-17 mg/d	trace-103 µmol/d
Plasma volume			
Plasma	Male	25-43 ml/kg	0.025-0.043 L/kg
	Female	28-45 ml/kg	0.028-0.045 L/kg
Platelet count (thrombocyte count)			
Whole blood (EDTA)	Newborn (After 1 week, same as adult)	$84\text{-}478 \times 10^3/mm^3$ (µl)	$84\text{-}478 \times 10^9/L$
	Adult	$150\text{-}400 \times 10^3/mm^3$ (µl)	$150\text{-}400 \times 10^9/L$
Potassium*			
Serum	Newborn	3.0-6.0 mEq/L	3.0-6.0 mmol/L
	Thereafter	3.5-5.0 mEq/L	3.5-5.0 mmol/L
Plasma (heparin)		3.4-4.5 mEq/L	3.4-4.5 mmol/L
Urine, 24 hr		2.5-125 mEq/d varies with diet	2.5-125 mmol/L
Protein			
Serum, total	Premature	4.3-7.6 g/dl	43-76 g/L
	Newborn	4.6-7.4 g/dl	46-74 g/L
	1-7 years	6.1-7.9 g/dl	61-79 g/L
	8-12 years	6.4-8.1 g/dl	64-81 g/L
	13-19 years	6.6-8.2 g/dl	66-82 g/L

Modified from Behrman RE et al: *Nelson's textbook of pediatrics*, ed 14, Philadelphia, 1992, WB Saunders. In Wong DL: *Whaley & Wong's essentials of pediatric nursing*, ed 5, St Louis, 1997, Mosby.

TABLE I-2 Selected Neonatal and Pediatric Reference Values—cont'd

Test/Specimen	Age/Sex/ Reference	Conventional Units	International Units (SI)
		Normal Ranges	
Protein—cont'd			
Total			
Urine, 24 hr		1-14 mg/dl	10-140 mg/L
		50-80 mg/d (at rest)	50-80 mg/d
		<250 mg/d after intense exercise	<250 mg/d after exercise
Total			
CSF		Lumbar: 8-32 mg/dl	80-320 mg/L
Prothrombin time (PT)			
One-stage (Quick)			
Whole blood (Na citrate)	In general	11-15 s (varies with type of thromboplastin)	11-15 s
	Newborn	Prolonged by 2-3 sec	Prolonged by 2-3 sec
Two-stage modified (Ware and Seegers)			
Whole blood (Na citrate)		18-22 sec	18-22 sec
RBC count, see erythrocyte count			
Red blood cell volume			
Whole blood	Male	20-36 ml/kg	0.020-0.036 L/kg
	Female	19-31 ml/kg	0.019-0.031 L/kg
Reticulocyte count			
Whole blood	Adults	0.5%-1.5% of erythrocytes or 25,000-75,000/mm^3 (μl)	0.005-0.015 (number fraction) 25,000-75,000 × 10^6/L
Capillary	1 day	0.4%-6.0%	0.004-0.060 (number fraction)
	7 days	<0.1%-1.3%	<0.001-0.013 (number fraction)
	1-4 weeks	<0.1%-1.2%	<0.001-0.012 (number fraction)
	5-6 weeks	<0.1%-2.4%	<0.001-0.024 (number fraction)
	7-8 weeks	0.1%-2.9%	0.001-0.029 (number fraction)
	9-10 weeks	<0.1%-2.6%	<0.001-0.026 (number fraction)
	11-12 weeks	0.1%-1.3%	0.001-0.013 (number fraction)
Salicylates			
Serum, plasma	Therap. conc.	15-30 mg/dl	1.1-2.2 mmol/L
	Toxic conc.	>30 mg/dl	>2.2 mmol/L
Sedimentation rate: see erythrocyte sedimentation rate			
Sodium			
Serum or plasma	Newborn	136-146 mEq/L	134-146 mmol/L
	Infant	139-146 mEq/L	139-146 mmol/L
	Child	138-145 mEq/L	138-145 mmol/L
	Thereafter	136-146 mEq/L	136-146 mmol/L
Urine, 24 hr		40-220 mEq/L (diet dependent)	40-220 mmol/L
Sweat	Normal	<40 mEq/L	<40 mmol/L
	Indeterminate	45-60 mEq/L	45-60 mmol/L
	Cystic fibrosis	>60 mEq/L	>60 mmol/L

Continued

TABLE I-2 Selected Neonatal and Pediatric Reference Values—cont'd

Test/Specimen	Age/Sex/Reference	Conventional Units		International Units (SI)	
		Normal Ranges			
Specific gravity					
Urine, random	Adult	1.002-1.030		1.002-1.030	
	After 12 hour fluid restriction	>1.025		>1.025	
Urine, 24 hr		1.015-1.025			
Theophylline					
Serum, plasma	Therap. conc.				
	Bronchodilator	10-20 µg/ml		56-110 µmol/L	
	Premature apnea	6-10 µg/ml		28-56 µmol/L	
	Toxic conc.	>20		>166 µmol/L	
Thrombin time					
Whole blood (Na citrate)		Control time ± 2 sec when control is 9-13 sec		Control time ± 2 sec when control is 9-13 sec	
Thyroxine, total (T_3)					
Serum	Cord	8-13 µg/dl		103-168 nmol/L	
	Newborn	11.5-24 (lower in low-birth-weight infants)		148-310 nmol/L	
	Neonate	9-18 µg/dl		116-232 nmol/L	
	Infant	7-15 µg/dl		90-194 nmol/L	
	1-5 years	7.3-15 µg/dl		94-194 nmol/L	
	5-10 years	6.4-13.3 µg/dl		83-172 nmol/L	
	Thereafter	5-12 µg/dl		65-155 nmol/L	
	Newborn screen (filter paper)	6.2-22 µg/dl		80-284 nmol/L	
Tourniquet test (capillary fragility)		<5-10 petechiae in 2.5 cm circle on forearm (halfway between systolic and diastolic); pressure for 5 min; 0-8 petechiae in 6 cm circle (50 torr for 15 min); 10-20 petechiae in 5 cm circle (80 mm Hg)		<5-10 petechiae in 2.5 cm circle on forearm (halfway between systolic and diastolic); pressure for 5 min; 0-8 petechiae in 6 cm circle (50 torr for 15 min); 10-20 petechiae in 5 cm circle (80 mm Hg)	
Triglycerides (TG)					
Serum, after ≥12-hour fast					
		mg/dl		g/L	
		M	F	M	F
	Cord blood	10-98	10-98	0.10-0.98	0.10-0.98
	0-5 years	30-86	32-99	0.30-0.86	0.32-0.99
	6-11 years	31-108	35-114	0.31-1.08	0.35-1.14
	12-15 years	36-138	41-138	0.36-1.38	0.41-1.38
	16-19 years	40-163	40-128	0.40-1.63	0.40-1.28
Triiodothyronine, free					
Serum	Cord	20-240 pg/dl		0.3-3.7 pmol/L	
	1-3 days	200-610 pg/dl		3.1-9.4 pmol/L	
	6 weeks	240-560 pg/dl		3.7-8.6 pmol/L	

Modified from Behrman RE et al: *Nelson's textbook of pediatrics,* ed 14, Philadelphia, 1992, WB Saunders. In Wong DL: *Whaley & Wong's essentials of pediatric nursing,* ed 5, St Louis, 1997, Mosby.

TABLE I-2 Selected Neonatal and Pediatric Reference Values—cont'd

Test/Specimen	Age/Sex/ Reference	Conventional Units	International Units (SI)
		Normal Ranges	
Triiodothyronine, total (T_3-RIA)			
Serum	Cord	30-70 ng/dl	0.46-1.08 nmol/L
	Newborn	72-260 ng/dl	1.16-4.00 nmol/L
	1-5 years	100-260 ng/dl	1.54-4.00 nmol/L
	5-10 years	90-240 ng/dl	1.39-3.70 nmol/L
	10-15 years	80 210 ng/dl	1.23-3.23 nmol/L
	Thereafter	115-190 ng/dl	1.77-2.93 nmol/L
Urea nitrogen			
Serum or plasma	Cord	21-40 mg/dl	7.5-14.3 mmol urea/L
	Premature (1 week)	3-25 mg/dl	1.1-9 mmol urea/L
	Newborn	3-12 mg/dl	1.1-4.3 mmol urea/L
	Infant/child	5-18 mg/dl	1.8-6.4 mmol urea/L
	Thereafter	7-18 mg/dl	2.5-6.4 mmol urea/L
Urine volume			
Urine, 24-hour	Newborn	50-300 ml/d	0.050-0.300 L/d
	Infant	350-550 ml/d	0.350-0.500 L/d
	Child	500-1000 ml/d	0.500-1.000 L/d
	Adolescent	700-1400 ml/d	0.700-1.400 L/d
WBC, see leukocyte			

Appendix

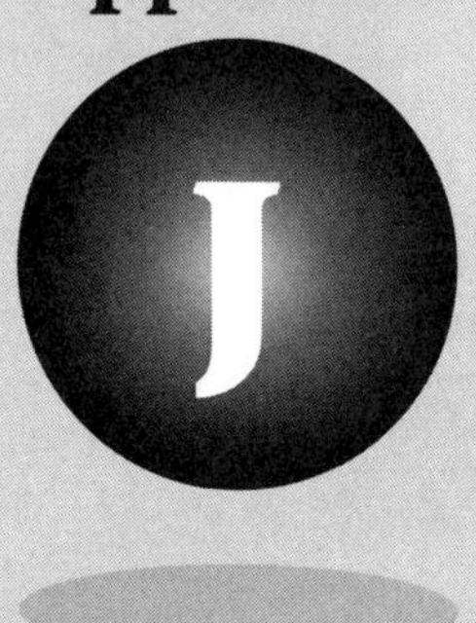

Nonsteroidal Antiinflammatory Drugs (NSAIDs)

NSAIDs are effective analgesic and anti-inflammatory drugs, but they cause adverse effects in susceptible patients. Careful evaluation of the risks and benefits, and monitoring of adverse effects is important. Discussion of the various nonsteroidal antiinflammatory drugs (NSAIDs) is included, along with suggestions for safe clinical use.

Characteristics of NSAIDs:

- Not effective for severe pain due to ceiling effect
- Analgesic at lower doses, and antiinflammatory at higher doses
- Non-addicting
- Little to no sedative effect or respiratory depression
- Increase risk for drug interactions due to high protein binding
- Block platelet aggregation (Amadio P, Cummings D, Amadio PL: NSAIDs revisited, *Postgrad Med* 101(2): 259, 1997.)

Recommendations for safe clinical use:

- NSAIDs should be included as part of a therapeutic plan, not the only treatment.
- Analgesic dose is ½ of antiinflammatory dose.
- Consider using acetaminophen to provide initial analgesia initially as inflammation resolves.
- Consider using once a day formulations to increase compliance.
- Prescribe only one NSAID at a time to avoid increased side effects. Always ask about over-the-counter use.
- Anticipate drug interactions: warfarin (Coumadin), oral hypoglycemics, and anticonvulsants.
- Be aware of PMH that may impact the use of NSAIDs: peptic ulcer disease (PUD), renal disease, hepatic dysfunction, or cardiovascular disease. Elderly patients may be at higher risk for toxic effects.
- Take NSAIDs with/after meals or with antacid. Cytoprotective agents may be necessary in those with a history of PUD.
- Teach patients about the signs of gastrointestinal bleeding.
- Be aware of interaction of NSAIDs with some antihypertensive agents.
- Do not use in pregnancy.

Drug by Class	Dose	Maximum Dose	Comments
Salicylates			
ASA OTC	325-650 mg q4h	4 gm/d	GI irritation ++++, peptic ulcer ++, tinnitus +++, hepatitis ++, CNS and renal + Pregnancy: Not recommended SE: Gastric upset, prolonged bleeding, asthma, rhinitis, urticaria
Diflunisal (Dolobid)	0.5-1 g initially, then 250-500 mg q8-12h		GI irritation, peptic ulcer, tinnitus, hepatitis, CNS, renal effects + Pregnancy: C SE: PUD, GI bleeding, nausea, dyspepsia, nephritis
Magnesium salicylate (Doan's Extra Strength, etc) OTC	500-1000 mg initially, then 500 mg q4h	3.5 g in 24 hr period	Same as ASA

+, Below-average risk; ++, average risk; +++, ++++, above-average risk.
ASA, Aspirin; *CNS*, central nervous system; *ER*, extended release; *GI*, gastrointestinal; *OA/RA*, osteoarthritis/rheumatoid arthritis; *OTC*, over-the-counter; *PUD*, peptic ulcer disease; *SE*, side effects; *SGPT/SGOT*, serum glutamic pyruvic transaminase/serum glutamic oxaloacitic transaminase.

Drug by Class	Dose	Maximum Dose	Comments	Cost
Naphthylalkanone				
Nabumetone (Relafen)	500-750 mg tab 500 mg BID or 1 g QD	2000 mg/d	Not indicated for pain; used for OA/RA GI ++, diarrhea, peptic ulcer, CNS effects, tinnitus, hepatitis, renal: + Pregnancy: C SE: Photosensitivity, fatigue, dry mouth, somnolence, pruritus	
Propionic Acid Derivatives				
Carprofen (Rimadyl)	Not currently marketed		GI irritation, hepatitis: ++ Peptic ulcer, CNS effects, tinnitus +	
Flurbiprofen (Ansaid)	200-300 mg in 2-4 divided doses	max single dose 100 mg	Used for OA/RA GI irritation, hepatitis, renal effects ++, peptic ulcer, CNS effects, tinnitus + Pregnancy: B SE: Elevated SGPT/SGOT, headache, depression, rhinitis accentuated hypotensive effects with beta blockers (except atenolol)	
Ibuprofen (Advil, Motrin IB, Nuprin, etc) OTC	200 mg q4-6h	1.2 g/day	GI irritation, hepatitis, renal effects ++, peptic ulcer, CNS effects, tinnitus + Pregnancy: Not recommended	
Ketoprofen (Orudis, Oruvail) OTC	25-75 mg TID	300 mg/day	Appropriate for pain for OA/RA; GI irritation, hepatitis, renal effects ++, peptic ulcer, CNS effects, tinnitus + Pregnancy: B SE: flatulence, rash, visual disturbances	
Naproxen (Naprelan, Naprosyn)	ER: 375-500 mg tablet; 375-1000 mg/day	1500 mg/day	Appropriate for pain for OA/RA; GI irritation, hepatitis, renal effects, peptic ulcer, CNS effects, tinnitus ++ Pregnancy: B SE: constipation, insomnia, rash, myalgia, dizziness	
Naproxen sodium (Aleve, Anaprox) OTC	≤65 y/o: 220 mg q8-12h; may increase to 400 mg q4-6h	1.2 g/day	GI irritation, hepatitis, renal effects ++, peptic ulcer, CNS effects, tinnitus +	
Oxaprozin (Daypro)	1200 mg/day	1200 mg/day	Not for acute pain; used for OA/RA; GI irritation, hepatitis, renal effects ++, peptic ulcer, CNS effects, tinnitus + Pregnancy: C SE: Constipation, blurred vision, rash, dysuria	
Indoles				
Indomethacin (Indocin)	25 mg BID/TID	200 mg/day	Moderate to severe pain; OA/RA; GI irritation, CNS effects ++++; peptic ulcer, renal effects +++; hepatitis ++, tinnitus + Pregnancy: Not recommended SE: Headache, corneal deposits, drowsiness	
Sulindac (Clinoril)	150 mg BID	400 mg/day	Moderate to severe pain: OA/RA; hepatitis ++. GI irritation, peptic ulcer, CNS effects, tinnitus, renal effect + Pregnancy: Not recommended SE: Dyspepsia, edema, jaundice	

Continued

Drug by Class	Dose	Maximum Dose	Comments	Cost
Fenamates				
Mefenamic acid (Ponstel)	500 mg initially, then 250 mg q6h	Take for max of 1 week	Moderate pain, menstrual cramps; renal effects ++; GI irritation, peptic ulcer, CNS effects + Pregnancy: C SE: Dizziness, urticaria, depression, abdominal pain	
Naphthylakanone				
Nabumetone (Relafen)	500 mg BID or 1 g QD	2000 mg/day	Not for acute pain; used for OA/RA; GI irritation ++, peptic ulcer, CNS effects, tinnitus, hepatitis, renal effects + Pregnancy: C SE: Diarrhea, dry mouth	
Phenylacetic Acids				
Diclofenac potassium (Voltaren)	50 mg BID or TID 100 mg ER 1 QD	150 mg/day	For pain and OA/RA; ER for chronic therapy of OA/RA; check SGPT/SGOT within 8 wks and then periodically; hepatitis +++, GI irritation, peptic ulcer, renal effects ++, CNS effects, tinnitus + Pregnancy: B SE: Edema	
Diclofenac (Cataflam)	50 mg BID/TID	150 mg/day	For OA/RA; check SGPT/SGOT within 8 wks and then periodically; hepatitis +++, GI irritation, peptic ulcer, renal effects ++, CNS effects, tinnitus + Pregnancy: B SE: Constipation, headache, edema	
Pyrrolo-pyrrole				
Ketorolac	30-60 mg q6h intramuscularly 10 mg QID	120 mg/day 40 mg/day	For acute pain only; restricted to 5 days' use	
Tromethamine (Toradol)			GI irritation, peptic ulcer, renal effects +++, hepatitis ++, CNS effects, tinnitus + Pregnancy: C SE: Purpura, sweating, rash, constipation	
Pyranocarboxylic Acid				
Etodolac (Lodine)	200-400 mg q6-8h	1200 mg/day	Used for acute pain and OA/RA; less inhibition of gastric prostaglandins; GI irritation, peptic ulcer, CNS effects, tinnitus, hepatitis, renal effects + Pregnancy: C SE: Malaise, urinary frequency, rash, pruritus	
Other				
Piroxicam (Feldene)	20 mg QD		Used for OA/RA; GI irritation, peptic ulcer +++, hepatitis, renal effects ++, CNS effects, tinnitus + Pregnancy: Not recommended SE: Peripheral edema, jaundice	

+, Below-average risk; ++, average risk; +++, ++++, above-average risk.
ASA, Aspirin; *CNS*, central nervous system; *ER*, extended release; *GI*, gastrointestinal; *OA/RA*, osteoarthritis/rheumatoid arthritis; *OTC*, over-the-counter; *PUD*, peptic ulcer disease; *SE*, side effects; *SGPT/SGOT*, serum glutamic pyruvic transaminase/serum glutamic oxaloacitic transaminase.

Appendix

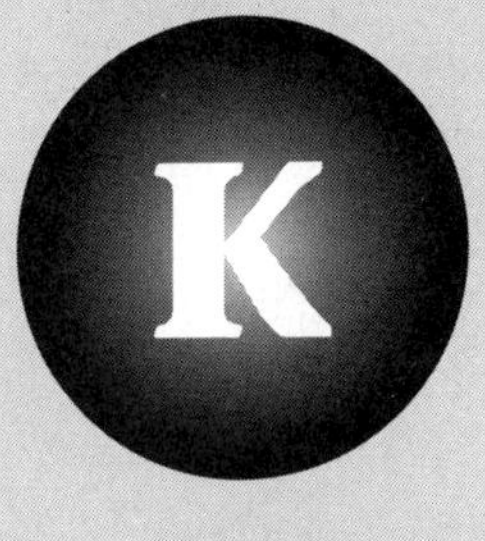

Oral Contraceptive Drug Interactions*

Drug Class	Generic (Trade)	Effect	Recommendation
Anti-infectives	Erythromycin (*E-Mycin,* etc) Griseofulvin (*Grisactin,* etc) Penicillins Rifampin (*Rifadin,* etc) Tetracycline (*Achromycin V,* etc)	Oral contraceptive action may be decreased. Erythromycin, penicillins and tetracyclines may kill GI bacteria, which decreases serum levels of OC by interfering with enterohepatic recirculation. Griseofulvin or rifampin may increase OC metabolism.	Use alternative method of contraception during the anti-infective course of treatment and for at least one week after stopping the anti-infective (and for one month after stopping rifampin).
Anti-infective	Troleandomycin (*Tao*)	Increased risk of cholestasis.	Use alternative antibiotic.
Anticonvulsants	Carbamazepine (*Tegretol,* etc) Felbamate (*Felbatol*) Phenobarbital Phenytoin (*Dilantin,* etc) Primidone (*Mysoline,* etc)	Oral contraceptive action may be decreased due to increased metabolism.	Use alternative method of contraception or consider a higher dose product (e.g., ethinyl estradiol 50 mg daily). Sodium valproate (*Depakene*) does not appear to interact with OCs.
Antiviral	Ritonavir (*Norvir*)	Action of OC may be decreased due to increased metabolism.	Use alternative method of contraceptive.
Azole Antifungal Agents	Fluconazole (*Diflucan*) Itraconazole (*Sporanox*) Ketoconazole (*Nizoral*)	Oral contraceptive action may be decreased.	Use alternative method of contraception.
Benzodiazepines	Alprazolam (*Xanax,* etc) Chlordiazepoxide (*Librium,* etc) Diazepam (*Valium,* etc) Flurazepam (*Dalmane,* etc) Triazolam (*Halcion,* etc)	Metabolism of benzodiazepines that undergo oxidation may be decreased, increasing their CNS effects.	It may be necessary to decrease the dose of the benzodiazepine if the CNS effects are increased
Bronchodilator	Theophylline	The metabolism of theophylline may be decreased, increasing theophylline side effects.	Monitor serum theophylline levels when starting or stopping OCs and adjust the dose as needed.

*David S. Tatro, Pharm.D., Drug Information Analyst

Reprinted with permission from Prescriber's Letter. Prescriber's Letter is a totally independent newsletter providing unbiased drug information to physicians and other prescribers who subscribe.

References: 1. Tatro DS: Oral contraceptive drug interactions; *Drug Newsletter* 15:66-69, 1996. 2. Bolt HM: Interactions between clinically used drugs and oral contraceptives, *Environ Health Perspect* 102(suppl 9):35-38, 1994. 3. Fazio A: Oral contraceptive drug interactions: important considerations; *South Med J* 84:997-1002, 1991. 4. Baciewicz AM: Oral contraceptive drug interactions, *Ther Drug Monit* 7:26-35, 1985. 5. Back DJ et al: Pharmacokinetic drug interactions with oral contraceptives, *Clin Pharmacokinet* 18:472-484, 1990.

Continued

Drug Class	Generic (Trade)	Effect	Recommendation
Corticosteroids	Hydrocortisone Methylprednisolone (*Medrol,* etc) Prednisolone (*Delta-Cortef,* etc) Prednisone (*Deltasone,* etc)	The effects of the corticosteroid may be increased due to inhibition of metabolism by the OC.	Monitor the response of the patient for several weeks after starting or stopping the contraceptive. Adjust the dose of the corticosteroid as needed.
Lipid Lowering Agent	Clofibrate *(Atromid-S)*	Metabolism of clofibrate may be increased, decreasing the effect.	Monitor serum lipoprotein when starting or stopping OCs. Adjust clofibrate dose as needed.
Tricyclic Antidepressants	Amitriptyline (*Elavil,* etc) Imipramine (*Tofranil,* etc)	The metabolism of the TCA may be decreased, increasing the side effects.	Monitor TCA levels and decrease the dose if needed.

David S. Tatro, Pharm.D., Drug Information Analyst

Reprinted with permission from Prescriber's Letter. Prescriber's Letter is a totally independent newsletter providing unbiased drug information to physicians and other prescribers who subscribe.

References: 1. Tatro DS: Oral contraceptive drug interactions; *Drug Newsletter* 15:66-69, 1996. 2. Bolt HM: Interactions between clinically used drugs and oral contraceptives, *Environ Health Perspect* 102(suppl 9):35-38, 1994. 3. Fazio A: Oral contraceptive drug interactions: important considerations; *South Med J* 84:997-1002, 1991. 4. Baciewicz AM: Oral contraceptive drug interactions, *Ther Drug Monit* 7:26-35, 1985. 5. Back DJ et al: Pharmacokinetic drug interactions with oral contraceptives, *Clin Pharmacokinet* 18:472-484, 1990.

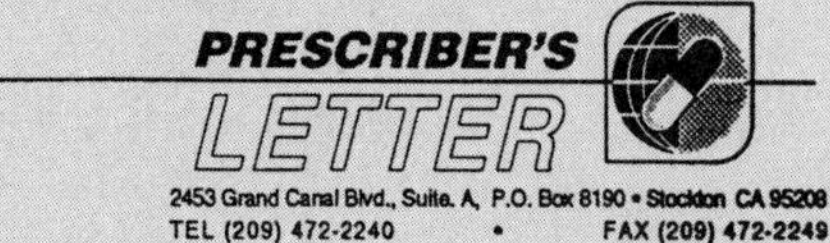

2453 Grand Canal Blvd., Suite A, P.O. Box 8190 • Stockton CA 95208
TEL (209) 472-2240 • FAX (209) 472-2249

Appendix

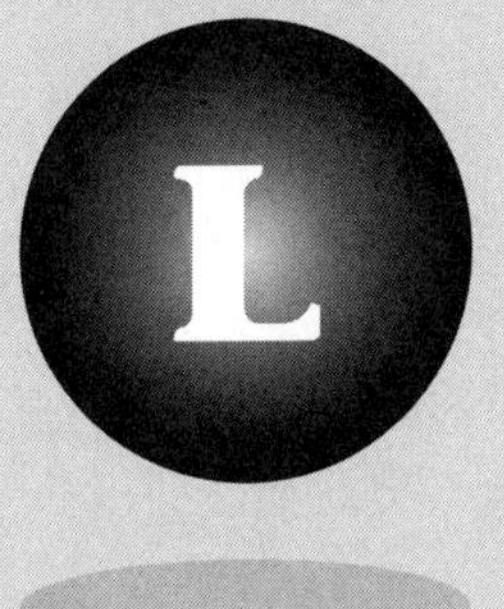

Normal Predicted Average Peak Expiratory Flow (liters per minute)

Normal Males*

Age (Years)	Height (in) 60″ (cm) 152	65″ 165	70″ 176	75″ 191	80″ 203
20	554	575	594	611	626
25	580	603	622	640	656
30	594	617	637	655	672
35	599	622	643	661	677
40	597	620	641	659	675
45	591	613	633	651	668
50	580	602	622	640	656
55	566	588	608	625	640
60	551	572	591	607	622
65	533	554	572	588	603
70	515	535	552	568	582
75	496	515	532	547	560

Normal Females*

Age (Years)	Height (in) 55″ (cm) 140	60″ 152	65″ 165	70″ 178	75″ 191
20	444	460	474	486	497
25	455	471	485	497	509
30	458	475	489	502	513
35	458	474	488	501	512
40	453	469	483	496	507
45	446	462	476	488	499
50	437	453	466	478	489
55	427	442	455	467	477
60	415	430	443	454	464
65	403	417	430	441	451
70	390	404	416	427	436
75	377	391	402	413	422

Normal Children and Adolescents†

Height (in)	Height (cm)	Males & Females	Height (in)	Height (cm)	Males & Females
43	109	147	55	140	307
44	112	160	56	142	320
45	114	173	57	145	334
46	117	187	58	147	347
47	119	200	59	150	360
48	122	214	60	152	373
49	124	227	61	155	387
50	127	240	62	157	400
51	130	254	63	160	413
52	132	267	64	163	427
53	135	280	65	165	440
54	137	293	66	168	454

The National Asthma Education and Prevention Program recommends that a patient's "personal best" be used as his/her baseline peak flow. "Personal best" is the maximum peak flow rate that the patient can obtain when his/her asthma is stable or under control. These tables are intended as guidelines only.

*Nunn AH, Gregg I: *Br Med J* 298:1068-1070, 1969.

†Polgar G. Promadhal V: *Pulmonary Function Testing in Children: Techniques and Standards.* Philadelphia, 1971, WB Saunders.

NOTE: All tables are averages and are based on tests with a large number of people. The peak flow rate of an individual can vary widely. Individuals at altitudes above sea level should be aware that peak flow readings may be lower than those at sea level, which are provided in the tables.

Appendix

Pediatric Dosages

Table M-1 Pediatric Antibiotic Dosing Chart

Weight (lb)	Amoxicillin 45 mg/kg/day Divided BID or 25 mg/kg/day	Augmentin 45 mg/kg/day Divided BID or 40 mg/kg Divided TID	Biaxin 15 mg/kg/day q12h Divided BID	Ceftin* (cefuroxime) 30 mg/kg Divided BID (20 mg/kg/day)	Cefzil (cefprozil) 15 mg/kg BID for OM (7.5 mg/kg BID)
Bacteria affected by:	*S. pneum, B. lactamase-H. flu, B. lactamase M. Cat, Strep,* ?anerobes	*S. pneum, H flu, M. cat, Strep, Staph aureus,* ?anerobes	Gram +, *M. cat, Legionella,* Mycoplasma Pneumo (macrolide)	*S. Pneum, ? B. lactam + H. Flu* and *M. cat, Strep, ? Staph,* no anerobes (second-generation ceph	*S. Pneum, ? B. lactam + H. Flu* and *M. cat, Strep, ? Staph,* no anerobes (second-generation ceph)
Illness approp. For:	OM, bites, Lyme disease, sinusitis, pneumonia, urinary tract infection, wound infection	Second line OM, lower respiratory tract, skin and soft tissue, urinary tract infection	Upper/lower respiratory tract, skin	Pharyngitis, max. sinusitis, OM, uncomplicated skin, urinary tract infection, gonorrhea, early Lyme disease	Pharyngitis, bronchitis, sinusitis, skin and skin structures, OM
5 kg (11)	125/5 ml 1 tsp	125/5 ml 1 tsp	Not used for <6 mos of age	125/5 ml ½-¾ tsp	Not used for under 6 mos
10 kg (22)	250/5 ml 1 tsp	250/5 ml 1 tsp	½ tsp 125/5 ml	125/5 ml 1 tsp	125/5 ml ½ tsp
15 kg (33)	250/5 ml 1¼ tsp	250/5 ml 1¼ tsp	¾ tsp	250/5 ml 1 tsp	125/5 ml ¾ tsp
20 kg (44)	250/5 ml 1¾ tsp	250/5 ml 1¾ tsp	1 tsp	250/5 ml 1¼ tsp	125/5 ml 1¼ tsp
25 kg (55)	250/5 ml 2¼ tsp	2¼ tsp	1½ tsp	250/5 ml 1½ tsp	125/5 ml 1½ tsp
30 kg (66)	250/5 ml 2¾ tsp	2¾ tsp	1¾ tsp	250/5 ml 1¾ tsp	250/5 ml 1 tsp
35 kg (77)	250/5 ml 3 tsp	3 tsp	2 tsp or 1 tsp 250/5 ml	250/5 ml 2 tsp	250/5 ml 1 tsp
40 kg (88)	Same (>40 kg-adult)	Same (>40 kg-adult)		Same	Same
45 kg (100)	500/5 ml 2 tsp	500/5 ml 2 tsp	1¼ tsp 250/5 ml	Same (>12 yr-adult)	Same (>13 yr-adult)

Calculated doses given for most common use: Otitis media. Calculated for fewest doses per day. Other doses are indicated in parentheses but are not calculated.
CAP, Community acquired pneumonia; *ceph,* cephalosporin; *OM,* otitis media; *?,* indicates questionable coverage.
*Take with food.

Diclox 62.5/5c 12.5-25 mg/kg/d Divided QID	Duricef 30 mg/kg Divided BID	Erythro Estolate (Ilosone) 30-50 mg/kg BID, TID, or QID	Erythro Ethyl Succinate (EES) 30-50 mg/kg/ day Divided BID, TID, QID	Keflex (cephalexin) 75-100 mg/kg/day Divided QID (25-50 mg/ kg/day)
Staph, Strep	Gram +, *Staph, Strep* (first-generation ceph)	*S. Pneum, H. Flu, M. cat, Strep, Staph,* ? anerobes	*S. Pneum, H. flu, M. cat, Strep, Staph,* ? anerobes	Gram +, *Staph, Strep* (first generation ceph)
Impetigo, furuncle	*Strep* pharyngitis, OM, skin, bone, respiratory tract, urinary tract infection	Wound, *Strep*, penicillin allergy, impetigo, OM, atypical	Wound, *Strep*, penicillin allergy, impetigo, OM, atypical *Pneumonia*, bites	*Strep* pharyngitis, OM, skin, bone, respiratory tract, urinary tract infection
62.5/5 ml ¼-½ tsp	125/5 ml ½ tsp	125/5 ml ½-1 tsp BID	200/5 ml ¼-¾ tsp BID	250/5 ml ¼-½ tsp
½ 1 tsp	1 tsp	1¼-2 tsp BID	¾-1¼ tsp BID	¾-1 tsp
¾-1½ tsp	1¾ tsp	1¾-3 tsp BID	1-1¾ tsp BID	¾-1½ tsp
1-2 tsp	250/5 ml 1¼ tsp	250/5 ml 1¼-2 tsp BID	1½-2½ tsp BID	1½-2 tsp
1¼-2½ tsp	250/5 ml 1½ tsp	1½-2½ tsp BID	1¾-3 tsp BID	1¾-2½ tsp
1½-3 tsp	1¾ tsp	1¾-3 tsp	400 mg/5 ml 1-1¾ tsp BID	2¼-3 tsp
1¾-3.5 tsp	2 tsp	2-3½ tsp	1¼-2 tsp BID	2½-3½ tsp
Same	Same	Same	1½-2¾ tsp BID	Same (>15 yr-adult)
2-4½ tsp	2½ or 1¼ of 500/5 ml	2¾-4½ tsp	Same	

Continued

TABLE M-1 Pediatric Antibiotic Dosing Chart—cont'd

Weight (lb)	Lorabid 30 mg/kg/day Divided BID (15 mg/kg/day)	Macrodantin 5-7 mg/kg/day QID	PCN Benzathine IM (lasts 2-4 wks)	Pediazole (200 mg Erythro + 600 Sulfisoxazole) q8h
Bacteria affected by:	*S. Pneum, B. Lactam-H. Flu* and *M. cat, Strep, Staph,* no anerobes	(Macrobid not for children) *E. coli, Enterococcus, Klebsiella*	*Strep.*	*S. Pneuma, H. Flu, M. Cat, Strep, Staph aureus,* no anaerobes
Illness approp. For:	Second or third line for OM, URI, empty stomach	UTI, with food, also suspension	*Strep* throat, scarlet fever, syphilis	Second line OM, pneum
5 kg (11)	100 mg/5 ml ¾ tsp	Not for children less than 1 month	600,000 U <30 lb	½ tsp
10 kg (22)	1½ tsp	25 mg/5 ml ½ tsp	Same	Same
15 kg (33)	2¼ tsp	¾ tsp	900,000 U 30-60 lb	1 tsp
20 kg (44)	200 mg/5 ml 1½ tsp	1 tsp	Same	Same
25 kg (55)	2 tsp	1¼ tsp	Same	2 tsp QID
30 kg (66)	2¼ tsp	1½ tsp	900,000 U 60-90 lb	Same
35 kg (77)	2½ tsp	1¾ tsp	Same	2½ tsp
40 kg (88)	Same	2 tsp	Same	Same
45 kg (100)	3¼ tsp	2¼ tsp	>90 lbs 1.2 million U	Same

Calculated doses given for most common use: Otitis media. Calculated for fewest doses per day. Other doses are indicated in parentheses but are not calculated.
*Take with food.

PEN V K 25-50 mg/kg/ day Divided TID	Septra (Bactrim) 160 TMP/800 SMX	Suprax 8 mg/kg/day QD	Zithromax 10 mg/kg First Day, Then 5 mg/kg Days 2-5 for OM and CAP
Strep	*? S. Pneum, H. Flu, M. Cat, ? Strep, Staph,* no anerobes	*S. Pneum, H. Flu, M. Cat, Strep,* no anerobes (third-generation Ceph)	*S. Pneum, H. Flu, M. Cat, Strep, Staph,* anerobes (macrolide)
Strep throat, scarlet fever, cellulitis, dental abscess	OM, sinusitis, penicillin allergies, pneumonia, UTI	Second line OM, sinusitis, penicillin allergies	Pneumonia, strep, pharyngitis, skin, chlamydia/gonorrhea
125 mg/5 ml 1 tsp TID	2.5 ml BID	100 mg/5 ml ½ tsp	>6 mos of age
Same	5 ml BID	¾ tsp	100 mg/5 ml: 1 tsp for day 1, then day 2-5 ½ tsp
Same	7.5 ml BID	1¼ tsp	100 mg/5 ml: 1½ tsp for day 1, then day 2-5 ¾ tsp
Same	10 ml BID	1½ tsp	200 mg/5 ml day 1, 1 tsp day 2-5 ½ tsp
Same	12.5 ml BID	2 tsp	200 mg/5 ml day 1: 1¼ tsp; day 2-5: ½ tsp
250 mg/5 ml; 1 tsp	15 ml BID	2½ tsp	200 mg/5 ml day 1: 1½ tsp; day 2-5: ¾ tsp
Same	17.5 ml BID	2¾ tsp	Same
Same	20 ml or 2 reg tabs or 1 DS	Same	40 kg: 200 mg/5 ml; day 1: 2 tsp; day 2-5: 1 tsp
Same	Same	Over 110 kg or age 12 = adult	Same

Continued

Table M-1 Pediatric Antibiotic Dosing Chart—cont'd

Classification	Bacteria
Gram + aerobic cocci	*Staph epidermidis, Staph aureus, Streptococcal species: S. pneumonia, S. pyogenes (Group A), S. agalactiae (Group B), enterococcus (Group D)*
Gram + aerobic bacilli	*Bacilus antrhacis, Corynebacterium diphtheriae, Listeria monocytogenes, Erysipelothrix rhusiopathieae, Lactobacillus, Nocardia*
Gram – aerobic diplococci	*Neisseria gonorrhea, Neisseria meningitidis, Moraxella catarrhalis*
Gram – aerobic coccobacilli	*Hemophilus influenzae, Hemophilus ducreyi*
Gram – aerobic bacilli	*Pseudomonas aeruginosa, Campylobacter jejuni, Campylobacter fetus, Hellicobacter pylori, Legionella pneumophilia, Bordatella pertussis, Enterobacteriaceae: E. coli, Citrobacter, Salmonella, Shigella, Klebsiella, Enterobacter, Serratia, Porteus, Providencia*
Anaerobes	*Bacteroides fragilis, Peptostreptococcus, Clostriudium tetani, Clostridium perfringens, Clostridium botulinusm, Clostridium difficile*
Defective cell wall bacteria	*Mycoplasma pneumonia, Chlamydia trachomatis, Chlamydia psittaci, Chlamydia pneumoniae, Rickettsia*
Spirochetes	*Treponema pallidum, Borrelia burgdorferi, Leptospira*
Mycobacteria	*M. tuberculosis, M. leprae, M. avium-intracellulare, M. kansasii*

Calculated doses given for most common use: Otitis media. Other doses are indicated in parentheses but are not calculated.

Table M-2 Pediatric Acetaminophen Dosing Chart

Age	Weight in lb (kg)	Drops 80 mg/0.8 ml (15 ml) $1.80	Suspension 160 mg/ 5 ml (100) $2	Chewable tablets 80 mg (24) $4	Junior Strength Chewable Tablets 160 mg	Caplets 325 mg (24) $3
0-3 mos	6-11 (2.5-5.4 kg)	½ dppr (0.4 ml)				
4-11 mos	12-17 (5.5-7.9 kg)	1 dppr (0.8 ml)	½ tsp			
12-23 mos	18-23 (8-10.9 kg)	1½ dppr (1.2 ml)	¾ tsp			
2-3 yrs	24-35 (11-15.9 kg)	2 dppr (1.6 ml)	1 tsp	2 tabs		
4-5 yrs	36-47 (12-21.9 kg)		1½ tsp	3 tabs		
6-8 yrs	48-59 (22-26.9 kg)		2 tsp	4 tabs	2 tab	
9-10 yrs	60-71 (27-31.9 kg)		2½ tsp	5 tabs	2½ tab	
11-12 yrs	72-95 (32-43.9 kg)		3 tsp	6 tabs	3 tab	>96 lbs (44 kg) 1 or 2 caps/tabs

Fever reducer and pain reliever in children 6 mos to 12 years of age. Dose every 4-6 hours. Do not exceed 5 doses in 24 hours. Do not use longer than 3 days for fever.

TABLE M-3 Pediatric Ibuprofen Dosing Chart

Age	Weight in lb (kg)	Drops 40 mg/ml	Suspension 100 mg/5 ml (120 ml) $6		Chewable Tablets 50 mg (100) $19	Chewable Tablets 100 mg (100) $19	Caplets 100 mg
		Increase dose if temp >102.5°	Fever 102° or below (5 mg/kg)	Fever over 102.5° (10 mg/kg)	Increase dose if temp >102.5°	Increase dose if temp >102.5°	Increase dose if temp >102.5°
6-11 mos	13-17 (5.5-7.9 kg)	½-1 dropper	¼ tsp	½ tsp			
12-23 mos	18-23 (8-10.9 kg)	1-2 dropper	½ tsp	1 tsp	1-2 tabs	½-1 tab	
2-3 yrs	24-35 (11-15.9 kg)	1½-3 dropper	¾ tsp	1½ tsp	1½-3 tabs	¾-1½ tab	
4-5 yrs	36-47 (12-21.9 kg)		1 tsp	2 tsp	2-4 tabs	1-2 tab	1-2 caps
6-8 yrs	48-59 (22-26.9 kg)		1¼ tsp	2½ tsp	2½-5 tabs	1¼-2½ tab	1¼-2½ caps
9-10 yrs	60-71 (27-31.9 kg)		1½ tsp	3 tsp	3-6 tabs	1½-3 tab	1½-3 caps
11-12 yrs	72-95 (32-43.9 kg)		2 tsp	4 tsp	4-8 tabs	2-4 tab	2-4 caps

Fever reducer and pain reliever in children 6 mos to 12 years of age. Dose every 6-8 hours. Maximum daily dose is 40mg/kg.

Appendix

Patient in Need of Surgery

From Liebowitz R: *Perioperative evaluation.* In Greene HL, Johnson WP, Lemcke D: *Decision making in medicine,* ed 2, St Louis, 1998, Mosby.

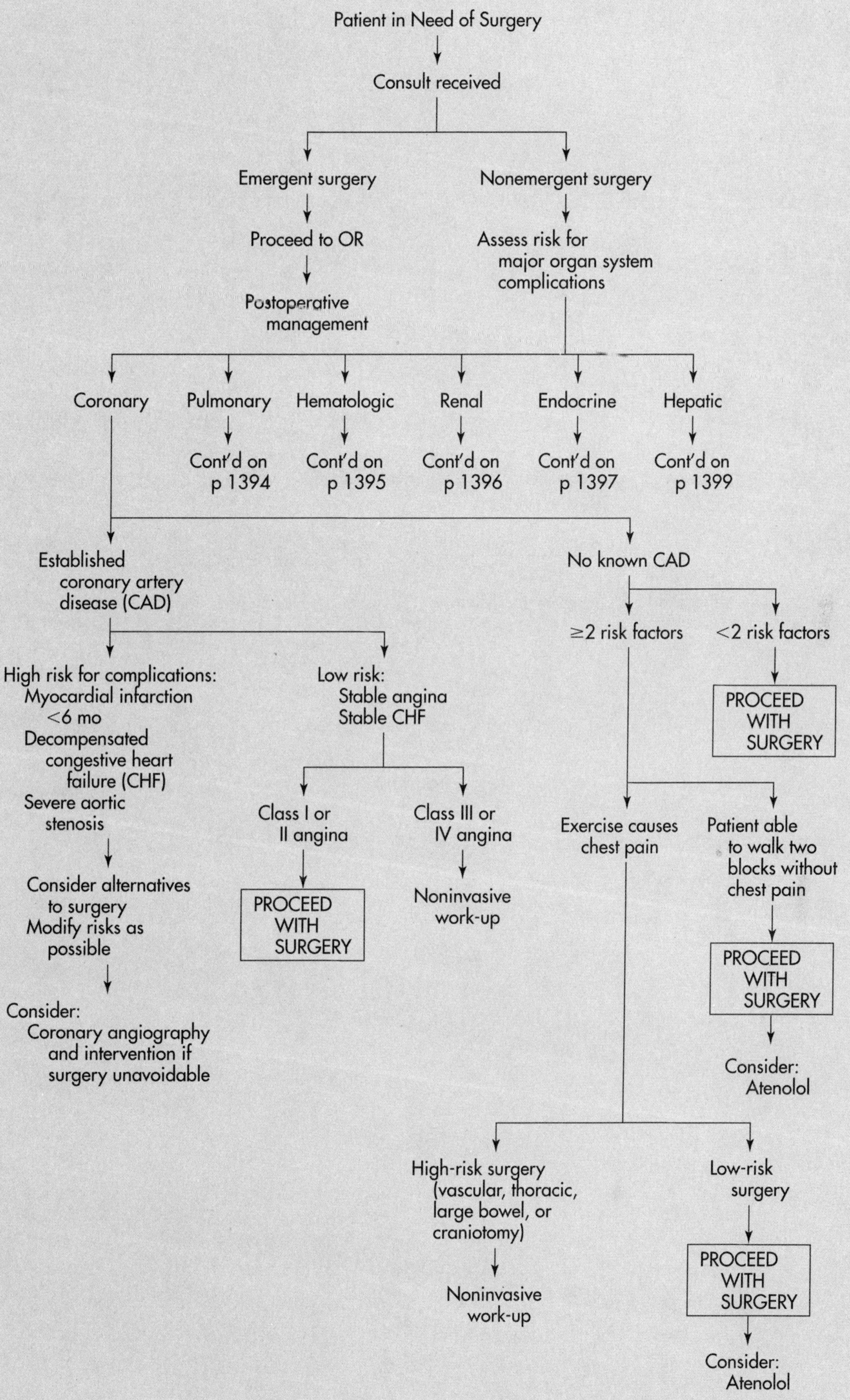
Patient in Need of Surgery
Consult received
Emergent surgery
Proceed to OR
Postoperative management
Nonemergent surgery
Assess risk for major organ system complications
Coronary
Pulmonary
Cont'd on p 1394
Hematologic
Cont'd on p 1395
Renal
Cont'd on p 1396
Endocrine
Cont'd on p 1397
Hepatic
Cont'd on p 1399
Established coronary artery disease (CAD)
High risk for complications: Myocardial infarction <6 mo Decompensated congestive heart failure (CHF) Severe aortic stenosis
Consider alternatives to surgery Modify risks as possible
Consider: Coronary angiography and intervention if surgery unavoidable
Low risk: Stable angina Stable CHF
Class I or II angina
PROCEED WITH SURGERY
Class III or IV angina
Noninvasive work-up
No known CAD
≥2 risk factors
<2 risk factors
PROCEED WITH SURGERY
Exercise causes chest pain
Patient able to walk two blocks without chest pain
PROCEED WITH SURGERY
Consider: Atenolol
High-risk surgery (vascular, thoracic, large bowel, or craniotomy)
Noninvasive work-up
Low-risk surgery
PROCEED WITH SURGERY
Consider: Atenolol

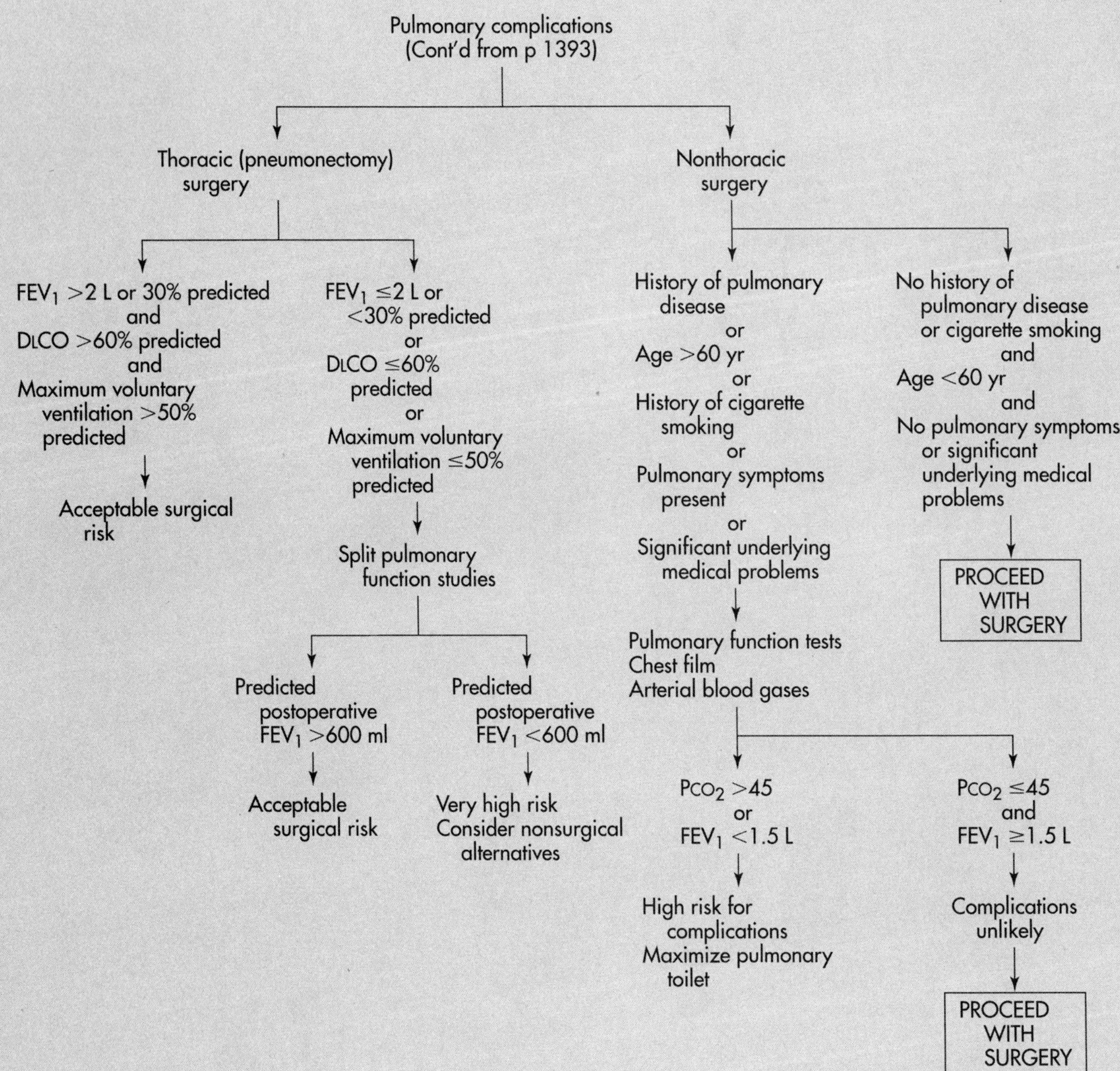
Pulmonary complications
(Cont'd from p 1393)
Thoracic (pneumonectomy) surgery
Nonthoracic surgery
FEV1 >2 L or 30% predicted and DLCO >60% predicted and Maximum voluntary ventilation >50% predicted
Acceptable surgical risk
FEV1 ≤2 L or <30% predicted or DLCO ≤60% predicted or Maximum voluntary ventilation ≤50% predicted
Split pulmonary function studies
Predicted postoperative FEV1 >600 ml
Acceptable surgical risk
Predicted postoperative FEV1 <600 ml
Very high risk
Consider nonsurgical alternatives
History of pulmonary disease or Age >60 yr or History of cigarette smoking or Pulmonary symptoms present or Significant underlying medical problems
Pulmonary function tests
Chest film
Arterial blood gases
PCO2 >45 or FEV1 <1.5 L
High risk for complications
Maximize pulmonary toilet
PCO2 ≤45 and FEV1 ≥1.5 L
Complications unlikely
PROCEED WITH SURGERY
No history of pulmonary disease or cigarette smoking and Age <60 yr and No pulmonary symptoms or significant underlying medical problems
PROCEED WITH SURGERY

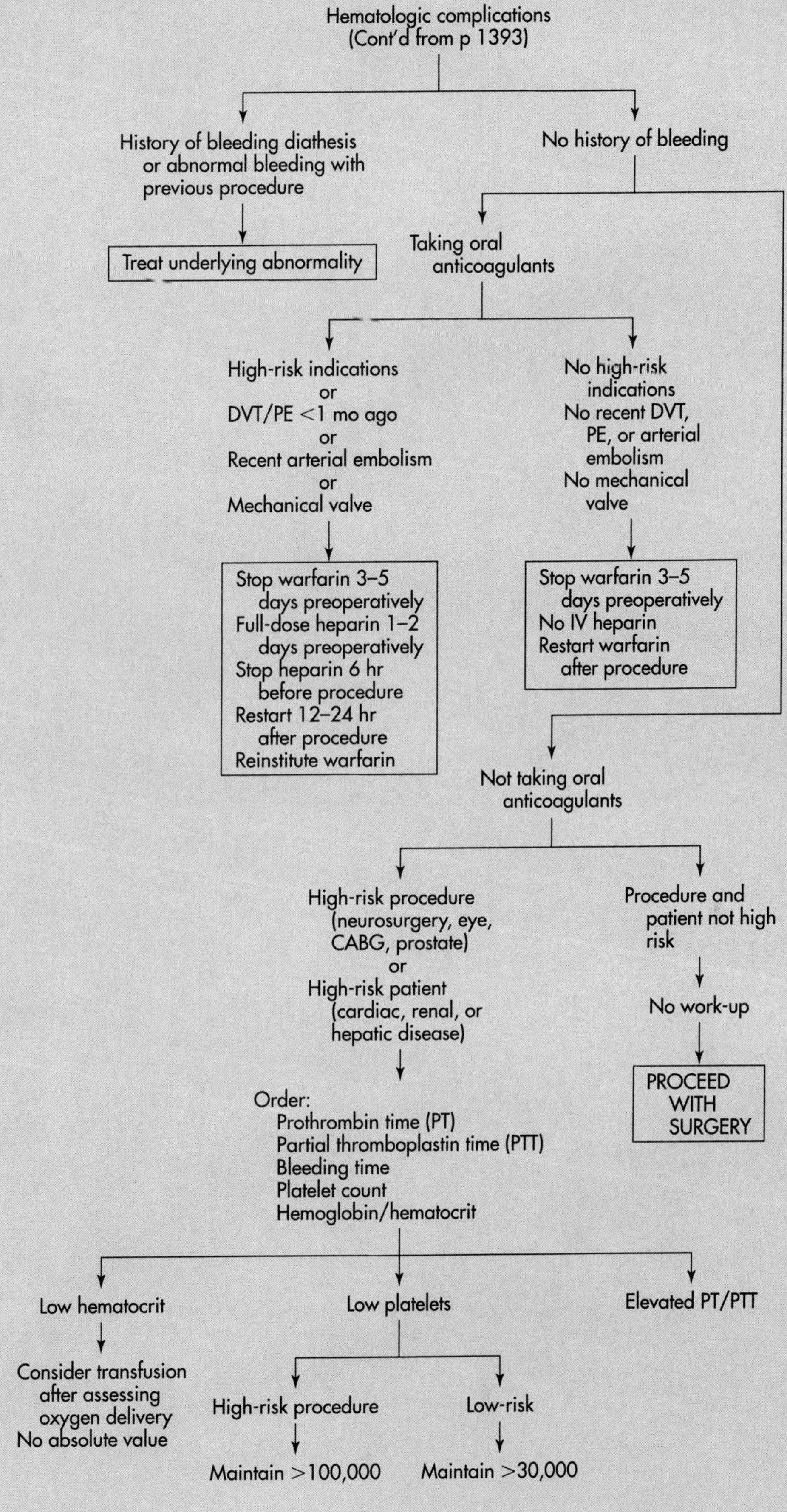
Hematologic complications
(Cont'd from p 1393)
History of bleeding diathesis or abnormal bleeding with previous procedure
Treat underlying abnormality
No history of bleeding
Taking oral anticoagulants
High-risk indications
or
DVT/PE <1 mo ago
or
Recent arterial embolism
or
Mechanical valve
Stop warfarin 3–5 days preoperatively
Full-dose heparin 1–2 days preoperatively
Stop heparin 6 hr before procedure
Restart 12–24 hr after procedure
Reinstitute warfarin
No high-risk indications
No recent DVT, PE, or arterial embolism
No mechanical valve
Stop warfarin 3–5 days preoperatively
No IV heparin
Restart warfarin after procedure
Not taking oral anticoagulants
High-risk procedure (neurosurgery, eye, CABG, prostate)
or
High-risk patient (cardiac, renal, or hepatic disease)
Order:
Prothrombin time (PT)
Partial thromboplastin time (PTT)
Bleeding time
Platelet count
Hemoglobin/hematocrit
Procedure and patient not high risk
No work-up
PROCEED WITH SURGERY
Low hematocrit
Consider transfusion after assessing oxygen delivery
No absolute value
Low platelets
High-risk procedure
Maintain >100,000
Low-risk
Maintain >30,000
Elevated PT/PTT

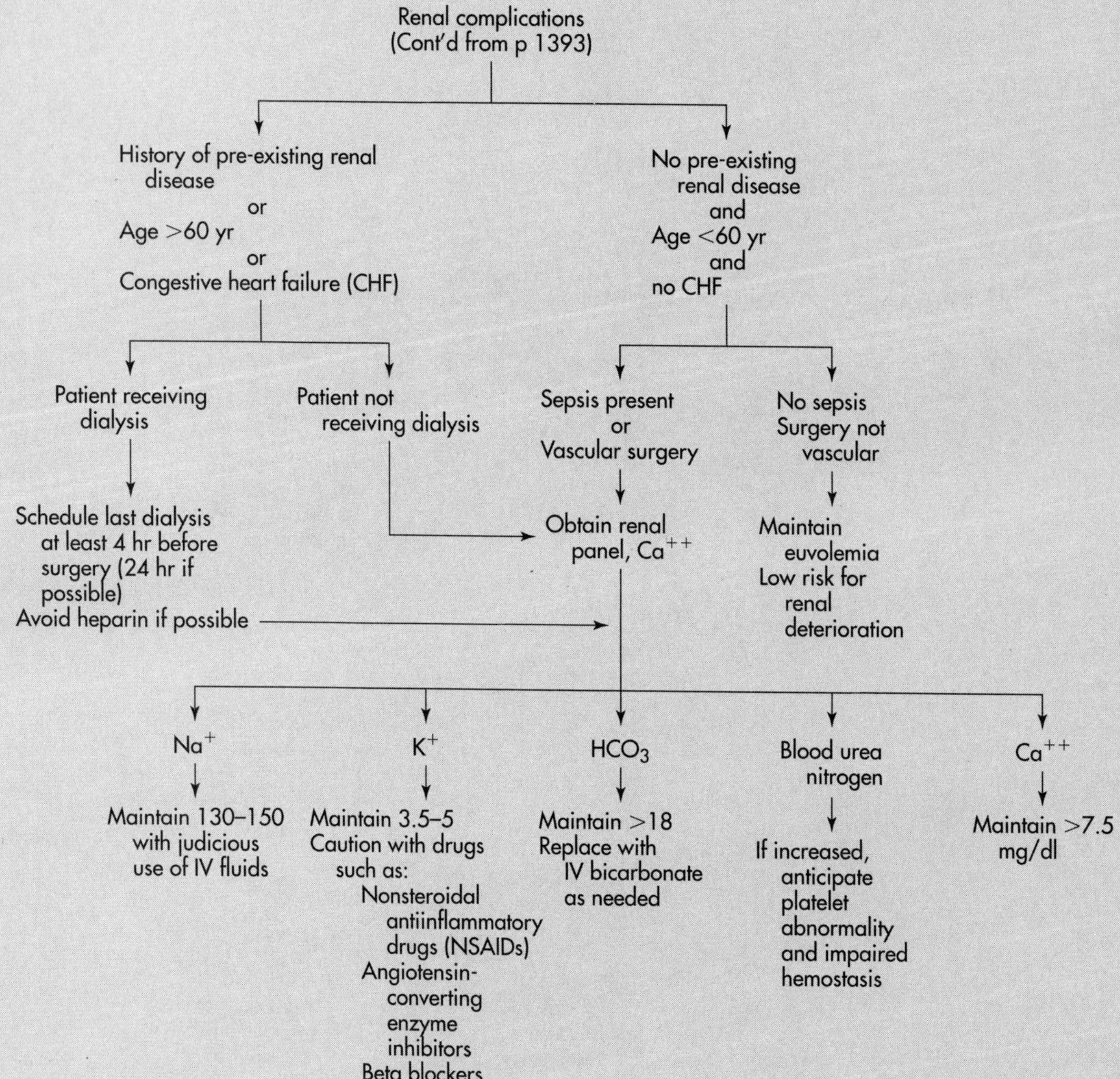
Renal complications
(Cont'd from p 1393)
History of pre-existing renal disease
or
Age >60 yr
or
Congestive heart failure (CHF)
No pre-existing renal disease
and
Age <60 yr
and
no CHF
Patient receiving dialysis
Patient not receiving dialysis
Sepsis present
or
Vascular surgery
No sepsis
Surgery not vascular
Schedule last dialysis at least 4 hr before surgery (24 hr if possible)
Avoid heparin if possible
Obtain renal panel, Ca++
Maintain euvolemia
Low risk for renal deterioration
Na+
K+
HCO3
Blood urea nitrogen
Ca++
Maintain 130–150 with judicious use of IV fluids
Maintain 3.5–5
Caution with drugs such as:
Nonsteroidal antiinflammatory drugs (NSAIDs)
Angiotensin-converting enzyme inhibitors
Beta blockers
Maintain >18
Replace with IV bicarbonate as needed
If increased, anticipate platelet abnormality and impaired hemostasis
Maintain >7.5 mg/dl

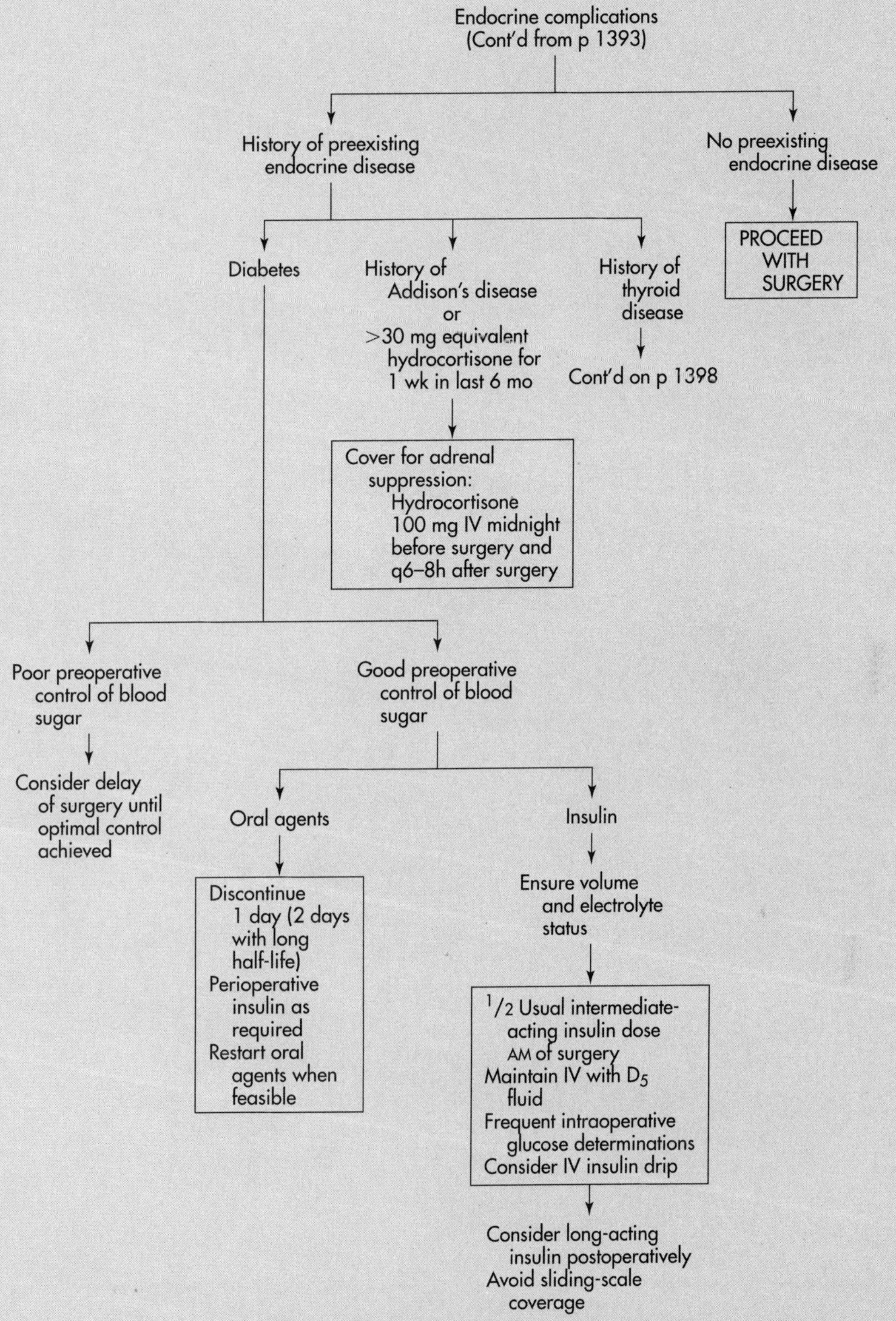
Endocrine complications
(Cont'd from p 1393)
History of preexisting endocrine disease
No preexisting endocrine disease
PROCEED WITH SURGERY
Diabetes
History of Addison's disease or >30 mg equivalent hydrocortisone for 1 wk in last 6 mo
History of thyroid disease
Cont'd on p 1398
Cover for adrenal suppression: Hydrocortisone 100 mg IV midnight before surgery and q6–8h after surgery
Poor preoperative control of blood sugar
Good preoperative control of blood sugar
Consider delay of surgery until optimal control achieved
Oral agents
Insulin
Discontinue 1 day (2 days with long half-life)
Perioperative insulin as required
Restart oral agents when feasible
Ensure volume and electrolyte status
1/2 Usual intermediate-acting insulin dose AM of surgery
Maintain IV with D5 fluid
Frequent intraoperative glucose determinations
Consider IV insulin drip
Consider long-acting insulin postoperatively
Avoid sliding-scale coverage

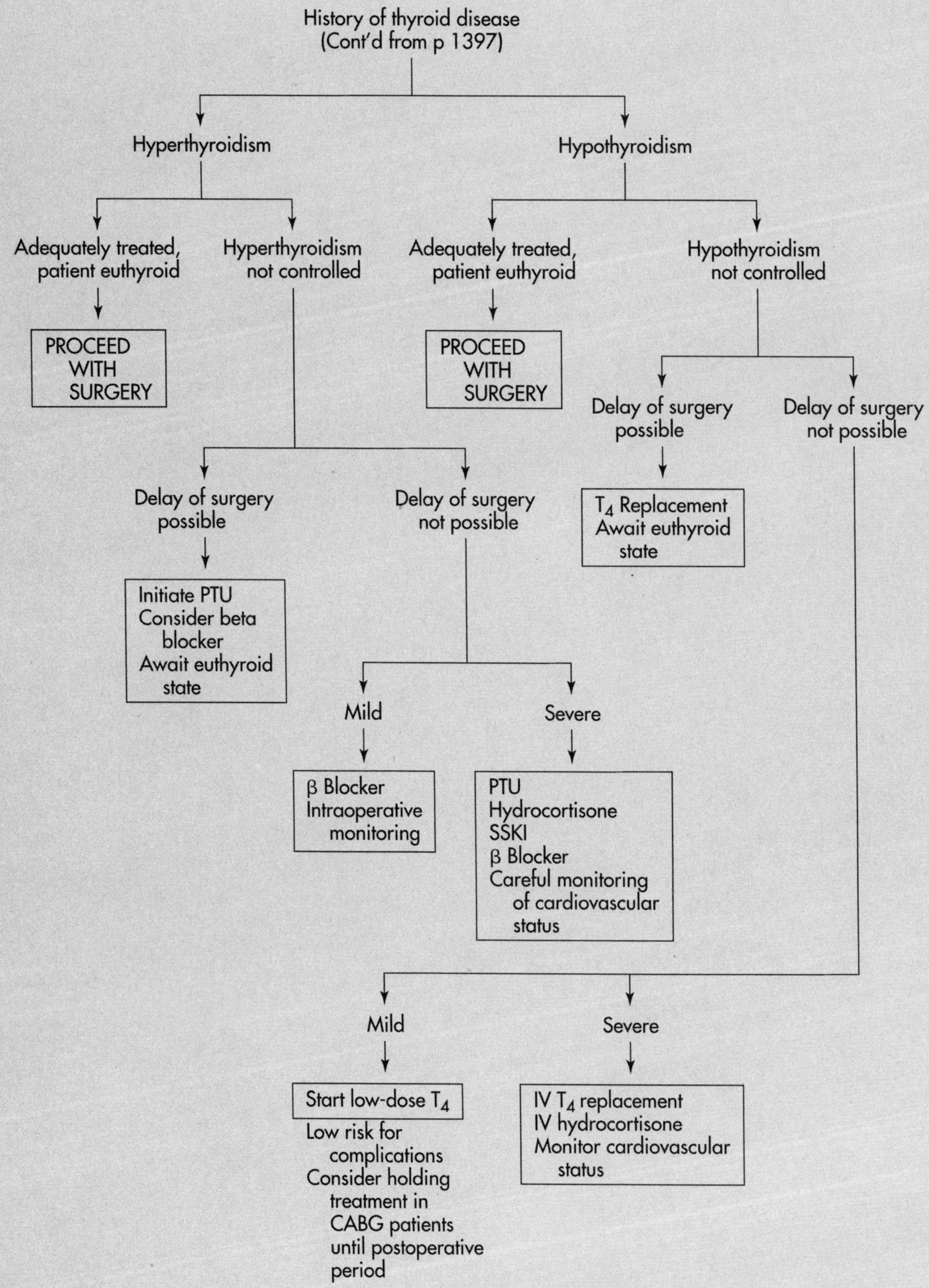
History of thyroid disease
(Cont'd from p 1397)
Hyperthyroidism
Hypothyroidism
Adequately treated, patient euthyroid
Hyperthyroidism not controlled
Adequately treated, patient euthyroid
Hypothyroidism not controlled
PROCEED WITH SURGERY
PROCEED WITH SURGERY
Delay of surgery possible
Delay of surgery not possible
Delay of surgery possible
Delay of surgery not possible
T_4 Replacement
Await euthyroid state
Initiate PTU
Consider beta blocker
Await euthyroid state
Mild
Severe
β Blocker
Intraoperative monitoring
PTU
Hydrocortisone
SSKI
β Blocker
Careful monitoring of cardiovascular status
Mild
Severe
Start low-dose T_4
Low risk for complications
Consider holding treatment in CABG patients until postoperative period
IV T_4 replacement
IV hydrocortisone
Monitor cardiovascular status

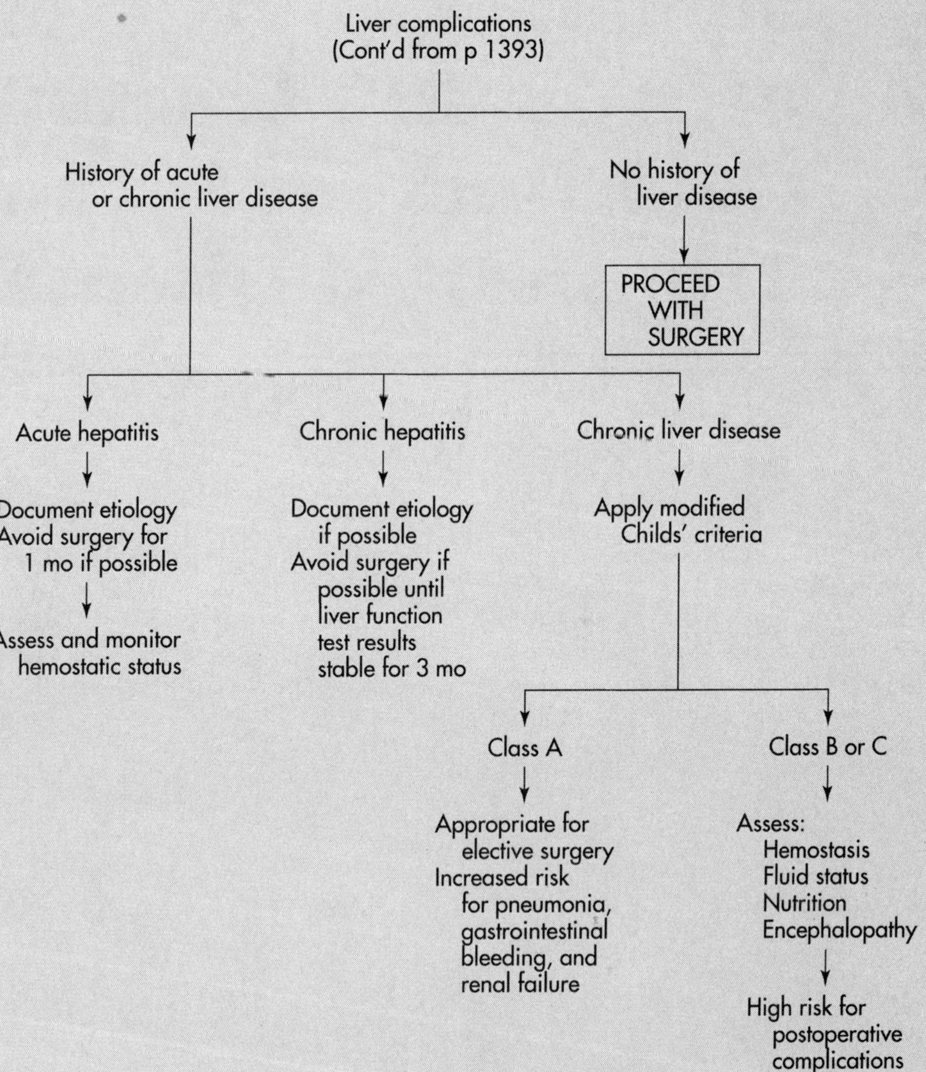
Liver complications
(Cont'd from p 1393)
History of acute
or chronic liver disease
No history of
liver disease
PROCEED
WITH
SURGERY
Acute hepatitis
Chronic hepatitis
Chronic liver disease
Document etiology
Avoid surgery for
1 mo if possible
Assess and monitor
hemostatic status
Document etiology
if possible
Avoid surgery if
possible until
liver function
test results
stable for 3 mo
Apply modified
Childs' criteria
Class A
Class B or C
Appropriate for
elective surgery
Increased risk
for pneumonia,
gastrointestinal
bleeding, and
renal failure
Assess:
Hemostasis
Fluid status
Nutrition
Encephalopathy
High risk for
postoperative
complications

Appendix

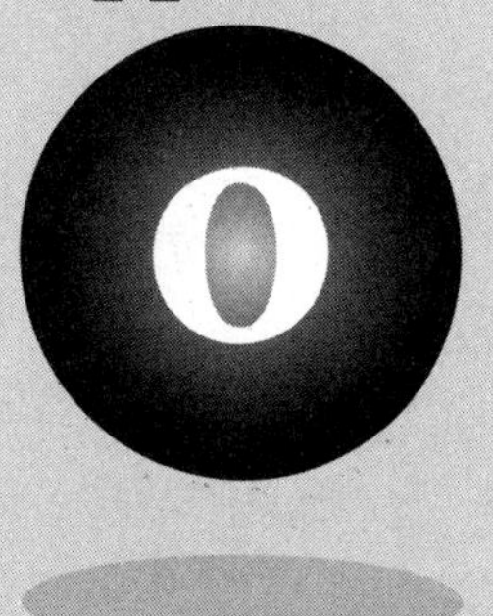

Summary Chart of 1998 CDC Treatment Guidelines for Sexually Transmitted Diseases

This is a summary of the 1998 Centers for Disease Control and Prevention Treatment Guidelines for STDs and is not intended as a replacement for review of the actual publication. Patients should abstain from sexual activity or use condoms until STDs are cured. Evaluation and treatment of partners is indicated for all diagnoses except for bacterial vaginosis and vulvovaginal candidiasis. For information regarding identification and management of at-risk sex partners, refer to the complete CDC guidelines. Unless otherwise indicated, treatment recommendations for HIV-positive individuals are the same as for HIV-negative individuals.

Disease (causative organism)	Specific Indication	Primary Therapy	Alternative Therapy	Special Notes
BACTERIAL VAGINOSIS (BV) (*Prevotella* sp, *Mobiluncus* sp, *G. vaginalis*, *Mycoplasma hominis*)	Nonpregnant females	**Metronidazole** 500 mg bid × 7 days (avoid alcohol during or 24 hours after) *OR* **Clindamycin cream (2%),** one applicator full (5 gm) intravaginally qhs × 7 days *OR* **Metronidazole gel (0.75%),** one applicator full (5 gm) intravaginally bid × 5 days	**Metronidazole** 2 gm po × 1 dose *OR* **Clindamycin** 300 mg po bid × 7 days	Only women with symptomatic disease need treatment. Treatment of male partners has **not** been shown to alter course or relapse/reinfection rate of BV. Single dose metronidazole less effective than other regimens. Flagyl ER (metronidazole 750 mg) po qd × 7 days also FDA approved for BV; no comparative data with other regimens available. Patients allergic to oral metronidazole should not be given vaginal gel. Recent meta-analysis of metronidazole does not indicate teratogenicity in humans. Intravaginal route may be preferred due to ↓ systemic side effects.
	Pregnancy	**For high or low risk:** **Metronidazole** 250 mg po tid × 7 days	**Metronidazole** 2 gm po × 1 dose *OR* **Clindamycin** 300 mg po bid × 7 days *OR* **Metronidazole gel (0.75%),** one applicator full (5 gm) intravaginally bid × 5 days **[low risk only]**	BV has been associated with adverse outcomes of pregnancy. Treatment of high-risk pregnant women (previous premature delivery) who are asymptomatic might reduce premature delivery. Screening and treatment suggested early in second trimester. Low risk pregnant women who have symptomatic BV should be treated. Lower doses recommended to minimize exposure to fetus. Clindamycin vaginal gel not recommended; use associated with increase in premature deliveries.
CHANCROID (*H. ducreyi*)		**Azithromycin** 1 g po × 1 dose *OR* **Ceftriaxone** 250 mg IM × 1 dose *OR* **Ciprofloxacin** 500 mg po bid × 3 days *OR* **Erythromycin base** 500 mg po qid × 7 days		Patients should be tested for HIV at time of diagnosis. HSV and *T. pallidum* must be ruled out. Erythromycin regimen suggested for HIV patients. Ciprofloxacin contraindicated in pregnancy

Reprinted with permission from Prescriber's Letter. Prescriber's Letter is a totally independent newsletter providing unbiased drug information to physicians and other prescribers who subscribe. Prepared for subscribers of Pharmacist's Letter and Prescriber's Letter—by M. Sharm Steadman, Pharm.D., BCPS, Member Research and Review Board

Disease (causative organism)	Specific Indication	Primary Therapy	Alternative Therapy	Special Notes
CHLAMYDIAL INFECTIONS (*C. trachomatis*)	Adolescents and adults	**Azithromycin** 1 gram po single dose *OR* **Doxycycline** 100 mg po bid × 7 days	**Erythromycin base** 500 mg po qid × 7 days *OR* **Erythromycin ethylsuccinate** 800 mg po qid × 7 days *OR* **Ofloxacin** 300 mg po bid × 7 days	Screen sexually active adolescents on annual basis. Screen women ages 20-24 years with new or multiple partners and who do not use barrier contraceptives. Sequelae from untreated infection may include PID, ectopic pregnancy, and infertility. Ofloxacin cannot be used in pregnancy and in patients <17 years old. Azithromycin 1 g sachets are less expensive than using 250 mg tablets or capsules. No test of cure indicated. HIV positive patients receive same treatment as HIV negative.
	Pregnancy	**Erythromycin base** 500 mg po qid × 7 days *OR* **Amoxicillin** 500 mg po tid × 7 days	**Erythromycin base** 250 mg po qid × 14 days *OR* **Erythromycin ethylsuccinate** 800 mg po qid × 7 days *OR* **Erythromycin ethylsuccinate** 400 mg po qid × 14 days *OR* **Azithromycin** 1 gram po single dose	Erythromycin estolate is contraindicated in pregnancy. Doxycycline and ofloxacin are contraindicated during pregnancy. Insufficient data to recommend routine use of azithromycin in pregnancy. **Repeat cultures** 3 weeks after therapy completed because of high noncompliance rates and lower efficacy of erythromycin regimens.
	Ophthalmia neonatorum	**Erythromycin** 50 mg/kg/day po divided into 4 doses for 10-14 days		Neonatal ocular prophylaxis with silver nitrate or antibiotic ointments does not prevent perinatal transmission of *Chlamydia*. Prophylactic antibiotics not indicated; treat only if symptomatic. Topical antibiotic treatment is ineffective and unnecessary if systemic antibiotics are used. Erythromycin is 80% effective; might need second course of therapy. Treat mother and partner(s).

	Infant pneumonia	**Erythromycin** 50 mg/kg/day po divided into 4 doses 10-14 days		
	Children	**Children who weigh <45 kg:** **Erythromycin** 50 mg/kg/day po divided into 4 doses for 10-14 days **Children who weigh ≥45 kg, but are <8 years old:** **Azithromycin** 1 gram po single dose **Children ≥8 years old:** **Azithromycin** 1 gram po single dose or **Deoxycycline** 100 mg po bid × 7 days		Consider sexual abuse in preadolescent children.
EPIDIDYMITIS (*N. gonorhoeae, C. trachomatis*, Gram-negative enteric)		**Ceftriaxone** 250 mg IM single dose *PLUS* **Doxycycline** 100 mg po bid × 10 days	**For enteric organisms and cephalosporin and/or tetracycline allergic:** **Ofloxacin** 300 mg po bid × 10 days	Enteric organisms more common in men >35 years old, recent urinary tract instrumentation or surgery, or with anatomical abnormalities. Ofloxacin is not indicated for use in children <17 years old. Fungal and mycobacterial causes are more common in HIV+ patients.
GENITAL HERPES SIMPLEX VIRUS (HSV-2 usually)	First clinical episode of genital herpes	**Acyclovir** 400 mg po tid for 7-10 days or until clinically resolved *OR* **Acyclovir** 200 mg po 5×/day for 7-10 days or until clinically resolved *OR* **Famciclovir** 250 mg po tid for 7-10 days or until clinically resolved *OR* **Valacyclovir** 1 g po bid for 7-10 days or until clinically resolved		Topical acyclovir is less effective than oral; use is discouraged. First clinical episode during pregnancy may be treated with acyclovir. Safety of valacyclovir and famciclovir in **pregnancy** not established; benefits must outweigh risks.
	First clinical episode of herpes proctitis or oral infection (stomatitis or pharyngitis)	**Acyclovir** 400 mg po 5×/day tor 7-10 days or until clinically resolved		Valacyclovir and famciclovir probably effective but clinical experience lacking.

Continued

Disease (causative organism)	Specific Indication	Primary Therapy	Alternative Therapy	Special Notes
GENITAL HERPES SIMPLEX VIRUS—cont'd	Recurrent episodes	**Acyclovir** 400 mg po tid × 5 days *OR* **Acyclovir** 200 mg po 5×/day × 5 days *OR* **Acyclovir** 800 mg po bid × 5 days *OR* **Famciclovir** 125 mg po bid × 5 days *OR* **Valacyclovir** 500 mg po bid × 5 days		Treatment must be initiated during prodrome or within 1 day of onset of lesions for patient to experience benefit from therapy.
	Daily suppressive therapy	**Acyclovir** 400 mg po bid *OR* **Famciclovir** 250 mg bid *OR* **Valacyclovir** 250 mg bid *OR* **Valacyclovir** 500 mg qd *OR* **Valacyclovir** 1 gram qd		Reduces frequency of HSV recurrences by at least 75% in patients with 6 or more recurrences/year. Safety and efficacy documented with daily use of acyclovir for up to 6 years, and with valacyclovir and famciclovir for 1 year. After year of suppressive therapy, discontinuation should be considered to assess rate of recurrent episodes. Valacyclovir 500 mg po qd less effective than other valacyclovir regimens in patients with >10 episodes/yr.
	Severe infection	**Acyclovir** 5-10 mg/kg body weight IV q8h for 5-7 days or until clinical resolution		
	HIV+ or immunocompromised	**Acyclovir** 400 mg po 3-5×/day until clinically resolved (if severe, see above) *OR* **Famciclovir** 500 mg po bid	If resistance suspected, **foscarnet** 40 mg/kg IV q8h until clinical resolution attained *OR* topical **cidofovir 1% gel** applied to lesions qd × 5 days	All acyclovir-resistant strains are resistant to valacyclovir and most are resistant to famciclovir.
	Neonatal herpes	**Acyclovir** 30-60 mg/kg/day for 10-21 days		Available data does not support routine use of acyclovir for asymptomatic infants exposed during birth process.

GENITAL WARTS (Human papillomavirus, HPV)	External genital/ perianal warts	**Patient Applied:** **Podofilox 0.5% solution or gel** (apply bid × 3 days, then off 4 days. May repeat cycle total of 4 times) *OR* **Imiquimod 5% cream** (apply qhs 3 × week; wash off after 6-10 hours. May use up to 16 weeks; may clear in 8-10 weeks or sooner) **Provider-Administered:** Cryotherapy with liquid nitrogen or cryoprobe *OR* **Podophyllin** 10%-25% in compound tincture of benzoin (wash off thoroughly in 1-4 hours after application. Repeat weekly if necessary.) *OR* **Trichloroacetic acid (TCA) 80%-90%,** apply only to warts. Powder with talc or baking soda to remove unreacted acid. Repeat weekly if necessary. *OR* Surgical removal	Intralesional interferon *OR* Laser surgery	No therapy has been shown to eradicate or effect natural history of HPV. **Imiquimod, podofilox and podophyllin are contraindicated in pregnancy.** Some experts advocate removal of visible warts during pregnancy. Scarring in the form of hypo- or hyperpigmentation is common with ablative therapies. If warts persist after one type of therapy, other therapies should be considered. Most experts believe combining modalities does not increase efficacy but may increase complications. Examination of sex partners is not necessary for management due to minimal risk for reinfection. Screening for subclinical genital HPV infection using DNA or RNA tests or acetic acid is not recommended. Patients with HIV may not respond as well to treatment.
	Cervical warts	Dysplasia must be excluded before treatment started. Consult with expert for management.		
	Vaginal warts	Cryotherapy with liquid nitrogen (cryoprobe is not recommended) *OR* **Trichloroacetic acid (TCA) 80%-90%,** apply only to warts. Powder with talc or baking soda to remove unreacted acid. Repeat weekly if necessary. *OR* **Podophyllin 10%-25%** in compound tincture of benzoin. Apply to treatment area, which must be dry before removing speculum. Treat <2cm² per session. Repeat weekly.		**Podophyllin is contraindicated in pregnancy,** due to systemic absorption.

Continued

Disease (causative organism)	Specific Indication	Primary Therapy	Alternative Therapy	Special Notes
GENITAL WARTS—cont'd	Urethral meatus warts	Cryotherapy with liquid nitrogen *OR* **Podophyllin 10%-25%** in compound tincture of benzoin. Treatment area must be dry before contact with normal mucosa. Wash off in 1-2 hours. Repeat weekly if necessary.		**Podophyllin is contraindicated in pregnancy,** due to systemic absorption.
	Anal warts	Cryotherapy with liquid nitrogen *OR* Surgical removal *OR* **Trichloroacetic acid (TCA) 80%-90%,** apply only to warts. Powder with talc or baking soda to remove unreacted acid. Repeat weekly if necessary.		Warts on rectal mucosa should be referred to an expert.
	Oral warts	Cryotherapy with liquid nitrogen *or* Surgical removal		
GONOCOCCAL INFECTIONS (*N. gonorrhoeae*)	Uncomplicated gonococcal infections (cervicitis, urethritis, rectal)	**Cefixime** 400 mg po single dose *OR* **Ceftriaxone** 125 mg IM single dose *OR* **Ciprofloxacin** 500 mg po single dose *OR* **Ofloxacin** 400 mg po single dose ***PLUS*** A regimen effective against possible coinfection with *C. trachomatis:* **Azithromycin** 1 gram po single dose *OR* **Doxycycline** 100 mg po bid × 7 days	**Spectinomycin** 2 gm IM × 1 dose *OR* **Ceftizoxime** 500 mg IM × 1 dose *OR* **Cefotaxime** 500 mg IM × 1 dose *OR* **Cefotetan** 1 gm IM × 1 dose *OR* **Cefoxitin** 2 gm IM × 1 dose with **probenecid** 1 g po *OR* **Lomefloxacin** 400 mg po × 1 dose *OR* **Enoxacin** 400 mg po × 1 dose *OR* **Norfloxacin** 800 mg po × 1 dose	Azithromycin 2 grams po single dose effective but expensive and cause GI distress; 1 gram dose insufficient. **Pregnancy-** Quinolones and tetracyclines contraindicated. If cephalosporins cannot be tolerated by pregnant woman, treat with spectinomycin 2 gm IM × 1 dose along with effective chlamydia regimen. **Pharyngeal infections-** Recommended regimens are ceftriaxone or ciprofloxacin. **Alternative therapy-** A regimen effective against possible coinfection with *C. trachomatis* (see: Chlamydial infections) **must** be included.

Gonococcal pharyngitis	**Ceftriaxone** 125 IM single dose *OR* **Ciprofloxacin** 500 mg po single dose *OR* **Ofloxacin** 400 mg single dose ***PLUS*** **Azithromycin** 1 gram po single dose *OR* **Doxycycline** 100 mg po bid × 7 days		If unable to tolerate cephalosporins or quinolones, use spectinomycin 2 g IM (only 52% effective).
Disseminated gonococcal infection (DGI, adults)	**Ceftriaxone** 1 gm 1M or IV q 24h	**Cefotaxime** 1 gm IV q8h *OR* **Ceftizoxime** 1 gm IV q8h *OR* **Spectinomycin** 2 gm IM q12h (if beta-lactam allergic)	Hospitalization is recommended for initial therapy. Continue parenteral regimen for 24-48 hours after improvement; may then switch to one of the following to complete a full week of therapy: **Cefixime** 400 mg PO bid, **Ciprofloxacin** 500 mg po bid, or **Ofloxacin** 400 mg po bid. Quinolones not recommended for use in pregnant or lactating women, or in children <17 years old. Treat presumptively for concurrent *C. trachomatis* infection.
Disseminated gonococcal infection (DGI, infants)	**Ceftriaxone** 25-50 mg/kg/day IM/IV qd × 7 days, up to 10-14 days if meningitis is documented *or* **Cefotaxime** 25 mg/kg IM/IV q12h × 7 days, up to 10-14 days if meningitis is documented		
Gonococcal meningitis and endocarditis	**Ceftriaxone** 1-2 gm IV q12h		Therapy for meningitis should be continued for 10-14 days and at least 4 weeks for endocarditis.
Gonococcal conjunctivitis	**Ceftriaxone** 1 gm IM × 1 dose **plus** Lavage of infected eye with saline solution once		

Continued

Disease (causative organism)	Specific Indication	Primary Therapy	Alternative Therapy	Special Notes
GONOCOCCAL INFECTIONS—cont'd	Ophthalmia neonatorum prophylaxis	**Silver nitrate (1%) aqueous solution** × 1 application *OR* **Erythromycin (0.5%) ophthalmic oint.** × 1 application *OR* **Tetracycline (1%) ophthalmic oint.** × 1 application		Not effective for prophylaxis of chlamydial eye disease. Prophylaxis should occur for both vaginal and caesarian deliveries. Bacitracin is not effective. Povidone iodine has not been adequately studied.
	Ophthalmia neonatorum treatment	**Ceftriaxone** 25-50 mg/kg IM/IV × 1 dose (max 125 mg)		Topical antibiotic therapy alone is inadequate and unnecessary if systemic therapy is administered. Simultaneous infection with *C. trachomatis* is possible. Use ceftriaxone cautiously in infants with elevated bilirubin levels. Treat until cultures negative at 48-72 hours.
	Prophylaxis for infants	**Ceftriaxone** 25-50 mg/kg IM/IV × 1 dose (max 125 mg)		Use in infants born to untreated mothers. Simultaneous infection with *C. trachomatis* is possible. Use ceftriaxone cautiously in infants with elevated bilirubin levels. Treat mother.
	Gonococcal infections in children	**Children who weigh ≥45 kg:** See adult regimens. **Children who weigh <45 kg:** **Ceftriaxone** 125 mg IM × 1 dose (*for uncomplicated gonococcal vulvovaginitis, cervicitis, urethritis, pharyngitis, or proctitis*) *OR* **Ceftriaxone** 50 mg/kg IM/IV qd (max dose 2 gm >45 kg and 1 g <45 kg) × 7 days (*for bacteremia, arthritis, or meningitis*)	**Children who weigh <45 kg:** **Spectinomycin** 40 mg/kg (max 2 gm) IM × 1 dose (*for uncomplicated gonococcal vulvovaginitis, cervicitis, urethritis, pharyngitis, or proctitis*)	Sexual abuse is the most common cause. For meningitis, increase duration of treatment to 10-14 days. Only parenteral cephalosporins are recommended for use among children; oral cephalosporins have not been adequately evaluated in children. Cefotaxime is only approved for gonococcal ophthalmia. Simultaneous infection with *C. trachomatis* is possible.

MUCOPURULENT CERVICITIS (*C. trachomatis, N. gonorrhoeae*)		Treat according to therapies for chlamydia or gonorrhea		Treat according to suspicion for chlamydia and/or gonorrhea. Wait for test results if prevalence of both organisms is low and chance for follow-up is good.
NONGONOCCAL URETHRITIS (NGU) (*C. trachomatis, Ureaplasma urealyticum, Mycoplasma genitalium, Trichomonas vaginalis*)		**Azithromycin** 1 gram po single dose *OR* **Doxycycline** 100 mg po bid × 7 days **Recurrent/Persistent Urethritis:** **Metronidazole** 2 grams po single dose ***PLUS*** **Erythromycin base** 500 mg po qid × 7 days *OR* **Erythromycin ethylsuccinate** 800 mg po qid × 7 days	**Erythromycin base** 500 mg po qid × 7 days *OR* **Erythromycin ethylsuccinate** 800 mg po qid × 7 days *OR* **Ofloxacin** 300 mg po bid × 7 days **If high dose erythromycin cannot be tolerated: Erythromycin base** 250 mg po qid × 14 days *OR* **Erythromycin ethylsuccinate** 400 mg po qid × 14 days	If symptoms persist and patient non-compliant or exposed to untreated partner, re-treat with initial regimen. In compliant or unexposed patients, perform wet mount and culture for *T. vaginalis*, then follow with recurrent/persistent regimen.
PARASITIC INFECTIONS (Pediculosis pubis, *Sarcoptes scabiei*)	Pediculosis pubis (pubic lice)	**Permethrin 1% creme rinse,** applied to affected areas and washed off after 10 minutes *OR* **Lindane 1% shampoo,** applied for 4 minutes then thoroughly washed off *OR* **Pyrethrins with piperonyl butoxide,** applied to affected areas and washed off after 10 minutes.		Lindane is not recommended for use in pregnant/lactating women or children <2 years of age. Toxicity related to prolonged exposure to lindane (>4 minutes) includes seizures and aplastic anemia. Permethrin has less potential for toxicity. Decontaminate clothing and bedding or remove from body contact for at least 72 hours. Fumigation is not necessary. Evaluate and retreat in 1 week if symptoms persist and lice are observed. Sexual partners within preceding month should be treated.

Continued

Disease (causative organism)	Specific Indication	Primary Therapy	Alternative Therapy	Special Notes
PARASITIC INFECTIONS—cont'd	Scabies	**Permethrin cream (5%),** applied to all areas of the body from the neck down and washed off after 8-14 hours	**Lindane (1%),** 1 oz of lotion or 30 gm of cream applied thinly to all areas of the body from the neck down and washed off thoroughly after 8 hours *OR* **Sulfur (6%) precipitated in ointment,** applied thinly to all areas nightly for 3 consecutive nights; wash off previous application before new ones applied. Thoroughly wash off 24 hours after the last application.	Do not use lindane after a bath, in patients with extensive dermatitis, in pregnant or lactating women, or children <2 years old. Decontaminate clothing and bedding. Pruritus may persist for several weeks; some experts recommend retreatment after 1 week if still symptomatic. Both sexual and close personal or household contacts within preceding month should be examined and treated. Control of scabies epidemic requires treatment of entire population at risk. Scabies among children is usually not sexually transmitted.
PELVIC INFLAMMATORY DISEASE (PID) (*N. gonorrhoeae, C. trachomatis, G. vaginalis, H. influenzae*, etc.)	Inpatient Management	**Regimen A: Cefoxitin** 2 gm IV q6h *OR* **Cefotetan** 2 gm IV q12h ***PLUS*** **Doxycycline** 100 mg IV/po q12h ***followed by*** **Doxycycline** 100 mg po bid for 14 days total **Regimen B: Clindamycin** 900 mg IV q8h ***PLUS*** **Gentamicin** 2 mg/kg IV/IM loading dose then 1.5 mg/kg maintenance dose q8h (Single daily dosing may be substituted) ***followed by*** **Doxycycline** 100 mg po bid for 14 days total **or** **Clindamycin** 450 mg po qid for 14 days total	**Ofloxacin** 400 mg IV q12h *PLUS* **Metronidazole** 500 mg IV q8h *OR* **Ampicillin/Sulbactam** 3 g IV q6h *PLUS* **Doxycycline** 100 mg IV/po q12h *OR* **Ciprofloxacin** 200 mg IV q12h *PLUS* **Doxycycline** 100 mg IV/po q12h *PLUS* **Metronidazole** 500 mg IV q 8h	Parenteral therapy may be discontinued 24 hours after clinical improvement. When tubo-ovarian abscess is present, clindamycin may be preferred for continued therapy. Other 2nd or 3rd generation cephalosporins may be effective but clinical data is limited. Azithromycin 500mg IV × 2 days, followed by 500mg po for total of 10 days recently FDA approved. **Pregnancy:** Women should be hospitalized and treated with parenteral therapy. HIV+ women should be hospitalized and treated aggressively.

	Outpatient Management	**Regimen A: Ofloxacin** 400 mg po bid × 14 days ***PLUS*** **Metronidazole** 500 mg po bid × 14 days **Regimen B: Ceftriaxone** 250 mg IM × 1 dose *OR* **Cefoxitin** 2 gm IM plus **Probenecid** 1 gm po × 1 dose *OR* Other parenteral 3rd generation cephalosporin ***PLUS*** **Doxycycline** 100 mg po bid × 14 days		Patients who do not respond within 72 hours to therapy should be hospitalized. Alternative oral regimens suggested include amoxicillin/clavulanic acid plus doxycycline. Insufficient data to recommend azithromycin as part of treatment regimens.
PROCTITIS (*N. gonorrhoeae, C. trachomatis, T. pallidum,* and HSV)		**Ceftriaxone** 125 mg IM (or other agent effective against anal and genital gonorrhea) ***PLUS*** **Doxycycline** 100 mg po bid × 7 days		For patients with herpes proctitis, see HSV section. HIV positive patients may not respond to recommended therapy and need to be evaluated for other causative organisms
SEXUAL ASSAULT (*C. trachomatis, N. gonorrhoeae, T. vaginalis,* and HSV)		**Ceftriaxone** 125 mg IM × 1 dose ***PLUS*** **Metronidazole** 2 gm po × 1 dose ***PLUS*** **Azithromycin** 1 g po single dose ***or*** **Doxycycline** 100 mg po bid × 7 days	For alternative treatments, refer to sections in this chart that specifically address those agents.	Hepatitis B vaccine should be administered with follow-up doses at 1-2 and 4-6 months after first dose. Testing for HIV and possible antiretroviral prophylaxis should be considered. Presumptive treatment for children is not recommended.
SYPHILIS (*T. pallidum*)	Primary and secondary syphilis Early latent syphilis (<1 year)	**Adults: Benzathine penicillin** G 2.4 million units IM × 1 dose **Children: Benzathine penicillin** G 50,000 units/kg IM × 1 dose (up to 2.4 mil units) **If penicillin allergic:** **Tetracycline** 500 mg po qid × 14 days *OR* **Doxycycline** 100 mg po bid × 14 days	**If penicillin allergic:** **Erythromycin** 500 mg po qid × 14 days *OR* **Ceftriaxone** 1 gram daily (must provide 8-10 days treponemicidal levels)	If titers not ↓ 4× by 6 months after tx for primary or secondary, **re-treat** with 3 weekly injections of benzathine penicillin G 2.4 mil units IM. Erythromycin regimen less effective than other regimens. Optimal dose and duration for ceftriaxone have not been established. **Single dose ceftriaxone is not effective.** Test for HIV.

Continued

Disease (causative organism)	Specific Indication	Primary Therapy	Alternative Therapy	Special Notes
SYPHILIS—cont'd	Late latent or latent syphilis of unknown duration Late (tertiary) syphilis (gumma and cardiovascular syphilis)	**Adults: Benzathine penicillin G** 2.4 mil units IM/week × 3 weeks (7.2 mil units total) **Children: Benzathine penicillin G** 50,000 units/kg IM (up to 2.4 million units) for 3 total doses (150,000 units/kg or 7.2 million units) **If penicillin allergic:** **Tetracycline** 500 mg po qid × 4 weeks *or* **Doxycycline** 100 mg po bid × 4 weeks		Patients are seroreactive with no other evidence of disease and should be evaluated for evidence of tertiary disease. Some recommend CSF evaluation before treatment for latent syphilis, and if treatment fails, neurosyphilis should be considered. Pregnant women and HIV positive patients should receive only penicillin regimens.
	Neurosyphilis	Aqueous crystalline penicillin G 18-24 million units IV qd, administered as 2-4 million units IV q4h × 10-14 days	**If compliance assured:** Procaine penicillin 2.4 million units IM qd *plus* probenecid 500 mg po qid × 10-14 days	May occur at any stage of syphilis. Some experts add benzathine penicillin 2.4 mil units IM following treatment in order to complete regimen for late syphilis. Follow CSF q6 months until cell count is normal. If not ↓ at 6 months or normal in 2 years, re-treat. If penicillin allergic, desensitize.
	HIV and syphilis	**Primary/secondary/early latent syphilis:** Treat as above. Some experts recommend other supplemental antibiotics in addition to standard therapy or **benzathine penicillin G** as dosed for late syphilis. **Late Latent syphilis or unknown duration:** CSF exam, then treat as above for late latent or neurosyphilis based on exam results.		Neurosyphilis must be considered in differential for HIV patients with mental status changes. Evaluate at 3, 6, 9, 12 and 24 months for treatment failure. If failure, examine CSF and re-treat as previously recommended. **Penicillin must be used to treat;** penicillin allergic must be desensitized.

	Pregnancy and syphilis	Treat for appropriate stage of syphilis. Some experts recommend a second dose of **benzathine penicillin** 2.4 mil units IM one week after initial dose for women with primary, secondary or early latent syphilis **If penicillin allergic:** Desensitize patient to penicillin.	**Doxycycline** and **tetracycline** are contraindicated in pregnancy. **Erythromycin** cannot be relied upon to treat infected fetus. Insufficient data on **azithromycin** or **ceftriaxone**	Routine screening for syphilis at time of first prenatal visit. High risk should also be screened at 28 weeks and at delivery. Titers should be repeated in 3rd trimester and at delivery (monthly for high risk). Penicillin is effective in preventing transmission to and established infection in fetuses. Women treated in second half of pregnancy are at risk for premature labor and/or fetal distress. All patients who have syphilis should be offered testing for HIV.
	Congenital syphilis	**For newborns: Aqueous crystalline penicillin G** 100,000-150,000 units/kg/day IV (50,000 units/kg IV ql2h for first 7 days of life and q8h thereafter for total of 10 days) *or* **Procaine penicillin G** 50,000 units/kg IM qd (single dose) × 10 days **For children identified at >1 month: Aqueous crystalline penicillin G** 200,000-300,000 units/kg/day IV or IM (as 50,000 units/kg q4-6h) × 10 days	Insufficient data regarding use of other antibiotics	Routine screening of newborn sera or cord blood not recommended; check mother's serum. All infants born to mothers with syphilis should be evaluated with VDRL; not FTA or MHA. Treatment decisions should be based on ID of syphilis in mother, adequacy of maternal therapy, evidence of syphilis in infant, and comparison of infant's VDRL with mother's VDRL. If more than one day of therapy is missed, the entire course must be restarted. Followup every 2-3 months until titers decline or become nonreactive in VDRL positive infants.
TRICHOMONIASIS (*T. vaginalis*)		**Metronidazole** 2 gm po single dose	**Metronidazole** 500 mg bid × 7 days	If treatment fails, use 500 mg bid × 7 day regimen. If repeated failure, use 2 gm qd × 3-5 days. **Flagyl 375** mg po bid × 7 days FDA approved; no clinical data available comparing its efficacy with 500 bid × 7 days regimen. May treat pregnant women with 2 gm single dose.

Continued

Disease (causative organism)	Specific Indication	Primary Therapy	Alternative Therapy	Special Notes
VULVOVAGINAL CANDIDIASIS (VVC) (*C. albicans*, other *Candida* sp, *Torulopsis* sp. or other yeasts)		**Butoconazole 2% cream** 5 gm intravaginally × 3 days*† *or* **Clotrimazoie 1% cream** 5 gm intravaginally × 7-14 days*† *or* **Clotrimazole** 100 mg vaginal tablet × 7 days*† *or* **Clotrimazole** 100 mg vaginal tablet, two tabs × 3 days* *or* **Clotrimazole** 500 mg vaginal tablet × 1 dose* *or* **Miconazole 2% cream** 5 gm intravaginally × 7 days*† *or* **Miconazole** 200 mg vaginal suppository, 1 dose × 3 days* *or* **Miconazole** 100 mg vaginal suppository, 1 dose × 7 days*† *or* **Nystatin** 100,000 unit vaginal tablet qd intravaginally × 14 days		**VVC:** Topical azole products more effective than nystatin. Self-medication with OTC products advised only if diagnosed previously with VVC and same symptoms recur. Uncomplicated VVC responds to all regimens. Oral azoles, itraconazole and ketoconazole, might be as effective topical agents, but potential toxicity and drug interactions must be considered. Complicated VVC (severe local or recurrent VVC inpatient with uncontrolled diabetes or infection caused by less susceptible organism) requires 10-14 days of topical or oral therapy. Treatment of **sex partners** has not been shown to ↓ frequency of recurrences. VVC may occur more frequently in HIV+ women; treatment is the same. **Pregnancy:** Only topical azole therapies should be used. Most effective are butoconazole, clotrimazole, miconazole, and terconazole. 7 day regimens preferred.

or

Tioconazole 6.5% ointment 5 gm intravaginally × 1 dose*†

or

Terconazole 0.4% cream 5 gm intravaginally × 7 days*

or

Terconazole 0.8% cream 5 gm intravaginally × 3 days*

or

Terconazole 80 mg suppository, 1 dose × 3 days*

Oral agent:

Fluconazole 150 mg po single dose

**Oil based; may weaken latex condoms and diaphragms*

†Available as an OTC preparation

Recurrent vulvovaginal candidiasis (RVVC): Defined as four or more episodes of symptomatic VVC per year. Risk factors for RVVC: uncontrolled diabetes, immunosuppression and corticosteroid use. Optimal treatment has not been established. Initial intensive regimen of 10-14 days, followed by a maintenance regimen for 6 months is recommended. Ketoconazole 100 mg po qd for up to 6 months reduces frequency of episodes. Studies are evaluating a weekly fluconazole regimen. All cases of RVVC should be confirmed by culture before initiating maintenance therapy. Management of HIV+ women should be same as other women with RVVC.

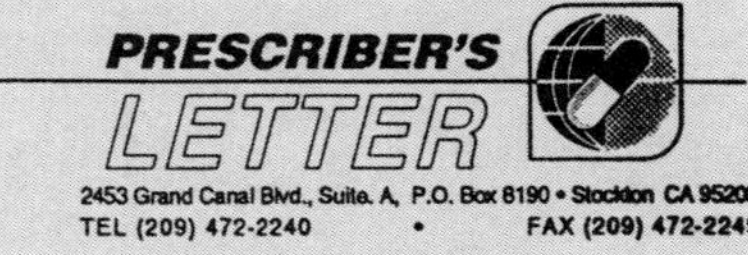

2453 Grand Canal Blvd., Suite A, P.O. Box 8190 • Stockton CA 95208
TEL (209) 472-2240 • FAX (209) 472-2249

Appendix

Surgical/Nonsurgical Antimicrobial Prophylaxis

From Erstad BL: Antimicrobial prophylaxis in surgical patients. In Greene HL, Johnson WP, Lemcke D: *Decision making in medicine,* ed 2, St Louis, 1998, Mosby; and Freeman C: Nonsurgical antimicrobial prophylaxis. In Greene HL, Johnson WP, Lemcke D: *Decision making in medicine,* ed 2, St Louis, 1998, Mosby.

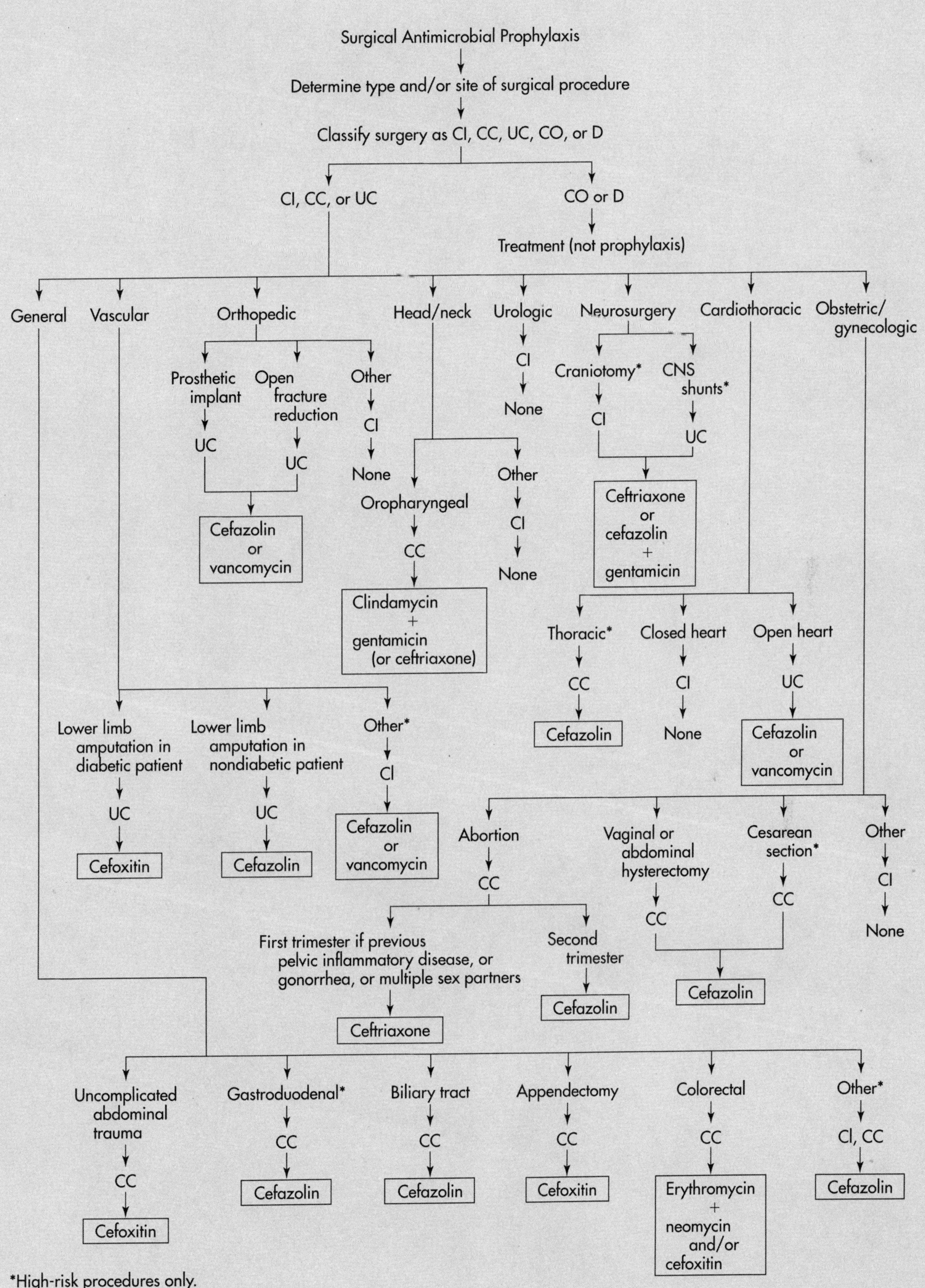

*High-risk procedures only.

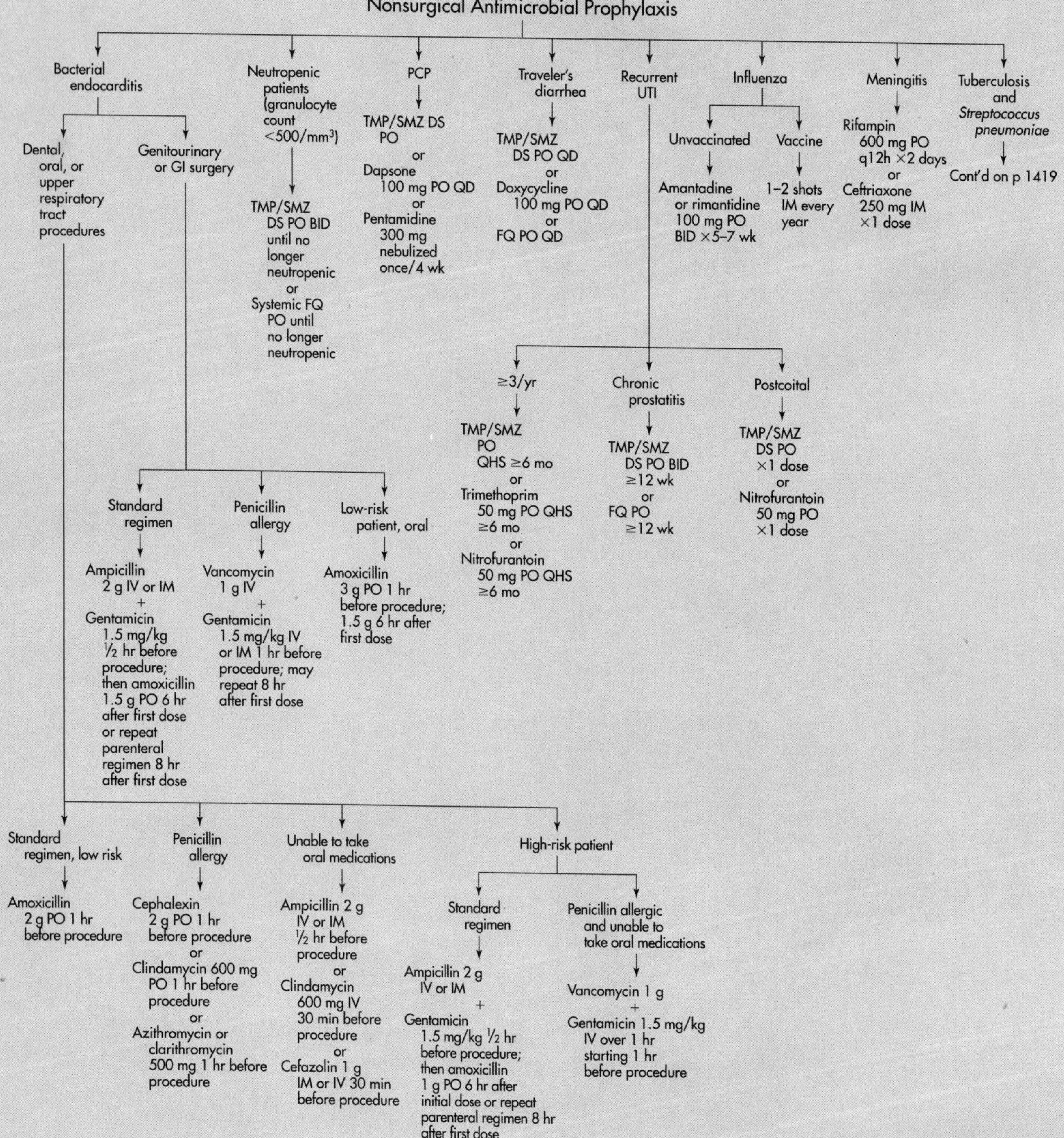
Nonsurgical Antimicrobial Prophylaxis
Bacterial endocarditis
Dental, oral, or upper respiratory tract procedures
Genitourinary or GI surgery
Neutropenic patients (granulocyte count <500/mm3)
TMP/SMZ DS PO BID until no longer neutropenic or Systemic FQ PO until no longer neutropenic
PCP
TMP/SMZ DS PO or Dapsone 100 mg PO QD or Pentamidine 300 mg nebulized once/4 wk
Traveler's diarrhea
TMP/SMZ DS PO QD or Doxycycline 100 mg PO QD or FQ PO QD
Recurrent UTI
Influenza
Unvaccinated
Amantadine or rimantidine 100 mg PO BID ×5–7 wk
Vaccine
1–2 shots IM every year
Meningitis
Rifampin 600 mg PO q12h ×2 days or Ceftriaxone 250 mg IM ×1 dose
Tuberculosis and Streptococcus pneumoniae
Cont'd on p 1419
≥3/yr
TMP/SMZ PO QHS ≥6 mo or Trimethoprim 50 mg PO QHS ≥6 mo or Nitrofurantoin 50 mg PO QHS ≥6 mo
Chronic prostatitis
TMP/SMZ DS PO BID ≥12 wk or FQ PO ≥12 wk
Postcoital
TMP/SMZ DS PO ×1 dose or Nitrofurantoin 50 mg PO ×1 dose
Standard regimen
Ampicillin 2 g IV or IM + Gentamicin 1.5 mg/kg ½ hr before procedure; then amoxicillin 1.5 g PO 6 hr after first dose or repeat parenteral regimen 8 hr after first dose
Penicillin allergy
Vancomycin 1 g IV + Gentamicin 1.5 mg/kg IV or IM 1 hr before procedure; may repeat 8 hr after first dose
Low-risk patient, oral
Amoxicillin 3 g PO 1 hr before procedure; 1.5 g 6 hr after first dose
Standard regimen, low risk
Amoxicillin 2 g PO 1 hr before procedure
Penicillin allergy
Cephalexin 2 g PO 1 hr before procedure or Clindamycin 600 mg PO 1 hr before procedure or Azithromycin or clarithromycin 500 mg 1 hr before procedure
Unable to take oral medications
Ampicillin 2 g IV or IM ½ hr before procedure or Clindamycin 600 mg IV 30 min before procedure or Cefazolin 1 g IM or IV 30 min before procedure
High-risk patient
Standard regimen
Ampicillin 2 g IV or IM + Gentamicin 1.5 mg/kg ½ hr before procedure; then amoxicillin 1 g PO 6 hr after initial dose or repeat parenteral regimen 8 hr after first dose
Penicillin allergic and unable to take oral medications
Vancomycin 1 g + Gentamicin 1.5 mg/kg IV over 1 hr starting 1 hr before procedure

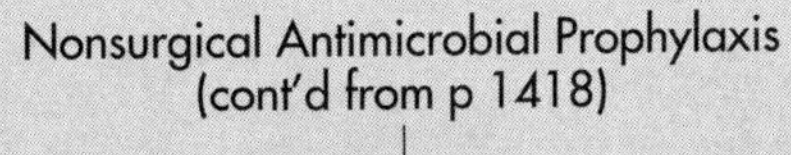
Nonsurgical Antimicrobial Prophylaxis
(cont'd from p 1418)

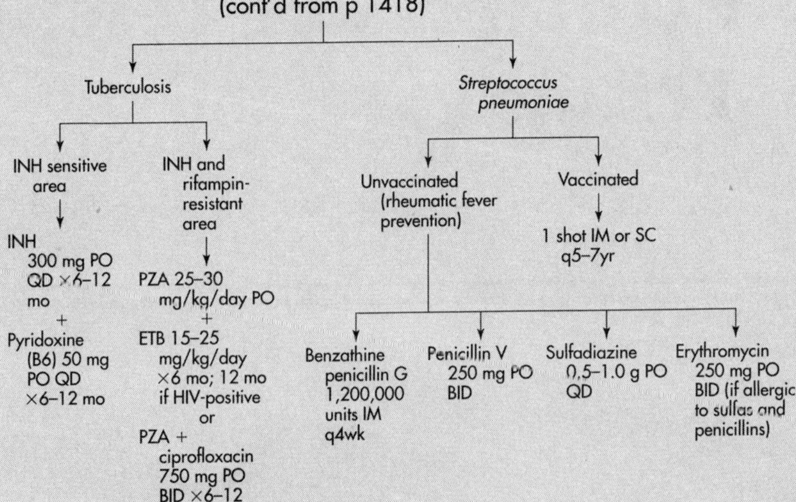
Tuberculosis
INH sensitive area
INH 300 mg PO QD ×6–12 mo
+
Pyridoxine (B6) 50 mg PO QD ×6–12 mo
INH and rifampin-resistant area
PZA 25–30 mg/kg/day PO
+
ETB 15–25 mg/kg/day ×6 mo; 12 mo if HIV-positive
or
PZA + ciprofloxacin 750 mg PO BID ×6–12 mo
Streptococcus pneumoniae
Unvaccinated (rheumatic fever prevention)
Benzathine penicillin G 1,200,000 units IM q4wk
Penicillin V 250 mg PO BID
Sulfadiazine 0.5–1.0 g PO QD
Erythromycin 250 mg PO BID (if allergic to sulfas and penicillins)
Vaccinated
1 shot IM or SC q5–7yr

Appendix

Principles of Telephone Triage

The concept of triage means "sorting out." Triage with patients in the office can be difficult due to multiple complaints and numerous medical conditions; when using the telephone to conduct triage for patients, triage becomes even more tricky. Sorting patients according to the urgency of their condition, and making appropriate recommendations regarding that care over the telephone requires an organized, consistent process.

- Telephone triage background
  - Most calls from patients deal with minor problems
  - Calls requiring some kind of counseling are also common
  - Very few lawsuits on record for health care professionals giving telephone advice
  - No standards of practice established for telephone triage
  - Once advice is begun with a patient, appropriate advice or a referral must be given; termination of the call without referral or advice may be considered abandonment
  - Accountability for following the advice remains with the caller
  - Warn the patient about noncompliance, since failure to give adequate warning is an important theory in lawsuits involving telephone advice
  - Use clear and unambiguous terms to warn such as, "Serious injury or death could result if the advice is not followed"
- Issues related to telephone triage
  - Advice given based on information provided by untrained observer
  - Caller may not know what are pertinent and critical symptoms, and may not recognize what is normal or abnormal
  - Absence of visual cues with total reliance on verbal communication
  - Young and old patients may not present with "Classic" symptoms for serious illnesses
  - Algorithms or protocols should be used to help identify which calls require immediate care
  - Protocols or guidelines should include information to obtain to help classify when the patient needs to be seen; these protocols also should include critical information to obtain related to the symptoms the caller has; numerous publications are available that provide detailed information for call triage
  - Collect baseline information: Age, medications, allergies, chronic illnesses (see documentation sample on p. 1422)
  - Provide clear documentation of the call
  - The following information is needed to accurately document triage calls:
    - Date and time of call
    - Name of caller/patient
    - Demograpic information
      - Medications prescribed or OTC taken
      - PMH
      - Allergies
    - History of present illness
    - Brief statement of advice given or protocol followed
    - Warnings or referrals given
  - Documentation should be included in the patient's chart to provide a record of what was discussed
  - Sample documentation guide follows:

SUGGESTED READINGS

Blanchford K, Schwarzentnub L, Reisinger P: Development of telephone triage nurse practice standards, *Nurse Economics* 15(5):265-267, 1997.

Brown J: *Pediatric telephone medicine,* ed 3, Philadelphia, 1997, JB Lippincott.

Crouch R et al: Telephone assessment and advice: a training program, *Nurs Standards* 11(47):41-47, 1997.

Edwards B: Seeing is believing: picture building: a key component of telephone triage. *J Clin Nurs* 7(1):51-57, 1998.

Poole S et al: After hours telephone coverage, *Pediatrics* 92:670-679, 1993.

Ottoline M, Greenburg S: Development and evaluation of CD-ROM computer program to teach residents telephone management, *Pediatrics* 101(3Pt.1):E2, 1998.

Reisinger P: Experiences of critical care nurses in telephone triage, *Dimen Crit Care Nurs* 17(1):20-27, 1998.

Robinson D, Anderson M, Erpenbeck P: Telephone Advice for Nurse Practitioners, *Nurse Pract* 22(3):179-192, 1997.

Robinson D, Anderson M, Acheson P: Telephone advice: lessons learned and consideration for starting programs, *J Emerg Nurs* 22(5):409-415, 1996.

Tennenhouse D: Minimizing liability for telephone advice, *Calif Nurs* 2:24-26, 1991.

Wheeler S: *Telephone triage,* New York, 1993, Delmar.

Wheeler S, Siebelt B: Calling all nurses: how to perform telephone triage, *Nurs* 27(7):37-41, 1997.

Woodke D: *Telephone triage protocols,* Indianapolis, 1991, Methodist Hospital of Indiana.

SAMPLE TELEPHONE TRIAGE DOCUMENT

Date:		Name: DOB:		Allergies:
T:	P:	B/P:	Weight:	
Chief Complaint:			LMP:	Medications:

History:
☐ Hospitalizations ________
____
____
____
☐ Illnesses: chronic ________
____
____
____
____

Referrals:
☐ 911
☐ ED
☐ Crisis line
☐ Dentist
☐ Poison control

Telephone Protocol Used/Advice Given:
____
____
____
____
____

FH:
☐ HTN ☐ MI
☐ CAD ☐ CVA
☐ DM ☐ CA
☐ Resp. ☐ Depression
☐ ETOH ☐ Seizures

Warnings Given:
☐ Recommend that you seek emergency treatment or serious illness or death could result

☐ Follow-up with NP/MD ________
Signature: ________

Appendix

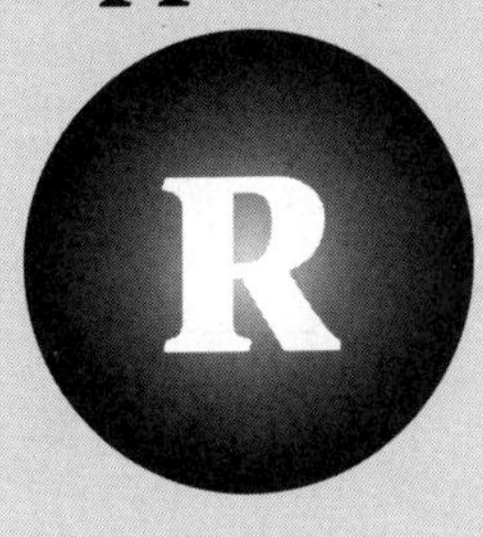

Topical Steroid Potency Ranking

Some commonly used topical steroids listed by potency group. Group I is the super-potent category descending to Group VII, which is the least potent. There is no significant difference between agents *within* Groups II through VII (compounds simply listed alphabetically). *However,* within Group I, Temovate Cream and ointment are more potent than the others.

Group	Brand Name	Generic Name	Sizes (g, unless otherwise noted)
I	Temovate cream 0.05%	Clobetasol propionate	15, 30, 45
	Temovate ointment 0.05%		15, 30, 45
	Diprolene ointment 0.05%	Betamethasone diproprionate	15, 45
	Diprolene AF cream 0.05%		15, 45
	Psorcon ointment 0.05%	Diflorasone diacetate	15, 30, 60
	Ultravate cream 0.05%	Halobetasol proprionate	15, 45
	Ultravate ointment 0.05%		15, 45
II	Cyclocort ointment 0.1%	Amcinonide	15, 30, 60
	Diprosone ointment 0.05%	Betamethasone diproprionate	15, 45
	Elocone ointment 0.1%	Mometasone furoate	15, 45
	Florone ointment 0.05%	Diflorasone diacetate	15, 30, 60
	Halog cream 0.1%	Halcinonide	15, 30, 60, 240
	Halog ointment 0.1%		15, 30, 60, 240
	Halog solution 0.1%		20, 60 ml
	Lidex cream 0.05%	Fluocinonide	15, 30, 60, 120
	Lidex gel 0.05%		15, 30, 60, 120
	Lidex ointment 0.05%		15, 30, 60, 120
	Lidex solution 0.05%		20, 60 ml
	Maxiflor ointment 0.05%	Diflorasone diacetate	15, 30, 60
	Maxivate cream 0.05%	Betamethasone diproprionate	15, 45
	Maxivate Ointment 0.05%		15, 45
	Topicort cream 0.25%	Desoximetasone	15, 60, 120
	Topicort gel 0.05%		15, 60
	Topicort ointment 0.25%		15, 60

This listing is adapted with permission from Richard B. Stoughton, M.D. Reproduced with permission from Ferndale Laboratories, Inc., 780 West Eight Mile Road, Ferndale, MI 48220.

Group	Brand Name	Generic Name	Sizes (g, unless otherwise noted)
III	Aristocort A ointment 0.1%	Triamcinolone acetonide	15, 60
	Cyclocort cream 0.1%	Amcinonide	15, 30, 60
	Cyclocort lotion 0.1%		20, 60 ml
	Diprosone cream 0.05%	Betamethasone diproprionate	15, 45
	Florone cream 0.05%	Diflorasone diacetate	15, 30, 60
	Lidex E cream 0.05%	Fluocinonide	15, 30, 60, 120
	Maxiflor cream 0.05%	Diflorasone diacetate	15, 30, 60
	Maxivate lotion 0.05%	Betamethasone diproprionate	60 ml
	Valisone ointment 0.1%	Betamethasone diproprionate	15, 45
IV	Aristocort ointment 0.1%	Triamcinolone acetonide	15, 60, 240, 2400
	Cordran ointment 0.05%	Flurandrenolide	15, 30, 60, 225
	Elocon cream 0.1%	Mometasone furoate	15, 45
	Elocon lotion 0.1%		30, 60 ml
	Kenalog cream 0.1%	Triamcinolone acetonide	15, 60, 80, 240
	Kenalog ointment 0.1%		15, 60, 80, 240
	Synalar ointment 0.025%	Fluocinolone acetonide	15, 30, 60, 120, 425
	Topicort LP cream 0.05%	Desoximetasone	15, 60
V	Cordran cream 0.05%	Flurandrenolide	15, 30, 225
	Kenalog lotion 0.1%	Triamcinolone acetonide	15, 60 ml
	Kenalog ointment 0.025%		15, 60, 80, 240
	Locoid cream 0.1%	Hydrocortisone butyrate	15, 45
	Locoid ointment 0.1%		15, 45
	Synalar cream 0.025%	Fluocinolone acetonide	15, 30, 60, 425
	Tridesilon ointment 0.05%	Desonide	15, 60
	Valisone cream 0.1%	Betamethasone valerate	15, 45, 110, 430
	Valisone lotion 0.1%		20, 60 ml
	Westcort cream 0.2%	Hydrocortisone valerate	15, 45, 60, 120
	Westcort ointment 0.2%		15, 45, 60
VI	Aclovate cream 0.05%	Alclometasone diproprionate	15, 45
	Aclovate ointment 0.05%		15, 45
	Aristocort cream 0.1%	Triamcinolone acetonide	15, 60, 240, 2520
	Kenalog cream 0.025%	Triamcinolone acetonide	15, 60, 80, 240, 2520
	Kenalog lotion 0.025%		60 ml
	Locoid solution 0.1%	Hydrocortisone butyrate	20, 60 ml
	Locorten cream 0.03%	Flumethasone pivolate	15, 60
	Synalar cream 0.01%	Fluocinolone acetonide	15, 45, 50, 425
	Synatar solution 0.01%		20, 60 ml
	Tridesilon cream 0.05%	Desonide	15, 60
VII	Hytone cream 1.0%	Hydrocortisone	30, 120
	Hytone cream 2.5%		30, 60
	Hytone lotion 1.0%		120
	Hytone lotion 2.5%		60
	Hytone ointment 1.0%		30
	Hytone ointment 2.5%		30
	Pramosone cream 1.0%	Hydrocortisone Acetate & Pramoxine HCl 1%	1, 2, 4 oz
	Pramosone cream 2.5%		1, 2, 4 oz
	Pramosone lotion 1.0%		2, 4, 8 oz
	Pramosone lotion 2.5%		2, 4 oz
	Pramosone ointment 1.0%		1, 4 oz
	Pramosone ointment 2.5%		1, 4 oz
	and others containing dexamethasone, flumetholone, prednisolone, and methylprednisolone		

Appendix

Vital Signs: Normal Ranges

	Pulse	Respirations	Blood Pressure
Newborn	120 to 160	30 to 50	60 to 96/30 to 62 mm Hg
Toddlers (1-3 years)	90 to 140	20 to 30	78 to 112/48 to 78 mm Hg
Preschool (4-6 years)	80 to 110	18 to 26	78 to 112/50 to 82 mm Hg
School age (7-11 years)	75 to 110	16 to 22	85 to 114/52 to 85 mm Hg
Adolescent (12-16 years)	60 to 100	14 to 20	94 to 136/58 to 88 mm Hg
Adult	60 to 110	12 to 20	100 to 140/60 to 90 mm Hg

From Thompson JM: *Quick reference for clinical nursing,* ed 2, St Louis, 1997, Mosby.

Index

B

C

E

H

I

J

K

M

N

T

U

X

Z

ISBN 0-323-00148-3

LIFESPAN

Infant

Child

Adolescent

Adult

Geriatric

All Ages